Pages

Med-Surg 1–902

Psychiatric 903–980

Maternity 981–1060

Pediatric 1061–1464

Index Appendixes

THE LIPPINCOTT MANUAL OF NURSING PRACTICE

LILLIAN SHOLTIS BRUNNER

R.N., M.S.N., Sc.D., F.A.A.N.

Consultant in Nursing, Schools of Nursing:
Presbyterian-University of Pennsylvania Medical Center,
Philadelphia, Pennsylvania; and
The Bryn Mawr Hospital, Bryn Mawr, Pennsylvania;
formerly Assistant Professor of Surgical Nursing,
Yale University School of Nursing, New Haven, Connecticut

DORIS SMITH SUDDARTH

R.N., B.S.N.E., M.S.N.

Formerly Consultant in Health Occupations,
Job Corps Health Office, U.S. Department of Labor; and
Formerly Coordinator of the Curriculum, Alexandria
Hospital School of Nursing, Alexandria, Virginia

Bette Bonine Faries, R.N., M.S.—Maternity Nursing Section
Formerly Maternal and Infant Health Professor of Department of Nursing,
Montgomery Community College, Takoma Park, Maryland

Anne Schwalenstocker Klijanowicz, R.N., M.S.—Pediatric Nursing Section
Assistant Professor and Clinician II (Pediatrics),
University of Rochester School of Nursing,
Rochester, New York

Donnajeanne Bigos Lavoie, R.N., M.S.N.—Pediatric Nursing Section
Assistant Professor, College of Nursing, Department of Maternal and Child Health, Howard University, Washington, D.C.; and
Neonatology Nurse Consultant;
formerly Neonatology Nurse Consultant, Children's Hospital
National Medical Center, Washington, D.C.

Gertrude K. Ramseier McFarland, R.N., D.N.Sc.—Psychiatric Nursing Section
Nurse Consultant, Nursing Education Branch, Division of Nursing,
Health Resources Administration, Department of Health and
Human Services, Hyattsville, Maryland

Evelyn L. Wasli, R.N., D.N.Sc.—Psychiatric Nursing Section
Psychiatric Nursing Coordinator, Saint Elizabeths Hospital,
National Institute of Mental Health, Department of Health and Human Services, Washington, D.C.

CONTRIBUTORS

Herbert H. Butler, M.D.
Emergency Department Physician, Underwood-Memorial Hospital, Woodbury, New Jersey; Past President, New Jersey
Chapter American College of Emergency Physicians

James F. Elam, Ph.D.
Clinical Biochemist, Pathology Department, Alexandria Hospital, Alexandria, Virginia

Joseph B. Mizgerd, M.D.
Director, Department of Pulmonary Medicine, Washington Adventist Hospital, Takoma Park, Maryland

Kathleen C. Morton, M.D., F.A.A.P.
President, New York Medical College, Valhalla, New York; formerly Dean for Primary Care Education, Johns Hopkins School
of Medicine

Alfred Munzer, M.D.
Director, Critical Care, Washington Adventist Hospital, Takoma Park, Maryland

Becky A. Winslow, R.N., M.S.N.
Assistant Director, Nursing Education Programs, School Health Services, Johns Hopkins University, Baltimore, Maryland

THE LIPPINCOTT MANUAL OF NURSING PRACTICE

3RD EDITION

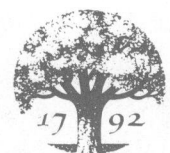

J. B. LIPPINCOTT COMPANY

Philadelphia • Toronto

Third Edition

Copyright © 1982, by J. B. Lippincott Company
Copyright © 1978, 1974 by J. B. Lippincott Company
All rights reserved. No part of this book may be used
or reproduced in any manner whatsoever without written permission except in
the case of brief quotations embodied in critical articles and reviews.
Printed in the United States of America. For information address
J. B. Lippincott Company, East Washington Square, Philadelphia, Penna.
19105

654321

Library of Congress Cataloging in Publication Data

Brunner, Lillian Sholtis.
    The Lippincott manual of nursing practice.

    Includes bibliographies and index.
    1. Nursing—Handbooks, manuals, etc. I. Suddarth,
Doris Smith. II. Title. [DNLM: 1. Nursing care—
Handbooks. WY 100 B897L]
RT51.B78   1982   610.73   81-8278
ISBN 0-397-54352-2   AACR2

The authors and publisher have exerted every effort to ensure that drug selection and dosage set forth in this text are in accord with current recommendations and practice at the time of publication. However, in view of ongoing research, changes in government regulations, and the constant flow of information relating to drug therapy and drug reactions, the reader is urged to check the package insert for each drug for any change in indications and dosage and for added warnings and precautions. This is particularly important when the recommended agent is a new or infrequently employed drug. It is assumed that treatment is given under the supervision of a physician.

CONTENTS

LIST OF GUIDELINES

PSYCHIATRIC NURSING

MATERNITY NURSING

PEDIATRIC NURSING

HEALTH EDUCATION/PATIENT EDUCATION

PREFACE

Because we live in an uncertain world, today's nurse needs ever-increasing knowledge, skill, and understanding of the human condition to make sound clinical nursing decisions.

The authors have sought new developments, research findings, and feasible innovations from authoritative resources and experiences which have an impact on nursing. To utilize and demonstrate these findings, every clinical condition and guidelines section in the book has been reviewed, amplified, and updated. Nursing principles and accountability are stressed along with the basic rationale for optimum patient management. Health promotion and disease prevention are given special emphasis throughout. Early recognition and management of complications and their consequences receive attention, since mastery of this knowledge is essential in the promotion of optimum patient well-being and safety. Cognizance of the rights of patients/clients as delineated by the National League for Nursing and the American Hospital Association are assuumed throughout the Manual. The caring functions of the nurse involving feelings, emotions, values, and skills are identified to assist patients toward ultimate self-care where possible.

Since persons with mental health problems are now remaining in the community and those with long-term mental health conditions are being discharged into the community, a section on Psychiatric Nursing has been added to help meet the special challenges and needs of these individuals.

Cost-effectiveness continues to be a significant concern in health care. In this regard it must be emphasized that not all tests, for example, that are presented for various conditions are expected to be performed. The selection of tests is determined by the needs of the patient and the judgment of health care personnel.

This book is organized so that the nursing process can be used as a framework to facilitate formulation of nursing care plans. Current references representing authoritative opinions and research are included. The bibliographic citation formats have been revised to conform with those of the American National Standards Institute.

The authors continue to be grateful for the input of their nursing colleagues and for the continued enthusiastic reception of this Manual.

Lillian Sholtis Brunner and
Doris Smith Suddarth

ACKNOWLEDGMENTS

Edward G. Abramson, M.D.
Instructor in Urology,
George Washington University Medical Center,
    Washington, D.C.; and
Chief, Urology Service, Alexandria Hospital,
Alexandria, Virginia

Marjorie H. Baer, R.N., B.S., M.N.
Assistant Director, School of Nursing,
The Bryn Mawr Hospital,
Bryn Mawr, Pennsylvania

Brenda G. Bare, R.N., M.S.N.
Curriculum Cordinator,
Alexandria Hospital School of Nursing,
Alexandria, Virginia

Elizabeth W. Bayley, R.N., M.S.N., M.S.
Clinical Specialist in Burn Nursing, Department of
    Nursing,
Crozer-Chester Medical Center,
Chester, Pennsylvania

Stephen J. Bednar, M.D.
Assistant Professor of Medicine,
Georgetown University School of Medicine,
Washington, D.C.

Abraham A. Coster, D.P.M.
Chairman, Department of Podiatry,
Jefferson Memorial Hospital,
Alexandria, Virginia

Jean E. DeVries, R.N., C.N.O.R.
Assistant Director of Nursing for Surgical Services,
Alexandria Hospital,
Alexandria, Virginia

Joan B. DiBianco, R.N., M.S.N.
Nursing Coordinator, Cardiovascular Step-Down
    Unit,
Georgetown University Hospital,
Washington, D.C.

Robert DiBianco, M.D.
Assistant Chief, Cardiology Section,
Veterans Administration Medical Center; and
Assistant Professor of Medicine
Georgetown University School of Medicine,
Washington, D.C.

Melvyn L. Elgart, M.D.
Professor and Chairman, Department of
    Dermatology,
George Washington University Medical Center,
Washington, D.C.

Beverly Z. Faro, R.N., M.S.
Instructor and Clinician II (Pediatrics),
University of Rochester School of Nursing,
Rochester, New York

Anne B. Fletcher, M.D.
Associate Professor of Child Health and
    Development,
George Washington University School of Medicine;
    and
Associate Director of Neonatology, Children's
    Hospital
National Medical Center, Washington, D.C.

Patricia S. Goode, R.N., M.S.N., E.T.
Director, Nursing Education,
Cooper Green Hospital, Birmingham, Alabama; and
Assistant Editor, *Journal of Enterostomal Therapy*

George W. Gregory III, M.D.
Associate Clinical Professor of Cardiothoracic
    Surgery,
University of California; and
Chairman, Department of Cardiothoracic Surgery,
Naval Regional Medical Center, San Diego,
    California

Robert L. Hanson, R.N., M.N.
Research Associate, School of Nursing, University of
    Washington; and
Owner and Consultant, Health Systems Management
    Services,
Seattle, Washington

Elizabeth S. Harding, R.N., B.S.N., M.S.N.
Director, School of Nursing,
The Bryn Mawr Hospital,
Bryn Mawr, Pennsylvania

Marilyn B. Hartsell, R.N., M.S.N., N.S.
Co-ordinator Infant Apnea Program and
Pediatric Pulmonary Nurse Specialist,
Children's Hospital National Medical Center,
Washington, D.C.

Martha N. Hill, R.N., M.S.N.
Assistant Professor, Division of Nursing, Johns
    Hopkins University; and
Nurse Specialist, Hypertension Clinic, Johns Hopkins
    Hospital,
Baltimore, Maryland

Joan Holihan, R.N., M.S.N.
Clinical Unit Coordinator—Burn Unit,
Children's Hospital National Medical Center,
Washington, D.C.

Nancy Tillotson Jacobson, R.N., M.S.N.
Formerly Nutrition Support Service Nursing
    Coordinator/
Staff Development, Hospital of the University of
    Pennsylavania; and
Instructor, Holy Family College of Nursing,
    Philadelphia, Pennsylvania

Harvey Gordon Klein, M.D.
Chief of Blood Services Section,
Clinical Center Blood Bank, National Institutes of
    Health,
Bethesda, Maryland

Louis J. LaBorwit, Ph.D.
Chief Speech Pathologist,
Department of Physical Medicine and Rehabilitation,
Georgetown University Hospital,
Washington, D.C.

Dorothy Leonard, R.N., B.S.Ed., M.S.N.
Nurse Recruiter, Veterans Administration Medical
    Center,
Wilmington, Delaware

Stephen M. Levin, M.D.
Assistant Clinical Professor of Orthopedic Surgery,
Howard University,
Washington, D.C.

Edwina A. McConnell, R.N., M.S.
Consultant, Medical-Surgical Nursing, Nursing
   Management,
Madison, Wisconsin

Catherine D. McMahon, R.N., C.C.R.N.
Associate Clinical Unit Co-ordinator, Pediatric
   Intensive Care Unit, Children's hospital National
   Medical Center,
Washington, D.C.

Irene C. Morelli, R.N., M.S.
Associate Executive Director,
Maryland Nurses Association,
Bethesda, Maryland

James M. Moss, M.D.
Clinical Professor of Medicine,
Georgetown University School of Medicine,
Washington, D.C.

A. E. Parrish, M.D.
Director, Division of Renal Diseases,
George Washington University Medical Center,
Washington, D.C.

Donald M. Poretz, M.D.
Chief of Infectious Diseases,
The Fairfax Hospital,
Falls Church, Virginia

James W. Preuss, M.D.
Associate Professor of Neurosurgery,
Georgetown University School of Medicine; and
Chief, Neurosurgery,
Alexandria Hospital, Alexandria, Virginia

Mary Evans Robinson, Ph.D.
Pediatric Psychologist, Children's Hospital National
   Medical Center,
   Washington, D.C.

Howard E. Sullivan, Jr., M.D.
Chief, Section of Allergy, The Bryn Mawr Hospital,
Bryn Mawr, Pennsylvania

RESEARCH/LIBRARY

**Albert M. Berkowitz, Chief of Reference Services Division,
   and the Reference Staff,**
National Library of Medicine, Bethesda, Maryland

Martin M. Cummings, M.D., Director,
National Library of Medicine, Bethesda, Maryland

Carol Ditzler, Supervisor Librarian, and staff,
National Library of Medicine, Bethesda, Maryland

Leslie D. Gundry, Chief Medical Librarian,
The Bryn Mawr Hospital and School of Nursing,
Bryn Mawr, Pennsylvania

Joan Konrad, Catalog Librarian, Scott Memorial Library,
The Thomas Jefferson University, Philadelphia,
   Pennsylvania

Alexander G. Kulchar, Medical Librarian,
The Bryn Mawr Hospital and School of Nursing,
Bryn Mawr, Pennsylvania

Alice Mackov, Reference (Head), Scott Memorial Library,
The Thomas Jefferson University,
Philadelphia, Pennsylvania

Jacqueline van de Kamp, Technical Information Specialist,
National Library of Medicine, Bethesda, Maryland

ILLUSTRATIONS

William Burke
Neil O. Hardy
Lynn Ellen Waldo

The authors express appreciation to
Barton H. Lippincott, Edward T. Hutton, and David
   T. Miller for their unique assessment of nursing
   trends, their complete faith in the Brunner/
   Suddarth author team, and their unwavering
   genuine support.

Diana Intenzo, Jeanne Wallace, and their associates
   in the editorial department, including Mary
   Murphy, secretary, and manuscript editors Darlene
   Pedersen and Kathy Dunn, for their dedication to
   accuracy and quality, concern for important detail,
   and consideration of author personalities.

Tracy Baldwin, Carol Kerr, and their colleagues in
   the art department for their creativity and
   sensitivity in implementing and presenting the art
   work.

John Cooke and members of the production staff for
   their early projected time plan and conscientious
   adherence to it.

Lastly, but definitely most importantly, our deep
appreciation to Mathias J. (Mat) and Hilton for their
many years of love and understanding.

THE LIPPINCOTT MANUAL
OF NURSING PRACTICE

MEDICAL-SURGICAL NURSING

PART 1

THE NURSING PROCESS

The *nursing process* is a systematic, decision-making process that involves assessment (data collection), planning, and implementation and uses evaluation and subsequent modifications as feedback mechanisms that promote the ultimate resolution of the patient's nursing problems. The process as a whole is cyclic, the steps being interrelated, interdependent, and recurrent.

Steps of the Nursing Process

1. *Assessing*—systematic assessment of the patient's problems for the purpose of establishing nursing diagnoses. (Analysis of data is included as part of the assessment. For those who wish to emphasize its importance, analysis may be identified as a separate step of the nursing process.)
2. *Planning*—development of a plan of care to resolve the problems.
3. *Implementing*—implementation of the plan of care or supervision of others who implement the plan.
4. *Evaluating*—evaluation of the effectiveness of the plan of care in resolving the assessed problems.

Assessing

Assessment begins with the nurse's first encounter with the patient. It involves the systematic collection of data about the patient's nursing needs and the use of this data to formulate nursing diagnoses.

A. *The Nursing History* (see details, p. 12)

1. Is carried out for the purpose of determining the patient's state of wellness or illness and is best accomplished as part of a planned interview.
2. Provides the nurse with the opportunity to collect data and also to convey interest, support, and understanding to the patient.

B. *The Physical Examination* (see details, p. 18)

1. To determine the patients's physical alterations and limitations.
2. To determine the patient's assets, which may serve to complement his limitations.

C. *Other Sources of Assessment Data*

1. Patient's family and/or significant others
2. Members of the health team
3. Patient's health record

D. *Nursing Diagnoses*

Those health problems that have the potential for resolution by means of nursing actions.
1. Organize, analyze, synthesize, and summarize the collected data.
2. Identify the patient's nursing problem(s), its particular characteristic(s) and etiology(ies).
3. State nursing diagnoses concisely and precisely.

Planning

See Example of a Nursing Care Plan, page 4.
1. Assign priorities to the nursing diagnoses. Highest priority is given to problems that are the most urgent and critical.

2. Establish goals of nursing actions.
   a. Specify short-term, intermediate, and long-term goals as established by nurse and patient together.
   b. State goals in realistic and measurable terms.
3. Identify nursing actions appropriate for goal attainment.
4. Establish expected outcome criteria.
   a. State outcomes in terms of patient behaviors.
   b. Outcomes must be realistic and measurable.
   c. Identify critical time periods for the attainment of outcomes.
5. Formulate the nursing care plan (see sample nursing care plan, p. 4).
   a. Include nursing diagnoses in order of priority, goals, nursing actions, outcome criteria, and critical time periods.
   b. Write entries precisely, concisely, and systematically.
   c. Keep the plan current and flexible to meet the patient's changing problems and needs.
   d. Involve the patient, his family and/or significant others, nursing team members, other health team members, and community agencies in all aspects of planning.

Implementing

1. Put the nursing care plan into action.
2. Coordinate the activities of the patient, his family and/or significant others, nursing team members, and other health team members.
3. Delegate specific nursing actions to other members of the nursing team, as appropriate.
   a. Consider the capabilities and limitations of the members of the nursing team.
   b. Supervise the performance of the nursing actions.
4. Record the patient's responses to the nursing actions.
   a. Record the responses precisely, concisely, and objectively.
   b. Recordings should be related to the nursing diagnoses.
   c. Include any additional pertinent assessment data.

Evaluating

1. Collect objective data.
2. Compare the patient's behavioral outcomes to the outcome criteria. Determine the extent to which the goals were achieved.
3. Include the patient, his family and/or significant others, nursing team members, and other health team members in the evaluation.
4. Identify alterations that need to be made in the nursing care plan.

Continuation of the Nursing Process

1. Continue all steps of the nursing process: assessing, planning, implementing, and evaluating.
2. Continuous evaluation provides the means for maintaining the viability of the entire nursing process and for demonstrating accountability for the quality of nursing care rendered.

Example of a Nursing Care Plan

Mrs. Joanne Collins, a 48-year-old secretary, was admitted to the hospital with a diagnosis of thrombophlebitis of the right lower leg. She stated that she had noticed slight swelling of her right calf for several days and then experienced redness and tenderness of the calf on the day of admission. The *nursing history* revealed no significant health problems except for a 2-year history of "some problems with varicose veins." *Physical examination* revealed slight redness and tenderness of the right calf and several large, tortuous leg veins bilaterally. The physician's requests upon admission included bedrest with bathroom privileges, foot of bed elevated 15 cm. (6 inches), heparin therapy, and Tylenol for pain. Several days after admission, the physician indicated that Mrs. Collins would receive Coumadin therapy after discharge.

Nursing Diagnosis:	Inflammation of right calf veins related to varicose veins and sedentary life-style.
Goals—Short-term:	Increased venous return from lower extremities.
Intermediate:	Resolution of inflammation.
Long-term:	Altered life style to include measures that promote venous return from lower extremities. Compliance with anticoagulant therapy regimen.

Nursing Orders	Outcome Criteria	Critical Time*	Outcome
Promote venous return from lower extremities:			
Encourage bedrest with foot of bed elevated 15 cm. (6 inches)	Complies with activity restriction and with elevation of lower extremities	24 Hr.	Remains in bed with legs elevated except when out of bed to bathroom; uses TV, books, and needlework to prevent boredom
Prevent pressure on calves and popliteal areas	Calves and popliteal areas free of excessive pressure	24 hr.	Assumes proper position in bed with calves and popliteal areas free of excessive pressure; avoids crossing legs
Encourage active exercises of lower extremities for 5 minutes every 2 hours—simulate walking when lying on back and bicycling when on side	Exercises lower extremities for 5 minutes every 2 hours	24 hr.	Assumes responsibility for active exercises—5 minutes every 2 hours
Continue assessment of venous circulation:			
Inspect legs from groin to feet:			
Observe for asymmetry, edema, hardness; measure circumference of calves daily	Legs symmetrical and free of edema	3 days	Right (R) calf circumference, 37.5 cm., Left (L) calf circumference, 36.5 cm., on admission; circumference on both calves, 36.5 cm., 2 days after admission
Compare temperature of both legs: ankles, calves, knees	Temperature of both legs equal and normal	3 days	Temperature of both legs equal and normal 2 days after admission
Assess for side effects of heparin therapy:			
Check APTT (activated partial thromboplastin time) prior to administration. (APTT is used to monitor the anticoagulation effects and dosage of heparin)	APTT between 1½ and 2½ times the normal control	48 hr.	APTT stabilized at 1½ to 2 times the normal control
Observe for bleeding: Urine—note evidence of hematuria Stool—check for tarry color Gums—check emesis basin after toothbrushing for pink or bloody return Monitor vital signs q.i.d.	Free from bleeding	48 hr.	No evidence of blood in urine or stool; gums not bleeding; vital signs stable: BP 108/66, P 70, R 16
Encourage food and fluid intake that promotes normal nutrition, digestion, and elimination: Regular diet fiber foods 1500–2000 ml. fluid/day	Tolerates regular diet Maintains normal bowel elimination Intake of 1500–2000 ml. fluid/day	3 days	Selects and eats a balanced diet; bowel movement daily; no constipation or diarrhea; fluid intake 1800–2200 ml./day
Teaching: anticoagulant therapy regimen	(See teaching plan, p. 8.)		

*These times have not been standardized, but are individualized according to the patient's needs.

BIBLIOGRAPHY

Books

Brunner LS and Suddarth DS. Textbook of Medical-Surgical Nursing. Philadelphia, JB Lippincott, 1980
Campbell C. Nursing Diagnosis and Intervention in Nursing Practice. New York, John Wiley & Sons, 1978
Duke University Hospital Nursing Services. Quality Assurance. Guidelines for Nursing Care. Philadelphia, JB Lippincott, 1980
LaMonica EL. The Nursing Process: A Humanistic Approach. Menlo Park, Addison-Wesley Publishing Co, 1979
Yura H and Walsh MB. Human Needs and the Nursing Process. New York, Appleton-Century-Crofts, 1978
Yura H and Walsh MB. The Nursing Process. New York, Appleton-Century-Crofts, 1978

Articles

Bruce GL et al. Implementation of ANA's quality assurance program for clients with end-stage renal disease. Adv Nurs Sci 1980 Jan; 2(2):79–95
Bruce JA. Implementation of nursing diagnosis. Nurs Clin North Am 1979 Sept; 14(3):509–15
Dalton JM. Nursing diagnosis in a community health setting. Nurs Clin North Am 1979 Sept; 14(3):525–31
Field L. The implementation of nursing diagnosis in clinical practice. Nurs Clin North Am 1979 Sept; 14(3):497–508
Fortin JD and Rabinow J. Legal implications of nursing diagnosis. Nurs Clin North Am 1979 Sept; 14(3):553–61

Gordon M. The concept of nursing diagnosis. Nurs Clin North Am 1979 Sept; 14(3):487–96
Gordon M and Sweeney MA. Methodological problems and issues in identifying and standardizing nursing diagnosis. Adv Nurs Sci 1979 Oct; 2(1):1–15
Gordon M et al. Nursing diagnosis: Looking at its use in the clinical area. Am J Nurs 1980 Apr; 80(4):672–4
Hausman KA. The concept and application of nursing diagnosis. J Neurosurg Nurs 1980 Jun; 12(2):76–80
Jones PE. A terminology for nursing diagnosis. Adv Nurs Sci 1979 Oct; 2(1):65–72
Kneedler JA. Perioperative role in three dimensions. AORN J 1979 Nov; 30(5):859–74
Kritek PB. Commentary: The development of nursing diagnosis and theory. Adv Nurs Sci 1979 Oct; 2(1):73–9
McKeehan KM. Nursing diagnosis in a discharge planning program. Nurs Clin North Am 1979 Sept; 14(3):517–24
Miller BK and White NE. Diabetes assessment guide. Am J Nurs 1980 Jul; 80(7):1314–16
Porter-O'Grady T and Carter JA. Bringing the nursing process into the OR. AORN J 1979 Nov; 30(5):898–9,902–3
Price MR. How nursing diagnosis helps focus your care: The patient is starving—but why? RN 1979 Nov; 42(11):45–8
Price MR. Nursing diagnosis: Making a concept come alive. Am J Nurs 1980 Apr; 80(4):668–71
Weber S. Nursing diagnosis in private practice. Nurs Clin North Am 1979 Sept; 14(3):533–9

HEALTH EDUCATION AND THE NURSING PROCESS

HEALTH EDUCATION

Health education is an essential component of nursing care and is directed toward promotion, maintenance, and restoration of health, as well as adaptation to the residual effects of illness.

OBJECTIVE: to teach people to live as healthy a life as possible—that is, to strive toward achieving one's maximum health potential.

Principles of Teaching and Learning

1. The teaching–learning process requires the active involvement of both the teacher and the learner.
2. The desired outcome of the teaching–learning process is a change in the learner's behavior.
3. The teacher serves as a facilitator of learning.
4. Learning is facilitated by progressing from the simple to the complex and from the known to the unknown.
5. Learning is facilitated when the learner is aware of his progress toward the learning goals.

Variables that Affect Learning Readiness

A. *Physical Readiness*

1. Physical distress that absorbs the patient's attention prevents effective learning.
2. Readiness to learn can be promoted by alleviating or at least minimizing as much as possible the patient's physical distress.

B. *Emotional Readiness*

1. Motivation to learn depends upon
   a. Acceptance of the illness or acceptance of the fact that illness is a threat.
   b. Recognition of the need to learn.
   c. A therapeutic regimen compatible with the patient's life-style or altered life-style.
2. Motivation to learn can be promoted by
   a. Creating a warm, accepting, positive atmosphere.
   b. Encouraging the patient to participate in the establishment of realistic, attainable learning goals.
   c. Providing feedback about progress, i.e., positive reinforcement when the patient is successful, constructive criticism when he is unsuccessful.

C. *Experimental Readiness*

1. The patient's previous experiences, especially learning experiences, affect the learning process.

a. Success in past learning experiences usually serves to motivate future learning.
b. Failure in past learning experiences often causes the learner to be hesitant to make new attempts to learn; this learner must be helped to gain confidence in his ability to learn.

2. Learning is dependent upon attainment of those behaviors that are prerequisites to the specific learning task, e.g., knowledge of the basics of normal nutrition is a prerequisite to understanding a special diet.

The Learning Atmosphere

1. The physical environment should be conducive to learning: quiet, uninterrupted, and comfortable. Consider the following variables:
   a. temperature
   b. lighting
   c. noise level
   d. traffic
   e. seating facilities and arrangement
2. The time of the teaching–learning session should be scheduled to meet the patient's needs.
   a. Encourage the patient and his family to participate in the scheduling of the teaching–learning session.
   b. Select a time when the patient is most alert, most comfortable, and least fatigued.
   c. Select a time when the patient is not anticipating immediate diagnostic or therapeutic procedures.
   d. Select a time when family members who are to be included in the teaching plan are available.

Teaching Strategies

Learning is facilitated by selecting teaching modes and media that are most appropriate to meet the individual patient's needs.

A. *Lecture*

1. Is most useful in teaching groups of patients who share the same learning needs.
2. Should always be accompanied by discussion, which allows the individual patient to
   a. Express his feelings and concerns.
   b. Ask questions.
   c. Clarify information.

B. *Group Discussion*

1. Is most useful for patients who relate well in groups.
2. Allows patients to experience security through being a member of a group of patients with similar problems or learning needs.
3. Provides patients with the opportunity to gain support, assistance, and encouragement from group members.

C. *Demonstration and Practice*

1. Is most useful when skills are to be learned.
2. Ample opportunity must be provided for practice sessions.
3. Equipment should be the same as that which the patient will use after leaving the hospital.

D. *Teaching Aids*

1. Are useful to supplement the nurse in helping the patient to learn.

2. Include books, pamphlets, pictures, films, slides, tapes, and models.
3. Must be reviewed prior to presentation to ensure that they are appropriate for meeting the patient's individual learning needs.

E. *Reinforcement and Follow-up*

1. Allow ample time for the patient to learn and to have his learning reinforced.
2. Follow-up sessions promote the patient's confidence in his ability to retain his newly learned behaviors.
3. Evaluate patient's progress, which is imperative, and plan additional teaching sessions, as necessary.
4. Follow-up sessions after discharge may be needed to assist the patient in transferring what he has learned in the hospital to his home setting.

THE NURSING PROCESS IN PATIENT TEACHING

The teaching–learning process is an integral part of the nursing process. With a focus on learning and with regard for the principles, variables, techniques, and strategies of teaching and learning, the steps of the nursing process—assessing, planning, implementing, and evaluating—are used for the purpose of meeting the teaching and learning needs of the patient and his family.

Assessing

1. Assess the patient's learning needs and his physical, emotional, and experiential readiness for health education.
   a. What are his health beliefs and behaviors?
   b. What psychosocial adaptations is he making?
   c. Is he ready to learn?
      (1) Is he able to learn these behaviors?
      (2) What are his expectations?
      (3) What additional information is needed about him?
2. Use appropriate assessment guides to facilitate data collection.
      Adapt such guides to the individual responses, problems, and needs of the patient.
3. Formulate nursing diagnoses that relate to the patient's learning needs.
   a. Organize, analyze, synthesize, and summarize the collected data.
   b. Identify the patient's learning problem(s), its particular characteristic(s) and etiology(ies).
   c. State nursing diagnoses concisely and precisely.

Planning

1. Assign priority to the nursing diagnoses.
2. Specify the short-term, intermediate, and long-term learning goals established by both the nurse and patient.
3. Identify teaching actions appropriate for goal attainment.
4. Establish expected outcome criteria.
5. Identify critical time periods for the attainment of outcomes.

6. Develop a written teaching plan (see sample teaching plan, p. 8).
   a. Include diagnoses (in order of priority), goals, teaching actions, outcome criteria, and critical time periods.
   b. Write entries precisely, concisely, and systematically.
   c. Include a topical outline of the information to be presented.
   d. Select appropriate teaching modes and media.
   e. Keep the plan current and flexible to meet the patient's changing learning needs.
7. Involve the patient, his family and/or significant others, nursing team members, and other health team members in all aspects of planning.

Implementing

1. Put the teaching plan into action.
2. Know the material to be presented.
3. Provide an atmosphere conducive to learning.
4. Use language the patient can understand.
5. Use appropriate teaching modes and media.
6. Use the same equipment that the patient will use after discharge.
7. Encourage the patient and his family to actively participate in learning.
8. Coordinate the activities of the patient, his family and/or significant others, nursing team members, and other health team members.
9. Record the patient's responses to the teaching actions.

Evaluating

1. Collect objective data.
   a. Observe the patient.
   b. Ask questions to determine if the patient understands.
   c. Use rating scales, checklists, anecdotal notes, and written tests when appropriate.
2. Compare the patient's behavioral outcomes to the outcome criteria. Determine the extent to which the goals were achieved.

Example of a Teaching Plan (For background information see nursing care plan example, p. 4.)

Assessment of Mrs. Collins' teaching and learning needs revealed the following: Basic knowledge about the relationship between sedentary life-style and impairment of venous circulation ● Definitive plans for scheduled short walks during work hours ● Definitive plans for walking and other exercises when at home; also, plans to minimize activities that involve prolonged standing and sitting ● Acceptable practices of foot and leg care to prevent complications related to impairment of circulation ● Inadequate knowledge about anticoagulant therapy regimen

Nursing Diagnosis:	Potential noncompliance with anticoagulant therapy regimen related to inadequate understanding of the regimen.
Goals—Short-term:	Describes action, use, and correct administration of Coumadin.
Intermediate:	Identifies signs of side effects of Coumadin and measures to prevent complications. Observes for side effects of Coumadin. Uses precautions to prevent complications of Coumadin therapy.
Long-term:	Complies with anticoagulant therapy regimen.

Nursing Orders	Outcome Criteria	Critical Time*	Outcome
Explain and discuss the action and use of Coumadin and the need to take the correct amount at the prescribed time.	Explains in her own words the necessity for and the action of Coumadin and the need for administering the accurate dose at the prescribed time.	4 days	Stated explanation accurately.
Explain and discuss the necessity for recording daily dose of Coumadin taken; provide patient with dosage calendar.	Explains in her own words the necessity for recording daily dose of Coumadin.	4 days	Stated explanation accurately.
	Records daily dose of Coumadin on dosage calendar.	4 days	Assumes responsibility for recording daily dose of Coumadin.
Explain and discuss the necessity for observing and reporting immediately any signs of bleeding:	Explains in her own words the necessity for observing and reporting bleeding immediately.	6 days	Stated explanation accurately.
hematuria, tarry stools, hematemesis, bleeding gums, easy bruising, epistaxis, hemoptysis, abdominal or lumbar pain, prolonged bleeding from any injury, faintness, dizziness, or unusual weakness.	Identifies signs of bleeding that must be reported.	6 days	Accurately identifed signs of bleeding.
	Observes for signs of bleeding.	6 days	Assumes responsibility for observing for signs of bleeding and has conscientiously reported that no signs are evident.
Explain and discuss the necessity for using a soft toothbrush and electric razor.	Uses soft toothbrush and electric razor.	6 days	Uses soft toothbrush and electric razor.
Explain and discuss the reason why over-the-counter drugs should not be taken without prescription, e.g., aspirin, cold medicines, antacids, mineral oil, vitamin K.	Explains in her own words the reason for avoiding unprescribed over-the-counter drugs.	6 days	Stated explanation accurately; does take over-the-counter aspirin at home—will now use Tylenol after discharge.
Explain and discuss the necessity for maintaining well-balanced diet and abstaining from alcohol.	Explains in her own words the necessity for well-balanced diet and abstinence from alcohol.	6 days	Stated explanation accurately; does not drink alcohol.
	Selects well-balanced diet from menu.	6 days	Uses basic principles of nutrition to select well-balanced diet.
Explain and discuss the reasons for informing dentist, podiatrist, and any other physicians about Coumadin therapy.	Explains in her own words reasons for informing other medical personnel about Coumadin	6 days	Stated explanation accurately; notified dentist of Coumadin therapy and postponed dental exam for 1 month.
Encourage to wear Medic Alert bracelet and carry medication identification on her person.	Wears Medic Alert bracelet.	6 days	Obtained Medic Alert bracelet and wears at all times.
	Carries medication identification on her person.	6 days	Filled out medication identification card and placed it in visible place in wallet.
Explain and discuss the necessity for keeping all physician and laboratory test appointments.	Explains in her own words the reasons for keeping all appointments with physician and for laboratory tests.	6 days	Stated explanation accurately.
	Keeps all appointments with physican.	after discharge	
	Keeps all appointments for laboratory tests.	after discharge	

* These times have not been standardized, but are individualized according to the patient's needs.

3. Include the patient, his family and/or significant others, nursing team members, and other health team members in the evaluation.
4. Identify alterations that need to be made in the teaching plan.
5. Make referrals to appropriate resource persons or agencies for reinforcement of learning after discharge.
6. Continue all steps of the teaching–learning process: assessing, planning, implementing, evaluating.

BIBLIOGRAPHY

Books

Redman BK. The Process of Patient Teaching in Nursing. St. Louis, CV Mosby, 1980
Zander KS et al. Practical Manual for Patient Teaching. St. Louis, CV Mosby, 1978

Articles

Chaisson GM. Patient education: Whose responsibility is it and who should be doing it? Nurs Admin Q 1980 Winter; 4(2):1–11
Clark MD. The utilization of theoretical concepts in patient education. Nurs Admin Q 1980 Winter; 4(2):55–60
Condon MB Sr, Dannen CJ and Hall MA. The teaching resource unit: A comprehensive approach to patient education. Nurs Admin J 1980 Winter; 4(2):69–73
Fitzgerald S. Utilizing Orem's self-care nursing model in designing an educational program for the diabetic. Top Clin Nurs 1980 Jul; 2(2):57–65
Frantz RA. Selecting media for patient education. Top Clin Nurs 1980 Jul; 2(2):77–83
Hochbaum GM. Patient counseling vs patient teaching. Top Clin Nurs 1980 Jul; 2(2):1–7
Huckabay LMD. A strategy for patient teaching. Nurs Admin Q 1980 Winter; 4(2):47–54
Johnson-Saylor MT. Seize the moment: Health education for the young adult. Top Clin Nurs 1980 Jul; 2(2):9–19
McCulloch C, Boggs BJ and Varner CF. Implementation of educational programs for patients. Nurs Admin Q 1980 Winter; 4(2):61–8
Nowakowski L. Health promotion/self-care programs for the community. Top Clin Nurs 1980 Jul; 2(2):21–7
Phippin ML. Perioperative nurses use patient teaching conference. AORN J 1979 May; 29(6):1046–51
Pyle N. Health education for the aging. J Gerontol Nurs 1979 May/June; 5(3):24–9
Toth JC. Effect of structured preparation for transfer on patient anxiety on leaving coronary care unit. Nurs Res 1980 Jan/Feb; 29(1):28–34
Walters J. Four practical questions to ask when organizing preoperative classes. Am J Nurs 1979 Jun; 79(6):1090–1
Whitehouse R. Forms that facilitate patient teaching. Am J Nurs 1979 Jul; 79(7):1227–9

DATA COLLECTION AND RECORD KEEPING: PATIENT HISTORY AND PROBLEM ORIENTED RECORDS

DATA COLLECTION

Purpose
1. Data collection is the first step in the process of defining problems.
2. A thorough and accurate assessment of a patient's problems or condition depends on the completeness and accuracy of the data collected.

Types of Data Collected
A. *The Patient's History* (see details, p. 12)

1. Is elicited in an interview.
2. The history, in final written form, logically presents the *patient's views* of:
   a. His health problems
   b. General health condition
   c. Past medical history
   d. Family health history
   e. A profile of the patient's personal and social life and well-being
3. The patient history will also reveal what the patient knows about his health, what is important in terms of health care, and expectations of the health care being sought.
   This may be supplemented by information from the patient's hospital record, conversations with other care-givers, parents (in the case of children and infants), or consultants.
4. The patient history is always *subjective* information in that it is presented from the point of view of the person reporting to the interviewer rather than directly observed by the interviewer.

B. *The Physical Examination* (see details, Chapter 4)—is performed by the practitioner for the following purposes:

1. To corroborate the patient's history.
2. To observe any findings not reported in the history.
3. To obtain *objective* information about the individual's health state and/or status of a health problem.
   Objective information is that body of data about a person which can be perceived by another person.

C. *Laboratory Data*—from test results

It is important to know that laboratory data constitute another source of *objective data* which is important in assessing many health problems and conditions; these must be considered by all nurses engaged in caring for and understanding patients.

Principles of Data Collection
1. All data collection should be well organized and should follow a format that promotes thoroughness.
2. There is no room for bias in data collection since the practitioner's mind must be open to clues and cues that might otherwise be missed.
3. Understanding the techniques of interviewing is basic to collecting accurate data in the patient history and to establishing the basis for a working relationship with the patient.
4. Information gathered must be organized and recorded so that it has meaning for members of the health care team and can guide patient assessment and care.

RECORDING THE DATA GATHERED

General Guidelines
1. Keep in mind the purpose of recording the information and the audience for whom it is intended. This serves to guide the form and content of the record.
2. Remember that the patient's record is a legal document.
   The record must present the information about the patient as completely, concisely, and accurately as possible, without unnecessary duplication of material.
3. Avoid redundancy.
   Redundancy obscures important information and makes careful reading of the record unnecessarily time-consuming. As a result, the record is not read carefully.

General Principles

1. *When to record:*

    As soon as the information is gathered—to minimize omission and distortion of facts.

2. *Organization*

    Information must be organized and recorded systematically. (This applies to complete history, physical examination, or progress notes.)

    a. The history, or subjective information, is recorded first.

    b. Then the physical examination, or objective data, is recorded.

    c. From a systematic recording of the facts must stem a logical assessment of the subjective and objective data.

    d. Therefore, facts must be reported so that their meaning is clear and they tell a connected story.

3. *Detail*

    Describe the data gathered, using the appropriate vocabulary.

4. *Language*

    a. The written record must be succinct, yet understandable to the reader.

    b. Avoid using abbreviations.

5. *Legal considerations*

    a. Since the patient's record is a legal document, facts must be identified and must be stated precisely and objectively.

    b. Both inaccuracy and interpretation must be avoided.

    c. Assessment or judgment can be made only after facts are obtained and recorded with great care.

    d. The document must be signed and dated.

Recording the History

(The general principles listed above apply to recording the history.)

1. The present illness must be recorded chronologically, beginning with the onset of the problem.

Often it is helpful to think of a beginning phrase such as "The patient was well until. . . ." Each paragraph should then describe events in sequence up to the time that the patient is being interviewed.

2. Quantify anything related to measurement.

    For example: "the patient has *frequent* headaches" is less accurate than "the patient has an average of 3 headaches a week . . ."

Recording the Physical Examination

(It is important to follow the above principles.) Other specific guidelines include the following:

1. Describe any abnormality in detail.

2. Carefully describe a normal finding in conditions where one might expect the normal to be abnormal.

    For instance, in the patient with hypertension, it would be important to report the absence of hemorrhages and exudates in the fundoscopic examination report.

3. If there are any laboratory results, they are recorded after the physical examination and before the assessment and plan.

Progress Notes

1. Progress notes are records of the patient's health status from visit to visit, day to day, or shift to shift as the case may be.

2. They are usually written in relation to a specific problem or condition and report the relevant subjective (history) and objective (physical exam and lab results) data that bring the record up to date.

3. Progress notes also include an assessment of the data and a plan dealing with the problem.

    (The Problem Oriented Medical Record format developed by Dr. Lawrence Weed is an extremely useful and instructive guide in organizing and recording the initial data base and the progress notes.)

THE PROBLEM ORIENTED RECORD (POR)

A *problem oriented record* is a patient's health record organized so that specific problems are defined, numbered, and then referred to by number throughout the record. Problems are identified and numbered after the initial data base is collected.

Components of the POR

These may vary according to the particular setting in which the system is used. However, every system includes the following:

A. *Initial Data Base*

Consists of:

a. The patient's comprehensive health history

b. A complete physical examination

c. Available laboratory data

B. *Problem List*

1. Consists of a numbered list of medical, social, psychological problems derived from the initial data base.

2. Includes active and inactive problems, date of onset, and date of resolution when applicable.

a. Often this list appears at the very beginning of the record and serves as an index.

b. A number is never used twice even though new problems arise, some old ones are resolved, or several problems are found to be related to one common problem.

3. It is important to remember that the numbered problem list should serve as an index to the record, so that information can be systematically ordered around a problem and not get lost or be misinterpreted as the volume of the record grows in the course of many visits.

C. *Progress Notes*

See Sample Progress Note, page 12.

1. Organization of the progress note varies, but the basic format remains the same.

2. The note begins with the problem and its number and then continues as follows:

    S = *Subjective* data (history, consultation) concerning the problem and covering the time interval since the last entry.

    O = *Objective* data (physical examination, laboratory

reports) concerning the problem and covering the same time period.

A = *Assessment* of the *S* and the *O*. Includes, as appropriate, statements about probable etiology; course of the problem; the patient's response to therapy and his coping ability; general diagnostic, therapeutic, and health education plans; and a rationale for the entire plan. It should include a statement about the patient's participation in planning and his reaction to the plan.

P = *Plan*—This is a statement *specifying* what is to be done regarding the problem, who is to do

it, and when it is to be done. A timetable is provided when possible. The plan stems directly from the rationale in the assessment and may include any or all of the following:
1. *Diagnostic plan*—states what is to be done to make the data base more complete.
2. *Therapeutic plan*—indicates projected methods for curing, improving, or palliating the patient's problem.
3. *Health education plan*—outlines content of health teaching concerning the problem and the diagnostic and/or therapeutic plan.

Sample Progress Note

#3 Hypertension

S.   The patient has felt well since he was seen 3 months ago. He has had no headaches; no visual or gastrointestinal problems; no chest pain or palpitations, no shortness of breath. His activity is unchanged; he sleeps on one pillow; has no nocturia or ankle swelling. He is taking his medications, knows their names and dosages. Drinks orange juice with fluid pill qd. He is following a diet that has "no added" salt; drinks 5 beers a week; lunchmeat sandwiches for lunch. He thinks he is gaining weight—his "clothes are tighter."

O.   P.   72 regular
Wt.   82.5 kg. (182 pounds)
BP   148/95 right arm lying
        140/100 right arm standing

Respiratory: Chest expands/symmetrically; fremitus (perceptible vibration) normal bilaterally; bronchovesicular sounds present; no adventitious (not natural) sounds.

Cardiovascular: No heaves or thrills; point of maximal impulse (PMI) at 5th intercostal space in midclavicular line; normal sinus rhythm without murmurs, gallops or extrasystoles; trace pedal edema.

A.   BP is fairly well controlled. Weight is up 2.3 kg. (5 pounds). The patient is taking his medication. However, his diet contains a lot of sodium, even though none is "added." If he can cut out some of the high-salt foods and lose 2.3–4.5 kg. (5–10 pounds), his pressure will no doubt be under better control. He seems motivated to lose some weight, since his clothes are tighter. He needs to know about sodium content of food, and his wife needs instruction too, since she does the shopping. Will continue the same medications and try having the patient lose weight to bring BP under better control. The patient comprehends the consequences of uncontrolled hypertension and the need for sustained weight control and medical follow-up. His wife sounds very supportive. Patient will need routine yearly blood work and cardiogram by next visit.

P.   1. Diet instruction for patient and wife. Patient will call to suggest a convenient time and will set up appointment then.
2. Continue same medications: Aldomet 250 mg. tid; hydrochlorothiazide 50 mg. qd with dietary K^+ supplement.
3. Return visit in 3 months to check BP and weight.
4. Blood work before next visit (Na^+, K^+, CO_2, urea-N, glucose, creatinine).
5. Electrocardiogram before next visit.

THE PATIENT HISTORY

General Principles

1. The first step in caring for a patient and in soliciting his active cooperation is to gather a careful and complete history.
   a. In *all* patient concerns and problems, an accurate history is the foundation on which data collection and the process of assessment are based.
   b. The comprehensiveness of the history elicited will depend on the information available in the patient's record.
2. Time spent early in the nurse-patient relationship gathering detailed information about what the patient knows, thinks, and feels about his problems will prevent time-consuming errors and misunderstandings later.

3. Skill in interviewing will affect both the accuracy of information elicited and the quality of the relationship established with the patient.
   This point cannot be overemphasized; the reader is encouraged to consult other sources for detailed discussion of techniques of health interviewing.
4. The purpose of the interview is to encourage an interchange of information between the patient and the nurse.
   a. The patient must feel that his words are understood and that his concerns are being listened to and dealt with sensitively.
   b. Some basic techniques for achieving these ends include the following:
      (1) Provide privacy for the patient in as quiet a place as possible and see that he is comfortable.
      (2) Begin the interview with a courteous greeting and an introduction. Explain who you are and why you are there.
      (3) Be sure that facial expressions, body movements, and tone of voice are pleasant, unhurried, and nonevaluative, and that they convey the attitude of a sensitive listener, so that the patient will feel free to express his thoughts and feelings.
      (4) Avoid reassuring the patient prematurely (before you have adequate information about the problem). This only serves to cut off discussion; the patient may then be unwilling to bring up a problem causing concern.
      (5) At times a patient gives cues or suggests information, but does not tell enough. It may be necessary to probe for more information in order to obtain a thorough history; the patient must realize that this is done for his benefit.
      (6) Guide the interview so that the necessary information is obtained, without cutting off discussion. Controlling the rambling patient is often difficult, but with practice it can be done skillfully, without jeopardizing the quality of the information gained.

Identifying Information

A. Purposes

1. To eliminate confusion about the patient's identity; to obtain the information required for contacting him if the need arises.
2. To provide an introduction to the patient and some indication of his habits, life-style, and beliefs, which may be explored in greater depth in the personal and social history.
3. To initiate a relationship based on recognition of the importance of the informant's role in sharing in the care of the patient (when this is the case).

B. Types of Information Needed

1. Date and time
2. Patient's name, address, phone number, race, religion, birthdate, and age
3. Name of referring practitioner
4. Insurance data
5. Name of informant—the patient may be the person giving this history; if not, record the name, address, phone number, and relationship to patient of the person giving the history
6. Accuracy and reliability of informant—this is a judgment based on the consistency of responses to questions and on a comparison of information in the history with your own observations in the physical examination

C. Method of Collecting Data

1. Careful interviewing of the patient or his "care person" will provide most of the information.
2. The patient's hospital or clinic record may also be a valuable source.
3. Repeat information when necessary to verify accuracy (e.g., to assure that there has been no change in address or phone number).
4. Assume a direct and courteous manner.
5. Explain the reasons why the information is needed— to help put the patient at ease.

Chief Complaint

A. Purposes

1. To allow the patient to describe his own problems and expectations with little or no direction from the interviewer.
2. To identify the overriding problem for which the person is seeking help.
   a. Adults with chronic conditions often have numerous complaints.
   b. If possible, focus on a single problem or concern— the one most important to the patient.
3. To identify the patient's feelings about his symptoms. The patient may show fear, guilt, defensiveness in this first statement.

B. Types of Information Needed

The patient's primary problem(s) or concern in his own words. A statement describing the duration of the complaint.

C. Method of Collecting Data

1. Ask the patient a direct question, e.g., "How may I help you?" or "For what reason have you come to the hospital (clinic, etc.)?"
2. Avoid confusing questions, e.g., "What brings you here?" ("The bus.") or "Why are you here?" ("That's what I came to find out.")
3. Ask how long the concern or problem has been present. If necessary, establish the time of onset precisely by offering such clues as "Did you feel this way a month (6 months or 2 years) ago?"
4. Let the patient speak freely without offering your opinion until he has had an opportunity to identify the problem as clearly as possible.
5. Write down what the patient says, using quotation marks to identify his words.

History of Present Illness

A. Purposes

1. To amplify the description of the chief complaint and to clarify its relationship to other symptoms and events.
2. To carefully describe a symptom or problem that may be a clue to future diagnosis.

B. Type of Information Needed

1. A *detailed chronological* picture beginning with the time the patient was last well (or, in the case of a problem with an acute onset, the patient's condition just prior to the onset of the problem) and ending with a description of the patient's current condition.
2. If there is more than one important problem, each is described in a separate, chronologically organized paragraph in the written history of present illness.

3. The outline for reporting the present illness will vary with each case.

C. *Method of Collecting Data*

1. For each problem investigate the following:
   a. Quality (e.g., sharp, dull, knife-like—referring to pain)
   b. Quantity (e.g., $\frac{1}{2}$ cup sputum)
   c. Location of symptoms, intensity, periodicity (e.g., epigastric area; daily; after meals)
   d. Aggravating and alleviating factors (e.g., medications, prescribed and over-the-counter; rest; diet)
   e. Associated phenomena (e.g., shortness of breath)
2. Date the onset of the problem as accurately as possible since chronology is of the utmost importance (see Chief Complaint, p. 13).
3. Describe the character of the symptoms and state whether they have changed over time.
4. In the case of acute infections, inquire about possible exposure or an incubation period.
5. When the present illness has been characterized by attacks separated by free intervals, obtain the history of a typical attack.
   Onset, duration, and associated symptoms—pain; fever; chills; relation to any activity, either physical or emotional, or to such factors as diet, medication, etc.
6. In both acute and chronic illnesses note whether and when the patient stopped working and/or went to bed.
7. Get the patient's subjective appraisal of whether the symptom or problem is getting better or worse.
8. When a particular organ or system is disturbed, ask for a review of that system and related systems so that important negative and positive information may be included in the written history.
   For instance, if a patient complains of chest pain, ask about both the respiratory and cardiac systems as well as the musculoskeletal history of the chest.
9. Questioning may reveal that other systems must also be reviewed.
10. Ask about previous treatment, including medications, prescribing physician or practitioner, and place where treatment was obtained (name of hospital, clinic, etc.).
11. At the end, review the chronology and specifics with the patient and ask him to affirm or correct the information.
12. Organize the information for recording or presentation.

Past Medical History

A. *Purposes*

1. To determine any change in the patient's normal patterns of living that may or may not be caused by illness.
2. To identify clues that may aid in diagnosing the present illness.
3. To participate in gathering and recording information that may be helpful in making a diagnosis, even though the nurse may not have the final responsibility for diagnosing the patient's particular problem.

B. *Type of Information Needed*

1. *General health and strength*—sleeping patterns, appetite, stability of weight, usual activities.

2. *Acute infectious diseases*—measles, mumps, whooping cough, chickenpox, pneumonia, pleurisy, tuberculosis, scarlet fever, acute rheumatic fever, rheumatic heart disease, tonsillitis, hepatitis, polio, venereal disease, tropical or parasitic diseases, any other acute infectious problem the patient describes.
3. *Immunization*—polio, diphtheria, pertussis, tetanus, influenza, last PPD or other skin test, any abnormal or unusual reactions. Give date when possible.
4. *Operation*—indications, diagnosis, dates, hospital, surgeon, complications.
5. *Previous hospitalizations*—doctor, hospital date (year), diagnosis, treatment.
6. *Injuries*—type; resulting disabilities.
7. *Major illnesses* (any prolonged illnesses not requiring hospitalization)—dates, symptoms, course, treatment.
8. *Allergies* (may appear in review of systems)—asthma, hay fever, hives, food allergies, drug reactions, previous treatment with penicillin and any reactions.
9. *Obstetrical history* (may appear in review of systems)
   a. Pregnancies, miscarriages, abortions.
   b. Describe course of pregnancy, labor, and delivery; date, place of delivery.
10. *Psychiatric history* (may appear in review of systems)—treatment by a psychiatrist or psychologist, indications, date, place, medications for "nerves."

C. *Method of Collecting Data*

1. Begin by explaining the purpose and type of questions you will be asking; e.g., "I am now going to ask you some questions about your past health."
2. Explain that these questions are important in order to obtain an accurate picture of all the events that affected or that *did not* affect the patient's health in the past.
3. Use direct questions, e.g., "How would you describe your general health?" and then proceed with more specific queries, such as "Has your weight been stable over the past 5 years?"

Family History

A. *Purposes*

1. To present a picture of the patient's family health, including that of grandparents, parents, brothers, and sisters specifically.
   It also involves the health of close relatives, since some diseases show a familial tendency or are hereditary.
2. To describe the health of the patient's spouse and children, since this may give clues about possible communicable disease problems.
   Also it will be important in determining what sort of condition a family is in and how this affects the patient.

B. *Type of Information Needed*

1. Age and health status of (or age at and cause of death of) parent, sibling.
2. History, in immediate and close relatives, of heart trouble, high blood pressure, stroke, diabetes, gout, kidney disease or stones, thyroid disease, asthma or other allergies, blood problems, cancer (types).
3. Hereditary diseases such as hemophilia or sickle cell disease.
4. Age and health status of spouse and children.

C. *Method of Collecting Data*

1. Begin with an explanation of what you are asking and why, since the patient may not understand the purpose of your questions. Example:

   "I am going to ask now about the health of your immediate family and relatives. It is important to know if there are any conditions which tend to or could occur in your family, or in you as a member of the family."

2. Ask direct questions.

   a. Begin with the patient's siblings.

      "Do you have any brothers and sisters?" "How old are they and what is the state of their health?"

   b. List each sibling separately, giving age and state of health.

Review of Systems

A. *Purpose*

To obtain detailed information about the current state of the patient and any past symptoms, or lack of symptoms, he may have experienced related to a particular body system.

B. *Type of Information Needed*

Subjective information about what the patient feels or sees with regard to the major systems of the body.

1. *Skin*—rash, itching, change in pigmentation or texture, sweating, hair growth and distribution, condition of nails.
2. *Skeletal*—stiffness of joints, pain, deformity, restriction of motion, swelling, redness, heat. If there are problems, ask the patient to specify any activities of daily life that he finds difficult or impossible to perform.
3. *Head*—headaches, dizziness, syncope, head injuries.
4. *Eyes*—vision, pain, diplopia, photophobia, blind spots, itching, burning, discharge, recent change in appearance or vision, glaucoma, cataracts, glasses worn, date of last refraction, infection.
5. *Ears*—hearing acuity, earache, discharge, tinnitus, vertigo.
6. *Nose*—sense of smell, frequency of colds, obstruction, epistaxis, postnasal discharge, sinus pain or therapy, use of nose drops or sprays (type and frequency).
7. *Teeth*—pain; bleeding, swollen or receding gums; recent abscesses, extractions; dentures; dental hygiene practices.
8. *Mouth and tongue*—soreness of tongue or buccal mucosa, ulcers, swelling.
9. *Throat*—sore throats, tonsillitis, hoarseness, dysphagia.
10. *Neck*—pain, stiffness, swelling, enlarged glands or lymph nodes.
11. *Endocrine*—goiter, thyroid tenderness, tremors, weakness, tolerance to heat and cold, changes in hat or glove size, changes in skin pigmentation, libido, bruisability, muscle cramps, polyuria, polydypsia, polyphagia, hormone therapy.
12. *Respiratory*
    a. Pain in the chest and relationship to respirations.
    b. Dyspnea, wheezing, cough, sputum (character, quantity), hemoptysis.
    c. Night sweats (Does the patient have to change his bed clothes?)
    d. Last chest x-ray and result; (indicate where obtained).
    e. Exposure to tuberculosis.
13. *Cardiac*
    a. Presence of pain or distress and location (have patient point to location); radiation of pain; precipitating/aggravating causes; alleviating measures; timing and duration.
    b. Palpitations, dyspnea, orthopnea (note number of pillows required for sleeping), edema, cyanosis.
    c. Exercise tolerance (determine in relation to patient's regular activities—how much can he do before stopping to rest?)
    d. Blood pressure (if known); last ECG and results (indicate where obtained).
14. *Hematologic*—anemia (if so, treatment received), tendency to bruise or bleed, thromboses, thrombophlebitis, any known abnormalities of blood cells.
15. *Lymph nodes*—enlargement, tenderness, suppuration, duration and progress of abnormality.
16. *Gastrointestinal*
    a. Appetite and digestion, intolerance to certain classes of foods.
    b. Pain associated with hunger or eating, eructation, regurgitation, heartburn, nausea, vomiting, hematemesis.
    c. Regularity of bowel movement; (describe normal bowel habits and whether they have changed recently or not); diarrhea, flatulence, stools (color—brown, black, clay; tarry, fresh blood, mucus, etc.).
    d. Hemorrhoids, jaundice, dark urine, use of laxatives—type; frequency. (This should be included under past medical history with medications, but may be repeated here.)
    e. History of ulcer, gallstones, polyps, tumors.
    f. Previous x-rays—where, when, results.
17. *Genitourinary*—dysuria, pain, urgency, frequency, hematuria, nocturia, polydipsia, polyuria, oliguria, edema of the face, hesitancy, dribbling, loss in size or force of stream, passage of stones, stress incontinence, hernias.
    a. Males
       (1) Puberty—onset, voice change, erections, emissions
       (2) Libido—satisfaction with sexual relations
    b. Females
       (1) Menses—onset, regularity, duration of flow, dysmenorrhea, last period, intermenstrual bleeding or discharge, dyspareunia
       (2) Libido—satisfaction with sexual relations
       (3) Pregnancies (see past medical history)
       (4) Methods of contraception
       (5) Breasts—pain, tenderness, discharge, lumps, mammograms, breast self-examination—techniques and timing with regard to menstrual cycle
18. *Neuromuscular*
    a. Mental status—orientation to time, place, person, and distance. "How far is your home from the hospital?" (Interviewer must be able to verify the answer.)
    b. Memory—distant memory shown by recalling past medical history.
       —recent memory shown by recalling what was eaten for breakfast.
    c. Cognition, or ability of patient to conceptualize

(very useful information in determining a health education plan for the patient).

   d. Patient's description of his personality—how he views himself.
   e. Presence of tics, twitching, weakness, paralysis, tremor, wasting of muscles, incoordination, fatigue, sensory loss with respect to pain, temperature, touch, muscle pain, cramps.
   f. Psychiatric history may be entered here.
19. *General Constitutional Symptoms*—Fever, chills, malaise, fatigability, recent loss or gain of weight.

C. *Method of Collecting Data*

1. Begin by explaining to the patient—"I am going to ask you many questions about your body which will help in understanding your present problem."
2. Ask direct questions about each system, using terms that the patient understands.
3. Whenever the patient complains or suggests a symptom, ask the questions outlined under method of collecting data about the present illness (onset, duration, etc.).
4. Never assume that things are "OK" if the patient fails to mention something.
   a. Ask about every aspect of the function of a particular system and be sure to record the patient's responses.
   b. Often the fact that a body system has been free of any symptoms is as important as any symptoms that have been experienced.
5. If necessary, memorize a list of questions for each system or use a list when interviewing the patient. Knowing what to ask about each system is based on knowledge of the function of each body system and of the way that normal function manifests itself.

Personal and Social History

A. *Purposes*

1. To describe the patient's life situation—may have bearing on the present condition and/or the patient's ability to cope with this problem.
2. To develop a plan of care that "fits" the patient. Here the interviewer finds out the many personal and family resources an individual has to aid him in coping with the situation—both long-term and short-term.
3. To have some idea of how the patient patterns his life.
   a. Certain habits and patterns are more easily assimilated and changed than others, when necessary.
   b. Knowing the patient's patterns is useful in helping to organize hospital routine in ways that will be least disruptive to the patient.
4. To help the patient develop a workable plan of care at home, based on knowledge of home conditions.

5. To determine if the patient's occupation is directly or indirectly related to his condition.
6. To determine if the patient's religious affiliation may affect therapy.

B. *Type of Information Needed*

1. *Personal status*—birth place, education, armed service affiliation, position in the family, satisfaction with life situations (home and job), personal concerns
2. *Habits/Patterns*
   a. Sleeping, activities/hobbies, nutrition/eating habits (diet for a typical day)
   b. Consumption of alcohol, coffee, tea, drugs (marijuana, over-the-counter medications)
   c. Tobacco (what form; how long)
   d. Sexual habits (can be part of GU history)—relationships, frequency, satisfaction
3. *Home Conditions*
   a. Marital status, nature of family relationships
   b. Economic conditions—source of income; health insurance, Medicare, Medicaid
   c. Living arrangements and housing (owning/renting, heating, sewage, pets, etc.)
   d. Involvement with agencies (name, case worker, etc.)
4. *Occupation*
   a. Past and present employment and working conditions, including exposure to stress/tension, noise, pollution
   b. Working hours
   c. Job satisfaction
5. *Religion*—name, whether practicing or not, any stipulations with regard to health practices

C. *Method of Collecting Data*

1. Begin by explaining that you are now going to ask questions about the patient's life situation in order to gain a clearer perspective of the patient's condition and of how you might help him.
2. Your manner should be matter-of-fact, yet concerned. If you are uncomfortable asking the questions, most likely the patient will sense that and be uneasy answering them.
3. A sensitive interviewer can ask most of the questions listed above in an initial interview without alienating the patient. For instance, ask "What has been your education?" instead of "How far have you gone in school?"

Ending the History

When you have completed the history, it is often helpful to say: "Is there anything else you would like to tell me?" or "What do you think is the matter with you?" This allows the patient to end the history by saying what is on his mind and what concerns him most.

BIBLIOGRAPHY

DATA COLLECTION AND RECORD KEEPING

Books

Accreditation Manual for Hospitals. Chicago, Joint Commission on Accreditation of Hospitals, Feb 1978
Enelow AJ and Swisher SN. Interviewing and Patient Care. London, Oxford Press, 1979

Froehlich RE and Bishop FM. Clinical Interviewing Skills, 3rd ed. St. Louis, CV Mosby, 1977
Prior JA and Silberstein JS. Physical Diagnosis: The History and Examination of the Patient. St. Louis, CV Mosby, 1977
Robinson J (ed). Documenting Patient Care Responsibly. Horsham, Intermed Communications, 1978
Walker JB et al (eds). Dynamics of Problem-Oriented Ap-

proaches: Patient Care and Documentation. Philadelphia, JB Lippincott, 1976

Weed L. Medical Records. Medical Education and Patient Care. Cleveland, Case Western Reserve University Press, 1968

Yura H and Walsh MB (eds). The Nursing Process: Assessing Planning, Implementing and Evaluating, 3rd ed. New York, Appleton-Century-Crofts, 1978

Articles

Austin E. How your nursing notes can rob your patients of benefits. Nursing '78 1978 Sept; 8(9):58–59

Bartos LT and Knight MR. Documentation of nursing process. Super Nurse 1978 July; 9(7):41–48

Cassell EJ. Listen: "Illogical" patients often make sense. Patient Care 1980 Jan 15: 14(1):91–106

Dossey B. Perfecting your skills for systematic patient assessments. Nursing '79 1979 Feb; 9(2):42–45

Eggland ET. Charting: How and why to document your care daily and fully. Nursing '80 1980 Feb; 10(2):39–43

Farrell J. The human side of assessment. Nursing '80 1980 April; 10(4):74–75

Friedman RB, Huhta J and Cheung S. An automated verbal medical history system. Arch Intern Med 1978 Sept; 138(9):1359–1361

Gooding M. If you think care plans are a nuisance, read this. RN 1978 Oct; 41(10):95–102

Mandell HN. A revolution in nurse's notes. Postgrad Med 1980 Dec; 68(6):22–23

McCaman B and Hirsh HL. Medical records—legal perspectives. Primary Care 1979 Sept; 6(3):681–691

O'Sullivan AL. Privileged communication. Am J Nurs 1980 May; 80(5):947–950

Raymer MC. Improving patient teaching with an all-in-one program (documenting). Nursing '80 1980 Aug; 10(8):18–19

Reilly MM. Let's set the record straight. Nursing '79 1979 Jan; 9(1):56–61

Schneggenberger C. History taking skills. How do you rate? Nursing '79 1979 March; 9(3):97–101

Sharing records to share the onus of care. Patient Care 15 Nov 1979; 13(19):166–181

Shuler C. Documenting patient teaching. Super Nurse 1979 June; 10(6):43–49

Tucker G. Record sharing: Lawyer's viewpoint. Patient Care 15 Nov 1978: 13(19):182–193

Vasey EK. Writing your patient's care plan . . . efficiently. Nursing '79 1979 April; 9(4):67–71

Want to share records with patients? Here's how. Patient Care 15 Jan 1980; 14(2):124–138

ADULT PHYSICAL EXAMINATION

General Principles

1. A complete or partial physical examination is conducted following a careful comprehensive or problem-related history.
2. It is conducted in a quiet, well-lit room with consideration for patient privacy and comfort.

Approach to the Patient

1. When possible, begin with the patient in a sitting position so that both front and back can be examined.
2. Completely expose the part to be examined but drape the rest of the body appropriately.
3. Conduct the examination systematically from head to foot so as not to miss observing any system or body part.
4. While examining each region consider the underlying anatomical structures, their function, and possible abnormalities.
5. Since the body is bilaterally symmetrical, for the most part, compare findings on one side with those on the other.
6. Explain all procedures to the patient while the examination is being conducted—to avoid alarming or worrying the patient and to encourage his cooperation.

Techniques of Examination and Assessment

Use the following techniques of examination as appropriate for eliciting findings.

Inspection

1. Begins with first encounter with the patient and is the most important of all the techniques.
2. Is an organized scrutiny of the patient's behavior and body.
3. With the knowledge and experience, the examiner can become highly sensitive to visual clues.
4. The examiner begins each phase of the examination by inspecting the particular part with the eyes.

Palpation

1. Involves touching the region or body part just observed and noting what the various structures feel like.
2. With experience comes the ability to distinguish variations of normal from abnormal.
3. Is performed in an organized manner from region to region.

Percussion

1. By setting underlying tissues in motion, percussion helps in determining whether the underlying tissue is air-filled, fluid-filled, or solid.
2. Audible sounds and palpable vibrations are produced which can be distinguished by the examiner.

There are 5 basic notes produced by percussion which can be distinguished by differences in the qualities of sound, pitch, duration, and intensity.

	Relative Intensity	Relative Pitch	Relative Duration	Example Location
Flatness	Soft	High	Short	Thigh
Dullness	Medium	Medium	Medium	Liver
Resonance	Loud	Low	Long	Normal lung
Hyperresonance	Very loud	Lower	Longer	Emphysematous lung
Tympany	Loud	*	*	Gastric air bubble or puffed out cheek

* Distinguished mainly by its musical timbre.
(From Bates, B.: A Guide to Physical Examination. Philadelphia, J. B. Lippincott, 1979.)

3. The technique for percussion may be described as follows:
   a. Hyperextend the middle finger of your left hand, pressing the distal portion and joint firmly against the surface to be percussed.
     (1) Other fingers touching the surface will damp the sound.
     (2) Be consistent in the degree of firmness exerted by the hyperextended finger as you move it from area to area or the sound will vary.
   b. Cock the right hand at the wrist, flex the middle finger upwards, and place the forearm close to the surface to be percussed. The right hand and forearm should be as relaxed as possible.
   c. With a quick, sharp, *relaxed* wrist motion, strike the extended left middle finger with the flexed right middle finger, using the tip of the finger, not the pad. (A very short fingernail is a must!)
     Aim at the end of the extended left middle finger (just behind the nail bed) where the greatest pressure is exerted on the surface to be percussed.
   d. Lift the right middle finger rapidly to avoid damping the vibrations.
   e. The movement is at the wrist, not at the finger, elbow, or shoulder; the examiner should use the lightest touch capable of producing a clear sound.

Auscultation

1. Is a method that uses the stethoscope to augment the sense of hearing.
2. The stethoscope must be constructed well and must fit the user. Earpieces should be comfortable, the length of the tubing should be 25–38 cm. (10–15 inches), and the head should have a diaphragm and a bell.
   a. The bell is used for low-pitched sounds such as certain heart murmurs.
   b. The diaphragm screens out low-pitched sounds and is good for hearing high frequency sounds such as breath sounds.
   c. Extraneous sounds can be produced by clothing, hair, and movement of the head of the stethoscope.

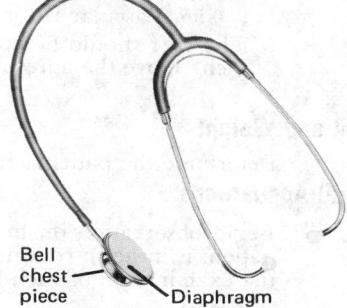

Bell chest piece   Diaphragm

Equipment Thermometer
Sphygmomanometer
Oto-ophthalmoscope
Flashlight
Tongue depressor
Cotton applicator stick
Stethoscope
Reflex hammer
Tuning fork
Safety pin

Additional items include disposable gloves and lubricant for rectal examination and a speculum for examination of female pelvis.

Vital Signs Importance—Many major therapeutic decisions are based on the vital signs; therefore, accuracy is essential.

TECHNIQUE	**FINDINGS**

TEMPERATURE

1. Routinely, where accuracy is not crucial, an oral temperature will suffice.
2. A rectal temperature is the most accurate.
3. Unless contraindicated (as in a patient with a severe cardiac arrhythmia), a rectal temperature is often preferred.

Temperature—may vary with the time of day.
Oral: 37°C. (98.6°F.) is considered normal. May vary from 35.8°C. to 37.3°C. (96.4°F. to 99.1°F.)
Rectal: Higher than oral by 0.4°C. to 0.5°C. (0.7°F. to 0.9°F.)

PULSE

1. Palpate the radial pulse and count for at least 30 seconds.
2. If the pulse is irregular, count for a full minute and note the number of irregular beats/minute.
3. Note whether the beat of the pulse against your finger is strong or weak, bounding or thready.

Pulse—Normal adult pulse is 60–80 beats/minute; regular in rhythm. Elasticity of the arterial walls, blood volume, and mechanical action of the heart muscle are some of the factors that affect strength of the pulse wave, which normally is full and strong.

RESPIRATION

1. Count the number of respirations taken in 15 seconds and multiply by 4.
2. Note rhythm and depth of breathing.

Respiration—Normally 16–20 respirations/minute.

BLOOD PRESSURE

1. Measure the blood pressure in both arms.
2. Palpate the systolic pressure before using the stethoscope in order to detect an auscultatory gap.*
3. Apply cuff firmly; if too loose, it will give a falsely high reading.
4. Use cuff in appropriate size: a pediatric cuff for children; a leg cuff for obese people (see p. 355, Vascular Disorders).
5. The cuff should be approximately 2.5 cm. (1 inch) above the antecubital fossa.

Normal range
Systolic—95–140 mm. Hg.
Diastolic—60–90 mm. Hg
A difference of 5–10 mm. Hg between arms is common.
Systolic pressure in lower extremities is usually 10 mm. Hg higher than reading in upper extremities.
Going from a recumbent to a standing position can cause the systolic pressure to fall 10–15 mm. Hg and the diastolic pressure to rise slightly (by 5 mm. Hg).

Height and Weight

Determine the patient's height and weight.

General Appearance

Begin observation on first contact with the patient (in the waiting room or while the patient is in bed); continue throughout the interview systematically—as the first step in the examination of each body part.

Inspection

Observe for: race, sex, general physical development, nutritional state, mental alertness, evidence of pain, restlessness, body position, clothes, apparent age, hygiene, grooming.

Careful observation of the general state of the individual provides many clues about a person's body image and how he behaves and also some idea of how well or ill he is.

Skin

1. Examination of the skin is correlated with the information obtained in the history and other parts of the physical examination.
2. Examine skin as you proceed through each body system.

* Auscultatory gap:
  1. The first sound of blood in the artery is usually followed by continuous sound until nothing is audible with the stethoscope.
  2. Occasionally the sound is not continuous and there is a gap after the first sound, after which the sound of blood in the vessel is heard again.
  3. If one uses only the auscultatory method and pumps the cuff up until the sound is no longer heard, it is possible, when there is a gap in the sound or when the sound is not continuous, to get a falsely low systolic reading.

TECHNIQUE	FINDINGS

Inspection

Observe for: skin color, pigmentation, lesions (distribution, type, configuration, size), jaundice, cyanosis, scars, superficial vascularity, moisture, edema, color of mucous membranes, hair distribution, nails.

Palpation

Examine skin for temperature, texture, elasticity, turgor.

1. "Normal" varies considerably depending on racial or ethnic background, exposure to sun, complexion, pigmentation tendencies (e.g., freckles).

2. The skin is normally warm, slightly moist, and smooth and returns quickly to its original shape when picked up between two fingers and released. There is a characteristic hair distribution over the body associated with gender and normal physiologic function. Nails are present and smooth and cared for in some way.

Head

TECHNIQUE	FINDINGS

Inspection

Observe for: symmetry of face, configuration of skull, hair color and distribution, scalp.

Palpation

Examine: hair texture, masses, swelling or tenderness of scalp, configuration of skull.

1. Normally, the skull and face are symmetrical, with distribution of hair varying from person to person. (However, determine by history if there has been any change.)

2. The scalp should be free of flaking, with no signs of nits (small, white louse eggs), lesions, deformities, or tenderness.

Eyes and Vision

Equipment

Ophthalmoscope

Anatomical Landmarks

Globes	Sclerae
Palpebral fissures	Pupils
Lid margins	Iris
Conjunctivae	

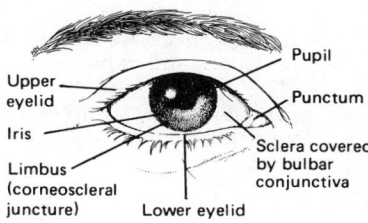

Inspection

1. *Globes*—for protrusion.
2. *Palpebral fissures* (longitudinal openings between the eyelids)—for width and symmetry.

3. *Lid margins*—for scaling, secretions, erythema, position of lashes.

4. *Bulbar and palpebral conjunctivae*—for congestion and color.
   Bulbar conjunctiva—membranous covering of the sclera (contains blood vessels).
   Palpebral conjunctiva—membranous covering of the inside of the upper and lower lids (contains blood vessels).
5. *Sclerae*—for color; *iris* for color.

2. *Palpebral fissures*—appear equal in size when the eyes are open.
   a. Upper lid: covers a small portion of the iris and cornea.
   b. Lower lid: margin is just below the junction of the cornea and sclera (limbus).
   c. *Ptosis:* drooping of eyelids.
3. *Lid margins*—are clear; the lacrimal duct openings (puncta) are evident at the nasal ends of the upper and lower lids.
   Eye lashes—normally are evenly distributed and turn outward.
4. *Bulbar conjunctiva* (cover of sclera)—consists of transparent, red blood vessels which may become dilated and produce the characteristic "bloodshot" eye.
   Palpebral conjunctivae—are pink and clear.
   Conjunctivitis—inflammation of the conjunctival surfaces.
5. *Sclerae*—should be white and clear.

TECHNIQUE

6. *Pupils*—for size, shape, symmetry, reaction to light and accommodation (ability of the lens to adjust to objects at varying distances).

7. *Eye movement*—extraocular movements, nystagmus, convergence.
   (Nystagmus: rapid, lateral, horizontal or rotary movement of the eye.)
   (Convergence: ability of the eye to turn in and focus on a very close object.)
   (See neurologic examination, p. 45.)

8. *Gross visual fields*—by confrontation.
   (See neurological examination, p. 44.)

9. *Visual acuity*
   Check with a Snellen chart (with and without glasses).

Palpation

1. Determine strength of upper lids by attempting to open closed lids against resistance.

2. Palpate globes through closed lids for tenderness and tension.

Fundoscopic Examination (ends eye examination).

1. *Red retinal reflex*—check the transparency of the anterior and posterior chambers.

2. *Cornea*—check for transparency.

3. *Lens*—check for transparency.

4. *Retina*—check for color, pigmentation, hemorrhages, and exudates.

5. *Optic disc*—check for color, distinction of margins, pigmentation, degree of elevation, cupping.

FINDINGS

6. *Pupils*—normally constrict with increasing light and accommodation. Pupils are normally round and can range in size from very small ("pinpoint") to large (occupying the entire space of the iris).

7. *Extraocular movement*—Movement of the eyes in conjugate fashion. (Six muscles control the movement of the eye.) Eyes normally move in conjugate fashion, except when converging on an object which is moving closer.
   Nystagmus—May be seen normally as a result of eye fatigue.
   Convergence—fails when double vision occurs, usually 10–15 cm. (4–6 inches) from nose.

8. *Peripheral vision*—is full (medially and laterally, superiorly and inferiorly) in both eyes.

9. *Normal vision*—20/20.
   Myopia—nearsightedness.
   Hyperopia—farsightedness.

1. The examiner should not be able to open the lids when the patient is squeezing them shut.

2. Globes normally are not tender when palpated.

1. *Red retinal reflex* can be spotted by the examiner while standing 30 cm. (12 inches) from the eye. The anterior and posterior chambers should be transparent.

2. *Cornea*—should be transparent.

3. *Lens*—should be transparent (i.e., retina can be seen).

4. *Retina*—color varies according to the amount of pigment present. There should be no hemorrhages or exudates.

5. *Optic disc*—is circular and has a yellowish-pink color. Although disc appearance may vary, the margins are normally distinct and regular, with varying amounts of pigment.

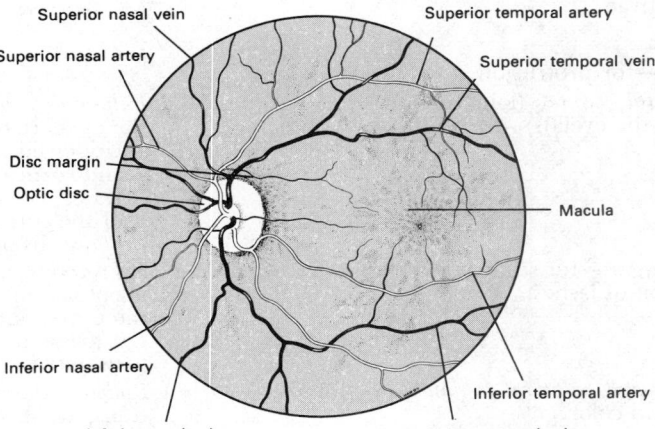

6. *Macula*—check for color. (Lies at a distance of 2 optic disc diameters laterally from the optic disc.)

7. *Blood vessels*—check for diameter; arteriovenous (A/V) ratio; origin and course; venous-

6. *Macula*—since it is free of blood vessels, it is lighter in color than the rest of the retina.

7. *Retinal arteries and veins*—arteries are approximately ⅘ the size of the veins and lighter in

TECHNIQUE

arterial crossings. (Both arteries and veins are present and move outward from the disc nasally and temporally.)

Use of the Ophthalmoscope

1. Hold the instrument in your right hand and use your right eye to examine the patient's right eye.
   a. Reverse the procedure to examine the patient's left eye.
   b. This approach allows you to get close to the patient without bumping noses.
2. Hold the instrument so that your last 2 fingers are straight, rather than curved around the handle.
   You can place these fingers against the patient's cheek to steady the instrument and to avoid hitting the patient with it.
3. Begin the fundoscopic examination standing about 30 cm. (a foot) from the patient. The room should be darkened.
4. Turn the dial on the head of the ophthalmoscope to +8 or +10 (black numbers.)
5. Turn on the ophthalmoscope light and place the eyepiece up to your eye.
   If you wear glasses or contact lenses, it is best to wear them during the examination so that you do not have to accommodate for your vision by turning the dial on the ophthalmoscope.
6. Aim the light at the pupil of the eye. You should see the red reflex immediately.
7. Slowly move in toward the patient, continuing to look through the eyepiece and keeping the light directed at the pupil, beyond which is the fundus.
8. With the index finger of the hand holding the ophthalmoscope, turn the dial toward zero as you move in.
   a. This allows you to focus on the various chambers of the eye.
   b. A way to find the eye and pupil is to put your hand on top of the patient's head and your thumb at the outer corner of the eye. If you lose the fundus, you can return to your thumb and get your bearings by moving medially from the thumb nail.
9. Once your hand is resting on the patient's cheek, continue to turn the dial until you can focus on the retina and the blood vessels and the optic disc appear sharp.
10. Once you are focused on the optic disc, it is possible to follow the blood vessels out from the disc inferiorly and superiorly, medially and laterally.
    (See Chapter 15, [Eye] for visual fields, color vision tests, refraction, gonioscopy, tonometry.)

FINDINGS

color. Where arteries and veins cross, there is usually no disturbance in the course of either. Pulsations may occur in the vein near the optic disc.

Ears and Hearing

Equipment
Tuning fork, otoscope

To Examine with Otoscope

1. Hold the helix of the ear and gently pull the pinna upward and back toward the occiput to straighten the external canal.
2. Gently insert the lighted otoscope using an earpiece that is a comfortable size for the patient.
3. Once otoscope is in place, put eye up to eyepiece and examine external canal.

Examination Techniques

Inspection

1. *Pinna*—examine for size, shape, color, lesions, masses.
2. *External canal*—examine with otoscope for discharge, impacted cerumen, inflammation, masses, or foreign bodies.

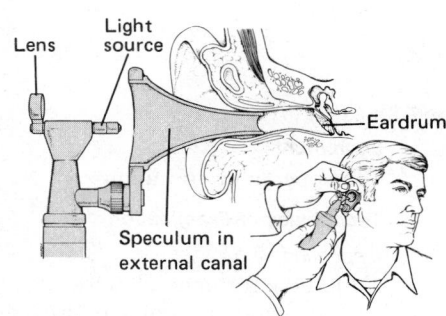

2. *External canal*—is normally clear with perhaps minimal cerumen.

TECHNIQUE	**FINDINGS**

TECHNIQUE

3. *Tympanic membrane*—examine for color, luster, shape, position, transparency, integrity, and scarring.
4. *Landmarks*—note cone of light, umbo, handle and short process of the malleus, pars flaccida, and pars tensa.
   Gently move the otoscope to observe the entire drum. (Cerumen may obscure visualization of the drum.)

Palpation

   Pinna—examine for tenderness, consistency of cartilage, swelling.

Mechanical Tests

1. Test each ear for gross hearing acuity using whispered word or watch. Cover the ear not being tested.
2. *Weber test*—test for lateralization of vibration. Place tuning fork in the center of the scalp near the forehead (*A*).
   (Also see Chapter 16 [Ear], p. 688).
3. *Rinne Test*—compares air and bone conduction.
   a. Place vibrating tuning fork on the mastoid process behind the ear and have the patient tell you when the vibration stops (*B*).
   b. Then quickly hold the buzzing end of the tuning fork *near* the ear canal and ask if patient can hear it (*C*).
   (See p. 190 for Audiogram.)

FINDINGS

3. *Tympanic membrane and landmarks.*

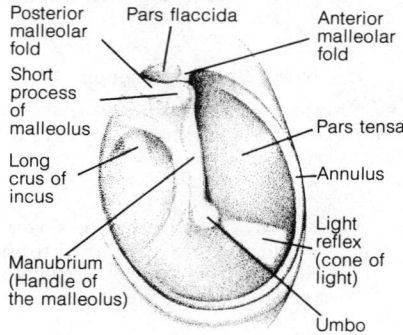

Posterior malleolar fold — Pars flaccida — Anterior malleolar fold — Short process of malleolus — Long crus of incus — Pars tensa — Annulus — Manubrium (Handle of the malleolus) — Light reflex (cone of light) — Umbo

1. A person with normal hearing can hear whispered word from approximately 4.5 meters (15 feet) and a watch from 30 cm. (12 inches).

   The patient should hear the sound equally well in both ears; i.e., there is no lateralization.

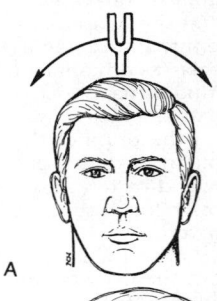

A

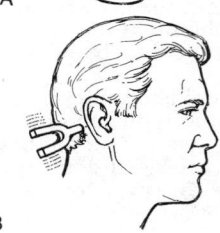

B

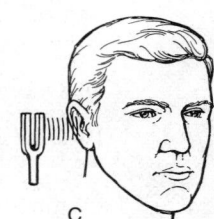

C

Normally, sound should be heard after vibration can no longer be felt; i.e., air conduction is greater than bone conduction.

Lateralization and conduction findings are altered by damage to the 8th cranial nerve and damage to the ossicles in the middle ear.

Nose and Sinuses

Equipment

Otoscope, nasal speculum

Techniques of Examination

Inspection

1. Observe for general deformity.
2. With nasal speculum (otoscope, if speculum unavailable) examine for:
   a. Nasal septum (position and perforation).

   b. Discharge (anteriorly and posteriorly).
   c. Nasal obstruction and airway patency.
   d. Mucous membranes for color.
   e. Turbinates for color and swelling.

Nasal septum—is normally straight and not perforated.
Discharge—none should be present
Airways—are patent.
Mucous membranes—are normally pink.
Turbinates—3 bony projections on each lateral

TECHNIQUE

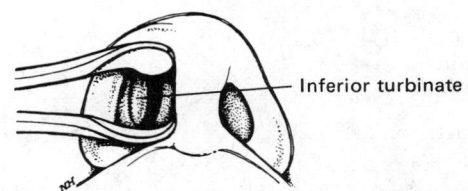

—Inferior turbinate

Palpation

Sinuses (frontal and maxillary) for tenderness.
Frontal: direct manual pressure upward toward wall of sinus. Avoid pressure on eyes.
Maxillary: with thumbs, direct pressure upward over lower edge of maxillary bones.

FINDINGS

wall of the nasal cavity covered with well vascularized mucus-secreting membranes. They serve to warm the air going into the lungs and may become swollen and pale with colds and allergies.

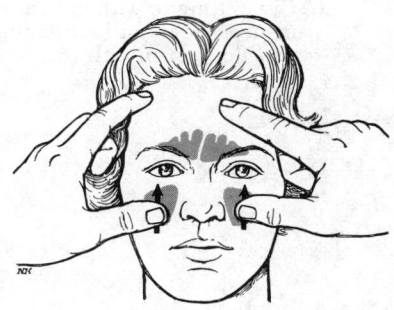

Mouth

Equipment

Flashlight, tongue depressor, gloves, gauze sponges

Soft palate—
Palatopharyngeal arch—
Hard palate
Uvula
Tonsil
Tongue

Techniques of Examination

Inspection

1. Observe lips for color, moisture, pigment, masses, ulcerations, fissures.
2. Use tongue depressor and penlight to examine:
   a. *Teeth*—number, arrangement, general condition.
   b. *Gums*—for color, texture, discharge, swelling, or retraction.

   c. *Buccal mucosa*—for discoloration, vesicles, ulcers, masses.
   d. *Pharynx*—for inflammation, exudate, and masses.
   e. *Tongue* (protruded)—for size, color, thickness, lesions, moisture, symmetry, deviations from midline, fasciculations.

   f. *Salivary glands*—for patency.
      Parotid glands.

      Sublingual and submaxillary glands.

   g. *Uvula*—for symmetry when patient says "ah."
   h. *Tonsils*—for size, ulceration, exudates, inflammation.
   i. *Odor of breath.*
   j. *Voice*—for hoarseness.

Teeth—the normal adult has 32 teeth.

Gums—commonly recede in adults.
      —bleeding is fairly common and may result from trauma, gingival disease, or systemic problems (less common).

Tongue—is normally midline and covered with papillae, which vary in size from the tip of the tongue to the back. (The circumvallate papillae are large and posterior.)

Parotid glands—open in the buccal pouch at the level of the upper teeth halfway back.
Sublingual and submaxillary glands—open underneath the tongue.

Lingual tonsils—can often be seen on the posterior portion of the tongue.
Odor of breath—may indicate dental caries.

TECHNIQUE

FINDINGS

Palpation

a. Examine oral cavity with gloved hand for masses and ulceration. Palpate beneath tongue and explore laterally the floor of the mouth (*A*).

b. Grasp tongue with gauze sponge to retract; inspect sides and undersurface of tongue and floor of mouth (*B*).

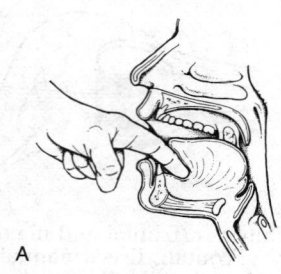

A

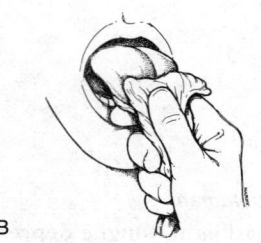

B

Neck

Equipment

Stethoscope

Techniques of Examination

Inspection

1. Inspect all areas of the neck anteriorly and posteriorly for muscular symmetry, masses, unusual swelling or pulsations, and range of motion.

2. *Thyroid*—Ask the patient to swallow and observe for movement of an enlarged thyroid gland at the suprasternal notch.

3. *Muscular strength*

    a. *Cervical muscles*—have patient turn his chin forcefully against your hand.
    b. *Trapezius muscles*—exert pressure on the patient's shoulders while having him shrug his shoulders.

4. *External jugular veins*—observe with patient sitting and then lying at 30–40 degree angle; patient's neck should not be flexed.

1. *Range of Motion*—normally the chin can touch the anterior chest, the head can be extended at least 45 degrees from the vertical position and can be rotated 90 degrees from midline to side.

2. *Thyroid*—is not usually visible, except in extremely thin persons.

3. *Strength*—See Findings, 11th cranial nerve, p. 45.

Jugular veins. When the patient is lying with head elevated 30–40 degrees, the jugular veins are approximately at the level of the right atrium, and pulsations that are transmitted from the right atrium can normally be seen with tangential lighting. Veins are not distended when the patient is sitting.

This serves as a fairly constant and therefore reliable landmark, when patient is supine or sitting, for estimating venous pressure; i.e., the height in cms. measured from level of distended internal jugular veins to level of sternal angle.

Note the sternal angle, the point on the surface anatomy which is approximately 5–7 cm. (2–2.75 inches) above the right atrium.

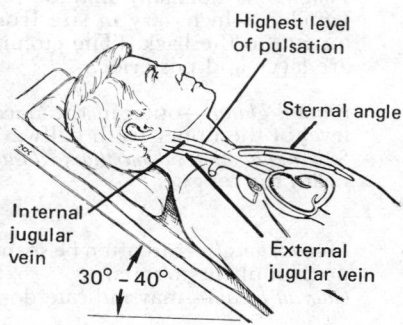

Highest level of pulsation

Sternal angle

Internal jugular vein

External jugular vein

30° – 40°

TECHNIQUE	**FINDINGS**

Palpation

1. *Cervical nodes and salivary glands.*

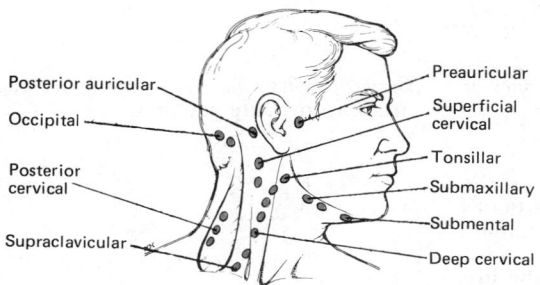

Cervical nodes. In the adult, the cervical lymph nodes are not normally palpable unless the patient is very thin, in which case the nodes are felt as small, freely movable masses.

2. *Trachea*—palpate at the sternal notch. Stand behind (or in front of) patient and allow the middle finger of each hand to glide off the head of the clavicle into the sternal notch. Palpate for deviation and tracheal tug.

2. *Trachea* should be midline.
Landmarks are easy to identify utilizing this procedure.

This is the downward pull synchronous with cardiac pulsation; usually the result of aneurysm of aorta.

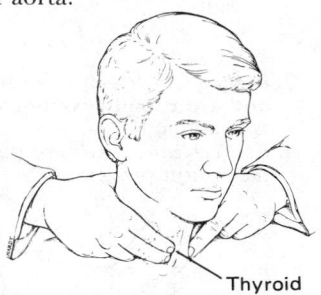

3. *Thyroid*
   a. Stand behind the patient and have him flex his neck to relax the cervical muscles.
   b. Place the fingertips of left hand behind the left sternocleidomastoid muscle adjacent to the trachea just below larynx.
   c. Palpate area over trachea and to left of trachea to discern outline of isthmus of left lobe of thyroid gland.
   d. Note any enlargement, nodules, masses, consistency.
   e. Reverse the procedure and examine the right lobe of the thyroid.
   f. Since the thyroid gland moves upward upon swallowing, have patient swallow to facilitate examination.

4. *Carotid arteries*
   a. Palpate the carotids 1 side at a time.
   b. The carotids lie anterolaterally in the neck—avoid palpating the carotid sinuses at the level of the thyroid cartilage just below the angle of the jaw since this may cause slowing of heart rate.
   c. Note symmetry of pulsations, strength, and amplitude.

If the thyroid is palpable, it is normally smooth, without nodules, masses, or irregularities, or bruits (gushing sound produced by blood moving through a narrow vessel).

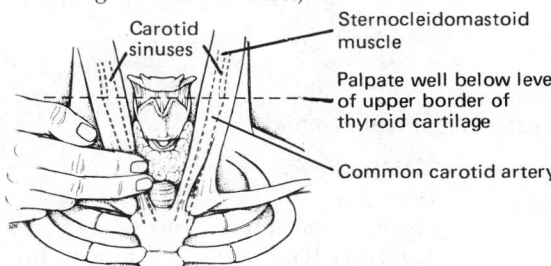

Lymph Nodes

1. It is important at some point in the examination to palpate all areas where lymphadenopathy might appear.
2. Often this is done as each region of the body is examined; e.g., the cervical nodes are examined when the neck is examined.
3. However, in the record, the condition of the lymph nodes is described under a separate heading.

TECHNIQUE

Techniques of Examination

Inspection

Note size, shape, mobility, consistency, tenderness, and inflammation.

Palpation

1. Palpate the *cervical, supra-* and *infraclavicular nodes.*
2. *Axillary nodes*
   a. Examine while patient is sitting.
   b. Place patient's arm at his side and insert the examining fingers to the apex of the patient's axilla. (Use fingers of right hand to examine left axilla and vice versa.)
   c. Rotate the examining hand so that the fingers can palpate the anterior and posterior axillary fossae pressing against the chest wall. Press against the humerus bone in the axilla to examine the lateral fossa for nodes. Conclude the axillary examination by moving the fingers from the apex of the axilla downward in the midline along the chest wall.

3. *Inguinal nodes*—are located in inguinal canal and are usually examined when the abdomen is examined.
4. *Epitrochlear nodes*—are palpated just above the olecranon process.

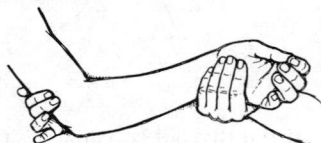

FINDINGS

Cervical nodes and supra- and infraclavicular nodes are not normally palpable.

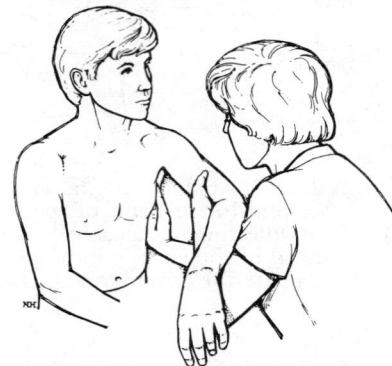

Axillary nodes are not normally palpable.
Inguinal nodes—a few may be felt, but are small, movable, and nontender.

Epitrochlear nodes—not usually palpable.

Breasts (Male and Female)

FEMALE BREAST

Inspection

(With patient sitting, arms relaxed at sides.)

1. Inspect the areolae and nipples for position, pigmentation, inversion, discharge, crusting, and masses.

   Extra, or supernumerary, nipples may occur normally, most commonly in the anterior axillary region or just below the normal breasts.
2. Examine the breast tissue for size, shape, color, symmetry, surface, contour, skin characteristics, and level of breasts. Note any retraction or dimpling of the skin.
3. Ask the patient to elevate her hands over her head; repeat the observation.
4. Have patient press her hands to her hips; repeat the observation.

1. The *nipples* should be at the same level and protrude slightly.
   An inverted nipple (one that turns inward), if present since puberty, may be normal.
   A *supernumerary nipple* usually consists of a nipple and a small areola and may be mistaken for a mole.
2. *Breast size*—In the female it is not uncommon to find a difference in the size of the 2 breasts. Normal asymmetry has usually been present since puberty and is not a recent phenomenon.
3. If there is a mass attached to the pectoral muscles, contracting the muscles will cause retraction of the breast tissue.

TECHNIQUE

Palpation

This is best done with the patient recumbent.

1. The patient with pendulous breasts should be given a pillow to place under the ipsilateral scapula of the breast being palpated so that the tissue is distributed more evenly over the chest wall.
2. The arm on the side of the breast being palpated should be raised above the patient's head.
3. Palpate one breast at a time, beginning with the "asymptomatic" breast if the patient complains of symptoms.
4. To palpate, use the palmar aspects of the fingers in a rotating motion, compressing the breast tissue against the chest wall. (This is done quadrant by quadrant until the entire breast has been palpated—including the "tail" of the breast tissue which extends into the axillary region in the upper outer quadrant of the breast.)
5. Note skin texture, moisture, temperature, or masses.

6. Gently squeeze the nipple and note any expressible discharge.
7. Repeat examination on opposite breast and compare findings.

MALE BREAST

Examination of the male breast can be brief and should never be omitted.

1. Observe the nipple and areola for ulceration, nodules, swelling, or discharge.
2. Palpate the areola for nodules and tenderness.

Thorax and Lungs

General Information

1. Methodical inspection of the thorax requires reference to established "landmarks" in order to locate specific structures and to report significant findings.
2. The same structural landmarks are used in examining both the lung and the heart.
3. It is important to visualize the underlying structures and organs when examining the thorax.

FINDINGS

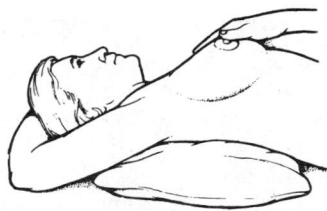

3. This allows the examiner to palpate the "normal" breast first and then compare the "symptomatic" breast to it.
4. *Breast texture*—varies according to the amount of subcutaneous tissue present.
   a. In young females, tissue is fairly soft and homogeneous; in postmenopausal women, tissue may feel nodular or stringy.
   b. Consistency also varies with menstrual cycle, being more nodular and edematous just prior to menstruation.*
5. *Masses*—If a mass is palpated, its location, size, shape, consistency, mobility, and associated tenderness are reported.
6. *Discharge*—In the normal nonpregnant or nonlactating female, there is no nipple discharge.

1. There should be no discharge.

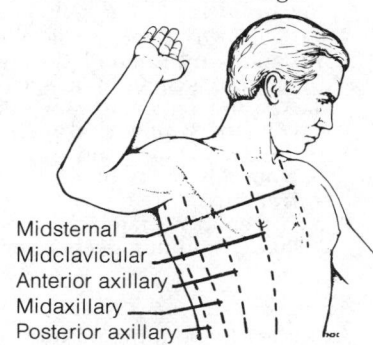

Midsternal
Midclavicular
Anterior axillary
Midaxillary
Posterior axillary

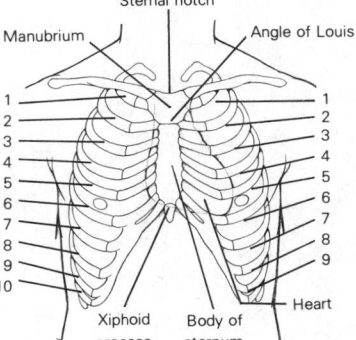

Sternal notch
Manubrium
Angle of Louis
1 1
2 2
3 3
4 4
5 5
6 6
7 7
8 8
9 9
10
Heart
Xiphoid process
Body of sternum

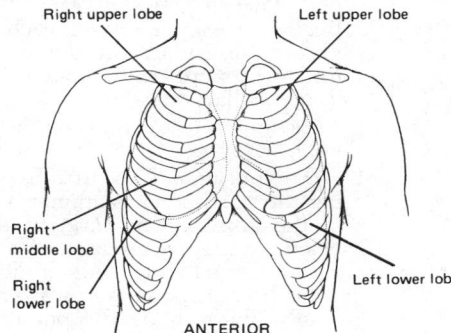

Right upper lobe
Left upper lobe
Right middle lobe
Right lower lobe
Left lower lobe
ANTERIOR

* In teaching women about breast self-examination, explain that the best time for performing the examination is a week after the menstrual period, when the breasts are least engorged and tender.

TECHNIQUE

Techniques of Examination

POSTERIOR THORAX AND LUNGS

Begin the examination with the patient seated; examine posterior chest and lungs.

FINDINGS

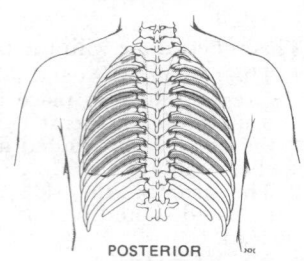

POSTERIOR

Inspection

1. Inspect the spine for mobility and any structural deformity.
2. Observe the symmetry of the posterior chest and the posture and mobility of the thorax upon respiration. (Note any bulges or retractions of the costal interspaces upon respiration or any impairment of respiratory movement.)
3. Note the anteroposterior diameter in relation to the lateral diameter of the chest.

2. The thorax is normally symmetrical; it moves easily and without impairment upon respiration. There are no bulges or retractions of the intercostal spaces.

3. The anteroposterior (AP) diameter of the thorax in relation to the lateral diameter is approximately 1:2.

Palpation

1. Palpate the posterior chest with the patient sitting; identify areas of tenderness, masses, inflammation.
2. Palpate the ribs and costal margins for symmetry, mobility, and tenderness and the spine for tenderness and vertebral position.
3. To assess respiratory excursion—place the thumbs at the level of the 10th vertebra; with hands held parallel to the 10th ribs as they grasp the lateral rib cage, ask the patient to inhale deeply. Observe the movement of the thumbs while feeling the range, and observe the symmetry of the hands.
4. To elicit vocal and tactile fremitus (palpable vibrations transmitted through the broncho-pulmonary system upon speaking).
   a. Ask the patient to say "99"; palpate and compare symmetrical areas of the lungs with the ball of one hand.
   b. Note any areas of increased or decreased fremitus.
   c. If fremitus is faint, ask the patient to speak louder and in a deeper voice.

2. On palpation there should be no tenderness; chest movement should be symmetrical and without lag or impairment.

4. Posteriorly, fremitus is generally equal throughout the lung fields.
   It may be increased near the large bronchi.
   It may be decreased or absent anteriorly and posteriorly when vocal loudness is decreased, when posture is not erect, or when excessive tissue or underlying structures are present.
   One must distinguish the various normal causes of increased or decreased fremitus from the pathological causes.

Percussion

As with palpation, the posterior chest is percussed with the patient sitting.

1. Percuss symmetrical areas, comparing sides.
2. Begin across the top of each shoulder and proceed down between the scapulae and then under the scapulae, both medially and laterally in the axillary lines.
3. Note and localize any abnormal percussion note.
4. For diaphragmatic excursion, percuss by placing the pleximeter (stationary) finger parallel to the approximate level of the diaphragm below the right scapula.
   a. Ask the patient to inhale deeply and hold his breath; percuss downward to the point of dullness. Mark this point.
   b. Let the patient breathe normally and then ask him to exhale deeply; percuss upward from the mark to the point of resonance.

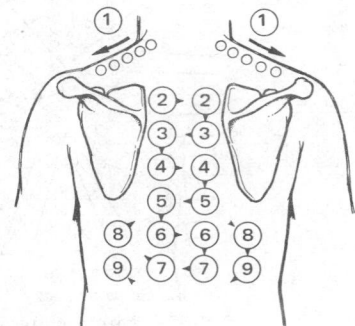

TECHNIQUE

FINDINGS

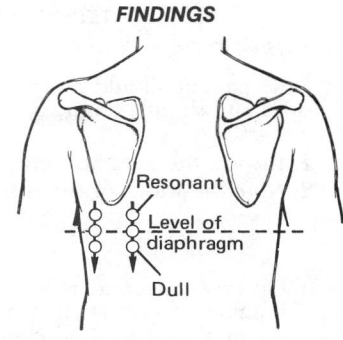

c. Mark this point and measure between the 2 marks—normally 5–6 cm. (2–2.3 inches).

d. Repeat this procedure medially and laterally on the right and left sides of the chest.

The lower border of the lungs on normal respiration is approximately at the level of the 10th thoracic spinous process.

Percussion normally reveals resonance over symmetrical areas of the lung.

Percussion sound may be altered by poor posture and/or presence of excessive tissue.

Auscultation

Aids in assessing air flow through the lungs, the presence of fluid or mucus, and the condition of the surrounding pleural space and lungs.

1. Have patient sit erect.*

2. With stethoscope, listen to lungs as patient breathes somewhat more deeply than normal with mouth open. (Let the patient pause as needed to avoid hyperventilation.)

3. Place the stethoscope in the same areas on the chest wall as those percussed, and listen to a complete inspiration and expiration in each area.

4. Compare symmetrical areas methodically from the apex to the lung bases.

5. It should be possible to distinguish 3 types of normal breath sounds as indicated in the following table.

Breath Sounds

On auscultation, breath sounds vary according to proximity of large bronchi.

a. They are louder and coarser near the large bronchi and over the anterior.

b. They are softer and much finer (vesicular) at the periphery over the alveolae.

Breath sounds also vary in duration with inspiration and expiration.

Sounds may normally decrease in obese individuals.

Pathology will alter the normal bronchial, bronchovesicular, and vesicular breath sounds. (Abnormal breath sounds or adventitious sounds are to be noted and localized.)

Breath Sounds	Duration of Inspiration and Expiration	Pitch of Expiration	Intensity of Expiration	Sample Location
Vesicular	Insp. > Exp.	Low	Soft	Most of lungs
Bronchovesicular	Insp. = Exp.	Medium	Medium	Near the main stem bronchi, i.e., below the clavicles and between the scapulae, especially on the right.
Bronchial or tubular	Exp. > Insp.	High	Usually loud	Over the trachea.

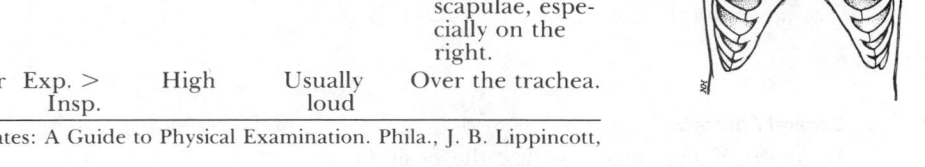

Bronchial (tracheal) breath sounds   Bronchovesicular breath sounds

(From Bates: A Guide to Physical Examination. Phila., J. B. Lippincott, 1979)

* Note: if patient is unable to sit with or without assistance for examination of the posterior chest and lungs, position the patient first on one side and then on the other as you examine the lung fields.

TECHNIQUE

FINDINGS

ANTERIOR THORAX AND LUNGS

(The patient should be recumbent with arms at sides and slightly abducted.)

Inspection

1. Inspect the chest for any structural deformity.
2. Note the width of the costal angle.

3. Observe rate and rhythm of breathing, any bulging or retraction of intercostal spaces on respiration, use of accessory muscles of respiration (sternocleidomastoid and trapezius on inspiration and abdominal muscles on expiration).
4. Note any asymmetry of chest wall movement on respiration.

Palpation

(Serves the same purposes in examining the anterior chest as in the posterior chest.)

1. To assess diaphragmatic excursion, place hands along the costal margins and note symmetry and degree of expansion as the patient inhales deeply.
2. Palpate for fremitus anteriorly and laterally with the ball of the hand.
   (Underlying structures, e.g., heart, liver, etc., may damp, or decrease, fremitus.)
3. Compare symmetrical areas.
4. Displace the female breast gently if necessary.

Percussion

1. With patient's arms resting comfortably at his sides, examiner percusses the anterior and lateral chest.
   Begin just below the clavicles and percuss downward from one interspace to the next, comparing the sound from the interspace on one side with that of the contralateral interspace.
2. Displace the female breast so that breast tissue does not damp the vibration. Continue downward noting the intercostal space where hepatic dullness is percussed on the right and cardiac dullness on the left.
3. Note effect of underlying structures.

Auscultation

Listen to the chest anteriorly and laterally for the distribution of resonance and any abnormal or adventitious sounds.

2. Angle at the tip of the sternum is determined by the right and left rib margins at the xiphoid process. Normally the angle is less than 90 degrees.
3. The thorax is normally symmetrical and moves easily without impairment on respiration. There are no bulges or retractions of the intercostal spaces.

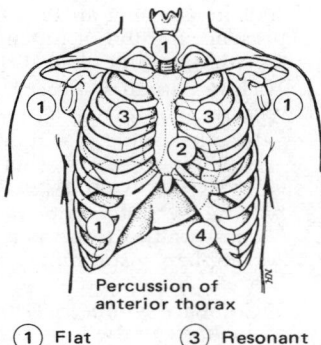

Percussion of anterior thorax

① Flat ③ Resonant

② Dull ④ Tympanic

2. A tympanic sound is produced over the gastric air bubble on the left somewhat lower than the point of liver dullness on the right.

3. Percussion over heart will produce a dull sound.
   Upper border of the liver will be percussed on the right side, producing a dull note.

Heart

General Approach

1. The examiner must visualize the position of the heart under the sternum and the ribs and know certain landmarks for identification of certain structures and significant findings.
2. It is also important to identify those "areas" on the chest wall which will yield the most infor-

TECHNIQUE	**FINDINGS**

mation initially about the function of the heart and its valves.

 a. In locating the intercostal spaces, begin by identifying the Angle of Louis, which is felt as a slight ridge approximately 2.5 cm. (1 inch) below the sternal notch where the manubrium and the body of the sternum are joined.

 b. The 2nd ribs extend to the right and left of this angle.

 c. Once the 2nd rib is located, palpate downward and obliquely away from the sternum to identify the remaining ribs and intercostal spaces.

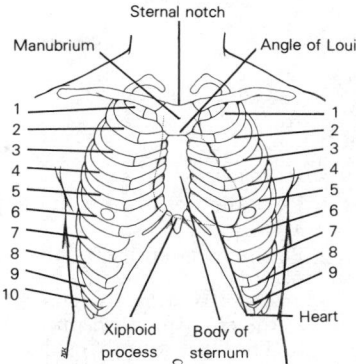

Inspection

1. Inspect the precordium for any bulging, heaving, or thrusting.

2. Look for the apical impulse approximately in the 5th or 6th intercostal space at or just medial to the midclavicular line.

3. Note any other pulsations. Tangential lighting is most helpful in detecting pulsations.

Palpation

1. Use the ball of the hand to detect vibrations, or "thrills," which may be caused by murmurs. (Use the fingertips and/or palmar surface to detect pulsations.)

2. Proceed methodically through the examination so that no area is omitted. Palpate for thrills and pulsations in each area (aortic, pulmonic, tricuspid, mitral).

 a. Begin in the aortic area (2nd right intercostal space close to the sternum) and proceed downward to the apex of the heart. (The mitral area is considered the apex of the heart.)

 b. In the tricuspid area, use the palm of the hand to detect any heaving or thrusting of the precordium (tricuspid area—5th intercostal space next to the sternum).

 c. In the mitral area (5th intercostal space at or just medial to the midclavicular line) palpate for the apical beat; identify the point of maximal impulse (PMI) and note its size and force.

Percussion

1. Outline the border of the heart or area of cardiac dullness.

 a. The left border generally does not extend beyond 4, 7, and 10 cm. left of the midsternal line in the 4th, 5th, and 6th intercostal spaces respectively.

 b. The right border usually lies under the sternum.

2. Percuss outward from the sternum with the stationary finger parallel to the intercostal space until dullness is no longer heard. Measure the distance from the midsternal line in centimeters.

FINDINGS column:

1. Normally there are no bulges.

2. An apical impulse may or may not be observable.

3. There should be no other pulsations.

1. There should be no thrills or other pulsations. (Thrills are vibrations [caused by turbulence of blood moving through valves] which are transmitted through the skin. Feels similar to a purring cat.)

Ordinarily no heaving of the ventricle is felt, except possibly in the pregnant female.

The apical pulse should be felt approximately in the 5th intercostal space at or just medial to the midclavicular line. In the young and thin person it is a sharp, quick impulse no larger than the intercostal space. In the older person the impulse may be less sharp and quick.

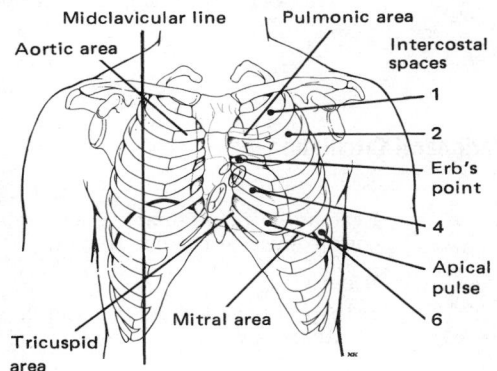

TECHNIQUE

FINDINGS

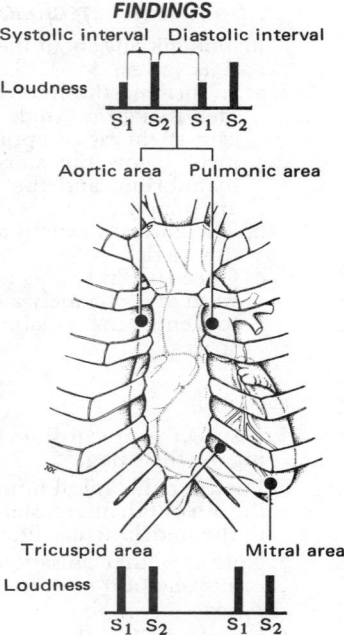

Auscultation

1. Place the stethoscope in the pulmonic or aortic area.
2. Begin by identifying the 1st and 2nd heart sounds.
   a. The 1st sound is caused by the closing of the tricuspid and mitral valves.
   b. The 2nd sound results from the closing of the aortic and pulmonary valves.

   The 2 sounds are separated by a short systolic interval; each pair of sounds is separated from the next pair by a longer diastolic interval. Normally 2 sounds are heard—"lub," "dub."
   a. In the aortic and pulmonic areas, S_2 is usually louder than S_1. In this way each of the paired sounds can be distinguished from the other.
   b. In the tricuspid area, S_1 and S_2 are of almost equal intensity, and in the mitral area S_1 is often slightly louder than S_2.

3. Once the heart sounds are identified, count the rate and note the rhythm as discussed under vital signs.

   If there is an irregularity, try to determine if there is any pattern to the irregularity in relation to the intervals, heart sounds, or respirations.

Normally the heart sounds are regular, with a rate of 60–80 beats/minute (in the adult). In the athlete or jogger the resting pulse may be between 40 and 60 beats/minute.

4. Once rate and rhythm are determined, listen in each of the 4 areas and at Erb's point (3rd left interspace close to the sternum) systematically, first with the diaphragm (detects higher pitched sounds) and then with the bell (detects lower pitched sounds).
   a. In each area, listen to S_1 and then to S_2 for intensity and splitting.

   a. Occasionally there may be a splitting of S_2 in the pulmonary area. This is normal. Splitting of S_2 (2 contiguous sounds are heard instead of 1) is best heard at the end of inspiration when right ventricular stroke volume is sufficiently increased to delay closure of the pulmonic valve *slightly* behind closure of the aortic valve.
   b. There are usually no extra sounds.

   b. Listen to the intervals 1 at a time and note any extra sounds or murmurs.

Peripheral Circulation

JUGULAR VEINS

Evaluation of jugular venous distention is most useful in patients with suspected compromise of cardiac function.

Inspection

1. Inspect neck for internal jugular venous pulsations.

1. Jugular venous pulsations can be distinguished from carotid pulsations by the following chart:

TECHNIQUE	*FINDINGS*
Internal Jugular Pulsations	**Carotid Pulsations**
Rarely palpable	Palpable
Soft undulating quality usually with 2 or 3 outward components (a, c, and v waves)	A more vigorous thrust with a single outward component
Pulsation eliminated by light pressure on the vein just above the sternal end of the clavicle	Pulsation not eliminated
Level of pulsation usually descends with inspiration	Pulsation not affected by inspiration
Pulsations vary with position	Pulsations are unchanged by position

(From Bates: A Guide to Physical Examination, 2nd ed.)

2. Identify the highest point at which the pulsations can be seen and measure the vertical line between the point and the sternal angle.
   With the head raised to 45 degrees, the internal jugular venous pulsations should not be visible above 3 cm. (1.18 inch).

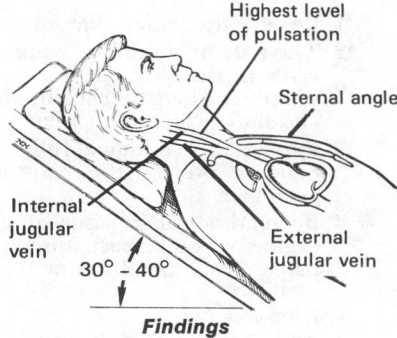

Findings

EXTREMITIES

Inspection

1. Observe skin over extremities for color, pallor, rubor, hair distribution.
2. Inspect for any superficial vessels.

1. Extremities should be symmetrically even in color, warmth, and moisture, without swelling.
   a. Swelling of feet may occur after prolonged standing or sitting, but will disappear readily when extremity is elevated.

Palpation

1. Note temperature of skin over extremities, comparing one side to the other.
2. Palpate pulses (radial, femoral, posterior tibial, dorsalis pedis) comparing symmetry from side to side.

2. There should be no arterial bruits.

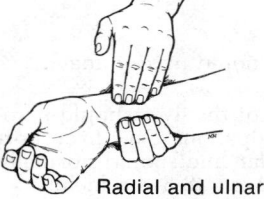

Radial and ulnar

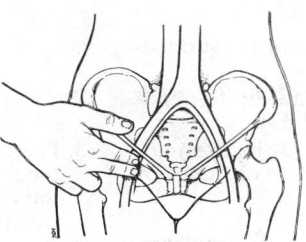

Femoral

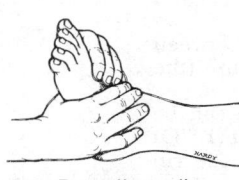

Posterior tibial

Dorsalis pedis

TECHNIQUE

3. Palpate skin over the tibia for edema by pressing skin between thumb and index finger for 30 seconds to 1 minute.
Then run pads of fingers over the area pressed and note indentation.
If indentation is noted, repeat procedure, moving up the extremity, and note the point at which no more swelling is present.

Abdomen

General Approach

1. Be sure the patient has an empty bladder.
2. The patient should be lying comfortably with arms at the side. Often, bending the knees slightly will help to relax the abdominal muscles and make palpation easier.
3. Expose the abdomen fully. Make sure your hands as well as the stethoscope diaphragm are warm.
4. Be methodical in visualizing the underlying organs as you inspect, auscultate, percuss, and palpate each quadrant or region of the abdomen.

Inspection

1. Observe the general contour of the abdomen (flat, protuberant, scaphoid, or concave; local bulges). Also note symmetry, visible peristalsis, aortic pulsations.
2. Check the umbilicus for contour or hernia and the skin for rashes, striae, and scars.

Auscultation

1. This is done before percussion and palpation since the latter may alter the character of bowel sounds.
2. Note the frequency and character of bowel sounds (pitch, duration).
3. Listen over the aorta and renal arteries (either side of the umbilicus) for bruits.

Percussion

1. Percussion provides a general orientation to the abdomen.
2. Proceed methodically from quadrant to quadrant, noting tympany and dullness.
3. In right upper quadrant (RUQ) in the midclavicular line percuss the borders of the liver.

a. Begin at a point of tympany in the midclavicular line of the right lower quadrant (RLQ) and percuss upward to the point of dullness (the lower liver border); mark the point.
b. Percuss downward from the point of lung resonance above the RUQ to the point of dullness (the upper border of the liver) and mark the point.
c. Measure in centimeters the distance between the 2 marks in the midclavicular line (the liver span).
d. Tympany of the gastric air bubble can be percussed in the left upper quadrant (LUQ) over the anterior lower border of the rib cage.

FINDINGS

3. Edema is usually graded from trace to 3+ or 4+ pitting (note scale used when recording data). Trace is a slight indentation which disappears in a short time. Grade 3+ or 4+, depending on the scale, is *deep* pitting which does not disappear readily. At best, these are subjective measurements which are tried and confirmed through practice and comparison of findings with associates.

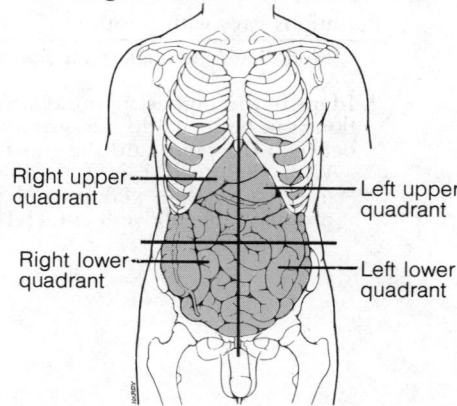

Right upper quadrant / Left upper quadrant / Right lower quadrant / Left lower quadrant

The abdomen may or may not have any scars and should be flat or slightly rounded in the nonobese person.

2. Anywhere from 5–35 bowel sounds/minute. May have familiar sound of "growling."
3. There should be no bruits or rubs.

2. Tympany should predominate.

3. Percussion of the liver should help guide subsequent palpation. The liver border in the midclavicular line should normally range between 6–12 cm. (2.3–4.6 inches).

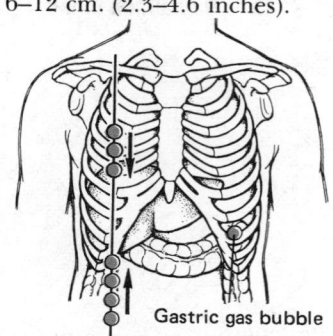

Gastric gas bubble
Midclavicular line

TECHNIQUE

e. Location of the spleen is often difficult. It may be obscured by gastric or colonic air. However, it may be percussed just posterior to the midaxillary line near the left 10th rib.

Light Palpation

1. Using palmar surfaces of the fingers of one hand, palpate the 4 quadrants lightly and smoothly, without jerking or poking.
2. While palpating, observe the patient's facial expression for any sign of discomfort.

Deep Palpation

1. Instruct the patient to relax the abdominal muscles.
2. Use the palmar surface of the fingers of one hand and systematically move through the 4 quadrants. (It may be necessary to use one hand on top of the other to palpate the abdomen of an obese individual or of a patient whose muscles are taut.)
3. Identify any masses and note any tenderness by observing the patient's facial expressions while palpating.

LIVER

1. Begin by placing the left hand under the patient's back at the level of the 11–12th rib. Place the right hand, with fingers angled and slightly facing the costal margin, just below the percussed lower border of the liver.
2. During palpation with the right hand, press upward with the left hand to move the liver anteriorly (to facilitate palpation).
3. Have the patient inspire, and on expiration press the fingers of the right hand inward. On deep inspiration by the patient, do not change the position of the right hand; feel for the liver edge moving over the fingers. If nothing is felt on inspiration, palpate more deeply, then on each subsequent inspiration, move the finger upward toward the costal margin.

SPLEEN

1. Reach over the patient and place the left hand behind the left rib cage. Place the palmar surface of the right hand so that the fingertips face the left costal margin in the LUQ. Right hand should be far enough away from costal margin to avoid missing an enlarged spleen and to allow mobility of the right hand.
2. Ask the patient to take a deep breath, and feel for the edge of the spleen.
3. This procedure may be repeated with the patient lying on his right side, since gravity may bring the spleen forward into a palpable location.

FINDINGS

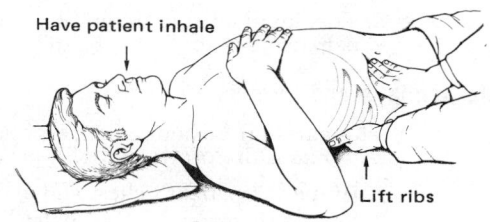

Light palpation of the abdomen is helpful in determining muscle tension and resistance, tenderness, and superficial masses or organ enlargement.

It is only with deep palpation that organs can be delineated and deeper masses of the abdomen felt.
Identify any masses (size, shape, consistency, mobility) and note location—whether they are in the musculature or deep (obscured by contracting abdominal muscles).

The liver border, if felt, should be firm and smooth.

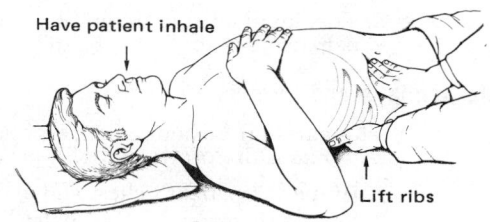

With each new position of the fingers, have the patient breathe deeply and feel for the liver.

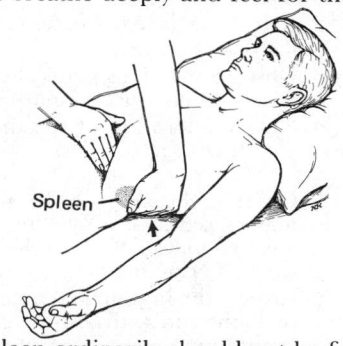

The spleen ordinarily should not be felt.

TECHNIQUE	FINDINGS
KIDNEY	
1. Next palpate for the left and right kidneys.	
2. Place the left hand under the patient's back between the rib cage and the iliac crest.	
3. Support the patient while you palpate the abdomen with the right palmar surface of the fingers facing the left side of the body.	
4. Palpate by bringing the left and right hands together as much as possible slightly below the level of the umbilicus on right and left.	4. The kidney is usually felt only in persons with very relaxed abdominal muscles (very young, aged, multiparous women). The right kidney is slightly lower than the left. The kidney, if felt, is a solid, firm, smooth elastic mass.
5. If the kidney is felt, describe its size, shape, and any tenderness.	
6. Costal vertebral angle (CVA) tenderness is palpated with the patient sitting—usually during the examination of the posterior chest. Locate the costal vertebral angle in the flank region and strike firmly with the ulnar surface of your hand. Note any tenderness over the area.	6. There should be no costal vertebral tenderness.
AORTA	
1. Next, palpate for the aorta with the thumb and index finger.	The aorta is soft and pulsatile.
2. Press deeply in the epigastric region (roughly in the midline) and feel with the fingers for pulsations as well as for the contour of the aorta.	
OTHER FINDINGS	
1. Palpation of the RLQ may reveal the part of the bowel called the cecum.	1. The cecum will be soft.
2. The sigmoid colon may be palpated in the LLQ.	2. The sigmoid colon is rope-like and vertical and, if filled with feces, may be quite firm.
3. The inguinal and femoral areas should be palpated bilaterally for lymph nodes.	3. Often small inguinal nodes are present; they are nontender, freely movable, and firm.

Male Genitalia and Hernias

This part of the examination, especially for hernias, is best done with the patient standing. (A *hernia* is the protrusion of a portion of the intestine through an abnormal opening.)

1. Drape the patient's chest and abdomen.	
2. Expose the groin and genitalia.	
Inspection	
1. Inspect pubic hair distribution and the skin of the penis.	
2. Retract or have the patient retract the foreskin if present.	2. The foreskin of the penis, if present, should be easily retractable.
3. Observe the glans penis and the urethral meatus. Note any ulcers, masses, or scars.	3. The skin of the glans penis is smooth, without ulceration.
4. Note the location of the urethral meatus and any discharge.	4. The urethral meatus normally is located ventrally on the end of the penis. Normally, there is no discharge from the urethra.
5. Observe the skin of the scrotum for ulcers, masses, redness, or swelling. Note size, contour, and symmetry. Pick up the scrotum to inspect the posterior surface.	5. The scrotum descends approximately 4 cm. (1.5 inches) in the adult; the left side is often larger than the right side.
6. Inspect the inguinal areas and groin for bulges (without and with the patient bearing down— as though having a bowel movement).	

TECHNIQUE	FINDINGS

Palpation

Use gloves if there are any inflammatory lesions present.

1. Palpate any lesions, nodules, or masses, noting tenderness, contour, size, and induration. Palpate the shaft of the penis for any induration (firmness in relation to surrounding tissues).

2. Palpate each testis and epididymis separately between the thumb and first 2 fingers, noting size, shape, consistency, and undue tenderness (pressure on the testis normally produces pain).

   2. The testes are usually rubbery and of equal size. The epididymis is located posterolaterally on each testis and is most easily palpable on the superior portion of the testis.

3. Also palpate the spermatic cord, including the vas deferens within the cord, from the testis to the inguinal ring. Note any nodules or tenderness.

4. Palpate for inguinal hernias, using the left hand to examine the patient's left side and the right hand to examine the patient's right side.
   a. Insert the right index finger laterally, invaginating the scrotal sac to the external inguinal ring.
   b. If the external ring is large enough, insert the finger along the inguinal canal toward the internal ring and ask the patient to strain down, noting any mass that touches the finger.

   4. Normally there is no palpable herniating mass in the inguinal area.

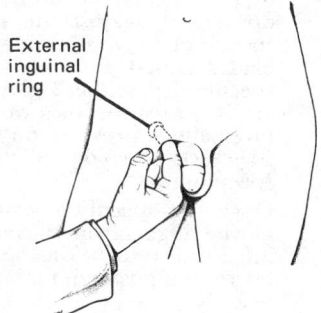

External inguinal ring

5. Also palpate the anterior thigh for a herniating mass in the femoral canal. Ask patient to strain down. (Femoral canal—not palpable, but is a potential opening in the anterior thigh medial to the femoral artery below the inguinal ligament.)

   Ordinarily, there is no palpable mass in the femoral area.

Female Genitalia

Equipment

Disposable gloves, lubricant, speculum of appropriate size, excellent direct lighting, cervical scraper, glass slide, fluid for fixing Papanicolaou smear, cotton tip applicator

General Approach

1. The patient's bladder should be empty.
2. The patient should lie in the lithotomy position with her buttocks extending slightly over the end of the examining table.
3. Her thighs are flexed and abducted; her feet are in the stirrups.
4. Her arms are at her side or crossed over her chest.
5. If a male is performing the examination, a female attendant must be present.
6. The examination will be most successful if the patient is relaxed. This can best be accomplished by draping the patient well so that the drape extends over the knees.
7. Explain each step of the procedure and avoid any quick, unexpected movements.
8. Be sure that your hands and the speculum are warm.

Inspection and Palpation

(These are performed almost simultaneously through the course of the examination.)

1. Begin with inspection of the pubic hair distribution.

   1. Normally the pubic hair is distributed in an inverted triangle over the symphysis pubis.

2. Inspect the labia majora, the mons pubis, and the perineum (tissue between the anus and the vaginal opening).

   2. In the virgin, the labia majora are full and rounded. They become thinner in older and multiparous women.

3. With gloved hand, separate the labia majora and inspect the clitoris, urethral meatus, vaginal opening. Note skin color, ulcerations, nodules, discharge, or swelling.

   3. The labia minora and the prepuce around the clitoris are pinkish.

TECHNIQUE	FINDINGS

4. Note area of the Skene's and Bartholin's glands. If there is any history of swelling of the latter, palpate the glands by placing the index finger in the vagina at the posterior end of the opening and the thumb outside the posterior portion of the vagina. Palpate between the finger and thumb for nodules, tenderness, or swelling. Repeat on each side of the posterior vaginal opening.

4. The hymen, or membranous fold which may partially occlude the vaginal opening, may or may not be present.

Speculum Examination

1. Have the appropriate size speculum available and lubricated with warm water. (Other lubricants may interfere with cytologic studies.)

2. Begin by inserting the first 2 fingers of the gloved hand into the vagina; locate the cervix, noting the angle of the fingers and the distance from the vaginal opening to the cervix.

2. Normally, the uterus is positioned forward with the cervix at almost a right angle to the vagina.

3. Proceed by removing the 2 fingers to the edge of the vaginal opening. Press the 2 fingers downward against the perineum. Take the speculum in your other hand and with the blades closed and held obliquely guide the speculum past the 2 gloved fingers while exerting pressure downward. (This avoids putting painful pressure on the anterior urethral structures.) Avoid pinching the vagina with the speculum.

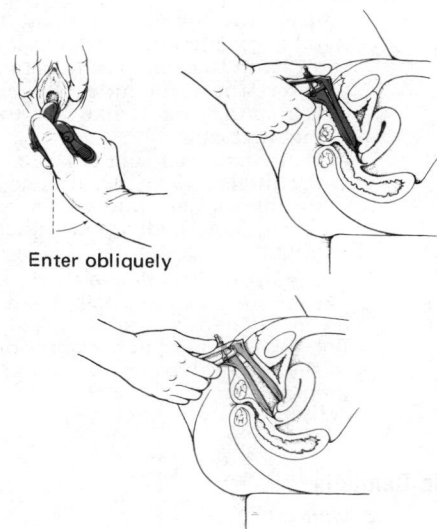

Enter obliquely

4. Once the speculum is inserted, remove the gloved fingers from the introitus (vaginal opening) and return the speculum blades to a horizontal position, maintaining pressure posteriorly.

5. Next, open the speculum blades and with direct light visualize the cervix. Maneuver the speculum so that the cervix comes into full view.
   (The cervix lies within the *fornix*, or posterior portion of the vagina, dividing the fornix into the anterior, posterior, right, and left fornices.)

6. Inspect the cervix and its opening (os), noting position, color, and shape of the os, ulceration, nodules, bleeding, and discharge. (For Papanicolaou smear, see page 530.)

6. The cervix of the nonpregnant woman is pink and smooth.

7. As you slowly pull the speculum out of the vagina, inspect the vaginal mucosa for color, inflammation, ulcers, masses, or discharge.

7. A small amount of clear lubricating mucus is normal in the vagina. Normally there is no bleeding from the nonmenstruating female.

8. Close the blades before reaching the introitus, and remove the speculum without pinching the vaginal wall. (Also see Guidelines in Chap. 11, p. 531.)

Palpation (Bimanual Examination)

1. Lubricate the index and middle fingers of the gloved hand and insert them into the vagina, noting nodules, masses, or irregularities anteriorly and posteriorly.

2. Locate the cervix and fornices and note tenderness, shape, size, consistency, regularity, and mobility of the cervix.

3. Place the gloved finger in the posterior fornix and the ungloved hand on the abdomen approximately midway between the umbilicus and the symphysis pubis.

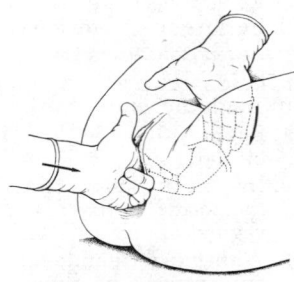

4. Press the 2 hands toward one another and palpate the uterus, noting its size, shape, reg-

The cervix of the nonpregnant woman is smooth, firm, and slightly movable. It is non-

TECHNIQUE

ularity, consistency, mobility, tenderness, and any masses.

5. Next, place the gloved fingers in the right lateral fornix and the ungloved hand in the right lower quadrant. Palpate the ovaries if possible, noting shapes, size, consistency, regularity, mobility, pain (the ovary is usually tender) or masses. Repeat the procedure on the left side.

6. Next, withdraw the gloved hand, leaving the index finger in the vagina and placing the middle finger in the rectum. Repeat the procedure of the bimanual examination.

7. If possible, press the uterus downward toward the rectal finger so that as much of the posterior surface of the uterus as possible can be examined.

8. Proceed with the rectal examination (see below).

9. Upon completing examination, wipe genitalia and perineum with a tissue or offer the patient one so that she may do it herself.

FINDINGS

tender.

The uterus is firm, smooth, and nontender.

5. The ovaries vary in size considerably, but average about 3.5 × 2 × 1.5 cm (1.4 × 0.8 × 0.6 inches). The fallopian tubes are generally not palpable.

6. Explain what you are doing since this is uncomfortable for the patient and may produce the sensation of wanting to defecate.

Rectum

Equipment

Glove, lubricant

Techniques of Examination

MALE

General Approach

1. If the patient is ambulatory, have him stand and bend over the edge of the table.

2. It is also possible to examine the anus and rectum with the patient lying on his left side, knees drawn up and buttocks close to the edge of the table. (This is generally an uncomfortable position and the patient should be told that he may feel as though he wants to move his bowels.)

3. The patient should be draped so that only his buttocks are exposed.

Inspection

1. Spread the buttocks and inspect the anus, perianal region, and sacral region for inflammation, nodules, scars, lesions, ulcerations, rashes. Ask the patient to bear down; note any bulges.

Palpation

1. Palpate any abnormal area noted on inspection.

2. Lubricate the index of the gloved hand. Rest finger over the anus as the patient bears down and, as the sphincter relaxes, insert finger slowly into the rectum.

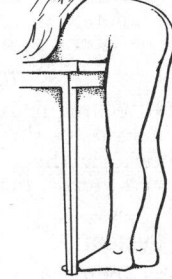

1. In males and females the perianal and sacrococcygeal areas are dry, with varying amounts of hair covering them. In the sacrococcygeal region it is not uncommon to find a small opening or sinus surrounded by a tuft of hair. This is a *pilonidal cyst;* it should be nontender and noninflamed.

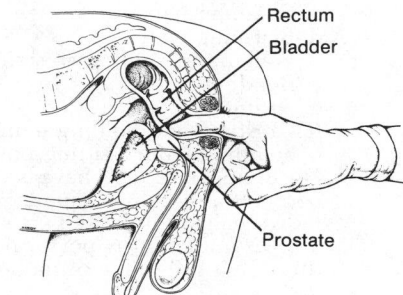

Rectum
Bladder
Prostate

3. Note sphincter tone, any nodules or masses, or tenderness.

3. The anal canal is approximately 2.5 cm. (1 inch) long; it is bordered by the external and internal anal sphincters, which are normally firm and smooth.

TECHNIQUE	*FINDINGS*
4. Insert the finger further and palpate the walls of the rectum laterally and posteriorly while rotating your index finger. Note irregularities, masses, nodules, tenderness.	4. The wall of the rectum in males and females is smooth and moist.
5. Anteriorly, palpate the 2 lateral lobes of the prostate gland and its median sulcus for irregularities, nodules, swelling, or tenderness.	5. The male prostate gland is approximately 2.5 cm. (1 inch) long, smooth, regular, nonmovable, nontender, and rubbery.
6. If possible, palpate the superior portion of the lateral lobe, where the seminal vesicles are located. Note induration, swelling, or tenderness.	6. The seminal vesicles are generally not palpable unless swollen.
7. Just above the prostate anteriorly, the rectum lies adjacent to the peritoneal cavity. If possible, palpate this region for peritoneal masses and tenderness.	
8. Continue to insert the finger as far as possible and have the patient bear down so that more of the bowel can be palpated.	
9. Gently withdraw your finger. Any fecal material on the glove should be tested for occult blood (see p. 414).	9. There is normally no occult blood in the stools.

FEMALE

General Approach

1. The examination is usually performed following the pelvic examination with the patient still in the lithotomy position.
2. If only the rectal examination is done, the patient may be positioned laterally, as for examination of the male.
   The lateral position permits better visualization of the sacral region.

TECHNIQUE	*FINDINGS*
1. The technique is basically the same for the female as for the male.	
2. Anteriorly the cervix, and perhaps a retroverted uterus, may be felt.	2. Anteriorly, the cervix is round and smooth.

Musculoskeletal System

General Approach

1. Examine the muscles and joints, keeping in mind the structure and function of each.
2. This discussion will center on the technique for examining the patient who is asymptomatic and, therefore, will not present in detail the techniques for inspecting and palpating joints that are symptomatic or deformed.
3. It is important to ask in the history and to note in the examination whether the patient has difficulty performing activities of daily living:
   a. Bathing
   b. Dressing (buttoning, using zippers, tying shoelaces)
   c. Combing hair
   d. Brushing teeth
   e. Walking up and down stairs
   f. Bending
   g. Sitting
   h. Grasping and holding items without dropping them
   i. Standing from a sitting position, unaided
4. Once the above facts have been ascertained, the examination proceeds. The examiner observes and palpates joints and muscles for symmetry and then examines each joint individually as indicated.
5. The examination is performed with the joints both at rest and in motion—moving through a full range of motion; joints and supporting muscles and tissues are noted.

Inspection

1. Inspect the upper and lower extremities for size, symmetry, any deformity, muscle mass.
2. Inspect the joints for range of motion (in degrees), enlargement, redness.

For the purpose of this text, it is sufficient to say that in the course of the history and examination the examiner should not find any compromise or restriction of the patient's activities of daily

TECHNIQUE

3. Note gait and posture; observe the spine for range of motion, lateral curvature, or any abnormal curvature.
4. Observe the patient for signs of pain during the examination.

Palpation

1. Palpate the joints of the upper and lower extremities and the neck for tenderness, swelling, temperature, and range of motion.
2. Hold the palm of the hand over the joint as it moves, or move the joint through the fullest range of motion and note any crepitation (crackling feeling within the joint).
3. Palpate the muscles for size, tone, strength, and tenderness.
4. Palpate the spine for bony deformities and crepitation. Gently hit the spine with the ulnar surface of your fist from the cervical to the lumbar region and note any pain or tenderness.

FINDINGS

living or any other normal activities. If any activity is restricted because of muscular or skeletal problems, the reader is referred to a more detailed book on physical examination.

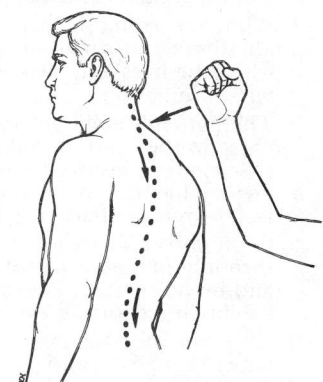

Neurological System

Equipment

Pin, cotton, tuning fork, reflex hammer, flashlight, tongue blade

General Information

1. The examination described in this section is a screening neurological examination.
   a. It is performed on individuals without specific neurological complaints.
   b. There is a more detailed examination for patients with specific signs and symptoms.
   c. The student is referred to another text for the content and technique of a detailed neurological examination.
2. The examination is performed with the patient in either the sitting or supine position.
3. Much of the neurological examination can be performed as different regions of the body are being examined. This facilitates the flow of the entire examination.
   Example: The cranial nerves can be examined at the same time as the head and neck.
   A mental status evaluation can be done while the history is elicited and while the entire physical examination is performed.

Components of the Neurological Examination

There are 6 components of the neurological examination:
1. Mental status (cerebral function)
2. Cranial nerve function
3. Cerebellar function
4. Motor function
5. Sensory function
6. Deep tendon reflexes (DTRs)
The screening neurological examination involves testing all of these components at least superficially. Learning these components in order will help in organizing the examination and in avoiding the omission of any part.

Basic Principles

1. Symmetry of function and findings on both sides of the body is important to note.
   Always compare one side of the body with the other side (e.g., compare degree of motor strength of the right biceps with that of the left biceps).
2. Integrating the neurological examination into the examination of the various body regions is advisable, although the results of the neurological findings should be recorded together as an entity.

Carrying Out the Examination

MENTAL STATUS

Components of the mental status examination include the following:
   —State of consciousness (alert, somnolent, stuporous, comatose)

In a screening examination, mental status is evaluated by observing the patient's affect during the history and the content of what he or she says.

TECHNIQUE

—Memory (short-term, long-term, intermediate)
—Cognition (calculations, current events)
—Affect (mood)
—Ideational content (hallucinations)

1. While recording the history ask the patient for identifying information (how to spell his name, where he lives), and ask what the date is. This tests orientation.

2. The patient's ability to remember is also evaluated as the history is taken—by asking for his past medical history (long-term memory) and dietary habits: "What did you eat for breakfast?" (intermediate memory).

3. Cognition and ideational content are evaluated throughout the history by what the patient says and by his articulateness, consistency, and reliability in reporting events.

4. Affect or mood is evaluated by observing the patient's verbal and nonverbal behavior in response to questions asked, to sudden noises, to interruptions—i.e., does the patient laugh or smile when talking about normally sad events; is he easily startled by unexpected noises?

CRANIAL NERVE FUNCTION

First (Olfactory) Nerve

(Is not usually tested unless the patient complains of a disturbance in sense of smell.)

1. The airway must be patent.

2. Occlude 1 nostril; ask the patient to close his eyes and then present various substances to smell (e.g., coffee, tobacco). Occlude the other nostril and repeat.

3. Use substances which do not have a lingering effect.

Second (Optic) Nerve

(Includes tests of visual acuity and of gross visual fields and examination of the optic disc with a fundoscope.)

Visual acuity:

Is tested with the use of a Snellen Chart (patient uses glasses if required).

1. Have the patient cover 1 eye at a time and read the smallest print possible on the chart from a distance of 6 meters (20 feet).

Visual fields:

1. Measure by having patient cover his right eye with his right hand. (You cover your left eye with your left hand.)

2. Stand approximately 60 cm. (2 feet) from the patient and have him fix his gaze on your nose.

3. Bring 2 wagging fingers in from the periphery (in a plane equidistant from the patient and you) in all quadrants of the visual field and ask patient to tell you when he sees your wagging fingers.

Optic disc:

Is visualized as part of the fundoscopic examination (see p. 22).

FINDINGS

1. Normally the individual is alert, knows who he is and where he lives and can tell you the date.

2. The patient remembers recent and past events consistently, and willingly admits forgetting something.
Elderly people often have much better long-term memory than recent memory.

4. Mood should be appropriate to the content of the conversation.

1. Normal vision and corrected vision should be 20/20.

3. Assuming your visual fields are grossly normal, the patient and you should see the wagging fingers approximately simultaneously. (The patient's peripheral vision should approximate the examiner's, assuming that it is normal.)

TECHNIQUE

Third (Oculomotor), Fourth (Trochlear), and Sixth (Abducens) Nerves

(Are tested together.) These nerves control the movements of the extraocular muscles of the eye—the superior and inferior oblique and the medial and lateral rectus muscles.

The oculomotor nerve also controls pupillary constriction.

1. Hold your index finger approximately 30 cm. (1 foot) from the patient's nose. Ask the patient to hold his head steady.
2. Ask patient to follow your finger with his eyes.
3. Move your finger to the right as far as the patient's eye moves. Before bringing your finger back to the center, move it up and then down, so that the patient glances up and peripherally and then down and peripherally.
4. Repeat the test, moving your finger to the left.

Fifth (Trigeminal) Nerve

(Has motor component which controls muscles of mastication and a sensory component which controls sensations of the face.)

Motor:

1. Have patient bite down on tongue depressor with one side of his mouth while you try to pull the blade out.
2. Repeat the test on the other side of the mouth and compare muscle strength of the 2 sides.

Sensory:

(Sensation to light touch.)

1. Have patient close eyes.
2. Touch first one side of the patient's face and then the other (forehead, cheek, and chin), asking patient if the sensation is present and feels the same on both sides.
3. Sensation to pain (pinprick) is also tested similarly.

Seventh (Facial) Nerve

(Motor function is tested by observing facial expression and symmetry of facial movement.) Ask the patient to frown, close his eyes, and smile.

Eighth (Acoustic) Nerve

(Has 2 branches.)

Cochlear (mediates hearing). See ear examination, pp. 23.
Vestibular (helps control equilibrium).

Romberg test: Have the patient stand erect with his eyes closed and feet close together.

Ninth (Glossopharyngeal) and Tenth (Vagus) Nerves

(Are tested together since both have a motor portion innervating the pharynx.)

1. Ninth: Test the presence of the gag reflex.
2. Tenth: Ask the patient to say "ah" and observe movement of the uvula and palate for deviation and asymmetry.

Eleventh (Spinal Accessory) Nerve

(Mediates the sternocleidomastoid and upper portion of the trapezius muscles.)

FINDINGS

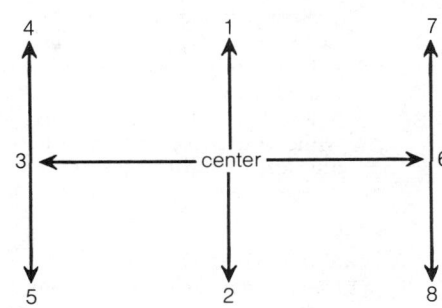

Muscle strength in the face should be present and should be symmetrical.

Sensation should be present and symmetrical. Always demonstrate to the patient how and with what you are testing sensation—to avoid startling the patient and to encourage cooperation.

The facial muscles should look symmetrical when the patient frowns, closes his eyes, and smiles. Notice particularly the symmetry of the nasolabial folds.

Slight swaying may occur, but the patient should not fall. (Stand close to the patient so that you can assist if he begins to fall.)

The gag reflex should be present and there should be no difficulty in swallowing.
The palate and uvula should move symmetrically without deviation.

TECHNIQUE	FINDINGS

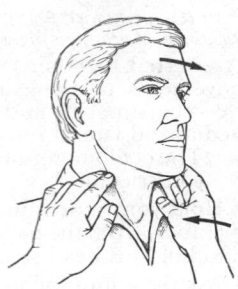

1. Ask the patient to turn his head to the side against resistance while your fingers apply pressure to the jaw.
2. Palpate the sternocleidomastoid muscle on the opposite side.
3. Then have the patient shrug his shoulders while you place your hands on his shoulders and apply slight pressure.

Neck and shoulder muscle strength should be symmetrical.

Twelfth (Hypoglossal) Nerve
(Innervates muscles of the tongue.)
  Test by noting articulation and by having the patient stick out his tongue, noting any deviation or asymmetry.

The tongue should be symmetrical and should not deviate.

CEREBELLAR FUNCTION

(Purpose: to screen for coordination.)
1. Observe posture and gait.
2. Ask patient to walk forward (and then backward) in a straight line.
3. To test for muscle coordination in the lower extremities, have patient run his right heel down his left shin and vice versa.
4. To test coordination in upper extremities have patient touch his nose with his index finger (starting position: arms outstretched) first left, then right, in rapid succession.

The patient should be able to perform all the tests described with smooth, even movement and without losing balance.

The normal person can do this with rapid, smooth movements without undershooting or overshooting the target.

MOTOR FUNCTION

(Tested in conjunction with skeletal system since any bony deformity will affect motor function.)
  Evaluate muscle mass, tone, strength, and any abnormal movements (tics, fasciculations, twitching).
Muscle mass: Note symmetry between sides of the body and distribution distally and proximally.
Tone: Test by noting the resistance the muscle offers to movement upon passive motion.

Muscle mass is usually considered in relation to sex and body build and to use of various muscle groups.
Tone: Generally there is slight resistance to passive movement of muscles as opposed to flaccidity (no resistance) or rigidity (increased muscle tone).
Strength: Will vary from person to person.

Strength:
  Lower extremity—have the patient do deep knee bends; walk on his toes and then his heels; hop on 1 foot and then the other.
  Upper extremity—have patient squeeze your fingers with both hands; compare sides of the body.
  Also, apply resistance (1) to the patient's outstretched arms and (2) when the patient flexes the wrist and elbow; compare sides.
Unusual muscle movements: If present, are noted both when muscle is at rest and when it is moving.

Normally, tremors, tics, or fasciculations are not present either at rest or with movement.

TECHNIQUE	FINDINGS

TECHNIQUE

SENSORY FUNCTION

(Should test sensitivity to light touch [cotton]; pain [pinprick]; vibration [tuning fork]; and position.) Compare both sides of body.

Light touch:

Ask the patient to close his eyes. Brush his skin with a piece of cotton (on back of hands, forearms, upper arms, dorsal portion of foot laterally and medially; and along the tibia and thigh laterally and medially). Ask the patient to indicate when he feels the cotton and to compare the sensation bilaterally.

Pain: Use a safety pin; touch the skin as lightly as possible to elicit a sharp sensation.

Vibration sense: Test by placing a vibrating tuning fork on a bony prominence (wrist, medial and lateral malleoli). Ask the patient to tell you when he no longer feels vibration. Stop the vibration with your hand.

Position sense:

1. Have the patient close his eyes.
2. Move the patient's digit (finger, great toe) up or down and ask patient to say in what direction his finger or toe is pointing.
3. Place your thumb and index finger on either side of the digit being moved so that the patient will not sense any pressure from your finger in the direction in which you are moving the digit.

DEEP TENDON REFLEXES

1. Have the patient relax; provide support for the extremity being tested.
2. Compare reflex amplitude of the same tendons on either side of the body.

Upper Extremities

Biceps:

1. Place your right thumb on the patient's right biceps tendon (located in the antecubital fossa).
2. Rest the patient's forearm on your left hand and strike your thumb with the pointed end of the hammer head. (Hold the hammer loosely so that it pivots in your hand when it is moved with a wrist action.)

3. Strike your thumb with the least amount of pressure needed to elicit the reflex.

Triceps tendon:

1. Hold the patient's arm abducted and bent at the elbow.
2. Posteriorly, about 2.5 cm. (1 inch) above the olecranon process, strike the tendon directly using the pointed end of the hammer.

FINDINGS

The patient should normally feel no vibration within a very short time.

Normally the patient can tell you without hesitation in what direction his digit is pointing.

Amplitude of the reflex may vary for different tendons.

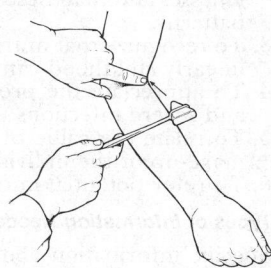

The forearm may move and your thumb should feel the tendon jerk.

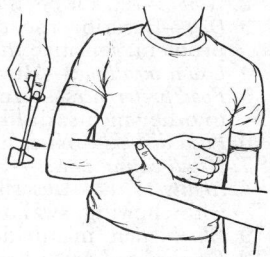

The forearm should move slightly.

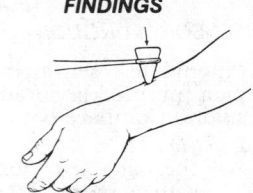

TECHNIQUE   **FINDINGS**

Brachioradialis tendon:
1. Strike the forearm with the hammer about 2.5 cm. (1 inch) above the wrist over the radius.
2. Be sure the forearm is supported and relaxed.

The thumb may be observed moving downward.

Lower Extremities

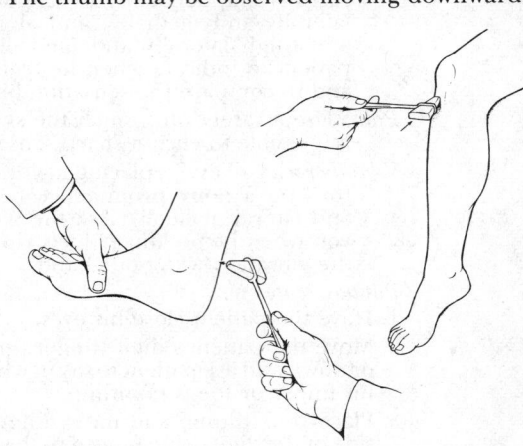

Quadriceps reflex:
1. Strike the tendon just below the patella.
2. Have the patient sitting with his legs hanging over the edge of the table or lying down while you support the legs at the knee (slightly bent).
3. If reflexes are difficult to elicit, have the patient interlace the fingers of both hands and then have him try to pull his hands apart. While he is thus distracted, inhibition of the quadriceps reflex is diminished and the reflex can be elicited more easily. If such a distraction is used to elicit the reflex, record this fact with the physical findings.

Achilles reflex:
1. Support the foot in dorsiflexed position.
2. Tap the Achilles tendon with the hammer head.

The foot should move downward into your hand.

Nutritional Assessment

Purposes

1. To determine the nutritional status of the patient, which may directly or indirectly affect his state of health.
2. To note that different populations in different geographic areas suffer from different illnesses and that these factors, along with mobility of populations, are changing disease patterns.
3. To recognize that nutritional patterns may have lifelong effects, e.g., victims of famine in early childhood can have permanent alterations in physical size and behavior.
4. To appreciate the profound effect (catabolism) on the body from surgery, trauma, and severe infections when there is little intake of nutrients.
5. To relate the value of clinical nutrition to the whole biophysiologic and psychologic make-up of the individual.
6. To refer potential nutritional problems to the nutritionist or metabolic specialist.

Types of Information Needed

Specific information about the patient's nutritional pattern and the correlation of this information with pertinent physical findings and laboratory determinations. Age and health status should already be known.

1. *Appetite*—How is it described by the patient: good, fair, poor, too good?
2. *Weight*—Has it been stable? How has it changed?
3. *Diet*—Describe the type: regular, special. If not regular, why not? (e.g., teeth a problem, sensitive mouth?)
4. *Usual mealtimes*—How many meals a day? When? Which are heavy meals?
5. *Food preferences*—Size of servings; any imbalance such as craving for salt; prefers beef to other meats; dislikes seafood; prefers desserts but not fruit
6. *Food dislikes*—What and why? Culture related?
7. *Usual eating places*—Home, snack shops, restaurants
8. *Ability to eat*—Describe inabilities—dental problems; ill-fitting dentures; difficulties with chewing, swallowing
9. *Elimination* (micturition and defecation)—Nature, frequency, problems
10. *Exercise and physical activity*—How extensive or deficient?
11. *Psychosocial—cultural factors*—Review any having a bearing on proper nutrition.
12. *Medications*—May be obtained from nursing or medical history
13. *Laboratory determinations*

Blood: hemoglobin
       hematocrit
       protein
       albumin
       cholesterol

Urine: protein
      glucose
      acetone

14. *Specific physical examination information*
   Height
   Weight   Desired or preferred weight
   Body type: Small   Medium   Large

15. *Anthropometric Measurement**
   a. Mid-upper arm circumference (MUAC)
      1. Locate midpoint between acromial process of scapula (bony protrusion on posterior of upper shoulder) and olecranon process of the elbow (bony point of elbow).
      2. Place tape measure around upper arm at previously marked midpoint: Tighten snugly (do not pinch) and note measurement in centimeters.
   b. Triceps/subscapular skinfold (TSF)
     This is an objective estimate of subcutaneous fat reserves.
     With patient standing with left arm hanging by his side, examiner grasps a vertical pinch of skin and subcutaneous fat about 1 centimeter above midpoint mark. An adipometer (caliper) is placed over the skin fold using left hand while right hand maintains grasp of skinfold. Three readings are taken and averaged.
   c. Arm muscle circumference (AMC)
     This is determined using above calculations in centimeters as follows:
     $AMC = MUAC - (3.14 \times TSF)$

Method of Obtaining Data

1. Eating and food usually are topics that can be talked about easily. Items listed above under "Types of Information Needed" are readily adapted to a conversational type interview.
2. As in all history taking, ensure the privacy of the patient. The use of the caliper in obtaining anthropometric measurements can serve as a conversation piece.
3. Be alert for questions that this assessment may stimulate in the patient.
4. After obtaining information, summarize your findings and determine the nutritional diagnosis and nutritional plan of care.

BIBLIOGRAPHY

Books

Assessing Your Patients (Nursing Photobook). Horsham, Intermed Communications, 1980

Bates B. A Guide to Physical Examination, 2nd ed. Philadelphia, JB Lippincott, 1979

Berger K and Fields W. Pocket Guide to Health Assessment, Reston, Reston Publishing Co, 1979

Bernstein L and Bernstein R. Interviewing, 3rd ed. New York, Appleton-Century-Crofts, 1980

Brown MS, Bernneman J and Walsh K. Student Manual of Physical Examination. Philadelphia, JB Lippincott, 1977

Bruner JMR. Handbook of Blood Pressure Monitoring. Littleton, PSG Publishing Co, 1978

Judge RD and Zuidema GD (eds). Methods of Clinical Examination. Boston, Little, Brown & Co, 1974

Kraytman M. The Complete Patient History. New York, McGraw-Hill, 1979

Malassanos L et al. Health Assessment. St. Louis, CV Mosby, 1977

Nursing Skillbook Series. Assessing Vital Functions Accurately. Horsham, Intermed Communications, 1977

Patient Assessment Series—18 units. New York, Educational Services Division, American Journal of Nursing Co

Prior JA and Silberstein JS. Physical Diagnosis: The History and Examination of the Patient, 5th ed. St. Louis, CV Mosby, 1977

Sherman JL and Fields SK. Guide to Patient Evaluation, 3rd ed. Flushing New York, Medical Examination Publishing Co, 1978

Stromborg MF and Stromborg PM. Primary Care Assessment and Management Skills for Nurses. Philadelphia, JB Lippincott, 1979

Thompson JM and Bowers AC. Clinical Manual of Health Assessment. St. Louis, CV Mosby, 1980

Articles

Bauman DJ. Nine ways to improve your cardiovascular examination. Consultant 1979 Nov; 19:25–26

Bluestone R et al. Four diagnosticians show their pearls. Patient Care 1979 Feb 15; 13(3):20–48

Farrell J. The human side of assessment. Nursing '80 1980 Apr; 10(4):74–75

Gordon M and Sweeney MA. Methodological problems and issues in identifying and standardizing nursing diagnoses. Adv Nurs Sci 1979 Oct; 2(1):1–15

Hayden GF. Olfactory diagnosis in medicine. Postgrad Med 1980 April; 67(4):110–118

Prager D. Evaluating the mouth and the hypopharynx during the routine physical examination. CA 1980 Nov/Dec; 30(6):322–323

Roach LB. Dark skins; recognizing and interpreting color changes. Crit Care Update 1977 Oct; 4(10):5–15

*Courtesy of Ross Laboratories, Columbus, Ohio.

Rubin BA. Black skin. RN Mag 1979 March; 42(3):31–35

Watts RJ. Dimensions of sexual health. Am J Nurs 1979 Sept; 79(9):1568–1572

Nutritional Assessment

Blackburn GL et al. Nutritional and metabolic assessment of the hospitalized patient. J Parent Nutri Assessment 1977; 1(1):11–22

Hirsch J. Nutrition. Medicine in the '80s. Drug Ther 1980 Feb; 10(2):119–138

Keethley JK. Proper nutritional assessment can prevent hospital malnutrition. Nursing '79 1979 Feb; 9(2):68–72

Kaminski MV and Jeejeebhoy KN. Nutritional assessment—diagnosis of malnutrition and selection of therapy. J Surg Pract 1979 May/June; 8(3):45–62; July/Aug; 8(4):31–38

Salmond SW. How to assess the nutritional status of acutely ill patients. Am J Nurs 1980 May; 80(5):922–924

Zikria BA and King TC. Gastrointestinal function and nutrition in surgical patients. Contemp Surg 1979 June; 14(6):37–41

REHABILITATION CONCEPTS

5

REHABILITATION NURSING

Rehabilitation involves an active, dynamic program aimed at enabling an ill or disabled person to achieve the highest level of physical, mental, social, and economic self-sufficiency of which he is capable.

Objective of Rehabilitation

To enable an ill or disabled person to achieve optimum functional efficiency by the use of an individualized approach.

Rehabilitation Team

Rehabilitation is a creative process; it calls for a team of health care professionals working together and contributing the specialized services that may be required to help the patient function as well as possible. In group sessions the team members evaluate the patient's progress and make necessary program changes.

1. *Patient*—key member of the health care team.
2. *Rehabilitation nurse*—responsible for developing a plan of patient care directed toward defined patient goals and for coordinating the actions of other team members toward these goals. Included in the rehabilitation nurse's responsibilities are the following:
   a. Prevention of complications.
   b. Restoration and maintenance of optimal physical and psychosocial health.
   c. Application of nursing care plan, with interventions in skin care, positioning, transfer techniques, bladder and bowel management, nutrition, psychosocial support, and patient education.
3. *Physician*—makes the medical diagnosis so that ther-

apy can be directed toward realistic goals; designs patient program, and directs the team.
4. *Physiatrist*—a physician who is a specialist in physical medicine and rehabilitation.
   a. Tests the patient's physical functioning.
   b. Determines the potential functional goal.
   c. Supervises the rehabilitation program.
5. *Physical therapist*—strengthens weak muscles and prevents deformity; teaches and supervises the patient during his prescribed exercise program, teaches new ways of locomotion, transportation, and daily activities; uses physical agents and materials as aids to restoration of bodily function after illness and injury.
6. *Psychologist*—helps patient in exploring and expressing feelings about himself; assesses the patient's motivation, values, and attitude towards his disability; may also work with the family to help them cope with problems that have arisen as a result of patient's disability.
7. *Occupational therapist*—develops skills which can be transferred to home and work situations; devises practical projects for the patient to pursue that will develop his coordination and maintain his interest.
8. *Social worker*—investigates patient's background and socioeconomic status and assists patient and family as patient adjusts to home and social environment.
9. *Vocational counselor*—tests patient to determine his interests and aptitudes so that vocational training can be instituted.
10. *Rehabilitation engineer*—uses technology in designing and constructing devices that help severely and multiple handicapped persons to function despite their disabilities.

CAUSES OF DISABILITY

Primary Disability—the result of a pathologic process (congenital disorders, disease, injury).
Secondary Disability—the result of either inactivity or contraindicated and injurious activity.
Disuse Syndrome—disabilities due to inactivity.

DISUSE PHENOMENA*

Condition	Cause	Prevention
1. Muscle atrophy (diminution in muscle strength and size)	Lack of exercise	Exercise
2. Joint contracture (limited range of motion)	Lack of joint motion	Passive range of motion; splinting; proper positioning
3. Metabolic disturbances		
Osteoporosis	Lack of weight-bearing ability Postmenopausal problem	Tilt table (p. 70) and stand-up exercises
Urinary tract stones	Demineralization of bone Immobilization Dehydration/urine concentration	Mobilization High fluid intake No excess vitamins or minerals
	Urinary tract infection	Prompt treatment of urinary infections; minimal use of catheter
4. Circulatory disturbances		
Orthostatic hypotension	Recumbent position	Tilt table and stand-up exercises
Venous thrombosis	Slowing of venous return Lack of motion in lower extremities	Change of position; exercise; elastic stockings
Hypostatic pneumonia	Poor position/prolonged rest in one position	Change of position Prone position to drain bronchial tree; exercise and deep breathing
Pressure sores	Pressure Immobility	Frequent change of position (p. 53)
5. Sphincter disturbances		
Urinary incontinence	Lack of opportunity	Urinal or bedpan instead of indwelling catheter Increased sensory input (p. 76)
Bowel incontinence/constipation	Improper diet Lack of activity Lack of opportunity	Regular bowel routine (p. 76) Adequate fluids; diet
6. Psychological deterioration	Inactivity Isolation	Maximum activity Active participation in planning own care
	Separation from accustomed environment	Participation in decision making
	Institutional routine	Increase sensory input; build self-esteem with meaningful activity

* Adapted from Hirschberg et al. Rehabilitation, 2nd ed. JB Lippincott, 1976.

PSYCHOLOGICAL IMPLICATIONS OF A DISABILITY

Disability has a tremendous impact on the patient's body image (physical appearance, bodily sensations, beliefs and emotions about the body). A patient with a disability has normal needs which must sometimes be met in different ways.

Nursing Objectives

1. To be aware of the factors influencing the patient's behavior.
2. To help the patient feel worthwhile.

Nursing Insight

The mode of the patient's interpersonal relations will be altered by the changes he makes concerning his body image.

Emotional Reactions of the Patient to Newly Acquired Disability

A. *Period of Confusion, Disorganization, and Denial*

1. Is in a state of conflict; has to cope with problems of

forced dependence, with loss of self-esteem and with feeling that personal and family integrity are threatened.
2. Uses mechanisms of denial by refusing to accept new limitations.
   a. May have false hopes of a speedy and complete recovery.
   b. Likely to be self-centered and childlike.
   c. May attempt to remain "normal" and nondisabled.
   d. Denial is the mechanism used by those who have placed great value on strength and attractive appearance.

B. *Period of Depression and Grief; a Period of Situational Reaction*

1. Appears to mourn for his lost function or missing body part.
2. May have body-image distortions.
3. Depression is also due to sensory deprivation and restricted environmental stimulation.

4. Limited mobility and sensory stimulation may produce behavioral disruptions.

C. *Period of Adaptation and Adjustment*

1. Redirects energies toward coping with physical functioning, etc.
2. Revises his body image and modifies his former picture of himself; has a reorientation of values.
3. Accepts a degree of dependency.
4. Accepts limitations imposed by the disability.
5. Begins to develop realistic goals for the future.

D. *Nursing Implications*

1. Realize that every patient will not progress in an orderly fashion through these stages.
   a. Assess patient's reaction to his disability.
   b. Work with him, emphasizing his assets, while, at the same time, listening, encouraging, and sharing his problems and triumphs.
2. Encourage the patient to assume some responsibility for his own therapy.

SEXUALITY: A PART OF THE REHABILITATION PROGRAM

Sexuality is part of a person's self-concept and involves feelings of self-worth, acceptance, sharing, affection, and intimacy as well as feelings of masculinity or femininity. It is reflected in everything a person says and does.

The handicapped person is also a sexual human being.

Implications for Nursing

1. Be comfortable with your own sexuality; avoid imposing your values onto the patient.
2. Establish an atmosphere that is conducive to acceptance and open discussion.

3. Help the patient to feel positive about and to value him- or herself to accept his or her own sexuality.
4. Recognize that feelings of warmth, approval, and friendship as well as sharing and touching are important.
5. Be aware that patients with long-standing disabilities may need training in communication and assertiveness skills.
6. Understand that the disabled may have need for more sex education and specialized services; there are alternative techniques for the severely handicapped.
7. See bibliography at the end of the chapter.

PREVENTING COMPLICATIONS AND DEFORMITIES

Deformities and complications of illness or injury can often be prevented by *frequent changes of position, proper positioning in bed*, and *exercise*.

POSITIONING

Purposes for Changing Positions

1. To prevent contractures.
2. To stimulate circulation and to help prevent thrombophlebitis, pressure sores, and edema of the extremities.
3. To promote lung expansion and drainage of respiratory secretions.
4. To relieve pressure on a body area.

Principles of Body Alignment in Body Positioning

A. *Dorsal or Supine Position*

1. The head is in line with the spine, both laterally and anteroposteriorly.
2. The trunk is positioned so that flexion of the hips is minimized.

3. The arms are flexed at the elbow with the hands resting against the lateral abdomen.
4. The legs are extended with a small, firm support under the popliteal area.
5. The heels are suspended in a space between the mattress and the footboard.
6. The toes are pointed straight up.
7. Trochanter rolls are placed under the greater trochanters in the hip joint areas (see Fig. 5-1).

B. *Side-lying or Lateral Position*

1. The head is in line with the spine.
2. The body is in alignment and is not twisted.
3. The uppermost hip joint is slightly forward and supported by a pillow in a position of slight abduction.
4. A pillow supports the arm, which is flexed at both the elbow and shoulder joints.

C. *Prone Position*

1. The head is turned laterally and is in alignment with the rest of the body.
2. The arms are abducted and externally rotated at the shoulder joint; the elbows are flexed.

3. A small, flat support is placed under the pelvis, extending from the level of the umbilicus to the upper third of the thigh.
4. The lower extremities remain in a neutral position.
5. The toes are suspended over the edge of the mattress.

THERAPEUTIC EXERCISES

Exercise involves the function of muscles, nerves, bones, and joints as well as the cardiovascular and respiratory systems. The return of function depends on the strength of the musculature that controls the joint.

Objectives

1. To develop and retrain deficient muscles.
2. To restore as much normal movement as possible to prevent deformity.
3. To stimulate the functions of various organs and body systems.
4. To build strength and endurance.

Accomplishments of Exercise Programs

1. Maintain and build muscle strength
2. Maintain joint function
3. Prevent deformity
4. Retrain for neuromuscular coordination
5. Stimulate circulation
6. Build tolerance and endurance

Types of Exercises

1. Passive
2. Active assistive
3. Active
4. Resistive
5. Isometric or muscle-setting

A. *Passive*—an exercise carried out by the therapist or the nurse without assistance from the patient.

1. Purpose: to retain as much joint range of motion as possible.
   to maintain circulation.
2. Action
   a. Stabilize the proximal joint and support the distal part.
   b. Move the joint smoothly, slowly, and gently through its full range of motion (pp. 59–63).
   c. Avoid producing pain.

B. *Active Assistive*—an exercise carried out by the patient with the assistance of the therapist or the nurse.

1. Purpose: to encourage normal muscle function.
2. Action
   a. Support the distal part and encourage the patient to take the joint actively through its range of motion.
   b. Give only the amount of assistance necessary to accomplish the action.
   c. Short periods of activity should be followed by adequate rest periods.

C. *Active*—an exercise accomplished by the patient without assistance.

1. Purpose: to increase muscle strength.
2. Action
   a. When possible, active exercise should be done against gravity.
   b. The joint is moved through full range of motion without assistance.

c. The patient should not substitute another joint movement for the one intended.
d. Other active forms of exercise include turning from side to side, turning from back to abdomen, and moving up and down in bed.

D. *Resistive*—an active exercise carried out by the patient working against resistance produced by either manual or mechanical means.

1. Purpose: to provide resistance in order to increase muscle power.
2. Action
   a. The patient moves the joint through its range of motion while the therapist provides slight resistance at first and then progressively increases resistance.
   b. Sandbags and weights can be used and are supplied at the distal point of the involved joint.
   c. The movements should be done smoothly.

E. *Isometric or Muscle-Setting*—alternately contracting and relaxing a muscle while keeping the part in a fixed position. This exercise is performed by the patient.

1. Purpose: to maintain strength when a joint is immobilized.
2. Action
   a. The patient contracts or tightens the muscle as much as possible without moving the joint.
   b. He holds for several seconds, then "let's go" and relaxes.
   c. He breathes deeply during the contraction phase.

RANGE-OF-MOTION EXERCISES

Range of motion is the movement of a joint through its full range in all appropriate planes. It may be passive, active, or resistive.

Objectives

1. To maintain function and prevent deterioration.
2. To maintain or increase the maximal motion of a joint.

Underlying Principles

1. Range-of-motion testing is done by the physician to determine the movement that exists at the joint areas. Testing helps set realistic and positive goals.
2. The patient's range of motion is affected by his physical condition, the disease process, and his genetic makeup.
3. Each joint of the body has a normal range of motion (Table 5–1).
4. Joints may lose their normal range of motion, stiffen, and produce a permanent disability; frequently seen in neuromuscular conditions—hemiplegia.
5. Range-of-motion exercises are individually planned since there is wide variation in the degrees of motion of which patients of varying body builds and age groups are capable.
6. Range-of-motion exercises should be carried out whenever there is physical inactivity provided the patient's clinical status allows such activity.

Techniques of Range of Motion

1. Place the patient in a supine position with his arms to the side and the knees extended.
2. Hold the extremity at the joint, e.g., elbow, wrist, or

TABLE 5–1. RANGE OF MOTION*

SHOULDER

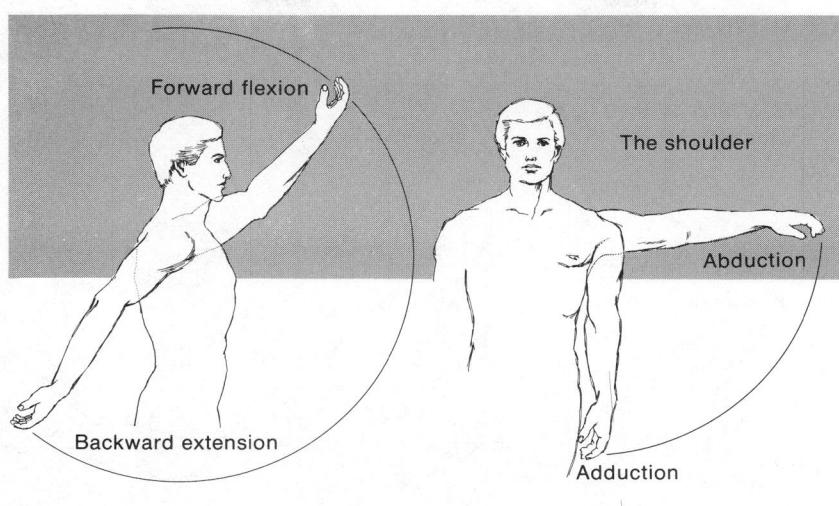

ELBOW

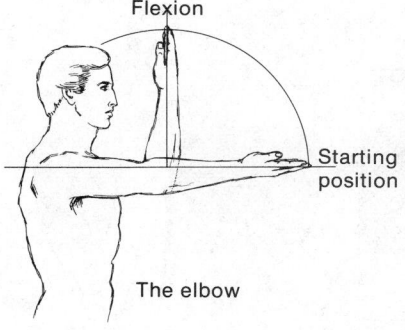

FOREARM

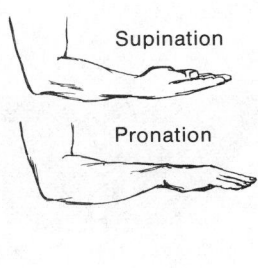

WRIST

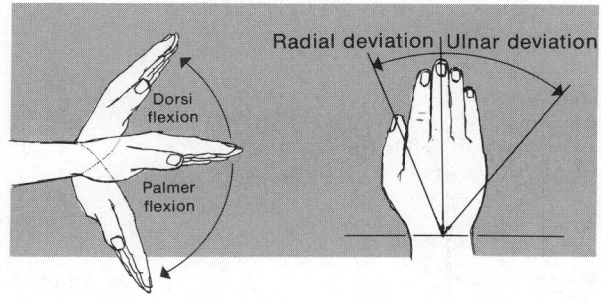

THUMB

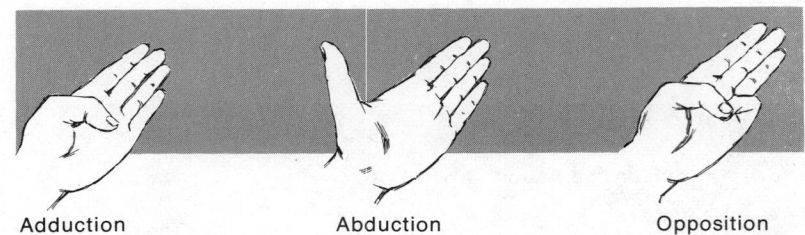

Adduction   Abduction   Opposition

FINGERS

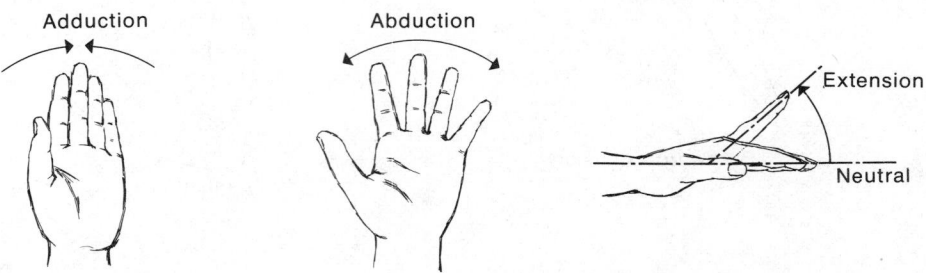

Adduction   Abduction

Extension

Neutral

ANKLE   **FOOT**

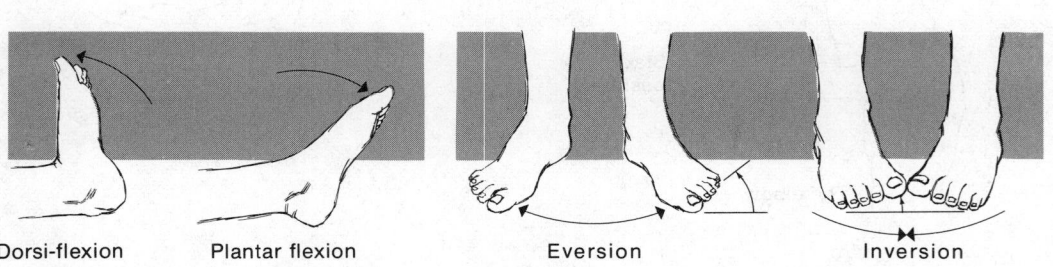

Dorsi-flexion   Plantar flexion   Eversion   Inversion

TOES

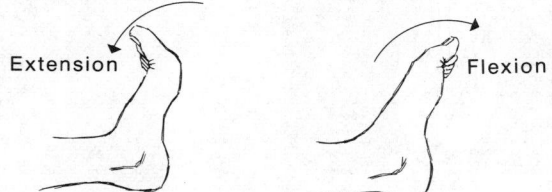

Extension   Flexion

Adduction   Abduction

HIP

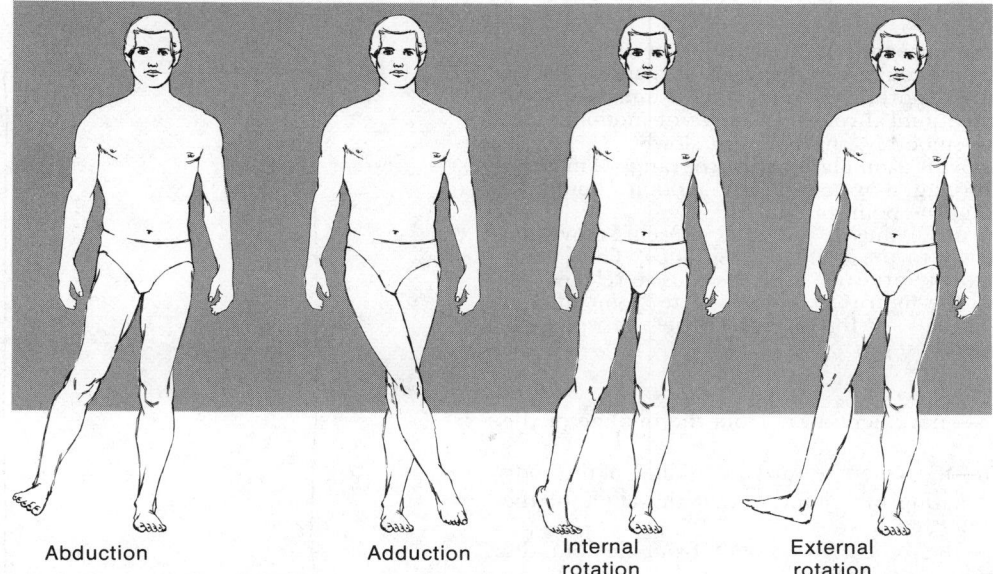

Abduction   Adduction   Internal rotation   External rotation

KNEE

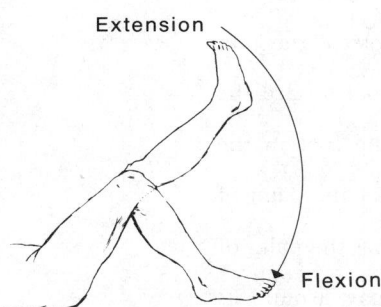

Extension

Flexion

CERVICAL SPINE

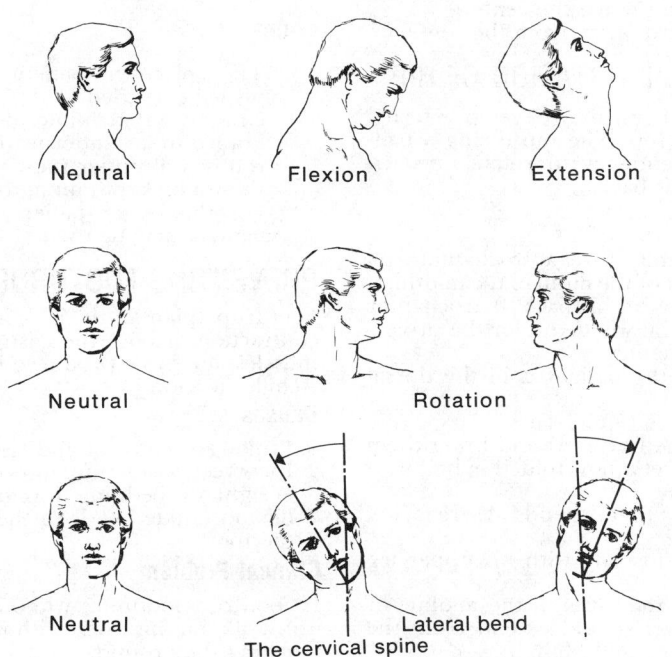

Neutral   Flexion   Extension

Neutral   Rotation

Neutral   Lateral bend

The cervical spine

knee, and move the joint smoothly, slowly, and gently through its range. If the joint is painful (as in arthritis) support the extremity in the muscular area.

3. Move each joint through its range of motion about 3 times—smoothly, rhythmically, slowly.
4. Avoid moving a joint beyond its free range of motion; avoid forcing movement. The motion should be stopped at the point of pain.
5. When painful muscle spasm is present, move the joint slowly to the point of resistance. Then exert gentle, steady pressure until the muscle relaxes.
6. Refer to the figures in Table 5–1 for joint motion and in Table 5–2 for pictorial review of range-of-motion exercises.

Definitions

Abduction—movement away from the midline of the body

Adduction—movement toward the midline of the body

Flexion—bending of a joint so that the angle of the joint diminishes

Extension—the return movement from flexion; the joint angle is increased

Inversion—movement that turns the sole of the foot inward

Eversion—movement that turns the sole of the foot outward

Dorsiflexion—flexing or bending the foot toward the leg

Plantar flexion—flexing or bending the foot in the direction of the sole

Pronation—rotating the forearm so that the palm of the hand is down

Supination—rotating the forearm so that the palm of the hand is up

Rotation—turning or movement of a part around its axis
  Internal: turning inward toward the center
  External: turning outward, away from the center

PREVENTING EXTERNAL ROTATION OF HIP

Patients on prolonged bed rest may develop external rotation deformity of the hip. The hip (being a ball-and-socket joint) has a tendency to rotate outward when the patient lies on his back.

Nursing Management

1. To prevent this deformity, use a trochanter roll extending from the crest of the ilium to the midthigh when the patient is lying on his back. A trochanter roll serves as a mechanical wedge under the projection of the greater trochanter.
2. Use a footboard when the patient is in the dorsal position.
3. To make a trochanter roll (Fig. 5-1):
   a. Take both ends of the towel (A) and bring them to the center. The towel is now folded in half with the edges at the center.
   b. Turn the towel over so that the ends (A) are facing downward.
   c. Turn the patient on his side with his upper leg flexed.
   d. Place one side (B) of the towel in the midline of the buttock. The towel should extend from the crest of the ilium to the midthigh.

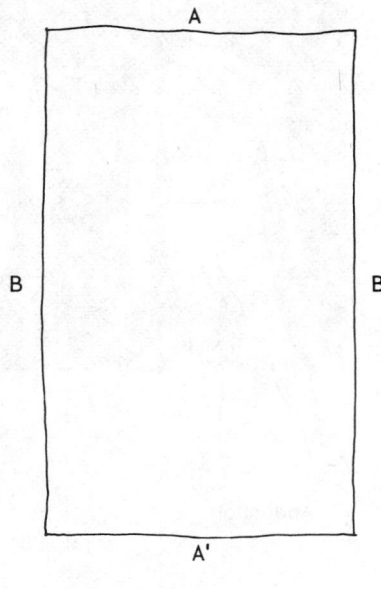

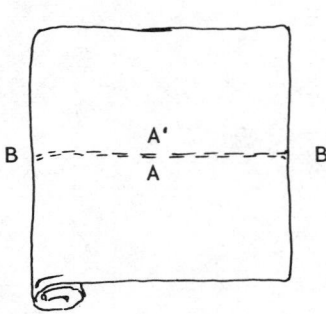

FIGURE 5-1.

e. Then place the patient in a dorsal position with his leg extended.
f. Grasp the remaining side (B) of the towel and roll inward in an underneath fashion until the entire roll is well under the patient's buttocks. The roll should be kept taut and smooth.
g. For the larger patient, a drawsheet or a bath blanket may be used.

PREVENTING FOOTDROP

Footdrop (plantar flexion) is a deformity caused by contraction of both the gastrocnemius and the soleus muscles; it may be produced by loss of flexibility of the Achilles tendon.

Causes

1. Prolonged bed rest and lack of exercise
2. Incorrect positioning in bed
3. Weight of bedding forcing the toes into plantar flexion (ankle bends in the direction of the sole of the foot)

Clinical Problem

If footdrop continues without correction, the patient will walk on his toes without the heel of his foot touching the ground.

TABLE 5-2. RANGE OF MOTION EXERCISES*

SHOULDER: Flexion

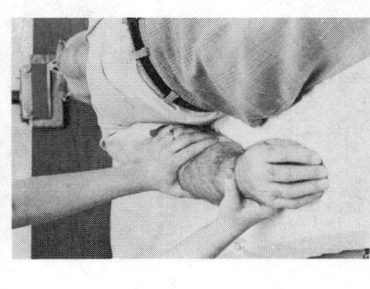
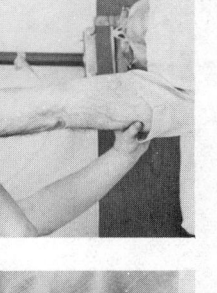
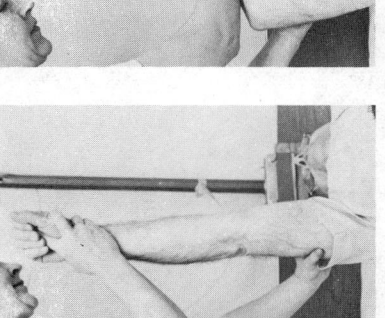
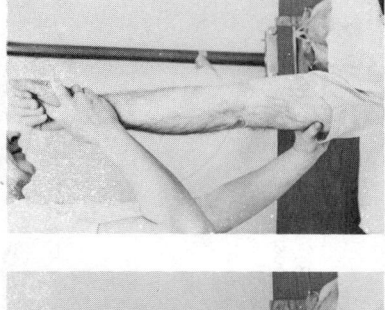

1. Start by placing one hand above the patient's elbow. Hold the patient's hand with your other hand.

2. Lift his arm up from the side of his body.

3. Move the arm slowly and gently toward his head as far as possible without causing pain.

4. If the headboard prevents full forward flexion, bend the arm at the elbow.

5. Lift arm again before returning to side or neutral position. Repeat the exercise.

SHOULDER: Abduction and Adduction

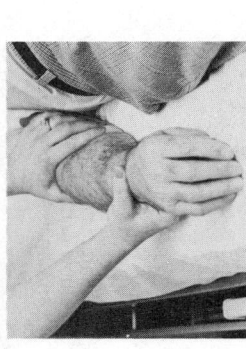
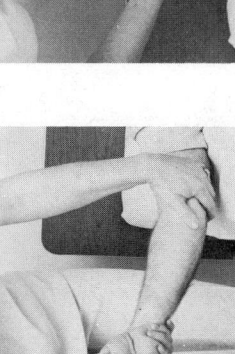
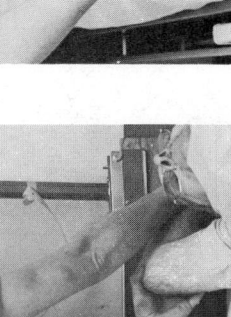
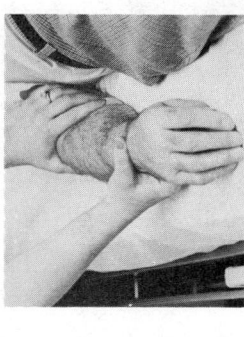

1. Place one hand above the patient's elbow. Hold his hand with your other hand.

2. Keeping his arm straight, move it sideways away from his body.

3. Bend and move the arm slowly around toward the patient's head. Move his arm back as far as possible without pain.

4. Return the arm to the side or neutral position. Repeat the exercise.

* From Nursing '72, April, 1972.

TABLE 5-2. (continued)

SHOULDER: Internal and External Rotation

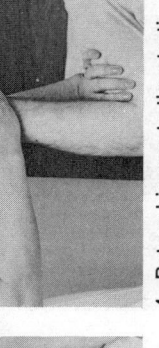
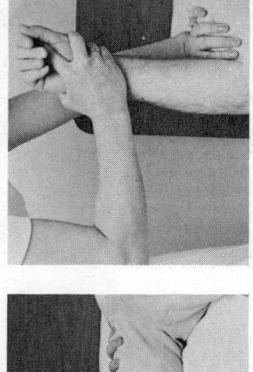
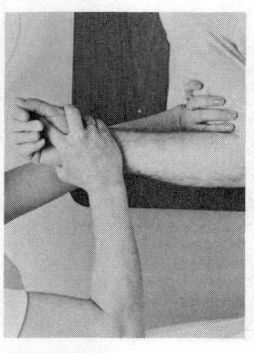

1. Place the patient's arm pointed away from his body, elbow bent. Hold his upper arm against the mattress.

2. Lift his lower arm and hand.

3. Move his lower arm and hand slowly and gently back toward his head as far as possible without causing pain.

4. Return his arm to the starting position. Repeat exercise.

SHOULDER: Cross Adduction

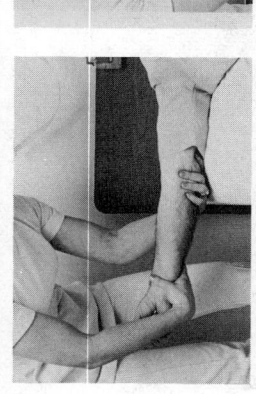
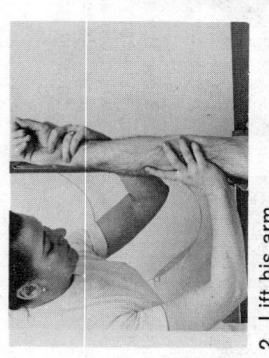
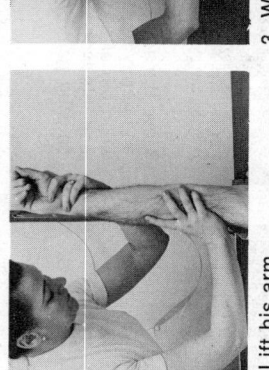
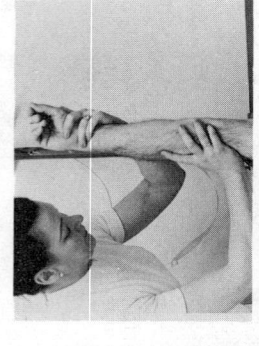
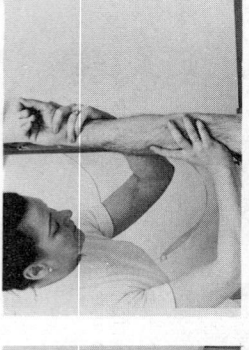
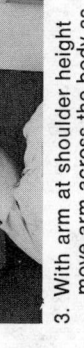

1. Place one hand on the patient's arm above his elbow. Hold his hand with your other hand.

2. Lift his arm.

3. With arm at shoulder height move arm across the body as far as possible toward the other shoulder.

4. Return the arm to the starting position. Repeat the exercise.

FOREARM: Supination and Pronation

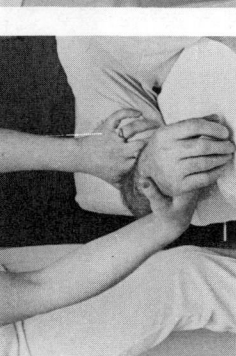
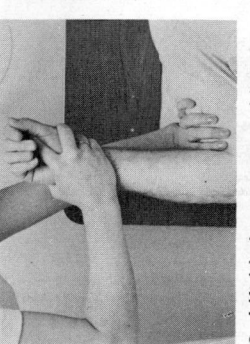
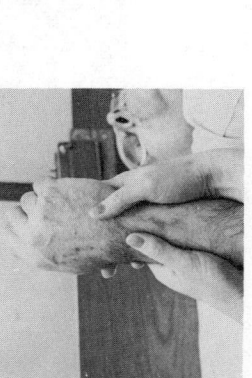
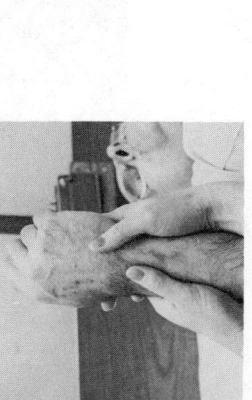
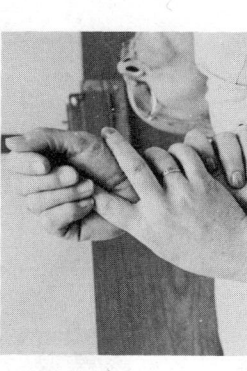

1. Starting position: Note the position of the patient's hand and the nurse's hands.

2. Twist the palm of the patient's hand toward his face.

3. Then, twist the palm of his hand back toward his feet. Repeat.

WRIST AND FINGER: Extension and Flexion

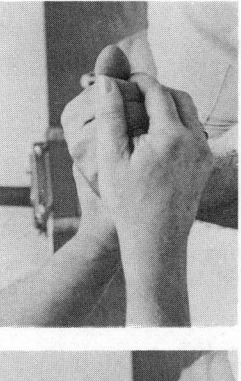

1. Hold the patient's wrist with one hand and his hand with your other hand.

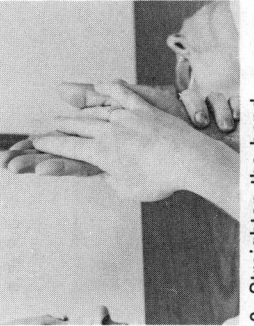

2. Bend his hand backward while keeping his fingers straight.

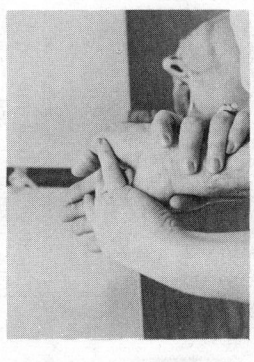

3. Straighten the hand.

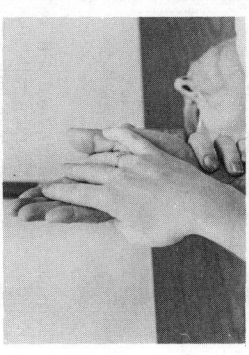

4. Bend his hand forward, closing his fingers to make a fist. Open his hand and repeat the exercise.

THUMB: Flexion and Extension

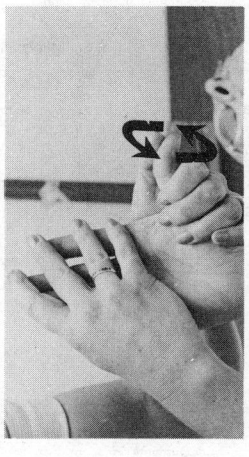

1. Hold the patient's fingers straight within one of your hands. Bend the patient's thumb into the palm of his hand with your other hand.

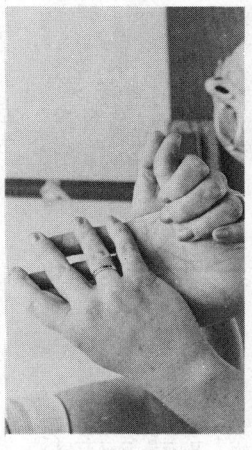

2. Pull his thumb back so that it points away from his palm. Repeat the exercise.

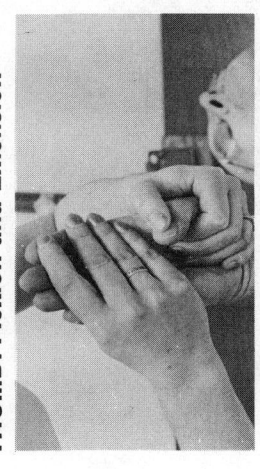

3. Move his thumb around in a circle. (circumduction)

KNEE AND HIP: Flexion and Extension

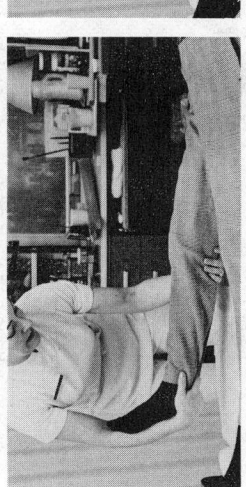
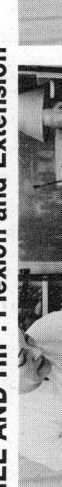

1. Place one of your hands under the patient's knee. Place your other hand on the heel of his foot.

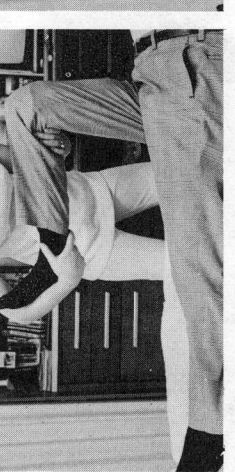

2. Lift his leg and bend it at the knee. Move his leg slowly back toward his head as far as it will go without hurting him.

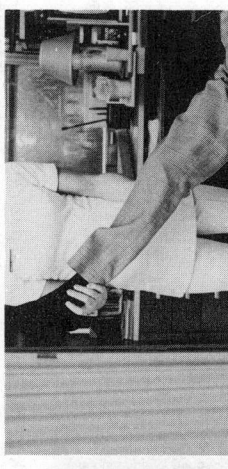

3. Then straighten his knee by lifting the foot upward. Lower his leg to the starting position and repeat the exercise.

TABLE 5-2. (continued)

HIP: Internal and External Rotation

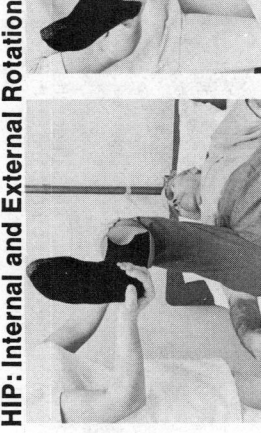
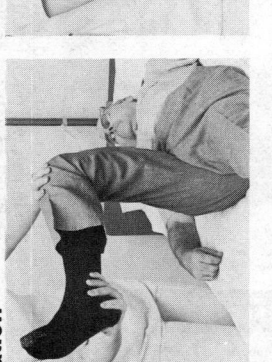
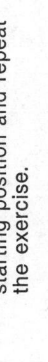
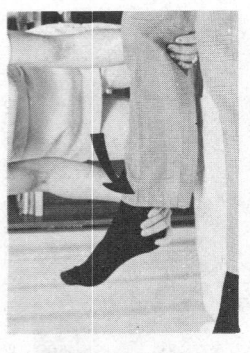

1. Place one hand under the patient's knee and your other hand on the heel of his foot. Lift his leg and bend it to a right angle at the knee.

2. Hold his knee in place and pull his foot toward you.

3. Move his foot back to the starting position.

4. Then push his foot away from you. Move his foot back to the starting position and repeat the exercise.

HIP: Abduction and Adduction

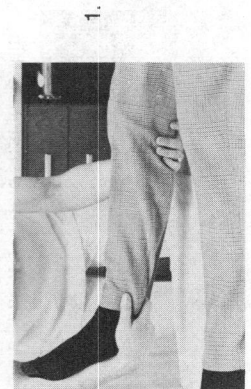
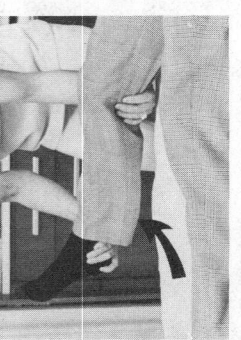

1. Place one hand under the patient's knee. Place your other hand under his heel. Hold the leg straight and then lift it up about 2 inches from the mattress.

2. Pull the leg out toward you (abduction).

3. Push the leg back to the starting position (adduction). Repeat the exercise.

ANKLE: Dorsiflexion and Plantar Flexion

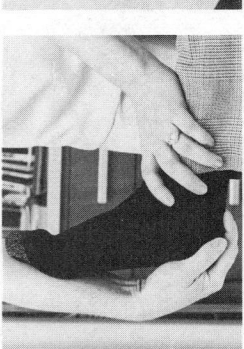
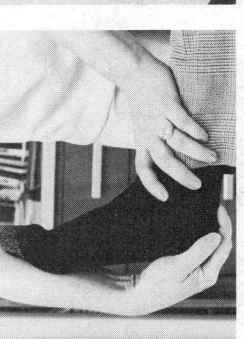
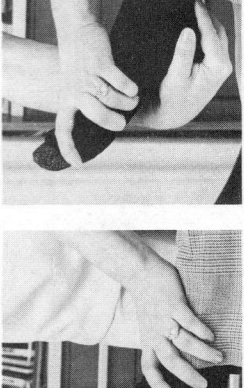

1. Hold the patient's heel with your hand, letting the sole of his foot rest against your arm.

2. Press your arm against the bottom of the foot, moving it back toward the leg (dorsiflexion). At the same time, pull on the heel.

3. Move your arm back to the starting position.

4. Move your hand up to the top of the foot, below the toes. Push down on the foot to point the toes and at the same time, push up against the heel (plantar flexion).

FOOT: Eversion and Inversion

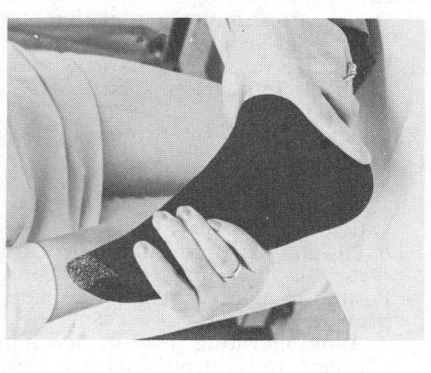

1. Start by turning the whole foot so that the sole is facing outward (eversion).

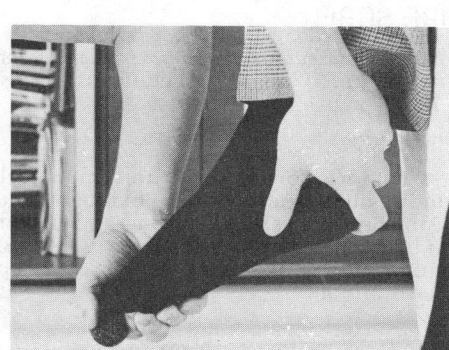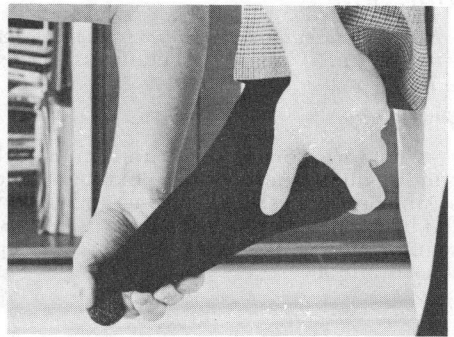

2. Then turn the foot so that the sole is facing inward (inversion).

TOE: Extension and Flexion

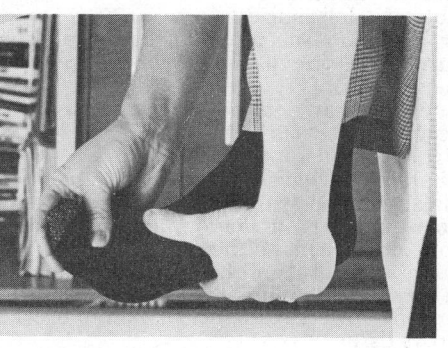

1. Start by pulling up on the toes.

2. Then push down on the toes.

Nursing Management

1. Use a footboard or pillows to keep feet at right angles to the legs when the patient is lying on his back.
   a. Position the feet with the entire plantar surface firmly against the footboard.
   b. Maintain the legs in a neutral position. Use a trochanter roll.
2. Encourage the patient to flex and extend (curl and stretch) his feet and toes frequently.
3. Have the patient rotate ankles clockwise and counterclockwise several times each hour.

PREVENTING AND TREATING PRESSURE SORES

Pressure sores (decubitus ulcers; bedsores) are localized areas in which necrosis of skin and subcutaneous tissues has been produced by pressure.

Altered Physiology

Pressure → compression of small nutrient vessels of skin and underlying tissue → tissue anoxia and ischemia → necrosis of tissue cells → sloughing and ulceration → invasion by microorganisms → infection → sepsis → involvement of underlying body structure → rapidly irreversible condition.

Causes

A. *Pressure*—exerted on skin and subcutaneous tissues by bony prominences and by the object on which the body part rests (mattress, cast, etc.); pressure interferes with the blood supply of the tissues and if prolonged will cause tissue death.

B. *Contributing Factors*

1. Immobilization and lack of normal movement—from neurologic, orthopedic, circulatory inadequacies and other conditions.
2. Sensory and motor deficits
   a. Sensory loss—produces lack of awareness of pain and pressure
   b. Motor paralysis with associated muscular atrophy—causes lack of movement and reduction in amount of padding between overlying skin and underlying bone
3. Circulatory deficiencies
4. Poor nutrition—negative nitrogen, phosphorus, sulfur, and calcium balance will produce wasting of tissue, osteoporosis, and loss of weight
   a. Anemia—may determine whether hypoxia and necrosis will occur
   b. Hypoproteinemia
   c. Vitamin deficiencies (particularly ascorbic acid)
   d. Malabsorption syndromes
5. Edema—impairs circulation and interferes with supply of nutrients to the cells.
6. Friction, moisture, and heat—irritate skin, making it less resistant to injury
7. Infection—lowers resistance of skin to breakdown; destroys tissue.
8. Shearing force—caused by gravitational forces that pull patient's body down towards the foot of the bed and by resisting forces created by friction taking place on the skin surface.
   a. Pulls tissues so that tissues and blood vessels are stretched and injured

   b. Occurs when patient is pulled up in bed, is allowed to slump in bed or chair, or moves in bed by digging heels or elbows into the mattress
9. Changes in the skin (especially in aged, because of reduced production of sebum)
10. Equipment—traction, casts, restraints, improper bedding and seats.

Sites

A. *Weight-bearing bony prominences covered only by skin and small amounts of subcutaneous fat*—75% of all pressure sores located at such sites.

1. Ischial tuberosities—especially in patients who sit for prolonged periods.
2. Trochanters
3. Sacrum

B. *Other bony prominences*—knees, malleoli, heels, and elbows.

Signs and Symptoms

1. Redness (a danger sign); redness will blanch on pressure
2. Dusky, cyanotic blue-gray area (fails to blanch on pressure)—shows capillary occlusion and subcutaneous weakening
3. Vesiculation (blistering)
4. Break in skin, progressing to deep, penetrating necrosis; may involve deeper soft tissues, bursae, muscles, tendons, bone and/or joints.

Nursing Assessment

1. Inspect each pressure area for erythema.
   a. Press on the area; look for blanching.
   b. Note how long hyperemia persists following removal of pressure.
2. Inspect for dry skin, moist skin, and breaks in the skin.
3. Palpate for warmth.
   Is the skin temperature increased? Compare with other parts of the body.
4. Palpate peripheral pulses to evaluate circulatory status.
5. Check patient's record for hematocrit, hemoglobin, and serum albumin levels.

Preventive Measures (Fig. 5-2)

OBJECTIVES: to relieve or remove pressure.
to stimulate circulation.
to keep the skin dry.

1. Recognize those patients in whom pressure sores are likely to develop. *Pressure sores may appear in a matter of hours.*
2. Relieve pressure by encouraging the patient to keep active.
   a. Turn the patient hourly or at 2-hour intervals—shifting of weight allows blood to flow back into tissues and helps tissues to recover from pressure.
   b. Position patient on all four sides (laterally, prone, dorsally) in sequence unless contraindicated.
3. Position patient with pillows, pads, etc. to relieve pressure.
   a. Avoid elevating head of bed more than 30 degrees—to reduce shearing forces.
   b. Avoid the use of rubber rings or doughnuts—they merely increase pressure around bony prominences.
   c. Keep foundation sheet dry and tightly stretched to prevent wrinkles.

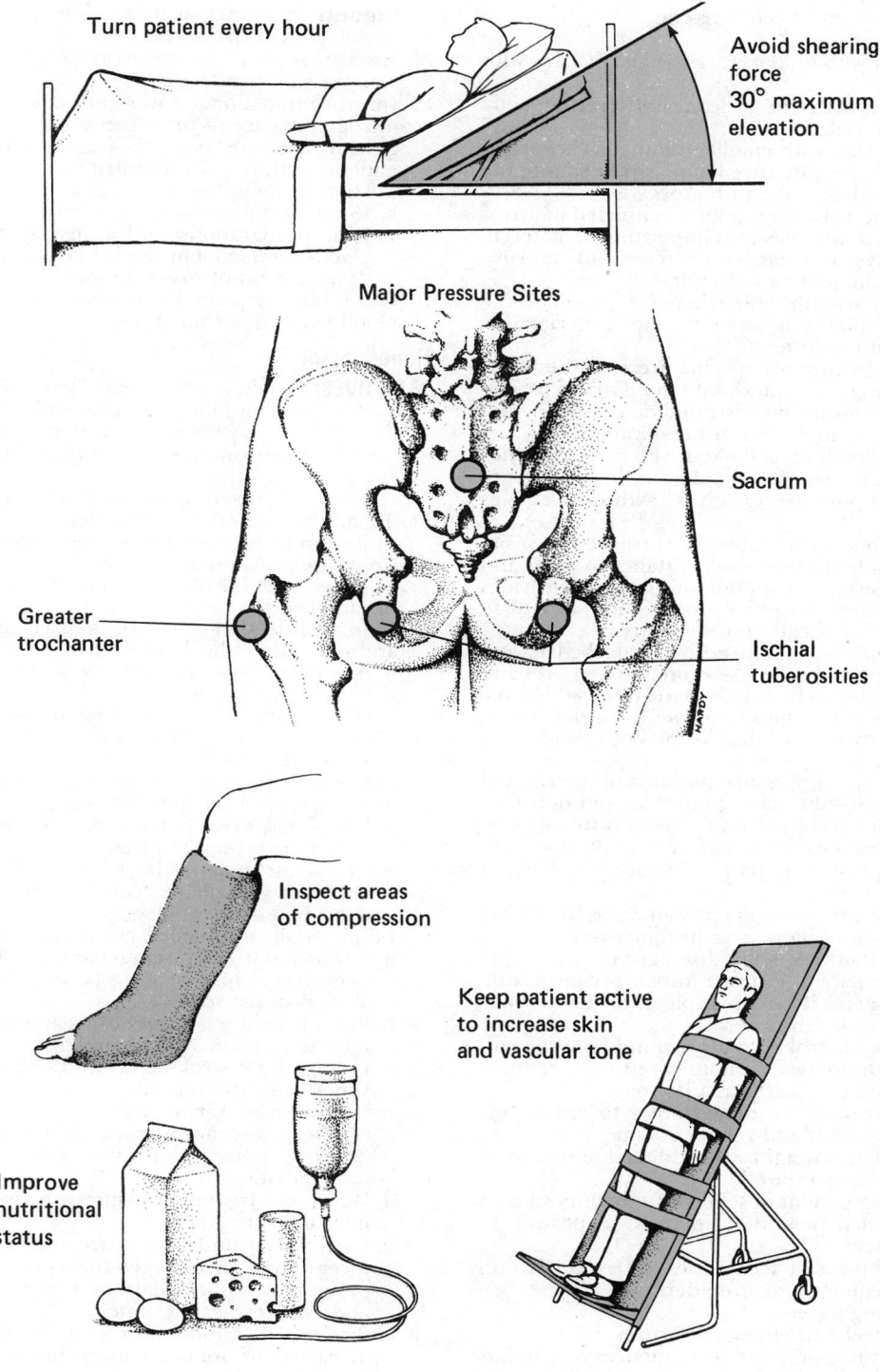

Turn patient every hour

Avoid shearing force 30° maximum elevation

Major Pressure Sites

Sacrum

Greater trochanter

Ischial tuberosities

HARDY

Inspect areas of compression

Keep patient active to increase skin and vascular tone

Improve nutritional status

FIGURE 5-2. *Prevention of pressure sores.*

4. Maintain meticulous skin hygiene.
   a. Inspect skin daily.
   b. Wash skin with mild soap, rinse and *blot* dry with soft towel.
   c. Keep local areas dry, clean, and free of body waste material.
   d. Lubricate skin with emollient lotion to keep skin soft and pliable. Be sure lotion is rubbed into the skin around coccyx and buttocks.
5. Avoid placing patient on poorly ventilated mattress that is covered with plastic or impermeable material.
6. Employ active and passive exercises—to improve muscular, skin, and vascular tone.
7. Ambulate or use tilt table whenever possible—the degree of mobility is an important criterion for prognosis and treatment.
8. Use devices to support specific areas of the body; the supporting medium should mold to the patient to ensure uniformly distributed pressure and should allow evaporation of perspiration.
   a. Gel-type flotation pad—reduces pressure since the gel-like material (similar in consistency to human adipose tissue) "gives" with the patient's weight.
   b. Natural sheepskin padding—softness and resilience of padding provides resistance to shear and results in even distribution of pressure; provides freedom from wrinkles and friction and dissipation and absorption of moisture.
   c. Fluid-supported mattresses (waterbeds) and fluid-supported seats—eliminates pressure points; as the body sinks into the fluid, additional surface area becomes available for weight-bearing, thereby further decreasing body weight per unit area.
9. Use of alternating pressure mattress or alternating pressure chair—alternating inflation and deflation of pad produces constriction of vessels followed by dilation of superficial blood vessels of the skin; pressure on any one part is reduced and blood supply is increased.
10. Relieve pressure over bony prominences by correct positioning with pillows and bridging techniques.
11. Inspect the skin frequently for signs of pressure.
    a. Teach the patient to use a mirror for inspecting posterior areas if he is paraplegic or has another neuromuscular disorder.
    b. Massage and stroke lightly around bony prominences—promotes venous return, reduces edema, and increases vascular tone.
    c. Massage around reddened areas to reduce venous congestion and relieve edema.
    d. Keep patient's weight off reddened area until it has completely cleared.
12. Avoid placing patient in semi-recumbent positions; discourage activities that increase exposure to shearing forces.
    a. Use good transfer techniques to reduce friction and consequent loss of epidermis.
    b. Use turning sheets.
    c. Employ heel and elbow protectors.
13. Relieve pressure on bony prominences of patients sitting in wheelchairs for prolonged periods—use foam-padded seat boards that are cut out posteriorly over ischial areas. Teach paraplegic patient to raise himself from his wheelchair for a few seconds every half-hour for intermittent relief of pressure from ischial tuberosities and prevention of ischial pressure sores.
14. Inspect, adjust, and pad casts, braces, splints, and compression bandages.
15. Improve nutritional status and maintain a positive nitrogen balance—pressure sores develop more quickly and are more resistant to treatment in patients suffering from nutritional disorders.
    a. High protein diet
    b. Vitamins and protein supplements
    c. Iron preparations and transfusions of whole blood—hemoglobin level a critical factor in the development of pressure sores
16. Carry out frequent hemoglobin, hematocrit, and blood sugar determinations.

Management

OBJECTIVES: to relieve all pressure from the area.
to continue with preventive measures of a more vigorous nature.
to encourage restoration of circulation and cellular function.
to prevent necrosis of deeper structures.

1. Treat the underlying disorder—underlying conditions must be managed to allow ulcer to heal.
2. Continue preventive measures (see page 64).
3. Improve general health of patient to provide optimum healing.
4. Control infection—may be a precipitating cause and may inhibit healing of ulcer.
   a. Assess for systemic infection—fever, cellulitis, lymphangitis.
   b. Give systemic antimicrobial therapy based on identification of pathogens and antimicrobial sensitivity determinations.
5. Debride ulcer—devitalized tissue promotes infection, delays granulation, and impedes healing.
   a. Use sharp dissection (scalpel blade) to remove eschar covering the ulcer.
   b. Cross-hatching of the eschar with the scalpel blade may facilitate penetration of enzymatic debriding agent (collagenase therapy).
6. Employ daily mechanical cleansing of ulcer—clears up sepsis and stimulates regeneration of epithelium. Deep ulcers may need to be irrigated with prescribed sterile solution.
7. Utilize physical modalities of treatment.
   a. Expose ulcer to air and sunlight.
   b. Employ light stroking around lesion—promotes venous return and reduces edema.
   c. Use ultraviolet irradiation—
      (1) Clean discharges from surface of ulcer.
      (2) Cover normal skin surrounding ulcer during irradiation.
   d. Whirlpool treatments—increase circulation and have debriding action.
   e. Use oxygen under pressure applied directly on ulcer (hyperbaric oxygen therapy)—directs more oxygen to tissues; hastens metabolic processes and reduces healing time.
8. Utilize topical applications as directed. There is a wide variety of opinion concerning these agents.
   a. Drying agents
   b. Skin barriers—Karaya powder, Stomahesive, etc.
   c. Antiseptic plastic sprays
   d. Aerosol spray containing a corticosteroid and an antibiotic

e. Absorbable gelatin sponges (Gelfoam)—placed at base of ulcer

f. Enzymatic debriding agents (collagenase therapy, e.g., Santyl)—digests necrotic tissue and purulent exudate and is applied using the following procedure:

   (1) Remove eschar covering ulcer or crosshatch eschar with scalpel blade to allow enzyme to come in contact with the material to be digested.

   (2) Remove loose debris with forceps.

   (3) Irrigate with prescribed sterile solution.

   (4) Assess wound for inflammation, pus, odor.

   (5) Apply enzymatic debriding ointment in thin, even layer over surface of ulcer.

   (6) Cover with dry sterile dressing secured with hypoallergenic tape or gauze bandage.

g. Dextranomer (Debrisan)—useful when depth of ulcer exceeds 2 mm. or for a moist sloughing wound.

   (1) Cleanse ulcer thoroughly with prescribed solution for each treatment and damp-dry.

   (2) Apply Debrisan directly onto lesion—Debrisan contains dry porous beads with hydrophilic (water absorbing) properties; also absorbs debris, allowing granulation tissue to develop.

   (3) Cover with dry porous dressing and secure with a gauze bandage.

9. Ensure good nutrition—patient may lose large amounts of protein from a draining ulcer.

a. High-protein feedings may be employed to correct protein deficiency.

b. Iron and ascorbic acid (Vitamin C) given as directed—Vitamin C is necessary for collagen formation. (Wound healing is dependent on collagen.)

10. Prepare patient for surgical intervention if ulcer does not respond to conservative measures.

a. Incision and drainage—if ulcer is not draining properly, is suppurating, or is not undermined.

b. Grafting procedures—different types of grafts used according to size of ulcer.

c. Closure of defect—removal of ulcer, surrounding scar, underlying bursa, affected bone.

SUPPORTING THE PATIENT IN DAILY SELF-CARE

ACTIVITIES OF DAILY LIVING

Activities of daily living are those self-care activities which must be accomplished each day in order for the patient to care for his own needs and participate in society. They include:

1. Getting in and out of bed (transfers)
2. Personal hygiene
3. Dressing
4. Eating
5. Using a wheelchair (if necessary)
6. Ambulating (when possible)
7. Performing manual tasks

Patient Objective

To care for himself in his daily routine within the boundaries of his physical limitations.

Role of Nurse

To teach, support, and supervise patient while he performs these activities.

Patient Teaching

1. Study each component motion of the desired activity.
2. Ascertain what methods can be used to accomplish the task. (Example: There are several ways of putting on a given garment.)
3. Determine what the patient can do by watching him perform.
4. Encourage the patient to exercise the muscles used in performing the motions involved in the activity.
5. Select activities that encourage gross functional movements of the upper and lower extremities (e.g., bathing, holding larger objects).
6. Gradually include activities that use finer motions, e.g., buttoning clothes, eating with a spoon.
7. Extend the period of activity as much and as fast as the patient can tolerate.
8. Have the patient perform and practice the activity in a real life situation.
9. Encourage the patient to perform every activity up to his maximal capabilities within the framework of his disability.
10. Support the patient by giving justifiable praise for effort put forth and for acts accomplished.

The Activities of Daily Living (ADL) Sheet

This is an information sheet for those who are caring for the patient. It is a guide to the assessment of the patient's functional capabilities (see p. 69).

PURPOSES: to inform each member of the rehabilitation team what activities the patient can carry out.

to serve as an index of progress.

Nurse's Responsibility in Using ADL Sheet

1. Review the ADL sheet each morning to know what the patient is capable of doing and what activities he is learning,
2. Avoid doing for the patient what he can do for himself.

Self-help Devices

Self-help devices include adaptive equipment that can help a patient to carry out his daily activities (Fig. 5-3). They may be devised and made by the patient, nurse, or family or purchased readymade. Publications are available offering extensive information on self-help devices.

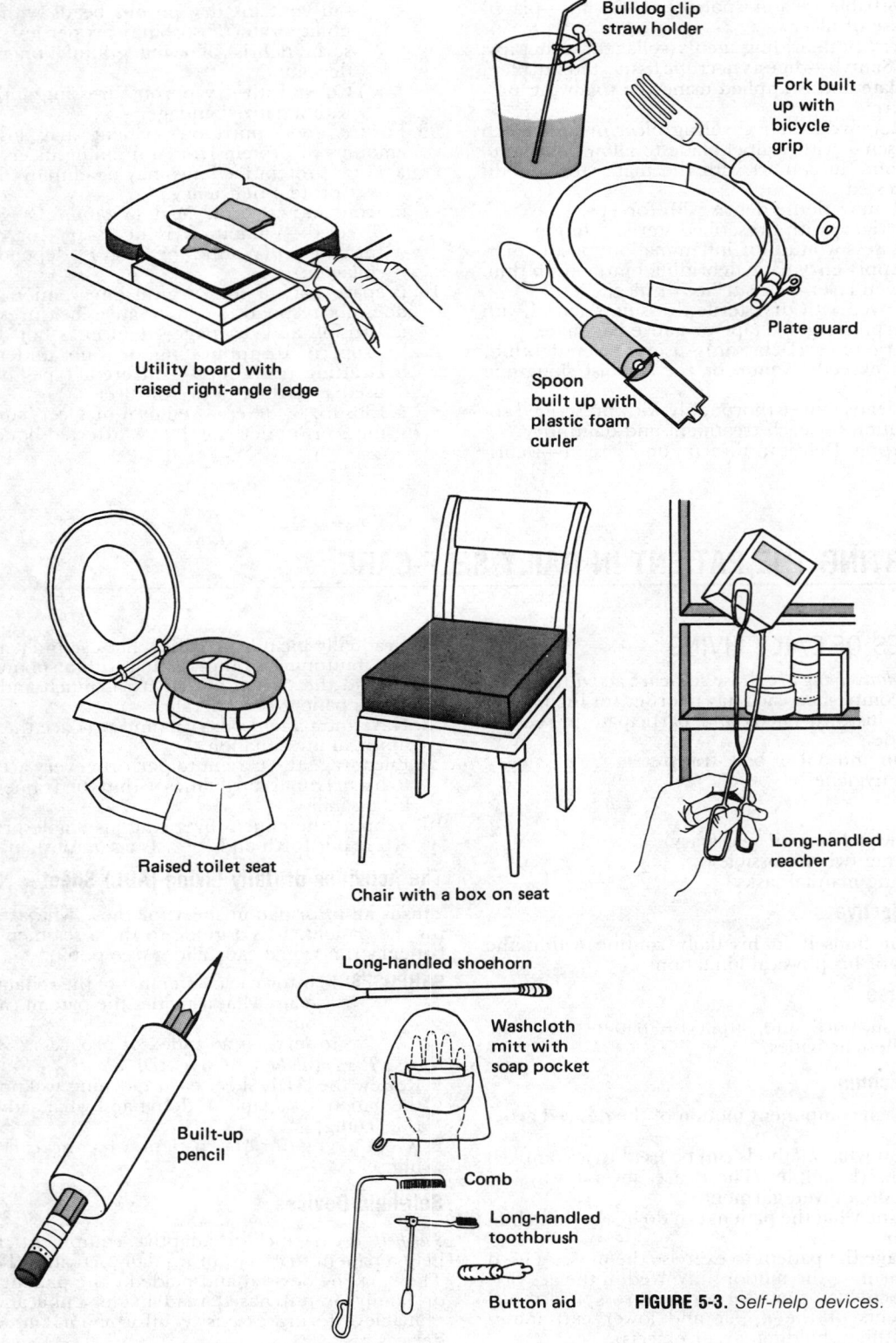

Bulldog clip straw holder

Fork built up with bicycle grip

Plate guard

Spoon built up with plastic foam curler

Utility board with raised right-angle ledge

Raised toilet seat

Chair with a box on seat

Long-handled reacher

Built-up pencil

Long-handled shoehorn

Washcloth mitt with soap pocket

Comb

Long-handled toothbrush

Button aid

FIGURE 5-3. *Self-help devices.*

Activities of Daily Living (ADL) Sheet

	Evaluation of the Patient's Functioning		
	Total Assistance	Partial Assistance	Independent

Prescribed Activities:

Range of Motion

Positioning

Use of Tilt Table

  Degree

  How long

Exercises

  Breathing

  Balancing

  Crutch Training

  Parallel Bars

  Steps

Other Information:

Appliances or Prosthesis

Ambulation

Time Permitted Up

Bladder/Bowel Program

Bathing/Grooming Schedule

Speech Problems

Activities Being Learned

Functional Capabilities:

1. Flexes neck
2. Raises hand to head
3. Raises hand behind head
4. Reaches out at shoulder level to side
5. Pronates/supinates forearm
6. Grasps objects
7. Begins grasp ability
8. Closes fist
9. Opens fist
10. Flexes and extends knee joint
11. Touches floor while seated
12. Crosses leg over opposite knee while sitting (with or without help of hands)
13. Transfers from sitting to standing (with or without holding to support)
14. Walks

Name:

Diagnosis:

Doctor:

ASSISTING THE PATIENT WITH AMBULATION

GUIDELINES: Using a Tilt Table

A *tilt table* is a board or table that can be tilted gradually from a horizontal to a vertical (upright) position.

Purposes
1. To help patient adjust gradually to varying degrees of the upright posture and ultimately to complete upright position.
2. To help patient start weight-bearing activities.
3. To increase standing tolerance.
4. To prevent disuse syndrome.
5. To prevent demineralization of bone and development of urinary tract stones.
6. To condition the vascular system.

Clinical Usefulness

Spinal cord injuries
Orthostatic hypotension
Brain damage

Equipment

Tilt table with footboard
Straps
Sphygmomanometer and stethoscope
Abdominal binder, elastic stockings or venous pressure gradient leotard*

Procedure

NURSING ACTION	RATIONALE/AMPLIFICATION
Preparatory Phase	
1. Apply snug-fitting abdominal binder, elastic compression bandages from toes to groin on both legs or a leotard (waist-high venous pressure gradient support*).	1. Compression of abdomen prevents pooling of blood in splanchnic area and subsequent postural hypotension and inadequate cerebral circulation. Compression of legs restricts the vascular walls of the blood vessels and prevents pooling of blood in the legs with development of edema.
Performance Phase	
1. Transfer the patient to tilt table by 3-person carry method. Place the patient in a dorsal position with his feet placed firmly against the footboard. Position the body in correct alignment.	
2. Fasten the straps across the pelvis, knees, chest, and abdomen.	
3. Apply the blood pressure cuff to the arm and take and record the blood pressure while the patient is lying flat.	3. This serves as a baseline recording for future comparisons.
4. Tilt the table 15–30 degrees. Take the blood pressure every 3–5 minutes.	4. Tilting the patient from a supine to upright position causes a decrease in systolic pressure.
5. Evaluate patient constantly and assess for a drop in blood pressure. If the patient feels dizzy and the blood pressure drops, return him to a flat position.	
6. Observe for pallor, diaphoresis, tachycardia, and nausea.	6. These are signs and symptoms of insufficient cerebral circulation.
7. Increase the standing tolerance by 5- to 10-degree increments.	7. The angle of tilt will be determined by the patient's tolerance, blood pressure stability, and the desired amount of weight-bearing.
8. Continue the procedure until the patient tolerates the desired tilt (usually between 45–80 degrees).	
9. Avoid allowing the patient to stand for prolonged periods.	9. Prolonged standing may cause pressure ulceration on plantar surfaces of feet.
10. Do not leave patient unattended.	
Follow-up Phase	
1. Place the patient back in bed at the end of the prescribed period or when his condition indicates.	
2. Record degree of tilt, amount of time on tilt table, and reaction of patient.	

* Jobst Venous Pressure Gradient Support.

TRANSFER ACTIVITIES

A *transfer* is the movement of the patient from one piece of furniture or equipment to another (from bed to chair, bed to commode, bed to wheelchair).

Weight-bearing transfers—carried out by patients who have at least one stable lower extremity (hemiplegics, unilateral lower extremity amputees, patients with hip fractures).

Nonweight-bearing transfers—done by double lower-extremity amputees, or paraplegics who are not wearing braces (Fig. 5-4).

Preparation for Transfers

OBJECTIVE: to develop ability to raise and move the body in different positions.

A. Exercises to Strengthen Arm and Shoulder Extensors

1. Have the patient sit upright in bed.
2. Place a book under each hand.
3. Instruct the patient to push down on the book thus raising his body weight.

B. Technique for Moving the Patient to the Edge of the Bed

1. Move the patient's head and shoulders toward the edge of the bed.
2. Move his feet and legs to the edge of bed. (The patient is now in a crescent position giving good range of motion to the lateral trunk muscles.)
3. Place both of your arms well under the patient's hips. (Before the next maneuver tighten or set the muscles of your back and abdomen.)
4. Straighten your back while moving the patient toward you.

C. Technique for Sitting the Patient on the Edge of the Bed

1. Place one hand under the patient's shoulders.
2. Instruct the patient to push his elbow into the bed while you lift his shoulders with one arm and swing his legs over the edge of the bed with the other. (Gravity pulls the legs downward, which aids in raising the patient's trunk.)

D. Technique for Assisting the Patient to Stand

1. Place the patient's feet well under him.
2. Face the patient and firmly grasp each side of his rib cage.
3. Push your knee against one of the patient's knees.
4. Rock the patient forward as he comes to a standing position. (Your knee is pushed against the patient's knee as he comes to the standing position.)
5. Ensure that the patient's knees are "locked" (full extension) while he is standing. (Locking the patient's knees is a safety measure for those patients who are weak or who have been in bed for a period of time.)
6. Give the patient enough time to balance himself.
7. Pivot the patient, positioning him to sit in the chair.

E. Technique for Transfer by Sliding Board

1. A *sliding board* (or transfer board) is a polished lightweight board that is used to bridge the gap between the bed and the chair (or chair and tub, etc.).
2. When the muscles that the patient uses to lift himself off the bed are not strong enough to overcome the resistance of body weight, use the following maneuver:
   a. Place one side of the sliding board under the patient's buttocks and the other side on the surface of the chair, bed, toilet, etc., to which the transfer is being made.
   b. Instruct the patient to push up with his hands, to shift his buttocks, and to slide across the board to the other surface.

CRUTCH WALKING

Crutches are artificial supports that assist patients who need aid in walking because of disease, injury, or a birth defect.

Preparation for Crutch Walking

OBJECTIVES: to develop power in the shoulder girdle and upper extremities that bear the patient's weight in crutch walking.
to strengthen and condition the patient.

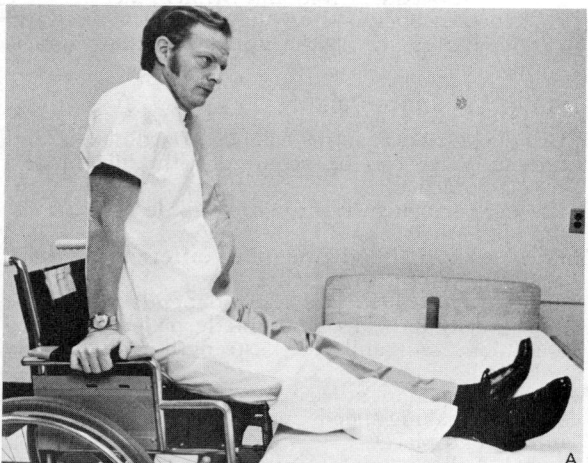 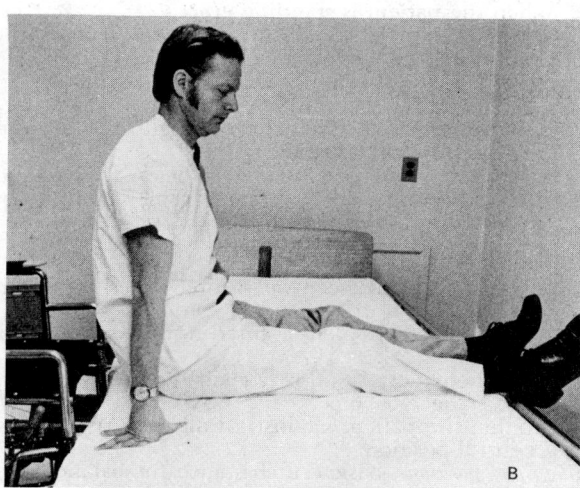

FIGURE 5-4. *Vertical transfer of a paraplegic patient. A. Place the wheelchair facing the bed as close to the bed as possible. Lock brakes. Instruct the patient to push up on his hands and arms and slide his body forward onto the bed. B. This is a nonweight-bearing transfer in which the patient learns to transfer on the same level. Later this type of nonweight-bearing transfer can be done to a higher and lower level by the push-up method.*

A. *To Strengthen the Muscles Needed for Ambulation*

Instruct the patient as follows:
1. For *quadriceps setting*
   a. Contract the quadriceps muscle while attempting to push the popliteal area against the mattress and raise the heel.
   b. Maintain the muscle contracture for the count of 5.
   c. Relax for the count of 5.
   d. Repeat this exercise 10 to 15 times hourly.
2. For *gluteal setting*
   a. Contract or pinch the buttocks together for the count of 5.
   b. Relax for the count of 5.
   c. Repeat 10 to 15 times hourly.

B. *To Strengthen the Muscles of the Upper Extremities and Shoulder Girdle*

Instruct the patient as follows:
1. Flex and extend arms slowly while holding traction weights; gradually increase poundage of weight and number of repetitions to increase strength and endurance.
2. Do pushups while lying in a prone position.
3. Squeeze rubber ball—increases grasping strength.
4. Raise head and shoulders from bed; stretch hands forward as far as possible.
5. Sit up on bed or chair.
   a. Raise body from chair by pushing hands against chair seat (or mattress).
   b. Raise body out of seat. Hold. Relax.

C. *To Measure for Crutches*

1. When the patient is lying down (an approximate measurement)
   a. Instruct the patient to wear the shoes he will be using for walking.
   b. Measure from the anterior fold of the axilla to the sole of the foot. Then add 5 cm. (2 inches).
   c. Or subtract 40 cm. (16 inches) from the patient's height.
2. When the patient is standing erect.
   a. Stand the patient against the wall with feet slightly apart and away from the wall.
   b. Mark 5 cm. (2 inches) out to the side from the tip of the toe.
   c. Measure 15 cm. (6 inches) straight ahead from the first mark. Mark this point.
   d. Measure from 5 cm. (2 inches) below the axilla to the second mark. This measurement is the approximate crutch length.

D. *Crutch Stance*

1. Have the patient wear well-fitting shoes with firm soles.
2. The crutches should be fitted with large rubber suction tips.
3. Have the patient stand by a chair on the unaffected leg to achieve balance.
4. Position the patient against a wall with his head in a neutral position.
5. *Tripod position*—basic crutch stance for balance and support
   a. Crutches rest approximately 20–25 cm (8–10 inches) in front of and to the side of patient's toes. (Fig. 5–5)
   b. Taller patient requires a wider base, whereas shorter patient needs a narrower base.

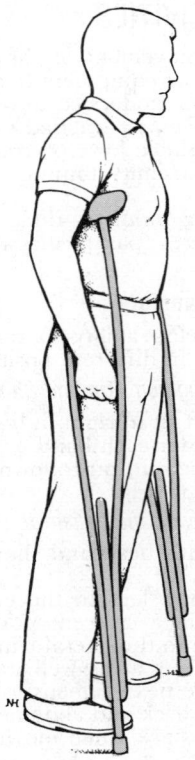

FIGURE 5-5. *Crutch stance.*

6. Teach the patient to support his weight on his hands; weight borne on the axillae can damage the brachial plexus nerves and produce "crutch paralysis."
   a. The hand piece should be adjusted to allow a 30-degree elbow flexion.
   b. There should be a 2-finger-width insertion between the axillary fold and the arm piece.
   c. A foam-rubber pad on the underarm piece will relieve pressure on the upper arm and thoracic cage.

Teaching the Crutch Gait

1. Crutch walking requires balance, coordination, and timing; these can be acquired with diligent and regular practice.
2. Practice balancing with crutches while leaning against the wall.
3. Practice shifting body weight in different positions, while standing with crutches.
4. The selection of the crutch gait depends on the type and severity of the disability and the patient's physical condition, arm and trunk strength, and/or body balance.
5. Teach the patient at least 2 gaits—a faster gait to be used for making speed, and a slower one to be used in crowded places.
6. Instruct the patient to change from one gait to another—relieves fatigue since a different combination of muscles is used.
7. Make sure the patient is bearing weight on his hands—If the weight is borne on the axilla, the pressure of the crutch can damage the brachial plexus and produce crutch paralysis.

FIGURE 5-6. *Four-point gait.*

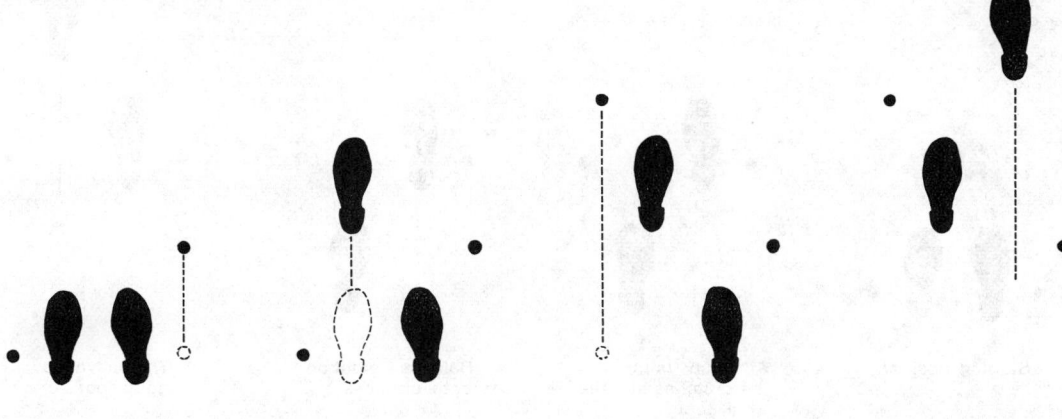

Right crutch forward   Advance left foot   Left crutch forward   Advance right foot

Crutch Gaits

A. *4-Point Gait* (4-point alternate crutch gait)

1. This is a slow but stable gait; the patient's weight is constantly being shifted.
2. 4-point gait can be used only by patients who can move each leg separately and bear a considerable amount of weight on each of them.

Crutch-foot sequence (Fig. 5-6)
1. Right crutch
2. Left foot
3. Left crutch
4. Right foot

B. *2-Point Gait* (2-point alternate crutch gait)

1. This is a faster gait but requires more balance since there are only 2 points of contact with the floor.

Crutch-foot sequence (Fig. 5-7)
1. Right crutch and left foot
2. Left crutch and right foot simultaneously

C. *3-Point Gait*

1. This is a fairly rapid gait but requires more strength and balance.

2. The patient's arms must be strong enough to support his entire body weight.

Crutch-foot sequence (Fig. 5-8)
1. Both crutches and the weaker lower extremity are moved forward simultaneously.
2. Then the stronger lower extremity is moved forward.

D. *Tripod Crutch Gaits*

1. The patient constantly maintains a tripod position.
2. At the start, both crutches are held fairly widespread out front while both feet are held together in the back.
3. These gaits are slow and labored.

Tripod Alternate Crutch Gait

Crutch-foot sequence
1. Right crutch
2. Left crutch
3. Drag body and legs forward.

Tripod Simultaneous Crutch Gait

Crutch-foot sequence (Fig. 5-9)
1. Both crutches
2. Drag body and legs forward.

FIGURE 5-7. *Two-point gait.*

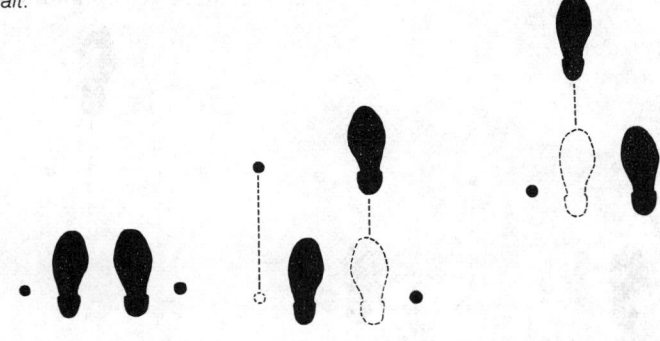

Starting position   Advance right foot and left crutch   Then advance left foot and right crutch simultaneously.

FIGURE 5-8. *Three-point gait.*

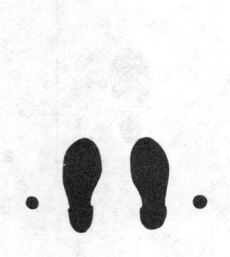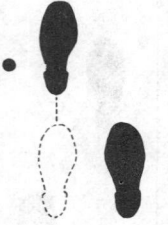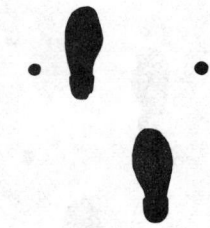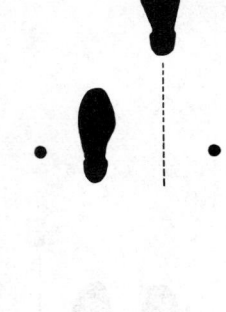

Starting position	Advance both of the crutches and the weak foot	Balance weight on both crutches	Then advance good foot

E. *Swinging Crutch Gaits*

1. In the swinging crutch gaits, both legs are lifted off the ground simultaneously and swung forward while the patient pushes up on the crutches.

Swinging-to Gait

Crutch-foot sequence
1. Both crutches forward
2. Then lift and swing body up *to* crutches.
3. Place crutches in front of body and continue.

Swinging-through Gait

Crutch-foot sequence
1. Both crutches forward
2. Lift and swing body *beyond* crutches.
3. Place crutches in front of body and continue.

Other Crutch Maneuvering Techniques

A. *To Stand Up*

1. Place one or both feet in a wide stance under the chair or as close to the chair as possible.
2. Grasp the handpieces of the crutches (either in each hand or both hand pieces in one hand.)
3. Push down on the hand pieces while raising the body to a standing position.

B. *To Sit In A Chair*

1. Grasp the crutches at the hand pieces for control and bend forward slightly while assuming a sitting position.

FIGURE 5-9. *Tripod simultaneous crutch gait.*

C. *To Go Up Stairs*

1. Advance the stronger leg first up to the next step.
2. Then advance the crutches and the weaker extremity.

D. *To Go Down Stairs*

1. Place feet forward as far as possible on the step.
2. Advance crutches to the lower step. The weaker leg is advanced first and then the stronger one—the stronger extremity shares the work of raising and lowering the body weight with the patient's arms.

NOTE: Strong leg goes up stairs first and down stairs last.

AMBULATION WITH A CANE

Purposes

A cane is used for balance and support:
1. To assist the patient to walk with greater balance and support and less fatigue.
2. To compensate for deficiencies of function normally performed by the neuromuscular skeletal system.
3. To relieve pressure on weight-bearing joints.
4. To provide forces to push or pull the body forward or to restrain the forward motion of the patient while walking.

Underlying Principles

1. An adjustable aluminum cane, fitted with a 3.75 cm. (1½-inch) rubber suction tip to provide traction while walking, gives optimum stability to the patient.

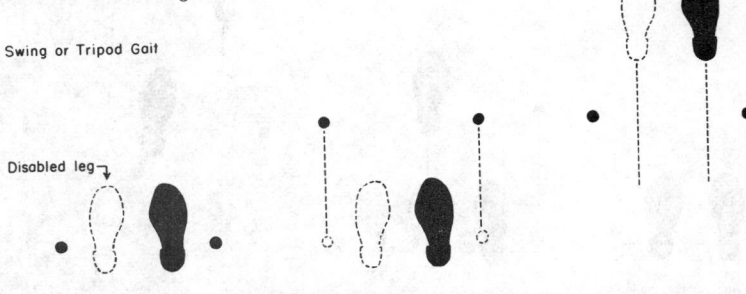

Swing or Tripod Gait

Disabled leg

Starting position	Put both crutches some distance in advance with weight on good leg	Then swing forward with weight on good leg again

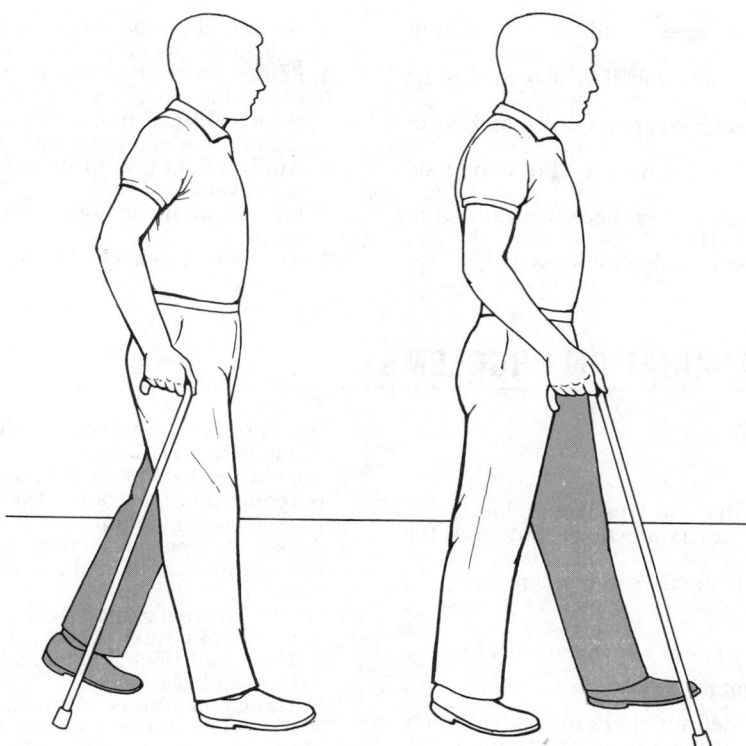

FIGURE 5-10. *Walking with cane.*

2. To fit for a cane
   a. Have patient flex his elbow at a 30 degree angle and hold the cane 15 cm. (6 inches) lateral to the base of his fifth toe.
   b. Adjust the cane so that the handle is approximately level with the greater trochanter. (Fig. 5-10)

Technique for Walking with a Cane

Instruct the patient as follows:
1. Hold the cane in the hand opposite to the affected extremity, i.e., the cane should be used on the good side.
2. Advance the cane at the same time the affected leg is moved forward.
3. Keep the cane fairly close to the body to prevent leaning.
4. To go up and down stairs
   a. Step up on *unaffected* extremity.
   b. Then place cane and affected extremity on the step.
   c. Reverse this procedure for descending steps.
   d. The strong leg goes up first and comes down last.

PROSTHETIC AND ORTHOTIC DEVICES

A *prosthesis* is an artificial replacement for a missing portion of the body. An *orthosis* is an orthopedic appliance/device used to provide support and alignment, prevent or correct deformities, and to improve the function of the body (includes braces and splints).

Preprosthetic Nursing Management*

1. Help the patient to develop an attitude of realistic hopefulness.
2. *Prevent deformities*—to limit the time between the healing of tissues and the fitting of a prosthesis.
3. Bandage an extremity stump correctly so that proper shrinkage and shaping of the stump occur.

Support and Health Education of the Patient Using Braces

A *brace* is a support that protects weakened muscles, prevents and corrects deformities, aids in controlling involuntary muscle movements, and immobilizes and protects a diseased or injured joint.

The following are the main points to emphasize in teaching the patient to care for his brace:
1. Place the brace on a table or the floor, or prop it against the wall when it is not in use; hanging may cause distortion of its position.
2. Twisting of the brace may occur with use; check alignment frequently. Look down the full length of the brace. The joints should coincide with the body joints.
3. Before putting a brace on, check carefully for worn

* Specific prostheses are described in this volume under the clinical conditions requiring such devices. Information concerning prosthetic and orthopedic appliances may also be obtained from the American Orthotic and Prosthetic Association, 1440 N. Street, N.W., Washington, D.C. 20005.

areas, missing or loose screws, and the condition of straps and buckles.
4. Pressure areas may occur if metal or plastic rubs the skin.
5. Check the skin for reddened areas immediately after removing the brace.
6. Keep the heels and soles of the shoes in good condition.
7. Clean and dry the brace, when necessary, at night.
8. To clean the plastic parts:
    a. Wipe the plastic parts with a damp cloth.

b. Do not oil plastic surfaces and joints.
 To clean the metal parts:
    a. Remove rust or corrosion spots with steel wool.
    b. Clean dirt out of metal joints and locks with a pipe cleaner dipped in a solvent.
    c. Clean the metal parts with a solvent.
    d. Apply a light coat of paste wax to the metal parts to prevent rust.
    e. Put oil in metal joints with an eyedropper or toothpick.
9. Have the brace checked periodically.

OVERCOMING ELIMINATION PROBLEMS

BLADDER TRAINING

Objectives

1. To keep the patient dry and free from odor.
2. To prevent urinary tract infections and preserve renal function.
3. To help the patient maintain social acceptance.

Neurogenic Bladder

See page 512 for discussion of neurogenic bladder.

Bladder Training Regimen

1. Set up a schedule of definite times for patient to try to empty his bladder using a toilet or commode.
2. Give patient a measured amount of fluid to drink at regularly scheduled times.
3. Have patient wait 30 minutes and then ask him to attempt to void; *regularity is the key to success.*
    a. Position patient with thighs flexed and feet and back supported; sufficient daily fluid intake (2500 ml.) is essential.
    b. Instruct him to press or massage over bladder area or increase intra-abdominal pressure by *leaning forward*—helps to initiate evacuation of bladder.
    c. Have the patient concentrate on voiding.
    d. Have patient try to void every 2 hours; interval may be lengthened as control is gained.
        (1) Set alarm clock at 2-3 hour intervals during the daytime.
        (2) Set alarm clock 2 times during night.
        (3) Curtail or limit fluids after 5 p.m.
4. Have patient keep a voiding calendar—a continuous record of time and amount of fluid ingested and time and amount of each voiding.
5. Encourage the patient to hold his urine until specified voiding time if possible.
6. Assess for signs of urinary retention; test (catheterize) for residual urine as directed.
7. Encourage patient to continue self-care and exercise programs; encourage patient to wear his own clothing.
8. Stress the abilities (not the disabilities) of the patient.
9. Have a positive approach; the patient needs an atmosphere of encouragement and support.

Management of Incontinent Patient

(Not due to neurogenic bladder impairment)
1. Assist patient to bathroom at a regularly scheduled time—delay in responding to call for bedpan or urinal or for assistance to toilet is a common cause of incontinence.
2. Encourage patient to perform self-care activities—boredom and frustration lead to incontinence.
3. Give adequate amounts of fluids.
4. Avoid overt encouragement of incontinence such as the routine use of pads, diapers, and other depersonalizing procedures.
5. Create an environment which keeps sensory monotony to a minimum.
    a. Have wall clock and calendar to orient patient to time and place.
    b. Hang wall posters, pictures, etc. for visual stimulus.
    c. Use telephone, radio, and television selectively.
    d. Encourage patient to make decisions (menu selection, keeping intake/output chart)—improves self-esteem.
    e. Have patient do meaningful tasks (sort mail, straighten his bureau drawers, etc.).
    f. Extend patient's environment beyond the confines of his room.
    g. Increase patient's social contacts
6. Encourage patient to wear his own clothes—enhances his self-esteem and dignity and is a strong deterrent to regressive behavior.

BOWEL TRAINING

Objectives

1. To develop regular bowel habits.
2. To prevent fecal incontinence, impaction, irregularity.

Bowel Training Program

1. Secure a bowel history; bowel schedule should be normal and comfortable for the patient.
2. Establish a *specific and definite time* for the bowel movement; *regularity is necessary to establish reflex assistance.*
    a. The exact time period depends on the patient's schedule.
    b. Attempts at evacuation should be made within 15 minutes of this same time daily.
    c. Establish bowel evacuation after a regularly scheduled meal—utilizes the stimulation of peristalsis and the gastrocolic and duodenocolic reflexes.
    d. Stimulate anorectal reflex if necessary.
        (1) Insert a glycerine suppository into the rectum 15–30 minutes before the scheduled bowel time.

(2) Eventually patient may evacuate without any stimulation.

(3) If glycerine suppository is not effective, a suppository of bisacodyl (Dulcolax) may be tried.

e. Have patient use a normal posture for defecation—a toilet seat or commode most nearly approximates the physiologic position for defecation.

(1) Instruct patient to bear down and contract the abdominal muscles.

(2) Have patient lean forward to increase intra-abdominal pressure by compression against the thighs.

3. Ensure adequate roughage and fluid intake 2-4 L. (2.1–4.2 quarts) daily.

a. Give 120 ml. (4 oz.) of prune or fig juice at the same time daily (i.e., 30 minutes before breakfast)—helps establish regularity.

b. Encourage high residue diet (vegetables, fruits, salads, bran, cereals)—to prevent hard stools and to stimulate peristalsis.

4. Encourage patient to exercise—good abdominal muscle tone and muscular activity is helpful in bowel training.

DISCHARGE PLANNING AND REFERRAL FOR FOLLOW-UP CARE

OBJECTIVES: to improve the future quality of the patient's life.

to maintain continuity of care as patient is transferred from the health care facility to his home or an extended-care facility.

1. Plan for care at home as soon after hospital admission as possible.

2. Gather information about the patient's home environment (from patient, social worker, community health nurse).

3. Estimate the patient's functional potential; make plans with this in mind.

4. Plan, with the patient, ways and methods of coping with problems that may arise; and make realistic plans for the future.

5. Teach the family as much about the patient's condition as possible, so that they will not fear his return home.

a. Encourage family to ask questions.

b. Assess family's attitude toward patient, his disability, and his return home.

6. Send referral form to local community health agency so nurse can evaluate the home environment.

a. Review patient's ADL sheet with community health or visiting nurse—so community nurses will know exactly what activities patient can perform.

b. Determine what modifications will be necessary in the home (for wheelchair, for self-care activities).

c. Inquire how patient expects to be transported for clinic visits, special therapy, etc.

7. Send referral to State Vocational Rehabilitation Agency if patient will require additional educational or job training.

8. Assist with transfer of patient to extended-care facility if he is unable to return to home situation.

a. Recognize that not all families can be expected to carry on the rehabilitation program that the patient may require.

b. Send ADL sheet to extended-care facility with patient to help orient staff to patient's goals and programs.

BIBLIOGRAPHY

Books

American Medical Association. Guides to the Evaluation of Permanent Impairment. Chicago, American Medical Association, 1977

Basmajian JV. Therapeutic Exercise, 3rd ed. Baltimore, Williams & Wilkins, 1978

Bender M, Velletutti PJ, and Bender R. Teaching the Moderately and Severely Handicapped, Vols I, II, III. Baltimore, University Park Press, 1976

Bolton B and Cook DW. Rehabilitation Client Assessment. Baltimore, University Park Press, 1980

Bower FL and Brown MS (eds). Nursing and the Concept of Loss. New York, John Wiley & Sons, 1980

Galka G and Fraser BA. Gross Motor Management of Severely Multiply Impaired Students. Baltimore, University Park Press, 1979

Goldenson RM, Dunham JR and Dunham CS. Disability and Rehabilitation Handbook. New York, McGraw-Hill, 1978

Hopkins HL and Smith HD. Willard and Spackman's Occupational Therapy, 5th ed. Philadelphia, JB Lippincott, 1978

Ince LP (ed). Behavioral Psychology in Rehabilitation Medicine: Clinical Applications. Baltimore, Williams & Wilkins, 1980

Kernaleguen A. Clothing Designs for the Handicapped. Edmonston, University of Alberta Press, 1978

Marinelli RP and Dell Orto AE (eds). Psychological and Social Impact of Physical Disability. New York, Springer Pub. Co., 1977

McDaniel JW. Physical Disability and Human Behavior. New York, Pergamon Press, 1976

Murray R and Kijek JC. Current Perspectives in Rehabilitation Nursing. St. Louis, C.V. Mosby, 1979

Nichols PJR. Rehabilitation Medicine. Boston, Butterworth & Co, 1980

Rusk H. Rehabilitation Medicine, 4th ed. St. Louis, C.V. Mosby, 1977

Sloan AW. The Physiological Basis of Physiotherapy. London, Baillière Tindall, 1979

Sexuality and the Disabled

Comfort A. Sexual Consequences of Disability. Philadelphia, George F Stickley Co, 1978

Craft M and Craft A. Sex and the Mentally Handicapped. London, Routledge & Kegan Paul, 1978

Gochros HL and Gochros JS (eds). The Sexually Oppressed. New York, Association Press, 1977

Marinelli RP and Dell Orto AE. The Physiological and Social Impact of Physical Disability. New York, Springer Pub. Co., 1977

Mims FH and Swenson M. Sexuality: A Nursing Perspective. New York, McGraw-Hill, 1980

Robinault IP. Sex, Society and the Disabled. New York, Harper & Row, 1978

Wolman BB. Handbook of Human Sexuality. Englewood Cliffs, Prentice-Hall, 1980

Woods NW. Human Sexuality in Health and Illness. St. Louis, C.V. Mosby, 1979

Sex and the handicapped. In Kolodny RC et al (eds). Textbook of Human Sexuality for Nurses, pp 247–277. Boston, Little, Brown & Co, 1979

Articles

Sexuality and the Disabled

Cole TM and Glass DD. Sexuality and physical disabilities. Arch Phys Med Rehabil 1977 Dec; 58(12):585–586

Hoch Z. Sex therapy and marital counseling for the disabled. Arch Phys Med Rehabil 1977 Sept; 58(9):413–415

McNab WL. The sexual needs of the handicapped. J Sch Health 1978 May; 48(5):301–306

Reinstein L, Ashley J and Miller KH. Sexual adjustment after lower extremity amputation. Arch Phys Med Rehabil 1978 Nov; 59(11):501–504

Rosenbaum R. Sexuality and the physically disabled: The role of the professional. Bull NY Acad Med 1978 May; 54(5):501–509

Sexuality and Disability. A journal devoted to the study of sex in physical and mental illness. New York, Human Sciences Press,

Thornton CE. A nurse-educator in sex and disability. Sexuality and Disability 1979 Spring; 2(1):28–32

Pressure Sores

Ameis A et al. Management of pressure sores: Comparative study in medical and surgical patients. Postgrad Med 1980 Feb; 67(2):177–184

Blicharz M. Interventions that promote decubiti healing. Current Practices in Nursing Care of the Adult 1979; 1:115–152

Coker KE. The intermittent air-fluidized bed and the neurologically impaired patient. J Neurosurg Nurs 1979 March; 11(1):31–33

Denne WA. The objective assessment of the sheepskins used for decubitus prophylaxis. Rheumatol Rehabil 1979 Feb; 18(1):23–29

DiMascio S. Debrisan for decubitus ulcers. Am J Nurs 1979 April; 79(4):684–685

Drimmer MA and Goldflies M. Treating decubiti and non-healing wounds of the lower extremities. Am Fam Physician 1980 March; 21(3):148–151

El-Toraei I and Chung B. The management of pressure sores. J Dermatol Surg Oncol 1977 Sept–Oct; 3(5):507–511

McClemont EJW, Shand IG and Ramsay B. Pressure sores: A new method of treatment. Br J Clin Pract 1979 Jan; 33(1):21–25

Meissner JE. Which patient on your unit might get a pressure sore? Nursing '80 1980 June; 10(6):64–65

Mikulic MA. Treatment of pressure ulcers. Am J Nurs 1980 June; 80(6):1125–1128

Nierman MM. Treatment of dermal and decubitus ulcers. Drugs 1978 March; 15(3):226–230

Parish LC and Collins E. Decubitus ulcers: A comparative study. Cutis 1979 Jan; 23(1):106–110

Parish LC and Witowski JA. The decubitus ulcer. Int J Dermatol 1979 April; 18(3):211–212

Principles and Practice of Rehabilitation Nursing

Beber CR. Freedom for the incontinent. Am J Nurs 1980 March; 80(3):482–484

Ciuca R, Bradish J and Trombly S. Passive range-of-motion exercises. A handbook. Nursing 78 1978 July; 8(7):59–65

Fenwick AN. An interdisciplinary tool for assessing patient's readiness for discharge in the rehabilitation setting. J Adv Nurs 1979 Jan; 4(1):9–21

Gonnella JS and Herman MW. Continuity of care. JAMA 1980 Jan; 243(4):352–354

Johnson JE (ed). Rehabilitation nursing. Nurs Clin North Am 1980 June; 15(2):221–320

Newman CE. Rehabilitation can be a cost containment device. Hospitals 1979 March; 53(5):45–46

O'Connell KM. Promoting normal bowel function in the patient on bed rest. Current Practice in Nursing Care of the Adult 1979; 1:77–85

Stonnington HH. Physical medicine and rehabilitation. JAMA 1979 March; 231(13):1380–1381

Ziegler JC. Physical reconditioning—for the convalescent patient. Nursing '80 1980 Aug; 10(8):67–69

CARE OF THE SURGICAL PATIENT

6

TYPES OF SURGERY

1. *Optional*
   Surgery is scheduled completely at the preference of the patient, e.g., cosmetic surgery.
2. *Elective*
   The approximate time for surgery is at the convenience of the patient; failure to have surgery is not catastrophic, e.g., superficial cyst.
3. *Required*
   The condition requires surgery within a few weeks, e.g., eye cataract.

4. *Urgent*
   Surgical problem requires attention within 24 to 48 hours, e.g., cancer.
5. *Emergency*
   Requires immediate surgical attention without delay, e.g., intestinal obstruction.

REGIONS AND INCISIONS OF THE ABDOMEN

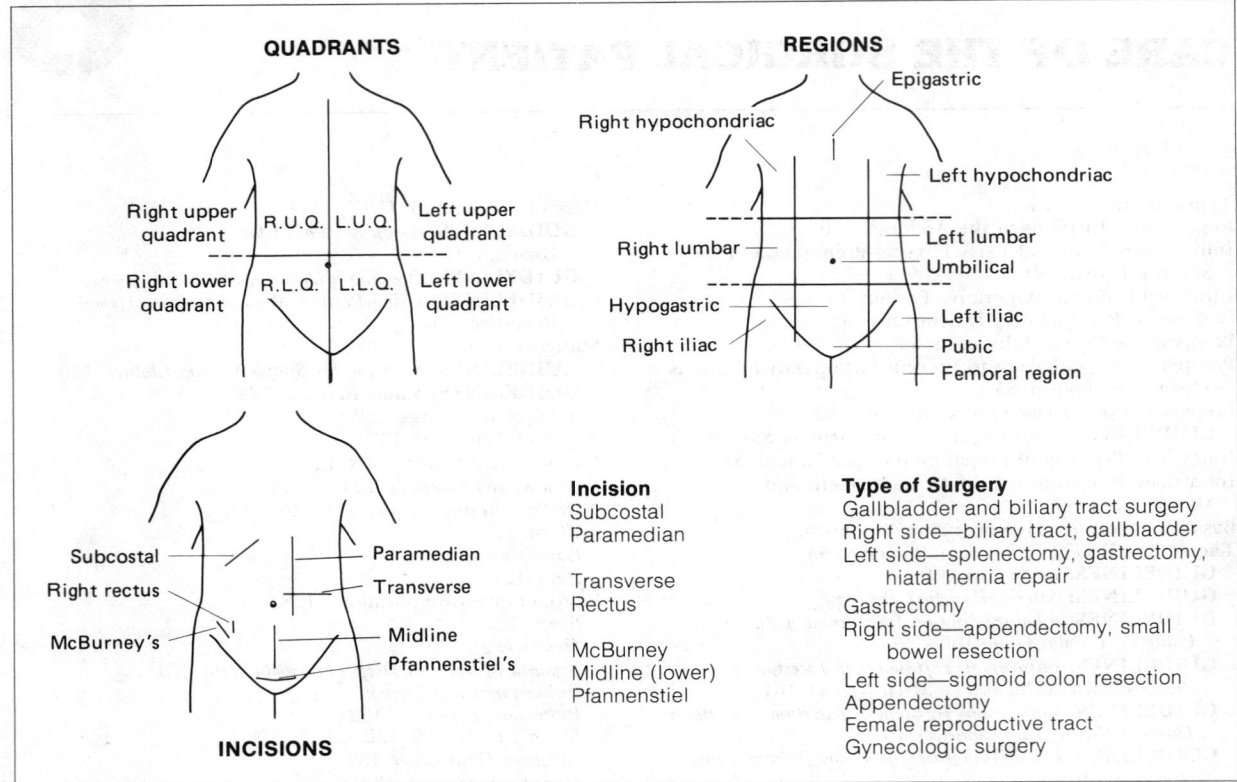

FIGURE 6-1. *Regions and incisions of the abdomen.*

INITIAL ASSESSMENT AND EARLY PHYSICAL PREPARATION OF THE SURGICAL PATIENT

General Physical Examination and Diagnostic Determinations

1. Observe the patient for skin lesions, rashes, pressure sores, and other abnormalities.
2. Engage the patient in conversation to determine his reaction to and concerns about hospitalization and the forthcoming operation.
3. Prepare him for various diagnostic tests by telling him why and how they are done and how he may contribute to the success of the test.
4. Record his reactions to tests as well as the outcome of such tests.
5. Assess his nutritional status (such as weight-loss history, albumin and transferrin levels, total protein, midarm muscle circumference, triceps skin fold). (See p. 48.)

Risk Factors and Preventive Strategies

A. *Obesity*
1. Danger
   a. Increases difficulty involved in technical aspects of performing surgery (e.g., sutures are difficult to tie because of fatty secretions); wound dehiscence is greater.
   b. Increases likelihood of infection because of lessened resistance.
   c. Postoperatively, more difficult to turn and ventilate the patient when he is lying on his side. This leads to hypoventilation, pneumonia, and other pulmonary problems.
   d. Increases demands on the heart, leading to cardiovascular embarrassment.
   e. Increases possibility of renal, biliary, hepatic, and endocrine disorders
2. Therapeutic Approach
   Encourage weight reduction if time permits.

B. *Fluid, Electrolyte, and Nutritional Status*
1. Danger
   Dehydration and malnutrition have adverse effects in terms of a general anesthetic, the shock of surgery, and postoperative recovery—can disturb fluid and electrolyte balance and lead to shock.

2. Therapeutic Approach
   a. Administer fluids (parenteral) as prescribed.
   b. Keep a detailed input and output record.
   c. Provide high calorie diet to alleviate malnutrition; supplement with protein and vitamin C—helps repair tissue and serves as a deterrent to infection.
   d. Recommend repair of dental caries and proper mouth hygiene to prevent respiratory tract infection.
   e. Assist with administration (and surveillance) of blood transfusion, protein hydrolysates, or blood plasma if there is a protein deficiency.
   f. Assist with hyperalimentation.
   g. Monitor for evidence of electrolyte imbalance (Na^+, K^+, Ca^{++}, etc.)

C. Aging

1. Danger
   a. Recognize that reactions to injury are not as obvious and are slower in appearing.
   b. Be aware that the cumulative effect of medications is greater in the older person than it is in younger people.
   c. Note that such medications as morphine and barbiturates in the usual dosages may cause confusion and disorientation; morphine may cause respiratory depression.
2. Therapeutic Approach
   a. Consider using lesser doses for desired effect.
   b. Anticipate problems from long-standing chronic disorders such as anemia, obesity, diabetes, hypoproteinemia.
   c. Adjust nutritional intake to conform to higher protein and vitamin needs.
   d. When possible cater to set patterns in older patients (sleeping and eating patterns, use of alcohol and laxatives).

D. Presence of Disease

1. Cardiovascular
   a. Increased diligence is required when surgical problem is complicated by a cardiovascular problem.
   b. Avoid overloading the body with fluids (oral, parenteral, blood) because of possible congestive failure and pulmonary edema.
   c. Prevent prolonged immobilization, which results in stasis of circulating fluids.
   d. Encourage change of position but avoid sudden exertion.
   e. Note evidence of hypoxia and initiate therapy.
2. Diabetes
   a. Be aware that hypoglycemia due to inadequate carbohydrate intake or insulin overdosage is life-threatening in uncontrolled diabetes.
   b. Recognize the signs and symptoms of ketoacidosis

and glucosuria (p. 643) which can threaten an otherwise smooth surgical experience.
   c. Reassure the diabetic patient that when his disease is controlled, the surgical risk may be no greater than it is for the nondiabetic person.
3. Alcoholism
   a. Anticipate the additional problem of malnutrition in the presurgical alcoholic patient.
   b. Recognize that the acutely intoxicated person is susceptible to injury and may receive serious injuries without being aware of them.
   c. Be prepared to perform gastric lavage on the intoxicated patient if surgery cannot be postponed; this may lessen the chance of vomiting and aspiration during anesthesia induction.
   d. Note that risk due to surgery is greater for the individual who is a chronic alcoholic.
   e. Anticipate the acute withdrawal syndrome (delirium tremens).
4. Pulmonary and Upper Respiratory Disease
   a. Surgery may be contraindicated in the patient who has an upper respiratory infection because an acute upper respiratory infection may be the forerunner of more serious illness, such as pneumonia.
   b. Patients with chronic pulmonary problems such as emphysema, bronchiectasis, etc. should be treated for several days preoperatively with bronchodilators, aerosol medications, and conscientious mouth care, along with a reduction in weight and smoking, and methods to control secretions.
5. Concurrent or Prior Pharmacotherapy
   a. Hazards exist when certain medications are given concomitantly with others; therefore, an awareness of prior drug therapy is essential. (Example: interaction of some drugs with anesthetics can lead to arterial hypotension and circulatory collapse.)
   b. Notify anesthesiologist if the patient is taking any of the following drugs:
      (1) Certain antibiotics*—may, when combined with a curariform muscle relaxant, interrupt nerve transmission, causing respiratory paralysis and apnea.
      (2) Antidepressants, particularly monoamine oxidase inhibitors (MAO), increase hypotensive effects of anesthesia.
      (3) Phenothiazines increase hypotensive action of anesthetics.
      (4) Diuretics, particularly thiazides, cause electrolyte imbalance and respiratory depression during anesthesia.

   * Neomycin, streptomycin, dihydrostreptomycin, polymyxin A and B, colistin, viomycin, paromomycin, and kanamycin.

INFORMED CONSENT (Operative Permit)

An *informed consent* (operative permit) is a form signed by the patient (and witnessed), granting permission to have the operation performed as described by the patient's physician; this is a medicolegal requirement.

The consent form should be written using short words and brief, simple sentences. Such forms should be reviewed by patients and hospital attorney prior to being adopted as a standard form.

Purposes

1. To ensure that the patient understands the nature of the treatment, including potential complications.
2. To indicate that the patient's decision was made without pressure.
3. To protect the patient against unauthorized procedures.
4. To protect the surgeon and hospital against legal action by a patient who claims that an unauthorized procedure was performed.

Prior to signing an informed consent, the patient should:
1. Be told in clear and simple terms by the surgeon what is to be done (drawings or audiovisual aids may help).
2. Be aware of the risks, possible complications, disfigurement, and removal of parts.
3. Have a general idea of what to expect in the early and late postoperative periods.
4. Have a general idea of the time frame involved from surgery to recovery.
5. Have an opportunity to ask any questions.
6. Sign a separate form for each operation.

Informed Consent and the Adolescent Patient

1. An *emancipated minor* is usually recognized as one who is not subject to parental control or regulation.
   a. Married minor
   b. Those in military service
   c. College student who is under age 18 but living away from home
2. Most states have enacted *minor-treatment statutes*.
   a. This applies to persons 14 to 18 years of age (statutes vary widely)

3. Standards of informed consent are the same for adolescents and adults.
   a. If patient of any age does not understand all material facts, the consent given will be held legally insufficient; no treatment should be given without parental consent except in an acute emergency.

Circumstances Requiring a Permit

1. Any surgical procedure where scalpel, scissors, suture, hemostats, or electrocoagulation may be used.
2. Entrance into a body cavity—paracentesis, bronchoscopy, cystoscopy.
3. General anesthesia, local infiltration, and regional block—e.g., for reduction of a fracture.

Obtaining Informed Consent

1. *Written* permission is best and is legally acceptable.
2. Signature is obtained with the patient's complete understanding of what is to occur; it is obtained before he receives sedation and is secured without pressure or duress.
3. A witness is desirable—nurse, physician, or other authorized person.
4. In emergency, permission via telephone or telegram is acceptable.
5. For a minor (or one who is unconscious or irresponsible), permission is required from a responsible member of the family—parent or legal guardian.
6. For a married minor, permission from the husband or wife is acceptable.
7. If the patient is unable to write, an "X" to indicate his sign is acceptable if there are 2 signed witnesses to his mark.

CONCEPT OF PERIOPERATIVE PATIENT CARE

Perioperative role in operating room nursing is a term used to describe the nursing functions in the total surgical experience of the patient: preoperative, intraoperative, and postoperative.

Preoperative phase—from the time the decision is made for surgical intervention to the transference of the patient to the operating room.

Intraoperative phase—from the time the patient is received in the operating room until he is admitted to the recovery room.

Postoperative phase—from the time of admission to the recovery room to the follow-up home/clinic evaluation.

Examples of nursing activities in the perioperative role are presented in the chart on page 83.

PREOPERATIVE PATIENT EDUCATION

Preoperative patient education is the giving of information to the patient who is scheduled to have an operation; such instruction may be offered through conversation, discussion, the use of audiovisual aids, demonstrations, and return demonstrations. It is designed to help the patient understand what he is about to experience so that he can participate intelligently and recover more effectively from surgery and anesthesia.

NOTE: Parts of this program may be initiated before hospitalization.

Examples of Nursing Activities in the Perioperative Role

Preoperative phase	Intraoperative phase	Postoperative phase

Preoperative assessment
Home/clinic
1. initiates initial preoperative assessment
2. plans teaching methods appropriate to patient's needs
3. involves family in interview
Surgical unit
1. completes preoperative assessment
2. coordinates patient teaching with other nursing staff
3. explains phases in perioperative period and expectations
4. develops a plan of care
Surgical suite
1. assesses patient's level of consciousness
2. reviews chart
3. identifies patient
4. verifies surgical site
 	
Planning
1. determines a plan of care
 	
Psychological support
1. tells patient what is happening
2. determines psychological status
3. gives prior warning of noxious stimuli
4. stands near/touches patient during procedures/induction
5. communicates patient's emotional status to other appropriate members of the health care team
	Maintenance of safety
	1. assures that the sponge, needle, and instrument counts are correct
	2. positions the patient
	  a. functional alignment
	  b. exposure of surgical site
	  c. maintenance of position throughout procedure
	3. applies grounding device to patient
	4. provides physical support
	Physiological monitoring
	1. calculates effects on patient of excessive fluid loss
	2. distinguishes normal from abnormal cardiopulmonary data
	3. reports changes in patient's pulse, respirations, temperature, and blood pressure
	Psychological monitoring (prior to induction and if patient conscious)
	1. provides emotional support to patient
	2. continues to assess patient's emotional status
	3. communicates patient's emotional status to other appropriate members of the health care team
	Nursing management
	1. provides physical safety for the patient
	2. maintains aseptic, controlled environment
	3. effectively manages human resources
		Communication of intraoperative information
		1. gives patient's name
		2. states type of surgery performed
		3. provides contributing intraoperative factors, ie, drain, catheters
		4. states physical limitations
		5. states impairments resulting from surgery
		6. reports patient's preoperative level of consciousness
		7. communicates necessary equipment needs
		
		Postoperative evaluation
		Recovery area
		1. determines patient's immediate response to surgical intervention
		Surgical unit
		1. evaluates effectiveness of nursing care in the OR
		2. determines patient's level of satisfaction with care given during perioperative period
		3. evaluates products used on patient in the OR
		4. determines patient's psychological status
		5. assists with discharge planning
		Home clinic
		1. seeks patient's perception of surgery in terms of the effects of anesthetic agents. Impact on body image, distortion, immobilization
		2. determines family's perceptions of surgery

(Source: Operating room nursing: Perioperative role, AORN 1978 May; vol. 27) (Reprinted with permission)

Value to Patient

1. Approach to surgery is more positive.
2. Recuperation is more rapid.
3. There is less need for medications for pain and discomfort.
4. Complications are lessened.
5. Participation in self-care is enhanced.
6. Ability to communicate with health professionals is facilitated.
7. Hospitalization is shortened—thus, the program is cost-effective.

Approach to Patient Education (May include family or significant others)

A. *Obtain data base and plan modus operandi.*

1. Determine what patient already knows and what he wishes to know. This can be accomplished by reading the patient's chart, by interviewing the patient, and by communicating with his physician, family, and other members of the health team.

2. Plan this presentation or series of presentations for this individual patient or a group of patients.
3. Encourage active participation of patients in their care and recovery.
4. Not only should essential techniques be demonstrated, but opportunity should be provided for return demonstration by the patient.
5. Provision should be made for the patient to ask questions and express his concerns; every effort is made to answer all questions truthfully and in basic agreement with the medical plan of therapy.

B. *Constantly assess needs of patient as teaching progresses.*

1. Begin at his level of understanding and proceed from there.
2. Correct misinformation—provide opportunity for him to express himself.
3. Provide general information and be alert for patient needs as intercommunication takes place. Assess his ability to absorb, his curiosity or lack of it.
  a. Explain details of preoperative preparation.

b. Offer general information on his specific surgery. (Physician is the resource person.)
c. Tell when surgery is scheduled (if known) and how long it will take; explain that afterwards he will go to the Recovery Room.
d. Let him know that his family will be kept informed and that they will be told where to wait and when they can see him; note visiting hours.
e. Explain to him how a procedure or test may *feel* during or after.
f. Describe the Recovery Room; anticipated equipment to expect: drains, tubes, monitors.
g. Explain the importance of his participation in his postoperative recovery. Tell him you will demonstrate to him some of the activities he will be doing postoperatively.
h. Utilize other resource persons; physicians, therapists, chaplain, interpreters, and so forth.
i. Document in outline form what has been taught and patient's reaction.

NURSING ALERT: Touch is a useful modality in preoperative teaching of patients that appears to reduce anxiety significantly.

C. *Utilize audiovisual aids if available.*

1. Videotapes with sound or film strips with narration are effective in giving basic information to a single patient or group of patients.
2. Booklets and brochures, if available, are helpful.
3. Demonstrate any equipment which will be specific for the particular patient. Examples:
   Drainage equipment   Monitoring equipment
   Side rails   Incentive spirometer
   Ostomy bag

NURSING ALERT: The extent of preoperative patient teaching is determined on an individual basis; determinants are the patient's previous knowledge, his desire to learn and willingness to use this new knowledge, his psychoemotional and physical condition, the amount of time available, and the quality of teaching. Effectiveness is greater when time is provided for patient discussion.

Preoperative Practice of Postoperative Activities

Activities which the patient will practice and do postoperative include the following:

A. *Diaphragmatic Breathing.*

This is a mode of breathing in which the dome of the diaphragm is flattened during inspiration resulting in enlargement of the upper abdomen as air rushes into the chest. During expiration, abdominal muscles and the diaphragm relax. (See p. 166.)
For the patient:
1. Assume bed position similar to that most likely to be used postoperatively; (semi-Fowler's).
2. Place both hands over lower rib cage; make a loose fist and rest the flat surface of the fingernails against the chest (to feel chest movement).
3. Exhale gently and fully; ribs will sink downward and inward toward midline.
4. Inhale deeply through mouth and nose; permit abdomen to rise as lungs fill with air.
5. Hold this breath through a count of 5.
6. Exhale and let *all* air out through mouth and nose.
7. Repeat 15 times with a brief rest following each group of five.
8. Practice this twice each day preoperatively.

B. *Incentive Spirometry.*

This is a method by which a patient preoperatively uses a spirometer to measure his deep breaths (inspired air) while exerting his maximum effort. (See pp. 183–184.)
This amount becomes the objective to be achieved as soon as possible postoperatively.
1. Postoperatively, the patient is encouraged to use the incentive spirometer about 10–12 times an hour. (He does this on his own.)
2. Atelectasis and other pulmonary complications can be prevented when alveoli are patent.
3. Commercial incentive spirometers are available.
4. There is less pain with inspiratory concentration than with expiratory concentration, such as with coughing and using blow bottles.

C. *Coughing*—to promote the removal of chest secretions.
1. Interlace the fingers and place the hands over the proposed incision site; this will act as a splint during coughing.
2. Lean forward slightly while sitting in bed.
3. Breathe, using the diaphragm as described under diaphragmatic breathing.
4. Inhale fully with the mouth slightly open.
5. Let out 3 or 4 sharp "hacks."
6. Then, with mouth open, take in a deep breath and quickly give 1 or 2 strong coughs.
7. Secretions should be readily cleared from the chest; splinting the incision will reduce pain and will not harm the incision.

D. *Turning*—circulation is stimulated, deeper breathing encouraged, and pressure areas are relieved when the patient is encouraged to move from his back to the side-lying position.
1. The patient may require assistance to move onto his side; pillows have to be readjusted.
2. Place the uppermost leg in a more flexed position than that of the lower leg and place a pillow comfortably between the legs.
3. Patient is turned from one side to his back and onto other side every 2 hours.

E. *Leg Exercises*—to improve circulation.
1. While lying on the back, bend the knee and raise the foot—hold it a few seconds, extend the leg and lower it to the bed.
2. Repeat above for about 5 times with 1 leg and then do it with the other. Repeat the set 5 times every 3–5 hours.
3. While lying on the side, exercise the legs by pretending to pedal a bicycle.
4. As a foot exercise, trace a complete circle with the great toe.

PREOPERATIVE PROPHYLAXIS TO PREVENT POSTOPERATIVE VENOUS THROMBOEMBOLISM*

Low-dose heparin administered to all *hemostatically competent* patients over the age of 40 who are to undergo major elective abdominal or thoracic surgical procedures will effect an 80% reduction in postoperative pulmonary emboli.

Significance

This could prevent 4,000–8,000 postoperative deaths annually.

Preoperative Screening

1. Administer no aspirin or other platelet antiaggregating drugs for 5 days prior to an operation.
2. Administer no coumarin therapy at time of operation.
3. Hematocrit, prothrombin time, partial thromboplastin time, and platelet count should be within normal range prior to operation.

Dose and Duration of Prophylaxis

1. Administer 5,000 USP units of heparin (s.c.) 2 hours before operation.

> * Council on Thrombosis of The American Heart Association. Special Report—Prevention of Venous Thromboembolism in Surgical Patients by Low-dose Heparin. Circulation 1977 Feb.; Vol. 55, No. 2.

2. Repeat above dosage every 12 hours until discharge from hospital.

Limitations and Contraindications

1. Of limited value in:
   a. Repair of femoral fracture
   b. Hip and knee joint reconstruction
   c. Open prostatectomy
2. Not recommended for operations:
   a. On the eye
   b. On the brain
   c. With spinal anesthesia
3. *The regimen is ineffective in patients with an active thrombotic process.*

Monitoring of Heparin Therapy

1. No laboratory test (whole blood clotting time, partial thromboplastin time, thrombin time, antithrombin III assay) is necessary during therapy to determine drug dosage or to prevent hemorrhage.
2. With this regimen, there may be a *slight increase in minor wound hematoma.* Report this immediately.
3. Employ adjunctive measures—early ambulation, leg exercises, and elastic stockings.
4. Avoid positioning of legs that could compromise venous return.
5. This regimen is followed at the discretion of the physician.

PREPARATION OF SPECIFIC OPERATIVE AREAS

Head surgery: Obtain specific instructions from surgeon concerning the extent of shaving.
Other surgery: See Figure 6-2 (pages 86–87).

GUIDELINES: Preparing the Patient's Skin for Surgery

Purpose To cleanse the skin and reduce the number of organisms on the skin so as to eliminate as far as possible the transference of such organisms into the incision site.

> **NURSING ALERT:** Unless contraindicated, it may be desirable for the nonemergency patient to bathe with a bacteriostatic soap for several days prior to surgery.

Pharmacophysiologic Emphasis

1. Human skin normally harbors transient and resident bacterial flora, some of which are pathogenic.
2. Skin cannot be sterilized without destroying skin cells.
3. Friction enhances the action of detergent antiseptics.
4. No existing antiseptic produces instant skin disinfection.

Equipment Disposable tray with essentials, or a tray containing
  2 bowls for detergent-germicide
  1 emesis basin
  2 applicator sticks
  6 or 8 (4 × 4-inch) gauze squares
  Razor and blades
  Scissors for cutting long hair, if required

GUIDELINES: Preparing the Patient's Skin for Surgery (cont.)

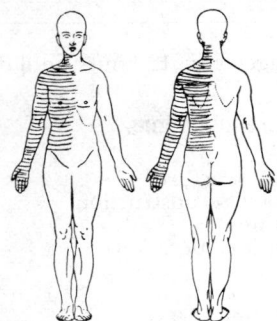 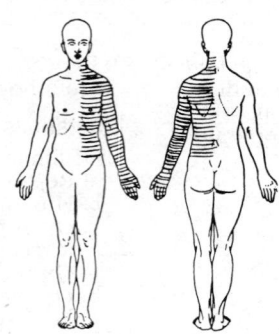 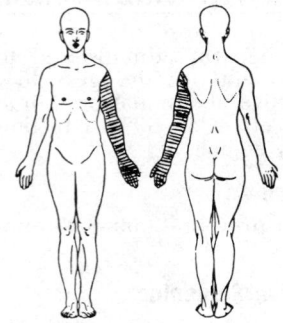

Shoulder prep. Shave fingertips to hairline, midline chest to midline spine on operative side and to iliac crest, including axillae.

Upper arm prep. Shave fingertips to neckline (hairline), on operative side from midline chest to midline spine on operative side from axilla to iliac crest. Trim and clean fingernails. Use brush on hand and nails.

Hand prep. Shave fingertips to shoulder. Trim and clean fingernails. Use brush on hand and nails.

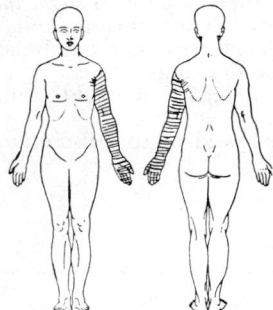 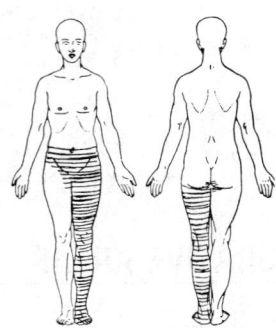 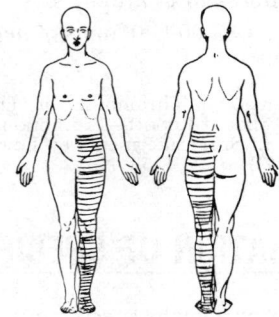

Forearm and elbow prep. Shave from fingernails to shoulder including axilla. Trim and clean fingernails. Use brush on hand and nails.

Saphenous vein ligation prep. Shave from umbilicus to toes of affected leg, or both legs. Include pubis and perineal area. Prep entire leg posteriorly.

Thigh prep. Shave from toes to 3 inches above the umbilicus, midline front and back. Complete pubic shave. Clean and trim toenails. Use brush on foot and nails.

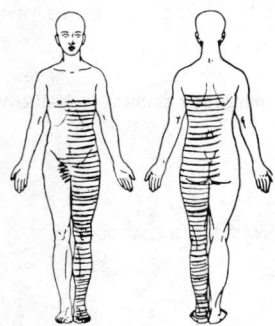 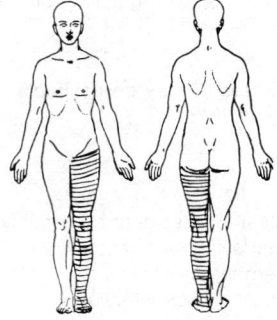 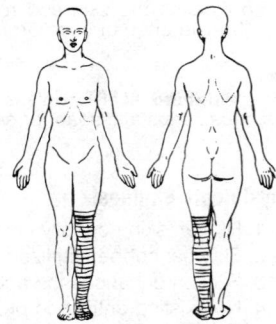

Hip prep. Shave toes to nipple line to at least 3 inches beyond midline back and front. Complete pubic shave. Clean and trim toenails. Use brush on foot and nails. Hip fractures—all preps done in the operating room.

Knee and lower leg prep. Shave entire leg, toes to groin. Clean and trim toenails. Use brush on foot and nails.

Ankle and foot prep. Shave entire leg, toes to 3 inches above the knee. Clean and trim toenails. Use brush on foot and nails.

FIGURE 6-2. *Preoperative preparation of the patient. (From Manual on Control of Infection in Surgical Patients, Philadelphia, JB Lippincott Co., 1977).*

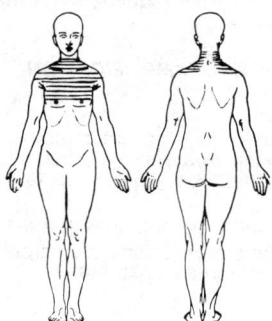

Thyroid prep. Shave from chin line to nipples, including axillary region. Extend to back of neck and upper shoulder as sketched.

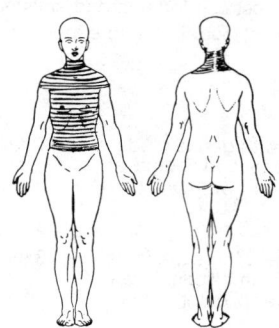

Parathyroid prep (as for sternal splitting). Shave from chin line to umbilicus, shoulder to shoulder in the front. Extend to back of neck and upper shoulder in back as shown. Prep laterally for chest tubes if so ordered.

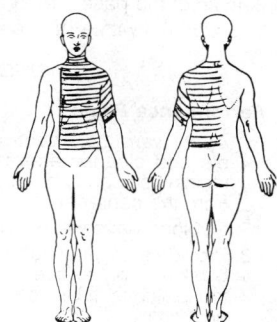

Thoracotomy prep. Shave from chin line to iliac crest, from nipple on unaffected side to at least 2 inches beyond the midline in back. Include axilla and entire arm to elbow.

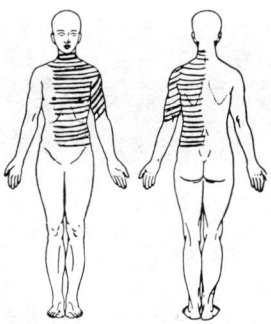

Mastectomy prep. Shave from upper neck to iliac crest, from nipple line on unaffected side to midline of back (affected side). Prep axilla and entire arm to elbow on affected side.

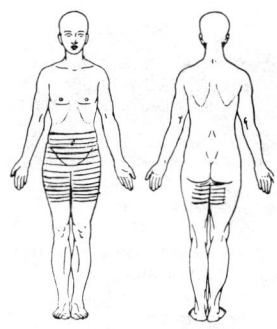

Lower abdominal prep (as for hernia, femoral vein ligation, femoral embolectomy). Shave from 2 inches above the umbilicus to mid-thigh, including the pubic area. Femoral ligation—shave to midline of thigh posteriorly. Hernia and embolectomy—shave to costal margin and down to knee as ordered.

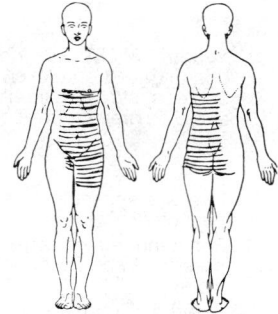

Flank prep (as for renal procedures, adrenalectomy, sympathectomy). Shave from nipple line to pubis and 3 inches beyond the midline in back. Shave pubic area. Shave upper thigh on the affected side.

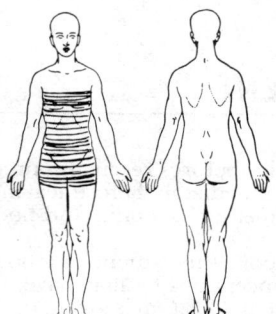

Abdominal prep. Shave from 3 inches above the nipple line to upper thighs, including pubis.

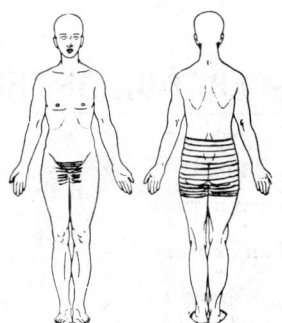

Perineal prep (as for hemorrhoidectomy, fistula-in-ano). Shave pubis, perineum, and perianal area. Shave from the waist in back to at least 3 inches below the groin.

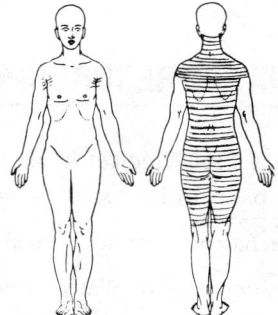

Spine prep. Shave entire back including shoulders and neck to hairline and down to knees and to both sides, including axillae.

FIGURE 6-2. *(continued)*

(Guideline continues on p. 88)

Procedure **Preparatory Phase**
1. Explain to the patient the purpose of the activity.
2. Instruct the patient to assume the most comfortable and satisfactory position for the required skin preparation.
3. Cover him with a bath blanket, protect bedding, and expose the area to be shaved.

NURSING ACTION	RATIONALE/AMPLIFICATION
Performance Phase	
1. Apply warm detergent-germicide with gauze pledgets and cleanse area using light friction; begin at incision site and, in a circular pattern, work outward from the center.	1. Oils, soil, and organisms are removed from skin surface. Working away from incision site prevents the clean area from becoming recontaminated.
2. Cut long hairs with scissors.	2. Much easier and quicker than with a razor.
3. Provide extra attention to areas where there are folds of skin, e.g., axillae, pubic area, umbilicus. Draw loose skin taut. Use cotton-tipped applicators where necessary.	3. Greater numbers of organisms are harbored in folds of skin; removal requires extra effort.
4. If the operative area includes calloused areas or the nails, use a brush.	4. Facilitates cleansing in out-of-the-way areas.
5. Soak hairy areas about 4 minutes before shaving.	5. Provides time allowing the keratin of the hair to absorb fluid, which makes the hair softer.
6. Shave with the direction of hair growth—not the opposite direction of hair growth.	6. This leaves a blunt rather than a sharp end that could penetrate the wall of the hair follicle and inject itself into the skin (risking postoperative pseudofolliculitis).

NURSING ALERT: *Pseudofolliculitis barbae* is a papulopustular inflammation of hair follicles in areas that have been shaved so closely that the sharp-pointed tip may inject itself into the side of the hair follicle, carrying bacteria into the skin. It simulates folliculitis barbae, which develops in bearded areas. Note above items 5 and 6 to prevent this condition.

7. Use a disposable or sterilized razor and a sharp new blade.	7 Avoids risk of infectious hepatitis from contaminated razor.
8. For denuded or sensitive areas, soak gently with detergent and flush thoroughly with saline or sterile water.	8. Prevents additional trauma.
9. Avoid nicking the skin; report any skin abrasions.	9. An opening in the skin increases the hazard of infection.
10. Scrub the skin area after the shaving is completed; rinse carefully and blot dry.	10. Prevents irritation and chapping.

Follow-up Phase
1. Remove all equipment and dispose of expendable materials according to local policy.
2. Remind the patient of the necessity for keeping the prepared area clean for surgery; provide for his comfort.

IMMEDIATE PRESURGICAL PREPARATION OF THE PATIENT

Physical and Psychological Attention to the Patient

1. Provide patient with a short gown to be worn to the operating room.
2. Remove hairpins; braid women's long hair; cover hair with a cap.
3. Remove dentures or plates (unless anesthesiologist requests that they be left in to reduce respiratory tract obstruction); inspect mouth for foreign material such as chewing gum.
4. Remove jewelry, identify properly, and place in the hospital safe; if wedding ring cannot be removed, tie with gauze bandage fastened around wrist.
5. Remove contact lenses; have patient place them in properly marked receptacle (left and right), identify properly, and deposit in the hospital safe.
6. Have patient void before receiving preoperative medication and immediately before leaving for the operating room; measure amount and note time of voiding; record.
7. Continue to support the patient emotionally and correct any misconceptions he may have.
8. After preoperative medication is given, raise the side rails. Instruct patient to call for assistance if necessary.

Preanesthetic Medication

(prescribed to meet individual needs)

Purposes
1. To facilitate the administration of any anesthetic and to relax the patient.

2. To minimize respiratory tract secretions and changes in heart rate and to reduce anxiety.

NURSING ALERT: Administer preanesthetic medication precisely at the time it is prescribed. If given too early, the maximum potency will have passed before it is needed; if given too late, the action will not have begun before anesthesia is started.

"On Call" Medications
1. Have medication ready and administer as soon as call is received.
2. Proceed with remaining preparation activities.
3. Indicate on the chart or preoperative check list the time when medication was administered.

Transporting Patient to the Operating Room

1. Adhere to the principle of maintaining the comfort and safety of the patient.
2. Accompany operating room attendants to patient's bedside for introduction and proper identification.
3. Assist in transferring patient from bed to stretcher (unless bed goes to O.R. floor).
4. Complete chart and preoperative check list; include laboratory reports and x-rays as required in the operating room.
5. Recognize importance of coordinating team effort to ensure arrival of the patient in the operating room at the proper time.

The Patient's Family

1. Direct patient's family to the proper waiting room where magazines, television, and coffee may be available.
2. Inform them that the surgeon will probably come to this room immediately after surgery to inform them of the operation.
3. Acquaint the family with the fact that a long interval of waiting does not mean the patient is in the operating room all the while; anesthesia preparation and induction take time, and after surgery the patient is taken to the Recovery Room.
4. Tell the family what to expect postoperatively when they see the patient—tubes, monitoring equipment, and blood transfusion, suctioning, and oxygen equipment.

IMMEDIATE POSTSURGICAL NURSING ASSESSMENT AND MANAGEMENT

Objective

To assist the patient in recovering from the operation and from the effects of the anesthetic agent as quickly, safely, and comfortably as possible (See Postanesthesia Recovery Room Scoring Guide, p. 90.)

NURSING ALERT: This phase of nursing care is geared to *recognizing* the significance of signs and *anticipating* and *preventing* postoperative difficulties.

Carefully monitor the patient coming out of general anesthesia until
1. Vital signs are stable for at least 30 minutes and are within *his* normal range.
2. He is breathing easily.
3. Reflexes have returned to normal.
4. He is out of anesthesia, responsive, and oriented to time and place.

For the patient who had regional anesthesia, observe carefully until
1. Sensation has been recovered.
2. Reflexes have returned.
3. Vital signs have stabilized for at least 30 minutes.

Immediate Nursing Assessment

Upon receiving a patient in the Recovery Room from the anesthesiologist and circulating nurse, the following determinations are made:
1. Appraise the air-exchange status of the patient and note his skin color.
2. Verify the patient's identity, the operative procedure, and the surgeon who performed the procedure.
3. Request a briefing on problems encountered in the operating room and those that may arise in the recovery period.
4. Determine vital signs and establish with the anesthesiologist an agreement as to their meaning.
5. Examine the operative site and check dressings for drainage.
6. Perform safety checks to verify that padded side rails are in place and restraints properly applied for infusions, transfusions, etc.

Nursing Management

A. *Ensure the Maintenance of a Patent Airway and Adequate Respiratory Function*

1. Place the patient in the lateral position with neck extended (if not contraindicated)—this permits the best possible expansion of the lungs.
2. Allow metal, rubber, or plastic airway to remain in place until the patient begins to waken and is trying to eject the airway.
   a. The airway keeps the passage open and prevents the tongue from falling backward and obstructing the air passages.
   b. Leaving the airway in after the pharyngeal reflex has returned may cause the patient to gag and vomit.

NOTE: Many seriously ill patients return from the operating room with a tracheal tube in place; this may be left in place for hours or days and requires special management.

3. When patient is partially awake and the airway is removed, he may show signs of gagging, nausea, or

Postanesthesia Recovery Room Scoring Guide*

Many hospitals use a scoring system to determine the patient's general condition and his readiness to be released from the Recovery Room. As the patient progresses through the recovery period, his physical signs are observed and evaluated by means of an objective scoring guide.

Objective:
To provide the Recovery Room staff with a guideline to the patient's condition following surgery and anesthesia. This evaluation system is a modification of the Apgar score.

Physical Signs and Criteria for Their Assessment
1. Activity
   Muscle activity is assessed by observing the ability of the patient to move his extremities spontaneously or on command.
   Score: 2—able to move all extremities
         1—able to move 2 extremities
         0—not able to control any extremity

2. Respiration
   Respiratory efficiency evaluated in a form that permits accurate and objective assessment without complicated physical tests.
   Score: 2—able to breathe deeply and cough
         1—limited respiratory effort (dyspnea or splinting)
         0—no spontaneous respiratory effort

3. Circulation
   Use changes in arterial blood pressure from preanesthetic level.
   Score: 2—systolic arterial pressure between plus or mi-
   nus 20% of preanesthetic level (Riva-Rocci method)
         1—systolic arterial pressure between plus or minus 20% to 50% of preanesthetic level
         0—systolic arterial pressure between plus or minus 50% or more of the preanesthetic level

4. Consciousness
   Determination of the patient's level of consciousness.
   Score: 2—full alertness seen in patient's ability to answer questions and acknowledge his/her location
         1—aroused when called by name
         0—failure to elicit a response upon auditory stimulation
   Physical stimulation should not be considered reliable since even a decerebrated patient might react to it.

5. Color
   This is an objective sign that is easy to recognize.
   Score: 2—normal skin color and appearance
         1—any alteration in skin color: pale, dusky, blotchy, jaundiced, etc.
         0—frank cyanosis

Implications of Score
1. The patient's score is taken at stated intervals such as every 15 or 30 minutes, and totaled on the official scorecard (Fig. 6-3).
2. Patients with a total score of less than 7 must remain in Recovery Room until improved or transferred to an intensive care area.
3. This guide permits a more objective evaluation of the patient's physical condition in the recovery area (Fig. 6-3).

* Margaret Furay Rozman. Introduction to Recovery Room Nursing. Denver, Association of Operating Room Nurses, 1977.

vomiting; place him in the lateral position with the upper arm supported on a pillow.
   a. This will promote chest expansion.
   b. Turn the patient every hour or two to facilitate breathing and ventilation.
4. Aspirate excessive secretions when they are heard in the nasopharynx and oropharynx.
   a. Using a Y-connecting tube with catheter, turn suction machine on, insert catheter into pharynx 15–20 cm. (6–8 inches), then close Y-tube outlet with finger to activate suction; withdraw slowly while rotating catheter.
   b. If secretions are lower in the tracheobronchial tree, intratracheal suctioning may be necessary. (See procedure for tracheal suctioning, p. 167.)
5. Encourage patient to take deep breaths to aerate lungs fully and prevent hypostatic pneumonia; use incentive spirometer to aid in this function (p. 183).
6. Administer humidified oxygen if required.
   a. Heat and moisture are normally lost during exhalation.
   b. Dehydrated patients may require oxygen and humidity because of higher incidence of irritated respiratory passages in these patients.
   c. Secretions can be kept soft to facilitate removal.
7. Employ mechanical ventilation to maintain adequate pulmonary ventilation if required (see p. 193).

B. *Assess Status of Circulatory System*
1. Take vital signs (blood pressure, pulse, and respiration) frequently, as clinical condition indicates, until patient is well stabilized. Then check every 4 hours thereafter.
   a. Know patient's preoperative blood pressure in order to make significant comparisons.
   b. Report immediately a falling systolic pressure.
   c. Variations in blood pressure and cardiac arrhythmias are reportable.
   d. Respirations over 30 should be reported.
   e. Evaluate pulse pressure to determine status of perfusion.
2. Recognize the variety of factors which may alter circulating blood volume.
   a. Reactions to anesthesia and medications
   b. Blood loss and organ manipulation during surgery
   c. Moving the patient from one position on the operating table to another on the stretcher
3. Monitor temperature hourly to be alert for malignant hyperthermia and to detect hypothermia. Over 37.7° C. (100° F.) or under 36.1° C. (97° F.) is reportable.
4. Be cognizant of early symptoms of shock or hemorrhage.
   a. Cool extremities, decreased urine output, and narrowing of pulse pressure may be indicative of decreased cardiac output.

Patient: Smith, Raymond
Room: B 1083
Date: 3/7/-

POST-ANESTHESIA RECOVERY ROOM
SCORING CARD

Final Score: 10
Physician: Dr. J. Evans
Nurse: Mrs. Peggy Fay, R.N.

Physical Signs → TIME ↓	ACTIVITY		RESPIRATION		CIRCULATION		CONSCIOUSNESS		COLOR		TOTAL SCORE
	Score	Comment	Score	Comment	Score	Comment	Score	Comment	Score	Comment	
Admission 11:15 A.M.	1	Spinal anesth.	1	chest & abdom. pain	1		1	Semi-conscious	1		5
½ Hour 11:45 A.M.	1		1		2		1		1	slight pallor	6
½ Hour A.M. P.M.											
Dismissal 12:15 P.M.	2		2		2		2	alert verbally responsive	2	color improved	10
FINAL SCORE A.M. P.M.	2		2		2		2		2		10

FIGURE 6-3. *Recovery room scoring card.*

b. Rapid, thready pulse and a falling blood pressure may indicate hemorrhage, leading to a decrease in blood volume.
c. Initiate oxygen therapy to increase oxygen availability from the circulating blood.
d. Place patient in shock position with feet elevated (uness contraindicated).
e. See page 128 for more detailed consideration of shock.

C. Promote Comfort and Maintain Safety

1. Provide a therapeutic environment with proper temperature and humidity; remove unnecessary blanket which might cause loss of body fluid through excessive perspiration; when cold, provide warm blankets.
2. Place side rails in protecting position until patient is fully awake.
3. Protect extremity into which intravenous fluids are running so that needle will not become accidentally dislodged.
4. Turn patient frequently and maintain good body alignment.
5. Avoid nerve damage and muscle strain by properly supporting and padding pressure areas.
6. Assess pain by observing behavioral and physiological manifestations.
7. Administer analgesics (low blood pressure may be result of pain.)

D. Continue Constant Surveillance of the Patient Until He Is Completely Out of Anesthesia

1. Be aware of the fact that the patient cannot complain of injury such as the pricking of an open safety pin, a clamp that is exerting pressure, a burn from a hot-water bottle.
2. Examine dressings for unexpected drainage or bleeding.
3. Check dressings for constriction.
4. Observe drainage tubes and catheters for proper connection and patency.

5. Note proper functioning of monitoring and suctioning devices, oxygen therapy equipment, etc.
6. Observe the patient for bladder distention (see Fig. 11-9, p. 490).
7. Inspect skin and tissue surrounding intravenous needles to detect early infiltration.
8. Evaluate periodically the patient's status of orientation—how he responds to being addressed by his name or performs simple movements upon receiving a command.

NOTE: Alterations in cerebral function may suggest impaired oxygen delivery to tissues.

9. Determine return of motor control following spinal anesthesia—indicated by how the patient responds to a pinprick or a request to move a part.

E. Recognize Stress Factors That May Affect the Patient in the Recovery Room and Attempt to Minimize These Factors.

1. Know that the ability to hear returns more quickly than other senses as the patient emerges from anesthesia.
2. Avoid saying anything in the patient's presence that may disturb him; he may appear to be sleeping but still consciously hears what is being said.
3. Explain procedures and activities at his level of understanding.
4. Minimize his exposure to emergency treatment of nearby patients by drawing curtains and lowering voice and noise levels.
5. Treat him as a person who needs as much attention as the equipment and monitoring devices.
6. Respect his feeling of sensory deprivation and simultaneous bombardment of sensory stimuli; make any necessary adjustments to minimize this problem.
7. Make every effort to demonstrate concern for and understanding of this patient—anticipate his needs and feelings.
8. Tell him repeatedly that the surgery is over and that he is in the recovery room.

BASIC POSTOPERATIVE HEMODYNAMIC MONITORING*

Critically ill patients or the postoperative trauma patient may require monitoring utilizing invasive techniques.

> **NURSING ALERT:** The most advanced electronic monitoring system cannot substitute for conscientious clinical surveillance.

Arterial Catheter (Cannula)

The radial artery is the usual site.

A. *Purpose*
1. Obtaining continuous blood pressure readings
2. Blood gas determination
3. Cardiac output measurement

B. *Complications*
1. Major
   a. Local obstruction with distal ischemia
   b. External hemorrhage
   c. False aneurysm
   d. Massive ecchymosis
   e. Dissection
2. Minor
   a. Pain
   b. Ecchymosis
   c. Temporary loss of pulse
   d. Infection

C. *Special Nursing Considerations*
1. *Allen Test*—this is done to assess ulnar palmar circulation. (Also see p. 350, Fig. 9-58.)
   Method:
   a. Compress radial artery at wrist.
   b. Simultaneously, have patient open and close hand a few times.
      Normal Reaction—slight transitory ischemia noted; this disappears rapidly when hand is kept still and compression maintained.
      Abnormal Reaction—ulnar artery does not adequately support palmar circulation, hence persistent signs of ischemia noted.
NOTE: During final part of test, fingers should not be hyperextended since this may result in a false-positive reaction.
2. Aseptic technique is mandatory.
3. Smaller catheter size relative to artery is probably associated with lower risk of thrombus formation.
4. Intermittent high volume irrigation of radial artery catheters may result in distal and even proximal embolization.
5. Removal of cannula should be followed by compression of puncture site for 5–10 minutes.

Central Venous and Pulmonary Artery Catheters

A. *Definitions*
1. *Central Venous Pressure (CVP)* is obtained via a catheter in the superior vena cava; it reflects right atrial pressure (see Guidelines, p. 271)

* Adapted from Horowitz and Luterman. Postoperative monitoring following critical trauma. Heart and Lung 1975 Mar–Apr; 4:269.

2. *Pulmonary Artery (PA)* and *Capillary Wedge Pressure (PCWP)*
   a. Swan-Ganz catheter is positioned in pulmonary artery to measure pulmonary artery pressure.
   b. When balloon is inflated, with catheter advanced to a wedge position, the pressure transmitted measures pressure changes in left atrium. (In absence of valvular heart disease, this PCWP also reflects left ventricular end-diastolic filling pressure.)

B. *Indications for Pulmonary Artery Catheters*
PAP indicates how efficiently the right ventricle is clearing the venous return presented to the right side of the heart at the time of measurement.
1. Increased pulmonary vascular resistance—chronic obstructive pulmonary disease (COPD)
2. Coronary artery disease requiring complicated intravenous fluid regimen
3. Cardiac surgery and trauma
4. Decreased left ventricular function secondary to anoxia, acidosis, or electrolyte imbalance
5. Decompensated cirrhosis, severe pancreatitis, generalized peritonitis, and severe multi-system trauma
6. Massive transfusions
7. High CVP in the presence of underperfusion of peripheral tissues

C. *Complications Associated with Central Venous and Pulmonary Artery Catheters*
1. CVP Catheters
   a. Infection, loss of catheter, thromboembolic complications
   b. Complications specific to insertion site
   c. Air embolism
   d. Perforation of right ventricle
2. PA Catheter
   a. Pulmonary artery perforation
   b. Pulmonary ischemic lesions
   c. Catheter kinking and intracardiac knotting
   d. Heart murmurs

D. *Guides to Safe Use of CVP Catheter* (See Guidelines, p. 271.)
1. Avoid venous cannulation in the leg in all patients except infants.
2. Carry out surgical skin preparation for all cannulations whether percutaneous or by direct cutdown.
3. Assure proper adapter-catheter fit prior to insertion.
4. Place the patient's head down when inserting subclavian or jugular catheters to avoid air embolism.
5. When subclavian puncture is unsuccessful, obtain x-ray of chest before attempting puncture on the contralateral side.
6. Use only radiopaque catheters.
7. Continuous dilute heparin infusions should be used to maintain patency in all intravenous monitoring cannulas.
8. When catheter does not advance through the needle with ease, remove needle and catheter together. Never attempt to withdraw the catheter through the needle.
9. Remove catheter when there is unexplained fever or local inflammation, or at the earliest date that catheter does not contribute to patient's care.
10. Submit the distal catheter tip for culture.

THE PATIENT RECEIVING INFUSION THERAPY

Objectives

1. To maintain or replace body stores of water, electrolytes, vitamins, proteins, calories, and nitrogen in the patient who cannot maintain an adequate intake by mouth.
2. To restore acid-base balance.
3. To replenish blood volume.
4. To provide avenues for the administration of medications.

Physiological Assimilation of Infusion Solutions

A. Principles

1. Blood cells (erythrocytes, etc.) are surrounded by a semipermeable membrane.
2. Osmotic pressure is the pressure demonstrated when a solvent moves through the semipermeable membrane from weaker to stronger concentrations.
3. Osmotic characteristics of different solutions are often determined by the way they affect red blood cells.

B. Types of Fluids

1. *Isotonic*—a solution which has the same osmotic pressure externally as that found across the semipermeable membrane within the cell.
   a. Normal saline 0.9%
   b. Dextrose 5% in water
   c. Lactated Ringers
   d. Balanced isotonic
2. *Hypotonic*—a solution which has less osmotic pressure than that of blood serum; this causes the cells to expand or swell.
   Sodium chloride 0.45%
3. *Hypertonic*—a solution which has higher osmotic pressure than that of blood serum; this causes the cells to shrink.
   a. Dextrose 5% in saline
   b. Dextrose 10% in saline
   c. Dextrose 10% in water
   d. Dextrose 5% in ½ strength saline
   e. Dextrose 20% in water

C. Composition of Fluids

1. Saline solution—fluids and electrolytes (Na^+ Cl^-)
2. Dextrose—fluid and calories
3. Lactated Ringers—fluid, electrolytes (Na^+, K^+, Cl^-, Ca^{++}, Lactate)
4. Balanced isotonic—fluid, electrolytes, some calories (Na^+, K^+, Mg^{++}, Cl^-, HCO_3^-, gluconate)
5. Blood-related fluids
   a. Whole blood
      (1) Approximately 45% cellular—red cells, white cells, blood platelets
      (2) Approximately 55% plasma
         (a) 90% water
         (b) 7% protein (albumin, globulin, fibrinogen)
         (c) 2% lipids, vitamins, carbohydrates, inorganic salts
      (3) Whole blood is used to replace blood lost in acute hemorrhage.
   b. Packed cells—red blood cells obtained by centrifuging whole blood and drawing off the plasma
      Packed cells are used in treatment of anemia or for the patient in whom there is a risk of circulatory overload (congestive heart failure); also used to combat shock

c. Fresh frozen plasma
   (1) To restore blood volume in shock
   (2) To correct hypoproteinemia
   (3) To treat coagulation disorders (see also p. 259)
6. Plasma expanders: albumin, dextran, plasminate
   To improve circulating blood volume
7. Parenteral hyperalimentation nutrients
8. Administration of a particular medication or combination of medications

Nursing Assessment

A. Diagnosis and Need for Fluid Therapy

It is important to know the major and minor medical problems of the patient as indicated in the physician's diagnostic evaluation and the nurse's assessment of the patient.

1. Can the patient's illness affect his fluid balance?
2. What medication or treatment is he receiving that can affect fluid components? How?
3. What is the relation of his fluid intake to fluid output?
4. Does he have dietary restrictions?
5. Is he taking adequate fluids by mouth?
6. What is the physician's plan of treatment?

B. Evidence of Fluid Imbalance in the Patient

1. Determine body temperature—febrile conditions suggest loss of body fluids through perspiration.
2. Is he thirsty? Possible dehydration.
3. Observe for dry, warm skin, cracked lips—signs of dehydration.
4. Check skin for elasticity—lightly pull up a pinch-fold of skin, release it. Does it rapidly resume its normal position?
   a. In elderly patient, check for tongue furrows—this may be more significant than skin turgor.
5. Note color and amount of urine—concentrated, scanty urine indicates lack of fluids.
6. Compare present weight with admission weight—it may indicate fluid change.
7. Absence of moisture in axillae or groin may indicate dehydration.

C. Inspection of Prescribed Fluid and Equipment to be Used for the Infusion

1. Observe fluid for discoloration, foreign particles, cloudiness, film—if present, do not use.
2. Fluid in a bag:
   Gently squeeze and observe for leakage.
3. Fluid in a glass bottle:
   a. Hold flask up to light.
   b. Slowly rotate flask in upright position and then on its side; carefully inspect for a flash of light that could indicate a crack.
4. Check IV tubing for discoloration or defects; if noted, secure new equipment.
5. Follow instructions for assembling equipment, using aseptic technique when inserting drip chamber spike into flask; flush equipment with 20–30 ml. of fluid from receptacle before using.
   (See Guidelines p. 100.)
6. Return defective equipment with a note describing defect to the proper department.

Criteria for Selecting a Suitable Vein for Venipuncture

1. Use distal branches of a large vein rather than the best sites—these are then available for emergencies.

> **NURSING ALERT:** Select lowest good vein on hand or arm initially for venipuncture or infusion. If, with subsequent venipunctures, this site is difficult to enter, move up higher on the arm. Conversely, if the antecubital fossa area is used first, and if later there is difficulty entering at this site, none of the lower veins can be used.

2. Convenient veins include the following:
   a. Back of the hand—basilic or cephalic vein (see Fig. 6-4A).
      (1) The advantage of this site is that it permits arm movement.
      (2) If later a vein problem develops at this site, another vein higher up the arm may be used.
   b. Forearm—basilic or cephalic vein (Fig. 6-4B).
   c. Inner aspect of elbow, antecubital fossa—median basilic and median cephalic for relatively short-term infusion.
      (1) These veins are large and easily accessible.
      (2) Note, however, that this site precludes arm movement.
      (3) Choose site below elbow crease for patient's comfort.
3. Otherwise, select other available veins
   a. Thigh—great saphenous and femoral veins
   b. Ankle—great saphenous
   c. Foot—venous plexus of dorsum, dorsal venous arch, medial marginal vein

> **NURSING ALERT:** Avoid leg veins if there are marked degrees of varicosity at or above proposed site of injection. Otherwise, injected solutions may stagnate along varicosed vessels.

4. Central veins are used
   a. When medications are hypertonic or highly irritating requiring rapid high-volume dilution to prevent systemic reactions and local venous irritation, e.g., protein hydrolysate, hypertonic sodium chloride. (See Table 6-1.)
   b. During shock or cardiac arrest; peripheral blood flow is diminished.

Methods of Distending a Vein

1. Apply manual compression above site where needle is to be inserted.
2. Have patient periodically clench his fist (if arm is used).
3. Massage area in direction of venous flow.
4. Apply sphygmomanometer cuff (keep pressure just below systolic pressure).
5. Fasten soft rubber tubing with a hemostat.
6. Tie soft rubber tubing as a slip knot.
7. Lightly slap vein site; this is to be done gently so that the vein is not injured.
8. Allow extremity to be dependent for a few minutes.

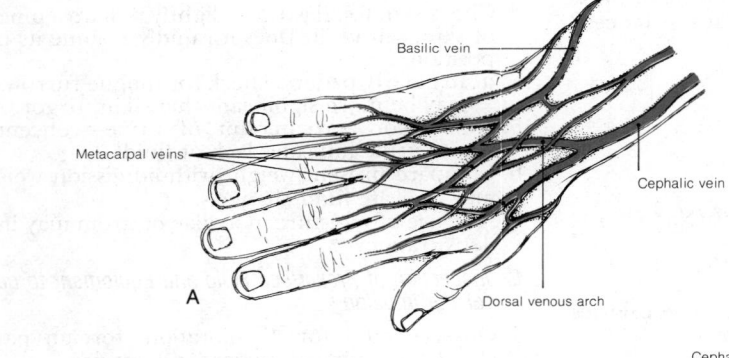

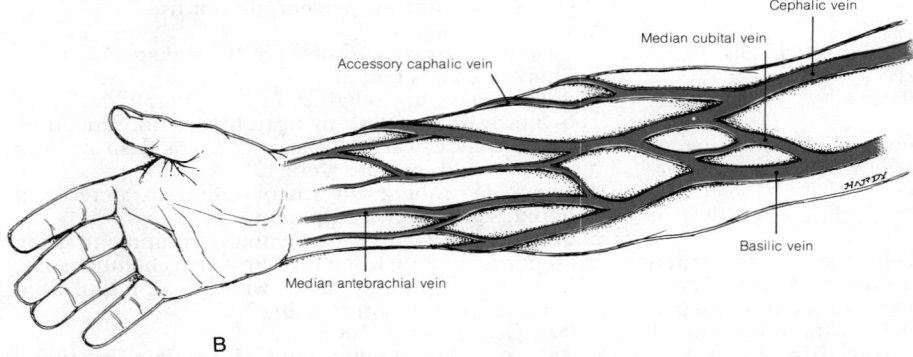

FIGURE 6-4. A. *Superficial veins, dorsal aspect of hand.* B. *Superficial veins, forearm.*

TABLE 6-1 FACTORS IN THE SELECTION OF PERIPHERAL OR CENTRAL SITES FOR INTRAVENOUS INSERTION

Factor	Peripheral Veins		Central Veins	
	Suitable	*Unsuitable*	*Suitable*	*Unsuitable*
Type of drug or solution	Most drugs Isotonic fluids	Irritating drugs or hypertonic fluids which require maximal dilution	Irritating drugs or hypertonic fluids	Drugs which if injected centrally could cause arrhythmias, shock or other complications
Duration of therapy	Short-term or intermittent therapy; is less hazardous	Long-term therapy, in which all available veins would be used up	Moderate to long-term continuous therapy	Short-term therapy; the patient is subjected to greater risks
Accessibility of veins	Patients with adequate peripheral veins	Very obese patients; I.V. drug abusers; conditions which impair peripheral circulation	When peripheral veins inaccessible, especially if intravenous line is needed in an emergency	At times not accessible after repeated use (e.g. pacemaker). May be accessible, but increased risks due to location near lung
Cooperation of patient	Extremity can usually be restrained sufficiently to allow insertion and maintenance of line	Disoriented or agitated adult or child may be more likely to attempt removal of intravenous line located in upper extremity	Central lines, especially subclavian, are less likely to be disrupted once inserted	Patient must lie absolutely still during the insertion to prevent pneumothorax and other complications

Source: Sager DP and Bomar SK. Intravenous Medications, p 40. Philadelphia, JB Lippincott Co. 1980

9. Apply moist heat by wringing out turkish towel and wrapping the part.
   Apply water-resistant wrapper externally and place a warm-water bottle or 2 along extremity. Leave in place from 10 to 20 minutes.
10. Apply external heat to extremity using a thermostatically controlled electric blanket.
    Hand-operated hair dryer can be used to direct heat to a possible needle site.

NOTE: Should the above measures fail, it may be necessary to perform a "cutdown"—this is a surgical procedure exposing the vein for venipuncture; the incision site is treated as a surgical wound.

Stabilizing Extremity with a Padded Armboard

1. This is done if the patient is restless, disoriented, elderly, or a child and if motion could result in infiltration into tissues or phlebitis.
2. Various kinds of armboards are available; an armboard should be padded.

NURSING ALERT: If hand and arm are to be immobilized, place in normal functional position. *Contractures may occur if hand is immobilized in flat position.*
For hand: (Fig. 6-5) Dorsiflexion of wrist about 20–25 degrees.
Flexion of metacarpophalangeal joint about 45–50 degrees.
Palm slightly cupped with finger flexion increasing from index to little finger.
Thumb should be extended in relaxed position and not flexed under fingers.

3. Prevent compression of nerves or blood vessels; check pulse and ask patient if pressure is too great.

Cleansing Infusion Site

1. Use a good surgical soap to thoroughly cleanse the infusion site. Dirt, dead skin, blood, mucus, and oil

are to be removed so that action of antiseptic is not hindered.
2. Rinse the area with an alcohol swab.
3. Apply an iodine-base antiseptic; 1 or 2% iodine in water or in 70% alcohol is effective. After 30 seconds, iodine can be washed off with alcohol.
   a. In patients sensitive to iodine, iodophors may be used. Do not wash off an iodophor, since it provides sustained release of free iodine which may enhance the germicidal action.
   b. If iodine preparations are not available, 70% alcohol is an alternative if it is applied vigorously for 1 minute after the area has been cleansed.
4. Wait until area is dry before inserting needle; this is done to prevent carrying antiseptic solution into the vein.

NURSING ALERT: In applying antiseptic, swab the infusion site first; then, covering an ever-widening circular area, move out to the periphery.

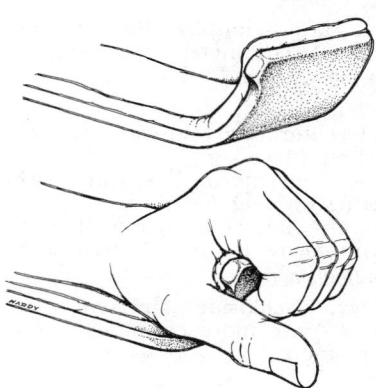

FIGURE 6-5. *Immobilization of hand and arm during infusion.*

TABLE 6-2 COMPARISON OF DIFFERENT TYPES OF INTRAVENOUS CANNULAE

Type of Cannula	Indications for Use	Advantages	Disadvantages
A. Needles 1. Straight needles	Cooperative, adult patients who require very short-term (1–3 days) therapy	Ease of insertion. Less likely to cause phlebitis	Rigid, difficult to secure so more prone to infiltration especially in active or agitated patients Less comfortable
2. Winged-needle unit (scalp-vein needle)	Short-term therapy for any patient, especially for infants and children; geriatric and other patients with fragile or rolling veins	Wings enable easy insertion and securing to prevent movement and dislodgement Less likely to cause phlebitis	Needle rigid and short so may infiltrate if patient very active or if needle not securely taped
3. Intermittent winged needle unit (heparin-lock)	Intermittent administration of drugs such as heparin, antibiotics; frequent blood sampling; or to keep vein open when no fluids are needed	Allows prompt access to the vein without giving fluids Economical; greater comfort and mobility for the patient	Will clot if not flushed with heparinized saline; part of clot can be injected into the patient when the next dose of drug is given
B. Plastic Catheters 1. Over-the-needle catheter	Active or moderately agitated patients who require a secure venous line for uninterrupted delivery of drugs and/or fluids	Easy to insert More comfortable for the patient Less prone to infiltration than needles	More likely to cause phlebitis, particularly if not changed every 48–72 hours Can kink if inserted near an area of flexion (such as elbow)
2. Over-the-needle catheter with resealable cap	Patients on intermittent drugs without need for fluids, yet who require a secure device	Combines advantages of over-the-needle catheter with those of intermittent winged-needle unit (heparin lock)	Same as those of other over-the-needle catheters Will clot unless flushed with heparinized saline periodically
3. Through-the-needle catheter	Administration of hypertonic fluids or irritating drugs which must be given via a central vein to insure adequate dilution; for monitoring of CVP; emergencies in which life-sustaining drugs and fluids must be given rapidly and accurately	Very secure Available in many sizes and lengths so it can be inserted directly into a central vein or via a peripheral vein	Greater risk of infection and other complications especially when inserted into central vein Insertion requires a high degree of skill; incorrect insertion or guarding of needle can cause severing and embolization of catheter fragment
4. In-lying (cutdown) catheter	Patients in whom percutaneous access to veins is unsuccessful such as those in shock or cardiac arrest; those with sclerosed veins due to IV drug abuse; markedly obese patients	Provides access to superficial or deep veins May be the only means of establishing an intravenous line during emergencies Once inserted is very secure	Must be inserted by a physician Creates a surgical wound so the risk of infection is greater

Source: Sager DP and Bomar SK. Intravenous Medications, p 37. Philadelphia, JB Lippincott Co., 1980

Providing Local Anesthesia for Infants or Unusually Sensitive Patients

1. Raise a wheal in the skin just over the vein by injecting 0.5 ml. procaine hydrochloride 1.0% solution.
2. Advance the needle close to the wall of the vein so that this area is also anesthetized.

Equipment

A. *Needle or Catheter.*

Infusion may be administered through a needle (short-term) or through a catheter (long-term.) (See Table 6-2 and also Figs. 6-6 and 6-7.)

B. *Bevel*

To facilitate entering a vein with least injury to skin, the bevel should face—

1. Upward—when entering a vein lumen which is larger than the needle (Fig. 6-8A).
2. Downward—when entering a small vein with lumen which approaches the size of the needle (Fig. 6-8B).

C. *Solution Container*

1. Soft polyvinyl chloride* and semi-rigid polyolefin containers** are more convenient and safer than glass containers.

* Life Care—Abbott; Viaflex—Travenol
** Accumed—McGaw

2. Polyolefin containers—less likely to leak; do not introduce DEHP (di-2-ethylhexyl phthalate) into IV solution.
3. Polyolefin containers require more storage space.
4. When plastic containers are used, adsorption of added medications may be greater than when glass bottles are used.

Rate of Flow of Fluid in Infusion Therapy

Physician prescribes flow rate. However, the nurse is responsible for regulating and maintaining the proper rate.

A. *Patient Determining Factors*

1. Surface area of the patient
   The larger the person, the more fluid he requires and the faster he utilizes it.
2. Patient condition
   If patient has cardiovascular or renal problems, the rate should be specified by the physician.

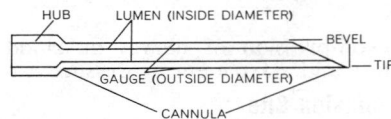

FIGURE 6-6. *Diagram of a hollow metal intravenous needle. (Abbott Laboratories)*

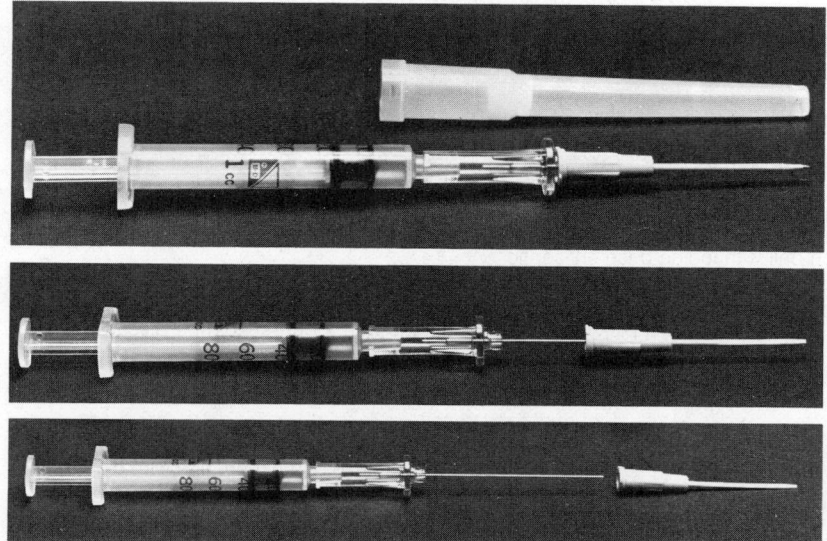

FIGURE 6-7. (top) *A catheter-threaded needle. The needle's protective sheath (above the needle in this photo) has been removed.*

(center) After the needle and catheter have been introduced into the vein, the needle and syringe are carefully withdrawn, leaving the catheter in place in the vein.

(bottom) After the needle is withdrawn completely, the tubing from the intravenous solution is connected to the catheter.

(Lewis LW. Fundamental Skills in Patient Care. Philadelphia, JB Lippincott, 1980)

3. Age of patient
   Administer fluid more slowly to elderly patient to prevent increase in venous pressure.
4. Tolerance to solutions
   Example—Test protein sensitivity by administering protein hydrolysates slowly.
5. Fluid composition for this particular patient
   When drugs are administered via infusion, the effect desired often depends on speed of administration
6. Patient movement and activity

B. *Factors Affecting Rate of Flow*

1. Pressure gradient—the difference between 2 levels in a fluid system
2. Friction—the interaction between fluid molecules and surfaces of inner wall of tubing
3. Diameter and length of tubing; kinking of tubing
4. Height of column of fluid
5. Size of opening through which fluid leaves receptacle
6. Characteristics of fluid
   a. viscosity
   b. temperature—refrigerated fluids may cause diminished flow and vessel spasm; bring fluid to room temperature.
7. Vein trauma, clots, plugging of vents, venous spasm, vasoconstriction, etc.
8. Flow-control-clamp derangement
   a. Some clamps may slip and loosen resulting in a very rapid, or "runaway," infusion.

b. Plastic tubing may distort causing "creep" or "cold flow"—the inside diameter of tubing will continue to change long after clamp is tightened or relaxed.
   c. Marked stretching of tubing may cause distortions of tubing and render clamp ineffective (may occur when patient turns over and pulls on a short tubing).
9. If there is any question regarding rate of fluid administration, check with physician.

C. *Calculation of Flow Rate**

1. Drops per milliliter vary with commercial parenteral sets. (Check directions on set or calculate by timing for 1 minute.) (Also see Table 6-3, Calibrating IV Fluids, p. 99.)
2. Utilize the following formula:

$$\text{Drops/min.} = \frac{\text{Total volume infused} \times \text{drops/ml.}}{\text{Total time for infusion in minutes}}$$

   Example:
   Infuse 1000 ml. of 5% D/W in 2½ hours
   (Set indicates 10 drops in 1 ml.)

$$\frac{1000 \times 10}{150 \text{ min}} = 60 \text{ drops/min.}$$

NOTE: Convenient calculators are available from manufacturers of parenteral solutions.

* Metheny NM and Snively WD, Jr. Nurse's Handbook of Fluid Balance, 3rd ed. Philadelphia, JB Lippincott Co., 1979.

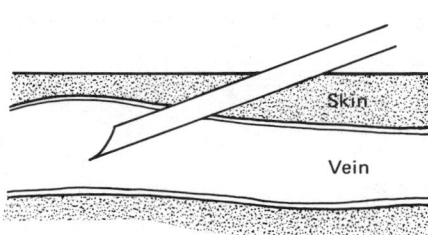

A.

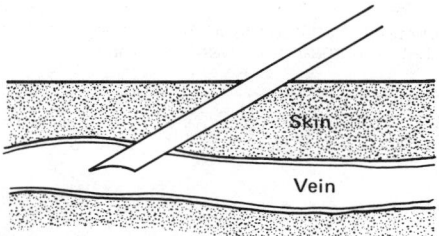

B.

FIGURE 6-8. *Position of needle in vein.*

GUIDELINES: Venipuncture

Venipuncture is the puncturing of a vein with a needle (steel or plastic) attached to a syringe.

Purpose
1. To obtain blood samples for analysis, cross matching
2. To administer fluids, blood, medications
3. To perform tests requiring a needle in a vein

Equipment
Tourniquet, usually rubber tubing or flat latex rubber, approximately 37.5 cm. (15 in.). (Blood pressure cuff is effective because it can be pumped to the desired 100 mm. Hg.)
Sterile gauze squares or cotton ball with iodine-base antiseptic
Sterile syringe: 10 or 20 ml. depending on amount of blood desired
No. 18 needle—with disposable needles, the likelihood of a burr is practically nonexistent. If there is any question, draw needle through sterile gauze—a burr will pick up threads. A needle with a burr should be discarded.

Procedure

NURSING ACTION	RATIONALE/AMPLIFICATION
Preparatory Phase	
1. Wash hands thoroughly.	
2. Explain procedure to patient.	2. Most patients have had experience with blood drawing.
3. Select site: The back of the hand, the back of the arm, or the antecubital vein is used (in order of preference). Vein selection is determined by size, elasticity, and distance below skin. (Shave hair if necessary.) Vein should be distinct, easily observable, and palpable; it should be large enough for a needle to enter.	
4. Ascertain if there is satisfactory distention of the vein.	4. This is done by observation or by drawing the skin tight over the vein.
5. Make decision about whether to use a tourniquet or not.	5. Pulling the skin taut over the vein, usually makes the vein prominent enough.
6. If tourniquet is used, do not apply too tightly—venous flow should be stopped but arterial flow should continue (radial pulse should be palpable).	6. Improperly applied tourniquet may cause blood stasis and may result in blood chemistry alterations. This is why some prefer to apply a blood pressure cuff to 100 mm. Hg.
7. Scrub area with iodine-base antiseptic. Allow to dry.	7. To reduce number of skin microorganisms.
8. If vein is prominent, it is not necessary to request patient to make a fist.	8. Fist-making may increase ammonia concentration in the blood.
Performance Phase	
1. Insert the needle, bevel up, through the skin, parallel to the vein.	1. Usually a single sliding stroke can be use to enter skin and vessel.
2. If vessel rolls, it may be necessary to penetrate the skin first at a 30-degree angle and then apply a second thrust parallel to the skin to enter the vessel.	2. Satisfactory penetration is evidenced by appearance of blood coming back into syringe.
3. Direct needle into vein; this usually means a slight change in direction to avoid going through the other side of the vessel.	3. If tourniquet was used, remove at this time to prevent extravasation of blood.
4. For blood sampling: Draw desired amount of blood into syringe.	4. Blood should flow easily; if suction is required, reposition needle to avoid hemolysis.
Follow-up Phase	
1. Place a cotton sponge over vein at site of puncture and withdraw needle.	1. Instruct patient to hold cotton ball in place with slight pressure for 2–3 minutes. If oozing continues, apply a strip of adhesive tape over a fresh sterile cotton ball.
2. Slowly inject blood specimen into proper receptacle, label, and see that specimen is deliverd to proper laboratory.	2. Record venipuncture and purpose of blood specimen.

GUIDELINES: Arterial Puncture

An *arterial puncture* is the entering of an artery for the purpose of drawing blood for blood gas determination or for other laboratory study.

Equipment
Iodine-base antiseptic
Lidocaine (0.5%) 0.5 ml. in a 1.0 ml. syringe
Heparinized syringe with No. 25 gauge needle (radial puncture)
Heparinized syringe with No. 22 gauge needle (femoral or brachial puncture)

Procedure

NURSING ACTION	RATIONALE/AMPLIFICATION
1. Wash hands carefully.	1. To minimize possibility of infection.
2. Check arm for color, temperature, and pulses for adequacy of circulation.	2. Particularly note brachial, radial, and ulnar pulses. If there is any question regarding circulation, check with physician.
3. Inform patient that a local anesthetic will be injected first so that the drawing of blood will cause little discomfort.	3. If patient's concern is not alleviated, hyperventilation could produce atypical blood values.
4. Have patient in a comfortable position.	4. Sitting in a chair or semi-Fowler's position in bed is acceptable.
5. Cleanse puncture site; then follow with iodine-base antiseptic.	5. Be sure site is free of soil, dead skin, or debris which would interfere with action of antiseptic.
6. Dorsiflex patient's wrist slightly—determine strongest pulse.	6. To determine best puncture site.
7. Puncture artery, entering at a 45-degree angle over strongest pulse area.	7. Holding needle with bevel up, pierce skin and artery using same technique as for venous puncture (p. 98).
8. Note "flashback," keep needle steady, and withdraw required sample; remove needle.	8. This indicates entrance into artery.
9. Apply constant pressure over puncture site for at least 5 or 6 minutes.	9. Time can be increased if there is a coagulation problem; pressure is applied until bleeding stops.
10. Hold syringe and needle in a vertical position and eject all air; cap needle with needle cover.	10. Air would alter gaseous content of blood.
11. Transport syringe and needle with blood specimen to laboratory immediately.	11. If the analysis will not take place within 5 minutes, entire syringe is placed in ice to preserve condition of blood.

TABLE 6-3. CALIBRATING IV FLUIDS

Prescription	Regular (15 drops/ml.)		Microdrip (60 drops/ml.)		Macrodrip (10 drops/ml.)	
	Drops/min.	Drops/¼ min.	Drops/min.	Drops/¼ min.	Drops/min.	Drops/¼ min.
40 ml./hr.	10	2¼	40	10	7	2
50 ml./hr.	12	3	50	12½	8	2
60 ml./hr.	15	4	60	15	10	2½
80 ml./hr.	20	5	80	20	13	3
100 ml./hr.	25	6	100	25	16	4
125 ml./hr.	30	7½	125	30	20	5
150 ml./hr.	38	9½	150	38	25	6

24-Hour Fluids	
ml./24 hours	ml./hour
1000	40
1500	60
2000	80
2500	100
3000	125
3500	145

Source: Norcross MB. Am J Nurs 1975 Nov; 75:2003

GUIDELINES: Administering an Intravenous Infusion Using the Cubital Fossa

Procedure

NURSING ACTION	RATIONALE/AMPLIFICATION
Preparatory Phase	
1. Place patient in bed in semi-Fowler's position.	1. This is comfortable for the patient and permits arm to assume a flexed comfortable position.
Inform him of the procedure and its purpose.	To secure his understanding and cooperation.
2. Remove patient's arm from sleeve of garment.	2. To permit removal of gown or pajama top if necessary while infusion is in progress (without cutting sleeve).
3. Position (but do not tighten) tourniquet under lower end of upper arm (5 cm. [2 inches] above joint).	3. To immobilize arm while needle or catheter is in vein; this will prevent dislodging of needle and injury to vein.
4. Place padded splint under arm; fix arm to splint by bandaging firmly (see p. 95).	4. Padding will prevent constriction of nerves or blood vessels.
5. Connect intravenous material; hang fluid receptacle after checking label for proper solution.	5. Intravenous fluids are considered medications; labeling must be verified.
6. Allow fluid to flow through the system; tighten the clamp; lay sterile needle on sterile surface until arm is prepared.	6. To eliminate air bubbles which could cause air emboli in the circulatory system.
Performance Phase	
1. Tighten tourniquet.	1. To distend veins (for better visualization) by preventing blood flow back to heart.
Ends of tubing should be opposite or away from infusion site.	To prevent contaimination of injection area by tubing ends.
2. Request patient to open and close his fist. Palpate and note suitable vein for injection.	2. Contracting muscles of lower arm forces blood into veins, which distends them further.
3. Cleanse skin thoroughly, using an antiseptic (at room temperature) on a cotton ball; apply friction in a circular pattern outward from injection site.	3. To remove skin pathogens and sebum which might otherwise be drawn into the subcutaneous tissue or vein as the needle is advanced. Avoid application of cold antiseptic solution particularly if patient has very small veins; cold application would further constrict the vessels.
4. Use thumb to apply tension on tissue and vein about 5 cm. (2 inches) distal to injection site.	4. To aid in anchoring the vein as the needle is introduced.
5. Hold the needle at a 45-degree angle alongside the wall of the vein in the direction of and near the intended site of injection; pierce skin.	5. This angle permits greatest ease and accuracy in entering the vein.
6. Decrease angle of needle until it is nearly parallel with the skin and slightly to one side of the vein; apply pressure in same direction as puncture and enter the vein.	
7. If there is a backflow of blood through the needle, the vein has been entered; advance the needle slowly about 2½ cm. (1 inch) while lifting the vein.	7. To prevent the needle from becoming dislodged and puncturing the posterior wall of the vein.
8. Release tourniquet.	8. To permit infusion solution to enter circulatory system.
9. Release clamp on infusion tubing and relax skin tension.	9. To allow flow of solution and to prevent blood from clotting in the needle.
10. Slip a sterile gauze square (3 x 3-inch) under the needle (double if necessary) to anchor it in the proper position.	10. To prevent needle orifice from pressing against vein wall and the needle from piercing vein wall.
11. Anchor needle in position using dressing and adhesive strips (Fig. 6-9); fasten a loop of tubing to prevent pull on needle (Figs. 6-10 and 6-11).	11. Effective taping allows some mobility for the patient and retains safe inflow of solution.
12. Regulate flow rate of solution.	12. Proper monitoring of solution will prevent overloading of the circulatory system.

Follow-up Phase

1. Gently loosen adhesive tape and fixation near injection site.
2. Place a sterile gauze square over needle or cannula where it enters vein; withdraw needle (or cannula) and *exert pressure at site.* If bleeding persists, apply a gauze square or Band-Aid and elevate part.
3. Remove adhesive marks with solvent.
4. Record
   a. Nature of therapy and time given
   b. Type of solution and rate of flow
   c. Total amount of solution
   d. Any problems
   e. Patient's reaction

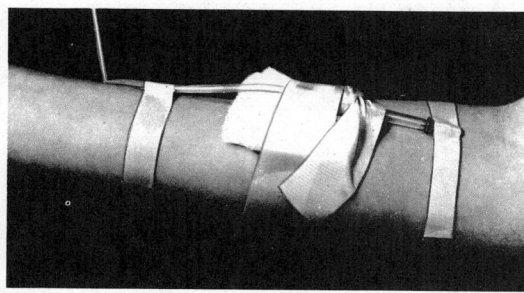

FIGURE 6-9. *Method for securing needle and tubing for IV infusion or blood transfusion. Needle is inserted into antecubital vein with arm secured to padded board. After the needle is inserted, it is secured with 1.3 cm. (½-inch) wide strips of tape. A sterile gauze pad may be used to build up the angle of insertion.*

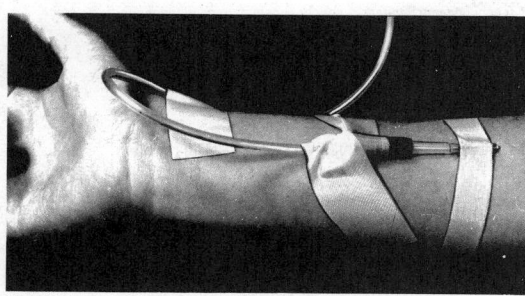

FIGURE 6-10. *Simple method of holding needle and tubing in forearm vein with tape to prevent traction on needle.*

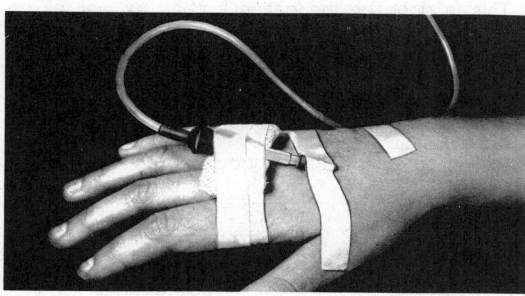

FIGURE 6-11. *Method of securing needle and tubing in vein on back of hand with tape.*

FIGURES 6-9, 10, 11. © *Johnson & Johnson. (Used by special permission of Johnson & Johnson, the copyright owners, and not to be reproduced for any purpose without Johnson & Johnson's permission.)*

GUIDELINES: Intravenous Infusion with Insertion of Plastic Catheter (Mounted on Metal Needle)

Equipment   Infusion Set containing (sterile)
Rubber tourniquet
Gauze squares
Foil wrapped alcohol sponges or iodine-base antiseptic
Hollow intravenous needle with catheter (Teflon, Silastic or polyvinylchloride) attached to rigid hub.

NOTE: Thorough hand washing followed by donning of sterile gloves is recommended.

Procedure   As described on page 98, then as follows:

NURSING ACTION	RATIONALE/AMPLIFICATION
1. When needle has punctured vein wall, gently push needle 1.2 cm. (½ inch) farther.	1. To ensure entry of catheter into vein lumen.
2. Hold needle in place; slowly advance catheter hub until it is in desired place.	2. Caution: After catheter is advanced, do not reinsert metal needle since it could cut catheter.
3. Slowly remove needle while holding catheter hub in place.	3. If catheter is not held in place, it is possible to pull catheter out of vein.
4. Apply pressure on vein beyond catheter with the small or ring finger (Fig. 6-12).	4. This will reduce blood leakage while removing needle and connecting tubing to infusion set.
5. Connect infusion tubing to hub of catheter.	
6. Apply iodine-base ointment.	6. To prevent infection.

GUIDELINES: Intravenous Infusion with Insertion of Plastic Catheter (Mounted on Metal Needle) (cont.)

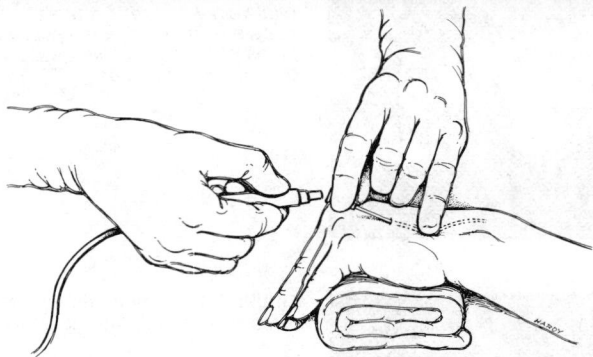

FIGURE 6-12. *Finger palpation of dorsal venous arch.*

Procedure (cont.)

NURSING ACTION	RATIONALE/AMPLIFICATION
7. Tape catheter after covering injection site with a sterile dressing.	7. To prevent catheter movement which could irritate vein and lead to phlebitis.
8. Loop tubing and fasten to arm. (see Fig. 6-11).	8. To prevent any tension on tubing from affecting or moving catheter in the vein.

Follow-up

1. Frequent inspection of venipuncture site.	1. To ensure proper functioning of infusion.
2. Record date of insertion, size and type of catheter.	2. This is done on the patient's chart as well as on adhesive tape near infusion puncture site.
3. Change dressing and apply antiseptic ointment every 24 hours.	3. To minimize possibility of infection.
4. Change catheter every 24 hours.	4. Preferably the entire set is changed every 24 hours; the longer an intravenous set is in use, the greater the possibility of contamination by either airborne microorganisms or those introduced via manipulation of equipment.

GUIDELINES: Intravenous Infusion by Insertion of Catheter Through Needle (IntraCatheter)

Equipment   Infusion Set containing: (sterile)
    Rubber tourniquet
    Gauze squares
    Foil wrapped alcohol sponges or iodine-base antiseptic
    Intravenous needle with plastic catheter through needle
NOTE: Thorough hand washing followed by donning of sterile gloves is recommended.

Procedure   As described on page 98, then as follows:

NURSING ACTION	RATIONALE/AMPLIFICATION
1. When needle has punctured vein wall, gently thread catheter through needle until desired length of catheter in vein has been achieved.	1. To ensure entry of catheter into vein.
2. Place index finger over vein (with catheter in place) and withdraw needle.	2. To hold catheter in proper position.
3. Apply pressure at puncture site for several seconds.	3. To control bleeding.
4. Slide needle shield to cover bevel of needle.	4. This will prevent cutting of the catheter by the needle.
5. An effective splint for the needle (and its junction with catheter) is made by taping a wooden tongue blade to needle and catheter.	5. This will prevent kinking of catheter and possibility of its breaking at bevel of needle.
6. Apply dressing and tape.	

NURSING ALERT: If insertion of catheter through the needle is unsuccessful, remove both catheter and needle *at the same time*. Otherwise, if catheter is pulled through needle, *it may break and slip into the circulatory system*.

Procedure (cont.)

NURSING ACTION	RATIONALE/AMPLIFICATION

Follow-up

1. Frequent inspection of venipuncture site will ensure proper functioning of infusion.
2. Record date of insertion, size and type of catheter.
3. Change dressing and apply antiseptic ointment every 24 hours.
4. Change catheter every 24 hours.

2. This is done on the patient's chart as well as on adhesive tape near puncture site.
3. To minimize infection possibility.
4. Preferably the entire set is changed every 24 hours; the longer an intravenous set is in use the greater the possibility of contamination either by airborne micro-organisms or via manipulation of equipment.

GUIDELINES: Use of Winged Infusion Set (Venipuncture) ''Butterfly''

Winged Infusion is the puncturing of a vein with a needle which has a pair of plastic wings attached to a flattened hub (Fig. 6-13).*

Advantages

1. Wings can be folded upward for easy manipulation and control of needle during insertion into vein.
2. The absence of a hub allows needle to be maneuvered close to skin surface.
3. Usually this type of commercially prepared set has a shorter needle with a short bevel that lessens possibility of puncturing the opposite vein wall.
4. Following insertion of the needle, the wings are released; they spread flat against patient's skin and provide 2 anchor surfaces for taping. Absence of hub reduces possibility of pressure irritation.

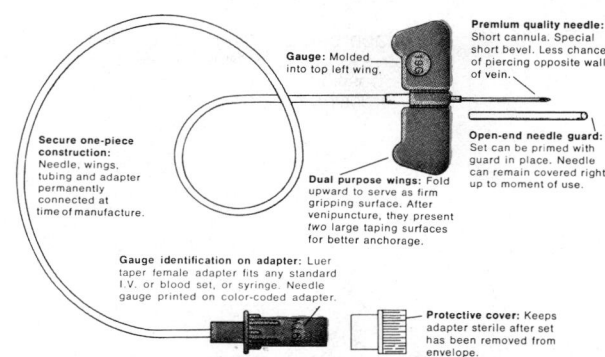

FIGURE 6-13. *''Butterfly'' winged infusion set.*

Procedure

As described on p. 98, then as follows:

NURSING ACTION	RATIONALE/AMPLIFICATION

1. Position wing set so that bevel of needle is up.
2. Note gauge of needle on left wing.
3. Pinch wings firmly together between thumb and index finger.

   Needle is held firmly and comfortably for insertion.

1. This permits proper introduction of needle through skin into vein.
2. Most sets are marked for easy recognition of needle gauge.

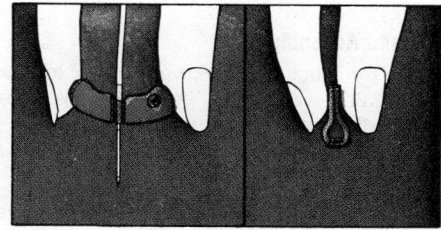

4. Follow usual procedure, described on p. 98, for inserting needle.
5. Advance needle cautiously into vein; simultaneously, lift wings up slightly—to avoid piercing opposite vein wall.

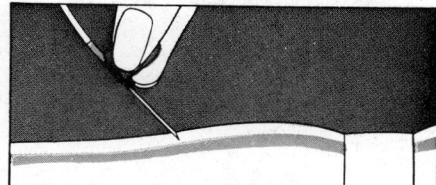

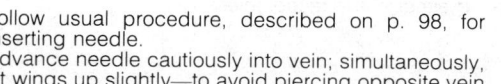

* Figures courtesy Abbott Laboratories.

GUIDELINES: Use of Winged Infusion Set (Venipuncture) "Butterfly" (cont.)

Procedure (cont.)

NURSING ACTION	RATIONALE/AMPLIFICATION

6. Release tourniquet and release wings; hold flat against patient's skin and permit fluid to flow temporarily.

   This will anchor needle in vein and permit checking of flow of fluid.

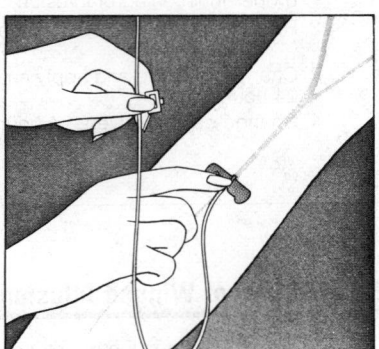

7. Apply tape parallel to needle on each side. Make a protective loop and fasten to arm with tape—to anchor needle position.
8. Apply dressing over site, and tape.

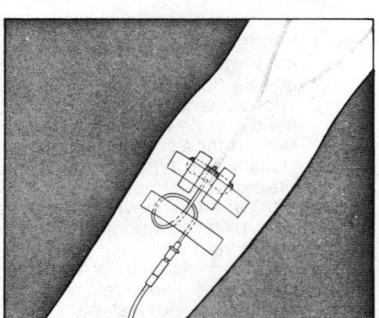

GUIDELINES: Setting Up An Automatic IV "Piggyback"

"Piggyback" intravenous administration is a means of administering medication via the fluid pathway of an established primary infusion line.

Features and Advantages

1. Drugs may be given on an intermittent basis through a "keep-open" infusion.
2. The secondary bottle contains the medication; this may be single dose or multiple dose.
3. When desired, the primary infusion is clamped off and the prescribed amount of medication from the secondary bottle is administered.
4. A check-valve performs the following functions:
   a. Permits the primary infusion to flow after the medication has been administered
   b. Prevents air from entering the system
   c. Prevents secondary fluid from "running dry"
   d. Permits less mixing of primary fluid with secondary solution
5. Higher flow rates can be achieved by elevating either of the receptacles.

Equipment
Infusion set (Primary)
Infusion set with admixture (Secondary)
Gauze squares and iodine-base antiseptic
Tourniquet
Tape

Procedure
Follow procedure of particular manufacturer of "Piggyback" infusion set.
In general, most procedures are similar to the following:

Procedure (cont.)

NURSING ACTION	RATIONALE/AMPLIFICATION
1. Wash hands thoroughly.	1. Minimizes possibility of infection.
2. Set up primary infusion set as described on p. 100; this should have a check-valve (Fig. 6-14A).	2. The primary set should be functioning effectively before the Secondary (Piggyback) set can be attached.
3. Lower the Primary flask on the IV pole; usually an extension hook accompanies the set.	3. This will permit check-valve to function (Fig. 6-14A).
4. Prime secondary set; hang it on IV pole.	4. This may be a partial-fill bottle or special additive container. Priming allows all air to escape from the system.
5. Use antiseptic swab to carefully cleanse injection site.	5. Usually this is a Y-connection on the Primary site.
6. Open clamp on Secondary set; check the check-valve to ensure that it closes off the flow of solution from the Primary source (Fig. 6-14C).	6. Pressure is greater from the Secondary source since it is more elevated; increased pressure forces the disc upward in the check-valve. This closes off the flow from the Primary source.
7. When fluid from Secondary source reaches level of fluid in Primary set drip chamber, hydrostatic pressure between the two sets equalizes (Fig. 6-14D).	7. This releases check-valve (Fig. 6-14B) and flow will then resume automatically from Primary source.

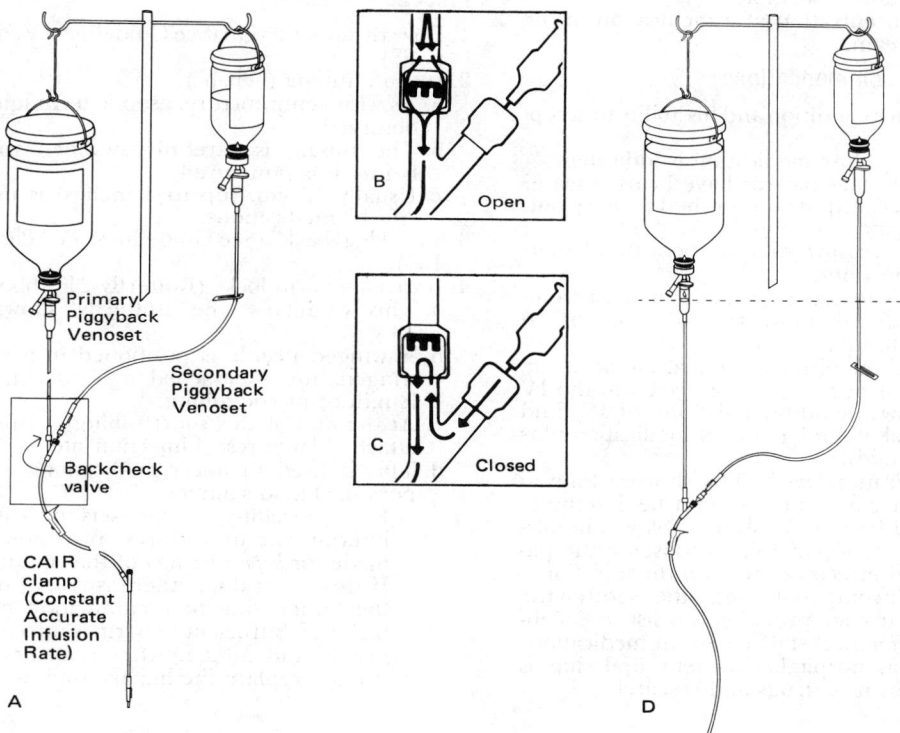

FIGURE 6-14. A. *"Piggyback" IV. On left is the Primary Infusion flask. Note use of extension hook (hanging from IV pole) to suspend Primary flask. Backcheck valve is seen more clearly in B and C. Secondary "piggyback" source is seen on the right.*
B. Open check-valve. Fluid from Primary source flows down on either side of movable disc. Fluid from Secondary source is closed off with clamp (not visible).
C. Closed check-valve. Note that fluid source from Secondary flask (where pressure is greater because flask source is higher) is forcing movable disc upward, thereby closing off fluid from Primary source.
D. When last of fluid from Secondary source reaches the level of the fluid in the Primary set drip chamber (as indicated by broken line), hydrostatic pressure between both sets will equalize. This releases check-valve; flow will shift from Secondary to Primary source. (Adapted from Abbott Laboratories)

Follow-up
1. Follow specific instructions on manufacturer's set for secondary replacement.
2. Discontinuation of primary source is as for conventional infusion set.

INTRAVENOUS "PUSH"

IV "Push" refers to the administration of a medication from a syringe and needle directly into an ongoing intravenous infusion. It may also be given directly into a vein or heparin lock. Although called "push," it is administered *slowly*, and the patient is carefully observed throughout the procedure.

NOTE: IV "push" medication is usually restricted to intensive care units and administered by especially prepared personnel.

Advantages

1. Avoids incompatibility problems that may occur when several medications are mixed in one bottle.
2. Reduces patient discomfort because there are fewer IM and IV injections.
3. Provides for immediate absorption of drugs; the effects are rapid and observable.
4. Permits rapid concentration of a medication in the patient's bloodstream.

Precautions and Recommendations

1. Determine patient's condition and his ability to accept the drug.
   Perhaps a more dilute medication is indicated.
     For example: Does patient have heart disease? limited cardiac output? diminished urinary output? pulmonary congestion?
2. Most medications require dilution because of their irritating effect on veins.
   A good policy is to use a syringe that can accommodate about 3 ml. more than the prescribed amount of medication.
     Example: If 2 ml. of medication are to be given, use a 5 ml. syringe. When connected to the IV line, withdraw the additional 3 ml. of IV fluid making a total of 5 ml. (2 ml. of medication plus 3 ml. of IV fluid).
3. Administer medication *slowly.* The shortest time to spend in emptying a syringe should be 1 minute; the longest could be 6 or 7 minutes. Slow administration provides an opportunity to observe the patient; if untoward effects occur, stop the injection.
4. Check the list of incompatible medications; often the local hospital pharmacy prepares this list in collaboration with the medical staff based on medications used by the local hospital. Frequent updating is needed because of new drugs and research.

5. Watch for major patient reactions such as anaphylaxis, respiratory distress, tachycardia, bradycardia, seizures. Also note "minor" side effects such as nausea, flushing, vomiting, skin rash, confusion, gastrointestinal distress.
   If a major reaction occurs or if a minor one is increasing in severity, stop the medication and notify the physician.
6. Be familiar with antidotes for side effects and be prepared to administer them if prescribed:
     Examples: Skin reactions—Benadryl
               Anaphylaxis—Epinephrine
               Vomiting—Tigan
               Diarrhea—Lomotil
       Emergency medications should be available in "crash carts"
7. Cardiopulmonary resuscitative procedures should be familiar to nurses giving IV "push" medications.

Procedure Methods

1. Directly into the vein (See Guidelines: Venipuncture, p. 98)
2. Into IV tubing ("Push")
   a. As with venipuncture, aseptic technique is rigidly observed.
   b. The tubing is carefully swabbed with alcohol before it is punctured.
   c. Usually 10 cm. (up to 4 inches) is used for IV "push" medications.
3. Via "Piggyback" (See Guidelines: IV "Piggyback," p. 104)
4. Into a "heparin lock" (Butterfly-21 Abbott)
   a. This is similar to the "Butterfly" shown in Fig. 6-13.
   b. A winged needle is positioned in a vein; to the winged hub is attached a 9–10 cm. (3½ inch) length of plastic tubing.
   c. At the end of this short tubing is a permanently attached latex reseal injection site.
   d. This is used to inject medications or withdraw periodic blood samples.
       For indwelling needle sets or catheters for intermittent procedures, provision should be made for *heparinization* of the venipuncture set. If this is not done, there is risk of occlusion of the lumen due to accumulation of fibrinous material. Sufficient heparin is injected to fill the needle and tubing. After each drug administration, replace the heparinized saline.

GUIDELINES: Heparin Lock

Heparin lock is an intermittent infusion reservoir that permits administration of periodic intravenous medications/solutions without continuous fluid administration (Fig. 6-15).

Equipment   #21 gauge intermittent infusion reservoir, or catheter infusion device
Foil-wrapped alcohol sponges or iodine-based antiseptic
Rubber tourniquet
Antimicrobial ointment
2 × 2-inch gauze squares
½-inch tape
Tuberculin syringe containing prescribed 0.5 ml. heparin solution (100 U./ml.) or other prescribed amount of heparin.
One 6-ml. syringe containing normal saline with #25 gauge needle.

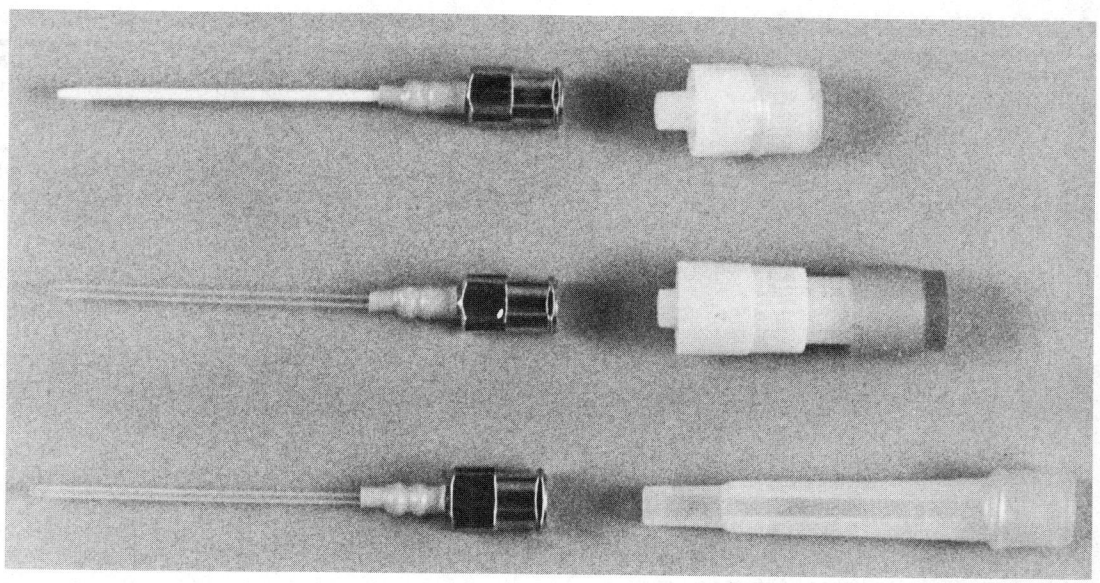

FIGURE 6-15. *Heparin lock. Several types of adaptor plugs that can be used to convert a standard over-the-needle cannula into a heparin lock. (From Sager DP and Bomar SK. Intravenous Medications, Philadelphia, JB Lippincott Co., 1980)*

Procedure

NURSING ACTION	RATIONALE/AMPLIFICATION
1. Explain nature and purpose of heparin lock to patient.	1. His understanding will facilitate proper functioning of the lock.

2. Follow Guidelines: Use of Winged Infusion Set, p. 103, using #21 gauge intermittent infusion reservoir:
  a: Prepare selected site for infusion reservoir as described on p. 98 in Guidelines: Venipuncture.
  b. Apply tourniquet to patient's arm.	

3. Cleanse rubber injection port of heparin lock.	3. Firmly rub using alcohol sponge.
4. Insert #25 gauge needle of syringe containing normal saline into injection port.	4. Small-gauge needle will prevent large puncture openings.
5. Hold wing-tip end higher than syringe and needle; flush reservoir with 1 ml. normal saline.	5. This will release air bubble from reservoir.
6. Perform venipuncture as described on p. 98 (Guidelines: Venipuncture).	
7. After confirming the position of the needle in the vein, secure wings with adhesive.	7. Carefully aspirate blood to verify needle position.
8. Inject 2 ml. of normal saline.	8. Observe site for evidence of infiltration.
9. Remove saline syringe with needle from injection port.	9. Continue to observe site for evidence of infiltration.
10. Apply antimicrobial ointment to insertion site; cover with 2 × 2-inch gauze square; secure with ½-inch tape.	10. To reduce possibility of infection.
11. Replace with needle and syringe containing heparin-holding solution.	11. Strict asepsis is observed in making this switch.
12. Inject 0.5 ml. heparinized saline (or other prescribed dose).	12. Heparin solution will keep the line open for the next injection.
13. Remove needle and syringe from injection port.	

To Administer Medication

1. Prepare the medication to be administered by drawing it into the appropriate syringe.	
2. Draw 4 ml. of normal saline into another syringe.	2. 2 ml. of normal saline will be used to flush the reservoir before and after the prescribed medication.
3. Draw 0.5 ml. of heparinized saline into a tuberculin syringe.	
4. Explain to the patient what are you about to do.	

GUIDELINES: Heparin Lock (cont.)

Procedure (cont.)

NURSING ACTION	RATIONALE/AMPLIFICATION
5. Cleanse injection port of the heparin lock with alcohol. Insert normal saline syringe needle into port and aspirate slightly.	5. This is done to determine that infusion needle is in the vein; aspirated blood will be evident.
6. Inject normal saline to flush reservoir of heparinized saline.	6. Note any signs of inflammation or infiltration; also observe patient for signs of discomfort. If such signs are present, discontinue injection.
7. Detach syringe from needle; attach medication syringe to needle and administer drug.	7. Keep syringe sterile between flushings by capping with a sterile needle.
8. Detach medication syringe; reattach saline syringe to flush reservoir.	8. Saline will clear the reservoir of medication and prepare the way for heparinized saline.
9. Detach saline syringe and reattach tuberculin syringe; inject 0.5 ml. heparinized saline into reservoir.	9. This will keep lock patent until it is time for the next dose of medication.
10. Remove heparin syringe and needle from injection port.	10. Treatment is completed.

Follow-up Phase

NURSING ACTION	RATIONALE/AMPLIFICATION
1. Check patency of heparin lock every 8–12 hours by aspirating and flushing with 3 ml. of normal saline.	1. This is done when medications are not given frequently via the lock.
2. Refill lock with 0.5 ml. of heparinized saline.	
3. Record all actions and medications.	
4. Heparin lock should not be left in place longer than 48 hours.	7. To do so enhances risk of infection.

Discontinuance of Heparin Lock

If patient is no longer
1. receiving antibiotics, heparin, chemotherapeutic agents, ACTH
2. receiving blood transfusion or blood derivatives
3. on telemetry

MANUAL FLOW RATE REGULATORS

Types

1. *Screw or Roller*—These are the most common types of devices used to control rate of fluid flow.
The roller clamp is easier to adjust with one hand.
NOTE: Slide clamps come with some sets but are not to be used to control rate; these are used to stop flow temporarily when changing container.
Many factors affect flow rate; even the best of these manual devices produce inaccurate and inconsistent rates.
2. *Dial-a-Flo®, Master IV Dial Lock™*—Simple devices allowing greater accuracy in regulating gravity-fed infusions; can be set to regulate flow between 5 and 250 ml./hr.
Advantages:
   a. More consistent than screw, or roller clamp.
   b. Economical and simple.
Disadvantages:
   a. Limited to standard solutions.
   b. Cannot be used with very viscous fluids such as blood and TPN solutions.

ELECTRONIC FLOW RATE REGULATORS

Types

1. *Controller*—An electronic device that is mechanically simpler than the pump (described next); it regulates by electronically monitoring drop rate* or regulating fluid passage by a magnetically activated metal ball valve.**

   * IVAC 230, IVAC Corporation, LaJolla, California 92038
   ** Epic 100, Burton Medical Products, Bethlehem, Pennsylvania 18018

Advantages:
   a. More accurate than nonelectronic regulators.
   b. Simpler than pumps, easily assembled and maintained.
   c. Takes care of a wide range of fluid and medication needs of patients.
2. *Infusion Pump*—An electronic device that exerts pressure (1) on tubing, or (2) on fluid.
By pumping against pressure gradients, a constant, accurate, and preselected fluid rate and volume can be maintained.
Types:
   a. Peristaltic—Moves fluid by exerting externally applied forces on tubing.
      (1) Linear   (2) Rotary
   b. Piston–cylinder—Exerts pressure on fluid in a cylinder by pumping action of a piston.
   c. Syringe—A motor-driven device in which plunger is depressed at a constant preset rate to eject medication.
   d. Volumetric—A device that uses the piston–cylinder principle. Chief advantage is that most models will not pump air (a safeguard against air emboli).

Advantages of Electronic Flow Rate Regulators

1. Ability to infuse large volumes of fluid (usually through a micropore filter).
2. Usually an alarm warns of problems.
3. Can be used with any type container.
4. Can be used for intra-arterial infusions.
5. Reduces complications: restarts, infiltration, "runaways."

Disadvantages of Electronic Flow Rate Regulators

1. Cost is high; however, studies (Rapp et al) have demonstrated that not only are these devices cost-

effective, but complications (such as infiltration, post-infusion phlebitis, and the necessity for infusion restarts) are reduced significantly.
2. Requires special tubing.
3. Requires more inservice time.

Indications for Use of Controlled Infusions

1. Intra-arterial infusions.
2. Critical care fluid and medication management.
3. Forcing fluids—TPN, enteral alimentation.
4. Closed wound irrigation.
5. Antacid titration via nasogastric tube.
6. Continuous heparin administration.
7. Minute doses of medications for systemic use.
8. Chemotherapy and oxytocic drugs.
9. Regional arterial perfusion.
10. Antiarrhythmic drugs; pressor agents.
11. Bronchoactive and hypoglycemic agents.

Considerations When Selecting Infusion Devices

(Also see Pediatric Techniques, Infusion Pumps p. 78.)
1. Cost vs. budget.
2. Specific needs of institution.
3. Inservice facilities.

COMPLICATIONS OF INTRAVENOUS THERAPY

Infection

A local reaction due to contamination; this may spread systemically.
1. Causes (Fig. 6-16)
   a. Fluid contamination; this may be due to faulty preparation, crack in flask, puncture in plastic container, fluid additives.

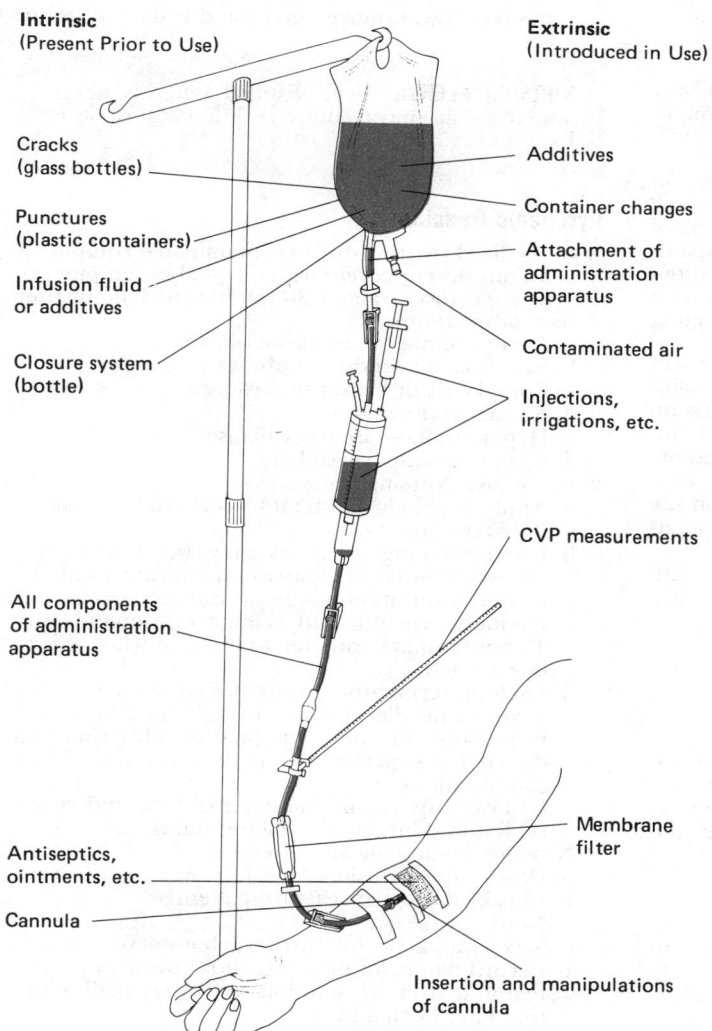

Intrinsic (Present Prior to Use)

Cracks (glass bottles)

Punctures (plastic containers)

Infusion fluid or additives

Closure system (bottle)

All components of administration apparatus

Antiseptics, ointments, etc.

Cannula

Extrinsic (Introduced in Use)

Additives

Container changes

Attachment of administration apparatus

Contaminated air

Injections, irrigations, etc.

CVP measurements

Membrane filter

Insertion and manipulations of cannula

FIGURE 6-16. *Potential mechanisms for contamination of IV infusion systems. (Maki DG. Preventing infection in intravenous therapy. Hospital Practice)*

b. The longer the IV catheter is left in the patient, the greater is the risk of infection.

c. Failure to cleanse skin rigorously—to remove dead skin, dirt, mucus, etc., before applying antiseptic agent to infusion site.

d. Failure to wash hands thoroughly before and after every patient contact by hospital personnel.

e. Use of contaminated hand lotion following hand washing by personnel coming in contact with patient.

f. May be transmitted within the patient from another infected part of his body to the catheter site.

g. The practice of irrigating or otherwise manipulating an occluded, leaking, or infiltrated catheter may provide the opportunity for introducing contaminants.

2. Preventive Nursing Measures

a. Practice rigid aseptic technique in starting an infusion; use sterile disposable gloves and consider the procedure a minor operation.

b. Thoroughly cleanse the infusion site; follow this with an iodine-base antiseptic.

c. Avoid the use of aqueous benzalkonium chlorides since they have been demonstrated to be ineffective against some gram-negative organisms, especially *Pseudomonas*.

d. Take care to anchor the catheter/cannula firmly in order to prevent excessive movement that might traumatize the cannulated vein and possibly facilitate entry of organisms at infusion site.

e. Record date of catheter or cannula insertion on patient's chart and also near dressing. This will serve to indicate how long the set has been in place and when it should be replaced. (1) In hospitals with low rates of intravenous contamination, changing administration sets every 48 hours is an acceptable policy (no benefits result from changing administration sets every 24 hours).

f. Check (daily) the cannulated vein by gentle palpation to detect evidence of tenderness or pain; note any unexplained fever. If these are present, remove dressings and examine for signs of inflammation. Discontinue infusion if they are present.

g. Apply antimicrobial ointment (containing neomycin, bacitracin, and polymyxin) to infusion site at time of insertion and at periodic intervals thereafter.

h. The use of winged (scalp-vein) needles with smaller bores appears to be associated with less infection than use of plastic catheters.

Mechanical Failures

(Solution flow slowing down or stopping, etc.)

1. Causes

a. Needle may be lying against the side of the vein, cutting off fluid flow. (Patient may have moved his arm.)

b. Level of intravenous receptacle may change rate of flow (gravity):
(1) Higher—more rapid
(2) Lower—less rapid

c. Needle may be clogged due to clotting.

d. Regulator of flow rate may be faulty; the clamp with a tapered v-shaped groove seems to provide greater dependability than the regular clamp.

2. Nursing Assessment and Approach

a. Note whether there is swelling at needle site; if edema is present, it suggests infiltration (see below).

b. Remove tape and check for kinking of tubing.

c. Rotate needle slightly—the bevel of the needle may be lying against wall of vein.

d. Move the patient's arm to a new position.

e. Elevate or lower needle to prevent occlusion of bevel of needle; if necessary to maintain a slightly different position use a gauze pad or cotton ball as a prop and maintain position by placing a few adhesive straps.

f. Try pulling the needle or catheter back a short distance since it may be occluded at a bifurcation.

g. Check patency of needle by lowering the receptacle below level of needle; a flashback of blood from the patient into the intravenous tubing indicates patency.

h. Never flush out a cannula or needle by injecting sterile saline with a syringe and needle directly into tubing since it may force a blood clot into circulation.

i. If none of the preceding steps produces the desired flow, remove needle and restart infusion.

NURSING ALERT: Sterile distilled water is never added to an intravenous set-up because it is hypotonic.

Pyrogenic Reaction

A generalized reaction due to contaminated equipment or solutions (less apparent with disposable equipment).

1. Symptoms (occur about 30 minutes to 1 hour after start of infusion)

a. Abrupt temperature elevation, chills

b. Face flushing, sudden pulse rate change

c. Complaints of backache, headache

d. Nausea and vomiting

e. Hypotension—vascular collapse

f. Cyanosis—vascular collapse

2. Preventive Nursing Measures

a. Apply antibiotic ointment to skin where needle or catheter enters.

b. Use indwelling catheters only when absolutely necessary; infection increases significantly with the length of duration of venous catheterization.

c. For long-term infusions, change infusion site every 48 hours; mark catheter to indicate when it is to be changed.

d. For long-term catheterization, a larger needle (i.e., a No. 14 needle with No. 16 catheter 20 cm. or 8 inches long) in external jugular or subclavian vein directed to superior vena cava seems to minimize complications.
(1) Less disparity in diameters of tube and vessel
(2) Rapid dilution of irritating fluids

3. Nursing Treatment Measures

a. Discontinue infusion.

b. Check vital signs; reassure patient.

c. Notify physician.

d. Save equipment for further laboratory study.

e. Record name, lot number, and information—i.e., manufacturer of solution and any medications that have been added.

Infiltration

Dislodging of needle will cause fluid to infiltrate tissues.
1. Symptoms at Site
   a. Edema, blanching of skin—also check undersurface of arm for puffiness.
   b. Discomfort, depending on nature of solution.
   c. Fluid flows more slowly or stops.
   d. Note temperature of skin; since solution is much cooler than patient, infiltration site will feel cool to touch.
   e. With a vasoconstrictor, such as norepinephrine (Levophed), infiltration can cause serious injury leading to necrosis and sloughing of tissues.
2. Preventive Nursing Measures
   a. Fasten needle securely.
   b. Limit arm movement by splinting properly.
   c. Check tubing for kinking.
   d. Avoid looping of tubing below bed level.
3. Nursing Treatment Measures
   a. Stop infusion.
   b. Notify intravenous therapist, physician, etc.
   c. Place a sterile 3 × 3-inch gauze pad over needle and vein; withdraw needle and apply firm pressure over venipunture site for several minutes.
   d. Apply warm compresses to increase fluid absorption.
   e. Restart infusion elsewhere.
   f. Use plastic cannula to reduce trauma when site is moved.
   g. If norepinephrine (Levophed) was used:
      (1) Notify physician of infiltration.
      (2) Prepare antidote—phentolamine (Regitine). When this is injected liberally into site, tissue necrosis and sloughing may be prevented.

Circulatory Overload

Patient receives an excessive amount of solution (happens more frequently in elderly patients or in infants).
1. Symptoms
   a. Headache, flushed skin, rapid pulse
   b. Venous distention
   c. Increased blood pressure
   d. Increased venous pressure
   e. Coughing, shortness of breath, increased respirations
   f. Syncope, shock
   g. Pulmonary edema leading to dyspnea and cyanosis
2. Preventive Nursing Measures
   a. Know whether patient has existing heart condition—more prone to develop acute pulmonary edema.
   b. Monitor solution flow.
   c. Place patient in semi-sitting position during infusion.
   d. Be especially attentive to the elderly or the infant.
3. Nursing Treatment Measures
   a. Stop the infusion; notify physician.
   b. Raise patient to sitting position—will ease the breathing problem.

Drug Overload

Patient receives an excessive amount of fluid containing drugs.
1. Toxic concentrations of drug are collected in main organs: brain and heart.

2. Symptoms
   a. Dizziness, fainting leading to shock.
   b Specific symptoms related to the offending drug.
3. Preventive Nursing Measures—monitor flow rate carefully.
4. Nursing Treatment—related to the nature of the medication.

Superficial Thrombophlebitis

1. Causes
   a. Overuse of a vein, which may cause vasospasm; this may lead to an inflammatory process.
   b. Irritating infusion solution (strong acids or alkalies, hypertonic glucose solutions, and certain drugs such as cytotoxic agents, methacillin, barbiturates).
   c. Clot formation in an inflamed vein.
   d. Anatomic location—veins of the lower extremity (relatively sluggish blood flow) are more vulnerable than cephalad vessels.
   e. Length of time the cannula is in place—the longer the cannulation, the greater the possibility of infection.
   f. Polyvinylchloride catheters appear to be associated with infection more often than steel needles.
   g. Catheter diameter; large-bore catheters are more often associated with phlebitis than small-bore.
2. Symptoms
   a. Tenderness at first, then pain along course of the vein
   b. Edema and redness at injection site
   c. Arm feels warmer than other arm
3. Preventive Nursing Measures
   a. When cephalothin is to be given for several days via infusion, change veins used.
   b. Add a small volume (20 ml.) of sterile 1% sodium bicarbonate* immediately prior to infusion to raise pH level to an acceptable level (on physician's prescription).
4. Nursing Treatment Measures
   a. Apply cold compresses immediately to relieve pain and inflammation.
   b. Later follow with moist warm compresses to stimulate circulation and promote absorption.

Air Embolism

Air manages to get into the circulatory system.

NURSING ALERT: Recognize the high possibility of air embolism when a physician pumps in blood (e.g., 500 ml.—1 pint in 10 minutes) since this builds high pressure in blood receptacle.

1. Symptoms
   a. Hypotension, cyanosis, tachycardia
   b. Increased venous pressure, loss of consciousness
2. Nursing Preventive Measures
   a. Replace initial bottle before it is completely empty with a fresh, full bottle; check attachment to be certain it is tight.

* Pederson BM. A solution for post-infusion thrombophlebitis. Am J Nurs 1970 Feb; 70:325.

b. In "Y" type sets, tightly clamp the nearly empty bottle to prevent air from being sucked into the tubing.
c. Allow fluid to flow through tubing and needle or catheter to force air out—before starting infusion.

3. Nursing Treatment Measures
Unless prompt action is taken, patient may die within minutes.
a. *Immediately* turn patient on left side with head down—air will rise into right ventricle and allow blood to pass into the lungs. The trapped air will be slowly dissipated through pulmonary system.
b. Administer oxygen.

Nerve Damage

May result from tying the arm too tightly to the splint.
1. Symptoms
   Numbness of fingers or hands.
2. Nursing Preventive Measures
   Place padding around arm where bandage is to be applied.
3. Nursing Treatment Measures
   a. Massage arm and move shoulder through its range of motion.
   b. Instruct patient to open and close hand several times each hour.
   c. Physical therapy may be required.

CARE OF THE WOUND

A *wound* is an injury to the tissues of the body causing disruption of the normal tissue pattern; such an injury is caused by physical means.

Classification

According to the manner in which it is made
Incised—made by a clean cut with a sharp instrument; e.g., a surgeon's incision with a scalpel.
Contused—made by blunt force, which does not break through the skin but causes considerable soft tissue damage; e.g., a rock when thrown bruises a person.
Lacerated—made by an object which tears tissues, producing jagged irregular edges; e.g., blunt knife, jagged wire, glass.
Puncture—made by a pointed instrument, such as an ice pick, bullet, knife stab, nail.

Surgical Classification

Clean—an aseptically made wound, as in surgery, in which all bleeding vessels have been ligated (tied).
Contaminated—exposed to excessive amounts of bacteria; e.g., unprepared colon surgery, dirty laceration. These wounds are not grossly infected but have been exposed to bacteria (contaminated) and have higher risk of infection.
Infected—a wound which may not be closed may contain devitalized or infected material.
Debridement—the process whereby devitalized or necrotic tissue is cut out and flushed clean with saline solution.

Physiology of Wound Healing

A. *First Intention Healing (Primary Union)*

Healing which takes place aseptically with a minimum of tissue damage and tissue reaction; this is the ideal sought by the surgical staff; surgically closed (sutures or surgical tapes).

B. *Second Intention Healing (Granulation)*

Wounds which are left open to heal spontaneously; not surgically closed. They need not be infected.
1. If infected, pus forms; drainage is accomplished by incision and perhaps insertion of drains.
2. Necrotic material disintegrates and sloughs off.
3. Cavity fills with a red, soft, sensitive tissue which bleeds easily.
4. Buds, called granulation tissue, enlarge to fill area formerly destroyed and thus form a scar (cicatrix).

C. *Third Intention Healing (Secondary Suture)*

1. Occurs when a wound breaks down and is resutured or when a wound has been kept open and fills with granulation tissue and then is closed with sutures (2 faces of granulation tissue are brought together in apposition).
2. Scar tissue formation is deeper, wider, and more pronounced.

Assessment of Factors that Affect Wound Healing

1. What type of surgery did patient have?
2. Where is the wound? How extensive?
   a. Was hemostasis in the operating room effective?
   b. What is nature of vascularity? e.g., adequate blood supply
   c. Evidence of edema? Inflammation?
3. How is the wound held together?
   a. butterfly tapes, wire sutures, tension sutures, clips?
4. Are there drains in place? What kind? How many? Portable suction?
5. What kinds of dressings are being used?
   a. Are they saturated with exudate?
   b. Is drainage consistent with nature of surgery?
6. How does the patient appear?
   a. Signs or complaints of wound pain or discomfort? Fever?
7. How old is the patient?
   a. What is his nutritional status?
   b. Has his intake of protein and vitamin C been adequate? (These are needed for wound healing.)
8. Was he given packed cells to maintain adequate levels of red blood cells?
9. What conditions does patient have, and what medications is he taking that could affect wound healing?
   a. Check his medications—steroids, etc.
   b. Note all listed diagnoses—diabetes mellitus, etc.
10. How long has patient been in the hospital preoperatively?
    (Longer preoperative hospitalization increases risk of nosocomial infections.)

The Purpose of Dressings

1. To protect the wound from mechanical injury.
2. To splint or immobilize the wound (Fig. 6-17).
3. To absorb drainage and fluid wastes.
4. To promote homeostasis and minimize accumulation of fluid, as in a pressure dressing.
5. To prevent contamination from bodily discharges.
6. To provide physical and psychological comfort for the patient as well as a physiological environment conducive to wound healing.
7. To debride a wound by combining capillary action and the entwining of necrotic tissue within its mesh.
8. To inhibit or kill organisms by using dressings that contain antiseptic medications.
9. To support a fractured or reconstructed area.
10. To provide information about the nature of the underlying wound.

Wound Healing Without Dressings

Preferred by some surgeons; may be desirable for a simple, clean wound.

A. *Advantages*

1. Permits better observation and early detection of problems.
2. Promotes cleanliness and facilitates bathing.
3. Eliminates conditions necessary for growth of organisms.
   a. Warmth
   b. Moisture
   c. Darkness
4. Avoids adhesive tape reaction.
5. Facilitates patient activity.
6. Is economical.

B. *Disadvantages*

1. Psychologically, a patient may object to an exposed wound.
2. Wound is more vulnerable to injury.
3. Bedding and clothing may catch on stitches.

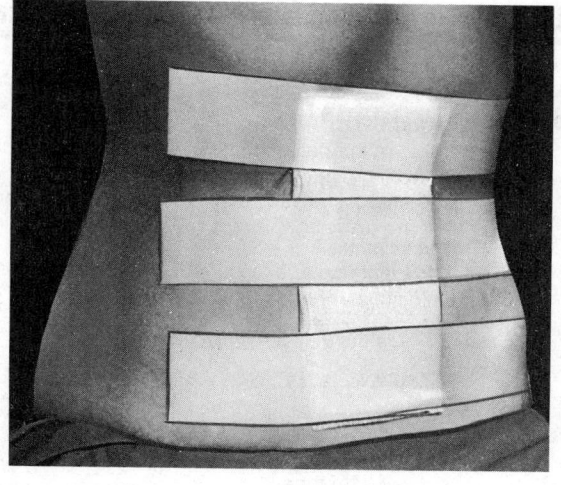

FIGURE 6-17. *Laparotomy dressings. Laparotomy dressings are of many types, depending on the nature of the operation; the most frequent use of adhesive tape on the abdomen is in the application of postoperative dressings.*
For the ordinary laparotomy, 5 or 8 cm (2" or 3") wide strips of adhesive tape are usually applied transversely in close arrangement over the dressing; the ends of these strips should extend at least to the midaxillary line in order to provide good support and fixation. The illustration shows an effective method of securing a standard abdominal dressing.
Some surgeons cover the dressing solidly with adhesive tape, but others question this practice on the grounds that it interferes with transpiration of water vapor from the area around the wound and thus may produce maceration and aid in the development of infection. (© Johnson & Johnson. Used by special permission of Johnson & Johnson, the copyright owners, and not to be reproduced for any purpose without Johnson & Johnson's permission.)

GUIDELINES: Assisting with a Change of Surgical Dressings

Surgical Dressing Technique

The procedure of changing dressings, examining and cleansing the wound, utilizing principles of asepsis.
1. A team works together to change a patient's dressing—nurse with surgeon or nurse with a colleague.
2. The condition of the wound is noted in order to better understand the nature of the patient's surgical recovery.
3. The healing process is facilitated by keeping the wound clean.
4. Stitches or clips are removed after the 5th or 6th day since wound edges have begun to knit together.

Equipment   *Sterile*

Gloves—disposable
Pack containing scissors, forceps, grooved director, dressings, cotton tipped swabs, solution cup
Antiseptic solution, sterile saline
Culture tubes
For draining wound: add sterile safety pin, packing, irrigation set

Unsterile

Plastic bag for discarded dressings
Adhesive, proper size
Pads to protect patient's bed
Gown for nurse, if wound is purulent

GUIDELINES: Assisting with a Change of Surgical Dressings (cont.)

Procedure   *Preparatory Phase*

1. Inform the patient that his dressing is to be changed. Explain procedure to him. Have him lie in bed.
2. Avoid changing dressings at mealtime.
3. Ensure his privacy by drawing the curtains or closing the door; expose the dressing site.
4. If the dressings have a foul odor, perhaps they can be changed in a separate treatment area that is adequately ventilated.
5. Prevent undue exposure of the patient; respect his modesty and prevent him from being chilled.
6. Wash your hands thoroughly; this should be done before and after each patient.

NURSING ACTION	RATIONALE/AMPLIFICATION
REMOVING ADHESIVE TAPE	
1. Remove tape along longitudinal axis, slowly and gently.	1. Removing tape in same plane is less injurious and less painful.
2. Peel back edges by holding skin taut and pushing away from tape.	2. It is less traumatic to push skin away from tape than to pull tape from skin.
3. Remove tape near a wound by pulling toward the wound.	3. Pulling away from a wound may tear some of the delicate newly formed tissues.
4. Using a suitable solvent such as baby oil if the tape does not pull away easily.	4. Oil is safe, works as well as true solvents, and, in addition, lubricates and soothes the sensitive skin beneath.
REMOVING OLD DRESSING	
Method A (Using disposable gloves)	
1. Don sterile disposable gloves; remove top dressings carefully and discard into plastic bag.	1. Dressings are not to be handled by ungloved hands because of the possibility of transmitting pathogenic organisms.
2. Gradually loosen last dressing and observe skin and wound site.	2. If dressings adhere, moisten them with sterile saline and slowly withdraw dressing.
3. Remove and discard disposable gloves into plastic bag.	3. This will go to the incinerator later.
Method B (Using a sterile plastic bag)	
1. After washing hands, open package containing sterile plastic bag.	1. Bag should extend several centimeters (inches) above wrist.
2. Put right hand into sterile bag being careful not to touch outside of bag (this bag acts as a sterile glove).	2. Bag acts as a glove to protect hand from the dressings.
3. Pick up all soiled dressings as above and hold them in right hand; use left hand to grasp top edge of bag and pull it down over the hand and dressings.	3. This encloses soiled dressings in a plastic container; this bag can be used to receive soiled cotton balls or dressings used to clean wound.

CLEANSING THE SIMPLE WOUND AND OBTAINING A WOUND CULTURE

ASSISTANT NURSE	NURSE OR SURGEON	RATIONALE
1. Use aseptic technique		1. To prevent contamination of a clean wound or to prevent further contamination of a "dirty" wound. Also to prevent transmission of pathogenic organisms to clean areas.
2. Open sterile package of gloves.	2. Don sterile gloves.	
3. Open package containing sterile syringe and needle.	3. Aspirate generous amount of liquid material into syringe; inject into anaerobic tube.	3. Collect specimen before wound is cleansed to obtain true sample of microorganisms present.
4. If liquid material is not obtainable, use cotton applicator swab.	4. Swab desired area attempting to get maximum saturation of cotton applicator with tissue fluid.	4. Used when there is insufficient liquid material to aspirate with a syringe.
5. Receive specimen and see that it gets to the laboratory.		
6. Open a sterile pack containing a scissors, forceps, a grooved director, dressings, and solution container.	6. Pick up dressing with forceps and hold it over emesis basin.	

ASSISTANT NURSE	NURSE OR SURGEON	RATIONALE
7. Pour antiseptic solution over dressing.	7. Clean wound gently but thoroughly.	
	8. Use forceps to pick up each stitch, cut with scissors and pull stitch out. Deposit in emesis basin or on a sterile gauze square.	8. After 5th or 6th day, stitches serve no useful purpose. If they remain in place, they can act as wicks carrying pathogenic organisms from the skin.

COMPLETION OF DRESSING

1. Select proper size and type of adhesive for securing dressing; rubber-based or acrylate adhesive.	1. Place minimal dressing over wound.	1. *Rubber-base* (cloth-backed or plastic-backed) dressing used principally for heavy support and where a high level of adhesion is required. *Acrylate* (nonwoven or fabric backing) usually used for surgical taping because of hypoallergenic quality.
2. A thin layer of "Skin Prep" may be applied.	2. This is sprayed on area before tape is applied.	2. This enhances sticking of tape.
3. Apply minimum amount of taping necessary to keep dressing in place (Fig. 6-18).	3. Remove gloves and complete dressing fixation with adhesive.	
4. Avoid placing adhesive in areas where sweat glands are numerous.		4. Adhesive does not adhere easily; when it is removed it is more traumatizing.

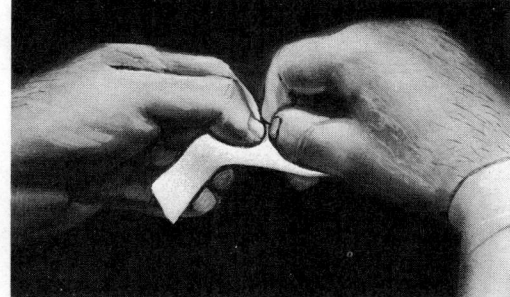 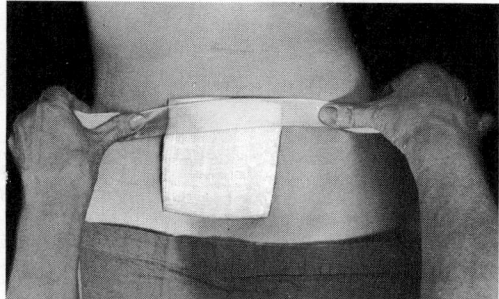

FIGURE 6-18. *Applying tape. When scissors are not at hand, adhesive tape can be readily torn by holding the strip of tape between the thumbnail and forefingers, as illustrated. Tearing is started by a quick rotary twist of the hands in opposite directions.*
To avoid undue traction on the skin beneath adhesive tape, thus lessening trauma and reducing the possibility of irritation, place tape on the dressing and affix to the skin on either side so that tension is applied evenly away from the midline of the dressing. (© Johnson & Johnson. Used by special permission of Johnson & Johnson, the copyright owners, and not to be reproduced for any purpose without Johnson & Johnson's permission.)

NURSING ACTION	RATIONALE/AMPLIFICATION
FOLLOW-UP CARE	
1. Make patient comfortable.	
2. Remove emesis basin and dispose of soiled dressings in proper receptacle. Discard disposable items and clean equipment which is to be reused.	2. To prevent transmission of pathogenic organisms.
3. Record nature of procedure and condition of wound as well as patient reaction.	

GUIDELINES: Dressing a Draining Wound

Reinforcement of Dressings

Draining wounds may require frequent changes of dressings.

Outer layers may be removed and fresh dressings applied without disturbing wound site.
   a. Saturated dressings cause discomfort to the patient.
   b. Dressing edges may become dry, hard, and scratchy.
   c. Odor may be unpleasant.

Auxiliary Aids to Facilitate Dressing Changes

Montgomery Straps

Strips of adhesive tape, the edges of which have been folded back for a short distance with a small hole cut in the folded portion and threaded with gauze strips or cotton tape. Two opposing strips are brought together and the tapes tied (Fig. 6-19).

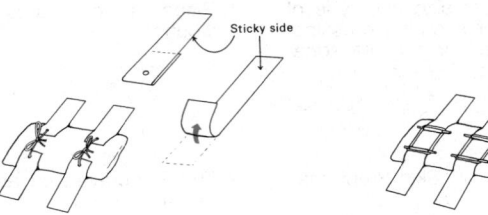

FIGURE 6-19. *Montgomery straps; two styles are shown.*

Scultetus Binder

A many-tailed binder which when applied snugly (starting at the lower end) produces a comfortable and conforming support for the patient (Fig. 6-20).

The binder should be placed low enough on abdomen to provide abdominal support without impeding respiration.

Commercially available wound drainage systems (such as Hollister, Squibb) are also available.

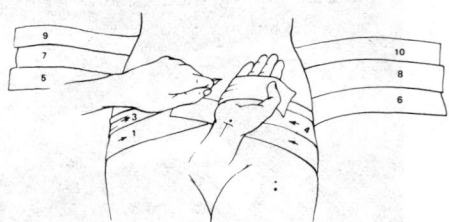

FIGURE 6-20. *Procedure for applying a many-tailed binder. (From Fuerst EV and Wolff L. Fundamentals of Nursing, 6th ed. Philadelphia, JB Lippincott Co.)*

Removal of Adherent Dressings

1. To prevent the discomfort of removing dry, sticking dressings, moisten the dressing with sterile saline or hydrogen peroxide using an asepto bulb syringe.
2. Provide an emesis basin to catch excess fluid.

Anchoring and Gradual Withdrawal of Drainage Tubes

1. With each dressing change, the drainage tube is often pulled out of the wound a few centimeters and the excess tube is cut.
2. Hollow hard rubber or polyethylene tubes are used occasionally to drain a cavity. After the tube is anchored with a suture, the tube is taped to the skin.
   a. Cut a 5-cm. (2-inch) length of adhesive tape; trifurcate the tape lengthwise to the middle.
   b. Place right half of tape on skin up to emerging rubber drain; allow 2 end tails to straddle tube and neatly fasten middle tail around drain in a spiral fashion.
   c. Repeat process in opposite direction. Then place 2 cross strips of 5-cm (2-inch) adhesive tape on either side of drain.

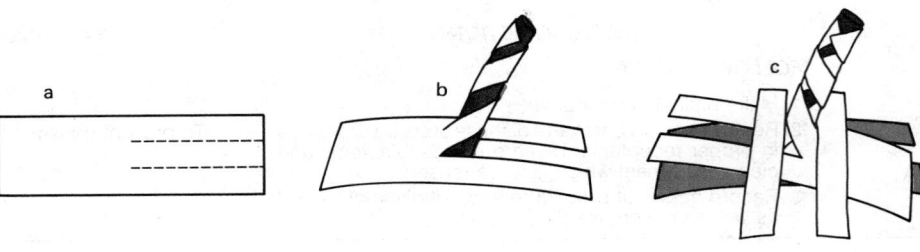

3. Penrose tube with a safety pin or a Taut "Safety Klip".

For the drain, such as a penrose, which is drawn out of the wound a few centimeters each day, a safety pin or Taut "Safety Klip" is positioned to prevent the drainage tube from slipping back into the wound (see Fig. 6-21).

Pin or clip should be placed in its new position *prior* to cutting the drain.

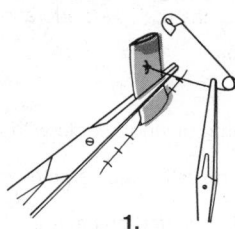

1.

Grasp pin with a hemostat, and the drain with a dressings forceps or another hemostat. Insert pin into drain distal to where it is being held by forceps.

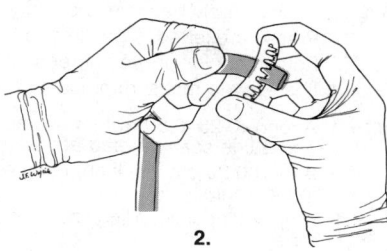

2.

Bend Taut sterile "Safety Klip" to spread teeth. Push drain through opened teeth.

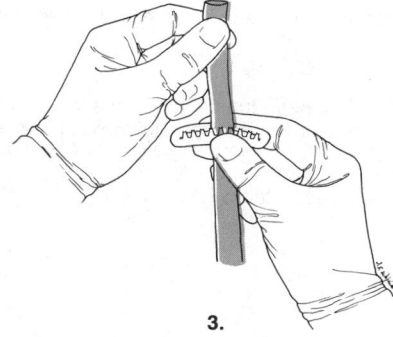

3.

Pull drain through "Safety Klip" evenly to desired position.

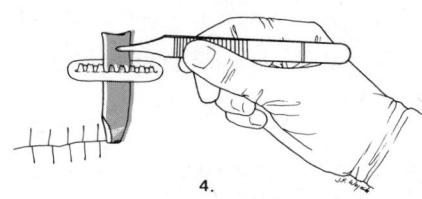

4.

Advance drain with a dressing forceps.

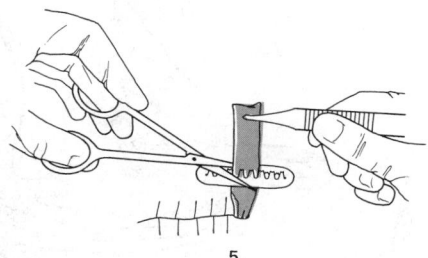

5.

Using opened surgical scissors, slide down "Safety Klip." A dressing can be placed between "Klip" and wound.

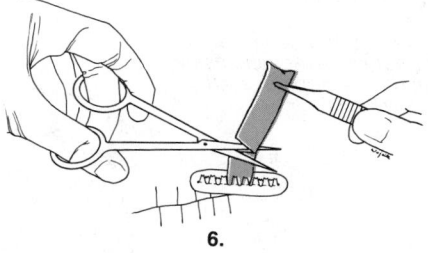

6.

Cut excess drain.

FIGURE 6-21. *Anchoring a drainage tube with a safety pin (1) or with a Taut "Safety Klip." (Courtesy Taut, Inc. for American Hospital Supply)*

Skin Care

1. Drainage is often irritating to surrounding skin tissues, particularly if it contains gastrointestinal secretions.
2. Apply protective ointment if prescribed (caution—ointments may cause maceration and may prevent drainage)
   a. Petrolatum gauze
   b. Zinc oxide ointment
   c. Stomahesive (by Squibb).
3. Recognize value of portable wound suction in maintaining cleanliness of surrounding tissues (see below).
4. Attach drainage tubing to suction bottle.
   Check tubing frequently for kinking or looping which would restrict flow of drainage.

GUIDELINES: Using Portable Wound Suction (HemoVac, Porto-Vac)

Portable wound suction is a suction system which gently removes adventitious fluid and debris from a wound by means of a perforated catheter connected to a portable suction apparatus.

Purpose   To speed healing of the wound by removing fluids that could retard tissue granulation and by exerting negative pressure which permits two layers of tissue to adhere and thus eliminates dead space.

Advantages   1. Tubing rarely becomes occluded because it is siliconized and has multiple perforations.
2. Pressure exerted is gentle and even; suction is quiet.
3. Equipment is lightweight, permitting patient to move easily.
4. It is easy to measure amount of wound drainage.

Equipment   1. A long (0.25–0.5 cm.) (⅛–¼ inch) malleable stainless steel introducing needle with a cutting edge on one end and a fine screw thread at the other.
2. A long 0.25 cm. (⅛ inch) calibre, siliconized, noncollapsible, polyethylene catheter with many small perforations in the center.
3. A noncollapsible, siliconized, polyethylene connecting tube. The wound catheter fits snugly into the lumen of this tube.
4. A vacuum source (evacuator) consisting of an unbreakable plastic container with rigid ends and collapsible sides (may be a size to collect 200, 400 or 800 ml. of fluid).
   Box has 1 cuffed hole into which the connecting tube fits snugly and an airhole supplied with a plug. This box may be of accordion-like collapsible plastic or it may have steel coil springs on the inside to hold the ends of the box apart.
5. A plastic Y-connector which fits between wound catheters and connecting tube and allows 2 wound tubes to be connected to 1 evacuator if desired.

Method of Inserting Drainage Tube(s)

1. In the operating room, the surgeon places the perforated drainage tubing in the desired wound area.
2. A stab wound is made with the needle and excess tubing is drawn through the wound (stab wound is preferred because a more tightly sealed porthole is created; if the wound opening is used, drainage may seep through the incision line).
3. Needle is cut off and tubing is attached via adaptor to evacuator tubing (Fig. 6-22).

FIGURE 6-22. A. *Two perforated catheters are draining the incisional area following a radical neck dissection. By means of a Y-tube, drainage is drawn into a portable wound suction receptacle. When full, open top plug of receptacle and empty.*
   B. To reestablish negative pressure, compress receptacle as indicated and replace plug; suction drainage will resume.

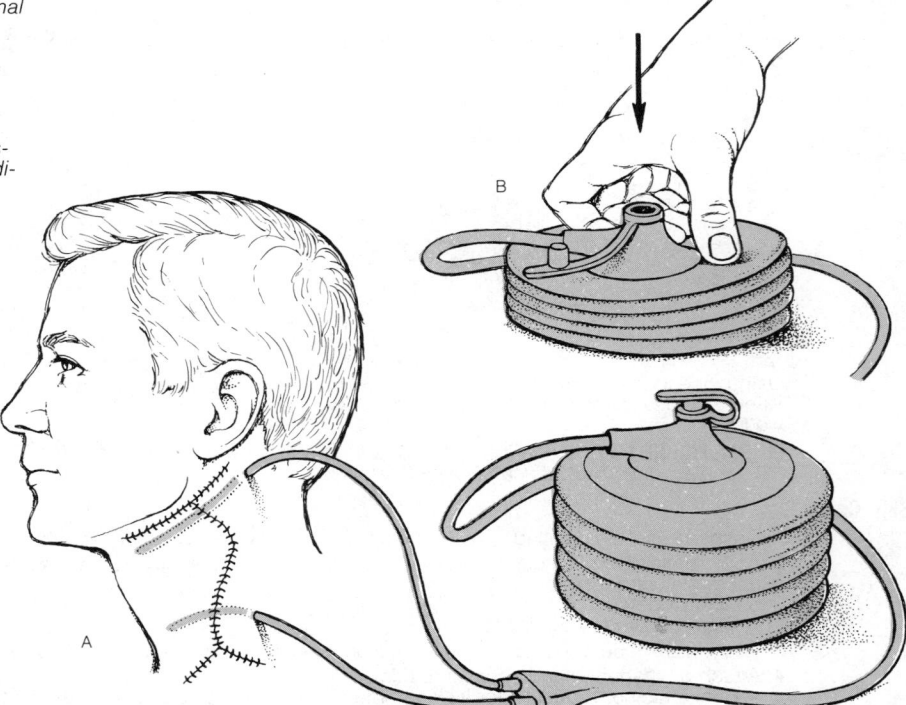

Method of Initiating Suction

NURSING ACTION	*RATIONALE/AMPLIFICATION*

1. Connect tubes to evacuator.
2. Squeeze ends of box together.
3. Plug air hole.
4. As spring expands, a negative pressure of approximately 45 mm. Hg is produced.

5. When evacuator is full (200, 400, or 800 ml.—depending on size of evacuator), it is time to empty. A good rule is to empty every 8 hours, or more frequently if necessary.

2. This will expel air.
3. To create a negative pressure.
4. Any fluid and blood in tissues is sucked into evacuator. Negative pressure is not great enough to suck the soft tissues into the holes of the catheters.
5. Negative pressure has been fully dissipated.

EMPTYING EVACUATOR

1. Carefully remove plug, maintaining its sterility.
2. Empty contents of evacuator into calibrated container.
3. Place evacuator on flat surface.
4. Cleanse opening as well as plug with an alcohol sponge.
5. Compress evacuator completely (Fig. 6-22).
6. Replace plug while evacuator is compressed.
7. Check system for proper operation.
8. Secure evacuator to bedding; if patient is ambulatory, fasten evacuator to his clothing.
9. Record character and amount of drainage.

2. Measure drainage.
3. To permit adequate compression.
4. To maintain cleanliness of outlet.

5. To remove air.
6. To reestablish negative pressure (suction).
7. Look for fluid entering receptacle.
8. This permits patient to move without disturbing closed suction.

Wound Irrigation Combined with Portable Wound Suction

1. Perforated wound tubes are placed side by side in wound (Fig. 6-23A). One is connected to irrigating fluid (or antibiotic solution), the other to portable wound suction.
2. At least 30% of the perforated section of one tube should be positioned parallel to the perforated area of the other.
3. If tubes are to remain for some time, a suture (usually stainless steel wire) is used (note arrow in Fig. 6-23B).
4. Having the drainage tube exit through a stab wound (away from main incision line) makes it convenient to manipulate, inspect, and remove the drainage tube without disturbing the wound dressing.
5. After drip fluid has been stopped, all remaining tubes should have suction applied for at least 48 hours.

Tube Removal

1. At conclusion of use, discard tubing and evacuator by placing in a paper bag and depositing in trash container for incineration.
2. See Guidelines: Assisting with a Change of Surgical Dressings (p. 113).

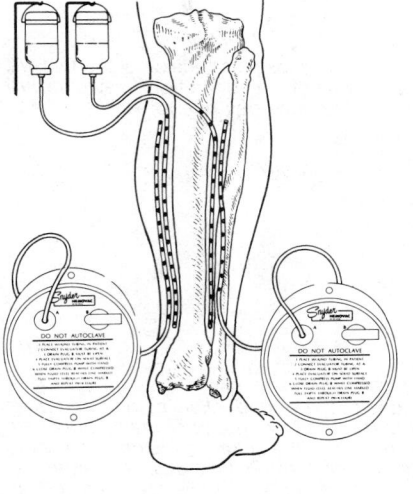
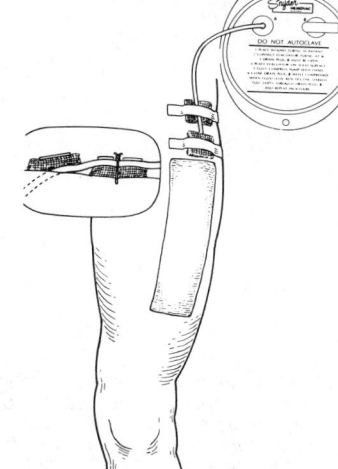

A   B

FIGURE 6-23. A. *An example of an efficient antibiotic drip and suction system. Note that the perforated wound tubes lie parallel to each other (intake and output).*
   B. *When drainage of long duration is anticipated, the wound-drainage tubing can be fixed (so that it will not slip out of the wound) by a stainless steel wire suture (size 40 or 50) as the magnified drawing indicates. The drainage tubing is cushioned on a pad of gauze. (Courtesy Zimmer, U.S.A., Warsaw, Ind)*

SUTURING

GUIDELINES: Suturing for Simple Wound Closure

Purpose   To close a small wound using nonabsorbable sutures such as black silk or dermal suture.

Equipment   Sterile gloves
Sterile suture set containing:
  Drape with aperture
  Needle holder for curved needles
  Needles: cutting edge—straight and/or curved
  Toothed forceps
  Scissors to cut sutures
  Suture material
  Dressings
Saline solution to cleanse suture line
Antiseptic solution or soap and water to cleanse area surrounding wound

Procedure

NURSING ACTION	RATIONALE/AMPLIFICATION
1. Thoroughly cleanse small wound using detergent-germicidal soap.	1. To remove foreign bodies, debris, crusted blood; to minimize the possibility of contamination.
2. Apply an antiseptic which will be nonirritating to exposed subcutaneous tissues.	2. To reduce microbial contamination.
3. Don sterile gloves and apply drape with opening centered over wound.	3. This will present a sterile field.
4. Usually a straight cutting edge-needle is preferable for suturing skin.	4. Less motion is required with a straight needle; if wound is deeper, a curved needle is more effective.

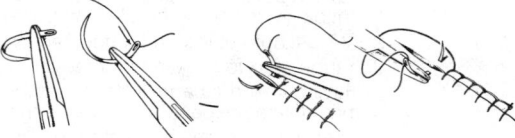

5. Thread needle with desired suture material. 37.5 cm. (15 inches) is a convenient suture length; when threaded, allow 30 cm. (12 inches) on one side of needle and 7.5 cm. (3 inches) on the other. A curved needle is threaded from inner curve outward. This method helps prevent suture from falling out of needle.	
6. Grasp wound edge gently with toothed forceps.	6. This will anchor tissue when needle is forced through.

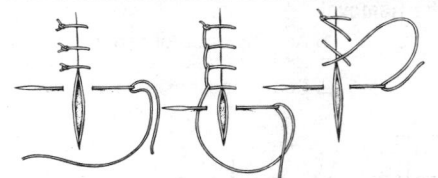

7. Stitches may be interrupted or continuous. Interrupted stitches are independent of each other; continuous sutures are applied more rapidly but if there is a break in the suture line, the entire wound is affected. Figure shows straight cutting edge needle, which is held by gloved fingers (not in needle holder).	
8. Space stitches evenly; tie a square knot (Fig. 6-24, p. 121). *Tissues need only be approximated.*	8. Do not tie knots with excess tension since this will traumatize the wound. If tied too tightly, stitches will be even tighter the next day due to edema.

FIGURE 6-24. *(1) After the suture is drawn through both sides of the wound, allow a short end of suture to remain. (2) Remove curved needle from holder and with the long end of the suture make a loop around the needle holder, starting with the holder in front of the suture. (3) Grasp the short end of the suture with the needle holder, which is through the loop. (4) Pull the suture through the loop and carefully tie the first part of the knot using the needle holder to pull one end. Traction is exerted parallel to the skin, with short end toward you. (5) To complete the square knot, reverse the suture ends so that the short end is away from you. (6) Tie second part of knot. (7) Again tighten by pulling ends parallel to skin. (8) Square knot is completed.*

Procedure (cont.)

NURSING ACTION	RATIONALE/AMPLIFICATION
9. When cutting sutures, hold scissors almost closed in right hand; hold suture ends taut and at right angle to skin. Glide scissors down along suture, holding scissors parallel to skin.	9. This will provide control when cutting and prevent cutting of skin or tissue.

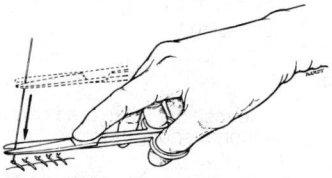

10. Cut stitch, leaving 0.65 cm (¼ inch) tails extending from knot.	10. To prevent knot from becoming undone; such a cut stitch will be easy to grasp when it is time for stitch removal.
11. Continue with stitches to close wound.	
12. Cleanse suture line with saline dampened gauze; apply dressing and tape.	12. Remove dried blood to lessen irritation to skin.

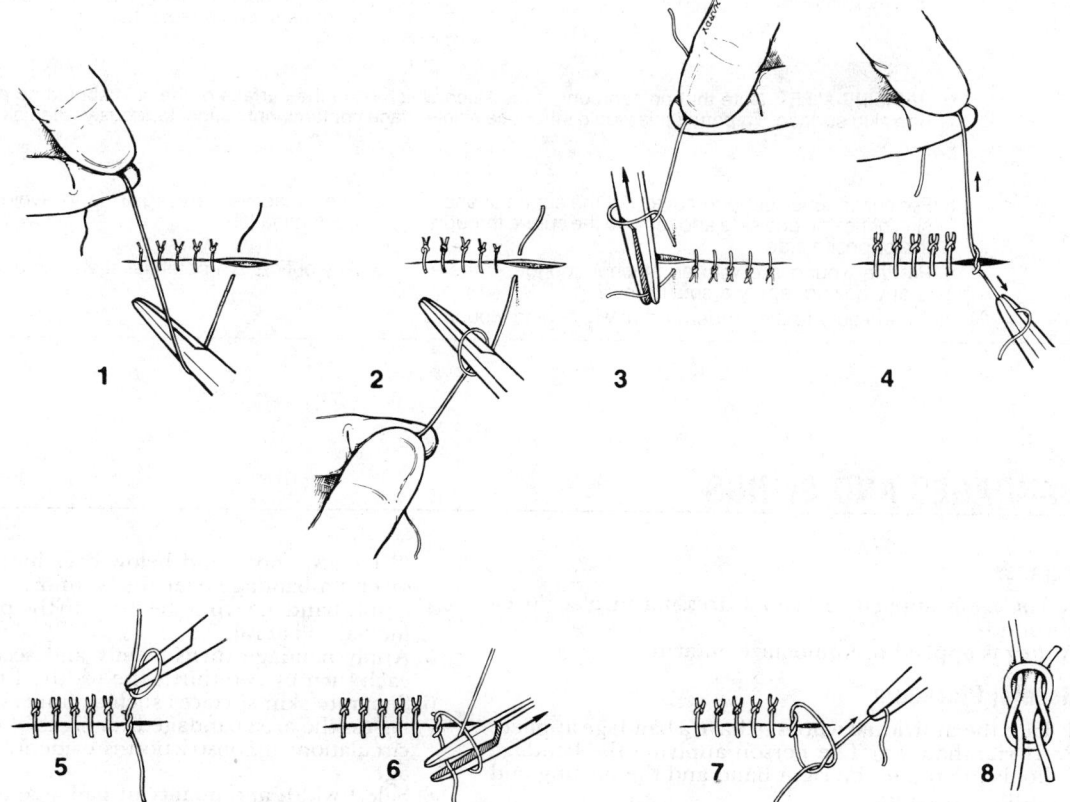

1 2 3 4

5 6 7 8

GUIDELINES: Suture Removal

The timing of stitch removal (of nonabsorbable stitches) depends on the location of the stitch on the body: head and neck, 3–5 days; chest and abdomen, 5–7 days; lower extremities, 7–10 days.

Equipment Stitch removal tray containing:
Antiseptic pledgets
Smooth forceps
Scissors
Dressings

Procedure

NURSING ACTION	RATIONALE/AMPLIFICATION
1. Cleanse the stitch area carefully and thoroughly using alcohol sponges.	1. Stitches provide pathways for microorganisms to invade tissues; therefore, skin surface must be rendered as clean as possible.
2. Use hydrogen peroxide if there are dried blood encrustations.	2. In the process of liberating oxygen, peroxide will loosen dried serum.
3. Grasp the knot of the suture with a pair of smooth forceps and gently pull upwards.	3. This will pull stitch away from skin.

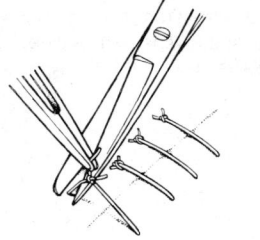 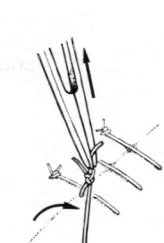

4. Cut the shortened end of the stitch as close to the skin as possible.	4. This will allow the stitch to be pulled free of wound so that only that part of the stitch which is under the skin touches subcutaneous tissues.

NURSING ALERT: Note that no segment of the stitch which is on the surface of the skin should be drawn below the skin surface. To permit this would introduce skin surface contaminants subcutaneously with risk of infection.

5. For continuous suture removal, cut the suture at each skin orifice on one side and remove the suture through the opposite side.	5. The objective here again is to avoid subcutaneous contamination.
6. Pat the wound site with an alcohol sponge. If there is any oozing, apply a small dressing.	6. Any orifice is a potential site for infection.
7. Avoid injury to the tender and newly healed wound.	

BANDAGES AND SLINGS

Purpose

A *bandage* is applied to keep a dressing in place over a wound.
A *sling* is applied to immobilize an arm.

General Procedure

1. Face the individual who is to have a bandage applied.
2. (If righthanded) The person applying the bandage holds the roll in the right hand and the starting end in the left hand.
3. Cover a dressing with a bandage that extends 5 cm. (2 inches) above and below dressing: do not begin or end a bandage over the wound.
4. Apply bandage from the distal to the proximal; from medial to lateral.
5. Apply bandage turns evenly and securely; overlap each turn by two thirds the width of the bandage.
6. Separate skin surfaces such as fingers.
7. Assess the area bandaged for signs of constriction of circulation; if constriction is evident, reapply bandage.
8. Select width and quality of bandage to suit the area being bandaged. (See Figs. 6-25–6-29.)

TYPES OF BANDAGES

Butterfly Strip

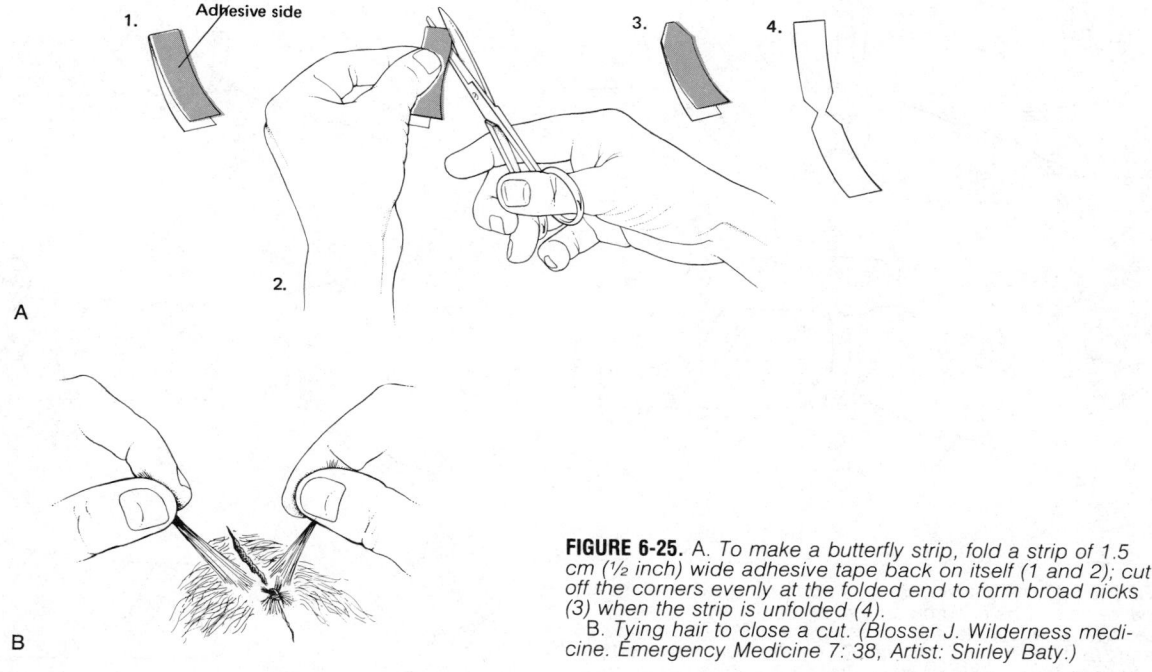

FIGURE 6-25. A. To make a butterfly strip, fold a strip of 1.5 cm (½ inch) wide adhesive tape back on itself (1 and 2); cut off the corners evenly at the folded end to form broad nicks (3) when the strip is unfolded (4).
B. Tying hair to close a cut. (Blosser J. Wilderness medicine. Emergency Medicine 7: 38, Artist: Shirley Baty.)

Finger Bandage

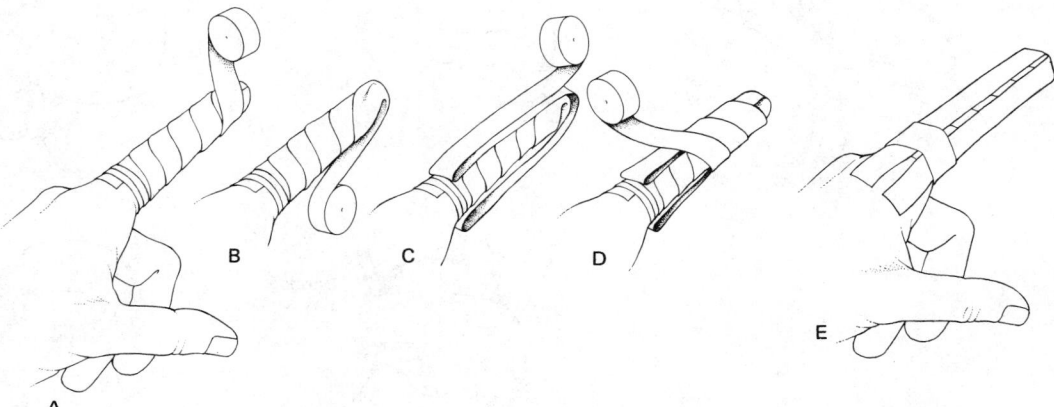

FIGURE 6-26. Bandaging a finger is effectively done using a spiral and recurrent loop technique. Note that the final dressing E is completed using narrow strips of adhesive.

Spiral Reverse Bandage for Arm and Leg

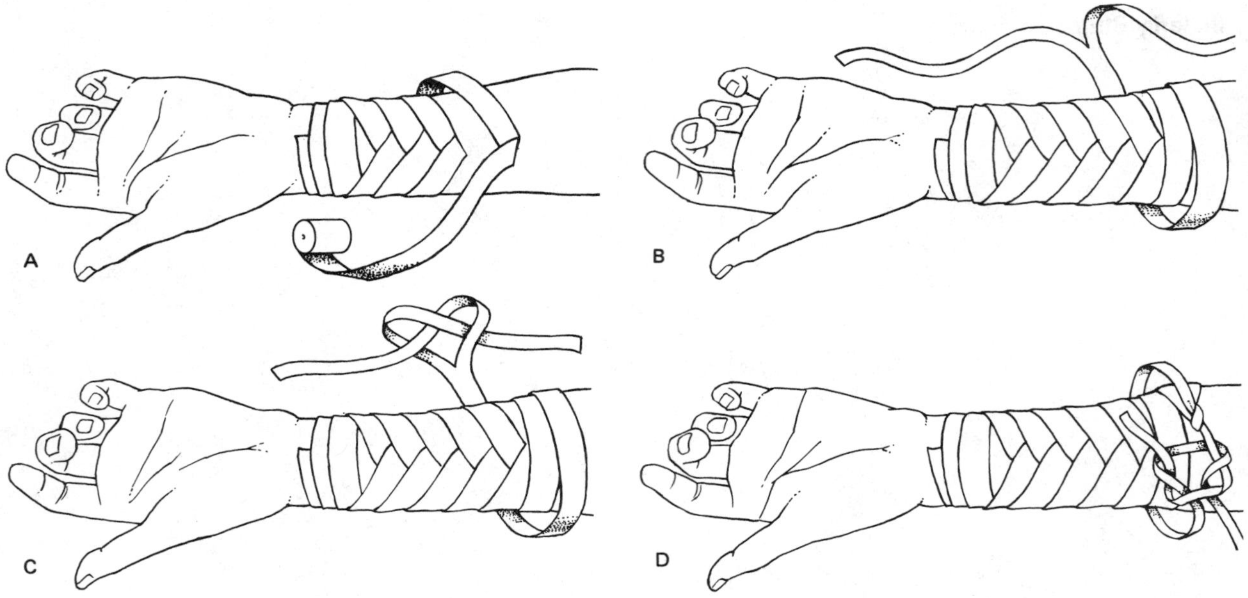

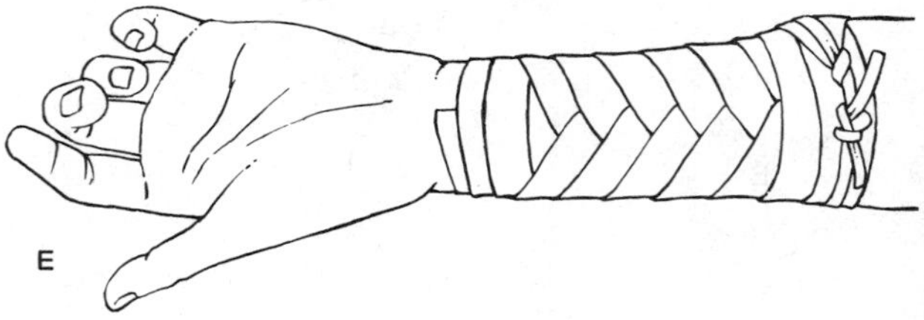

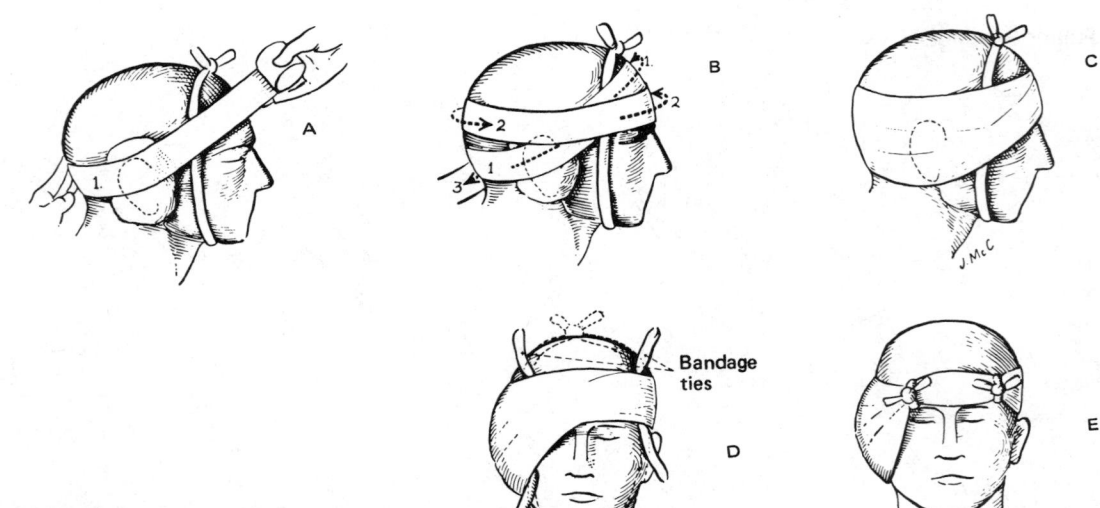

FIGURE 6-27. A. The technique of applying a spiral reverse bandage can be used on an arm or leg. B. After applying the bandage, cut the end tail down the middle to provide 2 ends for tying around the arm. C. A simple tie prevents the bandage from splitting further. D. The 2 ends are used to encircle the arm and are tied in a square knot. E. The final knot is placed so that the weight of the extremity is not resting on it, thereby causing pressure.

Pressure Bandage of Ear

FIGURE 6-28. Application of pressure bandage of ear. (Ferguson LK. Surgery of the Ambulatory Patient. Philadelphia, JB Lippincott Co.)

Triangular Sling

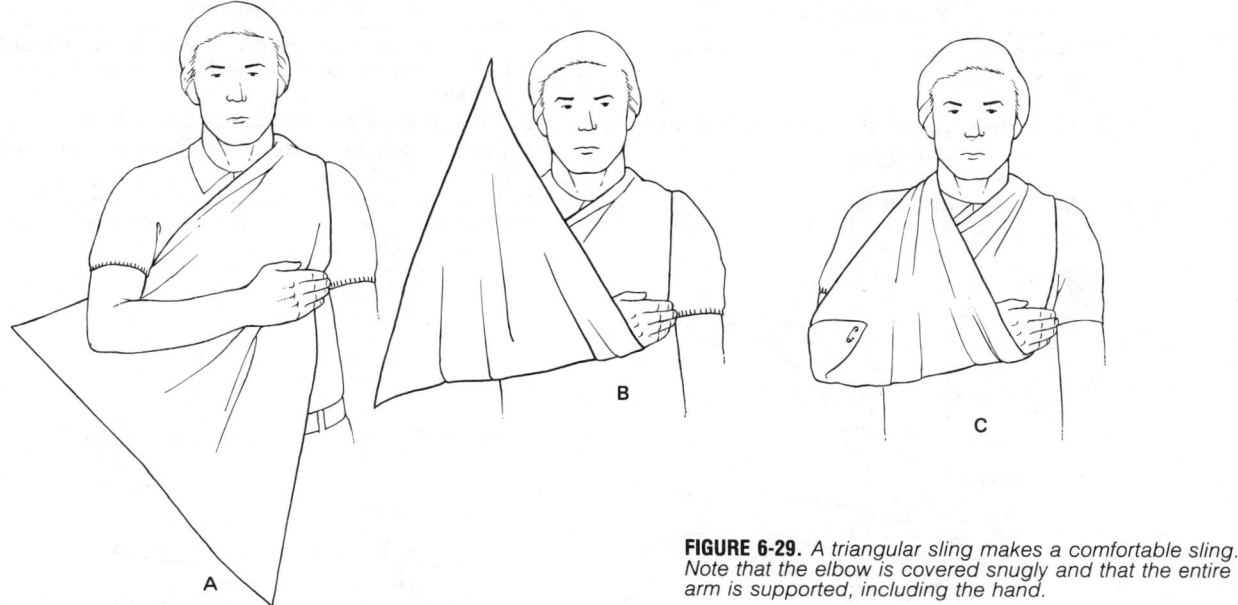

FIGURE 6-29. *A triangular sling makes a comfortable sling. Note that the elbow is covered snugly and that the entire arm is supported, including the hand.*

POSTOPERATIVE DISCOMFORTS

NAUSEA AND VOMITING

Incidence

1. Occurs in many postoperative patients.
2. Results from an accumulation of fluid or food in the stomach before peristalsis returns.
3. May occur as a result of abdominal distention which follows manipulation of abdominal organs.
4. Induced during anesthesia from inadequate ventilation.
5. Likely to occur if the patient believes preoperatively that he will vomit (psychological induction).
6. May be a side effect of narcotics.

Preventive Measures

1. Insert nasogastric tube preoperatively for operations on gastrointestinal tract to prevent abdominal distention which triggers vomiting.
2. Determine whether patient is sensitive to morphine and meperidine (Demerol) since they may induce vomiting in some patients.
3. Be alert for any significant comment such as "I just know I will vomit under anesthesia." Report such a comment to the anesthesiologist who may prescribe an antiemetic drug and also talk to the patient before the operation.

Treatment and Nursing Management

1. Encourage patient to breathe deeply to facilitate elimination of anesthetic.
2. Support the wound during retching and vomiting; turn head to side to avoid aspiration.
3. Discard vomitus and refresh patient—mouthwash for mouth, clean linens for bed, etc.
4. Suspect idiosyncratic response to a drug if vomiting is worse when a medication is given (but diminishes thereafter).
5. Administer antiemetic medication such as prochlorperazine (Compazine).
6. Offer hot tea with lemon or small sips of a carbonated beverage such as ginger ale, if tolerated.
7. Report excessive or prolonged vomiting so that the cause may be investigated.
8. Detect presence of abdominal distention, hiccups, suggesting gastric retention.
9. Suspect the possibility of paralytic ileus.

RESTLESSNESS AND SLEEPLESSNESS

Promoting Factors	Relief Measures
1. Discomfort such as back pain, headache, and thirst	1. Massage the back gently using an emollient lotion. Administer acetylsalicylic acid as prescribed.
2. Tight dressings or drainage-soaked dressings	2. Change dressings and check for tightness.
3. Urinary retention	3. Utilize nursing measures to initiate voiding (see p. 132).
4. Abdominal distention	4. Ambulation; insert rectal tube to relieve flatus—stimulates peristalsis and propels gas to rectum (Fig. 6-30).

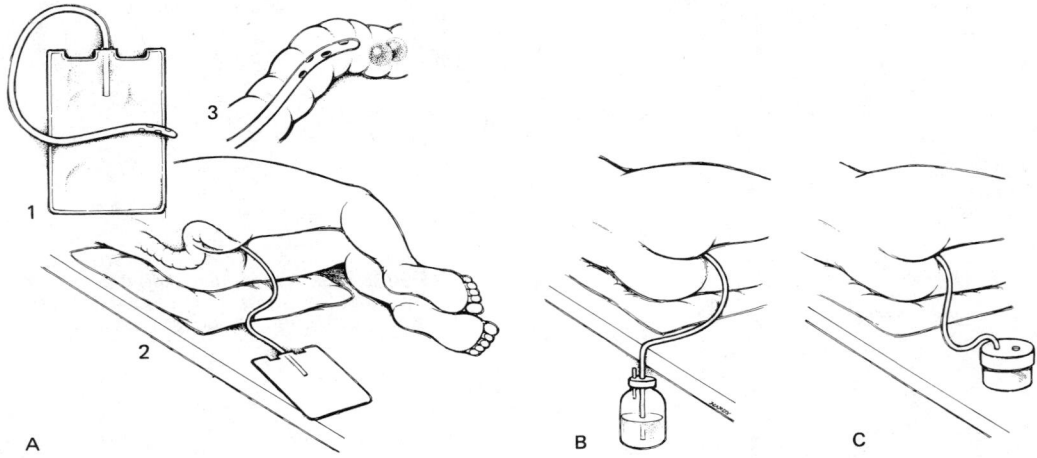

FIGURE 6-30. *Rectal intubation. A. (1) rectal tube attached to plastic bag; (2) tube in place, patient lying on left side; (3) enlargement of lower colon showing gas bubbles which will be tapped by rectal tube. B. Tubing connected to a water bottle with vent. C. Tubing connected to a plastic receptacle.*

5. Noise and environmental stimuli	5. Keep noise level at a minimum. Limit visitors to those who may promote rest in the patient. For rest periods provide privacy, darkness, and quiet. Schedule treatments with this in mind.
6. Worry and anxiety	6. Attempt to find cause of concern. Provide time to talk with the patient and permit him to vent his feelings. Seek advice of spiritual counselor or psychologist if necessary. Offer sedatives or hypnotics as required.

THIRST

Causes

1. Inhibition of secretions by preoperative medication with atropine.
2. Fluid lost via perspiration, blood loss, and dehydration due to preoperative fluid restriction.

Nursing Management

1. Administer fluids by vein or by mouth if tolerated.
2. Offer sips of hot tea with lemon juice to dissolve mucus.
3. Apply a moistened gauze square over lips occasionally to humidify inspired air.
4. Allow patient to rinse mouth with mouthwash; lemon juice and glycerin swabbing of the mouth is also refreshing.
5. Obtain hard candies or chewing gum to help in stimulating saliva flow and in keeping the mouth moist.

CONSTIPATION

Causes

1. Trauma and irritation to the bowel during surgery.
2. Local inflammation, peritonitis, or abscess.
3. Long-standing bowel problem: This may lead to fecal impaction.

Preventive Measures

1. Early ambulation to aid in promoting peristalsis.
2. Adequate fluid intake to keep stool soft and promote hydration.
3. Proper diet to promote peristalsis and maintain adequate fluid balance.
4. Query patient as to his usual remedy for constipation; try this.

Treatment (Fecal Impaction)

(See also p. 444.)
1. Insert a gloved finger and break up the impaction manually.
2. Administer an oil enema of 180–200 ml. to help soften the mass and facilitate evacuation.

PAIN

Pain is a subjective symptom in which the patient exhibits a feeling of distress caused by stimulation of certain nerve endings; usually it indicates that tissue damage is beginning to take place or has taken place as a result of surgery.

Clinical Manifestations

1. Autonomic
   a. Outpouring of epinephrine
   b. Elevation of blood pressure
   c. Increase in heart and pulse rate
   d. Rapid and irregular respiration
   e. Increase in perspiration
2. Skeletal muscle
   Increase in muscle tension or activity
3. Psychological
   a. Increase in irritability
   b. Increase in apprehension
   c. Increase in anxiety
   d. Attention focused on pain
   e. Complaints of pain

Patient's reaction depends upon:
1. Previous experience
2. Anxiety or tension
3. State of health
4. His ability to concentrate away from the problem or be distracted
5. Meaning that pain has for him.

Physiological and Psychological Assessment

1. Pain is one of the earliest symptoms which the patient expresses upon return to consciousness.
2. Maximal postoperative pain occurs between 12 and 36 hours after surgery and usually disappears by 48 hours.
3. Anesthetic agents which are soluble are slow to leave the body and therefore control pain for a longer time than agents which are insoluble; the latter produce rapid recovery, but the patient is more restless and complains more of pain.
4. Older persons seem to have a higher tolerance for pain than younger or middle-aged persons.
5. There is no documented proof that one sex tolerates pain better than the other.
6. Psychological conditioning of the patient affects pain tolerance.
7. The quality of nurse-patient interaction may have a greater influence on relief from pain than does the medication.
8. The nurse may reduce the patient's need for pain relief by making him more comfortable physically; frequent change of position, back rubs, talking with him, and letting him express his concern can help lower his anxiety level.
9. Patients who have had abdominal or chest surgery are more likely to need narcotics. The exchange of respiratory gases can be reduced by pain that causes reflex chest-muscle contraction.
10. Potent drugs such as morphine may produce depression of the patient's respiratory center thereby reducing rate and depth of breathing; also, such drugs tend to constrict bronchiolar smooth muscles and increase tracheal bronchial secretions—leading to atelectasis and pneumonia.

Nursing Management

1. Assess the nature, location, quality, intensity, and duration of pain and record these evaluations.
   a. Ask the patient to point to the pain center.
   b. Find out what the patient *means* by pain.
   c. Determine whether the pain is associated with an activity, such as turning or taking a deep breath.
   d. Encourage the patient to describe the pain in his own words, e.g., stabbing, consistent, dull.; involve him in controlling his pain.
   e. Investigative possible causes of pain such as bandage or adhesive which is too tight, full bladder, cast which is too snug, or elevated temperature suggestive of inflammation or infection.
2. Evaluate the patient's response to his pain.
   a. Observe the patient's facial expression and bodily movements as he experiences the pain.
   b. Is he pain-free when distracted by visitors or television?
   c. Does he appear to complain in anticipation of the next dose of medication?
   d. Help patient to express his angry feelings about pain and discomfort.
3. Employ comfort measures in caring for the patient.
   a. Provide therapeutic environment—proper temperature and humidity, ventilation, visitors.
   b. Increase patient's bodily comfort by adding blanket if he is cold, and vice versa.
   c. Massage his back in soothing strokes—move him easily and gently.
   d. Offer diversional activities, soft radio music, or favorite quiet television program.
   e. Provide for fluid needs by giving a cool drink, offering a bedpan.
4. Initiate measures to reduce the likelihood of pain.
   a. Encourage the patient to turn frequently.
   b. Massage pressure areas; support vulnerable areas—strategic placement of pillow, anchoring a footboard, placing a pillow between legs in the Sims's lateral position.
   c. Determine patient's need to void and need for relief from intestinal distention.
   d. Loosen constricting dressings.
   e. Keep bedding clean, dry, and free from crumbs.
   f. Maintain the patient in correct physiological position.
   g. Encourage patient to verbalize—to ease pain reaction, raise threshold.
   h. Give analgesic drugs as prophylaxis to prevent pain.
5. Relieve localized pain.
   a. Carefully support the painful area and elevate painful extremities.

b. Apply medications or counterirritants gently; use hot or cold applications as prescribed.

c. Encourage and assist the patient to follow pre-scribed exercise program.

6. Recognize the power of suggestion; mention that relief of pain will take place when a "reasonable" method is selected and used.

a. Combine chosen method of pain relief with verbal assurance that it will help.

b. Explain why the method chosen will help in relieving pain—positive assurance has been recognized as enhancing the effect of the "reasonable" action.

c. Indicate to the patient that you understand that he has pain, that you have time to listen and to help him, and that you care.

7. Be selective in administering pain-relieving agents; recognize individual differences.

a. First determine patient's respiratory rate and level of activity (arousal); use this information in making subsequent assessments.

b. Administer tranquilizers to relieve anxiety.

c. Use narcotic analgesics when postoperative pain justifies such medication.

d. Give narcotic agonist-antagonist (capable of reversing effects of narcotics, but in absence of narcotic, they produce a narcotic-like action) when prescribed.

e. Provide soporifics for sleep induction.

f. Administer muscle-relaxant and antispasmodic medications for uncontrolled muscle tension.

g. Utilize specific medications for specific conditions such as relief of nausea, relief of undesirable coughing, relief of headache.

h. Administer Narcan to relieve significant respiratory depression when brought about by a narcotic or narcotic agonist-antagonist.

> **NURSING ALERT:** "Potentiators" (hydroxyzine, promethazine) appear to sedate the patient, but it has not been proven that they are effective in potentiating the effects of an analgesic.

8. Recognize desired effects and untoward reactions of all medications given.

a. Observe patient for desired effect of medication.

b. Note respiratory rate; compare it with rate noted before medication was given. Assess the difference. A narcotic is more likely to cause respiratory depression.

c. Be alert to toxic manifestations and hypersensitivity reactions.

(1) Unpleasant psychic reactions (anxiety, hallucinations) may occur in some patients after taking a narcotic agonist-antagonist.

d. Be knowledgeable about drug interactions.

e. Note signs of respiratory embarassment, adverse vital signs, rashes.

POSTOPERATIVE COMPLICATIONS

SHOCK

Shock is a response of the body to a decrease in the circulating volume of blood; tissue perfusion is impaired culminating eventually in cellular hypoxia.

Classification

1. *Oligemic* (hematogenic)—shock resulting from loss of plasma or whole blood; this may be external or internal. When 10% of the blood volume is lost, *hypovolemic* shock occurs.

2. *Bacteremic* (septic or toxic shock)—characterized by a change in the capillary endothelium, permitting loss of blood and plasma through capillary walls into surrounding tissues; no actual fluid volume is lost from the body.

3. *Cardiogenic*—observed when there is interference with heart pumping action, as might occur in myocardial infarction, cardiac tamponade, which results in inadequate vascular circulation.

4. *Neurogenic* (vasogenic)—marked vasodilation and reflex inhibition which results in a sluggish circulating system, depriving vital centers of proper blood supply.

5. *Psychic*—results from extreme pain or deep fear.

Altered Physiology and Clinical Manifestations

1. Loss of effective circulating blood volume—initiates metabolic and physiologic reactions resulting in poor tissue perfusion. (See Table 6-4.)

2. Hyperventilation, caused by stress, leads to respiratory alkalosis; this is the earliest acid–gas change of shock.

3. Pituitary hormones are released

ACTH (adrenocorticotropic)—stimulates the adrenal cortex to secrete glucocorticoids.

ADH (antidiuretic)—stimulates kidney tubules to absorb more fluid.

ASH (aldosterone-stimulating)—stimulates potassium excretion by kidney, stimulates sodium chloride retention and water retention.

4. Epinephrine and norepinephrine promote capillary vasoconstriction—increases flow through vital organs but diminishes flow through peripheral tissues. Later, peripheral vasoconstriction produces *pale, cold, clammy skin.*

5. Acidemia causes lung to compensate—increased rate (tachypnea) and volume.

6. Heart rate accelerates; diastole lessens.

Coronary perfusion during diastole; with lessened perfusion, cardiac output falls, resulting in *reduced systolic pressure, lowered pulse pressure,* and generalized vasoconstriction.

7. Weak, thready pulse and subnormal temperature.

8. Lip cyanosis, circumoral pallor; decreased salivary secretions.

9. At first patient appears *nervous* and *apprehensive;* later, *apathy develops* and *sensations are dulled.* Muscle weakness and fatigue become apparent.

TABLE 6-4. CORRELATION OF MAGNITUDE OF VOLUME DEFICIT AND CLINICAL PRESENTATION.

Approximate Deficit	Decrease in Blood Volume	Shock	
		Degree	*Signs*
ml.	%		
0–500	0–10	None	None
500–1200	10–25	Mild (compensated)	Slight tachycardia Mild hypotension Mild peripheral vasoconstriction
1200–1800	25–35	Moderate	Thready pulse, 100–120 beats/min. Blood pressure, 90–100 mm. Hg systolic Marked vasoconstriction Diaphoresis Anxiety, restlessness Decreased urinary output
1800–2500	35–50	Severe	Thready pulse, 120 beats/min. Blood pressure, 60 mm. Hg systolic Marked vasoconstriction Marked diaphoresis Obtundation No urinary output

Source: Wilkins EW Jr (ed). MGH Textboook of Emergency Medicine, p 40. Baltimore, Williams & Wilkins Co. 1978.

Effects of Shock

1. Anoxia—lack of oxygen in the body
2. Anoxemia—decreased amount of oxygen in the blood
3. Hyperpyrexia—an excessive fever, about 42.2 to 42.8° C. (108–109° F.), which occurs shortly before death
4. Oliguria—decreased kidney secretion and urinary output
5. Anuria—absence of urinary secretion
6. Thrombosis with subsequent emboli due to blood stasis

Treatment and Nursing Management

Chief Objective: to restore circulating blood volume.

A. *Prevention*

1. Prepare adequately the mental as well as the physical condition of the patient.
2. Anticipate any complications that may arise during and after surgery.
3. Have blood available if there is any indication that it may be needed.
4. Measure accurately any blood loss.
5. Keep operative trauma to a minimum; minimize postoperative disturbance of the patient.
6. Anticipate progression of symptoms upon earliest manifestation.
7. Monitor vital signs frequently until they are stable.
8. Assess vital sign deviations; evaluate blood pressure in relation to other parameters.
9. Institute therapy immediately following an injury, etc., which is likely to lead to shock.
10. Recognize that blood pressure limits vary with individuals; in some patients 90/60 may be normal whereas in others it may indicate severe shock.
11. Prevent infection; this will prevent septic shock.

B. *Definitive Management*

1. KEEP THE AIRWAY PATENT
   a. Use an airway or place an endotracheal tube.
   b. Remove oral and tracheal secretions.
   c. Institute resuscitative measures if necessary.
2. Arrest hemorrhage (not present in septic shock).
   Ascertain where hemorrhage is occurring; if external, utilize pressure control.

3. Place patient in most physiologically desirable position for shock (Fig. 6-31).
   a. Elevate the head on a pillow.
   b. Keep the trunk horizontal.
   c. Elevate lower extremities about 20 to 30 degrees, keeping knees straight.

NURSING ALERT: Do not use Trendelenburg head-low position because (1) after initial increase of blood to the head, a reflex compensatory action takes place causing vasoconstriction and thereby decreasing blood supply to the brain; and (2) viscera tend to fall against the diaphragm causing increased resistance to breathing and inadequate ventilation.

4. Ensure an adequate venous return.
   a. Insert intravenous catheter for infusion in upper extremities; 2 may be required.
   b. Place a central venous pressure (CVP) catheter in or near right atrium (see Fig. 9-3 and Guidelines, p. 271).
      (1) Note direction and degree of change from initial reading.
      (2) Utilize route established by CVP catheter for emergency fluid volume and electrolyte replacement.
   c. Start plasma expanders if needed until whole blood is available.
   d. Begin blood transfusion when blood is available.
5. Obtain blood for determinations of pH, PO_2, PCO_2 and hematocrit; correct deviations.
   a. pH—may indicate acidosis resulting from anaerobic metabolism.
   b. PCO_2—assesses function of pulmonary alveolar membrane.
   c. PO_2—determines level of oxygen tension.
   d. Hematocrit—reveals losses due to obstruction or peritonitis.
6. Insert a urinary catheter to monitor hourly urinary output.
   Objective is to maintain a 1 ml./kg./hr. urinary

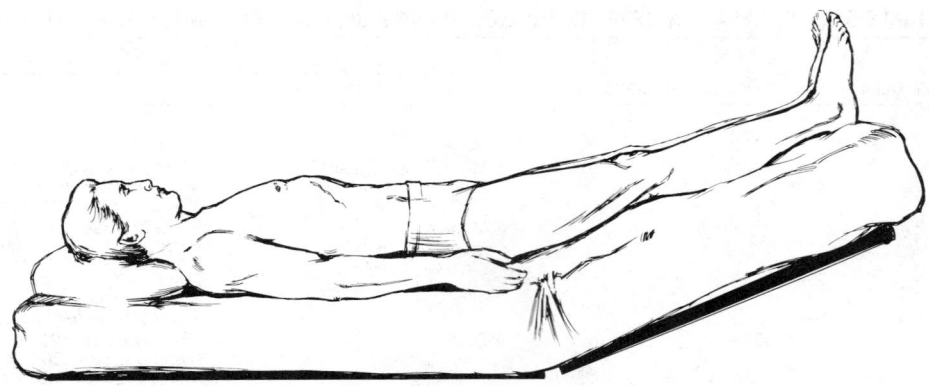

FIGURE 6-31. *Proper positioning of the patient who shows signs of shock. Elevate the lower extremities about 20 degrees keeping the knees straight, trunk horizontal, and head slightly elevated.*

volume output to ensure adequate kidney perfusion.

7. Administer antimicrobials in order to offset infection which can occur due to stagnant hypoxia in wounds and in peripheral tissues.
   Utilize large doses of penicillin, streptomycin, or broad-spectrum chemotherapeutic agents.
8. Support the defense mechanisms of the patient.
   a. Comfort and reassure patient if he is conscious.
   b. Resort to sedation and analgesia with discriminating judgment.
   c. Keep the patient warm, but do not apply too much external covering since it will produce unnecessary vasodilation resulting in more fluid loss.
9. Recognize signs of impending cardiac failure—increasing CVP, distended neck veins, pulmonary rales, etc.
   Initiate prophylactic inotropic drugs.
      Use rapid-acting medications in the very young and very old (dopamine, isoproterenol)
10. If the patient does not respond to fluid loading and inotropic drugs, expect steroids to be prescribed.
11. If response to conventional methods fails, it may be necessary to resort to mechanical assistance, such as use of intra-aortic balloon pump to increase diastolic aortic pressure.
12. Throughout entire panorama of impending shock, continue flow sheet, recording of vital signs, observations, and interventions.
13. Septic shock is most often due to gram-negative infection: peritonitis, meningitis; it may have a direct toxic effect on the heart resulting in depressed cardiac function.

HEMORRHAGE

Hemorrhage is copious escape of blood from a blood vessel.

Classification

A. *General*

1. *Primary*—occurs at the time of operation.
2. *Intermediary*—occurs within the first few hours after surgery.
   Blood pressure returns to normal and causes

loosening of poorly tied vessels and flushing out of weak clots from untied vessels.
3. *Secondary*—occurs some time after surgery.
   a. Ligature slips from blood vessel.
   b. Erosion of blood vessel.

B. *According to Blood Vessels*

1. *Capillary*—slow general oozing from capillaries.
2. *Venous*—bleeding which is dark in color and bubbles out.
3. *Arterial*—bleeding which spurts and is bright red in color.

C. *According to Location*

1. *Evident or External*—visible bleeding on the surface.
2. *Concealed or Internal*—bleeding which cannot be seen.

Clinical Manifestations

1. Apprehension, restlessness, thirst; cold, moist, pale skin.
2. Pulse increases, respirations become rapid and deep ("air hunger"), temperature drops.
3. With progression of hemorrhage.
   a. Decrease in cardiac output.
   b. Rapidly decreasing arterial and venous blood pressure as well as hemoglobin.
   c. Circumoral pallor, spots appear before the eyes, ringing in the ears.
   d. Patient grows weaker until death occurs.

Treatment and Nursing Management

1. Treat the patient as described for shock (p. 129).
2. Inspect the wound as a possible site of bleeding.
   If an extremity is bleeding, apply a gauze-pad pressure dressing.
3. Administer blood (typed) or blood substitute until blood is available

NURSING ALERT: In giving fluids by vein recognize that, in the case of hemorrhage, giving too large a quantity or administering fluids too rapidly may elevate the blood pressure sufficiently to recycle the hemorrhaging process.

FEMORAL PHLEBITIS OR DEEP THROMBOPHLEBITIS

Phlebitis often occurs after operations on the lower abdomen or during the course of septic conditions such as ruptured ulcer or peritonitis. (See p. 341, Chap. 9.)

Causes

1. Injury
   a. Damage to vein resulting from tight straps or leg holders during surgery.
   b. Compression of a blanket roll under the knees.
2. Fluid loss or dehydration leading to concentration of blood.
3. Lowered metabolism and circulatory depression after surgery leading to slowing of blood flow.
4. Combinations of the above.

Clinical Manifestations

1. Left leg appears to be affected more frequently than right.
2. Pain or cramp in the calf, progressing to painful swelling of entire leg.
3. Slight fever, chills, perspiration.
4. Marked tenderness over anteromedial surface of thigh.
5. Intravascular clotting without marked inflammation may develop leading to phlebothrombosis.

> **NURSING ALERT:** A complaint of slight soreness of the calf is never ignored. The danger inherent in femoral thrombosis is that a clot may be dislodged and produce an embolus.

Treatment and Nursing Management

A. *Prophylaxis*

1. Hydrate the patient adequately postoperatively to prevent blood concentration.
2. Encourage leg exercises and ambulate the patient as soon as permitted by the surgeon. (Exercises are taught preoperatively—see p. 84.)
3. Avoid any restricting devices such as tight straps that can constrict and impair circulation.
4. Prevent the use of bed rolls, knee gatches, even "dangling" over the side of the bed, because there is danger of constricting the vessels under the knee.

B. *Active Therapy*

1. Initiate anticoagulant therapy either intravenously, intramuscularly, or by mouth (see p. 85).
2. Prevent swelling and stagnation of venous blood by wrapping the legs from the toes to the groin with elastic bandage or elastic stockings.
3. Control pain in the extremities by bandaging.

PULMONARY COMPLICATIONS

Preventive Measures

1. Report any evidence of upper respiratory infection to the surgeon.
2. Postoperatively, initiate measures to prevent chilling.
3. Aspirate secretions that might cause respiratory embarrassment.
4. Recognize the predisposing causes of pulmonary complications:
   a. Infections—mouth, nose, throat.
   b. Aspiration of vomitus
   c. History of heavy smoking, chronic respiratory disease
   d. Obesity

Complications

1. *Atelectasis*—collapse of pulmonary alveoli caused by a mucous plug closing a bronchus.
2. *Bronchitis*—inflammation of bronchi causing a cough with considerable mucous secretion.
3. *Bronchopneumonia*—a chest complication with elevated temperature, pulse, and respiratory rate plus a productive cough.
4. *Lobar pneumonia*—onset of a chill followed by a high temperature, pulse and respiration elevation, flushed cheeks, respiratory embarrassment.
5. *Hypostatic pulmonary congestion*—more common in the debilitated or elderly patient whose weakened heart and vascular system permit stagnation of secretions at base of lungs.
6. *Pleurisy*—knife-like pain in the chest on the affected side, particularly on intake of a deep breath, and elevated temperature, pulse, and respirations.
   (For greater detail see Chapter 7, Conditions of the Respiratory System.)

Treatment and Nursing Management

1. Appraise the patient's progress very carefully on a daily basis for the first postoperative week to detect early signs and symptoms of respiratory difficulties.
   a. Slight temperature, pulse, and respiration elevations.
   b. Apprehension and restlessness
   c. Complaints of chest pain, signs of dyspnea or cough
2. Promote full aeration of the lungs.
   a. Turn the patient frequently.
   b. Encourage the patient to take 10 deep breaths hourly.
   c. Utilize a spirometer or any device which encourages the patient to ventilate. Inspiratory exercises are more effective than expiratory.
   d. Assist the patient in coughing in an effort to bring up mucous secretions.
   e. Assist the patient to ambulate as early as the physician will allow
3. Initiate specific measures for particular pulmonary problems.
   a. Provide cool mist or steam (electric vaporizer) for the patient who exhibits signs of bronchitis.
   b. Encourage the patient to take fluids and expectorants if he appears to be developing pneumonia.
   c. Administer antibiotics to patients with pulmonary infections.
   d. Prevent abdominal distention—causes pulmonary and circulatory embarrassment.
   e. Provide analgesics for discomfort.
   f. Note that the patient who has pleurisy with effusion may need chest aspiration; have a thoracentesis tray ready and be prepared to assist.
   g. Be prepared to administer oxygen to assist in aeration of the lungs for oxygenation of blood.

PULMONARY EMBOLISM

An *embolus* is a foreign body in the bloodstream—usually a blood clot that has become dislodged from the original site. When such a clot is carried to the heart, it is forced into the pulmonary artery or one of its branches. (See also p. 211.)

Clinical Manifestations

1. Sharp, stabbing pains in the chest
2. Anxiousness and cyanosis
3. Pupillary dilation, profuse perspiration.
4. Rapid and irregular pulse becoming imperceptible—leads rapidly to death
5. Dyspnea

Immediate Treatment

1. Administer oxygen and inhalations with the patient in an upright sitting position.
2. Reassure and quiet the patient.
3. Administer morphine to control panic.

URINARY DIFFICULTIES

Retention of Urine

1. *Incidence*—occurs most frequently after operations on the rectum, anus, vagina, or lower abdomen; caused by spasm of bladder sphincter.
2. *Nursing Measures*
   a. Assist patient to sit or even stand up (if permissible) since many patients are unable to void while lying in bed.
   b. Provide the patient with privacy.
   c. Use the psychological aid of running the tap water—frequently the sound or sight of running water relaxes the spasm of the bladder sphincter.
   d. Catheterize only when all other measures are unsuccessful.
      (1) May lead to possible bladder infection.
      (2) Subsequent catheterizations are often required.

NURSING ALERT: Recognize that when a patient voids small amounts (30–60 ml. every 15–30 minutes) this may be a sign of overdistended bladder ("overflow of retention").

Urinary Incontinence

1. *Cause*—loss of tone of the bladder sphincter.
2. *Incidence*—occurs as a complication in the aged after surgery or shocking injury.
3. *Recovery*—disappears as patient gains strength and muscle tone.
4. *Management*
   a. Offer a bedpan hourly.
   b. Provide extra padding under patient; use special disposable pants.
   c. Initiate a consistent plan for special care of the skin to avoid skin breakdown.

INTESTINAL OBSTRUCTION

Causes

1. May occur following surgery on lower abdomen and pelvis, especially when there is drainage.
2. A loop of intestines may kink because of inflammatory adhesions.
3. A loop of intestine may become involved in the drainage tract.

Clinical Manifestations

1. Most commonly occurs between the 3rd and 5th postoperative day.
2. Sharp, colicky abdominal pains with pain-free intervals.
3. Pain is localized and should be noted since it may become more generalized later; location may pinpoint source of difficulty.
4. Peristaltic activity can be assessed by listening to the abdomen with a stethoscope.
5. Pain-free intervals grow shorter as time advances.
6. With completion of obstruction, intestinal contents back up into stomach and cause vomiting.
7. Abdominal distention and perhaps hiccups occur, but no bowel movements, if obstruction is complete; if obstruction is partial or incomplete, diarrhea may occur.
8. Following simple enema, returns are clear, indicating very small amount of intestinal contents has reached large intestines.
9. If obstruction is not relieved, vomiting continues, distention become more pronounced, pulse increases, shock develops, and death occurs.

Management

1. Relieve abdominal distention by passing a nasoenteric suction tube.
2. Administer body-deficient electrolytes per intravenous infusion.
3. Consider surgical intervention if obstruction continues unresolved (see p. 434–436).

HICCUPS (SINGULTUS)

Hiccups are intermittent spasms of the diaphragm causing a sound ("hic") that results from the vibration of closed vocal cords as air rushes suddenly into the lungs.

Cause

Irritation of phrenic nerve between spinal cord and terminal ramifications on undersurface of diaphragm.
   a. *Direct*—distended stomach, peritonitis, abdominal distention, chest pleurisy, tumors pressing on nerves, or surgery performed near the diaphragm
   b. *Indirect*—toxemia, uremia
   c. *Reflex*—exposure to cold, drinking very hot or very cold liquids, intestinal obstruction

Management

1. Remove the cause if possible.
   a. Gastric lavage for gastric distention
   b. Adhesive strapping in pleurisy
   c. Removal of drainage tubes causing irritation
2. When removal of cause is not possible, favorite simple remedies may be tried.
   a. Holding breath while taking large swallow of water.
   b. Applying finger pressure on the eyeballs through closed lids for several minutes.
   c. Inhaling carbon dioxide (breathing in and out of a paper bag).

3. Medications may be prescribed (chlorpromazine, Benzedrine, quinidine, or barbiturates). The degree of success with these drugs varies widely.
4. Introduce a cathether (No. 16 Fr.) into the patient's pharynx about 7–10 cm. (3–4 inches); rotate gently and jiggle back and forth; this action interrupts impulses from vagus nerve and hiccups stop (Fig. 6-32).
5. For intractable hiccups, an extreme procedure is surgical crush of the phrenic nerve.

WOUND INFECTION

Infection in a wound occurs when there is growth of bacteria; infection may be limited to a single area or may affect a patient systemically.

A. *Causative Organisms*

1. *Staphylococcus aureus*
2. *Escherichia coli*
3. *Proteus vulgaris*
4. *Pseudomonas aeruginosa*
5. Anaerobic bacteria, e.g., *Bacteroides fragilis*. Anaerobes have become more prominent in wound infections, particularly following bowel surgery; a characteristic odor can be detected. Often this infection is detected only if anaerobic cultures are performed.

B. *Factors Affecting the Extent of an Infection*

1. The kind, virulence, and quantity of contaminating microorganisms
2. Presence of foreign bodies or devitalized tissue
3. Location and nature of the wound
4. Amount of dead space or presence of hematoma
5. Immune response of the patient
6. Presence of ischemia leading to wound compression
7. Condition of the patient, such as whether he is elderly, alcoholic, diabetic, malnourished

C. *Prophylaxis*

1. Strict asepsis when wound is made and later during wound management.
2. Housekeeping cleanliness and pertinent patient instruction concerning dressings.

D. *Clinical Manifestations*

1. Local
   Induration (hardening of area), erythema, pain
   Wound tenderness and swelling—apparent in 36 to 48 hours
2. Systemic
   Elevated temperature and pulse

NURSING ALERT: A useful rule of thumb is that an elevated temperature occurring within 24 hours suggests a pulmonary infection; within 48 hours suggests a urinary tract infection; after 72 hours suggests a wound infection.

Preventive Medical and Nursing Measures

A. *Preoperative*

1. Encourage patient to achieve an optimum nutritional level
   If hypoproteinemic with weight loss, provide oral or parenteral alimentation.

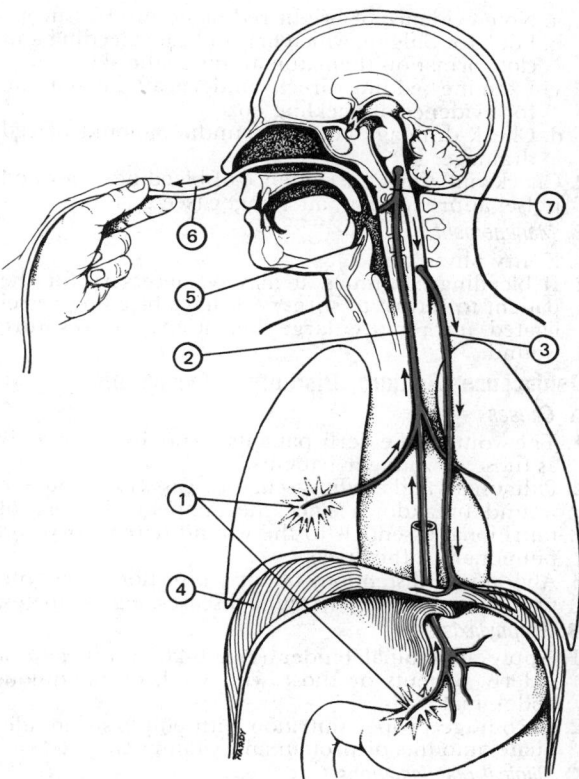

FIGURE 6-32. *Controlling hiccups. Irritations in chest or abdomen (1) are transmitted by the vagus nerve (2). The reflex arc is completed by the transmission of the impulses to the diaphragm by the phrenic nerve (3). This causes contraction of the diaphragm (4) resulting in sudden intake of breath, which in turn is suddenly interrupted by rapid closure of the glottis (5). This is the hiccup.*
Introduction of the No. 16F catheter into the nasopharynx about 7.5–10 cm. (3 to 4 inches) (6) stimulates the pharyngeal branches of the vagus nerve (7) and interrupts the reflex arc, stopping the hiccups.

2. Reduce preoperative hospitalization to barest minimum to avoid acquiring "hospital infection" (nosocomial infection).

B. *Postoperative*

1. Surgeon removes one or more stitches, separates wound edges, and examines for infection using a hemostat as a probe.
2. A culture is taken and sent to the bacteriology laboratory.
3. Wound irrigation may be done; have asepto syringe and saline available.
4. A drain (rubber or gauze) may be inserted.
5. Antibiotics are prescribed.
6. Hot wet dressings may be suggested.

WOUND COMPLICATIONS
Hemorrhage and Hematoma

A. *Manifestations*

1. Inspect dressings frequently during first 24 hours postoperatively.

a. Note evidence of bright red blood on dressings.
b. Look for bulging which may indicate bleeding and clot formation (hematoma) under the skin.
c. Examine bedding directly underneath incision site for evidence of trickling ooze.
d. Check drainage bottle for undue amount of red drainage.
2. Check vital signs for evidence of bleeding—elevated pulse, apprehension, air hunger (see p. 130).

B. *Management*
1. Notify physician.
2. If bleeding continues, it may be necessary for the patient to return to surgery to have bleeding vessel ligated, to remove large hematoma, to resuture wound.

Dehiscence (Rupture, Disruption, Evisceration)

A. *Causes*
1. The wounds of elderly patients do not heal as readily as those of younger patients.
2. Pulmonary and cardiovascular diseases contribute to wound breakdown since they impede delivery of nutritional essentials to the wound (circulatory and pulmonary difficulties).
3. Abdominal distention, obesity, infection, poor nutritional status, and systemic diseases, e.g., diabetes.

B. *Prophylaxis*
1. Apply abdominal binder (Fig. 6-20) for heavy or elderly patients or those with weak or pendulous abdominal walls.
2. Encourage proper nutrition with emphasis on adequate amounts of protein and vitamin C.

C. *Clinical Manifestations*
1. Patient complains that something suddenly gave way in his wound.
2. In an intestinal wound, the edges of the wound may part and the intestines may gradually push out—observe for drainage of peritoneal fluid on dressings (clear or serosanguineous fluid).

D. *Management*
1. Stay with the patient and have someone notify the surgeon immediately.
2. If intestines are exposed, cover with sterile moist dressings.
3. Keep patient on absolute bed rest.
4. Instruct patient to bend his knees—relieves tension on abdomen.
5. Assure the patient that his wound will be properly cared for; keep him quiet and relaxed.
6. Prepare patient for surgery and repair of the wound.

POSTOPERATIVE PSYCHOLOGICAL DISTURBANCES

Delirium is a mental aberration which occurs only occasionally in some postoperative patients.

Classification

A. *Toxic*
1. Incidence—occurs in combination with symptoms of general toxemia, e.g., peritonitis, sepsis.
2. Symptoms—acutely ill, restless patient with elevated temperature and pulse, flushed face, bright and roving eyes—indicates mental confusion.
3. Management
a. Administer fluids to aid in elimination of toxins.

NOTE: Not all delirious patients can tolerate fluids. It is also inappropriate to administer fluids if it may lead to cerebral fluid retention and delirium; treatment in this instance is fluid restriction.

b. Control infection by giving the proper antibiotics.

B. *Traumatic*
1. *Incidence*—develops following sudden trauma, particularly in the highly nervous person.
2. *Symptoms*—manifests itself by wild excitement, hallucinations, delusions, or melancholic depression.
3. Management
a. Administer tranquilizing medications; chloral hydrate, paraldehyde.
b. This state of delirium begins and ends abruptly.

C. *Delirium Tremens*
1. Incidence—patients who have used alcohol excessively are poor surgical risks and take anesthetic agents poorly.
2. Symptoms—postoperatively, after continued abstinence from alcohol, patient shows signs of delirium tremens.
a. Restless, nervous, easily irritated.
b. Sleeps poorly, disturbed by unreal dreams, momentarily appears to be in a strange place and does not know nursing or medical staff.
c. Later, loses control of mental functions; his mind is filled with haunting hallucinations that torment him constantly.
d. Additional symptoms include sleeplessness, excessive perspiration, and marked tremor of the limbs. Patient eventually becomes stuporous.
3. Medical and Nursing Management
a. Administer sedatives to keep the patient quiet and comfortable; stimulation may be required by older alcoholics.
b. Give glucose intravenously and concentrated vitamins by mouth to control nutritional deficiencies.
c. Recommend that the patient remain in bed; it may be necessary to restrain him so that injuries are minimized. (Bear in mind that restraining should be a last resort since this often makes such a patient quite rebellious.)
d. Encourage ambulation as soon as the surgical condition permits.
e. See also pages 896–897.

BIBLIOGRAPHY

Books

Altemeier WA et al (eds). Manual on Control of Infections in Surgical Patients. Philadelphia, JB Lippincott, 1976
American College of Surgeons Committee on Preoperative and Postoperative Care. Manual of Preoperative and Postoperative Care. Philadelphia, WB Saunders, 1977

Association of Operating Room Nurses. Standards of Nursing Practice: Recovery Room, Denver, AORN, 1980
Atkinson LJ and Kohn ML. Berry and Kohn's Introduction to Operating Room Techniques, 5th ed. New York, McGraw-Hill, 1978
David DL et al. The Surgical Experience: A Model for

Professional Nursing Practice in the Operating Room. Denver, AORN, 1978

Drain CB and Shipley SB. The Recovery Room. Philadelphia, WB Saunders, 1979

Dubay EC and Grubb RD. Infection: Prevention and Control, 2nd ed. St Louis, CV Mosby, 1978

Grubb, RD and Ondov G. Planning Ambulatory Surgical Facilities. St. Louis, CV Mosby, 1979

Gruendemann BJ et al. The Surgical Patient, 2nd ed. St. Louis, CV Mosby, 1977

Le Maitre GD and Finnegan JA. The Patient in Surgery, 4th ed. Philadelphia, WB Saunders, 1980

McCaffery M. Nursing Management of the Patient with Pain, 2nd ed. Philadelphia, JB Lippincott, 1979

Metheney NM and Snively WD Jr. Nurses' Handbook of Fluid Balance, 3rd ed. Philadelphia, JB Lippincott, 1979

Metzger RS and Robertson PA. Intraoperative Learning. Denver, AORN, 1977

Millar S (chief editor). Methods in Critical Care. The AACN Manual by the American Association of Critical-Care Nurses. Philadelphia, WB Saunders, 1980

Nealon TF. Fundamental Skills in Surgery, 3rd ed. Philadelphia, WB Saunders, 1979

Nursing 78 Books. Monitoring Fluid and Electrolytes Precisely. Horsham, Intermed Communications, 1978

Nursing 79 Books. Nursing Critically Ill Patients Confidently. Horsham, Intermed Communications, 1979

Nursing 80 Photobook. Managing I.V. Therapy. Horsham, Intermed Communications, 1980

Reinarz JA. Nosocomial Infections. Clinical Symposia. Vol 30, No. 6. Summit, CIBA Pharmaceutical Co, 1978

Rhodes MJ et al. Alexander's Care of the Patient in Surgery, 6th ed. St. Louis, CV Mosby, 1978

Sager DP and Bomar SK. Intravenous Medications. Philadelphia, JB Lippincott, 1980

Thompson MA. Shock Syndrome: Mechanisms and Manifestations, Nursing Assessment, Intervention, and Evaluation. Menlo Park, Addison-Wesley Publishing Co, 1978

Vandam LD (ed). To Make the Patient Ready for Anesthesia: Medical Care of the Surgical Patient. Menlo Park, Addison-Wesley Publishing Co, 1980

Walraven G et al. Manual of Advanced Prehospital Care. Bowie, Robert J Brady, 1978

PREOPERATIVE PATIENT CARE
Articles

Antimicrobial prophylaxis for surgery. The Med Letter 1979 Sept 7; 21(18):73–76

Cassileth BR et al. Informed consent—why are its goals imperfectly realized? N Engl J Med 1980 April 17; 302(16):896–900

Chamberlain SL. Low-dose heparin therapy. Am J Nurs 1980 June; 80(6):1115–1117

Copeland WM. Informed consent and the nurse. AORN J 1980 April; 29(5):928–944

Dean WF. Surgical evaluation of volume and ventricular function. Crit Care Q 1979 Sept; 2(2):43–50

Dickman RL. The ethics of informed consent. Nurse Pract 1980 May/June; 5(3):25–26, 32

Gargaro WJ Jr. How much to tell the patient. Cancer Nurs 1978 April; 1(2):167–168

Gargaro WJ Jr. Informed consent. Cancer Nurs 1978 Feb; 1(1):81–82

Gotto AM Jr et al. Obesity—risk factor No 1. Heart Lung 1978 Jan/Feb; 7(1):132–136

Groah L. Do patients value preoperative assessments? AORN J 1979 June; 29(6):1250–1256

Grundner TM. On the readability of surgical consent form. N Engl J Med 1980 April 17; 302(16):900–902

Hansen AE. Planning to implement preoperative interviews. AORN J 1979 Oct; 30(4):792–805

Hewitt D. Is that pre-op patient terrified? RN 1979 Sept; 42(9):44–47

Howard RB. More on informed consent. Postgrad Med 1979 Jan; 24(1):25

Hurley DL, Howard P Jr and Hahn HH III. Perioperative prophylactic antibiotics in abdominal surgery; a review of recent progress. Surg Clin North Am 1979 Oct; 59(5):919–934

Kakkar VV. Prevention of fatal postoperative pulmonary embolism by low doses of heparin: An international, multicentre trial. Lancet 1975 July; 2(7925):45–51

Kemp M. Dealing with depression after radical surgery. Nursing '79 1979 Feb; 9(2):47–51

Luce JM. Perioperative evaluation and perioperative management of patients with pulmonary disease. Postgrad Med 1980 Jan; 67(1):201–207

McConnell EA. Preop teaching helps. Nurs '80 1980 March; 10(3):90–92

Preop nutrition factor in postop complications. AORN J 1980 Jan; 31(1):134

Rayder M. Problem: A new nurse asks why preoperative teaching isn't done. Am J Nurs 1979 Nov; 79(11):1992–1995

Risser NL. Preoperative and postoperative care to prevent pulmonary complications. Heart Lung 1980 Jan/Feb; 9(1):57–67

Sandusky WR. Use of prophylactic antibiotics in surgical patients. Surg Clin North Am 1980 Feb; 60(1):83–92

Schrankel DP. Pre-operative teaching. Supervisor Nurse 1978 May; 9(5):82–90

Standards for infection control in recovery room nursing. AORN J 1979 June; 29(7):1305–1312

Tkach JR, Shannon AM and Beastron R. Pseudofolliculitis due to preoperative shaving. AORN J 1979 Nov; 30(5):881–884

Voshall B. The effects of preoperative teaching on postoperative pain. Top Clin Nurs 1980 April; 2(1):39–43

Walters J. Four practical questions to ask when organizing preoperative classes. Am J Nurs 1979 June; 79(6):1090–1091

Whitcher SJ and Fisher JD. Multidimensional reaction to therapeutic touch in a hospital setting. J Pers Soc Psychol 1979 Jan; 37(1):87

Wolfe BM, Phillips GJ and Hodges RE. Evaluation and management of nutritional status before surgery. Med Clin North Am 1979 Nov; 63(6):1257–1269

INTRAOPERATIVE NURSING CARE
Articles

Altman BJ. BMET (biomedical equipment technician): New Member on the OR team. AORN J 1979 Sept; 30(3):435–441

Copeland WM. Informed consent and the OR nurse. AORN J 1979 April; 29(5):928–944

Foster CG et al. Effects of surgical positioning. AORN J 1979 Aug; 30(2):219–232

How do nurses control stress in the OR? AORN J 1979 Sept; 30(3):442–446

Humphries SM. Nurturing the nurse: OR orientation. AORN J 1979 July; 30(1):64–75

Kneedler JA. Perioperative role in three dimensions. AORN J 1979 Nov; 30(6):859–874

Larke GA. Perioperative charting. OR nursing on display. AORN J 1980 Feb; 31(2):194–198

Lindeman CA. How to work with nursing schools for OR experience (guest editorial). AORN J 1980 Jan; 30(1):17–20

Ngai SH. Current concepts in anesthesiology. Effects of anesthetics on various organs. N Engl J Med 1980 Mar 6; 302(10):564–566

Ozuna JM and Foster C. Hypothermia and the surgical patient. Am J Nurs 1979 April; 79(4):646–648

Phippen ML. Perioperative nurses use patient teaching conference. AORN J 1979 May; 29(7):1046–1051

Porter-O-Grady T and Carter JA. Bringing the nursing process into the OR. AORN J 1979 Nov; 30(5):898–914

Ryan P. Reusables vs disposables? Defending your position. AORN J 1979 Sept; 30(3):415–423

POSTOPERATIVE NURSING CARE

Articles

Albanese AJ and Riley JM. Caring for the intubated patient. RN Mag 1980 April; 43(4):38–43, 98–100

Allen P. Applying standards to practice. AORN J 1980 April; 31(5):805–813

Armstrong ME. Current concepts in pain. AORN J 1980 Sept; 32(3):383–390

Boguslawski M. Therapeutic touch: A facilitator of pain relief. Top Clin Nurs 1980 April; 2(1):27–37

Calderwood SB and Moellering RC Jr. Common adverse effects of antibacterial agents on major organ systems. Surg Clin North Am 1980 Feb; 60(1):65–81

Dean WF. Surgical evaluation of volume and ventricular function. CCQ 1979 Sept; 2(2):43–50

Eickhoff TC. Pulmonary infections in surgical patients. Surg Clin North Am 1980 Feb; 60(1):175–183

Eisendrath SJ and Dunkel J. Psychological issues in intensive care unit staff. Heart Lung 1979 July/Aug; 8(4):751–758

Felton CL. Hypoxemia and oral temperatures. Am J Nurs 1978 Jan; 78(1):56–57

Finn KL. How's your post-op ambulation technique? RN 1979 Sept; 42(9):69–72

Fletcher MM. Airway obstruction. Med Times 1978 Sept; 106(9):74–81

Fowler E, Jeter KF and Schwartz AA. How to cope when your patient has an enterocutaneous fistula. Am J Nurs 1980 March; 80(3):426–429

Frain M and Valiga TM. The multiple dimensions of stress. Top Clin Nurs 1979 April; 1(1):43–52

Gelin LE et al. Septic shock. Surg Clin North Am 1980 Feb; 60(1):161–174

Graff C. Warning—don't jump to conclusions when a patient's in shock. RN 1979 Aug; 42(8):23–28

Halpern LM. Anxiety and pain in postoperative patients. Hosp Pract (special report) 1977 Jan; 12(1):31–33

Kirilloff LH and Maszkiewicz RD. Guide to respiratory care in critically ill adults. Am J Nurs 1979 Nov; 79(11):2005–2012

Lewis KP and Cressey I. Nursing care of postanesthesia shivering. AORN J 1979 Aug; 30(2):357–366

Lidocaine may prevent postoperative laryngospasm. AORN J 1980 Jan; 31(1):76

Love-Mignogna S. Taping and splinting. Nursing '80 1980 April; 10(4):88–92

McConnell E. Toward complication-free recoveries for your surgical patients. RN 1980 June; 43(6):31–33, 75–90

McDonnell DE. How to relieve pain with injectable narcotics. Nursing '80 Oct; 10(10):34–39

McDonnell DE. TENS (transcutaneous electrical nerve stimulation) in treating chronic pain. AORN J 1980 Sept; 32(3):401–410

Moorthy SS, LaSasso AM and Gibbs PS. Respiratory failure in patients following surgery and trauma. CCQ 1979 March; 1(4):15–25

Myers AM. Evaluation of the hemorrhage-prone patient. Postgrad Med 1980 April; 67(4):161–170

Promisloff RA. A spirometry update. Nursing '78 1978 Nov; 8(11):90–92

Regan WA. Is RR (recovery room) nurse liable for patient injury in understaffed unit? AORN J 1980 Sept; 32(3):465–468

Rhoads JE. The impact of nutrition on infection. Surg Clin North Am 1980 Feb; 60(1):41–47

Risser NL. Preoperative and postoperative care to prevent pulmonary complications. Heart Lung 1980 Jan/Feb; 9(1):57–67

Robusto N. Advising patients on sex after surgery. AORN J 1980 July; 32(1):55–61

Ruiz CE, Weil MH and Carlson RW. Treatment of circulatory shock with dopamine. JAMA 1979 July 13; 242(2):165–168

Salmond SW. How to assess the nutritional status of acutely ill patients. Am J Nurs 1980 May; 80(5):922–924

Sandroff R. The potent placebo. RN 1980 April; 43(4):35–37, 88–96

Smith BJ. Safeguarding your patient after anesthesia. Nursing '78 1978 Oct; 8(10):53–56

Sos J and Cassem NH. Managing postoperative agitation. Drug Ther 1970 March; 10(3):103–106

Standards of Nursing Practice: Recovery Room. AORN J 1980 April; 31(5):800–804

Strandness DE Jr. Prevention of deep venous thrombosis in general surgery patient. Contemp Surg 1979 Feb; 14(2):55–64

Sweeney SS. OR observations: Key to post-op pain. AORN J 1980 Sept; 32(3):391–392

Sutterley DC. Stress and health: A survey of self-regulation modalities. Top Clin Nurs 1979 April; 1(1):1–21

White SJ and Williamson K. Narcotic analgesics. RN 1980 April; 43(4):31–33

Wyman JB and Wick MR. The vomiting patient. Am Fam Physician 1980 Feb; 21(2):139–143

WOUND CARE—INFECTION

Articles

Altemeir WA. Perspectives in surgical infections. Surg Clin North Am 1980 Feb; 60(1):5–13

Aspinall MJ. Scoring against nosocomial infection. Am J Nurs 1978 Oct; 78(10):1704–1707

Besst JA and Wallace H. Wound healing—intraoperative factors. Nurs Clin North Am 1979 Dec; 14(4):701–712

Brachman PS et al. Nosocomial surgical infections: Incidence and cost. Surg Clin North Am 1980 Feb; 60(1):15–25

Bruno P. The nature of wound healing. Nurs Clin North Am 1979 Dec; 14(4):667–682

Buchanan L et al. Guidelines for supervised wound care by emergency nurse practitioners. Nurse Prac 1979 May/June; 4(3):20–25

Castle M et al. Outbreak of a multiply resistant *Actinobacter* in a surgical intensive care unit: Epidemiology and control. Heart Lung 1978 July–Aug; 7(4):641–644

Castle M and Watkins J. Fever: Understanding a sinister sign. Nursing '79 1979 Feb; 9(2):26–33

Chang LF. How to succeed with wet-to-dry dressings. RN 1979 Jan; 42(1):63–66

Chavigny KJ. The scope of hospital epidemiology. Top Clin Nurs 1979 July; 1(2):77–84

Choice of antimicrobial drugs. Med Letter 1978 Jan 13; 20(1):1–

Cooper DM and Schumann D. Postsurgical nursing intervention as an adjunct to wound healing. Nurs Clin North Am 1979 Dec; 14(4):713–726

Crow S. Control of surgical nosocomial infections. AORN J 1978 July; 28(1):148–158

Cruse PJE and Foord R. The epidemiology of wound infection. Surg Clin North Am 1980 Feb; 60(1):27–40

Current concepts in healing wounds (symposium). Contemporary Surg 1978 Oct; 13(4):73–98

Dellinger EP. A protocol for managing surgical infections. Drug Ther 1979 May; 9(5):30–50

DuPont HL. Rational antibiotic therapy. Top Clin Nurs 1979 July; 1(2):45–51

Fahlberg WJ. Environmental control of transmission of hospital-acquired infection. Top Clin Nurs 1979 July 1(2):35–43

Farber BF and Wenzel RP. Postoperative wound infection rates: Results of prospective statewide surveillance. Am J Surg 1980 Sept; 140(3):343–346

Finegold SM. Anaerobic infections. Surg Clin North Am 1980 Feb; 60(1):49–64

Fisher PC. 12 (at least) incredibly simple tips on how you can control infection. RN 1978 Nov; 41(11):57–60

Gallucci BB and Reheis CE. Infection, nutrition and the compromised patient. Top Clin Nurs 1979 July; 1(2):23–33

Goldman PL and Petersdorf RB. Prophylactic antibiotics:

Controversies give way to guidelines. Drug Ther 1979 June; 9(6):57–77

Keith CF. Wound management following head and neck surgery. Nurs Clin North Am 1979 Dec; 14(4):761–778

Kellerhals SA. Isolation for person–environment protection: Rationale and utilization. Top Clin Nurs 1979 July; 1(2):67–75

Krause SL and Pappas SA. The nurse epidemiologist: Role and responsibilities. Top Clin Nurs 1979 July; 1(2):1–6

Kunin CM and Edelman R. The impact of infections on medical care in the United States. Ann Intern Med 1978 Nov; 89(4):Part 2:737–66

Larson E. Hands: The healers and killers. Top Clin Nurs 1979 July; 1(2):59–65

Mackey C and Hopefl AW. Keeping infections down when risks go up. Nursing '80 1980 June; 10(6):69–78

Magnussen MH. Aminoglycoside therapy. Nursing '80 1980 Feb; 10(2):82–87

Maki DG. Control of colonization and transmission of pathogenic bacteria in the hospital. Ann Intern Med 1978 Nov; 89(5)Part 2:777–780

Meakins JL et al. The surgical intensive care unit: Current concepts in infection. Surg Clin North Am 1980 Feb; 60(1):117–132

Meshelany CM. Post-op wound dressings. Your guide to impeccable technique. RN 1979 May; 42(5):22–33

Miles SAA. The inflammatory response in relation to local infections. Surg Clin North Am 1980 Feb; 60(1):93–105

O'Byrne C. Clinical detection and management of postoperative wound sepsis. Nurs Clin North Am 1979 Dec; 14(4):727–742

O'Malley P. Managing the difficult draining wound. Nursing '79 1979 Dec; 9(12):40–41

Pietsch JB and Meakins JL. Predicting infection in surgical patients. Surg Clin North Am 1979 April; 59(2):185–197

Polk HC. Prevention of surgical wound infection. Ann Intern Med 1978 Nov; 89(5):Part 2:770–773

Postoperative wound sepsis rate can be cut by simple measures. JAMA 1978 Jan 2; 239(1):9–10

Schumann D. How to help wound healing in your abdominal surgical patient. Nursing '80 1980 April; 10(4):34–40

Schwartz SI (Moderator). Symposium: Surgical wounds. Contemp Surg 1979 Oct; 15(4):116–147

Smith G. Primary postoperative wound infection due to Staphylococcus pyogenes. Curr Probl Surg 1979 July; 16(7):1–56

Standards for infection control in recovery room nursing. AORN J 1979 June; 29(7):1305–1312

Stuver L. Wound management: How teamwork and innovation met a dying patient's needs. Nursing '79 1979 June; 9(6):38–42

Taylor V Sr. Meeting the challenge of fistulas and draining wounds. Nursing '80 1980 June; 10(6):45–51

Wineland MD. Invasive procedures and infection control. Top Clin Nurs 1979 July; 1(2):53–57

INFUSIONS AND FLUID BALANCE

Articles

Adlard JM and George JM. Hyponatremia. Heart Lung 1978 July–Aug; 7(4):587–593

An update on low-dose heparin. Am Fam Physician 1979 Sept; 20(3)170

Barber HRK. Fluid, electrolyte and nutritional management of the gynecologic patient. Curr Probl Obstet Gynecol 1979 Sept; 3(1):1–32

Bannister B and Harvard CWH. Setting up a drip. Br J Med 1980 Feb 16; (6212):463–465

Blust J. Preventing hematomas after venipuncture. Am J Nurs 1978 Oct; 78(10):1675–1676

Boylan A and Marbach B. Dehydration: Subtle, sinister, preventable. RN 1979 August; 42(8):37–41

Flomenbaum N. Acid–base disturbances. Emergency Medicine 1980 Oct 15; 12(17):24–45

Habel M. What you need to know about infusing plasma expanders. RN 1980 Aug; 43(8):31–33

Kangaroo + venoset = more accurate flow rates. Nursing '80 1980 March; 10(3):31

Lamb J. Intra-arterial monitoring. Nursing '77 1977 Nov; 7(11):65–71

Lumb PD et al. Aggressive approach to intravenous feeding of the critically ill patient. Heart Lung 1979 Jan–Feb; 8(1):71–80

Menzel LK. Clinical problems of fluid balance. Nurs Clin North Am 1980 Sept; 15(3):549–558

Menzel LK. Clinical problems of electrolyte balance. Nurs Clin North Am 1980 Sept; 15(3):559–576

Milhorn HT. Understanding arterial blood gases. Am Fam Physician 1980 March; 21(3):112–120

Pflaum SS. Investigation of intake–output as a means of assessing body fluid balance. Heart Lung 1979 May–June; 8(3):495–498

Plastic containers for intravenous solutions. Med Letter 1980 May 16; 22(10):43–44

Rapp RP, Grant K and Piecoro JJ Jr. Guidelines for the administration of commonly used intravenous drugs. Drug Intell and Clin Pharm 1976 April; 10(4):206–215

Rapp RP et al. Effects of electronic infusion control on the efficacy, complications, and cost of IV therapy. Hosp Forum 1979 Nov; 14(11):975–982

Rothrock R. Two-tape method. Nursing '79 1979 Feb; 9(2):86

Satterwhite BE. What to do when adriamycin infiltrates. Nursing '80 1980 Feb; 10(2):37

Sumner SM. Refining your technique for drawing arterial blood gases. Nursing '80 1980 April; 10(4):65–69

Upon J, Mulliken JB and Murray JE. Major intravenous extravasation injuries. Am J Surg 1979 April; 137(4):497–506

White SJ. IV fluids ad electrolytes: How to head off risks. RN 1979 Nov; 42(11):60–63

Wineland MD. Invasive procedures and infection control. Top Clin Nurs 1979 July; 1(2):53–57

Zeluff GW, Suki WN and Jackson D. Hypokalemia—cause and treatment. Heart Lung 1978 Sept–Oct; 7(5):854–860

HEPARIN LOCK

Articles

Couchonnal G et al. Complications with heparin-lock needles. JAMA 1979 Nov 9; 242(19):2098–2100

Huxley VD. Heparin Lock. RN 1979 Oct; 42(10):36–41

Managing IV Therapy. Horsham, Pennsylvania. Intermed Communications, 1980

Millam DA. How to insert an IV. Am J Nurs 1979 July; 79(7):1268–1271

CONDITIONS OF THE RESPIRATORY TRACT

7

1   CONDITIONS OF THE NOSE AND THROAT

PROBLEMS OF THE NOSE

EPISTAXIS (NOSEBLEED)

Causes

1. May result from injury
   a. "Picking" nose, or other trauma
   b. Crusting of nasal mucosa—initiated by dry air
   c. Deviated septum, perforated septum
2. May result from disease
   a. Acute rheumatic fever
   b. Acute sinusitis
   c. Arterial hypertension and hemorrhagic diseases
   d. Cancer

Kinds of Epistaxis and Therapeutic Management

A. *Anterior Epistaxis*

1. Applying pressure
   a. Have patient sit facing the nurse or examiner; instruct patient to tilt head slightly forward so that blood does not seep into nasopharynx.
   b. Instruct patient to pinch the soft lobular portion of his nose for a few minutes.
2. Suctioning and packing
   a. If above measures do not control bleeding, remove blood clots by suction or request patient to blow his nose.
      (1) Saturate a cotton ball with 1:1000 aqueous epinephrine and insert immediately on the bleeding side; apply pressure;
         or
      (2) Gently spray nasal mucosa with 2% cocaine; this will provide comfort and act as a vasoconstrictor.
   b. Almost always, bleeding will be controlled by above method.
3. Cauterization
   a. Utilizing a head mirror, nasal speculum, and suction, the examiner can locate the bleeding area and cauterize it with a silver nitrate applicator stick.
   b. If an electric cautery is used, local anesthetic must be injected.
4. Submucous resection
   If septum is deviated considerably, a submucous resection may be necessary. (See p. 141.)

B. *Anterior Ethmoidal Arterial Bleeding*

This is bleeding from the anterior ethmoidal artery, which is high and posterior; bleeding site cannot be seen.
1. Packing
   a. Apply packing (pack saturated with petrolatum and about the size of a small marble) to the crevice between septum and middle turbinate.
   b. Reinforce small pack by applying additional packing; keep packing in place for 2–3 days.
   c. If not successful the first time, repeat the process.
2. Bone realignment
   a. X-ray may be required to determine extent of bone displacement and skull involvement.
   b. Local or intravenous anesthesia may be required to realign bones.

   c. Usually nasal packing is inserted and external splints applied.
   d. Inform patient that a partial vacuum forms in the throat when he swallows, due to presence of nasal packing.
   e. Administer analgesics for comfort and antihistamines for symptomatic relief of sneezing and itching. Antimicrobials may be prescribed to prevent infection.
3. *Discharge Planning and Health Education*
   a. Explain to the patient that splinting may be necessary for up to two weeks (during which time collagen fibers continue to strengthen the wound).
   b. Instruct the patient in proper application of tape splint for the night, according to physician's preference; such splinting will prevent swelling of tissues at night when patient is lying down.
   c. Tell patient to soften crusts around nostrils by applying petrolatum.
   d. Inform patient that his ability to smell may be impaired the first few weeks; this may affect his appetite; therefore encourage him to maintain an adequate diet.
   e. Instruct patient to take precautions to prevent head colds and nose trauma.
   f. Remind patient of follow-up visits to the physician.

C. *Posterior Epistaxis*

This bleeding is often heavier and occurs more often in the elderly; usually the source cannot be seen, since it is posterior.

> **NURSING ALERT:** Because posterior nasal packing depresses the soft palate so that it causes airway resistance, CO_2 retention and hypoxemia may occur; observe patient closely, assess vital signs, recognize need for blood gas determinations, note level of consciousness, and listen to chest sounds. Do not oversedate patient.

1. Postnasal packing
   a. Treat by applying a postnasal pack after initial anesthetic spray or application of cocaine-saturated pledgets to area.
   b. While anesthesia is taking effect, determine nursing history—is bleeding due to an injury? does patient have arteriosclerotic heart disease? is he on anticoagulants?
   c. Insert a small No. 12 or 14 Fr. catheter through the nose and withdraw tip through the mouth.
   d. Prepare nasal pack by lubricating it with antimicrobial ointment.
   e. Attach nasal pack (to which 3 strings are attached) to catheter and pull catheter back through the nose; pack, which follows, is positioned in postnasal area. Two strings emerge from nose; fasten these over a wad of gauze or a dental cotton roll at tip of nose. The other string is brought out through the mouth and taped to the side of the face (Fig. 7-1).

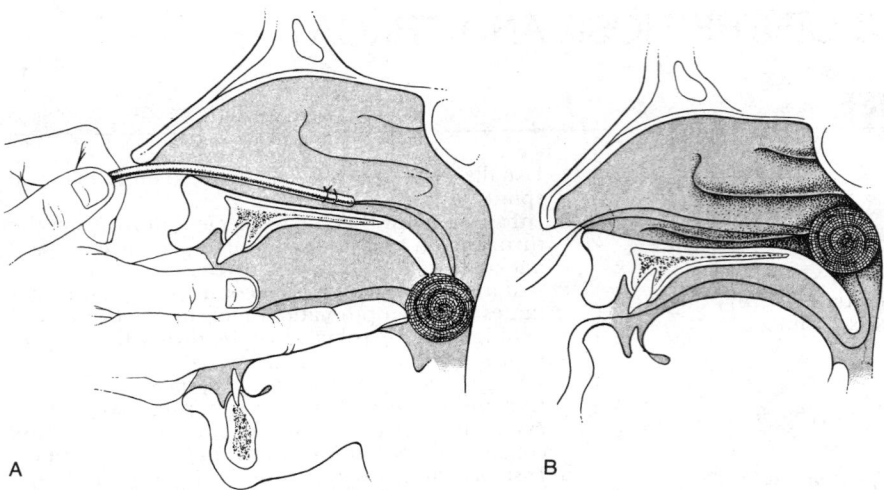

FIGURE 7-1. *Placing a postnasal pack for posterior epistaxis. Pass a catheter through the nose into the oropharynx and tie the posterior pack to its end. Then pull the catheter back through the nose while guiding the pack around the soft palate with your forefinger (A) and into place in the nasopharynx (B). Tie the two strings that emerge from the nose over rolls of cotton or gauze to keep the pack from sliding back into the oropharynx and tape the third string which emerges from the mouth, to the side of the face; this string will be used later when you remove the pack from the nasal cavity. (From Donald PJ: Leading with the nose. Emergency Medicine 7 (11):29)*

f. Keep packing in place for 2–4 days.

g. Permit liquid diet and other light sedation as prescribed for comfort.

h. Remove packing via oropharynx by grasping string with a clamp. (See Nursing Management, which follows.)

i. If bleeding continues, repeat the entire process.

NOTE: If postnasal packing is unsuccessful, it may be necessary to ligate surgically the internal maxillary artery.

2. Nursing Management in Postnasal Packing

a. Place patient in a semi-Fowler's position; recumbent position may permit blood to seep into the back of the throat, causing patient to gag.

b. Assess condition of patient to determine extent of hemorrhage, his general condition, and any evidence of shock.

c. Initiate first aid measures as described and evaluate for their effectiveness.

d. For posterior epistaxis, which requires postnasal packing, hospitalization is mandatory.

e. Observe patient for level of consciousness; if he appears faint, lower his head.

f. Be sure packs handed to the physician have strings tightly tied (2 on one end, 1 on the other).

g. Change the pad of gauze at the nostril area whenever it becomes necessary. Bright red blood indicates continued hemorrhage; dark, dry blood stains mean bleeding is controlled.

h. Inform patient that he will be breathing through his mouth; a sucking noise may be heard when he swallows, but this will disappear when packing is removed.

i. Encourage refreshing mouth care frequently because of the need to breathe through the mouth.

j. Provide subtle deodorizers in the room since packing often emits an offensive odor after 48 hours.

k. Monitor vital signs frequently in an effort to detect continued hemorrhage or early signs of infection due to prolonged packing.

l. If packing obstructs eustachian tubes, otitis media may develop; assess for early signs of earache.

m. Recognize that hematocrit and hemoglobin readings may be falsely high due to hypovolemia.

n. Assist physician when packing is removed; have patient in sitting position in bed, with towel draped and fastened at neck.

(1) Have emesis basin ready to receive packs.

(2) Instruct patient to close his eyes if he feels that seeing the packing may upset him.

(3) Permit the patient to be up and about if there is little or no bleeding. He may expect some trickling or oozing of blood in the back of his throat. Any excess bleeding (spitting of excess amounts of fresh blood) should be reported.

o. *Health Teaching*

Advise patient to avoid activities which increase pressure in the nose, causing fresh bleeding; i.e., sneezing hard, blowing the nose hard, lifting heavy objects, performing strenuous exercises. (This admonition applies to a 2-week period.)

E. *Ligation of Internal Maxillary and Ethmoidal Arteries*

1. Many otolaryngologists prefer this method of managing posterior epistaxis.

2. First, during patient evaluation, temporary control of bleeding with a nasal balloon is recommended (Fig. 7-2). This is followed by surgery.

3. Patients appear to prefer this method to packing.

RHINITIS

Rhinitis is an inflammation of the mucous membrane of the nose.

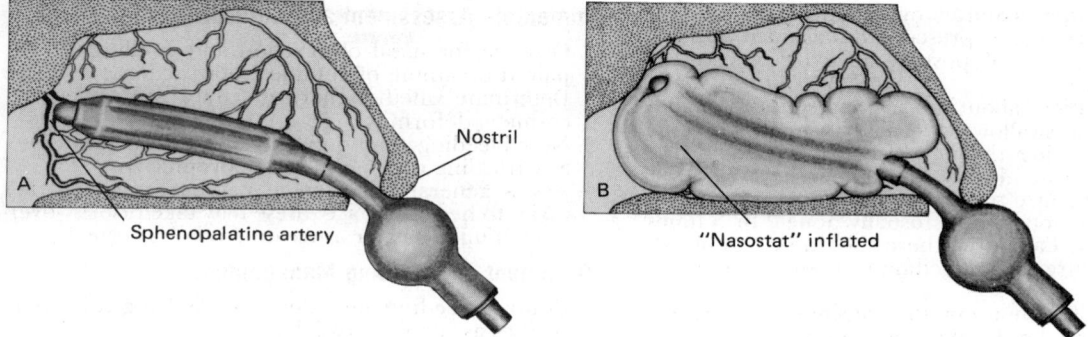

FIGURE 7-2. A. *This is a disposable, self-retaining nasal balloon for control of epistaxis. The "Nasostat" is inserted through the nostril and is positioned. There is an external shut-off valve for inflating and deflating that is designed to accept a Luer syringe tip.*
B. The balloon is designed so that when inflated as shown it compresses the sphenopalatine artery as it enters the nasal cavity (visible in A but not in B). The outside bulb is soft and is noncollapsible, to prevent the device from slipping posteriorly. (Courtesy of developer, G. Howard Gottschalk, M.D.; marketed by Sparta Instrument Corp.)

Clinical Manifestations

1. From allergic reaction, in infection (coryza), or early stages of viral infection
2. Congested and swollen mucous membranes; when persistent → "chronic catarrh"
3. Chronic rhinitis → abnormally large amounts of connective tissue → spurs, polyps, and hypertrophies on nasal septum → atrophy of mucous membrane and cartilage → abundant foul-smelling exudate (ozena)

NURSING ALERT: Instruct patient as follows:
1. Do not blow nose too frequently or too hard; doing so causes infection to spread, sinuses to become infected, and eardrum to be perforated, in some cases.
2. Blow through both nostrils at the same time to equalize pressure.

Management

1. Fundamental therapy is antihistamine administration, e.g., chlorpheniramine maleate. This may be supplemented with a decongestant, such as pseudoephedrine hydrochloride.
2. Also see Allergic rhinitis, p. 620, Allergy Problems)

NASAL OBSTRUCTION

Causes

1. Deflected septum
2. Hypertrophy of turbinate bones
3. Polyps
4. Tumors
5. Common cold
6. Foreign bodies
7. Fractures
8. Allergic rhinitis
9. Adenoid hypertrophy

Related Problems

1. Chronic infection of nose, such as nasopharyngitis
2. Sinusitis, which may include pain in sinus regions
3. Recurrent otitis media

Primary Care Nurse as a Case Finder

School and community nurses particularly will be able to detect children with nasal obstruction; these should be referred to the physician.

Management

1. Nasal obstruction should be removed.
2. Measures employed to curb chronic infection:
   a. Nasal allergy corrected
   b. Nasal sinuses drained (may be an operating room procedure)
   c. Nasal polyps clipped
   d. Hypertrophied turbinates shrunk with astringent solutions
   e. Hypertrophied adenoids removed
   f. Submucous resection or nasal septal reconstruction may be performed to remove deflected bone and cartilage (See following.)

SUBMUCOUS RESECTION (SMR) OR NASAL SEPTAL RECONSTRUCTION (NSR)

Submucous resection of the septum is an operation in which cartilaginous and/or osseous portions of the septum that lie between the flaps of the mucous membrane and perichondrium are removed or straightened—to establish an adequate partition between the right and left nasal cavities in order to provide a clear nasal airway.

Nasal septal reconstruction involves resection or removal of cartilaginous (or bony septum) followed by reconstruction of all parts of the septum that may produce nasal airway obstruction.

Postoperative Nursing Management

1. Raise head of bed to promote drainage—to make the patient more comfortable and to lessen edema.

2. Maintain patient comfort by administering meperidine or morphine as prescribed, inasmuch as there is a fair amount of postoperative discomfort for several hours.
3. Reassure patient about the sucking sound he experiences as he swallows; the nasal packing prevents air from moving through his nose and a partial vacuum is created in his throat when he swallows.
4. Change the gauze pad under his nose as it becomes soaked with blood; this is usually done 2 or 3 times the first day. Each time there should be less blood. Notify the surgeon if bleeding increases rather than decreases.
5. Administer frequent mouth care since the patient is forced to breathe through his mouth.
6. Administer a sedative—to make the patient more comfortable.
7. Apply cold compresses for first 24 hours—to lessen edema and discoloration, and to promote comfort.

FRACTURE OF THE NOSE

Cause

Results from direct trauma, e.g., a blow inflicted by an object (ball or fist), or an injury sustained in an automobile collision.

Immediate Assessment and Clinical Manifestations

1. Observe for nasal obstruction and swelling → impaired breathing or complete obstruction.
2. Determine whether there is nasal displacement → cosmetic deformity.
3. Note bleeding—not only external bleeding, but also any trickling of blood into the oropharynx.
4. Assess general condition of patient for related injuries to head and face; these may take priority over a nasal injury as far as treatment is concerned.

Treatment and Nursing Management

1. Control bleeding and edema by applying cold compresses as soon as possible.
2. Place patient in a comfortable position with head somewhat elevated to control bleeding; if in sitting position, the patient might faint during manipulation of nasal fracture.
3. The physician will determine whether fracture reduction can be maneuvered without anesthesia; often pressure can be exerted on the convex side of the nose and the bones and septum manipulated into position.

SPECIFIC INFECTIONS OF THE UPPER RESPIRATORY TRACT

General Considerations

A. *Predisposing Conditions*

Nasal septum and turbinate pathology, allergy, emotional problems

B. *Preventive Hygienic Measures*

1. Intended to support body defenses and reduce susceptibility to infection.
2. Patient should set up a conscientious health regimen—adequate exercise, plenty of sleep, nutritious diet, relaxing hobbies.
   a. Avoid chilling, particularly of the feet, since this lowers resistance.
   b. Employ humidifying measures indoors during winter months.
   c. Avoid emotionally upsetting experiences.
   d. Minimize indulgence in alcohol, smoking, drugs.
   e. Avoid inhaling irritating substances such as hair or other sprays, dust, chemicals, smoke, etc.

STREPTOCOCCAL SORE THROAT

Clinical Manifestations

1. Rapid onset of sore throat, chills, temperature above 38.3° C. (101° F.), headache, general malaise.
2. Children may have (in addition to the above) acute abdominal pain, nausea, perhaps repeated vomiting.
3. Red pharynx, enlarged tonsils and tonsillar nodes below angle of the mandible, edematous uvula.
4. Tonsils and pharynx may be covered with an exudate.
5. Throat pain may prevent swallowing.
6. Patient may present with a flushed face and leukocyte count over 12,000.

Treatment and Nursing Management

Early intervention with chemotherapeutic agents is important to prevent serious complications such as acute rheumatic fever, acute glomerulonephritis.
1. Obtain throat culture. (See p. 143.)
2. Initiate penicillin therapy for 24 hours.
3. If culture is positive in 24 hours for group A β-hemolytic *Streptococci,* continue treatment for 10 days.
4. If culture is negative and if there is no significant clinical improvement in the patient, discontinue penicillin.
5. If culture is negative and patient has improved clinically, continue penicillin for 10 days. (This means penicillin is effective; discontinuing penicillin too soon may cause a return of infection.)
6. If throat culture shows other microbial infection, utilize specific antimicrobial agent.

NOTE: See also page 294 for role of streptococcal infection in rheumatic heart disease—treatment and nursing management, page 294.

If patient is hypersensitive to penicillin, he may be treated with erythromycin.

GUIDELINES: Obtaining a Throat Culture

Purpose To determine the nature of microbial throat infection, secretion or material from the mucous surface of the throat may be transferred to a medium that encourages the growth of microorganisms. This growth is subsequently studied in the laboratory.

Equipment Tongue blade
Sterile cotton or Dacron swab
Blood agar plate or required culture medium
Adequate light source

Procedure (Fig. 7-3)

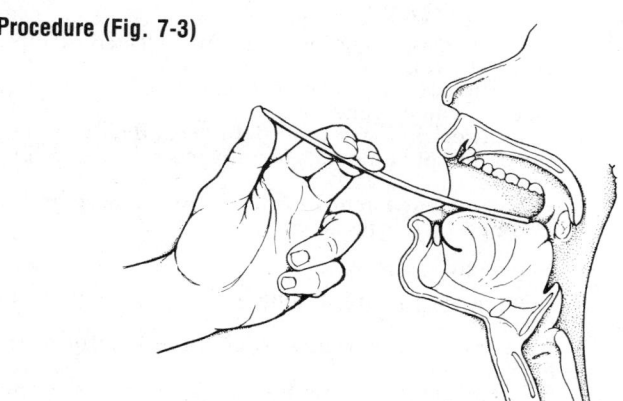

A. Grasp the tongue blade so that the thumb pushes the end upward (as a fulcrum) while the fingers push the middle section downward.

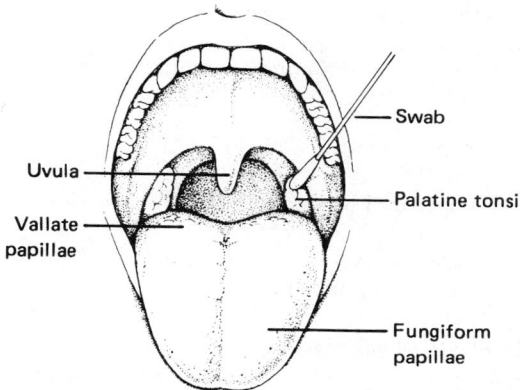

B. Vigorously rub a cotton or dacron swab over each tonsillar area and posterior pharynx.

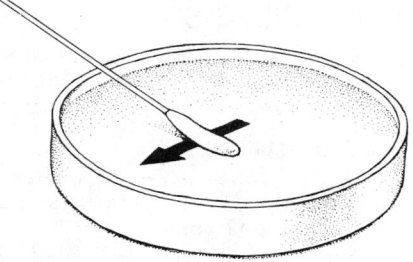

FIGURE 7-3. Throat culture.

C. Streak the swab on a blood agar plate and place in an incubator for 24 hours. Plate can then be read grossly.

NURSING ACTION	RATIONALE/AMPLIFICATION
1. Inform the patient of the need for a throat culture.	1. When patient is cooperative, procedure is facilitated and is more acceptable to him.
2. Place patient in a comfortable sitting or lying position; instruct him to tilt the head backward.	
3. Have patient open his mouth wide; direct maximum lighting toward back of throat.	3. A good light source illuminates back of throat and assists nurse in identifying structures.
4. Depress the tongue as shown in Fig. 7-3A. (Some patients object to the use of a tongue blade; if such a patient can relax his tongue while panting, this may be satisfactory.)	4. This permits access of the swab to the tonsillar area and posterior pharynx. (The tongue blade may stimulate the gag reflex.)
5. Vigorously swab the involved tonsillar area and posterior pharynx with the cotton or Dacron swab (Fig. 7-3B).	5. *Avoid* swabbing the tongue. Use aseptic technique in handling swab.
6. Immediately streak the swab on the plate or follow directions of the laboratory for transport medium (Fig. 7-3C).	6. In some instances, it may be required to submit the swab; in this instance, swab must not be allowed to dry, but should be brought to the laboratory in transporter-handling medium.
7. All specimens are to be labeled—include patient's name and unit; nature and source of specimen; date	7. This is recorded on label attached to specimen and also on patient's chart.
8. Patient is permitted to resume activity.	

ADENOVIRAL INFECTIONS

Types

A. *Acute Respiratory Disease (ARD)*

Symptoms
  Cold
  Sore throat
  Headache
  Temperature elevation
  Malaise

B. *Pharyngoconjunctival Fever*

1. Duration—1 to 10 days
2. Symptoms (common in summer in children who swim in pools)
   Fever
   Sore throat
   Cold
   Large and tender cervical lymph nodes
   Headache
   Hoarseness
   Acute conjunctivitis
   Malaise

C. *Rhinoviral Infections*

Examples: Common cold, croup, and bronchitis, which may lead to bronchopneumonia.

Management

1. Symptomatic
2. No specific antimicrobial or chemotherapy

HERPES SIMPLEX INFECTION

This infection produces common herpes labialis (fever blisters, cold sores, cankers).

Clinical Manifestations

1. Small vesicles, single or in groups, located on lips, tongue, cheeks, or pharynx.
2. Sore ruptures and becomes shallow ulcer covered with gray membrane.
3. Signs associated with other febrile conditions: pneumococcus pneumonia, meningococcal meningitis, malaise.
4. Virus remains latent in cells of lips or nose and is activated by febrile illnesses.

Management

1. Chemotherapy and antimicrobials appear to be of no value.
2. Analgesics and perhaps codeine are helpful in relieving pain.
3. Spirits of nitre or Campho-Phenique applied locally are helpful in drying the lesion.

SINUSITIS

Sinusitis is an inflammation of the sinuses. (Sinuses are often involved in upper respiratory tract infections.) Recovery is based on the condition that the nasal passage be clear. If passage is obstructed (blocked by deviated septum, polyps, spurs, enlarged turbinates) sinusitis may become chronic.

ACUTE SINUSITIS

Clinical Manifestations

1. Pain
   a. Frontal headache—related to frontal sinusitis
   b. In and about eyes—related to ethmoidal sinusitis
   c. Lateral to nose, upper teeth—related to maxillary sinusitis
   d. Occipital headache—related to sphenoidal sinusitis
2. Nasal congestion and discharge may or may not be present
3. Mild fever; anosmia
4. Acute suppurative infection
   If frontal sinus involved, this can be serious because it may rupture posteriorly and lead to brain abscess.
5. Nasal mucosa may be red and edematous

Medical and Nursing Management

1. Bed rest; analgesics for pain; hot compresses to midface and forehead
2. Nonsurgical drainage of sinuses
   a. Instill vasoconstrictor: Neo-Synephrine ¼% spray or drops.
   b. Use penicillin to speed recovery and lessen possibility of complications.
   c. Administer an antihistaminic.

CHRONIC SINUSITIS

Chronic sinusitis is a suppurative inflammation of the sinuses with chronic irreversible change in the musoca and sinus bony area.

Clinical Manifestations

1. Persistent nasal obstruction; purulent nasal discharge
2. Cough—produced by constant dripping of discharge back into nasopharynx
3. Headache—more noticeable in the morning

Medical and Nursing Management

1. Administration of vasoconstricting drugs to promote drainage
   Recognize danger of prolonged use of nasal decongestants. It may lead to *rhinitis medicamentosa*, which is a recurring cycle of: nasal congestion → use of decongestants → relief → leading to nasal congestion → more decongestants, etc.
2. Repair of structural deformities
   a. Polyps excised or cauterized
   b. Deviated septum removed
3. Draining of sinuses
   a. Frontal—incision through eyebrow
   b. Maxillary—*Caldwell-Luc operation,* in which the incision is made along the upper gum line above canine teeth under the upper lip. An opening is made into the anterior wall of the sinus to permit stripping out of infected contents. A "window" is created between maxillary sinus and nose.
   (1) Postoperative nursing management is similar to that for a patient who has had a submucous resection. (See p. 141.)

(2) Be prepared to support the patient and assist the physician when sinus packing is withdrawn through nose.
   (a) Drape patient, who is in a sitting position in bed.
   (b) Place emesis basin under nasal area.
   (c) Observe for bleeding while instructing patient to keep his eyes closed if he appears squeamish.
(3) Administer mouth care carefully; limit this to mouth rinses at first; when a toothbrush is used it should be of the soft type. Care is taken not to injure the incision area.
(4) Apply cold compresses over lip to help in reducing edema.
(5) Inform patient that swelling and a "black-eye" are often in evidence for a week or two; the latter is due to extravasation of blood into soft tissues under the eye.
(6) Offer liquid diet for the first few days and then progress to soft diet.

Health Education

1. Advise patient that numbness in the operative area may be present for several weeks or months.
2. Instruct patient not to blow his nose for at least 2 weeks after packing has been removed to avoid forcing nasal secretions back into the maxillary sinus.
3. Prevent irritation along incision line for several weeks; upper dentures should not be worn, since they could injure the operative area.

PHARYNGITIS

ACUTE PHARYNGITIS

Acute pharyngitis is an inflammation of the mucous membranes of the pharynx.

Clinical Manifestations

1. Reddened pharyngeal membrane
2. Edema of lymphoid follicles of throat
3. Enlarged and tender cervical lymph nodes
4. Temperature elevation
5. Mild sore throat
6. Difficulty swallowing

Clinical Course

1. Viral; uncomplicated—patient may recover in 3 to 10 days
2. Bacterial (beta hemolytic *Streptococcus*, hemolytic *Staphylococcus aureus*, *Haemophilus influenzae*); leads to more severe illness and danger of serious complications:
   Sinusitis, otitis media, mastoiditis, rheumatic fever, nephritis

Diagnostic Evaluation

Primarily by throat culture. Gram stain of throat secretions is proposed as an accurate method of early diagnosis of group A beta hemolytic streptococcal pharyngitis.

Nursing Management

1. Promote rest for the patient.
   a. Keep patient in bed during febrile stage.
   b. Encourage rest periods while he is ambulant.
2. Examine skin twice a day for telltale rashes indicating onset of a communicable disease.
3. Maintain medical asepsis to prevent spread of infection.
4. Assist in diagnostic evaluation by obtaining throat cultures, nasal swabbings, blood specimens.
5. Provide warm saline gargles or irrigations that approach the limit of heat tolerance for the individual— not to exceed 48.8° C. (120° F.)—to reduce pharyngeal muscle spasm and relieve throat soreness.
6. Offer symptomatic relief.
   a. Ice collar
   b. Analgesic medications—aspirin, or acetaminophen and codeine
   c. Antitussive medications to control cough
   d. Soporific at bedtime
7. Provide adequate mouth care for comfort and for prevention of secondary infection.
8. Suggest a soft diet if the patient is able to swallow comfortably.
9. Encourage fluids, up to 2500 ml. a day, if possible.

Convalescent Regimen and Health Education

1. Assess morning and evening temperature to detect low-grade infection or advent of a complication.
2. Promote rest and gradual resumption of full activity; advise patient to avoid overexertion, chilling, fatigue, etc. Watch for the onset of a complication such as glomerulonephritis or rheumatic fever (onset occurs 2 to 3 weeks after pharyngitis subsides if it is of streptococcal origin).
3. Recognize onset of infections adjacent to the pharynx which might indicate extension of disease to the mastoid, ear, lymph nodes, etc.

CHRONIC PHARYNGITIS

Types

1. Hypertrophic—general thickening and congestion of pharyngeal mucous membrane
2. Atrophic—characterized by a glistening, thin, whitish, wrinkled membrane
3. Chronic granular—numerous swollen lymph follicles

Clinical Manifestations

1. Sense of fullness in throat, persistent irritation
2. Collection of mucus, expelled by coughing
3. Swallowing difficulty

Management and Health Education

1. Tobacco and alcohol should be eliminated.
2. Patient should keep voice at rest.
3. Related problems (chest or upper respiratory) that may cause coughing should be corrected.
4. Humidification equipment should be used since this tends to liquefy secretions, making it easier to expel them; a humidifier connected to the forced air system in the home is effective.

DISEASE OF THE TONSILS AND ADENOIDS

(For children, see page 1262.)

TONSILS

Tonsils are paired structures of lymphatic tissue, one lying on either side of the oropharynx; they are a common site of focal infection. Occasionally they grow to such a size that normal respiration is hampered.

Clinical Manifestations

1. Throat pain, ranging from mild to severe and accompanied by difficulty in swallowing, fever, swollen lymph glands under the mandible
2. Muscle, joint pain, and frequently headache may accompany tonsillitis
3. Inflamed edematous tonsillar area
4. White or yellow spots on tonsils, which are exudate

Treatment

1. Analgesics, such as codeine and aspirin or acetaminophen; rest
2. Warm throat irrigations
3. Antimicrobial therapy, which should be continued for 2 days after symptoms abate (otherwise there is a possibility of recurrence)

Indications for Removal of Tonsils

1. Frequent infections, acute and/or chronic, the recurrent rate of which is uncontrolled by antibiotics.
2. Hypertrophy that causes significant obstruction

ADENOIDS

Adenoids consist of a mass of lymphatic tissue which when enlarged may obstruct nasal passages and cause headaches. Enlarged adenoids commonly accompany tonsillitis.

Chronic Adenoiditis

Produces frequent head colds, bronchitis, tonsillitis, nasal and eustachian-tube obstruction.
    a. Mouth breathing, fetid breath
    b. Voice impairment, snoring
    c. Earaches, draining ears, mastoid infection

Indications for Removal of Adenoids

1. Persistent nasal obstruction
2. Recurring middle-ear infection

CANCER OF THE LARYNX

Incidence

1. Occurs in men over 50; ratio of men to women is 10:1.
2. Greater predisposition to laryngeal cancer in some families and in people who smoke heavily or use their voices excessively.
3. In North America, about ⅔ of carcinomas of the larynx arise in the glottis, almost ⅓ arise in the

TONSILLECTOMY AND ADENOIDECTOMY

Nursing Management

A. *Immediate Nursing Concerns*
1. Reduce the possibility of postoperative bleeding and aspiration of blood; maintain a patent airway.
    a. Assess blood clotting time before surgery to determine possible needs during and after surgery.
    b. Place the patient in the sitting position postoperatively if he has had local anesthesia.
    c. Place the patient on the side, with head extended and turned, to allow drainage through nose and mouth (postgeneral anesthesia).
    d. Observe vital signs and recognize the changes which might indicate bleeding. (Watch for excessive swallowing—indicates bleeding.)
    e. Keep the patient as quiet as possible; excess activity will increase blood-flow rate, which may overtax suture line.
2. Minimize secretions in the throat during and after surgery and control pain.
    a. Administer atropine preoperatively.
    b. Give acetaminophen (Tylenol) or codeine, if prescribed.
    c. Place an ice collar around neck for comfort and to constrict blood vessels.

B. *Nursing Support During Convalescence; Health Education*
1. Promote healing and be alert for evidence of postoperative complications.
    a. Suggest bland diet: ices, ice cream, fruit gelatin, custards, soft-boiled egg, mashed potatoes, soft milk toasts, etc.
    b. Avoid serving excessively hot or cold beverages, spices, etc.
    c. Encourage rest and quiet activities during the first week.
    d. Add cooked vegetables, ground meat, as tolerated.
    e. Report any evidence of bleeding, particularly if it occurs on the 5th or 6th postoperative day; call the physician.
    f. Note any temperature elevation; if over a degree above normal, check with the physician.
2. Maintain cleanliness of the mouth to minimize infections and odors.
    a. Have the patient use mouth rinse frequently for comfort.
    b. See that patient brushes teeth at least 3 times daily.
3. Provide comfort as the tonsillar and adenoidal beds heal.
    a. Utilize prescriptions for analgesics since the throat will be sore for several days.
    b. Recognize that occasionally this patient may experience earache; this is a referred pain which can be controlled by analgesics.

supraglottic region and about 3% in the subglottic region of the larynx.

Clinical Expectations

1. When treated early, the likelihood of cure is great.
2. When limited to the vocal cords (intrinsic), spread is slow because of lessened blood supply.
3. When cancer involves the epiglottis (extrinsic), cancer

spreads more rapidly because of abundant supply of blood and lymph and soon involves the lymph nodes of the neck.

Clinical Manifestations

1. Hoarseness or voice change is usually the earliest sign; this symptom is apparent because the vocal cords are inhibited from approximating (coming close together) by the diseased tissue.
2. A feeling that there is a lump in the throat, dyspnea, dysphagia.
3. Pain in laryngeal prominence (Adam's apple), enlarged cervical nodes, cough.
4. Persistent sore throat (6 weeks).

Diagnostic Evaluation

1. Laryngoscopy, either indirect (mirror) or direct (using a laryngoscope), can be effective for early diagnosis.
2. Biopsy under local or general anesthesia.
   a. Toluidine blue contrast medium may be used to stain the larynx and pinpoint biopsy site (cancer cells have an affinity for the contrast medium).
3. Other diagnostic modalities are roentgenographic, such as
   (a) Anesthetizing larynx with cocaine and injecting Lipiodal for roentgenogram visualization
   (b) Tomography
   (c) Barium esophagogram

Medical Management

A. *Endoscopic Removal of Early Malignancy*

1. By means of an endoscope, the earliest cancer, or carcinoma in situ, is removed without an incision.
2. This does not affect the voice, and there are usually no other problems.
3. Close supervision is required (through follow-up visits to the physician).

B. *Radiation*—treatment is effective in controlling early cancers that are not deeply invasive and are without nodal metastasis.

1. The greater the extent of malignancy, the more likely radiation therapy will be used in conjunction with surgery.
2. Surgeons and radiologists vary as to the role of radiation therapy pre- and postoperatively; the quality of life is a strong consideration.

C. *Partial Laryngectomy*—for early intrinsic cancer

1. A small lesion on true cord may be removed on one side along with a substantial margin of healthy tissue.
2. *Laryngofissure* (thyrotomy) is used to remove tumor limited to one vocal cord.

NOTE: This operation is being replaced by x-ray therapy as a means of controlling early cordal lesions. Laryngofissure and radiation therapy have similar survival rates, but x-ray treatment gives a better voice. (This accounts for the less frequent use of laryngofissure.)

   a. An opening is made into the larynx through the thyroid cartilage; the involved cord and tumor are then removed. This approach is preferred if:
      (1) Muscles are not affected by the tumor
      (2) Vocal cord motility is normal
   b. Tracheostomy tube is inserted during surgery; removed when tissue edema subsides.

   c. Special nursing considerations:
      (1) Administer food and fluids for the first 48 hours by nasogastric tube or intravenous methods because of the possibility of difficulty in swallowing.
      (2) Gradually offer fluids by mouth.
      (3) Encourage slow, gradual resumption of vocal sounds; have patient begin with a whisper, until healing is complete, and then add more substantial sounds. He will have to occlude his tracheostomy tube to speak.
      (4) Usually there is no swallowing or airway problem.
      (5) Be sure patient knows that the tracheostomy tube is only a temporary measure.
      (6) Watch for evidence of subcutaneous emphysema since this occurs occasionally.
2. Horizontal (supraglottic laryngectomy)
   a. Hyoid bone, epiglottis, and false vocal cords are removed.
   b. Tracheostomy is done to maintain an adequate airway. (See p. 188.)
   c. Voice is normal.
   d. Watch for aspiration of fluids and difficulty in swallowing; this is due to liquids spilling into trachea.
   e. Often a radical neck dissection is done along with supraglottic laryngectomy.
3. Vertical (hemi-laryngectomy)
   a. Removal of one true vocal cord, false cord, one-half thyroid cartilage, arytenoid cartilage
   b. Voice may be hoarse
   c. No problem with airway or swallowing

D. *Partial and Subtotal Laryngectomy* is being performed more frequently to fulfill several objectives:

1. To remove tumor and nearby tissue.
2. To provide an airway that permits respiration and optimum sound production.
3. To preserve "glottic valve" function so that intrathoracic pressure may be increased during coughing, bowel function, etc.
4. To protect swallowing function without aspiration

E. *Conservation Laryngectomy*

1. Used on selected patients with extrinsic tumors.
2. Diseased parts of larynx are removed, but sufficient segments are salvaged to permit function.
3. Radical neck dissection (removal of lymph nodes and tissue adjacent to affected larynx) may be done on involved side.

F. *Total Laryngectomy* (Fig. 7-4B)

1. The entire larynx (epiglottis, false and true cords), cricoid cartilage, hyoid bone, and 2 or 3 tracheal rings are usually removed when there is extrinsic cancer of the larynx (extension beyond the vocal cords).
2. Often a radical neck dissection is also done because of metastasis to cervical lymph nodes.
3. See p. 148 for Nursing Management.

G. *Total Laryngectomy with Laryngoplasty*

1. Voice rehabilitation may be attempted through the *Asai operation.*
   a. A dermal tube is made from the upper end of the trachea into the hypopharynx.
   b. The tracheostomy opening is closed off with a finger.

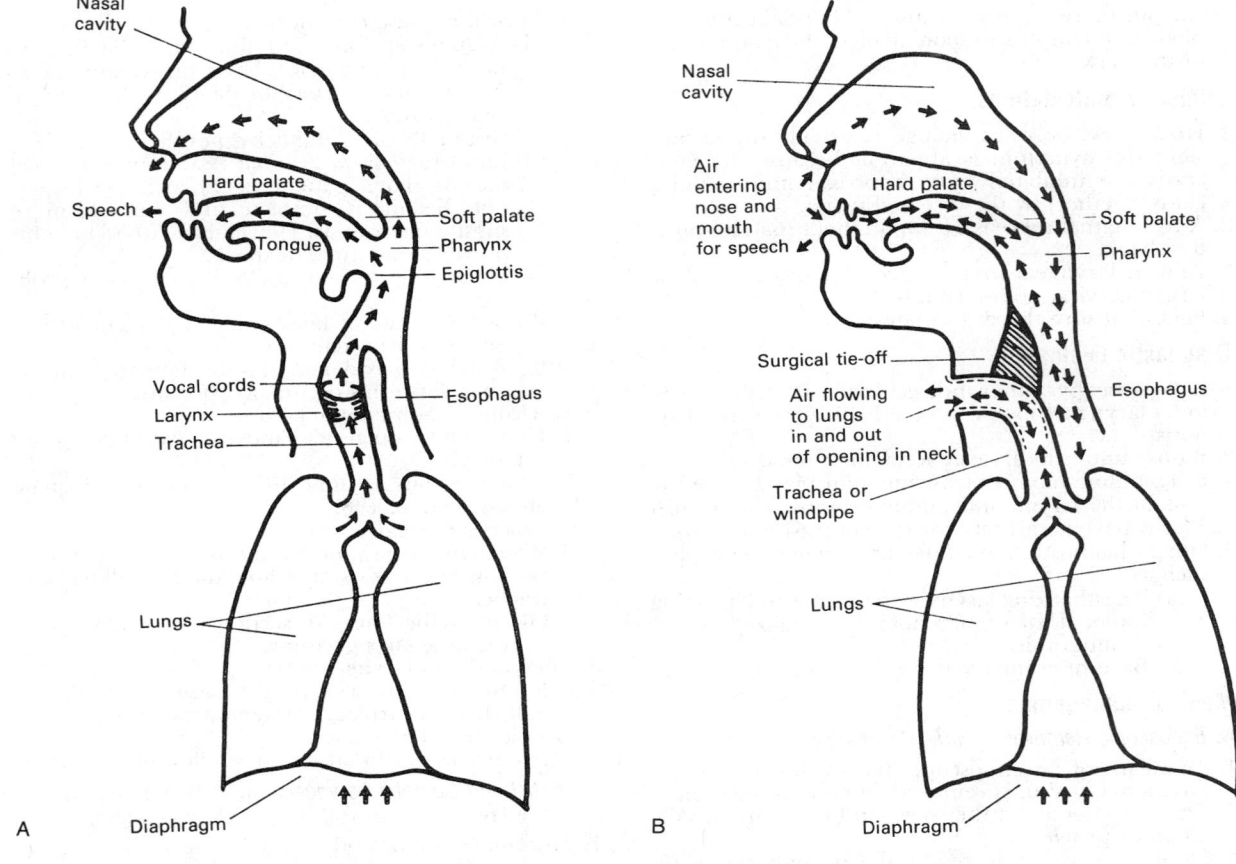

FIGURE 7-4. A. *Normal physiology of respiration and speech—note* arrows *indicating flow of air.* B. *This diagram illustrates the effect of a laryngectomy on the physiology of respiration and speech— again note air-flow patterns.* (American Cancer Society)

c. Then the patient expires air up the dermal tube into the pharyngeal cavity.
d. The sound produced is transformed into almost normal speech.

H. *Palliative Therapy*—For even more advanced cancer, palliative therapy may be initiated in the form of intra-arterial infusion with chemotherapeutic agents followed by deep roentgen ray therapy. (See p. 848.)

I. *CO_2 Laser* is being used endoscopically to re-establish airways blocked by tumor in order to de-bulk tumor mass prior to radiation and/or chemotherapy.

Advantage—Patient may return home on first postoperative day, eat, have a serviceable voice, no tracheostomy, and treatment is significantly cost-effective.

Nursing Management (for the Patient with a Total Laryngectomy)

A. *Psychosocial Preparation of the Patient for a Total Laryngectomy*

1. Collaborate with the physician in preparing the patient; amplify and interpret what the surgeon has already told the patient.

2. Inform him that he will breathe through an opening made in his neck.
3. Apprise him of the fact that his speech will be altered by surgery.
4. Expect reactions of depression, since the above informaton has a direct effect on his future.
5. Arrange for him to be visited by a laryngectomee (one who has had his larynx removed either totally or partially); such a person is able to transmit hope and encouragement to the patient.
6. Inform him of the services available for speech rehabilitation. Many patients make remarkable adjustments and pursue normal activities.
7. Practice a means of communication which is comfortable for the patient, i.e., sign language, pictures, word cards, pad and pencil.
8. Maintain good mouth hygiene; suggest that male patient shave his beard to allow for easier and safer postoperative care.

B. *Postoperative Nursing Management.*

(See postoperative care, Tracheostomy Patient, p. 188.)
1. Laryngectomy Management
    a. The laryngectomy tube is shorter but thicker than the tracheostomy tube. Care is similar to that for a tracheotomized patient. (See p. 188.)

b. Usually a laryngectomy tube is worn for a week or 10 days until the stoma heals.

c. Thereafter, observe the stoma area for crusting; crust can be softened and removed with a thin coating of petrolatum, antimicrobial ointment, and perhaps moist gauze over the opening; proper room humidification is helpful.

2. Nutritional Management

a. A nasogastric tube is passed by the physician postoperatively to prevent breakdown of suture line. This is kept in place until the pharyngeal suture line is healed—about 7–10 days.

b. If necessary, the stomach can be aspirated with low suction via the nasogastric tube.

c. Early feedings consist of skim milk and low-calorie gastrostomy fluids; observe patient for tolerance of feedings.

d. Follow feedings with water, up to 100 ml.; this rinses the tubing and provides additional fluids.

e. About 10 days after surgery, oral feedings are begun.

f. The patient's diet is supplemented with vitamins and infusions to maintain proper fluid, electrolyte, and nutritional balance.

NOTE: Some physicians do not employ a nasogastric tube postoperatively but begin early oral feedings.

3. Infection Control

a. Aseptic technique is practiced to avoid tracheal and respiratory infection.

b. If there is danger of incisional contamination, antimicrobial therapy may be prescribed.

C. *Discharge Planning and Health Education*

1. Speech Rehabilitation

a. Reassure the patient that speech rehabilitation can be very successful; laryngeal or esophageal speech or one of the artificial larynxes can be used.

b. Through the combined efforts of the surgeon, nurse, patient, family, other persons who have had laryngectomies, and a speech therapist, a plan of speech rehabilitation is initiated.

c. About 75% of postlaryngectomy patients utilize the technique of taking in a bolus of air as an energy source and then, by compression of the lips, simulating sounds by "plosive" speech. Esophageal speech is similar, but utilizes a belch to create a speech sound.

d. Various mechanical aids are available; it becomes a matter of selecting the best aid for the particular patient.

e. Tracheo-esophageal puncture (TEP) is a relatively new technique utilizing a prosthetic device (duck-bill).

(1) a fistula is made at the posterior trachea and anterior esophageal wall; a one-way valve is formed through the fistula. The finger is used to close the stoma during speech.

f. Motivation, determination, and relaxation are necessary for the patient to learn a new means of communication. He needs encouragement and support, which the nurse and his family can provide.

g. Affiliation with a group of similar individuals promotes the patient's progress. Addresses of organizations that offer assistance follow:

American Speech–Language–Hearing Association
10801 Rockville Pike
Rockville, Maryland 20852

International Association of Laryngectomees
American Cancer Society
777 Third Avenue
New York, New York 10017

Local groups of "Lost Chord Clubs"
"New Voice Clubs"

2. Stoma Cleanliness
Instruct the patient as follows:

a. Wash hands before touching stoma to prevent infection.

b. Wet wash cloth with warm water; wring dry, spread it over the stoma to cleanse tissue.

c. Do not use soap, tissues, or loose cotton since these substances may get into the airway.

d. Apply petrolatum thinly around exterior of (but not in) stoma. Wipe away excess lubricant.

3. Stoma Bib

a. A bib acts as a filter and warms the air about to enter the stoma. A crocheted cover or a cotton cloth that hangs over the stoma may be used. The bib can be fastened with ties around the neck.

b. For men: Ascot or turtle neck sweaters may be worn. When a regular shirt is worn, the second button from the top can be sewed over the buttonhole as though it were fastened—this leaves a wide opening through which a handkerchief can be inserted when coughing.

For women: A variety of fashionable scarves, jewelry, high-neck dresses, and turtleneck sweaters can be worn.

4. Mouth Care

a. Oral mucosa is not "aired" as before, and the patient's ability to detect mouth odors is lessened; therefore, special mouth care is required.

b. In addition to normal dental cleaning, a soft toothbrush is used to scrub the tongue and sides of the mouth; a turkish wash cloth is also effective in cleaning.

c. The mouth can be rinsed with a deodorizing mouthwash.

5. Drugs and Medications
Instruct the patient as follows:

a. Because many drugs tend to dry the stoma, always check with the physician before taking any medication.

b. Avoid undiluted alcohol since it has a tendency to dry the stoma; alcohol is also an irritant.

6. During a "cold"

a. Use steam inhalation—place a container of steaming water on a stool and sit in front of it with a towel draped around the neck and shoulders to form a hood. A steam inhalator can be used.

7. Complications to Avoid
Instruct the patient as follows:

a. Fistula. Observe suture line daily to note preliminary signs of redness, swelling, and possible secretions. If the temperature rises, this may be indicative of infection.

(1) Protect skin around stomal orifice, since secretions can cause breakdown of dermal tissues.

(2) Use a nasogastric tube for feedings; otherwise, whatever is eaten would leak through fistula and delay healing.

(3) Maintain intake and output records and be alert for signs of dehydration.

b. Occlusion of Opening.

(1) Protect stoma when showering by wearing a protective plastic cover.

(2) Swimming is not recommended.

(3) Protect stoma during a haircut and when powdering to prevent dust and hair from entering stoma.

(4) When shaving, use a dry towel around the neck to prevent hairs from entering stoma.

(5) In the event of an obstruction to the stoma, see Emergency First Aid next.

GUIDELINES: Emergency First Aid for the Laryngectomee

Nature of the Problem

Clogging or obstruction of the neck stoma is a life-threatening problem.

Equipment (if available):

Suction equipment	Sterile gloves
Sterile disposable catheter	Sterile saline
#14–16 Fr. (adult)	Portable mask and bag
#8–10 Fr. (child)	

Procedure for Total Neck Breather

One who breathes ONLY through the neck opening

1. There is no connection between lungs and nose or mouth.
2. A tracheostomy or laryngectomy tube may or may not be in the neck opening.

NURSING ALERT: No air can get through the mouth or nose of a total laryngectomee when stoma is clogged.

NURSING ACTION	RATIONALE/AMPLIFICATION
1. PLACE PATIENT ON HIS BACK, head straight, chin up. Bare the neck down to the sternum (Fig. 7-5A).	1. Access to the laryngeal stoma and observation of thoracic movement are facilitated.

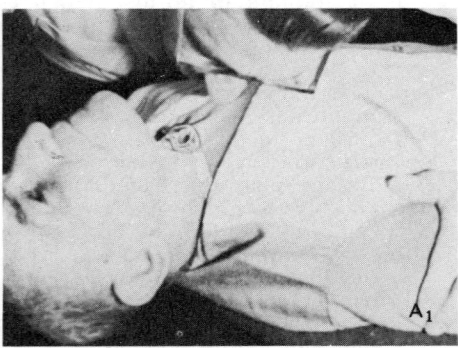

FIGURE 7-5. A$_1$. *Patient in proper position with laryngectomy tube in place.*

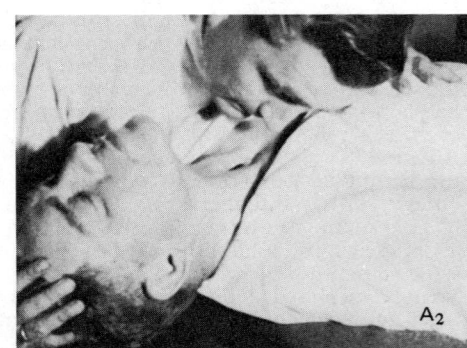

FIGURE 7-5. A$_2$. *Without laryngectomy tube.*

2. Position a blanket or any article of clothing under the shoulders.	2. This promotes hyperextension of the neck area, permitting access.
3. Make a rapid assessment of the situation: a. Is victim wearing a tracheostomy or laryngectomy tube? b. Has he been operated on recently? c. Check for tracheal obstruction. Clean stomal opening of mucus and encrusted matter.	3. a. In a laryngectomee, tube removal cannot cause immediate danger. b. If so, tracheostomy tube cannot be removed. c. Mucus, etc. may account for obstruction. Use a clean cloth or handkerchief—never tissue.
4. START MOUTH-TO-NECK BREATHING PROMPTLY Position yourself at side of victim; place your mouth and lips tightly over neck opening, or around the tracheal tube if the person is wearing one.	4. SECONDS COUNT. Do Not Remove the Tube.
5. If suction equipment is available, insert a soft rubber tube 7.5–12.5 cm. (3–5 in.) into opening for a few seconds (Fig. 7-5B).	5. A partially open airway transporting air to the victim is infinitely better than a clean airway that does not supply air at this crucial time.

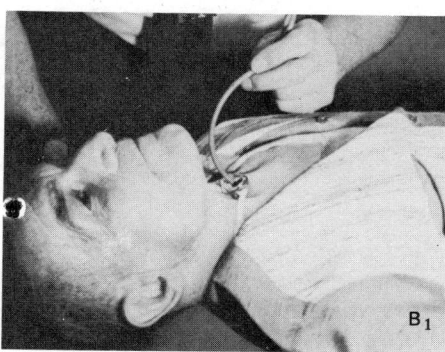

FIGURE 7-5. B₁. *Insert rubber catheter into laryngectomy tube.*

6. Blow in a sufficient amount of air to see chest rise (Fig. 7-5C & D).

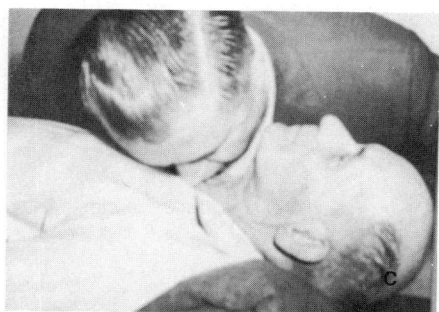

FIGURE 7-5. C. *Blow in sufficient amount of air to see chest rise.*

7. For the first 5 seconds repeat every 1–2 seconds; then slow down to a steady pace of every 4–5 seconds (12–20 times per minute).
8. Continue until spontaneous breathing returns.

Follow-up Phase

1. When victim recovers, provide oxygen from a portable supply.
2. If breathing fails again, resume mouth-to-neck breathing.
3. You can also use mechanical resuscitation with the rubber or plastic inflatable bag and mask combination (Fig. 7-5E).
4. Watch the chest rise.

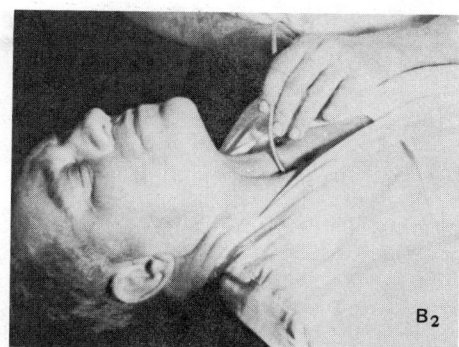

FIGURE 7-5. B₂. *Insert catheter directly into neck opening.*

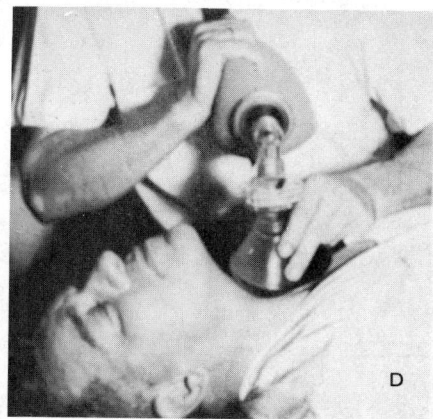

FIGURE 7-5. D. *Mechanical resuscitation can be employed.*

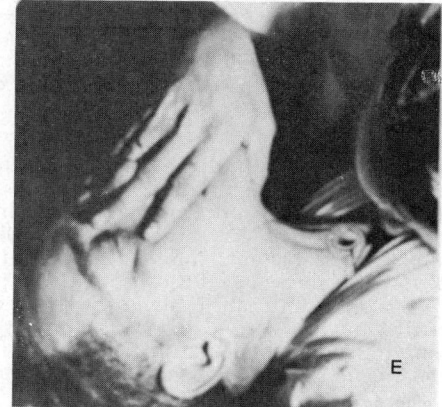

FIGURE 7-5. E. *Place palm of your hand over lips and mouth. (Courtesy of International Association of Laryngectomees, sponsored by the American Cancer Society, Inc.)*

3. Attach baby-sized mask; be sure there is a tight seal against neck opening.

4. Because a tight seal is difficult to maintain, and because pressure of the mask on the major blood

GUIDELINES: Emergency First Aid for the Laryngectomee (cont.)

NURSING ACTION	RATIONALE/AMPLIFICATION
5. Observe patient constantly.	vessels of the neck may interfere with blood supply to the brain, mouth-to-neck breathing is safer and better.

Procedure for Partial Neck Breather

One who breathes MAINLY through the neck opening.
1. A connection between the lungs and the nose and mouth still exists.
2. The larynx may or may not be present.
3. A tracheostomy or laryngectomy tube may or may not be in the neck opening.

NURSING ALERT: With mouth-to-neck breathing, FAILURE OF THE CHEST TO RISE is reliable proof that the patient is a partial neck breather. The rescuer may hear or feel air escaping from the victim's nose or mouth but it is not getting into the lungs.

NURSING ACTION	RATIONALE/AMPLIFICATION
1. a. Immediately place the palm of your hand (the one nearest to the patient's head) over the lips and mouth (Fig. 7-5E).	1. This will close the area between the trachea and throat and, at the same time, raise the base of the tongue against the palate and pharynx.
b. Pinch the nose shut between your third and fourth fingers.	
c. Place your thumb in the soft space under the chin and firmly press upward and backward.	
2. Remove patient's dentures	2. To ensure better lip closure and effective underchin thumb closure.
3. Now mouth-to-neck breathing will fill the lungs, and the chest will rise.	

2   CONDITIONS OF THE CHEST

MAJOR MANIFESTATIONS OF BRONCHOPULMONARY DISEASE

Cough and Sputum Production

A. *Causes*
1. Coughing is a protective mechanism that serves to clear the airway.
2. Cough-producing stimuli may be inflammatory, mechanical, chemical, or thermal.
3. Clinical problems producing cough are infection, inflammation, neoplasms, cardiovascular disorders, trauma, physical agents, and allergic disorders.
4. Violent coughing may cause bronchial obstruction and syncope, and cause further irritation of the bronchi.
5. Thick, mucopurulent sputum which is difficult to remove is more apt to cause violent coughing.

B. *Nursing Assessment*
1. Evaluate the character of the cough.
   a. Throat-clearing cough—postnasal drip.
   b. Dry and hacking—may be due to nervousness, viral infections, bronchogenic carcinoma, early congestive heart failure
   c. Loud and harsh—irritation in upper airway.
   d. Wheezing—associated with bronchospasm
   e. Severe or changing in character or with position—may be bronchogenic cancer (cough, chest pain, hemoptysis)
   f. Loose—indicates problems in peripheral bronchi and lung parenchyma
   g. Painful—may indicate pleural involvement, chest wall disease
   h. Chronic, productive—sign of bronchopulmonary disease
2. Note relationship of cough to time, to patient's position, and to environmental exposure.
   a. Coughing paroxysms at night—may indicate bronchial asthma or left-sided heart failure
   b. Cough that worsens when patient is supine—may be due to postnasal drip from sinusitis, bronchiectasis
   c. Cough associated with food intake—may be the result of aspiration into tracheobronchial tree
   d. Cough of recent onset—usually from acute infectious process.
   e. Smoking history: Current? Past?
   f. Environmental or occupational exposure to dusts, fumes, or gases?
   g. Allergies, asthma, sinusitis, upper respiratory infection?
3. Observe character and quantity of expectorated material.
   a. Clear or mucoid—stems from viral infection, chronic bronchitis, postnasal drip

b. Thick yellow or green sputum—due to primary or secondary bacterial infections.

c. Rusty—may indicate bacterial pneumonia (if patient not receiving antibiotics)

d. Malodorous—due to lung abscess, infection from fusospirochetal or anaerobic organisms

e. Frothy pink sputum—indicates acute pulmonary edema

f. Note amount of sputum produced daily. A sudden decrease in the quantity of sputum may indicate inspissation (drying and thickening) in tracheobronchial tree and may lead to respiratory insufficiency and failure.

g. Layering of sputum in sputum cup occurs in lung abscess or bronchiectasis.

C. Nursing Interventions

1. Make sure the patient is adequately hydrated to liquefy sputum.
2. Assist patient to cough productively by controlled coughing, postural drainage, and chest percussion.
3. Discourage smoking—interferes with lung defense mechanisms: paralyzes ciliary action, increases bronchial secretions, causes inflammation and hyperplasia of mucous glands, reduces production of surfactant, impairs function of alveolar macrophages (scavenger cells).
4. Encourage oral hygiene—odor and taste of sputum depresses appetite.

Dyspnea

(Shortness of breath)
May be acute, chronic, progressive, recurrent, or paroxysmal

A. Causes

1. In lung disease, shortness of breath is due to change in lung rigidity or increased airway resistance.
2. Lung disease places strain on right ventricle—may cause right ventricular failure.

B. Nursing Assessment

Ascertain circumstances that cause dyspnea
1. Relation to exertion, position, or environmental exposure.
2. Quantify exertion and specify type producing dyspnea (housework, mowing lawn, walking a set distance).
3. Mode of onset? Sudden? Gradual?
4. Quantify change in dyspnea. (What could patient do a year ago, a month ago that he cannot do now?)
5. At what time of day/night is it obvious?
6. Is there associated cough?
7. Is there expiratory wheeze?
8. Is dyspnea associated with other symptoms?

C. Nursing Interventions

The treatment depends on alleviating the cause
1. Place the patient at rest with his head elevated.
2. Administer oxygen as prescribed.

D. Clinical Implications

1. In general, the acute lung diseases produce a more severe grade of dyspnea than do the chronic diseases.
2. Sudden dyspnea in a healthy person may indicate pneumothorax (air in pleural cavity).
3. Sudden dyspnea in ill or postoperative patient may indicate pulmonary embolus; pneumothorax.
4. Orthopnea—characteristic of cardiogenic pulmonary congestion.

5. Expiratory wheeze—arises from obstructive disease in peripheral airways (asthma, chronic bronchitis, emphysema).
6. Wheezing respirations—related to localized obstruction of major branches, tumor, foreign body, or narrowing of smaller airways.
7. Inspiratory stridor—indicates partial obstruction at laryngeal or tracheal level.
8. Paroxysmal wheezing unrelated to exertion—may arise from bronchial (allergic) asthma or bronchitis.

Hemoptysis

(Expectoration of blood or bloodstained sputum from the respiratory tract)

A. Causes

1. Chronic bronchitis
2. Tumor
3. Bronchial or parenchymal infections
4. Cardiovascular conditions

B. Nursing Assessment

1. Recognize the patient's fear and apprehension due to this threatening symptom and give him understanding and support.
2. Ascertain whether blood is coming from nose or throat, gastrointestinal tract or lungs.
   a. Nose (epistaxis)—usually there is a discharge of blood from nose.
      (1) During severe epistaxis, patient may swallow or aspirate blood.
      (2) Look for dried blood in nose or nasopharynx.
   b. Gastrointestinal tract (hematemesis)
      (1) Usually preceded by nausea and accompanied by retching and vomiting.
      (2) Blood appears dark red in color; may contain food particles.
      (3) Blood is acid in reaction (pH less than 7.0).
   c. Lungs (hemoptysis)
      (1) Blood is *coughed* up; patient may have tickling in throat, salty taste, burning or bubbling sensation in chest.
      (2) Usually bright red and frothy.
      (3) Blood is alkaline in reaction (pH greater than 7.0).

C. Nursing Interventions

1. Place the patient on bed rest and give mild sedation as prescribed.
   a. Place on affected side (if known)—to avoid flooding the contralateral lung.
   b. Maintain a calm reassuring approach—fright in a patient promotes hyperventilation.
2. Record quantity, color, and character (mixed with mucus, pure blood).
3. Save all coughed up blood for inspection by physician.
4. Have equipment for emergency bronchoscopy/laryngoscopy in readiness—for removal of blood clots and identification of bleeding site.
5. In event of asphyxia or massive hemoptysis, prepare for balloon catheter insertion and inflation to occlude bleeding site and/or for surgical intervention.

Chest Pain

A. Causes

1. Parietal pleura has rich supply of sensory nerves coming from intercostal nerves to the diaphragm.

These nerve endings may be stimulated by inflammation and stretching of membranes and by respiratory movements—produces a characteristic sharp, knifelike pain.
2. Pleuropulmonary pain—bacterial pneumonia, infarction, spontaneous pneumothorax.

B. *Clinical Manifestations and Nursing Assessment*

1. Pleural pain is a common manifestation of inflammatory and malignant disease, but also accompanies pneumothorax and pulmonary embolism.
2. Pleural pain (usually well localized, sharp, and stabbing) occurs at end of inspiration.
3. Assess quality, intensity, and radiation of pain.
4. Note factors that precipitate pain.
5. Evaluate whether position of patient changes character of pain.
6. Determine the effect of inspiration and expiration on patient's pain.
7. Note other symptoms.

C. *Nursing Interventions*

1. Should be directed towards relieving underlying causes.
2. Give prescribed analgesic taking care not to depress respiratory center or productive cough.
3. Assist with regional anesthetic block—procaine is injected along the intercostal nerves that supply the painful area in cases where pain is intractable.

Hoarseness

A. *Causes*

1. Acute
   When associated with febrile episode suggests viral laryngotracheobronchitis
2. Persistent
   May indicate intrinsic neoplasm of vocal cord, bronchogenic cancer, mediastinal lesion

Constitutional Manifestations of Bronchopulmonary Disease

A. *Constitutional Symptoms of Bronchopulmonary Disease*

1. Anorexia
2. Fever
3. Weight loss
4. Fatigue, malaise, weakness } related to duration and severity of disease
5. Sweats
6. Chills

B. *Constitutional Signs of Bronchopulmonary Disease*

1. Cyanosis
2. Clubbing of fingers
3. Wasting

DIAGNOSTIC STUDIES*

Radiography

A. *Chest Roentgenogram*

1. Normal pulmonary tissue is radiolucent. Thus densities produced by tumors, foreign bodies, etc. can be detected.
2. Shows position of normal structures, displacement, and presence of abnormal shadows.
3. Chest x-rays may reveal extensive pathology in the lungs in the absence of symptoms.

B. *Tomography* (planigraphy)

1. Provides films of sections of lungs at different levels within the thorax.
2. Useful in demonstrating presence of small, solid lesions, calcification or cavitation within a lesion.

C. *Computed Tomography* is an imaging method in which the lungs are scanned in successive layers by a narrow beam x-ray. A computer printout is obtained of the absorption values of the tissues in the plane that is being scanned.

It may be used to define pulmonary nodules, small tumors adjacent to pleural surfaces (which may be invisible on routine roentgenograms), and to demonstrate mediastinal abnormalities and hilar adenopathy.

D. *Fluoroscopy*

Enables roentgenologist to view heart, lungs, and diaphragm in the dynamic (moving) state.

E. *Barium Swallow*

Outlines the esophagus, revealing displacement of esophagus and encroachment on its lumen, since cardiac, pulmonary, and mediastinal abnormalities can be seen as deviations of the esophagus.

F. *Bronchography*

A radiopaque medium is instilled directly into the trachea and bronchi and the entire bronchial tree or selected areas may be visualized. This is a diagnostic test for any disease that alters the caliber or patency of the bronchial tree or that causes its displacement.

1. Patient is assessed for allergic reaction to anesthetic agent or contrast media before the test is started.
2. Patient is kept fasting—to avoid aspiration of gastric contents.
3. Preoperative medication may include atropine to decrease secretions and vagally mediated reflex bradycardia and diazepam (Valium) for sedation/tranquilization.
   a. Topical anesthesia is sprayed in the mouth, on tongue and posterior pharynx.
   b. Local anesthetic is injected into the larynx and tracheal tree to prevent gagging and coughing when the tube is passed.
      (1) Extreme caution indicated in patients with respiratory insufficiency, since these patients may experience temporary problems with ventilation and diffusion.
      (2) Oxygen, antispasmodic agents, and cortisone should be available.
4. *Nursing Responsibilities after Bronchogram*
   a. Withhold fluids and food until patient demonstrates a cough reflex.
   b. Encourage patient to cough and clear his tronchial tree; postural drainage may be required.
   c. A slight elevation of temperature is common following a bronchogram.

* For physical examination of lungs and thorax, see page 29.

G. *Angiographic Studies of Pulmonary Vessels*

Radiopaque medium is rapidly injected into vasculature of the chest for radiographic study of pulmonary vessels.

1. It can be performed by
   a. Venous injection into one or both arms (simultaneously) through a needle or catheter, OR
   b. Introducing a catheter into main pulmonary artery or its branches.
2. Films are taken in rapid sequence after injection.

H. *Aortography*—opacification studies of either thoracic aorta or abdominal aorta; taken when aneurysm of thoracic aorta is suspected.

Endoscopic Procedures

A. *Bronchoscopy*—the direct inspection and observation of the larynx, trachea, and bronchi through a flexible or rigid bronchoscope; has both diagnostic and therapeutic uses in pulmonary conditions.

1. *Diagnostic Uses*
   a. To collect secretions for cytologic/bacteriologic studies.
   b. To determine location and extent of a pathologic process, and biopsy for diagnosis.
      (1) *Tissue biopsy*—use of small biopsy forceps to obtain sample of tissue for examination.
      (2) *Brush biopsy*—target bronchus is brushed using a small wire with brush on one end that is introduced through bronchoscope. Material (cells and secretions) can be examined cytologically or cultured to look for pathogenic organisms.
   c. To determine whether a tumor can be resected surgically.
   d. To diagnose bleeding sites (source of hemoptysis).
2. *Therapeutic Uses*
   a. To remove foreign bodies from tracheobronchial tree.
   b. To remove secretions obstructing the tracheobronchial tree when patient is unable to clear them.
   c. To fulgurate and excise lesions.

B. *Flexible Fiberoptic Bronchoscopy*—passage of thin, flexible bronchofiberscope that can be directed into segmental bronchi; by its smaller size, flexibility, and excellent optical system it allows increased visualization of peripheral airways.

1. May be done transnasally, transorally, or through an endotracheal tube; allows for brush biopsy (see above).
2. Causes very little patient discomfort; better patient acceptance even under local anesthetic.
3. Clinical applications for flexible fiberoptic bronchoscopy: allows diagnostic visualization of airways to segmental bronchi; therapeutic removal of secretions; localization of source of hemoptysis.
4. Possible complications: reaction to anesthetic agent, pneumothorax, arrhythmias, bronchospasm.

C. *Rigid Bronchoscopy*—hollow metallic tube with light at its end used for removal of foreign bodies, suctioning thick secretions, or investigating source of massive hemoptysis, or for endobronchial surgical procedures (resection of tumors, dilation of strictures, etc.).

1. May be done under local or general anesthesia.

2. Rigid bronchoscope preferred in following instances: small children, endobronchial tumor resection, massive hemorrhage, foreign body retrieval; otherwise it is being replaced by flexible fiberoptic bronchoscopy.
3. *Nursing Interventions*
   a. See that Informed Consent has been signed.
   b. Administer medication to reduce secretions and block the vasovagal reflex and relieve anxiety. Give encouragement and nursing support.
   c. Restrict fluid and food for 6 hours before procedure—to reduce risk of aspiration when reflexes are blocked.
   d. Remove dentures, contact lenses, and other prostheses.
   e. After the procedure, wait until patient demonstrates that he can cough before giving him cracked ice or fluids. A return to his usual diet is resumed in a few hours.
   f. Following bronchoscopy watch patient for
      (1) Cyanosis
      (2) Hypotension
      (3) Tachycardia and arrhythmia
      (4) Hemoptysis
      (5) Dyspnea

D. *Mediastinoscopy* (See p. 156.)

Radioisotope Diagnostic Procedures

A. *Perfusion Lung Scan*

Following injection of a radioactive isotope, scans are made with a scintillation camera.
1. Measures blood perfusion through the lungs; evaluates lung function on a regional basis
2. Useful in perfusion (vascular) abnormalities—pulmonary embolism

B. *Ventilation Scan*

1. Inhalation of radioactive gas (Xenon, Krypton), which diffuses throughout the lungs
2. Useful in detecting ventilation abnormalities (emphysema)

C. *Gallium Scan*

Radioisotope lung scan used to detect inflammatory conditions of the lungs.
1. Normal lung takes up little or no gallium.
2. Fibrotic lung takes up little or no gallium.
3. Acutely inflamed or infected lung takes up gallium.

Examination of Sputum

A. *Purpose*

1. Sputum is obtained for evaluation of gross appearance, for microscopic examination, for gram staining and culture to identify the predominant organisms, and for cytologic examination.
   a. Direct smear—shows presence of white blood cells and intracellular (pathogenic) bacteria and extracellular (mostly non-pathogenic) bacteria.
   b. Sputum culture—to make diagnosis, to determine drug sensitivity, and to serve as a guide for drug treatment (choice of antibiotic)
   c. Sputum cytology (exfoliative cytology)—used to identify tumor cells
2. Patients receiving antibiotics, steroids, and immunosuppressive agents for prolonged periods may have periodic sputum examinations since these agents may give rise to opportunistic pulmonary infections.

B. *Methods of Obtaining Sputum*

1. By deep breathing and coughing
   a. Clear nose and throat and rinse mouth—to decrease sputum contamination.
   b. Instruct patient to take several deep breaths, exhale, and perform a series of short coughs.
   c. Cough deeply and expectorate the sputum into a sterile container.
   d. See that specimen is transported to laboratory immediately; allowing it to stand in a warm room will result in overgrowth of organisms making identification of pathogen difficult; also alters cell morphology.
   e. Give oral hygiene frequently especially if patient has foul sputum.
2. By ultrasonic and/or heated hypertonic saline nebulization
   a. Patient inhales through mouth slowly and deeply for 10–20 minutes.
   b. Increases the moisture content of air going to lower tract; particles will condense on tracheobronchial tree and aid in expectoration.
3. Tracheal aspiration (see Guidelines, p. 167)
4. Bronchoscopic removal (p. 155)
5. Bronchial brushing guided by fluoroscopy (p. 155)
6. Gastric aspiration (rarely necessary since advent of ultrasonic nebulizer).
   a. Nasogastric tube is inserted into the stomach to siphon out swallowed pulmonary secretions.
   b. This test is useful only for culture of tubercle bacilli, but not for direct examination.
7. Transtracheal aspiration (see Fig. 7-7). See Guidelines, page 159.

Examination of Pleural Fluid and Pleural Biopsy

A. *Pleural Fluid*

Pleural fluid is continuously produced and reabsorbed, with a thin layer of fluid normally in the pleural space; abnormal accumulation of pleural fluid (effusion) occurs in diseases of the pleura, heart, or lymphatics. The pleural fluid is studied along with other tests to determine underlying cause.

1. Pleural fluid is obtained by aspiration (thoracentesis, p. 161) or by tube thoracotomy.
2. Pleural fluid is examined for cell count, differential, specific gravity, cytology, protein, glucose, pH, LDH, and amylase.
   a. Pleural fluid usually light straw color
   b. Purulent fluid—suggests empyema
   c. Blood-tinged fluid—pulmonary infarction; neoplastic disease
   d. Milky fluid (chylothorax)—invasion of thoracic duct by tumor or inflammatory process; traumatic rupture of thoracic duct
3. Observe and record total amount of fluid withdrawn, nature of fluid, and its color and viscosity.
4. Prepare sample of fluid for laboratory evaluation if prescribed.

B. *Pleural Biopsy*

Accomplished via needle biopsy of pleura or via pleuroscopy (visual exploration of pleural space through a bronchofiberscope inserted into pleural space).

Biopsy Procedures of the Lung

OBJECTIVE: to obtain histological material from lung to aid in diagnosis.

A. *Transbronchoscopic Biopsy*—flexible forceps inserted through bronchoscope and specimen of lung tissue obtained

B. *Percutaneous* (through the skin) *Needle Biopsy*

1. Skin site cleansed and anesthetized.
2. Small skin incision is made and a needle is advanced preferably under fluoroscopic control to the desired site.
3. With the needle in the periphery of the lesion, the stylet is removed, the syringe attached, and suction applied.
4. Specimen is smeared and fixed on a slide; makes immediate cytologic diagnosis possible; gives knowledge of cell type.
5. Observe for possible complications—pneumothorax, pulmonary hemorrhage, and empyema.

C. *Transcatheter Bronchial Brushing*

D. *Open Lung Biopsy*

1. Used in making a diagnosis when other biopsy methods fail.
2. Usually done by a small anterior thoracotomy; does not usually involve a rib resection.
3. Subsequent pneumothorax controlled by chest tube connected to a water-seal drainage system.

Lymph Node Biopsy (Scalene or Cervicomediastinal Nodes)

OBJECTIVE: to detect lymph node spread of pulmonary disease. It is used as a diagnostic and prognostic measure.

1. Scalene lymph nodes are enmeshed in deep cervical pad of fat; these nodes drain lungs and mediastinum and may show histologic changes from intrathoracic disease.
2. Mediastinoscopy—endoscopic examination of the mediastinum for evaluation of tumor spread and biopsy of mediastinal nodes.
   a. Incision is usually made in suprasternal notch below isthmus of thyroid.
   b. The edges of incision are spread with forceps; the tissues overlying the trachea are dissected and a channel is prepared for introduction of the mediastinoscope.
   c. Useful in diagnosing and staging bronchogenic cancer and to obtain tissue for diagnosis in other conditions.
3. Mediastinotomy—surgical resection of second anterior costal cartilage for access to anterior mediastinum to evaluate lung lymphatic drainage.
   Procedure most frequently used to evaluate left upper lobe disease processes.

Pulmonary Function Studies

Pulmonary function studies (Ventilatory Function Tests [Table 7-1]) are done to detect and measure abnormalities in respiratory function.

A. *Ventilatory Studies* (Spirometry)

1. Most commonly used test.
2. Requires water spirometer, electronic spirometer, or wedge spirometer that plots volume against time (*timed vital capacity*).
3. Patient is asked to take as deep a breath as possible and then to exhale into spirometer as completely and as forcefully as possible. Results are compared with normals for patient's age, height, and sex (see Table 7-1).

TABLE 7-1. VENTILATORY FUNCTION TESTS

Description	Term Used	Symbol	Remarks
The maximum volume of air exhaled from the point of maximum inspiration	Vital capacity	VC	Slow vital capacity may be normal or reduced in COPD*
Vital capacity performed with a maximally forced expiratory effort	Forced vital capacity	FVC	Forced vital capacity is often reduced in COPD due to air trapping
Volume of air exhaled in the specific time during the performance of forced vital capacity	Forced expiratory volume (qualified by subscript indicating the time interval in seconds)	FEV_t, usually FEV_1	A valuable clue to the severity of the expiratory airway obstruction.
FEV_T expressed as a percentage of the forced vital capacity	Ratio of timed forced expiratory volume to forced vital capacity	$FEV_t/FCV\%$, usually $FEV_1/FVC\%$	Another way of expressing the presence or absence of airway obstruction.
Mean forced expiratory flow between 200 and 1200 ml of the FVC	Forced expiratory flow	$FEF_{200-1200}$	Formerly called maximum expiratory flow rate (MEFR). An indicator of large airway obstruction.
Mean forced expiratory flow during the middle half of the FVC.	Forced mid-expiratory flow.	$FEF_{25-75\%}$	Formerly called maximum mid-expiratory flow rate. Slowed in small airway obstruction.
Mean forced expiratory flow during the terminal portion of the FVC.	Forced end-expiratory flow.	$FEF_{75-85\%}$	Slowed in obstruction of smallest airways.
Volume of air expired in a specified period during repetitive maximal effort.	Maximal voluntary ventilation.	MVV	Formerly called maximum breathing capacity. An important factor in exercise tolerance.

From American Lung Association. Chronic Obstructive Pulmonary Disease, 5th ed. 1977
* Chronic obstructive pulmonary disease

4. A reduction in the vital capacity *alone* may indicate a restrictive form of lung disease (disease due to increased lung stiffness).
5. A reduction in several parameters usually indicates an obstructive form of lung disease (obstruction to flow due to bronchial obstruction or loss of lung elastic recoil).

B. *Lung Volumes*

1. Are determined by asking patient to inhale known concentration of inert gas such as helium or 100% oxygen and measuring concentration of inert gas or nitrogen in exhaled air (dilution method). May also be measured in plethysmograph (body box).
2. Yields thoracic gas volume (total lung capacity, plus any unventilated blebs or bullae).
3. An increased residual volume is found in air-trapping due to obstructive lung disease.
4. A reduction in several parameters usually indicates a restrictive form of lung disease or chest wall abnormality.

C. *Diffusing Capacity*

1. Measures lung surface effective for the transfer of gas in the lung.
2. Requires patient to inhale gas containing known low concentration of carbon monoxide.
3. Measures carbon monoxide concentration in exhaled air (difference between inhaled and exhaled concentrations is related directly to uptake of carbon monoxide across alveolar-capillary membrane).

4. Is reduced in parenchymal lung disease, possibly severe anemia, and in some forms of heart disease.

Arterial Blood Gas Studies

A. *Purpose*

1. A measurement of partial pressure of oxygen and carbon dioxide in arterial blood, as well as the pH of the blood.
2. The partial pressure of oxygen together with hemoglobin is a measurement of the *amount* of oxygen in the arterial blood.
3. Provide a means of assessing the adequacy of oxygenation and ventilation, i.e., the lungs supplying O_2 to the body and removing CO_2.
4. Helps assess the acid-base status in the body—whether acidosis or alkalosis is present and to what degree.

B. *Clinical Uses of Arterial Blood Gas Studies*

Arterial blood gas studies are helpful in diagnosis and treatment in the presence of the following:
1. Unexplained tachypnea, dyspnea (especially in patients with cardiopulmonary disease).
2. Unexplained restlessness and anxiety in bed patients.
3. Drowsiness and confusion in patients receiving oxygen therapy.
4. Assessment of surgical risk.
5. Before and during prolonged oxygen therapy and during ventilator support of patients.
6. Progression of cardiopulmonary disease.

GUIDELINES: Assisting with Arterial Puncture for Blood Gas Analysis

Purpose   To obtain a sample of arterial blood for blood gas analysis.

Terminology

Partial Pressure—pressure exerted by each type of gas in a mixture of gases.
The following is a reference list of expressions related to partial pressure:

P = pressure

PO_2 —partial pressure of oxygen

PCO_2 —partial pressure of carbon dioxide

P_AO_2 —partial pressure of alveolar oxygen

P_ACO_2 —partial pressure of alveolar carbon dioxide

P_aO_2 —partial pressure of arterial oxygen

P_aCO_2 —partial pressure of arterial carbon dioxide

P_vO_2 —partial pressure of venous oxygen

P_vCO_2 —partial pressure of venous carbon dioxide

P_{50} —oxygen tension at 50% hemoglobin saturation

Equipment   (Disposable kit is available)

2-ml. glass syringe with No. 25 gauge needle

10-ml. glass syringe with No. 20 or 21 gauge needle (adult) (22 or 25 needle, child)

Sodium heparin

Stopper or cap

Procaine

Sterile sponges and skin germicide

Basin containing ice

Procedure

NURSING ACTION	RATIONALE/AMPLIFICATION
Preparatory Phase	
1. Take patient's temperature and respiratory rate.	1. These measurements are taken into consideration when the laboratory results are evaluated.
2. Note the amount of oxygen administered.	
3. Heparinize the syringe.	
a. Withdraw a sufficient amount of heparin into the syringe to wet the plunger completely and to fill the dead space of the syringe and needle.	a. This action coats the interior of the syringe with heparin to prevent the blood from clotting.
b. Hold syringe in upright position and expel excess heparin and air bubbles.	b. Air in the syringe may affect measurement of PO_2.
Performance Phase (by physician, respiratory therapist)	
1. Palpate the radial, brachial, or femoral artery.	1. Arterial puncture is performed on areas where a good pulse is palpable. (Radial or brachial arteries are preferred.)
2. Palpate for the presence of the ulnar artery before puncturing the radial artery.	
3. Perform the Allen test.	3. The Allen test is done by expressing the blood from the hand, occluding the radial artery, and watching the blood flow to the hand by way of the ulnar artery. This insures collateral circulation even if thrombosis of the radial artery should occur.
In the conscious patient:	
a. Obliterate the radial and ulnar pulses simultaneously at the wrist.	
b. Ask the patient to clench and unclench his fist until blanching of the skin occurs.	
c. Release pressure on ulnar artery (while compressing radial artery) and watch for return of skin color.	
In the unconscious patient:	
a. Obliterate the radial and ulnar pulses simultaneously at the wrist.	
b. Elevate patient's hand above his heart and squeeze or compress his hand until blanching occurs.	
c. Lower patient's hand while compressing radial artery (release pressure on ulnar artery) and watch for return of skin color.	

Procedure (cont.)

NURSING ACTION	RATIONALE/AMPLIFICATION

4. Feel along the course of the radial artery and palpate for maximum pulsation with the middle and index fingers. Prepare the skin with germicide. The skin and subcutaneous tissues are infiltrated with a local anesthetic agent (procaine).

4. The wrist may be stabilized to allow for finer control of the needle.

5. The needle is at a 45–60° angle (Fig. 7-6) and is inserted into the artery. Once the artery is punctured, arterial pressure will push up the hub of the syringe and a pulsating flow of blood will easily fill the syringe.

5. In most patients the artery is located close to the surface of the skin.

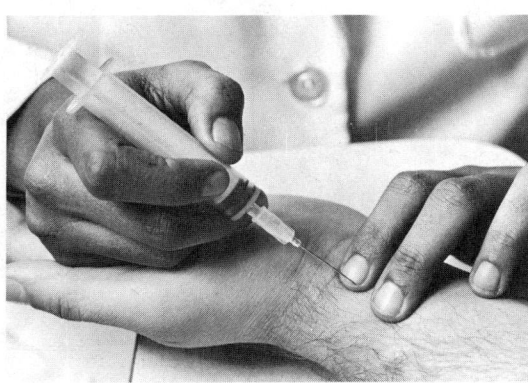

FIGURE 7-6. *Technique of arterial puncture for blood gas analysis.*

6. After blood is obtained, withdraw needle and apply firm pressure over the puncture.

7. Remove the needle carefully and cap the syringe tightly or plunge it into a rubber stopper.

7. Immediate capping of the needle prevents room air from mixing with the blood specimen.

8. Place the capped syringe in the container of ice.

8. The lower temperature reduces metabolism and minimizes the alteration of the true values of oxygen, carbon dioxide, and pH.

9. *Maintain firm pressure on the puncture site for 5 minutes* (by the clock).
   a. If the patient is on anticoagulant medication, apply direct pressure over puncture site for 15 minutes and then apply a firm pressure dressing.

9. Firm pressure on the puncture site prevents further bleeding and hematoma formation.

10. For patients requiring serial monitoring of arterial blood, an arterial catheter (connected to a flush solution of heparinized saline), is inserted into the brachial or radial artery.

10. All connections must be tight to avoid disconnection and rapid blood loss. The arterial line also allows for direct pressure monitoring in the critically ill patient.

Follow-up Phase

1. Record ventilator settings, oxygen flow on the patient's record at the time the arterial blood is drawn. Note the type and settings of the respiratory therapy equipment being used.

1. The PO_2 results will dictate whether to maintain, increase, or decrease F_IO_2. The PCO_2 and pH results dictate whether changes are necessary in tidal volume or rate in patients on ventilators.

2. Send the basin of ice with the syringe containing blood to the laboratory immediately.

2. Blood gas analysis should be done as soon as possible since gas tension and pH can change rapidly.

3. Palpate the pulse (distal to the puncture site), inspect the puncture site, and assess for cold hand, numbness, tingling, and discoloration.

3. Hematoma, arterial thrombosis, and ulnar nerve puncture are complications following this procedure.

GUIDELINES: Assisting with Transtracheal Aspiration

Transtracheal aspiration involves a transtracheal puncture with a needle through the cricothyroid membrane and the introduction of a fine catheter through the needle into the trachea. (Fig. 7-7.)

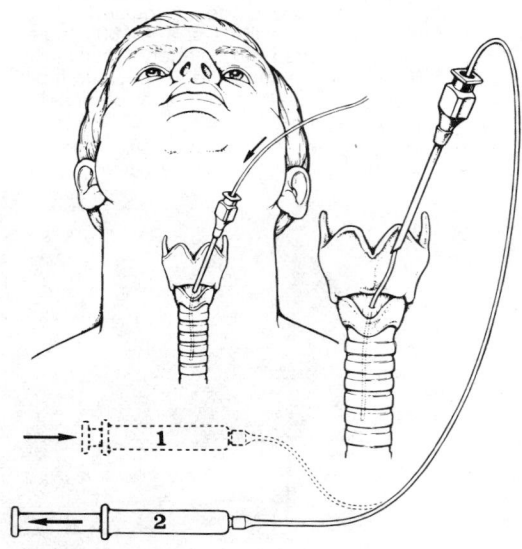

FIGURE 7-7. *Transtracheal aspiration.*

Purposes
1. To obtain an uncontaminated sputum specimen for culture and sensitivity studies.
2. To promote coughing in the patient with an absent cough reflex.

Equipment
Sterile transtracheal set:
 No. 14, No. 16, and No. 18 gauge needles
 Polyethylene catheter
 Syringe
 Skin germicide
 Local anesthetic
 Sterile gloves

Procedure

NURSING ACTION	RATIONALE/AMPLIFICATION
Preparatory Phase	
1. Explain the procedure and give reassurance by skilled and empathetic attention to the patient's needs.	1. Inform the patient that the procedure will cause coughing.
2. Extend the patient's neck and place a pillow under his shoulders.	2. This is the optimum position for cricothyroid puncture.
Performance Phase (by the physician)	
1. The skin over the cricothyroid area is cleansed and the area infiltrated with local anesthetic.	1. The cricothyroid membrane is less vascular and offers more safety in preventing posterior wall puncture than other areas.
2. A 14, 16, or 18 gauge needle is inserted through the cricothyroid membrane into the trachea and a polyethylene catheter is inserted through the needle into the trachea.	2. Caution the patient against swallowing or talking while the needle is introduced through the cricothyroid membrane.
3. The needle is withdrawn leaving the catheter in place.	
4. A small amount of sterile saline (2–5 ml.) is injected into the trachea through the catheter.	4. Saline loosens secretions and initiates a paroxysm of coughing.
5. The secretions and exudates are aspirated into the syringe.	
6. The catheter is withdrawn and pressure applied over the puncture site.	6. Gentle firm pressure over the site for about 5 minutes will help prevent subcutaneous or mediastinal emphysema.
7. The contents of the syringe may be expressed into a sterile culture tube.	7. Transtracheal aspiration bypasses the oropharynx and avoids specimen contamination by mouth flora.
Follow-up Care	
1. Instruct the patient to rest quietly for an hour or so.	
2. Observe for the following complications: pneumomediastinum, subcutaneous emphysema, tracheal bleeding, cardiac arrhythmias.	2. Assess for hoarseness after the procedure; this may be from a submucosal tracheal hematoma which can cause suffocation.

GUIDELINES: Assisting the Patient Undergoing Thoracentesis

Thoracentesis is the aspiration of fluid or air from the pleural space. It may be a diagnostic or a therapeutic procedure (Fig. 7-8).

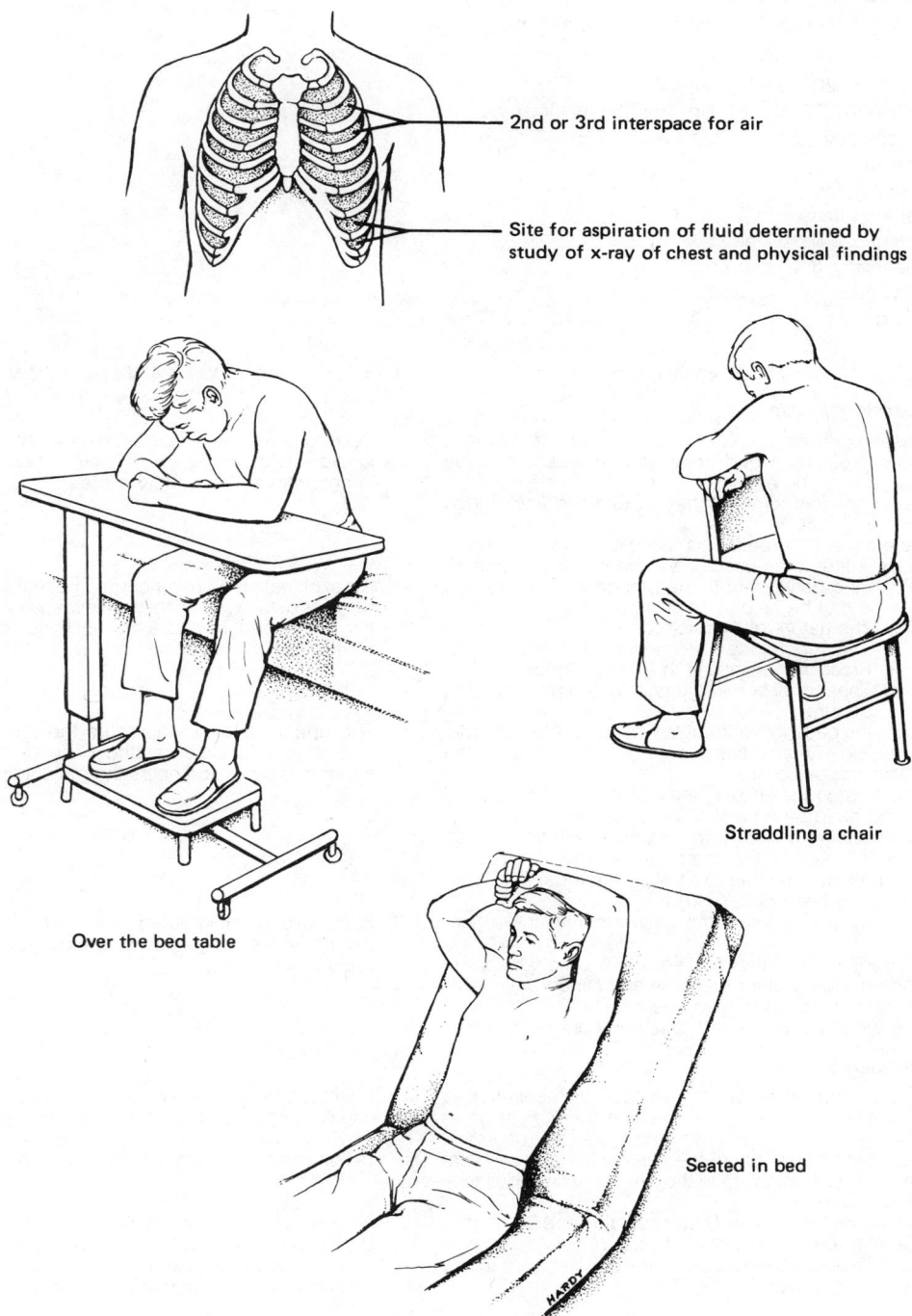

2nd or 3rd interspace for air

Site for aspiration of fluid determined by study of x-ray of chest and physical findings

Over the bed table

Straddling a chair

Seated in bed

FIGURE 7-8. *Selecting site and positioning patient for thoracentesis.*

GUIDELINES: Assisting the Patient Undergoing Thoracentesis (cont.)

Purposes
1. To remove fluid and air from the pleural cavity.
2. To obtain diagnostic aspiration of pleural fluid.
3. To obtain pleural biopsy.
4. To instill medication into the pleural space.

Equipment
Syringes: 5, 20, 50 ml. syringes
Needles: No. 22, No. 26, No. 16 (7.5 cm. long)
Stopcock and rubber tubing
Hemostat
Biopsy needle
Local anesthetic
Sterile gauze dressings
Sterile towels and drape
Sterile specimen container
Sterile gloves

Procedure

NURSING ACTION	RATIONALE/AMPLIFICATION
Preparatory Phase	
1. Ascertain in advance if chest roentgenograms have been prescribed and completed. These should be available at the bedside.	1. Posteroanterior and lateral chest x-rays are used to localize fluid and air in the pleural cavity and to aid in determining the puncture site.
2. See if consent form has been explained and signed (see p. 81).	
3. Determine if the patient is allergic to the local anesthetic agent to be used. Give sedation if prescribed.	
4. Inform the patient about the procedure and indicate how he can be helpful. Explain: a. The nature of the procedure b. The importance of remaining immobile c. Pressure sensations to be experienced d. That no discomfort is anticipated after the procedure	4. An explanation helps orient the patient to the procedure, assists him to mobilize his resources, and gives him an opportunity to ask questions and verbalize anxiety.
5. Make the patient comfortable with adequate supports. If possible place him upright and in one of the following positions: a. Sitting on the edge of the bed with feet supported and head on a padded over-the-bed table b. Straddling a chair with his arms and head resting on the back of the chair c. If patient is unable to sit in a chair or side of bed, elevate head of bed 30–45°.	5. The upright position facilitates the removal of fluid that usually localizes at the base of the chest. A comfortable position helps the patient to relax.
6. Support and reassure the patient during the procedure. a. Prepare the patient for sensations of cold from skin germicide and for pressure and sting from infiltration of local anesthetic agent. b. Encourage the patient to refrain from coughing.	6. Sudden and unexpected movement by the patient can cause trauma to the visceral pleura with resultant trauma to the lung.
Performance Phase	
1. Expose the entire chest. The site for aspiration is determined from chest x-rays and by percussion. If fluid is in the pleural cavity the thoracentesis site is determined by study of the chest x-ray and physical findings, with attention to the site of maximal dullness on percussion.	1. If air is in the pleural cavity, the thoracentesis site is usually in the 2nd or 3rd intercostal space in the midclavicular line. Air rises in the thorax because the density of air is much less than the density of liquid.
2. The procedure is done under aseptic conditions. After the skin is cleansed, the physician slowly injects a local anesthetic with a small caliber needle into the intercostal space.	2. An intradermal wheal is raised slowly; rapid intradermal injection causes pain. The parietal pleura is very sensitive and should be well infiltrated with anesthetic before the thoracentesis needle is passed through it.
3. The physician advances the thoracentesis needle with the syringe attached. When the pleural space is reached, suction may be applied with the syringe.	

Procedure (cont.)	*NURSING ACTION*	*RATIONALE/AMPLIFICATION*
	a. A 20 ml. or 50 ml. syringe with a 3-way adapter (stopcock) is attached to the needle. (one end of the adapter is attached to the needle and the other to the tubing leading to a receptacle that receives the fluid being aspirated.)	a. When a large quantity of fluid is withdrawn, a 3-way adapter serves to keep air from entering the pleural cavity.
	b. If a considerable quantity of fluid is to be removed, the needle is held in place on the chest wall with a small hemostat.	b. The hemostat steadies the needle on the chest wall. Sudden pleuritic pain or shoulder pain may indicate that the visceral or diaphragmatic pleura are being irritated by the needle point.
	4. After the needle is withdrawn, pressure is applied over the puncture site and a small sterile dressing is fixed in place.	
	Follow-up Phase	
	1. Place the patient on bed rest. A chest x-ray is usually obtained following thoracentesis.	1. Chest x-ray verifies that there is no pneumothorax.
	2. Record the total amount of fluid withdrawn and the nature of the fluid, its color and viscosity. If prescribed, prepare samples of fluid for laboratory evaluation (usually bacteriology, cell count and differential, determinations of protein, glucose, LDH, specific gravity). A small amount of heparin may be needed for several of the specimen containers, to prevent coagulation. A specimen container with formalin may be needed if a pleural biopsy is to be obtained.	2. The fluid may be clear, serous, bloody, purulent, etc.
	3. Evaluate the patient at intervals for increasing respirations, faintness, vertigo, tightness in the chest, uncontrollable cough, blood-tinged frothy mucus, and rapid pulse and signs of hypoxemia.	3. Pneumothorax, tension pneumothorax, hemothorax, subcutaneous emphysema, or pyogenic infection may result from a thoracentesis.

CHEST PHYSICAL THERAPY

POSTURAL DRAINAGE EXERCISES

Postural drainage is the use of specific positions so that the force of gravity can assist in the removal of bronchial secretions from the affected bronchioles into the bronchi and trachea by means of expectoration (Fig. 7-9).

Underlying Principles

1. The patient is positioned so that the diseased area(s) are in a near vertical position, and gravity is used to assist drainage of the specific segment(s).
2. The positions assumed are determined by the location, severity, and duration of mucus obstruction.
3. The exercises are usually performed 2 to 4 times daily, before meals and at bedtime.
4. Discontinue the procedure if tachycardia, palpitations, dyspnea, chest pain, or other symptoms occur—may indicate hypoxemia.

Nursing Management

1. Make the patient comfortable before the procedure starts and as comfortable as possible while he assumes each position.
   a. Bronchodilators, broncholytic agents, water, or saline may be nebulized and inhaled before postural drainage to reduce bronchospasm, decrease thickness of mucus and sputum, and combat edema of the bronchial walls.
   b. Use a folding cot to prop up patient to desired height if his bed is not adjustable; have an emesis basin ready for draining mucus.
2. Use a stethoscope to determine the areas of needed drainage.
3. Upper lobes are generally drained by upright positions; lower and middle lobes are drained by head-down positions.
4. Have patient assume left prone and left oblique positions (simultaneously)—this will give additional drainage to middle lobe and lateral segments of the right lower lobe; assuming the right prone and right oblique position (simultaneously) will give additional drainage to middle lobe and lateral segments of the left lower lobe.
5. Encourage the patient to cough after he has spent the allotted time in each position.
6. Encourage diaphragmatic breathing (p. 166) throughout postural drainage exercises; this helps widen airways so that secretions can be drained.
7. Chest wall percussion may be desirable to loosen and propel sputum in the direction of gravity drainage.

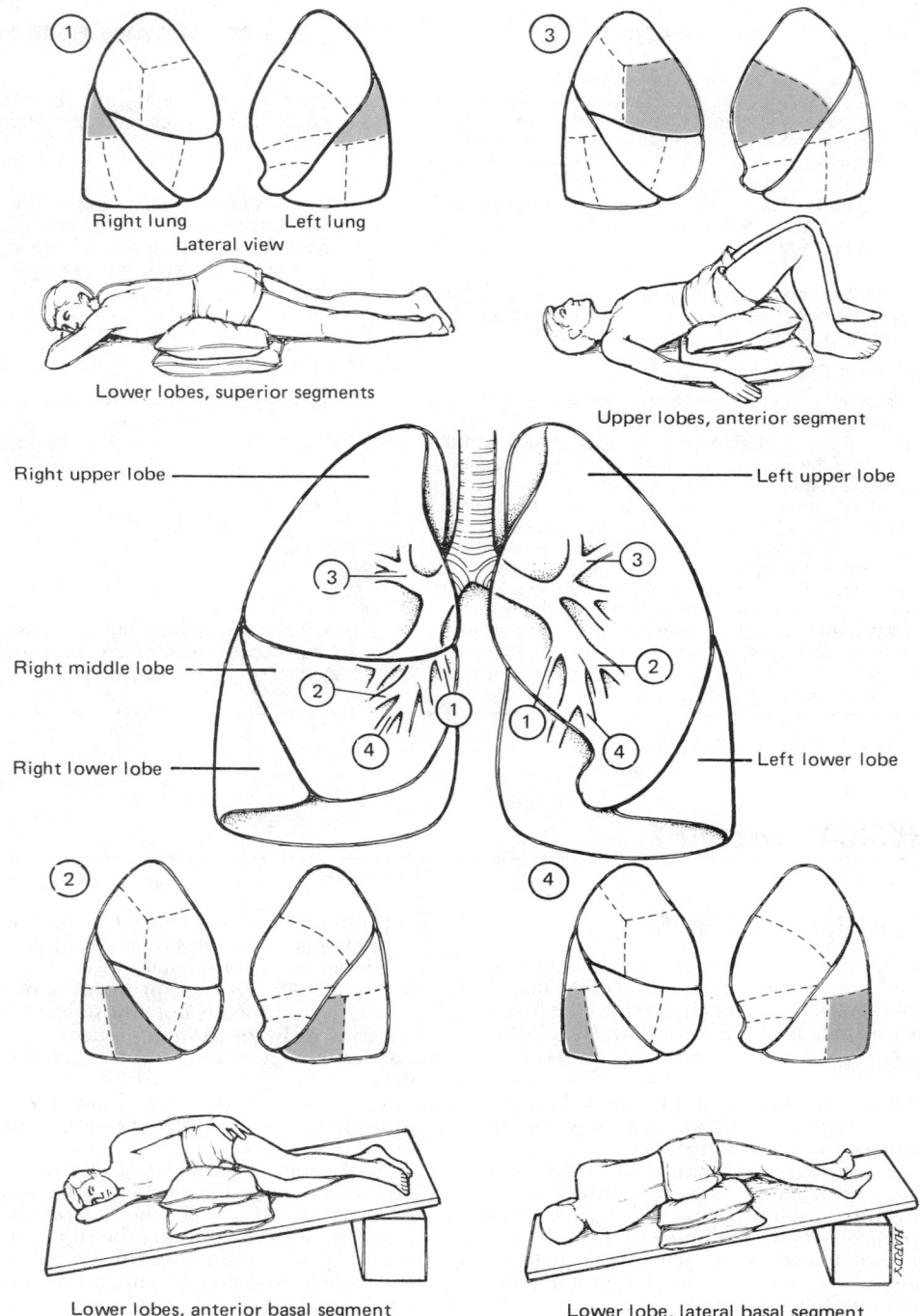

Right lung Left lung
Lateral view
Lower lobes, superior segments

Upper lobes, anterior segment

Right upper lobe — — Left upper lobe

Right middle lobe —

Right lower lobe —

— Left lower lobe

Lower lobes, anterior basal segment

Lower lobe, lateral basal segment

FIGURE 7-9. *Postural drainage.*

GUIDELINES: Percussion (Clapping) and Vibration

Percussion and vibration are manual techniques designed to loosen secretions and promote drainage of mucus and secretions from the lungs while the patient is in the position of postural drainage indicated for his specific lung problem. The procedure requires trained personnel.

1. *Percussion*—Movement done by striking the chest wall in a rhythmical fashion with cupped hands over the chest segment to be drained. The wrists are alternately flexed and extended so that the chest is cupped or clapped in a painless manner.
2. *Vibration*—Technique of applying manual compression and tremor to the chest wall during the exhalation phase of respiration.

Purposes

1. To dislodge mucus adhering to the bronchioles and bronchi.
2. To help mobilize secretions.

Clinical Indications

Lung conditions that cause increased production of secretions:

Bronchiectasis
Empyema
Cystic fibrosis
Chronic bronchitis

Contraindications

1. Lung abscess or tumors
2. Pneumothorax
3. Diseases of the chest wall

4. Lung hemorrhage
5. Painful chest conditions
6. Tuberculosis

NURSING ALERT: Postural drainage and chest percussion may result in hypoxia and should only be used if secretions are believed to be present.

Procedure

NURSING ACTION	RATIONALE/AMPLIFICATION
Performance Phase	
1. Instruct the patient to use diaphragmatic breathing (p. 166).	1. Diaphragmatic breathing helps the patient to relax and helps to widen airways.
2. Position the patient in prescribed postural drainage position(s) (p. 164). The spine should be straight to promote rib cage expansion.	2. The patient is positioned according to the area of the lung that is to be drained.
3. Percuss (or clap) with cupped hands over the chest wall for 1 or 2 minutes from: a. The lower ribs to shoulders in the back b. The lower ribs to top of chest in front	3. This action helps to dislodge mucous plugs and mobilize secretions toward the main bronchi and trachea. The air trapped between the operator's hand and chest wall will produce a characteristic hollow sound.
4. Avoid clapping over the spine, liver, kidneys, spleen, breast, scapula, clavicle, or sternum.	4. Percussion over these areas may cause injuries to the spine and internal organs.
5. Instruct the patient to inhale slowly and deeply. Vibrate the chest wall as the patient exhales slowly through pursed lips. a. Place one hand on top of the other over affected area or place one hand on each side of the rib cage. b. Tense the muscles of the hands and arms while applying moderate pressure and vibrate hands and arms. c. Relieve pressure on the thorax as the patient inhales. d. Encourage the patient to cough, using his abdominal muscles, after 3 or 4 vibrations.	5. This sets up a vibration that carries through the chest wall and helps free the mucus. b. This maneuver is performed in the direction in which the ribs move upon expiration. d. Contracting the abdominal muscles while coughing increases cough effectiveness. Coughing aids in the movement and expulsion of secretions.
6. Allow the patient to rest several minutes.	
7. Listen with a stethoscope for changes in breath sounds.	7. The appearance of moist sounds (rales, rhonchi) indicates movement of air around mucus in the bronchi.
8. Repeat the percussion and vibration cycle according to the patient's tolerance and his clinical response; usually 15 to 20 minutes.	

GUIDELINES: Teaching the Patient Breathing Exercises

Breathing exercises are techniques utilized to compensate for respiratory deficits by increasing efficiency of breathing. They are aimed at conserving energy through controlled breathing.

Purposes
1. To relax muscles and relieve anxiety.
2. To eliminate useless uncoordinated patterns of respiratory muscle activity.
3. To slow the respiratory rate.
4. To decrease the work of breathing.

General Instructions
1. Clear the nasal passages before beginning breathing exercises.
2. Always inhale through the nose—permits filtration, humidification, and warming of air.
3. Breathe slowly in a rhythmical and relaxed manner—permits more complete exhalation and emptying of lungs; helps overcome anxiety associated with dyspnea and decreases oxygen requirement.
4. Avoid sudden exertion.
5. Practice breathing exercises in several positions, since air distribution and pulmonary circulation vary according to position of the chest.

Diaphragmatic Breathing

Purposes:
1. to strengthen the diaphragm as the diaphragm is the main respiratory muscle
2. to decrease the use of the accessory muscles of respiration

TEACHING PROCEDURE	RATIONALE/AMPLIFICATION
Instruct the patient as follows: 1. Place one hand on stomach just below the ribs and the other hand on the middle of the chest.	1. This helps the patient to become aware of the diaphragm and its function in breathing.
2. Breathe in slowly and deeply through the nose, letting the abdomen protrude as far as it will (Fig. 7-10A). The abdomen enlarges during inspiration and decreases in size during expiration.	2. Slow inhalation provides ventilation and hyperinflation of the lungs.

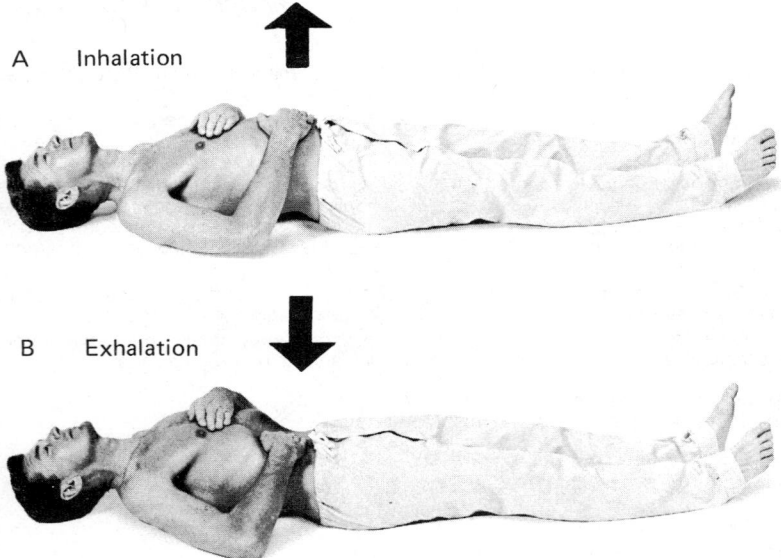

A   Inhalation

B   Exhalation

FIGURE 7-10. *Breathing exercises for inhalation and exhalation. (From Living with Asthma, Chronic Bronchitis, and Emphysema. Riker Laboratories, Inc., Northridge, California)*

3. Breathe out through pursed lips while contracting (tightening) the abdominal muscles. Press firmly inward and upward on the abdomen while breathing out (Fig. 7-10B).	3. Contracting the abdominal muscles assists the diaphragm in rising to empty the lungs.

TEACHING PROCEDURE	**RATIONALE/AMPLIFICATION**
4. The chest should not move; attention is directed at the abdomen, not the chest.	4. Contraction of the abdominal muscles should take place during expiration.
5. Repeat for approximately 1 minute (followed by a rest period of 2 minutes). Work up to 10 minutes, 4 times daily.	
6. Learn to do diaphragmatic breathing while lying, then sitting, and ultimately standing and walking. a. Coordinate diaphragmatic breathing with stair climbing, lifting, etc. b. Carry out activity (lifting) during the prolonged expiration phase.	6. Diaphragmatic breathing helps the patient breathe in a controlled manner during activities that produce dyspnea. If the patient becomes short of breath have him stop the exercises until his breathing pattern comes under control.

Pursed-lip Breathing

Purposes
1. To slow the respiratory rate
2. To assist in emptying the lungs
3. To combat dyspnea due to exertion

TEACHING PROCEDURE	**RATIONALE/AMPLIFICATION**
Instruct the patient as follows: 1. Inhale through the nose.	
2. Exhale slowly and evenly against pursed lips while contracting (tightening) the abdominal muscles. a. Count to 7 while prolonging expiration through pursed lips.	2. Pursing the lips increases intrabronchial pressure (helps maintain the bronchi in an open position) as well as intra-alveolar pressure. The pursed-lip maneuver also prolongs the expiratory phase of breathing, makes it easier to empty the air in the lungs and promotes carbon dioxide elimination.
3. Sit in a chair. Fold the arms across the abdomen. a. Inhale through the nose. b. Bend over and exhale slowly through pursed lips while counting to 7.	b. Leaning forward pushes the abdominal organs upward.
4. While walking: a. Inhale while walking 2 steps. b. Exhale through pursed lips while walking 4 steps.	4. Try any similar combinations according to breathing tolerance of patient.

Other Exercises

LOWER SIDE RIB BREATHING

1. Place hands on sides of lower ribs.
2. Inhale deeply and slowly while sides expand moving hands outward.
3. Exhale slowly through pursed lips and feel the hands and ribs move inward.
4. Rest.

LOWER BACK AND RIB BREATHING

1. Sit in a chair. Place hands behind back; hold flat against lower ribs.
2. Inhale deeply and slowly while rib cage expands backward; the hands will move outward.
3. Keep hands in place. Blow out slowly; hands will move in.

SEGMENTAL BREATHING

1. Place hands on sides of lower ribs.
2. Inhale deeply and slowly while concentrating on moving the right hand outward by expanding the right rib cage.
3. Ensure that the right hand moves outward more than the left hand.
4. Keeping hands in place, exhale slowly and feel the right hand and ribs moving in.
5. Repeat, concentrating on expanding left side more than the right side.
6. Rest.

GUIDELINES: Nasotracheal Suctioning

Purposes
1. To clear secretions from trachea and bronchi when the patient is unable to do so.
2. To collect a sputum specimen.

Equipment
Tracheal aspiration set
   Sterile catheter (No. 14 Fr.), gloves,
     cup, water, connecting tubing

Water soluble lubricant
Oxygen
Cardiac monitoring equipment (if appropriate)

NOTE: Tracheal suctioning requires knowledge and clinical practice under expert supervision.

Procedure

NURSING ACTION	RATIONALE/AMPLIFICATION
1. Explain the procedure to the patient.	1. Explanation and encouragement of verbalization of anxiety helps the patient to cope with stress.
2. Determine baseline vital signs. Auscultate the chest with a stethoscope.	2. A knowledge of these parameters is fundamental for assessing for *changes*. Chest auscultation helps determine when suctioning is required.
3. Occlude the tubing and check the suction pressure (on machine or wall suction).	
4. Oxygenate the patient before and after each passage of the catheter.	4. Suctioning can produce hypoxia and vagal stimulation and subsequent cardiac arrhythmias.
5. Don sterile gloves. Lubricate the catheter with water soluble lubricant or sterile water.	5. To facilitate passage of the suctioning catheter.
6. With the suction turned off, pass the catheter through the nose directing it in a smooth motion along the floor of the nasal cavity.	6. The tip of the catheter should point downward.

7. Pass the catheter to the larynx at a point above the hypopharynx.
  a. Tilt the patient's head back slightly as the catheter is passed into the hypopharynx.
  b. Listen for the sound of air at the proximal end of the catheter.
	7. The hypopharynx lies below the upper edge of the epiglottis and opens into the larynx and esophagus.
	
	  b. If the catheter inadvertently enters the esophagus, air flow will not be heard.

8. Have the patient take a few gentle deep breaths and advance the catheter into the trachea during inspiration.	8. Irritation of the trachea by the catheter usually stimulates forceful coughing that mobilizes secretions.
9. Apply intermittent suction by rotating the catheter between the thumb and forefinger.	9. Intermittent suctioning and rotating of the catheter aspirates secretions more effectively and minimizes mucosal damage.
10. Do not suction the patient more than 10–15 seconds without resting the patient and providing further oxygenation.	10. Arterial blood oxygenation may be diminished during suctioning and results in hypoxemia and vagal stimulation.
11. Suction while gently withdrawing the catheter.	
12. Withdraw the catheter immediately if patient becomes dyspneic, cyanotic, or develops an arrhythmia.	12. Complications of this procedure include laryngospasm, respiratory arrest, and cardiac arrest.
13. Re-oxygenate the patient. Auscultate the chest after suctioning.	13. Auscultation confirms presence or absence of secretions and the presence of air exchange.

RESPIRATORY FUNCTION AND THERAPY

Basic Terminology

1. *Ventilation*—movement of air in and out of the lungs by means of inspiration and expiration.
2. *Tidal volume*—total volume of each breath.
  a. Normal: 7–8 ml./kg. of body weight.
  b. Not all of the tidal volume reaches the alveoli to participate in oxygen and carbon dioxide exchange.
  c. *Dead space*
    (1) Portion of inspired air that remains in conducting airways from nose and mouth to bronchioles (not included in gas exchange).
    (2) Normal dead space: 150 ml.
    (3) Diseases that cause alveoli to lose venous blood flow add to dead space (pulmonary embolism, hemorrhage, hypotension, emphysema).
3. *Minute volume*—total volume of air expired through the nose and mouth each minute. Consists of (1) alveolar ventilation ($\frac{2}{3}$); and (2) dead space ventilation ($\frac{1}{3}$).
4. *Vital capacity*—maximum volume of gas that can be expelled from lungs by forceful effort following a maximal inspiration.
  a. Indicates patient's ability to take a deep breath.
  b. Normal: 70 ml./kg. of body weight.
  c. Reduction in vital capacity is important index of respiratory failure.
5. *Inspiratory force*—maximum negative pressure that the patient can exert against the occluded airway. (Minimum safe level is -25 cm. H_2O.)
6. *Diffusion*—transfer of a gas from alveoli to blood.
  Occurs when tension exerted by gas in alveoli differs from that in the blood.
7. *Perfusion*—Filling of the pulmonary capillaries with venous blood which has returned to the heart from the general circulation and is pumped via the right ventricle to the lungs.

8. *Shunting*
   a. Normally 2% of the blood that is pumped to the lungs by the right ventricle bypasses the alveoli and does not participate in blood-gas exchange.
   b. This blood is returned unoxygenated to the left heart and mixes with arterial blood.
   c. Increase in shunting occurs in atelectasis, pneumonia, pulmonary edema.

Abbreviations

P_ACO_2—partial pressure of alveolar carbon dioxide
P_aCO_2—partial pressure of arterial carbon dioxide
P_AO_2 —partial pressure of alveolar oxygen
P_aO_2 —partial pressure of arterial oxygen
F_IO_2 —fractional concentration of oxygen in the inspired air (ambient air 21% or 0.21)

For ventilatory function test symbols see Table 7-1, p. 157.

Respiratory Failure and Insufficiency

A. *Terminology*

1. *Respiratory insufficiency*—altered function of the respiratory system which produces clinical symptoms—usually includes dyspnea.
2. *Chronic respiratory failure*
   a. Hypoxemia (decreased P_aO_2) or hypercapnia (increased P_aCO_2).
   b. Due to disorder of any component of the respiratory system.
   c. Occurs usually over a period of months to years—allows for activation of compensatory mechanisms.
3. *Acute respiratory failure*
   a. Hypoxemia (P_aO_2 less than 50 or 60 mm.Hg) or hypercapnia (P_aCO_2 greater than 50).
   b. Occurs rapidly, usually in minutes to hours or days.
4. *Ventilatory failure*
   a. Respiratory failure due to decreased alveolar ventilation
   b. Characterized by elevated P_aCO_2
   c. Relationship to *minute volume* (amount of air inhaled and exhaled in one minute)
      (1) Alveolar ventilation + *dead space ventilation* = minute volume. (Dead space is amount of air moving in and out of conducting airways and other areas of lung which are ventilated but not perfused with blood)
      (2) Ventilatory failure may be present even if minute volume is normal or even high. The lung disorder causes an increase in dead space ventilation.
      (3) In ventilatory failure due to disorders of the respiratory control center or disorders of the thoracic cage and muscles, the minute volume and alveolar ventilation are reduced.
5. *Oxygenation failure*
   a. Consists purely of a decreased P_aO_2 with initial decrease of P_aCO_2.
   b. Found primarily in localized or diffuse infiltrative or vascular pulmonary disorders.
6. *Obstructive disorder*
   a. Ventilatory insufficiency or failure due to impaired airflow in conducting airways.
   b. Results from airway narrowing (bronchitis, asthma) or loss of lung elasticity required to expel air (emphysema).
7. *Restrictive disorder*—ventilatory insufficiency or fail-

ure due to impaired movement of the thoracic cage or musculature or to increased lung stiffness.

B. *Causes of Respiratory Failure*

1. Disorders of the respiratory control center
   a. Drug intoxication (general anesthetics, narcotics, barbiturates, hypnotics, excessive oxygen administration to patients with chronic obstructive pulmonary disease)
   b. Vascular disorders (brainstem infarction and hemorrhage, decreased perfusion due to shock)
   c. Trauma (head injury, increased intracranial pressure)
   d. Infection (meningitis, encephalitis)
   e. Others ("primary alveolar hypoventilation," myxedema coma, status epilepticus)
2. Disorders of impulse transmission
   a. Drug intoxication (curariform drugs, anticholinesterases)
   b. Degenerative disorders (amyotrophic lateral sclerosis, multiple sclerosis)
   c. Infection (poliomyelitis, Guillain-Barré syndrome, tetanus, rabies)
   d. Trauma (transection of the spinal cord)
   e. Others (myasthenia gravis)
3. Disorders of the thoracic wall and musculature
   a. Skeletal (scoliosis, flail chest, multiple rib fractures, thoracotomy)
   b. Muscular (polymyositis, muscular dystrophies)
   c. Pleural (effusion, hemothorax, empyema, fibrothorax, pneumothorax)
4. Disorders of conducting airways
   a. Upper airways (foreign body, epiglottitis, laryngitis, smoke and noxious gas inhalation, acute laryngeal edema, tumor)
   b. Peripheral airways (chronic bronchitis, emphysema, asthma)
5. Disorders involving the alveolar-capillary membrane
   a. Infection (lobar, aspiration, or interstitial pneumonia)
   b. Vascular (thromboemboli, fat emboli, polyarteritis, Wegener's granulomatosis, pulmonary edema)
   c. Neoplasm (lymphogenous spread of carcinoma)
   d. Others (interstitial fibrosis, uremic pneumonitis, shock lung, noncardiac pulmonary edema)

C. *Clinical Manifestations of Respiratory Failure (See p. 170)*

NURSING ALERT: 1. Any of the abnormalities outlined above should point to the possibility of actual or impending respiratory failure.

2. Arterial blood gases should be obtained whenever the nursing history or patient assessment suggests respiratory insufficiency or failure.

3. Even if arterial blood gas studies are normal, respiratory insufficiency may still be present and may progress to respiratory failure.

4. Bedside measurements of the vital capacity at frequent intervals is helpful in following the progress of patients with disorders of the respiratory control center, or impulse transmission, or of the thoracic musculature.

D. *Treatment of Respiratory Insufficiency and Failure*

1. Ventilatory insufficiency and failure
   a. *Without lung disease*

Clinical Manifestations of Respiratory Failure

Nursing History	Interpretation
Cough, dyspnea, wheezing, sputum production and color	*Any* recent *change* should point to an abnormality of the lung and raise suspicion of respiratory insufficiency or failure.
Drug usage	May point to depression of the respiratory control center and raise the likelihood of ventilatory failure.
Oxygen administration	Oxygen administration, particularly in patients with chronic bronchitis or emphysema who are dependent on hypoxemia as a stimulus to breathing and who have grown insensitive to carbon dioxide as a stimulus to breathing, may bring about ventilatory failure.
Weakness or paralysis	Weakness or paralysis in any other part of the body indicates the possibility of weakness or paralysis of the thoracic muscles and actual or impending ventilatory failure.
State of responsiveness	Coma occurs early in disorders of the respiratory control center but may be a late manifestation of other causes of respiratory failure; *any otherwise unexplained change in the level of consciousness should raise the possibility of respiratory failure.*
Respiratory rate	Reduced in disorders of the respiratory control center; rapid respiratory rate occurs early in disorders of the thoracic cage and musculature and of the lung proper.
Pattern of respiration	Abnormalities of rhythm (Cheyne-Stokes respiration, Biot's respiration) are found in disorders of the respiratory control center.
Depth of respiration	Shallow in disorders of the respiratory control center, disorders of impulse transmission, and weakness of the thoracic musculature; *may be deceptively normal* in disorders of the lung.
Use of accessory muscles of breathing (scalene, sternomastoid, and pectoralis) and intercostal retraction.	Labored breathing usually seen in disorders of the lung parenchyma, skeletal deformities.
Pulse	Usually rapid in acute respiratory failure, but may be deceptively normal in disorders of the respiratory control center (drug intoxication) and disorders of impulse transmission (Guillain-Barré syndrome).
Cyanosis	Useful only when present; absence of cyanosis, however, does not exclude respiratory failure.
Chest auscultation	Abnormalities may indicate lung disease; *breath sounds may be decreased in intensity or deceptively "normal" in severe airway obstruction.*

(1) Specific treatment for cause of respiratory failure (i.e., narcotic antagonist for narcotic or narcotic analogue intoxication, pyridostigmine for myasthenia gravis).

(2) Ventilatory support with mechanical ventilator if P_aCO_2 is elevated, or if vital capacity is 1 liter or less, *or if there is rapid progression of signs and symptoms.*

b. *With underlying lung disease* (usually emphysema or chronic bronchitis)

(1) Treat the cause of exacerbation (i.e., antibiotics for respiratory infection).

(2) Restore airflow in conducting airways.
  (a) Bronchodilators for bronchospasm.
  (b) Mucolytics to liquefy mucus plugs.
  (c) Chest physiotherapy to remove mucus plugs.

(3) Increase alveolar ventilation.
  (a) Remove respiratory depressants such as drugs or excessive oxygen.
  (b) Encourage deep breathing.
  (c) Administer IPPB with monitoring of tidal volume.

(4) Give ventilatory support with mechanical ventilator *if*:

(a) pH is less than 7.25 and P_aCO_2 is greater than 60 *or* if
(b) P_aCO_2 rises by 5 mm.Hg or more per hour—*or*
(c) If patient cannot cooperate with other therapeutic modalities.

2. Oxygenation failure
  a. Give specific treatment for underlying disorder (i.e., antibiotics for pneumonia; diuretics for pulmonary edema due to left ventricular failure).
  b. Administer oxygen to maintain P_aO_2 of 60 mm.Hg using devices that provide increased oxygen concentrations (cannula, aerosol mask, partial rebreathing mask, nonrebreathing mask).
  c. If P_aO_2 of 60 mm.Hg cannot be achieved with devices described above or if inspired oxygen concentration required is greater than 60% for 24 hours, patient may require intubation and the use of Positive End Expiratory Pressure (PEEP) with mechanical ventilation or Continuous Positive Airway Pressure (CPAP) without mechanical ventilation.

E. *Pharmacology*

For commonly used nebulized drugs see Table 7-2.

TABLE 7-2. COMMONLY USED NEBULIZED DRUGS

	Pharmacologic Effects	Indications	Undesired Effects	Nursing Implications
Bronchodilators and decongestants Racemic epinephrine	Sympathomimetic acting on alpha (vasoconstrictor), beta$_1$ (cardiac stimulation) and beta$_2$ (bronchial smooth muscle relaxation) receptors	Bronchospasm in asthma or bronchitis, laryngeal or tracheal edema	Tachycardia, arrhythmias, elevation of blood pressure, headache, nausea, vomiting, tachyphylaxis (fastness), paradoxical increase in bronchospasm	Use extreme caution in patients who are elderly, or who have heart or thyroid disease; discontinue treatment and observe pulse and blood pressure closely if major undesired effects occur.
Isoproterenol	Sympathomimetic acting on beta$_1$ and beta$_2$ receptors	Bronchospasm	Tachycardia, arrhythmias, headache, nausea, excitement, tremors	Use caution in patients who are elderly or who have heart or thyroid disease; discontinue and observe pulse if arrhythmias or other major undesired effects occur.
Isoetharine	Sympathomimetic, claimed to act more selectively on beta$_2$ than on beta$_1$ receptors	Bronchospasm	Tachycardia, headache, excitement	Although safer than the preceding drugs, caution should still be used in patients with heart disease.
Terbutaline	Sympathomimetics with selective beta$_2$ activity	Bronchospasm	Rare	Probably safer than other less selective agents.
Proteolytics Acetylcysteine	Derivative of naturally occurring protein; breaks disulfide bonds in mucoproteins and thus lowers viscosity of mucus; liquefaction starts 1 minute following nebulization and reaches maximum in 5 minutes; action is immediate in direct instillation	Abnormally thick or inspissated secretions in airways	Nausea, bronchospasm	Should be used with caution in patients with asthma or other bronchospastic disorders and should probably be administered with a bronchodilator; should be used with caution in patients who cannot cough up secretions and should be followed by vigorous suctioning to prevent "drowning" patient in liquefied secretions.
Antifoaming Agent Ethyl alcohol	Reduces surface tension and therefore collapses foam that may obstruct airways	Pulmonary edema due to left ventricular failure	None	None
Corticosteroids Beclomethasone	Synthetic corticosteroid with potent anti-inflammatory activity; effective when administered by inhalation	Patients with steroid-dependent asthma	Oral moniliasis	Should *not* be used in patients with status asthmaticus or other acute episodes of asthma.
Miscellaneous Cromolyn sodium	Inhibits release of histamine from mast cells in the respiratory tract when inhaled as a dry powder; prevents acute attacks *only*, and must be used for 2–4 weeks to demonstrate effectiveness	Asthma	Cough, bronchospasm	Should *not* be used in patients with status asthmaticus or other acute episodes of asthma; may have to be given in combination with bronchodilator if administration brings about bronchospasm.

OXYGEN THERAPY

General Considerations

1. Oxygen is an odorless, tasteless, colorless transparent gas that is slightly heavier than air.

2. Oxygen supports combustion, so there is always danger of fire when oxygen is being used.
   a. Avoid using oil or grease around oxygen connections.

b. Eliminate antiseptic tinctures, alcohol, and ether in immediate oxygen environment.

c. Do not permit any electrical devices (radios, heating pads, electric razors) in or near an oxygen tent.

d. Keep the oxygen cylinder (if used) secured in an upright position away from heat.

e. Post NO SMOKING signs on the patient's door and in view of the patient's visitors.

f. Have fire extinguisher available.

3. Oxygen is dispensed from a cylinder or piped-in system and requires:

a. *Reduction gauge*—reduces pressure to that of the atmosphere.

b. *Flow meter* (flow gauge, flow control)—regulates control of oxygen in liters per minute.

4. Oxygen is given to relieve hypoxia, either local or generalized.

a. *Hypoxia*—a state in which there is an insufficient amount of oxygen available in the tissue cells to meet the requirements of an organ or tissue at that moment.

b. *Hypoxemia*—a decrease in the oxygen content of the blood.

5. Measurement of the arterial blood gases is the best method of determining the need for and adequacy of oxygen therapy (p. 158).

Clinical Assessment

1. A change in the patient's respiration is often evidence of the need for oxygen therapy.

2. Other signs of hypoxia, such as cyanosis, may or may not be present.

3. The *goal* in administering oxygen is to treat the hypoxemia while decreasing the work of breathing and stress on the myocardium.

4. The appropriate form of oxygen therapy is best ascertained after obtaining arterial blood gases, which will indicate the patient's oxygenation status and acid-base balance.

5. Oxygen must be given with extreme caution to some patients. In certain conditions (chronic obstructive lung disease) the administration of a high oxygen concentration will remove the respiratory drive that has been created largely by the patient's low oxygen tension.

a. Ventilation is reduced.

b. Acute acidosis and carbon dioxide narcosis may follow.

NOTE: Oxygen toxicity should always be of concern in the patient receiving inspired concentrations over 60% for over 24 hours.

Oxygen Delivery Systems

1. Oxygen may be administered by nasal cannula, oropharyngeal catheter (nasal catheter), various types of face masks, and tent. It may also be applied directly to endotracheal or tracheal tube via T-piece or hyperinflation bag.

2. The method selected depends on the concentration of oxygen required.

Monitoring Oxygen Therapy

NURSING ALERT:

1. Arterial blood gas evaluations are the best means of gauging the effectiveness of oxygen therapy and guiding appropriate changes. Of particular importance is the effect of oxygen therapy on the patient who has chronic obstructive lung disease and who may retain carbon dioxide if given too much oxygen. Frequent blood gas evaluations may be necessary in this type of patient to make sure that his respiratory drive is not suppressed.

2. Various types of oxygen analyzers are available which allow the nurse to measure the concentration of oxygen delivered to the patient. Oxygen analyzers are especially useful in measuring the amount of oxygen delivered by the various types of masks.

GUIDELINES: Administering Oxygen by Nasal Cannula (Fig. 7-11)

Purpose To administer a low-to-medium concentration of oxygen, when precise accuracy is not essential.

Equipment Oxygen source
Plastic nasal cannula with connecting tubing (disposable)
Humidifier filled with sterile distilled water to indicated level
Flowmeter
NO SMOKING signs (2)

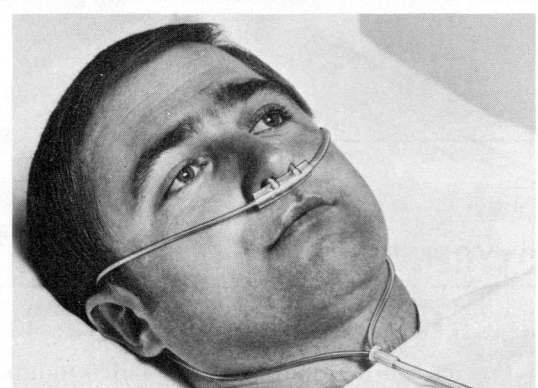

FIGURE 7-11. *Administering oxygen by nasal cannula. (Courtesy of Hudson Oxygen Therapy Sales Company)*

Procedure   ***Preparatory Phase***

1. Post NO SMOKING signs on patient's door and in view of patient and visitors.
2. Show the nasal cannula to the patient and explain the procedure.
3. Make sure the humidifier is filled to the appropriate mark. If the humidifier bottle is too full, the bubbling water will overflow into the gauges.
4. Attach the connecting tube from the nasal cannula to the humidifier outlet.
5. Set the flow rate at 2 liters/minute. Feel to determine if oxygen is flowing through the nasal tips of the cannula.

NURSING ACTION	RATIONALE/AMPLIFICATION
Performance Phase	
1. Place the tips of the cannula in the patient's nose.	1. Position the cannula so that the tips do not extend more than 2.5 cm. (1 inch) into the nares.
2. Adjust flow rate to prescribed rate.	2. A flow of ½–6 liters/minute should provide an inspired oxygen concentration of 22–35%, depending on the patient's breathing pattern. (The greater the Minute Volume, the less the oxygen enrichment.) Flow rates in excess of 6 liters/minute may lead to air swallowing and cause irritation to the nasal and pharyngeal mucosa. If higher concentrations are required, consider an alternate form of therapy.

> **NURSING ALERT:** Patients who require low, constant concentrations of oxygen and whose breathing pattern varies greatly may need to use the Venturi mask particularly if they are carbon dioxide retainers.

3. Fasten tubing to the pillow and bed clothing.	
Follow-up Phase	
1. Change cannula, humidifiers, tubing, and other equipment exposed to moisture daily.	1. Contaminated equipment may cause virulent infections in debilitated patients.
2. Assess patient's condition and the functioning of equipment at regular intervals.	2. Assess the patient for mental aberration, disturbed consciousness, abnormal color, perspiration, changes in blood pressure, and increasing heart and respiratory rates.

GUIDELINES: Administering Oxygen by Oropharyngeal Catheter*

Purpose   To administer moderate to moderately high concentrations of oxygen.

Equipment   Oxygen source
Flowmeter
Humidifier filled with sterile distilled water to appropriate mark
Oropharyngeal catheter
    No. 8–10 Fr. for children
    No. 10–12 Fr. for women
    No. 12–14 Fr. for men
Connecting tubing
Tongue depressor, water-soluble lubricant, gauze squares
Flashlight
Hypoallergenic tape
NO SMOKING signs

Procedure   ***Preparatory Phase***

1. Post NO SMOKING signs on door of room and in view of patient and visitors.
2. Explain the advantages of oxygen therapy to the patient.
3. Attach flowmeter to humidifier and then to wall outlet or oxygen cylinder.
4. Attach tubing to humidifier and the catheter to the connecting tube.

NURSING ACTION	RATIONALE/AMPLIFICATION
Performance Phase	
1. To measure the depth of catheter insertion.	
a. Measure the catheter from the tip of the patient's nose to the tragus (lobe) of the ear. Mark this with tape.	1. a. This is only an approximation of the correct distance to insert the catheter.

* Oropharyngeal catheters are used infrequently.

GUIDELINES: Administering Oxygen by Oropharyngeal Catheter (cont.)

Procedure (cont.)

NURSING ACTION	RATIONALE/AMPLIFICATION

2. To insert oropharyngeal catheter:
  a. Lubricate the catheter with a small amount of water-soluble lubricant.
  b. Start the flow of oxygen at 2–3 liters/minute.
	2. b. This assures the patency of the catheters and its apertures. If some of the holes in the catheter become plugged, the stream of oxygen flowing on a localized area of mucous membrane will cause a burning sensation.

c. Determine the natural droop of the catheter.
  d. Tilt the patient's head back.
  e. Slide the lubricated catheter along the floor of either nare into the oropharynx.
  f. Inspect the oropharynx, using the tongue depressor and flashlight to see the position of the catheter.
  g. *Pull the catheter back slightly until the tip cannot be seen.*
	f. The tip of the catheter should rest approximately opposite the uvula.
	  g. This is done to prevent aspiration of oxygen.

3. Use the opposite nare if insertion is difficult.	3. Nasal pathology (deviated septum, mucosal edema, mucus drainage, polyps) may interfere with catheter insertion.
4. Adjust flow rate to prescribed rate.	4. A flow rate of 4–8 liters/minute should provide an inspired oxygen concentration of 30–50%.
5. Secure the catheter to the bridge of the nose or the side of the face with 1.25 cm (½-inch) hypoallergenic tape.	5. Proper fixation is essential to prevent downward displacement of the catheter.
6. Attach the connecting tube to the bed, leaving enough slack so that the patient can move about comfortably.	
7. Observe and palpate the epigastrium to see if distention develops.	7. In patients with depressed glottal reflexes or epiglottal paralysis (coma, post stroke, etc.) the oxygen stream may be directed into the esophagus and may cause gastric distention or rupture (if the catheter is positioned too deeply).
8. Stay with the patient for a period of time to make sure he does not swallow, gag, or cough.	

Follow-up Phase

NURSING ACTION	RATIONALE/AMPLIFICATION
1. Remove old catheter and insert a fresh catheter into opposite nostril every 8–12 hours.	1. Frequent changes of the oropharyngeal catheter are necessary to prevent catheter encrustation and ulceration of the nasal mucosa.

2. Observe and examine the patient hourly to see if:
  a. Catheter is unobstructed and positioned correctly (use flashlight).
  b. Oropharynx is free from irritation.
  c. Humidifier bottle contains water.
  d. Leaks are occurring around humidifier and tubing connections.
  e. Oxygen cylinder contains enough oxygen.
	c. Oxygen dehydrates tissues unless moistened.

3. Assess the patient's condition frequently.	3. Assess the patient for mental aberration, disturbed consciousness, abnormal color, perspiration, changes in blood pressure, and increasing heart and respiratory rates.

GUIDELINES: Administering Oxygen by Venturi Mask

A *venturi mask* is a face mask designed to administer precisely controlled low oxygen concentrations (24%, 28%, 31%, 35%, 40%, and 50%). It is used primarily to increase the comfort and breathing efficiency of the patient with chronic lung disease (Fig. 7-12).

Underlying Principles

1. The venturi mask mixes a fixed flow of oxygen with a high but variable flow of air so as to produce a constant oxygen concentration regardless of breathing rate.
2. Excess gas leaves the mask through the perforated cuff, carrying with it the expired carbon dioxide; this virtually eliminates rebreathing of carbon dioxide.
3. This mask maintains an oxygen concentration sufficient to relieve the hypoxia of patients with chronic lung disease without inducing hypoventilation and CO_2 retention (Fig. 7-13).

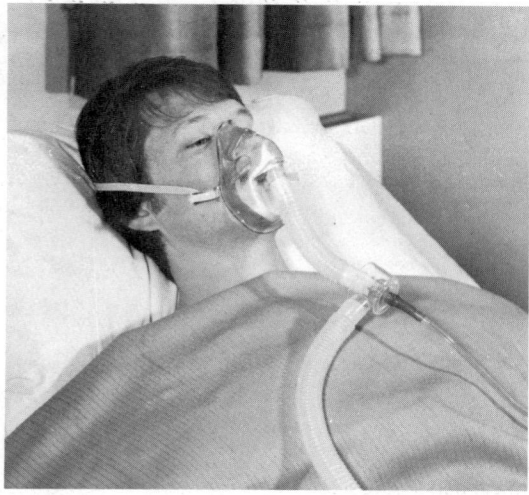

FIGURE 7-12. *Venturi mask with humidity enrichment.*

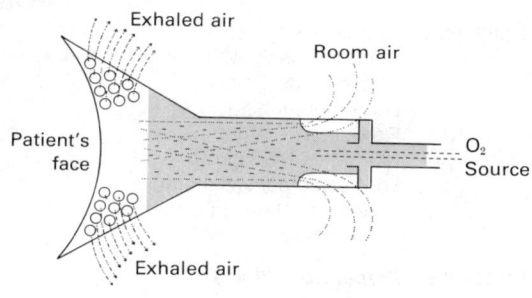

FIGURE 7-13. *The principle of high airflow with oxygen enrichment (HAFOE).*

Equipment Oxygen source
Flowmeter
O_2 nipple adaptor to attach connecting tubing to flowmeter
    If high humidity is desired:
        Nebulizer with sterile distilled water
        Large bore tubing
        Compressed air source and flowmeter to power nebulizer
Venturi mask with lightweight tubing and correct concentration adaptor if the venturi mask with interchangeable
    color-coded adaptors is used.
NO SMOKING signs.

Procedure ***Preparatory Phase***

1. Post NO SMOKING signs on the door of patient' room and in view of patient and visitors.
2. Explain the benefits of therapy to the patient.
3. Connect the mask by lightweight tubing to the oxygen source.
4. Turn on the flowmeter and adjust to the prescribed rate (usually indicated on the mask). Check to see that oxygen is flowing out the vent holes in the flexible face piece.

NURSING ACTION	RATIONALE/AMPLIFICATION

Performance Phase

1. Place venturi mask over patient's nose and mouth and under the chin. Mold the mask to fit the patient's face.
2. Adjust elastic strap around the patient's head and position strap below the ears and around the neck.
3. If high humidity is used, attach large bore tubing to nebulizer and connect it to the fitting for high humidity at the base of the venturi mask.

Follow-up Phase

1. Assess patient's condition at frequent intervals.

    1. Assess the patient for mental aberration, disturbed consciousness, abnormal color, perspiration, changes in blood pressure, and increasing heart and respiratory rates.

2. Change mask and tubing preferably daily.

GUIDELINES: Administering Oxygen by Aerosol Mask

Purpose To provide oxygen in concentrations of 35% or greater with high humidity by administering aerosol mist either heated or unheated, or when high humidity compressed air therapy is desired.

Equipment Oxygen source
Nebulizer bottle with sterile distilled water
Plastic aerosol mask
Large bore tubing
Flowmeter
NO SMOKING signs
For heated aerosol therapy:
   Nebulizer heating element
   Thermometer

Procedure **Preparatory Phase**

1. Post NO SMOKING signs on patient's door and in view of patient and visitors.
2. Show the aerosol mask to the patient and explain the procedure.
3. Make sure the nebulizer is filled to the appropriate mark.
4. Attach the large bore tubing from the mask to the nebulizer outlet.
5. Set desired oxygen concentration of nebulizer bottle and adjust thermostat if heating element is used.
6. If patient is tachypneic and concentration of 50% oxygen or greater is desired, two nebulizers and flowmeters should be yoked together.

NURSING ACTION	RATIONALE/AMPLIFICATION
Performance Phase	
1. Adjust the flow rate until the desired mist is produced (usually 8–10 liters/minute). The oxygen (or air) flow should be adjusted to that point at which the column of aerosol mist in the tubing is not completely withdrawn on the inspiratory phase.	1. This assures the patient of receiving flow sufficient to meet his inspiratory demand and maintains a constant accurate concentration of oxygen.
2. Apply the mask to the patient's face and adjust the straps so that the mask fits securely and there are no leaks.	
Follow-up Phase	
1. Change mask, tubing, nebulizer, and other equipment exposed to moisture daily.	1. Contaminated equipment may cause virulent infections in debilitated patients.
2. Assess patient's condition and the functioning of equipment at regular intervals.	2. Assess the patient for mental aberration, disturbed consciousness, abnormal color, perspiration, changes in blood pressure, and increasing heart and respiratory rates.
3. Drain the tubing frequently. If a heating element is used, the tubing will have to be monitored and drained more often.	3. The tubing must be kept free of condensate. Condensate allowed to accumulate in the delivery tube will block flow and alter oxygen concentration.
4. If a heating device is used, the temperature must be checked often.	4. Excessive temperatures can cause airway burns; patients with elevated temperatures should be humidified with an unheated device.
5. If the patient appears tachypneic, increase flow rate and monitor the oxygen concentration with an oxygen analyzer.	5. Inadequate flow rates may cause inaccurate oxygen concentrations in patients who are tachypneic.

GUIDELINES: Administering Oxygen by Partial Rebreathing Mask (Fig. 7-14)

A *rebreathing bag permits* the patient to inhale a moderately high concentration of oxygen from a reservoir bag. Perforations on both sides of the mask serve as exhalation ports. High concentrations of oxygen are indicated in the acute phase of some diseases (pneumonia, pulmonary edema, pulmonary embolism).

Purpose To administer a moderately high oxygen concentration (50–60%)

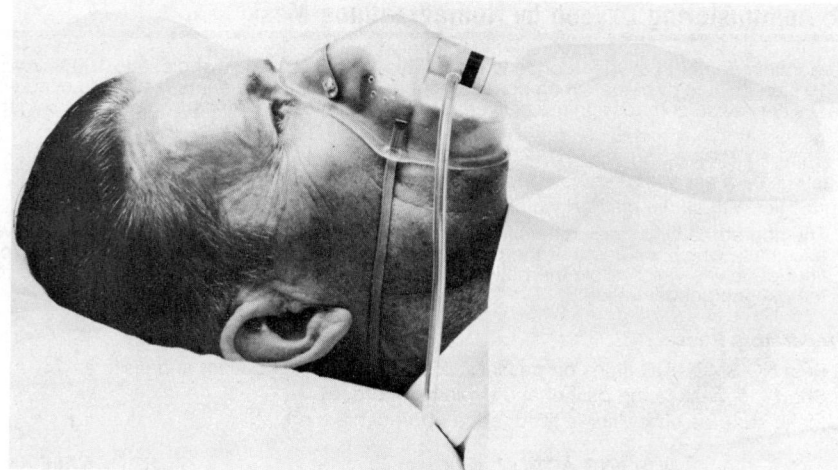

FIGURE 7-14. *Disposable face mask that is anatomically sculptured for patient comfort. There is a flexible aluminum strip at the nose portion of the mask that prevents oxygen leakage into the patient's eyes. (Courtesy of Hudson Oxygen Therapy Sales Company.)*

Equipment
Oxygen source
Plastic face mask with reservoir bag and tubing
Humidifier with distilled water

Flowmeter
NO SMOKING signs

Procedure
Preparatory Phase

1. Post NO SMOKING signs on patient's door and in view of patient and visitors.
2. Fill humidifier with sterile distilled water.
3. Attach tubing to outlet on humidifier.
4. Attach flowmeter.
5. Explain the benefits of the oxygen therapy to the patient.
6. Flush the reservoir bag with oxygen to inflate the bag partially and adjust flowmeter to 6–10 liters/minute.

NURSING ACTION	RATIONALE/AMPLIFICATION
Performance Phase	
1. Place the mask on the patient's face and adjust liter flow so that the rebreathing bag will not collapse during the inspiratory cycle, even during deep inspiration.	1. Be sure the mask fits snugly since there must be an airtight seal between the mask and the patient's face.
	With a well-fitting rebreathing bag adjusted so that the patient's inhalation does not deflate the bag, inspired oxygen concentrations of 50–60% can be achieved. Some patients may require flow rates higher than 10 liters/minute to insure that the bag does not collapse on inspiration.
2. Attach the tubing to the pillow and bed clothes. Keep the tubing free of kinks.	
3. Stay with the patient for a period of time to make him comfortable and observe his reactions.	3. Be sure that oxygen is not escaping from the top of the mask and blowing into the patient's eyes.
Follow-up Phase	
1. Remove mask periodically (if patient's condition permits) to dry the face around the mask. Powder skin and massage face around the mask.	1. These actions reduce moisture accumulation under the mask. Massage of the face stimulates circulation and reduces pressure over the area.
2. Observe for change of condition. Assess equipment for malfunctioning and low water level in humidifier.	2. Assess the patient for mental aberration, disturbed consciousness, abnormal color, perspiration, change in blood pressure, and increasing heart and respiratory rates.

GUIDELINES: Administering Oxygen by Nonrebreathing Mask

Purpose   To administer a high oxygen concentration. (This method can deliver close to 100% oxygen at flows of 10 liters/minute or higher when correct technique is used.) The same method is used when tanked gases of precise composition are delivered (e.g., helium-oxygen or carbon dioxide-oxygen mixtures).

Equipment   Oxygen source
Plastic face mask with reservoir bag and tubing
Humidifier with sterile distilled water

Flowmeter
NO SMOKING sign

The nonrebreathing mask differs from the partial rebreathing mask in that it has a one-way valve between the bag and mask which insures that the patient receives only 100% oxygen from the reservoir bag. The mask has two flapper valves which allow the patient to exhale but which do not allow him to inhale room air and thereby dilute the oxygen concentration.

Procedure   *Preparatory Phase*

1. Post NO SMOKING signs on patient's door and in view of patient and visitors.
2. Show the mask to the patient and explain the procedure.
3. Make sure the humidifier is filled to the appropriate mark.

NURSING ACTION	RATIONALE/AMPLIFICATION
Performance Phase	
1. Place the mask on the patient's face and adjust liter flow so that the reservoir bag will not collapse during the inspiratory cycle, even during deep inspiration.	1. Since the patient is receiving all of his ventilation from the reservoir bag, the flow rate must be sufficient to provide the patient's minute ventilation.

NURSING ALERT: If oxygen flow is not sufficient to keep reservoir bag filled, oxygen concentration will be reduced as room air is drawn in through flapper valves.

2. Be sure the mask fits snugly since there must be an airtight seal between the mask and the patient's face.	
Follow-up Phase	
1. Remove mask periodically (if patient's condition permits) to dry the face around the mask. Powder skin and massage face around the mask.	1. These actions reduce moisture accumulation under the mask. Massage of the face stimulates circulation and reduces pressure over the area.
2. Pay particular attention to see that the reservoir bag never completely collapses as the patient's ventilatory pattern varies.	2. Assess the patient for mental aberration, disturbed consciousness, abnormal color, perspiration, change in blood pressure, and increasing heart and respiratory rates.
3. Observe for change of condition. Assess equipment for malfunctioning and low water level in humidifier.	

GUIDELINES: Administering Oxygen via Endotracheal and Tracheostomy Tubes

A T-tube is a device which connects directly to the patient's endotracheal or tracheostomy tube; it delivers oxygen and humidity from a nebulizer source (see Fig. 7-24, p. 198).

Purpose   To administer oxygen in conjunction with humidity to the patient whose upper airway (and its humidification) has been bypassed either by a tracheostomy or by an endotracheal tube.

Equipment   Oxygen or compressed air source
Flowmeter
Nebulizer and sterile distilled water (heating element may be used as described in aerosol masks)
Large bore tubing
T-piece and 15.2–30.5 cm. (6–12 inch) reservoir tubing (a venturi tube system may be substituted for the T-piece and nebulizer if precise O_2 concentrations are required, but it is always used with humidity enrichment in patients with a tracheostomy or endotracheal tube)
NO SMOKING signs

Procedure   1. Post NO SMOKING signs on patient's door and in view of patient and visitors.
2. Show the T-tube or venturi tube to the patient and explain the procedure.
3. Make sure the nebulizer is filled to the appropriate mark.

Procedure (cont.)

4. Attach the large bore tubing from the T-tube to the nebulizer outlet.
5. Set desired oxygen concentration of nebulizer bottle and adjust thermostat if heating element is used.

NURSING ACTION	RATIONALE/AMPLIFICATION
Performance Phase	
1. Adjust the flow rate until the desired mist is produced and meets the patient's inspiratory demand.	1. The aerosol mist in the reservoir tube should not be completely withdrawn on the patient's inspiration.
2. The tubing should be positioned so that it is not pulling on the tracheostomy tube and so that it allows a comfortable range of movement for the patient.	
Follow-up Phase	
1. Change mask, tubing, nebulizer, and other equipment exposed to moisture daily.	1. Contaminated equipment may cause virulent infections in debilitated patients.
2. Assess patient's condition and the functioning of equipment at regular intervals.	2. Assess the patient for mental aberration, disturbed consciousness, abnormal color, perspiration, changes in blood pressure, and increasing heart and respiratory rates.
3. Drain the tubing frequently. If a heating element is used, the tubing will have to be monitored and drained more often.	3. The tubing must be kept free of condensate. Condensate allowed to accumulate in the delivery tube will block flow and alter oxygen concentration.
4. If a heating device is used, the temperature must be checked often.	4. Excessive temperatures can cause airway burns; patients with elevated temperatures will be better humidified with an unheated device.
5. If the patient appears tachypneic, increase flow rate and monitor the oxygen concentration with an oxygen analyzer.	5. Inadequate flow rates may cause inaccurate oxygen concentrations in patients who are tachypneic.

GUIDELINES: Administering Oxygen by Tracheostomy Collar

A *tracheostomy collar* is a device that fits over the tracheostomy and delivers humidity and oxygen (Fig. 7-15).

Purpose

To administer moisture to increase humidity (either with or without oxygen) to the tracheostomized patient. If the patient does not require either precise or high concentrations of oxygen he is usually more comfortable with a tracheostomy collar than with a T-tube (blow-by) or venturi tube.

Equipment

Oxygen or compressed air source
Flowmeter
Nebulizer and sterile distilled water (heating element may be used as described in aerosol masks)
Large bore tubing
Tracheostomy collar
NO SMOKING signs

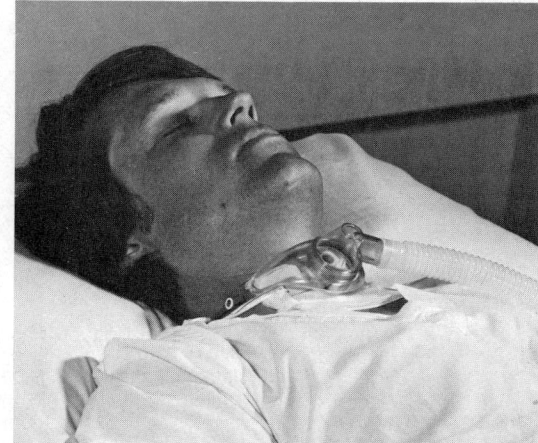

FIGURE 7-15. *Administering oxygen by tracheostomy collar.*

Procedure

NURSING ACTION	RATIONALE/AMPLIFICATION
Performance Phase	
1. Adjust the flow rate until the desired mist is produced and meets the patient's inspiratory demand.	1. The aerosol mist in the tracheostomy collar should not be completely withdrawn on the patient's inspiration.
Follow-up Phase	
1. Change mask tubing, nebulizer, and other equipment exposed to moisture daily.	1. Contaminated equipment may cause virulent infections in debilitated patients.

GUIDELINES: Administering Oxygen by Bag-Mask and Bag-Airway Systems

A *bag-mask* is used when a patient is not intubated. This situation usually occurs only during a cardiopulmonary arrest episode (Fig. 7-16).

Bag-airway systems are used on an intubated patient and commonly are used to hyperinflate ventilator patients during suctioning and when being transported (Fig. 7-17).

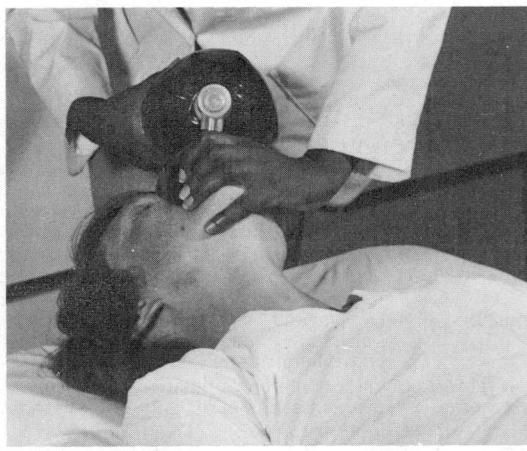

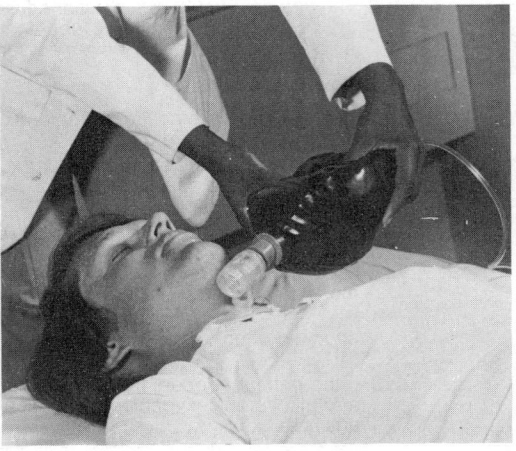

FIGURE 7-16. *Technique of using resuscitator bag with a mask.*

FIGURE 7-17. *Bag airway: the patient, who is on a ventilator, is hyperventilated with a resuscitator bag directly attached to the tracheostomy prior to suctioning.*

Equipment
Oxygen source
Resuscitation bag and mask
O_2 connecting tubing
Nipple adaptor to attach flowmeter to connecting tubing
Flowmeter

Procedure

NURSING ACTION	RATIONALE/AMPLIFICATION
Performance Phase	
1. Attach connecting tubing from flowmeter and nipple adaptor to resuscitation bag.	1. A humidifier bottle is not used since the high flow rates of oxygen required would force water into the tubing and clog it.
2. Turn flowmeter to "flush" position.	2. A high flow rate or "flush" position is necessary to meet the minute ventilation of the patient.
3. If the patient is not intubated, attach mask to the bag, insert an oral airway, and while tilting back the patient's head, place the mask over the patient's face.	3. In a cardiopulmonary arrest situation, every effort should be made to establish a patent airway in the comatose patient.
4. Squeeze resuscitation bag with sufficient force and at the rate necessary to maintain adequate minute ventilation.	4. If cardiac massage is being given, breaths will have to be quickly interposed between cardiac compressions. If the patient needs only respiratory assistance, watch for chest expansion, and listen with the stethoscope to insure adequate ventilation.
5. Continue squeezing bag at appropriate intervals until CPR (cardiopulmonary resuscitation) is no longer required or until the hyperinflation accompanying suctioning has ceased.	5. A rate of approximately 14–18 breaths per minute is used unless the patient is being given external cardiac compressions (see page 864).

GUIDELINES: Using Oxygen with CPAP

Continuous positive airway pressure (CPAP) is used in the spontaneously breathing patient in conjunction with oxygen. It maintains the alveoli in an "open" state to allow adequate oxygenation of the patient.

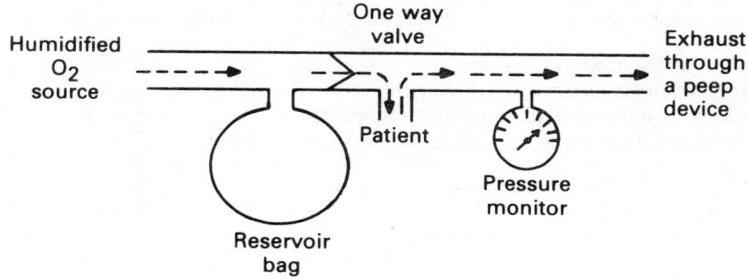

FIGURE 7-18. *CPAP schematic.*

Equipment

O₂ source—usually an oxygen blender

Large bore tubing

Reservoir bag

T-piece → system → patient's endotracheal or tracheostomy tube

Nebulizer with sterile distilled water

CPAP valves or premeasured water bottle and underwater CPAP of desired pressure is used

Pressure manometer

One-way valve

Procedure

NURSING ACTION	RATIONALE/AMPLIFICATION
Performance Phase	
1. Connect various pieces of equipment as shown in illustration (Fig. 7-18).	
2. Turn on oxygen source and adjust flowrate so that it is sufficient to meet the patient's inspiratory demand.	2. The patient will be receiving all of his minute ventilation from this "closed system," so it is essential that the flowrate be adequate to meet changes in the patient's breathing pattern.
3. Connect the T-piece to the patient and observe the patient's respiratory rate and effort.	3. If the CPAP level is too high for a particular individual (CPAP is usually not used in levels above 10 cm.), the patient's work of breathing may actually be increased rather than diminished.
Follow-up Phase	
1. Change tubing, nebulizer, and other equipment exposed to moisture daily.	1. Contaminated equipment may cause virulent infections in debilitated patients.
2. Assess patient's condition and functioning of equipment at regular intervals.	2. The pressure manometer should be checked frequently to determine that the correct level of CPAP is being maintained. Tubing should be drained frequently so that condensate does not build up and block flow to the patient. The patient's respiratory rate and effort of breathing should be assessed regularly to determine adequacy of the therapy.

OTHER RESPIRATORY THERAPEUTIC MODALITIES

GUIDELINES: Assisting the Patient Undergoing Intermittent Positive Pressure Breathing (IPPB)*

The intermittent positive pressure breathing unit is a piece of equipment that supplies air or oxygen under positive pressure (above atmospheric) during inspiration. It should only be used to augment ventilation in patients who because of weakness, chest wall deformity, or lethargy are unable to take voluntary deep breaths and use simpler modalities, such as a slipstream or compressor nebulizer.

Purposes
1. To administer aerosolized medication
2. To mobilize secretions and aid expectoration
3. To improve alveolar ventilation and prevent atelectasis
4. To assist respiration via positive pressure on inspiration

Contraindications
1. Untreated pneumothorax
2. Mediastinal and subcutaneous emphysema
3. Untreated active tuberculosis
4. Use with caution in patients with gastrointestinal surgery, hemoptysis, bullous disease

Equipment   According to the type of machine used (each machine has different controls and settings)
NO SMOKING signs

Procedure

NURSING ACTION	RATIONALE/AMPLIFICATION
Preparatory Phase	
1. Post NO SMOKING signs. Explain the procedure to the patient.	1. Proper explanation of the procedure helps to ensure the patient's cooperation.
2. Measure the heart rate before and after the treatment for patients using bronchodilator drugs for the first time.	2. Bronchodilators accelerate cardiac action. They may produce precordial distress, palpitation, dizziness, nausea, and excessive perspiration.
3. Place the patient in a comfortable sitting or semi-Fowler's position.	3. The diaphragmatic excursion is greater in this position, and the upright position helps prevent air-swallowing.
4. Turn on the pressure source (oxygen, compressed air).	
5. Place the prescribed medication in the nebulizer/or sterile distilled water.	5. An IPPB treatment should not be given with dry gas.
6. Adjust all controls on tentative settings (usually 15). Select the inspiratory flow rate according to the machine being used (and physician's request).	6. Positive pressure is measured in cm. of water pressure; the pressure delivery is usually in the range of 10–20 cm. H_2O. Each unit should be tested to see whether the predetermined setting is accomplished before treating the patient.
7. Check the nebulizer for mist.	7. Adequate fog and particle size is essential to effective distribution of medication.
Performance Phase	
1. Instruct the patient to bite down gently on the mouthpiece and to seal the mouthpiece with his lips.	1. The mouthpiece (or mask) must constitute a closed circuit if the unit is to cycle. (If the patient exhales through his nose while using the mouthpiece the unit will not reach the desired pressure.)
2. Tell the patient to breathe slowly and normally and let the machine do the work.	2. A slight inspiratory effort will activate the positive pressure phase, and the lungs will be inflated with a rapid rate of flow until the predetermined pressure is reached and pressure expiration takes place.
3. Observe expansion of the patient's chest and measure exhaled tidal volume to ensure adequate ventilation. a. Patient should take 8–10 breaths per minute. b. Instruct him to hold his breath 3–4 seconds at the end of each inspiration.	3. Measurement of tidal volumes is particularly useful in the patient who has a high arterial PCO_2 and needs high tidal volumes to lower it. a. The machine will exert a regulated pressure on inhalation, helping him to breathe more deeply. b. This ensures settling of aerosol particles on bronchiolar mucosa.
4. Remind the patient to exhale completely and slowly in a relaxed manner. The patient controls exhalation.	4. This type of breathing encourages good diaphragmatic motion and reduces residual air volume.
5. After several breaths, tell the patient to push all the air out, count 1, 2, 3, and stop inhaling (on the	5. The treatment should take 10–20 minutes depending on the clinical problem.

* IPPB is being supplanted by other forms of therapy, e.g., slipstream nebulizer and incentive spirometer.

Procedure (cont.)	NURSING ACTION	RATIONALE/AMPLIFICATION
	machine) for a few seconds to assess extent of improvement.	
	6. Encourage the patient to continue this type of breathing until all the medication is given.	6. The medication should be completely nebulized to ensure effectiveness of treatment.
	Follow-up Phase	
	1. Record medication used, patient's respiratory rate and effort, and description of secretions expectorated (also pressure limit and flow rate).	1. Note the patient's tolerance of the treatment.
	2. Disassemble and clean the exhalation unit and nebulizer after each use. Keep this equipment in the patient's room. This equipment is changed every 24 hours.	2. Each patient has his own breathing circuit (exhalation valve, nebulizer, and tubing, mouthpiece, and mask). By proper cleaning, sterilization, and storage of equipment, infection can be prevented from entering already diseased lungs.

GUIDELINES: Assisting the Patient Undergoing Nebulizer Therapy Without Positive Pressure (Slipstream Nebulizer)

The *slipstream nebulizer* is a piece of equipment which allows for the nebulization of medication without positive pressure. The nebulizer is powered by either oxygen or compressed air (air compressor or piped compressed air at 4–5 liters/minute).

Purposes
1. To administer aerosolized medication
2. To mobilize secretions and aid expectoration

Contraindications
1. Inability of patient to cooperate in taking deep breaths
2. Adverse reactions encountered with medication

Equipment
Air compressor or oxygen or air flowmeter
O_2 nipple adaptor

O_2 connecting tubing
Nebulizer manifold

Procedure	NURSING ACTION	RATIONALE/AMPLIFICATION
	1. Explain the procedure to the patient.	1. Proper explanation of the procedure helps to ensure the patient's cooperation. This therapy depends on patient effort.
	2. Measure the heart rate before and after the treatment for patients using bronchodilator drugs for the first time.	2. Bronchodilators accelerate cardiac action. They may produce precordial distress, palpitation, dizziness, nausea, and excessive perspiration.
	3. Place the patient in a comfortable sitting or semi-Fowler's position.	3. The diaphragmatic excursion is greater in this position.
	4. Connect the nebulizer and connecting tubing to flowmeter and set flow at 4–5 liters/minute.	
	Performance Phase	
	1. Instruct the patient to exhale.	
	2. Tell the patient to take in a deep breath from the mouthpiece.	2. This will ensure that medication is deposited below the level of the oropharynx.
	3. Nose clips are sometimes used if the patient has difficulty breathing only through his mouth.	
	4. Instruct the patient to breathe slowly and deeply until all of the medication is nebulized.	4. Medication usually will be nebulized in 10–15 minutes at a literflow of 4–5 liters/minute.
	5. Observe expansion of the patient's chest to ascertain that he is taking deep breaths.	
	6. Encourage the patient to cough after several deep breaths.	6. The deep lung inflation may loosen secretions and facilitate their expectoration.
	Follow-up Phase	
	1. Record medication used, patient's respiratory rate and effort, and description of secretions.	1. Note the patient's tolerance of the treatment.
	2. Disassemble and clean nebulizer after each use. Keep this equipment in the patient's room. This equipment is changed every 24 hours.	2. Each patient has his own breathing circuit (nebulizer manifold, tubing, and mouthpiece). By proper cleaning, sterilization, and storage of equipment, infections can be prevented from entering already diseased lungs.

GUIDELINES: Assisting the Patient Using Incentive Spirometry

The *incentive spirometer* is a piece of equipment that maximizes voluntary lung inflation; for this reason it is used in the prevention and treatment of atelectasis (Fig. 7-19).

Purpose   To prevent and treat atelectasis, especially in the postoperative patient.

Equipment   According to the type of device used.

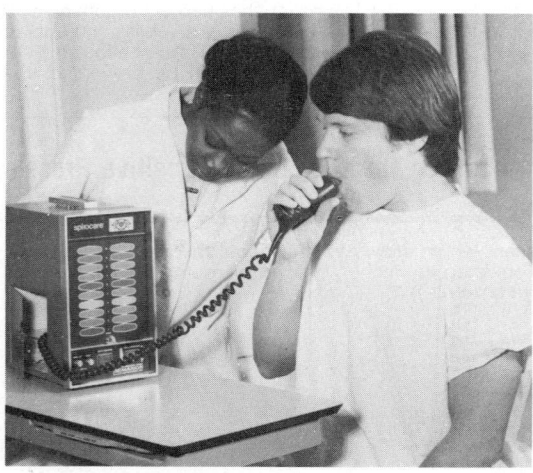

FIGURE 7-19. *Incentive spirometry.*

Procedure

NURSING ACTION	RATIONALE/AMPLIFICATION
Preparatory Phase	
1. Explain the procedure and its purpose to the patient.	1. Optimum results are achieved when the patient is given preoperative instructions.
2. Place the patient in a comfortable sitting or semi-Fowler's position.	2. The diaphragmatic excursion is greater in this position; however, if the patient is medically unable to be in this position, the exercise may be done in any position.
3. Set the incentive spirometer for the desired tidal volume (500 ml. is often used to start). The tidal volume is set according to the manufacturer's instructions.	3. The initial tidal volume may be prescribed by the physician, but the purpose of the device is to measure the patient's gradually increasing tidal volumes as he takes deeper breaths.
Performance Phase	
1. Instruct the patient to exhale.	
2. Tell the patient to take in a deep breath from the mouthpiece.	2. Nose clips are sometimes used if the patient has difficulty breathing only through his mouth—this will ensure him full credit for each breath measured.
3. When the desired goal is reached, ask the patient to try holding that level of inflation for a few seconds.	3. By pausing at peak inflation, the alveoli are held open longer and do not collapse as easily.
4. Instruct the patient to relax and exhale. He should take several normal breaths before attempting another one with the incentive spirometer.	4. Usually one incentive breath per minute minimizes patient fatigue.
5. Continue to monitor the patient's spirometer breaths, periodically increasing the tidal volume as the patient tolerates it.	
6. Encourage the patient to cough after a deep breath.	6. The deep lung inflation may loosen secretions and enable the patient to expectorate them.
Follow-up Phase	
1. Have the patient take the prescribed number of breaths and record the tidal volumes. Describe any secretions expectorated.	1. Ten breaths per hour while awake is a frequent request. A counter on the incentive spirometer indicates the number of breaths the patient has taken.

GUIDELINES: Assisting the Patient Using an Ultrasonic Nebulizer

An *ultrasonic nebulizer* delivers very small aerosolized particles into the lungs at atmospheric pressure (Fig. 7-20).

Equipment
Ultrasonic nebulizer and nebulizer cup
Large bore tubing 30.4 cm. (12 inches)
Large bore tubing 1.8 m. (6 feet)
One-way valve (placed between blower and nebulizer cup)
Disposable aerosol mask

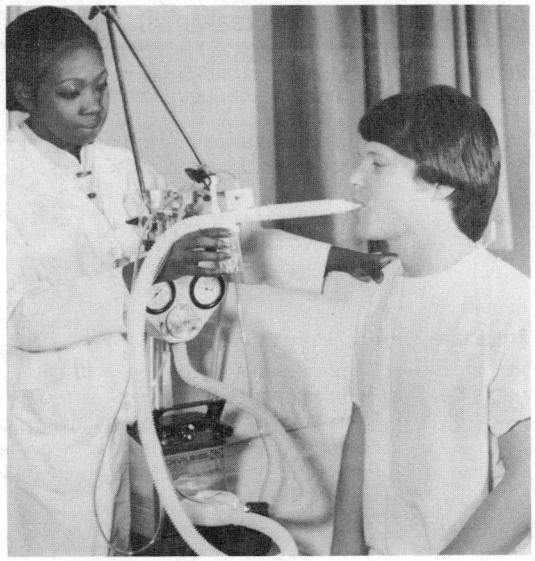

FIGURE 7-20. *IPPB treatment with ultrasonic nebulizer in line.*

Procedure

NURSING ACTION	RATIONALE/AMPLIFICATION
Preparatory Phase	
1. Fill the couplant compartment (water reservoir) of the machine with tap water.	
2. Place nebulizer cup in couplant compartment and fill with prescribed fluid.	2. Sterile distilled water or normal saline is used.
3. Connect 30.4 cm. (12") large bore tubing to blower, add one-way valve to the other end, and connect to the nebulizer cup.	3. If oxygen source is desired, connect large bore tubing from oxygen powered nebulizer to the ultrasonic nebulizer cup.
4. Connect 1.8 m. (6-foot) large bore tubing to the other side of the nebulizer cup.	
5. Connect the mask to the other end of the 1.8 cm. (6-foot) tubing.	
6. Plug in the machine and adjust the setting until the desired amount of mist is obtained.	
Performance Phase	
1. Instruct the patient to breathe in slowly through his mouth and to exhale the same way.	1. This allows maximum particle deposition.
2. Have the patient continue to breathe in this manner for the prescribed length of the treatments.	2. The procedure lasts usually 15–30 minutes.

3. Observe the patient for any adverse reactions to the treatment.
    a. Wheezing (bronchospasm)
    b. Excessive fluid deposition ("drowning") causing suffocation.
	3. The patient may develop wheezing or may not be able to expectorate delivered fluid or his secretions. He may need assistance in draining his secretions by suctioning or postural drainage.

4. Encourage the patient to periodically expectorate any secretions loosened during the treatment.	
Follow-up Phase	
1. Record medication used, patient's respiratory rate and effort, and description of secretions expectorated.	1. Note any adverse reactions.
2. Keep this equipment in the patient's room. The equipment should be changed every 24 hours.	2. Ultrasonic nebulizers have a high contamination rate when not used properly. It is desirable that each patient have his own machine in his room.

ARTIFICIAL AIRWAY MANAGEMENT

GUIDELINES: Endotracheal Intubation (Fig. 7-21)

Purpose An endotracheal tube may be inserted via the nose or mouth to facilitate suctioning, to bypass an upper airway obstruction, and to permit connection of the patient to a resuscitation bag or mechanical ventilator.

Equipment
1. Laryngoscope with curved or straight blade and working light source. (Check batteries and bulb periodically.)
2. Endotracheal tubes with low-pressure cuffs and adaptor to connect tube to ventilator or bag
3. Stylet to guide endotracheal tube
4. Oral airway (assorted sizes), tongue blade to keep patient from biting into and occluding endotracheal tube
5. Adhesive tape
6. Lubricant jelly
7. Syringe

Procedure **_Preparatory Phase_**
1. Remove dental bridgework and plates.
2. Remove headboard of bed.
3. Make sure light source of laryngoscope is working.
4. Select endotracheal tube of appropriate size (7.5–9 mm. for average adult).
5. Inflate and deflate cuff to make sure it is intact.
6. Lubricate endotracheal tube.
7. Insert stylet if tube is very flexible.

NURSING ACTION	RATIONALE/AMPLIFICATION
Performance Phase	
1. If cervical spine is not injured, place head in a "sniffing" position, flexed at the junction of the neck and thorax and extended at the junction of the spine and skull.	1. Upper airway is open maximally in this position and mouth of unconscious patient will often open.
2. Ventilate and oxygenate the patient with resuscitation bag before intubation.	2. This decreases the likelihood of cardiac arrhythmias secondary to hypoxia.
3. Hold the handle of the laryngoscope in the left hand and hold patient's mouth open with the right hand by crossing fingers.	3. Leverage is improved by crossing thumb and index fingers when opening the patient's mouth.
4. Insert blade of laryngoscope along the right side of the tongue, pointing tongue to the left, and use right thumb and index finger to pull patient's lower lip away from lower teeth.	4. Rolling lip away from teeth prevents injury by being caught between teeth and blade.
5. Lift laryngoscope forward (toward ceiling) to expose epiglottis.	
6. Lift laryngoscope upward and forward at 45-degree angle to expose glottis (vocal cords).	6. This stretches the hypoepiglottis ligament, folding the epiglottis upward and exposing the glottis.
7. As the epiglottis is lifted forward (toward ceiling) the vertical opening of the larynx between the vocal cords will come into view.	7. Do not use wrist; use shoulder and arm to lift epiglottis—to avoid using teeth as a fulcrum, which could lead to dental damage.
8. Once vocal cords are visualized, insert tube into the right corner of the mouth and pass the tube—guided by blade but keeping cords in constant view.	8. Make sure you do not insert tube in esophagus; the esophageal mucosa is pink and the opening is horizontal rather than vertical.
9. Gently push the tube through the triangular space formed by the vocal cords.	9. If the vocal cords are in spasm (closed), wait a few seconds before passing tube.
10. Stop insertion just after the tube cuff has disappeared from view beyond the cords.	10. Advancing tube further may lead to its entry into a mainstem bronchus (usually the right bronchus) causing collapse of the unventilated lung.
11. Withdraw laryngoscope, holding endotracheal tube in place.	
12. Inflate cuff with the minimal amount of air required to occlude trachea.	12. The amount of air used for cuff inflation depends on the size of the cuff and the diameter of patient's trachea.
13. Insert oral airway or bite block.	13. This keeps patient from biting down on the tube and obstructing the airway.
14. Observe expansion of both sides of the chest by observation and auscultation of breath sounds.	14. Observation and auscultation help in determining that tube remains in position and has not slipped into right mainstem bronchus.

Procedure (cont.)

NURSING ACTION	RATIONALE/AMPLIFICATION
15. Mark proximal end of tube with marking pen or tape.	15. This will allow for detection of any later change in position.
16. Secure tube with adhesive tape to the patient's face.	
17. Take chest x-ray to verify tube position.	

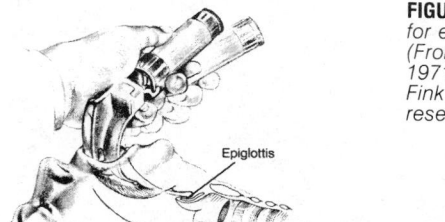

FIGURE 7-21. *Sequence of steps for endotracheal intubation. (From Patient care, 15 June 1971. Copyright 1971, Miller and Fink Corp., Darien, CT. All rights reserved.)*

A. Positioning of head and insertion of laryngoscope blade for endotracheal intubation.

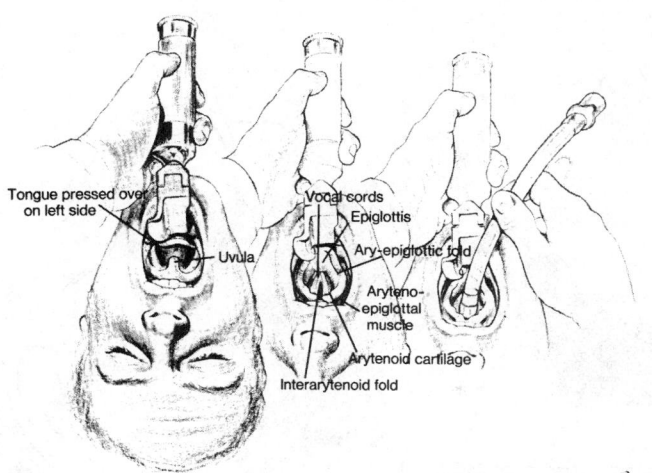

B. The landmarks to identify when advancing the laryngoscope.

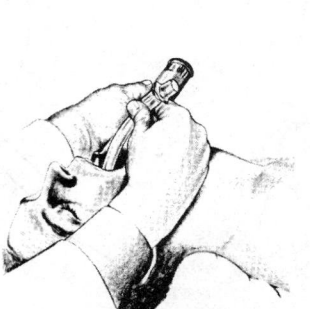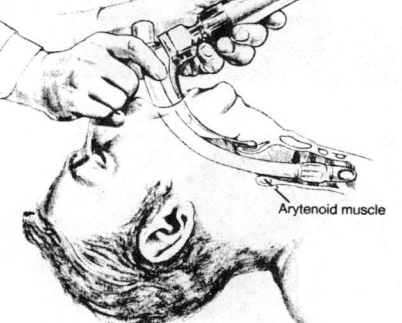

C. Positioning the endotracheal tube and removing the laryngoscope.

TRACHEOSTOMY

A *tracheostomy* is an external opening made into the trachea.

Purposes

1. To provide and maintain a patent airway.
2. To enable the removal of tracheobronchial secretions when the patient is unable to cough productively.
3. To permit the use of positive pressure ventilation.
4. To prevent aspiration of secretions in the unconscious (or paralyzed) patient by closing off the trachea from the esophagus.

5. To replace an endotracheal tube when such an airway is needed for more than 5–7 days.

Kinds of Tracheostomy Tubes

1. Plastic (nylon, polyvinyl chloride, or silastic) tracheostomy tubes are available with or without inner tubes and usually with attached low pressure cuffs.
2. Silver tracheostomy tube* consists of 3 parts: obturator (pilot), inner cannula, and outer cannula.
3. Jackson silver tracheostomy tube* with Morch adaptor—similar to No. 1 with a screw-on swivel adaptor (on the inner cannula) to connect with a ventilator. Suction is permitted without disturbing ventilator.

* Rarely used.

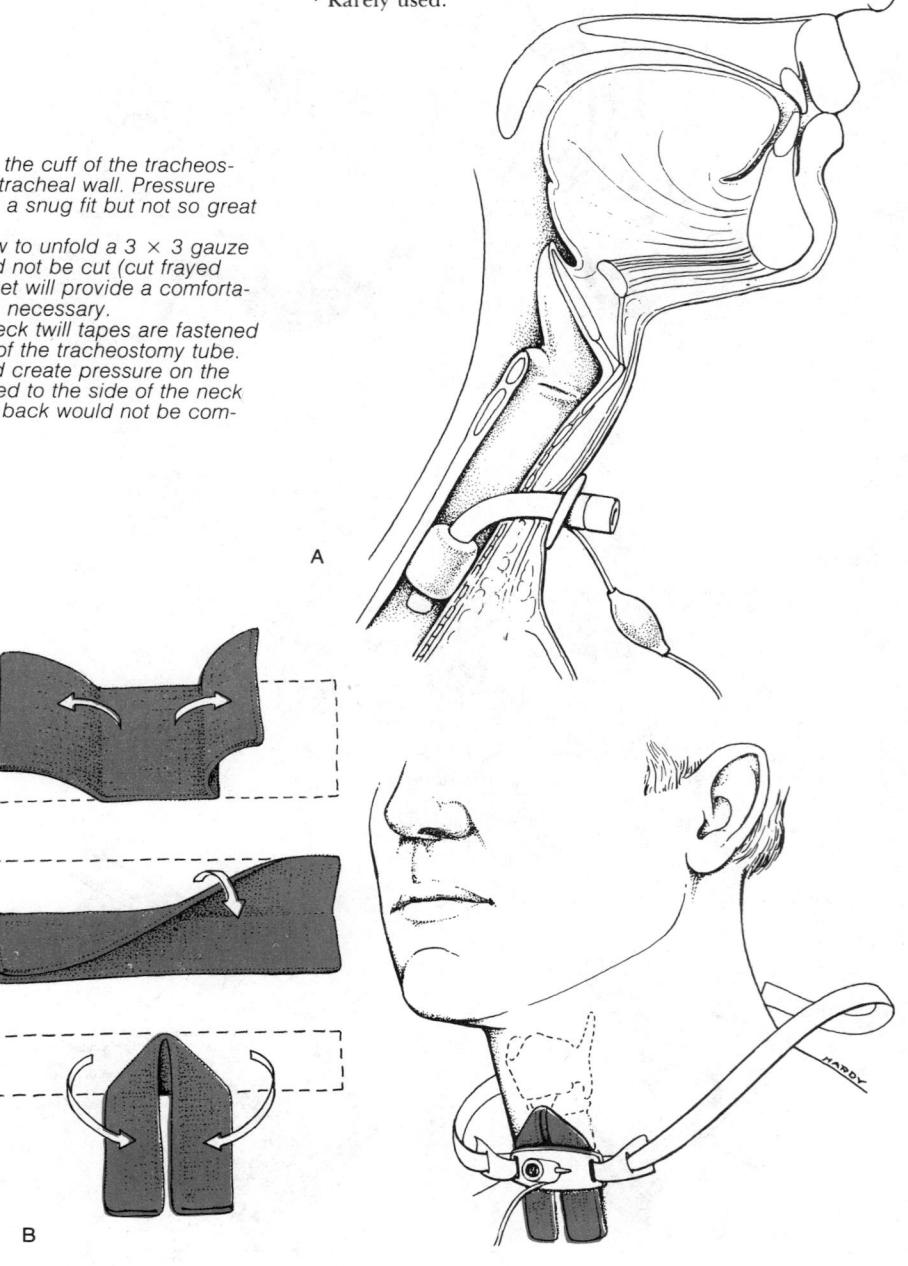

FIGURE 7-22. A. *Part A shows how the cuff of the tracheostomy tube fits smoothly within the tracheal wall. Pressure should be great enough to ensure a snug fit but not so great as to produce a stenosis.*
B. *The lower illustration shows how to unfold a 3 × 3 gauze square and refold it so that it need not be cut (cut frayed threads could be aspirated) and yet will provide a comfortable neck pad. Change as often as necessary.*

  Note the manner in which the neck twill tapes are fastened to the openings in the neck plate of the tracheostomy tube. This eliminates a knot which would create pressure on the neck. Twill tape ends should be tied to the side of the neck rather than in back. (A knot at the back would not be comfortable to lie on.)

4. Endotracheal cuff may be attached to the cannula to provide a closed system.

Performing a Tracheostomy (By the Physician)

1. Practice sterile aseptic technique throughout.
2. Inject local anesthetic.
3. Vertical incision preferred; control bleeding before trachea is opened to prevent patient from aspirating blood.
4. Perform high tracheostomy preferably, so that tip of cannula is well above carina.
5. Remove a segment of 3rd tracheal ring. (In children, ring is split but segment is not removed.)
6. Insert a dilator to permit insertion of No. 7 or No. 8 (adult) tracheostomy cannula.

Nursing Management

A. *Physical Care of Patient*

1. Provide adequate humidity since natural humidifying pathway of the oropharynx is no longer used.
2. Aspirate secretions since the patient's own cough mechanism is not as effective.
3. Suction gently to avoid injuring the epithelium; limit each suctioning time to between 10–15 seconds.
4. Introduce *sterile* aspirating tubes to prevent infection.
5. Recognize patient's ability to breathe comfortably; if he has difficulty, assess need for ventilatory assistance.
6. Elevate him to semi-Fowler's or sitting position if not contraindicated since this is usually more comfortable and makes breathing easier.
7. Observe stomal site for bleeding or irritation; when the outer tracheostomy tube is changed (by physician for first 4 or 5 days), apply small amount of antibiotic ointment before reinserting tube. Place unfrayed sterile dressing around collar of tracheostomy tube (Fig. 7-22).

B. *Psychological Care of Patient*

1. Recognize that the patient is usually apprehensive, particularly about choking, about being unable to remove secretions, and about his ability to communicate.
2. Explain and demonstrate the procedure carefully, using tracheostomy equipment; proceed according to the patient's ability to absorb information and his desire to learn; instruction may be divided into several sessions.
3. Inform the patient and his family that he will not be able to speak; determine with the patient the best method of communication, e.g., sign language, writing, etc.; supply him with note paper, pencil, "Magic slate," and call bell.
4. Anticipate some of his questions by providing the answer to "Is it permanent?" "Will it hurt to breathe?" "Will someone be with me?"
5. Provide an attendant for the first 24–48 hours, particularly if patient is fearful.

Equipment

1. Sterile gloves and duplicate sterile tracheostomy set including Trousseau dilator and 2 tracheal retractors (or hooks), 1 tissue forceps, 1 grooved director, 2 hemostats, petrolatum gauze or antibiotic ointment, sterile dressing
2. Humidifying equipment
   a. For the room—a heated aerosol machine
   b. For the patient—ultrasonic mist unit, nebulizer attached to tracheostomy tube, or a high humidity tracheal collar
3. Suction equipment (see following, Guidelines: Aspirating the Tracheostomy Tube)
4. Communication materials; pencil, paper, etc., call bell
5. Mirror—for use when patient is beginning self-care

GUIDELINES: Aspirating (Suctioning) through the Tracheostomy Tube

NOTE: For high-risk patient, see procedure immediately following.

Purpose To remove secretions when audible in the tracheobronchial tree, so that a patent airway is maintained.

Equipment Aseptic Technique
Sterile disposable catheter
  No. 14 or 16 (adult)
  No. 8 or 10 (child)
Sterile gloves, individually wrapped
Sterile saline
Sterile syringe—5 ml.

General Nursing Considerations

1. Administer analgesics and sedatives with caution so that the respiratory center is not depressed.
2. Suction trachea when necessary (may be every 5 or 10 minutes for the first several postoperative hours and less frequently when need is less).

NURSING ALERT: Need for aspiration is expressed by noisy, moist respirations, increased pulse and respirations. Encourage patient to cough to bring up and expel secretions; use suction if coughing is not productive.

3. Use stethoscope to check patency of airway.
4. Avoid unnecessary suctioning which is irritating to mucosa and may initiate infection.

GUIDELINES: Aspirating (Suctioning) through the Tracheostomy Tube (cont.)

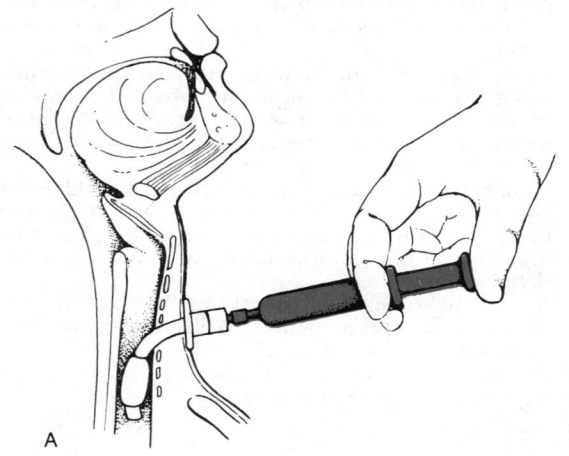

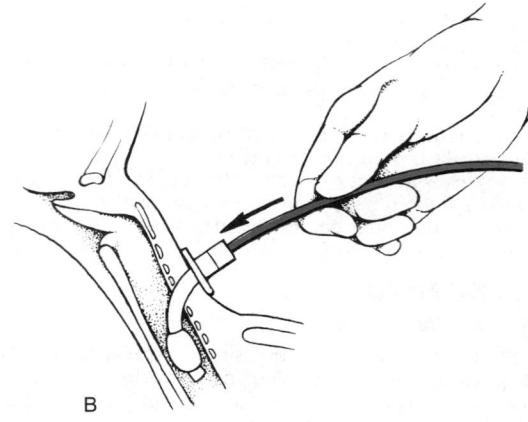

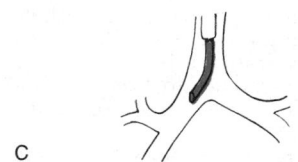

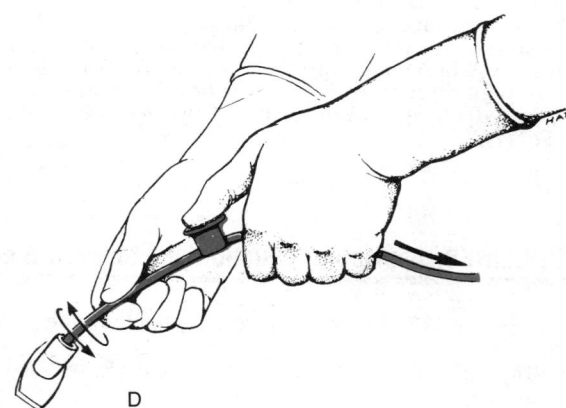

FIGURE 7-23. *Care of the tracheostomy patient. (A) After the tracheostomy cuff is deflated (note that cuff does not touch sides of trachea), 3–5 ml. of sterile saline can be instilled into the tube to loosen secretions. (B) After donning sterile gloves, the nurse introduces a sterile catheter without applying suction. (C) To remove secretions from the bronchus, insert tube 20–30 cm. (7.5–11.5 inches). (D) Suction is applied by sealing the button outlet with the thumb. Gradually withdraw the catheter with a rotating motion.*

Procedure (Fig. 7-23)

NURSING ACTION	RATIONALE/AMPLIFICATION
1. Lubricate catheter with normal saline.	1. To facilitate passage of tube.
2. Insert catheter with suction turned off.	2. So as not to suction the wall of the cannula or irritate the mucous membrane wall.
3. Pass tube into bronchus for 20 to 30 cm. (8–12 inches), unless contraindicated, and then gradually open suction.	3. To stimulate coughing and to loosen secretions even beyond the cannula.
4. Remove catheter when patient coughs.	4. Catheter obstructs cannula and interferes with expulsion of secretions.
5. For tenacious secretions, instill sterile saline solution as prescribed.	5. Saline aids in dissolving mucus. It is helpful to have patient take a deep breath.
6. Have tissue or container ready to receive expelled secretions.	
7. Rotate catheter between thumb and forefinger; move it up and down gently as it is withdrawn with suction on.	

Procedure (cont.)

NURSING ACTION	RATIONALE/AMPLIFICATION
8. Do not suction patient more than 15 seconds at a time (rest at least 3 minutes between suctionings). Administer oxygen and ventilate patient between aspirations to relieve hypoxia and prevent arrhythmias.	8. There is the danger of hypoxia if suctioning is prolonged.
9. Use a stethoscope along bronchial tree to detect gurgling mucous sounds.	9. Auscultation will determine effectiveness of suctioning; respiration should be quiet and essentially effortless at end of aspiration.

Aftercare of Equipment

1. When inner silver cannula is clogged with mucus, remove to clean.
2. Soak in a cold solution of half water and half hydrogen peroxide to loosen adhering particles (some prefer 2% sodium bicarbonate solution). Hot water would cause protein in mucus to coagulate.
3. A brush may be used to scrub interior of tube with soap and water. A pipe cleaner may be used for small tubes.
4. Disinfect tube by boiling for 5 minutes; cool.
5. Suction outer cannula in patient before reinserting cleaned inner cannula.

GUIDELINES: Caring for Patient with a Cuffed Tube (Tracheostomy or Endotracheal)

A *cuff* is the inflatable balloon of a tracheostomy or endotracheal tube which is designed to provide the snug fit required for ventilators. It prevents leakage of air and of secretions around the tube and aspiration of vomitus and oropharyngeal secretions.

General Nursing Considerations

1. Inform the patient that he will not be able to talk normally when the endotracheal cuffed tube is in place because no air passes over the larynx. (Speaking may be resumed when the tube is removed.)
2. Maintain the neck in a comfortable position.
3. Recognize the importance of frequent and adequate mouth care.

Procedure (May require a physician's request: Usually the cuff is initially inflated by the physician.)

NURSING ACTION	RATIONALE/AMPLIFICATION
Deflating a Cuff	
1. Suction pharynx—oral and nasal.	1. Removes secretions which could be aspirated during the process of deflation.
2. Deflate cuff slowly.	2. On endotracheal tube, a small test balloon at end of tubing remains inflated as long as cuff is inflated.
3. Suction through the tracheostomy or endotracheal tube.	3. Removes secretions which may have been present above inflated cuff and around exterior of tube and may now have seeped downward. The coughing reflex may be stimulated during deflation, which helps to mobilize secretions.
4. Provide adequate ventilation while cuff is deflated.	
a. If the patient does not require assisted ventilation: provide humidified warm air.	a. Continue observation of patient: pulse, color, etc. If any signs of distress, place patient back on mechanical ventilator.
b. If the patient requires assisted ventilation: provide a manually inflating breathing bag or respirator if patient has been on a mechanical ventilator.	b. If patient is apneic, cuff should not be deflated more than 30 or 45 seconds.
Inflating a Cuff (Slowly)	
1. Stipulations:	
a. To be done when patient requires mechanical ventilation or is being fed.	a. To prevent aspiration of food into lungs.
(1) Semi-Fowler's position is most comfortable if permissible, and is required for a half hour after feeding.	(1) Gravity assists in moving food into the stomach.
(2) On right side.	(2) To prevent regurgitation of feeding.
b. Inflate cuff during inspiration (positive pressure phase)	
2. Method A	
a. Inject air into cuff until complete seal is achieved or to selected pressure, following directions on package insert. By listening with a stethoscope placed just below chin (submental) one may determine that no leak exists.	a. The pressure-cycled ventilator will turn off; air will not escape around tube or from nose or mouth. In the conscious patient, a leak-free system is present when he is aphonic.
b. Clamp tube leading to cuff.	

GUIDELINES: Caring for Patient with a Cuffed Tube (Tracheostomy or Endotracheal) (cont.)

Procedure (cont.)	NURSING ACTION	RATIONALE/AMPLIFICATION

	3. Method B (minimal leak inflation)
	   a. Inject air until full seal is acquired; withdraw 0.5 ml. of air and clamp tube.
	   b. Note and record amount of air required to inflate cuff.
		a. A partial leak is purposely created so that ventilator can be set to compensate for it.
		b. If at subsequent times more air is required to inflate cuff, tracheal dilatation or other serious problem (erosion of a large blood vessel or tracheoesophageal diverticulum or fistula) may be the cause.

	Suctioning (done with *sterile* equipment). 1. Tracheobronchial secretions are suctioned as frequently as necessary—5 or 10 seconds at a time and not oftener than once every 3 minutes.	*To Minimize Possibility of Infection* 1. This is a nursing judgment based on recognition of signs suggesting accumulation of secretions.

	2. Via endotracheal tube
	   a. Insert catheter (for an adult) approximately 45–50 cm. (18–20 inches)
	      (1) If impossible to pass suction tube this distance, a mucus plug may be in the way; inject 5 ml. saline.
	3. Via tracheostomy tube (See Guidelines, p. 189)
	4. Oropharyngeal with endotracheal tube in place. Suction oropharynx frequently. (Patient is taking nothing by mouth.)
	5. Oropharyngeal with cuffed tracheostomy tube in place.
	(Patient is able to swallow and have a normal intake.)
		a. Tube inserted deep since this patient has difficulty mobilizing deep secretions.
		   (1) Injecting saline helps in liquefying mucus.
		
		4. Volume of secretions is greater due to irrigation caused by such a tube.

	Feeding the Patient
	NOTE: The nurse must decide which of the following 2 methods to use:
	   a. Cuff inflated during feeding
	   b. Cuff deflated during feeding
	
	Test: Feed patient colored gelatin; if color from gelatin appears in aspirated material, inflate tube.
		Depends on individual patient and the nurse's assessment of the situation.
		   a. To prevent aspiration
		   b. To prevent bulging into esophagus, which makes swallowing more difficult.
		   If color from gelatin does not appear in aspirated material, there is little chance of aspiration during feeding, hence cuff may be deflated.

	Maintaining Humidified Warm Inspired Air 1. Provide continuous flow of mist.	1. To prevent drying of secretions and irritation of mucous membrane.
	Complications 1. Laryngeal irritation and damage to vocal cord due to movement of endotracheal tube. 2. Laryngeal edema 3. Tracheal stenosis 4. Hemorrhage	*Means of Avoiding Complications* 1. Prevent movement or jarring of tube. 2. Supply mist during and after extubation. 3. Proper nursing care includes humidity, suction, etc.

GUIDELINES: Preparing for Tracheostomy Tube Removal

Purpose To preserve tracheostomy while training the patient to breathe through his mouth.

Procedure	NURSING ACTION	RATIONALE/AMPLIFICATION
	1. Determine patient's ability to breathe deeply and cough effectively. 2. Check the patient's reflexes for swallowing, gagging, coughing. 3. Observe patient's ability to bring up tracheobronchial secretions without assistance for 24 hours. 4. Cork tracheostomy tube intermittently with cuff deflated. 5. Remove tracheostomy tube as soon as safe. 6. Tape skin edges together.	1. Clinical assessment of respiratory exchange over a period of time helps in determining time of weaning. 4. Increase the time of occlusion as much as patient can tolerate. 5. This is determined by tolerance of the individual patient with no respiratory difficulties. 6. Tract closes spontaneously in a few days.

MECHANICAL VENTILATION

A *mechanical ventilator* is a positive pressure breathing device which can maintain respiration automatically for prolonged periods of time. It is indicated when the patient is unable to maintain safe levels of arterial carbon dioxide or oxygen by spontaneous breathing.

Types of Ventilators

1. *Pressure-cycled*—the ventilator delivers a predetermined pressure, then turns off.
   a. Gas flows result from this pressure and increase lung volume.
   b. Volume delivered is dependent on lung compliance and varies from breath to breath.
   c. Blockage at any point between machine and lungs will not stop the on-off cycling of the ventilator—but the patient will receive *no volume*.
   d. Volume-based alarms should always be used with this ventilator.
2. *Volume-cycled*—the ventilator delivers a predetermined volume of air to the patient regardless of any changing lung condition.
   If machine is unable to deliver such volume, the operator is alerted by an audible and visible alarm.

Modes of Operation

Ventilators are used as assistors, controllers, or as assist-controllers.
1. *Assist mode*—used for patient who is making an inspiratory effort, but who, for various reasons, cannot achieve an adequate tidal volume.
   The patient initiates each breath, which is then augmented by the ventilator to achieve a preset volume.
2. *Control mode*—used for patient whose respiratory drive is absent or excessive.
   a. If respiratory effort is absent, machine initiates breaths at a predetermined rate.
   b. If rate is excessive for maintenance of adequate acid-base status, the rate can be controlled—machine will not respond to any attempt by the patient to breathe spontaneously.
3. *Assist-Control mode*—used for patient whose respiratory rate is erratic.
   a. If patient maintains adequate rate, the ventilator functions as an assistor.
   b. If respiratory rate falls below a preset level, machine takes over and initiates breathing at a predetermined rate.
   c. The patient can resume regulation of his own respiratory rate at any time.

Special Mechanical Ventilator Techniques

A. *PEEP* (Positive End Expiratory Pressure)—refers to maintenance of a pressure above atmospheric level throughout the entire ventilatory cycle.
1. Purpose
   PEEP prevents collapse of alveolar units during exhalation and thus increases the surface for oxygen transfer.
2. Mechanisms of operation
   a. Mechanical ventilation and spontaneous ventilation are exactly alike—each allows a passive exhalation phase.
   b. The diaphragm relaxes (or ventilatory pressure is removed), intrapulmonary pressure falls until it *equals* atmospheric pressure, and gas flow out of the lung ceases.
   c. PEEP prevents intrapulmonary pressure from falling to atmospheric level—*a positive intrapulmonary pressure is maintained during inhalation and exhalation.*
3. Benefits
   a. Positive intrapulmonary pressure may be helpful in reducing the effects of pulmonary edema by diminishing the rate of transudation of fluid from the pulmonary capillaries to the alveoli.
   b. Since a greater surface area for diffusion is available and shunting is reduced, it is often possible to use inspired oxygen concentrations much lower than would otherwise be required to obtain adequate arterial oxygen levels. This reduces the risk of oxygen toxicity.
4. Hazards
   a. Since the mean intrathoracic pressure is increased by PEEP, venous return and cardiac output may be impeded.
   b. High PEEP levels (above 15–20 cm. H_2O) may possibly cause alveolar rupture with a resulting tension pneumothorax.
5. Precautions
   a. Chest auscultation must be performed very frequently. Diminished or absent breath sounds require immediate notification of the physician.
   b. Suctioning must never exceed 15 seconds from disconnection to reconnection of the ventilator. Presuctioning hyperventilation should be done on the ventilator with 100% oxygen or by a hand resuscitator capable of providing PEEP.

B. *CPAP*—Continuous Positive Airway Pressure (See Fig. 7-18)
1. Gives the same end results as PEEP but without the use of a ventilator.
2. Generally used if a patient is capable of maintaining an adequate rate and tidal volume but has some pathology which prevents maintenance of adequate levels of tissue oxygenation.
3. CPAP has the same purposes, benefits, hazards, and precautions noted with PEEP.

Underlying Principles

1. Variables that control ventilation and oxygenation:
   a. The ventilator *rate*—measured with a watch. (Some ventilators have respiratory rate marked on respirator and adjusted by a rate knob.)
   b. The *tidal volume*—measured as expired volume with a gas meter.
   c. The *inspired oxygen concentration*—measured with an oxygen analyzer.
2. Tidal volume and rate together control the elimination of carbon dioxide.
3. The inspired oxygen concentration is controlled to produce normal arterial oxygen tension.
4. The duration of inspiration should not exceed expiration. Obstruction of venous return by prolonged inspiration lowers cardiac output and decreases the rate of oxygen transport to body tissues.
5. The inspired gas delivered to the patient must be

fully saturated with sterile, distilled water at body temperature to prevent thickening of tracheobronchial secretions. Water is added by either a heated humidifier or nebulizer.

Clinical Indications

1. Respiratory failure (see p. 169)
2. Chronic obstructive pulmonary disease
3. Administration of respiratory depressants
4. Neuromuscular disorders
5. Drug intoxication
6. Cardiac arrest
7. Chest injury
8. Left ventricular failure and pulmonary edema
9. Pulmonary embolus

Complications

Airway obstruction (secretions, inadequate humidification)
Damage to the trachea (necrosis or malacia)
Infection
Gastrointestinal bleeding
Tension pneumothorax
Inability to wean from ventilator
Pulmonary oxygen toxicity

GUIDELINES: Managing the Patient Requiring Mechanical Ventilation

NURSING ACTION	RATIONALE/AMPLIFICATION
Performance Phase	
1. Obtain baseline samples for blood gas determinations (see p. 158) (pH, PO_2, PCO_2, HCO_3) and chest x-ray.	1. Baseline measurements serve as a guide in determining progress of therapy.
2. Give a brief explanation to the patient.	2. Emphasize that mechanical ventilation is a temporary measure. The patient should be prepared psychologically for weaning the day the ventilator is first used.
3. Establish the airway by means of a cuffed endotracheal tube.	3. Endotracheal intubation provides access to the lower part of the airway for removal of secretions. The cuffed tube prevents leakage of air into mouth during ventilation and permits control of pressure and lung inflation.
a. Inflate the cuff to achieve a proper seal. Inflation pressure should not normally exceed 20 mm. Hg as measured by a cuff pressure manometer. (See Cuff Inflation, p. 195.)	a. Pressure greater than 20 mm. Hg can compromise circulation in the trachea. Insufficient cuff pressure may allow gas leakage and a diminished volume of air may be delivered to the patient.
b. Secure the tube in place with surgical adhesive. Insert an oral airway as a bite block to prevent the patient from occluding an orotracheal tube.	b. Securing the tube prevents dislodgement into the right or left main-stem bronchus.

4. Prepare ventilator according to manufacturer's directions:
   a. Turn on machine.
   b. Adjust volume control; establish tidal and minute volumes as determined by the physician.
   c. Set the oxygen concentration.
	4. Maintenance of ventilation depends on correct machine settings.
	
	   b. Arterial blood pH, carbon dioxide, and oxygen tensions serve as guides in adjusting the ventilator.
	   c. This is generally based on the arterial oxygen levels obtained as a baseline.

d. Adjust respiratory rate of ventilator to 12–14 respirations/minute.	d. This setting approximates normal respiration. The patient who has respiratory stimulus will cycle machine by himself; set the control to a rate slightly lower than the patient's actual rate. These machine settings are subject to change according to patient's condition and response and the make of the machine being used.
e. Adjust flow state (velocity of gas flow during inspiration) to 30–40 liters/minute.	e. The slower the flow the lower will be the pressure required to deliver the patient's gas volume. This results in a lower intrathoracic pressure and less impedance of venous return and cardiac output.
f. Couple the patient's endotracheal tube to the ventilator.	f. Be sure connections are secure. Watch for accidental disconnection between the patient's airway and the ventilator; observe for separation of ventilator tubings from nebulizer, electrical wall-plug slippage, etc.
5. Carry out arterial blood gas determinations approximately 20 minutes after patient is on ventilator. Arterial blood sampling is carried out repeatedly during the acute period.	5. The only effective way to attain and maintain normal oxygen and carbon dioxide tensions is to measure these tensions frequently in arterial blood and adjust the settings of the ventilator accordingly. Arterial blood gases are monitored to assess the effectiveness of therapy. There are no reliable clinical signs of CO_2 retention or alkalosis.
6. *The patient is never left unattended or unobserved*	

Procedure (cont.)

NURSING ACTION	RATIONALE/AMPLIFICATION

Positioning

1. Turn patient from side to side hourly.
2. Lateral turns of 120 degrees are desirable; from right semiprone to left semiprone.
3. Sit the patient upright at regular intervals.
4. Position the patient in postural drainage positions as requested (p. 164).

3. Upright posture increases ventilation of lower lobes.
4. Adequate postural drainage decreases the need for deep tracheobronchial catheter aspiration by preventing retention of secretions in the periphery of the lungs.

5. Carry out passive range of motion exercises of all extremities (p. 54).

Deep Breaths

1. Augment the patient's spontaneous tidal volume by periodically giving him 6–8 deep breaths with a hand resuscitator bag or use sigh mechanism available on some ventilators. Provide patient with adequate oxygenation during this maneuver.

1. Periodic sighing with greater than normal tidal volumes helps to prevent alveolar collapse. Provision of deep breaths by mechanical hyperinflation also helps to promote coughing and reveals the presence of retained secretions.

Aspiration of Secretions

1. Aspirate secretions from the trachea using sterile technique.
2. Oxygenate patient for 1 to 2 minutes prior to each suctioning episode and before second passage of the catheter.
3. Note the amount, color, and consistency of tracheal secretions obtained.
4. Inform the physician if there is appreciable change.

1. Ventilation and nebulization liquefy secretions, causing them to rise into the upper airways.
2. Do not prolong aspiration more than 15 seconds because cardiac arrest may ensue in patients with borderline oxygenation.

Chest Auscultation

1. Listen with a stethoscope to the chest from bottom to top on both sides (hourly).

1. Auscultation of the chest is a means of assessing airway patency and ventilatory distribution. It also confirms the proper placement of the endotracheal or tracheostomy tube.

2. Determine whether breath sounds are present or absent, normal or abnormal, and whether a change has occurred.
3. Observe the patient's diaphragmatic excursions and changes in the use of accessory muscles of respiration.

Humidification

1. Check the water level in the humidification reservoir to ensure that the patient is never ventilated with dry gas. Empty the water that condenses in the delivery tubing.
   Humidifier or nebulizer and tubing must be changed every 24 hours.

1. Water condensing in the delivery tubing may cause obstruction and sudden flooding of the trachea.

   Warm, moist tubing is a perfect breeding area for bacteria.

Airway Pressure

1. Check the airway pressure gauge at frequent intervals in patients on volume-limited ventilators.

1. Since these ventilators deliver a fixed volume, a sudden drop in pressure indicates a leak in the system. A sudden rise in pressure indicates obstruction of the delivery of gas to the patient. Could indicate (1) blockage by secretions; (2) tube slippage into a main-stem bronchus; (3) pneumothorax; or (4) pulmonary edema.

Tidal Volumes

1. Measure the tidal volume with a respirometer for patients on pressure-limited ventilators.

1. An abrupt fall in tidal volume indicates increase in airway resistance (e.g., bronchospasm or other obstruction), an increase in tissue resistance (pulmonary edema), or a leak in the patient circuit of the ventilator.

Cuff Inflation

1. Clean the pharynx and larynx of accumulated secretions by either suction or postural drainage.
2. Release air slowly from the cuff, using a syringe, while maintaining positive pressure via the ventilator or a self-inflating manual resuscitator.

3. Reinflate the cuff with just enough air to prevent gross leakage when positive pressure is again applied to airway.

1. If the tube becomes blocked the patient will not be able to breathe.
2. The cuff is deflated periodically to prevent necrosis of the tracheal mucosa. However, with soft cuffs or atmospheric seal cuffs, deflation of cuffs is not usually necessary.
3. Excessive cuff inflation may cause pressure necrosis over a period of time.

GUIDELINES: Managing the Patient Requiring Mechanical Ventilation (cont.)

Procedure (cont.)

NURSING ACTION	RATIONALE/AMPLIFICATION
Tracheostomy 1. Tracheostomy care should be given as needed, using sterile technique.	1. To continue ventilation while the inner cannula is removed, a substitute sterile inner cannula or adapter should be inserted into the outer cannula and connected to the ventilator.

Bacteriologic Specimens
1. Aspirate tracheal secretions into a sterile container and send to laboratory for culture and sensitivity tests.
  a. This is done immediately after endotracheal intubation.
  b. Daily gram staining of secretions is also done.
	1. This technique allows the earliest detection of infection or change in infecting organisms in the tracheobronchial tree.

Circulatory Measurements 1. Monitor pulse rate and arterial blood pressure; intra-arterial pressure monitoring may be carried out.	1. To accomplish intra-arterial pressure monitoring a catheter is introduced into an artery, usually the radial or femoral, and the pressure at the catheter tip is transmitted to a pressure transducer that converts the pressure wave into an electrical signal that is displayed for continuous visual observation on an oscilloscope.
2. Use Swan–Ganz catheter (p. 268) to monitor pulmonary capillary wedge pressure, mixed venous PO_2, and cardiac output.	2. Intermittent and continuous positive pressure ventilation may reduce left ventricular function and cardiac output, which are reflected by a decrease in mixed venous PO_2 and wedge pressure.
Sedation and Muscle Relaxants 1. Administer morphine and curare, etc., as directed.	1. Sedatives and muscle relaxants eliminate spontaneous breathing efforts between ventilator cycles and reduce oxygen consumption. Morphine and curare (or similar drugs) produce vasodilation. Measure arterial blood pressure before their administration to detect hypotension.
2. Explain procedures to patient and provide reassurance.	2. The patient may be awake although not capable of any motor response while these drugs are being given.
Fluid Balance 1. Record intake and output precisely and obtain an accurate daily weight.	1. Positive fluid balance resulting in increase in body weight and interstitial pulmonary edema is a frequent problem in patients requiring mechanical ventilation. Prevention requires early recognition of fluid accumulation. Average adult who is dependent on parenteral nutrition can be expected to lose 0.25 kg. (½ lb.)/day; therefore, *constant body weight indicates positive fluid balance.*
Nutrition 1. Offer patient oral fluids and food if he is able to swallow. If aspiration occurs, stop the feeding and place patient in a semiprone position with head down; tilt and institute chest physical therapy to remove aspirated material. a. Start nasogastric feeding if oral intake is not adequate (p. 404).	1. Starvation is a frequent and serious complication of patients in respiratory failure.
Abdominal Complications 1. Test all stools and gastric drainage for occult blood.	1. About ¼ of patients requiring mechanical ventilation develop gastrointestinal bleeding; many of these patients require blood transfusions.
2. Measure abdominal girth daily.	2. Abdominal distention occurs frequently with respiratory failure and further hinders respiration by elevation of the diaphragm. Measurement of abdominal girth provides objective assessment of the degree of distention.
Communication 1. Provide writing paper and pad. A patient on mechanical ventilation with tracheostomy tube is unable to talk. 2. Establish some form of nonverbal communication if patient is too sick to write. Give patient the call light. 3. Reassure patient and family that normal speech will return upon removal of tracheal tube. 4. Ensure that the patient has adequate rest and sleep. 5. Keep the patient in touch with reality; explain that mechanical ventilation is only temporary.	
Recording 1. Maintain a flow sheet to record ventilation patterns, arterial blood studies, venous chemical determinations, hematocrit, status of fluid balance, weight, and assessment of patient's condition.	

GUIDELINES: Weaning the Patient from the Mechanical Ventilator

Weaning—the process by which the patient is gradually allowed to resume the responsibility for regulating his own breathing.

Weaning Modalities

A. *Intermittent Mandatory Ventilation (IMV)*

A process in which the rate of ventilator-delivered breaths/minute decreases. The patient is allowed to breathe spontaneously from a reservoir in line with the ventilator circuit between machine-controlled breaths.

NURSING ACTION	RATIONALE/AMPLIFICATION
1. Install IMV setup in ventilator circuit.	1. Explain procedure to patient.
2. Set ventilator to control mode.	2. This is done to assure that the patient's tidal volume will be the result of his inspiratory effort instead of simply initiating a machine-delivered breath.
3. Set IMV interval.	3. This determines the time period between machine-delivered breaths during which the patient will breathe on his own from the reservoir bag.
4. Observe reservoir bag.	4. The gas flow rate into the bag must be adequate to prevent the patient from collapsing it during inspiration. Flow rates of 4–6 liters per minute are usually adequate.
5. Stay with patient.	5. Constant reassurance, especially during initial weaning stages, is crucial.
6. Observe respiratory rate and pulse rate.	6. Dramatic increases in either respiration or pulse could indicate that the patient is not yet ready for weaning.
7. Obtain arterial blood gas analysis.	7. Blood gas analysis, especially the parameters of carbon dioxide and oxygen, are direct indicators of the ability of the patient to adequately ventilate himself. A dramatic rise in carbon dioxide levels indicates inadequate ventilation.
8. If step 7 results in adequate blood gases, then the IMV interval may be gradually increased and F_1O_2 levels may be decreased until the patient no longer needs any ventilator support.	8. With each increase of IMV interval or decrease in F_1O_2, blood gases should be obtained.

B. *Intermittent Demand Ventilation (IDV)*

Differs from IMV in that the patient must trigger the machine-assisted breaths.

C. *Synchronized Intermittent Mandatory Ventilation (SIMV)*

Differs from IMV in that the machine-controlled breaths are synchronized to augment the patient's spontaneous breaths.

NURSING ACTION	RATIONALE/AMPLIFICATION
1. Same principles apply in IDV and SIMV as in IMV but operation is simpler.	1. Breathing circuit is part of ventilator and not external reservoir.
2. For IDV, follow instructions supplied with ventilator and IDV timer.	2. Precise mode operation varies with different manufacturers and/or models.
3. For SIMV, set ventilator to SIMV mode and desired ventilator rate.	3. On many newer ventilators SIMV is simply another mode and therefore easiest to initiate.

D. *Briggs Adapter (T-Tube)*

This system provides oxygen enrichment and humidification to a patient with an endotracheal or tracheostomy tube while allowing completely spontaneous respiration (see Fig. 7-24). For further amplification see Oxygen Therapy Section.

NURSING ACTION	RATIONALE/AMPLIFICATION
1. Explain the procedure to patient.	
2. Install the equipment.	2. Oxygen levels are usually those used during IMV.
3. Observe patient closely.	3. Dramatic increases in pulse and respiratory rate may indicate the patient is not ready for this stage of weaning.
4. Obtain arterial blood gases in 30–60 minutes.	4. Same as #7 under IMV.
5. If step 4 above produces adequate blood gases the oxygen levels may be gradually decreased until the patient is breathing room air.	5. Repeat blood gas analysis after each change.

NOTE: It is not within the scope of this book to establish criteria for the use of one weaning modality as opposed to another.

GUIDELINES: Weaning the Patient from the Mechanical Ventilator (cont.)

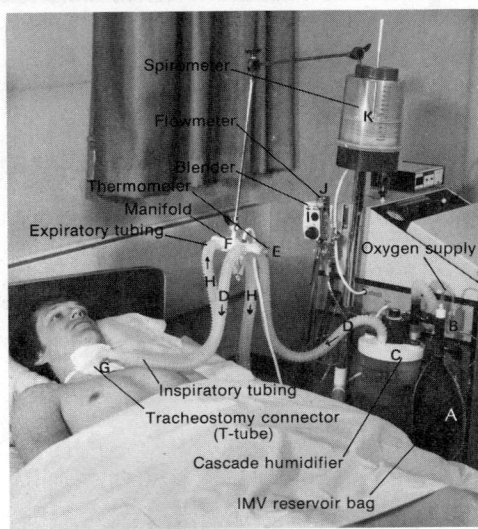

FIGURE 7-24. *Mechanical ventilation with IMV modality. Detail of T-tube.*

Stages of Weaning

A. *Preweaning Assessment*

1. Tidal volume—about 300–400 ml.
2. Forced vital capacity
   It is desirable to have an FVC of 1 liter or 2 times tidal volume.
3. Inspiratory effort
   a. This measures the ability of the respiratory muscles to develop subatmospheric pressure within the respiratory system.
   b. 20 cm. H_2O is generally deemed adequate.
4. Respiratory drive
   Patient must be breathing spontaneously.
5. Blood gas analysis
   a. Patient should be close to what is for him a "normal" acid-base state.
   b. Arterial CO_2 levels should also be close to "normal" for the patient.

NOTE: Steady-state values for a young, healthy adult are not the same as those of a 75-year-old person with severe COPD.
   c. Failure to adhere to guidelines a and b, above, may result in rapid alterations of pH and unsuccessful weaning attempts.

B. *Weaning from Mechanical Ventilator*

1. IMV (see p. 197), IDV, SIMV
2. T-tube (see p. 197)

C. *Weaning from Tracheostomy or Endotracheal Tube*

1. The patient must be able to maintain adequate blood gases when breathing spontaneously.
2. Sit patient upright and deflate tracheostomy or endotracheal cuff.
3. Test patient's ability to swallow without aspiration before cuff is deflated.
   a. Clear trachea, nasopharynx, and oropharynx of secretions.
   b. Deflate the cuff.
   c. Have the patient drink dilute methylene blue solution.
   d. Aspirate the trachea immediately; absence of blue dye in tracheal aspirate indicates the ability to swallow without aspiration.

D. *Weaning from the Tracheostomy Stoma*

1. A fenestrated tracheostomy tube (uncuffed tube with window in greater curvature to decrease resistance to air flow) may be used after mechanical ventilator has been discontinued.
2. Plug the external orifice of fenestrated tracheostomy tube.
   a. Evaluate the patient's ability to breathe spontaneously for long periods.
   b. Assess ability to cough and mobilize secretions without aid of tracheal aspiration.
   c. Have the patient drink dilute methylene blue solution.
   d. Aspirate the trachea immediately; absence of blue dye in tracheal aspirate indicates the ability to swallow without aspiration.

3. The tube is usually removed when tracheal aspiration has been unnecessary for 24 hours.
4. Cover the stoma with a sterile dressing; stoma is allowed to close.
E. *Weaning from Supplementary Inspired Oxygen*
   Supplementary inspired oxygen may be required for an additional period until patient can maintain adequate O_2 and CO_2 tensions while breathing room air.

Patient Education for Prevention of Recurrences of Respiratory Failure

Instruct the patient as follows:
1. Avoid and treat respiratory infections promptly.
2. Avoid respiratory irritants, particularly smoking.
3. Take oral and nebulized bronchodilators on prescribed basis.
4. Ensure adequate hydration.
5. Carry out a program of gradually increasing exercise tolerance.

CLINICAL CONDITIONS

THE PNEUMONIAS

Pneumonia is an infection of the lung parenchyma. (See Table 7–3, pages 200–201.)

Mode of Transmission

May be spread by droplets coughed up by infected patients or carriers; more often pneumonia arises from aspiration of endogenous flora by patients whose resistance has been lowered.

Causes

1. Lowered resistance of host
2. Upper respiratory infection, influenza
3. Excessive intake of alcohol—alcohol suppresses macrophage function and white cell mobilization
4. Depression of central nervous system (drugs, head injury, etc.)
5. Cardiac failure
6. Chronic illness (diabetes)
7. Superinfection in hospitalized patients; contaminated equipment
8. Any bronchial obstruction (chronic obstructive pulmonary disease, cancer, asthma, etc.) associated with mucus formation and impaired clearance of bacteria from lungs
9. Prolonged immobilization of patients

Unique Characteristics of Pneumonia

1. Pathogens producing pneumonia may be carried in nasopharynx of a healthy person.
2. Pathogens may invade tissues when the host's natural resistance is lowered.
3. Colds and upper respiratory tract infections lead to more serious illnesses by allowing bacterial invasion of lower respiratory tract.
4. A wide variety of pulmonary infections may develop in patients receiving corticosteroids or other immunosuppressive drugs (aerobic and anaerobic gram-negative bacilli, *Staphylococcus, Nocardia,* fungi, *Candida,* viruses [including cytomegalovirus], *Pneumocystis carinii,* reactivation of tuberculosis, and others).
5. Patients on high dosages of corticosteroids have a reduced resistance to infections.
6. Any condition interfering with normal drainage of the lung will predispose the person to pneumonia (e.g., cancer of the lung).
7. Postoperative patients may develop bronchopneumonia, since anesthesia impairs respiratory defenses and decreases diaphragmatic movement.
8. Persons over 50 have a higher fatality rate even with appropriate antimicrobial therapy.

> **NURSING ALERT:** Recurring pneumonia often indicates underlying disease (cancer of the lung, multiple myeloma).

Health Maintenance and Preventive Measures

1. Natural resistance should be maintained (adequate nutrition, rest, exercise).
2. Avoid contact with people who have upper respiratory infections.
3. Obliteration of cough reflex and aspiration of secretions should be avoided.
4. Adequate bronchial hygiene should be employed.
5. Immobilized patients should be turned every 2 hours and encouraged to breathe deeply, sigh, and cough.
6. Use every measure to reduce bacterial colonization and superinfection of hospitalized patient.
7. Highly susceptible persons (elderly and chronically ill) should be immunized against influenza.
8. Pneumococcal vaccine should be given to those at greatest risk—persons over 50 with chronic systemic diseases, COPD, sickle cell anemia, absence of spleen, immunosuppression patients who have had a pneumonectomy.

Clinical Manifestations

See Table 7–3, pages 200–201.

Diagnostic Evaluation

1. Chest auscultation and percussion—listen for dullness to percussion, bronchial breath sounds, crackles
2. Lateral and posteroanterior chest x-rays—to localize the process and determine presence or absence of fluid
3. Gram stain, culture, and sensitivity studies of sputum
4. Blood culture—to recover causative organism; blood

TABLE 7-3. COMMONLY ENCOUNTERED PNEUMONIAS

Type	Organism Responsible	Manifestations
Pneumococcal pneumonia	*Streptococcus pneumoniae*	May be history of previous respiratory infection Sudden onset, with shaking and chills Rapidly rising fever Cough, with expectoration of rusty or green (purulent) sputum Pleuritic pain aggravated by cough Chest dull to percussion; rales, bronchial breath sounds Confusion may be only presenting feature in the elderly
Staphylococcal pneumonia	*Staphylococcus aureus*	Often prior history of viral infection Insidious development of cough, with expectoration of yellow, blood-streaked mucus Onset may be sudden if patient is outside hospital Fever Pleuritic chest pain Pulse varies; may be slow in proportion to temperature
Klebsiella pneumonia	*Klebsiella pneumoniae* (Friedländer's bacillus—encapsulated gram-negative aerobic bacillus)	Onset sudden with high fever, chills, pleuritic pain, hemoptysis Dyspnea, cyanosis Dark brown-red gelatinous sputum expectorated Profound prostration and toxicity
Pseudomonas pneumonia	*Pseudomonas aeruginosa*	Apprehension, confusion, cyanosis, bradycardia, reversal of diurnal temperature curve
Legionnaires' disease	*Legionella pneumophila*	Prodromal period of abdominal pain and diarrhea High fever, chills, cough (dry or productive) Tachypnea; tachycardia
Mycoplasmal pneumonia (Atypical pneumonia)	*Mycoplasma pneumoniae*	Gradual onset, headache, irritating hacking cough productive of scanty, mucoid sputum Anorexia; malaise Fever, nasal congestion, sore throat
Viral pneumonia	Influenza viruses Parainfluenza viruses Respiratory syncytial viruses Adenovirus Varicella, rubella, rubeola, herpes simplex, cytomegalovirus, Epstein-Barr virus	Cough Constitutional symptoms may be pronounced (severe headache, anorexia, fever, and myalgia)
Pneumocystis carinii pneumonia (Interstitial plasma cell pneumonia)	*Pneumocystis carinii*	Insidious onset Increasing dyspnea and nonproductive cough Tachypnea; progresses rapidly to intercostal retraction, nasal flaring, and cyanosis Lowering of arterial oxygen tension Chest x-ray will reveal diffuse, bilateral interstitial pneumonia
Fungal pneumonia	*Aspergillus fumigatus*	Hectic fever, productive cough, chest pain, hemoptysis Chest x-ray reveals broad range of abnormalities from infiltration to consolidation, cavitation, and empyema

stream invasion (bacteremia) occurs frequently with bacterial pneumonia
5. Thoracentesis—if pleural effusion is present
6. Testing for cold agglutinin antibody titer—persons with *Mycoplasma pneumoniae* pneumonia will have elevated titer
7. Other serologic tests for *Legionella pneumophila*, psittacosis, etc.

Objectives of Treatment and Nursing Management

For patient with bacterial pneumonia

A. *To take a careful history to help establish etiologic diagnosis.*
1. What was the mode of onset?
2. Number and frequency and duration of chills
3. Description of chest pain

TABLE 7-3. COMMONLY ENCOUNTERED PNEUMONIAS (continued)

Clinical Features	Treatment	Complications
Herpes simplex lesions often present Usually involves one or more lobes	Penicillin G Alternate drug therapy in penicillin-allergic patient (erythromycin, or a cephalosporin)	Shock Pleural effusion Superinfections Pericarditis
Frequently seen in hospital setting Staphylococcal pneumonia is a necrotizing infection Treatment must be vigorous and prolonged due to disease's tendency to destroy the lungs Organism may develop rapid lung resistance Prolonged convalescence usual	Methicillin, nafcillin, clindamycin, cephalothin, vancomycin	Effusion/pneumothorax Lung abscess Empyema Meningitis
Tends to attack chronically ill, debilitated, alcoholic and elderly men or those with chronic obstructive pulmonary disease Tissue necrosis occurs rapidly in lungs May be rapidly fulminating, progressing to fatal outcome High mortality rate	Gentamicin, kanamycin, cephalosporins, chloramphenicol, polymyxin B, or colistin	Multiple lung abscesses with cyst formation Persistent cough with expectoration remains for prolonged period Empyema Pericarditis
Susceptible persons: those with preexisting lung disease, cancer (particularly leukemia); those with homograft transplants, burns; debilitated persons; patients receiving prolonged courses of antibiotics, endotracheal intubation, IPPB	Aminoglycoside antibiotics (gentamicin, tobramycin, amikacin)	Multiple lung abscess formation High fatality rate
Peak incidence in persons over 50 who are cigarette smokers and have underlying diseases that increase susceptibility to infection. Patients acutely ill High mortality rate in patients with respiratory failure	Erythromycin	Respiratory failure
Occurs most commonly in children and young adults Cold agglutinin antibody titer elevated in mycoplasmal complement fixation test	Erythromycin; tetracycline	Meningoencephalitis Polyneuritis Monoarticular arthritis Pericarditis; myocarditis
In majority of patients influenza begins as an acute coryza; others have bronchitis, pleurisy, etc., while still others develop gastrointestinal symptoms Risk of developing influenza related to crowding and close contact of groups of individuals	Treat symptomatically Does not respond to treatment with presently available antimicrobials Prophylactic vaccination recommended for high risk persons (over 65; chronic cardiac or pulmonary disease, diabetes and other metabolic disorders)	May develop a superimposed bacterial infection Bronchopneumonia Pericarditis; endocarditis
Usually seen in host whose resistance is compromised Organism invades lungs of patients who have suppressed immune system (from cancer, leukemia) or following immunosuppressive therapy for cancer, organ transplant, or collagen disease Frequently associated with concurrent infection by viruses, (cytomegalovirus) bacteria, and fungi	Combination of trimethoprim and sulfamethoxazole	Patients are critically ill Prognosis is guarded as it usually is a complication of severe underlying disorder
Neutropenic individual most susceptible May develop *Asperigillus* as superinfection	Amphotericin B	High fatality rate Invades blood vessels and destroys lung tissue by direct invasion and vascular infarction

4. Patient taking any recent antimicrobial drugs?
5. Any family illness?
6. Alcohol, tobacco, drug abuse?

B. *To identify the etiologic agent causing the pneumonia and to determine the drug sensitivity.*

1. Obtain freshly expectorated sputum for direct smear (gram stain) and culture.
2. Be sure patient *coughs* up sputum, not saliva.
3. Instruct patient to expectorate into sterile container for culture.
4. Utilize percussion (p. 165) with or without IPPB treatment as directed; tenacious sputum may be liquefied by inhaling nebulized aerosol of water or saline solution by mask.
5. Aspirate trachea with catheter if patient is too ill to raise sputum. (See Guidelines, p. 167.)

6. Sputum may also be collected by transtracheal aspiration (p. 159).

C. *To give prescribed antimicrobial agent*—the therapy of pneumonia depends on laboratory identification of the agent causing the infection and on the drainage of purulent secretions.

D. *To listen for crackles, rales, signs of consolidation or pleural effusion.*

E. *To clear the bronchi of collected secretions*—retained secretions interfere with gas exchange and may cause slow resolution (subsidence).

1. Encourage high level of fluid intake within limits of patient's cardiac reserve—adequate hydration thins mucus and serves as an effective expectorant; replaces fluid losses due to fever, diaphoresis, dehydration, and dyspnea.
2. Humidify air to loosen secretions and improve ventilation.
3. Encourage patient to cough; avoid suppressing the cough reflex, especially in patients who sound "bubbly."
4. Employ chest wall percussion (p. 165) and postural drainage (p. 164) to mobilize secretions.
5. Utilize tracheal aspiration in patients with poor cough response.
6. Assist in bronchoscopic removal of inspissated (thickened) mucus plugs if patient is too weak to cough effectively.
7. Control cough when coughing is non-productive and paroxysms cause serious hypoxemia; give moderate doses of codeine as prescribed.
8. Avoid hypoxemia especially in patients with existing heart disease.

F. *To observe the patient carefully and continuously until clinical condition improves.*

1. Remember that fatal complications may develop during the early period of antimicrobial treatment.
2. Monitor temperature, pulse, respiration, and blood pressure at regular intervals to assess patient's response to therapy.
3. Listen to lungs and heart—heart murmurs or friction rub may indicate acute bacterial endocarditis, pericarditis, or myocarditis.
4. Assess for resistant fever or return of fever from:
   a. Drug allergy. Usually skin eruptions appear 7–10 days after the beginning of treatment.
   b. Drug resistance or slow response to therapy.
   c. Inadequate or inappropriate antimicrobial therapy.
   d. Inadequate lung drainage.
   e. Superinfection (infection with a second organism resistant to antibiotics used).
   f. Failure of pneumonia to resolve; raises suspicion of underlying carcinoma of bronchus.
   g. Pneumonia caused by unusual bacteria, fungi, tuberculosis, or *Pneumocystis carinii*.
5. Obtain chest x-rays to follow resolution (subsidence) of pneumonic process.

G. *To utilize supportive modalities of treatment.*

1. Do blood gas analysis to determine oxygen need, give precise oxygen guidance and evaluate oxygen effectiveness.
   An arterial oxygen tension (PO_2) below 55 mm.Hg indicates hypoxemia.
2. Administer oxygen at concentration to maintain PO_2 at acceptable level.

3. Avoid high concentrations of oxygen in patients with chronic obstructive pulmonary disease (chronic bronchitis, emphysema)—*the use of high oxygen concentrations may worsen alveolar ventilation by removing patient's only remaining ventilatory drive.*
4. Observe patient for cyanosis, dyspnea, hypoxemia.
5. Patients with pneumonia and coexisting chronic ventilatory insufficiency may require mechanical ventilation.
6. Relieve the pleuritic pain.
   a. Avoid suppressing a productive cough.
   b. Avoid narcotics in patient with history of COPD.
   c. Administer moderate doses of analgesics to relieve pleuritic pain.
   d. Treat dry cough and laryngospasm with aerosolized water produced by an ultrasonic nebulizer.
   e. Evaluate patient's sensorium before administering sedatives or tranquilizers to assess for signs and symptoms suggestive of meningitis.

NURSING ALERT: Restlessness, confusion, aggressiveness may be due to cerebral hypoxia. In such instances sedatives are inappropriate.

7. Maintain adequate hydration since fluid loss is high from fever, dehydration, dyspnea, and diaphoresis.
8. Encourage modified bed rest during febrile period.
9. Treat abdominal distention which may be due to swallowing of air during intervals of severe dyspnea.
   a. Pass nasogastric tube for acute gastric distention.
   b. Use a rectal tube and give neostigmine methylsulfate to facilitate intestinal decompression.

H. *To observe for complications.*

1. Patients should respond to treatment within 24–48 hours. However, be on the alert for complications such as the following:
   a. Pleural effusion
   b. Sustained hypotension and shock, especially in gram-negative bacterial disease, particularly in the elderly
   c. Delayed resolution
   d. Superinfection: pericarditis, bacteremia, meningitis
   e. Atelectasis—from obstruction of bronchus by accumulated secretions; may occur at any stage of acute pneumonia.
   f. Delirium—*this is considered a medical emergency*
   g. Congestive heart failure, cardiac arrhythmias, pericarditis, myocarditis
   h. Peripheral thrombophlebitis, with or without pulmonary emboli
   i. Acute respiratory insufficiency
2. Employ special nursing surveillance for patients with the following conditions:
   a. Alcoholism or chronic obstructive pulmonary disease; these persons as well as elderly patients may have little or no fever.
   b. Chronic bronchitis. It is difficult to detect subtle changes in condition, since patient may have seriously compromised pulmonary function.
   c. Epilepsy; pneumonia may result from aspiration following a seizure.
   d. Delirium, which may be caused by hypoxia, meningitis, delirium tremens of alcoholism.

(1) Prepare for lumbar puncture; meningitis may be lethal.
(2) Assure adequate hydration and give mild sedation.
(3) Give oxygen.
(4) Delirium must be controlled to prevent exhaustion and cardiac failure.
3. Assess these patients for *unusual behavior*, alterations in mental status, stupor, and congestive heart failure.

Discharge Planning and Health Education

1. Fatigue, weakness, and depression may be prolonged after pneumonia.
2. Encourage chair rest after fever subsides; gradually increase activities to bring energy level back to pre-illness stage.
3. Encourage breathing exercises (p. 166) to clear lungs and promote full expansion and function after the fever subsides.
4. Explain that a chest x-ray is taken 2–4 weeks after discharge; should show cleared lungs.
5. It is wise to stop smoking. Cigarette smoking destroys tracheobronchial cilial action, which is first line of defense of lungs; also irritates mucosa of bronchi and inhibits function of alveolar scavenger cells (macrophages).
6. Advise patient to keep up natural resistance with good nutrition, adequate rest—one episode of pneumonia may make the individual susceptible to recurring respiratory infections.
7. Instruct patient to avoid fatigue, sudden changes in temperature, and excessive alcohol intake, which lower resistance to pneumonia.
8. Encourage patient to obtain influenza vaccine at prescribed times. Influenza increases susceptibility to secondary bacterial pneumonia.
9. Encourage patient to seek medical advice about receiving vaccine against *Streptococcus pneumoniae*, which is effective against the majority of bacteremic pneumococcal diseases.

ASPIRATION PNEUMONIA

Aspiration is the inhalation of oropharyngeal secretions and/or stomach contents into the lungs. It may produce an acute form of pneumonia.

Etiology

Patients at risk and factors associated with risk:
1. Loss of protective airway reflexes—swallowing, laryngeal, cough
   a. Altered state of consciousness (general anesthesia, head injury, stroke, coma, convulsions)
   b. Alcohol; drug overdose
   c. During resuscitation procedures
   d. Seriously ill, debilitated patients
2. Nasogastric tube feedings
3. Obstetrical patients—from general anesthesia, lithotomy position, delayed emptying of stomach from enlarged uterus, labor contractions
4. Esophageal disease—hiatal hernia
5. Delayed emptying time of stomach—intestinal obstruction, abdominal distention
6. Prolonged endotracheal intubation/tracheostomy—can depress glottic and laryngeal reflexes from disuse

Clinical Manifestations

1. Depends on volume and character of aspirated contents
   a. Food particles—mechanical blockage of airways and secondary infection
   b. Pathogenic bacteria—from oropharyngeal secretions containing bacteria
   c. Gastric juice—destructive to alveoli and capillaries; results in outpouring of protein-rich fluids into the interstitial and intra-alveolar spaces—impairs exchange of oxygen and carbon dioxide producing hypoxemia, respiratory insufficiency and failure
   d. Fecal contamination—endotoxins may be absorbed or thick proteinaceous material found in the intestinal contents may obstruct airway, leading to atelectasis and secondary bacterial infection
2. Tachycardia/tachypnea
3. Dyspnea and cough
4. Cyanosis
5. Rales, rhonchi, wheezing
6. Pink, frothy sputum (may simulate acute pulmonary edema)
7. Fever

Prevention

1. Be on guard constantly and monitor patients at risk as described above.
2. Elevate head of bed for debilitated patients, for those receiving tube feedings, and for those with motor diseases of the esophagus.
3. Place patients with impaired reflexes in a lateral position.
4. Be sure that nasogastric tube is patent.
5. Give tube feedings slowly with patient sitting up in bed. See page 404.
   a. Check position of tube in stomach before feeding.
   b. Check seal of cuff of tracheostomy or endotracheal tube before feeding.
6. Keep patients in a fasting state before anesthesia (at least 8 hours).
7. Place comatose patient on his side and elevate the foot of the bed 15–23 cm. (6–9 inches) unless medically contraindicated.

NURSING ALERT: The morbidity and mortality rate of aspiration pneumonia remains high even with optimum treatment. Prevention is the key to the problem.

Management

OBJECTIVE: to remove the factor(s) interfering with adequate gas exchange.
1. Clear the obstructed airway.
   a. If foreign body becomes lodged in throat, perform the Heimlich maneuver (p. 869) or remove object with forceps.
   b. Place patient in tilted head-down position on right side (right side more frequently affected if patient has aspirated solid particles).
   c. Suction trachea/endotracheal tube—to remove any particulate matter.
   d. Prepare for laryngoscopy/bronchoscopy if patient is asphyxiated by solid material.
2. Correct hypoxia by immediate ventilation.
   a. Give oxygen.
   b. Place patient on assisted ventilation—if adequate

PO_2 cannot be maintained with other means of administering oxygen. (See p. 194.)
   c. Give IV aminophylline or bronchodilators by nebulizer—to help relieve bronchospasm.
3. Correct hypotension (usually the result of hypovolemia and hypoxia) by fluid volume replacement.
4. Give supportive therapy as indicated.
   a. Corticosteroids (value uncertain; must be given immediately and in large doses)—may modify capillary permeability.
   b. Antimicrobials—if there is evidence of superimposed bacterial infection.
   c. Correct acidosis—respiratory acidosis and metabolic acidosis indicate a severe reaction due to aspiration of gastric contents
   d. Monitor arterial blood gases

PLEURISY

Pleurisy is a clinical term to describe *pleuritis*, (inflammation of the pleura).

Fibrinous pleurisy is deposition of a fibrinous exudate on the pleural surface.

Causes

May occur in the course of many pulmonary diseases:
1. Pneumonia (bacterial, viral)
2. Tuberculosis
3. Pulmonary infarction, embolism
4. Pulmonary abscess
5. Upper respiratory tract infection
6. Pulmonary neoplasm

Clinical Manifestations

1. Chest pain—becomes severe, sharp, and knife-like upon inspiration (pleuritic pain).
   a. Pain may become minimal or absent when breath is held.
   b. Pain may be localized or radiate to shoulder or abdomen.
2. Intercostal tenderness.
3. Pleural friction rub—grating or leathery sounds heard in both phases of respiration; heard low in the axilla or over the lung base posteriorly; may be heard only a day or so.
4. Evidence of infection; fever, malaise, increased white cell count.

Diagnostic Evaluation

1. Chest x-ray
2. Sputum examination
3. Examination of pleural fluid obtained by thoracentesis for smear and culture
4. Pleural biopsy (selected patients)

Treatment and Nursing Management

OBJECTIVE: to discover underlying condition.
1. Treat the underlying primary disease (pneumonia, infarction, etc.). Inflammation usually resolves when the primary disease subsides.
2. Relieve the pain.
   a. Give prescribed analgesics.
   b. Splint the rib cage (Fig. 7-26, p. 223) when the patient coughs.
   c. Apply heat or cold—to provide symptomatic relief.

   d. Instruct patient to lie on affected side occasionally—to splint chest wall.
   e. Assist with procaine intercostal block.
3. Watch for signs of development of pleural effusion (collection of fluid in pleural space): shortness of breath, pain, local decreased excursion of chest wall.

PLEURAL EFFUSION

Pleural effusion refers to a collection of fluid in the pleural space. It is rarely a primary disease, but is usually secondary to other diseases.

Etiology

Complication of:
1. Disseminated cancer (particularly lung and breast); lymphoma
2. Infection: tuberculosis, bacterial pneumonia, pulmonary infection
3. Congestive heart failure
4. Cirrhosis
5. Kidney disease
6. Others: Sarcoidosis, myxedema, peritoneal dialysis, etc.

Clinical Manifestations

1. Increasing dyspnea
2. Dullness or flatness to percussion (over areas of fluid) with minimal or absent breath sounds

Diagnostic Evaluation

1. Chest x-ray
2. Thoracentesis—biochemical, bacteriologic, and cytologic studies of pleural fluid
3. Physical examination
4. Pleuroscopy (visual exploration of pleural space through a thoracoscope inserted into the pleural space).

Treatment and Nursing Management

OBJECTIVES: to determine the cause.
   to remove fluid in order to relieve discomfort and dyspnea.
   to prevent fluid collection from recurring.
1. The treatment depends on the cause. Give specific treatment related to the underlying disease.
2. The following modalities of treatment have been advocated for malignant effusions.
   a. Thoracentesis (aspiration) for fluid removal and relief of dyspnea
      (1) In malignant diseases, thoracentesis may provide only transient benefits since effusion may return within a few days.
   b. Tube drainage (chest catheter) connected to underwater seal drainage system or suction; instillation into pleural space of cytotoxic or other chemical sclerosing agents.
      (1) Chest catheter helps to evacuate pleural space and re-expand lung.
      (2) Drug is introduced into catheter; tube is clamped; patient is helped to assume the following positions for at least 1 minute each to ensure uniform distribution of the drug and maximize drug contact with pleural surfaces: prone, left side down, supine, right side down, knee to chest (if able).
      (3) Tube is unclamped as prescribed.

(4) Nitrogen mustard may require aspiration within six hours—causes inflammatory reaction; may cause a systemic reaction (nausea, vomiting, etc.).

(5) Chest drainage continued several days longer.

c. Radiation of chest wall.

d. Surgical procedures to control malignant effusions—parietal pleurectomy; pleural abrasion.

LUNG ABSCESS

A *lung abscess* is a localized, pus-containing, necrotic lesion in the lung characterized by cavity formation.

Etiology

1. Aspiration of vomitus or infected material from upper respiratory tract
2. Aspiration of foreign body into lung
3. Bronchial obstruction (usually a tumor causes obstruction to the bronchus, causing distal stasis and infection of secretions, or there is necrosis within the tumor mass).
4. Necrotizing pneumonias
5. Tuberculosis
6. Pulmonary embolism

Clinical Features

1. The right lung is involved more frequently than the left—owing to dependent position of the right bronchus, the less acute angle which the right main bronchus forms within the trachea, and its larger size.
2. In the initial stages, the cavity in the lung may or may not communicate with the bronchus.
3. Eventually the cavity becomes surrounded or encapsulated by a wall of fibrous tissue, except at 1 or 2 points where the necrotic process extends until it reaches the lumen of some bronchus or pleural space and establishes a communication with the respiratory tract, the pleural cavity (bronchopleural fistula), or both.

Clinical Manifestations

1. Cough
2. Fever and malaise—from segmental pneumonitis and atelectasis
3. Headache, anemia, weight loss
4. Pleuritic chest pain—from extension of suppurative pneumonitis to pleural surface
5. Production of sputum—foul, yellow, green mucopurulent material which becomes profuse after abscess ruptures into bronchial tree
6. Clubbing of fingers and toes—may signify underlying bronchogenic carcinoma

Diagnostic Evaluation

1. History of patient
2. X-ray of chest—for diagnosis and location of lesion
3. Direct bronchoscopic visualization—to exclude possibility of tumor or foreign body; bronchial washings and brush biopsy may be done for cytopathologic study
4. Bronchogram—may be necessary to differentiate between lung abscess and bronchiectasis
5. Leukocytosis in acute stage
6. Sputum culture and sensitivity—to determine causative organism(s) and antimicrobial sensitivity

7. Dullness and bronchial breath sounds—may be heard over diseased segment

Management

OBJECTIVES: to establish adequate drainage.
to eradicate the infection.

1. Carry out drainage procedures.
   a. Postural drainage (hastens resolution)—positions to be assumed depend on the segmental localization of the abscess. (See p. 164.)
   b. Therapeutic bronchoscopy—to drain abscess.
2. Give appropriate antimicrobial based upon culture and sensitivity studies of organisms—mixed infections are common and may require multiple antibiotics.
3. Measure and record the volume of sputum—to follow the course of healing.
4. Utilize supportive measures during the acute phase of illness.
   a. Give a high protein, high calorie diet—chronic infections are associated with catabolic state, which requires calories and protein to facilitate healing.
   b. Care of the patient having blood transfusions—anemia may be advanced in patient with infection.
5. Prepare patient for serial radiographs—to judge effectiveness of therapy.
6. Prepare for surgical intervention if indicated—done only if patient fails to respond to adequate medical treatment.
   a. Excision—usually lobectomy (occasionally segmental resection); done because infiltrative pneumonitis surrounding the lung abscess pocket usually extends beyond the segmental confines of the lung.
   b. Thoracotomy tube drainage—usually done for patients who cannot tolerate major thoracotomy (elderly patients, alcoholics, patients with low pulmonary functional reserve).
   c. See page 220 for care of the patient having thoracic surgery.

Discharge Planning and Health Education

1. Encourage the patient to have patience—it may take 10 days to several months for the chest x-ray to be clear and for the cavity to close.
2. Encourage patient to assume responsibility for attaining and maintaining an optimum state of health through a planned program of good nutrition, rest, and exercise.

BRONCHIECTASIS

Bronchiectasis is a chronic dilatation of the bronchi and bronchioles due to inflammation and destruction of their walls.

Causes

1. Pulmonary infections and obstruction of bronchi
2. Aspiration of foreign bodies, vomitus, or material from upper respiratory tract
3. Extrinsic pressure from tumors, dilated blood vessels, enlarged lymph nodes

Altered Physiology

Impairment of bronchial clearance → increased bronchial secretions → stasis → infection → weakening and further destruction of bronchial walls → increased dilatation → atelectasis → inflammatory scarring → fibrosis of involved areas → respiratory insufficiency → ventilation and perfusion imbalance → hypoxemia.

Health Maintenance and Prevention

1. Treat all respiratory infections promptly.
2. Teach family to seek medical treatment and ongoing surveillance if child has recurrent respiratory infections; more than half the cases start in childhood.
3. All stuporous or comatose patients should be turned (prone position to lateral)—to drain all bronchial segments.
4. Encourage individual immunization program to prevent pertussis and measles (which can lead to bronchiectasis).

Clinical Manifestations

The patient experiences symptoms when he has superimposed infection.
1. Persistent and/or productive cough with mucopurulent sputum
2. Hemoptysis
3. Recurrent fever and bouts of localized pulmonary infection/pneumonia
4. Crackles (rales) and rhonchi over involved areas
5. Dyspnea (depending upon amount of lung tissue involved)
6. Wheezing
7. Clubbing of fingers (long-standing disease)

Diagnostic Evaluation

1. Chest roentgenogram (may reveal areas of atelectasis with widespread dilatation of bronchi)
2. Bronchogram (to map the entire bronchial tree to determine the extent of bronchial dilation and disease).
3. Bronchoscopy—to rule out obstructive lesion
4. Sputum Examination

Management

OBJECTIVES: to prevent and control infection.
to rid the affected portion(s) of the lungs of excessive secretions.
to improve bronchial drainage.
1. Treat the patient during periods of acute infection.
   a. Employ judicious antimicrobial therapy guided by sensitivity studies upon organisms cultured from sputum.
   b. Patients with repeated infections may be given short courses of antimicrobials prophylactically during the winter months.
2. Empty the bronchi of their accumulated secretions.
   a. Use postural drainage suitable to segment(s) involved to drain the bronchiectatic areas by gravity, thus reducing degree of infection and amount of secretions (see p. 164).
      (1) Postural drainage should be done for 20 minutes twice daily or more frequently as clinical condition indicates.
      (2) Affected chest area may be percussed or "cupped" to assist in raising secretions (see p. 165).
   b. Encourage copious fluid intake to reduce viscosity of sputum and make expectoration easier.
   c. Utilize vaporizer to provide humidification and to keep secretions liquid.

d. Eliminate smoking and dusts, which are bronchial irritants that increase secretions.
   e. Give expectorants and bronchodilator drugs when indicated. (See treatment of patient with emphysema, p. 207.)
   f. Prepare patient for bronchoscopy when necessary to drain sputum and remove foreign body.
3. Employ surgical intervention when conservative treatment is inadequate.
   a. Segmental resection to spare as much healthy, functioning lung parenchyma as possible. (See p. 221 for principles of nursing following chest surgery.)
   b. Evaluate for postoperative complications.
      (1) Pneumonia
      (2) Empyema

Discharge Planning and Health Education

1. Instruct the patient to avoid noxious fumes, dusts, and other pulmonary irritants (cigarette smoking).
2. Teach patient to monitor sputum. Report to physician/clinic if change in quantity or character occurs.
3. Encourage regular dental care.
4. Instruct patient in postural drainage exercises. See pages 209–210 for other health teaching aspects (patient with emphysema).
5. Encourage patient to be immunized against influenza.

CHRONIC OBSTRUCTIVE PULMONARY DISEASE (COPD)

Chronic obstructive pulmonary disease (COPD) is a term that refers to a group of conditions associated with chronic obstruction of airflow entering or leaving the lungs.

COPD includes:
1. Bronchitis
2. Emphysema
3. Asthma (see p. 620)

Altered Physiology

1. Basically, the person with COPD has:
   a. Excessive secretion of mucus and chronic infection within the airways not due to specific causes (bronchitis)
   b. An increase in size of air spaces distal to the terminal bronchioles with loss of alveolar walls and elastic recoil of the lungs (emphysema)
   c. Narrowing of the bronchial airways that changes in severity (asthma, see page 620, since the triggering device in asthma is allergic in origin)
   d. There may be an overlap of these conditions.
2. As a result of these conditions there is a subsequent derangement of airway dynamics—e.g., obstruction to airflow.

Causes of COPD (Emphysema-Bronchitis Complex)

1. Cigarette smoking
2. Air pollution
3. Occupational exposure
4. Allergy
5. Autoimmunity
6. Infection
7. Genetic predisposition
8. Aging

CHRONIC BRONCHITIS

Chronic bronchitis is a chronic infection of the lower respiratory tract characterized by excessive mucus secretion, cough, and dyspnea associated with recurring infections of the lower respiratory tract. There is often reduced ability to ventilate the lungs.

Altered Physiology

Infection, irritation, hypersensitivity → local hyperemia → hypertrophy of mucous glands → increase in size and number of mucus-producing elements in bronchi (mucous glands and goblet cells) → inflammation and changes in bronchial and bronchiolar walls.

Health Maintenance and Prevention

1. Avoid respiratory irritants, particularly tobacco smoke; chronic bronchitis is most often a smoker's disease.
2. Persons who are prone to respiratory infections should be immunized against influenza and *Streptococcus pneumoniae*.
3. Acute respiratory infections should be treated.

Clinical Manifestations

Usually insidious, developing over a period of years
1. Persistent bouts of cough and sputum production
2. Recurrent acute respiratory infections followed by persistent cough
3. Production of thick, gelatinous sputum (greater amounts produced during superimposed infections)
4. Wheezing and dyspnea as disease progresses

Clinical Features

1. A wide range of viral, bacterial, and mycoplasmal infections can produce acute exacerbations of bronchitis.
2. Exacerbations of chronic bronchitis are most apt to occur during winter months—patients have bronchospasm due to inhalation of cold air.
3. Secretions must be expelled; otherwise they produce chronic bronchial obstruction, air trapping, hypoxemia, carbon dioxide retention, and localized infection.
4. Chronic bronchitis often progresses to emphysema.
5. Hypoxemia may lead to right ventricular failure (Cor pulmonale).

Diagnostic Evaluation

1. Chest roentgenogram—to exclude other diseases of the chest
2. Pulmonary function and arterial blood gas studies

Treatment and Nursing Management

OBJECTIVES: to maintain patency of peripheral bronchial tree.
    to facilitate removal of bronchial exudates.
    to prevent disability.
See below (emphysema) for treatment and health education.

PULMONARY EMPHYSEMA

Pulmonary emphysema is a complex lung disease characterized by destruction of the alveoli, enlargement of distal airspaces, and a breakdown of alveolar walls. There is a slowly progressive deterioration of lung function for many years before the development of illness.

Causes

(See Causes of Chronic Obstructive Pulmonary Disease, p. 206).

Clinical Manifestations

1. *Dyspnea;* slow in onset and steadily progressive
2. Cough—may be minimal except with respiratory infection
3. Weakness, lethargy, anorexia, weight loss—due to hypoxia, increased respiratory muscular effort, and respiratory acidosis.

Diagnostic Evaluation

1. Clinical assessment of patient
2. History of cough, exertional dyspnea, wheezing, smoking, exposure to dusts, fumes, gases
3. Pulmonary function tests
4. Chest roentgenogram—abnormal only in advanced disease
5. Arterial blood gas analysis (with exercise if possible) to detect hypoxemia
6. Alpha$_1$-Antitrypsin Assay—useful in identifying person at risk

Complications

1. Respiratory acidosis
2. Cor pulmonale
3. Congestive heart failure
4. Spontaneous pneumothorax
5. Overwhelming respiratory infections
6. Cardiac arrhythmias
7. Profound depression
8. Malnutrition

Objectives of Treatment and Nursing Management

OBJECTIVES: to improve the quality of life.
    to reduce progression of disease (when detected early).

A. *To remove bronchial secretions in order to improve pulmonary ventilation and gas exchange.*

1. *Eliminate all pulmonary irritants, particularly cigarette smoking.*
 a. Cessation of smoking usually results in decreased pulmonary irritation, sputum production, and cough.
 b. Avoid outside physical activities when air pollutants are high.
 c. Keep bedroom as dust-free as possible.
 d. Consider the use of air filters to remove particles and pollutants from air in areas where this is a problem.
 e. Use a room humidifier during winter months—allows dust particles to settle and makes air less irritating.
2. Control bronchospasm to decrease the work of breathing—many patients with chronic obstructive pulmonary disease have some degree of bronchospasm.
 a. Bronchospasm is detected by auscultation with a stethoscope.
 b. Administer prescribed bronchodilators, which dilate airways by relieving bronchial mucosal edema and smooth muscle contraction.
 (1) See page 171 for table of bronchodilators.

(2) Drugs may be administered orally, subcutaneously, intravenously, or rectally; or via nebulization (by pressurized aerosols, hand-held nebulizers, pump-driven nebulizers, metered-dose devices, ultrasonic unit, or IPPB).

(3) Assess patient for unwanted side effects—tremulousness, tachycardia, cardiac arrhythmias, central nervous system stimulation, hypertension.

(4) Avoid excessive use of bronchodilators.

(5) Auscultate the chest after administration of aerosol bronchodilators to assess improvement of air entry and reduction of adventitious breath sounds.

(6) Assess if patient has reduction in dyspnea.

3. Keep secretions liquid.
   a. Encourage high level of fluid intake (8–10 glasses; 2–2½ liters daily) within level of cardiac reserve.
   b. Give inhalations of nebulized water to humidify bronchial tree and liquefy sputum.

4. Use postural drainage positions to aid in clearance of secretions, since mucopurulent secretions are responsible for airway obstruction.
   a. Positions that drain lower and middle lobes appear to be most helpful in patients with COPD.
   b. Other patients achieve effective cough and sputum clearance while seated and leaning forward.
   c. Employ percussion of thorax (p. 165) to assist in propulsion of sputum through the bronchi when necessary.

5. Use controlled coughing.
   a. Inhale slowly and deeply.
   b. Exhale through pursed lips—empties lungs of residual volume.
   c. Cough in short bursts of "huffing" rather than vigorously forcing cough which causes airways to collapse.

6. Prepare patient for bronchoscopic removal of secretions if he is unable to cough and raise his sputum.

7. Prepare patient for endotracheal intubation or tracheostomy if indicated, to permit more effective suctioning of secretions and to provide ventilatory assistance.

NURSING ALERT: Patients with acute respiratory failure along with acute ventilatory failure and rapid CO_2 retention will require mechanical ventilation.

B. *To control infections in order to diminish inflammatory edema and allow bronchial mucosa to recover normal ciliary action—repeated respiratory infections contribute to progress of COPD.*

1. Recognize early manifestations of respiratory infection—increased dyspnea, fatigue; change in color, amount, and character of sputum; nervousness; irritability; low grade fever.

2. Obtain sputum for smear and culture.

3. Give prescribed antimicrobials (ampicillin; erythromycin; tetracycline) at first sign of respiratory infection to control secondary bacterial infection in the bronchial tree, thus clearing the airways.

4. Periodic sputum cultures for possible superinfection should be done for patients on long-term antibiotic therapy.

5. Advise patient to avoid exposure to persons with respiratory tract infections.

6. Give corticosteroids as prescribed; these drugs have an anti-inflammatory effect, and thus help to relieve airway obstruction.
   a. Short course of corticosteroids may be beneficial to persons who have acute attacks of bronchial obstruction, severe wheezing, or marked eosinophilia in sputum or blood.
   b. Antacids may be ordered to prevent development of an ulcer.

NURSING ALERT: Watch for increased susceptibility to infections, for gastrointestinal ulceration, and for bleeding tendencies.

C. *To maintain nutrition, since anorexia is a common problem.*

1. Dyspnea, with accompanying air swallowing, cough, and sputum production combined with intake of medications, contributes to loss of appetite and weight loss.

2. Encourage 6 small meals daily if patient is dyspneic.

3. Offer high protein diet with between meal snacks to improve caloric intake and counteract weight loss.

4. Avoid foods producing abdominal discomfort.

5. Give supplemental oxygen while patient is eating to relieve dyspnea (when directed).

D. *To relieve severe hypoxemia and related symptoms.*

1. Give low-flow oxygen to selected patients with severe, chronic, obstructive pulmonary disease—to correct hypoxemia in a controlled manner and thereby minimize CO_2 retention.
   a. In patients with COPD, poor exchange of gases may result in chronically elevated CO_2 (which is then a less effective stimulus to respiration). Giving a high concentration of oxygen may remove the hypoxic drive—leading to increased hypoventilation, respiratory decompensation, and the development of a worsening respiratory acidosis.
   b. Low-flow oxygen dosage is individualized and is given after analysis of arterial blood gases.
   c. Graded exercises with low-flow oxygen may be given to increase exercise capacity.

2. Avoid narcotics, sedatives, and tranquilizers. Watch for excessive somnolence, restlessness, aggressiveness, anxiety, or confusion; which is frequently caused by acute respiratory insufficiency.

E. *To utilize techniques of breathing retraining to strengthen diaphragm and muscles of expiration and to decrease the work of breathing.*

1. Relaxation exercises—to reduce stress, tension, and anxiety.

2. Teach lower costal, diaphragmatic, and abdominal breathing (p. 166), using a slow and relaxed breathing pattern to reduce respiratory rate and decrease energy cost of breathing.

3. Use pursed-lip breathing (p. 167) at intervals and during periods of dyspnea to control rate and depth of respiration and improve respiratory muscle coordination.

F. *To recondition patient and increase his physical activity.*

1. Employ graded exercise and physical conditioning

programs—walking, stationary bicycle. Portable oxygen system for low-flow oxygen may be used for ambulation in selected patients.
2. Encourage patient to carry out regular exercise training program to increase physical endurance and promote sense of well-being and independence.
3. Train patient in energy-saving methods.

G. *To support the patient emotionally.*

1. Understand that the constant shortness of breath and fatigue makes the patient irritable, apprehensive, anxious, and depressed.
2. Demonstrate a positive and interested approach to the patient.
   a. Be a good listener and show that you care.
   b. Be sensitive to his fears, anxiety, and depression; helps give emotional relief and insight.
3. Strengthen the patient's self-image.
4. Allow the patient to express his feelings and retain (within a controlled degree) the mechanisms of denial and repression.
5. Be aware that sexual dysfunction is common in patients with COPD.

Discharge Planning and Health Education

OBJECTIVE: to improve the quality of life.
1. Give the patient a clear explanation of his disease, what to expect, how to treat and live with it.
   Reinforce by frequent explanations, reading material, demonstrations and question and answer sessions.
2. Review with patient the objectives of treatment and nursing management (pp. 207–209).
3. Work with the patient to set goals—i.e., stair climbing, return to work, etc.
Instruct the patient as follows:
1. Avoid exposure to respiratory irritants—cigarette smoke, pollens, fumes, aerosols, dust, cold.
   a. Stop smoking and avoid smoke-filled rooms.
   b. Avoid sweeping, dusting, and exposure to paint, aerosols, bleaches, and other respiratory irritants.
   c. Keep kitchen ventilated.
   d. Stay out of extremely hot/cold weather to avoid aggravating bronchial obstruction and sputum production.
      (1) Keep a warming mask or scarf over nose and mouth to warm inspired air in cold weather.
      (2) Stay indoors with air conditioning when pollution level is high.
      (3) Try to avoid abrupt environmental changes.
   e. Humidify indoor air in winter; maintain 30–50% humidity for optimal mucociliary function.
2. Prevent and treat respiratory infections.
   a. Avoid exposure to persons with respiratory infections; a respiratory infection makes symptoms worse and can produce further irreversible damage.
   b. Avoid crowds and areas with poor ventilation.
   c. Take influenza immunization (if not allergic) to decrease likelihood of developing infection.
   d. Recognize and report evidence of respiratory infection *promptly* to the physician/clinic—chest pain, changes in character of sputum (amount, color, or consistency), increasing difficulty in raising sputum, increasing cough/wheezing, increasing shortness of breath.
   e. Take prescribed antimicrobial at first sign of infection.

(1) Have a home supply available.
(2) Have periodic sputum cultures when receiving long-term antimicrobial therapy.
3. Reduce bronchial secretions.
   a. Maintain an adequate fluid intake (8–10) glasses daily); mark down the amount of liquid consumed daily.
   b. Take bronchodilators only as directed.
   c. Follow postural drainage exercises as prescribed.
      (1) Stay in each position 5–15 minutes.
      (2) Utilize controlled cough after each position.
   d. Take medications prescribed for cough and expectoration.
   e. Avoid drugs that suppress cough and dry secretions (certain cough medicines, antihistamines).
4. Increase pulmonary ventilation.
   a. Use respiratory therapy treatment consistently and faithfully.
      (1) Learn how to assemble and disassemble equipment.
      (2) Do the procedure immediately upon arising in the morning, before retiring, and as prescribed. Use the *exact* amount of medication prescribed.
      (3) Inhale and exhale as evenly as possible during the treatment.
      (4) Try to cough *productively* (with *controlled coughing*) after the treatment.
         (a) Breathe slowly and deeply, using diaphragmatic breathing.
         (b) Hold breath several seconds.
         (c) Cough—2 short, forceful coughs with the mouth open; the first cough loosens mucus and the second cough moves it.
         (d) Pause and inhale by sniffing quietly. (Inhaling vigorously may initiate unproductive coughing, which is energy consuming.)
         (e) Rest.
      (5) Practice oral hygiene after each treatment.
      (6) Clean respiratory therapy equipment daily to prevent contamination and secondary infection and ensure equipment functioning.
         (a) Allow equipment to dry thoroughly before reassembling.
         (b) Do not re-use medications/solution/water left standing in a humidifier/nebulizer.
5. Do breathing exercises to strengthen muscles of expiration, to strengthen and coordinate muscles of breathing, and to lessen fatigue and to help empty lungs more completely.
   a. Learn the importance of slow and relaxed breathing (controlled breathing).
   b. Practice diaphragmatic breathing and pursed-lip breathing.
   c. Consciously use pursed-lip breathing during episodes of dyspnea and stress.
   d. Maintain muscle tone of the body by regular exercise.
6. Maintain general health at highest attainable level.
   a. Follow good habits of nutrition—patients with COPD may have loss of muscle mass with poor nutritional status, poor appetite, potassium depletion, sodium retention, and dehydration.
   b. Follow high-protein diet with adequate mineral, vitamin, and fluid intake.
   c. Avoid excessive hot or cold fluids/foods that may provoke an irritating cough.
   d. Avoid hard-to-chew foods (causes tiring) and gas-

forming foods, which cause distention and restrict diaphragmatic movement.
  e. Eat 5–6 small meals daily—to ease shortness of breath during and after meals.
  f. Have rest periods before and after meals if eating produces shortness of breath.
  g. Do not eat when upset/angry.
  h. Avoid potassium depletion—patients with COPD tend to have low potassium levels; also patient may be taking diuretics.
    (1) Watch for weakness, numbness, tingling of fingers, leg cramps.
    (2) Foods high in potassium include bananas, dried fruits, dates, figs, orange juice, grape juice, milk, peaches, potatoes.
  i. Restrict sodium as directed.
  j. Use community resources (Meals on Wheels) if energy level is low.
7. Avoid activities that produce excessive shortness of breath.
  a. Live within the limitations that emphysema imposes.
  b. Learn to relax and work at a slower pace.
  c. Obtain vocational counseling to secure a sedentary job if presently in a demanding manual job.
  d. Avoid overfatigue, which is a factor in producing respiratory distress.
  e. Adjust activities according to individual fatigue patterns.
  f. Use pursed-lip breathing in a slow and relaxed manner during periods of breathlessness and physical exertion.
  g. Try to cope with emotional stress as positively as possible—such stress triggers attacks of dyspnea.
  h. Study individual life-style and avoid energy-wasting activities.
  i. Exercise to improve physical condition.
8. Understand the importance of preserving existing function.
  a. Become familiar with the nature of emphysema and reasons for a therapeutic program.
  b. Accept the fact that therapy and medical supervision must be continued for a lifetime.

PULMONARY HEART DISEASE (COR PULMONALE)

Pulmonary heart disease (cor pulmonale) is an alteration in the structure or function of the right ventricle resulting from disease affecting lung structure or function or its vasculature (except when this alteration results from disease of the left side of the heart or from congenital heart disease). Cor pulmonale refers to heart disease caused by lung disease.

Etiology

1. Chronic obstructive pulmonary disease—chronic bronchitis, emphysema most common
2. Conditions that restrict ventilatory function—kyphoscoliosis
3. Pulmonary vascular disease—pulmonary emboli

Pathophysiology

Chronic obstructive pulmonary disease → hypoxia → hypercapnea → acidosis → circulatory complications → pulmonary hypertension → right heart enlargement → right heart failure.

Clinical Manifestations

1. Peripheral edema
2. Respiratory insufficiency; progressive dyspnea (orthopnea, paroxysmal nocturnal dyspnea), chronic cough
3. Right heart enlargement demonstrated by:
  a. Physical examination
  b. ECG changes
  c. Chest x-ray—may show change in heart size
4. Manifestations of carbon dioxide narcosis—headache, confusion, somnolence, coma

Clinical Evaluation

1. Arterial blood gas analysis
2. Pulmonary function tests

Treatment and Nursing Management

OBJECTIVES: to treat underlying lung disease.
 to correct hypoxemia.
 to treat manifestations of heart disease.

1. Improve ventilation.
  a. Use oxygen with mechanical ventilatory aids or continuous low-flow oxygen.
  b. Monitor arterial blood gases as a guide in assessing adequacy of alveolar ventilation.
  c. Avoid central nervous system depressants (narcotics, barbiturates, hypnotics)—have depressant action on respiratory centers.
  d. See page 169 for management of respiratory failure.
2. Combat respiratory infection, which commonly precipitates pulmonary heart disease—respiratory infection causes carbon dioxide retention and hypoxia, resulting in constriction of pulmonary arterioles and subsequent pulmonary hypertension.
3. Treat heart failure when it exists.
  a. Reverse the patient's hypoxemia and hypercapnia. (See above treatment first in order to improve cardiac action.)
  b. Limit physical activity.
  c. Restrict sodium intake.
  d. Give diuretics to reduce peripheral edema and reduce circulatory loan on right heart.
  e. Watch electrolyte levels, especially potassium, as hypokalemia increases risk of arrhythmias.
  f. Give digitalis as prescribed if right ventricular failure is present. Digitalis is given with caution, since digitalis toxicity is a serious problem in management of respiratory failure because of hypoxia, acidosis, and electrolyte abnormalities.
  g. Employ ECG monitoring when necessary—high incidence of arrhythmias in these patients.

Discharge Planning and Health Education

1. Emphasize the importance of stopping cigarette smoking; cigarette smoking is a major cause of pulmonary heart disease.
  a. Query patient about his smoking habits.
  b. Inform patient of risks of smoking and benefits to be gained when smoking is stopped.
2. Teach patient to treat infections immediately.
3. Inform the patient of interrelationship between infection, air pollution, and cardiopulmonary disease.
4. Explain to patient/family that restlessness, depression, and poor sleeping, as well as irritable and angry behavior may be characteristic; patient should improve with rise in O_2 and fall in CO_2 levels in arterial blood gas values.

PULMONARY EMBOLISM

Pulmonary embolism refers to the obstruction of one or more pulmonary arteries by a thrombus (or thrombi) originating somewhere in the venous system or in the right side of the heart, which becomes dislodged and is carried to the lungs.

Predisposing Factors

1. Stasis of venous circulation, especially in blood vessels with injury to the endothelial lining—leads to intravascular clotting.
   Bed rest, sitting, prolonged standing contribute to venous stasis of lower extremities.
2. Intimal damage.
3. Hypercoagulability of the blood.
4. Most emboli originate in veins of the lower extremities or pelvic area where they become detached and are carried to the lungs.

Health Maintenance and Prevention

1. Assess each patient with a high index of suspicion for pulmonary embolism.
2. Be aware of high-risk patients—trauma to pelvis (especially surgical) and lower extremities (especially hip fracture), obesity, history of thromboembolic disease, varicose veins, pregnancy, congestive heart failure, myocardial infarction, malignant disease, postoperative patients, elderly.
3. Prevent stasis of blood in extremities due to dependent position of legs, prolonged sitting, immobility, constricting clothing.
   a. Elevate legs 15–20 degrees at intervals—to minimize stasis and increase venous return.
   b. Apply fitted elastic stockings—to increase blood flow to deep leg veins.
   c. Instruct patient to wiggle toes, move feet, raise and lower legs frequently—to increase venous return.
   d. Do not allow patient's legs and feet to dangle in a dependent position; have the patient place his feet on a chair when sitting on the edge of the bed (if bed is in a high position). Instruct patient to avoid crossing the legs.
   e. Encourage mobilization and weight bearing.
4. Avoid hemoconcentration and immobilization of patients confined to bed.
5. Encourage higher levels of fluid intake during periods of immobility.
6. Avoid leaving catheters in veins (parenteral therapy, measurement of central venous pressure) for prolonged periods.
7. Examine patient's legs carefully as thrombi frequently originate in deep veins of legs, particularly those of the calf. Assess for swelling of leg, duskiness, pain upon pressure over gastrocnemius muscle, pain upon dorsiflexion of the foot (positive Homan's sign).
8. Use agents for preventing venous thrombi and pulmonary embolism in high-risk patients; the approach depends on the patient's status.
   a. Oral anticoagulants (warfarin sodium)—antithrombotic agent useful in hip surgery.
   b. Low dose heparin—for patients over 40 undergoing major surgery.
   c. Dextran—may be used for patients unable to take oral anticoagulant or minidose heparin.
      (1) Dextran provides hemodilution, reduces whole blood viscosity, improves microcirculation, decreases stasis, lowers abnormally high platelet adhesiveness, and reduces high fibrinogen level seen in hypercoagulable states.
      (2) Dextran should be started *slowly* and in presence of physician; anaphylactoid reaction may occur.

Clinical Manifestations

Underlying principles
1. The size and location of the embolus determines the physiologic effect. Symptoms therefore vary from none to cardiovascular collapse.
2. The physiological effects develop from pulmonary artery obstruction and heightened resistance to blood flow through partially obstructed vessels.
3. Small emboli tend to be multiple and recurrent.
4. Substernal pain with apprehension and a sense of impending doom; occurs when most of the pulmonary artery is obstructed
5. Dyspnea and tachypnea; pleuritic pain.
6. Subtle deterioration in patient's condition with no explainable cause
7. Pallor, cyanosis, tachyarrhythmias, clinical shock
8. Engorgement of neck veins
9. Pleural friction rub, accentuated pulmonic second sound, gallop rhythm

NURSING ALERT: Have a high index of suspicion if there is a subtle deterioration in the patient's condition and unexplained cardiovascular and pulmonary findings.

Diagnostic Evaluation

1. Physical findings: clinical signs and symptoms are elusive.
2. Arterial blood gases—systemic arterial hypoxemia is usually found.
3. Radioisotope lung scans—perfusion scan investigates regional blood flow to determine presence of perfusion defects.
4. Pulmonary angiogram (most definitive)—emboli seen as "filling defects."
5. ECG.
6. Contrast phlebography or impedance phlebography—for detecting deep vein thrombosis of the legs.

Objectives of Treatment and Nursing Management

OBJECTIVES: to support life during acute episode.
to promote resolution and prevent recurrence.

A. *To restore cardiopulmonary function.*
1. Provide respiratory assistance to eliminate hypoxia.
   a. Oxygen via face mask or nasal catheter.
   b. Monitor vital signs, ECG and arterial blood gases.
2. Maintain blood pressure by slow infusion of isoproterenol or dopamine.
3. Treat patient for heart failure when present.
4. Give analgesics and sedatives as directed for pain control and apprehension.

B. *To give anticoagulant therapy to prevent recurrence and extension of thromboembolism.*
1. Administer heparin (IV)—stops further thrombus

formation and extends the clotting time of the blood; it is an anticoagulant and antithrombotic.

  a. IV loading dose usually followed by continuous pump or drip infusion or given intermittently every 4–6 hours.

  b. Dosage adjusted to maintain the activated partial thromboplastin time (PTT) at 1.5 to 2.5 times the pretreatment value (if the value was normal).

  c. Assess patient for untoward bleeding; major bleeding may occur from G.I. tract, brain, lungs, nose, and GU tract.

  d. Have protamine available to neutralize heparin during episodes of acute bleeding.

2. Give warfarin sodium (Coumadin) as anticoagulant; may be given simultaneously at the beginning or after 5–6 days of heparin therapy.

  a. Dosage is controlled by monitoring serial tests of prothrombin time; desired prothrombin time is 2 to 2.5 times normal value.

  b. Have phytonadione (Mephyton) available to counteract effects of prothrombin depressant drugs (warfarin sodium)—bleeding is the most important side effect.

  c. Anticoagulants may be contraindicated in certain situations: recent brain, spinal cord, joint, or urinary surgery; certain bleeding tendencies; fracture of pelvis or extremity; recent bleeding from peptic ulceration.

  d. Be aware that many drugs interact with anticoagulants.

3. Give fibrinolytic (thrombolytic) agents (urokinase; streptokinase) as directed; they appear to increase rate of clot dissolution; may be useful in preventing/treating thromboembolism.

C. *To prepare patient for surgical intervention when anticoagulation is contraindicated or has failed, or when patient has a major embolization.*

1. Inferior vena cava interruption—reduces channel size to prevent passage of emboli and at the same time permits some blood to flow. One of the following may be done:

  a. Plication with suture or clips.

  b. Intraluminal obstruction achieved with umbrella filters, balloon catheters, trapping catheters.

  c. All methods of venacaval interruption may produce venous insufficiency of lower extremities with subsequent stasis and edema.

2. Transvenous suction catheter introduced into affected pulmonary artery—to aspirate emboli.

3. Pulmonary embolectomy—direct removal of embolus from pulmonary artery.

  Performed with cardiopulmonary bypass in patients with massive embolism with shock.

Discharge Planning and Health Education

1. See "Preventive Measures," page 211.
2. Patient may have to continue taking anticoagulant therapy for 6 weeks to 6 months following his initial episode.
3. Female patients who have experienced thromboembolism should be advised against taking oral contraceptives.
4. Instruct the patient to watch for signs of overanticoagulation: bleeding gums, nosebleeds, bruising, hematuria, blood in stools, etc.
5. Patient should avoid taking *any* medications unless approved by physician, since many drugs interact with anticoagulants.

6. Patient should notify the dentist that he is on an anticoagulant.
7. Avoid inactivity for prolonged periods or sitting with legs crossed.

SARCOIDOSIS

Sarcoidosis is a systemic granulomatous disease of unknown cause. It may involve almost any organ or tissue but most commonly the lungs, lymph nodes, liver, spleen, skin, eyes, phalangeal bones, and parotid glands.

Clinical Features

1. Patients with sarcoidosis may show altered immunological reactivity.
2. The onset usually occurs during third or fourth decade.
3. First clinical manifestations are usually thoracic, with hilar and mediastinal lymph node enlargement; may progress to diffuse involvement of lungs and then to fibrosis.

Clinical Manifestations

(Depend on size and extent of lesions and degree of fibrosis)

1. Pulmonary manifestations—dyspnea and cough (may appear late)
2. Skin lesions—nodules and infiltrations of face, ears, nose, extensor surfaces
3. Hypercalciuria and hyperglobulinemia
4. Uveitis, joint pain, fever—depending on whether acute or slowly progressive
5. Constitutional symptoms—fatigue, fever, anorexia, weight loss

Diagnostic Evaluation

1. Biopsy of skin and lymph nodes (most definitive diagnostic procedure) reveals noncaseating granulomas.
2. Kveim test:
  a. Intradermal injection of saline suspension of sarcoid tissue obtained from spleen or lymph nodes of patients with active sarcoidosis
  b. Produces a nodule at injection site (in 4–8 weeks).
  c. Area is biopsied and tissue examined.
3. Elevated serum globulin, calcium, and alkaline phosphatase
4. Chest x-ray—reveals hilar adenopathy; causes smooth hilar enlargement
5. Pulmonary function tests—give an indication of the degree of functional impairment
6. Slit-lamp eye evaluation—to determine eye abnormalities

Management

1. There is no specific treatment, the natural course of the disease is towards resolution.
2. Corticosteroid therapy in selected patients; has anti-inflammatory effect; used in patients with hypercalcemia, ocular and myocardial disease, extensive pulmonary disease with compromise of pulmonary function.
3. Isoniazid may be given to patients with positive tuberculin test.

Health Education

1. The majority of persons do not require treatment. Most patients improve spontaneously.

2. Measurements of pulmonary function are made at intervals to follow physiological impact of disease.

OCCUPATIONAL LUNG DISEASES

Diseases of the lungs can occur in a variety of occupations as a result of exposure to organic or inorganic (mineral) dusts and noxious gases.

Altered Physiology

1. Effects of inhaling noxious particles, gases, or fumes depends upon composition of inhaled substance, its antigenic (precipitating an immune response) or irritating properties, the dose inhaled, the length of time inhaled, and the host's response.
2. Exposure to inorganic dusts stimulates pulmonary interstitial fibroblasts resulting in pulmonary interstitial fibrosis.
3. Noxious fumes may cause acute injury to alveolar wall with increasing capillary permeability and pulmonary edema.
4. Occupational lung diseases usually develop slowly (20–30 years) and are asymptomatic in the early stages.

Prevention and Health Maintenance

OBJECTIVE: to reduce exposure of workers to industrial products.
1. Preserve the general health of the worker/miner exposed to occupational dusts in every way possible.
2. Enclose toxic substances, and reduce their concentration in the air.
   a. Engineering controls to reduce exposure
   b. Monitoring of air samples
3. Ventilate properly to reduce dust content of work atmosphere.
4. Have workers use protective devices (face masks, respirators, hoods, etc.)
5. Monitor workers who are exposed to high concentrations of industrial dusts.

Pneumoconioses

The *Pneumoconioses* refer to a non-neoplastic alteration of the lung resulting from exposure to inorganic dust (e.g., "dusty lung"). The most common pneumoconioses are silicosis, asbestosis and coal worker's pneumoconiosis.

Silicosis

Silicosis is a chronic pulmonary fibrosis caused by inhalation of silica dust.

A. Etiology and Altered Physiology

1. Exposure to silica dust is encountered in almost any form of mining because the earth's crust is composed of silica and silicates (gold, coal, tin, copper mining); also stone cutting, quarrying, manufacture of abrasives, ceramics, pottery, and foundry work.
2. When silica particles (which have fibrogenic properties) are inhaled, nodular lesions are produced throughout the lungs. These nodules undergo fibrosis, enlarge, and fuse.
3. Dense masses form in the upper portion of the lungs; restrictive and obstructive lung disease results.

B. Clinical Manifestations

1. Chronic productive cough
2. Dyspnea upon effort

3. Loss of weight; generalized weakness
4. Susceptibility to lower respiratory tract infections

C. Management
1. There is no specific treatment; the patient is treated symptomatically.
2. Give prophylactic isoniazid (INH) to patients with positive PPD skin tests; silicosis is associated with tuberculosis.
3. *Prevention:* See Prevention and Health Maintenance.

Asbestosis

Asbestosis is a diffuse pulmonary fibrosis caused by inhalation of asbestos dust and particles.

A. Altered Physiology

1. Asbestos fibers are inhaled and enter alveoli, which in time are eventually obliterated by fibrous tissue that surrounds the asbestos particles.
2. Fibrous pleural thickening and pleural plaque formation produce restrictive lung disease, decrease in lung volume, diminished gas transfer, and hypoxemia with subsequent development of cor pulmonale.

B. Etiology

1. Found in workers involved in manufacture, cutting, and demolition of asbestos-containing materials; there are over 4000 known uses of asbestos fiber (asbestos mining and manufacturing, construction, roofing, demolition work, brake linings, floor tiles, paints, plastics, shipyards, insulation).

NURSING ALERT: Asbestosis is strongly associated with bronchogenic cancer, also with mesotheliomas of the pleura and peritoneum and probably with gastrointestinal cancer.

C. *Clinical Manifestations* (may develop 20–40 years after exposure)

1. Dyspnea on exertion: severe, progressive, irreversible
2. Cough
3. Rales at lung bases
4. Clubbing of fingers and toes; cor pulmonale

D. Treatment

1. No treatment will affect the progressive fibrosis. Most of the asbestos fibers already in the lungs will remain there.
2. Persuade persons who have been exposed to asbestos fibers to stop smoking. The risk of developing lung cancer for an asbestos worker who smokes is considered to be 50–100 times greater than that for a nonexposed nonsmoker.
3. Keep worker under cancer surveillance; watch for changing cough, hemoptysis, weight loss, melena, etc.
4. *Prevention:* See Prevention and Health Maintenance.

Coal Worker's Pneumoconiosis

Coal Worker's Pneumoconiosis (CWP; black lung) is a variety of respiratory disease found in coal workers in which there is an accumulation of coal dust in the lungs causing a tissue reaction in its presence.

A. *Altered Physiology*

1. Dusts (coal, kaolin, mica, silica) are inhaled and deposited in the alveoli and respiratory bronchioles.
2. There is an increase of macrophages that engulf the particles and transport them to terminal bronchioles.
3. When normal clearance mechanisms no longer can handle the excessive dust load, the respiratory bronchioles and alveoli become clogged with coal dust, dying macrophages, and fibroblasts, which leads to the formation of the coal macule, the primary lesion of CWP.
4. As macules enlarge, there is dilation of the weakening bronchiole with subsequent development of focal or centrilobular emphysema.

B. *Clinical Manifestations*

1. Progressive dyspnea
2. Cough and sputum production; expectoration of varying amounts of black fluid.

C. *Management*

1. There is no specific treatment; the treatment is symptomatic (e.g., bronchodilator drugs, antibiotics for infection).
2. See also treatment of emphysema, page 207.
3. *Prevention:* See page 213.

CANCER OF THE LUNG (BRONCHOGENIC CANCER)

Bronchogenic cancer refers to a malignant tumor of the lung arising within the wall or epithelial lining of the bronchus. The lung is also a common site of metastasis from cancer elsewhere in the body via venous circulation or lymphatic spread. Cancer of the pleura is uncommon.

Classification (according to cell type)

1. Epidermoid (squamous cell)—most common
2. Small cell (oat cell) carcinoma—usually widespread and not as resectable as other types
3. Adenocarcinoma
4. Large cell (anaplastic) carcinoma

Predisposing Factors

1. Cigarette smoking—amount, frequency and duration of smoking have positive relationship to cancer of the lung
2. Industrial exposure to asbestos, arsenic, chromium, nickel, iron, radioactive substances, isopropyl oil, coal tar fumes, petroleum oil mists

Health Maintenance and Prevention

1. Encourage patients to abstain from cigarette smoking.
   a. Teach by example.
   b. Refer patients to anti-smoking helping agencies within the community.
2. Maintain close watch of patients who are smokers—disease is insidious and exists before producing symptoms.
3. Recognize the presence of the tumor before symptoms appear.
   a. Continuous surveillance of smokers, especially those over 40.

> **NURSING ALERT:** Suspect cancer of the lung in patients who belong to a susceptible age group and who have repeated unresolved respiratory infections.

Clinical Manifestatons

Usually occur late and are related to size and location of tumor, extent of spread, and involvement of other structures.

1. Cough—especially a new type or changing cough
2. Hemoptysis
3. Dyspnea; wheezing
4. Thoracic discomfort; chest pain
5. Repeated infections of upper respiratory tract
6. Neural or humoral manifestations; hypertrophic pulmonary osteoarthropathy, Cushing's syndrome; hypoglycemia
7. Constitutional symptoms; weight loss, fatigue, anorexia
8. Usual sites of metastases: liver, bone, central nervous system, adrenal glands.

Diagnostic Evaluation

1. Roentgenogram of chest—including fluoroscopy and tomography; lung cancers may be partly or completely hidden by other structures
2. Cytologic examination of sputum.
3. Bronchoscopy and biopsy; bronchial brushing; bronchial washings.
4. Lymph node biopsy; mediastinoscopy.
5. Lung, brain, and bone scans, if indicated.
6. Computed tomography—sensitive in detecting small pulmonary nodules.

Management

OBJECTIVE: to provide the maximum likelihood of cure. The treatment depends on the cell type, the stage of disease (anatomic extent), and the physiologic status (cardiac and pulmonary evaluation) of the patient. Cancer of the lung is treated by surgery, radiation, chemotherapy, and immunotherapy, used separately or in combination.

A. *Surgical Therapy*—surgical removal of cancer plus surrounding lung tissue and regional lymph nodes. Operation may be a lobectomy, pneumonectomy, or a segmental resection with removal of adjacent lymph nodes depending on state of disease and patient's clinical status.
See page 220 for preoperative and postoperative management of patient undergoing chest surgery.

B. *Radiation Therapy*

1. May be used with curative intent.
2. Oat cell and epidermoid tumors are usually sensitive to radiotherapy.
3. There is usually toxicity to normal tissue within radiation field.
   a. Esophagitis (substernal pain aggravated by eating).
   b. Radiation pneumonitis and progressive pulmonary fibrosis.
4. Radiation may be used as palliative treatment—to decrease tumor size and relieve pressure on vital structures.
   a. May be used to relieve pain, cough, hemoptysis,

neurological symptoms, superior vena caval and bronchial obstruction.
  b. Prophylactic cranial irradiation—may decrease incidence of brain metastases; only used in those patients with oat cell cancer.
5. See page 853 for nursing management of patient undergoing radiation.

C. Chemotherapy

1. Used to shrink tumor and prolong survival; may be used in patients with disseminated disease or in conjunction with surgery or radiation.
2. Chemotherapy used in various ways; single agent, two or more chemotherapeutic agents having different mechanisms of action, and/or a combination of chemotherapy and radiation.
3. See page 849 for nursing management of patient having chemotherapy.

D. Immunotherapy

1 Patients with lung cancer tend to be immunosuppressed; severe immunodeficiency may exist before operation.
2. Immunotherapy may be tried to reverse this immunosuppression; in theory this may lead to tumor rejection.
3. Objective of immunotherapy: to restore or augment the normal mechanisms of host defense against the tumor.
4. Immunotherapeutic Approaches:
  a. BCG (Bacille Calmette-Guérin), an immune stimulating agent, is injectd into pleural space (either into clamped pleural drainage system or via thoracentesis). Theoretical rationale: Immunostimulating agent is brought into contact with tumor antigens; also allows stimulation of regional lymph nodes draining tumor.
  b. Levamisole
  c. Transfer factors—material extracted from sensitized lymphocytes of lymphocyte donors; injected into patient to stimulate cell-mediated immunity.

Discharge Planning and Health Education*

A. Quality of Life

1. Focus on carrying on as normal a life as possible; an improved quality of life can be maintained.

B. Concerns About Pain

1. Realize that not every ache and pain is due to the results of lung cancer; some patients do not even experience pain.
2. Use aspirin or prescription medication as necessary. Do not be concerned about "addiction."
3. Radiation therapy may be used for pain control if tumor has spread to bone.
4. Report any new or persistent pain; it may be due to some other cause, such as arthritis.

C. Emotional Reactions

1. Shock, disbelief, denial, anger, and depression are all normal reactions to the diagnosis of lung cancer.
2. Try to have patient express any concerns; share these concerns with health professionals.

* Adapted from Cox BG et al. Living with Lung Cancer. Rochester, Mayo Foundation, 1977.
  See also care of patient receiving chemotherapy, page 843, and nursing support and action in radiation therapy, page 853.

3. Encourage patient to communicate feelings to significant persons in his life.
4. Expect some feelings of anxiety and depression to recur during illness.
5. Encourage patient to keep busy and remain in the mainstream. Continue with usual activities (work, recreation, sexual) as much as possible.
6. Secure services of a trained counselor if emotional stresses become overwhelming.

D. Coping with Nutritional Problems

1. Keep up nutritional status. A person with lung cancer must eat. Food is as important as any part of the treatment.
2. Meats seem to be distasteful to many patients; substitute milk, milk products, commercially prepared protein powders until appetite returns, but be sure protein intake is adequate.
3. Eat small amounts of food frequently rather than three scheduled meals daily.

E. Additional Support

1. Talk to social service worker about financial assistance as money problems are a major concern to many.
2. Be aware that the American Cancer Society offers services and support modes to persons with cancer.

CHEST TRAUMA

Chest trauma is an injury to the chest caused by any form of violence.
1. Chest injuries are potentially life-threatening because of (1) immediate disturbances of cardiorespiratory physiology, and hemorrhage; and (2) later developments of infection, damaged lung and thoracic cage.
2. Patients with chest trauma may have injuries to multiple organ systems.
3. Patient should be examined for intra-abdominal injuries, which must be treated aggressively.

Altered Physiology

1. In penetrating injuries, some air escapes into the pleural space. (Negative intrapleural pressure is replaced by atmospheric pressure.)
2. The loss of normal negative pressure within the pleural cavity causes collapse of the lung.

Emergency Management

The order of priority is determined by the clinical status of the patient.

OBJECTIVE: to restore normal cardiorespiratory function as quickly as possible.
  This is accomplished by performing effective resuscitation while simultaneously assessing the patient, restoring chest wall integrity, and re-expanding the lung.
1. Evaluate the patency of the airway.
  a. Examiner's ear is placed close to patient's mouth and nose, allowing him to listen at the airway, watch uncovered chest movements, and monitor pulse—this provides a rough estimate of the adequacy of ventilation.
  b. Assess for signs of obstruction, sternal retraction, stridor, wheezing, and cyanosis.
  c. Check neck for position of trachea, subcutaneous emphysema, and distended neck veins.

2. Establish and maintain an open airway.
   a. Aspirate secretions, vomitus, and blood from nose and throat via:
      (1) Tracheal aspiration, if patient is unable to clear the tracheobronchial tree by coughing (p. 167).
      (2) Utilize endotracheal tube if patient is bleeding from nasopharynx or if trachea is injured (short-term use).
      (3) Employ bronchoscopic aspiration if necessary.
      (4) Prepare for tracheostomy if necessary.
         (a) Tracheostomy helps to obtain clear, dry tracheobronchial tree, helps patient breathe with less effort, decreases amount of dead air space in the respiratory tree, and helps reduce paradoxical motion.
         (b) The use of a cuffed tracheostomy tube permits a closed system for air exchange when connected to a ventilator.
   b. Stabilize the chest wall.
   c. Free the pleural cavity of blood and air.
   d. Sucking chest wounds should be closed with an emergency dressing. The presence of lung injury and chest tube drainage must also be considered.
3. Control hemorrhage.
4. Treat for shock. (Shock may be due to blood loss, impairment of cardiorespiratory function.)
   a. Use one or more intravenous infusion lines; obtain blood for baseline studies.
   b. Restore blood volume to adequate levels—plasma, plasma expanders, electrolyte solutions.
   c. Give infusion rapidly.
   d. Monitor serial central venous pressure readings to prevent hypovolemia and circulatory overload. (p. 271).

Types of Chest Injuries

A. Hemothorax

Blood in the pleural space as a result of penetrating or blunt chest trauma.
1. Blood in the pleural cavity produces a compression of the lungs and can result in hidden blood loss causing signs and symptoms of shock.
2. Patient may be asymptomatic; or he may be dyspneic, apprehensive, or in shock.
3. Management
   a. Blood and air are aspirated via needle thoracentesis *or*
   b. An intercostal catheter (thoracotomy tube) is inserted and drainage instituted to accomplish more complete and continuous removal of blood—effects re-expansion of lung and permits monitoring of blood loss.
   The chest catheter is sutured in position and connected to a water-seal drainage-bottle.
   c. Prepare for immediate blood replacement and thoracotomy if bleeding continues.

B. Pneumothorax—Air in the pleural space occurring spontaneously from injury or disease. In patients with chest trauma it is usually the result of a laceration to the lung parenchyma, tracheobronchial tree, or esophagus.
Patient's clinical status depends on the rate of air leakage and size of wound.
1. *Spontaneous pneumothorax*
   a. May occur in healthy individuals; is usually due to rupture of a subpleural bleb of the lung.

b. Treatment is generally nonoperative if pneumothorax is not too extensive; needle aspiration or chest tube drainage may be necessary to achieve re-expansion of collapsed lung.
c. Surgical intervention (thoracotomy) advised for patients with recurrent spontaneous pneumothorax.
2. *Tension Pneumothorax*—build up of pressure in the pleural space resulting in compromise of ventilation; produces a collapse of the lung and decreased ventilation of other lung due to compression, and decreased venous return to the heart.
   a. Clinical picture is one of air hunger, agitation, hypotension and cyanosis.
   b. If tension pneumothorax is present, the pleural space is immediately decompressed with a syringe attached to a 16-18 gauge needle inserted into the second intercostal space.
   c. Chest-tube drainage (closed thoracotomy) of pleural space to evacuate air. (Chest tube connected to underwater-seal suction.)

C. Open Pneumothorax (sucking wound of chest)—implies an opening in the chest wall large enough to allow air to pass freely in and out of thoracic cavity with each attempted respiration; the rush of air through the hole in the chest wall produces a "sucking sound."

1. When there is a large open hole in the chest wall the patient will have a "steal" in ventilation of other lung.
2. A portion of the tidal volume will move back and forth through the hole in the chest wall rather than the trachea as it normally does.
3. *Management*
   a. Close the chest wound immediately to restore adequate ventilation and respiration.
   b. Instruct the patient to inhale and exhale forcefully against a closed glottis (Valsalva maneuver) as the pressure dressing (petrolatum gauze secured with elastic adhesive) is laid in place. (This maneuver helps to expand collapsed lung.)
   c. Prepare for chest tube insertion and drainage to permit evacuation of fluid/air. Surgical intervention may be necessary.
   d. If condition permits, place patient in semisitting position to permit greater ventilatory efficiency.

D. Fracture of Ribs and Sternum (most common chest injury)

NURSING ALERT: Rib fractures should be regarded as potentially serious because they may result in underlying lung contusion. Older individuals with pre-existing pulmonary disease may develop atelectasis and pneumonia following a rib fracture. If rib fragments are driven inward there may be lacerations of the pleura, a pneumothorax, hemothorax, or hemopneumothorax.

1. *Manifestations*
   a. Localized tenderness or crepitus (crackling) over fracture site.
   b. Chest pain referred to the fracture site.
   c. Painful, shallow respirations (due to splinting of involved chest).

2. *Management*
   a. Give analgesics (usually non-narcotic) to assist in effective coughing and deep-breathing.
   b. Encourage deep breathing; give local support to injured area with nurse's hands.
   c. Assist with intercostal nerve block (see below)—to relieve pain so that coughing and deep breathing may be accomplished.

E. *Flail Chest*

Loss of stability of chest wall, with subsequent respiratory impairment. This is usually the result of multiple rib fractures.

1. *Pathophysiology*
   a. When this occurs, one portion of the chest has lost its bony connection to the rest of the rib cage.
   b. During respiration, the detached part of the chest will be pulled in on inspiration and blown out on expiration (paradoxical movement).
   c. Normal mechanics of breathing impaired to a degree that seriously jeopardizes ventilation.
   d. Generally associated with some degree of lung contusion (see below).
2. *Clinical Manifestations*
   a. Pain, dyspnea, cyanosis
   b. Paradoxical (reverse of normal) movements of involved chest wall
3. *Management*
   a. Stabilize the flail portion of the chest with the hands; apply a pressure dressing and turn patient on his injured side, or place 10-pound sandbag at site of flail.
   b. If respiratory failure is present, prepare for immediate endotracheal intubation and ventilation therapy with controlled ventilation or positive-end expiratory pressure (PEEP)—treats underlying pulmonary contusion and serves to stabilize the thoracic cage for healing of fractures, improves alveolar ventilation, and restores thoracic cage stability and intrathoracic volume by decreasing work of breathing.
   c. See also treatment for lung contusion, which follows.

G. *Pulmonary Contusion* (lung contusion)

Damage to the lung parenchyma that results in leakage of blood and fluid into the interstial space of the lung.
1. *Clinical Manifestations*

   a. Tachypnea, tachycardia
   b. Crackles (rales) on auscultation
   c. Pleuritic chest pain
   d. Copious secretions
   e. Cough—constant, loose, rattling
2. *Management (for moderate lung contusion)*
   a. Employ endotracheal intubation and ventilatory support; place patient on ventilator with low concentration of oxygen and positive-end expiratory pressure (PEEP)—to maintain the pressure and keep lungs inflated.
   b. Administer diuretics—to reduce edema.
   c. Correct metabolic acidosis with IV sodium bicarbonate.
   d. Utilize pulmonary artery pressure monitoring.

H. *Cardiac Tamponade*

Compression of the heart as a result of accumulation of fluid within the pericardial space.
1. *Clinical Manifestations*
   a. Falling blood pressure
   b. Rising venous pressure/distended neck veins
   c. Distant heart sounds
   d. Pulsus paradoxus (systolic blood pressure drops and fluctuates with respiration)
   e. Dyspnea, cyanosis, shock

> **NURSING ALERT:** A rapidly developing effusion interferes with ventricular filling and causes impairment of circulation. Thus, there is a reduced cardiac output and poor venous return to the heart. Cardiac collapse can result. In the patient with hypovolemia due to associated injuries, the venous pressure may not rise, thus masking the signs of cardiac tamponade.

2. *Management*
   a. Pericardial aspiration (pericardiocentesis), aspiration or drainage of the pericardium (see p. 274); permits heart action to be resumed.
      (1) Repeated aspirations may be necessary.
   b. Open operation (thoracotomy) to control hemorrhage and to repair cardiac injury may be necessary.

GUIDELINES: Assisting with an Intercostal Nerve Block (Fig. 7-25)

An *intercostal nerve block* is the injection of a local anesthetic into the area surrounding the intercostal nerves to relieve pain temporarily following rib fracture(s), chest wall injury, or thoracotomy.

Purpose To decrease pain and improve patient's ability to cough.

Equipment Syringes, 10 ml. Luer-Lok
Needles, No. 22–30 gauge
Anesthetic solution (Xylocaine; bupivacaine; Pontocaine; procaine)
Skin germicide; sterile gloves

Procedure

NURSING ACTION	RATIONALE/AMPLIFICATION
Preparatory Phase	
1. Inform the patient that he will experience the prick of the needle and a slight sensation of pressure.	
2. Position the patient according to the physician's preference:	

GUIDELINES: Assisting with an Intercostal Nerve Block (Fig. 7-25) (cont.)

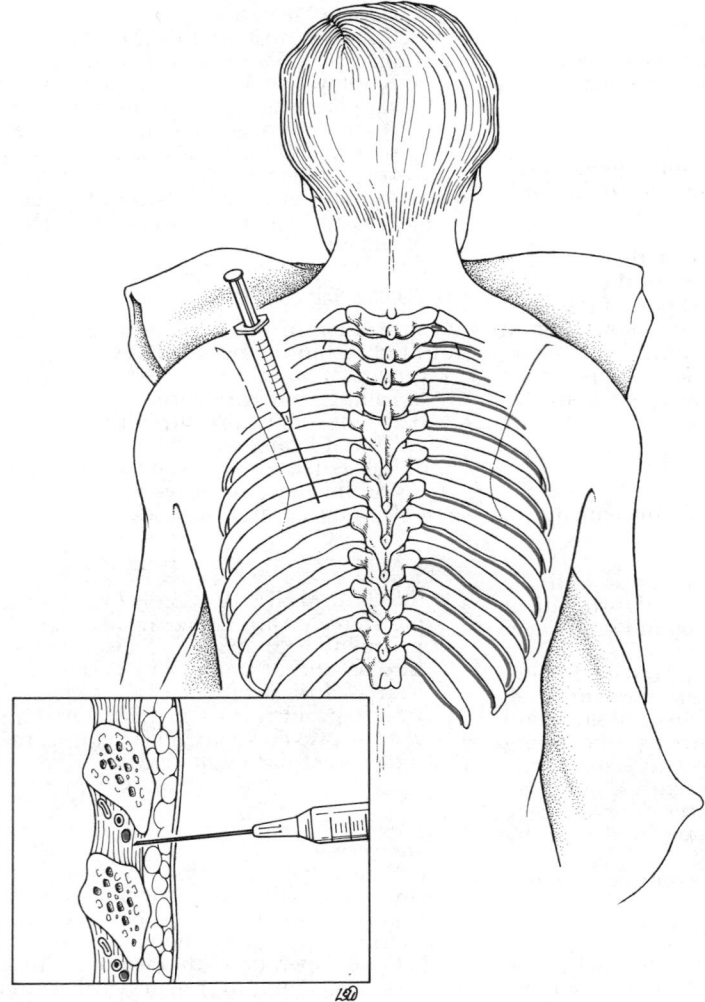

FIGURE 7-25. *Intercostal nerve block.*

Procedure (cont.)	NURSING ACTION	RATIONALE/AMPLIFICATION
	a. Have the patient sit up, bend forward and hug a pillow. OR	a. This posture moves the scapulae forward and out of the way.
	b. Place the patient prone with pillow under his chest. OR	b. The prone position helps immobilize the patient.
	c. Have the patient lie on his unaffected side with his upper arm hanging over the side of the table.	c. This pulls the scapula out of the way.
	3. Ask the patient to identify the site of pain.	3. To determine which intercostal nerves are to be injected.

Performance Phase *(by the physician)*

1. After the skin is prepared, the lower margin of the rib is palpated and a small skin wheal is raised using a 25–30 gauge needle.

2. Usually nerve blocks are done at the posterior angle of the ribs between the posterior axillary line and the spine.

1. This is infiltration anesthesia.

2. The posterior angle is the most prominent and accessible, and an injection at this area produces a block of the entire distal nerve.

Procedure (cont.)

NURSING ACTION	RATIONALE/AMPLIFICATION
3. A fine needle is advanced through the wheal and directed downward so that it slips under the edge of the rib into the upper portion of the interspace.	3. The intercostal nerve runs in a groove along the undersurface of the above rib.
4. The syringe (needle in place) is aspirated.	4. To ensure that the needle has not punctured the lung or that an intercostal vessel has been entered.
5. The local anesthetic (usually 3–5 ml.) is injected into the area.	5. Usually the local anesthetic is injected above and below the painful rib to obtain complete relief of pain as the sensory fields of intercostal nerves overlap.

Follow-up

1. Assess for relief of pain and less painful coughing.	1. This is the expected outcome.
2. Obtain a chest x-ray.	2. To ensure that a pneumothorax has not occurred.

GUIDELINES: Assisting with Tube Thoracostomy (Chest Tube Insertion)

A *tube thoracostomy* is the insertion of one or more flexible tubes into the pleural space to evacuate air, blood, or fluid collections.

Equipment   Tube thoracostomy tray:
Syringes
Needles/trocar
Basins/skin germicide
Sponges
Scalpel/sterile drape/gloves
Two large clamps
Suture material
Local anesthetic
Chest tube (appropriate size); connector
Chest drainage system—connecting tubes and tubing, collection bottles or commercial system, vacuum pump (if required)

Sites for Chest Tube Placement

For pneumothorax—2nd interspace along mid-clavicular or anterior axillary line
For pleural effusion or hemothorax—4th–6th interspace in anterior or mid-axillary line

Procedure

NURSING ACTION	RATIONALE/AMPLIFICATION
Preparatory Phase	
1. Assess patient for pneumothorax, hemothorax, presence of respiratory distress.	
2. Obtain a chest x-ray.	2. To evaluate extent of lung collapse or amount of bleeding in pleural space.
3. Assemble drainage system.	
4. Reassure the patient and explain the steps of the procedure. Tell the patient to expect a needle prick and a sensation of slight pressure during infiltration anesthesia.	4. The patient can cope by remaining immobile and doing relaxed breathing during tube insertion.
5. Position the patient as for an intercostal nerve block.	5. See page 217–218.
Performance Phase *(by the physician)*	
Needle or Intracath Technique	
A needle or IntraCath catheter is used for removal of small amounts of air or a minimal air leak from the lung.	
1. The skin is prepared and anesthetized with local anesthetic with a short 25-gauge needle. A larger needle is used to infiltrate the subcutaneous tissue, intercostal muscles, and parietal pleura.	1. The area is anesthetized to make tube insertion and manipulation relatively painless.
2. An exploratory needle is inserted.	2. To puncture the pleura and determine the presence of air/blood in the pleural cavity.
3. The IntraCath catheter is inserted through the needle into the pleural space. The needle is removed and the catheter is pushed several centimeters into the pleural space.	

GUIDELINES: Assisting with Tube Thoracostomy (Chest Tube Insertion) (cont.)

Procedure

NURSING ACTION	RATIONALE/AMPLIFICATION
4. The catheter is taped to the skin.	4. To prevent it from being pushed out of the chest during patient movement or lung expansion.
5. The catheter is attached to a connector/tubing and attached to a drainage system (underwater-seal or commercial system).	

Trocar Technique for Chest Tube Insertion

A trocar catheter is used for removal of a modest to large amount of air leak or for the evacuation of serous effusion.

1. A small incision is made over the prepared anesthetized site.	1. To admit the diameter of the chest tube.
2. The trocar is directed into the pleural space, the cannula removed, and a chest tube inserted into the pleural space and connected to a drainage system.	2. There is a trocar catheter available equipped with an indwelling pointed rod for ease of insertion.

Hemostat Technique Using a Large Bore Chest Tube

A large bore chest tube is used to drain blood or thick effusions from the pleural space.

1. After skin preparation and anesthetic infiltration, an incision is made through the skin and subcutaneous tissue.	1. The skin incision is usually made one interspace below proposed site of penetration of the intercostal muscles and pleura.
2. A curved hemostat is inserted into the pleural cavity and the tissue is spread with the clamp.	2. To make a tissue tract for the chest tube.
3. The tract is explored with an examining finger.	3. Digital examination helps confirm the presence of the tract and penetration of the pleural cavity.
4. The tube is held by the hemostat and directed through the opening up over the rib and into the pleural cavity.	
5. The clamp is withdrawn and the chest tube is connected to a chest drainage system.	5. The chest tube has multiple openings at the proximal end for drainage of air/blood.
6. The tube is sutured in place and covered with a sterile dressing.	

Follow-Up Care

1. Observe the drainage system for blood/air Observe that there is free fluctuation in the tube upon respiration. See water-seal drainage, page 226).	1. If a hemothorax is draining through a thoracostomy tube into a bottle containing sterile normal saline, the blood is available for autotransfusion.
2. Secure a follow-up chest x-ray.	2. To confirm correct chest tube placement and re-expansion of the lung.

THORACIC SURGERY

The Challenge: Meticulous attention must be given to the preoperative and postoperative care of patients undergoing thoracic surgery. These operations are wide in scope; obstructive pulmonary disease with compromised respiratory function may be present, and the margin of safety is apt to be narrow.

Preoperative Care

OBJECTIVES: to determine if patient can survive planned procedure.
to ensure optimal condition of patient for surgery.

A. *Determine the preoperative status of the patient, his physical assets and liabilities.*

1. Assist the patient undergoing diagnostic studies.
   a. History and physical examination
   b. Chest roentgenogram
   c. Pulmonary function studies to ascertain if patient will have adequately functioning lung tissue postoperatively; incidence of postoperative pulmonary complications is closely correlated with preoperative pulmonary disease.
   d. Special diagnostic studies as required; radionu-

clide lung scanning may show if gas exchange will be effected by procedure.
   e. Baseline studies to ascertain any unsuspected abnormalities and to serve as a baseline reference during the postoperative period
      (1) ECG—to disclose presence of atherosclerotic heart disease or conduction defect
      (2) Blood urea nitrogen, serum creatinine—to obtain a "rough" measurement of renal function
      (3) Blood sugar or glucose tolerance—to detect unrecognized diabetes
      (4) Blood electrolytes, serum protein studies, and blood volume determinations as indicated
      (5) Arterial blood gas studies to determine presence of hypoxemia/hypercapnia
2. Nursing assessment of the patient.
   a. What signs and symptoms are present? (cough, expectoration, hemoptysis, chest pain)
   b. What is his smoking history (amount and duration)? How much is he presently smoking?
   c. What is the patient's cardiopulmonary tolerance while bathing, eating, walking, etc.?
   d. What is the "physiologic age" of the patient?

(general appearance, mental alertness, behavior, degree of nutrition)
   e. What other medical conditions exist?
   f. What is his breathing pattern?
   g. How much exertion is required to produce dyspnea?
   h. What are his personal preferences and dislikes?

B. *Improve alveolar ventilation and overall respiratory function.*

1. Encourage the patient to stop smoking since this increases bronchial irritation.
2. Employ all measures to minimize pulmonary secretions.
   a. Measure sputum daily in patients with large volume of secretions to determine if volume of secretion is decreasing.
   b. Instruct the patient to cough against a closed glottis to increase intrapulmonary pressure.
   c. Humidify the air to loosen secretions.
   d. Administer bronchodilators for bronchospasm.
   e. Give antimicrobials for infection.
   f. Encourage deep breathing with the use of incentive spirometer or blow bottles.
   g. Teach diaphragmatic breathing preoperatively (see p. 166).
   h. Set up a schedule of breathing exercises that encourage the use of abdominal muscles.
   i. Carry out postural drainage in patients having increased mucus production (see page 163).

C. *Evaluate cardiovascular and pulmonary status so that complications may be anticipated and prevented.*

1. Study the results of diagnostic tests to learn of existing deviations from normal.
2. Observe the patient and his reactions to various activities of daily living.
3. Give cardiac drugs to patients with congestive heart failure.
4. Correct anemia, dehydration, and hypoproteinemia—intravenous infusions, tube feedings, blood transfusions as indicated.
5. Give prophylactic anticoagulant (low-dose heparin) as prescribed to reduce perioperative incidence of deep vein thrombosis and pulmonary embolism.

D. *Prepare the patient for the surgical experience by offering reassurance, explanations, and skillful preoperative nursing care.*

1. Orient the patient to events in the postoperative period.
   a. Cough and breathing routine
   b. Presence of chest tube and drainage bottles
   c. Oxygen therapy; ventilator therapy
   d. Measures used to control discomfort
   e. Leg exercises and range of motion exercises for affected shoulder
   f. Coping measures (breathing, turning, analgesics) for postoperative discomfort
2. Encourage expression of psychological and safety needs
3. See that consent form has been explained and signed

E. *Participate in preoperative preparations as indicated.*

1. Shaving of incision area
2. Antiseptic skin cleansing
3. Restriction of oral intake
4. Special medications
5. Placement of needed tubes as prescribed (IV lines, indwelling catheter, nasogastric tube)

Postoperative Care

OBJECTIVE: to restore normal cardiopulmonary function as quickly as possible.

1. Maintain an open airway.
   a. Look and listen at the patient's open mouth as he breathes for evidences of obstruction, and listen to his chest (auscultation) with a stethoscope.
   b. Monitor the arterial blood gases—a progressive fall in PO_2 is an indication for the use of the ventilator; an elevated PCO_2 also usually signifies need for ventilator support (except in patients with chronic obstructive airway disease).
   c. Patient may have endotracheal tube and be assisted by a ventilator until he demonstrates that he can support adequate respiration—initiating ventilator therapy at appropriate time may reverse the trend toward respiratory failure.
   d. Aspirate all secretions with suctioning until patient is able to raise secretions effectively—endotracheal secretions are present in excessive amounts in post-thoracotomy patients because of trauma to the tracheobronchial tree during operation, diminished lung ventilation, and diminished cough reflex.
      (1) Excessive secretions will produce airway obstruction; air in the alveoli distal to the obstruction will become absorbed and the lung will collapse.
      (2) Carry out tracheal aspiration on "wet" comatose patient to prevent atelectasis.
2. *Technique for tracheal suctioning if patient cannot clear rales or refuses to cough.*
   Sterile technique should be used. This procedure should be learned under expert clinical supervision.
      a. Place the patient in a sitting or semi-Fowler's position. Attach the sterile catheter to a "Y" or "T" tube that has been connected to a suction device.
      b. Oxygenate the patient several minutes before each suctioning procedure.
      c. Give patient a gauze square; instruct him to pull his tongue outward; this tilts the epiglottis forward (or have someone else do this).
      d. Pass the catheter (lubricated with water-soluble gel) through the nostril to the pharynx.
      e. Check the position of the tip of the catheter; it should be in the lower pharynx.
      f. Instruct the patient to take a deep breath—this action serves to open the epiglottis and also encourages the catheter to move in the direction of the negative pressure generated by inspiration.
      g. Advance the catheter into the trachea only during inspiration.
      h. Apply suction *intermittently* by closing the open end of the "Y" (or "T") catheter with the finger and slowly rotating between the thumb and forefinger.
      i. Suctioning must *never* be prolonged more than 5–10 seconds since cardiac arrest may ensue in patients with borderline oxygenation.
      j. While the catheter is being withdrawn, apply gentle suction to clear the tracheal walls of secretions.
      k. Ventilate the patient with oxygen for about 2–5 minutes prior to a second passage of the catheter (if this is necessary). Check the pulse rate.

NURSING ALERT: Look for changes in color and consistency of aspirated sputum. Colorless, fluid sputum is not unusual; opacification or coloring of sputum may mean dehydration or infection.

3. Maintain continuing nursing surveillance of the patient.
   a. Take blood pressure, pulse, and respiration 15 minutes or more frequently as indicated; extend the time intervals according to the patient's clinical status.
   b. Evaluate *character* of respirations and patient's color—depth of respiration is an important criterion in evaluating whether lungs are being adequately expanded.
   c. Monitor heart rate and rhythm via auscultation and ECG, since arrhythmias are more frequently seen after thoracic surgery.
      (1) Arrhythmias can occur anytime and contribute significantly to postoperative mortality rate.
      (2) *Rate of occurrence of arrhythmias increases with patients over 50 and with those undergoing pneumonectomy or esophageal surgery.*
      (3) Begin anti-arrhythmic measures immediately if indicated.
   d. Maintain an arterial line to facilitate frequent monitoring of blood gases, serum electrolytes, hemoglobin, hematocrit, and arterial pressure.
   e. Monitor the central venous pressure for prompt recognition of hypovolemia.
   f. Elevate the head of the bed 30–40 degrees when patient is oriented and his blood pressure stabilized.
4. Maintain surveillance and careful management of the chest drainage system, which is used to eliminate any residual air or fluid following thoracotomy.*
   a. Chest tube(s) inserted at time of surgery to prevent fluid and air from accumulating in pleural or mediastinal space and to assist in reexpansion of remaining lung tissue.
   b. Check amount and character of drainage immediately postoperatively and at necessary intervals thereafter—drainage should progressively decrease after first 12 hours.
   c. The drainage is usually bloody immediately after surgery but becomes serous in 24 hours or so.
   d. Persistence of bloody drainage indicates bleeding. Prepare for blood replacement and possible reoperation to achieve hemostasis.
   e. See page 226 for summary of the nurse's role in the management of water-seal drainage.
5. Give humidified oxygen in immediate postoperative period to assure maximum oxygenation—respirations are still depressed and residual secretions in the peripheral respiratory passages may partially block gas exchange. Monitoring by means of arterial blood gas analysis may be necessary.
   a. Assess for respiratory distress and a feeling of tightness in the chest.

* A patient with a pneumonectomy usually does not have water-seal chest drainage since it is desirable that the pleural space fill with an effusion which eventually obliterates this space. Some surgeons do use a "modified" water-seal system.

   b. Watch for restlessness—often the first sign of hypoxia.
6. Encourage and promote an effective cough routine (Fig. 7-26); a persistent and ineffective cough exhausts the patient, and retained secretions lead to atelectasis and pneumonia.
   a. Sit patient on side of bed with feet supported on a chair if his condition permits.
   b. Support the chest firmly over the operated side and against opposite side to lessen incisional pain or support the thorax with one hand pressing on the mid-sternum and the other arm around the back if there is a median sternotomy incision.
   c. Instruct the patient to take a deep breath (to increase cough pressure), to pull in his abdominal muscles, and to cough vigorously.
   d. Assist the patient to cough at least every 1–2 hours during the first 24 hours and when necessary thereafter.
      (1) Employ incentive spirometer as directed—stimulates deep and sustained inspiration.
      (2) Use ultrasonic-nebulization-mist inhalation—may increase inspiration and an effective cough by irritating airway mucosa.
         (a) If audible rales continue, it may be necessary to utilize chest percussion with cough routine until lungs are clear of rales.
         (b) If coughing and/or tracheal aspiration (suctioning) fail to clear rales, bronchoscopic removal of secretions may be necessary.
7. Listen to both lungs (anterior and posterior) with a stethoscope to determine if there are any changes in breath sounds since diminished breath sounds may indicate collapsed or hypoventilated alveoli.
   a. Are breath sounds normal, indicating free flow of air in and out of the lungs?
   b. Are breath sounds distant? Wheezing? Rales present?
8. Provide intelligent pain relief—pain limits chest excursions, thereby decreasing ventilation; pain also exhausts the patient.
   a. Severity of pain varies with type of incision and with patient's reaction to and ability to cope with pain. Usually a posterior-lateral skin incision is the most painful.
   b. Give narcotics (usually in frequent small doses) for pain relief, to permit patient to breathe more deeply and cough more effectively; place on oral analgesic (codeine) as soon as possible.
   c. Avoid depressing respiratory and vascular systems with too much narcotic; patient should not be so somnolent that he does not cough.
   d. Position in bed properly.
   e. Support chest tubes to avoid pull on chest wall.
   f. Assist patient having intercostal nerve block for pain control.
9. Monitor hourly urine output from indwelling catheter since urine volume reflects cardiac output and organ perfusion.
   a. Patient should excrete at least 30 ml. (1 oz.) of urine hourly.
   b. Decreasing urinary output is frequently secondary to decreased cardiac output.
   c. Urine specific gravity helps assess state of hydration.

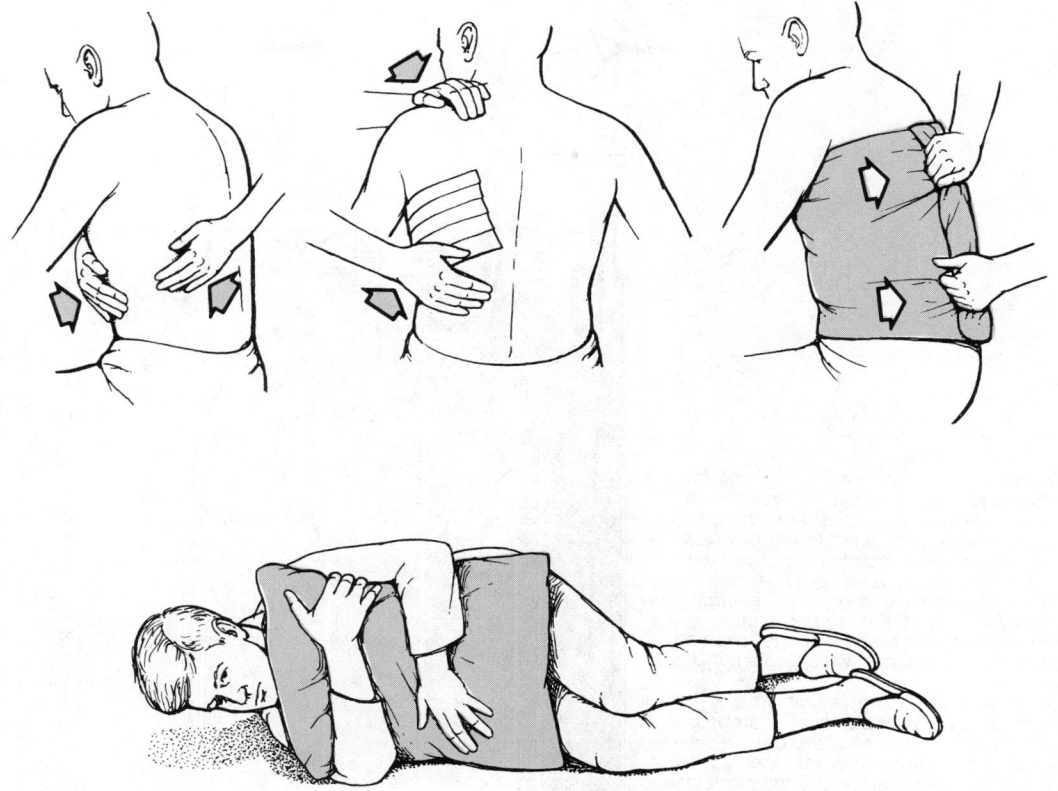

FIGURE 7-26. *Promotion of an effective cough.*

10. Continue to follow blood gas and serum electrolyte values—to detect early manifestations of ventilatory insufficiency or alterations in metabolic and acid–base status.
11. Administer blood and parenteral fluids at a slower rate after thoracic surgery—pulmonary edema due to transfusion/infusion overload is an ever-present threat; following pneumonectomy the pulmonary vascular system has been greatly reduced.
12. Maintain care in positioning the postoperative thoracotomy patient.
    a. Position patient upright (15–30°) if cardiovascular system is stable to facilitate optimal ventilation; this also helps residual air to rise in upper portion of pleural space where it can be removed by the chest tube.
    b. Patients with limited respiratory reserve may not be able to turn on unoperated side as this may limit ventilation of the operated side.
    c. Vary the position from horizontal to semierect; remaining in one position tends to promote the retention of secretions in the dependent portion of the lungs.
    d. Sit patient upright to cough.
13. Watch for evidences of acute gastric distention (not uncommon following thoracic surgery).
    a. Insert nasogastric tube for decompression.
    b. Keep nasogastric tube functioning to avoid vomiting and tracheobronchial aspiration (see p. 392).

14. Anticipate and forestall complications.
    a. Pulmonary insufficiency
    b. Hemorrhage
    c. Respiratory acidosis
    d. Pneumonitis; atelectasis
    e. Cardiac arrhythmias, myocardial infarction, pulmonary edema
    f. Renal failure
    g. Gastric distention
15. Restore normal range of motion and function of shoulder and trunk
    a. Encourage breathing exercises to mobilize thorax (p. 166).
    b. Encourage skeletal exercises to promote abduction and mobilization of the shoulder.
    c. Ambulate as soon as pulmonary and circulatory systems are compensated.
    d. Encourage progressive activities according to development of fatigue.

Discharge Planning and Health Education

1. There will be some intercostal pain for a period of time which can be relieved by local heat and oral analgesia.
2. Weakness and fatigability are common during the first 3 weeks following a thoracotomy.
3. Range of motion exercises for the arm and shoulder on the affected side should be carried out several times daily to avoid ankylosis of the shoulder ("frozen shoulder").

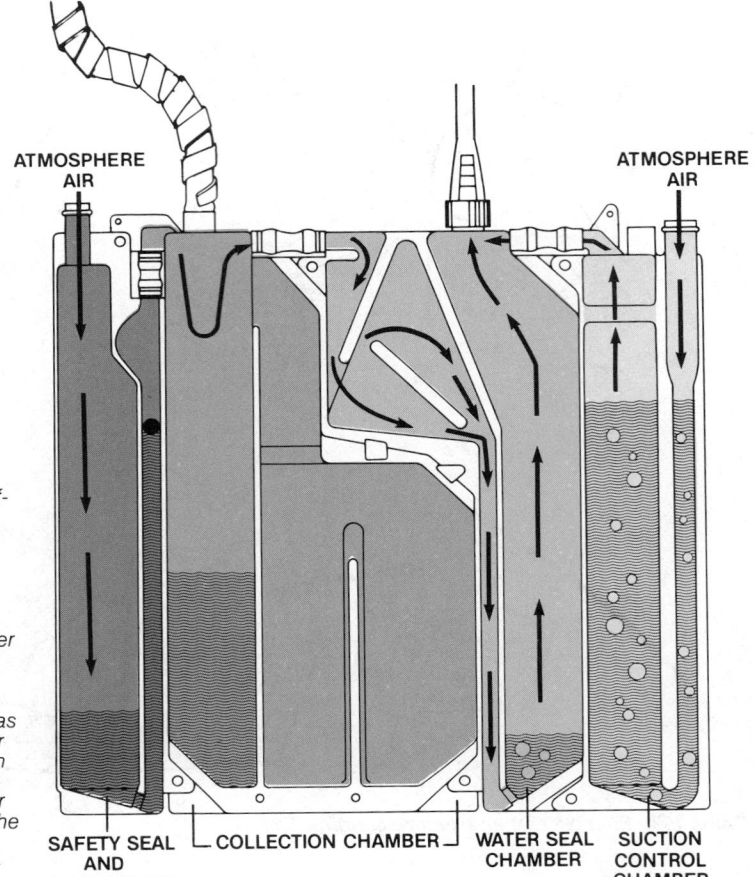

FIGURE 7-27. *The Argyle "Double Seal™" system consists of four chambers (whose sequence is different). Note that the second chamber is the collection chamber (reading from left to right), which is also divided into three subchambers. The next chamber to the right is the water seal chamber, whose shape is essentially that of a "U", except that the pathway through the chamber is more tortuous than in a Pleurevac unit. The last chamber is the suction control chamber, which again is U-shaped.*

The extra chamber in an Argyle unit is on the left. This chamber is also a water seal chamber, as is the third chamber. Customarily, the patient's air passes through the third chamber into the suction source. If, however, the passage into the suction source is accidentally obstructed, the patient's air can pass instead through the first chamber into the atmosphere. The first chamber thus provides a "safety" vent for the patient's air. (Courtesy of Argyle)

ATMOSPHERE AIR

ATMOSPHERE AIR

SAFETY SEAL AND MANOMETER

COLLECTION CHAMBER

WATER SEAL CHAMBER

SUCTION CONTROL CHAMBER

4. Carry out deep breathing exercises for the first few weeks at home.
5. Consciously practice good body alignment, preferably in front of a full-length mirror.
6. The chest muscles may be weaker than normal for 3 to 6 months following surgery. Avoid lifting more than 20 pounds until complete healing has taken place.
7. Alternate walking and other activities with frequent short rest periods. Walk at a moderate pace and gradually extend walking time and distance.
8. Stop any activity immediately that causes undue fatigue, increased shortness of breath, or chest pain.
9. Because all or part of one lung has been removed, stay away from respiratory irritants (smoke, fumes, high air pollution).
   a. Avoid anything that may cause spasms of coughing.
   b. Sit in non-smoking areas in public places.
10. Have an annual influenza injection (pneumonectomy patients)
11. Report for follow-up care by the surgeon or clinic as necessary

CHEST DRAINAGE

Pathophysiology

1. The normal breathing mechanism operates on the principle of negative pressure (the pressure in the chest cavity is lower than the pressure of the outside air, causing air to move into the lungs during inspiration).
2. Whenever the chest is opened, from any cause, there is loss of negative pressure, which can result in collapse of the lung. The collection of air, fluid, or other substances in the chest can compromise cardiopulmonary function and even cause collapse of the lung, because these substances take up space.
3. Pathologic substances that collect in the pleural space include: fibrin, or clotted blood, liquids (serous fluids, blood, pus, chyle) and gases (air from the lung, tracheobronchial tree, or esophagus).
4. Surgical incision of the chest wall almost always causes some degree of pneumothorax. Air and fluid collect in the intrapleural space, restricting lung expansion and reducing air exchange.
5. It is necessary to restore pleural negative pressure and prevent pneumothorax from happening. There-

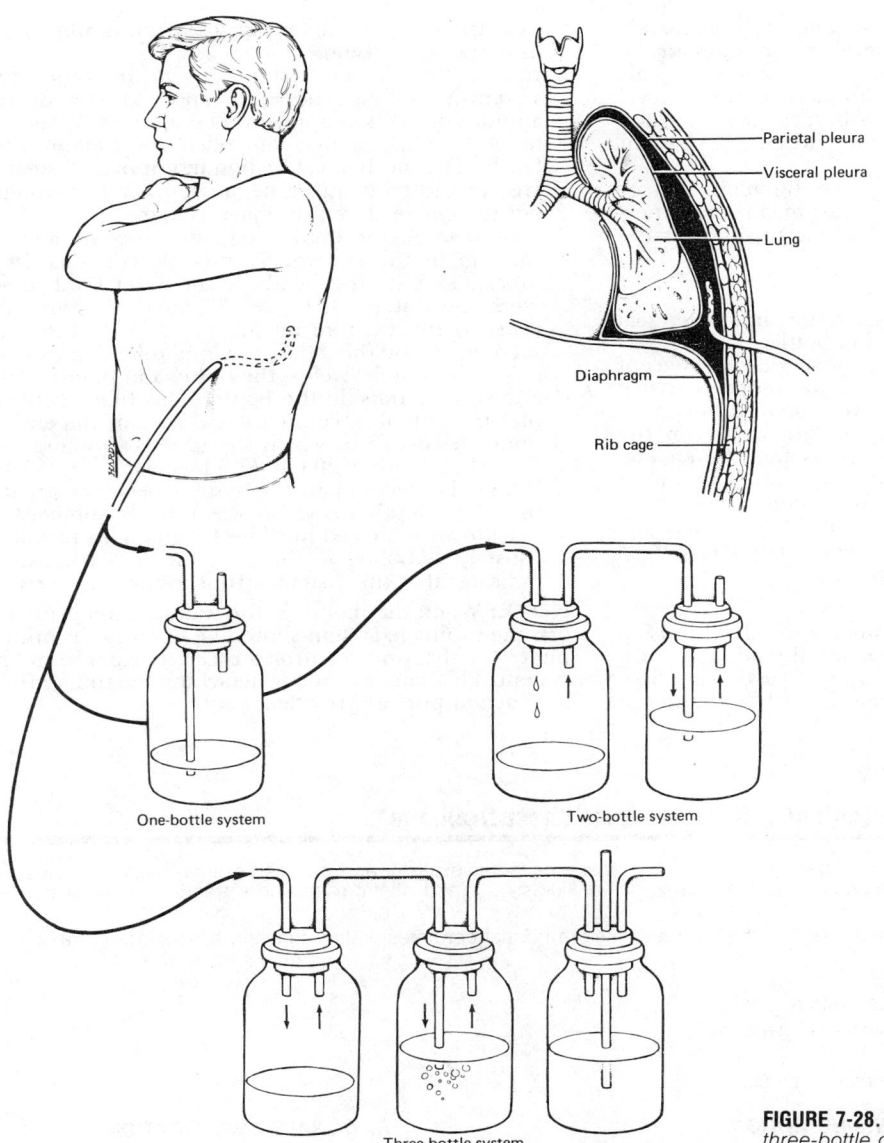

Parietal pleura

Visceral pleura

Lung

Diaphragm

Rib cage

One-bottle system

Two-bottle system

Three-bottle system

FIGURE 7-28. *One-, two-, and three-bottle chest drainage systems.*

fore, during or immediately after thoracic surgery, catheters are positioned strategically in the pleural space, sutured to the skin, and connected to some type of drainage apparatus to remove the residual air and drainage fluid from the pleural or mediastinal space. This assists in the reexpansion of remaining lung tissue.

Principles of Chest Drainage

1. A chest drainage system must be capable of removing whatever collects in the pleural space so that a normal pleural space and normal cardiopulmonary function may be restored and maintained.
2. There are many types of commercial chest drainage systems in use, most of which use the water-seal principle (Fig. 7-27). The chest catheter is attached to a bottle, using a one-way valve principle. Water acts as a seal and permits air and fluid to drain from the chest, but air cannot re-enter the submerged tip of the tube (Fig. 7-28).
3. Chest drainage can be categorized into three types of mechanical systems (Fig. 7-28.):

A. *The Single-Bottle Water-Seal System*

1. The end of the drainage tube from the patient's chest is covered by a layer of water which permits drainage of air and fluid from the pleural space, but does not allow air to move back into the chest. Functionally, drainage depends on gravity, on the mechanics of respiration, and, if desired, on suction by the addition of *controlled* vacuum.

2. The tube from the patient extends approximately 2.5 cm. (1 inch) below the level of the water in the container. There is a vent for the escape of any air that is drained from the lung. The water level fluctuates as the patient breathes; it goes up when the patient inhales and down when the patient exhales.

3. At the end of the drainage tube, bubbling may or may not be visible. Bubbling can mean either persistent leakage of air from the lung or other tissues or a leak in the system.

B. The Two-Bottle System

1. The two-bottle system consists of the same water-seal chamber, plus a fluid-collection bottle.
2. Drainage is similar to that of a single unit, except that when pleural fluid drains, the underwater-seal system is not affected by the volume of drainage.
3. Effective drainage depends on gravity or on the amount of suction added to the system. When vacuum (suction) is added to the system from a vacuum source, such as wall suction, the connection is made at the vent stem of the underwater-seal bottle.
4. The amount of suction applied to the system is regulated by the wall gauge.

C. The Three-Bottle System

1. The three-bottle system is similar in all respects to the two-bottle system, except for the addition of a third bottle to control the amount of suction applied.
2. The amount of suction is determined by the depth

to which the tip of the venting glass tube is submerged in the water.

3. In the three-bottle system (as in the other two systems), drainage depends upon gravity or the amount of suction applied. The amount of suction in the 3-bottle system is controlled by the manometer bottle. The mechanical suction motor or wall suction creates and maintains a negative pressure throughout the entire closed drainage system.

4. The manometer bottle regulates the amount of vacuum in the system. This bottle contains three tubes: (1) A short tube above the water level comes from the water-seal bottle; (2) another short tube leads to the vacuum or suction motor, or to wall suction; (3) the third tube is a long tube that extends below the water level in the bottle and opens to the atmosphere outside the bottle. This tube regulates the amount of vacuum in the system, depending upon the depth to which the tube is submerged—the usual depth is 20 cm. (7.6 inches).

5. When the vacuum in the system becomes greater than the depth to which the tube is submerged, outside air is sucked into the system. This results in constant bubbling in the manometer bottle, which indicates that the system is functioning properly.

NOTE: When the motor or the wall vacuum is turned off, the drainage system should be open to the atmosphere so that intrapleural air can escape from the system. This can be done by detaching the tubing from the suction port to provide a vent.

GUIDELINES: Managing the Patient with Water-Seal Chest Drainage*

Purposes
1. To remove liquids and gas from the pleural space or thoracic cavity and the mediastinal space. (Liquids are serous fluid, blood, pus, and occasionally other fluids; gas and air from the lung, tracheobronchial tree, or esophagus.)
2. To bring about reexpansion of the lung and restore normal cardiorespiratory function after surgery, trauma, or medical conditions.

Equipment
Closed chest drainage system
Holder for drainage system (if needed)
Vacuum motor
Sterile connector for emergency use

Procedure

NURSING ACTION	RATIONALE/AMPLIFICATION
1. Attach the drainage tube from the pleural cavity to the tubing that leads to a long tube with end submerged in sterile normal saline.	1. Water-seal drainage provides for the escape of air and fluid into a drainage bottle. The water acts as a seal and keeps the air from being drawn back into the pleural space.
2. Tape the places where the tubing is connected, if needed. Some connectors will hold without taping. a. The tube should be approximately 2.5 cm. (1 inch) below the water level. b. The short tube is left open to the atmosphere.	2. Taping the connecting points of the tubing will make certain that the tubing remains airtight to reestablish negative (intrapleural) pressure. a. If the tube is submerged too deep below the water level, a higher intrapleural pressure is required to expel air. b. Venting the short glass tube lets air escape from the bottle.
3. Mark the original fluid level with tape on the outside of the drainage bottle. Mark hourly/daily increments (date and time) at the drainage level.	3. This marking will show the amount of fluid loss and how fast fluid is collecting in the drainage bottle. It serves as a basis for blood replacement, if the fluid is blood. Grossly bloody drainage will appear in the bottle in the immediate postoperative period and if excessive may require reoperation. Drainage usually declines progressively after the first 24 hours.

* There are numerous commercial disposable chest drainage devices available that use the water-seal principle.

**Procedure
(cont.)**

NURSING ACTION

4. Fasten the tubing to the drawsheet with rubber bands and safety pins so that flow by gravity will occur. The tubing should *not* loop or interfere with the movements of the patient.

5. Allow the patient to assume a position of comfort. Encourage good body alignment. When the patient is in a lateral position, place a rolled towel under the tubing to protect it from the weight of the patient's body. Encourage the patient to change his position frequently.

6. Put the arm and shoulder on the affected side through range-of-motion exercises several times daily. Some pain medication may be necessary.

7. "Milk' the tubing in the direction of the drainage bottle hourly.

8. Make sure there is fluctuation ("tidaling") of the fluid level in the long glass tube.

9. Fluctuations of fluid in the tubing will stop when:
   a. the lung has re-expanded
   b. the tubing is obstructed from blood clots or fibrin
   c. a dependent loop develops (see #4)
   d. suction motor or wall suction is not operating properly.

10. Watch for leaks of air in the drainage system as indicated by contant bubbling in the water-seal bottle.
    a. Report excessive bubbling in the water-seal chamber immediately.
    b. "Milking" of chest tubes in patients with air leaks should only be done if requested by surgeon.

11. Observe and report immediately signs of rapid, shallow breathing, cyanosis, pressure in the chest, subcutaneous emphysema, or symptoms of hemorrhage.

12. Encourage the patient to breathe deeply and cough at frequent intervals. If there are signs of incisional pain, adequate pain medication is indicated.

13. Stabilize the drainage bottle on the floor or in a special holder.
    Caution visitors and personnel against handling equipment or displacing the drainage bottle.

14. If the patient has to be transported to another area, place the drainage bottle below the chest level (as close to the floor as possible) if he is lying on a stretcher.
    If the tube becomes disconnected, cut off the contaminated tips of the chest tube and tubing, insert a sterile connector in the chest tube and tubing and reattach to the drainage system.

15. When assisting the surgeon in removing the tube:
    a. Instruct the patient to perform the Valsalva maneuver (forcible exhalation against a closed glottis, holding one's breath)
    b. The chest tube is clamped and quickly removed
    c. Simultaneously, a small bandage is applied and made airtight with petrolatum gauze covered by 4 x 4 gauze and thoroughly covered and sealed with adhesive tape.

4. Kinking, looping, or pressure on the drainage tubing can produce back pressure, thus possibly forcing drainage back into the pleural space or impedes drainage from the pleural space.

5. The patient's position should be changed frequently to promote drainage and the body kept in good alignment to prevent postural deformity and contractures. Proper positioning helps breathing and promotes better air exchange. Pain medication may be indicated to enhance comfort and deep breathing.

6. Exercise helps to avoid ankylosis of the shoulder and assist in lessening postoperative pain and discomfort.

7. "Milking" the tubing prevents it from becoming plugged with clots and fibrin. Constant attention to maintaining the patency of the tube will facilitate prompt expansion of the lung and minimize complications.

8. Fluctuation of the water level in the tube shows that there is effective communication between the pleural cavity and the drainage bottle, provides a valuable indication of the patency of the drainage system, and is a gauge of intrapleural pressure.

10. Leaking and trapping of air in the pleural space can result in tension pneumothorax.

11. Many clinical conditions may cause these signs and symtoms, including tension pneumothorax, mediastinal shift, hemorrhage, severe incisional pain, pulmonary embolus, and cardiac tamponade. Surgical intervention may be necessary.

12. Deep breathing and coughing help to raise the intrapleural pressure, which allows emptying of any accumulation in the pleural space and removes secretions from the tracheobronchial tree so that the lung expands and atelectasis is prevented.

13. If any part of the apparatus is damaged, the closed system of drainage will be destroyed and the patient will be endangered by atmospheric pressure in the pleural space and resultant collapse of the lung. The drainage system must be kept airtight to reestablish negative intrapleural pressure.

14. The drainage apparatus must be kept at a level lower than the patient's chest to prevent backflow of fluid into the pleural space.

15. The chest tube is removed as directed when the lung is reexpanded (usually 24 hours to several days). During removal of the tube the chief priorities are prevention of entrance of air into the pleural cavity as the tube is withdrawn and prevention of infection.

BIBLIOGRAPHY

NOSE AND THROAT

Books

Adams GL, Boise Jr and Paparella M. Boles's Fundamentals of Otolaryngology, 5th ed. Philadelphia, WB Saunders, 1978

Ballantyne JC and Groves L. A Synopsis of Otolaryngology, 3rd ed. Chicago, Year Book Medical Publishers, 1978

Ballenger JJ. Diseases of the Nose, Throat and Ear, 12th ed. Philadelphia Lea & Febiger, 1977

DeWeese DD and Saunders WH. Textbook of Otolaryngology. St. Louis, C.V. Mosby, 1977

Pracy R et al. Ear, Nose and Throat Surgery. New York, John Wiley & Sons, 1977

Ritter FN. The Paranasal Sinuses, 2nd ed. St. Louis, CV Mosby, 1978

Snow JB Jr (ed). Controversy in Otolaryngology. Philadelphia, WB Saunders, 1980

Snow JB Jr. Introduction to Otorhinolaryngology. Chicago, Year Book Medical Publishers, 1979

Strong MS and Paparella MM. 1980 Yearbook of Otolaryngology. Chicago, Year Book Medical Publishers, 1980

Waite DE. Textbook of Practical Oral Surgery. Philadelphia, Lea & Febiger, 1978

Wood RP II, Northern JL and Jafek BW. Manual of Otolaryngology. Baltimore, Williams & Wilkins, 1979

Articles

General

Current care for pharyngitis. Patient Care 1980 Dec 15; 14(21):50–92

Current care for sinusitis. Patient Care 1980 Dec 15; 14(21):97–111

Sheffield RW et al. Complications of sinusitis. Postgrad Med 1978 March; 63(3):93

Stewart TW Jr. Common otolaryngologic problems of flying. Am Fam Physician 1979 Feb; 19(2):113–119

Wang RN. Streptococcal sore throat. Am J Nurs 1977 Nov; 77(11):1796–1798

Nose

Hayden GF. Olfactory diagnosis in medicine. Postgrad Med 1980 April; 67(4):110–118

Nasal hyperthermia may help cold symptoms. AORN J 1980 Jan; 31(6):72

Newman RK and Johnson JT. Nasal airway obstruction. Postgrad Med 1980 Aug; 68(2):184–191

Stewart TW Jr. Vasomotor rhinitis. Postgrad Med 1980 Jan; 67(1):171–178

Thomas JN. Submucous resection: A 2-year follow-up survey. J Laryngol Otol 1978 Aug; 92(8):661–666

Throat

Baker BM and Cunningham CA. Focal rehabilitation of the patient with a laryngectomy. Oncol Nurs Forum 1980 Fall; 7(4):23–36

Beukelman DR et al. Objective assessment of laryngectomized patients with surgical reconstruction. Arch Otolaryngol 1980 Nov; 106 (11):715–718

DeSanto LW et al. Cancers of the larynx: Glottic cancer. Surg Clin North Am 1977 June; 57(3):611–620

Gartside G. Mr. Smith's total laryngectomy. Nursing Times 1980 Oct 23; 76(43):1884–1885

Johnson JT, Newman RK and Olson JE. Persistent hoarseness. Postgrad Med 1980 May; 67(5):122–126

Lidocaine may prevent post-op laryngospasm. AORN J 1980 Jan; 31(1):76

Sherry D. The bond (terminal cancer of the larynx). Nursing '79 1979 Sept; 9(7):120

Sisson GA. Total laryngectomy and reconstruction of a pseudoglottis: Problems and complications. Laryngoscope 1978 April; 88(4):639–647

Sisson GA and Goldman ME. Pseudoglottis procedure: Updated secondary reconstruction techniques. Laryngoscope 1980 July; 90(7):1120–1129

Stallings JO, Daghestani A and Peterson C. Restoration of the voice after total laryngectomy. Ear Nose Throat J 1979 Jan; 58(1):83–89

Vaughan CW, Strong MS and Jako GJ. Laryngeal carcinoma: Transoral treatment utilizing the CO_2 laser. Am J Surg 1978 Oct; 136(4):440–443

Weaver AW and Fleming SM. Partial laryngectomy: Analysis of associated swallowing disorders. Am J Surg 1978 Oct; 136(4):486–489

INTENSIVE RESPIRATORY THERAPY

Books

Blodgett D. Manual of Respiratory Care Procedures. Philadelphia, JB Lippincott, 1980

Bushnell SS and Morrison ML. Respiratory Intensive Care Nursing, 2nd ed. Boston, Little, Brown & Co, 1979

DeKornfeld TJ. Selected Papers in Respiratory Therapy. Garden City, Medical Examination Publishing Co, 1979

Egan DF. Fundamentals of Respiratory Therapy, 3rd ed. St. Louis, C.V. Mosby, 1977

Haas A et al. Pulmonary Therapy and Rehabilitation: Principles and Practice. Baltimore, Williams & Wilkins, 1979

Harper RW. A Guide To Respiratory Care: Physiology and Clinical Applications. Philadelphia, JB Lippincott, 1981

Hechtman HB (ed). Acute Respiratory Failure: Etiology and Treatment. Boca Raton, Florida, CRC Press, 1979

Kacmarek RM, Dimas S and Mack CW. The Essentials of Respiratory Therapy. Chicago, Year Book Medical Publishers, 1979

Lehnert BE and Schachter EN. The Pharmacology of Respiratory Care. St. Louis, C.V. Mosby, 1980

Rau JL Jr. Respiratory Therapy Pharmacology. Chicago, Year Book Medical Publishers, 1978

Shapiro BA, Harrison RA and Trout CA. Clinical Application of Respiratory Care. Chicago, Year Book Medical Publishers, 1979

Simons NM (ed). The Psychological Aspects of Intensive Care Nursing. Bowie, Robert J Brady Co, 1980

Sweetwood HM. Nursing in the Intensive Respiratory Care Unit, 2nd ed. New York, Springer Pub. Co., 1979

Articles

Adams NR. The nurse's role in systematic weaning from a ventilator. Nursing '79 1979 Aug; 9(8):34–41

Kirilloff LH and Maszkiewicz RC. Guide to respiratory care in critically ill adults. Am J Nurs 1979 Nov; 79(11):2005–2012

Moody A. Oxygen therapy. JEN 1979 July–Aug; 5(4):15–20

Moore VB. Analyzing the ABG analysis. Nursing '79 1979 Sept; 9(9):28–33

Preventing and correcting tube and cuff problems in artificial airways. Nursing '80 1980 Jan; 10(1):65–67

Promisloff RA. Administering oxygen safely: When, why, how. Nursing '80 1980 Oct; 10(10):54–56

Shrake K. The ABCs of ABGs or how to interpret a blood gas value. Nursing '79 1979 Sept; 9(9):26–33

Sladen A. Emergency endotracheal intubation: Who can—who should. Chest 1979 May; 75(5):535–536

Sumner SM. Refining your technique for drawing arterial blood gases. Nursing '80 1980 April; 10(4):65–69

Welch MA Jr. Methods of intermittent positive pressure breathing. Chest 1980 Sept; 78(3):463–467

THE CHEST
Books

Bordow RA, Stool EW and Moser KM. Manual of Clinical Problems in Pulmonary Medicine. Boston, Little, Brown & Co, 1980

Burton GG, Gee GN and Hodgkin JE. Respiratory Care. Philadelphia, JB Lippincott, 1977

Chewing B. Staff Manual for Teaching Patients About Chronic Obstructive Pulmonary Disease. Chicago, American Hospital Association, 1979

Chicago Lung Association. Chronic Obstructive Pulmonary Disease. Chicago, Chicago Lung Association, 1977

Cordell RA and Ellison RG (eds). Complications of Intrathoracic Surgery. Boston, Little, Brown & Co, 1979

Cox BG, Carr TD and Lee RE. Living with Lung Cancer: A Reference Book for People with Lung Cancer and Their Families. Rochester, Mayo Foundation, 1977

Daughtry DC. Thoracic Trauma. Boston, Little, Brown & Co, 1980

Fishman AP. Pulmonary Diseases and Disorders. New York, McGraw-Hill, 1980

Forgacs P. Lung Sounds. London, Bailliere Tindall, 1978

Guenter CA and Welch MH. Pulmonary Medicine. Philadelphia, JB Lippincott, 1977

Hinshaw HC and Murray JF. Diseases of the Chest, 4th ed. Philadelphia, WB Saunders, 1980

Hodgkin JE. Chronic Obstructive Pulmonary Disease. Park Ridge, American College of Chest Physicians, 1979

Kacmarek RM, Dimas S and Mack CW. The Essentials of Respiratory Therapy. Chicago, Year Book Medical Publishers, 1979

Peterson BE. Cancer of the Lung. Littleton, PSG Publishing, 1979

Pinet F et al. Selective Bronchography and Bronchial Brushing. New York, Springer-Verlag, 1979

Ruppel G. Manual of Pulmonary Function Testing, 2nd ed. St. Louis, C.V. Mosby, 1979

Shapiro BA, Harrison RA and Trout CA. Clinical Application of Respiratory Care, 2nd ed. Chicago, Year Book Medical Publishers, 1979

Shibel EM and Moser KM. Respiratory Emergencies. St. Louis, C.V. Mosby, 1977

Tashkin DP and Cassan SM. Guide to Pulmonary Medicine. New York, Grune & Stratton, 1978

Articles

Assessment; Diagnosis

Blackburn NA and Cebenka DL. Honing your respiratory assessment techniques. RN 1980 May; 43(5):28–33

Brandstetter RD and Cohen RP. Hypoxemia after thoracentesis. JAMA 1979 Sept 17; 242(10):1060–1061

Editorial. Listening to the lungs. Br Med J 1978 Dec 2; 2(6151):1515–1516

Grossbach-Landis I and McLane AM. Tracheal suctioning: A tool for evaluation and learning needs assessment. Nurs Res 1979 July–Aug; 28(4):237–242

Herman PG. Needle biopsy of lung. Ann Thorac Surg 1978 Nov; 26(5):395–396

Hirsch A et al. Pleural effusion; laboratory tests in 300 cases. Thorax 1979 Feb; 34(1):106–112

Irwin RS, Demers RR. Management of the patient with cough. Compr Ther 1979 Oct; 5(10):43–49

Jones CC. Asepsis in pulmonary care: Improving old traditions. J Neurosurg Nurs 1979 June; 11(2):76–82

Kirillof LH and Maszkiewicz RC. Guide to respiratory care in critically ill adults. Am J Nurs 1979 Nov; 79(11):2005–2012

Moody LE, Martindale CL. Effect of pulmonary hygiene measures on levels of arterial oxygen saturation in adults with chronic lung disease. Heart Lung 1978 March–April; 7(2):315–319

Perrault JL. Hemoptysis: A major respiratory symptom. Compr Ther 1979 Oct; 5(10):50–54

Programmed Instruction. Pulmonary function tests in patient care. Am J Nurs 1980 June; 80(6):1135–1161

Richards V. Tube thoracostomy. J Fam Pract 1978 March; 6(3):629–635

Sagel SS et al. Percutaneous transthoracic aspiration needle and biopsy. Ann Thorac Surg 1978 Nov; 26(5):399–405

Sandham G and Reid B. Some Q's and A's about suctioning. Nursing '77 1977 Oct; 7(10):60–65

Sinner WN. Pulmonary neoplasms diagnosed with transthoracic needle biopsy. Cancer 1979 April; 43(4):1533–1540

Chronic Obstructive Pulmonary Disease

Bouhuys A, Beck GJ and Schoenberg JB. Priorities in prevention of chronic lung diseases. Lung 1979 May 18; 156(2):129–148

Broussard R. Using relaxation for COPD. Am J Nurs 1979 November; 79(11):1962–1963

Kaufman JS and Woody JW. For patients with COPD: Better living through teaching. Nursing '80 1980 March; 10(3):57–61

Petty TL (ed). Chronic obstructive pulmonary disease. Lung Biology in Health and Disease 1978; 9:1–244

Petty TL Outpatient oxygen therapy in chronic obstructive pulmonary disease. A review of 15 years' experience and an evaluation of modes of therapy. Arch Intern Med 1979 Jan; 139(1):28–32

Postma DS et al. Prognosis in severe chronic obstructive pulmonary disease. Am Rev Respir Dis 1979 March; 119(3):357–367

Skillman JJ. Terminal care in patients with chronic lung disease. Arch Intern Med 1979 Aug; 139(8):917–919

Taylor CM. Caring for the chronically ill—one day at a time. Nursing '78 1978 Sept; 8(9):59–61

White B et al. Pulmonary rehabilitation in an ambulatory group practice setting. Med Clin North Am 1979 March; 63(2):379–390

Lung Cancer; Thoracic Surgery

Adlkofer RM and Powaser MM. The effect of endotracheal suctioning on arterial blood gases in patients after cardiac surgery. Heart Lung 1978 Nov–Dec; 7(6):1011–1014

Bleeker JAC. Brief psychotherapy with lung cancer patients. Psychother Psychosom 1978; 29(1–4):282–287

Bricker PL. Chest tubes. the crucial points you mustn't forget. RN 1980 Nov; 43(11):20–26

Butler TP. 5-Fluorouracil, adriamycin and mitomycin-C (FAM) chemotherapy for adenocarcinoma of the lung. Cancer 1979 April; 43(4):1183–1188

Chang AE et al. Evaluation of computed tomography in the detection of pulmonary metastases: a prospective study. Cancer 1979 March; 43(3):913–916

Cohen MH et al. Thymosin fraction V and intensive combination chemotherapy. JAMA 1979 Apr 27; 241(17):1813–1815

Cooper JD, Nelems JM and Pearson FG. Extended indications for median sternotomy in patients requiring pulmonary resection Ann Thoracic Surg 1978 Nov; 26(5):413–420

Editorial. Choice of treatment in operable lung cancer. Br Med J 1979 Apr 14; 1(6169):970–971

Golomb HM and DeMeester TR. Lung cancer: A combined modality approach to staging and therapy. CA 1979 Sept–Oct; 29(5):258–275

Goodwin JO. Programmed instruction for self-care following pulmonary surgery. Int J Nurs Stud 1979; 16(1):29–40

Gracey DR, Divertie MB and Didier EP. Pre-op pulmonary preparation of patients with chronic obstructive pulmonary disease: A prospective study. Chest 1979 Aug; 76(2):123–129

Greco FA and Oldham RK. current concepts in cancer: Small-cell lung cancer. N Engl J Med 1979 Aug 16; 301(7):355–358

Greco FA et al. Small cell lung cancer. Am J Med 1979 April; 66(4):625–630

Harris CC (ed). Pathogenesis and therapy of lung cancer. Lung Biol Health Dis 1978; 10:653–700

Ioachim HL. Present trends in lung cancer. Monogr Pathol 1978; 19:192–214

Kemeny MM et al. Results of surgical treatment of carcinoma of the lung by stage and cell type. Surg Gynecol Obstet 1978 Dec; 147(6):865–871

Kirsh MM, Tashian J and Sloan H. Clinical presentation and management of patients with carcinoma of the lung: A 14-year experience. J Fam Pract 1979 June; 8(9): 1127–1131

Luce JM. Preoperative evaluation and perioperative management of patients with pulmonary disease. Postgrad Med 1980 Jan; 67(1):201–207

Mussia FM and Rozencweig M (eds). Lung cancer: Progress in therapeutic research. Progress in Cancer Research and Therapy 1979; 11:457

Panettiere FJ and Constanzi JJ. Advances in the chemotherapy and immunotherapy of lung cancer. Tex Med 1979 Feb; 75(2):95–97

Peters RM. Management of surgically treated patients with limited pulmonary reserve. Am J Surg 1979 Sept; 138(3):379–383

Seagren SL. A detailed guide to managing the patient with lung cancer. Med Times 1979 May; 107(5):31–38

Slawson Rg and Scott RM. Radiation therapy in bronchogenic carcinoma. Radiology 1979 July; 132(1):175–176

Van De Water JM. The chest tube. A procedure for proper placement. Postgrad Med 1980 July; 68(1):156–158

Occupational Lung Diseases

Irwin RS and Corrao WF. Sarcoidosis. Primary Care 1978 Sept; 5(3):447–464

Longley EO. Dust diseases of the lungs. Med J Aust 1978 Nov 4; 2(10):474–476

Redmond JB. Physician advisory—health effects of asbestos. Clin Toxicol 1978 Dec; 13(5):641–643

Schaefer GL. Asbestosis. West J Med 1979 July; 131(1):46–47

Wagner JC. Diseases associated with exposure to asbestos dusts. Practitioner 1979 July; 223(1333)28–33

Ziskind MM. Occupational pulmonary disease. Clin Symp 1978; 30(4):1–32

Pneumonia; Lung Abscess

Brown RB and Landis JN. Update on nonhospital-acquired pneumonias. Primary Care 1978 Sept; 6(3):463–481

Coyle N and Arbit E. How to protect your patients against aspiration pneumonia. Nursing '78 1978 Oct; 8(10):50–51

Cunha BA and Quintiliani R. The atypical pneumonias. Postgrad Med 1979 Sept; 66(3):95–102

Finland M. Pneumonia and pneumococcal infections with special reference to pneumococcal pneumonias. Am Rev Respir Dis 1979 Sept; 120(3):481–502

Green SL. Anaerobic pleuro-pulmonary infections. Postgrad Med 1979 Jan; 65(1):62–74

Hankins JR et al. Bronchopleural fistula. J Thorac Cardiovasc Surg 1978 Dec; 76(6):755–762

Jacobson JA. Pneumococcal pneumonia: Diagnosis, therapy and prevention. Compr Ther 1979 Oct; 5(10):55–60

Levine DP and Lerner AM. The clinical spectrum of Mycoplasma pneumoniae infections. Med Clin North Am 1978 Sept; 62(5):961–978

Pantell RH and Stewart TJ. The pneumococcal vaccine. JAMA 1979 May 25; 241(21):2272–2274

Rowe LD et al. Transbronchial drainage of pulmonary abscesses with the flexible fiberoptic bronchoscope. Laryngoscope 1979 Jan; 89(1):122–128

Tuazon CU. Aspiration pneumonia and anaerobic lung infections. Primary Care 1978 Sept; 5(3):487–501

Wallace RJ et al. Carcinomatous lung abscess. JAMA 1979 Aug 10; 242(6):521–522

Pulmonary Embolism

Atik M and Broghamer WL. The impact of prophylactic measures on fatal pulmonary embolism. Arch Surg 1979 April; 114(4):366–369

Baker RJ. Prophylaxis against pulmonary thromboembolism. Curr Surg 1979 May–June; 36(3):149–150

Doyle J. The intracaval filter: New nursing challenge. RN 1980 May; 43(5):38–42

Evarts CM. Thromboembolic disease. Instructional Course Lectures 1979; 28:67–71

Harvey-Smith W. Pulmonary embolism. Nurse Pract 1979 March–June; 4(2):43–44

Rosen RL. Heparin and warfarin: Use of anticoagulants in the prevention and treatment of venous thrombosis and pulmonary embolism. J Fam Pract 1979 May; 8(5):923–927

Sasahara A, Sharma GVRK and Parisi AF. New developments in the detection and prevention of venous thromboembolism. Am J Cardiol 1979 June; 43(6)1214–1224

Sharma GVRK and Sasahara AA. Diagnosis and treatment of pulmonary embolism. Med Clin North Am 1979 Jan; 63(1):239–250

Sigel B et al. Risk assessment of pulmonary embolism by multivariate analysis. Arch Surg 1979 Feb; 114(2):188–192

Wolfe WG and Sabiston DC Jr. Pulmonary embolism. Major Probl Clin Surg 1980; 25:1–175

Trauma

Budassi SA. Chest trauma. Nurs Clin North Am 1978 Sept; 13(3):533–541

Christensson P et al. Early and late results of controlled ventilation in flail chest. Chest 1979 April; 75(4):456–460

Corso P. Chest trauma. Primary Care 1978 Sept; 5(3):543–555

Goodwin JO. Programmed instruction for self-care following pulmonary surgery. Int J Nurs Stud 1979; 16(1):29–40

Griffith GL. Acute traumatic hemothorax. Ann Thorac Surg 1978 Sept; 26(3):204–207

Hancock EW. Cardiac tamponade. Med Clin North Am 1979 Jan; 63(1):223–237

Hankins JR et al. Management of flail chest: An analysis of 99 cases. Am Surg 1979 March; 45(3):176–181

Oparah SS and Mandal AK. Operative management of penetrating wounds of the chest in civilian practice. J Thorac Cardiovasc Surg 1979 Feb; 77(2):162–168

Programmed instruction: How to work with chest tubes. Am J Nurs 1980 April; 80(4):685–712

Sandra S. Management of penetrating stab wounds of the chest: an assessment of the indications for early operation. Thorax 1978 Aug; 33(4):474–478

Symbas PN. Acute traumatic hemothorax. Ann Thorac Surg 1978 Sept; 26(3):195–196

8

BLOOD DISORDERS

CELLULAR COMPONENTS OF NORMAL BLOOD

Erythrocytes (Red Blood Cells)

1. Comprise the vast majority of all blood cells; chiefly responsible for the color of blood.
2. Approximately 5 million erythrocytes per cu. mm. of blood.
3. Normal red cell has no nucleus; it is a biconcave disk.
4. Mature red blood cells consist primarily of hemoglobin, which makes up 95% of cell mass.
   a. Presence of a large amount of hemoglobin enables the cell to perform its principal function, the transport of oxygen between lungs and tissues.
   b. Iron is present in the heme portion of the molecule.
5. Whole blood normally contains about 15 gm. of hemoglobin per 100 ml. of blood.
6. Red blood cells are produced in red bone marrow, which also provides most of the blood's leukocytes and all of its platelets.
   Red cells of normal adults found in short and flat bones—ribs, sternum, skull, vertebrae, bones of the hands and feet, pelvis.
7. For normal erythrocyte production, the bone marrow requires iron, vitamin B_{12}, folic acid, pyridoxine (vitamin B_6), and other factors.
   If any of these factors is deficient during erythropoiesis (production of erythrocytes), decreased red blood cell production and anemia result.
8. Normal life expectancy of a red cell is between 115 and 130 days—then eliminated by phagocytosis in the reticuloendothelial system, predominantly in spleen and liver.

Leukocytes (White Blood Cells)

1. Normally the total leukocyte count is 5,000 to 10,000 cells per mm^3. Leukocytes can be differentiated from erythrocytes by the presence of a nucleus, their larger size, and different staining properties.
2. Three series of leukocytes are recognized: granulocytes, lymphocytes, and monocytes.
   a. *Granulocytes* (produced in marrow) comprise 70% of all white cells.
      (1) Called *granulocytes* because of the abundant granules contained in their cytoplasm or *polymorphonuclear leukocytes*, since their nuclei, when mature, are of a highly irregular, multilobed configuration.
      (2) Granulocytes are divided into 3 subgroups according to their staining properties: eosinophils, basophils, neutrophils.
   b. *Lymphocytes* comprise approximately 30% of white cells; produced primarily in the lymph nodes and lymphoid tissue.
   c. *Monocytes* comprise approximately 5% of total leukocytes; largest of the blood leukocytes; produced in bone marrow.
3. Function of the leukocytes is to protect the body from invasion by foreign cells (e.g., bacteria)—provide protection by phagocytosis, production of antibodies, and rejection of foreign tissue.
   a. The chief function of some granulocytes is phagocytosis; others (eosinophils and basophils) function as reservoirs of potent biological materials such as histamine, serotonin, and heparin. Release

of these compounds alters blood supply to the tissues and helps mobilize body defense mechanisms.

b. Lymphocytes produce substances (interferon, transfer factor, antibodies, etc.) that aid in attacking foreign material; responsible for the immunocompetence of an individual and for the long-term immunologic memory.

4. Loss of leukocyte activity causes patient to have diminished resistance to infections and reduction in number of leukocytes.

Platelets (Thrombocytes)

1. Are the smallest and most fragile of the formed elements; are small particles (devoid of nuclei) that arise as a result of budding from giant cells called *megakaryocytes* in the bone marrow.

2. Number approximately 150,000–300,000 platelets per cubic millimeter of blood.

3. Prime function to halt bleeding—important in the formation of clots at site of injury to blood vessels; maintain the integrity of the vascular epithelium.

a. Their granules contain adenosine diphosphate (ADP), calcium, serotonin, epinephrine, and other chemical substances.

b. After tissue injury, circulating platelets stick to the damaged blood vessel walls, release their granules, and form primary hemostatic plug.

c. The serotonin and epinephrine cause vasoconstriction at the site of injury, and the ADP promotes release of the granules from other platelets.

d. Additional substances released from platelets activate coagulation factors in the blood plasma.

COMMON PROBLEMS OF PATIENTS WITH BLOOD DISORDERS

The Problem	Nursing Management
Fatigue and weakness	Plan nursing care to conserve the patient's strength. Give frequent rest periods. Encourage ambulation activities as tolerated. Avoid disturbing activities, noise, stress, or any activity which ordinarily increases heart rate or cardiac output. Encourage optimal nutrition.
Hemorrhagic tendencies	Encourage patient to protect himself from injury. Avoid medications containing aspirin. Keep the patient at rest during the bleeding episodes. Apply gentle pressure to the bleeding sites. Apply cold compresses to the bleeding sites when indicated. Avoid disturbing clots. Use small gauge needles when administering medications by injection. Give a Popsicle to the patient who is bleeding orally—induces vasoconstriction. Observe for symptoms of internal bleeding. Check supine and standing blood pressure and pulse; if pulse or BP goes up, patient is not stable. Have a tracheostomy set available for the patient who is bleeding from the mouth or throat; observe for signs of asphyxiation. Support the patient during transfusion therapy.
Oral manifestations Bleeding gums, with sore mouth and difficulty in eating Thrush—from antibiotics altering mouth flora and general debility	Encourage regular dental visits—bleeding gums occur when there is gross tartar on teeth. Transfuse the patient with appropriate agents. Avoid irritating foods and beverages. Give frequent oral hygiene with mild, cool mouthwash solutions (sodium perborate and sodium hydrogen tartrate). Use cotton-tipped applicators or soft-bristled toothbrush. Use automatic toothbrush with an oscillating movement—exerts even pressure on gums, and small brush can reach all parts of mouth; appears to harden gums and control bleeding. Keep the lips lubricated. Give mouth care both before and after meals.
Dyspnea	Elevate the head of the bed. Use pillows to support the patient in the orthopneic position. Administer oxygen when indicated. Prevent unnecessary exertion. Avoid gas-forming foods.
Bone and joint pains	Relieve pressure of bedding by using a cradle. Administer either hot or cold compresses as prescribed. Provide for joint immobilization when prescribed.

The Problem	Nursing Management
Fever	Administer cool sponges.
	Give antipyretic drugs as prescribed.
	Encourage liberal fluid intake unless contraindicated.
	Maintain a cool environmental temperature.
Pruritus or skin eruptions	Keep the patient's fingernails short.
	Use soap sparingly.
	Apply emollient lotions in skin care.
	Give antihistamines as prescribed.
Anxiety of patient and his family	Explain the nature, the discomforts, and the limitations of activity associated with the diagnostic procedures and treatments.
	Encourage the patient to verbalize his *feelings*.
	Offer the patient the service of listening.
	Display an empathetic and accepting attitude.
	Promote the patient's relaxation and comfort.
	Remember the patient's individual preferences.
	Promote a sense of independence and self-care within the patient's limitations.
	Encourage the family to participate in the patient's care (as desired).
	Create a comfortable atmosphere for the family's visits with the patient.

BLOOD AND BONE MARROW SPECIMENS

Blood may be obtained by (1) skin puncture (finger, toe, heel, or ear lobe) or (2) venipuncture.*

A *skin puncture* is performed when only a small amount of blood is needed (for red and white cell counts, hemoglobin and hematocrit determinations,

* The most common hematologic tests are described in the Appendix, p. 1467.

reticulocyte counts, blood films for differential smear). However, the values for the red blood cells, hematocrit, hemoglobin, and platelets are lower in capillary blood than in venous blood.

A *venipuncture* is a puncture of a vein to obtain blood; used when larger amounts of blood are needed (preferred method).

GUIDELINES: Obtaining Blood by Skin Puncture

Equipment
Disposable lancet
Pipette and tubing
Slides
Alcohol sponges and dry sterile sponges

Procedure

NURSING ACTION	RATIONALE/AMPLIFICATION
Performance Phase	
1. Cleanse site (preferably ball of finger) with alcohol and dry with sterile gauze square.	1. If any alcohol remains, it will alter blood cell morphology; also it will not collect into a compact drop but will run down the patient's finger.
2. Create stasis by pressing on the distal joint of the finger to produce redness at the end the finger.	
3. Use a sterile disposable lancet, or an automated lancet.	3. This avoids the possibility of the transference of the hepatitis virus.
4. Prick the skin sharply and quickly with the lancet.	4. Pricking the skin sharply and quickly minimizes pain and produces a free-flowing sample.
5. Release pressure on the finger. Wipe off the first drop of blood.	5. Epithelial or endothelial cells may be found in the first drop of blood and render the count inaccurate. Also platelets will begin to clump immediately in the blood at the puncture site.
6. Allow the blood to flow freely with an adequate puncture.	6. Pressing out the blood dilutes it with tissue fluid.
7. Obtain the blood sample a. Fill the pipette. b. Make blood slides according to the study required.	
8. Apply pressure over the wound with a dry gauze sponge until bleeding stops	

GUIDELINES: Obtaining Blood by Venipuncture

Veins Used Antecubital area
Wrist
Dorsum (back) of hand
Top of foot

Equipment 70% alcohol and tincture of iodine
Dry sterile sponges
5 and 10-ml. syringe
No. 20 gauge needle(s)

Procedure

NURSING ACTION	RATIONALE/AMPLIFICATION
Performance Phase	
1. Reassure patient. Explain that relatively little blood will be taken.	1. The patient is reassured when the nurse displays self-assurance and competence in relating to people and when performing technical skills.
2. Instruct the patient to extend his arm; the arm should be held straight at the elbow.	
3. Apply the tourniquet directly above the elbow with just sufficient pressure to prevent venous return.	3. A tourniquet increases venous pressure and makes the vein more prominent and easier to enter.
4. Inspect the area to visualize the vein. Palpate the vein.	4. Select a vein that is visible, palpable, and well fixed to surrounding tissue so it does not roll away. (Not all veins are visible; some may be deep and can only be palpated.)
5. Cleanse the skin with iodine and alcohol. Dry.	5. Cleansing the skin reduces pathogens.
6. Fix chosen vein with the thumb and draw the skin taut immediately below the site before inserting needle to stabilize the vein.	6. The vein may roll beneath the skin when the needle approaches its outer surface (especially in elderly and extremely thin patients).
7. Hold the syringe between the thumb and last 3 fingers with the bevel up and directly in line with the course of the vein. Insert the needle quickly and smoothly under the skin and into the vein.	
8. Release the tourniquet.	
9. Obtain blood sample by *gently* pulling back on the plunger.	9. Use minimal suction to prevent hemolysis of blood and collapse of the vein.
10. Withdraw the needle slowly.	10. Slow withdrawal of the needle is less painful.
11. Gauze is applied with pressure over the puncture site for 2–4 minutes.	11. Firm pressure over the puncture site prevents leakage of blood into surrounding tissues with subsequent hematoma development. Merely flexing the arm may not prevent a hematoma as the vein can slip to the side of the area where pressure is applied.
12. Make the blood smear from the needle as desired.	
13. Remove the needle from the syringe. Gently eject the blood sample into a test tube containing an anticoagulant.	13. Slowly transfer the blood into the test tube *without* forming bubbles.
14. Place stopper on the test tube.	
15. Invert the tube gently several times to mix blood with anticoagulant.	
16. Label specimens correctly and send to laboratory immediately.	16. Specimens should go to the lab with a minimum of delay for optimum reliability.
17. Dispose of needle and syringe in appropriate containers to avoid possible spread of hepatitis. Clean all spills with alcohol and peroxide or other antiseptic agents according to agency policy.	

GUIDELINES: Bone Marrow Aspiration and Biopsy

Bone marrow aspiration or biopsy is done so that specimens of bone marrow and bone can be obtained for establishing a diagnosis.

Purposes 1. To diagnose hematologic disease—enables the precursors of cells in peripheral blood to be examined and their relative numbers determined; to evaluate for iron content.

2. To follow the course of disease and the patient's response to treatment.
3. To diagnose diseases other than pure hematologic disorders, such as primary and metastatic tumors, infectious diseases, certain granulomas, and parasitic infestations.
4. To isolate bacteria and other pathogenic agents by culture or animal inoculation.

Complications

1. Osteomyelitis (rare)
2. Bleeding and hematoma in patients with bleeding disorders
3. Puncture of vital organs if biopsy is too deep

Equipment

Bone marrow aspiration tray
  Marrow aspiration needles with stylets
  Sterile towels
  No. 25 and 22 gauge needles
  Two 20-ml. syringes
  Three 5-ml. syringes
Local anesthetic (1% procaine or xylocaine)
Gauze squares
Sterile gloves, drape
Skin antiseptic
Laboratory equipment
  Coverslips
  Microscopic slides
  Test tubes (plain and heparinized)
Scalpel blade and handle
Culture tubes when indicated

Procedure

NURSING ACTION

Preparatory Phase

1. Explain the procedure to the patient. Tell patient when the skin will be marked, antiseptic applied, and when the needle puncture will be performed.

2. Give medication (meperidine) or tranquilizer as requested; usually not necessary for aspiration.

3. Place the patient in prone or supine position.
4. Shave area. The following sites may be used:
   a. Iliac crest (posterior superior iliac spine)
   b. Spinous processes of vertebrae (usually 2nd or 3rd lumbar vertebra)
   c. Sternum
   d. Tibia—up to the age of 2 years

ILIAC CREST ASPIRATION/BIOPSY

Performance Phase *(by physician)*
Anterior Approach

1. Position the patient on his side with top knee flexed.
   a. The posterior superior iliac spine is located and marked.
   b. The skin area is prepared and draped. The marked area is infiltrated with local anesthetic through the skin and subcutaneous tissue to the periosteum of the bone.
   c. A small incision may be made.

   d. The bone marrow needle, with stylet in place, is introduced through the incision.

   e. The needle is advanced and rotated by using firm and steady pressure. When the needle is felt to enter the outer cortex of the bone marrow cavity, the stylet is removed and the syringe attached. Negative pressure is applied and a small volume of blood and marrow are aspirated.

RATIONALE/AMPLIFICATION

1. An explanation helps the patient to cope with anticipated stress. Tactile sensations (pressure, cold) can be misinterpreted as pain unless patient is forewarned.

2. Demerol may be used as an analgesic and sedative for apprehension. Anxiety may produce excessive discomfort.

b. The periosteum is the region of greatest sensitivity.

c. The biopsy needle is large, and a small incision facilitates insertion.
d. The needle is pointed toward the anterior superior iliac spine and brought into contact with the posterior iliac spine.
e. There is usually decreased resistance when the bone marrow cavity is entered.

  The actual aspiration may cause brief pain and the patient should be forewarned.

  Bone marrow appears rusty-red and normally has a thick, fluid-like consistency.

GUIDELINES: Bone Marrow Aspiration and Biopsy (cont.)

Procedure (cont.)	NURSING ACTION	RATIONALE/AMPLIFICATION

STERNAL ASPIRATION

***Performance Phase** (by physician)*

1. The skin is prepared and the site infiltrated with procaine or xylocaine.
2. The site selected is usually the midsternal line at the level of the 2nd interspace.
3. A small stab incision may be made before bone marrow needle insertion.
4. The marrow needle with stylet in place is inserted through the cortex of the bone with a slight rotating motion. The physician usually feels a "give" in the marrow needle when the marrow cavity has been penetrated.
5. The stylet is removed and a syringe attached to the hub of the needle. The plunger is withdrawn slowly until marrow appears in the syringe (0.2 ml. of fluid is aspirated).
6. Warn the patient that he will feel a brief episode of sharp pain.
7. The syringe and needle are removed and passed to a technician for preparation of smears.
8. Pressure is applied over the puncture site until bleeding (if any) ceases.
9. A small dressing is applied with pressure over the puncture site.

2. The sternum is thinner and marrow more plentiful between the sternal interspaces.
3. This technique avoids pushing the skin into the bone marrow.
4. A sternal puncture is considered more dangerous than other sites because of its proximity to vital structures in the mediastinum, it is not usually used for biopsy.
5. The marrow will appear as thick, dark reddish fluid.
6. The pain is caused by suction of the syringe and lasts only a few seconds.
7. Smears of aspirated marrow are made; technique is similar to that of preparing blood smears.
8. If the patient has thrombocytopenia, pressure should be applied 5 to 10 minutes.

Follow-up Phase

1. Give mild analgesic if needed.
2. Assess patient for discomfort, continued bleeding, and untoward symptoms.

Most patients have no discomfort after aspiration, but the site of a biopsy may ache for a day or so.

TRANSFUSION THERAPY

Blood transfusion is the introduction of whole blood or blood components directly into the circulatory system.

WHOLE BLOOD AND BLOOD COMPONENTS

Whole Blood

A unit of blood (drawn from a donor) consists of approximately 450 ml. of whole blood and 60–70 ml. of anticoagulant.
1. Used to restore or maintain blood's oxygen-carrying capacity as well as its intravascular volume.
2. Used clinically for acute massive blood loss and hypovolemic shock due to hemorrhage.

Blood Components

A blood component is administered when a specific component is needed; less risk to the patient than whole blood.
1. *Red cells* (packed red cells) are erythrocytes separated from a unit of whole blood by centrifugation or sedimentation; about 80% of the plasma is removed, leaving a hematocrit of 60–70%. The plasma is used for the preparation of various plasma fractions such as albumin, cryoprecipitate, or gamma globulin.
   a. Most useful of all the components; provides the same oxygen-carrying capacity as whole blood while minimizing potential hazards; less immunologic problems (most donor antibodies removed); fewer electrolyte problems as it contains less sodium, potassium, etc. than whole blood.
   b. Appropriate component for management of chronic anemia when transfusions are required.
   c. Administered through a large bore needle at a flow rate *slower* than whole blood, but may be diluted with normal saline when more rapid flow is desired.
   NOTE: Do not mix with Ringers, D_5W or other fluids or medications.
   d. *Washed red cells* have fewer sensitizing WBCs and platelets.
2. *Platelet Transfusion*—given to patients with dangerous degrees of thrombocytopenia (decrease of platelets in circulating blood) to control or prevent bleeding.

a. Platelets may be supplied in form of:
   (1) Fresh blood—replaces red cells and platelets; should be less than 12 hours old.
   (2) Platelet-rich plasma—contains 80–90% of original platelets in 200–250 ml.
   (3) Platelet concentrates—retain 70% of original platelets in viable state but reduced in volume; usually used in 4–8 unit batches.
b. The use of matched platelets is more advantageous and lessens the risk of antibody formation; more expensive and usually necessary only for refractory patients.
c. Platelet transfusions are given in the treatment of leukemia, aplastic anemia, and thrombocytopenia induced by chemotherapy or drugs.

3. *Granulocyte transfusion*—given to patients with severe and temporary bone marrow depression (granulocyte counts less than 500/cu. mm. and evidence of infection).
  a. Granulocytes are highly contaminated with RBCs and should generally be ABO compatible.
  b. Patients receiving granulocyte transfusions may experience acute reactions (fever and chills); patients with such reactions should receive antihistamines, steroids, etc. before transfusion.
  c. Usually given in a 10–14 day course of treatment.

4. *Whole Plasma*—fluid portion of the blood in which corpuscles are suspended
  a. Used for treatment of some clotting defects and correction of hypovolemia due to selective loss of plasma, mainly in burned patients.
  b. Must be ABO compatible.
  c. Largely replaced by other colloids such as albumin or electrolyte solutions (Ringer's lactate).

5. *Fresh Frozen Plasma*—plasma which has been separated immediately from freshly donated blood and then promptly frozen.
  a. Must be ABO compatible.
  b. Supplies clotting factors.

6. *Derivatives of Plasma*
  a. *Albumin*
    (1) Currently used to replace plasma in therapeutic plasma exchange procedures.
    (2) Used to expand blood volume in patients with hypovolemic shock; can be used to elevate the circulating albumin in patients with hypoalbuminemia; efficacy unproved.
    (3) Hepatitis free; no clotting factors; expensive.
  b. *Cryoprecipitate* (Factor VIII)—made from fresh frozen plasma; precipitate is separated and the rest of plasma can be used for other purposes.
    (1) Contains 60% of original factor VIII and 25% of original fibrinogen in 30 ml. Used in 6–12 bag units. Thaw at 37°C. water bath and infuse immediately.
    (2) Used for patients who are deficient in fibrinogen, factor VIII (hemophilia), von Willebrand's disease, and factor XIII.
  c. *Prothrombin Complex Concentrate*—contains prothrombin (factor II) and factors VII, IX, X.
    (1) Used for treatment of bleeding in congenital or acquired deficiencies of these factors, especially IX deficiency (Christmas disease).
    (2) High hepatitis risk; commercially available.
    (3) See package directives for diluting, storage; is reconstituted with *gentle agitation*.
  d. *Plasma Protein Fraction*
    (1) Used for volume expansion; does not have clotting factors; does not transmit hepatitis.
    (2) Commercially prepared and generally supplied by pharmacy; expensive.
  e. *Gamma globulin* (Immune serum globulin)
    (1) Given prophylactically for hepatitis B, inadvertent needle stick following use on someone suspected of having hepatitis B.
    (2) Given to attenuate (render less virulent) measles, hepatitis, poliomyelitis. Available as specific high titered globulin against hepatitis B (HBIG), Herpes Zoster (ZIG), tetanus toxoid

GUIDELINES: Administering Blood Transfusions

Blood transfusion is the introduction of blood and blood components into the body circulation.

Purposes
1. To restore circulating blood volume.
2. To stop bleeding due to coagulation factor deficiencies.
3. To improve oxygen-carrying capacity of the blood.
4. To combat infection due to decreased white cells.

Equipment
Blood administration set (disposable)
Needles, No. 22 and larger
Normal saline infusion
Blood as prescribed
Iodine-containing antiseptic
Tourniquet

Procedure

NURSING ACTION	RATIONALE/AMPLIFICATION
Preparatory Phase	
1. Make sure that the blood has been typed and cross matched. The ABO group and Rh type on the label of the blood container are checked to be certain of agreement with compatibility record.	1. Typing is done to establish the blood group (A, B, AB, or O) and Rh factor; a cross match is done to establish the compatibility between the patient's blood and the donor's.

GUIDELINES: Administering Blood Transfusions (cont.)

Procedure (cont.)

NURSING ACTION	RATIONALE/AMPLIFICATION
2. Give the blood immediately after taking it from the blood bank.	2. Storage at 1–6° C. (33.8–42.8 F.) should be maintained until just before administration. Rapid deterioration of the red blood cells can occur with uncooled blood.
3. Inspect the blood for gas bubbles and any abnormal color or cloudiness.	3. Gas bubbles may indicate bacterial growth; abnormal color or clouding may warn of hemolysis.

Performance Phase

NURSING ACTION	RATIONALE/AMPLIFICATION
1. *Check the labels identifying the donor and recipient blood (number and type) and confirm the identity of the patient who is to receive it.* Ask the patient to identify himself by his full name. Check his identification wrist band with the container identification; check his chart to make sure of his number and type.	1. Meticulous attention to detail is essential to avoid giving the wrong blood to the wrong patient (which may cause a fatal reaction).
2. Take the patient's TPR and blood pressure.	2. Baseline vital sign measurements are used for later comparisons.
3. Prepare the normal saline solution and clear the administration set of air.	3. The normal saline solution is connected to one lead of the Y infusion set.
4. Select a suitable vein (see p. 94). Cleanse skin thoroughly (alcohol and iodine). Allow to dry.	4. Skin cleansing is done to remove skin bacteria and sebum.
5. Perform the venipuncture (see p. 98).	5. Transfusion is given through a large needle or plastic catheter.
6. Allow 50 ml. of saline to run into the patient's vein.	6. Normal saline is used to flush the tubing before blood is started. Isotonic solutions are compatible with red blood cells.
7. Allow the blood to run through the blood transfusion set.	7. A filter is located between the container and the flow indicator to screen out particles that can embolize. Precipitation of platelets, leukocytes, and fibrin may clog the administration set.
8. Hang the unit of blood about a meter (3–4 feet) above the level of the patient's heart.	8. The rate of flow is determined by the height at which the bottle is suspended and the size of the needle.
9. Discontinue the saline infusion and start the blood.	
10. DO NOT GIVE MEDICATIONS IN THE BLOOD. DO NOT GIVE 5% DEXTROSE IN WATER OR RINGERS IN BLOOD. Only normal saline is compatible.	10. The addition of drugs to blood may cause a pharmacologic incompatibility between the blood or anticoagulant solution in the blood. Dextrose does not contain electrolytes and can cause hemolysis and clotting in the IV tubing. Also, bacterial contamination is a hazard whenever a unit of blood is entered.
11. Adjust the rate of blood flow to 5 ml. per minute during the first 10–30 minutes of the transfusion. Stay with the patient for at least 15–30 minutes after the start of the transfusion. If there are no signs of reaction and circulatory overloading, the infusion rate may be increased.	11. The rate of transfusion depends on the patient's condition and the product being transfused. Signs or symptoms of an untoward reaction are usually manifested during the initial 50–100 ml. of blood. If the transfusion is stopped early, acute renal failure and death rarely occur. The transfusion should be finished in about 1½ hours.
12. Give the blood at a slower rate if the patient is elderly or has heart disease.	12. Too rapid administration of blood may overload a precarious circulatory system and induce congestive heart failure and pulmonary edema. However, with severe blood loss, prompt and rapid replacement is essential.
13. Return after 15 minutes to check that the transfusion is proceeding uneventfully.	
14. Monitor central venous pressure through a separate infusion line for patients with circulatory overload problems.	
15. Watch the patient carefully. Monitor the vital signs hourly or more frequently as indicated.	15. A change in the condition of the patient may signal the development of a transfusion complication.
16. Change the administration set (tubing, filter) if another unit of blood is to be given. If another IV is to be given immediately after the transfusion, the infusion set should be rinsed with normal saline before starting solutions/drugs.	16. The filter may become clogged after a unit of blood has been given.
17. Record time started and discontinued; whether adverse effects occurred.	

Adverse Effects of Blood Transfusion

Circulatory Overloading

Due to administration of excessive volume or at a rate faster than the heart can accept. Causes a rise in venous pressure, increase in volume of blood in pulmonary blood vessels, and a diminution in lung compliance.

Clinical Manifestations:
a. Rise in venous pressure
b. Distended neck veins
c. Dyspnea
d. Cough
e. Rales heard in base of lungs

Prevention:
1. Prevent by using packed cells, proper spacing of transfusions; give at rate within circulatory reserve of patient.
2. Monitor CVP of patients with heart disease.

Management:
1. Stop transfusion immediately and keep IV open.
2. Place patient upright, with his feet in a dependent position.
3. Apply rotating tourniquets to extremities. (See p. 278.)
4. Prepare for phlebotomy.
5. Administer diuretics oxygen, morphine, aminophylline as directed.

Febrile Reaction

Due to hypersensitivity to donor white cells, platelets or plasma proteins; pyrogenic contamination of donor blood, unknown factors.

Clinical Manifestations:
(may occur after transfusion is discontinued)
a. Sudden chilling and fever
b. Headache
c. Flushing; tachycardia
d. Anxiety

Prevention:
1. Premedicate with antipyretic (acetaminophen or aspirin)

Management:
1. Stop transfusion and keep vein open. Notify physician and blood bank.
2. Save urine. Draw blood as directed. Return blood bags to bank.
3. Take temperature ½ hour after chill and as indicated thereafter.
4. Give antipyretics as prescribed; treat symptomatically.

Septic Reaction

Due to transmission of blood or components contaminated with bacteria.

Clinical Manifestations:
a. Rapid onset of chills
b. High fever
c. Vomiting; diarrhea
d. Marked hypotension

Prevention:
1. Do not allow blood to stand unnecessarily at room temperature—accelerates growth of any contaminating organism.
2. Do not warm containers of blood before transfusion.
3. Inspect blood for gas bubbles and change in color before starting transfusion.
4. Transfusions should be completed in less than 4 hours.

Management:
1. Stop transfusion immediately and keep IV open.
2. Obtain cultures of donor's blood (and recipient's blood)—send remainder of blood to lab.
3. Treat septicemia as directed—antibiotics, intravenous fluids, fresh transfusion, vasopressors, steroids. (See treatment of gram-negative shock, page 805.)

Immunologic (Allergic) Reactions

Cause of allergic reaction is thought to be sensitivity to a plasma protein in the transfused blood, or passive transfer of antibodies from the donor which react with some antigen to which the recipient is exposed.

Clinical Manifestations:
a. Flushing
b. Itching and rash
c. Urticaria (hives)
d. Asthmatic wheezing
e. Laryngeal edema

Prevention:
1. Ask patient whether he has history of allergy to blood products.
2. Give prescribed prophylactic antihistamine before blood is started to patients known to have allergic reactions to blood.

Management:
1. Stop the transfusion immediately and keep IV open.
2. Give diphenhydramine (Benadryl) as directed.
3. Observe for anaphylaxis.
4. Prepare epinephrine if respiratory distress is severe.
5. Blood is sometimes continued at a slower rate if the appearance of hives is the only clinical manifestation.

Acute Hemolytic Reaction (most severe)

Occurs when the donor blood is incompatible with that of the recipient.
(1) Antibodies in the recipient's plasma rapidly combine with the donor erythrocytes, and the cells are hemolyzed either in the circulation or in the reticuloendothelial system.
(2) May cause severe reaction accompanied by hemoglobinemia, hemoglobinuria, hypotension, disseminated intravascular coagulation, acute renal failure, death.

Clinical Manifestations:
a. Chilliness; fever
b. Low back pain
c. Feeling of head fullness; flushing
d. Oppressive feeling in chest
e. Distention of neck veins
f. Tachycardia; tachypnea
g. Fall in blood pressure and vascular depression
h. Hemoglobinuria (red urine)

Prevention:
1. Positively identify patient and blood before transfusion is started.
2. Stay with patient during the first 10–30 minutes that he is receiving the transfusion—if transfusion is stopped early, untoward (and possibly fatal) reaction may be averted.
3. Administer blood very slowly during this period.

Treatment and Nursing Management:
Objective: To correct hypotension and prevent renal damage which can follow hemoglobinuria.
1. Stop transfusion immediately—consequences are in proportion to the amount of incompatible blood given.
2. Keep IV open with saline.
3. Treat shock if present; support patient with intravenous colloid.
4. Start diuretics (furosemide) immediately to maintain urine flow, glomerular filtration, and renal blood flow.
5. Maintain volume with intravenous infusions if diuresis ensues.
6. Insert indwelling catheter; monitor hourly urinary output.
7. Suspect renal failure if diuresis does not occur—treat by fluid and electrolyte management, dialysis—at a center with these facilities.
8. Send sample of patient's blood and urine to lab for presence of hemoglobin and for tests for disseminated intravascular coagulation.

Delayed Hemolytic Reaction

1. See #1 above. Usually occurs 5–10 days after transfusion.

Clinical Manifestations:
Fever, mild jaundice, and decreased hematocrit.

Anaphylaxis

Due to anti-IgA antibody in patient who is IgA deficient.

Prevention:
Give only blood from other IgA deficient individual or frozen red cells.

Management:
As for any anaphylaxis.

Allergic Pulmonary Edema

Due to HLA antibodies in donor or recipient; seen most frequently with WBC transfusions.

Iron Overload

Iron deposition in heart, endocrine organs, liver, spleen, skin, etc. Patient develops arrhythmias, congestive heart failure, diabetes, decreased thyroid function, etc.

Seen when patient receives multiple long-term transfusions (aplastic anemia, thalassemia).

Transmission of Disease (delayed reaction)

Serum hepatitis, malaria, cytomegalovirus, syphilis (rare), and Epstein–Barr virus may be transmitted from donor to recipient via infected blood.

Prevention:
1. Screen donor carefully.
2. Reject donors with history of hepatitis or jaundice or if laboratory test is positive for hepatitis B antigen.

Summary of Nursing Responsibilities in Transfusion Reaction

1. Notify physician and blood bank immediately when a suspected transfusion reaction has occurred.
2. Stop the transfusion but keep the vein open with intravenous fluids infused through a new administration set in case intravenous medication should be needed rapidly.
3. Save the blood bag and tubing; send to blood bank for repeat typing and culture.
4. Have patient's blood drawn for plasma hemoglobin, culture, and retyping.
5. Collect urine sample and send to laboratory for a hemoglobin determination. Save subsequent voidings of urine.

BONE MARROW TRANSPLANTATION (Engraftment)

Bone marrow transplantation is the aspiration of bone by needle from multiple sites of a donor; bone marrow is then transfused intravenously into a recipient. The marrow cells travel to the marrow space which has been emptied by disease (aplastic anemia; leukemia) or by chemotherapy.

Indications for Bone Marrow Transplant

1. Aplasias with serious prognosis before patients are sensitized by transfusions.
2. Leukemias in remission and before sensitization by transfusions.
3. Immunodeficiency states.

Donor Selection

1. Syngeneic marrow grafts between identical twins (donor and recipient carrying same tissue antigens); no immunologic barrier to transplantation.
2. Matched siblings (siblings with histocompatible marrow).

3. Autologous marrow transplantation—marrow removed from patient while he is in remission from disease; frozen and then used to "rescue" patient by infusing his own stored marrow when he relapses.

Complications

1. Graft rejection
2. Graft vs. host disease
3. Infections (cytomegaloviral, gram-negative bacterial, and Candida)
4. Recurrence of original disease (i.e. leukemia)
5. Hemorrhage

Preparation of Recipient

OBJECTIVE: to prepare patient with immunosuppressive therapy so that he will not reject the marrow transplant (graft).

1. Recipient of a graft from an identical twin donor requires no immunosuppressive preparation.
2. *Preparation of Patient with Aplasia:*
   a. Cyclophosphamide given for prescribed number of days and followed 36 hours later by marrow infusion; some medical centers use total body irradiation as well.
   b. Maintain high urine flow with IV fluids and diuretics—to prevent severe cystitis due to cyclophosphamide metabolites excreted in urine.
3. *Preparation of Patient with Malignant Disorders:*
   a. Total body irradiation carried out—to kill leukemia cells.
   b. Immunosuppression with cyclophosphamide; also increases leukemia cell kill.

Technique of Marrow Transplantation (Fig. 8-1)

1. One unit of blood is obtained from marrow donor a few days before procedure; returned to donor during marrow aspiration to avoid risks of blood transfusion from another person.
2. Donor anesthetized; marrow is obtained by multiple aspirations from iliac bones.

3. Marrow aspirated, transferred into beaker, and diluted in tissue culture medium with heparin; the aspirated marrow (400–800 ml.) is passed through screens to prevent marrow emboli.
4. The marrow is infused intravenously into the recipient.
5. Chemotherapy is given for a period to prevent graft vs. host disease.

Supportive Care

OBJECTIVE: to support patient during period of marrow aplasia (no marrow function) until graft begins to function.

1. Provide an environment as pathogen-free as possible—marrow-depleted patient is prone to infection; infection accounts for the majority of deaths in transplant victims.
   a. Private room; meticulous handwashing; sterility of articles coming into room; sterilization of food; gowning and masking of personnel entering room.
   b. Laminar air-flow room when available.
2. Give nonabsorbable antibiotics (vancomycin; gentamicin; colistin)—for alimentary tract "sterilization" to minimize risk of endogenous infection.
3. Monitor for fever and other evidences of infection.
4. Give appropriate antibiotic (or antifungal) regimen after obtaining cultures of nasopharynx, oropharynx, axillae, stool, urine.
5. Prepare for granulocyte transfusion—indicated for serious bacterial or fungal infection developing in agranulocytopenic patient.
6. Continue giving immunosuppression therapy during post-transplant period—to prevent graft vs. host disease
7. Administer platelet transfusions and red blood cells—patient lacks blood cell products in immediate post-graft period and is in danger of hemorrhage.
8. Give psychological support to patient and family; acute phase of illness may last several weeks. HLA compatible relative may be required for platelet, WBC support.

ANEMIA

Anemia is a laboratory definition which implies a low red cell count and a below normal hemoglobin or hematocrit level. Physiologically anemia exists when there is an insufficient amount of hemoglobin to deliver oxygen to the tissues.

Altered Physiology

1. The appearance of anemia reflects (1) decreased production of red cells, (2) red cell loss, and (3) increased destruction.
2. Marrow failure may occur as a result of nutritional deficiency, toxic exposure, tumor invasion, or unknown causes.
3. Red cells may be lost through hemorrhage or hyperhemolysis (increased destruction).
   a. This problem may be rooted in some red-cell defect that is incompatible with normal red-cell survival or is explainable on the basis of some factor extrinsic to the red cell that promotes red-cell destruction.
   b. Red-cell lysis occurs mainly within the phagocytic cells of the reticuloendothelial system, notably within the liver and spleen.
   c. As a by-product of this process, bilirubin, formed from hemoglobin within the phagocyte, enters the bloodstream, and an increase in hemolysis is promptly reflected by an increase in total plasma bilirubin.

Clinical Manifestations

(Any manifestations are attributable to a decrease in the oxygen-carrying capacity of the blood, and are the same regardless of the cause of anemia.)

1. The more rapidly the anemia develops, the more severe its symptoms:
   a. Pallor
   b. Susceptibility to fatigue
   c. Shortness of breath
   d. Headache; disturbed cerebration; dizziness
   e. Predisposition to angina pectoris or congestive heart failure in susceptible individuals

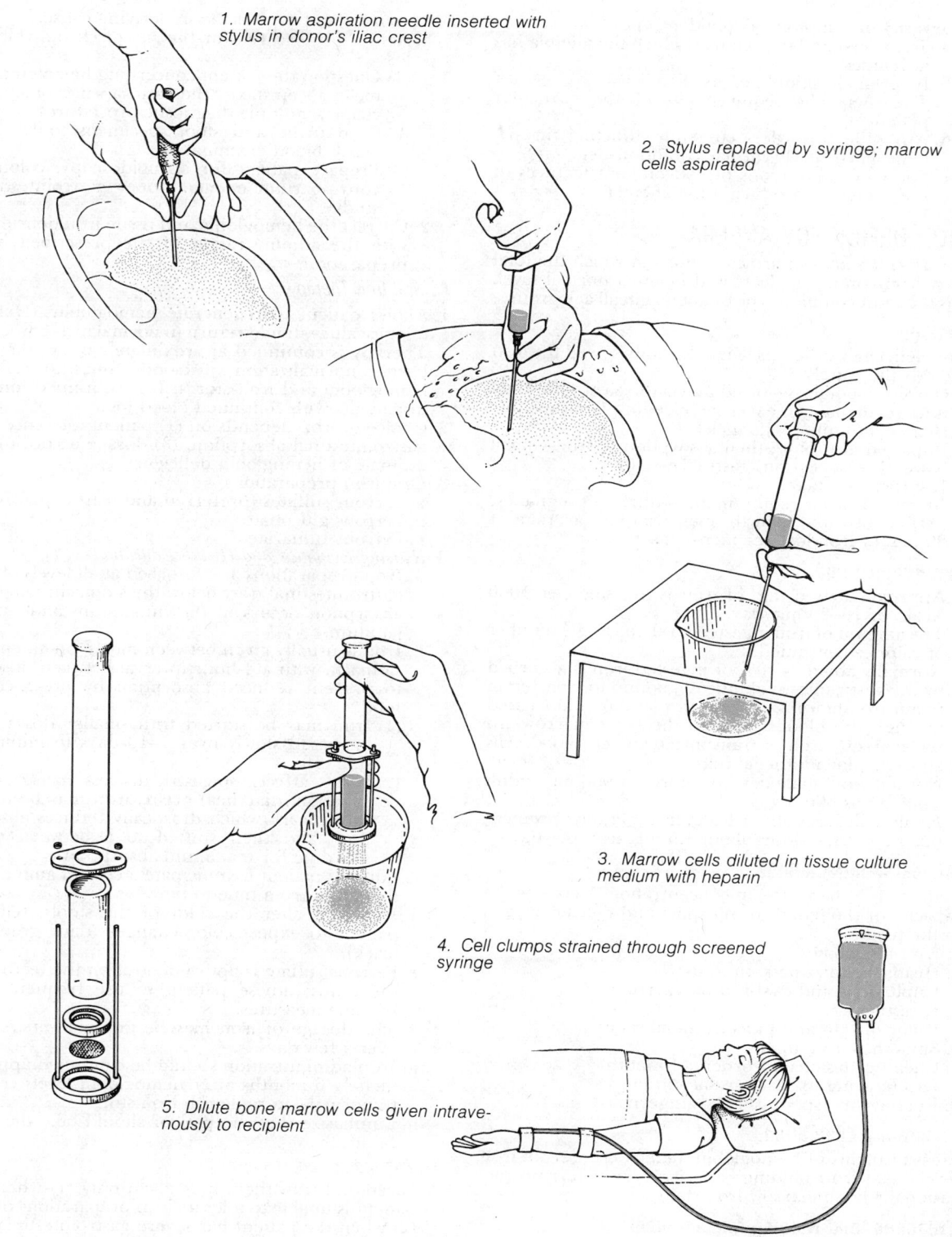

1. Marrow aspiration needle inserted with stylus in donor's iliac crest

2. Stylus replaced by syringe; marrow cells aspirated

3. Marrow cells diluted in tissue culture medium with heparin

4. Cell clumps strained through screened syringe

5. Dilute bone marrow cells given intravenously to recipient

FIGURE 8-1. *Bone marrow transplantation. (Redrawn from Medical Times 1978 Aug; vol. 106)*

2. Severity of symptoms dependent upon:
   a. The speed and degree with which the anemia has developed
   b. Its prior duration, i.e., its chronicity
   c. The metabolic requirements of the particular patient
   d. Any other disorders currently afflicting the patient, particularly cardiac conditions, etc.
   e. Special complications or concomitant features of the condition producing the anemia

IRON DEFICIENCY ANEMIA

Iron deficiency anemias are conditions in which the total body iron content is decreased below a normal level. It is the most common type of anemia in all age groups.

Etiology

Iron deficiency develops when the body's need for iron exceeds the supply.
1. Chronic blood loss—bleeding via the gastrointestinal tract (malignancy), excessive bleeding from menorrhagia, multiple pregnancies.
2. Impaired gastrointestinal absorption of iron—small bowel disease, certain gastric resections.
3. Insufficient intake.
4. Increased iron requirements—during pregnancy, periods of rapid growth, menstruation (average of 20 mg. of iron lost per menstrual cycle).

Iron Balance and Stores

1. Approximately 6 mg. of iron is ingested per 1000 Kcal.; or 16–20 mg./day.
2. The amount of iron ingested is related to the number of calories consumed.
   Normally about 5–10% of ingested iron is absorbed by the gastrointestinal mucosa, bound to transferrin (main iron-binding protein in plasma), and carried through the bloodstream to the bone marrow. In the marrow, iron is transported to red blood cells and reticuloendothelial cells.
3. Normal adult male has iron stores of 900 mg.; adult woman has 300 mg.
4. Adult male loses about 1 mg. iron per day; premenopausal woman loses about 1.5 mg. iron per day.

Clinical Manifestations

Reduction in hemoglobin concentration decreases the capacity of the blood to transport and deliver oxygen to the tissues.
1. Easy fatigability
2. Headache, dizziness, tinnitus
3. Palpitations and dyspnea on exertion
4. Paresthesias
5. Pallor of skin and mucous membranes
6. Smooth, sore tongue
7. Cheilosis (lesions at corners of mouth)
8. Pica (craving to eat unusual substances)
9. Koilonychia (spoon-shaped fingernails)

Laboratory Evaluation

Measurements of hemoglobin, hematocrit, serum iron level, total iron binding capacity, serum ferritin (occasionally bone marrow iron stain)

Treatment and Nursing Management

OBJECTIVE: to replenish the body's depleted iron stores and restore the circulating hemoglobin mass.

1. Recognize and correct the underlying cause.
   a. Assist in the search for the site of chronic blood loss.
      (1) Question the patient concerning hematemesis, melena, epistaxis, hematuria, menometrorrhagia, multiple diagnostic procedures.
      (2) Send urine and stool specimens to lab for occult blood examination.
      (3) Prepare patient for sigmoidoscopy, colonoscopy, barium enema, upper gastrointestinal studies.
2. Correct the hemoglobin and tissue iron deficiency with the administration of the prescribed iron preparation.

A. *Oral Iron Therapy*

1. Allows patient to regenerate hemoglobin. (Hematologic values should return to normal in 4–8 weeks.) Therapy is continued approximately 6 months following normalization of blood values to restore hemoglobin and iron stores. It is continued longer in patients with continued blood loss.
2. Choice of iron depends on (1) patient tolerance, (2) gastrointestinal absorption, (3) dosage according to estimate of hemoglobin deficiency.
3. Oral iron preparations
   a. Ferrous sulfates (preferred and least expensive)
   b. Ferrous gluconate
   c. Ferrous fumarate
4. *Nursing Emphasis and Health Education*
   a. Iron preparations are absorbed at all levels of the gastrointestinal tract below the stomach; maximal absorption occurs in the duodenum and upper jejunum.
   b. Iron is usually given between meals, on an empty stomach, with a 4-hour interval between doses—to prevent reduced absorption by presence of food.
      (1) Iron may be started with smaller doses and increased slowly over 7–10 days to minimize side effects.
      (2) If side effects (epigastric distress, nausea, constipation, diarrhea) occur, iron may be taken with meals (which drastically reduces absorption) and then shifted to a between meal schedule for maximum absorption.
   c. Educate patient to anticipate a certain amount of dyspepsia from time to time.
   d. Iron salts alter the color of the stools; tell the patient to expect color changes (dark green to black).
   e. Ferrous sulfate is apt to deposit on the teeth and the gums; advise patient to use frequent oral hygiene measures.
   f. The dosage of iron may be gradually increased over a few days.
   g. Iron administration should be continued approximately 6 months after hemoglobin levels return to normal—to replenish iron stores.
   h. Emphasize that the patient should take the iron faithfully.

B. *Parenteral Iron Therapy*

1. Parenteral iron therapy is given only (1) when the patient is unable to tolerate iron preparations orally, (2) when the patient has severe gastrointestinal disorders, or (3) when there is continuing negative iron balance while patient is taking maximum oral dose tolerated.

NURSING ALERT: Extravasation of iron medication results in painful local induration. An anaphylactic reaction may occur following either intramuscular or intravenous injection of iron dextran.

2. Parenteral iron preparations
   a. Iron dextran (Imferon)
   b. Iron sorbitex (Jectofer)—may cause patient's urine to turn black on standing, as about 50% of iron is excreted in the urine within 24 hours.
3. Technique of parenteral iron administration:
   a. Discard needle that is used to draw medication into syringe; use a fresh needle for injection—to avoid tracking medication through subcutaneous tissue.
   b. Allow a small amount of air in syringe.
   c. Use a needle 5 cm. (2 inches) long—medication is injected deep into upper outer quadrant of buttock.
   d. Retract the skin over the muscle *laterally* before inserting needle (Z track)—to prevent leakage along injection tract and staining of skin.
   e. Inject solution slowly followed by air in syringe. Wait a few seconds before withdrawing needle.

C. *Health Education*

1. Encourage the selection of a well-balanced diet. Adolescent girls should receive nutritional counseling.
2. Iron supplements should be given during pregnancy.
3. Keep iron medications out of reach of small children—iron tablets are dangerous when ingested by small children.

PERNICIOUS ANEMIA

Pernicious anemia is a megaloblastic anemia* due to vitamin B_{12} deficiency caused by lack of the intrinsic factor in the gastric juice. (B_{12} deficiency is also seen in diseases of the small intestine, i.e., malabsorption, blind loop syndrome, etc.)

Altered Physiology

1. Pernicious anemia is produced by a defect in the gastric mucosa; the stomach wall becomes atrophic and fails to secrete the intrinsic factor.
2. This substance ordinarily binds with the dietary vitamin B_{12} and travels with it to the ileum, where the vitamin is absorbed. Without intrinsic factor, no orally administered B_{12} can enter the body.
3. Therefore, after the body's stores of B_{12} are used up, the patient begins to show signs of the anemia.
4. Vitamin B_{12} is the extrinsic factor necessary for the maturation of red blood cells.

---

* Megaloblastic anemias
1. A megaloblast is a nucleated red cell with delayed and abnormal nuclear maturation.
2. The most common megaloblastic anemias are B_{12} deficiency anemia and folic acid deficiency.
3. Anemias due to deficiencies of the vitamins B_{12} and folic acid show identical bone marrow and peripheral blood changes. This is because both vitamins are essential for normal DNA synthesis.

Clinical manifestations

1. Symptoms due to anemia
   a. Pallor
   b. Dyspnea or orthopnea
   c. Angina pectoris
   d. Edema of legs
2. Symptoms due to physiologic changes in gastrointestinal tract
   a. Sore mouth with smooth, red, "beefy" tongue
   b. Loss of appetite
   c. Indigestion and epigastric discomfort
   d. Recurring diarrhea or constipation
   e. Weight loss
3. Symptoms due to neurologic changes (occurs in high percentage of untreated patients)
   a. Tingling and numbness or burning pain (paresthesia) involving hands and feet
   b. Loss of position sense, leading to disturbances of gait
   c. Disturbances of bladder and bowel function
   d. Irritability; depression
   e. Paranoia and delirium

Diagnostic Evaluation

1. Blood smear—reveals marked variation in size and shape of cells and a variable number of unusually large cells containing a normal concentration of hemoglobin.
2. Gastric analysis—the gastric juice lacks free hydrochloric acid (achlorhydria).
3. *Schilling Test*—a test for vitamin B_{12} absorption.
PURPOSE: to prove that the patient cannot absorb oral vitamin B_{12} unless intrinsic factor is added.
   a. The patient is given a small dose of radioactive B_{12} in water to drink followed by a large nonradioactive intramuscular dose.
   b. When the oral vitamin is absorbed, it will be excreted in the urine; the IM dose helps to flush it into the urine.
   c. A 24-hour urine specimen is collected and measured for radioactivity. All urine must be collected. Patients with renal disease may require longer periods of collection.
   d. If very little has been excreted, the test is repeated several days later (the "second stage") with a capsule of oral intrinsic factor added to the oral B_{12}.
   e. If the patient has pernicious anemia, this time much more radioactivity will be found in the 24-hour urine specimen.
4. Low B_{12} level in the serum.

Treatment and Nursing Management

OBJECTIVES: to support the patient during the acute phase of his illness.
to give enough antianemic factor (vitamin B_{12}) to produce a remission.
to help the patient accept that he must be on vitamin B_{12} maintenance for his lifetime.

A. *Treatment During Acute Stage*

1. Give cyanocobalamin (vitamin B_{12}) as directed.
   a. Reticulocytes begin to increase on 4th day after therapy is started; normal hemoglobin values are obtained in approximately 6 weeks.
   b. Patient begins to improve in general well-being and mental status in a few days.

c. Recent neurological changes will usually be reversed.
2. Give transfusion of packed cells very slowly (rarely necessary).
   a. Transfusions are only given to patients whose anemia is life-threatening (symptoms of hypoxia to heart or brain).
   b. Place the patient in a sitting position in bed.
      Too rapid administration of transfusion to patient with anemia may produce acute pulmonary or cerebral edema.
3. Support the patient with neurological involvement (see p. 512 for management of patient with neurogenic bladder).

B. *Maintenance Therapy*
1. Impress upon the patient that vitamin B_{12} must be continued for his lifetime.
   a. Maintenance dose schedule—vitamin B_{12} IM every 4 weeks.
   b. Teach patient and family or have community health nurse give maintenance therapy.
   c. Untreated pernicious anemia is fatal.
2. Instruct the patient to report for follow-up examinations every 6 months—for hematocrit and physical examination.
   a. Patient may develop hematologic or neurologic relapse if therapy is inadequate.
   b. Patients with pernicious anemia have a higher incidence of gastric cancer and thyroid problems; therefore, periodic stool examinations for occult blood and gastric cytology, along with thyroid function tests, should be made.
3. Following total gastrectomy (and occasionally subtotal gastrectomy) patient should receive maintenance dose of vitamin B_{12} as often as indicated—removal of gastric fundus deprives the patient of all intrinsic factor; may take as long as 10 years for clinical symptoms to appear, due to small amount of daily vitamin B_{12} required and the large body stores available for use.
4. Parenteral vitamin B_{12} therapy is preferred—greater reliability, better patient supervision, less expensive.

APLASTIC ANEMIA

Aplastic anemia is a form of organ failure characterized by reduced numbers of circulating red and white blood cells and platelets and which is associated with a hypoplastic bone marrow.

Causes

1. Idiopathic—approximately 50% of aplastic anemia cases are of unknown etiology.
2. Chemical compounds—benzene and benzene derivatives may induce permanent bone marrow damage.
3. Drugs—antimicrobials (chloramphenicol), antitumor agents, antidiabetic agents, phenothiazines, antihistamines, insecticides, antidepressants, thyroid medication, gold. (Almost any drug has potential.)
4. Ionizing radiation—therapeutic, industrial, or laboratory accidents.
5. Viral infections—viral hepatitis, mononucleosis, etc.
6. Congenital (Fanconi's anemia)—congenitally constituted defect in the bone marrow.

Clinical Manifestations

1. Anemia—resulting from depression of hemoglobin and rapidity of blood cell change

a. Pallor; weakness
b. Exertional dyspnea, palpitation
2. Infections with high fever—resulting from granulocytopenia
   a. Pharyngitis
   b. Sepsis via gastrointestinal tract or genitourinary tract
3. Abnormal bleeding—resulting from granulocytopenia
   a. Purpura; petechiae; ecchymoses
   b. Bleeding from gums, nose, gastrointestinal, and urinary tracts

Diagnostic Evaluation

1. Peripheral blood smear shows pancytopenia (deficiency in all the cellular elements of the blood).
2. Bone marrow aspiration and biopsy—bone marrow is hypoplastic or aplastic; reduction of its cellular elements occurs, and there is an almost complete absence of hemopoietic activity.

Clinical Course

1. The clinical course is variable and the overall mortality rate is high; patients with severe pancytopenia with totally aplastic marrow have a poor prognosis.
2. Approximately half of the patients with aplastic anemia die of the disease, usually from *infection, hemorrhage,* and *complications of chronic anemia.*

Treatment and Nursing Management

OBJECTIVES: to bring the patient to remission.
              to prolong his survival time with supportive therapy.
1. Attempt to identify and eliminate the underlying toxic agent(s)—gives marrow opportunity to recover before being damaged too severely. However, permanent damage often occurs.
   a. Question patient regarding all agents (drugs, chemicals) to which he has been exposed.
   b. Instruct patient to discontinue all unnecessary medications and eliminate exposure to toxins.
2. Support the patient undergoing bone marrow transplantation (see p. 241) (replacement of affected bone marrow with marrow from healthy donor—preferably matched sibling). This modality of treatment is performed at specialized transplant centers.
   a. Bone marrow transplantation should be carried out *early* since subsequent blood and platelet transfusions can cause irreversible sensitization of patient and result in graft rejection.
   b. Antilymphocyte globulin (ALG) is being used in patients who do not have histocompatible donor.
Supportive treatment for patient when bone marrow transplantation is not feasible:
1. Give blood components—to supply red cells, platelets, and granulocytes when bone marrow has ceased to produce them.
   a. Keep veins open—patient may require frequent transfusions for long periods; monitor IV sites carefully.
   b. Give packed red cell transfusions carefully—to maintain hemoglobin level compatible with patient's activities and to relieve symptoms of dyspnea, palpitation, and weakness.
   c. Give platelet transfusions from histocompatible donors when necessary—to arrest bleeding in patient hemorrhaging from thrombocytopenia.

(Hemorrhagic complications occur with platelet counts below 20,000/cu. mm.)

d. Keep patient who receives multiple transfusions over a period of time under careful nursing surveillance—transfusion complications usually develop with these patients.
   (1) Eventually, patient may develop antibodies to minor red cell antigens and to platelet antigens so that transfusions no longer raise the counts sufficiently.
   (2) Multiple transfusions decrease chance for successful bone marrow transplantation.

2. Give agents (androgenic steroids) to attempt to stimulate marrow regeneration and bring about a remission; may be indicated in a few patients.

3. Prepare patient for splenectomy (p. 260) if indicated—the spleen destroys large numbers of white cells and platelets; splenectomy may cause slight elevation of hemoglobin levels and decrease the transfusion requirements.

4. Maintain continuing surveillance for evidences of infection—infection is major cause of death.
   a. Organisms not usually pathogenic may become so, particularly those of the *Pseudomonas aeruginosa*, *Proteus* and *Klebsiella* species.
   b. Sources of infection in these patients are endogenous bacteria from gastrointestinal and upper respiratory tracts, particularly in those patients hospitalized for prolonged periods.

5. Attempt to reduce potential endogenous pathogens in the hospitalized patient.

a. Use reverse isolation procedures for patients with pronounced neutropenia.
b. Pay scrupulous attention to skin infections. Regard any small break in the skin as hazardous.
   (1) Use antiseptic soaps.
   (2) Encourage the use of an electric razor.
c. Examine axillae, and groin areas—apt to harbor pathogens and develop pustules.
d. Monitor temperature—fever implies bacterial, fungal, or viral infection.

6. Give antibiotics at first sign of infection.
   a. Oral antifungal agent may be administered before antibacterial drugs—to eradicate yeasts since absence of bacteria may encourage fungal overgrowth.
   b. Broad spectrum antibiotics usually given IV.
   c. Granulocyte transfusions may be given.

Discharge Planning and Health Education

Instruct patient as follows:
1. Be aware of drugs that may damage the bone marrow cell.
2. When taking drugs that can produce blood dyscrasias (chloramphenicol, phenylbutazone, sulfonamides), have regular blood counts; however, aplastic anemia may develop after drug has been discontinued.
3. Prevent minor infections. Any abrasion or wound of mucous membranes or skin is a potential site of infection.
4. Report any infection, no matter how trivial.
5. Avoid crowds or potential sources of infection.

POLYCYTHEMIA VERA

Polycythemia vera refers to a primary hyperplasia of bone marrow with increased numbers of circulating erythrocytes, granulocytes, and platelets. The underlying defect is unknown. It is a multiple organ system disease.

Altered Physiology

1. Increased blood volume because of increase in red cell mass
2. Increased supply of precursor cells (to the erythroid, myeloid, and megakarocytic line)
3. Striking increase in total blood volume; gradually increasing blood viscosity
4. Decreased marrow iron
5. Engorgement of all organs with blood
6. Hyperplasia of all bone marrow elements
7. Enlargement of spleen

Clinical Course

1. Insidious and gradual onset—probably measured in years.
2. Clinical course of long duration—up to 20 years.
3. More frequent in males; most common during middle and later years of life.
4. Peptic ulcers are common in these patients; cerebral, gastrointestinal, and nasal hemorrhages may occur at any time during the course of the disease.
5. Acute leukemia may be the terminal complication of polycythemia vera.

Clinical Manifestations

(Clinical manifestations are referable to increased blood volume and viscosity from erythrocytosis [increased red cells].)
1. Headache, dizziness, impaired mental ability, visual disturbances and paresthesias
2. Pruritus (worsens after bathing/showering)
3. Plethoric appearance (reddish-purple hue of skin and mucosa)
4. Splenomegaly, producing abdominal discomfort
5. Hypertension
6. Hepatomegaly
7. Hyperuricemia—from increased formation and destruction of erythrocytes and leukocytes and increased metabolism of nucleic acids
8. Weakness and easy fatigability

Diagnostic Evaluation

1. Increased red cell volume—measured by an isotopic technique, high hematocrit
2. Thrombocytosis; often abnormal platelet aggregation
3. Leukocytosis
4. Elevated granulocyte alkaline phosphatase activity
5. Increased serum B_{12}

Treatment and Nursing Management

(Opinion divided on optimum therapy.)

OBJECTIVES: to reduce the red cell volume and blood viscosity.

to control the proliferative process.

1. Assist with phlebotomy (venesection) to reduce viscosity of blood by removal of the excessive numbers of red blood cells and the decrease of blood volume, thereby alleviating symptoms and hemorrhagic and thrombotic complications.
   a. 250–500 ml. of blood removed every other day until hematocrit reaches desired level.
   b. Repeated phlebotomies may be performed to lower hemoglobin, hematocrit, and red cell mass to normal ranges.
   c. Elderly persons with compromised cardiovascular systems are phlebotomized with caution!
2. Myelosuppressive Therapy—radioactive phosphorus (^{32}P) either orally or intravenously—acts on hyperplastic bone marrow to suppress panmyelosis.
3. Chemotherapy—to control the proliferative process.
   a. Chlorambucil (Leukeran)
   b. Melphalan (Alkeran)
   c. Cyclophosphamide (Cytoxan)
   d. See page 843 for nursing support of patient receiving chemotherapy.
4. Administer allopurinol when necessary—to control hyperuricemia.
5. Support patient troubled with pruritus.
   a. May subside with myelosuppressive therapy.
   b. Antihistamine drugs or cholestyramine may give relief.
6. Keep patient ambulatory—likelihood of thrombosis increases when patient is on bed rest. Evaluate and treat for complications—the clinical course of polycythemia is determined by the development of complications.
   a. Thromboembolic complications—due to hyperviscosity which leads to reduced blood flow and subsequent infarction.
      Includes deep vein thrombophlebitis, myocardial and cerebral infarction, and thrombotic occlusion of the splenic, hepatic, portal, and mesenteric veins.
   b. Hemorrhagic tendency—bleeding occurs spontaneously from increasing blood volume and capillary and venous distention.
   c. Gout—from overproduction of uric acid (secondary to nucleoprotein turnover of marrow cells).
   d. Congestive failure—from increased blood volume and hypertension.
   e. Acute leukemia—may be a terminal complication.

Health Education

1. Report at prescribed intervals for follow-up blood studies.
2. Avoid taking *hot* baths/showers—worsens pruritus.

AGRANULOCYTOSIS (GRANULOCYTOPENIA)

Agranulocytosis (granulocytopenia) is an acute disease in which the white blood cell count drops to extremely low levels and neutropenia becomes pronounced.

Etiology

1. Hypersensitivity to certain drugs or chemicals—may suppress bone marrow activity and decrease production of white blood cells. Some agents occasionally associated with agranulocytosis include:
   a. Phenothiazines
   b. Antihistamines
   c. Analgesics (Butazolidin)
   d. Diuretics
   e. Tranquilizers
   f. Antithyroid drugs
   g. Sulfonamides and their derivatives (including hypoglycemic agents)
   h. Certain antibiotics (chloramphenicol)
   i. Anticonvulsants
   j. Agents that regularly depress leukopoiesis (alkylating agents, antimetabolites)
2. In some patients the cause cannot be identified
3. Hereditary

Clinical Manifestations

1. Sore throat, ulcerations of mucosa of mouth and pharynx (agranulocytic angina); throat becomes increasingly sore and eventually necrotic
2. Fever/chills
3. Extreme prostration
4. Vaginal and rectal ulceration—may occur as a result of local infection
5. Pneumonia, urinary tract infection, sepsis

Clinical Course

Spontaneous restoration of marrow function (except in patients with neoplastic disease) may occur in 1 to 3 weeks if death from infection can be averted.

Diagnostic Evaluation

Blood shows marked reduction in number of circulating neutrophils

Bone marrow examination

Treatment and Nursing Management

OBJECTIVES: to eliminate the factor responsible for the bone marrow suppression.

to prevent and treat infection until the bone marrow has returned to normal.

1. Question the patient concerning any drugs he has been taking, including over-the-counter drugs.
2. Take the patient off the offending drug. Warn the patient to avoid reexposure to offending drug.
3. Prevent and treat infection.

NURSING ALERT: Granulocytes are the first barrier to infection. In patients with agranulocytosis, infection develops rapidly and may soon become overwhelming.

   a. Patients with profound granulocytopenia may lack usual signs and symptoms of systemic infection. Assess for:

(1) Erythema and pain—in an area with no previous symptoms.
(2) Pulmonary infiltrates on chest x-ray with no evidence of rales or consolidation.
(3) Malaise; change in level of responsiveness.
(4) Fever greater than 38° C. (100.4° F.).
b. Physical examination is performed with attention to lungs and perianal, inguinal and axillary areas, and sites of intravenous therapy.
c. Take cultures (aerobic, anaerobic, viral, and fungal) of blood, urine, pharynx, rectum, and wounds daily as long as fever persists.
d. The therapy of suspected sepsis is started as soon as cultures are taken. It is undertaken with a combination of antibiotics, since at this time no single agent provides a spectrum broad enough to control all common pathogenic organisms usually involved. May include the use of a penicillin (carbenicillin or ticarcillin) and an aminoglycoside (gentamicin).
e. Granulocyte transfusions may be given if patient fails to respond to appropriate antibiotic therapy. Watch for adverse reaction to granulocyte transfusion—fever, chills, shortness of breath, hypotension, tachycardia, and hypoxia.
f. Patient may be placed in protective isolation (controversial); however, infection usually arises from patient's endogenous flora (in gastrointestinal tract, urinary tract) or from organisms in hospital environment. Careful handwashing and environmental cleanliness should be observed.
4. Administer androgen therapy (oxymetholone; fluoxymesterone) as directed—may stimulate the marrow stem cell; outcome is uncertain.
5. Utilize measures to support the patient and increase comfort.
a. Use nursing and therapeutic measures to relieve throat pain—gargles, ice collar, analgesics, anesthetic lozenges.
b. Encourage patient to remain on bed rest if fever is present.
c. Give high vitamin, high caloric, soft, or liquid diet.

Complications

1. Sepsis
2. Bronchial pneumonia
3. Hemorrhagic necrosis of mucous membrane lesions.

THE LEUKEMIAS

The *leukemias* are neoplastic disorders of the blood-forming tissues (spleen, lymphatic system, and bone marrow). The common features of the leukemias are an unregulated proliferation or accumulation of white cells in the bone marrow and replacement of normal marrow elements. There is also proliferation in the liver, spleen, and lymph nodes, and invasion of nonhematologic organs such as the meninges, gastrointestinal tract, kidney, and skin.

Classification

Classified according to:
1. The cell type involved (lymphocytic, granulocytic, or monocytic)
2. The maturity of malignant cells
   a. acute (immature cells)
   b. chronic (differentiated cells)

Predisposing Factors

Etiology unknown: several factors are associated with increase in incidence:
1. Exposure to radiation
2. Chemical agents—benzene
3. Infectious agents—viruses (currently being investigated)
4. Genetic abnormalities—increased risk of leukemia in patients with Down's syndrome (see p. 1439)
5. Chemotherapy treatment—
6. Myeloproliferative disorders—polycythemia vera, myelofibrosis (fibrosis of bone marrow)
7. Genetic influence—some families with incidence of leukemia

ACUTE LEUKEMIA*

Acute leukemia is a rapidly progressive disease involving primitive cells or blasts that continue to proliferate. It may be lymphocytic, granulocytic (or myelocytic), or monocytic (rare). The clinical course of the acute leukemias is similar for all types.

Clinical Manifestations

Produced by proliferation and infiltration of bone marrow and other organs by immature white blood cells of the lymphocytic, granulocytic, or monocytic group.
1. Easy fatigability and general malaise; pallor—from bone marrow failure and anemia
2. Fever or infection—secondary to granulocytopenia
3. Enlarged lymph nodes and spleen; abdominal discomfort—from organ infiltration
4. Bone pain, arthralgia—from expanding marrow in bone and gout of hyperuricemia
5. Bleeding of gums, epistaxis, petechiae, prolonged bleeding following a surgical procedure—from thrombocytopenia (lowered platelet count)
6. Tachycardia, weight loss, dyspnea on exertion, intolerance to heat—from increased metabolism
7. Leukemia infiltration of the skin—tendency for leukemic tissue to infiltrate other organs and tissues
8. Cerebral hemorrhage, cranial nerve paralysis, increased intracranial pressure—from neurological

* For discussion of acute leukemia in children, see page 1425.

complications (leukemia cells frequently invade the central nervous system—usually in patients in long remission)
9. Pain—from infarction, particularly the spleen

NURSING ALERT: Undiagnosed patients may appear in the Emergency Department for treatment of acute infections.

Diagnostic Evaluation

1. Blood evaluation—total peripheral white count varies widely (10,000–100,000/cu. ml.)
2. Bone marrow biopsy—characteristically large percentage of bone marrow's nucleated cells are immature leukocyte forms called "blasts"
3. Lymph node biopsy
4. Chest x-ray—to detect mediastinal node and lung involvement
5. Skeletal x-ray—to detect skeletal lesions

Treatment and Nursing Management

OBJECTIVES: to restore normal marrow function as quickly as possible.
to achieve complete remission.
to provide the patient with as long and as normal life as possible.

Initial treatment in a specially equipped medical facility that treats patients with leukemia with a multidisciplinary team approach gives the best promise for prolonged remission.

A. *Chemotherapy*

1. The drugs are classified on the basis of their effects on cell chemistry. (See p. 846 for complete list of drugs used in cancer chemotherapy.)
2. Objective of chemotherapy—to induce remission (disappearance of all abnormal cell forms in the bone marrow and peripheral blood).

B. *Underlying Principles of Chemotherapy*

1. Chemotherapy inhibits growth of leukemic cells by destroying or inactivating nucleic acids or by interfering with their synthesis; causes bone marrow depression and depresses the patient's immunological defense mechanism.
2. Drugs are usually given in combination (exert different biological effects) at high dose levels to produce greater leukemic cell damage.
3. The treatment regimen is designed to affect cells in different phases of miotic cycle.
4. Usually there is intensive treatment with multiple agents at the beginning of therapy (induction) to induce a remission, followed by long-term continuation (maintenance) therapy.
5. The drugs used to treat leukemia produce major toxicity to the hematopoietic system, resulting in prolonged periods of pancytopenia.
6. The nursing management of the patient with acute leukemia includes constant assessment of the patient for effects of drug toxicity.

C. *Chemotherapy in Adult Acute Leukemia*

The therapeutic strategy is to use combinations of drugs to induce a remission; then to maintain remission by cyclic administration of drugs and/or immuno-

therapy. A large number of drugs have an antileukemic effect. The drug protocol changes as research developments are received, and no one regimen produces successful responses in all patients.

Drugs used for acute lymphocytic leukemia

1. Combinations of an anthracycline derivative (daunorubicin or doxorubicin) and cytosine arabinoside; vincristine, and prednisone.
   Other combinations used include methotrexate, 6-mercaptopurine, cyclophosphamide, vincristine, and prednisone.

*Drugs used for acute nonlymphocytic leukemias**

2. Combinations of cytosine arabinoside and 6-thioguanine or 6-mercaptopurine.
   Other combinations used include cyclophosphamide, vincristine, cystine arabinoside, prednisone.
3. Patients usually given allopurinol, increased fluid administration, and urinary alkalinization for hyperuricemia which occurs as a result of drug-induced cell breakdown.

Nursing Management

A. *Constant Nursing Surveillance of Patient Receiving Chemotherapy*

1. Obtain baseline information before chemotherapy is started.
   a. Know the patient's "normal" TPR and BP.
   b. Follow the WBC, differential count, hemoglobin measurements, platelet counts—to be aware of the drug's effect on the body.
   c. Follow blood chemistry studies, electrolytes, urea nitrogen, creatinine, liver enzymes, bilirubin.
   d. Weigh the patient once or twice weekly.
   e. Assist with bone marrow aspirations as directed (see p. 234).
2. Watch for toxic manifestations during chemotherapy.
   a. Modifications of patient's chemotherapy regimen are based on laboratory and physical examinations before each course of treatment.
   b. Monitor intravenous infusion of drugs—may cause local irritation in the veins; patient may complain of burning sensations during infusions of methotrexate and prednisone.
      (1) Adjust infusion flow to a slower rate.
      (2) Change position of extremity to prevent muscular cramping
      (3) Patient may complain of nausea, vomiting, and burning sensation along the gastrointestinal tract during or immediately after drug infusion.
   c. Watch for mouth ulcers—frequently occur when patient is taking methotrexate. Offer medicated mouth rinses frequently to relieve oral discomfort.
   d. Expect the patient to experience loss of hair during anti-leukemic treatment—alopecia occurs in high percentage of patients receiving vincristine.
      Encourage the patient to experiment with wigs, hair pieces, head scarfs.
   e. Check deep tendon reflexes. Assess patient for footdrop, weakening hand grasp, ptosis of eyelids—vincristine may cause neuropathy.

* Acute nonlymphocytic leukemias include acute myelocytic, myelomonocytic, monocytic, progranulocytic and erythroleukemia.

f. Assess for constipation and abdominal pain—vincristine may produce adynamic ileus.

g. Watch for personality changes, fluid retention, hypertension, gastric ulcers, and diabetes mellitus—occur with prednisone therapy.

h. Watch for other drug side effects—diarrhea, maculopapular rash, stomatitis, phlebitis, bone marrow depression, evidences of cardiac toxicity (tachycardia, arrhythmias, tachypnea, dyspnea).

i. Take ECG readings as prescribed—cardiac toxicity is associated with certain chemotherapeutic agents.

j. See page 849 for nursing management of patient undergoing chemotherapy.

B. *Supportive Measures for Patient with Leukemia or Lymphoma*

Underlying Consideration: The therapy for leukemia causes severe bone marrow suppression. Failure to improve is usually due to complications—infection and hemorrhage.

OBJECTIVE: to control complications so that chemotherapeutic agents can demonstrate their effectiveness.

1. To prevent and treat infection, which is the major morbidity and mortality factor associated with leukemia—patient susceptible because of granulocytopenia (from leukemia and chemotherapy, from malnutrition, from patient's own endogenous flora, and from organisms acquired during hospitalization).

a. Monitor the concentration of circulating granulocytes. Concentrations below 500 cu. mm.—serious danger of infection.

b. Avoid venipuncture, subcutaneous and intramuscular injections unless absolutely necessary.

c. Recognize infection promptly.
   (1) Monitor temperature at regular intervals—fever is major symptom of infection.
   (2) Usual manifestations of infection are altered in patient with leukemia.

d. Obtain cultures (for both aerobes and anaerobes) of blood, urine, sputum, spinal fluid.

e. Obtain serial chest x-ray.

f. Broad spectrum antimicrobials are usually given until organism is identified; oral nonabsorbable antibiotic regimens may be given to prevent enteric colonization and systemic infection.

g. Watch for development of fungal infection (especially *Candida* and *Aspergillus*)—from indwelling catheters, antimicrobials, immunosuppressive effects of chemotherapy, and decreased resistance of patient.

h. Give irradiated granulocyte transfusions to patients with severe neutropenia.

2. To eliminate the morbidity and mortality resulting from hemorrhage.

a. Major cause of hemorrhage is thrombocytopenia (decrease in platelets).

b. Risk of hemorrhage is high at platelet levels below 15,000–20,000 platelets/cu. mm.

c. Prepare the patient for a transfusion of platelets or platelet concentrates—to prevent bleeding or treat hemorrhage.
   Platelet transfusion may have to be repeated 2–3 times weekly—average platelet half-life is 3–5 days.

3. To prevent infectious complications by control of environmental contamination.

a. Secure a private room and use protective isolation procedures (p. 799), meticulous handwashing, and hygienic care of the patient.
   (1) Special assessment and monitoring of axillary and inguinal areas with inspection of buttocks and perineum after each bowel movement. Avoid use of rectal thermometers—*perirectal abscess is a common complication.*
   (2) Inspect nose and mouth for evidence of infection.

b. Laminar air-flow room—a unidirectional air flow "barrier" that establishes an air environment in which the infection-prone patient is free from contact with exogenous microorganisms (See Fig. 21-1, p. 850) when available.

c. Antibiotic prophylaxis may be initiated before patient enters protected environment.

4. To support the patient receiving blood component therapy.

a. The myelosuppression (bone marrow) is profound from a combination of the disease and therapy. Transfusion requirements depend on the type of leukemia, state of the disease, and the intensity of chemotherapy.

b. Red cell transfusion (packed cells)—almost all patients have anemia.

c. Platelet transfusion—to prevent and treat hemorrhage.

d. Platelets and clotting factors—to treat disseminated intravascular coagulation (p. 259).

e. Granulocyte transfusion—may be used to treat infection in severely neutropenic patients.

5. To control the pain and discomfort.

a. Use milder analgesics when possible; change to a stronger narcotic as the patient's condition requires.

b. Give tranquilizers as directed to enhance the effects of narcotics.

c. Give antiemetic medication before meals—to help assuage the patient's nausea; sedatives may also be helpful.

6. To maintain oral intake between 3–4 liters daily—to prevent precipitation of uric acid crystals in the urine; overproduction of uric acid is due to the tremendous proliferation of blood cells and the destruction of these cells by antileukemic agents.

7. To control fever—employ fever sponges, increased fluid intake, antipyretic drugs.

8. To give frequent and special mouth care—to remove dried blood, combat odor, and soothe oral ulcerations.

a. Reduce the number of commensal organisms in mouth by:
   (1) prophylactic dental visits for regular removal of plaque and mucus.
   (2) regular toothbrushing (with small automatic toothbrush) except in presence of gross gingival hypertrophy with associated pain and bleeding.
   (3) use of mouthwashes (with sodium perborate, hydrogen peroxide, sodium bicarbonate)—effervescent action helps remove detritus and inspissated mucus from teeth, dentures, and ulcers.
   (4) use of analgesic mouthwash (benzocaine) for patients with painful gingival problems.

b. Watch for development of candidiasis and infective processes of the mouth—from corticosteroids and some antibiotics.

   c. Encourage patient to see dentist during period of remission—to eradicate plaque and for routine dental treatment.

9. To assist the patient to accept and participate in his therapeutic regimen.

   a. Give expert physical care and support—encourages the patient to endure discomfort associated with treatment.

   b. Help the patient to mobilize his defenses to cope with his physiologic and emotional distress.

     (1) Patient may react with shock and anger when disease is first recognized; anger may be directed at health care personnel.

     (2) Anger is a defense mechanism; patient realizes that death is inevitable; anger is also a defense against anxiety.

     (3) Develop ability to accept and deal with this anger—important for establishing a therapeutic patient-nurse relationship.

     (4) Allow patient and family to ventilate their emotions.

     (5) Patient may use mechanism of denial—denial may need to be supported or worked through.

Health Education

1. Avoid possible sources of infection—crowds, unnecessary hospital visits, etc.

   a. Employ good, frequent handwashing practices.

   b. Report any sign of infection to physician/clinic promptly.

   c. Report any exposure to varicella, measles, hepatitis, etc.

2. Pay careful attention to nutrition—undernourished person does not tolerate antileukemic drugs as well as well-nourished individual.

3. Monitor weight to be certain a significant amount of weight is not lost.

4. See your dentist—oral disease is frequently present.

5. Remember that leukemia is a treatable disease with continual advances being made; most side effects of antileukemic drugs are short-term and treatable.

CHRONIC LYMPHOCYTIC LEUKEMIA

Chronic lymphocytic leukemia is a type of leukemia characterized by a great increase in mature lymphocytes in the circulation and in the lymphoid organs of the body.

Clinical Features

1. Occurs most frequently between ages 45 and 60

2. Insidious onset; symptoms closely resemble those of chronic myelogenous type (see Clinical Manifestations, Chronic Granulocytic Leukemia).

3. The course is variable

Clinical Manifestations

(Related to infiltration of lymph nodes, bone marrow, liver and spleen with lymphocytes.)

1. Gradual appearance of generalized lymph node enlargement—cervical region, axillae, groin; splenomegaly

2. Anemia, fever, weight loss, and hemorrhagic features

3. Possible leukemic infiltrations in retinae of eyes and in skin. (Skin may become pruritic and bronzed.)

4. Ascitic and pleuritic infiltrations

5. White blood cells may be in excess of 100,000/cu.

ml. of blood; lymphocytes may comprise 90–99% of cells

6. Abnormalities of erythrocytes, granulocytes, and platelets are common

Treatment and Nursing Management

OBJECTIVES: to achieve a remission of symptoms.
to relieve symptoms.

A. *Asymptomatic patient with chronic lymphocytic leukemia*

1. May not require treatment for a period of years.

2. Support the patient with optimum nutrition, rest, exercise, recreation, and mental activity.

B. *Symptomatic patient* (with massive adenopathy, severe anemia, thrombocytopenia, skin involvement, recurring infections)

1. *Chemotherapy*—brings symptomatic relief; decreases size of lymph nodes and spleen

   a. Chlorambucil (Leukeran)

   b. Combination drug therapy (3 or 4 drug regimen) may be given to patients with poorly differentiated lymphocytes who are unresponsive to a single chemotherapeutic agent)—reduces white blood cell count, improves constitutional symptoms

2. For anemia—from blood loss; from replacement of bone marrow by leukemia cells

   a. Radiation therapy for local disease

   b. Corticosteroids (prednisone)

   c. Chemotherapy

   d. Transfusions: whole blood for hemorrhage; packed red cells when hemolysis or bone marrow failure exists

3. For adenopathy
Supervoltage x-ray therapy for localized nodes, masses, or splenomegaly

4. For hemorrhage—may occur when severe thrombocytopenia and purpura are present or when bleeding, secondary to peptic ulcer, occurs as a complication of corticosteroid therapy.
Transfusion to replace blood loss.

C. *See page 849 for nursing support of patient receiving chemotherapy and page 250 for other aspects of management of a patient with leukemia.*

CHRONIC GRANULOCYTIC LEUKEMIA

Chronic granulocytic (myelocytic, myelogenous) leukemia is a condition characterized by an increased proliferation of myeloid elements including WBCs, platelets, and occasionally red cells. It affects the granulocytes which are produced by the myeloid, or bone marrow. The condition is often associated with great enlargement of the spleen and liver. It may also occur in the acute form.

Clinical Features

1. Appears most often between ages 35–50 and 60–70

2. Gradual, insidious onset; the disease runs a progressive course over several years

3. The Philadelphia chromosome is present in cells of bone marrow origin in over 90% of cases

Clinical Manifestations

1. Pallor, palpitations, dyspnea—from anemia

2. Dragging sensation or enlargement of left side of abdomen—from splenic enlargement

3. Hematologic features: elevated platelet count, ele-

vated granulocyte count; blood smear shows pre-dominance of granulocytes at all stages of maturation
4. Weakness, loss of weight, loss of appetite—from increased metabolic rate due to progress of disease
5. Tenderness and pain in long bones (particularly tibia, ribs, sternum)—due to invasion by abnormal marrow

Treatment and Nursing Management

OBJECTIVES: to achieve a remission of symptoms.
to relieve symptoms related to the disease.
1. Chemotherapy
  a. Busulfan (Myleran)—will induce a complete or partial remission in majority of patients.
    (1) Following initial treatment patient may be placed on long-term, low-dose maintenance

therapy or high-dose therapy when evidence of disease recurs.
    (2) Eventually patient will no longer respond; the acute exacerbation phase is termed myelo-blastic or "blast" crisis which is refractory to treatment and is a terminal phase. The patient is then treated as for acute leukemia. (See p. 250.)
  b. Other chemotherapeutic agents (second line drugs) may be used.
2. Leukapheresis (removal of WBC from blood; blood retransfused into patient) may be used for patient who needs white blood count reduced rapidly.
3. See page 849 for nursing support of patient receiving chemotherapy.
4. See page 250 for other aspects of management of a patient with leukemia.

MALIGNANT LYMPHOMAS

The *lymphomas* are a group of neoplastic diseases of the lymphoreticular system and include Hodgkin's disease and the non-Hodgkin's lymphomas.
1. Lymphomas are classified, according to the predom-inant malignant cell, as lymphocytic lymphoma (pre-viously called lymphosarcoma), histiocytic lymphoma (previously reticulum cell sarcoma), or Hodgkin's disease.
2. These tumors usually start in lymph nodes, but can involve any lymphoid tissue in the spleen, gastroin-testinal tract (tonsils, walls of stomach), liver, or bone marrow.
3. They may spread to all these areas and to extralym-phatic tissues (lungs, kidneys, skin).
4. The etiology of these diseases is unknown.

HODGKIN'S DISEASE

Hodgkin's disease is a malignant disease of unknown etiology that originates in the lymphoid system and involves predominantly the lymph nodes. It may occur in nearly any lymphoid mass of tissues: spleen, bone marrow.

Altered Physiology

1. The malignant cell of Hodgkin's disease is the "Reed-Sternberg" cell, which is a gigantic, atypical tumor cell, morphologically unique and of uncertain lineage.
2. The different histopathologic types of Hodgkin's disease are associated with varying prognoses.
3. Hodgkin's disease shows a highly predictable pattern of spread—usually via the lymphatic channels from one chain of lymph nodes to another, often to the spleen, and ultimately to extralymphatic sites.
4. Hodgkin's disease may have a hematogenic spread as extra nodal sites involved include the gastrointes-tinal tract, bone marrow, skin, upper air passages, and other organs.

Clinical Manifestations

1. Painless enlargement of lymph nodes (usually on one side of neck)

2. Slight to high fever; chills, night sweats, weight loss
3. Pruritus (itching), (either local or generalized)
4. Progressive anemia
5. Enlargement of lymph nodes in other regions of the body
6. Enlargement of mediastinal and retroperitoneal lymph nodes produces pressure symptoms
  a. Dyspnea from pressure against the trachea
  b. Dysphagia from pressure against the esophagus
  c. Laryngeal paralysis due to pressure against the recurrent laryngeal nerve
  d. Brachial, lumbar, or sacral neuralgias due to pressure on the nerve
  e. Edema of the extremities due to pressure on the veins
  f. Enlargement of spleen and liver
7. Effusions into the pleura or peritoneum
8. Obstructive jaundice—from pressure on the bile duct

Diagnostic Evaluation

The extent of the disease is determined before treat-ment.
1. Biopsy of lymph node(s) to identify characteristic histologic features
2. Complete blood count
3. Chest x-ray and tomography—to detect mediastinal or hilar disease
4. Computed tomography—to determine precise lo-cation of nodal involvement and if tumor has invaded lungs; also used in diagnosing staging, treatment planning, and follow-up
5. Roentgenographic skeletal survey
6. Technetium bone scan
7. Bone marrow biopsy
8. Liver function tests and scan
9. Lymphangiogram
  a. Reveals size of lymph nodes
  b. Detects abdominal lymph node enlargements which may not be seen or felt by ordinary means
10. Surgical staging (laparotomy with splenectomy, liver biopsy, multiple lymph node biopsies)—to identify disease in the spleen and lymph nodes below the diaphragm

Staging of Hodgkin's Disease*

Staging is done to provide guidance in prognosis and to assist in therapeutic decisions.

Stage I: Involvement of a single lymph node region (I) or of a single extralymphatic organ or site (I_E)

Stage II: Involvement of two or more lymph node regions on the same side of the diaphragm (II) or localized involvement of extralymphatic organ or site and of one or more lymph node regions on the same side of the diaphragm (II_E)

Stage III: Involvement of lymph node regions on both sides of the diaphragm (III) which may also be accompanied by localized involvement of extralymphatic organ or site (III_E) or by involvement of the spleen (III_S) or both (III_{ES})

Stage IV: Diffuse or disseminated involvement of one or more extralymphatic organs or tissues with or without associated lymph node enlargement

Treatment and Nursing Management

(Depends upon stage, symptoms, and cell type)

OBJECTIVE: to provide treatment that gives best opportunity for cure or long-term survival.

A. *Concepts*

1. Radiotherapy and combination chemotherapy are the two primary therapeutic modalities.
2. Radiotherapy (delivery of a lethal dose of ionizing radiation to tumor cells) is the first choice of treatment in early Hodgkin's disease; potentially curable by radiotherapy. An important factor in treatment is the radiation dose administered.
3. Hodgkin's disease may be eradicated from any site that has received 4000–4500 rads within the space of 4 weeks. Megavoltage radiation techniques permit the delivery of such a dose to one or more entire lymph node chains.
4. Areas of the body in which the lymph node chains are located can tolerate doses of this magnitude without serious damage (as can the area of the spleen and the oronasopharynx); vital structures such as the lungs, liver and kidneys are protected by lead shields.
5. Radiotherapy usually given daily over a period of weeks.
6. *Complications of Intensive Radiotherapy*
   a. Pneumonitis, pericarditis, sterility, development of second malignancies (leukemia)—depending on site of irradiation and dose-related circumstances.
   b. Acute reactions to irradiation—dryness of mouth; loss of taste; dysphagia; nausea and vomiting; apathy and lassitude; skin redness, dry peeling in treatment fields; loss of hair at back of neck and under areas treated; reduction of white blood cells.

B. *Treatment of Patients with Localized Disease Plus Constitutional Symptoms*

OBJECTIVES: to produce tumor regression and remission.

* Committee on Hodgkin's Disease Staging Classification, *Cancer Research* 31 (November 1971): 1860–1861.

to relieve pressure on a vital organ (brain, bronchi, kidney).

1. Chemotherapy is used since Hodgkin's disease is considered a drug-responsive tumor.
   a. Combination chemotherapy—many variations are being used.
      (1) Chlorambucil, prednisone, vincristine, procarbazine, carmustine, bleomycin, doxorubicin.
      (2) Nitrogen mustard, vincristine, procarbazine, and prednisone (MOPP).
      (3) Three or four drugs may be used in monthly courses.
      (4) Dosage depends on patient's status and his response to treatment.
      (5) Intermittent maintenance therapy may be required to keep disease under control.
      (6) Toxic effects of these drugs often overlap, especially bone marrow depression.
      (7) See page 843 for discussion of patient undergoing chemotherapy.
   b. Combination chemotherapy in addition to extended field radiation may be used.

Nursing Management

1. Support the patient having toxic effects from chemotherapy.
2. Encourage the patient by saying that the therapy will end in "a period of time"—serves as an incentive for the patient to continue with therapy.
3. Give stool softeners to control constipation that accompanies chemotherapy or place on a bowel conditioning program. (See p. 76.) Offer bulk foods (bran) to maintain intestinal tone.
4. Anticipate that patients on chemotherapy will develop leukopenia, thrombocytopenia, and anemia.
5. Help patient cope with unpleasant side effects of radiation.
   a. Esophagitis—bland soft foods at mild temperatures, aspirin gum (use moderately), anesthetic lozenges, pain medication before eating if patient unable to eat.
   b. Loss of taste—serve palatable meals.
   c. Anorexia—encourage patient to make the effort to eat.
   d. Nausea—antiemetics given to cover peak time of nausea.
   e. Vomiting—reduction of radiation dose may be necessary.
   f. Diarrhea—anti-diarrheal medication.
   g. Skin reaction (sunburned/tanned appearance of treatment area)—avoid rubbing, heat, cold, application of lotions.
   h. Lethargy—rest/sleep to keep energy level up; diversional activities to prevent boredom.
   i. Tingling with numbness in hands, toes; weakness in knees, hands—use a cane for stability.
6. Prepare patient for surgical excision of localized lymph nodes if indicated (may be followed by radiation therapy).
   Surgery may also be used to alleviate complications caused by pressure or obstruction due to tumor masses.
7. Complications: susceptibility to infections; obstruction to vital structures—from enlarged nodes; pancytopenia—secondary to bone marrow failure; disseminated malignancies (cerebral, bone metastases, lung, kidney).

NURSING ALERT: There is an apparent increase in second malignancies (primarily leukemia) of patients who are long-term survivors of Hodgkin's disease.

Health Education

The control of the disease requires continuing observation by the patient.
1. Report fever or any sign of infection immediately as the disease and its treatment makes one susceptible to infection.
2. Use humidifier/throat lozenges for dry throat and to control desire to cough.
3. Express his feelings and anxieties; seek supportive persons and groups.
   a. Depression and fear are normal reactions to diagnosis, treatment, and stress of uncertain outcome.
   b. Expect to feel fatigued up to a year after therapy.
   c. Remain active and employed (if possible); seek to enjoy the present.
4. Expect some degree of hair loss if taking vincristine or nitrogen mustard; almost always reversible after therapy is completed.
5. Avoid taking alcohol, narcotics, antihistamines, tranquilizers, or sympathomimetic agents when taking procarbazine.

LYMPHOCYTIC LYMPHOMA

Lymphocytic lymphoma is a malignant growth of lymphocytes in lymphoid tissue characterized by progressive generalized lymphadenopathy and splenomegaly, often progressing to involvement of one or more nonlymphoid organ systems. Marrow damage, manifested by anemia and thrombocytopenia, and immune dysfunction, with heightened susceptibility to bacterial and mycotic infections, are also evident in these patients.

Clinical Manifestations

1. Prominent generalized lymphadenopathy
2. Fatigue—attributable primarily to anemia from impaired erythropoiesis and hemolysis
3. Malaise, anorexia, weight loss
4. Fever and sweating
5. Abdominal distention—due to enlargement of spleen

Diagnostic Evaluation

1. Bone scan
2. Reticuloendothelial (liver, spleen) scan
3. Intravenous pyelogram
4. Retroperitoneal lymphography
5. Bone marrow biopsy
6. Liver Biopsy
7. Laparotomy

Treatment and Nursing Management

OBJECTIVE: to induce a remission.
1. The treatment approach depends on the stage of the disease and histiopathologic classification. Many of these patients have disseminated disease at the time of diagnosis.
   a. Radiation therapy (may be curative) (See p. 852.)
   b. Chemotherapy—combinations of cyclophosphamide, prednisone, vincristine, procarbazine, bleomycin, doxorubicin. (See p. 846.)
2. Be on constant vigil for complications.
   a. Infection—by bacteria, viruses, fungi; due to deficiencies of cellular immunity.
   b. Anemia—from bone marrow invasion, hemorrhage, chemotherapy, hypersplenism, failure of bone marrow, hemolysis.
   c. Spinal cord compression—from lymphomatous infiltration.
   d. Hyperuricemia.
3. See also discussion of the care of patients with Hodgkin's disease (see above).

MYCOSIS FUNGOIDES

Mycosis fungoides is a neoplastic disease of the lymphorecticular system first manifested in the skin that may progress to involve the lymph nodes and other internal organs. The term "mycosis fungoides" describes the mushroom-like appearance of the skin tumors. The late stage of the disease closely resembles malignant lymphoma.

Clinical Manifestations

1. Generalized severe itching—may last for several years
2. Erythematous, urticarial, eczematous, or psoriasis-like lesions—there are exacerbations and remissions of these eruptions
3. Ulcerating and necrotic tumors of the skin—lesions become indurated and more fungoidal until they are mushroom-like growths (scarlet or purplish in color), varying in size from 1-5 cm.; the body may be covered with these lesions
4. After the disease involves extracutaneous sites (nodes, liver, spleen), there is usually a fatal outcome.

Diagnostic Evaluation

Biopsy of skin lesion—gives distinctive diagnostic pattern of mycosis fungoides.

Treatment and Nursing Management

OBJECTIVE: to bring about a remission.
(Selection of treatment is based on clinical staging.)
1. Topical (local) therapy used for cutaneous manifestations.
   a. Nitrogen mustard used as topical therapy—effective in certain stages of the disease—allergic dermatitis may develop as response to mustard.
   b. Other agents used include topical corticosteroids (under plastic occlusive dressings.)
2. Systemic chemotherapy—used when internal involvement is suspected, when skin tolerance limits further radiation therapy, or other methods fail to control the disease.
   a. A combination of topical therapy, radiotherapy, or systemic therapy may be used.
   b. Antimetabolites, cytoxic antibiotics, and corticosteroids may be used.
3. Radiation (ultraviolet light, photochemotherapy with psoralen, and long-wave ultraviolet light, grenz ray, electron beam, or x-ray).
4. Watch for evidences of infection (major cause of death, particularly septicemia, bacterial pneumonia).
5. Support the patient who has painful ulcerative lesions.

a. Place bed cradle over patient when he is unable to tolerate the weight of the bed clothing on his skin lesions.
b. Apply bacteriostatic ointment (as prescribed) to lesions as a prophylaxis against infection and to promote comfort by excluding air from open nerve endings.
c. Apply wet dressings to ulcerated or eczematous lesions.
d. Give analgesics for pain.
e. See page 254 for discussion of the nursing management of patients with Hodgkin's disease.

MULTIPLE MYELOMA

Multiple myeloma (plasma cell myeloma; plasmacytoma; myelomatosis) is a malignant disease of the plasma cell that infiltrates bone and soft tissues. The cause is not known. It is a disease of older people and is not classified as a lymphoma.

Altered Physiology

1. The malignant cell is the plasma cell; a widespread proliferation of immature plasma cells takes place in the bone marrow throughout the skeleton. (The plasma cell is derived from lymphocytes and produces immunoglobulins [antibodies]).
2. The bones most commonly affected are the vertebrae, skull, ribs, sternum, pelvis, upper ends of humerus. In later stages the lymph nodes, liver, spleen, and kidneys may become involved.
3. The malignant plasma cells usually produce abnormal amounts of an immunoglobulin or parts of an immunoglobulin protein (Bence Jones protein) that can usually be detected in the serum, and in urine by immunoelectrophoresis.
4. There is a constant threat of hypercalcemia, hypercalciuria, and hyperuricemia due to skeletal destruction, because myeloma cells stimulate osteoclasts.
5. Increased loss of bone substance leads to collapse of vertebral bodies, rib fractures, etc.

Clinical Manifestations

1. Constant severe bone pain, especially on movement—marrow is infiltrated with plasma cells and there are destructive bone lesions
   a. Low back pain—the most characteristic symptom
   b. Skeletal lesions—producing swelling, tenderness, pain, and *pathological fractures*
2. Anemia—due to malignancy and/or replacement of marrow with neoplastic plasma cells. May be associated with thrombocytopenia and granulocytopenia—causes increased susceptibility to infection and abnormal bleeding
3. Marked weight loss
4. Symptoms of renal failure—may be due to precipitation of the immunoglobulin in the tubules or to pyelonephritis, hypercalcemia, increased uric acid, infiltration of the kidney with plasma cells (myeloma kidney), renal vein thrombosis
5. Bleeding tendencies—due to thrombocytopenia and platelet dysfunction
6. Nausea, vomiting, constipation, lethargy (late stage)

Diagnostic Evaluation

1. Abnormalities present in basic hemogram—anemia, elevated sedimentation rate, leukopenia with diminished granulocytes; decreased platelets
2. Malignant plasma cells produce abnormal globulins which appear in serum electrophoresis as a paraprotein "spike"—fragments of these globulins are excreted in urine as Bence Jones proteins
3. Bone marrow biopsy—may show evidence of increased number of abnormal plasma cells in the marrow
4. Bony lesions may appear on x-ray; numerous areas of localized bone destruction may be visible; demineralization of skeleton (osteoporosis) may occur
5. Radioactive technetium bone scans—involved areas show increased uptake of technetium

Treatment and Nursing Management

OBJECTIVES: to suppress the plasma cell growth.
to control pain.

A. *Decrease the tumor mass and relieve bone pain.*

1. Give the appropriate chemotherapy (foundation of treatment).
   a. Combination drug therapy appears more effective than single dose therapy in most patients.
   b. See page 849 for supportive care of patient receiving chemotherapy.
2. Support patient receiving radiotherapy—given for relief of pain from large lesions (especially from nerve compression and fracture) and for reducing size of extraskeletal plasma cell tumors.

B. *Give attentive and supportive care.*

1. Keep the patient ambulatory and avoid immobilization unless lesions in spine (extradural plasmacytomas) produce danger of cord compression; ambulation prevents further bone resorption and hypercalcemia.
2. Control pain.
   a. Avoid excessive lifting and straining. Handle patient with smooth, unhurried movements.
   b. Try to *prevent* pain.
      (1) Administer pain-relieving medication at a scheduled time around the clock until pain control is attained.
      (2) Oral narcotic mixture—methadone or morphine, cocaine, alcohol with an antiemetic and flavorings (or other combinations) can be used to lower sensory dimension of pain and diminish fear.
      (3) Assess the effectiveness of pain intervention in order to decrease dosage or change medication until pain relief is achieved without sedation.
      (4) Radiation therapy, splinting, back brace, relaxation techniques—are other measures used for pain.
3. Evaluate for spinal cord compression—from invasion of canal by neoplastic tissue. Watch for bladder distention (spinal cord compression).
   a. Radiation therapy—to prevent paraplegia.
   b. Laminectomy for decompression—for cord compression or vertebral fractures.
4. Watch for recurrent infections—patient has impaired capacity for antibody production.
   a. Monitor temperature—patients on steroids may not have overt symptoms of infection. Assess for apathy, lethargy.
   b. Assess for symptoms of urinary tract infection and bronchopneumonia.
   c. Secure cultures from skin lesions, blood, sputum, and urine as indicated.

5. Assess the patient for signs and symptoms of renal insufficiency—abnormal proteins may exert a nephrotoxic effect at tubular level; or renal failure may develop from pyelonephritis; hypercalcemia (from bony destruction and immobilization), amyloidosis, hyperuricemia, myeloma kidney.
   a. Encourage liberal fluid intake—to prevent protein precipitation and to minimize hypercalciuria.
   b. Give allopurinol as prescribed—to control hyperuricemia.
   c. Watch for symptoms of hemorrhagic cystitis in patient taking Cytoxan; maintain on liberal fluid intake.
   d. Avoid dehydration—can precipitate acute renal failure; IV fluids may be necessary.
   e. Give prednisone as prescribed by physician—may be used in management of hypercalcemia. Weigh patient daily to monitor fluid retention.

NURSING ALERT: Patients with multiple myeloma should *not* have their fluid intake restricted prior to diagnostic tests, since dehydrating procedures can precipitate acute renal failure.

   f. Monitor renal status through blood studies and urinalysis.
   g. Dialysis may be employed for relief of uremic symptoms; kidney transplantation is also being used.
6. Treat concomitant anemia—occurs in most patients.
   a. Give packed red cell transfusions for patients with severe anemia.
   b. Administer chemotherapy, steroid hormones, and androgens—to stimulate erythropoiesis; may improve anemia.
   c. Determine methods to conserve patient's energy; note this on nursing care plan.
7. Be aware of the complications.

   a. Infection—from decrease in normal circulating antibodies due to proliferation of abnormal plasma cells which produce ineffective globulins; extensive bone marrow involvement causes leukopenia; chemotherapy and radiotherapy also cause marrow depression; steroid hormones increase susceptibility to opportunistic infection.
   b. Neurologic complications
      (1) Paraplegia—from collapse of supporting structures, from infiltration of nerve roots, or from cord compression of plasma cell tumors.
   c. Bone complications—pathologic fractures—may occur when patient turns; is placed on a bedpan, etc.
   d. Renal complications.
      (1) Renal failure—from plugging of renal tubules by proteinaceous casts.
      (2) Renal stones from hypercalcemia—due to bone destruction and increased bone resorption.
      (3) Infiltration of kidney from plasma cells, etc.
      (4) Hypercalciuria—excessive bone destruction creates increased excretion of calcium in urine.
      (5) Hyperuricemia—may produce renal failure.
   e. Acute leukemia.

Health Education and Emotional Support

1. Support the patient emotionally and demonstrate continuing interest.
   a. Reinforce the patient's understanding of treatment and its possible side effects.
   b. Take a positive approach emphasizing the benefits of therapy.
   c. Emphasize the patient's strengths.
      (1) Share and work through patient's anxieties.
      (2) Explore precisely what the patient fears.
      (3) Allow patient to talk about his problems. Give *specific* help (for pain, breathlessness, depression, etc.).
      (4) Anticipate patient's anxieties after leaving hospital.
2. Use diet supplement during periods of anorexia.

BLEEDING DISORDERS

Bleeding disorders may be classified as congenital or acquired and single or multifactorial.

History

1. Is there a history of abnormal or excessive bleeding? Following previous surgery? Dental extraction? Tonsillectomy? Family history of bleeding tendencies?
2. What medications is the patient taking? (Many drugs impair platelet function.) Taking aspirin? (More than 250 preparations contain aspirin.)
3. Has there been occupational exposure to toxic agents? Ionizing radiation?

Assessment

1. Mucocutaneous bleeding—petechiae or ecchymosis on skin, nosebleeding, gastrointestinal bleeding, lower urinary tract bleeding, hemorrhagic bullae in oral mucosa.
2. Bleeding into soft tissue, joints, viscera.

3. Palpable liver and spleen (hepatomegaly and splenomegaly).
4. Bleeding in central nervous system.

Nursing Management

1. Use every measure to prevent bleeding:
   a. Use electric razor.
   b. Avoid intramuscular injections when possible.
   c. Handle the skin gently; try to avoid use of adhesive tape.
   d. Rotate extremities for blood pressure measurement.
   e. Administer stool softeners—to prevent rupture of blood vessels from straining.
2. Measure blood loss; weigh linens, bandages, measure drainage.
3. Evaluate hemoglobin and hematocrit.
4. Conserve patient's strength during and after bleeding episodes.

VASCULAR PURPURAS

The term *purpura* refers to extravasation (escape) of blood into the skin and mucous membranes. Purpuric lesions may occur spontaneously as an isolated phenomenon or as an accompaniment of obvious disease.

Types of Purpura

1. *Petechiae*—small pinpoint hemorrhages under the skin.
2. *Ecchymoses*—escape of blood into tissues; producing a large bruise.
3. Petechiae and ecchymoses may occur as the result of vascular rupture, permitting the leakage of blood into the subcutaneous tissue of the mucous membranes.
4. *Symptomatic or secondary purpura*—certain types of bloodstream infections (e.g., meningococcemia and infective endocarditis) exhibit this phenomenon due to damage to the vascular walls by the infectious agent.
5. Severe arterial hypertension—may cause the patient to bruise easily; Valsalva maneuver may cause petechiae.
6. *Anaphylactoid purpura*—generally regarded as an allergic disorder in which there are various skin lesions (purpuric and otherwise) and episodes of arthritis, abdominal pain, hematuria, gastrointestinal hemorrhages, and fever.
   a. Attacks last several weeks and recur for years.
   b. Steroid therapy is often effective.
7. *Familial hemorrhagic telangiectasia*—a hereditary disorder manifested by an abnormal tendency to bleed and bruise.
   a. Precise nature of defect is obscure.
   b. Condition does not respond to any proved method of treatment.
8. *Toxic purpura*—a condition observed after exposure to certain drugs and poisons.
9. *Vitamin C deficiency*—a vascular purpura.
10. Senile purpura.
11. Collagen and vascular disease.
12. Steroid purpura.

THROMBOCYTOPENIA

Thrombocytopenia is a subnormal number of blood platelets. It is a common cause of abnormal bleeding.

Altered Physiology and Causes

Decreased platelet production (infiltrative diseases of bone marrow, radiation, myelosuppressive therapy, drugs, aplastic anemia, etc.)

Increased platelet destruction (infection, hemolytic reactions, disseminated intravascular coagulation, idiopathic thrombocytopenia purpura, drug induced, etc.)

Abnormal distribution or sequestration (entrapment)—(hypersplenism, hypothermia)

Loss of platelets from body (extracorporeal circulation, multiple blood transfusions)

Clinical Manifestations

When the platelet count drops below 20,000/mm^3:
1. Petechiae
2. Bleeding from mucosal surface, nose, uterus, gastrointestinal tract, urinary tract, respiratory tract, central nervous system (may be fatal)
3. Menorrhagia
4. Excessive bleeding after surgery or dental extractions

Treatment and Nursing Management

1. Treat the underlying disease (e.g. treat the leukemia, discontinue offending drugs, etc.).
2. Administer platelet transfusions if platelet production is impaired; if excessive destruction of platelets is the problem, transfused platelets will also be destroyed and will not raise the count.
3. Hormonal ablation of menstrual periods is usually carried out.

IMMUNE THROMBOCYTOPENIC PURPURA

Thrombocytopenic purpura refers to purpura (extravasation of blood into skin) which is accompanied by reduction in the number of circulating platelets. Antiplatelet antibodies are produced for unknown reasons, so that the platelet life span is markedly shortened.

Clinical Manifestations

1. Onset is usually sudden
2. Bleeding—mild to severe (thrombocytopenia not usually accompanied by bleeding unless the platelet count falls below 20,000/mm^3.)
   a. Skin lesions—small red hemorrhages; do not blanch on pressure
   b. Purpuric lesions may occur in vital organ (brain)
   c. Bleeding may occur from nose, mouth, genitourinary tract.

Laboratory Manifestations

1. Platelets may be absent or only slightly decreased in number; abnormalities may be seen in platelet size or morphologic appearance
2. Proteinuria and microscopic or gross hematuria present in majority of patients

Treatment and Nursing Management

OBJECTIVES: to search for possible causes of bleeding. to treat patient during spontaneous bleeding episodes.

1. Give adrenal corticosteroids (prednisone) for acute bleeding—may produce improvement by reducing bleeding (by affecting blood vessels, resulting in decreased capillary fragility; or by elevating the level of circulating platelets; or by suppression of phagocytic cells of reticuloentothelial system). This form of therapy is controversial.
2. Prepare the patient for a splenectomy (p. 260) if patient fails to respond to steroids.
   Splenectomy may bring about improvement by elevating the platelet levels and by removing major site of platelet sequestration.
3. Support the patient receiving red cell transfusions.
4. Give immunosuppressive therapy—used for patients who do not respond to corticosteroids or splenectomy.
5. Utilize other measures to help the patient.
   a. Avoid unnecessary trauma (IM injections, etc.).
   b. Keep patient on bed rest during periods of active bleeding.
   c. Administer iron salts for iron deficiency anemia from chronic blood loss.
   d. Suppress menstrual flow (by oral progestational-estrogenic agents) if patient has recurrent menorrhagia.
   e. Avoid aspirin—interferes with the hemostatic function of platelets.

BLEEDING DISORDERS DUE TO COAGULATION DEFECTS

DISSEMINATED INTRAVASCULAR COAGULATION (DIC)

Disseminated intravascular coagulation is an acquired hemorrhagic syndrome in which there is widespread clotting in small vessels of the body, leading to consumption of the clotting factors and platelets so that bleeding and thrombosis are occurring simultaneously. It is secondary to some underlying disease.

Clinical Features

1. Seen in a variety of diseases
   a. Infections; septicemia
   b. Obstetrical complications
   c. Malignancies
   d. Massive tissue injuries (burns)
   e. Vascular and circulatory complications; shock
   f. Anaphylaxis
   g. Hemolytic transfusion reactions
2. Hemorrhagic tendency is the consequence of the acute activation of the clotting mechanism of the blood—results in intravascular consumption of the plasma clotting factors
3. Clotting factors are consumed more quickly than they can be replenished by the liver

Clinical Manifestations

1. Bleeding or a tendency to bleed—from occult internal bleeding to profuse hemorrhaging from all orifices
2. Acrocyanosis (generalized sweating with cold, mottled fingers and toes)
3. Dyspnea, hemoptysis, crackles—from involvement of pulmonary circulation due to microcirculatory obstruction
4. Signs and symptoms of acute renal failure—from fibrin deposition in small vessels of kidneys

Diagnostic Evaluation

Coagulation profile—prolonged

Thrombocytopenia

Hypofibrinogenemia

Deficiencies in prothrombin factors V and VIII and elevated levels of fibrin degradation products

Treatment and Nursing Management

1. Remove the underlying condition responsible for DIC
   a. Correct any condition that exaggerates coagulopathy (shock, acidosis, sepsis).
   b. Give antisepsis treatment for coagulation changes produced by bacteremia.
2. Administer blood component replacement and other modalities of treatment as indicated by individual patient's condition.
3. Give heparin in initial stages (IV)—to stop the coagulation process and to permit normalization of clotting tests and a decrease in hemorrhagic manifestations (controversial).
   a. Heparin may be administered along with platelet and clotting factor replacements.
   b. See page 337 for administration of heparin.
   c. Heparin may be contraindicated in certain conditions (acute hepatic failure, intracranial hemorrhage).
4. Carry out ongoing nursing assessment for occult bleeding.
   a. Assess color of skin and mucosa, petechiae, cold mottled hands and feet, gingival bleeding, nose bleeding, bleeding/jaundice of conjunctivae and sclerae, hemoptysis.
   b. Ask about bone and joint pain, changes in vision (retinal hemorrhage).
   c. Evaluate cardiopulmonary function; assess for tachypnea, orthopnea, tachycardia, palpitations, orthostatic hypotension—reflect inadequacy of tissue oxygenation and/or fall in blood volume.
   d. Examine for abdominal tenderness.
   e. Check urine and stools for occult blood.
   f. Look for changes in mental status—from cerebral bleeding.

HEMOPHILIA

Hemophilia is a hereditary coagulation disorder. (See p. 128.)

VON WILLEBRAND'S DISEASE

Von Willebrand's disease is a common bleeding disorder inherited as a dominant character and affecting males and females equally. There are several genetic variants. It is due to a deficiency of a plasma protein associated with an impairment of platelet function.

Clinical Manifestations

1. Epistaxis; easy bruising
2. Gastrointestinal bleeding
3. Menorrhagia
4. Prolonged bleeding from cuts
5. Postoperative bleeding

Treatment and Nursing Management

OBJECTIVE: to give specific substitution therapy.
1. Administer cryoprecipitate.
2. Administer fresh plasma for patient not requiring intense substitution therapy.
3. Emphasize to the patient that aspirin is contraindicated.

ACQUIRED DEFECTS IN COAGULATION

Acquired defects in coagulation may be associated with many conditions, including:
1. Hypothrombinemia
2. Administration of coumarin-indanedione anticoagulant drugs
3. Heparin therapy
4. Diseases of the liver
5. Disseminated intravascular coagulation
6. Uremia
7. Transfusion-induced clotting factor deficiency
8. Chronic renal failure
9. Certain antibiotics—inhibit coagulation factors

SPLENECTOMY

Splenectomy is removal of the spleen.

Indications for Splenectomy

1. Staging procedure for Hodgkin's disease
2. Rupture of spleen
   a. History of injury
   b. Persistent abdominal pain
   c. Abdominal rigidity, rebound tenderness, shock
3. Hypersplenism (premature destruction of blood cells by the spleen)

Nursing Management

(New approaches are being tried to salvage a ruptured spleen.)

A. *Preoperative Care*

1. Carry out studies of coagulation status of patient.
   a. Have platelet donor packs available; have fresh frozen plasma available.
   b. Administer vitamin K for abnormalities of prothrombin time.
   c. Prepare for transfusion of packed red cells or fresh whole blood if patient has significant anemia.
2. Assist with preoperative pulmonary physical therapy—to reduce incidence of pulmonary complications; patient may be debilitated from hematologic disease, from immunosuppressants, etc.
3. *Preoperative Preparation for Patient with Rupture of Spleen*
   a. Administer whole blood if rupture of spleen has occurred.
   b. Evacuate stomach with nasogastric tube—to prevent aspiration.
   c. Check patient for pneumothorax/hemothorax—thoracotomy tube may be in place before anesthesia is started.

B. *Postoperative Care*

1. See page 89 for general aspects of nursing management following abdominal surgery.
2. Watch for the development of complications—related to location (anatomic) of spleen, the reason for its removal, and sequelae of splenectomy.

   a. Atelectasis of left lower lobe with pneumonia; pleural effusion—operations on left upper quadrant predispose to limited diaphragmatic movement.
   b. Subphrenic abscess/hematoma—assess for persisting fever.
   c. Infection—especially in children.
   d. Thrombocytopenia—if patient had thrombocytopenia before splenectomy, the condition may become extreme after splenectomy.
   e. Persistent or recurrent hemorrhage; measure abdominal girth.
   f. Thrombosis—may follow a few days after splenectomy; platelet count of 3–5 times normal values may occur; this postoperative physiological thrombocytosis may be conducive to thromboembolic complications.
      (1) Low-dose heparin regimen may be instituted.
      (2) Abdominal discomfort and fever may be caused by thrombi lodging in branches of portal system.
      (3) Mesenteric thrombosis—watch for postprandial cramping, abdominal pain; small bowel resection is indicated.

NURSING ALERT: Asplenic patients are at increased risk for infection. Those having combined modality therapy (radiotherapy and chemotherapy) are at increased risk of overwhelming sepsis.

Discharge Planning; Health Education

1. Emphasize that febrile illness should be reported immediately. An antimicrobial agent is usually given at the first sign of infection.
2. Encourage immunization with pneumococcal polysaccharide vaccine—an individual undergoing a splenectomy is at risk for pneumococcal infections and sepsis.

BIBLIOGRAPHY

Books

American Association of Blood Banks. Miller WV (ed). Technical Manual of the American Association of Blood Banks, 7th ed. Philadelphia, JB Lippincott, 1977

Erslev AJ and Gabuzda TG. Pathophysiology of Blood, 2nd ed. Philadelphia, WB Saunders, 1979

Geary CC. Aplastic Anemia. London, Bailliere Tindall, 1979

Hubbell RC (ed). Advances in Blood Transfusion. Arlington, American Blood Commission, 1979

Huestis DW, Bove JR and Busch S. Practical Blood Transfusion, 2nd ed. Boston, Little, Brown & Co, 1976

Lichtman MA (ed). Hematology for Practitioners. Boston, Little, Brown & Co, 1978

Mollison PL. Blood Transfusion in Clinical Medicine, 6th ed. Oxford, Blackwell Scientific Publications, 1979

Platt WR. Color Atlas and Textbook of Hematology, Philadelphia, JB Lippincott, 1979

Spivak JL (ed). Fundamentals of Clinical Hematology. Hagerstown, Harper & Row, 1980

Triplett DA (ed). Platelet Function. Chicago, American Society of Clinical Pathologists, 1978

Williams WJ et al. Hematology, 2nd ed. New York, McGraw-Hill, 1977

Wintrobe MM. Blood, Pure and Eloquent. New York, McGraw-Hill, 1980

Wintrobe MM. Clinical Hematology, 7th ed. Philadelphia, Lea & Febiger, 1974

Articles

Administration of Blood and Blood Components

Blajchman MA, Shepherd FA and Perrault RA. Clinical use of blood, blood components and blood products. Can Med Assoc J 1979 July; 121(1):33–42

Buickus BB. Administering blood components. Am J Nurs 1979 May; 79(5):937–941

Cullins LC. Preventing and treating transfusion reactions. Am J Nurs 1979 May; 79(5):935–936

Daly PA et al. Platelet transfusion therapy. JAMA 1980 Feb; 243(5):435–442

Kahn RA et al. Use of plasma products with whole blood and packed RBC's. JAMA 1979 Nov 9; 242(19):2087

Parker AL. Massive transfusions. Am J Nurs 1979 May; 79(5):945–948

Rice CL and Moss GS. Blood and blood substitutes: Current practice. Adv Surg 1979; 13:93–114

Rossman M. Slavin R and McCurdy PR. Pheresis therapy: Patient care. Am J Nurs 1977 July; 77(7):1135–1141

Scarlato M. Blood transfusions today. What you should know and should do. Nursing '78 1978 Feb; 8(2):68–72

Schiffer CA. Some aspects of recent advances in the use of blood cell components. Br J Haematol 1979 July; 39(3):289–294

Solanki D and McCurdy PR. Delayed hemolytic transfusion reactions. JAMA 1978 Feb 20; 239(8):729–731

Tenczynski J. Leukapheresis: The process. Am J Nurs 1977 July; 77(7):1133–1134

Zipursky A. The quiet revolution in blood transfusion therapy. Can Med Assoc J 1979 July; 121(1):14

Agranulocytosis

Berkman EM, Eisenstaedt RS and Caplan SN. Supportive granulocyte transfusions in the infected severely neutropenic patient. Transfusion 1978 Nov–Dec; 18(6):693–700

Freston JW. Cimetidine and granulocytopenia. Ann Intern Med 1979 Feb; 90(2):264–265

Golden W. Routine protective isolation: Worth the trouble in neutropenic patients? JAMA 1979 Nov 9; 242(19):2045

Hopefl AW. Empiric therapy of febrile granulocytopenic patients Am J Hosp Pharm 1979 Feb; 36(2):178—187

Lohner D et al. Comparative randomized study of protected environment plus oral antibiotics versus antibiotics alone in neutropenic patients. Cancer Treat Rep 1979 March; 63(3):363–368

Anemias

Brown JM et al. Helping the family withstand the stress of disease. Nursing '79 1979 Sept; 9(9):50–55

Camitta BM and Thomas ED. Severe aplastic anaemia. A prospective study of the effect of androgens or transplantation on haematological recovery and survival. Clin Haematol 1978 Oct; 7(3):587–595

Clift RA and Buckner CD. Supportive measures for patients with aplastic anemia. Clin Haematol 1978 Oct; 7(3):623–637

Coccia P et al. A primary overview of the anemias. Patient Care 1979 March; 13(5):114–115

Feig SA. Current approaches to the management of aplastic anemia. A summary. Transplant Proc 1978 March; 10(1):147–149

Gever LN. Thinking about parenteral iron supplements. Nursing '80 1980 Aug; 10(8):60

Muss HB and White DR. Iron deficiency anemia in adults. Am Fam Physician 1978 Feb; 17(2):174–185

Najean Y et al. Prognostic factors in acquired aplastic anemia. Am J Med 1979 Oct; 67(4):564–571

Savin MA. A practical approach to the treatment of iron deficiency. Ration Drug Ther 1979 Sept; 11(9):1–6

Bleeding Disorders

Ellison N. Diagnosis and management of bleeding disorders. Anesthesiology 1977 Aug; 47(2):171–180

Franco LM. Acute disseminated intravascular coagulation. Cardiovasc Nurs 1979 Sept–Oct; 15(5):22–27

Hardaway RM. Disseminated intravascular coagulation. Compr Ther 1978 Jan; 4(1):22–28

Jennings BM. Improving your management of DIC. Nursing '79 1979 May; 9(5):60–67

Nilsson IM and Holmberg L. Von Willebrand's Disease today. Clin Haematol 1979 Feb; 8(1):147–168

Saidi P. Diagnosis and management of bleeding disorders. Am Fam Physician 1980 Jan; 21(1):146–151

Bone Marrow Transplantation

Dreizen S et al. Oral complications of bone marrow transplantation in adults with acute leukemia. Postgrad Med 1979 Nov; 66(5):187–196

Edwards J. Bone marrow transplantation: Transatlantic comparisons. Nursing Mirror 1979 June; 148(23):31–32

Mathe G and Schwarzenberg L. Bone marrow transplantation (1958–1978): Conditioning and graft-versus-host disease, indications in aplasias and leukemias. Pathol Biol 1979 June; 27(6):337–343

Thomas ED et al. Bone marrow transplantation. N Engl J Med 1975 292 (16):Part I:832—843; Part II:292(17):895–902

Thomas ED. Marrow transplantation for nonmalignant disorders. N Engl J Med 1978 April 27; 298(17):963–946

Walker P. Bone marrow transplant: A second chance for life. Nursing '77 1977 Jan; 7(1):24–25

Winston DJ et al. Infectious complications of human bone marrow transplantation. Medicine 1979 Jan; 58(1):1–31

Leukemia

Bloomfield CD. Treatment of adult acute nonlymphocytic leukemia–1978. Arch Intern Med 1978 Sept; 138(9):1333–1334

Bodey GP et al. Treatment of acute leukemia in protected environmental units. Cancer 1979 Aug; 44(2):431–436

Canellos GP. Treatment of the leukemias. Med Times 1978 March; 106(3):42–45, 49

Cline MJ et al. Acute leukemia: Biology and treatment. Ann Intern Med 1979 Nov; 91(5):758–773

Desotell S. A brighter future for leukemia patients. Nursing '77 1977 Jan; 7(1):18–24

Dittmar K. Acute myeloblastic leukemia with polycythemia vera. NY State J Med 1979 April; 79(5):758–761

Gale RP. Advances in the treatment of acute myelogenous leukemia. N Engl J Med 1979 May 24; 300(21):1189–1199

Goldman JM. Modern approaches to the management of chronic granulocytic leukemia. Semin Hematol 1978 Oct; 15(4):420–430

Gouldstone J. Nursing care study: Leukaemia—to live or let die? A dilemma for the caring team. Nursing Times 1979 May; 75(22):914–918

Hoagland HC. Acute leukemia and its complications. Mayo Clin Proc 1978 April; 53(4):260–261

Peterson DE and Overholser CD. Dental management of leukemic patients. Oral Surg 1979 Jan; 47(1):40–42

Pinkel D et al. Exploring current leukemia therapies. Patient Care 1979 Dec; 13(21):54–78

Pippard MJ, Callender ST and Sheldon PWE. Infiltration of central nervous system in adult acute myeloid leukaemia. Br Med J 1979 Jan 27; 1(6158):227–229

Preisler HD and Higby DJ. Therapy of acute nonlymphocytic leukemia. I. Clinical aspects. NY State J Med 1979 May; 79(6):879–884

Preisler HD, Rustum YM and Epstein J. Biologic characteristics and prediction of response. NY State J Med 1979 May; 79(6):885–889

Sanders JE and Thomas ED. Bone marrow transplantation for acute leukaemia. Clin Haematol 1978 June; 7(2):295–311

Shepherd JP. The management of the oral complications of leukemia. Oral Surg 1978 April; 45(4):543–548

Thomas ED et al. Marrow transplantation for patients with acute lymphoblastic leukemia in remission. Blood 1979 Aug; 54(2):468–476

Wallace J and Freeman PA. Mouth care in patients with blood dyscrasias. Nursing Times 1978 June; 74(22):921–922

Wiernik PH. Treatment of acute leukaemia in adults. Clin Haematol 1978 June; 7(2):259–273

Woodruff R. The management of adult acute lymphoblastic leukaemia. Cancer Treat Rev 1978 June; 5(2):95–113

Lymphomas

Bergsagel DE et al. The chemotherapy of plasma-cell myeloma and the incidence of acute leukemia. N Engl J Med 1979 Oct 4; 300(14):743–768

Canellos GP. Diagnosis and treatment of Hodgkin's disease. Med Times 1978 March; 106(3):30–35

Canellos GP (ed). The lymphomas. Clin Haematol 1979 Oct; 8(3):531–698

Canellos GP. Treatment of the non-Hodgkin's lymphomas. Med Times 1978 March; 106(3):37–41

Cohen HJ et al. Combination chemotherapy with intermittent 1–3 Bis (2-chloroethyl) 1-Nitrosourea (BCNU), cyclophosphamide and prednisone for multiple myeloma. Blood 1979 Oct; 54(4):824–836

Davis AJ. Brompton's cocktail: Making good-byes possible. Am J Nurs 1978 April; 78(4):611–612

Desforges JF, Rutherford CJ and Piro A. Hodgkin's disease. N Engl J Med 1979 Nov 29; 301(22):1212–1222

Eckhardt S. Advances in the therapy of non-Hodgkin's lymphoma. Recent Results Cancer Res 1979; 69:63–75

Johnson WJ, Kyle R and Dahlberg PJ. Dialysis in the treatment of multiple myeloma. Mayo Clin Proc 1980 Feb; 55(2):65–72

LeBlanc DH. People with Hodgkin's disease: The nursing challenge. Nurs Clin North Am 1978 June; 13(2):281–300

Mann RB, Jaffe ES and Berard CW. Malignant lymphomas—a conceptual understanding of morphologic diversity. Am J Pathol 1979 Jan; 94(1):105–191

McIntyre OR. Current concepts in cancer: Multiple myeloma. N Engl J Med 1979 July; 301(4):193–196

Minna JD, Roenigk HH and Glatstein E. Report of the Committee on Therapy for Mycosis Fungoides and Sézary Syndrome. Cancer Treat Rep 1979 April; 63(4):729–736

Mullen JL, Reichman J and Rosato EF. Multiple carcinomas following therapy for Hodgkin's disease. J Surg Oncol 1979; 11(1):75–78

Ostchega Y et al. Nursing grandrounds: Achieving pain control in the patient with multiple myeloma: A team approach. Nursing '79 1979 Nov; 9(11):34–39

Valentine AS, Steckel S and Weintraub M. Pain relief for cancer patients. Am J Nurs 1978 Dec; 78(12):2055–2056

Wood RA. If I had Hodgkin's disease. Br Med J 1978 May 20; 1(6123):1329–1331

Polycythemia; Splenectomy

Meakins JL. Splenectomy for rupture of the spleen: A reappraisal. Can Med Assoc J 1979 July; 121(1):11–12

Traetow WD, Fabri PJ and Carey LC. Changing indications for splenectomy. Arch Surg 1980 April; 115(4):447–451

Walsh JR. Polycythemia vera: Diagnosis, treatment and relationship to leukemia. Geriatrics 1978 May: 33(5):61–63, 66–69

Wasserman LR. The treatment of polycythemia vera. Semin Hematol 1976 Jan; 13(1):57–78

9

CONDITIONS OF THE CARDIOVASCULAR SYSTEM

1 HEART DISORDERS

MANIFESTATIONS OF HEART DISEASE

The patient's symptoms of heart disease depend on:
1. Nature of cardiopathy
2. Resultant physiological disturbances of the circulation

Dyspnea

Dyspnea is undue breathlessness, an awareness of discomfort associated with breathing.

A. *General Features*

1. Dyspnea of cardiac origin—failure of left ventricle characterized by increased left atrial, pulmonary venous and capillary pressures; as left atrial pressure rises, the lungs become congested resulting in dyspnea.
2. The threshold (tolerance) for dyspnea varies with the individual.

B. *Types of Cardiac Dyspnea*

1. *Exertional dyspnea*—breathlessness upon moderate exertion, which is relieved by rest.
2. *Orthopnea*—shortness of breath when lying down which is relieved by promptly sitting upright.
3. *Paroxysmal nocturnal dyspnea*—sudden dyspnea at night while lying down.
4. *Cheyne-Stokes respiration*—periodic breathing characterized by gradual increase in depth of respiration followed by a decrease in respiration resulting in apnea; periods of hyperpnea alternating with periods of apnea.
   a. Cheyne-Stokes respiration is usually considered a serious sign.
   b. Associated with left ventricular failure (severe), cerebral vascular disease.

C. *Nursing Assessment of Dyspnea*

1. What precipitates or relieves the dyspnea?
2. What position does the patient assume?
3. What is the skin color? Pallor? Cyanosis?

Chest Pain

A. *Cardiac Causes of Chest Pain*

1. Ischemia caused by an increase in demand for coronary blood flow and oxygen delivery, which exceeds available blood supply; due to coronary artery disease (angina pectoris, myocardial infarction).
2. Excruciating pain radiating to back and flanks—from acute dissecting aneurysm of the aorta.
3. Sharp precordial pain (over heart area) radiating to left shoulder and upper back aggravated by respirations—indicates acute pericarditis.

B. *Assessment of Patient with Chest Pain*

1. Where is pain located? Does it radiate? To neck? face? back? abdominal area?
2. What is the character of the pain—dull, sharp, boring, crushing?
3. Are there associated symptoms and signs? Diaphoresis? Light-headedness? Nausea? Shortness of breath?
4. What are the time and mode of onset?
5. How long does the episode last?
6. What factors precipitate pain (breathing, coughing, swallowing, rapid walking, emotional stress, exposure to cold)?
7. What factors alleviate pain (rest, change in position, nitroglycerin)?

Palpitation

Palpitation is a rapid, forceful, or irregular heartbeat felt by the patient.

A. *General Features*

1. The patient complains of pounding, jumping, stopping sensations in his chest.

2. May be associated with heart disease—enlargement of heart, disturbances of rhythm.
3. Other causes—anxiety, fever, anemia, thyroid disturbances.

B. *Nursing Assessment.*

1. Notify physician and take ECG during episodes of palpitation—for later interpretation.
2. Compare apical and a peripheral pulse.
3. Note comcomitant symptoms—dizziness, chest pain, dyspnea.
4. Take blood pressure to check for hemodynamic changes.

Edema

Edema is an abnormal accumulation of serous fluid in the connective tissues.

A. *General Features*

1. Cardiac causes of edema—congestive heart failure
2. Other causes of edema—sodium retention, liver disease, renal disease, hypoproteinemia, venous or lymphatic obstruction

B. *Types*

1. Ascites—excessive fluid in peritoneal cavity
2. Pleural effusion—excessive fluid in the pleural cavity
3. Anasarca—gross generalized edema

C. *Nursing Implications*

1. In heart conditions the location of edema is influenced by gravity. Fluid collects in the lower parts of the body (dependent edema).
   a. Evaluate for edema of ankles and feet in the ambulatory patient.
   b. Evaluate for edema of sacral area and posterior thighs in patients confined to bed.
2. Avoid undue pressure on edematous areas. Edematous patients are prone to develop pressure sores.

Fatigue

1. Fatigue associated with heart disease is produced by low cardiac output.
2. As heart disease advances, fatigue is precipitated by less and less effort.

Dizziness and Syncope

May be caused by fall in cardiac output with resulting cerebral ischemia: may be secondary to arrhythmias, atrioventricular block, carotid-sinus sensitivity, and cerebrovascular obstructive disease.

Skin Color and Temperature

Examine for change in skin color: pallor, flushing, cyanosis, jaundice. *Cyanosis* is a bluish discoloration of the skin and mucous membranes.

A. *Types of Cyanosis*

1. Central cyanosis—low oxygen saturation of arterial blood.
2. Peripheral cyanosis—reduction of oxyhemoglobin in capillaries from restricted circulation (low output or vasoconstriction)

B. *Cardiac Causes of Cyanosis*

1. Congenital heart disease—due to mixing of arterial stream with venous blood.
2. Congestive heart failure and pulmonary edema—due to hypoxia resulting from low cardiac output and poor oxygenation of blood by lungs.

C. *Nursing Assessment*
1. Look at lobes of ears, fingernail beds, and palms.
2. Look in mouth—less color variation in mucous membranes.
3. Palpate for sweaty, cold, clammy, warm, or dry skin.
4. Evaluate for jaundice—may indicate congestive heart failure associated with severe liver congestion.

Hemoptysis

Hemoptysis is the coughing up of blood.
1. Small quantities of dark, clotted blood may indicate mitral stenosis, but more commonly associated with pulmonary embolism and pulmonary infarction.
2. Mixture of blood and pus—indicates pulmonary suppuration.
3. Pink, frothy sputum—indicates acute pulmonary edema.
4. Blood-streaked sputum—indicates acute pulmonary congestion.
5. Frank hemoptysis—due to lung pathology (see p. 153).

Abdominal Pain or Discomfort

1. Epigastric (upper abdominal) pain—due to myocardial infarction, distention of liver capsule from congestive heart failure.
2. Severe abdominal pain—may be due to dissection of the abdominal aorta or rupture of an aortic abdominal aneurysm.
3. Intermittent abdominal pain (related to food intake) may indicate circulatory insufficiency of mesenteric arteries or non-cardiac pain.

Other Manifestations of Heart Disease

1. Distention of neck veins—may be produced by pressure on liver (hepatojugular reflux), congestive heart failure, pericardial compression due to effusion, or constrictive pericarditis.
2. Digital clubbing (clubbing of fingers)—due to cyanotic congenital heart disease, bacterial endocarditis, certain forms of lung pathology; may also be familial.
3. Jaundice—congestive heart failure associated with severe liver congestion.

DIAGNOSTIC EVALUATION FOR HEART DISEASE

Physical Assessment

A. *Arterial Pulse*
1. Examine the pulses bilaterally; peripheral pulses should be equal.
   a. Note amplitude (fullness), which depends on pulse pressure (difference between systolic and diastolic pressures); this gives an estimate of stroke volume.
      (1) Small volume pulse may be from low stroke volume and peripheral vasoconstriction (myocardial infarction, shock, constrictive pericarditis, vasoconstrictive drugs).
      (2) Large volume pulse produced by large stroke volume (aortic regurgitation, pregnancy, thyrotoxicosis, bradycardia, patent ductus arteriosus).
   b. Palpate carotid artery—reveals character of pulse in the proximal aorta and provides indication of any abnormality causing disease of left ventricle.

B. *Blood Pressure*
1. Take on both arms; subsequently blood pressure is taken on right arm.
2. Measure blood pressure with patient supine and standing.
3. Document site of blood pressure measurement and position of patient. (See also page 20 for further discussion of technique.)

C. *Respiration*
Note rate, depth, and respiratory pattern.

D. *Jugular Venous Pulse*
1. Venous pulsation can be more easily seen than felt.
2. Identification of venous pulse permits assessment of height of venous pressure.
3. See page 34 for technique.

E. *Heart Auscultation*
1. Heart auscultation requires knowledge, experience, and a "listening ear" tuned to hear each event of the cardiac cycle.
2. Heart auscultation should be systematic, and the stethoscope should "inch" from one area to another.
3. Four main areas of auscultation: aortic area, pulmonary area, mitral area, and the tricuspid area.
4. Listen for rate and regularity of rhythm.
   a. Determine if an irregularity is related to respiratory movements.
   b. Evaluate the sequence in which an irregularity occurs.
5. During auscultation, the examiner assesses the venous pulse, feels the pulsation of the right carotid artery and the radial artery, feels precordial movement, and listens to the heart (Fig. 9-1).
6. See page 32 for a more complete discussion of heart examination and pages 35–36 for examination of abdomen and extremities.

Cardiographic Studies

A. *Electrocardiogram*—a visual representation of the electrical activity of the heart as reflected by changes in electrical potential at the skin surface.
1. ECG is obtained by placing leads on various body parts and recording the electrical impulse as a tracing on a strip of paper or on the screen of an oscilloscope.
2. Clinical usefulness—evaluation of conditions that interfere with normal electrophysiological function—disturbances of rhythm, disorders of cardiac muscle, enlargement of chambers of heart, presence of myocardial infarction, electrolyte disturbances.
3. See page 308 for a more detailed account.

B. *Echocardiography (Ultrasound Cardiography)*—a record of high frequency sound vibrations which have been sent into the heart through the chest wall. The cardiac structures return the echoes derived from the ultrasound. The motions of the echoes are traced on an oscilloscope and recorded on film.
1. Patient is placed in supine position and the transducer is placed on his chest.
2. Transducer applied (left sternal border) with ultra-

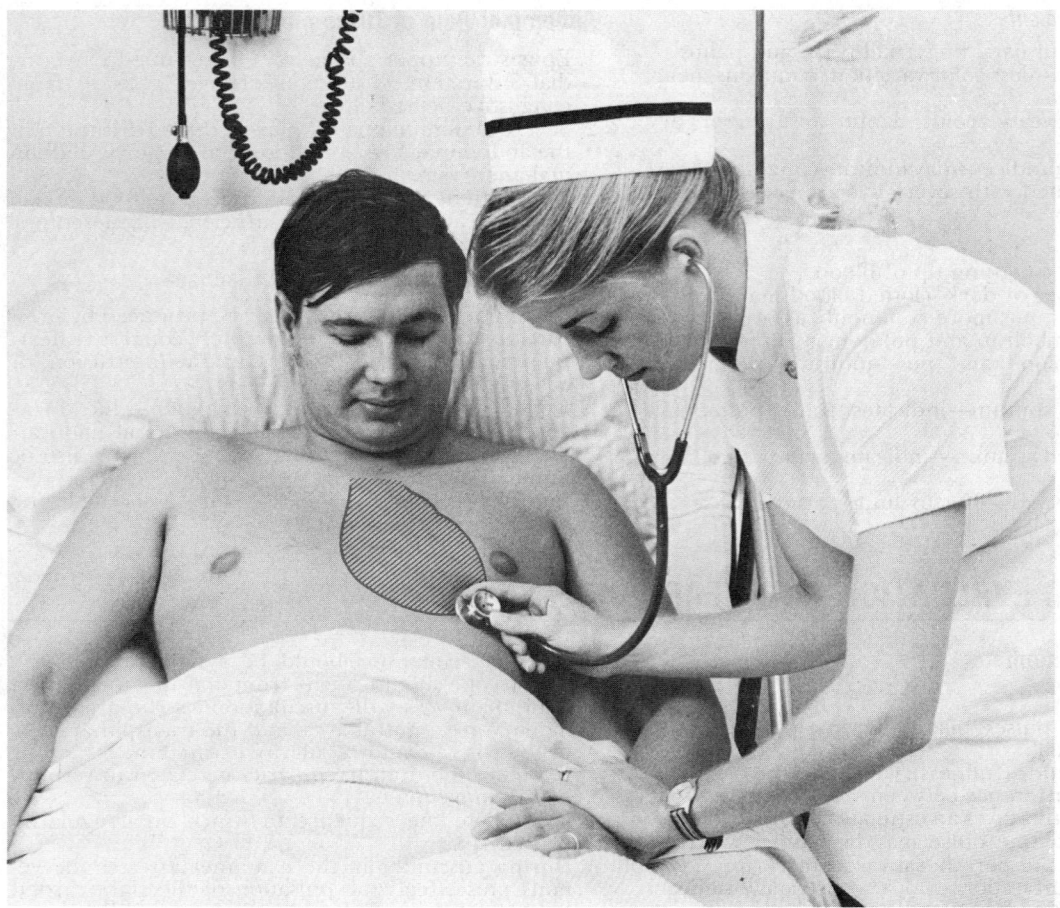

FIGURE 9-1. *Heart auscultation.*

sonic gel to maintain airless contact between skin and transducer.
3. ECG is recorded simultaneously to time the events within cardiac cycle. (Two-dimensional echocardiography now in use.)
4. *Clinical usefulness*
   a. Demonstration of valvular and other structural deformities
   b. Detection of pericardial effusion
   c. Evaluation of prosthetic valve function
   d. Diagnosis of cardiac tumors; asymmetric thickening of interventricular septum
   e. Diagnosis of cardiomegaly (heart enlargement)

C. *Ambulatory Electrocardiographic Monitoring*—continuous recording of an ECG to monitor the heart beat while the patient goes about his daily routine.

1. Patient wears miniaturized tape-recording device using a single or double lead system attached to belt or worn on a shoulder strap.
2. Patient keeps a diary—records his activities and any symptoms that are noted; useful when symptoms are provoked by specific activities (jogging, stress); used for assessing patients who suffer from transient dizziness, syncope, or near syncope; detecting ar-

rhythmias; assessing response to therapy; and evaluating patients after myocardial infarction.

D. *Exercise Stress Testing*—exercise testing on a treadmill or a bicycle-like device carried out to identify ischemic heart disease, to evaluate patients with chest pain, to assess results of therapy, and to aid in developing individual physical fitness programs.

1. Obtain informed consent—patient advised of purpose and risks of test.
2. ECG electrodes applied to patient and tracings made before, during, and after exercise testing.
3. Patient is exercised by increasing walking speed and the incline of the treadmill or by increasing the load against which he pedals.
4. Instruct patient to avoid smoking, eating, and drinking for 4 hours prior to test and to rest and avoid stimulants or extreme temperature changes after the test.

E. *Phonocardiography*—graphic recording of the heart sounds and pulse waves and their relation to time.

1. Helps to identify, to accurately time, and to differentiate various sounds and murmurs.
2. Provides a permanent record for future comparison.

F. *Vectorcardiography*—presents a three-dimensional view of the electrical forces of the heart.
1. Amplifies understanding of the ECG.
2. Gives more specific information in certain situations than the standard electrocardiogram.

Roentgenologic Studies

A. *Chest X-Ray*—shows heart size, contour, and position; reveals cardiac and pericardial calcifications and demonstrates physiologic alterations in pulmonary circulation.

B. *Fluoroscopy*—provides visual observation of the heart on a luminescent x-ray screen.
1. Shows heart and vascular pulsations; useful in the assessment of unusual cardiac contours and especially calcifications.
2. Useful in placement and positioning of intravenous electrodes and for guiding the catheter in cardiac catheterization.

C. *Angiocardiography*—injection of contrast medium into the vascular system (to outline the heart and blood vessels) accompanied by *cineangiograms* (rapidly changing films or movies on an intensified fluoroscopic screen), which record the passage of contrast media through the vascular tree.

Useful for providing information regarding coronary anatomy, structural abnormalities (occlusions, defects, fistulae) or abnormal heart-valve function.
1. *Selective angiocardiography*—contrast medium is injected through a catheter directly into one of the heart chambers, coronary arteries, or greater vessels, and the angiocardiogram is recorded by means of a rapid film changer or motion picture camera.
2. *Aortography*—a form of angiography that outlines the lumen of the aorta and major arteries arising from it.
3. *Coronary Arteriography* (most common form of selective angiocardiography)—a radiopaque catheter is introduced into the right brachial artery via open arteriotomy (or femoral artery via percutaneous puncture), passed into the ascending aorta, and manipulated into appropriate coronary artery under fluoroscopic control.
   a. Used as an evaluation tool before coronary artery surgery or myocardial revascularization and after surgery to evaluate graft patency.
   b. Used to study suspected congenital anomalies of the coronary arteries.
4. *Nursing Implications in Angiocardiography*
   a. Before angiogram
      Keep the patient in a fasting state prior to examination—to minimize danger of pulmonary aspiration should emesis occur.
   b. After angiogram
      (1) Record vital signs every 15 minutes (or more often as patient's condition indicates) until vital signs are stable.
      (2) Check for bleeding at puncture or cutdown site.
      (3) Check distal extremity for normal color and intact pulses.
      (4) The patient may complain of mild headache and/or discomfort in the groin or other site, depending on route by which contrast medium was administered.
      (5) Check for bed rest and special fluid directives from physician.

Cardiac Catheterization

Cardiac catheterization is a diagnostic procedure in which a catheter(s) is (are) introduced into the heart and blood vessels to (1) measure oxygen concentration, saturation, tension, and pressure in the various heart chambers; (2) detect shunts; (3) provide blood samples for analysis; and (4) determine cardiac output and pulmonary blood flow. Cardiac catheterization is also done to assess heart status before heart surgery.

Angiography is usually combined with heart catheterization for coronary artery visualization. During the procedure, the patient is monitored electrocardiographically by means of an oscilloscope.

A. *Right-heart Catheterization*—a radiopaque catheter is passed from an antecubital or femoral vein into the right atrium, right ventricle, and pulmonary vasculature under direct visualization with a fluoroscope.
1. Right atrium and right ventricle pressures measured; blood samples taken for hematocrit and oxygen saturation.
2. After entering the right atrium, the catheter is then passed through the tricuspid valve, and similar tests are performed on blood within the right ventricle.
3. Finally the catheter is passed through the pulmonic valve and as far as possible beyond that point; capillary samples are obtained and "capillary pressures" (wedge pressure) are recorded.
4. Complications: Cardiac arrhythmias, venous spasm, thrombophlebitis, infection of cutdown site, cardiac perforation, and cardiac tamponade.

B. *Left-heart Catheterization*—usually done by retrograde catheterization of the left ventricle or by transseptal catheterization of the left atrium.
1. Retrograde approach—catheter inserted under direct vision into right brachial artery and advanced under fluoroscopic control into the ascending aorta and into the left ventricle; or, catheter may be introduced percutaneously by puncture of femoral artery.
2. Transseptal approach—catheter is passed from the right femoral vein (percutaneously or by saphenous vein cutdown) into right atrium. A long needle is passed up through the catheter and is used to puncture the septum separating the right and left atria; needle is withdrawn and the catheter advanced under fluoroscopic control into left ventricle. Patient is monitored by ECG during both retrograde and transseptal techniques.
   a. Gives hemodynamic data—permits flow and pressure measurements of left heart.
   b. Most often performed to evaluate the function of the left ventricular muscle and mitral and aortic valves, or the patency of coronary arteries.
   c. Used to evaluate patients before and after cardiac surgery.
   d. Complications of left heart catheterization and implications for nursing assessment are
      (1) Arrhythmias (ventricular fibrillation), syncope, vasospasm
      (2) Pericardial tamponade, myocardial infarction, pulmonary edema
      (3) Allergic reaction to contrast medium
      (4) Perforation of great vessels of heart; systemic embolization (stroke, MI)
      (5) Loss of pulse distal to arteriotomy and possible ischemia of lower arm and hand.

C. *Nursing Management in Heart Catheterization*

1. Preceding Heart Catheterization
   a. Know which approach is to be used in order to anticipate possible complications.
   b. Withhold food and fluid 6 hours before procedure—to prevent vomiting and aspiration.
   c. Ascertain history of previous allergies.
   d. Mark distal pulses—for easy reference after catheterization.
   e. Explain to the patient that he will be lying on an examining table for a prolonged period and that he may experience certain sensations:
      (1) Occasional thudding sensations in the chest—from extrasystoles, particularly when the catheter is manipulated in ventricular chambers.
      (2) Strong desire to cough—may occur during contrast medium injection into right heart during angiography.
      (3) Transient feeling of heat, particularly in head—from injection of contrast medium.
   f. Remove dentures; give prescribed medication.
2. Following Heart Catheterization
   a. Record the blood pressure and apical pulse every 15 minutes (or more frequently) until vital signs are stable after the procedure—to discern arrhythmias.
   b. Check peripheral pulses in affected extremity (dorsalis pedis, posterior tibial pulse in the lower extremity, and radial pulse in upper extremity); evaluate extremity temperature, color, and complaints of pain, numbness, or tingling sensation—to determine signs of arterial insufficiency.
   c. Watch puncture (cutdown) sites for hematoma formation. Question patient about increase in pain/tenderness at site.
   d. Assess for complaints of chest pain and report occurrence immediately—myocardial infarction may occur and is a serious complication of cardiac catheterization.
   e. If protocol requires, see that the patient remains in bed with little movement of the involved extremity until the following morning.

Blood Studies

1. CBC
2. Blood electrolytes (potassium, sodium, chloride, carbon dioxide)—for patients treated with digitalis or diuretics
3. Blood urea nitrogen and creatinine—to evaluate cardiac output
4. Sedimentation rate, C-reactive protein and antistreptolysin O titer—to rule out inflammatory heart disease
5. Blood culture—to exclude bacterial endocarditis

Enzyme and Isoenzyme Tests

A. *Rationale of Tests*—the release of enzymes from cells into body fluids and into the circulation provides an indication of tissue damage and of changes taking place within the cells.

B. *Underlying Concepts*
1. Heart muscle is rich in enzymes that promote different biochemical reactions.
2. When myocardial tissue is damaged (myocardial infarction) certain cardiac enzymes are released into the blood stream and result in elevated peripheral blood enzyme levels:
   Creatine kinase (CK)
   Aspartate aminotransferase (AST)
   Lactic dehydrogenase (LDH)
3. However, these enzymes may be widely distributed in tissues and elevated in conditions not associated with myocardial infarction—i.e., damage to skeletal muscles, liver, brain, kidneys, and other organs.

C. *Isoenzymes*—forms of protein species that promote the same biochemical action as enzymes but differ chemically, physically, and/or immunologically.
1. Isoenzymes can be identified by laboratory methods to reveal the specific tissue that is damaged; Creatine kinase can be separated into 3 isoenzymes known as MM, MB, and BB.
2. An elevation of serum CK-MB activity signifies that an adverse effect on myocardial cells has taken place; thus, it is the most specific and sensitive enzymatic criterion of myocardial injury now available.

HEMODYNAMIC MONITORING

Hemodynamic monitoring is the assessment of the patient's circulatory status; it includes measurements of heart rate, intra-arterial pressure, pulmonary artery and pulmonary capillary wedge pressures (see below), central venous pressure (p. 271), cardiac output (p. 274), and blood volume.

GUIDELINES: Measuring Pulmonary Artery Pressure by Flow-Directed Balloon-Tipped Catheter (Swan-Ganz Catheter)

The *Swan-Ganz catheter* is a multipurpose catheter that permits monitoring of pressure in the pulmonary artery and measurement of pulmonary artery wedge pressure; it also has the capability to measure cardiac output.

Purposes*
1. To obtain precise hemodynamic data concerning pressures in the right atrium, right ventricle, pulmonary artery, and distal branches of the pulmonary artery (pulmonary capillary wedge pressure). The latter reflects the level of the pressure in the left atrium (or filling pressure in the left ventricle); thus, pressures on the left side of the heart are inferred from pressure measurements obtained on the right side of the circulation.

* With the placement of 2 or more fine wires into the catheter, additional functions such as intra-atrial electrocardiography as well as atrial and ventricular pacing may be achieved.

Purposes (cont.)
2. To evaluate the patient and permit rational selection of therapy when critical changes in cardiac dynamics occur.
3. To measure cardiac output.
4. To draw blood from the pulmonary artery.

Underlying Considerations

1. Left atrial pressure is closely related to left ventricular end-diastolic pressure (LVEDP) (filling pressure of the left ventricle) and is therefore an indicator of left ventricular function.
2. Swan-Ganz catheterization permits measurement of pulmonary capillary pressure. This is called pulmonary capillary wedge pressure (PCWP).
3. Pulmonary artery pressures are important in evaluating patients with cardiogenic shock, severe left ventricular failure with pulmonary edema, mitral regurgitaion, and/or ventricular-septal rupture, etc.

Equipment

Swan-Ganz catheter set
ECG; monitor and display unit
Defibrillator
Pressure transducer; transducer holder
Cutdown tray
Syringes: tuberculin; 2.5 ml. syringe
Sterile saline solution

Heparin
Antiarrhythmic drugs
Local anesthetic
Skin antiseptic
Elastoplast tape
Sterile drape/gloves

Procedure (Fig. 9-2)

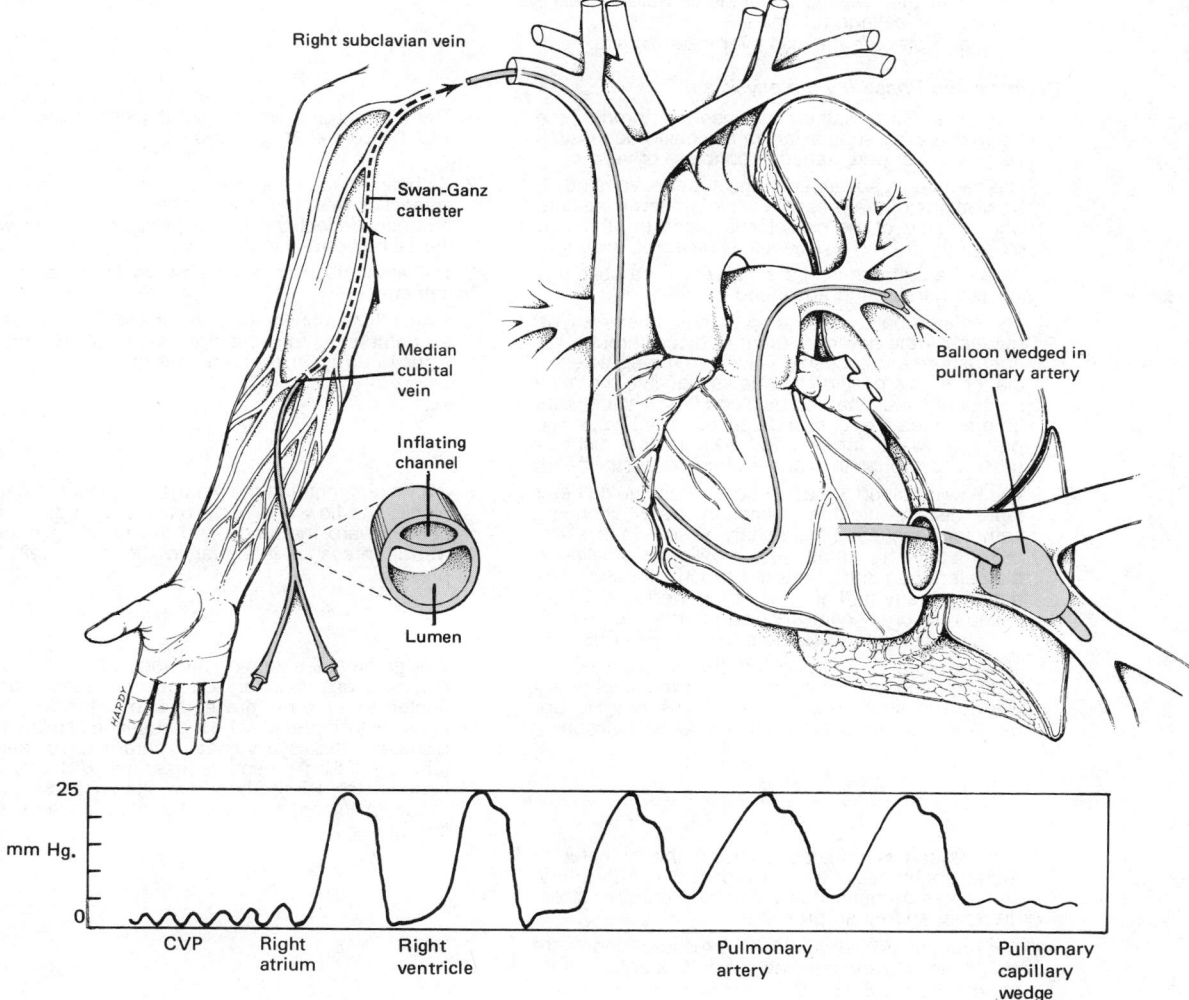

FIGURE 9-2. *Insertion of a Swan-Ganz catheter. The position of the catheter is reflected by the pressure tracings. Capillary wedge pressure is obtained by inflating the balloon.*

GUIDELINES: Measuring Pulmonary Artery Pressure by Flow-Directed Balloon-Tipped Catheter (Swan-Ganz Catheter) (cont.)

NURSING ACTION	**RATIONALE/AMPLIFICATION**

Procedure (cont.)

Preparatory Phase

1. Explain procedure to patient and family/significant other.
2. Check vital signs and apply ECG electrodes.
3. Place patient in a position of comfort; this is the baseline position.

4. Set up equipment according to manufacturer's directives:
   a. The pulmonary artery catheter requires a transducer; recording, amplifying, and flush systems.

   b. The pressure equipment is calibrated and flushed according to manufacturer's directives.
   c. The balloon is inflated with air and then deflated, or it is inflated with air under sterile water or saline to test for leakage (bubbles).
5. Shave and prepare the skin over insertion site.

Performance Phase (by the physician)

1. The Swan-Ganz catheter is inserted through the internal jugular, subclavian, or any easily accessible vein by either percutaneous puncture or venotomy.
2. The catheter is advanced to the superior vena cava. Oscillations of the pressure waveforms will indicate when the tip of the catheter is within the thoracic cavity (Fig. 9-2). The patient may be asked to cough.
3. When the catheter is in the superior vena cava it is inflated with air and advanced gently.
4. The inflated balloon at the tip of the catheter will be guided by the flowing stream of blood through the right atrium and tricuspid valve into the right ventricle. From this position it finds its way into the main pulmonary artery carried by blood flow. The catheter tip pressures are recorded continuously by specific pressure wave forms (Fig. 9-2) as the catheter advances through the various chambers of the heart.
5. The flowing blood will continue to direct the catheter more distally into the pulmonary tree. When the catheter reaches a pulmonary vessel that is approximately the same size or slightly smaller in diameter than the inflated balloon, it cannot be advanced any further. This is the wedge position, called pulmonary capillary wedge pressure (PCWP) or pulmonary artery wedge pressure (PAWP).
6. The pressure is recorded with the balloon wedged in the pulmonary vascular bed. A mean capillary wedge pressure between 14 and 18 mm. Hg appears to indicate optimal left ventricular function.

7. The balloon is deflated, causing the catheter to retract spontaneously into a larger pulmonary artery. This gives a continuous pulmonary artery systolic, diastolic, and mean pressure.

8. The normal systolic pulmonary pressure ranges are 15–25 mm. Hg and the diastolic pulmonary pressure ranges are 8–12 mm. Hg.

9. The normal mean pulmonary artery pressure (average pressure in pulmonary artery throughout the entire cardiac cycle) ranges from 10–20 mm. Hg.

1. Tell the patient he may feel the catheter moving through his vein and this is normal.

3. Note the angle of elevation if patient cannot lie flat as subsequent pressure readings are taken from this baseline position to ensure consistency.

   a. Monitoring systems may vary greatly. The complexity of equipment requires an understanding of the equipment in use.
   A constant microdrip is maintained except when reading pressures.
   b. Flushing of the catheter system ensures patency and eliminates air bubbles.
   c. To ensure that the balloon is intact.

1. The internal jugular vein establishes a short route into the central venous system.

2. Catheter placement may be determined by characteristic wave forms and changes. Coughing will produce deflections in the pressure tracing when the catheter tip is in the thorax.

3. The amount of air to be used is indicated on the catheter.

4. Watch ECG monitor for signs of ventricular irritability as catheter enters the right ventricle. Report any signs of arrhythmia to the physician.

5. With the catheter in the wedge position, the balloon blocks the flow of blood from the right side of the heart toward the lungs and the resulting capillary wedge pressure is equal to the mean left atrial pressure.

6. Wedge pressure reading provides information about the level of pulmonary congestion and is closely related to left atrial pressure and to left ventricular end-diastolic pressure (in the absence of mitral valve disease). This is a valuable parameter of cardiac function. Filling pressures less than 8–10 mm. Hg in an acutely injured heart are often associated with reduction in cardiac output, hypotension, and tachycardia.

Procedure (cont.)

NURSING ACTION	RATIONALE/AMPLIFICATION
10. The catheter is sutured in place.	10. An antibactericidal ointment may be placed around the site and covered with a sterile dressing.
11. The patency of the catheter is maintained with a low-flow continuous irrigation.	11. A chest x-ray to confirm catheter position and as a baseline for future reference is obtained after Swan-Ganz insertion.

To obtain a wedge pressure reading:

1. Close off the microdrip.	1. The transducer converts the pressure wave into an electronic wave that is displayed on a screen.
2. Inflate the balloon slowly until the contour of the pulmonary arterial pressure changes to that of pulmonary wedge pressure. As soon as a wedge pattern is observed, no more air is introduced. Do not introduce more air into balloon than specified.	2. Pulmonary capillary wedge pressure is only measured intermittently. Do not allow catheter to remain in the wedge position when patient is unattended or when not directly making the measurement.
3. Deflate the balloon as soon as the pressure reading is obtained.	3. Segmental lung infarction may occur if the catheter balloon is left inflated for long periods.

Follow-Up Phase

1. Inspect the insertion site daily. Look for signs of infection, swelling, and bleeding. Culture the site every 48 hours.	1. A foreign body (catheter) in the vascular system increases the risk of sepsis.
2. Record date and time of dressing change and IV tubing change.	
3. Assess the extremity for color, temperature, capillary filling, and sensation.	3. Ischemia (with possible loss of digits) may occur from inadequate arterial flow.
4. Evaluate pulse.	
5. Assess for complications: pulmonary embolism, arrhythmias, heart block, damage to tricuspid valve, intracardiac knotting of catheter, thrombophlebitis, infection, balloon rupture, rupture of pulmonary artery.	

For removal of the catheter:

1. Be sure that the balloon is not inflated.	
2. The catheter is removed without excessive force or traction; pressure dressing is applied over the site.	2. The site should be checked periodically for bleeding.

GUIDELINES: Central Venous Pressure*

Central venous pressure (CVP) is the pressure within the right atrium or in the great veins within the thorax.

Purposes
1. To serve as a guide to fluid replacement in seriously ill patients.
2. To estimate blood volume deficits.
3. To determine pressures in the right atrium and central veins.
4. To evaluate for circulatory failure (in context with total clinical picture of patient).
5. For drug administration (long-term chemotherapy).
6. To serve as a route for hyperalimentation.

Vein Sites for Catheter Placement

The most commonly used sites are:
Subclavian
Internal or external jugular
Median basilic

Equipment
Venous pressure tray
Cutdown tray
Infusion solution and infusion set
3- or 4-way stopcock (a pressure transducer may be used)
IV pole attached to bed; arm board; adhesive tape.
ECG monitor
Carpenter's level (for establishing zero point)

* Central venous pressure provides a guide to the assessment of left ventricular function only in the absence of cardiopulmonary disease.

GUIDELINES: Central Venous Pressure (cont.)

Procedure (Fig. 9-3)

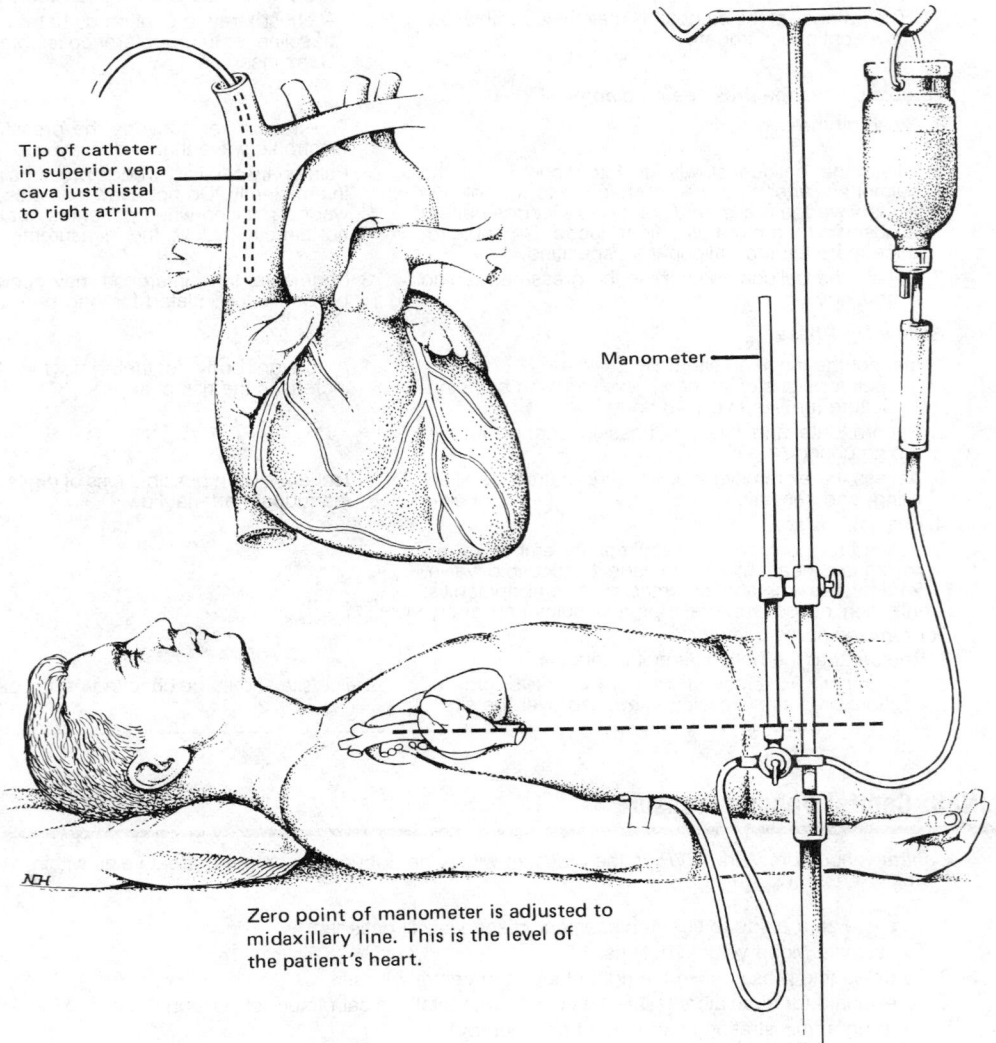

Tip of catheter in superior vena cava just distal to right atrium

Manometer

Zero point of manometer is adjusted to midaxillary line. This is the level of the patient's heart.

FIGURE 9-3. *Central venous pressure.*

NURSING ACTION	RATIONALE/AMPLIFICATION
Preparatory Phase	
1. Assemble equipment according to manufacturer's directions.	
2. Explain that the procedure is similar to an IV and that the patient may move in bed as desired after the passage of the CVP catheter.	
3. Place the patient in a position of comfort. This is the baseline position used for subsequent readings.	3. Serial CVP readings should be made with the patient in the same position. Inaccuracies in CVP readings can be produced by changes in position, coughing, or straining during the reading.

Procedure (cont.)

NURSING ACTION	RATIONALE/AMPLIFICATION

4. Attach manometer to the IV pole. The zero point of the manometer should be on a level with the patient's right atrium.

   Mark the midaxillary line on the patient with an indelible pencil.

4. The right atrium is at the midaxillary line, which is about ⅓ of the distance from the anterior to the posterior chest wall (Fig. 9-3).

   The midaxillary line is an external reference point for the zero level of the manometer (which coincides with the level of the right atrium).

5. The CVP catheter is connected to a 3-way stopcock which communicates to an open IV (e.g., saline and heparin) and to a manometer (the measuring device).

5. Or, the CVP catheter may be connected to a transducer and an electrical monitor with either digital or calibrated CVP wave readout.

6. Start the IV flow and fill the manometer 10 cm. above anticipated reading (or until the level of 20 cm. H_2O is reached). Turn the stopcock and fill the tubing with fluid.

7. The CVP site is surgically cleansed. CVP catheter (line) is introduced percutaneously or by direct venous cutdown and threaded through an antecubital, subclavian, or internal or external jugular vein into the superior vena cava just before it enters the right atrium.

7. If the catheter is inserted through the subclavian or internal jugular vein, place patient in a head down position to increase venous filling and reduce risk of air embolism. The correct catheter placement can be confirmed by fluoroscopy or chest x-ray.

8. When the catheter enters the thorax an inspiratory fall and expiratory rise in venous pressure are observed.

8. The fluid level fluctuates with respiration. It rises sharply with coughing, straining.

9. The patient may be monitored by ECG during catheter insertion.

9. When the tip of the catheter contacts the wall of the right atrium (or right ventricle) it may produce aberrant impulses and disturb cardiac rhythm.

10. The catheter may be sutured and taped in place. A sterile dressing is applied.

10. Label dressing with time and date of catheter insertion.

11. The infusion is adjusted to flow into the patient's vein by a slow continuous drip.

11. The infusion may cause a significant increase in venous pressure if permitted to flow too rapidly

To Measure the CVP

1. Place the patient in the identified position and confirm the zero point. (See #3 under "Preparatory Phase.") Intravascular pressures are measured to the atmospheric pressure at the middle of the right atrium; this is the zero point or external reference point.

1. The zero point or baseline for the manometer should be on a level with the patient's right atrium. The middle of the right atrium is the midaxillary line in the 4th intercostal space.

2. Position the zero point of the manometer at the level of the right atrium.

2. All personnel taking the CVP measurement use the same zero point.

3. Turn the stopcock so that the IV solution flows into the manometer filling to about the 20–25 cm. level. Then turn stopcock so that solution in manometer flows into patient.

4. Observe the fall in the height of the column of fluid in manometer. Record the level at which the solution stabilizes or stops moving downward. This is the central venous pressure. Record CVP and the position of the patient.

4. The column of fluid will fall until it meets an equal pressure, i.e., the patient's central venous pressure. The CVP reading is reflected by the height of a column of fluid in the manometer when there is open communication between the catheter and the manometer. The fluid in the manometer will fluctuate slightly with the patient's respirations. This confirms that CVP line is not obstructed by clotted blood.

5. The CVP may range from 5–12 cm. H_2O. (Absolute numerical values have not been agreed upon.)

5. The change in CVP is a more useful indication of adequacy of venous blood volume and alterations of cardiovascular function. CVP is a dynamic measurement. The normal values may change from patient to patient. The management of the patient is not based on one reading but on repeated serial readings in correlation with patient's clinical status.

6. Assess the patient's clinical condition. Frequent changes in measurements (interpreted within the context of the clinical situation) will serve as a guide to detect whether the heart can handle its fluid load and whether hypovolemia or hypervolemia is present.

6. CVP is interpreted by considering the patient's entire clinical picture; hourly urine output, heart rate, blood pressure, cardiac output measurements.
   a. A CVP near zero indicates that the patient is hypovolemic (verified if rapid IV infusion causes patient to improve).
   b. A CVP above 15–20 cm. H_2O may be due to either hypervolemia or poor cardiac contractility.

7. Turn the stopcock again to allow IV solution to flow from solution bottle into patient's veins.

7. When readings are not being made, flow is from a very slow microdrip to the catheter, bypassing the manometer.

GUIDELINES: Central Venous Pressure (cont.)

Procedure (cont.)	NURSING ACTION	RATIONALE/AMPLIFICATION

Follow-up Phase

1. Observe for complications.
   a. From catheter insertion: pneumothorax; hemothorax; hematoma; cardiac tamponade.
   b. Secondary to presence of indwelling venous catheter: air embolism; catheter embolization; colonization of organisms.
2. Carry out ongoing nursing surveillance of the insertion site and maintain aseptic technique.
   a. Inspect entry site twice daily for signs of local inflammation/phlebitis. Remove immediately if there are any signs of infection.
   b. Change dressings as prescribed.
   c. Label to show date/time of change.
   d. Send the catheter tip for bacteriological culture when it is removed.

1. The incidence of complications rises rapidly the longer the CVP catheter is left in place. The patient's complaint of a new or different pain should be assessed and acted upon.

> **NURSING ALERT:** A CVP line is a potential source of septicemia.

CARDIAC OUTPUT

Cardiac output is the amount (volume) of blood ejected during a given time period by the heart.

Clinical Assessment of Cardiac Output

A low cardiac output may be detected by:
1. Cyanosis or duskiness of buccal mucosa, nailbeds, and ear lobes
2. Cool, moist skin
3. Low urine output
4. Falling blood pressure

Underlying Concepts

1. Cardiac output depends on cardiac function, tone of the blood vessels, and blood volume.
2. Cardiac output is expressed in liters per minute divided by body surface, which yields the cardiac index in liters/minute/square meter of body surface. The body surface area is determined from standard charts.
3. Cardiac output is measured by a variety of techniques. In the clinical setting it is usually measured by the thermodilution technique used in conjunction with a flow-directed balloon catheter (Swan-Ganz catheter, p. 268).

Method

1. The triple-lumen Swan-Ganz catheter is positioned in its final position in a branch of the pulmonary artery; it has a thermistor (external heat-sensing device) situated 4 cm. from the tip of the catheter, which measures the temperature of the blood that flows by it.
2. Sterile dextrose or saline solution at 0° C is injected through one lumen of the catheter. The solution mixes with the blood in the right side of the heart and flows to the pulmonary artery where blood temperature is detected by the thermistor.
3. A small computer converts the temperature changes into a direct reading of cardiac output.

SPECIAL MEDICAL AND NURSING MEASURES

GUIDELINES: Assisting the Patient Undergoing Pericardiocentesis (Pericardial Aspiration)

Pericardiocentesis is the puncturing of the pericardial sac in order to aspirate fluid and thereby relieve cardiac tamponade.

Cardiac tamponade is compression of the heart by blood, effusion, or a foreign body in the pericardial sac which impairs normal heart action.

Clinical Manifestations of Cardiac Tamponade

1. Rising venous pressure
2. Falling arterial blood pressure
3. Small, quiet heart; muffled heart sounds (evidenced by fluoroscopy and chest auscultation)
4. Narrowing pulse pressure (difference between systolic and diastolic pressures)
5. Paradoxical pulse (abnormal degree of decline in systolic arterial blood pressure during inspiration) Assessment for paradoxical pulse (pulsus paradoxus).
   a. Place patient in a recumbent position.
   b. Inflate blood pressure cuff until Korotkoff sounds disappear; slowly release cuff pressure.

c. A decline in systolic blood pressure of 10 mm. Hg or more with each inspiration is considered indicative of a paradoxical pulse, or a decrease in amplitude (palpable at wrist) during inspiration may be evident if decline is 15 mm. Hg or more.

d. Indicates presence of significant pericardial effusion.

6. Distention of neck veins and inspiratory rise in venous pressure (Kussmaul's sign)
7. Apprehension; dyspnea
8. Tachypnea; pallor or cyanosis
9. Characteristic posture—sitting upright and leaning forward
10. Clinical shock

Purpose

1. To remove fluid from the pericardial sac caused by:
   a. Pericarditis
   b. Effusion from malignant neoplasm or lymphoma
   c. Trauma to heart/chest; cardiac surgery
   d. Infection
2. To obtain fluid for diagnosis
3. To instill certain therapeutic drugs

Equipment

Pericardiocentesis tray
Intracath set
Skin antiseptic
1–2% procaine
Sterile gloves
ECG for monitoring purposes
Sterile ground wire—to be connected between pericardial needle and V lead of ECG (use alligator clip type connectors)
Equipment for cardiopulmonary resuscitation

Sites for Pericardiocentesis (Fig. 9-4)

1. Subxiphoid—needle inserted in the angle between left costal margin and xiphoid
2. Near cardiac apex, 2 cm. (0.8 inch) inside left border of cardiac dullness
3. To the left of the 5th or 6th interspace at the sternal margin
4. Right side of 4th intercostal space just inside border of dullness

Procedure (Fig. 9-4)

NURSING ACTION	RATIONALE/AMPLIFICATION
Preparatory Phase	
1. Medicate patient as prescribed.	
2. Start a slow intravenous drip of saline or glucose.	2. This preserves a route for intravenous therapy in the event of an emergency.
3. Place the patient in a comfortable position with the head of the bed or treatment table raised to a 60-degree angle.	3. This position makes it easier to insert needle into pericardial sac.
4. Apply the limb leads of the ECG to the patient.	4. The patient is monitored during the procedure by ECG.
5. Have defibrillator available for immediate use.	5. In case the procedure has severe adverse effect.
6. Have pacemaker available.	
7. Open the tray, using aseptic technique.	
Performance Phase (by physician)	
1. The site is prepared with skin antiseptic; the area is draped with sterile towels and injected with procaine solution.	
2. The pericardial aspiration needle is attached to a 50 ml. syringe by a 3-way stopcock. The V lead (precordial lead wire) of the ECG is attached to the hub of the aspirating needle by a sterile wire and alligator clips or clamp.	2. There is danger of laceration of myocardium/coronary artery and of cardiac arrhythmias.
3. The needle is advanced slowly until fluid is obtained.	3. Fluid is generally aspirated at a depth of 2.5–4 cm. (1 to 1½ inches).
4. When the pericardial sac has been entered, a hemostat is clamped to the needle at the chest wall just where it penetrates the skin. Pericardial fluid is aspirated slowly.	4. This prevents movement of the needle and further penetration while fluid is being removed.
5. Monitor the patient's ECG, blood pressure, and venous pressure constantly.	5. a. The ST segment rises if the point of the needle contacts the ventricle; there may be ventricular ectopic beats. b. The PR segment is elevated when the needle touches the atrium. c. Large, erratic QRS complexes indicate penetration of the myocardium.

GUIDELINES: Assisting the Patient Undergoing Pericardiocentesis (Pericardial Aspiration) (cont.)

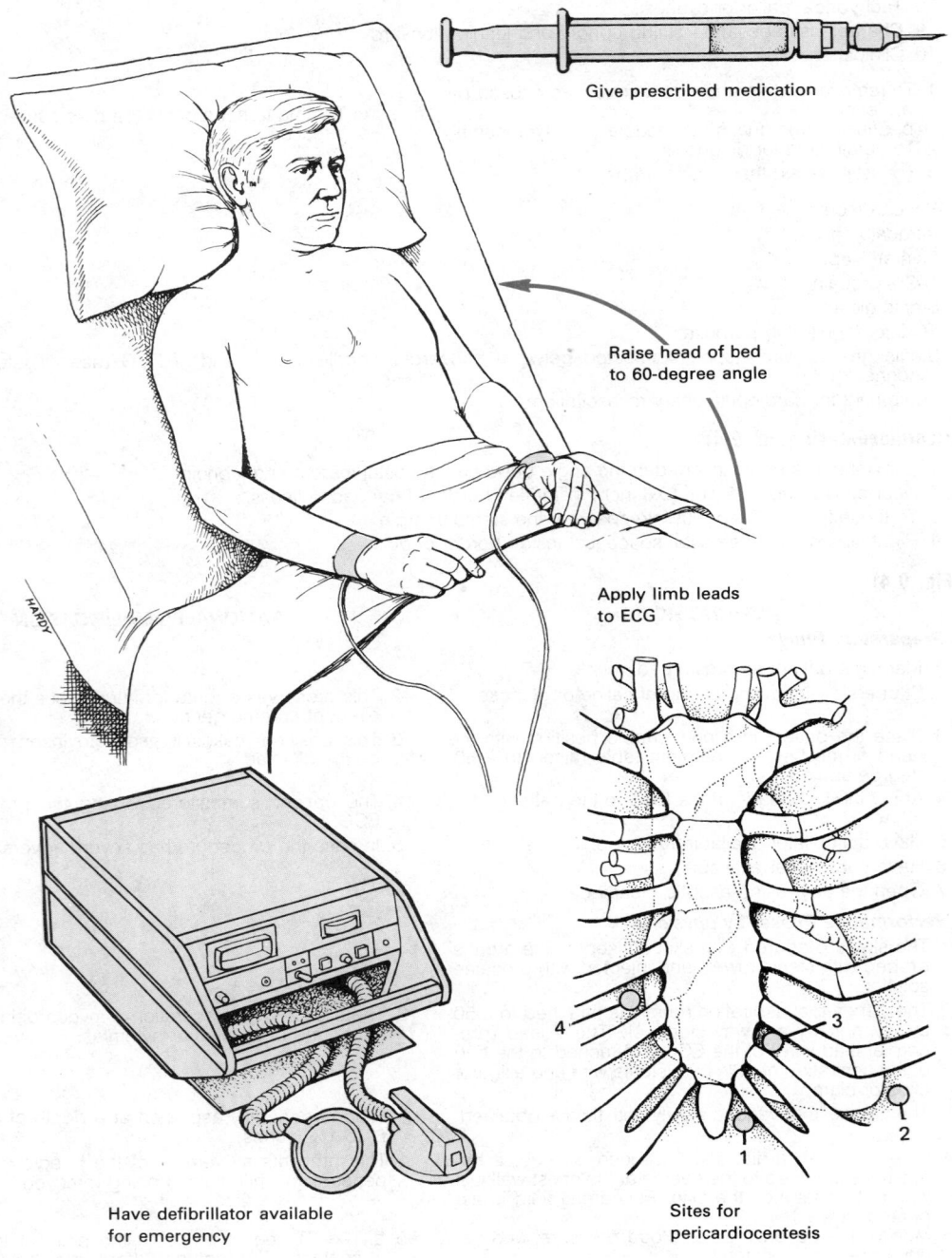

Give prescribed medication

Raise head of bed
to 60-degree angle

Apply limb leads
to ECG

Have defibrillator available
for emergency

Sites for
pericardiocentesis

FIGURE 9-4. *Preparing patient for pericardiocentesis.*

Procedure (cont.)

NURSING ACTION	RATIONALE/AMPLIFICATION
6. If a large amount of fluid is present, a polyethylene catheter may be inserted through a needle (an intracath) and left in the pericardial sac; it is then attached to a drainage bottle.	6. An indwelling catheter left in the pericardial space permits further slow drainage of fluid and prevents recurrence of cardiac tamponade.
7. Watch for presence of bloody fluid. If blood accumulates rapidly, an immediate thoracotomy and cardiorrhaphy (suturing of heart muscle) may be indicated.	7. Bloody pericardial fluid may be due to trauma. Bloody pericardial effusion fluid does not clot readily, whereas blood obtained from inadvertent puncture of one of the heart chambers *does* clot.

Follow-up Phase

NURSING ACTION	RATIONALE/AMPLIFICATION
1. Place patient in intensive care unit or cardiac care unit.	1. Following pericardiocentesis, careful monitoring of blood pressure, venous pressure, and heart sounds will be necessary to indicate possible recurrence of tamponade. A repeated aspiration is then necessary.
2. Watch for rising venous pressure and falling arterial pressure.	2. In the presence of these signs the patient is probably experiencing cardiac tamponade.
3. Auscultate the area over the heart.	3. Listen for decrease in intensity of heart sounds indicating recurring cardiac tamponade.
4. Prepare for surgical drainage of pericardium if: a. Pericardial fluid repeatedly accumulates or b. The aspiration is unsuccessful or c. Complications develop	
5. Assess for complications: Inadvertent puncture of heart chamber Arrhythmias Puncture of lung, stomach, or liver Laceration of coronary artery or myocardium	

Cardiopulmonary Resuscitation for Cardiac Arrest.

See Chapter 22, Emergency Nursing, p. 864.

GUIDELINES: Direct Current Defibrillation for Ventricular Fibrillation

Defibrillation (or countershock) is the passing of an electrical shock of short duration through the heart to terminate ventricular fibrillation.

A *defibrillator* is an instrument that delivers an electric shock to the heart to convert ventricular fibrillation to normal sinus rhythm. (Defibrillators are also used to convert other abnormal and rapid cardiac rhythms.)

Purpose   To terminate ventricular fibrillation.

Equipment   DC defibrillator with paddles
Interface material (saline-soaked gauze pads, electrode gels and pastes, disposable conductive gel pads)
Resuscitative equipment

Procedure

NURSING ACTION	RATIONALE/AMPLIFICATION
Performance Phase	
1. Expose the patient's anterior chest.	1. This procedure should be carried out immediately after ventricular fibrillation is detected to minimize cerebral and circulatory deterioration.
2. Start cardiopulmonary resuscitation immediately.	2. Cardiopulmonary resuscitation is essential before and after defibrillation to assure blood supply to the cerebral and coronary arteries.
3. Apply interface material (gel, paste, saline pads) to the paddles. The electrode paddles should be in firm contact with the patient's skin.	3. The interface material helps provide better contact and prevents skin burns. Do not allow any paste on the skin between the electrodes. If the paste areas touch, the current may short circuit (severely burning the patient) and may not penetrate the heart.
4. Disconnect the oxygen.	
5. A second person should turn on the defibrillator to the prescribed setting. A charge of 200–400 joules (or watt seconds) is delivered in 0.0025 seconds.	5. The shock is measured in joules or watt seconds (the dose is based on estimated body weight). The ideal energy dose for defibrillation remains controversial.

GUIDELINES: Direct Current Defibrillation for Ventricular Fibrillation (cont.)

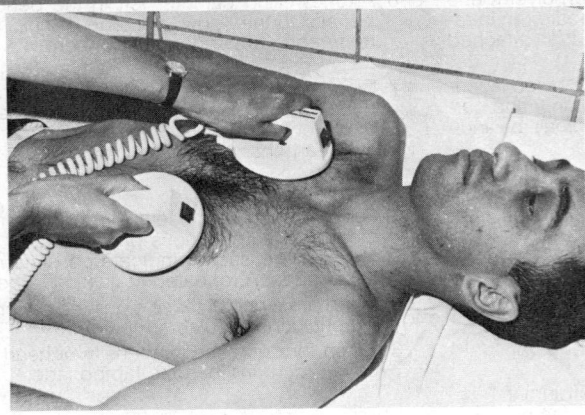

FIGURE 9-5. *Paddle placement in ventricular defibrillation.*

Procedure (cont.)

NURSING ACTION	RATIONALE/AMPLIFICATION
6. Apply one electrode just to the right of the upper sternum below the clavicle and the other electrode just to the left of the cardiac apex or left nipple (Fig. 9-5).	6. The paddles are placed so that the electrical discharge flows through as much myocardial mass as possible. If anteroposterior paddles are used, the anterior paddle is held with pressure on the middle sternum while the patient lies on the posterior paddle under the left infrascapular region. In this method the countershock more directly traverses the heart.
7. Grasp the paddles only by the insulated handles.	
8. GIVE THE COMMAND TO STAND CLEAR OF THE PATIENT AND THE BED.	8. If a person touches the bed, he may act as a ground for the current and receive a shock, especially if there are electrolyte solutions on the floor.
9. Push the discharge buttons in both paddles simultaneously.	
10. Remove the paddles from the patient *immediately* after the shock is administered (unless monitoring leads are in the paddles).	
11. Resume cardiopulmonary resuscitation efforts until stable rhythm, spontaneous respirations, pulse, and blood pressure return.	11. After discharge of the countershock, CPR efforts should be resumed; total delay should be no more than 5 seconds in order to oxygenate the patient and restore circulation.
12. Look at the ECG monitor to determine the specific therapy for the resultant electrical mechanism. Further high energy countershocks may be necessary.	

Follow-up Phase

1. After the patient is defibrillated and rhythm is restored, lidocaine is usually given to prevent recurrent episodes, and sodium bicarbonate administered to treat metabolic acidosis.	1. Any resultant arrhythmia may require appropriate drug intervention. Metabolic acidosis is due to accumulation of acidic products in blood because of cessation of respiration.
2. Continue with intensive monitoring/care.	

GUIDELINES: Application of Rotating Tourniquets or Automatic Inflating Cuffs

Rotating tourniquets refers to a technique whereby tourniquets are systematically rotated on the extremities to remove a volume of blood from the central circulation in order to decrease venous return and right ventricular output; this technique aids in decongesting the lungs.

Purpose   To pool the blood temporarily in the extremities in order to reduce venous return to the heart.

Underlying Principles

1. Three of the 4 extremities are compressed while 1 extremity is usually free at all times.
2. No single extremity should be compressed continuously for more than 45 minutes.
3. Tourniquets may have to be rotated at 5-minute intervals on the elderly patient to prevent gangrene and other complications.
4. These principles are important since they can reduce the risks of phlebothrombosis and fatal pulmonary embolism.

Equipment
Equipment for extremity compression
    4 sphygmomanometer cuffs or
    4 tourniquets, 61 cm. (2 feet) long with outside diameter 0.8–3.8 cm. (5/16 to 1½ inches) or
    Equipment designed to inflate and deflate blood pressure cuffs automatically (Danzer apparatus)
Small towels
Watch—to note time interval
Work sheet

Procedure

NURSING ACTION	RATIONALE/AMPLIFICATION

Performance Phase (Fig. 9-6)

1. Explain to the patient (if his condition permits) the purpose of the compression and that the skin of the extremities may become discolored.
2. Take the blood pressure. Mark the peripheral pulses if time permits.
3. Apply the 4 blood pressure cuffs (or Danzer apparatus if available) to extremities and inflate 3 to a pressure less than the systolic blood pressure; or
4. Apply tourniquets as high as possible on 3 extremities. Place tourniquets over gown or small towel in a definite rotation pattern.
5. Release 1 tourniquet every 15 minutes. Then apply a tourniquet to the previously free extremity.
6. Rotate tourniquets in a definite clockwise pattern.
7. Monitor blood pressure every few minutes after tourniquets have been applied.
8. Measure urinary output at frequent intervals. (Usually an indwelling catheter is used.)
9. At the completion of the rotation, remove 1 tourniquet at a time according to the specified time interval (usually 15 minutes).
10. Examine each extremity after tourniquet removal for color, warmth, and the presence of a palpable pulse.

1. To relieve anxiety.
2. Initial blood pressure reading serves as a baseline for future comparison.
3. Venous flow must be occluded but arterial flow must not be impeded.
4. Tourniquet should be placed in such a way that the arterial pulse can be palpated. One extremity should be free of a tourniquet during each time interval.
5. The venous outflow in any 1 extremity will be occluded for 45 minutes and unoccluded for 15 minutes. The time interval may be shorter if patient's condition indicates.
7. Application of tourniquets may precipitate hypotension in some patients.
8. Watch for sudden reduction in plasma volume with hypotension and oliguria after administration of rapid-acting diuretics (ethacrynic acid, furosemide).
9. Releasing the tourniquets 1 at a time prevents a sudden increase in circulatory blood volume and thus prevents circulatory overload.

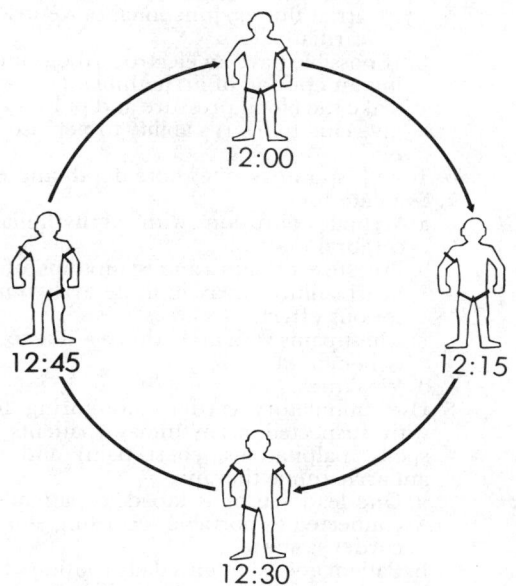

FIGURE 9-6. *One method of rotating tourniquets. This illustration shows a clockwise pattern.*

Follow-up Phase

1. Record starting time of procedure, rotation intervals, clinical response, medications given, and the time tourniquets were discontinued.

CARDIAC ARRHYTHMIAS

Arrhythmia is a clinical disorder of the heart beat; it may include a disturbance of rate, rhythm (sequence), or both. Arrhythmias are derangements of heart function and not of heart structure.

Etiology

1. Arrhythmias due to organic heart disease
   a. Inflammatory heart disease
   b. Degenerative heart disease (atherosclerosis)
   c. Congenital heart disease
   d. Hypertensive heart disease
2. Arrhythmias due to disturbances of other organ systems
   a. Disease of central nervous system—from sympathetic and vagal stimulation
   b. Pulmonary disease
   c. Endocrine disorders (hyper- and hypothyroidism, hypoglycemia, diabetic ketoacidosis)
   d. Gastrointestinal disorders (fluid and electrolyte imbalance)
   e. Renal disorders (renal failure)
3. Arrhythmias from other causes
   a. Drugs (digitalis intoxication, quinidine, procainamide)
   b. Infection
   c. Disturbances of electrolyte balance
   d. Anemia
   e. Following cardiac surgery

Classification of Arrhythmias Based on Disturbed Physiology

1. Disturbance of impulse formation—heartbeat activated for one or more beats by a pacemaker other than the SA node.
2. Disturbances of conduction—due to delayed transmission of impulses, to failure of some impulses to be conducted, or to a block of impulses at the affected site.
3. Combined disorders—combination of abnormally rapid impulse formation and decreased ability to conduct the impulses.

Clinical Manifestations

(Depends on ventricular rate, condition of heart, and patient's psychological reaction.)
1. Symptoms and signs of rapid arrhythmias
   a. Palpitation
   b. Dizziness and fainting
   c. Throbbing in head and neck
   d. Shortness of breath
   e. Precordial discomfort and pain
   f. Anxiety
2. Symptoms and signs of slow heart action (bradyarrhythmia)
   a. Shortness of breath
   b. Fatigue on exertion
   c. Dizziness and fainting—may indicate syncopal attacks, leading to convulsive seizures

Clinical Effects

1. Some arrhythmias are relatively harmless while others are harbingers of cardiac arrest.
2. Cardiac arrhythmias impair pumping action of the heart and reduce cardiac output, which has the effect of lowering the blood pressure and decreasing blood perfusion of the brain, heart, kidneys, gastrointestinal tract, muscles, and skin.
3. Cardiac arrhythmias often produce attacks of transient cerebral ischemia, which may result in stroke from reduction in cerebral blood flow.
4. Arrhythmias can precipitate congestive heart failure or angina pectoris in certain patients.
5. Bradyarrhythmias (rate below 60) predispose to electrical instability of the heart and decreased cardiac output.
6. A marked degree of disability may accompany an arrhythmia.

Nursing Assessment

1. Evaluate the patient's general appearance: pallor, cyanosis, sweating—may indicate peripheral arteriolar constriction.
2. How does the patient describe his symptoms?
3. What is the duration and frequency of the arrhythmia?
4. Observe carotid pulsation: Rapid and vigorous? Irregular with varying amplitude?
5. Listen to the heartbeat with a stethoscope.
   a. Listen for rate, presence of irregularity, increase in intensity of first heart sound.
      (1) 30 beats or lower—complete AV block, partial AV block, or sinus bradycardia.
      (2) 40–60 beats per minute—varying degrees of AV block, sinus bradycardia.
      (3) 60–110 beats per minute—sinus arrhythmia, premature beats, AV heart block, atrial fibrillation, atrial flutter, atrial tachycardia with block.
      (4) 140–180 beats per minute—atrial tachycardia, atrial flutter, junctional or ventricular tachycardia.
   b. If possible have an electrocardiogram taken during an episode of arrhythmia.
   c. Take the blood pressure and pulse—distal pulses give clue to heart's ability to perfuse the periphery.
6. Take respiratory rate: note depth and effort.
7. Evaluate for:
   a. Mental confusion with arrhythmia—indicates cerebral ischemia.
   b. Presence of signs and symptoms of congestive heart failure—may indicate arrhythmia causing serious effect.
   c. Chest pains with arrhythmia—due to myocardial ischemia.
   d. Weakness.
8. Use ambulatory cardiac monitoring for persons with suspected arrhythmias (patients with dizzy spells, palpitations, chest pain) and to evaluate antiarrhythmic therapy.
   a. One lead sensor is taped to patient's chest and connected to portable recording equipment. Recorder is started.
   b. Patient goes about his daily routine while keeping a diary of times and activities during which he feels his symptoms.
   c. After 8–30 hours the tape is put through a scanner for oscilloscope reading (computer scanning now available).

9. Offer calm explanations and convey optimism—patients with arrhythmias are apt fo be anxious and anxiety tends to aggravate symptoms; fear and anxiety can outweigh all other factors.
10. The treatment of arrhythmias includes pharmocologic, electrical (pacing; cardioversion), and surgical (excision of the "foci" etc.) therapy. See page 313 for a complete discussion of the most common arrhythmias, their ECG interpretations and treatment.

Health Education

Involve family in the teaching as follows:
1. Take prescribed medication on schedule
2. Stop smoking
3. Modification of the diet may be indicated; in general, avoid caffeine (coffee, cola, cocoa, chocolate, tea) and pain medications that contain caffeine or stimulants.
4. Notify physician if unusual symptoms or unexpected intolerance to exercise, emotional states, or cold occurs.

CARDIAC PACING

A *pacemaker* is an electronic device that provides repetitive electrical stimuli to the heart muscle for the control of heart rate. It initiates and maintains the heart rate when the natural pacemakers of the heart are unable to do so.

Pacemaker Design

Pacemakers consist of two component parts:
1. *Pulse generator,* which contains the circuitry and batteries that generate the electrical signal; the battery cells are usually lithium cell units with a projected life of 8–12 years, or less frequently, mercury–zinc batteries. Isotopic (nuclear) batteries are available.
2. *Pacemaker electrodes,* which transmit the pacemaker impulses to the heart. The stimuli from the pacemaker travel through a flexible catheter electrode (lead) that is threaded through a vein into the right ventricle (endocardial approach), or introduced by direct penetration of the chest wall (requires thoracotomy or upper abdominal surgical approach).

Clinical Indications

1. Bradyarrhythmias
   Heart block
   Arrhythmias and conduction defects following acute myocardial infarction
   Following open heart surgery; during coronary arteriography
2. Tachyarrhythmias—to break rapid rhythm disturbances

Pacing Modes

A. *Demand (synchronous; noncompetitive)*—most commonly used; has the advantage of working only when the heart rate goes below a certain level. Therefore it does not compete with the heart's basic rhythm. It stimulates the heart when a normal ventricular depolarization does not occur or if heart rate drops below a specified rate.

B. *Fixed rate (asynchronous; competitive)*—this unit stimulates the ventricle at a preset constant rate that is independent of the patient's rhythm. However, it can compete with the patient's own rhythm. Used infrequently, usually in patients with complete and unvarying heart block.

C. *New developments*
1. *Programmable pacemaker*—allows noninvasive adjustment (programming) of implanted pacemaker.
2. *Atrial-ventricular sequential pacing*—mode of choice for pacing patients with borderline cardiac function and selected dysrhythmias.

Temporary and Emergency Pacemaker Systems

Temporary pacing of the heart is usually an emergency procedure that permits observation of the effects of pacing on heart function so that an optimum pacing rate can be selected before a permanent pacer is implanted. Temporary pacing may be done for hours, days, or weeks; it is continued until the patient improves or a permanent pacemaker is implanted.

A. *Approaches*
   Accomplished by either an endocardial (transvenous) approach or a transthoracic approach to the myocardium.
1. The transvenous electrode is passed under fluoroscopic guidance through a peripheral vein (subclavian, femoral, jugular, brachial, etc.) and the catheter (electrode) is positioned in the apex of the right ventricle.
2. The pacing wire protrudes from the incision or percutaneous site and is connected to an external pulse generator attached to the patient or fastened to the bed linens. The catheter is anchored in place to allow motion of the extremity (Fig. 9-7). The external pacemaker is powered by standard batteries that require proper maintenance.

B. *Nursing Management*
1. *Preoperative*
   Reinforce explanation of procedure to patient and family. Explain that the patient will be awake (for transvenous pacing), will lie on a hard table 20–30 minutes, but discomfort will be minimal.
2. *Postoperative*
   a. Patient is monitored by continuous ECG for several days—usually permitted to walk around room and use bedside commode while being monitored.
      (1) Monitor blood pressure and hemodynamic status.
      (2) Question patient about his symptoms.
      (3) Observe for hiccups—may be caused by chest wall/diaphragmatic stimulation.
      (4) Use sterile technique at electrode insertion site; observe wound for bleeding, infection, phlebitis.
   b. Check to see that no metal parts are exposed and electrode insulation is intact—to prevent accidental ventricular fibrillation from stray electrical currents.
   c. Be sure that the patient is in an electrically safe environment.
      (1) All monitoring and other electrical equipment should be grounded with 3-pronged plugs inserted into a proper outlet.
      2) Avoid using electrocautery, electrocoagulating equipment, and electric razors—external interference may suppress output of temporary pacemaker.

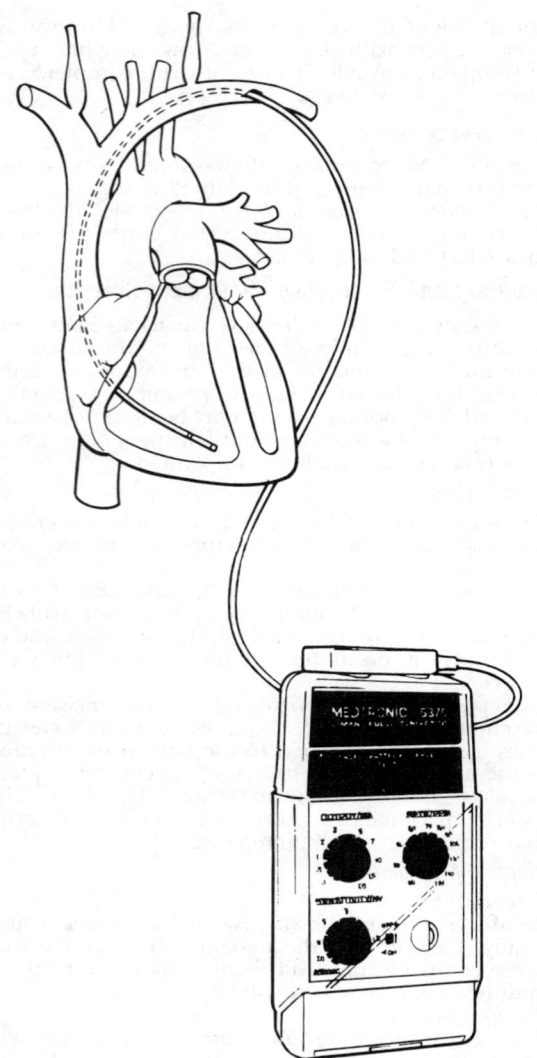

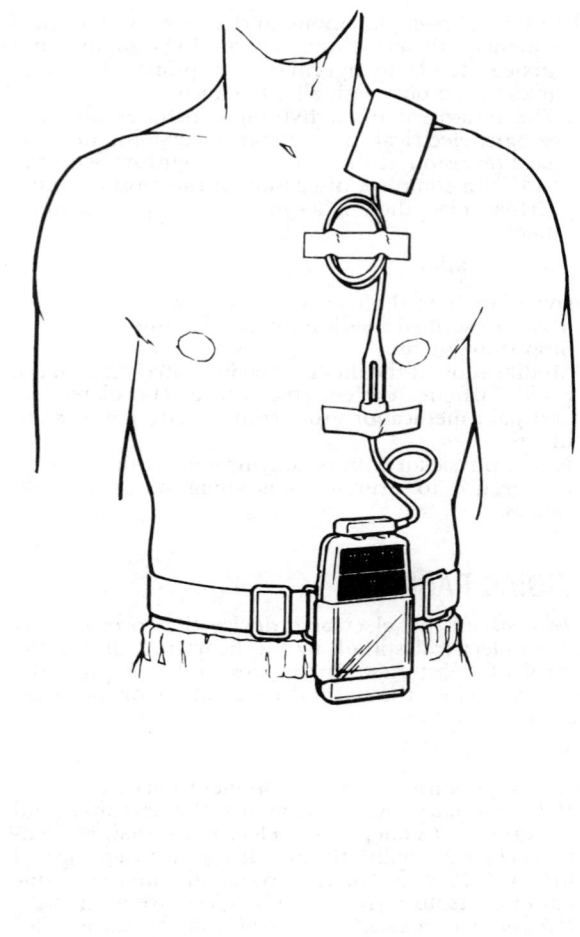

FIGURE 9-7. *External pacemaker. (Courtesy of MEDTRONIC, Inc.)*

(3) Know the proper and safe operation of the unit (see manufacturer's directives)—necessary before assessment of pacing malfunctions can be made.

d. Record time, date, pacing mode, and control settings for rate and output. Report and record changes in these parameters.

Permanent Pacemakers

A. *Approaches*

1. *Transvenous*—electrodes (unipolar or bipolar) are threaded through cephalic or external jugular vein and into the right ventricle. The peripheral end of the electrode is connected to the pulse generator which is implanted underneath the skin below the right or left pectoral region (Fig. 9-8).

2. *Myocardial Implantation*—electrodes are applied directly to the myocardium, and the pulse generator is usually placed underneath the skin of the subcostal area.

a. A variety of surgical approaches are used, including subxiphoid, transxiphoid, and subcostal or extrapleural approaches.

b. See page 221 for care of patient following chest surgery if patient has implantation via thoracotomy; incidence of arrhythmias is higher with thoracotomy.

B. *Nursing Management Following Permanent Pacemaker Implantation*

1. The patient is monitored by ECG following implantation of the pacemaker—high risk if electrode is displaced soon after insertion.

a. Take pulse for a full minute.

b. Assess for dizziness, light-headedness, chest pain, shortness of breath—may indicate pacemaker malfunction.

2. Note the data about the model, date of insertion, location of pulse generator, stimulation threshold, and pacer rate on the patient's record.

a. Place a card at the head of the bed indicating that the patient has a pacemaker.

b. Make sure the preset pacemaker rate remains constant.

3. Keep the intravenous infusion running—to have a readily accessible vein in the event of an arrhythmia and to combat dehydration.

4. Make sure all equipment is grounded with 3-pronged plugs inserted into a proper outlet—improperly grounded equipment can generate currents capable of producing ventricular fibrillation.

A clinical engineer, electrician, or other qualified person should make certain that the patient is in an electrically safe environment.

5. Inspect the incision site under the pressure dressings for bleeding and hematoma—hematoma appears to be a contributing factor to wound infection.

6. Observe the vein through which the pacing catheter has been placed for evidences of phlebitis.

7. Give analgesic drugs to relieve pain at implantation site.

8. Be aware that there is a high incidence of associated disease in elderly patients; the mean age of these patients is 70 years—have associated arteriosclerotic heart disease and heart failure, hypertension, and diabetes.

a. Assist patient in and out of bed when ambulatory—a fall can dislodge electrode.

Complications Following Pacemaker Implantation

1. *Complications arising from the presence of the pacemaker within the body*

    a. Local infection (sepsis or hematoma formation)—occurs at the site of venous cutdown or subcutaneous pacemaker placement.

    b. Arrhythmias; ventricular ectopic activity—from irritation of the ventricular wall by the electrode. (Pacemakers can create baffling arrhythmias.)

    c. Complications from electrode malposition, dislocation, dislodgment, or perforation.

    d. High ventricular threshold—may cause abrupt loss of pacing.

2. *Complications from pacemaker malfunction*

    a. Failure in one or more components of the pacing system

    b. Battery exhaustion

    c. Wire (electrode) fractures

    d. Failure to capture and/or sense properly

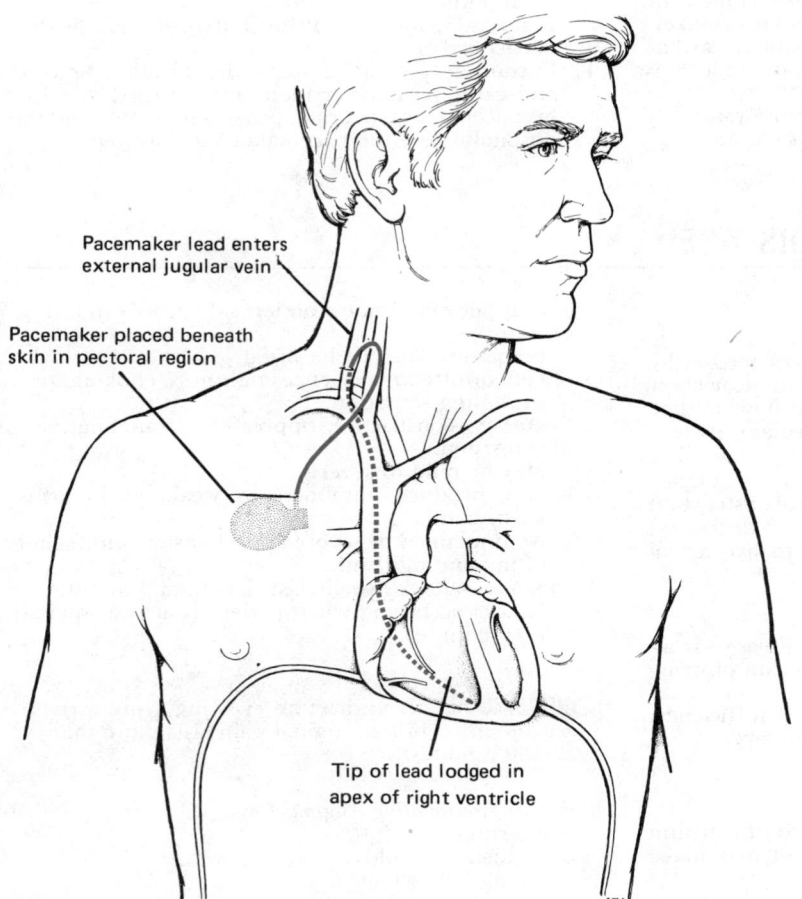

Pacemaker lead enters external jugular vein

Pacemaker placed beneath skin in pectoral region

Tip of lead lodged in apex of right ventricle

FIGURE 9-8. *Permanent pacemaker.*

Health Education

1. Reassure the patient so that he will develop confidence in his pacemaker and new life-style.
   a. Physical activity does not usually have to be curtailed because of an implanted pacemaker.
   b. Sexual activity may be resumed when desired.
   c. Caution patient not to manipulate pulse generator by twisting or retracting electrode catheter ("twiddler's syndrome").
2. Inform the patient that the pulse generator will have to be surgically removed for a variety of reasons (battery failure) and replaced; improved power sources and circuitry make reoperation less frequent.
   a. Relatively simple procedure performed under local anesthesia.
   b. Incision made; old generator disconnected from electrode catheter.
   c. New generator connected and placed in existing subcutaneous pocket; incision closed.
   d. Prophylactic antibiotics usually administered.
   e. Patient discharged from hospital 1–3 days postoperatively.
3. Give the patient the manufacturer's instructions (for his particular pacemaker) and help him to become familiar wth his pacemaker.
4. Encourage patient to have regular pacemaker checkup (preferably at a pacemaker clinic) for monitoring function and integrity of his pacemaker. Transtelephonic evaluation of implanted cardiac pacemakers for battery and electrode failure is available.
5. Teach the patient to check his own pulse rate daily to be certain that preset rate remains constant.
   a. Report *immediately* any sudden slowing of pulse greater than 4–5 beats per minute, or any increase in pulse rate.
   b. Report signs and symptom of dizziness, fainting, palpitation, prolonged hiccups, and chest pain to physician immediately—indicative of pacemaker failure.
   c. Take pulse while these feelings are being experienced.
6. See that the patient has a copy of his ECG tracing (according to agency policy)—for future comparisons.
7. Advise patient to wear loose-fitting clothing around the area of pacemaker implantation until healing has taken place.
8. Watch for signs and symptoms of infection around generator and leads—fever, heat, pain, skin breakdown at implant site.
9. Advise patient that improvements in pacemaker design have reduced problems of electromagnetic interference (EMI).
   a. Sources of electromagnetic interference that still affect a number of pulse generators include high-energy radar, television and radio transmitters, industrial arc welders, certain electrocautery machines used in hospitals. Avoid these sources of EMI.
   b. Move a few feet away from EMI sources if symptoms develop.
   c. Advise patient to inform dentist that he has pacemaker.
10. Encourage patient to wear identification bracelet and carry pacemaker identification card that lists his pacemaker type, rate, physician's name, and the hospital where the pacemaker was inserted.

ATHEROSCLEROTIC HEART DISEASE

ANGINA PECTORIS

Angina pectoris is a clinical syndrome characterized by paroxysms of pain or oppression in the anterior chest caused by insufficient coronary blood flow and/or inadequate oxygen supply to the myocardial muscle.

Altered Physiology

Atherosclerosis of major vessels → critical obstruction with diminution of coronary blood flow → decreased myocardial oxygen delivery in response to myocardial oxygen demand → anginal pain.

Etiology

1. Usually due to atherosclerotic heart disease—is almost invariably associated with a significant obstruction of a major coronary artery.
2. May be from severe aortic stenosis or insufficiency, aortitis, hyperthyroidism, anemia, tachycardia.

Clinical Manifestations

Pain—(caused by myocardial ischemia).
1. *Location*—behind middle or upper third of sternum (retrosternal) felt deep in chest. Patient may make a fist over site of pain.
2. *Radiation*—usually radiates to neck, jaw, shoulders, and upper extremities (on left side more often than on right).
   a. Frequently may be localized.
   b. Patient often experiences tightness, choking, or a strangling sensation.
3. *Character*—constrictive, oppressive, strangling, vise-like, insistent.
   a. May be mild to severe.
   b. May produce numbness or weakness in arms, wrist, hands.
   c. Accompanied by severe apprehension and feeling of impending death.
4. *Duration*—attack usually lasts less than 3 minutes. Attacks occurring when patient is at rest—persist 5–15 minutes.

NURSING ALERT: Suspect an evolving acute myocardial infarction if anginal pain lasts more than 20–30 minutes.

5. *Factors Precipitating Anginal Pain:*
   a. Exertion
   b. Exposure to cold
   c. Eating a heavy meal
   d. Emotion and excitement

Diagnostic Evaluation

1. Evaluation of clinical manifestations (pain).
2. Nitroglycerin test—positive response (relief of pain) to nitroglycerin.
3. ECG and stress testing—ST and T wave changes indicative of myocardial ischemia.

Assessment

A. *Record all facets of patient's activities that precede or precipitate attacks of anginal pain.*

1. When do attacks tend to occur? Following a meal? After engaging in certain activities? After physical activities in general? After visits of family/others?
2. Where is the pain located?
3. How does the patient describe the pain?
4. Was the onset of pain sudden? Gradual?
5. How long did it last—seconds? minutes? hours?
6. Was the pain steady and unwavering in quality?
7. Is the discomfort accompanied by other symptoms? Sweating? Light-headedness? Nausea? Palpitations? Shortness of breath?
8. How many minutes after taking nitroglycerin did the pain last?
9. What was the mode of abatement?

B. *Try to take an ECG during episodes of pain*—ECG may show transient ST segment shifts or T wave changes that revert to normal when pain is relieved.

Management

OBJECTIVES: to reduce the work load of the heart thereby decreasing myocardial oxygen demands.
to relieve pain.
to prevent myocardial infarction.

A. *Activity Considerations*

1. Help the patient to participate in self-assessment to determine the provoking factors/events that precipitate the onset of angina—including physical activity, emotional pressures, worries, family, financial problems.
2. Reduce activity to below the point where anginal pain occurs.
3. See Health Education, page 286.

B. *Drug Therapy to Prevent and Relieve Anginal Pain*

1. *Nitroglycerin* (mainstay of treatment)
   a. Purpose—to reduce myocardial oxygen consumption
   b. Effects—decreases ischemia and relieves anginal pain
   c. Mechanism of action (not clearly established)
      (1) Nitroglycerin has an effect on peripheral circulation—by increasing the capacity of the venous bed it causes venous pooling of blood throughout the body.
      (2) As a result, less blood is returned to the heart and there is a reduction in ventricular volume, stroke volume, and cardiac output.
      (3) Nitrates also relax the systematic arteriolar bed and thus may cause a fall in blood pressure.
   d. Nitroglycerin should be taken *before* pain develops. The patient regulates the drug usage, taking the smallest dose that relieves pain.
   e. Nitroglycerin is usually given sublingually (under tongue) or in buccal pouch while patient is seated. (See Health Education, p. 286).
      (1) Pain relief usually begins within 3 minutes.
      Caution patient not to take more than 2–3 sublingual nitroglycerin tablets over a 15-minute period.
      (2) If anginal pain undergoes a change in pattern, intensifying, lasting longer, or becoming more easily provoked, suspect an acute myocardial infarction.
      (3) Assessment of acute anginal attack:
         (a) How long did it take for the nitroglycerin to relieve discomfort?
         (b) Was the relief partial or complete?
         (c) Take blood pressure every 3 minutes (1–2 minutes after drug administration) to evaluate adequacy of drug effect (should be a moderate decline in systolic pressure).
         (d) Assess for dizziness and faintness after drug administration; check blood pressure and heart rate with patient in upright position.
   f. Nitroglycerin should be used prophylactically to avoid pain known to occur with certain activities (stair climbing, sexual intercourse, exposure to cold).
   g. Side effects: headaches, transient dizziness, weakness, syncope (may be caused by cerebral ischemia from postural hypotension); some side effects may subside with continued therapy.
2. *Nitroglycerine ointment*—appears to protect against anginal pain and promote its relief. Useful for patients experiencing nocturnal angina or whose angina occurs frequently.
   a. Ointment is measured with a calibrated strip of paper that comes with the product and is smoothed onto the skin in a thin uniform layer; can be applied on any convenient skin surface, since it is topically absorbed.
   b. May be covered with plastic wrap—protects clothing and enhances absorption.
   c. Appears to have beneficial effects persisting for up to 4–6 hours.
3. *Beta-adrenergic blocking drugs*—to decrease myocardial oxygen need
   a. Propanolol—reduces oxygen consumption by blocking sympathetic impulses to the heart. This produces a reduction in heart rate, systemic blood pressure, and myocardial contractility which is associated with a decrease in myocardial oxygen consumption. This allows patient to work or exercise while requiring less myocardial oxygen delivery.
   b. Given daily in divided doses at equally spaced intervals; dosage titrated to patient's symptoms.
   c. Side effects: fatigue, hypotension, severe bradycardia, mental depression, bronchospasm in susceptible individual; may precipitate congestive heart failure.
   d. Take blood pressure and heart rate with patient in upright position 2 hours after administration to assess for postural hypotension.
   e. Do not give if pulse rate drops below 50 per minute.
   f. Propanolol also used in conjunction with sublingual isosorbide dinitrate for antianginal and anti-ischemia prophylaxis.
   g. Exercise ECG testing may be used to determine when optimal therapy has been achieved.
4. *Sedatives and tranquilizers*—may be used to prevent attacks precipitated by aggravation, excitement, or tension.

C. *Other Therapeutic Interventions*
1. Correct other problems in order to decrease oxygen demands of myocardium—hypertension, hyperthyroidism, aortic stenosis, anemia.
2. Assess for development of unstable angina (progressive increase in frequency, intensity, and duration of anginal attacks); these patients are at high risk for myocardial infarction and sudden death; may be admitted to CCU.
3. Watch for development of congestive heart failure and arrhythmias.
4. Support patient having coronary arteriography to determine if surgical intervention is advisable.
5. Prepare for surgical intervention (coronary artery bypass surgery) to bring a new blood supply to ischemic myocardium when symptoms cannot be controlled. See page 303.

Health Education

Instruct the patient as follows:
1. Chest discomfort or pain can be provoked when doing any activity that puts too much load on the heart and increases heart rate and blood pressure.
2. Use moderation in all activities to prevent an episode of anginal pain.
   a. Participate in a normal daily program of activities that do not produce chest discomfort, shortness of breath, and undue fatigue.
   b. Avoid activities known to cause anginal pain—sudden exertion, walking against the wind, extremes of temperature, high altitude, emotionally stressful situations; may accelerate heart rate, raise blood pressure, and increase cardiac work.
   c. Refrain from engaging in physical activity for 2 hours after meals. Rest after each meal if possible.
   d. Do not undertake activities requiring heavy effort (carrying heavy objects).
   e. Try to avoid cold weather if possible; dress warmly and walk more slowly. Wear scarf over nose and mouth when in cold air.
   f. Reduce weight if necessary to reduce cardiac load.

g. Avoid overeating
   (1) Avoid excessive caffeine intake (coffee, cola drinks) that can increase the heart rate and produce angina.
   (2) Do not use "diet pills," nasal decongestants, or any over-the-counter medications that can increase the heart rate or stimulate high blood pressure.
3. Use prescribed nitroglycerin effectively.
   a. Carry nitroglycerin at all times.
      (1) Nitroglycerin is volatile and is inactivated by heat, moisture, air, light, and time.
      (2) Keep nitroglycerin in original dark glass container, tightly closed—to prevent absorption of drug by other pills or pillbox.
      (3) Do not carry nitroglycerin in a plastic or metal pillbox or mixed with other pills.
      (4) Renew supply every 5–6 months.
      (5) Nitroglycerin should cause a slight burning or stinging sensation under the tongue when it is potent.
   b. Place nitroglycerin under tongue at first sign of chest discomfort.
      (1) Stop all effort/activity; sit, and take nitroglycerin tablet—relief should be obtained in a few minutes.
      (2) Do not swallow saliva until tablet is dissolved.
      (3) Bite the tablet between front teeth and slip under tongue to dissolve if quick action is desired.
      (4) Repeat dosage in a few minutes for total of 3 tablets if relief is not obtained.
      (5) Keep a record of number of tablets taken—to evaluate any change in anginal pattern.
      (6) Take nitroglycerin prophylactically to avoid pain known to occur with certain activities.
4. If taking a beta blocker, do not interrupt therapy without first consulting the physician—abrupt withdrawal can produce exacerbation of angina, myocardial infarction.
5. Go to nearest health care facility if pain persists more than 20 minutes or becomes more intense or widespread. (Do not drive yourself.)

MYOCARDIAL INFARCTION (MI)

Myocardial infarction refers to the process by which myocardial tissue is destroyed in regions of the heart that are deprived of their blood supply because of a reduced coronary blood flow.

Causes

1. Critical narrrowing of a coronary artery—due to atherosclerosis or, less commonly, to a complete occlusion of an artery from embolus or thrombus.
2. Decreased coronary blood flow—causes a profound imbalance between myocardial oxygen supply and demand.

Clinical Manifestations

1. Chest pain—steady, constrictive pain (central portion of chest and epigastrium) not relieved by rest or nitrates; pain may radiate widely; may produce arrhythmias, hypotension, shock, cardiac failure
2. Profuse perspiration; moist, clammy skin with pallor

3. Drop in blood pressure
4. Dyspnea, weakness, and fainting
5. Nausea and vomiting
6. Anxiety and restlessness
7. Tachycardia or bradycardia

NURSING ALERT: Many patients do not have symptoms; these are the "silent myocardial infarctions." Nevertheless there is still resultant damage to the myocardium.

8. Atypical symptoms—extreme fatigue, epigastric or abdominal distress, shortness of breath.

Diagnostic Evaluation

1. Clinical history and findings from physical examination.

2. ECG changes (within 2–12 hours, but may take as long as 72–96 hours). See page 313 for ECG interpretation of MI.
3. Elevation of serum isoenzymes (CK-MB test). See page 268.
4. Radionuclide imaging—allows recognition of areas of decreased perfusion as "cold spots," which are seen in areas of ischemia and infarction.

Nursing Management (Fig. 9-9)

OBJECTIVES: to maintain adequate circulatory function.
to prevent death from arrhythmia, asystole, and cardiogenic shock.
to limit the size of the infarct.
to provide healing for the myocardium.
to facilitate rehabilitation.

A. *To provide constant nursing surveillance during the critical stage of the illness.*

1. Admit patient to cardiac care unit for constant monitoring and aggressive early treatment of arrhythmias—risk of ventricular fibrillation and death is greatest in first few hours following MI.
   a. Lift patient from stretcher to bed; place in position of comfort.
   b. Start an intravenous infusion running slowly—to keep vein open for administration of IV medications in event of an arrhythmia.
   c. Be vigilant for occurrence of any type of premature ventricular beats—may presage ventricular tachycardia and ventricular fibrillation. (See p. 313 for discussion of arrhythmias).
      (1) Correct arrhythmia immediately—may unfavorably alter the balance between oxygen supply and demand at the periphery of the infarct.
      (2) Lidocaine may be given prophylactically—to protect patient against ventricular fibrillation.
      (3) Other antiarrhythmic drugs include procainamide, quinidine, propranolol, atropine, etc.—selected by classification.
      (4) Prepare patient for prophylactic pacing (p. 281), if indicated.
2. Provide continuing nursing assessment of peripheral perfusion (blood supply to organs and tissues).
   a. Attach ECG monitoring electrodes to monitor the heart rhythm and to confirm clinical impression of MI.
   b. Measure and record vital signs—to determine presence of impending complications, especially arrhythmias and cardiogenic shock.
      (1) Note on record method of taking blood pressure (palpation/auscultation).
      (2) Evaluate both apical and radical pulse rates. Note strength of femoral pulse.
   c. Count respirations—tachypnea may indicate congestive heart failure, pulmonary embolism.
   d. Monitor body temperature—gives some indication of tissue perfusion.
   e. Assess skin temperature and color.
   f. Auscultate for breath sounds, rales.
   g. Auscultate the heart for gallop, friction rub, murmurs.
   h. Assess neck veins for distention—elevation of venous pressure may indicate failure of heart to pump effectively.
   i. Assess for changes in mental status (apathy, confusion, restlessness)—from inadequate cerebral perfusion.

j. Evaluate urine output (30 ml./hour)—decrease in urine volume reflects a decrease in renal blood flow.
3. Utilize hemodynamic monitoring for critically ill patient.
4. Place patient at rest—to lower heart rate and blood pressure and oxygen demands of heart and to maintain cardiac work at its lowest level.
5. Administer oxygen by nasal cannula (p. 172)—may decrease incidence of arrhythmias by allowing the myocardium to be less ischemic and thus less irritable; may reduce size of infarct.
6. Relieve patient's pain and anxiety—anxiety and fear increase the heart rate (which puts heart under more stress), raise the blood pressure, and cause the adrenal glands to release epinephrine which may produce an arrhythmia.
   a. Give analgesic (morphine or meperidine)—decreases sympathetic activity and reduces myocardial oxygen consumption with subsequent decreases in heart rate, blood pressure, and muscle tension.
   b. Give in small IV doses repeated every 15–20 minutes until relief is obtained (if vital signs are within safe parameters).

NURSING ALERT: Assess for persistent or recurring pain, which suggests an extension or threatened extension of infarct; urgent and aggressive intervention is required.

   c. Monitor blood pressure, pulse, and respiratory rate before administering narcotics—narcotics depress arterial pressure and may contribute to development of shock and arrhythmias. Do not leave patient in a sitting position.
   d. Administer antianxiety agents—anxiety is associated with increased sympathetic drive.
   e. Discuss CCU environment and what can be anticipated in the coming days with patient to allay anxiety and help him mobilize his resources for coping.
   f. Give intelligent reassurance and assist patient in establishing a positive attitude toward his illness.
      (1) Most persons use the mechanism of denial during initial stages of MI.
      (2) Depression is commonly encountered on about the 3rd day in CCU although it may not surface until the patient returns home.
         (a) Depression following MI is normal; patient is grieving over his losses—health, confidence, independence.
         (b) Patient may feel pressure from having to alter his life-style; i.e., eating, drinking, smoking.
      (3) Assess for maladaptive coping patterns—inappropriate denial, withdrawal, changes in usual communicative patterns, destructive behavior. Ask patient what he is thinking about and feeling; try to draw out specific concerns.
      (4) Involve family in support and education.

B. *To provide nursing surveillance and support of patient's activities.*

1. Diet (depends on patient's circulatory status)

a. Clear liquids and progressive diet depending on patient's lipid analysis, body weight, etc.
b. Restrict sodium if signs and symptoms of congestive heart failure are present.
c. Restrict coffee and cola beverages (substitute decaffeinated coffee)—caffeine can affect heart rate, rhythm, coronary circulation, and blood pressure.

2. Activities: patient management is individualized; trend toward earlier ambulation and discharge from hospital.
a. Apply antiembolism stockings.
b. Patient is usually allowed out of bed to use bedside commode—requires less cardiovascular work than using bedpan.

1. Monitor patient
ECG monitoring
Evaluation of blood pressure
Evaluation of apical pulse
Hemodynamic
monitoring

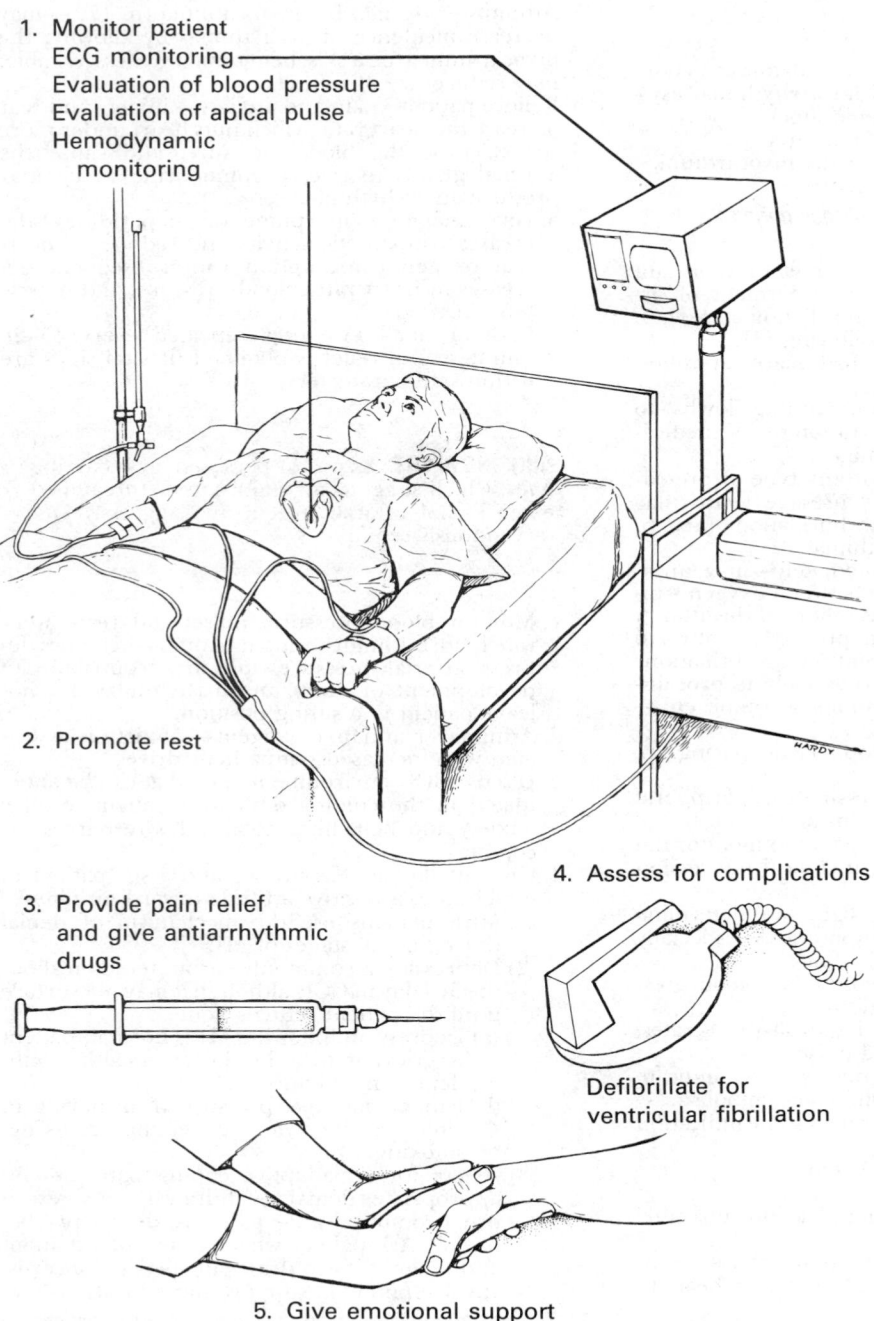

2. Promote rest

3. Provide pain relief and give antiarrhythmic drugs

4. Assess for complications

Defibrillate for ventricular fibrillation

5. Give emotional support

FIGURE 9-9. *Myocardial infarction.*

(1) Use stool softeners as directed.
(2) Avoid Valsalva maneuver (straining)—this form of isometric exercise can limit coronary flow, because it increases cardiac work.
c. Chair rest (after 1–3 days) if free of pain, arrhythmias, failure, and shock—work of heart is less when patient is sitting than when he is recumbent.
d. Usually permitted light reading, transistor radio for diversion.
e. Start physical activities as directed. Avoid exercise for at least 1 hour after meals.
f. Monitor pulse and patient response during and after exercise.
g. Instruct patient to avoid sudden effort.
h. Gradually increase patient's physical activity (walk around room, in hall, etc.)—to enable him to achieve the activity level required for self-care by the time he returns home.
i. Graduate to progressive cardiac care unit.

C. *To be alert for complications.*
1. Cardiogenic shock.
   a. Falling arterial blood pressure.
   b. Reduced urinary volume (30 ml./hour or less).
   c. Cool, moist skin; may be peripheral cyanosis—due to systemic vasoconstriction caused by reduction in cardiac output.
   d. Restlessness, apathy, lessening of responsiveness—from systemic vasoconstriction.
   e. See page 290 for management of cardiogenic shock. A patient with cardiogenic shock should ideally be transferred to cardiac center with hemodynamic monitoring capabilities.
2. Arrhythmias—occur frequently in first few days after infarction. The reduction in myocardial oxygenation produces myocardial ischemia. Ischemic muscle is electrically unstable and produces arrhythmias.
   a. Assess, prevent, and treat conditions which may initiate an arrhythmia—congestive heart failure, pulmonary embolus, inadequate pulmonary ventilation, electolyte disturbances, underoxygenation of blood.
   b. Draw arterial blood for blood gas analysis.
   c. Watch for ventricular fibrillation, ventricular tachycardia, AV block, asystole.
   d. See page 313 for management of arrhythmias.
3. Congestive heart failure—myocardial infarction reduces ability of left ventricle to eject blood, diminishes cardiac output, produces an elevation of left ventricular end pressure with ensuing pulmonary vascular complications.
   a. Assess for tachycardia and gallop rhythm, dyspnea, orthopnea, edema, hepatomegaly.
   b. Watch for development of pulmonary edema (see p. 302)—represents extreme left ventricular failure. Assess for extreme dyspnea, frothy, blood-stained mucus, tachycardia, distended neck veins, and diffuse rales.
   c. See page 299 and page 302 for treatment of congestive heart failure and acute pulmonary edema.
4. Other complications:
   a. Papillary muscle rupture, ventricular septal rupture, ventricular aneurysm.
   b. Postmyocardial infarction syndrome (Dressler's syndrome)—a recurrent febrile illness with pericarditis, pleuritis, and pneumonitis.
   c. Cerebral and peripheral emboli; pulmonary emboli.

D. *Prepare for surgical intervention if indicated*—insertion of intra-aortic counterpulsation device, coronary artery bypass, repair of ventricular septal defect, mitral valve replacement. (See nursing management of patient undergoing heart surgery, page 303.)

Health Education

OBJECTIVES: to restore patient to his optimal physiologic, psychologic, social, and work level.
to aid in restoring confidence and self-esteem.
to prevent progression of underlying disease (atherosclerosis).

1. Inform the patient about what has happened to his heart and explain that myocardial healing starts early but is not complete for 6–8 weeks.
2. A myocardial infarction may require some modification of life style.
3. Exercise tolerance testing will be done after myocardial healing to determine optimum level of activity and to plan rehabilitation program.
4. A program of exercise training will be prescribed at this time to improve cardiovascular functional capacity.
5. Physical limitations are usually only temporary. The following guidelines usually apply until the patient is reevaluated after complete myocardial healing:
   a. Expect to feel weak and tired for a period of time; depression is not uncommon.
   b. Walk daily, slowly increasing the distance and time.
   c. Avoid doing anything that tenses the muscles (isometric exercises, weight lifting, straining, lifting heavy objects, pushing/pulling heavy loads)—may place strain on coronary reserve.
   d. Rest after meals and before doing any exercise.
   e. Space activities throughout the day to alternate rest and work.
      (1) Stop as soon as fatigued.
      (2) Avoid tenseness and rushing.
   f. Avoid working with arms above shoulder level.
   g. Shorten work hours when first returning to work.
6. Advise the patient to eat 3–4 meals daily (each containing about the same amount of food).
   a. Avoid large meals.
   b. Avoid hurrying while eating.
   c. Limit caffeine intake (coffee and cola) and cigarettes.
   d. Stay with prescribed diet (modifications in calories, fats, and sodium).
7. Extremes in temperature and walking against the wind should be avoided.
   a. Stop immediately for shortness of breath.
   b. Sit down and take nitroglycerin for chest pain.
8. Sexual relations may be resumed upon advice of physician, usually after exercise tolerance is assessed.
   a. If patient can walk briskly or climb two flights of stairs, he can usually resume sexual activity with familiar partner; resumption of sexual activity parallels resumption of usual activities.
   b. Sexual activity should be avoided after eating a heavy meal, after drinking alcohol, or when tired.
9. Instruct patient to notify the physician when the following symptoms appear:
   a. Chest pressure or pain not relieved in 15 minutes by nitroglycerin or rest.
   b. Shortness of breath

c. Unusual fatigue
d. Swelling of feet and ankles
e. Fainting, dizziness
f. Very slow or rapid heart beat
10. Explain pharmacologic regimen.

CARDIOGENIC SHOCK

Cardiogenic shock (power failure), the end stage of left ventricular dysfunction, occurs when the left ventricle is extensively damaged by myocardial infarction. The heart muscle loses its contractile power and there is marked reduction in cardiac output with decreased perfusion (lack of blood and oxygen) to vital organs (heart, brain, and kidneys). The degree of pump dysfunction is related to the extent of damage to the heart muscle.

Cardiogenic shock now accounts for the majority of hospital deaths from myocardial infarction and has a high mortality rate.

Clinical Manifestations

1. Low systolic pressure (90 mm. Hg or 30 mm. Hg less than previous levels)
2. Oliguria—urine output less than 30 ml./hour—from impaired renal circulation
3. Cold, clammy skin, weak pulse, cyanosis—from circulatory insufficiency
4. Mental lethargy, confusion—from poor cerebral perfusion

Treatment and Nursing Management

OBJECTIVES: to maintain perfusion to vital organs while preserving the borderline areas of myocardium and limiting infarct size.
to improve the ability of the heart to pump blood throughout the body.
to determine effectiveness of treatment.

1. Start hemodynamic monitoring at the *first* indication of deterioration of patient's condition—hemodynamic monitoring is necessary for continuing patient evaluation and serves as a guideline for therapy. Measure left ventricular pressure—oxygen demands of ischemic myocardium are determined by left ventricular pressure and heart rate, myocardial contractility, size, shape, and wall thickness of left ventricle.
   a. Measurement of left ventricular end-diastolic pressure is estimated by the pulmonary arterial wedge pressure as measured by the Swan-Ganz catheter.
      (1) Values are elevated in patients with left ventricular failure, mitral valve disease, pulmonary hypertension.
      (2) See page 268 for technique.
   b. Pulmonary capillary wedge pressure (PCWP) provides an accurate estimate of left ventricular filling pressure only in the absence of mitral valve disease.
      (1) Used also as a guide for infusion therapy; pulmonary congestion is indicated by PCWP greater than 18 mm. Hg; the increase signifies that the left side of the heart is in failure.
      (2) See page 271 for technique.
   c. Evaluate cardiac output—pulmonary artery catheters are also used to evaluate cardiac output by thermodilution technique.
2. Measure intra-arterial pressure by direct arterial cannulization—more accurate measurement of blood pressure.
3. Administer continuous oxygen at percentages needed to combat hypoxemia.
4. Correct hypovolemia
   a. Administer IV fluids until left ventricular pressure increases to 18–20 mm. Hg (the value associated with highest cardiac output).
   b. Watch for development of pulmonary edema, which may occur abruptly.
5. Give appropriate drug therapy if patient is still in shock—to lessen ischemia and limit size of infarct and decrease the work of the heart.
   a. *Vasodilator therapy*—vasodilator drugs dilate capacitance vessels (veins and venules) and/or resistance vessels (arterioles), reducing impedance to left ventricular outflow and venous return to the heart; decreases myocardial oxygen consumption; improves perfusion to organs. Vasodilators in current use include sodium nitroprusside, phentolamine, nitroglycerin.
   b. *Inotropic agents*—used to increase cardiac output by direct effect on myocardium. Include digitalis, dopamine, and dobutamine.
   c. *Diuretics*—may reduce tissue edema at site of infarct and improve myocardial perfusion and oxygenation.
6. Measure urine volume via indwelling catheter every ½–1 hour—urine flow reflects renal blood flow and the status of central circulation.
7. Take arterial blood gases to assess for hypoxia and metabolic acidosis.
8. Utilize counterpulsation to decrease ventricular work of patient with severe shock. (See description of method, which follows.)
9. Prepare patient for surgical intervention to correct defects that are interfering with pump function and to reperfuse the heart.

COUNTERPULSATION (MECHANICAL CARDIAC ASSISTANCE)

Counterpulsation (diastolic augmentation) is a method of assisting the failing heart and circulation by mechanical support that may be accomplished by (1) intra-aortic balloon pump or (2) external counterpulsation pressure.

A. *Intra-aortic balloon pump*—introduction of a balloon catheter via the femoral artery or via a percutaneous route into the descending thoracic aorta; it is inflated and deflated in sequence with the cardiac cycle and acts as an auxiliary pump assisting forward blood flow (Fig. 9-10).

1. Using synchronization with the patient's ECG, the balloon is inflated at the onset of diastole ("diastolic augmentation"); this results in increased diastolic pressure, which increases coronary blood flow and myocardial nutrition.
2. The balloon is deflated at the onset of cardiac systole to lower the aortic blood pressure so that the work of the left ventricle is reduced (reduction in left ventricular impedance and afterload).
3. A bedside console provides gas for balloon inflation and controls the inflation/deflation cycle to accommodate variations in the patient's heart rate.
   It is timed by the ECG and monitored by the arterial pulse wave.

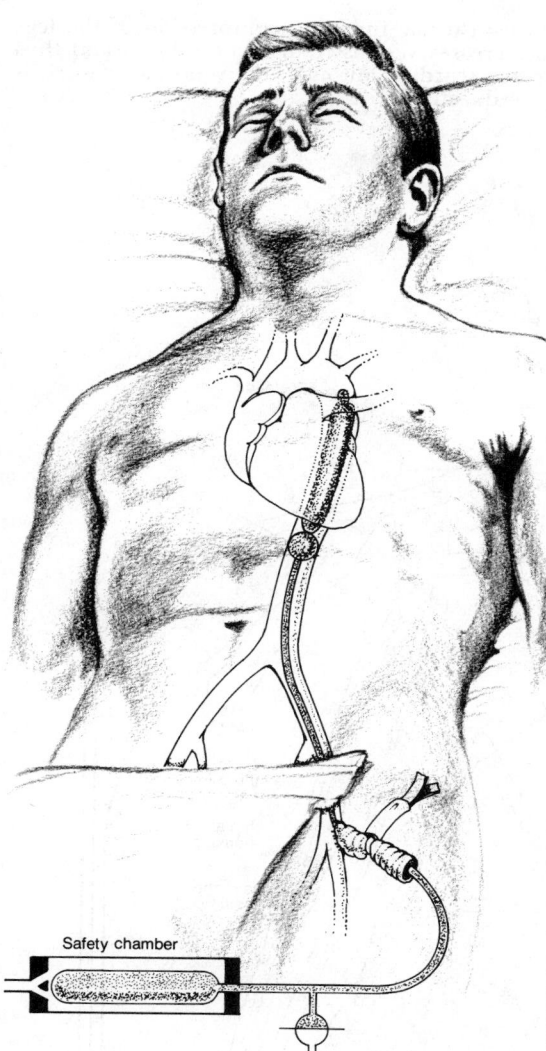

FIGURE 9-10. *Intra-aortic balloon pump. (From Lewis RP, Russell RO, and Williams DO. Therapies to brighten post-MI prospects. Patient Care 1 Jan 1976. Copyright © 1976, Miller and Fink Corp., Darien, Ct. All Rights Reserved)*

Counterpulsation with an intra-aortic balloon pump during the acute phase of MI eases the work load of a damaged heart and, if started before irreversible changes take place, limits infarct size by increasing coronary blood flow. The newer dual-chambered balloon shown here is twice as effective as the conventional single-chambered balloon in increasing coronary flow.

The balloon catheter is passed through a Dacron tube graft into one of the common femoral arteries, then threaded upward until the tip of the catheter is just below the left subclavian artery. A fail-safe bedside console (attached to safety chamber) supplies the CO_2 and controls the inflation/deflation cycle thus:

Diastole   The distal spherical chamber of the balloon is inflated slightly sooner than the cylindrical proximal chamber, which has the effect of obstructing aortic blood flow, pumping blood toward the aortic root and, most important, increasing coronary blood flow—"diastolic augmentation."

Systole CO_2 is evacuated from the balloon just prior to ventricular ejection, allowing the aorta to clear without reversing coronary blood flow.

The patient can be weaned from assistance when such hemodynamic parameters as pulmonary wedge pressure, cardiac output, and systolic pressure are satisfactory.

Safety chamber

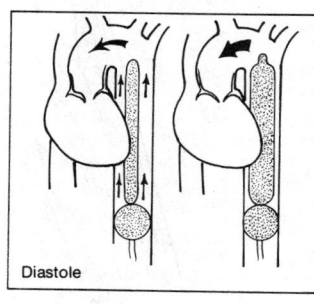

Diastole

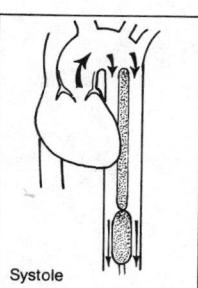

Systole

It augments diastole, which results in an increase in coronary blood flow and cardiac output, and it reduces left ventricular-end pressure (by causing a more complete emptying of the left ventricle). This decreases the resistance in the arterial tree against which the heart must pump and reduces myocardial oxygen requirements.

4. *Clinical Uses*
   a. Treatment of cardiogenic shock following myocardial infarction.
   b. Low cardiac output states—following open heart surgery; life-threatening arrhythmias.

B. *External counterpulsation pressure* (ECP) is a noninvasive method of assisting the circulation; it is designed to boost the heart temporarily during a period of pump failure. It helps maintain adequate perfusion of vital organs and tissues until the heart is able to resume its function (Fig. 9-11).

1. The counterpulsation device is positioned around the lower extremities from thighs to ankles; the legs are encased in 2 rigid troughs and the system is closed to make an airtight seal.
2. A pump is positioned between the patient's ankles.
3. Water is pumped through the system during diastole in response to an electronic signal triggered by the ECG; squeezing the legs during diastole forces a column of arterial blood back to the heart, which provides diastolic augmentation and improves coronary arterial filling pressure.
4. The pressure is released (application of negative pressure) during cardiac systole, which lowers the

systolic pressure (and thus the peak left ventricular pressure).

5. In cardiogenic shock, ECP increases the coronary blood flow by raising diastolic pressure, which may improve cardiac function; compression of the legs also increases venous return to the heart and thus increases cardiac output. Left ventricular work is thus reduced.

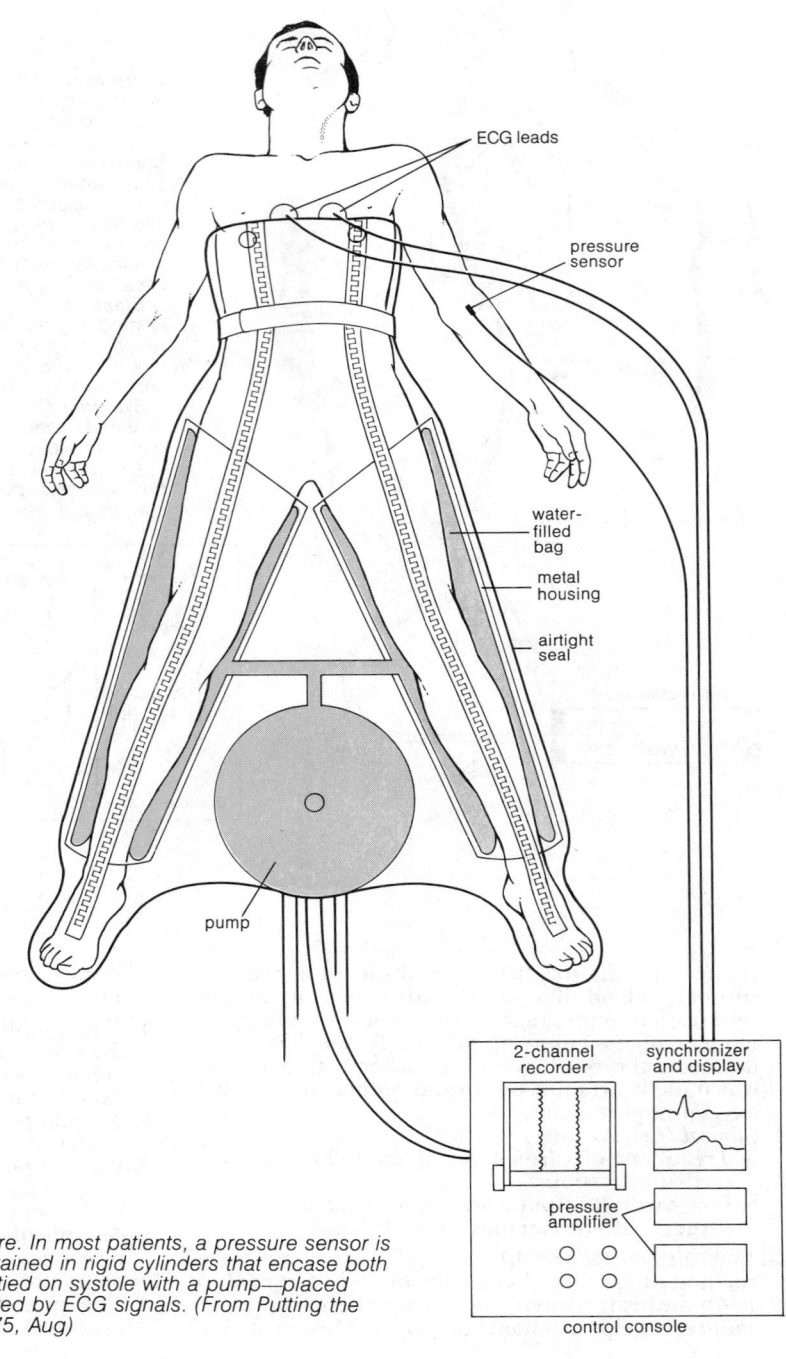

FIGURE 9-11. *External counterpulsation pressure. In most patients, a pressure sensor is threaded into a radial artery (right). Bags contained in rigid cylinders that encase both legs are filled with water on diastole and emptied on systole with a pump—placed between the patient's ankles—which is triggered by ECG signals. (From Putting the counterpressure on. Emergency Medicine 1975, Aug)*

ENDOCARDIAL DISEASE

Diseases Affecting the Endocardium

1. Infective endocarditis (see below)
2. Rheumatic endocarditis (complication of acute rheumatic fever, p. 294)
3. Chronic valvular heart disease (p. 297)

Altered Physiology

1. When an area of the endocardium becomes inflamed, a fibrin clot (vegetation) may form that in time becomes converted into a mass of scar tissue.
2. The scarred endocardium becomes thickened, stiffened, contracted, and deformed.
3. A fringe of vegetations along the free margins of the valve flaps represents the basic lesion of endocarditis and is the forerunner of chronic valvular heart disease.

INFECTIVE ENDOCARDITIS

Infective endocarditis (bacterial endocarditis) is an infection of the valves and inner lining of the heart caused by direct invasion of bacteria or other organisms; leading to deformity of the valve leaflets.

Prosthetic valve endocarditis—infection of previously inserted mechanical or biological heart valve.

Etiology

1. Bacteria (streptococci, pneumococci, staphylococci)
2. Fungi
3. Rickettsiae

Characteristics

1. Although infective endocarditis may develop on a heart valve already injured by other disease (rheumatic fever, congenital defects) or on abnormally vascularized valves, normal heart valves can become infected.
2. The vegetations on the affected endocardial surface may travel to various organs and tissues and cause emboli—spleen, kidney, coronary arteries, central nervous system and lungs.
3. May follow cardiac surgery, especially when prosthetic heart valves are used. (Foreign bodies, such as prosthetic valves, predispose to infection.)
4. High incidence among narcotic addicts in whom the disease mainly affects normal valves.
5. Hospitalized patients with indwelling catheters, those on prolonged intravenous therapy or prolonged antibiotic therapy, and those on immunosuppressive drugs or steroids may develop fungal endocarditis.
6. Rapid valvular destruction may lead to death.

Clinical Manifestations

A. *General Manifestations*

1. Fever, chills, sweats (fever may be absent in elderly or in patients with uremia)
2. Anorexia, weight loss, weakness
3. Cough; back and joint pain
4. Splenomegaly

B. *Skin and Nail Manifestations*

1. Petechiae—conjunctiva, mucous membranes
2. Splinter hemorrhages in nail beds

3. Roth's spots (hemorrhages with pale centers in the fundi of eyes)
4. Osler's nodes (painful red nodes on pads of fingers and toes)
5. Janeway's lesions (purplish macules on palms or soles)

C. *Heart Manifestations*

Murmur—appearance of a new murmur or change in an old one

D. *Central Nervous System Manifestations*

Headaches, transient cerebral ischemia, focal neurologic lesions, cerebrovascular accidents, encephalopathy, meningitis

E. *Embolic Phenomena*

Lung (recurrent pneumonia); kidney (hematuria); spleen; heart (myocardial infarction); brain (stroke); or peripheral vessels.

Diagnostic Evaluation

1. Blood culture—serial blood cultures are drawn to document the presence of continuous bacteremia and to determine etiologic agent.
2. Sensitivity studies—to determine the antibiotic for treatment.
3. Elevated sedimentation rate; anemia; mild leukocytosis
4. ECG
5. Echocardiography—to follow ventricular dimensions, progressive cardiomegaly

Treatment and Nursing Management

OBJECTIVES: to eradicate the invading organisms by adequate doses of appropriate agent to kill every organism in every vegetation. to prevent development of endocarditis in susceptible persons.

1. Determine the causative organism by obtaining serial blood cultures.
2. Treat with bactericidal (capable of destroying bacteria) or other appropriate drugs based on proven sensitivity of causative agent and allergies patient may have.
   a. Bactericidal serum levels of selected antibiotic are monitored by titering it against the causative organism; if the serum does not have adequate bactericidal activity, more antibiotic or a different antibiotic is given.
   b. Blood cultures are taken periodically—to monitor adequacy of therapy.
   c. Intravenous route usually used for long-term administration of parenteral antibiotics.
      (1) Apply antimicrobial ointment at needle entry site and cover with sterile dressing.
      (2) Note the date of needle or cannula insertion on nursing care plan.
   d. Adequate dosages are necessary to kill every organism in every vegetation.
   e. Combinations of drugs may be used if adequate serum levels are not achieved with one drug.
   f. Treatment with amphotericin B and surgery usually required for patient with fungal endocarditis.
3. Take temperature at regular intervals—course of fever is evaluated as one determinant of effectiveness of treatment.

4. Place patient in cardiac monitoring unit if patient is in congestive heart failure or to detect cardiac arrhythmias (secondary to involvement of heart conduction system or myocarditis).
5. Watch for development of complications—congestive heart failure, embolic phenomena, mycotic aneurysms, new heart murmurs, neurologic, renal, and hematologic complications.
6. Prepare for surgical intervention for:
   a. Acute destructive valvular lesion—excision of infected valves or removal of prosthetic valve.
   b. Hemodynamic impairment
   c. Recurrent emboli
   d. Infection that cannot be eliminated with antimicrobial therapy.
   e. Drainage of abscess/empyema—for patient with localized abscess or empyema.
   f. Repair of peripheral or cerebral mycotic aneurysm.

Preventive Management and Health Education

1. Treat all Group A beta-hemolytic streptococcal infections with suitable antibiotics.
2. Encourage patients with heart murmurs to receive pneumococcal vaccine and influenza vaccine—reduces risk of severe infections that may precipitate cardiac failure.
3. Educate persons at risk to look for and treat symptoms of illness indicating bacteremia—injuries, sore throats, furuncles, etc.
4. Antibiotic prophylaxis is recommended for persons at risk for the following procedures and circumstances:*
   a. Dental procedures causing gingival bleeding.
   b. Surgery or instrumentation of the respiratory tract (T & A, bronchoscopy) or procedures involving disruption of respiratory mucosa; surgery or instrumentation of the genitourinary tract (especially urethral procedures, including catheterization) or prostatic manipulation; surgery or instrumentation of the gastrointestinal tract and gallbladder.
   c. Cardiac surgery in which extracorporeal circulation is used, especially replacement of prosthetic valves.
   d. Surgical procedures on infected or contaminated tissues.
   e. Obstetrical infections (postpartum infection; septic abortion)

RHEUMATIC ENDOCARDITIS (RHEUMATIC HEART DISEASE)

Rheumatic endocarditis is damage done to the heart, particularly the valves, resulting in valve leakage (regurgitation) and/or obstruction (narrowing or stenosis). There are associated compensatory changes in the size of the heart's chambers and the thickness of chamber walls.

Role of Streptococcal Infection in Rheumatic Fever and Rheumatic Endocarditis

Rheumatic fever is a sequela to Group A streptococcal infection. It is a preventable disease through the de-

* From statement prepared by the Committee on Prevention of Rheumatic Fever and Bacterial Endocarditis of the American Heart Association. Circulation 1977 July; 56:139A–143A.

tection and adequate treatment of streptococcal pharyngitis.

A. *Symptoms of Streptococcal Pharyngitis*
1. Sudden onset of sore throat; throat reddened with exudate
2. Swollen, tender lymph nodes at angle of jaw
3. Headache and fever 38.9°–40° C. (101°–104° F).
4. Abdominal pain (children)

NURSING ALERT: Some cases of streptococcal throat infection are relatively asymptomatic.

B. *Diagnostic Evaluation*
Throat culture—to determine presence of streptococcal organisms

C. *Treatment of Streptococcal Infection*
1. Benzathine penicillin (single dose IM) or oral penicillin for full 10 days—to eradicate streptococci.
2. Erythromycin for patients sensitive to penicillin.

Clinical Manifestations of Rheumatic Fever

1. Polyarthritis; warm and swollen joints
2. Carditis
3. Chorea (irregular, jerky, involuntary, unpredictable muscular movements)
4. Erythema marginatum (wavy, thin red-line skin rash on trunk and extremities)
5. Subcutaneous nodules
6. Fever
7. Prolonged PR interval demonstrated by ECG
8. Heart murmurs; pleural and pericardial rubs

Laboratory Evaluation

1. Increased sedimentation rate; WBC and differential and C-reactive protein—increase during acute phase of infection
2. Elevated antistreptolysin titer

Treatment and Nursing

OBJECTIVES: to protect the heart.
1. Limit physical activity during the acute phase—patient should rest in bed as long as there is fever or signs of active carditis.
2. Utilize penicillin therapy—to eradicate hemolytic streptococcus; erythromycin may be used if patient is allergic to penicillin.
3. Give salicylates to suppress rheumatic activity by controlling toxic manifestations, to reduce fever, and to relieve joint pain.
4. Give liquid high carbohydrate diet during acute febrile period; diet is liberalized after fever subsides.
5. See Treatment of Rheumatic Fever in Children, page 300.
6. Teach patient the importance of preventing recurrences—to prevent rheumatic heart disease.
   a. Monthly IM injection of benzathine penicillin, or oral sulfadiazine or penicillin given daily.
   b. Continuous prophylaxis may have to be continued indefinitely.

Chronic Rheumatic Heart Disease as a Sequela of Rheumatic Fever (Complications)

Chronic rheumatic endocarditis is a complication of rheumatic fever, which frequently produces progressive disability and a shortened life span. Every structural component of the heart is likely to be the site of an inflammatory reaction.

1. Although the patient is symptom-free for a time, the damage to the valves (rigidity and deformity, thickening and fusion of the commissures, or shortening and fusion of chordae tendinae) will produce heart sounds that are characteristic of valvular stenosis, regurgitation, or both.
2. The myocardium will compensate for these valvular defects for a while, but in time it fails to compensate and the patient develops symptoms of congestive heart failure.
3. See page 297 for treatment of valvular heart disease and page 299 for treatment of congestive heart failure.
4. *Health Education*
   Persons with rheumatic heart disease should have prophylactic penicillin therapy before undergoing dental procedures or surgery of genitourinary tract and lower intestinal tract.

MYOCARDITIS

Myocarditis is an inflammatory process involving the myocardium.

Etiology

1. Infectious process—viral (particularly Coxsackie group B), bacterial, mycotic, parasitic, protozoal, rickettsial, and spirochetal infections.
2. Following drug administration (doxorubicin [Adriamycin]).
3. Other conditions—sarcoidosis, collagen diseases (rheumatic fever).
4. Immunosuppressive therapy.

Clinical Manifestations

A. *Symptoms*

1. Depend on type of infection, degree of myocardial damage, capacity of myocardium to recover, and host resistance.
   a. Fatigue and dyspnea
   b. Palpitations
   c. Occasional precordial discomfort

B. *Clinical Findings*

1. Cardiac enlargement
2. Cardiac murmur—abnormal heart sound; sounds like fluid passing an obstruction
3. Pericardial friction rub
4. Gallop rhythm—a tripling or quadrupling of heart sounds (resembling the galloping of a horse) heard upon auscultation
5. Pulsus alternans—a pulse in which there is regular alternation of weak and strong beats
6. Fever with tachycardia
7. Evidence of development of congestive heart failure

Treatment and Nursing Management

OBJECTIVE: to reduce the work of the heart

1. Give specific therapy for underlying disease (example: antimicrobial for hemolytic streptococci).
2. Place patient on bed rest to reduce heart rate, stroke volume, blood pressure, and heart contractility; also helps to decrease residual damage and complications of myocarditis, and promotes healing.
   a. Prolonged bed rest may be required—until there is reduction in heart size and improvement of function
   b. Assess for clinical evidence that disease is subsiding—evaluate pulse, heart sounds, temperature, etc.
3. Treat the symptoms of congestive heart failure (see p. 298).
   a. Restrict activity—to reduce systemic oxygen requirements.
   b. Give digitalis—augments myocardial contractility and slows heart rate.
   c. Administer diuretics—to control pulmonary or systemic congestion.

NURSING ALERT: Patients with myocarditis may be sensitive to digitalis—assess for toxic symptoms (see p. 300).

   (1) Evaluate patient's pulse and apical rate for signs of tachycardia and gallop rhythm—indications that congestive heart failure is recurring.
   (2) Evaluate for evidences of arrhythmia—*patients with myocarditis are prone to develop arrhythmias.*
       (a) Place patient in unit with continuous cardiac monitoring if evidences of an arrhythmia develop.
       (b) See page 313 for management of arrhythmias.
       (c) Have equipment for resuscitation, cardiac defibrillation, and cardiac pacing available in event of life-threatening arrhythmia.

Health Education

Instruct patient as follows:

1. There is usually some residual heart enlargement; physical activity may be *slowly* increased; begin with chair rest for increasing periods of time; follow by walking in the room and then outdoors.
2. Report any symptom involving rapidly beating heart.
3. Avoid competitive sports, alcohol, and other myocardial toxins (doxorubicin).
4. Pregnancy is not advisable for women with cardiomyopathies (diseases which affect structure and function of myocardium).
5. Prevention—prevent infectious diseases by means of appropriate immunizations.

PERICARDITIS

Pericarditis is an inflammation of the pericardium, the membranous sac enveloping the heart. It is often a manifestation of a more generalized disease.

Pericardial effusion is an outpouring of fluid into the pericardial cavity.

Constrictive pericarditis is a condition in which a chronic inflammatory thickening of the pericardium compresses the heart so that it is unable to fill normally during diastole.

Etiology

1. Acute idiopathic—most common and typical form; etiology unknown
2. Infection
   a. Viral (influenza; Coxsackie)
   b. Bacterial—staphylococcus, meningococcus, streptococcus, pneumococcus, gonococcus, *Mycobacterium tuberculosis*
   c. Fungal
   d. Parasitic
3. Disorders of connective tissues and allergies—lupus erythematosus, periarteritis nodosa
4. Myocardial infarction; early, 24–72 hours; or late, 1 week to 2 years (Dressler's syndrome)
5. Malignant disease; thoracic irradiation
6. Chest trauma, heart surgery, including pacemaker implantation
7. Drug induced (procainamide; daunorubicin)

Clinical Manifestations

1. Pain in anterior chest, aggravated by thoracic motion—may vary from mild to sharp and severe; located in precordial area (may be felt beneath clavicle, neck, scapular region)—may be relieved by leaning forward.
2. Pericardial friction rub—scratchy, grating, or creaking sound occurring in the presence of pericardial inflammation.
   Nursing implications: Place the diaphragm of the stethoscope firmly on the chest wall along the mid-to-lower left sternal border or at the apex. Listen with patient in different positions.
3. Dyspnea—from compression of heart and surrounding thoracic structures.
4. Fever, sweating, chills—due to inflammation of pericardium.
5. Arrhythmias.

Diagnostic Evaluation

1. Echocardiogram—most sensitive method for detecting pericardial effusion
2. Chest x-ray—may show heart enlargement

> **NURSING ALERT:** Normal pericardial sac contains less than 25–30 ml. of fluid; pericardial fluid may accumulate slowly without noticeable symptoms. However, a rapidly developing effusion can produce serious hemodynamic alterations.

3. ECG—to evaluate for myocardial infarction
4. WBC and differential
5. Antinuclear antibody serologic tests and lupus erythematosus cell preparation—to rule out lupus erythematosus
6. PPD test—for tuberculosis; ASO titers—for rheumatic fever
7. Pericardiocentesis—for examination of pericardial fluid for etiological diagnosis
8. Serum urea nitrogen (BUN)—to evaluate for uremia

Treatment and Nursing Management

OBJECTIVES: to determine the cause.
    to administer therapy for the specific cause (when known).
    to be on the alert for the complication of cardiac tamponade.

1. Utilize *anticipatory nursing:* Be alert to the possibility of cardiac tamponade. Intervention with pericardiocentesis (pericardial aspiration) is indicated immediately (see p. 274). Assess patient for distant heart sounds, falling arterial pressure, and rising venous pressure.
2. Give prescribed drug regimen for pain and symptomatic relief.
   a. Nonsteroid anti-inflammatory drugs (aspirin, indomethacin)—suppress inflammatory symptoms of acute pericarditis.
   b. Corticosteroids—for more severe symptoms.
3. Give specific therapy when the cause is known.
   a. Bacterial pericarditis—penicillin or other antimicrobial agents
   b. Rheumatic fever—procaine penicillin, prednisone
   c. Tuberculosis—antituberculosis chemotherapy (see page 813)
      (There is a high incidence of constriction in tuberculosis pericarditis)
   d. Fungal pericarditis—amphotericin B
   e. Disseminated lupus erythematosus—adrenal steroids
   f. Uremic pericarditis—dialysis, indomethacin, biochemical control of uremia
   g. Neoplastic pericarditis—intrapericardial instillation of chemotherapy; radiotherapy
   h. Postmyocardial infarction syndrome—bed rest, aspirin, prednisone
   i. Postpericardiotomy syndrome (after open heart surgery)—treat symptomatically
4. Encourage patient to remain on bed rest when chest pain, fever, and friction rub occur. *Nursing Assessment:* Pericardial pain is aggravated by breathing, turning in bed, and twisting the body.
   a. Elevate head of bed; position pillow on over-the-bed table so that patient can lean on it.
5. Be cognizant of complications of pericarditis—congestive heart failure, arrhythmias, cardiac tamponade.
6. Prepare patient for surgical intervention (direct pericardial decompression)—for patient with cardiac embarrassment associated with constrictive pericarditis.

ACQUIRED VALVULAR DISEASE OF THE HEART

Altered Physiology

1. The function of normal heart valves is to maintain the forward flow of blood from the atria to the ventricles and from the ventricles to the great vessels.
2. Valvular damage may interfere with valvular function by stenosis or by impaired closure that allows backward leakage of blood (valvular insufficiency, regurgitation, or incompetence).
3. Acquired valvular heart disease is often the result of previous rheumatic fever, which has damaged one or more heart valves; mitral valve is most commonly involved, followed by aortic, tricuspid, and pulmonary valves.
4. Patients with valvular disease usually develop congestive heart failure in time.

MITRAL STENOSIS

Mitral stenosis is the progressive thickening and contracture of valve cusps with narrowing of the orifice and progressive obstruction to blood flow. It is the most common of the late lesions produced by rheumatic fever.

Altered Physiology

1. Acute rheumatic valvulitis has "glued" the mitral valve flaps (commissures) together, thus shortening the chordae tendinae, so that the flap edges are pulled down, greatly narrowing the mitral orifice.
2. The left atrium has difficulty in emptying itself through the narrow orifice into the left ventricle; therefore, it dilates and hypertrophies. Pulmonary circulation becomes congested.
3. As a result of the abnormally high pulmonary arterial pressure that must be maintained, the right ventricle is subjected to a pressure overload and may eventually fail.

Clinical Manifestations

1. Progressive fatigue—result of low cardiac output
2. Dyspnea on exertion, cough, repeated respiratory infections
3. Hemoptysis—from pulmonary venous hypertension
4. Weak, irregular pulse; atrial fibrillation
5. Characteristic murmurs—increased 1st heart sound, opening snap, and low pitched rumbling diastolic murmur heard at the apex

Diagnostic Evaluation

1. ECG
2. Echocardiography—can demonstrate mitral valve thickening, calcification, and abnormal, slowed diastolic valve excursion
3. Cardiac catheterization and angiocardiography

Treatment

1. Medical treatment
   a. Prevent rheumatic recurrences with antimicrobial therapy.
   b. Treat the developing congestive failure—vasodilators, digitalis, sodium restriction, limitation of activity (see p. 299).
   c. Control arrhythmias (especially atrial fibrillation).

2. Surgical intervention may be accomplished by:
   a. Closed mitral valvotomy—introduction of a dilator through the mitral valve to split its commissures.
   b. Open mitral valvotomy—direct incision of the commissures.
   c. Mitral valve replacement.
   d. See page 303 for the management of the patient undergoing heart surgery.

MITRAL INSUFFICIENCY

Mitral insufficiency (regurgitaton) is the result of incompetence and distortion of the mitral valve so that the free margins can no longer come into apposition during systole. The chordae tendinae may become shortened, preventing complete closure of the leaflets.

Mitral insufficiency may be caused by mitral valve prolapse, chronic rheumatic heart disease, postinfarction mitral regurgitation, and infective endocarditis.

Clinical Manifestations

1. Palpitations; arrhythmias.
2. Shortness of breath on exertion; cough—due to pulmonary congestion.
3. Murmur—soft first sound and a blowing pansystolic murmur heard at the apex and transmitted to the axilla.

Diagnostic Evaluation

(same as for mitral stenosis)

Nursing Management

1. Management of congestive heart failure, see page 299.
2. Surgical intervention—mitral valve replacement or annuloplasty (retailoring of the valve ring).

AORTIC STENOSIS

Aortic stenosis is a narrowing of the orifice between the left ventricle and the aorta. The obstruction to the aortic outflow places a pressure load on the left ventricle that results in hypertrophy and failure. In adults it may be congenital or from cusp calcification.

Clinical Manifestations

1. Loud rough systolic murmur over aortic area; often associated with a palpable thrill
2. Exertional dyspnea and fatigue
3. Dizziness and fainting—from reduced blood supply to brain
4. Angina pectoris
5. Low blood pressure and low pulse pressure—from diminished blood flow
6. Arrhythmias
7. Symptoms of congestive heart failure

Diagnostic Evaluation

1. Chest x-ray—usually shows left ventricular enlargement
2. Cardiac catheterization — will reveal the pressures
3. Angiocardiography — in the left ventricle and aorta

Treatment

1. Surgical replacement of aortic valve—prosthetic or tissue valve.
   See page 303 for care of patient undergoing heart surgery.
2. Treat angina and congestive heart failure as dictated by patient's condition.

AORTIC INSUFFICIENCY

Aortic insufficiency (regurgitation) is caused by inflammatory lesions that deform the flaps so that they fail to completely seal the aortic orifice during diastole and thus permit a backflow of blood from the aorta into the left ventricle.

It may be caused by rheumatic endocarditis, infective endocarditis, or congenital malformation or from diseases which cause dilation or tearing of the ascending aorta (syphilitic disease, rheumatoid spondylitis, dissecting aneurysm).

Clinical Manifestations

1. Awareness of increased force of heartbeat
   a. Arterial pulsations visible and palpable over precordium
   b. Arterial pulsations visible in neck
2. Exertional dyspnea; easy fatigability, progressing to paroxysmal nocturnal dyspnea and orthopnea
3. Widened pulse pressure
4. Water-hammer (Corrigan's) pulse—pulse strikes palpating finger with quick, sharp stroke and then suddenly collapses
5. Murmur—high-pitched blowing decrescendo diastolic murmur audible along the left sternal edge

Diagnostic Evaluation

1. ECG—shows pattern of left ventricular hypertrophy
2. Chest x-ray—reveals varying degrees of cardiomegaly from left ventricular enlargement
3. Echocardiography—estimates size and thickness of left ventricle
4. Cardiac catheterization and angiography

Treatment

Surgical intervention—replacement of damaged aortic valve. See page 303 for nursing management of patient undergoing heart surgery.

TRICUSPID STENOSIS

Tricuspid stenosis is restriction of the tricuspid valve orifice due to commissural fusion and fibrosis usually following rheumatic fever. It is commonly associated with diseases of the mitral valve.

Clinical Manifestations

1. Dyspnea, nocturnal dyspnea, orthopnea
2. Hemoptysis
3. Visible pulsations of neck veins
4. Murmurs—similar to those of rheumatic mitral disease; blowing diastolic murmur along left sternal border
5. Symptoms of right-sided heart failure (late)

Diagnostic Evaluation

1. ECG—may reveal atrial fibrillation
2. Cardiac catheterization and angiocardiography—to confirm diagnosis

Treatment

1. Patient may have mitral and aortic disease which must be corrected.
2. Surgical treatment of accompanying tricuspid valve disease may be carried out at the time of operation after correction of mitral valve disease.

TRICUSPID INSUFFICIENCY (REGURGITATION)

Tricuspid insufficiency allows the regurgitation of blood from the right ventricle into the right atrium during ventricular systole.

Clinical Manifestations

1. Right-sided heart failure—from overload of right ventricle
2. Edema—with congestion of liver and hepatic malfunction, ascites, hydrothorax
3. Elevated venous pressure
4. Pansystolic murmur in tricuspid area

Nursing Management

Surgical treatment of associated mitral valve disease, tricuspid valvuloplasty, or tricuspid valve replacement.

CONGESTIVE HEART FAILURE

Heart failure is the inability of the heart to pump the amount of oxygenated blood necessary to effect venous return and to meet the metabolic requirements of the body.

Congestive heart failure is the occurrence of circulatory congestion due to decreased myocardial contractility; as a result, cardiac output is inadequate to maintain the blood flow to body organs and tissues. This ultimately causes sodium and water retention and elevation of left atrial pressure, which results in pulmonary vascular congestion.

Causes

1. Disorders of heart muscle resulting in decreased contractile properties of the heart; coronary heart disease leading to myocardial infarction; hypertension; valvular heart disease; congenital heart disease; cardiomyopathies; arrhythmias
2. Pulmonary embolism; chronic lung disease
3. Hemorrhage and anemia
4. Anesthesia and surgery
5. Transfusions or infusions
6. Increased body demands (fever, infection, pregnancy, arteriovenous fistula)
7. Drug induced (doxorubicin)
8. Physical and emotional stress
9. Excessive sodium intake

Clinical Manifestations

Initially there may be isolated left ventricular failure, but in time the right ventricle fails because of the additional workload. Combined left and right ventricular failure is usual.

A. *Left-sided Heart Failure* (forward failure)

1. Congestion occurs mainly in the lungs from backing up of blood into pulmonary veins and capillaries
   a. Shortness of breath, dyspnea on exertion, paroxysmal nocturnal dyspnea (due to reabsorption of dependent edema that has developed during day), orthopnea, pulmonary edema
   b. Cough—may be dry, unproductive; often occurs at night
2. Fatigability—from low cardiac output, nocturia, insomnia, dyspnea, catabolic effect of chronic failure
3. Insomnia
4. Tachycardia—S_3 ventricular gallop
5. Restlessness

B. *Right-sided Heart Failure* (backward failure)

Signs and symptoms of elevated pressures and congestion in systemic veins and capillaries:
1. Edema of ankles; unexplained weight gain
   Pitting edema—is obvious only after retention of at least 4.5 kg. (10 pounds) of fluid
2. Liver congestion—may produce upper abdominal pain
3. Distended neck veins
4. Abnormal fluid in body cavities (pleural space, abdominal cavity)
5. Anorexia and nausea—from hepatic and visceral engorgement
6. Nocturia—diuresis occurs at night with rest and improved cardiac output
7. Weakness

Complications

1. Intractable or refractory heart failure—patient becomes progressively refractory to therapy (not yielding to treatment)
2. Cardiac arrhythmias
3. Myocardial failure
4. Digitalis toxicity—from decreased renal function, potassium depletion, etc.
5. Myocardial failure
6. Pulmonary infarction; pneumonia

Diagnostic Findings

1. Cardiovascular findings
   a. Cardiomegaly (enlargement of the heart)—detected by physical examination and chest x-ray
   b. Ventricular gallop—evident on auscultation; ECG
   c. Rapid heart rate
   d. Development of pulsus alternans (alternation in strength of beat)
   e. Distended neck veins
   f. Hepatomegaly (enlargement of the liver)
2. ECG, echocardiography
3. Chest x-ray—to evaluate heart size, show lung fields (for pleural effusion) and vascular congestion
4. Arterial blood gas studies
5. Liver function studies—may be altered due to hepatic congestion

Treatment and Nursing Management

OBJECTIVES: to promote rest to reduce the work of the heart.
to administer pharmacologic agents to increase the force and efficiency of myocardial contraction.
to eliminate excessive accumulation of body water by use of diuretics and sodium restriction.

A. *Assist in identifying, eliminating, and treating the underlying causes.*

B. *Place patient at physical and emotional rest to reduce work of heart.*

1. Provide rest in semirecumbent position or in armchair in air-conditioned environment—reduces work of heart, increases heart reserve, reduces blood pressure, decreases work of respiratory muscles and oxygen utilization, improves efficiency of heart contraction; recumbency promotes diuresis by improving renal perfusion.
2. Raise head of bed 20–30 cm. (8–10 inches)—reduces venous return to heart and lungs; alleviates pulmonary congestion.
   a. Support lower arms with pillows—to eliminate pull of their weight on shoulder muscles.
   b. Sit orthopneic patient on side of bed with feet supported by a chair, head and arms resting on an over-the-bed table, and his lumbosacral area supported with pillows.
3. Provide bedside commode—to reduce work of getting to bathroom and defecation.
4. Relieve nighttime anxiety and provide for rest and sleep—patients with congestive heart failure have a tendency to be restless at night because of cerebral hypoxia with superimposed nitrogen retention.
   a. Give oxygen during acute stage—to diminish work of breathing and increase the comfort of the patient.
   b. Give appropriate sedation—to relieve insomnia and restlessness.
      (1) Give small doses of morphine as prescribed for extreme dyspnea.
      (2) Give mild sedation as needed for sleep. Use sedation carefully to prevent respiratory depression; detoxification of drugs is delayed because of hepatic congestion and immobility of patient.
   c. Keep a night light on in the room; the presence of a family member provides reassurance to some persons.
   d. Avoid restraints—resistance to restraints increases cardiac load.
5. Increase the patient's activities gradually.
   a. Alter or modify patient's activities—to keep within the limits of his cardiac reserve.
   b. Observe the pulse, symptoms, and behavioral response to increased activity.
   c. Observe for the complications of bed rest—pressure sores (especially in edematous patients), phlebothrombosis, pulmonary embolism.
6. Provide for psychological rest—emotional stress produces vasoconstriction, elevates arterial pressure, and speeds the heart.
   a. Promote physical comfort.
   b. Avoid situations that tend to promote anxiety/agitation.
   c. Offer careful explanations and answers to patient's questions.
7. Assess the patient's response to rest; are his symptoms alleviated?

C. *Digitalis Therapy*

Administer digitalis (a cardiac glycoside) as prescribed—to increase the force of myocardial contraction and produce a stronger systolic contraction of the heart and to slow the heart rate. This results in increased cardiac output; decreased heart size, venous pressure, and blood volume; diuresis and relief of edema. Digitalis is also used to slow the ventricular rate in the setting of supraventricular arrhythmias.

1. A loading (digitalizing) dose may be given in order to induce the full therapeutic effect of the drug when rapid digitalization is necessary.
2. Otherwise, the patient is started without a loading dose. The patient is then given a daily dose just adequate to replace the drug that is destroyed or excreted—to maintain digitalis effect without toxicity.
3. *Digitalis preparations* (Choice of drug depends on speed of onset and duration of action required and on individual patient response.)

ORAL

Digoxin
Digitalis
Digitoxin
Lanatoside C (Cedilanid)
Acetyldigitoxin (Acylanid)
Gitalin (Gitalgin)

PARENTERAL

Digoxin
Ouabain
Deslanoside (Cedilanid-D)
Digitoxin

4. Factors that may cause increased sensitivity to digitalis:
   a. Myocardial infarction, particularly ischemia
   b. Potassium depletion
   c. Kidney or hepatic disease
   d. Diuretic therapy
   e. Diarrhea
   f. Loss of appetite
   g. Advancing age
   h. Hypoxia and hypercapnia in pulmonary disease
   i. Acidosis; alkalosis
5. Serum concentration of digitalis (digitalis assay) may be measured (by laboratory) for therapeutic guidance and to assess for toxicity.
6. Serum potassium levels and ECGs are followed, and signs and symptoms are carefully monitored in patients receiving digitalis, especially those receiving both digitalis and diuretics.
7. *Nursing responsibilities in administration of digitalis*
   a. Assess clinical response of patient with respect to relief of symptoms (lessening dyspnea and orthopnea, decrease in rales, relief of peripheral edema).
   b. Watch for toxic effects—*arrhythmias* (most important toxic effect), *anorexia*, nausea, vomiting, diarrhea, bradycardia, headache, malaise, behavioral changes, increasing congestive failure.

NURSING ALERT: The incidence of digitalis toxicity is high because of the narrow margin between therapeutic and toxic doses. Toxic effects do not always appear in a predictable manner. Digitalis toxicity has a high mortality rate.

c. Take pulse and apical heart rate before administering each dose of digitalis.
d. Withhold digitalis and notify physician if following is noted:
   (1) Slowing of rate.
   (2) Change in rhythm—bradycardia, premature ventricular contraction, bigeminy (2 pulse beats following in rapid succession), atrial fibrillation.*
   (3) Dangerous cardiac arrhythmias require immediate treatment (see p. 313).
e. Assess for symptoms of electrolyte depletion—lassitude, apathy, mental confusion, anorexia, decreasing urinary output, azotemia.
f. Watch carefully patient who is being treated simultaneously with diuretics and digitalis—*there is a predisposition to arrhythmias if the state of potassium balance is not evaluated and corrected.*

D. *Diuretics*

Administer prescribed diuretic (agent which increases the rate of urine flow). See Table 9-1.
1. Type and dosage of diuretic administered depends on degree of heart failure and state of renal function.
2. *Nursing Responsibilities in Administration of Diuretics*
   a. Give diuretic early in the morning—nighttime diuresis disturbs sleep.
   b. Keep input and output record—patient may lose large volume of fluid after a single dose of diuretic
   c. Weigh patient daily—to determine if edema is being controlled; weight loss should not exceed 0.45–0.9 kg. (1–2 pounds) per day.
   d. Assess for weakness, malaise, muscle cramps—diuretic therapy may produce hypovolemia and electrolyte depletion, namely *hypokalemia*.
      Hypokalemia may cause weakening of cardiac contractions and may precipitate digitalis toxicity in the form of arrhythmias.
   e. Give oral potassium as prescribed.
   f. Be aware that problems associated with diuretic administration include disorders of potassium balance, hyperuricemia, volume depletion and hyponatremia, magnesium depletion, hyperglycemia, and diabetes mellitus.
   g. Watch for signs of bladder distention in the elderly male with prostatic hyperplasia.

E. *Vasodilator Therapy* (for heart failure unresponsive to usual therapy)

1. *Rationale:* Vasodilators are used to increase cardiac output by dilating the peripheral vascular vessels and reducing impedance (resistance) to left ventricular outflow.
   a. By relaxing capacitance vessels (veins and venules), vasodilators reduce ventricular filling pressures (preload) and volumes.
   b. By relaxing resistance vessels (arterioles), vasodilators can reduce impedance to left ventricular ejection and improve stroke volume.
2. Vasodilators used in congestive heart failure:
   a. Nitrates (nitroglycerin, isosorbide dinitrate, nitroglycerin ointment)—predominantly dilates systemic veins
   b. Nitroprusside—dilator effect in both arterial and venous beds.

* Regularization of the rate in patient with chronic atrial fibrillation should be a warning that digitalis intoxication may be present.

TABLE 9-1 COMMONLY USED DIURETICS

Definition: Diuretics are agents which increase the rate of urine flow.

Action: Dependent upon functionally active kidneys; most diuretics decrease the reabsorption of electrolytes (principally sodium) by the kidneys, promoting water loss as a secondary action.

    In the treatment of hypertension the naturetic (sodium excretion) effect is probably the action of importance.

    In edema states, the salt and water actions are both important.

Special Precaution: Some diuretics may produce electrolyte depletion including potassium loss, which causes weakness and induces cardiac arrhythmias. Vigorous diuresis can produce hypovolemia.

Dosage Determination: (1) Patient's daily weight; (2) clinical signs and symptoms; (3) physical examination; (4) state of renal function

Diuretic	Action	Nursing Implications
Thiazides and Related Drugs Chlorothiazide (Diuril) Hydrochlorothiazide (HydroDIURIL, Esidrix, Oretic) Methyclothiazide (Enduron) Polythiazide (Renese) Chlorthalidone (Hygroton) Quinethazone (Hydromox)	Increases renal excretion of sodium (natu-resis), potassium, chloride, bicarbonate (alkaline urine) with accompanying "os-motic" water loss. Used principally in states of edema and hypertension. Most widely used for prolonged administration.	Monitor for electrolyte depletion. Watch for signs and symptoms of electrolyte imbalance: hyponatremia, hypokalemia, hypochloremic alkalosis. Adverse reactions may occur, manifested by gastrointestinal, central nervous system, hematologic, and cardiovascular signs and symptoms. Supplementary potassium is usually given with these diuretics.
Potassium-Sparing Diuretics Spironolactone (Aldactone)	Inhibits action of aldosterone in distal tubule and reduces reabsorption of sodium and chloride. Gives gradual diuretic effect. Used in treatment of CHF, cirrhosis, and edema when other diuretics are toxic or ineffective.	Monitor for electrolyte depletion. Usually used in combination with thiazide diuretic. Watch for side effects—skin rash, gynecomastia.
Triamterene (Dyrenium)	Inhibits reabsorption of sodium ions in exchange for potassium and hydrogen ions in distal tubule.	Usually used as an adjunct to thiazide therapy. May cause elevation in blood uric acid. Watch for nausea, vomiting, diarrhea, weakness, headache, and skin rash.
Potent Diuretics Furosemide (Lasix) Ethacrynic Acid (Edecrin)	Usually reserved for patients who do not respond to classical thiazide diuretics. Blocks the reabsorption of sodium and water in proximal renal tubule and interferes with reabsorption of sodium in ascending limb of loop of Henle and in the most proximal portion of the distal tubule. Associated with sodium, potassium, chloride, and hydrogen ion loss (acid urine). Have an almost immediate action (within 5 minutes) when given IV.	Monitor for electrolyte depletion: may produce *profound diuresis* with hyponatremia, hypokalemia, hypochloremic alkalosis, and circulatory collapse. Potent and rapid-acting. Especially useful in acute pulmonary edema. Watch for nausea, vomiting, diarrhea, skin rash, pruritus, blurring of vision, postural hypotension, vertigo, hearing loss. Furosemide is chemically related to sulfonamides; consider cross allergies. Administer early in the day to avoid nocturia and consequent loss of sleep.

    c. Hydralazine—predominantly affects arterioles; reduces arteriolar tone

    d. Prazosin—balanced effects on both arterial and venous circulation

3. Invasive hemodynamic monitoring is often used to guide drug administration. (See page 268.)

NURSING ALERT: Watch for sudden unexpected hypotension, which can cause myocardial ischemia and decrease perfusion to vital organs.

4. Inotropic Agents

    a. Dobutamine—directly increases myocardial contractility

    b. Digitalis

5. Combinations of above drugs used.

F. *Dietary Support*

1. Diet may be limited in sodium—to prevent, control, or eliminate edema; may also be limited in calories.

    a. Patients on diuretics may not be on sodium-restricted diet.

    b. Caution patients to avoid added salt in food and foods with high sodium content.

2. Teach the patient the importance of adhering to the low sodium diet.

    a. Sodium is present in many types of natural foods and in varying amounts in processed foods.

3. Make the diet as palatable as possible.

    a. Use flavorings, spices, herbs, and lemon juice.

    b. Avoid salt substitutes in the presence of renal disease.

4. Offer small, frequent feedings—to avoid excessive gastric filling and abdominal distention with subsequent elevation of diaphragm that causes decrease in lung capacity.

5. Teach the patient to rinse the mouth well after using tooth cleansers and mouthwashes—some of these contain large amounts of sodium. Water softeners are to be avoided.

6. Teach the patient that sodium is present in alkalizers, cough remedies, laxatives, pain relievers, estrogens, etc.

7. Give the patient written dietary instructions.

Health Education

1. Explain the disease process to the patient; the term "failure" may have terrifying implications.

    a. Explain the pumping action of the heart—"to move blood through the body to provide nutrients and aid in the removal of waste material."

b. Explain the difference between "heart attack" and congestive heart failure.
2. Teach the signs and symptoms of recurrence.
   a. Ask patient to recall how he felt when he first became ill.
   b. Watch for:
      (1) Gain in weight—report weight gain of more than 2–3 pounds (0.9–1.4 kg.) in a few days. Weigh at same time daily to detect any tendency toward fluid retention.
      (2) Swelling of ankles, feet, or abdomen
      (3) Persistent cough
      (4) Tiredness; loss of appetite
      (5) Frequent urination at night
3. Review medication regimen.
   a. Label all medications.
   b. Give written instructions concerning digitalis and diuretic therapy.
   c. Inform patient not to substitute another brand of digitalis for the one he is taking.
      (1) Make sure patient has a check-off system that will show that he has taken his medications.
      (2) Teach patient to take and record his pulse rate.
      (3) Inform patient of the signs and symptoms of digitalis toxicity and potassium depletion.
      (4) If patient is taking oral potassium solution, it may be diluted with juice and taken after a meal.

d. Tell him to weigh himself daily and log his weight if he is on diuretic therapy.
4. Review activity program.
   Instruct the patient as follows:
   a. Increase walking and other activities gradually, provided they do not cause fatigue and dyspnea.
   b. In general, continue at whatever activity level you can maintain without the appearance of symptoms.
   c. Avoid excesses in eating and drinking.
   d. Undertake a weight reduction program until optimum weight is reached.
   e. Avoid extremes in heat and cold—which increase the work of the heart; air conditioning may be essential in a hot, humid environment.
   f. Keep *regular* appointment with physician or clinic.
5. Restrict sodium as directed.
   a. Give patient a booklet containing sodium content of common foods from local chapter of American Heart Association.
   b. Give patient written diet plan with list of permitted and restricted foods.
   c. Advise patient to look at all labels to ascertain sodium content (antacids, laxatives, cough remedies, etc.).
   d. Ascertain the amount of sodium in the local drinking water through inquiry to local department of health.
6. Advise patient to accept the fact that restricting sodium and taking digitalis will be a permanent part of his way of life.

ACUTE PULMONARY EDEMA

Acute pulmonary edema refers to the presence of excess fluid in the lung, either in the interstitial spaces or in the alveoli. It usually follows acute left ventricular failure.

NURSING ALERT: Acute pulmonary edema is a true medical emergency since it is a life-threatening condition.

Causes

1. Heart disease: acute left ventricular failure, myocardial infarction, aortic stenosis, severe mitral valve disease, hypertension, congestive heart failure
2. Circulatory overload—transfusions and infusions
3. Drug hypersensitivity; allergy; poisoning
4. Lung injuries—smoke inhalation, shock lung, pulmonary embolism or infarct
5. Central nervous system injuries—stroke, head trauma
6. Infection and fever

Clinical Manifestations

1. Coughing and restlessness during sleep (premonitory symptoms)
2. Extreme dyspnea and orthopnea—patient usually uses accessory muscles of respiration with retraction of intercostal spaces and supraclavicular areas

3. Cough with varying amounts of white- or pink-tinged frothy sputum
4. Extreme anxiety and panic
5. Noisy breathing—inspiratory and expiratory wheezing and bubbling sounds
6. Cyanosis with profuse perspiration
7. Distended neck veins
8. Tachycardia

Treatment and Nursing Management*

OBJECTIVES: to improve ventilation and oxygenation.
to reduce pulmonary congestion.
Take steps to reduce venous return to the heart.
1. Place patient in upright position, head and shoulders up, feet and legs hanging down—to favor pooling of blood in dependent portions of body by gravitational forces; to decrease venous return.
2. Give morphine in small titrated intermittent doses (IV) until dyspnea lessens—to allay acute anxiety and decrease respiratory effort, allowing better oxygen exchange; this also decreases peripheral resistance so that blood can be redistributed from the pulmonary circulation to the periphery.
   a. Morphine is *not* given if pulmonary edema is caused by cerebral vascular accident or occurs in the presence of chronic pulmonary disease or cardiogenic shock.
   b. Watch for excessive respiratory depression.

* Many of these therapeutic interventions are done simultaneously.

c. Monitor blood pressure, since morphine may intensify hypotension.
d. Have morphine antagonist available—naloxone hydrochloride (Narcan).
3. Give oxygen in high concentration—to relieve hypoxia and dyspnea.
   a. Oxygen may be given with high enough pressure to provide blood oxygenation and to overcome the pressure barrier of the edema fluid.
   b. This is accomplished by giving oxygen by intermittent or continuous pressure.
4. Give injections of diuretic (ethacrynic acid; furosemide) IV—to reduce blood volume and pulmonary congestion by producing prompt diuresis.
   a. Insert an indwelling catheter—large urinary volume will accumulate rapidly.
   b. *Watch for falling blood pressure, increasing heart rate, and decreasing urinary output—indications that the total circulation is not tolerating diuresis and that hypovolemia may develop.*
   c. Check electrolyte levels, since potassium loss may be significant.
   d. Watch for signs of urinary obstruction in men with prostatic hyperplasia.
5. Use rotating tourniquets or automatic inflating cuffs on extremities (p. 278)—to decrease venous return and right ventricular output and thus aid in decongesting lungs.
6. Or, use phlebotomy (rapid withdrawal of blood from a peripheral vein)—to decrease venous return and produce a corresponding decline in right ventricular output.
   a. Phlebotomy is usually done to reduce intravas-

cular pressure when attack is precipitated by overadministration of blood or infusion fluids.
   b. Save the blood, since it may be needed in the treatment of shock if there has been extension of infarction. Packed cells may be returned to patient if need arises.
7. Administer vasodilator if patient fails to respond to therapy—to reduce impedance (resistance) to left ventricular ejection of blood; allows more complete ventricular emptying and increases venous capacity so that left ventricular filling pressure is reduced. Patient monitored by measuring pulmonary artery pressure and cardiac output.
8. Administer dobutamine as prescribed.
9. Aminophylline may be given when indicated to relieve bronchospasm.
10. Give appropriate drugs for severe, sustained hypertension.
11. Stay with the patient and display a confident attitude—the presence of another person is therapeutic, since the acute anxiety of the patient may tend to intensify the severity of his condition. (Arterial vasoconstriction diminishes as anxiety is relieved.)

Health Education

During convalescence, instruct the patient as follows in order to prevent recurrences of pulmonary edema.
1. Ask: What symptoms did you have before the attack? (He should be aware of these.)
2. If coughing develops (a wet cough), sit with legs dangling over side of bed.
3. See Health Education, Congestive Heart Failure, page 301.

HEART SURGERY

Preoperative Nursing Management

OBJECTIVE: to bring the patient to the peak of his physical and psychologic capabilities.
1. Support the patient undergoing diagnostic studies to determine type and severity of specific lesions; tests also provide a baseline for postoperative evaluation.
   a. Cardiac catheterization and angiography
   b. Pulmonary function studies
   c. ECG, echocardiogram, phonocardiogram
   d. Exercise stress testing
   e. Chest x-ray
2. Assess laboratory studies
   a. Complete blood count; serum electrolytes; lipid profile; and nose, throat, sputum and urine cultures
   b. Antibody screen
   c. Preoperative coagulation survey (platelet count, prothrombin time, partial thromboplastin time)—extracorporeal circulation will affect certain coagulation factors.
   d. Renal and hepatic function tests
3. Review patient's record to learn past history and present condition, paying close attention to pulmonary, renal, hepatic, hematologic, and metabolic systems.
   a. Cardiac history; *history of cardiac arrhythmias.*

   b. Pulmonary health—patients with COPD may require prolonged postoperative respiratory support.
   c. Depression—can produce a serious postoperative depressive state and can affect postoperative morbidity and mortality.
   d. Ask about previous/present alcohol intake; smoking history.
4. Evaluate patient's emotional state and try to reduce his anxieties—patients undergoing heart surgery are more anxious and fearful than other surgical patients.
   a. Give support by being present, by listening, and by showing interest—patient is called upon to deal with a stressful and life-threatening crisis.
   b. Encourage the patient to express what he feels and thinks—ventilation of feelings and fantasies relieves sense of isolation and facilitates a growing and supportive relationship.
   (1) Try to elicit special concerns.
   (2) Patients with unusual degree of anxiety and history of mental illness may require psychiatric consultation.
   (3) Patients with low levels of anxiety may have stormy postoperative course—have not prepared themselves for stress of surgery.
   (4) Patients with characteristics of Type A personality (competitive striving for achievement,

sense of time urgency, aggressiveness and hostility) may be extremely anxious due to sudden role reversal; attempt to meet needs with explanations of objectives of surgery and probable postoperative experience.

c. Help the patient and family to mobilize defenses and cope with fears.

d. Clarify the information given him previously by the cardiovascular surgeon.

e. Anticipate and answer the patient's questions.
(1) Ask the patient what he wants to know.
(2) Establish a relationship of trust.

f. Reinforce and accelerate education of patient as day of operation approaches.

g. Expect some patients to have psychological and psychiatric problems from prolonged illness.

5. Prepare the patient for events in the postoperative period.

a. Take patient and family on tour of ICU—lessens anxiety about being in ICU.
(1) Introduce him to staff personnel who will be caring for him.
(2) Give family a schedule of visiting hours and times for phone contact.

b. Teach chest physical therapy procedures—to optimize pulmonary function.
(1) Have patient practice with incentive spirometer.
(2) Show and practice diaphragmatic breathing techniques.
(3) Have him practice effective coughing, leg exercises.

c. Prepare patient for presence of monitors, chest tubes, IVs, blood transfusion, endotracheal tube, nasogastric tube, pacing wires, arterial line, indwelling catheter.

6. Assess the patient's reactions to medications—these patients are usually on multiple drugs.

a. Digitalis
(1) Patient may be receiving large doses to improve myocardial contractility.
(2) Drug may be stopped several days before surgery—to avoid digitoxic arrhythmias from cardiopulmonary bypass.

b. Diuretics
(1) Assess patient for potassium depletion and volume depletion (weakness, postural hypotension)—diuretics may produce potassium loss, and severe diuresis may cause a decrease in blood volume.
(2) Give potassium supplement if patient is on prolonged diuretic therapy—to replenish body stores.
(3) Diuretics may be omitted several days preoperatively to avoid electrolyte imbalance and consequent arrhythmias postoperatively. Salt and water restriction may be advised.

c. Beta blockers (propranolol)—continue as directed.

d. Psychotropic drugs (diazepam; chlordiazepoxide)—postoperative withdrawal may cause extreme agitation.

e. Antihypertensives (reserpine)—omitted as far in advance of procedure as possible to allow norepinephrine repletion.

f. Alcohol—sudden withdrawal may produce delirium.

g. Anticoagulant drugs—discontinued several days before operation to allow coagulation mechanism to return to normal.

h. Determine if patient has taken corticosteroids within the year prior to surgery—patients on steroids are given supplemental doses to cover stress of surgery.

i. Prophylactic antibiotics may be given preoperatively.

j. Determine whether patient has any drug sensitivities.

7. Be aware of the preoperative conditions which predispose to postoperative respiratory complications.
a. Pulmonary hypertension
b. Pulmonary congestion or edema
c. Preexisting lung disease
d. Pulmonary sepsis
e. Elderly or debilitated patient

8. Encourage the patient to stop smoking—smoking increases incidence of postoperative respiratory complications.

9. Surgical preparation:
a. Shave anterior and lateral surfaces of trunk and neck; shave entire body down to ankles (for coronary bypass).
b. Shower/bathe with Betadine soap.

Postoperative Surgical Care and Nursing Management

OBJECTIVE: to evaluate patient closely and continuously to prevent complications.

A. *Immediate Nursing Interventions*

1. Secure all connections for lines and tubes (arterial, Swan-Ganz, CVP, chest tubes, urinary catheter to collecting bottle, endotracheal tube to ventilator, ECG to monitoring system, pacing wires, etc.).

2. Assure adequate oxygenation in early postoperative period; respiratory insufficiency is common following open heart surgery.

3. Employ hemodynamic monitoring* during immediate postoperative period, especially for cardiovascular and respiratory status and fluid and electrolyte balance—to prevent complications or recognize them as early as possible.

4. Examine sternotomy incision and leg dressings.

B. *Ongoing Nursing Surveillance and Interventions*

1. Provide for tissue oxygenation and assess respiratory status.
a. Employ assisted or controlled ventilation (see p. 193)—respiratory support is used first 24 hours to provide airway in the event of cardiac arrest, to decrease work of heart, to maintain effective ventilation.
(1) Adequacy of ventilation is assessed by patient's clinical status and by direct measurement of tidal volume and arterial blood gases.
(2) Check endotracheal tube placement.
(3) Auscultate chest for breath sounds—rales indicate pulmonary congestion; decreased or absent breath sounds indicate pneumothorax.
(4) Arterial blood gas analysis (see p. 158) usually performed first hour postoperatively and p.r.n. thereafter.

---

* Monitoring equipment is valuable only when it is understood and used correctly. The clinical assessment of the patient by the nurse is indispensable to patient care.

(5) Sedate patient adequately—to help him tolerate endotracheal tube and cope with ventilatory sensations.

(6) Utilize chest physiotherapy for patients with lung congestion to prevent retention of secretions and atelectasis.

    (a) Check chest x-ray and auscultate chest to determine problem areas.

    (b) Use percussion and vibrating techniques to loosen secretions.

    (c) Promote coughing, deep breathing, and turning—to keep airway patent, prevent atelectasis, and facilitate lung expansion.

(7) Suction tracheobronchial secretions carefully (see p. 195)—prolonged aspiration leads to hypoxia and possible cardiac arrest.

(8) Restrict fluids (per request) for first few days—danger of pulmonary congestion from excessive fluid intake.

(9) Chest x-ray taken immediately after surgery and daily thereafter—to evaluate state of lung expansion and detect atelectasis; to demonstrate heart size and contour, confirm placement of central line, endotracheal tube, and chest drains.

(10) See page 197 for weaning process and endotracheal tube removal.

2. Monitor cardiovascular status to determine effectiveness of cardiac output with hemodynamic monitoring. Serial readings of blood pressure and arterial pressure, heart rate, CVP and left atrial or pulmonary artery pressure from monitor modules are observed, correlated with patient's condition, and recorded.

a. Assess arterial pressure every 15 minutes until stable and as directed thereafter—blood pressure is one of the most important physiological parameters to follow.

Take direct measurement (arterial line, transducer)—most accurate blood pressure. Extreme vasoconstriction following extracorporeal circulation makes auscultatory blood pressure unobtainable.

b. Auscultate the heart for evidences of cardiac tamponade (muffled distant heart sounds), precordial rub (pericarditis), arrhythmias.

(1) Check peripheral pulses (pedal, tibial, radial) as a further check on heart action.

(2) Palpate the carotid, brachial, popliteal, and femoral pulses; if these pulses are absent it may be due to recent catheterization of the extremity.

c. Measure left atrial pressure or pulmonary artery wedge pressure—to determine the left ventricular end-diastolic volume and to assess cardiac output (see p. 268).

Rising pressures may indicate congestive heart failure or pulmonary edema.

d. Take central venous pressure readings hourly (see p. 271)—indicate blood volume, vascular tone, and pumping effectiveness of the heart.

(1) High CVP reading may result from hypervolemia, heart failure, cardiac tamponade. Ventilator may elevate CVP.

(2) If blood pressure drop is due to low blood volume, CVP will show corresponding drop.

(3) *Changes* in values are more important than isolated readings.

e. Watch ECG monitor—cardiac arrhythmias frequently occur after heart surgery.

(1) Premature ventricular contractions occur most frequently following aortic valve replacement and coronary bypass surgery. May be treated with pacing, lidocaine, potassium.

(2) Arrhythmias also apt to occur with ischemia, hypoxia, alterations in serum potassium, edema, bleeding, acid-base or electrolyte disturbances, digitalis toxicity, myocardial failure.

(3) Observe other parameters in correlation with monitor information—a low serum potassium makes the heart susceptible to ventricular arrhythmias.

(4) See page 313 for discussion of cardiac arrhythmias.

f. Check cardiac enzymes daily—elevations may indicate myocardial infarction.

g. Check urine output every ½ to 1 hour (from indwelling catheter)—urine output is an index of cardiac output and renal perfusion.

h. Continue with ongoing patient assessment.

(1) Observe buccal mucosa, nail beds, lips, ear lobes, and extremities for duskiness/cyanosis—signs of low cardiac output.

(2) Feel the skin; cool, moist skin reveals lowered cardiac output. Note temperature and color of extremities.

(3) Note fullness and tone of superficial veins of feet; evaluate pedal and femoral pulses.

(4) Assess for venous distention of neck veins or veins of dorsal surface of hands (raised above level of heart)—may signal a changing demand or diminishing capacity of heart.

(5) Evaluate temperature.

3. Maintain fluid and electrolyte balance—adequate circulating blood volume is necessary for optimum cellular activity; metabolic acidoses and electrolyte imbalance can occur after use of pump oxygenator.

a. Fluids may be limited to avoid overloading.

b. Keep input and output flow sheet—as a method of determining positive or negative fluid balance and patient's fluid requirements.

(1) IV fluids (including flush solutions through arterial and venous lines) considered as input.

(2) Assess hydration status of patient—evaluation of pulmonary wedge, left atrial pressure, and CVP readings; weight, electrolyte levels, hematocrit readings, distention of neck veins, tissue edema, liver size, breath sounds.

(3) Record urine output every ½ to 1 hour.

(4) Measure postoperative chest drainage—should not exceed 200 ml./hour for first 4–6 hours.

    (a) Watch for sudden cessation of chest drainage—from kinked or blocked chest tube.

    (b) See page 226 for management of patient with water-seal drainage.

4. Be alert to changes in serum electrolytes—a specific concentration of electrolytes is necessary in both extracellular and intracellular body fluids in order to sustain life.

a. *Hypokalemia* (low potassium)

(1) May be caused by inadequate intake, diuretics, vomiting, excessive nasogastric drainage, stress from surgery.

(2) Effects of low potassium—arrhythmias, digitalis toxicity, metabolic alkalosis, weakened myocardium, cardiac arrest.

(3) Watch for specific ECG changes.

(4) Give IV potassium replacement as directed.

b. *Hyperkalemia* (high potassium)

(1) May be caused by increased intake, red cell breakdown from the pump, acidosis, renal insufficiency, tissue necrosis, and adrenal cortical insufficiency.

(2) Effects of high potassium—mental confusion, restlessness, nausea, weakness, and paresthesia of extremities.

(3) Be prepared to administer an ion-exchange resin, sodium polystyrene sulfonate (Kayexalate), which binds the potassium, or give IV sodium bicarbonate or IV insulin and glucose to drive the potassium back into the cells from the extracellular fluid.

c. *Hyponatremia* (low sodium)

(1) May be due to reduction of total body sodium or to an increased water intake causing a dilution of body sodium.

(2) Assess for weakness, fatigue, confusion, convulsions, and coma.

d. *Hypocalcemia* (low calcium)

(1) May be due to alkalosis (which reduces the amount of Ca^{++} in the extracellular fluid) and multiple blood transfusions.

(2) Signs and symptoms of reduced calcium levels—numbness and tingling in the fingertips, toes, ear, and nose, carpopedal spasm, muscle cramps, and tetany.

(3) Give replacement therapy as directed.

e. *Hypercalcemia* (high calcium)

(1) May cause arrhythmias imitating those caused by digitalis toxicity.

(2) Assess for signs of digitalis toxicity.

(3) Institute treatment as directed—this condition may lead to asystole and death.

5. Relieve patient's pain—cardiac surgical patients experience pain caused by sternotomy incision and irritation of pleura by chest tubes.

a. Record nature, type, location, and duration of pain—pain and anxiety increase pulse rate, oxygen consumption, and cardiac work.

b. Differentiate between incisional pain and anginal pain.

c. Watch for restlessness and apprehension—may be from hypoxia or a low-output state; analgesics or sedatives do not correct this problem.

d. Medicate patient as often as prescribed—to reduce amount of pain and to aid patient in performing deep breathing and coughing exercises more effectively.

(1) Reassure patient that staff understands that treatment is painful and that it is "OK to be angry."

(2) Allow patient to talk about his experience.

6. Assess neurological status—the brain is dependent on a continuous supply of oxygenated blood and must rely on adequate and continuous perfusion by the heart.

a. Hypoperfusion or microemboli (air debris) may produce CNS damage after heart surgery.

b. Observe for symptoms of hypoxia—restlessness, headache, confusion, dyspnea, hypotension, and cyanosis.

c. Assess patient's neurological status hourly in terms of:

(1) Level of responsiveness

(2) Response to verbal commands and painful stimuli

(3) Pupillary size and reaction to light

(4) Movement of extremities; handgrasp ability

d. Treat postoperative convulsive seizures.

7. Give medications according to therapeutic directives—coronary vasodilators, antibiotics, analgesics, anticoagulants (patients with prosthetic valves).

8. Offer reassurance, orientation to time and place, and attention to patient's needs to avoid postcardiotomy delirium (p. 307).

Complications Following Cardiac Surgery

1. *Hypovolemia* (decreased circulating blood volume)

a. Low central venous pressure is an indication of hypovolemia.

b. Assess for arterial hypotension, low CVP, increasing pulse rate, and low left atrial and pulmonary artery wedge pressures.

c. Prepare to administer blood, IV solutions.

2. *Persistent bleeding*—from cardiac incision, tissue fragility, trauma to tissues, clotting defects; blood clotting disturbances usually transitory following cardiopulmonary bypass; however, a significant platelet deficiency may be present.

a. Watch for steady and continuous drainage of blood; watch CVP and left atrial pressures.

b. Treatment: protamine sulfate, vitamin K, or blood components.

c. Prepare for potential return to surgery for bleeding persisting (over 300 ml. per hour) for 4–6 hours.

3. *Cardiac tamponade*—results from bleeding into the pericardial sac or accumulation of fluids in the sac, which compresses the heart and prevents adequate filling of the ventricles.

a. Assess for signs of tamponade—arterial hypotension, rising CVP, rising left atrial pressure, muffled heart sounds, weak, thready pulse, neck vein distention, falling urinary output.

b. Check for diminished amount of drainage in the chest-collection bottle; may indicate that fluid is accumulating elsewhere.

c. Prepare for pericardiocentesis (see p. 274).

4. *Cardiac failure* (low-output syndrome)—causes deficient blood perfusion to different organs.

Observe for falling mean arterial pressure, rising filling pressures (CVP, PCW, or LAP), and increasing tachycardia; patient may exhibit signs of restlessness and agitation, cold and blue extremities, venous distention, labored respirations, tissue edema, and ascites.

5. *Myocardial infarction*

a. Symptoms may be masked by the usual postoperative discomfort.

(1) Watch for decreased cardiac output in the presence of normal circulating volume and filling pressure.

(2) Obtain serial ECGs and isoenzymes to determine extent of myocardial injury.

(3) Assess pain to differentiate myocardial pain from incisional pain.

b. Treatment is individualized. Postoperative activity level may be reduced to allow heart adequate time for healing.

6. *Renal failure*—urine output depends on cardiac output, blood volume, state of hydration, and condition of kidneys.

a. Renal injury may be caused by deficient perfusion, hemolysis, low cardiac output prior to and following open heart surgery; use of vasopressor agents to increase blood pressure.

b. Measure urine volume; less than 20 ml./hour can indicate decreased renal function.

c. Carry out specific gravity tests to determine kidneys' ability to concentrate urine in renal tubules.

d. Watch BUN and serum creatinine levels as well as urine and serum electrolyte levels.

e. Give rapid-acting diuretics and/or inotropic drugs (dopamine, dobutamine) to increase cardiac output and renal blood flow.

f. Prepare patient for peritoneal dialysis or hemodialysis if indicated. (Renal insufficiency may produce serious cardiac arrhythmias.)

7. *Hypotension*—may be caused by inadequate cardiac contractility and reduction in blood volume or by mechanical ventilation (when patient "fights" the ventilator or PEEP is used), all of which can produce a reduction in cardiac output.

a. Monitor vital signs, left atrial pressure, CVP and arterial pressure.

b. Note chest tube drainage—hypotension may be caused by excessive bleeding.

c. Give blood as directed to maintain left atrial pressure at a level which will provide an adequate circulating volume for good tissue perfusion.

8. *Embolization*—may result from injury to the intima of the blood vessels, dislodgement of a clot from a damaged valve, venous stasis aggravated by certain arrhythmias, loosening of mural thrombi, and coagulation problems.

a. Common embolic sites are lungs, coronary arteries, mesentery, extremities, kidneys, spleen, and brain.

b. Symptoms of embolization (vary according to site):

(1) Midabdominal or midback pain

(2) Pain, cessation of pulses, blanching, numbness, coldness of extremity

(3) Chest pain and respiratory distress with pulmonary embolus or myocardial infarction and

(4) One-sided weakness, pupil changes, as in stroke.

c. Initiate preventive measures: antiembolic stockings; omit pressure on popliteal space (leg crossing, raising knee gatch); start passive and active exercises.

9. *Postcardiotomy delirium*—may appear after a brief lucid period.

a. Psychic disturbances are more frequent after heart operations with extracorporeal circulation than after general surgery.

b. Signs and symptoms include delirium (impairment of orientation, memory, intellectual function judgment), transient perceptual distortions, visual and auditory hallucinations, disorientation, and paranoid delusions.

c. Symptoms may be related to sleep deprivation, increased sensory input, disorientation to night and day, prolonged inability to speak due to endotracheal intubation, age, preoperative cardiac status, etc.

d. *Nursing Management*

(1) Keep patient oriented to time and place; notify patient of procedures and expectations of his cooperation. Give repeated explanations of what is happening.

(2) Establish rapport with patient preoperatively; have patient visit ICU *before* surgery.

(3) Encourage family to come in at regular times—helps patient regain sense of reality.

(4) Plan care to allow rest periods, day-night pattern, and uninterrupted sleep.

(5) Encourage mobility as soon as possible.

(6) Keep environment as free as possible of excessive auditory and sensory input. Prevent bodily injury.

(7) Reassure patient and his family that psychiatric disorders following cardiac surgery are usually transient.

(8) Remove patient from ICU as soon as possible.

(9) Allow patient to *ventilate* events of his psychotic episode—helps him deal with and assimilate exerience.

10. *Postpericardiotomy syndrome*—a group of symptoms occurring following cardiac and pericardial trauma and myocardial infarction.

a. Cause is not certain—may be from anticardiac antibodies, viral etiology, etc.

b. Manifestations—fever, malaise, arthralgias, dyspnea, pericardial effusion, pleural effusion, friction rub.

c. Treatment is symptomatic (bed rest, aspirin), since condition is self-limiting but recurrence is not uncommon.

11. *Postperfusion syndrome*

a. Signs and symptoms—fever, splenomegaly, lymphocytosis.

b. Draw blood for culture—postperfusion syndrome can mimic bacterial endocarditis or hepatitis.

c. Treatment is symptomatic, since syndrome is self-limiting.

d. Reassure patient that this is only a temporary setback in his convalescence.

12. *Febrile complications*—probably from body's reaction to tissue trauma or accumulation of blood and serum in pleural and pericardial spaces.

a. Control higher degrees of fever by use of hypothermia mattress.

b. Evaluate for atelectasis, pleural effusion, or pneumonia if fever persists.

c. Evaluate for urinary tract infection/wound infection.

d. Bear in mind the possibility of infective endocarditis if fever persists (see p. 293).

13. Hepatitis

Health Education, Discharge Planning and Rehabilitation Following Cardiac Surgery

OBJECTIVE: to assume a normal life as promptly as possible.

1. Begin discussing long-range plans with patient during convalescence in order to help him make modifications in his life style.

2. Give written guidelines:

a. *Activities*

(1) Increase activities gradually within limits. Avoid strenuous activities until after exercise stress testing.

(2) Take short rest periods.

(3) Avoid lifting more than 20 pounds.

(4) Participate in activities that do not cause pain or discomfort.

(5) Increase walking time and distance each day.

(6) Stairs (1–2 times daily) the first week; increase as tolerated.

(7) Avoid large crowds at first.

(8) Driving: Avoid driving until after first post-operative checkup. At this time ask physician when you may drive.

(9) Sexual relations: Resumption of sexual relations parallels ability to participate in other activities.

(10) Return to work—after first postoperative checkup as advised by physician.

(11) Expect some chest discomfort.

b. *Diet*

(1) Some patients are placed on minimum salt restriction, e.g., no salt added at table; cholesterol may be limited.

(2) Weigh daily and report weight gain of more than 3–4 pounds per week.

c. *Medications*

(1) Label all medications; give purposes and side effects.

(2) Patients with prosthetic valves may continue warfarin indefinitely.

3. Patients with prosthetic valves:

a. Pregnancy usually discouraged in women with prosthetic valves.

b. Caution patient about need for antibiotic coverage following dental and surgical procedures.

c. Patients on anticoagulants should watch for bleeding and should avoid use of aspirin (and many other drugs)—interferes with action of warfarin.

4. Advise patient to carry an indentification card stating cardiac condition and medications being taken.

5. Patient may be placed on rehabilitation and exercise program after exercise stress testing.

6. Inform the patient whom to contact (and how) in case of an emergency.

7. See also page 289 (Health Education After MI).

2 ESSENTIALS OF BASIC ELECTROCARDIOGRAPHY*

THE ECG AND HEART PHYSIOLOGY

The Electrocardiogram (ECG)

1. Is nothing more than a recording of the heart's electrical impulse.

2. The heart is stimulated to contract and thus pump blood to the body organs by the electrical pulsation which originates at the top of the heart and travels downward.

3. To record the impulse, electrodes do not have to be placed directly on the heart, but can be placed on the extremities, where the heart's activity can be sensed (Fig. 9-12).

Clinical Use of ECG

An electrocardiogram can be helpful in diagnosing the following:

1. Myocardial infarction and arteriosclerotic heart disease

2. Cardiac arrhythmias

3. Cardiac enlargement

4. Electrolyte abnormalities (especially potassium and calcium)

5. Pericarditis (inflammation of the pericardial sac which surrounds the heart)

6. Pericardial effusion (fluid in the pericardial sac which can restrict the heart's pumping ability)

Heart Anatomy and Physiology (Fig. 9-13)

1. The normal electrical impulse of the heart, which inscribes the ECG and causes the heart to contract, begins in the SA node (also called sinoatrial node, sinus node, or normal physiological pacemaker).

2. The SA node occupies the superior aspect of the right atrium.

3. The impulse, after beginning in the SA node, travels across the atria, causing them to contract and pump blood into the ventricles.

4. The impulse then hits the AV node (atrioventricular node) which lies between the atria and ventricles.

5. The impulse is somewhat delayed in the AV node and then travels down the ventricles, causing them to contract and thus pump blood to the body organs.

6. Both the SA and AV nodes are connected to 2 main nerve systems which control the rate at which the heart beats.

a. Sympathetic nerves—cause the heart rate to increase.

b. Parasympathetic nerves (vagus nerve)—slow the heart rate.

Normal ECG

1. Figure 9-14 represents a normal ECG.

2. Each heart beat manifests as 3 major deflections.

a. P wave

b. QRS complex

c. T wave

3. The QRS complex is composed of 3 parts:

a. Q wave—the first downward deflection

b. R wave—the first upward deflection

c. S wave—the first downward deflection after the R wave

4. Beats come at regular intervals (normal sinus rhythm), indicating that the impulse is originating properly from the sinus node.

* Some illustrations in this section appeared also in RN magazine. Butler H. How to read an ECG. RN, vol. 36, 1973 (reproduced with permission of the artist)

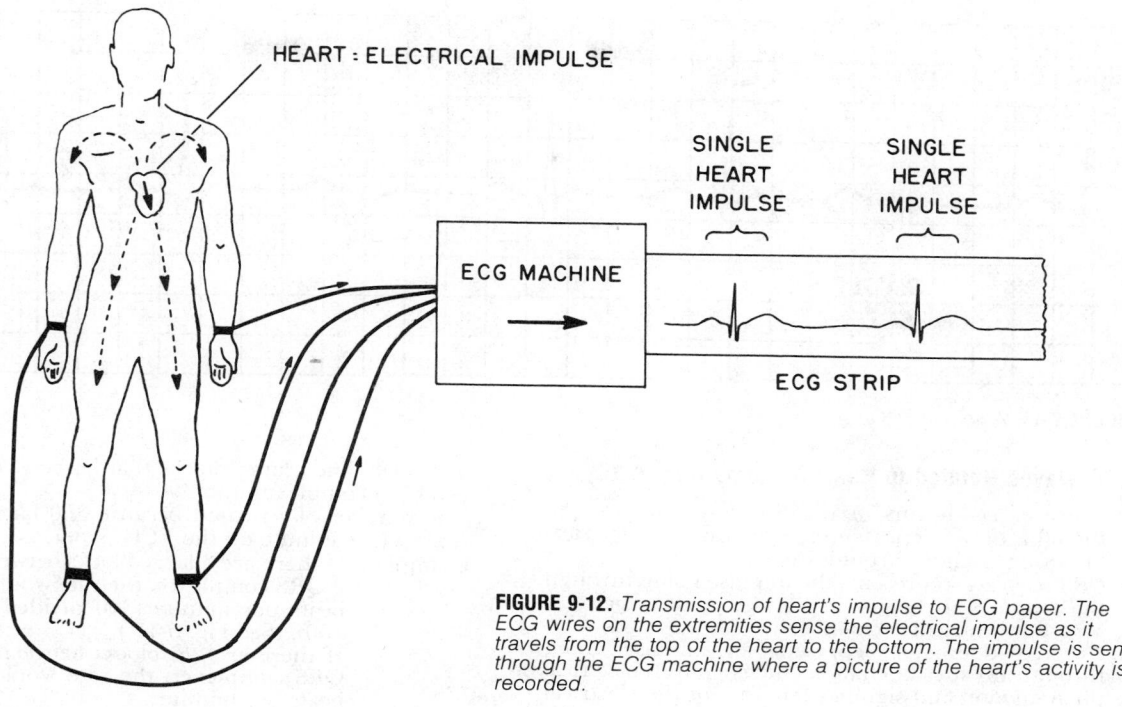

FIGURE 9-12. *Transmission of heart's impulse to ECG paper. The ECG wires on the extremities sense the electrical impulse as it travels from the top of the heart to the bottom. The impulse is sent through the ECG machine where a picture of the heart's activity is recorded.*

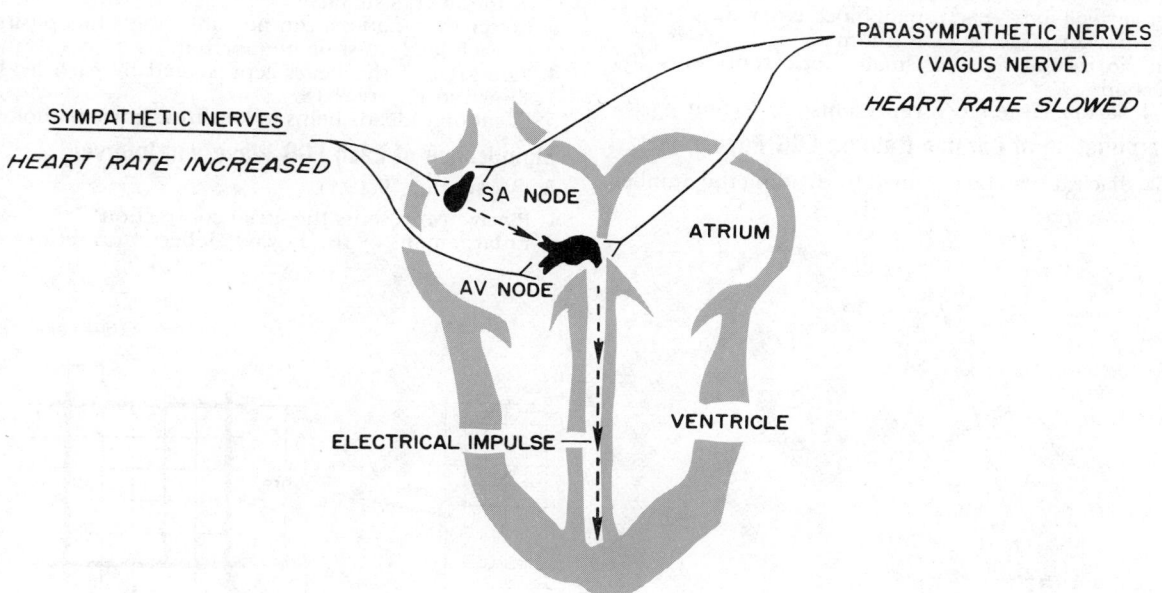

FIGURE 9-13. *Heart Physiology. Pictured is the pathway of the normal electrical impulse which inscribes the ECG and causes the heart to contract and pump blood. Also shown are the nerves which regulate the heart rate.*

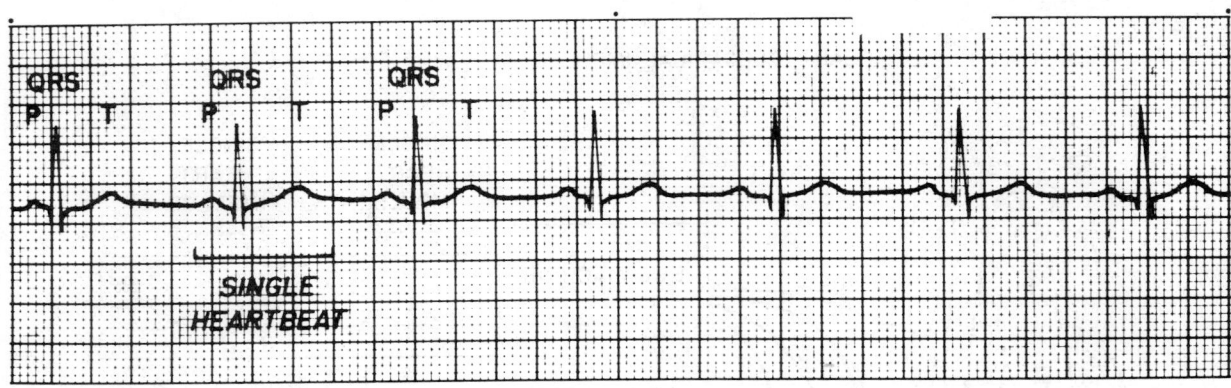

FIGURE 9-14. *A normal ECG.*

ECG Waves Related to Heart Anatomy (Fig. 9-15)

1. *The P wave*—begins in the SA node and can be thought of as representing the cardiac electrical impulse traveling through the *atria.*
2. *QRS complex*—represents the impulse going through the *ventricles.* It begins in the AV node which lies atop the ventricular chambers.
3. *T wave*—does not represent an impulse going through any specific chamber but is a purely electrical phenomenon and signifies recovery of the electrical forces (*repolarization*).

ECG Paper (Fig. 9-16)

1. Vertical lines—measure the *magnitude* of the electrical impulse.
2. Horizontal inscriptions—represent the *time* it takes for an impulse to travel over cardiac tissue.
3. In vertical axis—each small block is 1 mm.
    1 darker large block is 5 mm.
4. In horizontal axis—1 small block represents .04 second
    1 darker large block represents .20 second

Determination of Cardiac Rate on ECG Paper

1. Cardiac rate can be obtained by dividing the number

of heavily lined large blocks that lie between every two QRS complexes into 300.
2. The number 300 is used because 300 large blocks represent 1 minute on the ECG paper.
    Examples: If there are 3 large blocks between every 2 QRS complexes, the rate would be 100 beats per minute (300 divided by 3 = 100). (See Fig. 9-17.)
    If there are 2½ blocks between every 2 QRS complexes, the rate would be 120 beats per minute.

ECG Leads

1. Standard ECG machines have a dial which turns to 1 to 12 leads (I, II, III, AVR, AVL, AVF, V1, V2, V3, V4, V5, V6).
2. Each lead receives and records the heart's electrical impulse from a different anatomical position relative to the heart's surface.
3. Letter designations can be confusing; thus position of each lead must be memorized.
4. The area of the heart represented by each lead is shown in Figure 9-18.
5. Location of leads helps to localize cardiac pathology.

Significance of Each ECG Wave and Interval

A. *P Wave* (Fig. 9-19*A*)

1. P wave represents the atrial contraction.
2. Enlargement of the P-wave deflection indicates en-

FIGURE 9-15. *ECG waves related to heart anatomy. The electrical impulse is shown traveling through the chambers of the heart and thus inscribing the normal ECG of 1 heart beat. The P wave represents atrial activity and the QRS complex is derived from ventricular stimulation.*

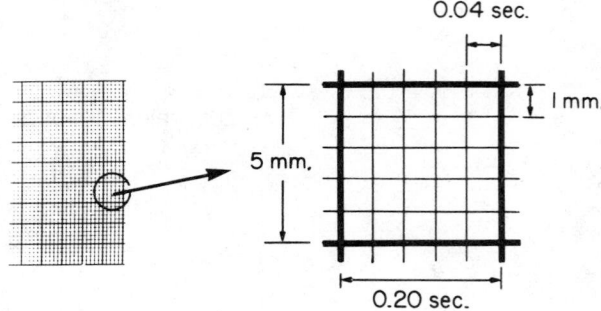

FIGURE 9-16. *Meaning of blocks on ECG paper. All one really needs to remember is that 1 small block is 1 mm. tall and .04 second wide.*

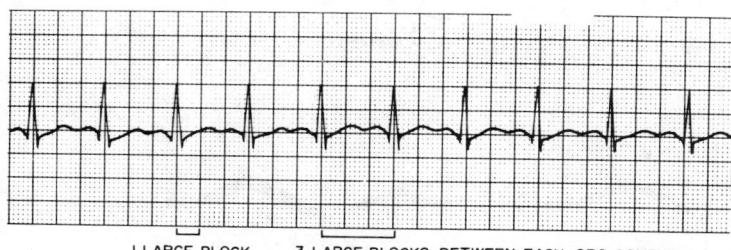

FIGURE 9-17. *Determination of rate. There are 3 large blocks between every 2 QRS complexes. By dividing 300 by 3, the rate is 100 beats per minute.*

largement of the atrium such as might occur in mitral stenosis. (The atrium enlarges in mitral stenosis because the mitral opening between the atrium and ventricle is small, causing blood to back up, which in turn forces the atrial wall to expand.)

3. P wave is considered enlarged it if it is over 3 mm. tall (3 small blocks) or .12 second wide (3 small blocks).

B. *PR Interval* (Fig. 9-19*B*)

1. Starts at the beginning of the P wave and extends to the onset of the Q wave.
2. At normal rates, the PR interval should not exceed .20 second (5 small blocks).
3. This interval increases in length in arteriosclerotic heart disease and in rheumatic fever.
4. The PR interval is prolonged because the area of heart tissue represented by the PR interval (namely the atrium and AV node area) is scarred or inflamed and the impulse is forced to travel at a slower rate.

C. *The QRS Complex* (Fig. 9-19*C*)

1. Q wave (first downward stroke)—when enlarged it is indicative of an old myocardial infarction.
2. The R wave (first upward deflection)
   a. Increases in amplitude when the ventricle enlarges, as in most types of heart disease. (Overwork of a specific part of the heart causes enlargement.)
   b. May become small when the heart is compressed by fluid, as in a pericardial effusion.

D. *The ST Segment* (Fig. 9-19*D*)

1. Begins at the end of the S wave (the first downward deflection after the R wave) and terminates at the beginning of the T wave.
2. Is elevated above the baseline of the ECG strip in an acute myocardial infarction or in pericarditis.
3. Becomes depressed when the heart muscle is getting a decreased supply of oxygen or when a patient is taking digitalis.

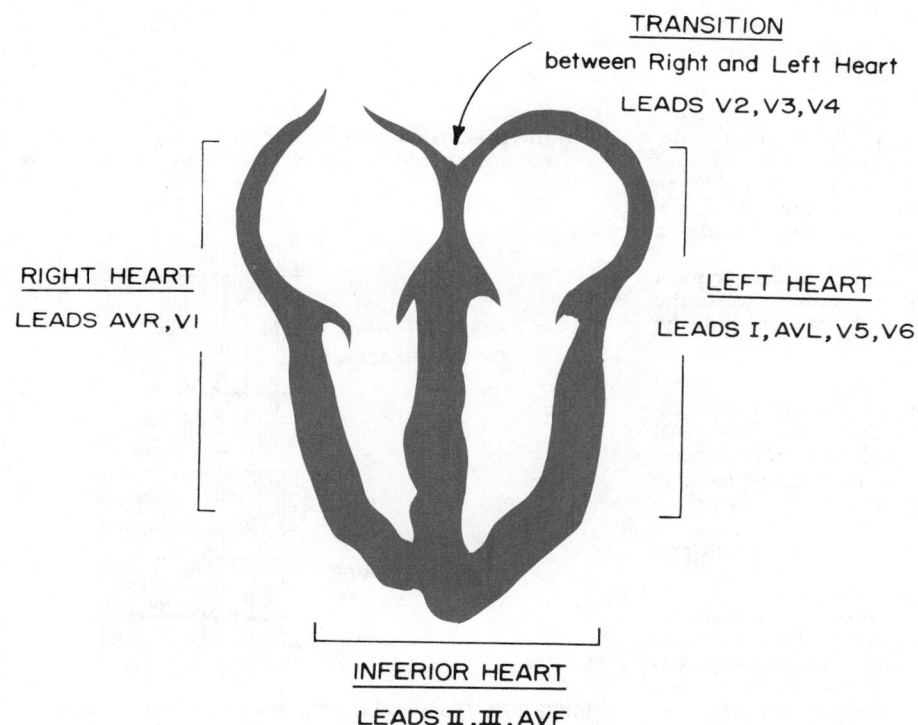

FIGURE 9-18. *ECG leads related to heart anatomy.*

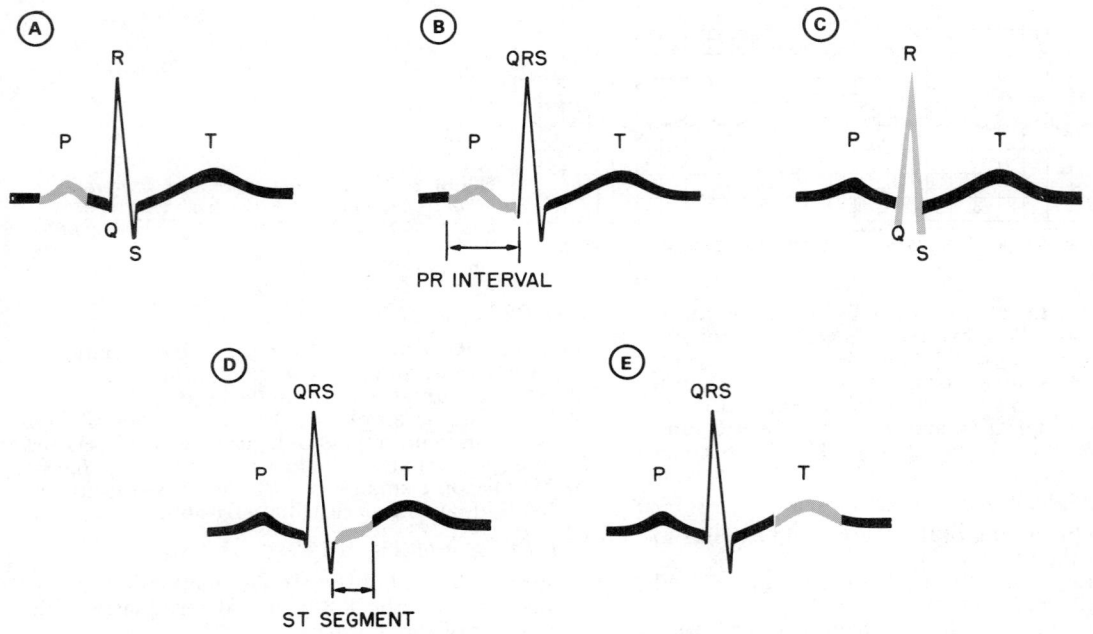

FIGURE 9-19. *Parts of a heartbeat. A. The P wave. B. The PR interval (extends from the beginning of the P wave to the onset of the Q wave). C. The QRS complex. (Even when the complex does not have a discrete Q or S wave, it is still referred to as the QRS complex to denote a ventricular impulse and to provide simplicity and uniformity.) D. The ST segment begins at the termination of the S wave and ends at the beginning of the T wave. E. The T wave.*

4. Becomes long in hypocalcemia. (Hypocalcemia occurs most commonly in chronic renal disease because the scarred kidneys cannot excrete phosphate. Since phosphate and calcium maintain a reciprocal balance in the body fluid, the elevated phosphate causes a depression in the calcium level.)
5. Becomes shorter in hypercalcemia, which is most commonly seen in metastatic carcinoma because the tumor erodes the bones and spills calcium into the serum.

E. *The T Wave* (Fig. 9-19*E*)

1. Represents no cardiac activity, but reflects the electrical recovery of the ventricular contraction. (An electrical impulse is the flow of electrons; the T wave is inscribed when these electrons migrate back to their resting position after traversing the heart muscle to make it contract.)
2. Is flat when the heart is not receiving enough oxygen (arteriosclerotic heart disease).
3. May be inverted in a myocardial infarction.
4. May be made tall by an elevated serum potassium.
   The most common cause of elevated serum potassium levels is renal disease; the most frequent ECG finding is a tall, peaked narrow-based T wave which begins to form when the potassium reaches levels of about 6 mEq./L. (Fig. 9-20).
5. Should not be over 10 mm. (10 small blocks) high

in the precordial leads (those that are placed on the chest) and should not be over 5 mm. in the remaining leads.

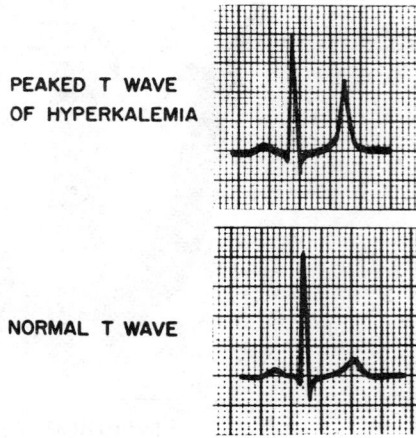

PEAKED T WAVE
OF HYPERKALEMIA

NORMAL T WAVE

FIGURE 9-20. *The above ECGs show the difference between the tall, peaked T wave of hyperkalemia and the normal rounded T wave.*

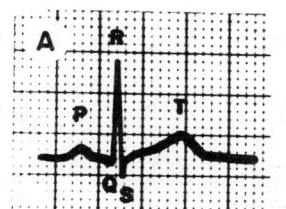 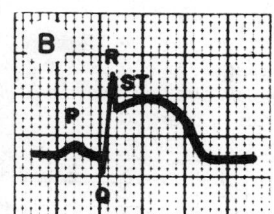 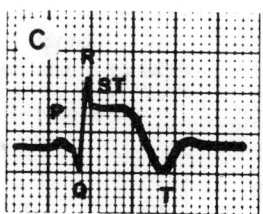

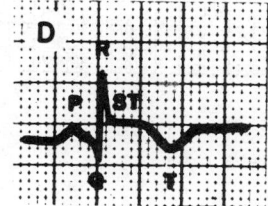 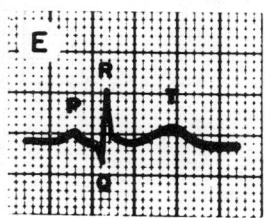

FIGURE 9-21. A. *Normal tracing. B. Hours after infarction, the ST segment becomes elevated. C. Hours to days later, the T wave inverts and the Q wave may become larger. D. Days to weeks later, the ST segment returns to near-normal. E. Lastly, the T wave becomes upright again, but the Q wave may remain permanently large.*

ECG INTERPRETATION OF MYOCARDIAL INFARCTION

ECG Interpretation (Fig. 9-21)

NOTE: The ECGs of some patients suffering myocardial infarctions may show *no specific changes* on the initial tracing. Therefore, if a person has symptoms compatible with a heart attack and has a normal ECG, he should nevertheless be admitted to the hospital for observation and further electrocardiograms.

1. Elevation of ST segment is first finding.
2. T wave inversion follows.
3. Then a large Q wave appears.
   a. As infarct heals, Q wave may remain as the only sign of an old coronary occlusion. (In AVR a large Q wave is normal.)
   b. Q wave can be considered abnormal if it is over .04 second wide (1 small block is .04 second) or if it is greater in depth than ⅓ the height of the QRS complex (Fig. 9-22).

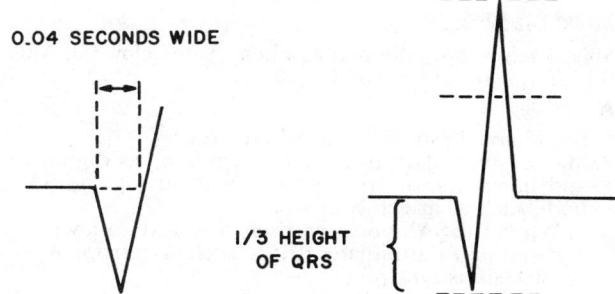

0.04 SECONDS WIDE

1/3 HEIGHT OF QRS

FIGURE 9-22. *Abnormal Q wave. A Q wave is considered abnormal when it is over .04 second (1 small block on the ECG paper) or over one-third the height of the QRS complex. This usually indicates an old myocardial infarction.*

ECG INTERPRETATION OF CARDIAC ARRHYTHMIAS

NOTE: The lower the ectopic focus resides in the heart, the more lethal the arrhythmia becomes.

Sinus Tachycardia

Sinus tachycardia can be defined as a cardiac rate of over 100 beats per minute. All the complexes are normal, but their rate is excessive.

A. *Altered Physiology*

The impulse begins normally in the SA node but comes at a faster rate secondary to increased sympathetic nerve stimuli.

B. *Causes*

1. Exercise
2. Anxiety
3. Fever
4. Shock

C. *Mechanism of Sinus Tachycardia*

The pathway of sinus tachycardia is the same as that of a normal sinus rhythm, but the number of impulses per minute is greater in sinus tachycardia. (See Fig. 9-23.)

RATE OF NODE INCREASED

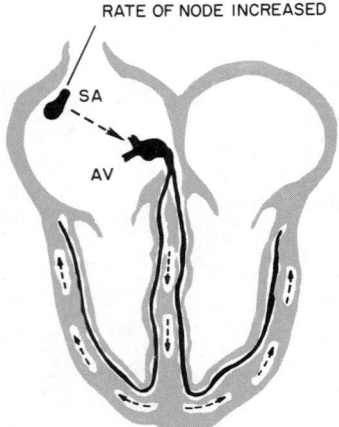

ECG of Sinus Tachycardia
The P wave, the QRS complex, and the T wave are all normal.
The only abnormality is a rate of over 100.

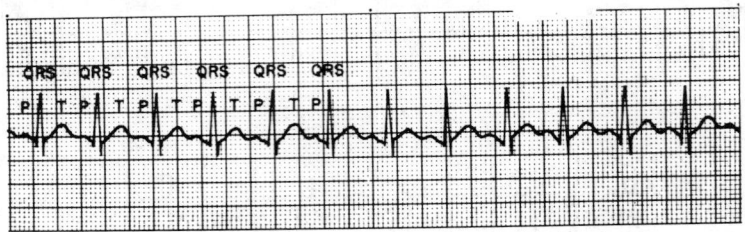

FIGURE 9-23. *Sinus Tachycardia Pathway*

D. *ECG of Sinus Tachycardia*

The P wave, the QRS complex, and the T wave are all normal. The only abnormality is a rate of over 100. (See Fig. 9-23).

E. *Treatment*

Since sinus tachycardia is usually a compensatory rhythm, treatment is directed at the primary causes, which usually are not cardiac.

Sinus Bradycardia

Sinus bradycardia is defined as a heart rate below 60. All the complexes are normal.

A. *Etiology*

1. Seen *normally* in well-trained athletes.
2. May be secondary to certain drugs such as digitalis and morphine or from processes involving the SA node such as arteriosclerosis.
   a. When the SA node is severely diseased it may not respond to stimulant drugs such as atropine— "sick sinus syndrome."

b. A tachycardia can so exhaust a diseased SA node that when the tachycardia ceases, the SA node fails to take up the rhythm at a respectable rate and the patient is left with a severe bradycardia. When this occurs, the "sick sinus syndrome" is called the "tachycardia-bradycardia syndrome." (See page 315)
3. Also seen in myocardial infarction in which instance it could be detrimental to the patient, who is already in a compromised cardiac state.

B. *Complications*

Slow rate and low cardiac output can cause:
Fainting (Stokes-Adams syndrome) or congestive heart failure (Heart cannot pump all the fluid presented to it, resulting in stasis or "congestion" of the blood in the lungs and other body tissues.)

C. *Mechanism of Sinus Bradycardia*

The pathway of sinus bradycardia is identical to that of normal sinus rhythm, but the rate is slower. (See Fig. 9-24)

RATE OF NODE DECREASED

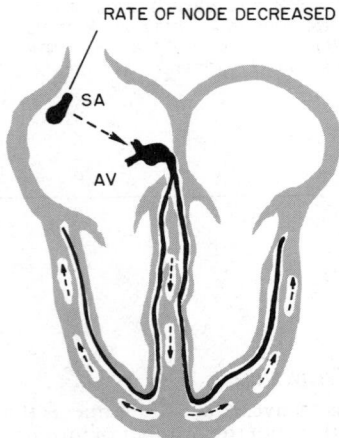

ECG of Sinus Bradycardia
The only abnormality is a rate below 60 beats per minute.

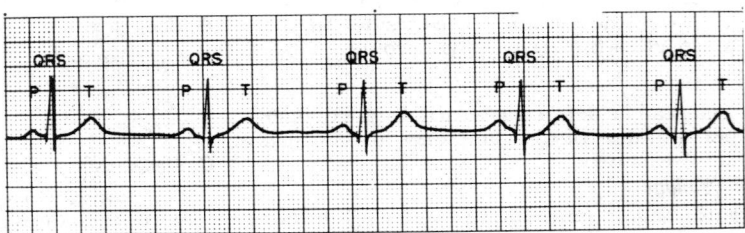

FIGURE 9-24. *Sinus Bradycardia Pathway*

D. *ECG of Sinus Bradycardia*

The only abnormality is a rate below 60 beats per minute. (See Fig. 9-24.)

E. *Treatment*

1. Rarely has to be treated.
2. If congestive failure or fainting occurs, treatment should be initiated immediately to increase the heart rate.
   a. Give 0.5–1 mg. of atropine by IV push (inhibits the vagal or "slowing" nerve and therefore makes the heart go faster).
   b. If patient becomes resistant to atropine, the rate can be increased by adding 1 mg. of isoproterenol (Isuprel) to 500 ml. of 5% glucose in water and initially running the solution at about 10 drops per minute. (Stimulates the sympathetic or "fast" nerve of the heart.) (Atropine can be prepared more quickly and is less toxic to the heart than Isuprel.)
   c. The heart rate can be increased or decreased by adjusting the rate of fluid administered.
   d. An electrical pacemaker may be necessary in refractory cases or when the fluid load becomes excessive.

Sinus Arrhythmia

Sinus arrhythmia is normally found in children and young adults and is characterized by a heart rhythm that is normal in every way except for irregularity.

A. *Etiology*

1. On inspiration the heart rate increases and on expiration the heart rate decreases.
2. Inspiration tends to inhibit the vagus nerve (slows the heart) and causes an acceleration of the cardiac rate.

B. *Mechanism of Sinus Arrhythmia*

The pathway of sinus arrhythmia is the same as that of the normal sinus rhythm; the only differential point is the regularity of the impulses. (See Fig. 9-25.)

C. *ECG of Sinus Arrhythmia*

All the complexes are normal; only the rate is irregular—varying with respiration. The rate in-

creases with inspiration and decreases with expiration. (See Fig. 9-25.)

D. *Treatment*

Since sinus arrhythmia is usually normal, no treatment is necessary.

Sick Sinus Syndrome

Sick sinus syndrome refers to a diseased SA node that conducts at a slow rate or fails to conduct completely for various periods of time. The most common cause of sick sinus syndrome is arteriosclerosis, which leads to ischemia.

A. *Clinical Manifestations*

Dizziness, fainting—from poor cerebral perfusion.

B. *Altered Physiology* (Fig. 9-26)

1. Sick sinus syndrome may be associated with a tachycardia, which may stop abruptly (either by cardioversion or spontaneously); since the sinus node is diseased, the heart may not begin to beat on its own.
2. This phenomenon is called the "tachycardia–bradycardia syndrome," which can be part of the sick sinus syndrome.
3. It is thought that the tachycardia precipitates the sinus arrest by constantly firing impulses into the sinus node (atrial fibrillation, for example, in which both ectopic foci originating in the atrium fire impulses *both* down into the ventricles and back into the SA node), which becomes depressed because of constant activation.

C. *Management*

1. The sick sinus syndrome with tachycardia is difficult to treat, because many drugs used to treat the tachycardia (propranolol or digitalis) will tend to further suppress the already compromised SA node leading further to asystole.
2. The treatment for a diseased sinus node associated with tachycardia is the implantation of a pacemaker.
3. With the pacemaker in place, the tachycardia is treated with depressant drugs. When the tachycardia abates, the pacemaker can activate the heart if the SA node fails.

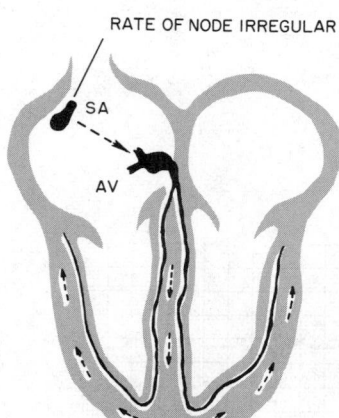

RATE OF NODE IRREGULAR

SA

AV

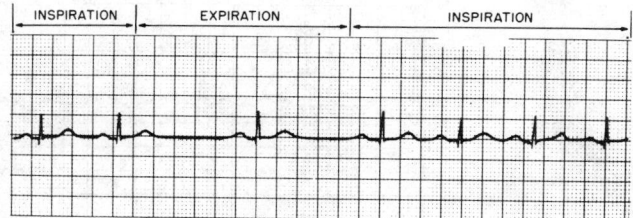

ECG of Sinus Arrhythmia
All the complexes are normal; only the rate is irregular—varying with respiration. The rate increases with inspiration and decreases with expiration.

INSPIRATION | EXPIRATION | INSPIRATION

FIGURE 9-25. *Sinus Arrhythmia Pathway*

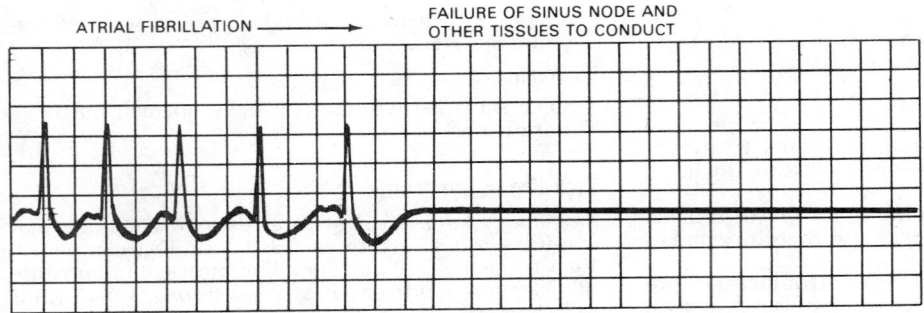

ATRIAL FIBRILLATION ⟶   FAILURE OF SINUS NODE AND
OTHER TISSUES TO CONDUCT

FIGURE 9-26. *In the ECG shown above atrial fibrillation has stopped abruptly and the diseased sinus node has failed—leaving the patient without a heartbeat. This ECG illustrates the importance of having a pacemaker in these patients. Drugs used to treat the atrial fibrillation further suppress the SA node, and there must be a backup system (pacemaker) to establish impulse formation.*

Premature Atrial Contractions (PACs)

PACs constitute a very common rhythm disturbance and are seen in both normal and abnormal hearts. They rarely cause symptoms and are felt to be of little consequence except when they occur frequently, at which time they tend to deteriorate into other more serious arrhythmias.

A. *Altered Physiology*

1. Beats occur *early* in the cycle; they begin in the atrium, but *outside* the sinus node where normal impulses originate.
2. Since the atrial pathway is abnormal, the P wave is distorted.
3. Since ventricular activation is undisturbed, the QRS is normal.

B. *Mechanism of a PAC*

    The PAC begins in the atrium outside the SA node. (See Fig. 9-27.)

C. *ECG of a PAC*

1. PAC comes early in the cycle.
2. P wave is abnormally shaped.
3. QRS complex is normal. (See Fig. 9-27.)

D. *Treatment*

1. Most of the time PACs do not need to be treated.
2. Quinidine, which is a good suppressant of atrial ectopic beats, may be used when the patient requires therapy.

Paroxysmal Atrial Tachycardia (PAT)

PAT is a common arrhythmia in young adults; it is usually found in normal hearts. There is a rapid heart rate which ranges from 140–250 beats per minute with an average of about 180 beats per minute.

A. *Clinical Manifestations*

    Patient will complain of a pounding or fluttering in the chest associated with shortness of breath and fainting—due to rapid heart rate.

B. *Altered Physiology*

1. Begins in an ectopic focus of the atrium outside the sinus node.
2. Its pathway over the heart is similar to that of a PAC. Thus PAT may be thought of as a rapid succession of PACs.
3. The P wave (atrial wave) is distorted because the pathway over the atrium is abnormal. (Most of the

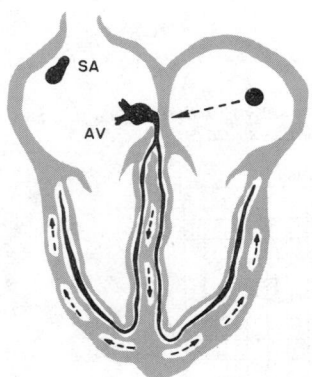

FIGURE 9-27. *PAC Pathway*

ECG of a PAC
1. PAC comes early in the cycle.
2. P wave is abnormally shaped.
3. QRS complex is normal.

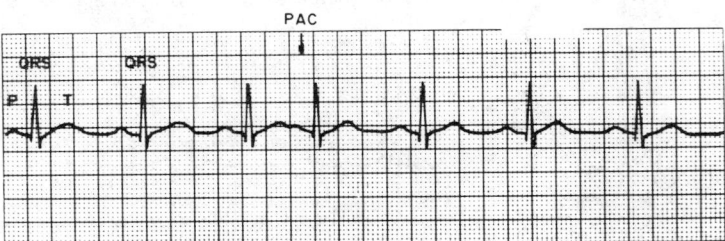

time the rate is so fast that the P wave is buried in the previous complex and is not seen.)

4. The QRS complex (ventricular wave) is normal because the route of the cardiac impulse after penetrating the AV node is undisturbed.

C. *Mechanism of PAT*

An impulse traveling along the abnormal PAT pathway produces an abnormal P wave and a normally shaped QRS complex (ventricular wave). Notice that the focus of the PAT is the same as that of a PAC. (See Fig. 9-28.)

D. *ECG of PAT*

1. The rate is very rapid—over 140 per minute (higher than in sinus tachycardia).
2. P waves cannot be seen because they are superimposed within the T wave of the preceding beat. If the P waves were seen they would be abnormal in configuration.
3. The QRS complex is normal. (See Fig. 9-28.)

E. *Treatment*

1. Since cardiac arrest can occur with any mode of treatment for PAT, an ECG machine should remain attached to the patient, an IV should be started, and appropriate resuscitation equipment, including a defibrillator, should be at hand.
2. If the patient is relatively asymptomatic and stable, with a normal blood pressure, giving a simple sedative and waiting 5–10 minutes may result in spontaneous conversion of PAT.
3. Start by stimulating the right carotid sinus (an area of dense nerve supply) of the carotid artery for several seconds or gagging the patient with a tongue depressor in an effort to terminate the arrhythmia. These maneuvers work by stimulating the vagus nerve, which puts a "brake" on the heart.
4. If the above procedure is not effective and if the blood pressure is low (many patients with PAT have a systolic pressure of about 90 mm. Hg), a slow drip of metaraminol (Aramine), IV, can be started.

a. Add 100 mg. of Aramine to 500 ml. of 5% glucose in water and run the IV initially at 10 drops per minute.
b. Gradually increase the rate of the infusion until the PAT terminates, at which time the IV should be stopped (usually a matter of seconds). (See Fig. 9-29.)
c. Do not raise the systolic blood pressure above 180. This drug increases the blood pressure, which in turn stimulates the vagus nerve to inhibit the ectopic focus of the atrium.
d. If the patient is already hypertensive (rare), Aramine should not be used.
e. Some authorities do not use a vasopressor such as Aramine because of the occasional report of a cerebral vascular accident, but this complication has usually occurred when the drug is used in bolus form. Instead of Aramine, they prefer a fast-acting digitalis preparation which works in part by stimulating the vagal nerve.
5. If raising the blood pressure is ineffectual, some clinicians would prescribe digoxin (Lanoxin) .25 mg. IV every 5 minutes up to 1 mg.
6. In an unusual case, in which the preceding steps are ineffective or contraindicated, 1–5 mg. of propranolol (Inderal)—a sympathetic nerve blocker—may be given by IV at a rate no greater than 1 mg./minute.
7. In the extreme case when the patient is in congestive heart failure, DC synchronized electrical shock (cardioversion) should be instituted (instead of giving Inderal).
a. Initial shock—can be 50–100 watt-seconds (joules).
b. Electrical shock stops the heart and allows the heartbeat to begin again normally at the SA node.

Atrial Flutter

Atrial flutter is a rapid, regular "fluttering" of the atrium.

A. *Altered Physiology*

1. P waves take on a "sawtooth" appearance because

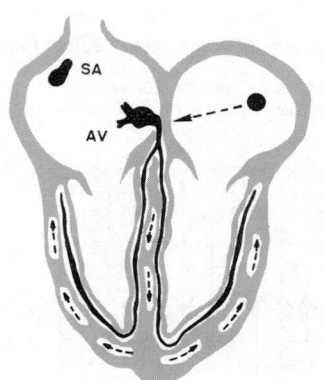

FIGURE 9-28. *PAT Pathway*

ECG of PAT
1. The rate is very rapid—over 140 per minute (higher than in sinus tachycardia).
2. P waves cannot be seen because they are superimposed within the T wave of the preceding beat. If the P waves were seen they would be abnormal in configuration.
3. The QRS complex is normal.

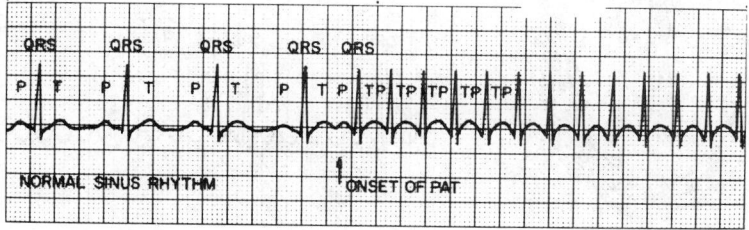

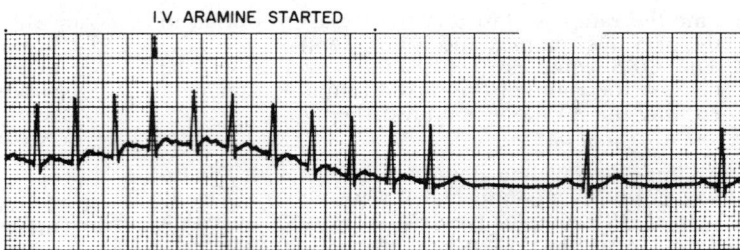

I.V. ARAMINE STARTED

FIGURE 9-29. *Termination of PAT. The ECG illustrates PAT being terminated with a slow IV infusion of Aramine.*

they are coming from a focus other than the sinus node and are coming at a very rapid rate.

2. As in PAC or PAT, the impulse comes from *one* ectopic focus in the atrium, but the *atrial* rate (not pulse or ventricular rate) is between 250 and 350 per minute for atrial flutter.

The following oversimplified arbitrary rule may be used to distinguish the atrial arrhythmias from each other:

Atrial rate in sinus tachycardia goes up to 140/minute.

Atrial rate in PAT is between 140–250/minute.

Atrial rate in atrial flutter is between 250–350/minute.

3. Atrial flutter generally occurs in a pathological heart (usually arteriosclerotic or rheumatic), as contrasted to PAT, which many times is associated with a normal heart.

4. Since the abnormality is above the AV node, the QRS complex (ventricular wave) is normal in configuration.

5. Since the P waves come so rapidly, the AV node cannot accept and conduct each one; therefore there is some degree of "blockage" at the AV node.

Example: If the atrial rate is 300, the ventricular rate (which is the same as the pulse rate) might be 150, since the AV node is not able to conduct every atrial impulse because of the excessive rapidity. In this instance, the "block" is said to be 2:1

since there are 2 atrial impulses per 1 ventricular response.

6. The 2:1 block is the most common block in atrial flutter.

7. Most cases of PAT do not exhibit a block since P waves do not occur as fast as in atrial flutter. Thus in PAT all the impulses are transmitted by the AV node to the ventricles.

B. *Mechanism of Atrial Flutter*

The pathways for atrial flutter are the same as for PAC and PAT, but in atrial flutter the ectopic impulse fires at a faster rate. (See Fig. 9-30)

C. *ECG of Atrial Flutter*

1. The arrows indicate the P waves generated by the fast-firing ectopic focus in the atrium.

2. Notice that not every P wave stimulates a QRS complex (ventricular wave).

3. Since the abnormality present in the heart is above the AV node, the QRS complexes that appear are normal in configuration. (See Fig. 9-30)

D. *Treatment*

1. Classic initial treatment is digitalis, which partially blocks the AV node; this allows fewer P waves to pass through the ventricles and thus slows the pulse rate.

Propranolol (Inderal) may also be effective by blocking the AV node.

2. The fast pulse rate must be slowed down (ventricular

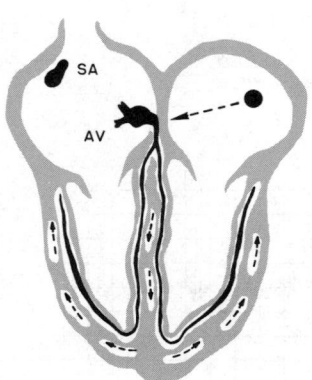

FIGURE 9-30. *Atrial Flutter Pathway*

ECG of Atrial Flutter
1. *The arrows indicate the P waves generated by the fast-firing ectopic focus in the atrium.*
2. *Notice that not every P wave stimulates a QRS complex (ventricular wave).*
3. *Since the abnormality present in the heart is above the AV node, the QRS complexes that appear are normal in configuration.*

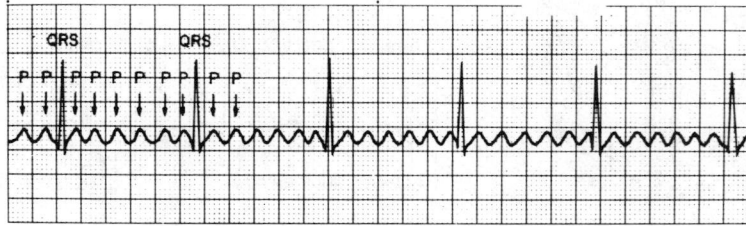

rate) because the heart is not given enough time to fill itself with blood when it is contracting rapidly; this causes the blood to back up in the body tissues, leading to congestive failure.
3. Cardioversion
   a. Tried when the patient is not tolerating the arrhythmia well.
   b. Atrial flutter responds well to cardioversion at a relatively low wattage (50–100 watts/second).

NURSING ALERT: When a patient is taking digitalis, cardioversion can be dangerous since a lethal arrhythmia may be precipitated.

Atrial Fibrillation

Atrial fibrillation is an atrial arrhythmia occurring at an extremely rapid and uncoordinated rate. The atria produce impulses so rapidly that the ventricles are not capable of responding to every atrial beat; therefore, only a small percentage of atrial stimuli excite the ventricles. Since the atrial rate is irregular, the ventricular (pulse rate) will also be irregular.

A. Etiology
Usually seen in patients with arteriosclerotic or rheumatic heart disease.

B. Altered Physiology
1. Arteriosclerosis leads to scarring of the atrium and thus to disruption of the normal course of the P wave (atrial wave).
2. P waves are replaced by irregular, rapid waves each of which is different in configuration from the other.
3. P waves (often called fibrillatory waves) assume different shapes because they come from different foci in the atrium. (In atrial flutter, the P waves are very regular and uniform since they come from one focus.)
4. Because P waves occur at variable intervals, the QRS

complexes assume an irregular rhythm, and thus the patient's pulse is irregular. (The configuration of the QRS is normal since the conduction tissue beyond the AV node has not yet become critically involved with the arteriosclerotic process.)
5. Since the P waves come so fast, all of them do not pass on to the ventricles, because of normal refraction of the AV node. Thus the atrial rate is usually much faster than the ventricular rate.
6. Occasionally, the ventricular rate is very fast because the AV node is blocking relatively fewer beats than is normal. If this is the case, atrial activity may not be seen, because the QRS complexes are so close together (since their rate is so rapid) that it is difficult to define the arrhythmia.

NOTE: General rule: If *normal* QRS complexes are present at a very rapid rate, so that atrial activity cannot be seen and the rhythm is *irregular*, the probable diagnosis is atrial fibrillation.

C. Mechanism of Atrial Fibrillation
1. In atrial fibrillation many ectopic foci are present in the atrium (left in Fig. 9-31).
2. Since each small atrial wave comes from a different focus and travels a different route, the shape of each atrial wave (P wave) is different.

D. ECG of Atrial Fibrillation
1. Note the small, irregular fibrillating P waves (right in Fig. 9-31 [arrows]).
2. As with atrial flutter, only an occasional P wave travels through the AV node to form a QRS complex, but since these complexes come at irregular intervals in atrial fibrillation, the ventricular rate is irregular.
3. Each P wave is different in shape because it comes from a different focus in the atrium.

E. Treatment
1. Depends on patient's clinical condition, cardiac rate, and drug status.
2. For the average patient who is not critical and not on digitalis, the following treatment is common:
   a. 0.25–0.5 mg. of IV digoxin, given over a 5-minute

ECG of Atrial Fibrillation
1. Note the small, irregular fibrillating P waves (arrow).
2. As with atrial flutter, only an occasional P wave travels through the AV node to form a QRS complex, but since these complexes come at irregular intervals in atrial fibrillation, the ventricular rate is irregular.
3. Each P wave is different in shape because it comes from a different focus in the atrium.

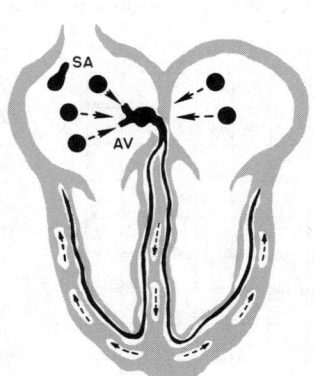

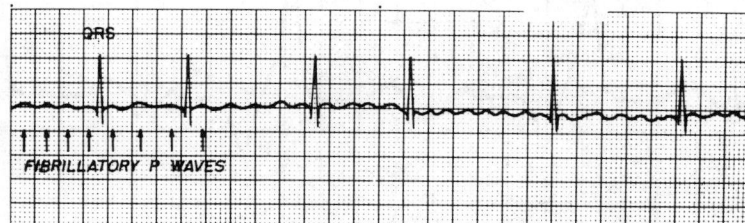

FIGURE 9-31. *Atrial Fibrillation Pathway*

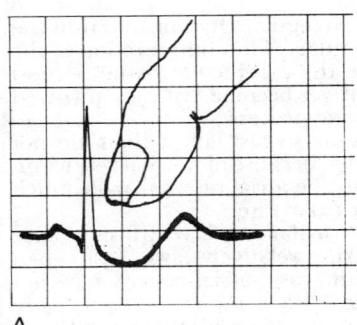
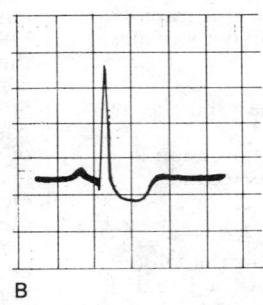
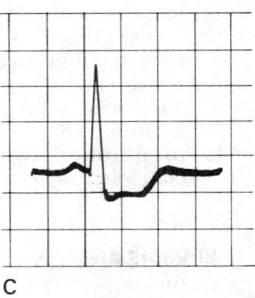

A   B   C

FIGURE 9-32. A. *The ST segment depression of digitalis often appears as if someone had dragged his finger through the end of the QRS complex into the T wave.*
B. *Digitalis effect: Notice the rounded scooped appearance of the ST segment.*
C. *Ischemic effect: In contrast to digitalis effect, the ST segment depression is horizontal.*

period under ECG control. Digitalis works by allowing fewer impulses from the rapidly contracting atrium to reach the ventricles by blocking the AV node.

  b. After 4 hours, an additional 0.25–0.5 mg. is given, depending on the ECG and the patient's condition. (Total IV dose before oral maintenance therapy is 0.5–1 mg.)

  c. If the ventricular rate continues to be rapid despite adequate doses of digitalis, propranolol (Inderal) may be added. Propranolol, as digitalis, also blocks the AV node to slow the ventricular rate.

3. If atrial fibrillation is an imminent, life-threatening emergency (rare):

  a. Cardioversion may be started with 100 watt-seconds.

  b. As with atrial flutter, cardioversion becomes somewhat of a risk when the patient is taking digitalis.

  c. In contrast to atrial flutter, atrial fibrillation is more difficult to correct to normal sinus rhythm with electric countershock.

Digitalis Toxicity

Digitalis toxicity—an abnormal cardiac rhythm produced by excessive digitalis. (Almost every arrhythmia can be produced by excessive digitalis.)

Digitalis effect—depression of ST segment from digitalis; does not represent toxicity.

A. *ECG of Digitalis Effect*

1. Normal levels of digitalis often produce a fairly

distinctive depression of the ST segment characterized by "scooping," said to look as if a finger had been dragged through the end of the QRS complex. (Fig. 9-32A)

2. This is in contrast to the "horizontal" ST segment depression frequently seen in myocardial ischemia. (Fig. 9-32B,C). Often the ST depression of digitalis and ischemia will be similar.

B. *Clinical Manifestations of Digitalis Toxicity*

Anorexia, followed by nausea and vomiting in 2–3 days. Green or yellow vision (uncommon).

C. *ECG of Digitalis Toxicity*

1. The most common arrhythmia associated with digitalis toxicity is *ectopic ventricular beats;* ectopic beats may be "multifocal," meaning they are coming from different locations in the ventricles and thus will take on different configurations in the ECG. (Fig. 9-33)

2. Probably the next most common serious arrhythmia in digitalis toxicity is junctional (AV nodal) rhythm.

  a. Frequently seen in patients being treated for atrial fibrillation. In this situation, digitalis is used to decrease the ventricular rate so the heart can have time to fill with blood and thus increase cardiac output.

  b. In this situation digitalis toxicity is identified by *regularization* of the previous irregular rate of atrial fibrillation. (The ventricular rate is regular because the AV node area is blocked from receiving atrial impulses by digitalis and sends its own impulses).

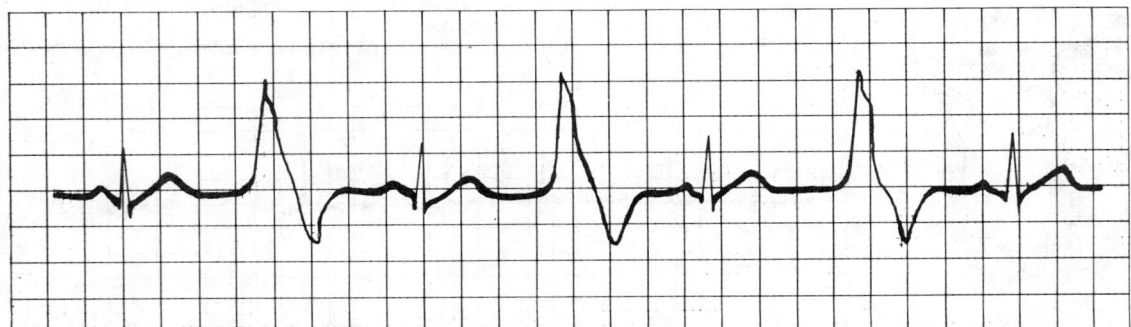

FIGURE 9-33. *The ectopic ventricular contractions shown above are secondary to digitalis toxicity.*

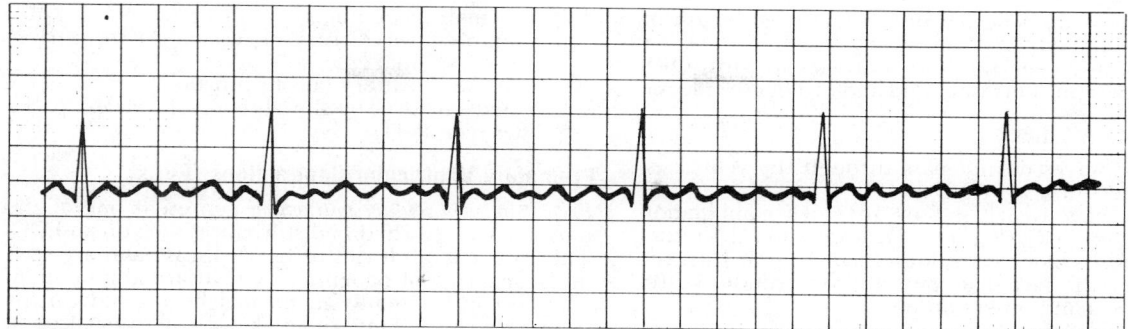

FIGURE 9-34. *Atrial fibrillation with a regular ventricular response which is often secondary to digitalis toxicity.*

c. Therefore, when one sees a regular rate in a patient with atrial fibrillation, the first thought should be digitalis toxicity because the ventricles are now being stimulated by the AV junction, which has a regular rate, and not by the irregularly beating atria. (Fig. 9-34)

3. Potassium and digitalis have a reciprocal relationship in their effect on the heart, so that if the serum potassium is low, digitalis will have a greater chance of causing toxicity.

D. *Treatment*

1. Withhold digitalis and await body excretion of the drug if the patient is hemodynamically stable.
   a. Replace potassium if the serum potassium level is low.
2. Administer potassium or phenytoin (Dilantin) as directed if the patient is doing poorly with his arrhythmia.
   a. Potassium (which prolongs impulse conduction) is contraindicated if the serum potassium is above a high normal level or if a significant AV block is present—potassium, in itself, tends to block the AV node as does digitalis.
   b. Average dose of potassium chloride is about 20–40 mEq. in IV fluid given over the prescribed time period.
   c. If potassium is not effective, give 50 mg. of phenytoin (Dilantin) IV every 5 minutes up to a total dose of 1 gm. under ECG control—phenytoin decreases myocardial excitability and increases rate of impulse formation through the AV node, both effects being opposite to that of digitalis.
3. Give lidocaine, propranolol (Inderal), or use pacing for digitalis toxicity not responsive to potassium and phenytoin.
4. Cardioversion is relatively contraindicated in digitalis toxicity—there is a propensity to convert relatively benign arrhythmias to more lethal ones.
5. Cardioversion or defibrillation should be attempted if all modalities fail and the situation seems terminal.

AV Block

AV block means that the AV node is diseased and has difficulty conducting the atrial waves (P waves) into the ventricles. Common causes are congenital and arteriosclerotic heart disease.

A. *Types of AV Block*

1st degree
2nd degree
3rd degree

B. *Mechanism of AV Blocks*

1. Abnormal tissue around and in the AV node causes physiological blockage affecting the entry of the atrial impulse into the ventricles. (Fig. 9-35)
2. In 1st degree block—the impules are merely slowed.
3. In 2nd degree block—only a portion of the atrial impulses penetrate to the ventricles.
4. In 3rd degree block—no atrial impulse enters the ventricles, so that the atria and ventricles beat independently.

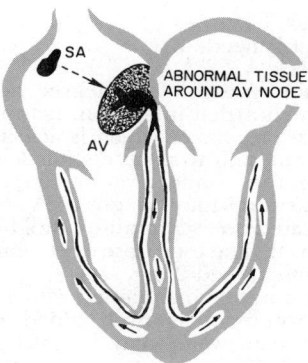

FIGURE 9-35. *AV Block*

1st Degree AV Block (Fig. 9-36)

1. The PR interval is prolonged. (The PR interval represents the impulse going through the atrium and the area of the AV node.) It should not exceed 0.20 second (5 small blocks on ECG paper when 1 block equals .04 second) at normal heart rates.
2. Since the atrial and AV nodal tissues are diseased, the electrical impulse takes a longer time to traverse

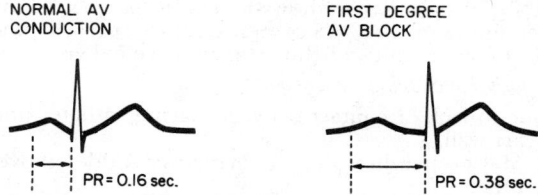

FIGURE 9-36. *1st degree AV block. Since the tissue around the AV node is abnormal, the impulse takes longer to traverse the area, which leads to a prolonged PR interval.*

its pathway (as reflected by the increased length of the PR interval).
3. All P waves penetrate the ventricles to form QRS complexes (in contrast to 2nd and 3rd degree block).

2nd Degree AV Block

1. Some P waves do not pass through the ventricles, but others do.
2. A ratio of 2:1, 3:1, 4:1 or any such combination appears on ECG. (Figure 9-37 represents a 2:1 ratio.)
3. 2nd degree block is distinguished from 3rd degree block by the fact that some P waves conduct QRS complexes and others do not.

3rd Degree AV Block

1. Also called a complete AV block.
2. *No* P waves penetrate the AV node and enter the ventricles; therefore, the P waves and QRS complexes are beating *independently.*
3. P waves are seen before the QRS complexes, but the PR interval varies and there is no constant relationship of the P waves to the QRS complexes (Fig. 9-38).
4. The pulse rate is usually slow since the ventricles are beating at their own inherent rhythm, which is about 35 beats per minute.

Treatment of AV Blocks

1. 1st degree block
   No treatment is needed.
2. 2nd degree block
   a. When certain types of 2nd degree heart block occur in a myocardial infarction, many cardiologists insert a pacemaker which is activated when the cardiac rate falls to unacceptable levels.
   b. To increase rate while awaiting a pacemaker, atropine (0.5 mg.) may be given IV. This dose may be repeated every 5 minutes until the desired rate is achieved. The total dose of atropine should generally not exceeed 2 mg.
   c. If the rate cannot be maintained with atropine, 1 mg. of isoproterenol (Isuprel) added to 500 ml. of 5% glucose in water may be infused by the "piggyback" technique to stimulate the heart to function at an acceptable rate.
3. 3rd degree heart block
   a. In myocardial infarction, 3rd degree block is frequently treated with a pacemaker.
   b. While awaiting insertion of the pacemaker, patient may be maintained on atropine or isoproterenol (Isuprel) as in 2nd degree block.

The Artificial Pacemaker

A. *Normally Functioning Pacemaker* (Fig. 9-39)

1. The ECG of a patient with a normally functioning artificial pacemaker shows a *vertical line* just at the beginning of the QRS complex. This represents the electrical stimulus of the artificial pacemaker.

B. *Poorly Functioning Pacemakers*

1. Due to lack of contact between pacing catheter and heart wall.
   a. May occur when patient performs a sudden movement.
   b. On the ECG the small vertical line denoting the pacemaker stimulus is *not* followed by a QRS complex (Fig. 9-40).

2. Due to malfunctioning:
   a. Examples: wires break or disconnect from pacemaker.
      battery fails to function.
   b. Noted on ECG by the absence of vertical pacer lines (Fig. 9-41).

Premature Ventricular Contractions (PVCs)

Premature ventricular contractions represent one of the most recognized rhythm disturbances seen on an ECG. They occur in all forms of heart disease and are seen in the majority of patients with myocardial infarction. They occur frequently in normal hearts and can be secondary to smoking, or intake of coffee or alcohol. While not usually symptomatic, PVCs, when frequent, may cause palpitations.

A. *Altered Physiology*

1. Contractions come early in the cycle and originate in the ventricle *below* the AV node.
2. QRS configurations are wide and bizarre, since a PVC does not begin normally and therefore does not follow the true conduction path in the ventricle.

B. *Mechanism of a PVC*

Since a PVC begins in the ventricle outside the AV node, a bizarre ventricular QRS complex will be inscribed (Fig. 9-42).

C. *ECG of PVCs*

PVCs occur early in the cycle and are wider than the normal beat. (See Fig. 9-42)

D. *Danger of PVCs*

PVCs can be especially dangerous when they:
1. Occur more frequently than once in 10 beats
2. Occur in groups of 2 or 3
3. Land near the T wave
4. Take on multiple configurations—this indicates that the PVCs come from different foci, which in turn means that the ventricle is more irritable.

E. *Treatment*

If a patient has an infarct, PVCs are treated vigorously since they *can precipitate ventricular fibrillation by hitting a T wave.*
1. Lidocaine (Xylocaine) can be given—PVCs are usually seen with a cardiac rate of over 60 per minute; lidocaine (suppressor of cardiac automaticity) is drug of choice because PVCs are most apt to come from an irritable focus such as an infarct.
   a. Dosage: 75–100 mg. IV as a bolus over a 2- to 3-minute period.
   b. If effective, a continuous IV drip of lidocaine should be started with a delivery of 1–4 mg. per minute.
      (1) Addition of 1 gm. of lidocaine to 500 ml. of 5% glucose in water will give a concentration of 2 mg. of lidocaine per ml. of fluid.
      (2) Most IV sets are calibrated to deliver 1 ml. in 10 drops of fluid.
      (3) If above concentration results in too much fluid for the patient, the amount of lidocaine in the IV solution should be increased.
   c. If lidocaine is ineffective, procainamide is the next drug of choice. The dose is indicated in the next section under "Ventricular Tachycardia."
2. If heart rate is *slow* secondary to a myocardial infarction involving the heart's normal physiological

FIGURE 9-37. *2nd degree AV block. Some P waves pass through to the ventricles, but others do not.*

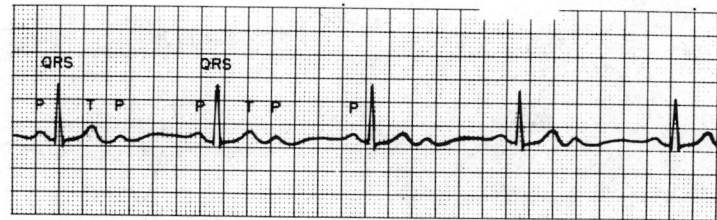

FIGURE 9-38. *3rd degree AV block. The P waves and QRS complexes are beating independently of each other.*

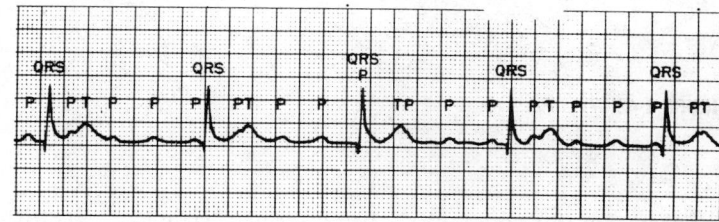

FIGURE 9-39. *Normal pacemaker function. In this ECG each QRS complex is preceded by a small vertical line (arrows), which represents the electrical stimulus of the artificial pacemaker.*

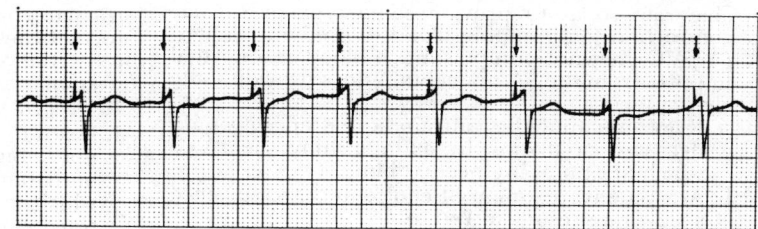

FIGURE 9-40. *Poor pacemaker contact. Notice that the first and last pacemaker stimuli are followed by ventricular complexes and that the other pacemaker deflections failed to produce a cardiac impulse because of the lack of pacemaker contact with the heart wall.*

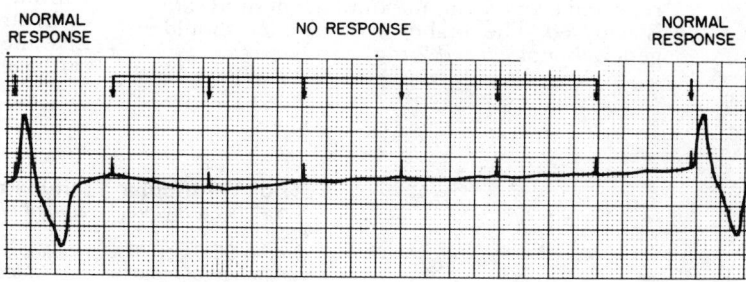

FIGURE 9-41. *Malfunctioning pacemaker. Notice the eventual absence of pacemaker stimuli which in this case resulted in cardiac standstill. This patient had a faulty pacemaker.*

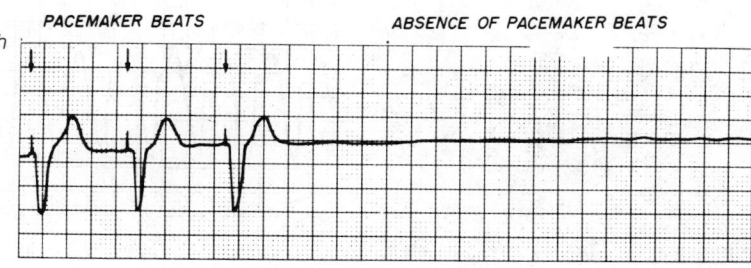

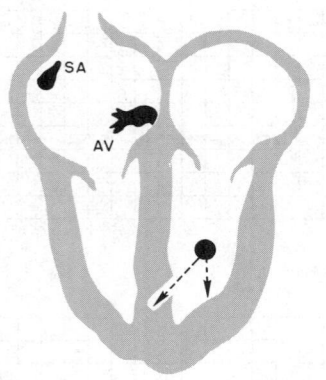

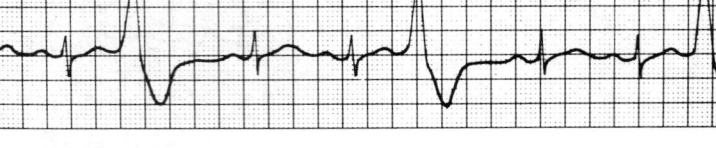

ECG of PVCs
PVCs occur early in the cycle and are wider than the normal beat.

FIGURE 9-42. *PVC Pathway*

pacemaker (SA node), PVCs (better termed "ectopic ventricular beats" since in this circumstance the beats are not "premature" but late in the cycle) may occur as a compensatory mechanism to maintain a reasonable rate so as to provide some type of cardiac contraction for pumping blood to the body tissues. (A PVC does not pump as much blood as a normal impulse from the SA node, but it does provide some circulation.)

a. Xylocaine would be contraindicated since it would decrease circulation by extinguishing the PVCs which are pumping needed blood.
b. Atropine is treatment of choice in this case (since a slow rate results in PVCs).
   (1) Increases the sinus node rate, which in turn terminates the inefficient ectopic beats by replacing them with normal impulses.
   (2) Dosage: 0.5–1.0 mg., IV. This dose may be repeated every 5 minutes until the desired rate is achieved. The total dose of atropine should generally not exceed 2 mg.

Ventricular Tachycardia

Ventricular tachycardia is one of the dreaded complications of a myocardial infarction and can be considered as multiple (3 or more), consecutive, premature ventricular contractions that originate from an ectopic focus below the AV node in the ventricles and thus cause the complexes to be wide and bizarre in configuration.

A. *Dangers of Ventricular Tachycardia*
1. Leads to a reduced cardiac output (the ventricles are not being stimulated normally from the AV node, but from a focus farther down in the ventricle wall, which leads to an incomplete and inefficient contraction of the heart muscle).
2. Is a precursor of ventricular fibrillation, in which there is no cardiac output.

B. *Mechanism of Ventricular Tachycardia*
1. Pathway is the same as for PVC since ventricular tachycardia can be thought of as a series of PVCs.
2. Like the PVCs, the complexes of ventricular tachycardia show a bizarre configuration. (See Fig. 9-43)

ECG of Ventricular Tachycardia
1. Since this arrhythmia begins below the AV node, the atria are beating independently.
2. On the ECGs of 20% of patients, when the ventricular rate is not too fast and the ventricular complexes are not too wide, P waves that are independent of the QRS complexes can be seen.
3. The rate is fast and the QRS complexes are wide. A width equivalent to 0.12 second (3 small blocks) or more is considered abnormal for a QRS complex.

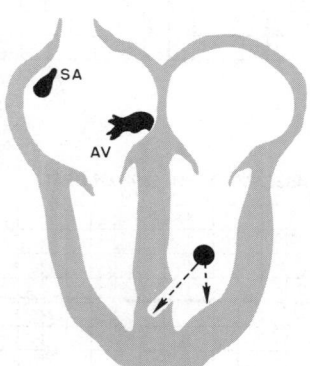

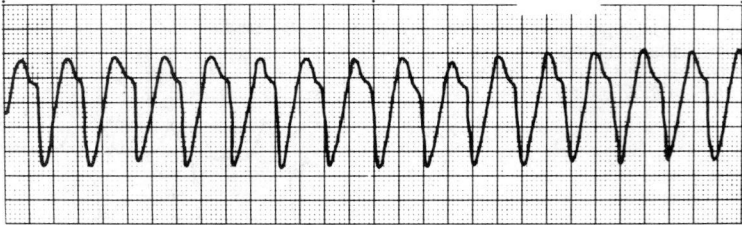

FIGURE 9-43. *Ventricular Tachycardia Pathway*

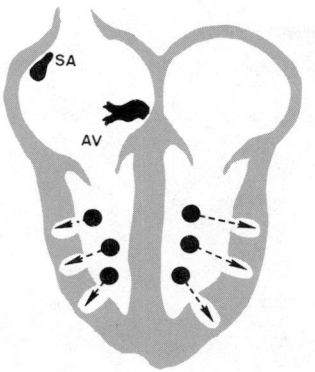

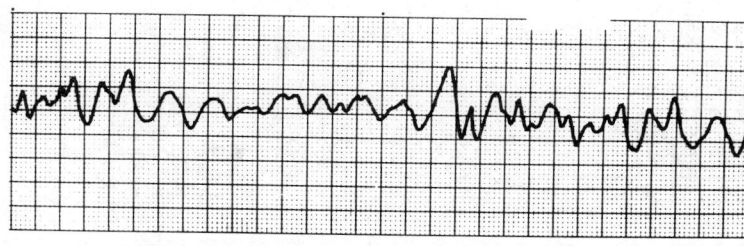

ECG of Ventricular Fibrillation
The complexes are completely distorted and irregular.

FIGURE 9-44. *Ventricular Fibrillation Pathway*

C. *ECG of Ventricular Tachycardia*
1. Since this arrhythmia begins below the AV node, the atria are beating independently.
2. On the ECGs of 20% of patients, when the ventricular rate is not too fast and the ventricular complexes are not too wide, P waves which are independent of the QRS complexes can be seen.
3. The rate is fast and the QRS complexes are wide. A width equivalent to 0.12 second (3 small blocks) or more is considered abnormal for a QRS complex. (See Fig. 9-43)

D. *Treatment*
1. If patient is tolerating the arrhythmia fairly well:
   a. Give lidocaine (Xylocaine)
      (1) 75-100 mg. IV as a bolus over a 2-minute period.
      (2) If effective, a continuous IV drip of lidocaine should be started (with delivery of 1–4 mg. per minute) and in 20 minutes another bolus of 50 mg. may be given to maintain a therapeutic blood level.
      (3) An addition of 1 gm. of lidocaine to 500 ml. of 5% glucose in water will give a concentration of 2 mg. of lidocaine per ml. of fluid.
   b. If lidocaine is ineffective and the patient is stable, then procainamide (Pronestyl) 100 mg. may be given every 5 minutes IV, not to exceed 1000 mg. If this is effective then a drip of 1–4 mg. per minute should be started.
   c. If the previous 2 drugs do not work and it is deemed that the patient is not critical enough to undergo cardioversion, bretylium (Bretylol) may be given as IV push at a dose of 5 mg./kg. with a constant infusion of 1–2 mg./ minute.
   d. Propranolol (Inderal) in a bolus of 0.5 mg. to 1 mg. every 5 minutes, up to 5 mg. over a 30-minute period, can be used.

NURSING ALERT: Because the heart muscle is weakened, the cardiac patient should not receive excessive fluid since this may precipitate congestive failure.

2. Cardioversion
   a. Used when lidocaine does not work or if patient is not tolerating the arrhythmia well.
   b. Start with about 200 watt-seconds.
   Cardioversion is a *timed* electric shock delivered by a machine which is set so that its electrical output does not hit a T wave, which is considered the vulnerable period on the cardiac cycle. If an electrical shock such as that from an external source or from an electrical impulse within the heart itself (such as a PVC) hits the T wave, ventricular fibrillation may ensue. If not terminated, ventricular fibrillation results in death.

Ventricular Fibrillation

Ventricular fibrillation is a lethal condition seen most commonly in the setting of a myocardial infarction. The patient will die within minutes if the arrhythmia is not terminated.

A. *Altered Physiology*
1. The heart is being stimulated simultaneously from numerous ectopic foci throughout the ventricles; therefore, there is no effective contraction of the cardiac musculature and thus no pulse.
2. Characterized by totally irregular appearance on ECG.

B. *Mechanism of Ventricular Fibrillation*

In ventricular fibrillation, the presence of multiple ectopic foci in the ventricle prohibits an effective heart beat. (See Fig. 9-44)

C. *ECG of Ventricular Fibrillation*

The complexes are completely distorted and irregular. (See Fig. 9-44)

NOTE: It is extremely important to be sure that the chaotic undulations on the ECG do not represent artifacts since movement by the patient or of the monitor wires can give the same appearance. If the patient is alert or has a pulse, the rhythm does *not* represent ventricular fibrillation.

1. *Treatment*

Electrical defibrillation at 200–400 watt-seconds. (In children, start with lower energies.)

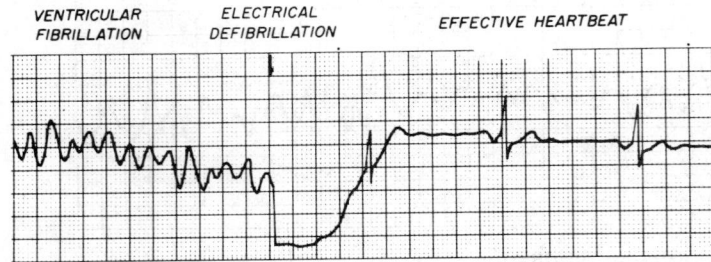

VENTRICULAR FIBRILLATION   ELECTRICAL DEFIBRILLATION   EFFECTIVE HEARTBEAT

FIGURE 9-45. *Electrical Defibrillation*

1. If successful, the defibrillation shock stops the erratic uncoordinated electrical activity of the ventricle. After a moment, the heart resumes its normal innate rhythm from the SA node (Fig. 9-45).
2. If defibrillation is unsuccessful, epinephrine 1 mg. may make the heart more susceptible to electrical shock. Also bretylium (Bretylol) may be effective. (See ventricular tachycardia, p. 324.)
3. Differs from cardioversion in that timing of the defibrillation shock is not necessary since there are no T waves in ventricular fibrillation.
4. Paddle placement (Fig. 9-46)
   a. The center of 1 paddle is applied just to the right of the upper sternum in the 2nd interspace.
   b. The rim of the other paddle is placed just below the left nipple.
   c. Paddles should be well lubricated and in firm contact with the skin.
5. See pages 277–278.

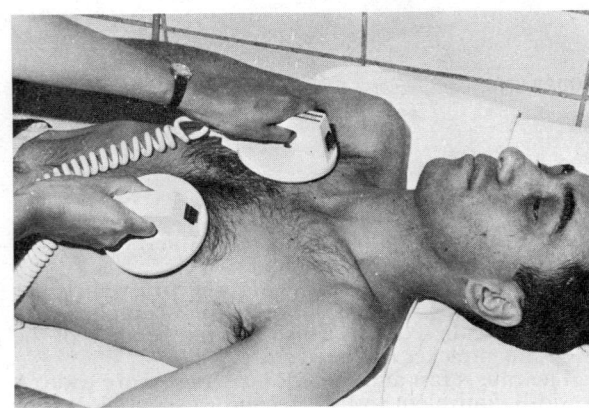

FIGURE 9-46. *Paddle placement in ventricular defibrillation.*

GUIDELINES: Synchronized Cardioversion

Synchronized cardioversion is a *timed* electrical shock to the heart for the purpose of terminating certain arrhythmias.

Asynchronized cardioversion is the same as defibrillation and is used principally for ventricular fibrillation.

Both types of cardioversion use the same type of electricity, but timed shock is not needed in ventricular fibrillation because there are no T waves. (Synchronized cardioversion is timed *not* to hit the T wave, since an electrical discharge during this phase of the cardiac cycle may cause ventricular fibrillation.)

Purpose

To stop the abnormal electrical activity of the heart and allow the SA node (heart's natural pacemaker) to resume normal sinus rhythm.

Contraindications

Synchronized cardioversion is relatively *contraindicated* when a patient has been taking a significant amount of *digitalis*, since more lethal arrhythmias may ensue after electrical discharge.

Equipment

Cardioverter and ECG machine
Conduction jelly and cardiac medications
Resuscitative equipment including:
    Endotracheal tubes
    Laryngoscopes

Equipment (cont.)

Suctioning equipment
Manual breathing bag
Pacing equipment

Procedure

NURSING ACTION	RATIONALE/AMPLIFICATION
1. If the procedure is elective it is advisable to have the patient "NPO" 12 hours before the cardioversion.	1. During sedation or the procedure, the patient may vomit and aspirate if the stomach is full.
a. Reassure patient and see that informed consent has been obtained.	a. Do not use word "shock" since this will increase the patient's apprehension.
b. Make sure patient has not been taking digitalis and that the serum potassium is normal.	b. Low potassium may precipitate post-shock arrhythmias
2. Make sure IV line is secure.	2. An IV line may be necessary for medications such as lidocaine and atropine.
3. Obtain a 12 lead ECG before and after cardioversion with the *ECG machine*. The ECG machine wires are best left on the patient since the ECG printout is of much better quality than that of the monitor. This fact is especially important when one is trying to dissect complicated arrhythmias.	3. An ECG is taken to ensure that the patient has not had a recent myocardial infarction (either just before or secondary to the cardioversion).

4. a. Allow patient to receive oxygen before and after cardioversion.
  b. Do *not* give oxygen during the procedure.
	4. a. Oxygen will help prevent unwanted arrhythmias after cardioversion.
	  b. An explosion could occur if a spark from the paddles should ignite the oxygen during the procedure.

5. Place the paddles in one of the following 2 positions:
  a. *Anterior-posterior position*
    One paddle—left infrascapular area
    Other paddle—upper sternum at 3rd interspace
  b. *Anterior position*
    One paddle—just to right of sternum at 2nd interspace
    Other paddle—just under left nipple	

6. Determine if the machine's synchronization mechanism is working before applying the paddles.
  a. The discharge should hit near the peak of the R wave.
  b. The R wave usually has to be of substantial height; if it is not, turn up the gain or change the lead. On many machines, the R wave must be upright before there is synchronization.
	a. If the electrical discharge hits the T wave, ventricular fibrillation may occur.
	  b. Synchronization is not used for ventricular fibrillation. (The machine will not work for *defibrillation* if the synchronization mode is on.)

7. Apply electrode paste to all of the paddle surface, but make sure there is no excess around the edges of the paddles.
  a. The paste should be rubbed into the skin very thoroughly, since this allows more electricity to penetrate the body surface.
  b. Make sure paddles are clean because surface material will interfere with the flow of electricity.
  c. Apply firm pressure to the paddle.
	7. If there is excess paste around the paddles, the discharge may run onto the skin, causing a burn. If there is not firm contact between the paddle and skin, a burn may occur; also, electricity is lost from the heart.

8. Set dial for lowest level of electrical energy that can be expected to convert the arrhythmia. Some arrhythmias (such as atrial flutter) can be converted with very low energies, such as 25 watt-seconds (joules).	8. Excessive energies cause myocardial damage.
9. Valium or a short-acting barbiturate should be given if the patient is conscious.	9. This helps produce amnesia concerning the cardioversion.
10. After the patient is in a light sleep from the IV medication and when no one is touching the bed or patient, discharge the cardioverter. If cardioversion does not occur, proceed to a higher energy level.	
11. Monitor the ECG after conversion occurs. Blood pressures should be recorded about every 15 minutes until the preshock blood pressure is reached.	11. The patient may revert to his previous arrhythmia after conversion.

Summary: Emergency Diagnosis and Treatment of Arrhythmias

Type of Arrhythmia	Appearance of ECG	Treatment	Pathway
Normal rhythm		None.	
Sinus tachycardia		Treat cause.	
Sinus bradycardia		Atropine, Isuprel, or pacemaker when condition is pathological.	
Sinus arrhythmia		None.	
PACs		Usually none. Quinidine may be used.	
PAT		Carotid sinus pressure or metaraminol (Aramine).	
Atrial flutter		Digitalis if rate above 100. Cardioversion is very effective. Inderal may be helpful.	
Atrial fibrillation		Digitalis if rate is above 100, and if fibrillation is not caused by too much digitalis. Cardioversion* may be effective. Inderal may be helpful.	
AV Blocks 2nd degree		Atropine, Isuprel, or pacemaker.	
3rd degree		Atropine, Isoprel, or pacemaker.	
PVCs		No treatment if benign. Lidocaine (Xylocaine) in most patients. Atropine if basic rhythm is slow.	
Ventricular tachycardia		Cardioversion* or lidocaine. Procainamide and/or bretylium if lidocaine is ineffective.	
Ventricular fibrillation		Electrical defibrillation. Epinephrine and/or bretylium in resistance cases.	

*Cardioversion can be very dangerous when a patient has a significant level of digitalis in his bloodstream since ventricular fibrillation or other lethal arrhythmias can be precipitated.

Drugs Commonly Used for Arrhythmias

TABLE 9-2. DRUGS COMMONLY USED FOR ARRHYTHMIAS

	Principal Indications	Dose	Principal Toxicity	Nursing Implications
Digoxin	Atrial fibrillation Atrial flutter PAT	Start with .25–0.5 mg. IV	Almost any cardiac arrhythmia, especially PVCs	Make sure that the patient has not been on digitalis previously, since this situation would decrease the dose. Give the drug very slowly and watch for arrhythmias. Remember that once the patient has received a significant amount of digitalis, cardioversion may produce a more serious arrhythmia than the digitalis-induced arrhythmia.
Lidocaine (Xylocaine)	PVCs Ventricular tachycardia	50–100 mg. by IV bolus followed by an infusion of 1–4 mg. per minute. The bolus dose may be repeated 15 minutes after the first to ensure a proper therapeutic blood level.	Seizures, cardiac arrhythmias, and hypotension	Watch very closely for signs of CNS toxicity that could lead to seizures, such as light-headedness, tinnitus, twitching, confusion, visual changes, vomiting, and lethargy. Watch for early signs of cardiac arrhythmias such as prolongation of the PR intervals or the QRS complex. Lidocaine is metabolized in the liver, and patients with hepatic disease need a lesser dose.
Procainamide (Pronestyl)	PVCs and ventricular tachycardia resistant to lidocaine	100 mg. IV q. 5 minutes not to exceed 50 mg. per minute or a total dose of 1 gm. May be followed by an infusion of 1–4 mg. per minute.	Hypotension, cardiac arrhythmias	Hypotension is a frequent complication, and vasopressors such as norepinephrine (Levophed) or metaraminol (Aramine) should be readied.
Propanolol (Inderal)	PAT Other arrhythmias such as atrial fibrillation, atrial flutter, and ventricular tachycardia not responsive to first line drugs. Digitalis-induced arrhythmias (potassium or phenytoin is preferred).	1–5 mg. IV, no faster than 1 mg. per minute.	Bradycardia Heart failure Hypotension Bronchospasm	Bradycardia can be neutralized with 0.5–1 mg. of atropine or isoproterenol (Isuprel), 1 mg. in 500 ml. of fluid, IV. Hypotension can be countered with norepinephrine (Levophed) or epinephrine. Bronchospasm may be treated with isoproterenol and/or aminophylline.
Phenytoin (Dilantin)	Digitalis-induced arrhythmias	25 mg. IV per minute, not to exceed 750 mg.	Cardiac depression such as sinus bradycardia and AV block Hypotension	Watch for cardiac toxicity and make sure the rate of administration is not too fast.
Atropine	Bradyarrhythmias	0.5 mg. IV	Tachycardia	Watch for PVCs and tachyarrhythmias.
Isoproterenol (Isuprel)	Bradyarrhythmias	Add 1 mg to 500 cc of fluid and titrate to appropriate rate	Tachycardia	Watch for PVCs and tachyarrhythmias.
Bretylium (Bretylol)	Ventricular tachycardia and ventricular fibrillation that have failed standard therapy.	5 mg/kg IV initially	Hypotension	Monitor for blood pressure drop and have dopamine (Intropin) or norepinephrine (Levophed) ready for a blood pressure drop below 75 mm. Hg, systolic. It should be noted that paradoxically bretylium is associated with a rise in blood pressure immediately after administration. Bretylium is more dangerous when a patient has been taking digitalis, hence simultaneous administration with digitalis should be avoided.

3. VASCULAR DISORDERS

Vascular disorders is a term that refers to conditions of the blood vessels.

Peripheral vascular disease (PVD) refers to disease affecting the blood vessels that supply the extremities: veins, arteries, and lymphatics.

Nature of the Disorder

1. Long-term. This is often discouraging to the patient: treatment may be painful and tedious; healing is slow.

2. Appears minor, but hospitalization or disability may last for months before healing takes place.
   Patient may have financial concerns and may worry about loss of job, separation from family, and community responsibilities.
3. Older people are especially prone to peripheral vascular disease.
4. This condition is often compounded by other medical problems, such as diabetes.
5. If lesions heal, recurrence of the condition, with concomitant incapacitation, is frequent.

Thrombus and Embolus Formation

1. *Thrombus*—a blood clot which partially or completely occludes a blood vessel.
   a. Thrombosed vessel—an occluded vessel
   b. Thrombosis—the condition of having a thrombosed vessel
2. Spontaneous clotting of the blood will usually not occur unless there is damage to the intimal surface of the vessel wall.
   a. Injury by trauma
   b. Inflammation
   c. Degenerative changes due to arteriosclerosis
3. Injured intima—causes platelets to collect, fibrin to form, and thrombus to develop.
4. *Embolus*—a fragment of a thrombus or a thrombus that has broken away from the point of formation.
   a. *Embolism*—occurs when an embolus moving through a blood vessel arrives at a narrowing of the vessel and thus occludes it.
   b. Air embolism—a bubble of air in the bloodstream
   c. Fat embolism—multiple droplets of fat in the bloodstream

Ischemia

Ischemia is a lack of blood supply sufficient to meet tissue needs. This can develop as a result of:
1. Gradual occlusion of the lumen of the artery by encroachment of the thickened wall (atherosclerosis).
2. More rapid development of ischemia due to formation of a blood clot (thrombus) at the atherosclerotic site.
3. Rapid occlusion of an artery when a free-flowing clot (embolus) lodges at a bifurcation or narrowing of the vessel.

ASSESSMENT AND PATHOPHYSIOLOGIC MANIFESTATIONS OF VASCULAR DISORDERS

Skin Color and Temperature

Objective determination of skin temperature—differences between 2 extremities are observed when individual is placed in a new environment: coolness of 1 extremity.

A. *Coldness*
1. Due to deficient blood supply to a part even though the environment is warm.
2. One extremity may be compared to another to note the difference.
3. The patient notices that the part feels uncomfortably cold.

B. *Pallor (Paleness)*
1. Normally the pink hue of the skin is due to adequate superficial circulation.
2. Diminished blood supply produces paleness, or lack of color.
3. Blanching occurs when the part is elevated above the level of the heart and the arterial pressure in that part is lower than normal.

C. *Rubor (Redness)*
1. Instead of a normal rosy-pink, the part may be red or reddish-blue. This is due to injury of superficial capillaries which causes them to remain dilated; it may also occur with chronic ischemia.
2. Circulation is impaired.
3. Anoxia or coldness may be the cause of rubor.

D. *Cyanosis (Blueness)*
1. Indicates that less than normal amount of oxygen is in the blood.
2. When localized, it implies very slow circulation in that part.

Pain

1. Due to inadequate blood supply.
2. This is common, but varies with the condition. May be constant and severe, e.g., ulceration.
3. When it occurs only after a certain amount of exercise it is called *intermittent claudication*. (This disappears after rest, but returns with exercise.)
4. When it occurs at rest (rest pain), it indicates a more severe degree of ischemia.

Exercise Tolerance

Measurement of the amount of exercise the involved part can tolerate before pain is experienced.

Pulse Volume

A useful method for recording peripheral pulse volume and is based on a scale from zero to +4, as follows:
0	not palpable—absent pulsations
+1	thready, weak, fades in and out—marked impairment of pulsations
+2	difficult to palpate, stronger than +1—moderate impairment
+3	easily palpable, not easily obliterated with pressure—slight impairment
+4	strong and bounding—normal pulsations

Capillary Refill Time

The capillary bed contains arterial blood and is called *microcirculation.* Capillary refill time is an indicator of peripheral perfusion and cardiac output.
1. This test can be done at the same time arterial pulses are checked.
2. Depress finger or toe nailbed until skin blanches.
3. Release pressure and note how rapidly color returns to the original appearance.
   a. Normally, capillaries fill within a fraction of a second
      (1) Acceptable—less than 3 seconds.
      (2) Abnormal or sluggish   more than 3 seconds.

Blood Pressure (See p. 20 and p. 354)

See Assessment of Acute Arterial Occlusion vs. Deep Vein Thrombosis, page 331.

Assessment of Acute Arterial Occlusion vs. Deep Vein Thrombosis

	Acute Arterial Occlusion	**Deep Vein Thrombosis**
Onset	Sudden	Gradual
Color	Pale: later—mottled, cyanotic	Slightly cyanotic; rubescent
Skin Temperature	Cold	Warm
Leg size—diameter	May be reduced from normal	Enlarged
Superficial veins	Collapsed	Appear enlarged and prominent
Arterial pulsation	Pulse deficit noted	Normal and palpable (except in marked edema)
Effect of elevating leg	Condition worsens	Condition improves

Diagnostic Evaluation of Vascular Conditions (Fig. 9-47)

A. *Oscillometry*

1. Degree of arterial occlusion may be measured by an oscillometer, which measures pulse volume. One extremity may be compared to the other.
2. An inflatable cuff is wrapped around the extremity, and the *oscillometric index* is determined by inflating the cuff and reading the dial.
3. Normal readings (points of pressure at which circulation ceases)
   a. Lower extremity

Midthigh	4– 16 mm./Hg
Upper third of leg	3– 12 mm./Hg
Above ankle	1– 18 mm./Hg
Foot	0.2–1.0 mm./Hg

   b. Upper extremity

Upper arm	4–16 mm./Hg
Elbow	3–12 mm./Hg
Wrist	1–10 mm./Hg
Hand	0.2– 2 mm./Hg

B. *Phlebography (Venography)*—an x-ray visualization of the vascular tree after the injection of a contrast medium (renografin).

1. Inform the patient that he may experience an intense burning sensation in the vessel where the solution is injected. This will last for only a few seconds.
2. Note any evidence of allergic reaction to the contrast medium; this may occur as soon as the contrast medium is injected or it may be delayed and occur when the patient reaches his room.
   a. Perspiring, dyspnea, nausea, vomiting
   b. Rapid heart rate, numbness of extremities
   c. Hives
   d. Management
      (1) Notify physician.
      (2) Have adrenalin available for injection, as well as antihistamine drugs and oxygen.
3. Nursing management
   a. Observe injection site for the following:
      (1) Signs of redness, swelling, bleeding; signs of thrombosis (loss of distal pulses).
          If above signs occur, notify physician.
      (2) Evidence of bleeding
          Therapy
          (a) Apply pressure dressing.
          (b) Notify physician.
   b. Check for arterial occlusion.
      (1) Note extremity pulses; check for quality.
      (2) Observe color (pallor or cyanosis).
      (3) Ask patient about sensation of pain, numbness.

4. Chief disadvantages: It is an expensive and invasive diagnostic method and may cause painful side effects.

C. *Intermittent Claudication Determination*

1. At rest, blood supply is adequate—but an exercised muscle may require 10 times more blood.
2. Following exercise such as walking, running, or climbing stairs, a severe cramping pain or sensation of tiredness develops in those muscle areas not receiving an adequate blood supply.
3. Upon resting, pain is relieved; metabolites are carried away and normal blood-to-tissue demand ratio is restored.
4. Measurement
   a. Have patient walk up steps, counting number of steps taken before pain occurs.
   b. Use a foot-pedal device which lifts a weight when pressed.
      (1) Normally, fatigue occurs in 5–10 minutes.
      (2) The person with arterial occlusion usually complains of pain in less than a minute.

D. *Lumbar Sympathetic Block*

1. Used to evaluate element of constriction in peripheral circulation in the legs.
2. Procedure
   a. Local anesthetic is injected into retroperitoneal space, blocking lumbar sympathetic trunk and thus the sympathetics to leg.
   b. Sympathetic nerves control tension of muscles in blood vessels; a block causes vasodilation of vessels.
   c. Arteriosclerotic vessels are not capable of dilating.

E. *Doppler Ultrasound*—a noninvasive test used to detect blood flow.

1. A beam of ultrasound is sent into the tissues through an acoustic gel on the skin. Reflected sound from moving blood cells is detected, amplified as audible sound, and recorded; velocity of blood flow has a direct effect on the waveforms.
2. Usually the posterior tibial, calf, popliteal, and common femoral veins are examined. Arterial flow can be detected by the pulsatile nature of the flow.
3. Signals are assessed for venous patency and valvular competence. Arterial flow is used as an indicator of patency, and the cuff pressure required to stop it indicates arterial pressure at that point.
4. Entire test takes about 5–10 minutes.
5. This technique when checked with arteriography has a reliability factor of 95%, and thus qualifies as a simple, inexpensive, highly reliable, and noninvasive diagnostic tool. (Fig. 9-48)

F. *Plethysmography*—a noninvasive measurement of

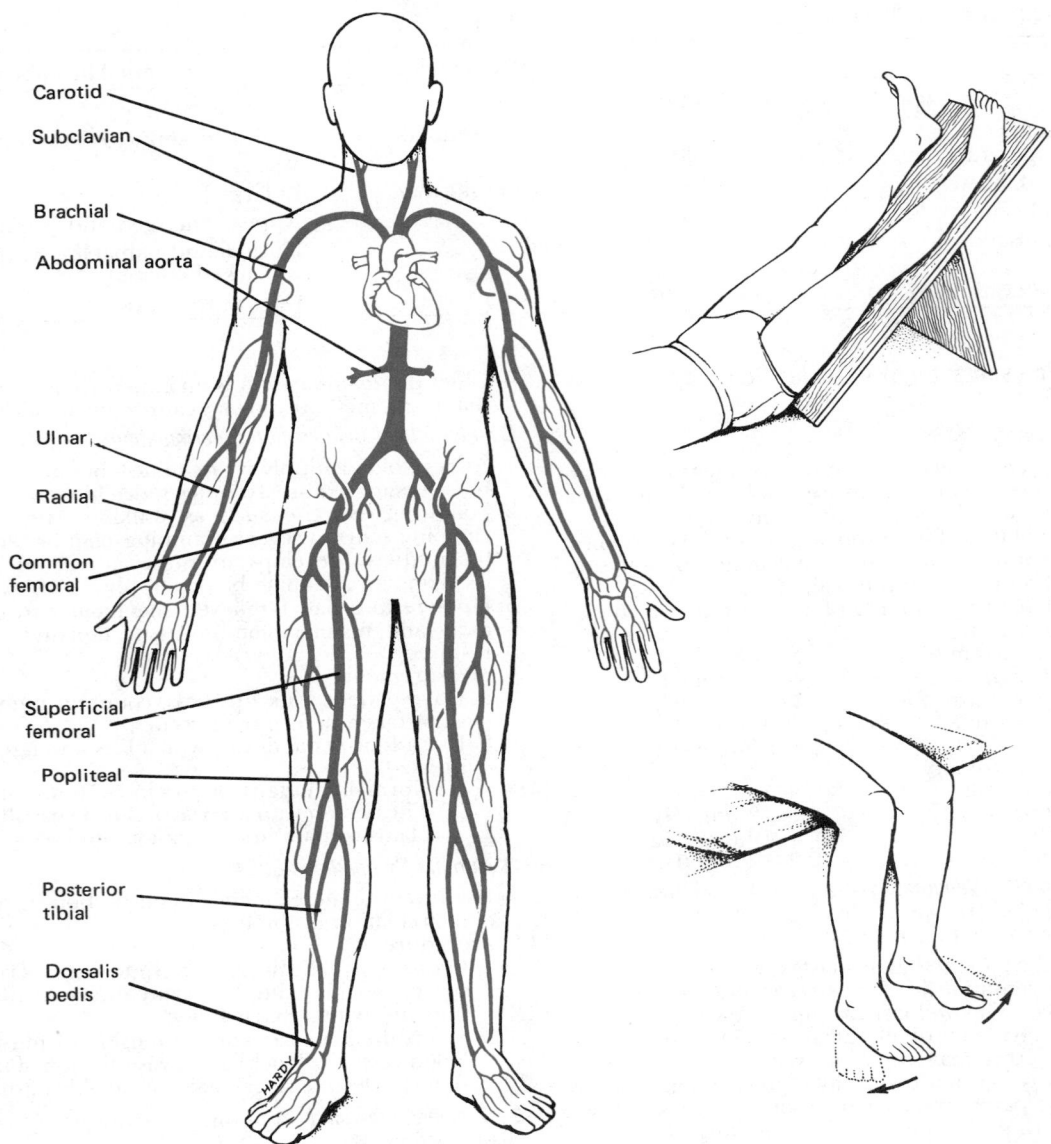

FIGURE 9-47. *Salient points in evaluating peripheral arterial insufficiency.*

changes in calf volume corresponding to changes in blood volume brought about by temporary venous occlusion with a high pneumatic cuff.

1. Variations of the above test are practiced in various clinics; some use a strain-gauge placed about the calf.
2. Temporary venous occlusion with a pneumatic cuff (50 mm. Hg) applied to the thigh results in an increase in circumference of the calf.
3. Sudden cuff deflation results in a decrease in calf circumference; this is proportional to rate of venous outflow from extremity.

G. ^{125}I *Fibrinogen Uptake Test*—an invasive radioactive test in which labeled fibrinogen given before a thrombus forms will be concentrated in the area of clot formation. Formation of clots may be detected with serial scanning and by comparing one leg with the other.

1. Disadvantages:
   a. It is not sensitive to thrombi high in the iliofemoral region.
   b. It is costly.
   c. It carries a minimal risk of hepatitis.

H. *Carotid Phonoangiogram (CPG)*—a noninvasive diagnostic test of the carotid artery.

1. Sound is greatly amplified and the instrument permits localization of the source of the bruit and provides a method of photographing the oscillographic tracing from which one can estimate the degree of stenosis.

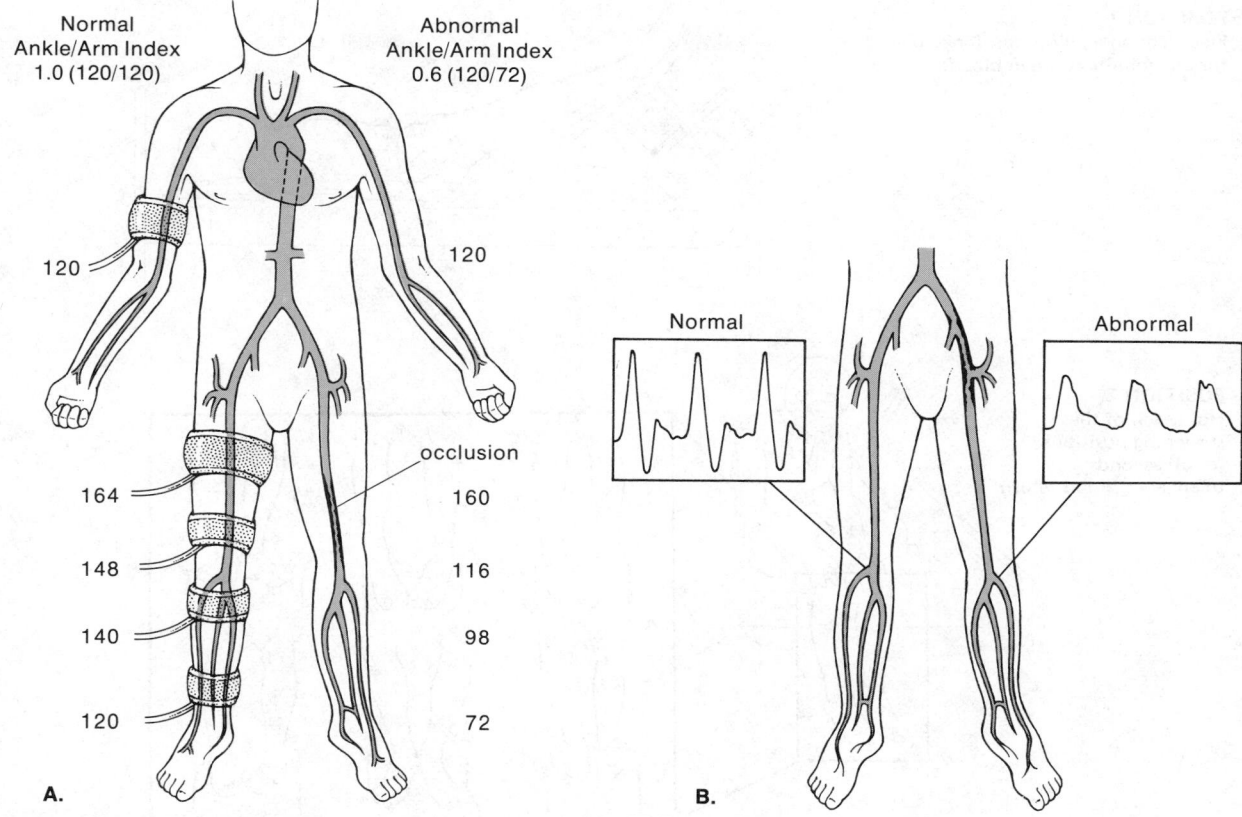

FIGURE 9-48. A. *The Doppler probe determines pressures over the brachial and posterior tibial or dorsalis pedis arteries. The cuff is inflated until the arterial segment disappears; the cuff is then slowly deflated until the arterial velocity signal returns at systolic pressure. NOTE: Normally, ankle pressure is equal to or slightly above arm pressure. In the presence of arterial occlusive disease (right side of diagrammed person), ankle and lower leg pressures are lower by an amount proportional to the degree of circulatory impairment.*

B. Diagram comparing the analogue wave tracings in a normal (left) and a diseased limb (right). Note the lack of diastolic deflection and the protracted systolic components in the tracing of the abnormal limb. (AbuRahma et al: Doppler testing in peripheral vascular occlusive disease. Surg Gynec Obstet 1980 Jan; 150 (1):27)

GENERAL MANAGEMENT OF PATIENTS WITH VASCULAR DISORDERS

THERAPEUTIC MODALITIES FOR INCREASING BLOOD SUPPLY TO TISSUES

Postural Therapy

OBJECTIVE: to increase blood flow through use of gravity by intermittent filling and emptying of capillaries, veins, and arteries.

Observation: Arterial blood supply to a section or part of the body can be increased by positioning it lower than the heart (gravity-assist).

A. *Walking*—a simple but very effective exercise.

1. A level surface is preferred.
2. Encourage patient to set realistic goals; each week these goals may be extended in keeping with his tolerance.
3. Use assistive devices as necessary—walker, cane, etc.
4. Evaluate patient's ability to climb stairs.

B. *Jogging*—a means of stimulating collateral blood flow not only to legs but also to the myocardium.

May be practiced as long as it is comfortable and pleasurable.

C. *Buerger's exercises*—prescribed according to condition of extremities and condition of patient.

1. Elevate extremity for a minute.
2. Place extremities in a dependent position until cyanosis or rubor becomes maximal.
3. Lie with extremities horizontal for a minute.
4. See Buerger-Allen exercises below.

D. *Buerger-Allen exercises*—exercises by which gravity alternately fills and empties the blood vessels (Fig. 9-49).

1. Procedure
   a. Begin with patient lying flat in bed. Elevate legs

POSITION 1
Place legs on a pillow-cushioned chair
for one minute to drain blood.

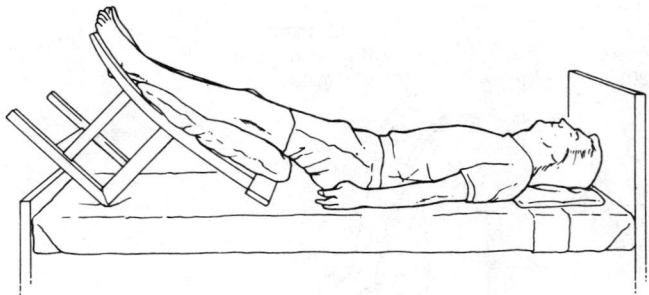

POSITION 2
Hold each of these
stretching positions
for 30 seconds
to enhance blood return.

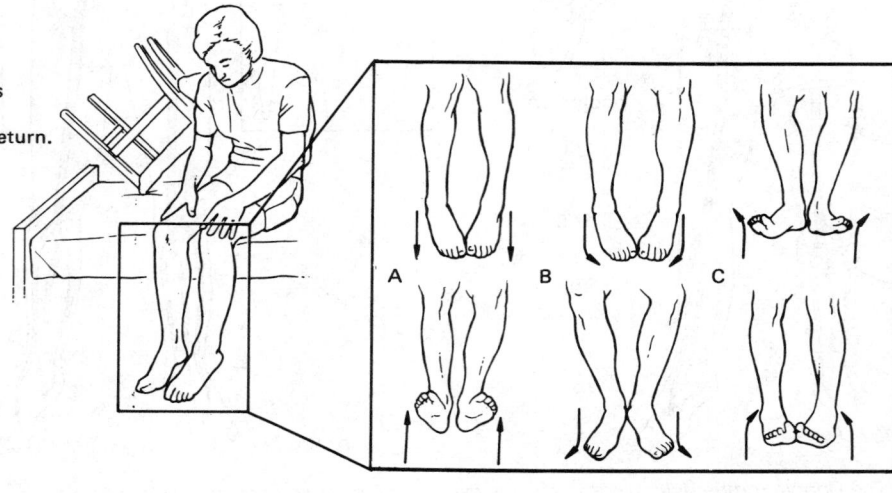

POSITION 3
Lie flat on back, with legs straight.
Hold position for one minute.

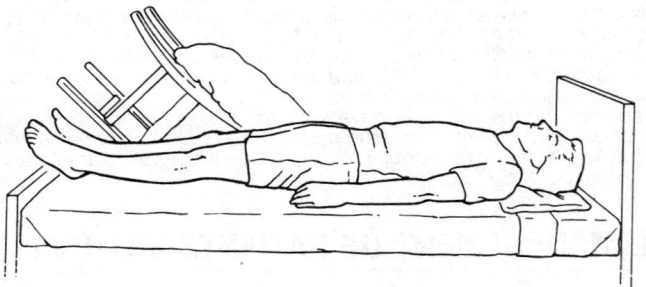

FIGURE 9-49. *Buerger-Allen exercises. Do exercise series 6 times, 4 times a day. (From Forshee T. and Minckley B. Lumbar sympathectomy. RN 1976 July)*

to above level of heart—2 minutes or until blanching takes place.
  b. Allow legs to be dependent; exercise feet—3 minutes or until legs are pink.
  c. Instruct patient to lie flat—5 minutes.
  d. Repeat a, b, and c 5 times; do entire set 3 times a day.
2. Tolerance and proper pacing
  a. Advise patient to rest when he feels pain.
  b. Avoid chilly environment since it causes vasoconstriction, which in turn further diminishes flow.
  c. Maintain stability, particularly if postural hypotension is a problem.

3. Comfort
  a. Improvise equipment that will provide comfortable support for the patient in the leg-elevated position.
  b. Well-padded straight-back chair can be placed on the bed so that the back of the chair supports the leg—top of chair is toward the top of the thigh.
  c. Overbed table may be used with a pillow.

E. *Oscillating bed*—provides postural exercises using a passive method.

1. Aids indirectly in prevention of pressure areas—pressure sores.

2. Prescribed according to patient needs.
3. Explain to the patient that the bed will assist in relieving his circulatory difficulty.
   a. Explain how the bed is turned on, regulated, and stopped.
   b. Advise him whether he can stop for meals, treatments, rest periods, etc.
4. Introduce motion of bed gradually in order to eliminate the possibility of headache, dizziness, or nausea.
5. Follow prescribed cycle for the individual patient.
   Cycle: Degree of angle and the length of time to be elevated
   Degree of angle and the length of time to be lowered
6. Prevent the patient from slipping downward by providing a padded footboard.

Thermotherapy

NURSING ALERT: When heat is applied externally to an extremity—demand for circulation is increased. When applied to diseased tissues—sensations are impaired; may result in damaging burn and necrosis.

A. Dry Heat

1. Warm water bottles
   a. Check temperature of water before filling bottle—not to exceed 48.8° C. (120° F.).
   b. Apply cover to bottle so that it does not come in direct contact with skin.
2. Heat cradle (thermostatically controlled or regulated with electric bulbs)
   a. Pad metal edges of cradle to prevent injury to extremities.
   b. Control temperatures so that it will not exceed 32.2° C. (90° F.).
   c. Ensure that bulbs are not likely to be touched by extremity (usually legs and feet).
   d. Higher temperatures would stimulate metabolism (not desired).
   e. Reduce temperature if patient complains of pain in extremity.
3. Ultrasound (acoustic vibration with frequencies beyond human ear perception)
   a. Useful in small areas where deeper penetration of heat is desired and where circulation needs to be stimulated.
   b. Application time is under 10 minutes.
   c. Avoid areas where metal sutures may be present.
4. Paraffin bath (see p. 788)

B. Moist Heat

1. Hydrotherapy
   a. Sitz bath—used for perineal therapy.
   b. Basin—for hands or feet with prescribed temperatures and for prescribed times.
2. Whirlpool bath
   a. In addition to moist heat, the effect of agitated water provides hydromassage.
   b. May be used for 1 or 2 extremities or the whole body.
3. Warm compresses
   a. Applied directly to the skin.
   b. When hot, apply over toweling.

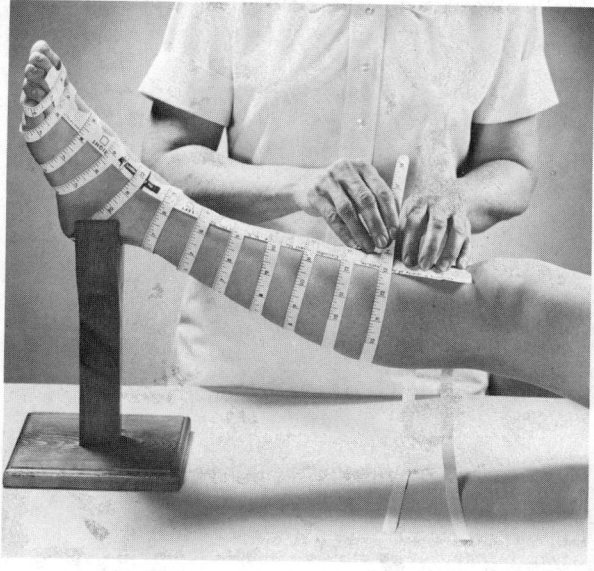

FIGURE 9-50. *By using a special measuring tape, exact measurements of the extremity can be obtained. Measurements are taken while the patient is lying down with the extremity slightly elevated. The foot is in a normal relaxed position. The horizontal spine of the measuring tape is placed anteriorly; key cross straps are fastened and then each succeeding strap is fastened. All straps are calibrated in centimeters. When properly and completely fastened, this measuring device can be cut according to directions and sent to the manufacturer for made-to-order support. (Courtesy of Jobst)*

Pressure Gradient Therapy (Compression Devices and Garments)

A. Cuffs, Sleeves, or Boots

1. Circulator—electrically produced air pressure alternately inflates and deflates a boot in which the extremity is encased.
   Rhythm of occlusion and release as well as pressure can be regulated to correspond to pulse.
2. Pressor sleeve or boot—a plastic tube filled with air.
   a. Can be maintained at low pressure for several hours.
   b. Can be regulated to function intermittently. (Useful in lymphedema of arm following mastectomy; see p. 563.)

B. Elastic Garments

1. Support for an extremity can be tailor-made: A unique measuring tape was devised by Jobst* so that exact "fabric pressures" are produced with their custom-made venous pressure gradient supports (Fig. 9-50).
2. Method of applying supporting hose is demonstrated in Figure 9-51.
3. Any type of support hose, if applied incorrectly (such as permitting rolling at the top), can act as a tourniquet. This will produce stasis rather than prevent it.

* The Jobst Institute, Box 653, Toledo, Ohio 43694.

Put on supports early in the morning, before swelling occurs.

Always begin with supports "inside-out" . . . as they are when you receive them.

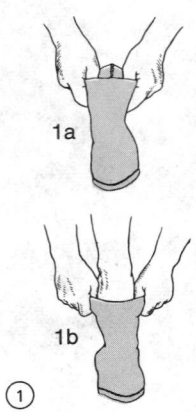

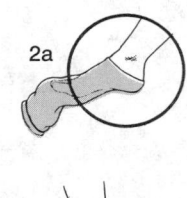

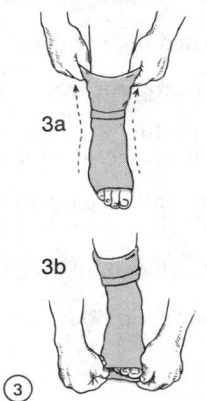

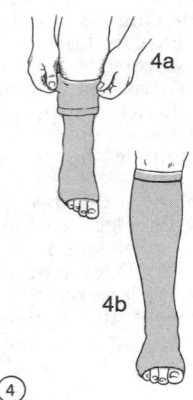

Sit with feet in easy reach. Support must be "inside out," with its foot inverted back to heel. Seam faces down (sketch 1a). Grasp each side firmly and pull onto foot (sketch 1b).

Pull past midpoint of heel (sketch 2a), so support will not slip back. Then, reach just beyond toes and grasp fabric between fingers and start pulling over foot. Pull from sides . . . never by seams.

Pull all the way up past ankle (sketch 3a). Seat heel in place. Pull foot portion of support out toward tips of toes (sketch 3b) to set fabric evenly on foot. Allow to settle back normally.

Using short (2 inches at a time) snappy pulls (sketch 4a) pull support up to point it was measured to end (sketch 4b). Smooth evenly down leg. **Never allow top to roll or turn down.**

FIGURE 9-51. *Method of applying supporting hose. (Courtesy of Jobst)*

4. Many question the effectiveness of elastic stockings; the nurse will be guided by the preferences of the patient's physician.
5. Elastic stockings with inflatable pneumatic bladders connected to an automatic air pump are available to help prevent deep-vein thrombi from forming in the calf and lower leg.
   a. The bladders in this device, called the *Pulsatile Anti-Embolism System,* expand and contract and are designed to stimulate circulation.

ANTICOAGULANT THERAPY

Anticoagulant therapy is the administration of medications

OBJECTIVES: to disrupt the blood's natural clotting mechanism
to prevent formation of a thrombus in postoperative patients
to intercept the extension of a thrombus once it has formed

NOTE: Anticoagulants cannot dissolve a thrombus that has already formed. Precise nursing assessment is required because of the delicate balance sought between too much clotting (thrombus formation) and too little clotting (hemorrhage).

Clinical Indications

(Authorities disagree about the justification of long-term use of anticoagulants in various disease entities.)
1. *Venous thrombosis*—because of the danger of extension and the danger of emboli.
2. *Pulmonary embolism*—prophylactically, if patient is known to be suspect; also indicated during recovery phase to prevent further clot formation.
3. *Patient susceptible to embolism*—such as a surgical patient who has rheumatic heart disease, one who has had valve surgery.
4. *Coronary occlusion with myocardial infarction.*
5. *Cerebral vascular accident caused by emboli or cerebral thrombi*—to reduce sludging of blood: useful in prevention and treatment of strokes.

Highest Risk

1. Patients whose prothrombin time has been difficult to control from the outset.
2. Men (not women) with aortic valve prostheses.
3. Patients treated with anticoagulants for more than 3 years.

Contraindications

1. May cause spontaneous bleeding—therefore not used when there is likelihood of bleeding because of increased capillary fragility or an aneurysm.
2. Individuals with peptic ulcer and chronic ulcerative diseases are considered poor risks, because of the possibility of bleeding.
3. Should not be given following neurosurgery because of danger of hemorrhage in brain or spinal cord.
4. Liver disease may present a problem because of interference with plasma protein clotting factors.
5. Liver and kidney insufficiency diseases may preclude use of anticoagulants because of difficulty in metabolizing and eliminating them—resulting in toxicity and difficulty in responding to antidotal medication (not true of heparin).
6. Poor follow-up by patients; unless the patient cooperates by reporting for blood tests, etc., he should not be on anticoagulants.
7. Severe diabetes, infections, or severe traumatic conditions are circumstances in which anticoagulant therapy may be contraindicated.

Types of Anticoagulants

	Generic Name	Proprietary Name
Heparin sodium	Heparin	Panheprin Lipo-Repin Liquaemin
Oral		
Coumarin derivatives	Bishydroxycoumarin Warfarin sodium	Dicumarol Coumadin Panwarfin
	Acenocoumarol Phenprocoumon	Sintrom Liquamar
Indandione derivatives	Anisindione Diphenadione Phenindione	Miradon Dipaxin Danilone Eridione Hedulin

Heparin Sodium

(Parenteral anticoagulant)

A. *Pharmacologic Action*

1. Affects coagulation time by its effect on the clotting mechanism.
2. Inactivates thromboplastin, which in turn interferes with changing of prothrombin to thrombin.
3. Inactivates any thrombin which manages to form.
4. May decrease adhesiveness of platelets.
5. May promote resolution of a newly formed clot.
6. Does not dissolve fibrin of a well established clot.

B. *Advantages*

1. Chief advantage is its rapid action which makes it the medication of choice in emergency situations and for short-term therapy.
2. When administered by vein, it acts within seconds and is both predictable and controllable (action time intramuscularly or subcutaneously is 30 minutes).
3. Its effect can be readily neutralized by injecting protamine sulfate or other heparin antagonists intravenously, and it is therefore the safest anticoagulant.
4. It has little cumulative effect and dissipates quickly (within 4 hours).
5. It is the most effective agent available in treatment of phlebitis.

C. *Disadvantages*

1. Chief disadvantage is that it must be given parenterally; it is unpleasant when used for long-term maintenance therapy.
2. For continued effectiveness, heparin must be given frequently.
3. Heparin is expensive—price varies greatly.

D. *Side Effects and Contraindications*

1. Bleeding may occur; therefore, heparin should not be given to those patients listed under Contraindications (p. 336), to those who have lost large areas of skin, or to those with clotting-factor deficiencies.
2. Allergic reactions may appear in patients sensitive to substances of animal origin (redness, itchy skin, utricarial wheals) but are uncommon.
3. Heparin sodium in full therapeutic doses is contraindicated when suitable blood coagulation tests, such as Lee-White whole-blood clotting time, activated

partial thromboplastin time (APTT), etc., cannot be performed at the required intervals.

> **NURSING ALERT:** All anticoagulants should be used with extreme caution in disease states in which there is increased danger of hemorrhage.

E. *Antidotes*

1. Protamine sulfate—this should be available in the department where the patient is receiving heparin anticoagulant therapy.
2. Blood transfusion.

Coumarin and Indanedione

(Oral anticoagulants)

A. *Most Commonly Used*

1. Bishydroxycoumarin (Dicumarol)
2. Warfarin sodium (Coumadin)

B. *Pharmacologic Action*

1. Acts to reduce blood coagulability by its effect on prothrombin activity.
2. Interferes with vitamin K absorption—the latter being required in the synthesis of prothrombin.
3. Failure of Factor VII leads to prolonged clotting time.
4. Has no effect on clotting factors already in circulation—hence the delayed action of these drugs is noted later and can be measured by prothrombin time tests.

C. *Prothrombin Time Testing*

1. Normal prothrombin time—11-13 seconds.
2. By lengthening prothrombin time to about 19-24 seconds, coagulability of blood is depressed sufficiently to lessen danger of thrombosis but not enough to cause spontaneous bleeding. This represents the *desired therapeutic range.*

D. *Prothrombin Activity*

Prothrombin range may also be reported in percents of normal—the activity of the plasma prothrombin.
1. Desired therapeutic range is 20–30% of normal.
2. Probability of hemorrhage exists when activity is less than 10% of normal. In other words, when prothrombin activity lessens, hypoprothrombinemia increases.

E. *Advantages*

1. Is convenient since it is given by mouth; efficient absorption from gastrointestinal tract.
2. Unnecessary to keep the patient in the hospital.
3. Since it is synthetically produced, dosage and strength are uniform; it is also less expensive than parenteral heparin.

F. *Disadvantages*

1. Effects are unpredictable; dosage varies from one person to another and even from one time to another in the same patient, i.e., decreased liver or kidney function and fever enhance or prolong response. Many drugs enhance or antagonize effects of oral anticoagulants.
2. Because the prothrombin level must be tested frequently, laboratory facilities must be available. (This is often a problem.)

3. There is a cumulative effect:
   Dicumarol has a slow effect (2–3 days) and extended cumulative effect (up to 9 days after last dose).
   Coumadin onset occurs within 18–24 hours; cumulative effect lasts up to 7 days.
   Phenindione onset is within 10–12 hours; effects disappear after 24–48 hours; however, there are side effects with which to reckon.
4. Cannot be quickly counteracted.

G. *Antidotes to Coumarin Anticoagulants*

1. Administer vitamin K—phytonadione (Aquamephyton) by vein, or Mephyton tablets by mouth. Usually brings prothrombin values back to safe levels within 8–24 hours.
2. Provide fresh whole blood if immediate antidote action is required, e.g., physical injury or other emergency.

Nursing Management

1. The preferred method of heparin administration is continuous infusion (using a pump) because of the low incidence of hemorrhagic complications.
2. Check patient's weight, since dosage is calculated on the basis of weight.
3. Be sure clotting profiles are obtained before treatment is initiated, to detect hidden bleeding tendencies.
4. Place pump out of reach of patient to prevent interference with its proper functioning.
   a. Check frequently to ensure that system is working properly: exact dosage, no leaks, no kinks.
5. Note that periodic coagulation tests are done; these include hematocrit and partial thromboplastin time (PTT).
6. Recognize that heparin may be given by *intermittent intravenous injection*. This may be facilitated by the use of a "heparin-lock" (see p. 106).
7. *Minidose heparin* is used in certain patients preoperatively to reduce postoperative thromboembolism (see p. 85).
8. Since heparin may be given along with longer lasting hypoprothrombinemic agents, for the first few days of treatment, each day's medication orders should be checked *after* reports of daily prothrombin time tests are known.
9. Have on hand the antidotes to anticoagulants being used:
   Heparin—protamine sulfate
   Coumarin—phytonadione (vitamin K_1, Aquamephyton, Konakion, Mephyton)
10. Note that the relatively long duration of action of oral anticoagulants makes it easier to maintain low prothrombin levels for long periods.
11. Observe carefully for any possible signs of bleeding and report immediately so that anticoagulant dosage may be reviewed and altered if necessary:
    a. Urine—note evidence of hematuria; indandione derivatives may turn alkaline urine a red orange color—acidifying this urine causes this color to disappear.
    b. Stool—check for tarry color; use Hemoccult test tape for easy rapid checking.
    c. Emesis basin following tooth brushing—note any pink or bloody return.
12. Be aware of the following with regard to sensitivity to coumarin derivatives:

May be intensified by

antibiotics
mineral oil
quinidine
salicylates
tolbutamide (Orinase)

May be decreased by

antacids
barbiturates
oral contraceptives
adrenal corticosteroids

NURSING ALERT: Drug interactions can alter the effect of anticoagulants. Review with the physician the effect of other medications the patient may be taking during anticoagulant therapy.

Patient Education

1. Information to be relayed to the physician before anticoagulant therapy is initiated:
   a. What medications are currently being taken? Note that barbiturates increase metabolism of coumarin medications—therefore an increased dose of anticoagulants is in order.
   b. What treatments are being done for problems other than circulatory problems?
   c. If female, whether a pregnancy is planned or confirmed?
   d. If other treatments are anticipated, such as major dental work, hemorrhoidectomy?
2. During anticoagulant therapy:
   a. Follow instructions carefully and take medications exactly as prescribed.
   b. Take medications at the same time each day and do not stop taking them even though symptomless.
   c. Wear a bracelet or carry a card indicating that anticoagulants are being taken; include name, address, and phone number of physician.
3. Notify the physician:
   a. If you have an accident, infection, or other significant illness that may affect blood clotting.
   b. If surgical care by another physician or dentist is needed. Inform him that you are on anticoagulants.
   c. If you have forgotten to take your anticoagulant. Do not take extra pills to make up for a skipped dose.
   d. If you have diarrhea, upset stomach, high fever.
4. Avoid:
   a. Taking any other medications without first checking with physician, particularly
      (1) vitamins
      (2) aspirin
      (3) mineral oil
      (4) cold medicines
      (5) antibiotics
      (6) phenylbutazone (Butazolidin)
   b. Excessive use of alcohol, since alcohol may affect clotting capacity; check on acceptable limits for social drinking.
   c. Participation in activities in which there is high risk or injury.
   d. Foods that may cause diarrhea or upset stomach.

5. Be alert for these warning signs:
   a. Excessive bleeding that does not stop quickly (such as following shaving, a small cut, teeth brushing with gum injury, nose bleed)
   b. Excessive menstrual bleeding
   c. Skin discoloration or bruises that appear suddenly.
   d. Black or bloody bowel movements; for questionable stool discoloration, use Hemoccult test tape.
   e. Blood in urine.

NOTE: Patients on phenindione produce orange or beige-colored urine; when the urine is acidified, this coloration disappears. With true hematuria, acid does not affect color.
   f. Faintness, dizziness, or unusual weakness.
6. A reminder:
   Later, when anticoagulant medication is stabilized, patient must be reminded to keep prothrombin test appointments as scheduled—once a week or however often they are required.

GUIDELINES: Subcutaneous Injection of Heparin

Purpose   When prolonged therapy is indicated, heparin may be given subcutaneously into fatty tissues (Fig. 9-52).

Equipment   1- or 2-ml. syringe or disposable tuberculin syringe
Fine sharp needle, No. 27, 1.6 cm. (⅝ inch) long (or premeasured Tubex cartridge-needle unit)
Skin antiseptic

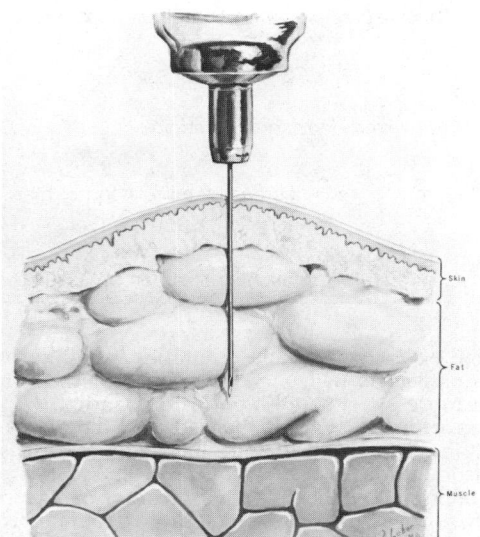

A

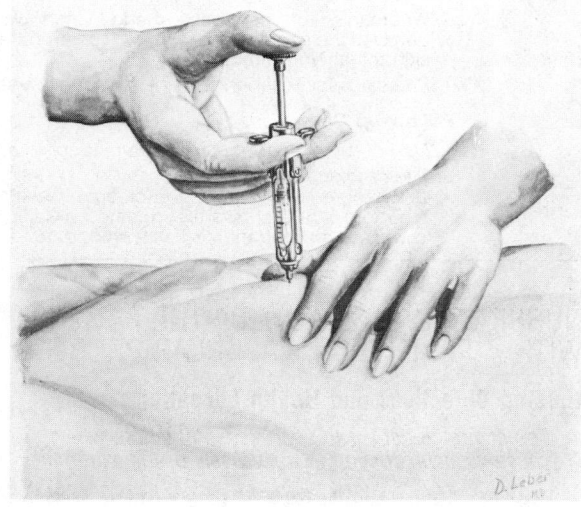

B

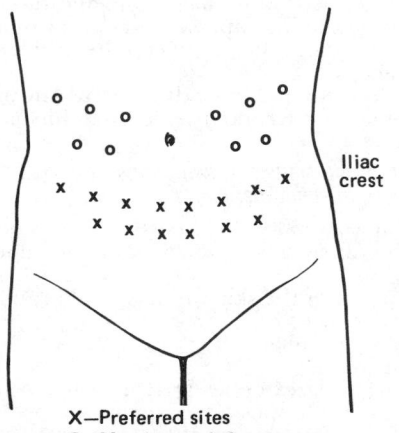

C

X—Preferred sites
O—May be used if necessary

FIGURE 9-52. *Subcutaneous injection indicating technique and sites for heparin therapy. A. When prolonged therapy is indicated, heparin is most conveniently given subcutaneously into the fatty tissue, which is a distinct layer beneath the skin. B. First stretch skin to empty vessels so that they are less apt to be pierced by needle. Then insert the needle directly through the skin at a right angle (see A). C. Since the site of injection of heparin must be changed each time heparin is administered, a suggested division of the abdomen into suitable areas is indicated. Do not inject into a bruised area or within 5 cm. (2 inches) of the umbilicus or any scar. (Courtesy of Wyeth Laboratories, Philadelphia, Pa)*

GUIDELINES: Subcutaneous Injection of Heparin (cont.)

Considerations

1. Most convenient sites are along lower abdominal fat pad—to avoid inadvertent intramuscular injection and hematoma formation.
   a. A common location site is the fatty area anterior to either iliac crest.
   b. Avoid injection sites within 5 cm. (2 inches) of the umbilicus because of possibility of entering a larger blood vessel.
2. Areas where subcutaneous layer is thin should be avoided.

Procedure

NURSING ACTION	RATIONALE/AMPLIFICATION
Performance Phase	
1. Sponge the area gently with alcohol. Do not rub!	1. Rubbing or pinching skin might initiate damage to the tissue; heparin would aggravate any bleeding.
2. Attempt to stretch skin out, using palm of left hand. Some prefer to (gently) pick up a well-defined fold of skin.	2. Try to empty vessels in local area to lessen likelihood of their being pierced by needle—with subsequent hematoma formation.
3. Holding the shaft of the syringe in dart fashion, insert needle directly through the skin at a right angle (Fig. 9-52A) just into the subcutaneous fatty layer.	
4. Move right hand into position to direct plunger. a. Do not move needle tip once it is inserted. b. Do not pull back plunger for testing.	4. Aspiration in a forcible manner can damage small blood vessels and frequently leads to bleeding and hematoma formation, especially in the presence of high local concentration of heparin.
5. Firmly push plunger down as far as it will go. (Fig. 9-52B)	5. This ensures administration of total dose of heparin.
6. When injection has been made, withdraw needle gently at the same angle at which it entered, releasing skin roll as you withdraw.	6. To minimize tissue damage.
7. Press an alcohol sponge to the site for a few seconds.	7. To minimize oozing or bleeding.
Follow-up Care	
1. *Do not rub the area. Instruct patient not to rub area.*	1. Rubbing would increase the likelihood of bleeding.
2. *Site of Injection* a. Change site of injection each time heparin is administered. b. Figure 9-52C shows a suggested division of abdomen into suitable areas. c. A chart can be marked with time, date, and measured dosage so that rotation of sites can be assured.	

NURSING MANAGEMENT OF THE PATIENT WITH A PERIPHERAL VASCULAR PROBLEM

Nursing Objectives and Health Education

A. *To encourage patient to avoid those practices which cause vasoconstriction in the vessels of the extremities.*

1. Impress the patient with the *dangers of smoking,* especially inhaling.
2. Promote an atmosphere that is devoid of emotional tension; restrict those visitors who appear to upset the patient.
3. Maintain a warm and properly humidified environment.
4. Advise the patient against wearing constrictive garments, such as panty girdles, garters, belts, and tight panty hose.
5. Utilize analgesic and tranquilizing medications as required to keep the patient comfortable.

B. *To encourage the following measures and activities to increase the blood flow to the patient's extremities.*

Instruct the patient as follows:
1. Put on warm clothing before going out into cool air; protect hands and feet with lamb's wool lining in gloves and boots to prevent vasoconstriction.
2. Take a warm bath to offset chilling; replace vigorous rubbing of the skin after a bath with gentle patting.
3. Avoid excessive heat to extremities (using hot water bottle, electric pad, etc.)—increases metabolism, so that more oxygenated blood is demanded.
4. Sleep with the head of the bed elevated about 20.3 cm. (8 inches)—if patient has pain at rest; wear bedsocks to keep feet warm if necessary.
5. Walking is the best form of exercise; otherwise, active or passive exercise of the extremities is recommended.
6. Take prescribed vasodilating medications even though they may not appear to help; at times they maintain the status quo and keep the problem from worsening.
7. Take prescribed antilipidic drugs to retard progress of concomitant sclerotic disease by reducing serum lipids.

C. *To recognize the signs and symptoms of circulatory disturbances affecting peripheral tissues.*

1. Pain in the extremity—(Note whether this occurs at rest, with limited activity, or with more pronounced exercise.)
2. Color changes of the skin or nails—pallor, pinkness, rubor, cyanosis
3. Impaired or peculiar growth of nails
4. Shiny, taut skin
5. Discrepancy in size of one extremity when compared to contralateral (opposite) extremity
6. Enlarged veins or abnormal pulsations of veins

7. Temperature variations—abnormally cold or abnormally warm
8. Ulcerations, necrosis, or gangrene

D. *To keep metabolic demands on the body at a minimum.*

Instruct the patient as follows:
1. Take precautions to prevent injury and infection, particularly of the extremities.
2. Practice daily hygienic cleanliness and care of the feet: trim nails properly, avoid strong medications, utilize lamb's wool for pressure areas, wear shoes and hosiery that fit correctly.
3. Avoid exposure to cold or excessive heat.
4. Exercise within recognized limits; set up a reasonable rest plan.
5. Remain in bed if there is evidence of necrosis, ulceration, or gangrene; consult physician.

E. *To encourage the patient to obtain a second opinion if lower-extremity amputation is suggested.*

1. Major vascular centers are reporting commendable results in vascular surgery as an alternative to amputation.
2. Various synthetic graft materials are available for very specific vascular needs.
3. Microsurgery is adding a new dimension to very fine surgical repair.

FOOT CARE IN THE PATIENT WITH A VASCULAR DISORDER

Patient Education

1. Keep the feet clean to prevent irritation and infection.
   a. Wash daily with a bland soap and warm water.
   b. Dry thoroughly, paying particular attention to areas between the toes; pat rather than rub dry.
   c. Apply lanolin or petrolatum to prevent drying and cracking of skin.
   d. Wear clean hose daily: woolen socks for winter, cotton for summer.
2. Avoid injury, excessive pressure, or other irritants to the feet.
   a. Shoes
      (1) Wear properly fitting shoes with a comfortable heel.
      (2) Check inside of shoe; avoid wearing shoes with protruding seams, torn lining, piercing nails, or faulty lumps.
      (3) Wear shoes when out of bed; avoid going barefoot.
      (4) Break in new shoes gradually; alternate with an older pair.
      (5) Leather is preferred to rubber or synthetics

because the latter interfere with proper circulation of air.
      (6) Allow wet or damp shoes to dry slowly on shoe trees to prevent misshaping.
   b. Hose
      (1) Wear proper length and size—if too short, toes are compressed; if too long, wrinkles form and exert pressure on skin.
      (2) Avoid seams, holes, or lumpy darned areas.
      (3) Use bedsocks rather than hot water bottle or heating pad if feet are cold in bed.
      (4) Use woolen or cotton hose; they absorb moisture; nylon is not as absorbent.
      (5) Avoid constricting garments—foundation garments, garters, and even support hose unless they are specifically prescribed.
   c. Pedicure
      (1) Trim toenails straight across after soaking the feet in warm water.
      (2) Place wisps of cotton under corner of great toenail if there is a tendency toward ingrown toenails.
      (3) Have a podiatrist cut corns and calluses; do not use corn pads or strong medications.
   d. Heat and cold
      (1) Keep feet warm; avoid exposure to cold for long periods of time.
      (2) Use heating devices only on advice of physician; excessive heat can be as damaging as insufficient warmth.
      (3) Rely on warm socks, fleece-lined boots or mitts, lightweight blankets, etc. rather than on heating extremities near a fire, oven or radiator.
   e. General measures
      (1) Avoid areas where injury to feet is likely, e.g., crowded subways, construction areas, sports shows, etc.
      (2) Prevent sunburn in the summer and avoid wading in very cold water.
3. Prevent pressure on feet; rest and exercise in moderation.
   a. Place a pillow under covers at end of bed to provide a footrest and prevent weight of top bedding from exerting pressure on toes.
   b. Avoid remaining in one position for long periods of time.
   c. Do not cross legs when sitting because of pressure on nerves and blood vessels.
   d. Elevate feet on a chair or footstool with proper support of leg; do this about 15 minutes every 2 hours.
4. If damage or injury occurs to any part of foot or leg, report to physician.
   a. Redness, swelling, irritation, blistering
   b. Itching, burning—athlete's foot
   c. Bruises, cuts, unusual appearance of skin.

CONDITIONS OF THE VEINS

PHLEBITIS, THROMBOPHLEBITIS, PHLEBOTHROMBOSIS

NOTE: While the terms do not necessarily represent identical pathologies, for clinical purposes they are used interchangeably when discussing the same process.

Phlebothrombosis is the formation of a thrombus or thrombi in a vein; in general the clotting is related to (1) stasis, (2) abnormality of the walls of the vein(s), and (3) abnormality of clotting mechanism. Deep veins of the lower extremities are most commonly involved.
Deep vein thrombosis (DVT) is the thrombosis of deep rather than superficial veins. Two serious complications

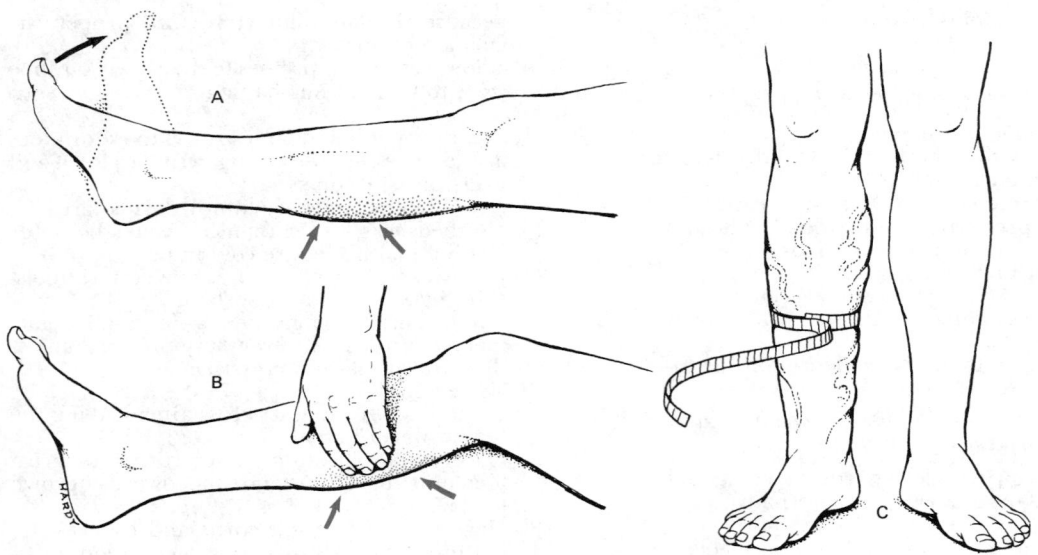

FIGURE 9-53. *Assessment of Signs and Symptoms of Phlebothrombosis. A. With the leg in extension, the patient may complain of pain in the calf on dorsiflexion (Homans' sign)—this was considered an unmistakable sign of early and subclinical thrombosis; it may or may not be present. B. Gentle compression reveals tenderness of the calf muscles (note arrow). C. The affected leg may swell; veins are more prominent and may be palpated easily.*

are pulmonary embolism (p. 344) and postphlebitic syndrome (p. 211).

Phlebitis is an inflammation of the walls of a vein.

Thrombophlebitis is a condition in which a clot forms in a vein secondary to phlebitis or because of partial obstruction of the vein.

Etiology

1. Venous stasis—following operations, childbirth, or bed rest for any chronic illness
2. Prolonged sitting or as a complication of varicose veins
3. Injury (bruise) to a vein; may result from direct trauma to veins from IV injections, indwelling catheters
4. Extension of an infection of tissues surrounding the vessel
5. Continuous pressure of a tumor, aneurysm, heavy pregnancy
6. Unusual activity in a person who has been sedentary
7. Hypercoagulability associated with malignant disease, blood dyscrasias

Basically, there are 3 causes: stasis, injury to a vessel wall, and hypercoagulability (or a combination of these factors).

Clinical Manifestations

1. For phlebothrombosis there are no clinical signs, since there is no inflammation.
2. Slight swelling around ankle; obvious prominence of leg veins in affected leg.
3. Calf pain may be aggravated when foot is dorsiflexed with the leg extended (Fig. 9-53A). Unfortunately, this is not a clear sign of early or positive thrombosis. In some patients with obvious thrombophlebitis, the sign is not present and in other kinds of involvement

(irritation of sciatic nerve roots and myositis) the sign may be positive.
4. Muscle ache—may be falsely assumed to result from wearing flat bedroom slippers postoperatively (Fig. 9-53B).

NURSING ALERT: Do not massage the leg; this may dislodge blood clot and cause pulmonary embolism.

Preventive Measures

1. Encourage early ambulation of surgical patients—encourage leg exercises for the bedridden patient, to prevent venous stasis.
2. Suggest deep breathing exercises that produce increased negative pressure in the thorax, which in turn assists in emptying large veins.
3. Recommend properly applied elastic stockings to increase deep venous blood circulation. (Remove twice daily and check for skin changes or calf tenderness.)
4. Electrical stimulation of calf and pneumatic compression of leg.
5. Use of oral anticoagulants preoperatively; not usually done because of fear of increasing possibility of hemorrhage during operation. Mini-doses of heparin may be prescribed.
6. Prophylactic measures for bedridden patients who are prone to develop thrombosis:
   a. Lie in bed in the slightly reversed Trendelenburg position because it is better for the veins to be full of blood than empty.

b. Place a footboard across the foot of the bed.
c. Instruct patient to press the balls of the feet against the footboard, just as if he were rising up on his toes.
d. Then have patient relax the foot.
e. Request that patient do this many times a day.

High-Risk Factors

1. Hip fracture
2. Prosthetic joint replacement
3. Malignancy
4. Major surgery after age 40
5. Acute myocardial infarction
6. Thrombotic cerebrovascular accident
7. Previous venous insufficiency
8. Contraceptives (oral)

Nursing Assessment

1. Inspect the lower extremities by removing top bedding from foot end up to patient's groin (remove any temperature-controlling devices such as heavy wool socks, ice bag, at least 10 minutes before clinical inspection.
2. Note symmetry or asymmetry
   Measure and record calf circumference daily (Fig. 9-53C)—mark on skin with felt tip pen where the measuring tape is used so that the same area is measured each time.
3. Observe for evidence of venous distention or edema, puffiness, stretched skin, hardness to touch.
4. Hand test extremities for temperature variations.
   a. The examiner's hands should be placed in cold water and then dried.
   b. Hands are then placed simultaneously on each leg—first compare ankles, then move to the calf and up to the knee.
5. Examine for signs of obstruction due to occluding thrombus:
Swelling, particularly in loose connective tissue of popliteal space, ankle, or suprapubic area

Nursing Management

OBJECTIVES: to achieve early resolution of thrombi and prevention of sequelae.
1. Avoid massaging or rubbing calf because of the danger of breaking up the clot, which can then circulate as an embolus.

2. Check with physician concerning proper position of the extremity, since there may be differences of opinion.
   a. Some recommend elevation—reduces venous congestion and edema.
   b. Others do not recommend elevation—because of possibility of releasing emboli.
3. If prescribed, apply heat in the form of hot wet dressings or a heat cradle to promote circulation and comfort.
4. Place the patient on anticoagulant therapy (see p. 336).

Health Education

OBJECTIVES: to increase venous return from lower extremities.
to avoid further injury to damaged vessel walls.

1. Prevent venous stasis by proper positioning in bed.
   a. Support full length of legs when they are to be elevated. (Fig. 9-54)
   b. Prevent bony prominence of one leg from pressing on soft tissue of other leg (in side-lying position, place a soft pillow between legs).
   c. Avoid hyperflexion at knee as in jackknife position (head up, knees up, pelvis and legs down); this promotes stasis in pelvis and extremities.
2. Initiate active exercises, *unless contraindicated,* in which case use passive exercises.
   a. If patient is on bed rest:
      (1) Simulate walking if lying on back—5 minutes every 2 hours.
      (2) Simulate bicycle pedaling if lying on side—5 minutes every 2 hours.
   b. If contraindicated, resort to passive exercises—5 minutes every 2 hours.
   c. If permissible, have patient sit up and move to side of bed in sitting position.
      Provide a foot support (stool or chair)—dangling of feet is not desirable, since pressure may be exerted against popliteal vessels and may cause obstruction to blood flow.
   d. If patient is permitted out of bed, encourage him to walk 10 minutes each hour; otherwise carry out passive exercises.
   e. Discourage crossing of legs because compression of vessels can restrict blood flow.

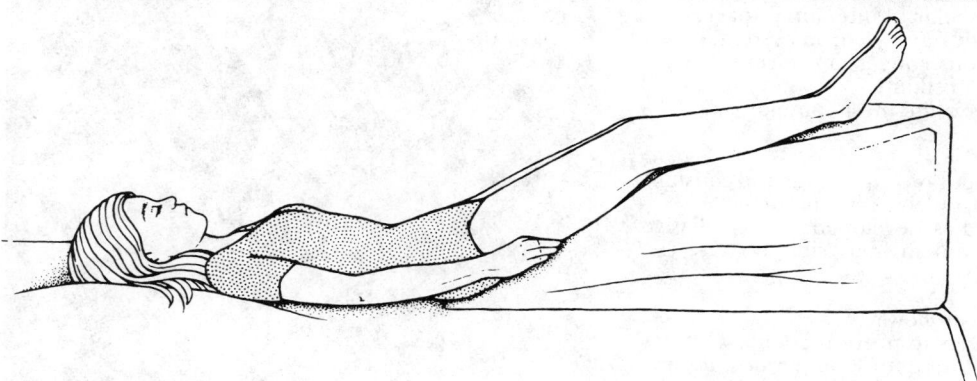

FIGURE 9-54. *This leg elevator is of foam construction with a removable cotton cover that may be machine washed. It is clamped to the lower end of the mattress. This position is anatomically correct and provides adequate support to all parts of the leg. Edema and stasis of the lower extremities can be controlled. (Courtesy of Jobst)*

3. Promote circulation and prevent stasis by applying elastic hose.
   Apply elastic hose or elastic bandage from the toes up the leg; support must be consistent along entire leg.

> **NURSING ALERT:** Elastic hose have no role in the management of the acute phase of deep venous thrombosis, but are of value once ambulation has commenced. Their use will minimize or delay the development of the postphlebitic syndrome.

4. Avoid straining or any maneuver that increases venous pressure in the leg.
   Eliminate the necessity to strain at stool by providing increased bulk in the diet, and administer stool softeners if necessary.
5. Also follow Nursing Objectives in Management of the Patient with Peripheral Vascular Disease (p. 340).

CHRONIC VENOUS INSUFFICIENCY (POSTPHLEBITIC SYNDROME)

Postphlebitic syndrome is a form of chronic venous stasis; it may be a residual effect of phlebitis. It results from chronic occlusion of the veins or destruction of the valves.

Etiology

1. Smaller vessels have dilated because main channel for returning blood from the leg to the heart was blocked by a thrombus.
2. Valves of diseased veins can no longer prevent backflow, thereby leading to → chronic venous stasis → swelling and edema → superficial varicose veins.
3. Lower leg becomes discolored due to venous stasis and pigmentation ulceration (postphlebitis).

Altered Physiology and Clinical Manifestations

1. Pressure in veins at ankle is much greater than normal when leg is dependent—leads to transudation of fluid from intravascular to interstitial space.
2. Stasis, intractable induration, chronic edema, discoloration, pain, venous congestion, ulceration, recurrent thrombosis → cellulitis.
3. The medial malleolus is the most common site.

Management

1. Best treatment is prevention of phlebitis and constant use of compression if phlebitis has occurred.
2. After this syndrome has developed, only palliative and symptomatic treatment is possible because the damage is irreparable.
3. Health Education
   Instruct the patient as follows:
   a. Wear elastic stockings to prevent edema.
   b. Avoid sitting or standing for long periods of time.
   c. Elevate legs on a chair 5 minutes every 2 hours.
   d. Elevate legs above level of head by lying down (2–3 times daily).
   e. Raise foot of bed 15–20 cm. (6–8 inches) at night to allow venous drainage by gravity.

f. Apply bland oily lotions to prevent scaling and dryness of skin.
g. Avoid constricting bandages.
h. Prevent injury, bruising, scratching, or other trauma to skin of leg and foot.

VARICOSE VEINS

Primary varicose veins—bilateral dilatation and elongation of saphenous veins; deeper veins are normal. As the condition progresses, because of hydrostatic pressure and vein weakness, the vein walls become distended with asymmetrical dilatation and some of the valves become incompetent. The process is irreversible.

Incidence

This is a common venous disorder of the lower extremity; 10% of the population is affected.

Etiology

1. Dilatation of the vein prevents the valve cusps from meeting; this results in increased back-up pressure, which is passed into the next lower segment of the vein. The combination of vein dilatation and valve incompetence produces the varicosity (Fig. 9-55).
2. Varicosities may occur elsewhere in the body (esophageal and hemorrhoidal veins) when flow or pressure is abnormally high.
3. Predisposing factors
   a. Hereditary weakness of vein wall or valves
   b. Long-standing distention of veins brought about by pregnancy, obesity, or prolonged standing.
   c. Old age—loss of tissue elasticity

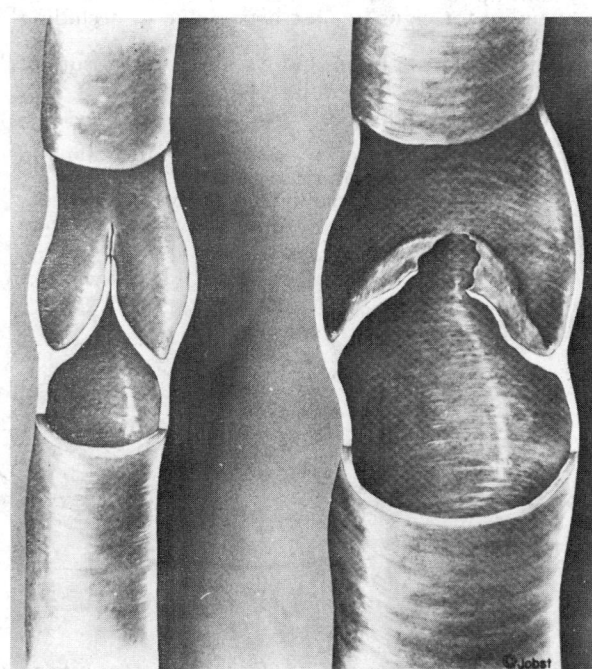

FIGURE 9-55. *Valve incompetence develops as dilatation of a vessel prevents effective approximation of the valve cusps. (Courtesy of Jobst)*

Clinical Manifestations

1. Disfigurement due to large, discolored, tortuous leg veins
2. Easy leg fatigue, cramps in leg, heavy feeling, increased pain during menstruation, nocturnal muscle cramps

Complications

1. Leg edema, pain from superficial thrombosis
2. Hemorrhage due to the weakening of the vein wall and pressure upon it
3. Skin infection and breakdown, producing ulcers (rare in primary varices)

Diagnostic Evaluation

A. *Trendelenburg Test*—for valvular competence

1. Have the patient lie down; elevate leg 65 degrees to allow veins to empty.
2. Apply tourniquet high on upper thigh to constrict superficial veins (not deep veins).
3. Instruct the patient to stand with tourniquet in place.
   a. Veins fill slowly from below in 20-30 seconds. Rate of filling is not accelerated when tourniquet is removed. This is considered normal.
   b. Veins fill rapidly from below. Lower-leg "blow-outs" may be evident. Rate of filling is not accelerated when tourniquet is removed. This indicates the incompetence of the communicating veins of the lower leg.
4. Remove tourniquet
   a. There is a rapid flow of blood down the saphenous vein from above. This is a sign of the incompetence of the valves of the saphenofemoral and superficial veins.
   b. Veins fill as in 3b; in addition, there is rapid flow of blood downward. This indicates the incompetence of the saphenofemoral veins, valves, superficial veins, and valves of communicating veins.

B. *Phlebography*—injection of radiopaque substance into veins, followed by observation of blood flow and valve action via x-ray.

1. If dorsal vein of foot is used, contrast medium usually remains in superficial veins unless tourniquet is used.
2. If dye injection is done directly into medial malleolus to the marrow cavity, regional or general anesthesia is required (because of pain).

Treatment and Nursing Management

OBJECTIVE: to decrease or eliminate blood flow in the affected vessels, forcing the blood to return through deep veins.

A. *Medical Treatment* (nonoperative) *and Health Education*

Patient is instructed to:
1. Avoid activities that cause venous stasis by obstructing venous flow.
   a. Wearing tight garters, tight girdle
   b. Sitting or standing for prolonged periods of time
   c. Crossing the legs at knees for prolonged periods while sitting (reduces circulation by 15%)
2. Control excessive weight gain.
3. Wear firm elastic support as prescribed, from toe to thigh when in upright position. Put elastic stockings on in bed before getting up.

4. Elevate foot of bed 15-20 cm. (6–8 inches) for night sleeping.
5. Avoid injuring legs.

B. *Surgical Treatment*

1. Indications
   a. Progressively advancing varicosities
   b. Stasis ulceration
   c. Cosmetic needs
2. Modalities—A single method or combination of methods is tailored to meet the needs of the individual:
   a. *Sclerosing injection*—not used as frequently today; may be combined with ligation or limited to treatment of isolated varicosities. The affected vessel may be sclerosed by injecting sodium tetradecyl sulfate or similar sclerosing agent. Compression bandage is then applied without interruption for 6 weeks; inflamed endothelial surfaces adhere by direct contact.
   b. *Multiple vein ligation*
   c. *Ligation and stripping* of the greater and/or lesser saphenous systems. This procedure is the most effective.
   d. Some physicians are using the *laser* beam in treating varicosities
3. Preoperative Patient Care
   a. Prepare the skin each day beginning 3 or 4 days prior to surgery by thoroughly cleansing the lower abdomen and legs with a detergent-germicidal soap.
   b. Have patient prepared on the day before surgery (and after his daily skin cleansing) for the surgeon to mark his skin with a felt tip pen (indelible). Usually the patient stands on a chair in proper light so that the incision sites, paths of veins, dilated tributaries, etc., can be marked to aid the surgeon during the operation.
4. Postoperative Nursing Care and Patient Support
   a. Elevate the legs about 30 degrees and provide adequate support of the entire leg.
   b. Observe the patient for complaints of pain in specific areas of the foot or ankle; if the elastic bandage is too tight, loosen the bandage—later, have it reapplied.
   c. Observe circulation to detect constriction or hemorrhage.
   d. Follow the individualized therapeutic plan for the following:
      (1) Permit ambulation according to the preoperative condition of the skin and subcutaneous tissues; if skin is healthy, bathroom privileges are usually permitted the day after surgery.
      (2) Discourage dangling of the legs because it causes stasis of blood in the lower leg.
      (3) Encourage the patient to walk with a normal gait; offer support if necessary; this activity should be progressive, depending on tolerance.
   e. At first the legs are encased in pressure bandages from the toes to the groin; this is followed by knee-level elastic stockings for 3-4 weeks after surgery.
   f. If there are significant trophic changes in the leg, due to long-term varicosities (past history), then postoperative care requires more bed rest and slow ambulation; in this event, leg and foot exercises in bed are helpful.
   g. Note that complaints of patchy numbness can be expected but should disappear in less than a year.

h. Recognize that varicosities may recur; therefore conservative measures, learned preoperatively, should be continued.

STASIS ULCERS

Stasis ulcer is an excavation of the skin surface produced by sloughing of inflammatory necrotic tissue usually caused by vascular insufficiency in the lower extremity.

Incidence

1. Occurrence is increasing, particularly in the older age group.
2. Postphlebitic syndrome and stasis account for most leg ulcers (Fig. 9-56).
3. Other causes include obstruction of one of the main veins by pregnancy or abdominal tumor, incompetency of valves of the ileofemoral vein, burns, sickle-cell anemia, neurogenic disorders.
4. Hereditary factors also play a role in the predisposition of certain individuals.

Prevention

1. Prevent edema
   In stasis dermatitis, pruritus and scaling pigmentation may be the only manifestations; bed rest and a 30-degree elevation of the lower extremity may alleviate the edema.
2. Avoid trauma.

Diagnostic Evaluation

   Phlebography
1. A radiopaque contrast medium is injected into a foot or ankle vein and forced into the deep system.
2. Films are taken before and after exercises.
3. Normal results show intact deep venous circulation and good valves.
4. Exercise clears contrast medium from the deep veins after the test is completed.
   (See also Diagnostic Evaluation of Vascular Conditions, p. 331)

Objectives of Treatment and Nursing Management

A. *To promote rest and reduce the inflammation.*

1. Elevate the leg and maintain bed rest.
2. Initiate proper cleansing routine.
   a. Handle leg very gently.
   b. Use mild soap, warm water, and cotton balls.
3. Remove devitalized tissue.
   a. Flush out necrotic materials with hydrogen peroxide.
   b. Apply enzymatic ointments such as fibrinolysin and desoxyribonuclease, combined-bovine (Elase), and proteolytic enzymes with neomycin (Biozyme) (prescribed in some clinics).

B. *To stimulate healing by reducing the infection and providing physiological and nutritional support.*

1. Again, elevation of the extremity is most important.
2. Participate in physiotherapy and maintain a regular exercise program.
3. Control excess weight and provide proper vitamin and protein dietary supplements.
4. Apply gold leaf (done in some clinics) directly over ulcer site to stimulate formation of granulation tissue.
5. Check with individual physician for specific therapy; treatment varies from clinic to clinic.

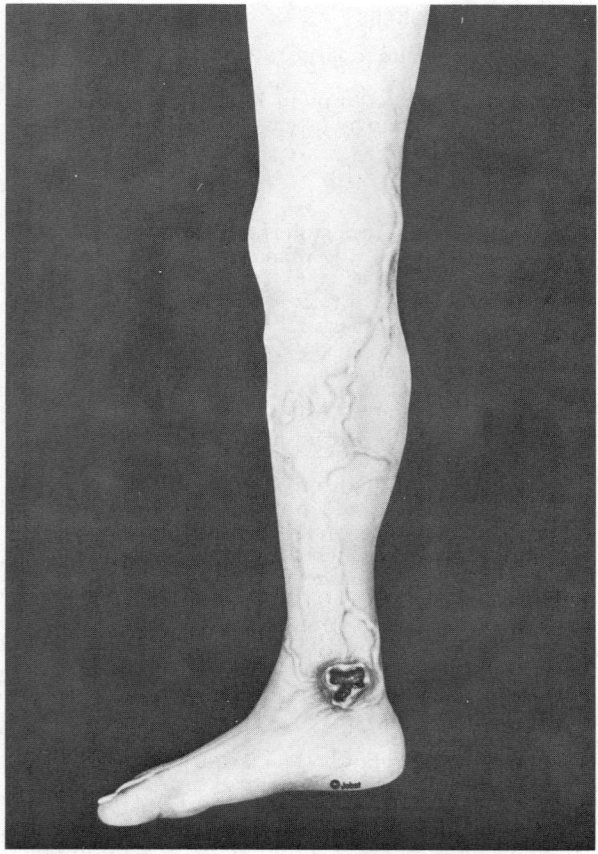

FIGURE 9-56. *Diagram showing leg ulcer resulting from concomitant postphlebitis and varicose veins. (Courtesy of Jobst)*

C. *To stimulate and maintain healthy tissue in the skin surrounding the ulcer.*

1. Use sterile saline compresses if area is inflamed or oozing.
2. Apply compression bandages to the leg (gelatin compression boot—Fig. 9-57).

D. *To encourage the patient who is likely to get discouraged during prolonged treatment.*

1. Stress the importance of following explicitly the recommendations of the physician-nurse team.
2. Explain the hazards of trying other remedies on his own at home.
3. Indicate that the treatment may be long but that patience is an important aspect.
4. Maintain healthy tissue when the ulcer is healed by continuing with the safeguards practiced before, because breakdown of healthy tissue unfortunately is frequent.

E. *Health Education.* (See Objectives A, B, C, D, above.)

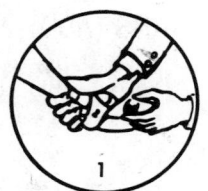 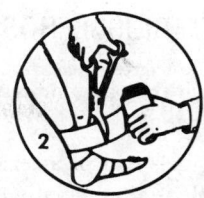 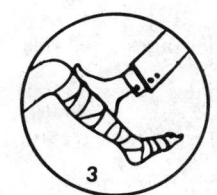 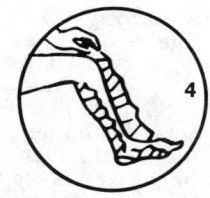

1. Apply right from can. Hold knee in slight flexion. Pad instep and ankle with cotton wad. Start at inner ankle. Make overlapping turns. Figure of eight turn around ankle joint. Use firm equal compression up to the knee.

2. If a turn does not fit snugly, nip the edges with scissors or cut bandage off and start a new turn.

3. Mold cast during application with free hand until cast appears even and smooth. Make a cut 5 cm. (2") long below knee to avoid constriction. Cover cast with loosely woven gauze bandage.

4. Patient can be fully ambulatory. Boot is usually changed once a week. Remove by cutting with scissors.

FIGURE 9-57. *Application of gelatin compression boot. (Manufactured by Graham-Field Surgical Co., Inc., New Hyde Park, NY)*

CONDITIONS OF THE ARTERIES

ARTERIAL EMBOLISM

Causes

1. Arterial emboli usually (about 85%) originate from thrombi in the heart chambers.
2. Arteriosclerosis may cause roughening or ulceration of atheromatous plaques which can lead to emboli.

Clinical Manifestations

1. May vary from the patient's being totally unaware of the event, to
2. Acute pain—severe
3. Loss of function—motor and sensory
   a. Paralysis of part ⎤ Due to embolic block of
   b. Anesthesia of part ⎬ artery
   c. Pallor and coldness ⎦ Due to associated vasomotor reflex

Treatment and Nursing Management

1. Heparin should be administered intravenously to reduce tendency of emboli to form or expand—useful in smaller arteries.
2. Protect the extremity by keeping it at or below the horizontal plane; protect leg from hard surfaces and tight or heavy overlying bed linens.
3. Administer analgesics as prescribed for relief of pain.
4. Prepare patient for surgery; surgical intervention (embolectomy) is essential when an embolus blocks a large artery, such as the iliac.

NOTE: This is an emergency and is life-threatening; it requires immediate operative intervention if the embolus has major effect.

5. Postoperative nursing management
   a. Encourage activity in the leg to prevent stasis—obtain specific recommendations from surgeon concerning type and duration of exercises.
   b. Administer anticoagulants with full knowledge of what to watch for.
      (1) Inspect for bleeding anywhere, including surgical wound; this may be indicative of overdose of heparin.
      (2) Monitor vital signs.
      (3) Recognize cardiovascular history of this patient; hence be able to assess cardiac and circulatory manifestations.

Prognosis

1. Arterial embolism is a threat not only to the extremity (5-25% possibility of amputation) but also to the patient (15-40% mortality rate).
2. Mortality rate increases because of cardiac disease; development of gangrene also contributes to increase in number of deaths.
3. Other cardiovascular difficulties compound the problem.

ARTERIOSCLEROSIS AND ATHEROSCLEROSIS

Arteriosclerosis is an arterial disease manifested by a loss of elasticity and a hardening of the vessel wall.

Atherosclerosis is the most common type of arteriosclerosis, manifested by the formation of atheromas (patchy lipoidal degeneration of the intima).

Significance

1. Arteriosclerosis is the chief cause of death in the U.S.
2. One of the major clinical manifestations of arteriosclerosis is coronary heart disease.
3. Studies indicate that arteriosclerotic heart disease is partially preventable if attention is paid to "risk" factors.

Etiology and Risk Factors

(A combination of many factors)
1. Predisposition to arteriosclerosis is thought by many authorities to be inheritable (genetics).
2. Other etiologic factors include metabolic disturbances, arterial hypertension, platelet capability of initiating formation of atherosclerotic lesions.

3. Risk Factors
   a. Age—death rate in white males (ages 25–34) is 10 per 100,000
      death rate in white males (ages 55–64) is 1000 per 100,000
   b. Sex—death rate (ages 35–44) is 6 times greater in white males than in females.
   c. Impaired glucose tolerance (diabetes mellitus)
   d. Hypertension
   e. A relatively large amount of cholesterol in the low-density lipoprotein fraction (serum).
   f. Obesity
   g. Cigarette smoking
   h. Physical inactivity—since substantial collateral circulation is not established.
   i. Emotional tension

Altered Physiology

1. Arteriosclerosis → narrowing of arterial vessels → malnutrition of tissue cells → ischemic necrosis → fibrosis → sclerosis.
2. Sclerosis → degeneration of major organs due to lack of blood supply (nutrition): brain, myocardium, kidney.
3. Calcium deposits in tunica media of arterial vessel cause loss of elasticity.
4. Atheromas (plaque-like deposits) of cholesterol, fatty acids, and often calcium form on intima of arterial vessels (atherosclerosis).
5. Dislodging of plaque may occur or a thrombus may be formed near the plaque; subsequent embolus may cause arterial occlusion and infarction in distant body sites.
6. After menopause, women are no longer protected by estrogen.

General Patient Assessment

1. Arteriosclerosis is a generalized vascular disease; however, it varies from patient to patient in that it may affect one area more than another.
2. Often it limits itself to a segment of the vascular tree.
3. Five areas which are the most dangerous and cause disturbing symptoms are:
   a. Brain—cerebroarteriosclerosis
   b. Heart—coronary artery disease
   c. Gastrointestinal tract
   d. Kidneys
   e. Extremities
4. Prognosis depends on extent of pathology and area of involvement.

Treatment

1. Since arteriosclerosis and atherosclerosis affect many different parts of the body, treatment is described where the major condition occurs. For example: angina pectoris and myocardial infarction are brought about by atherosclerosis of coronary arteries; treatment is discussed under the disease entity (p. 284).
2. Operative reconstruction of involved vessels.

Health Education

Attention is directed to reducing risk factors by avoiding tension, reducing excess weight, giving up cigarette smoking, controlling diabetes, and adjusting diet to reduce cholesterol intake (Table 9-3).

ARTERIOSCLEROSIS OBLITERANS (ASO)

Arteriosclerosis obliterans is a form of arteriosclerosis in which the vascular system of the leg becomes blocked.

Incidence

Parallels that of arteriosclerotic heart disease.

Clinical Manifestations

Symptoms appear gradually
1. Intermittent claudication (see p. 331)
2. Coldness of extremity
3. Color change—pallor
4. Decrease in size of leg
5. Tingling, numbness of toes
6. Later—pain, even when leg is at rest; occurs at night, requiring patient to get out of bed to walk to relieve pain
7. Cramp-like excruciating pain in calf muscles
8. Ulcers of toes and feet develop

Diagnostic Evaluation

1. Vascular physical examination
2. Doppler ultrasound probe
3. Segmental plethysmograph
4. Angiography

Treatment and Nursing Management

OBJECTIVES: to preserve the extremity.
to relieve the intermittent claudication.
See page 333, General Management of the Patient with a Peripheral Vascular Problem.
1. Where conservative measures clearly are not enough, grafting is the treatment of choice.
2. If the arteriogram does not show a suitable situation for grafting, a sympathectomy may be done.

VASOPASTIC DISORDER—RAYNAUD'S PHENOMENON

Raynaud's phenomenon is a condition in which there is an increased or unusual sensitivity to cold or emotional factors, and occurs primarily in the hands, rarely in the feet.

Etiology

1. Unknown; there appears to be a hereditary predisposition.
2. Vasoconstriction appears to be mediated through release of the catecholamines at neuro-arteriole junction.
3. An underlying problem such as a collagen vascular disease may exist.

Clinical Manifestations

1. Intermittent arteriolar vasoconstriction resulting in coldness, pain, pallor.
2. Occasionally there is ulceration of the finger tips.
3. The condition occurs most commonly in females between the age 16 and 40 years.
4. It occurs more frequently in cold climates and during winter months.
5. Involvement of the fingers appear to be asymmetric; thumbs are less often involved.
6. Characteristic color changes: Blue–white–red
   a. Blue—cyanotic, relatively stagnant blood flow

TABLE 9-3. FAT-CONTROLLED, LOW CHOLESTEROL DIET

A variety of foods may be selected from each of the Basic Four Food Groups.
Emphasize those foods listed in the left hand "Suggested" column.

Meat, poultry, fish, dried beans and peas, eggs. Adults may be allowed 2 or more servings (up to 6 to 8 oz) daily

Suggested	*Avoid or Use Infrequently*
Most often: 　Chicken, turkey, veal, fish, shellfish (except shrimp)	Duck, goose, shrimp (substitute shrimp for red meat or egg once a week if desired*)
A few times a week: 　Very lean beef, lamb, pork, ham 　All visible meat fat is discarded	Fatty meats, e.g., heavily marbled beef, spare ribs, frankfurters, sausage, bacon, bologna, and other lunch meats, regular hamburger. 　Organ meats (substitute liver for red meat or for egg once a week if desired*)
Dried peas, beans, lentils—prepared with allowed ingredients Peanut butter in moderation Egg whites as desired	Beans prepared with salt pork or bacon Egg yolks: limit to 3 per week*

Vegetables and fruit—at least 4 servings daily, including surces of vitamins C and A

Suggested	*Avoid or Use Infrequently*
All types of fruits and vegetables may be used (unless prepared with restricted ingredients): fresh, frozen, canned, dried	Vegetables in butter, cream, or cheese sauce Vegetables fried in saturated fat

---

Bread and cereals (whole grain, enriched, or fortified—at least 4 servings daily)

Suggested	*Avoid or Use Infrequently*
Breads: whole wheat, rye, pumpernickel, oatmeal, white enriched, French, Italian, raisin, English muffins, bagels, hard rolls Cereal (hot or cold), rice, bulghur, barley Pasta Melba toast, matzo, pretzels Biscuit, muffins, etc., made at home using allowed ingredients	Egg bread, cheese bread Commercial biscuits, muffins, donuts, butter rolls, sweet rolls Commercial granola, Cracklin' Bran Egg noodles Snack crackers Commercial mixes containing dried eggs, whole milk and/or shortening

---

Milk products. Adults should use 500 ml (2 or more cups) or the equivalent daily

Suggested	*Avoid or Use Infrequently*
Skim milk dairy products: fortified skim (nonfat) milk or milk powder, buttermilk, evaporated skim milk, chocolate flavored skim milk Acceptable in some cases: low fat milk and yogurt Cheeses made from skim milk: cottage cheese, farmer's, baker's, or hoop cheese, sapsago cheese Occasionally allowed: cheeses made from part-skim milk such as part-skim mozarella	Whole milk and whole milk products: chocolate milk, canned evaporated whole milk, ice cream, cream of any type, whole milk yogurt Most nondairy cream substitutes Cheeses made from cream or whole milk

---

Fats and oils (polyunsaturated).
Adults are often allowed about 30–60 ml (2–4 Tbsp) daily (depending on caloric needs), including oil used in cooking

Suggested	*Avoid or Use Infrequently*
Polyunsaturated vegetable oils: corn oil, cottonseed oil, safflower oil, sesame seed oil, soybean oil, sunflower seed oil Margarines and liquid oil shortenings made with an allowed oil and having a high P/S ratio (i.e., about 2:1 or above) Salad dressings made with allowed ingredients, mayonnaise	Solid fats and shortenings: butter, hard margarine and vegetable shortening with a low P/S ratio (i.e., 3:2 or lower), lard, salt pork, meat fat, coconut oil, palm oil (Peanut oil and olive oil are not saturated or polyunsaturated. They may be used occasionally for flavor.) Creamy and cheese salad dressings

---

Desserts, beverages, snacks, condiments

Acceptable If Calories Allow	*Avoid or Use Infrequently*
Cocoa powder, fruit whip, gelatin, puddings made with nonfat milk, water ice, sherbet Jelly, jam, marmalade, honey, hard candy, angel food cake, most types of nuts Homemade baked desserts using allowed ingredients Carbonated beverages, fruit drinks, wine,† beer,† whisky†	Chocolate, whole milk puddings, ice cream (ice milk is sometimes allowed) Chocolate candy, caramels, butterscotch Coconut, macadamia nuts, cashews Commercial cakes, pies, cookies, and mixes Potato chips and other commercial fried snacks

Negligible Calorie Content

Tea, herb tea, coffee,† decaffeinated coffee
Herbs, spices, vinegar, mustard, small amounts of ketchup and barbecue sauce, horseradish, meat sauce, soy sauce

---

* When allowed a total of 300 mg cholesterol or more daily
† With approval of physician
Suitor CW and Hunter MF. Nutrition: Principles and Application in Health Promotion pp 455–456 Philadelphia, JB Lippincott Co. 1980

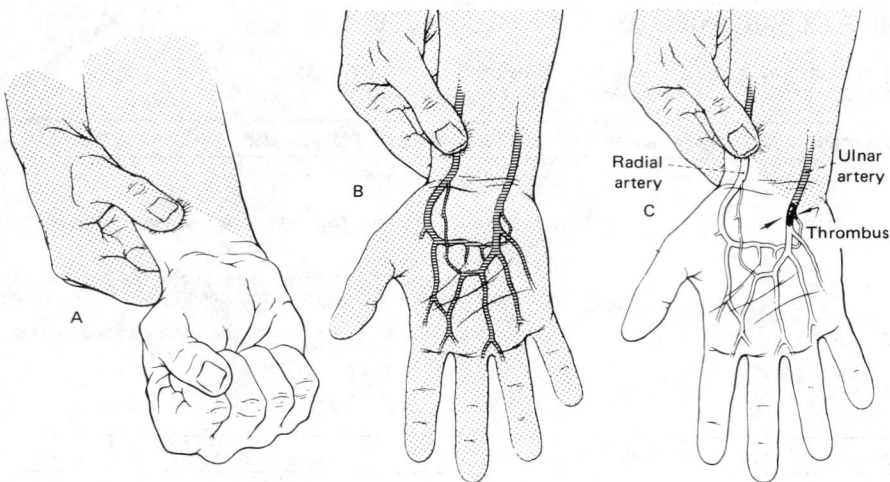

FIGURE 9-58. *Allen test: Diagrammatic representation of the procedure (A) for determining patency of occlusion of the ulnar artery distal to the wrist.*
B. The ulnar artery is patent as determined by the prompt return of color to the skin of the hand while the radial artery is still compressed.
C. Occlusion of the ulnar artery is demonstrated by persistence of pallor as long as the radial arterial inflow is blocked by the examiner's finger. (Modified from Juergens and Fairbairn. Arteriosclerosis Obliterans. Heart Bulletin 8:22–24. By permission of the American Heart Association)

  b. White—blanching, dead-white appearance if spasm is severe
  c. Red—a reactive hyperemia upon rewarming.
7. The Allen test may provide clues to circulatory problems. (Fig. 9-58)

Nursing Management

1. Prime objective is to avoid whatever provokes vasoconstriction.
2. Minimize exposure to cold, since this precipitates a reaction.
3. Suggest the wearing of warm clothing—boots, gloves, hooded jackets, when going out in cold weather.
  a. Turn heat on in automobile during travel.
  b. Shop in heated stores; avoid unheated buildings.
4. Avoid placing hands in cold water, the freezer, or the refrigerator unless protective gloves are worn.
5. Use extra precautions to avoid injuries to fingers and hands from needle pricks, knife cuts.
6. Varying benefits are reported with such medications as reserpine, methyldopa, tolazoline (Priscoline) and phenoxybenzamine (Dibenzyline).

Medication	Adverse Effects
1. Phenoxybenzamine Hydrochloride (Dibenzyline)	Headache, tachycardia, nasal congestion, orthostatic hypotension.
2. Cyclandelate (Cyclospasmol)	Headache, nausea, heavier than usual perspiration, vertigo, flushing, tingling.
3. Tolazoline Hydrochloride (Priscoline)	Gastrointestinal upset, orthostatic hypotension, chilliness, tachycardia, palpitations.

Health Education

1. Think through the possible causative factors which provoke a spasm; these should be avoided.
2. Utilize insulating clothing when it is necessary to go out into the cold: wool gloves and socks, fleece-lined boots and footwear, etc.
3. Avoid exposing hands to cold objects, e.g., reaching into the freezer, handling a cold, ice-filled glass, etc.
4. Give up smoking; consider moving to a warmer climate, if possible.

DISEASES OF THE AORTA

AORTITIS

Aortitis is inflammation of the aorta—usually of the aortic arch.

Types of Aortitis

A. *Arteriosclerotic Aortitis*

1. Accompanies the generalized disease of arteriosclerosis.
2. Appears after the age of 60, usually—may occur earlier.
3. May cause pain, dilatation (aneurysm), aortic valve insufficiency.
4. Degeneration and sclerosis of entire surface of intima occur.

B. *Syphilitic Aortitis*

1. Appears before age 50.
2. Begins at root of aorta and spreads in patch-like

areas over normal intima to involve aorta, aortic arch.
3. Symptoms are variable—may be severe or mild.
   a. Sensations of substernal oppression or weight (viselike pains).
   b. Sudden attacks of dyspnea may be agonizing and last 5–15 minutes.
      Accompanied by tachycardia, deep cyanosis, profuse perspiration.
   c. Symptoms lead to aortic insufficiency and aneurysms which may erode bone.

Diagnostic Evaluation

Aortic insufficiency without associated mitral lesion, paroxysmal dyspnea, anginal attacks, or aneurysm suggest syphilitic aortitis.

Management and Prognosis

1. Antisyphilitic therapy for syphilitic aortitis (see p. 823).
2. Damage cannot be repaired completely—may require graft and prosthetic valve.

AORTIC ANEURYSM

Aneurysm is a distention of an artery.

Types of Aneurysms

Morphologically, they may be classified as follows:
1. Saccular—distention of a vessel projecting from one side.
2. Fusiform—distention of the whole artery, i.e., entire circumference is involved.

Etiology

1. Local infection, pyogenic or fungal (mycotic aneurysm)
2. Congenital weakness of vessels
3. Arteriosclerosis
4. Syphilis
5. Trauma

Thoracic Aneurysm

A. *Clinical Manifestations*

1. Subjective Symptoms
   a. At first no symptoms; later symptoms may come from congestive heart failure or a pulsating tumor mass in the chest.
   b. Pain and pressure symptoms
      (1) Constant, boring pain because of pressure, or
      (2) Intermittent and neuralgic pain because of infringement on nerves
   c. Dyspnea causing pressure against trachea
   d. Cough, often paroxysmal and brassy in sound
   e. Hoarseness, voice weakness, or complete aphonia resulting from pressure against recurrent laryngeal nerve
   f. Dysphagia due to impingement on esophagus
2. Objective Signs
   a. Edema of chest wall—infrequent
   b. Dilated superficial veins on chest
   c. Cyanosis because of vein compression of chest vessels

d. Ipsilateral dilatation of pupils due to pressure against cervical sympathetic chain
e. Pulse difference in 2 wrists if aneurysm interferes with circulation in left subclavian artery
f. Abnormal pulsation may be apparent on chest wall—due to erosion of aneurysm through rib cage—in syphilis

B. *Management*

1. The prognosis is poor for untreated patients.
2. Surgical—remove aneurysm and restore vascular continuity.
   Aortic arch aneurysms are the most difficult to treat.

Abdominal Aneurysm

A. *Clinical Manifestations*

1. About ⅔ of these patients display symptoms; the rest are asymptomatic.
2. Abdominal pain is most common; persistent or intermittent—often localized in middle or lower abdomen to the left of midline.
3. Low back pain.
4. Feeling of an abdominal pulsating mass.
5. Hypertension may be in evidence.

B. *Diagnostic Evaluation*

1. Ordinarily the systolic blood pressure of the thigh exceeds that in the arm; in many of these patients, the opposite is true.
2. A palpable pulsating abdominal mass; fluoroscopy will reveal pulsating tumor.
3. Angioaortogram allows visualization of vessels and aneurysm.
4. Ultrasound allows visualization of vessels and aneurysm.
   This is the best test to confirm the presence of and check the size of abdominal aortic aneurysms. It is less expensive than other tests.
5. Computed tomography allows visualization of vessels and aneurysm.

C. *Treatment and Nursing Management*

1. If untreated, the prognosis is poor.
2. Abdominal aortic aneurysm
   a. Surgery to excise area affected.
   b. Replacement of excised segment by a bypass (synthetic) graft.

Dissecting Aneurysm of the Aorta

a. This is a type of aneurysm in which there is a tear in the intima of the aorta; as a result of pressure, blood splits the wall and may produce a large hematoma or may continue to rip the wall.
b. Symptoms may resemble coronary occlusion; diagnosis is confirmed by aortography.
c. Prognosis is poor, but surgical removal of involved aneurysm and replacement of segment with a graft may be effective.

Peripheral Vessel Aneurysms

a. May involve renal artery, subclavian artery, popliteal artery (knee) or any major artery.
b. These produce a pulsating mass and may cause pain or pressure on surrounding structures.
c. Replacement grafts are used to repair these aneurysms.

HYPERTENSION

Hypertension is a disease of regulation in which the mechanisms that control arterial pressure within the normal range are deranged. Predominant mechanisms are the central nervous system, the renal pressor system (renin–angiotensin–aldosterone system), extracellular fluid volume. Why these mechanisms fail is not known. Basic explanation is that blood pressure is elevated when there is increased cardiac output plus peripheral vessel resistance.

Essential hypertension refers to patients (over 90%) with high blood pressure of undetermined cause.

Community Health Concern

1. Undetected and uncontrolled hypertension can lead to heart attacks, heart failure, strokes, and renal failure.
2. Few patients with hypertension need to be hospitalized.
3. Most patients with hypertension do not have symptoms.
4. Most patients with hypertension need life-long treatment.
5. Early recognition and management of hypertension are essential in preventing end organ damage (brain, eye, heart, kidney).
6. The nurse is a prime agent in early detection of hypertension and patient education.

Normal Physiology

1. *Normal blood pressure* (normotension) is the pressure of the blood within the systemic arterial system. It ranges from 100/60 to 140/90.
2. *Systolic pressure* represents the greatest pressure of the blood against the wall of the vessel following ventricular contraction.
3. *Diastolic pressure* represents the least pressure of the blood against the wall of the vessel following closure of the aortic valve.
4. *Pulse pressure* represents the difference between the systolic and diastolic readings—the range of pressure in the arteries.
5. The *mean arterial pressure* is the average pressure attempting to push blood through the circulatory system.
   This can be determined electronically or mathematically as well as by using an intra-arterial catheter and mercury manometer.
   Mathematical determination. (Slightly less than average of systolic and diastolic.)
      Example: for a blood pressure of 130/85
      Mean arterial pressure is roughly 100 mm. Hg
      Kidney function requires a minimum of 70 mm. Hg (mean arterial pressure).
6. *Basal blood pressure* is the lowest blood pressure taken in supine position after several days of hospitalization without treatment.*

*Most hypertensive patients admitted to the hospital are admitted for nonhypertension-related problems, i.e., breast biopsy, total hip replacement, etc. These patients are not routinely taken off their antihypertensive medications. If patient is admitted for evaluation of secondary hypertension or refractory hypertension, then all antihypertensive medications are cancelled and basal pressures are obtained. All patients going on to investigational antihypertensive medication are, if possible, "washed out" (medications cancelled for several days); most studies are done with these persons as outpatients.

Basal sitting pressure and basal standing pressure are often taken for later comparison.

Factors Affecting Pressure of Blood

Blood volume, peripheral resistance, blood viscosity, cardiac output.
1. Blood pressure = cardiac output × total peripheral resistance.
   a. Pressure varies with exercise, emotional reaction, sleep, digestion, time of day.
   b. Renal, adrenal, vascular, and neurogenic functions affect blood pressure.
2. Higher blood pressure = increased cardiac output × greater total peripheral resistance (circulatory overload).
3. Lower blood pressure = lessened cardiac output × lesser total peripheral resistance.
4. Increased diastolic pressure due to peripheral resistance indicates decrease in diameter of arterioles: These are affected by sympathetic stimulation, hereditary factors, more vasopressor hormones in the blood.
5. Increased systolic pressure indicates increased cardiac output and systolic hypertension, which is always secondary.

Etiology and the Significance of Blood Pressure Elevation

1. Cause of essential hypertension is unknown; however, there are several areas of investigation:
   a. Hyperactivity of sympathetic vasoconstricting nerves
   b. Presence of blood component which contains a vasoconstrictor that acts on smooth muscle, sensitizing it to constrictor substances
   c. Increased cardiac output followed by arteriole constriction
   d. Prostaglandins affect regulatory mechanisms, which include the renin–angiotensin system, renal sodium and water excretion, and vascular smooth muscle tone.
   e. Familial (genetic) tendency.
   f. Hypertensive vascular disease: Modifications of both large elastic arteries (macroangiopathy) and small muscular arteries and arterioles (microangiopathy).
2. Individual tolerance of increased blood pressure varies; however, there is a direct correlation between increase in blood pressure and the rate at which atherosclerosis and arteriosclerosis develop.
3. Rising blood pressure adversely affects the brain, the heart, and the kidneys.
   a. Heart—myocardial infarction, congestive heart failure
   b. Kidney—nephrosclerosis, kidney failure
   c. Brain—headache (in some persons), encephalopathy, cerebral hemorrhage, cerebrovascular accident
   d. Eye—papilledema, swelling of optic disc
4. Emotional stress affects the central nervous system, and there may be increased cardiac output; increased catecholamines, etc., may account for increased peripheral vascular resistance.
5. Obesity and diabetes mellitus are associated with hypertension.

Prevalence and Risk Factors

1. Hypertension is one of the most prevalent chronic diseases for which treatment is available.
2. There is a higher incidence in the black race (2:1 ratio).
3. It appears that a high sodium intake is related to the development of hypertension; when sodium intake is decreased, blood pressure often decreases.
4. Increase in incidence is associated with the following risk factors:
   a. Age: between 30 and 70
   b. Race: black
   c. Birth control pills and estrogen supplements
   d. Overweight
   e. Medications with sodium-retaining properties
   f. History of smoking
5. Possible risk factors under investigation:
   a. Sodium intake
   b. Lack of activity
   c. Stress
   d. Industrialized societies
   e. Genetic factors

Prevention of Hypertension

1. *Sodium restriction* is important in the treatment of some hypertensive patients, but whether limiting sodium intake will prevent the disease is not known. Until more facts are available, it is recommended that restraint be exercised in sodium consumption. Recommendations include:
   a. Not using the salt shaker at the table.
   b. Cooking with only small amounts of salt.
   c. Avoiding salted prepared foods.
   d. Reducing the amount of sodium added to baby foods.
2. In the United States as persons age, they gain weight; arterial pressure rises with age. Excess body fat must work through some mechanisms to elevate arterial pressure. Although it is very difficult, attempts should be made to *keep weight under control*: behavior modification, group therapy programs.
3. There is increased prevalence of hypertension among subjects with poor physical fitness. Considering the benefits of exercise for weight control and general health, *emphasis on physical fitness* should be increased.

Classification of Hypertension

A. *Primary or Essential Hypertension* (approximately 90% of patients with hypertension)

1. When the diastolic pressure is 90 mm. Hg or higher and other causes of hypertension are absent, the condition is said to be *primary hypertension.*
   More specifically, an individual is considered hypertensive when the average of 3 or more blood pressures taken at rest several days apart exceeds the upper limits of the following chart:

Class	BP, mm. Hg
Stratum I (mild)	90–104
Stratum II (moderate)	105–114
Stratum III (severe)	≥115

2. "Mild" is used because of common usage; however, even for persons with so-called mild hypertension, the cardiovascular risk is twice that for individuals with normal blood pressure.
3. With the presence of target organ damage, the overall risk is increased.
4. Genetic factors appear to contribute to this condition; patterns of the patient indicate that he is hypersensitive to internal and external stimuli.
5. Hypertension may be present for years *without any symptoms.*
6. *Labile* is a term used to indicate intermittently elevated blood pressure.
7. *Accelerated* refers to a sudden and severe escalation in arterial pressure producing many symptoms and vascular damage.
8. *Resistant* is a reference to hypertension that is not responsive to usual treatment.

B. *Secondary Hypertension*

1. Occurs in approximately 5–10% of patients with hypertension.
2. Apparently follows other pathology.
   a. *Renal pathology* which may lead to hypertension
      (1) Congenital anomalies, pyelonephritis, renal artery obstruction, acute and chronic glomerulonephritis
      (2) Reduced blood flow to kidney (such as atherosclerotic plaque)—release of *renin*
         (a) Renin reacts with serum protein in liver (alpha-2-globulin) → angiotensin I; this plus an enzyme → angiotensin II → leads to increased blood pressure.
         (b) Symptoms: proteinuria, polyuria, elevated blood pressure.
         (c) Therapy—endarterectomy, bypass graft, nephrectomy; blood pressure may be reduced if the initial problem is corrected.
   b. *Coarctation of Aorta* (stenosis of aorta)
      (1) Blood flow to upper extremities is greater than flow to lower extremities—hypertension of upper part of body.
      (2) Correction—removal of stenosed section of vessel; anastomosis or graft to eliminate area.
   c. *Endocrine Disturbance*—elevated blood pressure may be due to pheochromocytoma
      (1) Pheochromocytoma—causes release of epinephrine and norepinephrine and a rise in blood pressure
      (2) Adrenal cortex tumors lead to an increase in aldosterone secretion and an elevated blood pressure
      (3) Cushing's syndrome leads to an increase in adrenocortical steroids and hypertension.
      (4) Hyperthyroidism.

C. *Accelerated Hypertension—A Hypertensive Emergency* (formerly called "malignant") (Fig. 9-59)

1. Blood pressure may elevate very rapidly with serious damage to vital organs.
   a. Hypertensive encephalopathy or cerebrovascular accident
      Progressive headache—stupor—convulsions
   b. Eye effect—visual impairment, hemorrhage, papilledema, exudates
   c. Kidney effect
      (1) Blood flow decreased, vasoconstriction
      (2) BUN more than 100 mg./dl.
      (3) Plasma renin activity

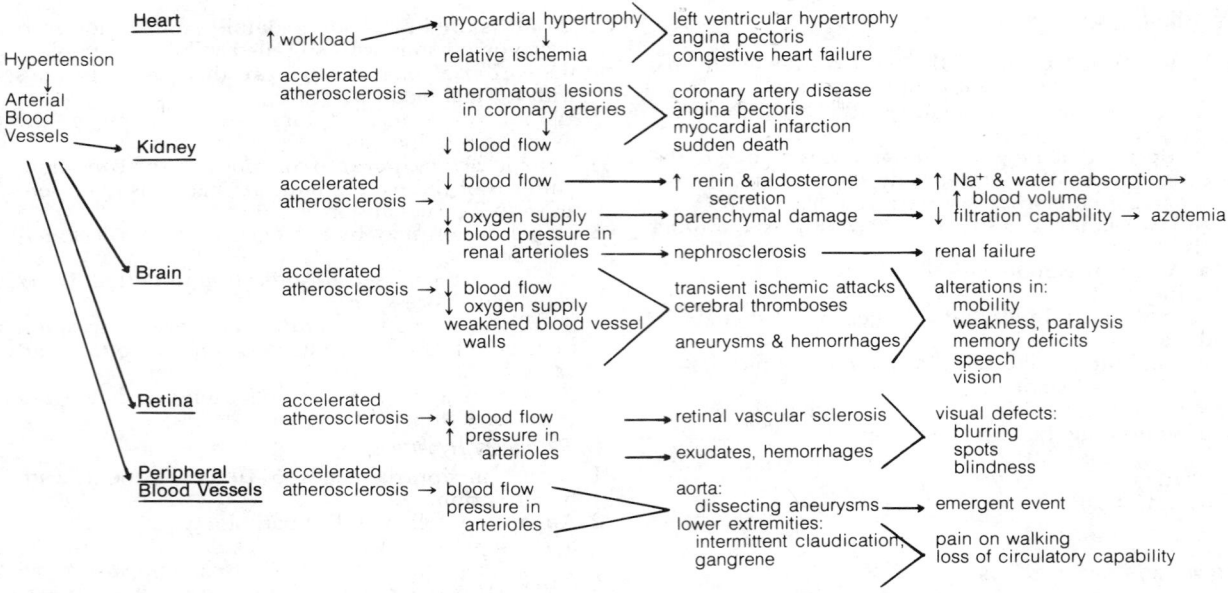

FIGURE 9-59. *Pathologic effects of sustained hypertension. (Massachusetts Nurse. Hypertension: The Scope of the Problem and the Role of the Nurse, MNA Bulletin, Special Edition, rev. 1980)*

(4) Specific gravity lowered
(5) Proteinuria
d. Epigastric pain
e. Left ventricular failure
f. Morning headache, nausea, and vomiting
2. Onset of Complications
a. Pathology
(1) Elevated diastolic pressure → strain on arterial wall → thickening and calcification of arterial media (sclerosis) → narrowed blood vessel lumen.
(2) Sclerosis of vessels → increased wall permeability → deposits placed on intima and media of vessels → cerebral, myocardial, or renal ischemia.
b. Cerebrovascular manifestations
Changes are determined by the type of onset of symptoms
(1) *Rapid*
(a) Cerebral hemorrhage → headache, increase in cerebrospinal pressure → papilledema → retinal hemorrhages → hemiplegia → coma
(b) Cerebral thrombosis → tingling sensations → numbness, limb paresis → aphasia
(c) Subarachnoid hemorrhage → stiffness of neck → pupil dilatation on side of hemorrhage → blood cells in cerebrospinal fluid → unconsciousness
(2) *Slow*
Gradual vascular insufficiency
(3) Neurologic changes with recovery in a few hours ("TIA"—transient ischemic attacks) → cerebrovascular spasms
c. Therapy:
(1) If exceeding 130 mm. Hg (diastole), hospital rest is recommended.

(2) Immediate treatment if the following are present:
(a) Convulsive movements
(b) Abnormal neurologic signs
(c) Severe occipital headache
(d) Pulmonary edema
(3) Watch blood pressure; reduce gradually and avoid wide pressure variations—note that bringing pressure down to the usual normal may not be tolerated.
(4) Measure and record urinary output.

NURSING ALERT: The actual blood pressure reading by itself is not the sole criterion for determining the severity or urgency of the person's condition. The patient/client must be assessed in terms of what, if any, evidence there is of end organ damage. For example: a person with a blood pressure of 140/105 and papilledema is at far greater risk than one with a reading of 170/115 with no evidence of papilledema. The nurse will respond accordingly.

Blood Pressure Determination

Measure the blood pressure of the patient under the same conditions each time.
1. Place patient in the desired position (sitting, standing, etc.) according to the routine of the agency or the preferences of the physician.
2. Support the arm (an unsupported arm may cause the reading to be higher and lead to a false diagnosis of hypertension).
3. Use the correct size of blood pressure cuff. (Table 9-4)

TABLE 9-4. RECOMMENDED BLADDER DIMENSIONS FOR BLOOD PRESSURE CUFF

Arm Circumference at Midpoint* (cm.)	Cuff Name	Bladder Width (cm.)	Bladder Length (cm.)
17–26	Small adult	11	17
24–32	Adult	13	24
32–42	Large adult	17	32
42–50**	Thigh	20	42

* Midpoint of arm is defined as half the distance from the acromion to the olecranon.
** In persons with very large limbs, the indirect blood pressure should be measured in the leg or forearm.
Source: Recommendations for Human Blood Pressure Determination by Sphygmomanometers. Am Heart Assoc, 1980

4. Record precisely the systolic and diastolic pressures:
   a. Systolic—the pressure within the pressure cuff indicated by the level of the mercury column at the moment when the first of two consecutive Korotkoff sounds is first heard (Fig. 9-60).
   b. Phase 4 (first diastolic)—the pressure within the compression cuff indicated by the level of the mercury column at the moment when the sound suddenly becomes muffled (beginning of Phase 4).
   c. Phase 5 (second diastolic)—the pressure within the compression cuff at the moment when the sound finally disappears (beginning of Phase 5), i.e., the onset of silence.

5. If required, mark the blood pressure reading to indicate patient's position and the arm used:
   L (lying)
   St (standing)
   Sit (sitting)
   R.A. (Right Arm)
   L.A. (Left Arm)
   Example: L.A. 152/78/68 St.
6. Average 2 readings or the second and third of 3 readings, if procedure requires.
7. Compare present reading with several previous readings to note differences and detect trends.
8. Alert physician if significant changes are apparent.

General Detection, Confirmation, and Referral of Patients with High Blood Pressure*

When there is group screening and measurement of blood pressure, resources for referral, confirmation, and follow-up should be provided.
1. Prior to blood pressure determination, ask the patient whether he has been or is currently under treatment for hypertension.
   a. Urge him to continue treatment even if blood pressure is normal.

* Based on the 1980 Report of the Joint National Committee on Detection, Evaluation, and Treatment of High Blood Pressure. Arch Intern Med 1980 Oct; 140 (10): 1280–1285

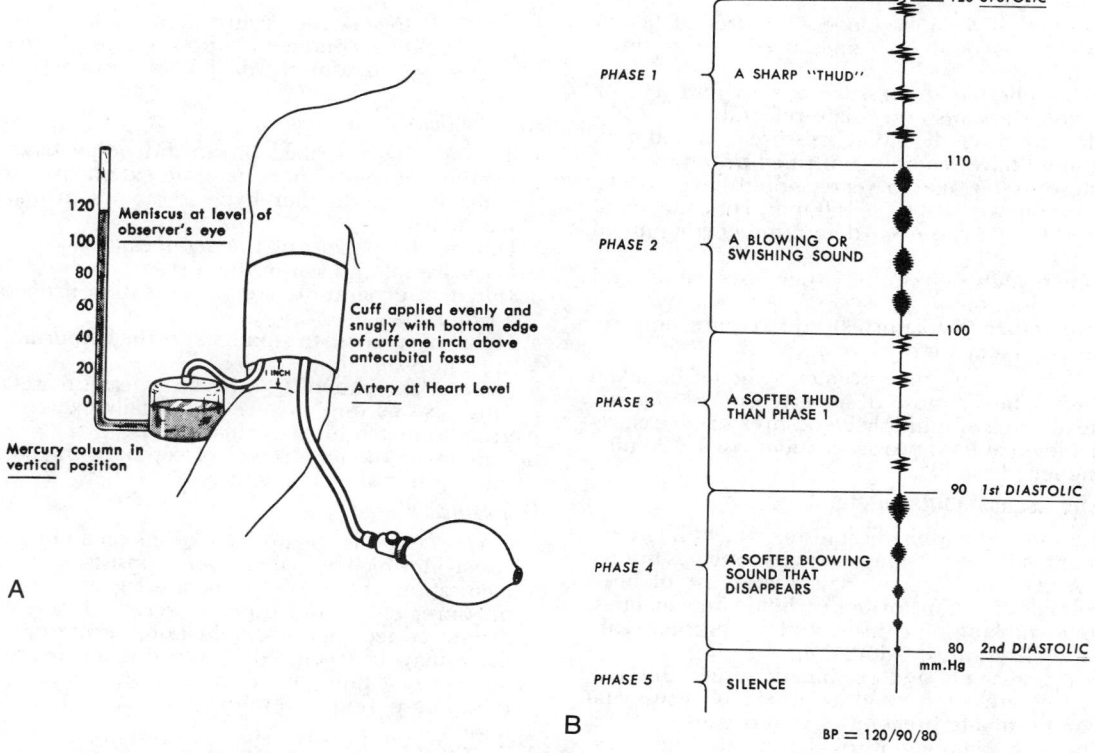

FIGURE 9-60. A. *Important "rules" for accurate recording of arterial blood pressure. B. The various phases of the Korotkoff sounds. Consult text for details. (From Burch GE and DePasquale NP. Primer of Clinical Measurement of Blood Pressure. St Louis, CV Mosby)*

b. Urge him to report an elevated blood pressure to his physician.
2. Take blood pressure with patient seated and resting comfortably with arm bared. (See p. 354.)
3. Record both systolic and diastolic pressure (diastolic—*disappearance of sound*)
4. Use a mercury sphygmomanometer preferably.
5. Use a larger size cuff for persons with obese arms and smaller cuff for persons with thin arms.
6. Discuss with the patient/client:
   a. previous treatment for high blood pressure
   b. the numerical value of current blood pressure
   c. the need for periodic remeasurement or further evaluation
   d. the desirability of blood pressure control and the potential dangers of uncontrolled hypertension
   e. the vital need to seek promptly and maintain antihypertensive therapy
7. Referral or confirmation cutoff levels are arbitrary; they may be modified by presence of risk factors:
   a. smoking
   b. hyperlipemia
   c. coronary or cerebrovascular disease
   d. cardiac or renal failure
   e. diabetes
8. The higher the blood pressure, the greater the urgency for follow-up management. (Early initial follow-up improves adherence to treatment plan.)
9. Adults with a diastolic blood pressure of 95 mm. Hg or above at screening or first visit should have the elevation confirmed promptly (within one month).
   a. Those with diastolic blood pressures of 90–95 mm. Hg should be remeasured within three months.
   b. A diastolic blood pressure of 115 mm. Hg or greater warrants immediate referral.
10. Adults with a systolic blood pressure over 160 mm. Hg should have reading confirmed promptly.
   a. Those under age 35 years should have systolic elevations greater than 150 mm. Hg confirmed.
11. *Confirmation:* Purpose is to determine whether initial elevations
   a. remain high or require closer observation and evaluation, or
   b. have returned to normal and require only remeasurement within 1 year.

NOTE: Two or more measurements should be taken at each visit. The diagnosis of hypertension is *confirmed* when the average of multiple blood pressure measurements made on at least two subsequent visits is 90 mm. Hg or higher (diastolic).

Diagnostic Assessment of Patient

1. Careful nursing and medical history (including family history of hypertension); note any previous history of hypertension, excessive salt intake, use of birth control pills or other hormones, lipid abnormalities, cigarette smoking, and history of headache, weakness, muscle cramps, palpitation, sweating.
2. Physical assessment and examination. (Fig. 9-61)
3. Blood pressure: supine and standing; also assess vital signs and evaluate function of vital organs.
4. Fundoscopic examination of the eye to detect vascular changes in the capillaries—note edema, spasm, hemorrhage.
5. Careful examination of the heart; examination of peripheral pulse disparities.
6. Listen for bruits over all peripheral arteries to determine presence of atherosclerosis; also listen for bruits in abdomen to note signs of renal arterial stenosis.
7. Chest x-ray to determine cardiac size; auscultation of lungs.
8. Neurologic tests to detect cerebral damage, neurological deficits.
9. Laboratory studies:
   a. Hematocrit reading
   b. BUN to determine renal excretory function
   c. Serum potassium concentration to determine hyperaldosteronism
   d. Electrocardiogram to establish a baseline
   e. Urinalysis for blood, protein, and glucose to determine renal parenchymal disease.

Therapeutic Guidelines

Virtually all patients with a diastolic pressure of 90 mm. Hg or greater should be treated. All patients with a diastolic pressure of 105 mm. Hg or greater should be on antihypertensive drug therapy.

OBJECTIVES: to individualize the therapeutic goal for each patient.
to achieve and maintain diastolic pressures at less than 90 mm. Hg.
to maintain the lowest diastolic pressure consistent with safety and tolerance.
to correct risk factors which directly affect the blood pressure.
to delay the progress of and to control the disease.
to slow the progression of atherosclerosis.
to recommend supportive psychotherapy in some form if it will lessen vasoconstriction.

A. *Initial Conservative Therapy*

1. Therapy is prescribed on an individual basis, depending on blood pressure, the extent of vascular damage, and whether hypertension is primary or secondary.
2. Inform the patient of the significance of avoiding excessive fat and salt in the diet.
3. Initiate a program of weight reduction if obesity is a problem.
4. Help the patient to understand the importance of giving up smoking.
5. Instruct the patient that he must learn to rest and must also become involved in a daily exercise program to match his particular needs.
6. Emphasize the importance of coping with and minimizing stressful situations.

B. *Pharmacotherapy*

"Stepped Care" is an approach (done on an individual basis) in which initial therapy consists of a single medication; if this fails to meet the goal of lowering pressure, either the dose is increased or another drug is added; upon reevaluation, perhaps another drug may be required. Increasing or decreasing dosages or adding or subtracting drugs is suggested following periodic reevaluation.

NOTE: When there is a choice of two medications, the one with fewer side effects, less patient inconvenience, less frequency of administration, and less cost is preferred. No one combination of drugs works in all patients.

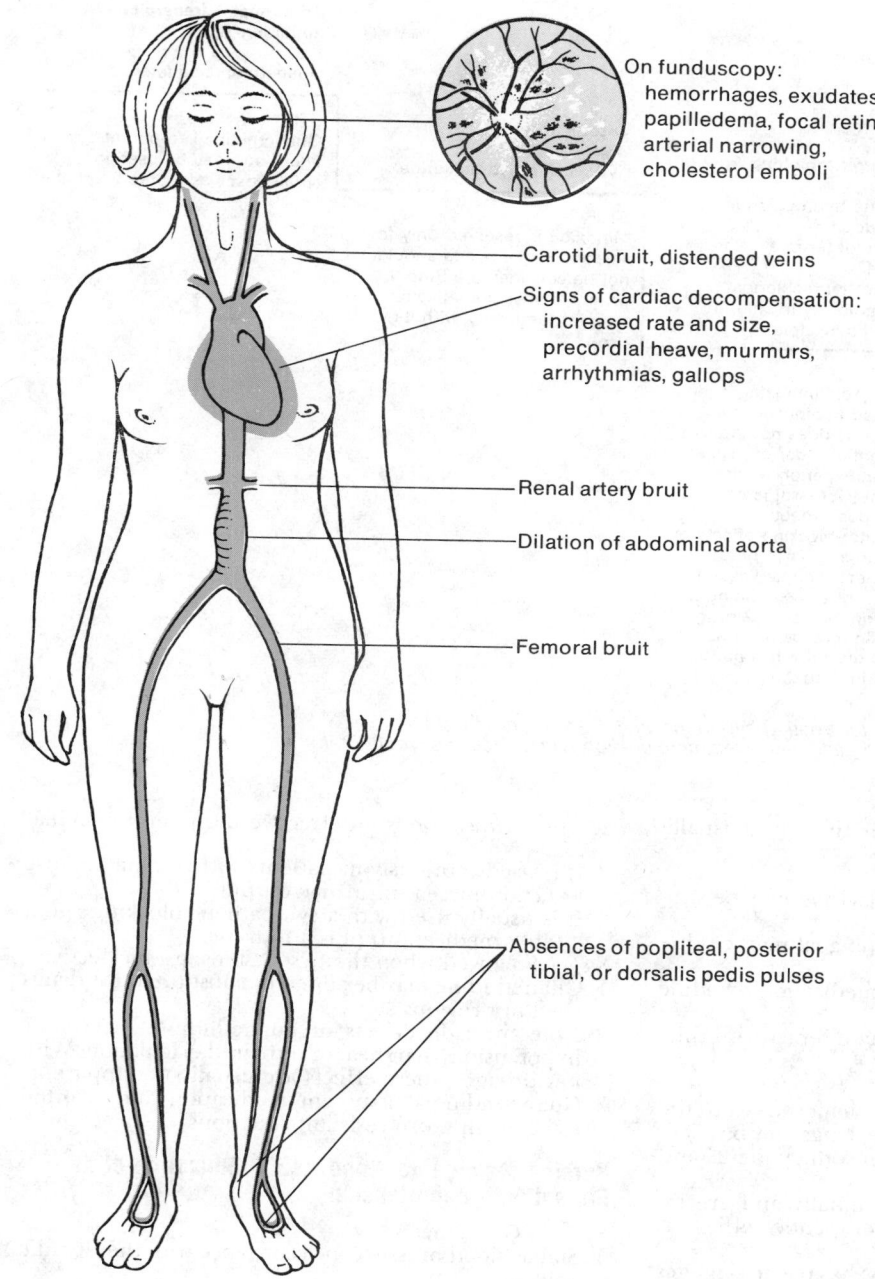

On funduscopy:
hemorrhages, exudates,
papilledema, focal retinal
arterial narrowing,
cholesterol emboli

Carotid bruit, distended veins

Signs of cardiac decompensation:
increased rate and size,
precordial heave, murmurs,
arrhythmias, gallops

Renal artery bruit

Dilation of abdominal aorta

Femoral bruit

Absences of popliteal, posterior
tibial, or dorsalis pedis pulses

FIGURE 9-61. *Physical assessment for hypertension. In addition to assessment of the central nervous system and a complete physical examination, the above specific observations are significant in detection of high blood pressure.*

Step 1—Thiazides (diuretics) (Fig. 9-62)
1. Unless contraindicated, thiazide-type diuretics are prescribed as initial therapy. This will control many patients.
2. Physiological effects may be anticipated from diuretics:
   a. Hypokalemia

(1) Provide diet adequate in postassium and controlled for sodium.
(2) The combination of a diuretic with digitalis requires attention, because hypokalemia induced by a diuretic potentiates the toxicity of digitalis.
   b. Hyperuricemia—when asymptomatic and low

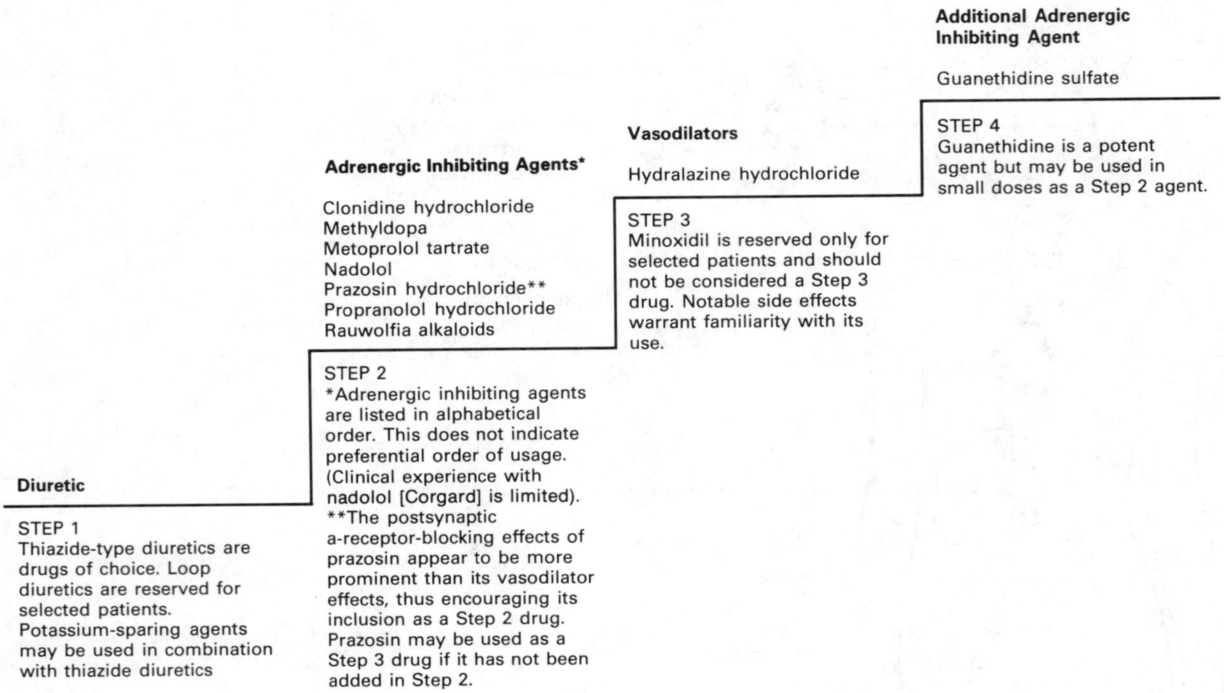

Additional Adrenergic Inhibiting Agent

Guanethidine sulfate

STEP 4
Guanethidine is a potent agent but may be used in small doses as a Step 2 agent.

Vasodilators

Hydralazine hydrochloride

STEP 3
Minoxidil is reserved only for selected patients and should not be considered a Step 3 drug. Notable side effects warrant familiarity with its use.

Adrenergic Inhibiting Agents*

Clonidine hydrochloride
Methyldopa
Metoprolol tartrate
Nadolol
Prazosin hydrochloride**
Propranolol hydrochloride
Rauwolfia alkaloids

STEP 2
*Adrenergic inhibiting agents are listed in alphabetical order. This does not indicate preferential order of usage. (Clinical experience with nadolol [Corgard] is limited).
**The postsynaptic a-receptor-blocking effects of prazosin appear to be more prominent than its vasodilator effects, thus encouraging its inclusion as a Step 2 drug. Prazosin may be used as a Step 3 drug if it has not been added in Step 2.

Diuretic

STEP 1
Thiazide-type diuretics are drugs of choice. Loop diuretics are reserved for selected patients. Potassium-sparing agents may be used in combination with thiazide diuretics

FIGURE 9-62. *Stepped-Care Regimens for treating hypertension. (The 1980 report of the Joint National Committee on Detection, Evaluation, and Treatment of High Blood Pressure. Arch Intern Med 1980 Oct; 140 (10):1282)*

grade (7 to 10 mg./dl.), specific therapy is usually not required.
  c. Hyperglycemia
    (1) When this occurs, spironolactone may be substituted as a diuretic.
3. Failure to achieve the therapeutic goal may be due to the following:
  a. Lack of patient adherence to medication schedule
  b. Excessive salt intake
  c. Use of other drugs which may interact with thiazides
Step 2
1. If the therapeutic goal is not achieved with the diuretic alone, several alternative drugs may be tried. One or more may be effective in some patients and not in others;
  a. Usually, low doses are used initially and are increased gradually until therapeutic effect is achieved.
  b. Reserpine (rauwolfia alkaloids) has the advantages of low cost and once-a-day administration (see Table 9-5).
  c. Clonidine hydrochloride (Catapres) and prazosim hydrochloride (Minipress) may be substituted for any Step 3 drug.
    (1) Clonidine side effects—dry mouth, drowsiness
    (2) Prazosim side effects—weakness, postural dizziness, sudden collapse
  d. Propranolol or other beta adrenergic blocking agents
  e. The patient needs to be monitored for occurrence of fluid retention.
Step 3 Usually hydralazine hydrochloride is added.

1. This medication is an effective peripheral vasodilator.
2. It is used cautiously in patients with angina because its action increases cardiac output.
3. It is usually used with a sympathetic blocking agent (Step 2 medication) plus a diuretic.
Step 4 Followed when the first 3 steps are ineffective.
1. Guanethidine may be added or substituted for drugs used in previous steps.
2. Note the side effects of guanethidine: orthostatic hypotension, diarrhea, or impaired ejaculation. With low dosages, these effects are usually not apparent.
3. Guanethidine is a potent medication and is often effective in more resistant situations.

Nursing Management and Health Education of the Patient with Hypertension

Patient Outcomes*
1. Stable blood pressure in accordance with therapeutic goal
2. Minimal therapeutic side effects
3. Minimal pathophysiological changes secondary to hypertension
4. Patient and family adjustment to health status and therapy
5. Maintenance of life-style compatible with personal and health care goals
6. Patient and/or family understand hypertension and treatment appropriate for self-care

* Guidelines for Educating Nurses in High Blood Pressure Control. U.S. Department of Health, Education, and Welfare. NIH Pub. No. 80-1241, March 1980

Statement on Hypertension in the Elderly*

Approved by the National High Blood Pressure Education Program Coordinating Committee September 1979

	Detection, evaluation, and drug therapy	Patient education
General	☐ Blood pressure should be measured in the sitting and standing positions at each visit. ☐ Three blood pressure determinations per visit should be made on multiple visits in elderly patients with initial elevated readings. ☐ Extensive diagnostic workup is not recommended unless abrupt exacerbation of stable hypertension or *de novo* onset after age 55 raises the level of suspicion. Then, secondary causes should be sought. ☐ Adjuncts to therapy such as weight loss, dietary sodium restriction, and judicious exercise can be employed for some elderly patients. ☐ A portion of one or more visits spent with the patient's spouse, close relative, or neighbor can build support for the total hypertension control regimen.	☐ Special adherence problems often result from the physical, psychological, and social limitations of elderly people. Professionals counseling elderly hypertensives may have to make innovative use of existing skills and available materials and resources to help these patients achieve high blood pressure control. ☐ Discussions with the patient should be very specific about what to do and how to do it. The initial session should be limited only to the task(s) essential to achieve high blood pressure control, e.g., pill-taking routine. ☐ Written material and memory aids which reinforce verbal instructions should be given to patients and family members for home use. These aids should be selected with attention to patients' hearing and sight impairments as well as educational background and present mental status. ☐ The patient living alone should be encouraged to identify a neighbor or an active friend who can offer reinforcement (even by phone) or provide transportation for office visits. ☐ Where appropriate, regular social service agencies, community or public health services/departments, or senior citizen programs should be identified to assist the elderly patient with other special needs such as benefits, meals, home nursing visits, transportation, and other services, many of which may be reimbursable through private insurance or public assistance.
Medication	☐ Antihypertensive agents known to produce severe orthostatic hypotention, such as guanethidine, should probably be avoided. ☐ Patients should be encouraged to bring all of their medications with them at each visit to facilitate identification. ☐ Containers without safety caps are recommended for elderly patients. ☐ Initial doses of chosen agents should be reduced by one-half the usual initial adult dose for elderly patients. ☐ Dosages should be increased very gradually over a period of weeks rather than days unless the blood pressure is very high. ☐ Follow-up visits should be scheduled every two to four weeks until the blood pressure has stabilized as the result of antihypertensive therapy. After control has been established, visits may be required no more often than every three or four months. ☐ *A CAVEAT.* Practitioners should be alert to the hazard of adverse drug interactions in older persons on multiple medications. Over-the-counter preparations may increase this hazard. Patients on multiple medications may require additional counseling to deal with adherence problems.	☐ The first few minutes of each visit should be used for reviewing medications and for specific questioning and listening to the patient for clues to problems such as side effects, forgetting medication, poor eating habits, or financial difficulties with acquiring medications. This is especially important when the stated treatment goal is not being achieved. ☐ The number of medications and the schedule for taking them should be as simple as possible to encourage adherence. ☐ Prescribing new medications in small quantities until the drug(s) of choice is/are established will reassure the patient with limited financial resources. ☐ Insofar as possible, providers should ensure that patients acquire and refill prescribed medications: Nursing and pharmacy personnel may facilitate the monitoring of adherence.

* Excerpts

TABLE 9-5. A QUICK GUIDE TO ANTIHYPERTENSIVE DRUG THERAPY

Agent	Range of Usual Daily Maintenance Dose	Hemodynamic Effects	Comments
Thiazides and Related Diuretics			
chlorothiazide (Diuril)	500–1.000 mg	At first, blood volume, renal blood flow, and cardiac output are decreased; then return toward normal as therapy continues. Peripheral vascular resistance is at first increased and then drops below normal.	All the thiazides are comparable in antihypertensive effect; they differ principally in potency and duration of effect. At optimum dosage—which is highly individual—a thiazide alone will control mild to moderate hypertension in 35% to 40% of patients. In combination therapy, thiazides permit smaller doses of other antihypertensive agents, enhancing control without side effects.
chlorthalidone (Hygroton)	50–100 mg**		
hydrochlorothiazide (Esidrix, HydroDIURIL, Oretic*)	25–100 mg		
hydroflumenthiazide (Saluron*)	50–100 mg		
methyclothiazide (Enduron*)	2.5–5 mg		
polythiazide (Renese)	2–4 mg		
Other Diuretics			
furosemide (Lasix)	40 mg b.i.d.	Comparable to the thiazide diuretics; antagonizes actions of aldosterone.	The diuretic of choice in patients with impaired renal function.
spironolactone (Aldactone)	25 mg q.i.d. (up to 100 mg q.i.d. with aldosteronism)	Blocks action of aldosterone on kidney, retains potassium.	A weak diuretic that potentiates other antihypertensives, counteracts potassium loss caused by other diuretics.
Antihypertensives			
clonidine (Catapres)	0.2–2.4 mg	Cardiac output decreases at first, then returns to normal. Peripheral vascular resistance and heart rate decrease. Renal blood flow unchanged.	To avoid rebound hypertension, discontinue drug gradually over 2 to 4 days; periodic eye exams recommended.
guanethidine (Ismelin)	25–50 mg for moderate hypertension. Up to 300 mg in severe cases	Venous pooling: pulse rate, cardiac output, and renal blood flow are all decreased	Dose is limited only by onset of intolerable side effects. Usually reserved for severe or intractable hypertension.
hydralazine (Apresoline)	40–200 mg	At first, pulse rate, cardiac output, and renal blood flow increase, then become normal. Peripheral vascular resistance decreases.	Given with diuretic for moderate and severe hypertension, especially in toxemias of pregnancy or acute glomerulonephritis.
methyldopa (Aldomet)	750 mg–3 Gm	Venous pooling may occur: pulse rate and peripheral vascular resistance, cardiac output decreased.	Used with a diuretic, particularly in severe hypertension. Interferes with catecholamine measurement.
prazosin (Minipress)	3–20 mg	Cardiac output and heart rate usually unchanged. Peripheral vascular resistance decreased. Renal blood flow may increase.	Combining with other antihypertensives may permit smaller doses and reduce side effects. Combining with beta blocker (e.g., propranolol) may cause hypotension.
propranolol (Inderal)	80–640 mg	Cardiac output, heart rate, renal blood flow, and peripheral vascular resistance reduced. Increased heart rate after exercise is blocked.	Used most effectively with diuretic. May be used with hydralazine to block reflex tachycardia.
reserpine (other rauwolfia alkaloids have similar clinical effects)	0.1–0.25 mg	Venous pooling may occur: pulse rate and peripheral vascular resistance are decreased.	Seldom used alone. Report side effects promptly. Depletes catecholamines, so stop drug 2 weeks before elective surgery.

* Not available in Canada
** NOTE: According to FDA Drug Bulletin, Vol. 11, No. 1, Mar 1981, the dosage of chlorthalidone has been reduced from 50 or 100 mg. per day to 25 mg. per day.
Source: Reprinted with permission from the October issue of NURSING 78. Copyright © 1978, Intermed Communications, Inc., Horsham, Pa. 19044

What to Tell Patients to Expect	Side Effects	Major Contraindications
Dry mouth, thirst, weakness, drowsiness, restlessness, muscle pains or cramps, hypotension, polyuria, tachycardia. GI disturbances. Warn patient that orthostatic hypotension may be potentiated by alcohol, barbiturates, or narcotics.	Hypokalemia, hyperglycemia, hyperuricemia, hypercalcemia, lethargy. (Order serum electrolytes, BUN, uric acid, CO_2, and blood sugar tests before therapy starts and at appropriate intervals thereafter.)	Known sensitivity to sulfonamide-derived drugs, anuria, oliguria, increasing azotemia, severely impaired renal function, severe hepatic disease, lactation. BUN 40 mg% or higher.
Same as for thiazides, plus sweet taste, oral and gastric burning, swelling.	Same as for thiazides, plus dehydration and vascular thrombosis and embolism in elderly.	Comparable to thiazides, not recommended for pregnant women.
Drowsiness, headache, GI symptoms, skin eruptions, urticaria, confusion, ataxia.	Hyperkalemia, hyponatremia, elevated BUN, mild feminizing effects. Monitor serum potassium.	Acute renal insufficiency, rapidly progressing impaired renal function, anuria, hyperkalemia.
Dry mouth, sedation, dizziness, constipation, headache and fatigue—which usually disappear with continued therapy. Warn against stopping drug abruptly.	Bradycardia (effect may be additive with propranolol, digitalis, and guanethidine). Sodium and fluid retention may last 3 to 4 days.	Not recommended for pregnant women. Tricyclic antidepressants may block drug's antihypertensive effect.
Postural hypotension accentuated by alcohol, exercise, or hot weather. Warn against standing suddenly, possible sexual dysfunction, fatigue, diarrhea, or edema.	Sodium and fluid retention. Combining with other agents may cause postural hypotension, bradycardia, occasional urinary incontinence.	Proven or suspected pheochromocytoma; not to be used with tricyclic antidepressants, MAOIs, or chlorpromazine. Contraindicated for CHF not secondary to hypertension.
This drug is usually well tolerated in small doses: headache, palpitation, anorexia, nausea, dizziness, sweating.	Headache, palpitation, flushing, dyspnea, tachycardia, and angina pectoris. May produce lupus-like syndrome after prolonged use.	Hypersensitivity, coronary artery disease, mitral valvular rheumatic heart disease.
Postural hypotension, sleepiness, bradycardia, and impotence (rare). Edema, decreased mental acuity.	Acquired hemolytic anemia (rare). Influenza-like illness, loss of libido. Drug fever. Sodium and fluid retention.	Active hepatic disease. Not recommended for pregnant women.
Dizziness and lightheadedness result from standing quickly. Headache, drowsiness, nausea, lethargy, palpitations may disappear with continued therapy.	Postural hypotension may cause syncope; often seen after first dose or dosage increase, or addition of another antihypertensive.	Not recommended for pregnant women.
Warn diabetics that signs of hypoglycemia (pulse rate and blood pressure changes) may be masked. Warn against abrupt withdrawal of drug.	Bradycardia, CHF, fluid retention, pulmonary edema, bronchospasm, hypoglycemia, fatigue, GI discomfort, insomnia, depression. Raynaud's syndrome. Serious side effects most likely in patients with asthma, bradycardia, or CHF.	Bronchial asthma, allergic rhinitis, bradycardia, with 2° or 3° heart block, right ventricular failure secondary to pulmonary hypertension, or CHF. Don't give with (or less than 2 weeks following) MAOI therapy.
Depression: tell patient to notify his doctor if "low mood" sets in.	Weight gain, nasal stuffiness, peptic ulceration, postural hypotension, drowsiness, sedation, constipation.	Mental depression, especially with suicidal tendencies; active peptic ulcer, ulcerative colitis.

7. Patient assumes responsibility for self-care within psychosocial and physical limitations

Ambulatory/Outpatient

Nursing Action

1. Explain the meaning of hypertension, risk factors, and their influences on the cardiovascular system; hypertension is a lifetime problem.
2. Usually there can never be total cure, only control of essential hypertension; emphasize the consequences of uncontrolled hypertension.
3. Stress the fact that there may be no correlation between high blood pressure and symptoms; the patient cannot tell by the way he feels whether his blood pressure is normal or elevated.
4. Recognize the various effects of certain factors on symptoms of a patient with primary hypertension.
   a. Age, sex, occupation, race, environment, emotional response of the individual, etc.
   b. Understanding of his problem and his rapport with physician, nurse, etc.
   c. Ability to adapt and adjust his activities in line with the prescribed therapeutic regimen.
5. Have patient recognize that hypertension is chronic and requires persistent therapy and periodic evaluation; effective treatment improves life expectancy, therefore follow-up visits to the physician are mandatory.
6. Enlist the patient's cooperation in redirecting his life-style in keeping with the guidelines of therapy.
   a. Present an instructional pattern to fit individual requirements.
   b. Reassure patient when encouragement is needed; the modifications required must appear meaningful to him.
7. Present a coordinated and complementary plan of guidance.
   a. Be available when the physician visits the patient so that his approach and instructions to the patient are known.
   b. Inform the patient of the meaning of the various diagnostic and therapeutic activities to minimize his anxiety and to obtain his cooperation.
   c. Solicit the assistance of the patient's wife or husband—provide information regarding the total treatment plan.
   d. Be aware of the dietary plan developed for this particular patient.
8. Practice supportive psychotherapy by observing the patient's reactions, appearance, and personality as he relates to the professional staff, visitors, ancillary personnel, etc.
   a. Permit him to express his feelings; promote positive reactions; analyze negative reactions in an attempt to avoid their recurrence.
   b. Note side-reactions which can be easily missed; investigate these.
      (1) Failure to make eye contact in conversation
      (2) Suggestion of uneasiness, nervousness, restlessness
      (3) Side remarks or "under-the-breath" comments
9. Measure the patient's blood pressure under the same conditions each day.
   Place patient in the desired position, sitting, standing, etc., according to the preferences of the physician.

10. If elevated blood pressure can be brought down to normal range, there is very clear evidence that congestive heart failure, strokes, and renal failure can be almost completely prevented; therefore treatment should continue in spite of medication cost or inconvenience.
11. Develop a plan of instruction which will be practiced by the patient at home.
   a. Instruct him regarding proper method of taking his blood pressure at home and at work if his physician so desires. (Some authorities recommend this practice.) Inform him of the readings which should be reported to the physician.
   b. Plan his medication schedule so that the many medications are given at proper and convenient times; set up a daily checklist on which he can record the medication he has taken.
   c. Determine recommended dietary plans, e.g., extent of salt restriction, exchange foods, etc.
12. Assist the patient in coping with the side effects of the therapeutic medications.
   a. Recognize that the drugs used to effectively control the elevated blood pressure will very likely produce side effects.
   b. Warn the patient of the possibility that hypotension may occur following the intake of certain drugs.
      (1) Instruct him to get up slowly to offset the feeling of dizziness.
      (2) Encourage him to lie down immediately if he feels faint.
   c. Alert patient to expect such effects as nasal congestion, asthenia (loss of strength), anorexia (loss of appetite), orthostatic hypotension (dizziness on changing position).
   d. Inform the patient that the goal of treatment is to control his blood pressure, reduce the possibility of complications, and utilize the minimum number of drugs with lowest dosage necessary to do the task.
13. Educate the patient to be aware of toxic manifestations and report them so that adjustments can be made in his individual pharmacotherapy.
   a. Note that dosages are individualized; therefore, they may need to be adjusted since it is often impossible to predict reactions.
   b. Remember that certain circumstances produce vasodilatation—a hot bath, hot weather, febrile illness, consumption of alcohol.
   c. Be aware that blood pressure is decreased when circulating blood volume is reduced—dehydration, diarrhea, hemorrhage.
   d. Suspect the presence of edema as a reportable symptom particularly when guanethidine is taken; these medications are less effective in the presence of edema.

Inpatient/Hospitalized Patient with Hypertensive Crisis

OBJECTIVE: to first reduce diastolic pressure toward, but not below 90 mm. Hg and then to initiate oral therapy.

Therapy and Nursing Management

1. Use parenteral medications in hypertensive emergencies.
   a. Diastolic blood pressure over 150 mm. Hg
   b. Pulmonary edema, cerebral hemorrhage, enceph-

TABLE 9-6. DRUGS FOR PARENTERAL TREATMENT OF HYPERTENSION

Drug	Action	Side Effects and Pertinent Points
1. Diazoxide (Hyperstat)	Orally—mildly antihypertensive Intravenously—strongly antihypertensive	Salt is restricted to prevent salt and water retention
2. Nitroprusside (Nipride)	Has immediate antihypertensive effect Reduces total peripheral resistance (vasodilator) Produces a relaxation of arteriolar and venular smooth muscle	Useful in patients with hypertensive emergencies complicated by cardiac and aortic disease
3. Trimethaphan camsylate (Arfonad)	Has immediate antihypertensive effect—its effect disappears when infusion is discontinued (Ganglion-blocking agent)	Extremely potent hypotensive drug requiring adequate facilities, equipment, and personnel for monitoring patient
4. Pentolinium (Ansolysen)	Administered intramuscularly, usually into deltoid muscles Acts within 3 minutes with maximal effects occurring in 15 minutes	Apply tourniquet above injection site if severe hypotension results Place patient in sitting position or with head elevated
5. Methyldopa (Aldomet)	Effective in lowering blood pressure in 4–6 hours—effect extends 10–16 hours after injection	Sedation sometimes occurs as a result of this medication but usually wears off in a few days when a maintenance dose is established Watch for kidney toxicity
6. Hydralazine (Apresoline)	Effective in treating hypertensive patients with acute glomerulonephritis Onset of action in 10–20 minutes Maximum response—1 hour Persists—12 hours	Monitor blood pressure every 15 minutes

alopathy in combination with diastolic pressure over 120 or 130.

2. Patient must be hospitalized and monitored constantly.
   a. Record blood pressure frequently.
      Some drugs such as trimethaphan, nitroprusside, and pentolinium require blood pressure to be taken every 5 minutes.
   b. Measure urine output accurately.
   c. Be prepared to administer vasopressors if severe hypotension develops.
   d. Administer diuretics such as furosemide and ethacrynic acid as adjuncts when prescribed.
      They serve to maintain sodium diuresis when the arterial pressure falls.
   e. Administer spironolactone when prescribed if hypokalemia is a problem.
3. Observe patient for signs of cerebral nervous system complications.
   a. Note signs of confusion, irritability, lethargy, disorientation.
   b. Listen for complaints of headache, difficulty with vision; be alert for evidence of nausea or vomiting.
   c. Be prepared to offer protection to the patient if he exhibits seizures—padded bed sides, nonrestrictive garments, anticonvulsive medications.
4. Prevent those reactions or activities which will increase arterial pressure.
   a. Avoid situations which might engender feelings of anxiety, anger, or annoyance in the patient. Psychological stress has a direct effect on physiological function.
   b. Prevent alterations in the ordinary functions of eating, sleeping, or elimination which might lead to discomfort or annoyance—physiological disturbance may increase stress reaction.
   c. Provide rest period and maintain a pleasant, comfortable environment.

(1) Advise patient to rest for a short time before and after eating.
(2) Remind him to rest during the waking hours for a full hour.
   d. Serve food in small quantities frequently rather than in 3 heavier meals.
      (1) Cardiac output increases with food intake.
      (2) Blood pressure is elevated with large intake of fluids.
      (3) Sodium intake may be restricted depending on severity of hypertension.
5. Pharmacotherapy
   a. Drugs which act in a few minutes but are not satisfactory for long-term management.
      (1) Diazoxide
      (2) Nitroprusside
      (3) Trimethaphan
      (4) Pentolinium
   b. Drugs which require 30 minutes or more to obtain full effects; they can later by used orally for long-term management of hypertension.
      (1) Methyldopa
      (2) Hydralazine
   c. See Table 9-6.

Long-term Control of Blood Pressure

Patient Behaviors Critical to Achievement of Long-term Blood Pressure Control*

Once hypertension is diagnosed, the patient must:
1. Make the decision to control his blood pressure
2. Take medication as prescribed
3. Monitor progress toward his blood pressure goal
4. Resolve problems that block his achieving blood pressure control (Table 9-7)

* Patient behavior for blood pressure control: Guidelines for professionals. JAMA 1979 June 8; 241:2535–2536

TABLE 9-7. FOUR CRITICAL BEHAVIORS WITH CONCOMITANT KNOWLEDGE, ATTITUDES, AND SKILLS

Knowledge	Attitude	Skill
Make Decision to Control Blood Pressure (BP) The patient is able to state:	The patient believes that:	The patient is able to:
His BP and normal limits	His BP exceeds normal	Differentiate between normal and abnormal
That high BP can be asymptomatic	His BP is high even if there are no symptoms	. . .
That untreated high BP can lead to stroke, kidney failure, or heart disease	Although consequences may not occur for years, they are nevertheless real and serious	. . .
That drug therapy can control high BP and reduce risk of these complications	Drug therapy and high BP control lessen risk of stroke, kidney failure, or heart disease	Explain the benefits of high BP control, eg, increased length and quality of life
The necessity of lifelong therapy for control of high BP	Potential problems can be resolved	Differentiate between control and cure
	The benefits of control outweigh the costs	Identify potential problems related to medication regimen, fear of medication, time, and money
Take Medication as Prescribed The patient is able to state:	The patient believes that:	The patient is able to:
Medical regimen: which pill to take, when to take it, what to do if doses are missed	Prescribed medicine will lower BP, is needed every day for BP control, should not be stopped without medical advice	Develop habit of taking medicine by tailoring plan to fit personal schedule
. . .	Folk remedies are not substitutes for prescribed medication	Cue medication taking (if necessary) by associating with daily activities, storing in a prominent place, marking medication calendar
. . .	. . .	Select accessible source to obtain medications
. . .	. . .	Make financial plan and arrangements to obtain medications
. . .	. . .	Renew prescription before supply exhaustion
Monitor Progress Toward BP Goal The patient is able to state:	The patient believes that:	The patient is able to:
His BP goal	As a partner with physician, he has the right to understand what is expected of him, follow own progress, interact with advisor concerning progress	Identify and communicate progress toward goal: state of health, problems encountered with therapy
That BP readings vary and the trend during time is the basis for therapeutic decisions	Accepts daily BP fluctuations (within range physician defines) without undue concern	Keep track of his BP trend (if the physician recommends home BP measurement, then additional skills need to be developed)
That medications may need to be changed	. . .	. . .
Date and time for next appointment	Continuous therapy is important, including appointment keeping	Make arrangements necessary to keep appointment: travel, time from work, financial, reminder systems
What to do if he cannot keep appointment	Continuous therapy is important, including appointment keeping	Reschedule appointment
Resolve Problems That Block Achieving BP Control A. Communication The patient is able to state:	The patient believes that:	The patient is able to:
That BP control requires a combined effort by both physician and patient	Physician is interested in his concerns	State concerns; ask questions
. . .	As a partner, he has responsibility to know what is expected, state what he expects of physician	With the physician: identify possible solutions, select and try out solutions, evaluate progress
That other health professionals can help solve problems	Others can assist him to solve problems	Select appropriate health professional
	Aforementioned attitudes apply here as well	Aforementioned skills apply here as well
That BP control requires emotional support from friends and relatives	He can ask and will gain empathy, support, and assistance with high BP therapy from friends and relatives	State when and how family members can help and ask for that assistance
. . .	. . .	Request instruction for friends and relatives about BP control and its management
. . .	. . .	Accept and use reinforcement and support
B. Medication regimen The patient is able to state:	The patient believes that:	The patient is able to:
Important side effects of his BP drugs	Side effects occur	Recognize symptoms as possibly being drug-induced
Action to be taken if symptoms occur	Physician will correct problems that pose danger to health	Consult physician about bothersome symptoms

TABLE 9-7. FOUR CRITICAL BEHAVIORS WITH CONCOMITANT KNOWLEDGE, ATTITUDES, AND SKILLS (cont.)

Knowledge	Attitude	Skill
Methods of minimizing side effects, eg, dosage scheduling, dietary supplements, activity precautions	. . .	Utilize methods when necessary
That other medications are available if side effects are intolerable	Living with minor side effects is more acceptable than consequences of uncontrolled BP	Request that other medication be prescribed if side effects are intolerable
That other drugs can interfere with BP goal, eg, over-the-counter medications such as decongestants	Drug interactions can interfere with BP goals	Inform all providers of current regimen
. . .	. . .	Seek advice before taking nonprescription medications
C. Costs		
Time required for follow-up visits, getting medicine	Time commitment to high BP therapy is as important as conflicting time demands	Inform physician of special time constraints
How this time will be built into his life	. . .	Request advice on how to minimize time spent on treatment of high BP
Dollar costs of medicine and follow-up visits	Treatment of high BP has high priority in budget	Inform physician of special financial problems
. . .		Request advice on resources to assist with cost

* National Institutes of Health, Bethesda, Md. 1979

THE LYMPHATIC SYSTEM

The *lymphatic system* is a network of vessels and nodes that are interrelated with the circulatory system. It removes tissue fluid from intercellular spaces and protects the body from bacterial invasion. Lymph nodes are located along the course of the lymphatic vessels and filter lymph before it is returned to the bloodstream.

Significance of Lymphangiography

Radiologic visualization of the lymphatic system is possible when a contrast medium is injected into a lymphatic vessel of the hands or feet.

It is a means of detecting lymph node involvement due to metastatic carcinoma, lymphoma, or infection in otherwise inaccessible sites (except by surgery) such as the pelvis, retroperitoneum, deep axilla.

LYMPHANGITIS

Lymphangitis is an acute inflammation of lymphatic channels.

Etiology

Arises most commonly from a focus of infection in an extremity.

Clinical Manifestations

1. Displays characteristic red streaks that extend up an arm or leg from an infection that is not localized and that can lead to septicemia.
2. Produces general symptoms: high fever, chills.
   Produces local symptoms: local pain, tenderness, swelling along involved lymphatics.
   Produces local lymph node symptoms: enlarged, red, tender (acute lymphadenitis).
   Produces an abscess: necrotic, pus-producing (suppurative lymphadenitis).

Treatment and Nursing Management

1. Administer antimicrobial agents since causative organisms usually are streptococci and staphylococci.
2. Treat affected part by rest, elevation, and the application of hot, moist dressings.
3. Incise and drain if necrosis and abscess formation take place.

ACUTE CERVICAL ADENITIS

Acute cervical adenitis is an acute infection of the lymphatic glands of the neck.

Etiology

1. Usually cervical adenitis is secondary to an infection of the mouth, pharynx, or scalp.
2. Occurs more frequently in children.
   a. Inspect teeth, tonsils, etc., since they are often foci of infection.
   b. Examine scalp for evidence of pediculosis

Clinical Manifestations

1. Swelling on one side of neck: markedly tender and edematous.
2. Systemic signs indicative of an infection: temperature elevation, malaise, increased pulse, etc.
3. Process may continue, leading to abscess formation and spontaneous rupture if not treated.

Treatment and Nursing Management

1. Determine the source of infection and treat it.
2. Administer antimicrobials.
3. Apply warm, moist compresses to localize infection.
4. Incise and drain; continue with moist, warm compresses until drainage ceases and infection is cleared.

LYMPHEDEMA

Lymphedema is a swelling of the tissues (particularly in the dependent position) produced by an obstruction to the lymph flow in an extremity.

Clinical Manifestations

1. Edema may be massive and is often firm.
2. Obstruction may be in lymph nodes as well as in the lymphatic vessels.
   Observed in arm following radical mastectomy (see pp. 561, 563)

Treatment and Nursing Management

1. Apply elastic bandages or stocking.
2. Keep patient at rest with affected part elevated, each joint higher than the preceding one.
3. Administer diuretics to control excess fluid.
4. Give antimicrobials as prescribed.
5. Recommend isometric exercises with extremity elevated.
6. Suggest moderate sodium restriction in diet.
7. Advise patient to avoid infection and trauma and to practice good hygiene to avoid super-imposed infections.

BIBLIOGRAPHY

HEART DISORDERS

Books

Adler JS and Francis GS. Manual of Coronary Care. Boston. Little, Brown & Co, 1977

American Heart Association. Pre-hospital Care of Cardiovascular Emergencies. Los Angles, American Heart Association,1979.

Behrendt DM and Austen WC. Patient Care in Cardiac Surgery. Boston, Little, Brown & Co, 1976

Cohn LH (ed). The Treatment of Acute Myocardial Ischemia: An Integrated Approach. Mt. Kisco, Futura Publishing Co, 1979

Comoss PM, Burke EAS and Swails SH. Cardiac Rehabilitation: A Comprehensive Nursing Approach. Philadelphia, JB Lippincott, 1979

Corday E and Swan HJC. Clinical Strategies in Ischemic Heart Disease. Baltimore, Williams & Wilkins, 1979

Cordell RA and Ellison RG (eds). Complications of Intrathoracic Surgery. Boston, Little, Brown & Co, 1979

Chung, EK. Cardiac Emergency Care, 2nd ed. Philadelphia, Lea & Febiger, 1980

Davis H and Nelson WP. Understanding Cardiology. Boston, Butterworth & Co, 1978

Davies, JA and Spillman SJ. Cardiac Rehabilitation for the Patient and Family. Reston, Reston Publishing Co, 1980

Fishman AP. Heart Failure. New York, McGraw-Hill, 1977

Fowler NO. Cardiac Diagnosis and Treatment, 3rd ed. Hagerstown, Harper & Row, 1980

Gentry WD and Williams RB Jr. Psychological Aspects of Myocardial Infarction and Coronary Care. St. Louis, CV Mosby, 1979

Helfant RH and Banka VS. A Clinical and Angiographic Approach to Coronary Heart Disease. Philadelphia, FA Davis, 1978

Hurst JW (ed). The Heart, 4th ed. New York, McGraw-Hill, 1978

Kaplan JA. Cardiac Anesthesia. New York, Grune & Stratton, 1979

Leatham A. An Introduction to Examination of the Cardiovascular System. New York , Oxford Medical Publishers, 1979

Monteiro LA. Cardiac Patient Rehabilitation. New York, Springer Pub. Co., 1979

Morse D and Steiner RM. The Pacemaker and Value Identification Guide. Garden City, Medical Exam Publishing Co, 1978

Narula OS (ed). Cardiac Arrhythmias. Baltimore, Williams & Wilkins, 1979

Nursing Skillbook: Combatting Cardiovascular Diseases Skillfully. Horsham, Intermed Communications, 1978

Nursing Skillbook: Giving Cardiovascular Drugs Safely. Horsham, Intermed Communications, 1978

Ochsner JL and Mills NL. Coronary Artery Surgery, Philadelphia, Lea & Febiger, 1978

Phillips RE. Cardiovascular Therapy; A Systemic Approach, Vol 1. Philadelphia, WB Saunders, 1979

Rose LB and Rose BK. Fundamentals of Mobile Coronary Care. Baltimore, Williams & Wilkins, 1979

Samet P and El-Sherif N (eds). Cardiac Pacing, 2nd ed. New York, Grune & Stratton, 1980

Simon NM (ed). The Psychological Aspects of Intensive Care Nursing. Bowie, Robert J. Brady Co, 1980

Sokolow M and McIlroy MB. Clinical Cardiology. Los Altos, Lange Medical Publications, 1979

Timmis GC. Cardiovascular Review. Baltimore, Williams & Wilkins, 1979

Vanden Belt RJ, Ronan JA and Bedynek JL. Cardiology. Chicago, Year Book Medical Publishers, 1979

Varriale P and Naclerio EA. Cardiac Pacing. Philadelphia, Lea & Febiger, 1979

Wenger NK and Hellerstein HK. Rehabilitation of the Coronary Patient. New York, John Wiley & Sons, 1978

Articles

Angina/Myocardial Infarction

Aronow WS. Clinical use of nitrates. I. Nitrates as antianginal drugs. Mod Concepts Cardiovasc Dis 1979 June; 48(6): 31–5

Cairns JA. Current management of unstable angina. Can Med Assoc J 1978 Sept 9; 119(5):477–480

Frishman W and Silverman R. Clinical pharmacology of the new beta-adrenergic blocking drugs. Am Heart J 1979 June; 97(6):797–807

Fuller EO. The effect on antianginal drugs on myocardial oxygen consumption. Am J Nurs 1980 Feb; 80(2): 250–254

Gazes PC, Gaddy JE. Bedside management of acute myocardial infarction. Am Heart J 1979 June; 97(6):782–796

Gerber SD et al. A diagnostic strategy for myocardial infarction. J Fam Pract 1979 Aug; 9(2):207–218

Gunnar R. Management of acute myocardial infarction and accelerating angina. Prog Cardiovasc Dis 1979 July–Aug; 22(1):1–30

Hansen MS and Woods SL. Nitroglycerin ointment—Where and how to apply it. Am J Nurs 1980 June; 80(6): 1122–1124

Hirsch AT. Postmyocardial infarction syndrome. Am J Nurs 1979 July; 79(7):1240–1241

Karsh DL et al. Prolonged benefit of nitroglycerin ointment on exercise tolerance in patients with angina pectoris. Am Heart J 1978 Nov; 96(5):587–595

Lester RM and Wagner GS. Acute myocardial infarction. Med Clin North Am 1979 Jan; 63(1):3–24

Navin TR and Hager DW. Creatine kinase MB isoenzyme in the evaluation of myocardial infarction. Curr Probl Cardiol 1979 March; 3(12):1–32

O'Flynn-Comiskey AI. The Type A individual. Am J Nurs 1979 Nov; 79(11):1956–1958

Plotnick GD. Approach to the management of unstable angina. Am Heart J 1979 Aug; 98(2):243–255

Resnekov L and DasGupta DS. Prevention of ventricular rhythm disturbances in patients with acute myocardial infarction. Am Heart J 1979 Nov; 98(5):653–659

Rossi LP and Haines VM. Nursing diagnoses related to acute myocardial infarction. Cardio-Vasc Nursing 1979 May–June; 15(3):11–15

Assessment/Diagnosis

Bauman DJ, Creatine phosphokinase isoenzymes and the diagnosis of myocardial infarction. Postgrad Med 1980 Jan; 67(1):103–116

Blewett CH. Dynamic electrocardiography. CVP 1979 Oct–Nov; 7(6):29–32

Burlina A. The clinical relevance of isoenzyme assays. Clin Biochem 1979 June; 12(3):71–76

Cannon C. Hands-on guide to palpation and auscultation. RN 1980 March; 43(3):20–27, 76

Finlayson JK, Kenmure ACF and Short DS. Cardiac signs for students: The wheat and the chaff. Br Med J 1978 June; 1(6125):1471–1473

Marmor A et al. Creatine kinase isoenzyme MB (CK-MB) in acute coronary ischemia. Am Heart J 1979 May; 97(5):574–577

Papenhausen P. Cardiovascular and respiratory assessment for critical care practitioners. Current Practice in Critical Care 1979, 1:30–63

Pelletier C, Dufort G and Fortier P. Cardiac output measurement by thermodilution. Can J Surg 1979 July; 22(4):347–350

Pepler C. Your finger on the pulse: Evaluating what you feel. Nursing '80 1980 Nov; 10(11):32–39

Wasserman AG and Rose AM. Advances in noninvasive cardiology: Nuclear imaging and two dimensional echocardiography. CVP 1979 Oct–Nov; 7(6):63–67

Winkle RA. Ambulatory electrocardiography. Mod Concepts Cardiovasc Dis 1980 Feb; 49(2):7–12

Cardiogenic Shock

Amsterdam EA et al. Mechanical circulatory assist in acute ischemic heart disease. Adv Cardiol 1978; 23:142–162

Amsterdam EA et al. Vasodilators in myocardial infarction: Rationale and current status. Drugs 1978 Dec; 16(6):506–521

Bregman D and Casarella WJ. Percutaneous intra-aortic balloon pumping: Initial clinical experience. Ann Thorac Surg 1980 Feb; 29(2):153–155

Bricker PL. The intense nursing demands of the intra-aortic balloon pump. RN 1980 July; 43(7):22–29

Chrzanowski AL. Intra-aortic balloon pumping: Concepts and patient care. Nurs Clin North Am 1978 Sept; 13(3):513–530

Geddes JS, Adgey AAJ and Pantridge JF. Prevention of cardiogenic shock. Am Heart J 1980 Feb; 99(2):243–254

Juhlin-Dannfelt A, Norlander R and Nyquist O. Peripheral hemodynamics in assisted circulation with intra-aortic balloon pumping in patients with cardiogenic shock. Acta Med Scand 1979; 205(6):505–508

Massie BM and Chatterjee K. Vasodilator therapy of pump failure complicating acute myocardial infarction. Med Clin North Am 1979 Jan; 63(1):25–31

Miller RR et al. Surgical treatment of myocardial infarction shock. Adv Cardiol 1978; 23(6):163–172

Phillips SJ et al. Cardiogenic shock. Treatment by augmentation with a pulsatile assist device. JAMA 1979 Sept 22; 240(13):1376–1377

Promisloff R. Therapy for cardiogenic shock. Compr Ther 1978 Nov; 4(11):49–56

Resnekov L. Cardiogenic shock. Br J Hosp Med 1978 Sept; 20(3):232–241

Sonnenblick EH, Frishman WH and LeJemtel TH. Dobutamine: A new synthetic cardioactive sympathetic amine. N Engl J Med 1979 Jan 4; 300(1):17–22

Wei JY, Hutchins GM and Bulkley BH. Papillary muscle rupture in fatal acute myocardial infarction: A potentially treatable form of cardiogenic shock. Ann Intern Med 1979 Feb; 90(2):149–152

Whitman G. Intra-aortic balloon pumping and cardiac mechanics: A programmed lesson. Heart Lung 1978 Nov–Dec; 7(6):1034–1050

Cardiovascular Surgery

Blacher RS. Heart surgery. JAMA 1979 Nov 30; 242(22):2463–2464

Bregman D, Spotnitz HM and Malm JR. Cardiac surgery. Current Cardiology 1979; 1:305–321

Cromwell V et al. Understanding the needs of your coronary bypass patient. Nursing '80 1980 March; 10(3):34–41

Derrick HF. How open heart surgery feels. Am J Nurs 1979 Feb; 79(2):276–285

Dubin WR, Field HL and Castfriend DR. Postcardiotomy delirium: A critical review. J Thorac Cardiovasc Surg 1979 April; 77(4):586–594

Fox AC, Glassman E and Isom OW. Surgically remedial complications of myocardial infarction. Prog Cardiovasc Dis 1979 May–June; 21(6):461–484

Korn R et al. Meeting the needs of your coronary bypass patient. Nursing '80 1980 March; 10(3):40–45

Ott DA and Cooley DA. Current status of cardiac valve surgery. J Fla Med Assoc 1979 Oct; 66(10):1034–1038

Romero PE. Preoperative teaching for cardiovascular surgical patients. Cardio-Vasc Nursing 1978 Nov–Dec; 14(6):27–32

Stuart EM et al. Nursing rounds: Care of the patient with a mitral commissurotomy. Am J Nurs 1980 Sept; 80(9):1611–1632

Cardiopulmonary Resuscitation/Defibrillation

Bander JJ. Defibrillation. Topics in Emergency Medicine 1979 July; 1(2):75–86

DeSilva RA and Lown B. Energy requirements for defibrillation of a markedly overweight patient. Circulation 1978 April; 57(4):827–830

Ewy G (ed). Cardiac arrest and resuscitation: Defibrillators and defibrillation. Curr Probl Cardiol 1978 Feb; 11(11):8–71

Goldfarb AL and Logudice A. Cardiopulmonary resuscitation in a general hospital—variations on a theme. CVP 1979 Aug–Sept; 7(5):15–18

National Conference on Standards and Guidelines for Cardiopulmonary Resuscitation (CPR) and Emergency Cardiac Care (ECC). Standards and guidelines for cardiopulmonary resuscitation. JAMA 1980 Aug 1; 244(5):453–509

Tyler ML. Basic cardiopulmonary resuscitation. Nurs Clin North Am 1978 Sept; 13(3):499–512

Walraven G and Kavanaugh M. Cardiac arrest: A review of the resuscitation process. Topics in Emergency Medicine 1979 July; 1(2):115–127

Congestive Heart Failure/Pulmonary Edema

Armstrong PW. Contributions of hemodynamic monitoring to the treatment of chronic congestive heart failure. Can Med Assoc J 1979 Oct; 121(7):913–918

Aronow WS. Clinical use of nitrates. II Nitrates in congestive heart failure. Mod Concepts of Cardiovasc Dis 1979 July; 48(7):37–42

Blonder RD. The use of vasodilator therapy for heart failure. AOA 1979 June; 78(10):753–756

Franciosa JA. The role of vasodilators in managing congestive heart failure. Postgrad Med 1980 Jan; 67(1):87–91, 94–98

Hall WD. Clinical use of diuretics in congestive heart failure. Med Times 1979 Jan; 107(1):24–32

Heggie J. Pulling your patient through congestive heart failure. RN 1980 Sept; 43(9):31–36, 131–132

Lakier JB, Khaja F and Stein PD. Rationale and use of vasodilators in the management of congestive heart failure. Am Heart J 1979 April; 97(4):519–526

Mason DT and Awan NA. Recent advances in digitalis research. Am J Cardiol 1979 May; 43(5):1056–1059

Mason DT (ed). Symposium on vasodilator and inotropic therapy of heart failure. Am J Med 1978 July; 65(1):101–216

Mason DT et al. Vasodilator therapy for chronic heart failure. Compr Ther 1979 July; 5(7):6–14

Overland ES and Severinghaus JW. Noncardiac pulmonary edema. Adv Intern Med 1978; 23:307–326

Parmley WW and Chatterjee K. Vasodilator therapy. Curr Probl Cardiol 1978 March; 11(12):8–75

Segal BL. New approaches to therapy of acute heart failure. Am Fam Physician 1980 Feb; 21(2):131–135

Smith-Collins A. Dobutamine. A new inotropic agent. Nursing '80 1980 March; 10(3):62–66

Von Hoff DD et al. Risk factors for doxorubicin-induced congestive heart failure. Ann Intern Med 1979 Nov; 91(5):710–717

White S and Williamson K. What to watch for when you give loop diuretics. RN 1979 Dec; 42(12):25–27

Endocarditis/Myocarditis/Pericarditis

Agner RC and Gallis HA. Pericarditis: Differential diagnostic considerations. Arch Intern Med 1979 April; 139(4):407–412

Bandt CM, Staley NA and Noren GR. Acute viral myocarditis. Clinical and histological changes. Minn Med 1979 April; 62(4):234–237

Breaux EP et al. Cardiac tamponade following penetrating mediastinal injuries; improved survival with early pericardiocentesis. J Trauma 1979 June; 19(6):461–466

Brown AK. Pericardial disease. Practitioner 1980 March; 224(1341):249–252

Cohen PS, Maguire JH and Weinstein L. Infective endocarditis caused by gram-negative bacteria: A review of the literature, 1945–1977. Prog Cardiovasc Dis 1980 Jan–Feb; 22(4):205–242

Dormer AE. The management of infective endocarditis. Practitioner 1980 March; 224(1341):225–259

Dracup KA. Managing and understanding the patient with infective endocarditis. Nursing '80 1980 May; 10(5):44–50

Gregoratos G and Karline R. Infective endocarditis. Med Clin North Am 1979 Jan; 63(1):173–199

Hancock EW. Cardiac tamponade. Med Clin North Am 1979 Jan; 63(1):223–237

Hancock EW. Management of pericardial disease. Mod Concepts Cardiovasc Dis 1979 Jan; 48(1):1–6

Kotler MN and Segal BL. The inflamed heart: Pericarditis in the elderly. Geriatrics 1980 Jan; 35(1):63–73

Krikorian JG and Hancock EW. Pericardiocentesis. Am J Med 1978 Nov; 65(5):808–814

McDonald A. Management of infective endocarditis. Br J Hosp Med 1979 May; 21(5):498–506

Moore SJ. Pericarditis after acute myocardial infarction: Manifestations. Heart Lung 1979 May–June; 8(3):551–558

Pankey GA. The prevention and treatment of bacterial endocarditis. Am Heart J 1979 July; 98(1):102–118

Petersdorf RG and Goldman PL. Changes in the natural history of bacterial endocarditis. J Chronic Dis 1979; 32(4):287–291

Phair JP (ed). Recent topics in endocarditis. Prog Cardiovasc Dis 1979 Nov–Dec; 22(3):135–204

Roberts WC. Cardiomyopathy and myocarditis: Morphologic features. Adv Cardiol 1979; 22:184–198

Robinson PH. Pericarditis. Med Times 1979 Jan; 107(1):73–78

Wong B et al. The risk of pericardiocentesis. Am J. Cardiol 1979 Nov; 44(6):1110–1114

Hemodynamic Monitoring

Arbitman M and Kart BH. Hemomediastinum after aberrant central venous catheter placement. Crit Care Med 1979 Jan; 7(1):27–29

Baigrie RS and Morgan CD. Hemodynamic monitoring: Catheter insertion techniques, complications and troubleshooting. Can Med Assoc J 1979 Oct; 121(7):885–892

Csanky-Treels JC. Hazards of central venous pressure monitoring. Anaesthesia 1978 Feb; 33(2):172–177

Dalen JE. Bedside hemodynamic monitoring. N Engl J Med 1979 Nov 22; 301(21):1176–1178

Editorial. Swan–Ganz catheters. Lancet 1978 Aug 12; 2(8085):357–358

Felices FJ et al. Use of the central venous pressure catheter to obtain blood cultures. Crit Care Med 1979 Feb; 7(2):78–79

Fisher RE. Measuring central venous pressure: How to do it accurately—and safely. Nursing '79 1979 Oct; 9(10):74–78

Gill BA. Hemodynamic monitoring setup. AORN J 1979 March; 29(4):756, 758, 760, 764

Gomez F, Spagna P and Lemole GM. Improved techniques in using the Swan–Ganz catheter. Ann Thorac Surg 1979 May; 27(5):468–471

Hathaway R. The Swan–Ganz catheter: A review. Nurs Clin North Am 1978 Sept; 13(3):389–407

Haughey B. CVP lines: Monitoring and maintaining. Am J Nurs 1978 April; 78(4):635–638

Lalli SM. The complete Swan–Ganz. RN 1978 Sept; 41(9):64–77

Lantiegne KC and Civetta JM. A system for maintaining invasive pressure monitoring. Heart Lung 1978 July–Aug; 78(4):610–621

Nichols WW, Nichols MA and Barbour H. Complications associated with balloon-tipped, flow-directed catheters. Heart Lung 1979 May–June; 8(3):503–506

Pego RF and Lurin MH. Left subclavian vein puncture for insertion of Swan–Ganz catheters. Heart Lung 1979 May–June; 8(3):507–510

Pelletier C, Dufort J and Fortier P. Cardiac output measurement by thermodilution. Can J Surg 1979 July; 22(4):347–350

Rettig FM. Appraisal of intracardiac monitoring. AORN J 1979 April; 29(5):839–844

Shipley SB. Pitfalls and perils of intracardiac monitoring. AORN J 1979 April; 29(5):845–855

Swan HJC and Ganz W. Hemodynamic monitoring: A personal and historical perspective. Can Med Assoc J 1979 Oct; 121(6):868–871

Cardiac Pacing

Bartecchi CE. Emergency transvenous subclavian cardiac pacing in elderly patients. J Am Geriatr Soc 1979 May, 27(5):208–211

Del Negro AA and Fletcher RD. Indications for use of artificial cardiac pacemakers: Part II. Curr Prob Cardiol 1978 Nov; 3(8):6–43

Furman S. Recent developments in cardiac pacing. Heart Lung 1978 Sept–Oct; 7(5):813–826

Jara FM et al. The infected pacemaker pocket. J Thorac Cardiovasc Surg 1979 Aug; 78(2):298–300

Smyth NPD. Cardiac pacing. Ann Thorac Surg 1979 March; 27(3):270–283

Smyth NPD et al. Clinical experience with the isotopic cardiac pacemaker. Ann Thorac Surg 1979 July; 28(1):14–21

Vera Z, Klein RC and Mason DT. Recent advances in programmable pacemakers. Am J Med 1979 March; 66(3):473–483

Rheumatic Heart Disease

deLeon AC Jr. Mitral valve prolapse. Postgrad Med 1980 Jan; 67(1):66–77

Selzer A. Nonrheumatic mitral regurgitation. Mod Concepts Cardiovasc Dis 1979 May; 48(5):25–30

Ward DC. A reappraisal of the clinical features in acute and chronic rheumatic heart disease: Etiological implications. Am Heart J 1979 Sept; 98(3):298–306

Wyse DG, McAnulty JH and Rahimtoola SH. Antibiotic prophylaxis in patients with rheumatic heart disease. Clin Cardiol 1978 Aug; 1(2):112–117

ESSENTIALS OF BASIC ELECTROCARDIOGRAPHY

Books

Andreoli K et al. Comprehensive Cardiac Care, 4th ed. St. Louis, C.V. Mosby, 1979

Castellanos A. Cardiac Arrhythmias: Mechanisms and Management. Cardiovascular Clinics. Philadelphia, F.A. Davis, 1980

Chou T. Electrocardiography In Clinical Practice. New York, Grune Stratton, 1979

Chung E. Electrocardiography. Hagerstown, Harper & Row, 1980

Chung E. Principles of Cardiac Arrhythmias, 2nd ed. Baltimore, Williams & Wilkins, 1977

Delman AJ and Stein E. Dynamic Cardiac Auscultation and Phonocardiography. Philadelphia, WB Saunders, 1979

Dubin D. Rapid Interpretation of EKGs, 3rd ed. Tampa, Cover Publishing Co, 1975

Ferrer J. The Sick Sinus Syndrome. New York, Futura Publishing Co, 1974

Friedman H. Diagnostic Electrocardiography and Vectorcardiography, 2nd ed. New York, McGraw-Hill, 1977

Goldman M. Principles of Clinical Electrocardiography, 9th ed. Los Altos, Lange Medical Publishers, 1976

Hurst, W. The Heart. New York, McGraw-Hill, 1978

Mangiola S and Ritota M. Cardiac Arrhythmias: Practical ECG Interpretation. Philadelphia, JB Lippincott, 1974

Marriott H. Practical Electrocardiography, 6th Ed. Baltimore, Williams, & Wilkins, 1977

Meltzer L, Pinneo R and Kitchell J. Intensive Coronary Care, 3rd ed. Bowie, Charles Press Publishers, 1977

Moss A and Emmanouilides G. Practical Pediatric Electrocardiography. Philadelphia, JB Lippincott, 1973

Phibbs B. The Cardiac Arrhythmias, 3rd ed. St. Louis, C.V. Mosby, 1978

Schamroth L. An Introduction to Electrocardiography, 5th ed. Oxford, Blackwell Scientific Publications, 1976

Stein E. The Electrocardiogram. Philadelphia, WB Saunders, 1976

Articles

Basta L. The ambulatory patient with ectopic beats and episodic tachyarrhythmias. Am Fam Physician 1977 Feb; 15(4):94–98

Bigger JT. Sick Sinus syndrome label for many cardiac problems. JAMA 1978 Feb 13; 239(7):597

Bretylium (Bretylol) for ventricular arrhythmias. Med Lett Drugs Ther 1978 Dec 1; 20(24):105–106

Chung E. Artificial cardiac pacing. Postgrad Med 1976 June; 59(6):83–90

Chung EK. Tachyarrhythmias in Wolff–Parkinson–White syndrome: Antiarrhythmic drug therapy. JAMA 1977 Jan 24; 237(4):376–379

Disopyramide (Norpace) for ventricular arrhythmias. Med Lett Drugs Ther 1977 Dec 16; 19(25):101–102

Dolgin M. The peculiarities of cardiac arrhythmias. Consultant 1976 May; 16(5):167–175

Furman S. Cardiac pacing and pacemakers. I. Indications for pacing bradyarrhythmias. Am Heart J 1977 Apr; 93(4):523–530

Galen R. Myocardial infarction: A clinician's guide to the isoenzymes. Resident & Staff Physician 1977 May; 23:67–72

Gallagher JJ, Svenson RH and Sealy WV et al. The Wolff–Parkinson–White syndrome and the preexcitation dysrhythmias. Medical and surgical management. Med Clin North Am 1976 Jan; 60(1):101–123

Glasser S and Martinez-Lopez J. Atrial flutter. Postgrad Med 1977 Aug; 62(2):61–67

Grace W. Protocol for the management of arrhythmias in acute myocardial infarction. Crit Care Med 1974 Sept–Oct; 2(5):235–242

Harrison DC. Should lidocaine be administered routinely to all patients after acute myocardial infarction. Circulation 1978 Oct; 58(4):581–584

Harrison DC, Miffin PJ and Winkle RA. Clinical pharmacokinetics of antiarrhythmic drugs. Prog Cardiovasc Dis 1977; 20(3):217–242

Josephson ME and Kastor JA. Supraventricular tachycardia: mechanism and management. Ann Intern Med 1977 Sept; 87(3):346–358

Kastor J. Atrioventricular-block. New Engl J Med 1975 Mar; 292(11):572–574

Kleiger R (ed). Arrhythmias, Part 1. Heart Lung 1977 Jan–Feb; 6(1):60–88

Kleiger R (ed). Arrhythmias, Part 2. Heart Lung 1977 Mar–Apr; 6(2):249–262

Krikler D. A fresh look at cardiac arrhythmias. Lancet May 4, 1(7862):851–854; May 11, 1(7863):913–918; May 18, 1(7864):974–976; May 25, 1(7865):1034–1037

McNeal GP. Tracing arrhythmias. Am J Nurs 1979 Jan; 79(1):98–100

Narula O. Sick sinus syndrome. Primary Cardiol 1978 Jan; 4(1):27–31

Tai A et al. Step-by-step protocols for arrhythmias. Patient Care 1977 Feb 25; 11(6):100–123

Treatment of cardiac arrhythmias. Med Lett Drugs Ther 1978 Dec 29; 20(26):113–120

Uhley H. Clinical application of electrocardiographic trend recording. Heart Lung 1976 Mar–Apr; 5(2):267–272

Winslow EF and Powell AH. Sick sinus syndrome. Am J Nurs 1976 Aug; 76(8):1262–1265

VASCULAR CONDITIONS

Books

Berger EC. The Physiology of Adequate Perfusion. St. Louis, C.V. Mosby, 1979

Berger JJ and Yao STJ. Venous Problems. Chicago, Year Book Medical Publishers, 1978

Bernstein EF. Noninvasive Diagnostic Techniques in Vascular Disease. St. Louis, C.V. Mosby, 1978

Brunner JMR. Handbook of Blood Pressure Monitoring. Littleton, PSG Publishing Co. 1978

Cooley DA and Wukash DC. Techniques in Vascular Surgery. Philadelphia, WB Saunders, 1979

Dardik H (ed). Graft Materials in Vascular Surgery. Chicago, Year Book Medical Publishers, 1978

Guyton AC. Arterial Pressure and Hypertension. Philadelphia, WB Saunders, 1980

Johnson PC (ed). Peripheral Circulation. New York, John Wiley & Sons, 1978

Kaplan NM. Clinical Hypertension. Baltimore, Williams & Wilkins, 1978

May R. Surgery of the Veins of the Leg and Pelvis. Philadelphia, WB Saunders, 1979

O'Brien B Mc. Microvascular Reconstructive Surgery. New York, Churchill Livingston, 1977

Rapaport E (ed). Current Controversies in Cardiovascular Disease. Philadelphia, WB Saunders, 1980

Rutherford RD. Vascular Surgery. Philadelphia, WB Saunders, 1977

Stehbens WE. Hemodynamics and the Blood Vessel Walls. Springfield, Charles C Thomas, 1979.

Articles

Diagnosis of Vascular Problems

AbuRahma AF, Diethrich EB and Reiling M. Doppler testing in peripheral vascular occlusive disease. Surg Gynecol Ostet 1980 Jan; 150(1):26–28

Cranley JJ and Hyland LJ. Diagnoses in peripheral vascular diseases. Contemp Surg 1979 April; 14(4):45–80

Cutler BS et al. Assessment of operative risk with electrocardiographic exercise testing in patients with peripheral vascular disease. Am J Surg 1979 April; 137(4):484–490

Miller KM. Assessing peripheral perfusion. Am J Nurs 1978 Oct; 78(10):1673–1674

Smith RN. Invasive pressure monitoring. Am J Nurs 1978 Sept; 78(9):1514–1521

Sphygmomanometer accuracy. Am J Nurs 1979 Nov; 79(11):2004

General Vascular Problems

AbuRahma AF, Diethrich EB and Reiling M. Doppler testing in peripheral vascular occlusive disease. Surg Gynecol Obstet 1980 Jan; 150(1):26–28

Balloon catheter successfully treats peripheral occlusion. AORN J 1980 Jan; 31(1):59–60

Cerkoney KA. The psychological effects of regular exercise on the health/illness continuum. Focus 1980 Sept/Oct; 7(4):27–31

Crawford DW and Blankenhorn DH. Regression of atherosclerosis. Ann Rev Med 1979; 30:289–300

Dardik H et al. Current status; valvular graft materials. Contemp Surg 1978 March; 12(3):9–20

DeBakey ME. The development of vascular surgery. Am J Surg 1979 June; 137(6):697–738

Diminished platelet survival is linked to atherosclerosis. Am Fam Physician 1980 March; 21(3):165

Dosick S and Blakemore WS. The role of Doppler ultrasound in acute deep vein thrombosis. Am J Surg 1978 Aug; 138(2):265–268

Deykin D. Antithrombotic therapy. Postgrad Med 1979 Jan; 65(1):135–146

Eddy ME. Teaching patients with peripheral vascular disease. Nurs Clin North Am 1977 March; 12(1):151–159

Fagan-Dubin L. Atherosclerosis: A major cause of peripheral vascular disease. Nurs Clin North Am 1977 March; 12(1):101–108

Gulhold GW. Prevention of thrombolism. Am Fam Physician 1979 March; 19(3):147–153

Hirsh J. Antiplatelet drugs in thromboembolism. Postgrad Med 1979 Sept; 66(3):119–126

Intermittent claudication. Lancet 1980 Feb 23; 1 (8165):404–405

Jordan H. Your fingers on the pulse—evaluating what you feel. Nursing '80 1980 Nov; 10(11):33–39

Kahn SB. Prevention of thrombosis with antiplatelet drugs. Am Fam Physician 1980 May; 21(5):166–168

Kannel WB, Castelli WP and Gordon T. Cholesterol in the prediction of atherosclerotic disease. Ann Intern Med 1979 Jan; 90(1):85–91

Metzler M and Silver D. Vasospastic disorders. Postgrad Med 1979 Feb; 65(2):79–81

Pierce PF. Gains and losses of vascular surgery patients. Nurs Clin North Am 1977 March: 12(1):119–127

Raines J and Traad E. Noninvasive evaluation of peripheral vascular disease. Med Clin North Am 1980 March; 64(2):283–302

Ryzewski J. Factors in the rehabiltation of patients with peripheral vascular disease. Nurs Clin North Am 1977 March; 12(1):161–168

Weiss RB and Shah S. When "lymphoma" is not lymphoma. Postgrad Med 1978 May; 63(5):101–109

Veins

Dosick S and Blackmore WS. The role of Doppler ultrasound in acute deep vein thrombosis. Am J Surg 1978 Aug; 138(2):265–268

Hyland DB and Kirkland VJ. Infrared therapy for skin ulcers. Am J Nurs 1980 Oct; 80(10):1800–1801

Kistner RB. Primary venous valve incompetence of the leg. Am J Surg 1980 Aug; 140(2):218–227

Lofgren KA. Varicose veins. Postgrad Med 1979 June; 65(6):131–139

O'Donnell TF et al. Diagnosis of deep venous thrombosis in the outpatient department by venography. Surg Gynecol Obstet 1980 Jan; 150(1):69–74

Sasahara AA, Ho DD and Sharma GVRK. When and how to use fibrinolytic agents (thromboembolism). Drug Ther 1979 Oct; 9(10):111–128

Straith RE, Lawson JM and Choi CS. Circumsuture treatment for varicosities. Postgrad Med 1980 Jan; 67(1):191–197

Weissberg D. Treatment of varicose veins by compression sclerotherapy. Surg Gynecol Obstet 1980 Sept; 151(3):353–356

Arteries

Biofeedback for patients with Raynaud's phenomenon. JAMA 1979 Aug 10; 242(6):509–510

Campbell HC, Hubbard SG and Ernst CB. Continuous heparin anticoagulation in patients with arteriosclerosis and arterial emboli. Surg Gynecol Obstet 1980 Jan; 159(1):54–56

Chang FC et al. Abdominal aortic aneurysms. Am J Surg 1978 Dec; 136(6):705–708

Fenn JE. Reconstructive arterial surgery. Nurs Clin North Am 1977 March; 12(1):129–142

Hardening of the arteries—1980. Harvard Medical School Health Letter 1980 Feb; 5(4):1–2; 5

Heyman A et al. Risk of stroke in asymptomatic persons with cervical arterial bruits; a population study in Evans County, Georgia. N Engl J Med 1980 April 10; 302(15):838

Kessro B. Peripheral arterial insufficiency. Nurs Clin North Am 1977 March; 12(1):143–149

Miller DC and Griepp RB. A modern view of the surgical treatment of peripheral arterial disease. JAMA Sept 29 1978; 240(14):1524–1527

Rich S. Percutaneous transluminal angioplasty. Postgrad Med 1980 Sept; 68(3):217–224

Satiani B and Evans WE. Immediate prognosis and five-year survival after arterial embolectomy following myocardial infarction. Surg Gynecol Obstet 1980 Jan; 150(1):41–44

Sexton DL. The patient with peripheral arterial occlusive disease. Nurs Clin North Am 1977 March; 12(1):89–99

Taggart E. The physical assessment of the patient with arterial disease. Nurs Clin North Am 1977 March; 12(1):109–117

Thompson JE and Garrett WV. Peripheral-arterial surgery. N Engl J Med 1980 Feb; 302(9):491–503

Anticoagulant Therapy

Campbell HC, Hubbard SG and Ernst CB. Continuous heparin anticoagulation in patients with arteriosclerosis and arterial emboli. Surg Gynecol Obstet 1980 Jan; 150(1):54–56

Chamberlain SL. Low-dose heparin therapy. Am J Nurs 1980 June; 80(6):1115–1117

Estes JW. Heparin in clinical practice. Drug Ther 1979 Sept; 9(9):47–59

Forfar J. A seven-year analysis of haemorrhage in patients on long-term anticoagulant treatment. Br Heart J 1979 July 42:128–132

Furie B. Using oral anticoagulants effectively. Drug Ther 1979 Sept; 9(9):77–83

Gelfand R and Mitani G. Surreptitious use of warfarin. J Nerv Ment Dis 1979 July; 167(7):447–449

Hand J. Keeping anticoagulants under control. RN 1979 April; 42(4):25–29

Lunden D. You can inject heparin subcutaneously. RN 1978 Dec; 41(12):51–54

McKee PA. The prevention of thromboembolism. Drug Ther 1979 Sept; 9(9):19–21

Rosenberg RD and Rosenberg JS. The anticoagulant function of heparin. Drug Ther 1979 Sept; (9):26–38

Zalunas JC and Simon C. Anticoagulants: Accepted treatment and current trends. Nurses' Drug Alert 1979 Sept; 3(12):105–112

HYPERTENSION

Books

American Heart Association. Cooking Without Your Salt Shaker. Cleveland, American Heart Association Northeast Ohio Affiliate, 1978

Capell P and Case DB. Hypertension, Ambulatory Care Manual for Nurse Practitioners. Philadelphia, JB Lippincott, 1976

Chewning B. Staff Manual for Teaching Patients about Hypertension. Chicago, American Hospital Association, 1978

Erfurt JC and Foote A Blood Pressure Control at the Work Site. Manual of Procedures for Blood Pressure Control Programs in Industrial Settings. Ann Arbor, University of Michigan-Wayne State University, 1979

Fighting High Blood Pressure in the Inner City. Washington,

D.C., Citizens for the Treatment of High Blood Pressure, 1979

Freis ED and Kolata GB. The High Blood Pressure Book: A Guide for Patients and Their Families. Sausalito, Painter Hopkins Publishers, 1979

High Blood Pressure and the Nurse, Bibliography. High Blood Pressure Information Center, National High Blood Pressure Education Program, 1979

High Blood Pressure—Risk Factors, Bibliography. High Blood Pressure Information Center, National High Blood Pressure Education Program, 1979

Hypertension and Oral Contraceptives, Bibliography, High Blood Pressure Information Center, National High Blood Pressure Education Program, 1979

Hypertension in the Elderly, Bibliography, High Blood Pressure Information Center, National High Blood Pressure Education Program, 1979

Kochar MS and Daniels LM. Hypertension Control for Nurses and other Health Professionals. St. Louis, C.V. Mosby, 1978

Margie J and Hunt JV. Living with High Blood Pressure: The Hypertension Diet Cookbook. Bloomfield, HLS Press, 1978

National High Blood Pressure Education Program. Washington, D.C., Audiovisual Aids for High Blood Pressure Education, DHEW, 1980

Studies and Statements

American Heart Association. Recommendations for Human Blood Pressure Determination by Sphygmomanometers, Pub No. 70–019–B, Dallas, American Heart Assoc., revised 1980

Guidelines for Educating Nurses in High Blood Pressure Control. U.S. Department of Health, Education, and Welfare, NIH Pub No 80–1241, March, 1980

National High Blood Pressure Education Program. California Conference on High Blood Pressure Control in the Spanish Speaking Community, April 1-2, 1978. Los Angeles, Cal. Summary Report, Washington, D.C., DHEW, 1979

National High Blood Pressure Education Program Coordinating Committee. Statement on Blood Pressure Measurement Devices Used by Consumers, April, 1980

The 1980 Report of the Joint National Committee on Detection, Evaluation, and Treatment of High Blood Pressure. Washington, D.C., DHHS, NIH Pub No 81–1088, 1980

Report of the Hypertension Task Force, National Institutes of Health, Vols. 1–9. NIH Pub No. 79–1623, September, 1979

Articles

A look at high blood pressure. Harvard Med School Health Letter, Part I 1979 June; 4(8):1–2, 5; Part II 1979 July; 4(9):1–2,5

Benson H et al. Stress and hypertension: Interrelations and management. Cardiovasc Clin 1978; 9(1):113–124

Berkson D et al. Evaluation of an automated blood pressure measuring device intended for general public use. Am J Public Health 1979 May; 69(5):473–479

Burke MD. Hypertension: Strategies for laboratory diagnosis. Postgrad Med 1980 June; 67(6):77–85

Caldwell JR. Practical approach to hypertension. Part I. Diagnostic evaluation. Postgrad Med 1979 May; 65(5):66–77; Part II. Treatment. Postgrad Med 1979 May; 65(5):81–92

Canessa M et al. Increased sodium–lithium countertransport in red cells of patients with essential hypertension. N Engl J Med 1980 April 3; 302(14):772–776

Catopril for hypertension. Med Letter 1980 May 2; 22(9):39–40

Clinical trials provide new information. JAMA 1980 May 2; 243(17):1706

Conomy JP. Impact of arterial hypertension on the brain. Postgrad Med 1980 Aug; 68(2):86–97

Daniels LM and Kochar MS. Monitoring and facilitating adherence to hypertension therapeutic regimens. Cardiovasc Nurs 1980 March–April; 16(2):7–12

Finnerty FA Jr. Hypertension in the elderly. Postgrad Med 1979 May; 65(5):119–125

Foster SB et al. Influence of side effects of antihypertensive medications on patient behavior. Cardiovasc Nurs 1978 May–June; 14(2):9–14

Frohlich ED. Special Report: Review of the WHO expert committee report on arterial hypertension. Hypertension 1979 Sept–Oct; 1(5):547–548

Gantt CL. Drug therapy of hypertension. Med Clin North Am 1978 Nov; 62(6):1273–289

Garay RP et al. Laboratory distinction between essential and secondary hypertension by measurement of erythrocyte cation fluxes. N Engl J Med 1980 Apr 3; 302(14):769–791

Gillum RF. Pathophysiology of hypertension in blacks and whites. Hypertension 1979 Sept–Oct; 1(5):468–475

Hartshorn JC. Hypertensive crisis. Nursing '80 1980 July; 8(7):37–45

Hill M. Helping the hypertensive patient control sodium intake. Am J Nurs 1979 May; 79(5):906–909

Hill MN. Hypertension: What can go wrong when you measure blood pressure? Am J Nurs 1980 May; 80(5):942–946

Hypertension detection and follow-up program: Five-year findings of the hypertension detection and follow-up program. JAMA 1979 Dec 7; 242(23):2562–2577

Hypertension—The Scope of the Problem and the Role of the Nurse. Massachusetts Nurses Association, 1980

Hypertension—Try a practical first step. Patient Care 1980 Sept 30; 14(16):17–46

Kotchen TA and Havlik RJ. High blood pressure in the young. Ann Intern Med 1980 Feb. 92(2):254

Loggie JMH. Identification and management of juvenile hypertension. Postgrad Med 1979 May; 65(5):103–114

Mainzer M. A reminder—fever due to methyldopa. N Engl J Med Jan 17 1980; 302(3):174

Maloney R. Helping your hypertensive patients live longer. Nursing '78 1978 Oct; 8(10):26–35

Marcinek MB. Hypertension: What does it do to the body? Am J Nurs 1980 May; 80(5):927–936

Minoxidil (Loniten). The Med Letter 1980 Mar 7; 22(5):21–22

Moore MA. Hypertensive emergencies. Am Fam Physician 1980 Mar; 21(3):141–146

Moser M. Hypertension: How therapy works. Am J Nurs 1980 May; 80(5):937–941

Nadolol (Corgard) a new beta-blocker. The Med Letter 1980 Apr 18; 22(8):33–34

Onesti G. Selection of drugs for hypertensive crisis. Am Fam Physician 1980 Dec; 22(6):141–142

Parker JC (ed). Hypertension and the red cell. N Engl J Med 1980 Apr 3; 302(14):804–805

Patient behavior for blood pressure control. JAMA 1979 June 8; 241(23):2534–2537

Rodman MJ. How to cope with those new antihypertensive drugs. RN 1979 Oct; 42(10):109–116

Schoof CS. Hypertension: Common questions patients ask. Am J Nurs 1980 May; 80(5):926–927

Segal JL. Hypertensive emergencies. Postgrad Med 1980 Aug; 68(2):107–125

Silverberg D, Shemesh E and Iaina A. The unsupported arm: A cause of falsely raised blood pressure readings. Br Med J 1977 Nov 19; 2: 1331

Stamler J et al. Prevention and control of hypertension by nutrition–hygienic means. JAMA 1980 May 9; 243(18):1819–1823

Treat mild hypertension. Amer Fam Physician 1980 Apr 21; (4):86–91

Wagner EG et al. Hypertension control in a rural biracial community: Successes and failures of primary care. Am J Public Health 1980 Jan; 70(1):48–55

Warren W et al. Clonidine and propranolol paradoxical hypertension. Arch Intern Med 1979 Feb; 139(2):253

Weiner EE. Nurse management of hypertension. Am J Nurs 1980 June; 80(6):1129

White SJ and Williamson K. What to watch for with peripherally acting antihypertensives. RN 1980 Jan; 43(1):51–58

DISORDERS OF THE DIGESTIVE SYSTEM

10

1 CONDITIONS OF THE MOUTH, NECK, AND ESOPHAGUS

MOUTH CONDITIONS

NURSING ASSESSMENT FOR EFFECTIVE MOUTH CARE

Psychosocial Significance

1. The person's comfort, good nutrition, and general well-being are promoted by maintaining clean and well cared for teeth and gums.
2. Personal attractiveness is enhanced.
3. Participation in community dental health programs promotes prevention, early detection, and correction of dental problems.

Client/Patient Self-Care Goals

1. To reduce bacterial count and prevent tissue infection by removing food and rinsing the mouth.
2. To prevent dental caries when plaque is removed periodically by the dentist.
3. To empasize importance of regular periodic dental examination to maintain good mouth health.
4. To maintain healthy mouth structures by tooth brushing, flossing between teeth and massaging gums.
5. To promote proper nutrition, since dentition and mouth tissue tone are directly affected.
6. To encourage topical application of fluoride as well as fluoridation of water, since this chemical significantly reduces dental caries.
7. To recognize that fatigue, emotional upsets, and injury lower resistance of dental tissue to infection.
8. To examine soft tissues of the mouth frequently for evidences of irritation, unusual growths, discoloration, encrustation, and leukoplakia, since abnormal manifestations may herald malignancy and early detection may achieve early correction.

Causes of Trauma to Oral Structures

1. *Mechanical:* Stiff-bristled toothbrush, hot pipe stem, ill-fitting dentures, carious or broken teeth, grinding of teeth, cheek and lower lip biting
2. *Thermal:* Smoking, hot liquids, hot foods
3. *Chemical:* Sucking hard candy, using full-strength antiseptic mouthwashes, chewing or smoking tobacco, drinking alcoholic beverages, chewing Aspergum, sucking mouth lozenges, using breath sweeteners, drinking citrus juices
4. *Bacterial:* Poor oral and nutritional attention that permits food to collect.
5. *Irradiation:* Exposure to sun, ultraviolet rays, radium, and x-rays

Assessment and Diagnostic Evaluation

A. *Assessment*

(See Physical Assessment of the Adult—Mouth, pp. 25.)

B. *Oral Cell Smear for Cytologic Examination*
1. Grasp the tongue with a 4″ × 4″ gauze square and gently move the tongue to expose the questionable area.
2. Using a moistened tongue depressor, scrape the area or lesion.
3. If a hyperkeratotic lesion is present, scrape off surface keratin so that deeper epithelial cells are available for a specimen (these are usually involved in early malignant change).
4. Smear cells on a glass slide, immerse carefully in alcohol, and send to laboratory.

LESIONS OF THE LIP

Actinic Cheilitis

(Heat-ray or sun-induced inflammation of the lip)
1. Often results from overexposure to sun radiation.
2. May lead to squamous-cell carcinoma.
3. *Clinical Manifestations*
   White hyperkeratosis, fissuring, erythema
4. *Management*
   a. Lips may be protected with sunscreen ointment.
   b. Local application of 1–5% 5-fluorouracil ointment for two weeks may be prescribed.
   c. Cryosurgery or electrosurgery may be required.

Contact Dermatitis

(Skin irritation produced by allergen)
1. Allergens from cosmetics, lipsticks, ointments, toothpaste, or chewing gum may be causative factors.
2. *Clinical Manifestations*
   Itching of lips, erythema, vesiculation, or burning may develop.
3. *Management*
   a. Eliminate irritant or suspected contactant.
   b. Apply corticosteroid ointment.
   c. Use hypoallergenic cosmetics.

Harelip and Cleft Palate (See Pediatrics, p. 1307)

LESIONS OF THE MOUTH

Herpes Simplex

(A viral infection commonly producing herpes labialis—cold sore, canker, fever blister)

1. *Clinical Manifestations*

   a. Small vesicles may erupt on lips (and/or tongue, cheeks, and pharynx).
   b. Vesicles then erupt to form sore shallow ulcers.
   c. This infection may be secondary to other febrile infections (meningococcus meningitis, malaria, and *Streptococcus pneumoniae* infections).

2. *Treatment and Nursing Management*
  a. Does not respond to chemotherapeutic agents that are available.
  b. Some relief is obtained from ointments containing benzocaine or lidocaine (note that there is the potential for allergic sensitization when used over long periods).
  c. Provide adequate fluids to combat dehydration.
  d. Antihistaminics such as diphenhydramine (Benadryl) and dyclonine (Dyclone) are helpful before meals to relieve discomfort and pain; either of these is normally applied in an aqueous rinse with cracked ice. (1 teaspoon elixir Benadryl mixed with 1 tablespoonful cracked ice.)

Gingivitis

(Inflammation of gums)
1. This is the most common infection of oral tissues.
2. *Clinical Manifestations*
  a. Inflammation and slight swelling of superficial gingivae and interdental papillae.
  b. With continued neglect, this may advance to chronic degenerative gingivitis and eventually to periodontal disease
3. *Nursing Management*
  a. Conscientious mouth hygiene
  b. Periodic professional dental cleaning

Acute Ulcerative Gingivitis

("Trench mouth," Vincent's gingivitis)
1. This is pseudomembranous painful ulceration affecting gums, inner dental papillae, mouth mucosa, tonsils, and pharynx, especially in young adults and adolescents.
2. *Etiology*
  a. Thought to be caused by both a spirochete and a fusiform bacillus.
  b. May be due to poor oral hygiene, low tissue resistance, and infection from complex microorganisms.
3. *Clinical Manifestations*
  a. Painful bleeding gums, mild fever, swelling of lymph nodes of neck.
  b. If infection spreads to tonsils and pharynx, swallowing and talking may be painful.
4. *Treatment and Nursing Management*
  a. Encourage mouth irrigations using dilute hydrogen peroxide or 2% sodium perborate (to combat anaerobic spirochetes) to treat infection, to control fetid breath, and to produce comfort.
  b. Administer antibiotics as prescribed to curb infection; give analgesics for pain and discomfort.
  c. Offer soft foods and liquids to reduce gum trauma.
  d. Instruct patient to avoid highly seasoned foods, alcoholic beverages, and smoking, all of which irritate infected oral tissues.
  e. Teach patient the importance of regular eating habits and sufficient rest.

CONDITIONS OF THE SALIVARY GLANDS

Salivary Calculus

(Sialolithiasis)
1. Salivary stones may form in the submaxillary gland following glandular infection or ductal stricture due to trauma or inflammation.
2. Salivary stones are usually mostly calcium oxalate.
  a. Stones found in the gland are irregularly lobulated.
  b. Stones found in the duct are small and oval in shape.
3. *Diagnostic Evaluation*
  Sialogram—x-ray with contrast medium
4. *Clinical Manifestations*
  a. None unless there is an infection.
  b. If calculus obstructs gland, the following conditions may occur:
    (1) Sudden, local pain, which is suddenly relieved by a gush of saliva.
    (2) Gland is swollen and tender.
    (3) Stone may be palpable.
    (4) Stone is visible with x-ray studies.
5. *Treatment*
  a. Surgical extraction of stone.
  b. Gland may have to be removed if condition occurs repeatedly.

DISTURBANCES OF THE TEMPOROMANDIBULAR JOINT

See Disturbances of the Temporomandibular Joint, page 375.

Exercise program for Temporomandibular Joint Disorders:*

1. Open and close mouth as widely and as rapidly as possible.
2. Open mouth against slight pressure applied by placing the open palm beneath the chin.
3. Close the mouth against slight pressure applied by placing the open palm above the chin.
4. Move the mandible from side to side without resistance; then move it from side to side with pressure from the palm of the hand against the side of the chin.
5. Protrude the jaw with and without resistance.
6. Chew a small piece of wax on each side and then in the center for 3–5 minutes.
  Repeat each exercise 5 times, twice a day. Increase at a rate of 5 times each week to a maximum of 25 exercises twice a day.

MAXILLOFACIAL FRACTURES

Fractures of the maxillofacial area usually include injury to the soft tissues and may occur as a result of a fall or if patient has been hit by a fist or a flying object.

Immediate Assessment and Management

1. Determine whether there is obstruction to the airway.
  a. Remove any obstruction from pharynx, such as broken teeth, dentures, blood clots, or broken bits of bone.
  b. Determine whether tongue has been displaced posteriorly; if so, insert index finger and pull tongue forward.
  c. Prepare for emergency tracheostomy if airway is obstructed.
2. Control hemorrhage by direct pressure on vessels supplying the area (see Fig. 22-4, p. 871).
  Prepare for fluid replacement.

   * English G: Otolaryngology: A Textbook. Hagerstown, Harper & Row, 1976, p. 766.

Disturbances of the Temporomandibular Joint

Problem	Possible Cause	Specific Management	General Management
Pain	Improper occlusion	Modify elevated areas of tooth fillings. Adjust dentures.	Effective in most instances: Soft or liquid diet.
Dislocation of condyle anteriorly beyond articular eminence	Sudden stretching or tearing of capsular ligament; mandible may be locked in open position.	Manual reduction. In chronic dislocation, surgery is necessary.	Conscious effort to avoid gritting or clenching teeth. Avoidance of wide yawning. In selected patients, application of heat to ligaments and muscles of jaw.
Arthritis of temporomandibular joint	Arthritic change due to trauma. Rheumatoid arthritis.	Intracapsular injection of corticosteroids. For ankylosis of joint, condylectomy.	Analgesics, antiinflammatory medications. In about 10%, intervention, such as dental adjustments, bite planes, grinding of teeth.
Temporomandibular joint syndrome (TMJ syndrome) Pain in ear or jaw with possible extension to neck and shoulder. Inability to open jaw fully.	Increased muscular tension and hyperexcitable reflexes possibly due to emotional tension.	Medication for pain; local anesthetics. Diazepam for muscle relaxation and to lessen cortical excitability. Use of *bite plane*, an acrylic mold that prevents teeth from meeting. Soft diet; exercises*	Lastly, resort to surgery.

* English G: Otolaryngology: A Textbook. Hagerstown, Harper & Row, 1976, p 766

3. Assess vital signs and note extent and involvement of other parts of the head and body.
4. Ascertain localization of pain to determine nerve injury.
5. Administer analgesics to relieve pain and anxiety but not to depress respirations.
6. Reassure patient that he is being given the best possible care.

Mandibular Fractures

1. Two thirds of significant facial fractures in the U.S. are of the mandible.
2. Most mandibular fractures can be treated with closed reduction and intermaxillary fixation.
3. Open reduction is preferred for certain patients:
   a. aged, senile, edentulous, and debilitated
   b. children and those who cannot tolerate intermaxillary fixation
   c. professional athletes
   d. patients who are psychotic or have a history of seizures
   e. the diabetic person with special nutritional needs
4. Objectives of Management
   a. to reduce the fracture
   b. to restore optimum dental occlusion
   c. to provide immobilization for healing
   d. to avoid complications: nonunion, malunion, infection

A. *Clinical Manifestations*
1. Malocclusion, asymmetry, abnormal mobility, and crepitus (grating sound with movement).
2. Tissue injury; note extent and involvement.

B. *Preoperative Medical and Nursing Intervention*
1. Determine priorities for repair.
   a. Irrigate laceration with copious amounts of normal physiologic saline.
   b. Prepare for debridement and suturing of lacerations.
   c. Apply sterile pressure dressings to control swelling, to prevent tension on stitches, and to maintain as clean an area as possible to minimize or prevent infection.
   d. Administer tetanus prophylaxis as prescribed.
   e. Give antibiotics as prescribed.
2. Prepare patient for roentgenograms to determine method of reducing and immobilizing fractures.
3. Reduce mandibular fractures first; maxillary fractures follow in positioning.
   Lower jaw is held tightly against upper jaw by cross-wires or rubber bands placed around arch bars wired to the teeth (intermaxillary fixation).

C. *Postoperative Nursing Care*
(Management of patient with intermaxillary fixation)
1. Immediately position patient on his side with head

slightly elevated to facilitate breathing and for ease of suctioning.
2. Note wire cutter or scissors taped to bandages or in some other obvious place.
   a. These cutters or scissors are to cut wires or rubber bands in the event the patient vomits; this will prevent aspiration.
   b. After the patient emerges from anesthesia, scissors or cutters must still be kept nearby for emergency use.
3. Suction drainage and stomach contents as required to lessen danger of aspiration.
   a. Connect nasogastric suction to low-pressure suction.
   b. Administer antiemetic medications as prescribed, if vomiting is anticipated.
   c. Insert small catheter into nasopharyngeal area for suctioning if a nasogastric catheter has not been inserted during surgery.
   d. Aspirate oral cavity; this is facilitated by inserting a tongue blade to move cheek away from teeth.
   e. Insert oral catheter behind third molar (or where a tooth may be missing) to aspirate within the oropharynx.
4. Modify care as patient emerges from anesthesia.
   a. Remind patient that his jaw is wired but that he can breathe and swallow.
   b. Provide a means of communication such as a "magic slate" (or chalk and chalkboard) or signal system.
   c. Elevate the head of the bed for comfort and to facilitate breathing.
   d. Continue to administer parenteral intravenous fluids as prescribed until nourishment can be taken by mouth.
   e. Administer medications to control pain and restlessness as well as to prevent nausea and infection.
5. Promote a climate to prevent complications and to promote recovery.
   a. Apply lubricant to the lips to prevent drying and cracking.
   b. Provide frequent and careful attention to the mouth.
      (1) Irrigate the mouth with tap water or normal saline after each feeding; use an Asepto syringe or irrigating set under low pressure.
      (2) Use a Water Pik if available, since it is effective in a gentle way.
      (3) Swab the area between teeth and cheek by using a tongue depressor to retract the cheek. Provide light with a flashlight.
6. Maintain adequate nutritional levels to promote healing.
   a. Provide privacy for the patient to eat, since he might be sensitive to his appearance and to the noisy sounds he makes as he tries to eat and drink.
   b. Provide a straw if the patient can manage it; the patient may suck soft foods from a demitasse spoon.
   c. Serve food attractively and arrange as pleasant an environment as possible (music, television, view from window) to encourage nutritional intake.
7. Set up a plan of instruction so that patient will be able to manage at home even with the jaw wired.
   a. Encourage exercise and proper diet to promote general good health, tissue healing, and to prevent constipation.

b. Develop a plan that is convenient for him to follow in maintaining mouth cleanliness.
c. Work with his family, if required, in determining interesting pursuits to counterbalance any worries he might have about appearance, cost of treatment, and other problems.
d. Remind him of follow-up visits to his physician.
e. Prepare him for possible reconstructive or orthodontic work if this is required.

PREMALIGNANT MOUTH LESIONS

Leukoplakia Buccalis

("Smoker's patch")
1. This condition is characterized by the appearance of one or more small, often crinkled pearly patches on the mucous membrane of tongue or mouth.
2. It is due to the keratinization of the mucosa and sclerosis of the underlying tissues.
3. *Manifestations and Nursing Management*
   a. If there are no symptoms other than appearance, emphasize importance of careful oral hygiene:
      (1) Recommend dental care and gingival treatment.
      (2) Advise patient to avoid alcohol, tobacco, coffee, and tea.
      (3) Suggest mouth rinses of half-strength milk of magnesia after meals and at bedtime.
      (4) Encourage increased vitamin intake, particularly of vitamin C.
   b. If in addition to appearance of white patches there is pain, induration, and ulceration, do the following:
      (1) Suggest biopsy to rule out cancer.
      (2) Follow above regime (3a).

CANCER OF THE LIP

Incidence

1. Cancer of the vermilion border of the lip is the most frequent (20–30%) of all mouth cancers (Fig. 10-1).
2. Most lip cancer is of squamous-cell type.
3. More men than women are affected.
4. This cancer usually occurs in the age group of 50–70.
5. The lower lip is most often the site; occasionally the upper lip is involved, and in this location more women than men are affected.

Predisposing Factors and Clinical Manifestations

1. Chronic irritation from actinic rays of sun accounts for most lip cancer; irritation from warm pipe stems may also be a factor.
2. The condition presents first as a well-differentiated small lesion that is infiltrating or ulcerating in character.
3. It continues to grow and may involve entire lip, progressing from there to the soft tissues of the chin.
4. Often it appears as a painless, indurated ulcer with raised edges.
5. Later it progresses to chronic labial fissures, particularly in the midline of the lower lip; repeatedly this fissure heals and breaks down.

Treatment

OBJECTIVE: to remove malignancy with best cosmetic result.

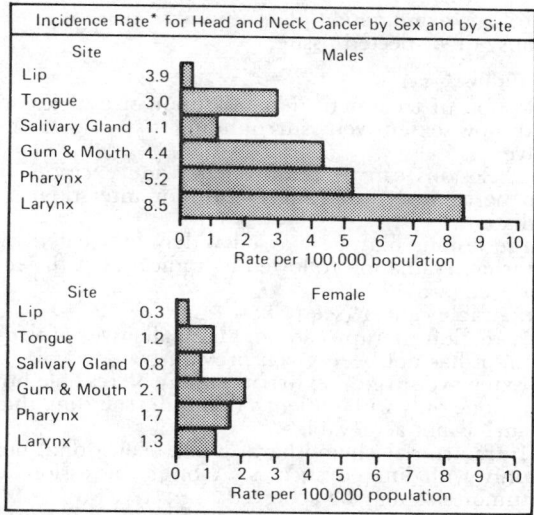

Incidence Rate* for Head and Neck Cancer by Sex and by Site

Site	Males
Lip	3.9
Tongue	3.0
Salivary Gland	1.1
Gum & Mouth	4.4
Pharynx	5.2
Larynx	8.5

Rate per 100,000 population

Site	Female
Lip	0.3
Tongue	1.2
Salivary Gland	0.8
Gum & Mouth	2.1
Pharynx	1.7
Larynx	1.3

Rate per 100,000 population

Source: National Cancer Institute SEER Program, 1973–1977

FIGURE 10-1. *Incidence rate for head and neck cancer by sex (at right) and by site (at left). (Courtesy American Cancer Society, Inc.)*

1. Small lesions are excised liberally. The lip is reconstructed by approximating the layers of the mucous membrane, the subcutaneous tissues, and the skin.
2. More extensive resection involves excising half of the lip or the entire lip.
3. If lesion involves more than one-third of lip, best treatment may be radiotherapy.
4. Metastases to cervical lymph nodes are uncommon; if lymph nodes are involved, a radical neck dissection is indicated (see p. 379).

Nursing Management

A. *For Small Excision*

1. Observe appearance of lip for uncontrolled bleeding that forms a hematoma. If untreated, the following may occur:
   a. Undue pressure on mucous membrane results in sloughing.
   b. Cosmetic results are poor.
2. Avoid trauma to incision when the patient eats.
   a. Keep a small dressing over lip.
   b. Feed patient liquids and blenderized foods through straw or nasal tube.
3. Observe for possible secondary infection.

B. *For More Extensive Resection*

(excision of half or entire lip)
1. Preoperative nursing management
   Provide meticulous oral hygiene (particularly in presence of infected teeth, gingivitis and a generally poor mouth condition)—to avert infection in the incision line, thereby interfering with proper healing.
2. Postoperative nursing management
   a. Observe incision to detect signs of inflammation or infection.
   b. Aspirate oral secretions frequently to keep mouth clean and to avoid crusting of secretions around sutures.

c. Note any swelling around incision which might indicate onset of infection or slow bleeding.
   d. Prevent the patient from exerting undue strain on operated lip when eating, talking, smiling, laughing or using other facial expressions.
   e. Feed patient preferably via a nasogastric tube to prevent strain on suture line.
   f. Offer sips of water, crushed ice, or tea to keep oral mucous membrane moist and free of drying secretions.
   g. Liberalize light liquid nourishment by mouth about the 5th day.
   h. Permit soft or semi-solid foods after 10 days.
3. *Health Education:*
   a. Cigarette smoking should be terminated.
   b. A sunscreening ointment should be applied to the lips when they are exposed to wind and sun.

CANCER OF THE TONGUE

Anterior Two Thirds of Tongue

A. *Incidence*

1. Occurs usually in males in the 40–80-year age group.
2. Strongly associated with history of heavy alcohol intake, smoking, and practicing poor mouth hygiene.

B. *Clinical Manifestations*

1. A small ulcer (or thickening) on the anterior undersurface of lateral aspects of tongue that has not healed in 3 weeks
2. Pain or soreness of tongue on eating hot or highly seasoned foods
3. Limitation of motion of tongue.
4. Spread of growth to neighboring structures leads to:
   a. Excessive salivation, blood-tinged sputum
   b. Slurred speech, trismus (contraction of mastication muscles)
   c. Pain on swallowing liquids
5. If untreated
   a. Inability to swallow
   b. Earache, face-ache and toothache
   c. Inability to eat or sleep
   d. Cervical lymph node metastasis
   e. Hemorrhage
   f. General debilitation

C. *Objectives of Treatment*

1. To remove the malignancy and salvage as much of the tongue as possible.
   a. When the lesion is small, particularly at the tip of the tongue, surgical excision is done because it is effective and produces minimal impairment of function.
   b. For more extensive lesions, irradiation, such as interstitial implantation of radium needles, is used.
   c. Radiation may be combined with surgical intervention.
   d. Cervical lymphadenectomy may be done prophylactically, since a high percentage of tongue cancers tend to metastasize.
2. To develop other lines of communication if patient is going to be unable to speak either for a short or a long period of time.
   a. Practice methods of communicating that the patient understands and can become adept at, such as use of magic slate, hand signals, eye blink code, and flash cards (words or pictures).

b. Include the family in using the most effective means of communications.

D. *Postoperative Medical and Nursing Management*

(See below, Cancer of the Mouth)

Posterior Tongue

A. *Manifestations*

Symptoms are less obvious
1. Slight dysphagia, sore throat
2. Salivation
3. Blood-tinged sputum

B. *Poor Prognosis*

1. It is a difficult site for effective radiation
2. Total glossectomy is very mutilating

C. *Postoperative Medical and Nursing Management*

(See below, Cancer of the Mouth, and p. 856, Advanced Cancer Nursing Care)

CANCER OF THE MOUTH

Incidence

1. Cancer of the mouth accounts for 3% of all male and 1% of all female cancer deaths in this country.
2. Males are afflicted 3 times more often than females.
3. Evidence suggests that the risk of cancer in the heavy smoker and drinker may be as much as 15 times greater than in those who neither smoke nor drink.

Clinical Manifestations

A. For precancerous mouth lesions—leukoplakia buccalis, keratosis labialis
   1. Pearly patches—1 or 2 small thin, often crinkled areas on mucous membranes of the tongue, mouth, or both, due to
      a. Keratinization of mucosa
      b. Sclerosis of underlying tissue
   2. Later, most of tongue and mouth may become covered
      a. Creamy white, thick, fissured mucous membrane
      b. Sometimes desquamates, leaving a beefy-red base
B. For cancerous lesions
   1. White patchy area, sore spot or ulcer on lips, gums, or mouth which fails to heal
   2. Swelling, numbness, or loss of feeling in the part
   3. An asymmetric, firm nodal enlargement or mass
   4. Erythroplakia—red plaques or well-defined velvety red patches, often with tiny areas of ulceration

Preventive Measures

1. Eliminate causes of chronic irritation.
2. Practice good oral hygiene.
3. Obtain proper dental care—remove or repair jagged, carious, and infected teeth.
4. Reduce or eliminate smoking and chewing tobacco; also eliminate pipe smoking if it irritates the lip.
5. Restrict or eliminate ingestion of highly spiced foods and reduce alcohol consumption.
6. If syphilis is suspected, seek treatment (see p. 823).

Diagnostic Evaluation

1. Roentgenogram of head and neck to determine involvement.

2. Cytologic examination of sputum (see p. 156).
3. Biopsy of suspected tissue.

Treatment

1. Selection of treatment depends upon size of lesion and how extensively surrounding tissues are involved.
2. Small lesions can be removed by wide excision or can be treated with radiotherapy or interstitial irradiation.
3. Large lesions may be excised widely or treated by external irradiation followed by radical neck dissection (see p. 379).
4. Inoperable cancer (see p. 856)
   a. Radiation therapy can be quite palliative, providing it has not been given previously.
   b. Extensive surgical extirpation may be feasible but is done only with patient's full understanding that cure is not achievable.
   c. Intra-arterial chemotherapy has been done, but only with limited success. A brief regression in tumor size may be achieved.
   d. Thalamotomy may be a useful palliative procedure for the patient with advanced malignancy and severe pain.

Nursing Management

(Principles applicable to any patient with a mouth problem)

A. *Preoperative Care*

1. Promote optimum physical condition and psychological adjustment.
   a. Assess patient's reaction to his condition.
      (1) Evaluate his apprehension and offer emotional support.
      (2) Correct any misinformation.
      (3) Determine therapeutic plan of care for patient's rehabilitation.
   b. Maintain a good nutritional level.
2. Provide optimum mouth care.
   a. Proper care of teeth because they are essential to mastication.
      (1) Stress regular dental care
      (2) Promote good nutrition
   b. Mouth cleanliness to reduce incidence of infectious disease such as mumps and surgical parotitis.
      (1) Brush teeth frequently.
      (2) Use oxygen-releasing and antimicrobial mouth-rinsing solutions.
      (3) Apply lanolin to dry and cracking lips.
      (4) Remove dentures and clean them frequently.
   c. Adequate fluid intake, particularly in debilitated patients who are prone to mouth infections.
   d. Stimulation of flow of saliva.
      (1) Offer chewing gum.
      (2) Encourage patient to suck lemon sour balls, a fresh lemon, or orange slices.
      (3) Administer antibiotics as prescribed to assist in control of infection.
3. Care for mouth lesions and control mouth odors.
   a. Feeding problems may be handled in the following way:
      (1) Use straws, teaspoon, feeders, etc.
      (2) Provide food that is soft, liquid, and nonirritating—not too hot or cold or highly seasoned.
      (3) Serve small, frequent meals attractively.
   b. Excessive salivation and mouth odors may be handled as follows:

(1) Insert gauze wick in corner of mouth; place basin conveniently to catch drippings.
(2) Use small rubber catheter and suction.
(3) Encourage use of mouthwashes, particularly oxidizing agents such as hydrogen peroxide half strength.
(4) Use power spray, if available.

4. Prepare for postoperative communication since patient may not be able to talk for a few days after surgery.

Practice lip reading, hand signals, magic slate, eye blink codes, and flash cards (words or pictures).

5. Provide regular preoperative care (see p. 80).

B. *Postoperative Care*

1. Maintain a patent airway.
   a. Recognize that the patient may have an airway, endotracheal tube, or tracheostomy to facilitate air exchange.
   b. Observe patient closely for signs of respiratory embarrassment such as changes in vital signs, dyspnea, and restlessness.
   c. Place patient in prone position, or in supine position with head turned to side, or laterally; position should facilitate drainage and prevent aspiration.
   d. Suction as required; precautions are necessary to avoid injury to suture line and sensitive tissues.
   e. When the patient is out of anesthesia, elevate head of bed for comfort, to facilitate deep breathing and coughing up of secretions, and to lessen edema.
2. Check pressure dressings that are used to control edema.
   a. Note whether dressings are hindering respirations.
   b. Observe surrounding tissues to determine whether dressings are constricting blood circulation.
   c. If portable suction is used, pressure dressings may not be applied.
3. Control pain so that respirations are not depressed. Employ nursing measures to make the patient comfortable so that narcotics for pain relief are not used unless absolutely required.
4. Maintain nutritional and electrolyte levels.
   Following intravenous therapy, administer tube feedings by nasogastric tube or gastrostomy (see p. 403).
5. Keep mouth clean for comfort and to assist in healing process.
   a. Mouth irrigations, using normal saline, diluted

hydrogen peroxide, sodium bicarbonate, or alkaline mouthwashes.
   b. Gentle lavaging, using a catheter between cheek and teeth to loosen mucus.
   c. Power spray to clean inaccessible spaces.
   d. Vaporizer to provide moisture to traumatized tissue and discourage crusting.
6. Encourage speech rehabilitation and social adjustment.
   a. Recognize that face and neck surgery can be disfiguring and the patient often is embarrassed, withdrawn, and depressed.
   b. Supply pad and pencil, magic slate, signal system (eye blinks or hand), so that patient can express his needs and thoughts. Note that if the patient usually wears glasses to read and write, he may not be able to put his glasses on because of dressings, skin flaps, etc.
   c. Allow patient to have his meals in privacy if he desires.
   d. Encourage his family and friends to visit so that he is aware others care for him.
   e. Assist him in caring for his personal appearance.
   f. Observe closely for indications of his needs which may be communicated in other ways.
   g. Refer him to a speech pathologist or therapist if the services of this specialist are indicated.
   h. Be consistent with emotional support.
7. Provide an environment conducive to the patient's recovery.
   a. Maintain proper humidification and aeration of room.
   b. Prevent odors by removing soiled dressings; use effective and pleasant deodorizers.
   c. Inform patient that his general throat discomfort is due to endotracheal anesthesia and will improve in a few days.
8. Prepare patient for convalescence and extended care at home.
   a. Provide detailed instructions to the patient or a member of his family.
   b. If suctioning is required, instruct as to method, type of equipment and where it can be obtained.
   c. Emphasize adequate nutrition—proper consistency, proper seasoning and right temperature. Suggest commercial baby foods or the use of a blender if available.
   d. Repeat the details of good mouth care and cleanliness of dressings.
   e. Review signs of obstruction, hemorrhage, infection and depression and what to do about them if they are evident.

RADICAL NECK DISSECTION FOR MALIGNANCY

OBJECTIVE: to remove all lymph-node-bearing tissue on the involved side of the neck.

Scope of Surgery—Removal of all tissue under the skin from the ramus of the jaw down to the clavicle; from midline back to the angle of the jaw. This includes: sternocleidomastoid muscle, other smaller muscles, jugular vein in the neck.

Concomitant Surgery—Tracheostomy (see p. 188)

Nursing Management
A. *Preoperative Care*

Preoperative care including diagnostic evaluation— see specific related condition, such as Cancer of Mouth, p. 378, Cancer of the Esophagus, p. 388, etc.

B. *Postoperative Care*

Postoperative nursing objectives are based on the following patient concerns:

1. His ability to breathe normally
   a. Place him in Fowler's position.
   b. Observe for signs of respiratory embarrassment, such as dyspnea, cyanosis, and edema.
2. His ability to avoid hemorrhage and infection
   a. Evaluate vital signs which may suggest hemorrhage or infection onset.
   b. Note condition of dressings to detect early signs of hemorrhage.
3. His ability to swallow
   a. Observe for throat irritation: edema, clearing of throat.
   b. Note how he accepts liquids: refusal may mean difficulty in swallowing, which in turn may be indicative of superior laryngeal nerve damage.
   c. Encourage his intake of fluids in order to "thin" secretions.
   d. Encourage coughing to remove secretions.
   e. Allow patient to assume sitting position to bring up secretions (the nurse should support his neck with her hands).
   f. Suction secretions if patient is unable to bring them up himself.
4. His wound healing
   a. Reinforce pressure dressings from time to time to assist in obliterating dead spaces and providing immobilization.
   b. Observe dressings for evidence of hemorrhage and constriction which may affect respiration.
   c. If suction drainage (Hemovac) is used, approximately 80–120 ml. of serosanguineous secretions are drawn off during the first postoperative day; this diminishes with each day.
   d. Apply Aeroplast or other antiseptic plastic sprays to protect the wound.
5. His ability to communicate
   a. Inform the patient that temporary hoarseness can be expected with extensive neck surgery and tracheostomy.
   b. Encourage him to write messages for first few days; if writing is a problem, it may be due to denervation of the trapezius muscle.
   c. Recognize that for this patient to nod "Yes" or "No" may be difficult because of the neck dissection.
   d. Manipulate his environment so that he is able to reach his call bell or other required articles without straining.
6. His appearance
   a. Respect his desire for privacy during treatments, dressing change, and feedings.
   b. Inform his visitors of his appearance before they see him so that their expressions do not cause him to be upset.
   c. Provide frequent aeration of the room and utilize deodorants to prevent unpleasant odors.
   d. Observe for lower facial paralysis, since this may indicate facial nerve injury.
   e. Watch for shoulder dysfunction which may follow resection of spinal accessory nerves.
      (1) Utilize postoperative muscle exercises and muscle re-education (see below).
      (2) Work with the patient to obtain good functional range of motion.
   f. Consult with the surgeon and patient in decisions on future cosmetic surgery or in use of a prosthetic device.
7. His prognosis

   a. Encourage the patient to verbalize his concerns and feelings.
   b. Consult the physician to determine the nature and extent of explanation and prognosis he has given to the patient.
   c. Encourage the patient to seek confirmation of his personal philosophy and religious beliefs if this would provide answers for him.
   d. Accentuate the positive.
   e. Encourage the patient to participate in his plan of care.
   f. Recognize that a great effort has to be made in behavior modification to change a life-style which included alcohol consumption and cigarette smoking. It is difficult to do.
8. His family
   a. Collaborate with the physician in informing the family of the nature and extent of the patient's disease and surgery.
   b. Help them to understand that without surgery, the patient's condition would be worse.
   c. Prepare them for the patient's postoperative appearance; how this will be done depends on the strengths and weaknesses of the family and the individual circumstances.
   d. If there is difficulty with a spouse or person close to the patient in accepting his appearance, refer the person to the physician, social worker, psychiatrist, or whatever resource seems advisable.

Rehabilitation Exercises Following Head and Neck Surgery

Exercises are recommended when the neck incision is sufficiently healed.

OBJECTIVE: to regain maximum shoulder function as well as head and neck motion following surgery.

1. Perform exercises morning and evening. At first, exercises are done only once; then the number is increased by one each day until each exercise is done ten times.
2. Following each exercise the patient is instructed to relax.
3. For neck:
   a. Gently rotate head to each side as far as possible.
   b. Tilt head to the right side as far as possible; repeat for left side.
   c. Drop chin to chest and then raise chin as high as possible.
4. For shoulder:
   a. Standing beside bed, place hand from unoperated side on bed for support.
   b. Gradually swing arm on operated side up and back as far as is comfortable for patient.
   c. Each day work toward finishing a complete circle.

HEMORRHAGE AS A MAJOR COMPLICATION FOLLOWING MOUTH SURGERY AND RADICAL NECK DISSECTION

Principal Causes of Sudden Hemorrhage Following Surgery

1. Loose ligature around a large vessel
2. Sudden distention of tied off blood vessel followed by rupture
3. Slipping of ligature that may occur in violent coughing spasm
4. Rupture of a vessel due to trauma incident during surgery

5. Rupture of a vessel weakened by erosion, tumor or slough
6. Sloughing associated with secondary infection

Treatment and Nursing Management

A. *Immediate Treatment for Sudden Hemorrhage*

1. Pressure over the common carotid and internal jugular vessels in the neck may be life saving.

2. Have someone notify surgery immediately.
3. Treat patient for shock.

B. *Definitive Treatment*

1. Surgical intervention to repair vessel defect
2. Correct fluid and blood loss with proper replacement
3. Initiate postoperative monitoring program until vital signs remain consistently normal.

CONDITIONS OF THE ESOPHAGUS

DIAGNOSTIC EVALUATION OF THE ESOPHAGUS

Nursing Assessment

During the taking of the nursing history, ask the following questions:

1. What problems or discomfort do you have when you eat? Do you have pain? Where? Is there food sticking in your throat or chest? Are you nauseated? How long does the discomfort last? Is it daily or intermittent?
2. How is your appetite? Are there any signs of anorexia (loss of appetite)?
3. Do you have to restrict the kinds of food you eat as determined by size or consistency (meat for example), as determined by seasoning, or as determined by spiciness or acidity (citrus fruits)? Do you have to limit food because of temperature (hot or cold)?
4. Do you experience any nausea, heartburn, dysphagia, regurgitation, reflux, or vomiting?
5. Does the position of your body (bending, stooping, lying down) affect the problem? Do you lie flat when sleeping or do you have the head of the bed elevated? Does assuming a particular position help or make the problem worse?
6. Do you have any gas formation? Eructation? Early satiety?
7. How has your weight been (stable, increasing, or decreasing)?
8. What relieves the discomfort?
9. Do you find food or saliva on your pillow in the morning on awakening?
10. How are your teeth? Do you have difficulty chewing?

Upper Gastrointestinal Roentgenography

(See p. 396)

Esophageal Endoscopy

This is the direct visualization of the entire mucosa of the esophagus to detect inflammation, ulceration, masses (tumors), or varices, and to obtain specimens for cytologic studies or biopsy.

A. *Nursing Management and Patient Instruction*

1. Give the patient nothing by mouth for 6 hours prior to test. This is done to decrease the possibility of aspiration and to be sure the esophagus is clear of particles that would block visibility.
2. Explain the procedure to the patient before it is done, and explain the steps during the examination.

3. Administer diazepam (Valium) or meperidine (Demerol) if prescribed for relaxation.
4. Spray the throat with local anesthetic to dull the effects of passing the esophagoscope and to reduce gagging.
5. If the esophagus is dilated (fluid-filled esophagus was seen on x-ray) first pass Ewald tube and then evacuate and irrigate esophagus.

NURSING ALERT: For *all* endoscopies, bouginage, and pneumatic dilatation procedures, have the following ready: oropharyngeal suction and emergency cardiopulmonary resuscitation equipment.

6. If a rigid scope is used, position the patient on his back. During insertion of esophagoscope, his neck is hyperextended and his head is supported.
7. With the flexible esophagofiberoscope, scope is passed with patient sitting, then examination is completed with patient lying on left side.

B. *Following Endoscopy*

1. Withhold fluid and foods until the patient's gag reflex has returned (about 2 hours). Test the patient's swallowing with sips of water before foods or fluids are given.
2. Offer anesthetic lozenges or normal saline gargles for throat discomfort.
3. Observe the patient for 24 hours for symptoms such as bleeding, dysphagia, fever, and neck pain (cervical area) that are suggestive of perforation. Check also for substernal or epigastric pain (thoracic area); shoulder pain, dyspnea, abdominal pain (diaphragmatic area), and subcutaneous emphysema.

Esophageal Biopsy and Exfoliative Cytology

1. Biopsy of tissue may be taken during esophagoscopy; prepare tissue for laboratory examination.
2. Cytology
   a. Usually an overnight fast is required (no food or fluids).
   b. A No. 12 or No. 16 French nasogastric tube is passed to the cardioesophageal junction (45 cm.).
   c. Residual contents are aspirated.
   d. Physiologic saline (50 ml.) or Ringer's lactate solution is forcefully instilled with a syringe and is immediately aspirated below the cardia; this procedure is repeated at various levels of the

esophagus (5-cm. intervals from 45 to 25 cm. from incisor teeth).
  e. Aspirated contents are collected in separate containers surrounded by ice; when all specimens are collected, take them *immediately* to laboratory for analysis (must be centrifuged and pallet spread on slide as soon as possible after aspiration).

ESOPHAGEAL TRAUMA

Esophageal trauma is injury to the esophagus caused by external or internal insult.
1. Externally—stab or bullet wounds, crush injuries, etc.
2. Internally—swallowed foreign bodies, i.e., metal objects, fishbones, dental appurtenances, poison (e.g., lye burn).

Treatment and Nursing Management

OBJECTIVES: to institute emergency life-saving treatment.
  to restore continuity of esophagus.
  to facilitate healing and prevent infection and constriction.
1. Assess condition of patient to determine his physiologic needs.
2. Maintain open airway. Often, difficulty in respiration is due to edema of throat or a collection of mucus in pharynx.
3. Control hemorrhage if present.
4. Treat for pain and shock. (Shock may be due to hemorrhage, impairment of cardiorespiratory function.)
5. Provide high fluid intake; may require parenteral therapy.
6. For external wound:
  a. Initiate emergency first-aid wound care and prepare for surgery (see p. 134).
  b. Maintain feeding through nasogastric tube.
7. For internal chemical damage, give specific antidote. If lye or other caustic or organic solvent is swallowed, do NOT try to induce vomiting.
  a. A gastrostomy may be performed, either as a temporary or a permanent means of feeding the patient (see p. 403).
  b. Resulting strictures may be relieved by dilating the narrow esophagus with bougies.
  c. Reconstructive surgery may be necessary to create a new passageway for food between pharynx and stomach.
8. For swallowed foreign bodies.
  a. When foreign body is made of metal, such as bobby and safety pins, needles, jacks, nails, and other similar objects, it is not considered safe to allow object to make its way through gastrointestinal tract.
  b. Usually these can be removed with the aid of an esophagoscope. A large-bore, rigid esophagoscope is best.
  c. A skilled operator is required; magnets can be used on end of retrieving instrument passed through esophagoscope.

ESOPHAGITIS

Esophagitis is an acute or chronic inflammation of the esophagus. Severity of symptoms may be unrelated to the degree of inflammation seen at endoscopy.

Clinical Manifestations

(Sudden or gradual in onset)
1. Hot burning pain (heartburn or pyrosis) behind xiphoid or sternum, → spreading to throat, jaw, arms, and back.
2. Pain with eructation or regurgitation of acidic or bitter fluid.
3. Symptoms aggravated by recumbency.
4. Symptoms may be precipitated by increases in intraabdominal pressure such as when patient bends over, lifts heavy objects, or has to strain to pass stool or urine (constipation or prostatism).
5. Dysphagia—worse at onset of meal. Food "sticking" in throat or chest—produced by spasm, edema, or narrow lumen. While swallowing bolus of food, patient may require "washing down" of food with liquids.
6. Pain on drinking citrus liquids, alcohol, or hot or cold fluids. Coffee often aggravates the pain.
7. Bleeding—acute or chronic; melena or hematemesis also occurs.
8. Relief may be obtained by taking water, milk, antacids, or by standing rather than lying.

Causative Factors

1. Fungal—*Candida*
2. Chemical—lye, ammonia, aerosols
3. Physical—alcohol, excessively hot liquids
4. Trauma—swallowing foreign body
5. Reflux esophagitis due to incompetent lower esophageal sphincter; condition appears to have no relationship to hiatal hernia
6. Malignancy associated with achalasia
7. Prolonged nasogastric intubation
8. Following gastric or duodenal surgery
9. Repeated vomiting (common in alcoholics)
10. Bending, stooping, coughing, and straining at stool

Diagnostic Evaluation

(For all esophageal disorders)
1. Cineradiographic esophagograms
2. Esophagoscopy (see p. 381) with cytology and biopsy may differentiate esophagitis from carcinoma
3. Esophageal manometry

Medical and Nursing Therapy

OBJECTIVES: to reduce gastric acidity and prevent regurgitation.
  to treat the basic problem.
1. Institute a feeding regime similar to that for gastric ulcer (see p. 399).
  a. Frequent feedings progressing to 5 meals—bland, low residue—no bedtime feedings.

NURSING ALERT: Milk actually is contraindicated for ulcer or esophagitis due to high calcium content which stimulates gastric acid secretion.

  b. Avoid foods high in residue, very hot foods, spices, alcohol, tobacco, and coffee (even decaffeinated).
  c. Avoid salicylates, phenylbutazone (Butazolidin), and anticholinergics.
  d. Do not give food within 2 hours of retiring.
  e. Chew food well and eat slowly.

2. Administer antacids, especially at bedtime.
3. Place 15–20 cm. (6–8 inch) bed blocks at head of bed. Be sure to remove wheels from bed.
4. Provide adequate mouth and dental care.
5. Administer cholinergic agents.
6. Promote a relaxing environment during mealtime.
7. For strictures, dilation therapy may be initiated; this is done initially several times weekly, then on a monthly basis.
8. Surgery is indicated when conservative measures fail.
   a. Fundoplication (Belsey or Nissen procedure) for reflux to throat—severe stricture
   b. Combined with vagotomy-pyloroplasty if associated with gastroduodenal ulcer.
   c. Stricture may need to be resected and an esophagogastrostomy may be required.

NURSING ALERT: Anticholinergics are contraindicated because they may further impair competence of lower esophageal sphincter.

ACHALASIA

Achalasia refers to a benign spasm of the lower esophageal sphincter often with marked dilatation of the esophagus. It is a neuromuscular disorder due to absent or defective nerves (of the myenteric plexus) going to the involuntary muscles in the esophagus.

Clinical Manifestations

1. Difficulty in swallowing both liquids *and* solids, substernal pressure, fullness and regurgitation, often heartburn appears.
2. Secondary pulmonary complications due to spillover of esophageal contents (aspiration pneumonia).
3. Loss of peristaltic activity and failure of esophageal sphincter to relax during swallowing process (detected by x-ray or manometry) may occur.
4. Emotional upsets, sudden shock, or dietary indiscretion may aggravate this disorder.
5. Weight loss is eventually noticed inasmuch as the patient has a decreased intake in order to avoid discomfort; eventually this can lead to emaciation.
6. Increased risk of esophageal carcinoma (8–10%). The patient may also have carcinoma at cardia invading esophagus, simulating achalasia.

Diagnostic Evaluation

1. Cineroentgenogram of esophagus with barium; this reveals weak or absent peristaltic waves and failure of sphincter relaxation.
2. Esophagoscopy with cytologic studies and biopsy.
3. Esophageal manometry with perfused open-tip catheters.
4. Nursing assessment
   a. Determine what the patient can and cannot swallow.
   b. Note location and kind of pain.
   c. Determine how relief is obtained.
   d. Ascertain what aggravates the problem.

Treatment and Nursing Management

OBJECTIVE: to enlarge the passageway so that contents pass more readily from esophagus to stomach

   a. Pneumatic (Mosher) bag dilatation (see p. 386)
   b. Surgical esophagomyotomy

A. *Nursing Management—Medical Therapy or Minor Surgical Therapy*

1. Direct patient to eat slowly, chew food thoroughly, and arch his back while swallowing to provide relief.
2. Suggest that the patient sleep with his head elevated to avoid reflux or aspiration.
3. Provide a bland diet and tell patient to avoid alcohol as well as spicy, very hot, and very cold foods in order to minimize symptoms.
4. Administer pharmacologic agents such as urecholine to increase lower esophageal sphincter tone.

NURSING ALERT: Anticholinergic drugs are contraindicated for achalasia because they further decrease esophageal peristalsis.

5. If pharmacotherapy fails, pneumatic dilatation is tried (see Guidelines: Pneumatic Dilatation, p. 386).

B. *Nursing Management—Major Surgical Therapy*

(Used only if pneumatic dilatation fails)
1. Esophagomyotomy—a division of muscular fibers enclosing the narrowed esophagus that permits mucosa to pouch out through the divided area in muscle layers.
2. Cardiomyotomy—when above operation is extended to include cardiac end of stomach.
3. Incisional approach determines nature of postoperative care; thus, an incision through chest implies nursing care similar to a thoracotomy (see p. 220).

DIFFUSE SPASM OF ESOPHAGUS

Diffuse esophageal spasm is a motor disorder of the esophagus.

Clinical Manifestations

(One or more of the following)
1. Pain on swallowing (odynophagia)
2. Dysphagia
3. Chest or back pain

Clinical Features

1. Diffuse spasm may be associated with achalasia, obstruction of the cardia by tumor, precipitation by reflux acid.
2. It is common in old age.
3. It may be an early stage of achalasia.

Treatment and Nursing Management

A. *Conservative*

1. Administer sedatives for pain.
2. Avoid food and beverages that precipitate symptoms.
3. Eliminate source of tension as a precipitating factor producing stress during mealtime.
4. Administer nitroglycerin or long-acting nitrites if reflux is not a factor.

B. *Later, if necessary*

Utilize pneumatic dilatation if manometric studies reveal increased lower esophageal sphincter pressure (providing gastroesophageal reflux is not part of the problem).

C. *See Guidelines:*
1. Feeding the Patient with Dysphagia (see below)
2. Teaching a Patient with Dysphagia How to Swallow
   p. 385

3. Esophageal Dilatation (Bougienage) p. 386
4. Pneumatic Dilatation p. 386

GUIDELINES: Feeding the Patient with Dysphagia

Dysphagia—difficulty or discomfort in swallowing; a bolus of food becomes impeded in its movement between the mouth and stomach.

Causative Factors

1. Circulatory disturbances of brain (stroke, brain stem vascular accidents)
2. Cranial nerve disturbances
3. Trauma to neck
4. Radiation therapy/surgery for head and neck tumors
5. Presence of tumors, inflammation
6. Disturbances of laryngeal sphincter
7. Psychological pathology

Clinical Manifestations

1. Patient complains of a sticking sensation behind sternum; relief is obtained by
   a. Retching
   b. Drinking liquids to dislodge bolus
2. Upper or thoracic esophageal discomfort noted in 3–5 seconds after attempting to swallow.
3. Lower thoracic discomfort noted in 5–15 seconds.

Assessment

1. Determine whether dysphagia occurs only with solid food. Does it occur with soft foods? liquids? warm liquids or cold liquids? saliva? Does it vary?
2. Has the patient lost weight? Evidence of cachexia?
3. Is hoarseness present? If so, it may be indicative of laryngeal lesion.
4. How long has the patient experienced this discomfort?
5. Did painful swallowing precede dysphagia? How long? Heartburn? How long? Hiccough?
6. Regurgitation—bringing up of undigested food or gastric acid into the mouth. Has this occurred?
7. In general, determine patient's eating habits and their relevance to this problem.

Procedure

NURSING ACTION	RATIONALE/AMPLIFICATION
1. Make a preliminary assessment of patient's problem (see above, Assessment). a. Determine his swallowing limitation.	1. By individualizing the approach, a more effective plan to meet particular needs will be achieved.
2. Prepare environment so that it will be well ventilated, uncluttered, and cheerful without distractions.	2. This will make patient's feeding experience more pleasant.
3. Place the patient in an upright sitting position (90°) for about 20 minutes before and after feeding. a. Provide adequate support and comfort.	3. This will provide time to adjust to this position thereby eliminating postural change disturbances during feeding.
4. Explain what you plan to do; sit rather than stand, and encourage conversation. Face patient and proceed in an unhurried manner. Encourage eating; allow time for chewing. Remove tray when patient is finished.	4. This procedure will more likely secure cooperation.
5. If food is difficult to manage, begin with liquids; if he continues to have trouble: a. Place tip and irrigation syringe in the back of the mouth cavity on the better side; gently squeeze bulb. b. When he is ready, allow patient to squeeze bulb himself. c. Frequent small feedings are offered initially.	5. Unclean or used tray may be psychologically distressing and may interfere with digestion. a. Proceed slowly and give patient time to swallow. b. Aim to involve the patient in his own care. c. Blenderized or commercially prepared liquid formula supplements are available.
6. If the patient has difficulty chewing: a. Manipulate jaw in an upward and downward motion. b. Encourage patient to close his lips after food is in his mouth; keep them closed until the food is swallowed. c. If patient does not swallow as soon as he should but appears to retain food in his mouth, place thumb on his chin and press downward toward his chest.	a. This not only stimulates jaw but will actually stimulate act of chewing. b. It may be necessary to manually close patient's lips, using your thumb and index finger. When lips are closed, the swallowing reflex is stimulated. c. This maneuver moves his larynx superiorly and anteriorly, thereby facilitating swallowing.

Procedure (cont.)

NURSING ACTION	RATIONALE/AMPLIFICATION
7. When one mouthful is swallowed, remove spoon at once. If patient drools, wipe his mouth before the next mouthful is presented.	7. Patient is more comfortable without the sensation of food trickling down his chin.

FEEDING THE PATIENT WITH AN AFFECTED SIDE OF THE MOUTH (FACIAL PARALYSIS, HEMIPLEGIA, HEMILARYNGECTOMY)

1. Turn patient to his unaffected side.	1. This provides better head and neck support.
2. Place food on the strong side of mouth rather than in the middle of the mouth.	2. Permits food to be managed more effectively.
3. Encourage patient to form a bolus by moving his tongue around inside of mouth.	3. This assists in placing food in a proper position for swallowing rather than permitting food to collect near cheek.

Follow-up Care

1. Record the amount of intake, patient's taste and food preferences, his progress, and any special tactics that were effective in helping him.	1. Progress notes will assist in moving patient toward self-care.
2. Encourage family members to participate in his feeding program.	

GUIDELINES: Teaching a Patient with Dysphagia How to Swallow

Purpose To assist the patient who has difficulty swallowing after injury/surgical correction of the oropharyngeal or upper esophagus, neurological deficit, stroke.

Equipment Baby bottle with nipple
Rubber glove for instructor's hand

Procedure

NURSING ACTION	RATIONALE/AMPLIFICATION
1. Explain to the patient that you plan to work with him in developing the sensation of swallowing.	1. His cooperation, concentration, and directed participation are essential to the success of this learning experience.
2. Demonstrate first how the lips pucker as you draw inward in sucking your gloved finger.	2. The patient's observation will assist him in imitating this action.
3. Wash your gloved hand and then put your gloved finger in the patient's mouth. When the patient demonstrates good sucking ability, proceed to the next step.	
4. The teacher re-demonstrates the sucking maneuver with one hand while placing the other hand on her throat to feel the motions caused by sucking and swallowing.	4. It becomes apparent that after sucking, a need to move whatever is in the mouth causes the complex swallowing process to be initiated.
5. Ask the patient to duplicate these motions.	5. It may help to have patient place his hand on the neck of the demonstrator to grasp the mechanisms of swallowing.
6. The swallowing function can be further stimulated as follows:	
a. Have patient suck on a fresh lemon, (if permissible), or use lemon glycerin swabs in his mouth; ice fruit popsicles may also help.	a. This will stimulate salivation reflexes.
b. If the sucking reflex is intact, a straw may be effective in initiating swallowing as he sucks on it. The straw may need to be placed further inside the mouth or patient's head may have to be tilted.	
c. Place a cup at corner of the lips and tilt slightly so that patient can take liquid slowly. Encourage patient to move toward cup.	c. This offers patient more control as he moves forward, swallowing reflex occurs more easily.
7. Use a baby bottle if it appears that it might help.	7. Recognize the psychological effect this might have—will patient feel he is regressing?

SPECIAL FOOD CONSIDERATIONS FOR THE PATIENT WITH DYSPHAGIA

1. Avoid milk and milk products, since they stimulate production of thick saliva which is difficult to swallow.
2. Serve liquids that are close to room temperature rather than cold or hot.
3. Diluted fruit juices are more palatable than concentrated juices.
4. Provide textured foods rather than foods that are too smooth (i.e., chopped cooked vegetables rather than pureed vegetables, baked rather than mashed potatoes.)
5. Avoid strong flavored foods, acids, or bitter tasting foods—excepting lemon juice added to food.

GUIDELINES: Esophageal Dilatation (Bougienage)

Purpose   To dilate the cardioesophageal sphincter so that food may pass from the esophagus into the stomach.

Equipment   Water-soluble lubricant
Bougies-flexible, woven silk-tipped or rubber, of various sizes
Dilators of the physician's preference

Procedure   *Preparatory Phase*

1. Cleanse dilators with povidone–iodine (Betadine) to prevent infection and bacteremia.
2. Explain the procedure to the patient and indicate why it is necesasry for him to fast and drink no fluids for 12 hours beforehand.
3. Administer sedative or narcotic as prescribed to allay apprehension and assist him in relaxation.
4. Have the patient in a sitting position in a chair or in bed elevated 30 to 45 degrees.
5. Place a drape bib-fashion around his chest and over shoulders to protect his clothing.
6. Provide him with an emesis basin; have suction equipment (oropharyngeal) available.
7. Remove dentures if present.

NURSING ACTION	RATIONALE/AMPLIFICATION
Performance Phase	
1. Spray the patient's throat with a local anesthetic (gargle may be preferred).	1. The spray or gargle will desensitize local tissues.
2. Lubricate bougie with water soluble lubricant (some bougies are weighted with mercury); remove excess lubricant.	2. Lubrication reduces friction between the mucous membrane and tube. Excess lubricant may be aspirated.
3. Assist the physician as he passes the tube and first dilator. Support the patient's head and encourage him to swallow.	3. The more relaxed the patient, the easier the bougie will descend to the cardiac sphincter.
4. Larger bougies are passed progressively until pain occurs. (For achalasia, a pneumatic or hydrostatic balloon is used with fluoroscopy.)	4. Sizes are increased to dilate progressively the stricture. By increasing the pressure of the balloon, under fluoroscopy the sphincter may be gradually dilated.

NOTE: If bougies do not pass the stricture, it will be necessary to pass a guide wire through the stricture via esophagoscope. The scope is then removed and metallic olive dilators are passed down the guide wire, progressively increasing the size.

Follow-up Phase	
1. Have the patient rest in bed following procedure.	1. Observe for 24 hours for evidence of esophageal perforation.
a. Give nothing by mouth for an hour after dilation.	a. NPO to prevent aspiration.
b. Check pulse and temperature at least hourly for 6 hours.	b. Elevated pulse and temperature plus chest pain and evidence of subcutaneous emphysema may indicate presence of air in the mediastinum.
c. Be attentive to complaints of chest pain.	c. It may be necessary to have x-ray verification.
d. Observe upper chest for signs of subcutaneous emphysema. Should any of the above occur, notify physician.	

GUIDELINES: Pneumatic Dilatation

Pneumatic dilatation is the introduction of a pneumatic dilator under fluoroscopic control to dilate a cardioesophageal sphincter (tightened by spasm) utilizing measured pressure control.

Equipment   Ewald tube (No. 34 Fr.)
Pneumatic dilators (usually 3 balloon sizes: 1⅛, 1½, and 1⅞ in.)
Guide wire

Procedure   *Preparatory Phase*

1. Explain procedure to patient; tell him some discomfort may be experienced but that he will be given medication to help combat this.
2. Intake is limited to fluids for at least 24 hours prior to dilatation.

Procedure (cont.)

a. Give nothing by mouth after midnight prior to treatment.
b. Medications are prescribed prior to treatment, usually meperidine (Demerol), atropine, and perhaps diazepam (Valium).
c. The throat is sprayed with a local anesthetic, which may also be given in the form of a gargle (viscous lidocaine can be swallowed).

3. Procedure is done with fluoroscope control (x-ray department).

MEDICAL ACTION	RATIONALE/AMPLIFICATION/NURSING SUPPORT
1. Place patient in sitting position and pass an Ewald tube.	1. This is to aspirate secretions and contents of esophagus.
2. Remove tube following aspiration.	
3. Pass pneumatic dilator and position to straddle cardioesophageal junction.	3. Done under fluoroscopic control.
4. Inflate balloon to 100 mm. Hg.	4. Keep at this pressure for 1 minute still under fluoroscopic control.
5. Note slight constriction of sphincter.	5. The constriction should be positioned in center of balloon.
6. Inflate balloon to 200 mm. Hg.	6. Keep the balloon inflated for 2–3 minutes; nurse to observe patient's response and provide support.
7. Inflate balloon to 300 mm. Hg.	7. Patient may experience moderate to moderately severe pain.
8. Release pressure and remove dilator.	8. A small amount of blood on balloon is frequently seen when it is deflated and removed.

(Procedure may be repeated over several days—gradually increasing pressure in balloon.)

NURSING ACTION	RATIONALE/AMPLIFICATION
Following Procedure	
1. Continue to keep patient fasting.	1. This is done until patient's condition is stabilized.
2. Monitor vital signs every 30 minutes for 2 hours.	2. When vital signs are stable, full fluids may be given.
3. Continue to monitor vital signs every 4 hours.	3. Monitor signs for an additional 16 hours.
4. Observe patient for vital sign changes and complaints of severe pain. Should changes or complaints occur, notify physicain and give patient nothing by mouth.	4. These may be indicative of bleeding or perforation; reassure patient.
5. Be prepared for physician to order CBC, typing, crossmatching, and chest x-ray.	5. These tests may be required to assist in assessing cardiovascular conditions.

ESOPHAGEAL DIVERTICULUM

An *esophageal diverticulum* is an outpouching of the wall, usually in the cervical posterior side.

Types

1. Pharyngoesophageal (pulsion)—also called Zenker's diverticulum; upper end of esophagus through cricopharyngeal muscle.
2. Midesophageal (traction)—near tracheal bifurcation.
3. Epiphrenic (traction-pulsion)—lower third of esophagus.

Clinical Manifestations

A. *Pharyngoesophageal*

1. Difficulty in swallowing, fullness in neck, a feeling that food stops before it reaches the stomach, and regurgitation of undigested food.
2. Belching, gurgling, or nocturnal coughing brought about by diverticulum becoming filled with food or liquid, which is regurgitated and may irritate the trachea.
3. Halitosis and foul taste in mouth caused by decomposing of food in pouch (diverticulum).
4. Weight loss.

B. *Midesophageal*

Generally no symptoms.

C. *Epiphrenic*

1. At times associated with achalasia or diffuse esophageal spasm (see p. 383).
2. No symptoms at first, but condition eventually may cause dysphagia, pain, and pulmonary complications.

Diagnostic Evaluation

1. Roentgenograms using barium should be taken.
2. Esophagoscopy is risky, because of danger of perforation of diverticulum, which may lead to mediastinitis.

Treatment

A. *Pharyngoesophageal*

Surgical intervention, usually with a vertical incision; however, some surgeons prefer a transverse cervical incision.

1. Caution taken to avoid injury to common carotid artery and internal jugular vein.
2. Sac is dissected free and then excised flush with esophageal wall.
3. If transthoracic approach is used, nursing management is similar to that described for chest operations (see p. 220).
4. Nasogastric tube inserted.

B. *Midesophageal*

Therapy is usually not required because of absence of symptoms and rarely does it cause complications.

C. *Epiphrenic*

Underlying primary condition must be treated.

Nursing Management

1. Institute nasogastric feedings utilizing fluids.
   a. Irrigate tube carefully with water following each feeding.
   b. Record kind and amount.
2. Observe wound for evidence of leakage from esophagus—may lead to fistula formation.
3. If patient is tolerating liquid diet well, consider offering a bland diet.

ESOPHAGEAL VARICES (see p. 456.)

ESOPHAGEAL PERFORATION

Esophageal perforation is an acute surgical emergency in which the esophagus is punctured by a swallowed foreign object (e.g., dental prothesis, open safety pin), by gunshot, which results in trauma, or by an esophagoscope or stiff tube.

Clinical Manifestations

1. Chest pain, usually substernal—may be mild or severe.
2. Temperature elevation occurring within 24 hours.
3. Abdominal pain and tenderness, and epigastric muscle spasm.
4. Subcutaneous emphysema and crepitus of neck, face, and chest wall—noted in cervical and thoracic esophageal perforations.

Diagnostic Evaluation

1. History of recent esophageal trauma.
2. Chest film to look for air in mediastinum.
3. Esophagogram.

Surgical Treatment and Nursing Measures

1. Utilize emergency resuscitative procedures.
2. Prepare for surgical intervention (may not be needed if diagnosed and treated early).
3. Administer parenteral fluids and antimicrobial agents as prescribed.

4. Pass nasogastric suction tubing to minimize pleural or mediastinal contamination. Give nothing by mouth.

NOTE: For Spontaneous Esophageal Perforation, see Figure 10-2, which shows clinical manifestations, operative findings, and treatment.

CANCER OF THE ESOPHAGUS

Incidence

1. Benign tumors and sarcomas of esophagus are unusual, except for leiomyomas.
2. About 80% of cancers of the esophagus involve men.
3. Middle third of esophagus is most involved.
4. Carcinoma of esophagus is responsible for 1.9% of all cancer deaths in the United States.
   a. Usually this is a geriatric patient who also has pulmonary and cardiovascular disorders.
   b. Proximity of lesion to vital body structures, e.g., heart and lungs; lymph-node-spread is easy and rapid.
   c. Before significant symptoms occur, the tumor may already have invaded surrounding structures.

Causes

Causative factors have not been proven; the condition is associated with achalasia.
1. Chronic trauma—frequent use of alcohol, tobacco, spicy foods, hot Oriental tea.
2. Poor mouth hygiene.

Clinical Manifestations

1. Progressively increasing difficulty in swallowing (dysphagia). At first, only solid foods give trouble; then, as growth progresses and obstruction becomes more complete, even liquids pass with difficulty into the stomach.
2. Pain on swallowing (odynophagia).
3. Possible hemorrhage—usually only occult bleeding.
4. Progressive loss of weight and strength due to starvation.
5. Later symptoms—vague substernal pain, hiccup, respiratory difficulty, foul breath, regurgitation of food and saliva.

PHYSICAL FINDINGS

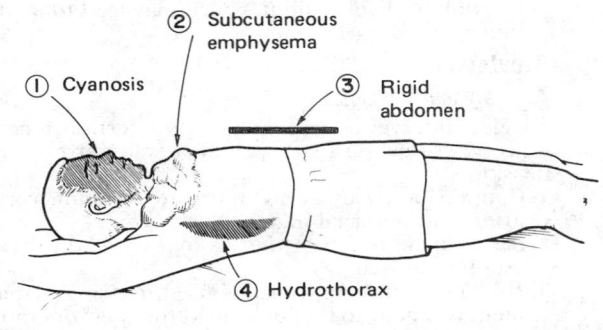

MANAGEMENT

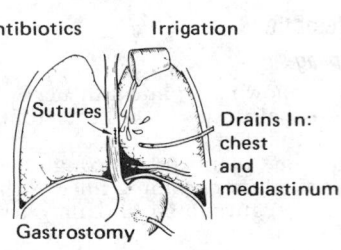

FIGURE 10-2. *Esophageal perforation. A. Characteristic physical findings with spontaneous rupture of the esophagus. B. Emergency operation to close perforation and drain mediastinum is indicated. (Adapted from Sawyers JL. Esophageal perforation and mediastinitis, AORN J, 15:42)*

Diagnostic Evaluation

1. Esophagogram.
2. Esophagoscopy.
3. Bronchoscopy—usually performed with lesions in the upper two-thirds of the esophagus in order to determine tracheal involvement and whether the lesion can be removed.
4. Cytologic examination and tissue biopsy.
5. Mediastinoscopy to determine involvement of nodes and other mediastinal structures.

Treatment

1. Lesions in middle and upper third, particularly, are not often suitable for excision.
   a. Irradiation is the preferred form of therapy.
   b. Some clinics report success with insertion of a prosthetic tube through the mouth to bridge the involved area and to facilitate swallowing. This insertion is done after dilatation of tumor-bearing portions of the esophagus.
2. Lesions of middle and lower esophagus are excised if there is no evidence of local or distant metastases.
   a. The portion of esophagus containing the tumor is removed.
   b. Continuity of gastrointestinal tract is restored by bringing the stomach (or a tube in stomach or a segment of colon) into the chest and implanting proximal end of esophagus into it.
   c. Chest drainage of pleural cavity is carried out (see p. 224).
3. If growth is inoperable, a gastrostomy (p. 403) may be performed as a palliative procedure to permit administration of food and fluids. This procedure does not appear to prolong life, since gastrostomy patients cannot swallow saliva either and are miserable from this problem.

Nursing Management

Principles are similar to those given for Radical Neck Dissection (p. 379) and Thoracic Surgery (p. 220).

2   GASTROINTESTINAL CONDITIONS

MAJOR MANIFESTATIONS OF GASTROINTESTINAL DISTURBANCE

ANOREXIA, NAUSEA, AND VOMITING

Normal Physiology

A. *Appetite*—a desire for food, or an agreeable attitude toward ingesting food, often specific kinds of food.
1. The frontal and parietal areas of the cerebrum, but especially the hypothalamus, are known to be associated with appetite.
2. Desire for food is acutely associated with increased rates of gastric hydrochloric acid secretion, with gastric hyperemia, and hypermotility.

B. *Hunger*—a strong sensation or urge to eat following a period of fasting.
1. Hunger is temporarily associated with rhythmic contractions of the stomach.
2. The precise mechanisms by which hunger is produced is unknown; it is related to a low blood-sugar level.

C. *Satiety*—a condition following consumption of sufficient food to meet present requirements; a feeling that one has had enough to eat.

Anorexia

Lack of appetite for food; lack of interest in all food.
1. Associated with a disinterest in consumption of even those foods which ordinarily one has great interest in and liking for.
2. Associated with decreased secretion of gastric hydrochloric acid.
3. Possible causes
   a. Unpleasant or upsetting experiences
   b. Apprehension, fear, and anxiety
   c. Excitement, both pleasurable and desirable.
   d. Systemic and local diseases, such as hepatic failure and uremia.

Nausea

A most unpleasant sensation usually associated with a distinct revulsion toward the ingestion of food; it may or may not precede vomiting.
1. Very often, anorexia is succeeded by nausea and vomiting. However, either of these states may occur without the others.
2. Associated with decreased motor activity of the stomach, pallor of gastric mucosa, and contraction of proximal duodenum.
3. Frequently associated with evidence of diffuse autonomic discharge: profuse watery salivation, sudden drenching perspiration, tachycardia.
4. Difficult to describe by many patients:
   a. Vague unpleasantness in epigastrium
   b. Distressing feelings in the throat
   c. Vague unpleasantness spread diffusely in abdomen (must be distinguished from mild visceral abdominal pain)

Vomiting

Sudden forceful expulsion of stomach contents through the mouth.
1. Vomiting center is located in the medulla.
2. May or may not be preceded by nausea and retching.
3. Exaggerated and often extreme vasomotor activities may immediately precede and accompany the vomiting act; watery salivation, sweating, pulse rate change, vasoconstriction, and pallor.
4. Tachycardia prior to vomiting becomes bradycardia during process.
5. Incited by neuromuscular "reverse peristalsis" or mechanical obstruction.

Nursing Management
1. Observe the preliminary symptoms.
   a. Patient is often lightheaded, weak, and dizzy.

b. Irregularity of respiration before and during vomiting.
c. Blood pressure may fall before and then fluctuate during vomiting.

2. Observe character and quantity of expectorated material.
   a. Yellowish or greenish color—may contain bile, which indicates pylorus is open.
   b. Fecal components—may indicate intestinal obstruction or infarction.
   c. Bright red (arterial) blood—may indicate hemorrhage from peptic ulcer. Dark red (venous) blood—may suggest hemorrhage from esophageal or gastric varices.
   d. "Coffee-grounds"—may indicate digested blood from slowly bleeding gastric or duodenal lesion.
   e. Undigested food—may indicate gastric tumor or ulcer obstruction.
   f. If taste is "bitter"—suggestive of bile.
      If taste is "sour" or "acid"—may indicate gastric contents.
   g. Odorless
   h. Sour-smelling
   i. Liquid
   j. Containing mucus or pus.

3. Be aware of progression of events when there is a diminution of intake and output—weight loss, dehydration, fluid and electrolyte imbalance:
   a. Skin becomes dry and loses turgor
   b. Poor mouth hygiene leading to halitosis

4. Recognize progression of events which might lead to shock, tachycardia, hypotension, oliguria.

Disturbances Associated with Anorexia, Nausea, and Vomiting

A. *Psychic and Neurologic Factors*

1. Life situations that evoke subjective manifestations of fear, frustration, depression, and anxiety may be associated with these symptoms.
2. *Anorexia* is commonly a manifestation of a depressed state which can lead to a profound impairment of food intake and possibly anorexia nervosa.
3. Nausea and Vomiting
   a. Occurring on a psychic basis
      (1) Frequently occurs during or shortly after meals
      (2) Often unaccompanied by nausea and retching
      (3) Frequently does not empty stomach
      (4) After vomiting, patient may desire to continue to eat
      (5) No recurrence of vomiting occurs.
   b. Projectile type associated with increasing intracranial pressure
      (1) Commonly not preceded by nausea.
      (2) May indicate meningitis, internal hydrocephalus, space-occupying lesion, cerebellar lesions.
   c. Accompanying migraine headache
      (1) Hypoxemia affecting the vomiting center
      (2) Vascular changes
      (3) Associated visual disturbances
   d. Caused by unusual stimulation of labyrinth of the ear Associated with vertigo
   e. Associated with systemic diseases, e.g., liver failure, uremia
   f. Associated with gastritis (alcohol, viruses, bacteria, or poisons)
   g. Associated with pyloric or intestinal obstruction
   h. Associated with cholecystitis, pancreatitis, or peptic ulcer

B. *Drugs and Toxic Agents*

1. Pathophysiologic Effect
   a. Medullary chemoreceptor zone may be stimulated.
   b. Direct effect on gastrointestinal organs brought about by mercury.
   c. Stimulation of hypothalamus nuclei brought about by alcohol, apomorphine, emetine, histamine, epinephrine.
2. Mucosal damage of upper gastrointestinal tract caused by mercury, ammonium chloride, copper sulfate, aminophylline, alcohol, aspirin.

C. *Intra-abdominal Disorders*

1. Mechanical obstruction in gastrointestinal tract (see p. 434)
2. Intra-abdominal inflammatory disorders—pancreatitis, peptic ulcer

D. *Nausea and Vomiting of Pregnancy* (see p. 994)

E. *Other Factors*

1. Febrile illness
2. Uremia (see p. 493)
3. Motion sickness
4. Ménière's disease (see p. 697)
5. Hepatocellular disease

Nursing Management

1. Observe and assess status of patient when he experiences anorexia, nausea, and vomiting. Note the effect of these symptoms on the patient generally:
   a. Food and fluid intake
   b. Balance between intake and output
   c. Effect on body weight, indicating malnutrition
   d. Character and amount of vomitus—measure and record
   e. Effect on patient's activity—malaise or apathy
   f. Changes in patient's skin color and turgor and in mucous membranes
   g. Note other fluid losses—perspiration, feces, urine, fluid and electrolyte balance which may result in dehydration
2. Improve psychological desire for food in order to overcome anorexia, nausea and vomiting.
   a. Determine patient's eating habits, cultural preferences, etc.
   b. Include patient's family in soliciting information.
   c. Encourage adequate rest before, during and after his meal; allay anxiety.
   d. Prepare patient for his meals by being certain he has had good oral hygiene, is comfortable and has clean bedding and clothing.
   e. Promote physical comfort of patient so that he may enjoy his food and not be distracted by discomfort during or after his meal.
   f. Protect his environment from noise, foul odors, confusion, too many visitors, etc.
   g. Serve food with attractive appearance and in appropriate quantity.
   h. Be sure that food is served at proper temperature.
3. If patient is nauseated but does not vomit:
   a. Reduce environmental stimuli
      Visual—other "sick" patients; soiled dressings
      Olfactory—drainage bottle
      Sensory—colostomy; cauterization; bedpan
      Auditory—noise
   b. Encourage rest and deep breathing.
   c. Cater to patient's preferences in food.
   d. Limit size of servings.

e. Remove meal tray as soon as he is finished.
f. If he does vomit, carefully observe vomitus and remove promptly; clean area and patient if necessary and offer mouthwash.
4. Provide opportunity for patient to express his feelings.
a. Keep channels of communication open.
b. Provide time to allow patient to talk.
5. Correlate administration of medication with needs of the patient.
a. If patient has pain, analgesics may be administered.
b. If patient is tired and exhausted, sedatives may be prescribed.
c. If patient appears tense and worried, tranquilizers may be indicated.
d. Specific antiemetic agents.
6. If secondary to intestinal obstruction, nasogastric suction or the insertion of a Miller-Abbott tube is indicated.

CONSTIPATION AND DIARRHEA

Constipation

Constipation is a decrease in the frequency, volume, or ease of stool passage.
Obstipation is absence of intestinal output (no stool).
1. Constipation is usually caused by altered routine in dietary and activity patterns; by drugs such as morphine, codeine, and atropine; by mechanical obstruction or surgery; by psychological factors resulting from restricted use of toilet facilities; and by old age. It may also occur as a result of chronic, strong-laxative abuse.
2. Manifestations of constipation include changes in color, consistency, and ease of expulsion of stools, which may be darker, harder, and difficult or painful to pass.

Diarrhea

Diarrhea is an increase in frequency, fluidity, and/or volume of stools.
1. It is a leading cause of death in developing countries where sanitation is poor and dietary deficiency widespread.
2. Acute diarrhea can be a serious problem in elderly and debilitated persons.
3. Chronic diarrhea is associated with malabsorption, malnutrition, anemia, and increased susceptibility to other diseases.

Nursing Assessment

1. Determine whether onset was sudden or gradual.
2. Find out how long the patient has had diarrhea—days?—weeks?—months?
3. Describe the character, consistency, and appearance of stools. Note that color changes are produced by presence of abnormal constituents.
a. "Tarry" stools—may indicate digested blood that usually originates in upper G.I. tract.
b. Bloody stools—may indicate hemorrhage, usually from lower G.I., tract.
c. Blood streaking on stool surface or on toilet paper—may indicate hemorrhoid or fissure.
d. Pale, pasty (clay-colored) stools—indicate totally obstructed biliary tract.
e. Foamy, foul smelling stools—indicates malabsorption or malabsorption syndrome.

f. Other color changes due to food or medication ingested indicates dietary excesses or effect of medication.
4. Learn when the bouts of diarrhea occur: in the daytime only, after meals, either day or night.
5. Determine whether diarrhea is associated with cramping or abdominal pain, fever, chills, nausea, weakness, travel exposure, etc.
6. Is pain in rectum or anus experienced at the time stools are passed?—may be indicative of tumor, inflammation, hemorrhoids, or anal fissure.
7. Has patient had any change in dietary habits, meals eaten away from home, etc?

NURSING ALERT: Alteration in bowel habits (such as constipation, then diarrhea, then constipation, then diarrhea) may mean partial obstruction.

8. Determine degree of dehydration. Look for signs of dehydration: weakness, postural hypotension, tachycardia, mucosal dryness, lethargy, poor skin, turgor.
9. Expect the need for laboratory evaluation: serum electrolytes, BUN, creatinine, hemoglobin, serum albumin, blood gases and pH, stool cultures, and stool for ova and parasites.

Nursing Management

A. *Constipation and Diarrhea*
1. Disturbances in elimination produce psychological discomfort; conversely psychologic deviation can produce elimination disturbances.
2. Assist patient in overcoming correctable problems by:
a. Affording privacy
b. Helping patient approach as near-normal position during evacuation as possible
c. Providing comfort measures such as warmed bedpan
d. Providing sufficient time and a schedule as close to the patient's own as possible.

B. *Constipation*
1. Correct dietary habits to include adequate fluids, fresh fruits, fiber (roughage)
2. Suggest a small glass of prune juice or lemon juice in warm water each morning.
3. If possible, encourage the patient to participate in active daily exercise: brisk walking, swimming.
4. Encourage a regular time for evacuation each day.
5. Suggest a bulk-forming laxative such as Metamucil that does not irritate the bowel. 1-2 heaping teaspoonfuls in a glass of water, once or twice daily, followed by a second glass of water.

C. *Diarrhea*
1. Consider hospitalization if diarrhea continues unresolved and there is significant dehydration.
2. Perform rectal examination to check for fecal impaction (common in the elderly, in mental patients, and in patients with neurologic disorders). If found, manually disimpact (see p. 444). Then give enemas.
3. Remove such causative factors as stress and food until cause is determined.
4. Encourage patient to take fluids such as Gatorade, juices, soups, and broths; avoid milk, fruits, and extreme roughage.

5. Prepare for fluid therapy and electrolyte replacement if dehydration is suspected. Administer prescribed medications.
   a. Kaolin-pectin (Kaopectate)—acts as an absorbent to bind gas and bacteria.
   b. Diphenoxylate (Lomotil)—decreases intestinal motility by acting on gastrointestinal smooth muscle (contraindicted when etiologic agent is *Shigella* or invasive bowel disease).
   c. Opiates—act to decrease bowel motility.

5. Prepare for fluid therapy administration if dehydration is suspected.

Health Education

1. Have required bathroom facilities readily available.
2. Pay particular attention to proper hand and body hygiene, since diarrhea may be infectious.
3. Use talcum powder or emollients to prevent skin excoriation.
4. Provide dry and clean bed linen and clothing.

DIAGNOSTIC STUDIES FOR GASTRODUODENAL CONDITIONS

GUIDELINES: Nasogastric Intubation—Levin Tube (Short Tube)

Purposes
1. To remove fluid and gas from the gastrointestinal tract (decompression).
2. To prevent or relieve nausea and vomiting.
3. To determine the amount of pressure and motor activity in the gastrointestinal tract (diagnostic studies).
4. To treat patients with mechanical obstruction and bleeding within the upper gastrointestinal tract.
5. To administer medications and feeding (gavage) directly into the gastrointestinal tract.
6. To obtain a specimen of gastric contents for laboratory studies.

Equipment
Nasogastric tube—usually Levin (rubber or plastic, No. 12 to 18 Fr.)—preferably disposable (plastic tubes are less irritating than rubber) or double-lumen sump tube
Water-soluble lubricant
Clamp for tubing
Towel and emesis basin
Glass of water and straw, or preferably ice chips
Adhesive tape (hypoallergenic)
Irrigating set with 20 ml. syringe
Stethoscope

Procedure *Preparatory Phase*

1. Explain procedure to patient and tell him how mouth breathing, panting, and swallowing can help in passing the tube.
2. Have patient in a sitting or high Fowler's position with neck flexed; place a towel across his chest.
3. Determine with the patient what sign he might use, such as raising his index finger, to indicate "wait a few moments" because of gagging or discomfort.
4. Remove dentures.
5. Place rubber tubing in ice-chilled water, making tubing firmer. Plastic tubing may already be firm enough; if too stiff, dip in warm water.
6. Mark distance tube is to be passed by measuring as indicated in Figure 10-3. This will ensure the passage of the tubing into the stomach.

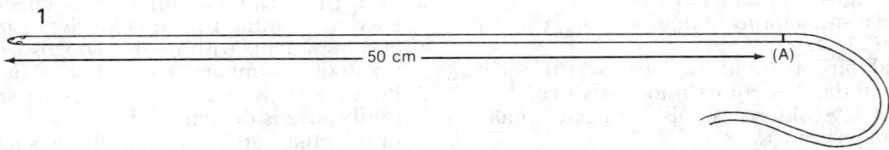

1

|— 50 cm —→| (A)

1. Mark the nasogastric tube at a point 50 cm. from the distal tip; call this point 'A'.

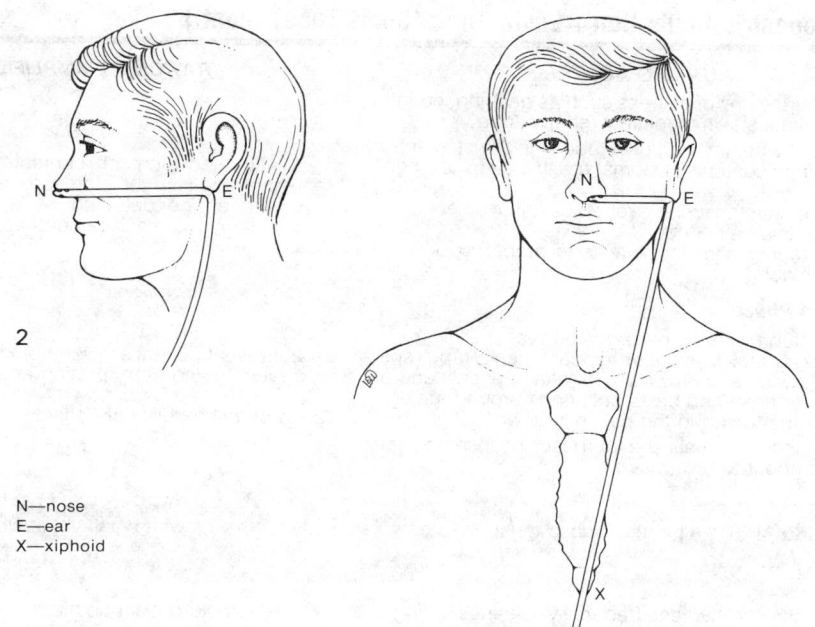

N—nose
E—ear
X—xiphoid

2. Have the patient sit in a neutral position with head facing forward. Place the distal tip of the tubing at the tip of the patient's nose (N); extend tube to the tragus (tip) of his ear (E), and then extend the tube straight down to the tip of his xiphoid (X). Mark this point 'B' on the tubing.

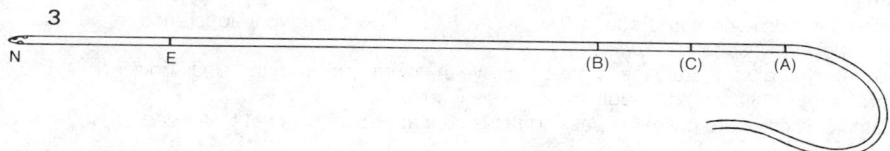

3. To locate point C on the tube, find the midpoint between points A and B. The nasogastric tube is passed to point C to ensure optimum placement in the stomach.

FIGURE 10-3. *The above diagram and steps (1, 2, 3) indicate how far a nasogastric tube is passed for optimum placement in the stomach. (From Hanson RL. Predictive criteria for length of nasogastric tube insertion for tube feeding. J Parenteral and Enteral Nutr 1979 May/June; 3 (3):160–163)*

	NURSING ACTION	RATIONALE/AMPLIFICATION
Procedure (cont.)	***Performance Phase***	
	1. Lubricate tube for about 15-20 cm. (6 to 8 inches) with thin coat of water soluble jelly.	1. Lubrication reduces friction between mucous membrane and tube.
	2. Lift head before inserting tube into nostril and gently pass it into the posterior nasopharynx aiming downward and backward.	2. Passage of tube is facilitated by following the natural contours of the body.
	3. When tube reaches the pharynx, the patient may gag; allow him to rest for a few moments.	3. Gag reflex is triggered by the presence of the tube.
	4. Have patient hold his head in a partially flexed position; offer him several sips of water sucked through a straw or permit him to suck on ice chips. Advance tube as he swallows.	4. Flexed head position makes swallowing easier and the tube less likely to enter trachea. Swallowing facilitates passage of tube. Actually, once the tube passes the cricopharyngeal sphincter into the esophagus, it can be slowly and steadily advanced even if the patient does not swallow.
	5. Continue to advance tube gently each time patient swallows.	
	6. If obstruction appears to prevent tube from passing, do *not* use force. Rotating tube gently may help. If unsuccessful, remove tube and try other nostril.	6. Avoid discomfort and trauma to patient.

GUIDELINES: Nasogastric Intubation—Levin Tube (Short Tube) (cont.)

Procedure (cont.)

NURSING ACTION	RATIONALE/AMPLIFICATION
7. If there are signs of distress such as gasping, coughing or cyanosis, immediately remove tube.	
8. To check whether the Levin tube is in the stomach: a. Aspirate contents of stomach with a 20-ml. syringe. b. Place a stethoscope over epigastrium; inject 5 ml. of air into Levin tube.	a. Aspirated stomach contents would indicate that the tube is in the stomach. b. Air can be detected by a "whooshing" sound entering stomach rather than the bronchus.
9. Adjust tubing after these tests to proper position in the stomach.	

Follow-up Phase

1. Anchor tube with hypoallergenic tape. a. Using 5 cm. (2 inches) hypoallergenic tape, split lengthwise and only halfway; attach unsplit end of tape to nose and cross split ends around tubing.	a. Prevent patient's vision from being disturbed; prevent tubing from rubbing against nasal mucosa.
2. Anchor the tubing to the patient's gown.	2. To permit mobility of patient.
3. Clamp the tube until the purpose for inserting the tube is about to take place.	

NURSING ALERT: All enteric tubes must be irrigated at regular intervals with small volumes of fluid to ensure patency.

4. Administer oral hygiene frequently. Cleanse tubing at nostril. Utilize a decongestant spray, if necessary.	4. To promote patient comfort.
5. Apply cream or lip pomade to lips and nostril to prevent encrustation.	5. To keep tissue soft.
6. If tube is to be in place for prolonged periods (beyond 12 hours), keep head of patient elevated at least 30 degrees.	6. To minimize gastroesophageal reflux.
7. Rotate tubing daily or more frequently.	7. To prevent adherence to mucosa.

Before Removing Nasogastric Tubing

1. Be certain that gastric drainage is not excessive in volume nor from the small bowel.
2. Ensure, by auscultation, that audible peristalsis is present.
3. Determine whether the patient is passing flatus so that abdomen is not distended.

NURSING ALERT: Recognize the potential for complications when intubation is prolonged—nasal erosion, sinusitis, esophagitis, and gastric ulceration. Pulmonary complications may occur postoperatively in patients with nasogastric intubation because of interference with coughing and clearing of the pharynx. (Fig. 10-4)

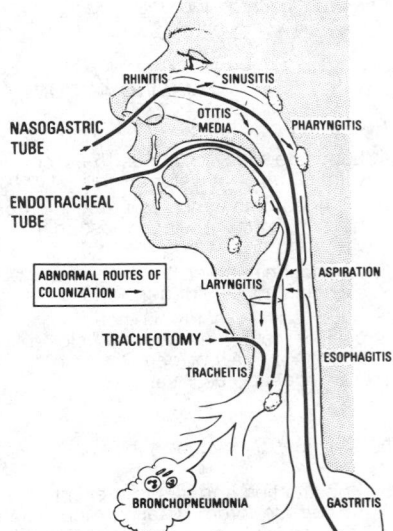

FIGURE 10-4. *This sagittal section demonstrates the points at which local defenses are altered or bypassed with the use of nasogastric or endotracheal tubes or in the presence of tracheostomy. Abnormal routes of colonization and sites of infection related to these different tubes are shown. (Meakins JL et al: The surgical intensive care unit: Current concepts in infection. Surg Clin North Am 1980 Feb)*

Procedure (cont.)

Removing Nasogastric Tubing

NURSING ACTION

1. Place a towel across patient's chest and inform him that the tube is to be withdrawn.
2. Rotate tubing and inject about 10 ml. of saline before clamping tubing.
3. Instruct patient to take a deep breath and exhale slowly.
4. Slowly but evenly withdraw tubing and cover it with a towel as it emerges.
5. Provide patient with materials for oral care and lubricant for nasal dryness.
6. Document time of tube removal and patient's reaction.

RATIONALE/AMPLIFICATION

1. No doubt patient will be happy to have progressed to this stage.
2. This will ensure its mobility. Tubing is clamped to prevent drainage within tube from being aspirated.
3. Slow exhalation will relax the pharynx and facilitate withdrawal of tubing.
4. Covering the tubing should dispel the momentary feeling of nausea.
5. Mouthwash and a nasal lubricant will be appreciated by the patient.

GUIDELINES: Gastric Analysis (Aspiration of Stomach Contents via Nasogastric Tube)

Purpose

1. To determine secretory activity of the gastric mucosa because of diagnostic significance.
2. To study the secretory component, hydrochloric acid.
3. To analyze gastric contents in patients suspected of having pyloric or intestinal obstruction.
4. To remove poisons.

Equipment

Rubber or plastic tube, No. 12–18 Fr. depending upon patient's size
Tube clamp
Syringe, 50 ml. or low-pressure intermittent suction apparatus
Water-soluble lubricant
Bowl of chipped ice for rubber tubing
Specimen containers

Procedure

NURSING ACTION

Preparatory Phase

1. Direct patient to fast (and take no fluids) for 8–10 hours preceding analysis.
2. Withhold anticholinergics for 48 hours.

3. Explain procedure to patient; cover his upper body with a drape to protect his clothing and provide an emesis basin for spittle and emesis.
4. Instruct patient to sit in a back-supporting chair or to assume Fowler's position in bed with neck flexed, leaning forward from the waist.
5. Establish with the patient a signal system to indicate when he wishes to rest a few minutes.
6. If dentures or bridges are present, they should be removed.
7. Chill tubing in ice water to make it firmer. If plastic tubing is too stiff, dip in warm water.

Performance Phase

Pass the nasogastric tube
(see Guidelines, p. 392).
1. Verify that the tube is in the stomach (for absolute assurance of tube position, fluoroscopic verification is required). Tip of the tube should be at least 50 cm. down from nose. When syringing air in and out, gurgling over stomach is audible with stethoscope.
2. Place patient semirecumbent in left lateral decubitus position.
3. Aspirate fasting stomach contents completely; then measure and record. If abnormal, notify physician before proceeding.

RATIONALE/AMPLIFICATION

1. An accurate sampling of stomach contents is ensured.
2. To permit normal emptying of the stomach and remove suppressive effect on gastric secretion.
3. Patient's understanding of how to breathe through his mouth and occasional swallowing will assist in passing the tube.
4. Gravity and this anatomic position will facilitate tubes passing into esophagus. If neck is hyperextended, tube is more likely to enter trachea.
5. Greater patient cooperation is obtained.

6. Dislodging of dentures could occur with risk of asphyxiation.
7. A manageable tube which droops naturally and is neither too stiff nor too limp is the objective.

1. Blue litmus turns pink in the presence of acid.

3. Normal: clear and watery; often contains green or yellow bile
Abnormal: see Nursing Alert

GUIDELINES: Gastric Analysis (Aspiration of Stomach Contents via Nasogastric Tube) (cont.)

Procedure (cont.)	NURSING ACTION	RATIONALE/AMPLIFICATION
	4. When tubing is properly positioned in the stomach, allow patient to rest for 20–30 minutes and continuously aspirate contents. This procedure allows patient to attain a basal state and to adjust to the tube in his throat.	4. Production of hydrochloric acid may be inhibited by the irritation of the tubing and by anxiety.

NURSING ALERT: In gastric analysis note the following:
1. Residual of 100 ml. or more, including undigested food particles may be indicative of gastric stasis or pyloric obstruction.
2. Fecal odor—suggests neoplasm or gastric fistula, intestinal obstruction.
3. Blood—indicates ulcerating lesion.
   Streaks of blood—suggests trauma from tubing.

Types of Analyses

A. *Basal Analysis*—A test to determine nature of secretions in the absence of stimuli.

1. Give no food or fluids from midnight on.
2. Obtain specimens as follows:
   1st specimen—label "residual."
   2nd specimen (30 minutes later)—label as to amount and time of collection.
   Then 4 additional specimens must be collected at 15-minute intervals—label as to amount and time of collection.
   > Continuous or frequent aspiration is required (manually or with suction apparatus) to avoid losses through pylorus.

B. *Stimulation Analysis* (betazole hydrochloride or pentagastrin) usually performed following basal study.

1. This is a test of gastric secretion following injection of a stimulant.
   a. Collect fasting specimen of gastric contents.
   b. Administer betazole hydrochloride (Histalog) or pentagastrin.
   c. Collect specimens every 15 minutes for 90 minutes or longer if physician desires.
2. Significance
   a. In presence of gastric ulcer visualized radiologically or endoscopically, the absence of any acid after stimulation (pH never falls below 6.0) suggests that ulcer is malignant and that surgical treatment is indicated.

NOTE: In absence of an ulcer, achlorhydria does *not* have the same significance (present in 40% of adults over age 60 without ulcer or cancer).

   b. In presence of a duodenal ulcer, basal output is greater than 20 mEq./hr. peak or maximal acid output greater than 50 mEq./hr. A basal/maximal ratio greater than 0.6 should strongly suggest Zollinger-Ellison syndrome.
   c. Otherwise, acid outputs, either basally or after stimulation, are of no diagnostic significance in peptic ulcer disease.

C. *Hypoglycemic Analysis* (Hollander test) A test that shows the vagal stimulation of parietal cells following a blood sugar drop to a hypoglycemic level of less than 50 mg./100 ml. (Hypoglycemia stimulates the secretory activity of the vagus nerve: if the nerve is divided, secretion will not occur. This test may be done postsurgically to determine effectiveness of vagotomy.)

1. Collect fasting specimen of gastric contents; label "residual."
2. Collect specimens every 15 minutes for 1 hour; label "basal secretion."
3. Administer prescribed insulin intravenously (calculated according to body weight).
4. Collect gastric specimens every 15 minutes for next 2 hours. Concomitantly, collect blood specimens every 15 minutes for determination of blood sugar. Measure, note characteristics, and record.

NURSING ALERT: Observe patient for signs of hypoglycemia; weakness, vertigo, tremors, perspiration, convulsions, unconsciousness. Have 50% glucose ready for intravenous administration if blood glucose level drops too low.

RADIOGRAPHY

Roentgenography of the Gastrointestinal Tract (Upper G.I. Series)

1. The entire gastrointestinal tract can be delineated by x-rays following the introduction of barium sulfate as the contrast medium. This procedure may be combined with cineradiography.
2. Barium is a tasteless, odorless, completely insoluble powder:
   a. It can be ingested in an aqueous suspension for upper gastrointestinal tract study (upper G.I. series); micronization of particles as well as chocolate or strawberry flavoring makes it more palatable.
   b. Effervescent fluids may also be administered to obtain air-contrast studies.
   c. Follow serially through small bowel over next 4–6 hours.
3. The fasting patient is required to swallow barium under direct fluoroscopic examination.
   a. Esophagus
      (1) Patency, caliber, and motility noted—may indicate anatomic and functional derangement.
      (2) Abnormally enlarged right atrium noted—indicates impingement on esophagus.
      (3) Esophageal varices noted—usually indicates liver cirrhosis.
   b. Stomach
      (1) Motility and thickness of gastric wall noted.
      (2) Spasms, ulcerations, malignant infiltrates and anatomic abnormalities noted.

(3) Pressure from outside of stomach detected.
(4) Patency of pyloric valve observed.
c. Small Intestine
Barium swallow or a continuous infusion of a thin barium sulfate suspension via duodenal tube may be done to visualize jejunum and ileum (small bowel enema).
4. During fluoroscopic examination, roentgenograms or movies are taken for permanent records.

Nursing Management and Patient Education

1. The patient is to receive nothing by mouth after midnight prior to the test.
2. During this interim, the patient is to receive no purgative, however mild, and no other medication unless specifically prescribed.
3. The patient remains in a fasting state until the last roentgenogram is taken.
4. Barium from prior barium enema must be fully evacuated before G.I. series or it will interfere with visualization of stomach and upper intestine. Cleansing enema is of particular value here.

Nursing Management

A careful nursing history may suggest patient high risk to contrast medium. (See chart below.)

UPPER GASTROINTESTINAL FIBEROSCOPY

Upper gastrointestinal fiberoscopy is the direct visualization of the gastric mucosa through a lighted endoscope (gastroscope). Fiberscopes are flexible scopes equipped with a fiberoptic lens through which colored photographs or motion pictures can be taken. This type of scope may be inserted with less discomfort to the patient, causes fewer perforations than the straight endoscope, and has thus completely replaced the older instrument.

Nursing Management and Patient Education

1. Explain the following to the patient:
a. What is about to happen.
b. That he must fast before the examination to prevent aspiration of gastric contents and to permit complete visualization of the stomach.
c. That dentures must be removed to facilitate passing the scope and to prevent injury.
d. That a topical anesthetic may be used for local comfort and to prevent gagging.
e. That a sedative or tranquilizer may be given to help him to relax.
f. That air will be pumped into the stomach during the procedure to permit visualization of the stomach.
2. Following a gastric examination, do this:
a. Check the gag reflex before offering food or fluids.
(1) Tickle the back of the patient's throat with a tongue depressor or cotton swab; usually 2–4

Reactions to Radiographic Contrast Material and Their Management

Reaction	Incidence	Manifestations	Medical and Nursing Management
Vasomotor	Up to 50% of patients	Mild flushing Warmth Tingling sensations Slight giddiness Metallic taste Nausea	Because these manifestations are mild and transient, treatment or pre-x-ray medication is not required
Anaphylactoid	Up to 4% of persons with history of allergy, hay fever, or bronchial asthma	Hives Sneezing Chest tightness Wheezing Angioedema Bronchoconstriction Hypotension Compensatory tachycardia	Check pulse frequently Vasopressors I. V. fluids Oxygen Antihistamines Steroids Pretreatment medication may help: Steroids (oral prednisone) 3x prior to x-ray Antihistamine (Benadryl) 1 hour before examination
Vagus		Apprehension Restlessness Hypotension Bradycardia—50 beats/ minute or less	Atropine—high doses I.V. fluids Monitor pulse rate since this indicates response to atropine Pretreatment—some recommend atropine

hours after the examination, the reflex functions return to normal.

    (2) If fluids are handled normally, patient may then be offered food.

  b. Check for signs of perforation: abdominal pain, subcutaneous emphysema, dyspnea, cyanosis, back pain, temperature elevation, hydrothorax, rigid abdomen.

  c. Offer throat lozenges or warm saline gargles to relieve throat soreness.

  d. Inform patient that he may pass gas by belching or passing flatus.

Gastric Biopsy

Obtaining a piece of gastric mucosa can be done through a gastroscope during endoscopy or fiberoscopy. Forceps extended through the scope may be used to bite tissue, or tissue may be obtained via suction as it pulls mucosa to excising blades within the scope. Tissue in one area may be representative of tissue in all sections of the stomach; however, by looking through the scope, the physician is discriminating in selection of specific tissue.

  Nursing management is similar to that for gastric endoscopy (see above).

GASTRODUODENAL CONDITIONS AND MANAGEMENT

PEPTIC ULCER

A *peptic ulcer* is an excavation found in the mucosal wall of the esophagus, the stomach, in the pylorus, or in the duodenum due to the erosion of a circumscribed area of its mucous membrane. Basically, the problem is too much secretion of hydrochloric acid in relation to the degree of protection afforded by both mucous secretion and the neutralization of gastric acid by duodenal, biliary, and pancreatic fluid.

Predisposing Factors

1. Emotional stress: anxiety, anger, resentment.
2. Drinking coffee and cola beverages and smoking cigarettes are associated with increased risk of ulcer development.
3. Drugs (salicylates, reserpine, phenylbutazone, aminophylline, and others) may be irritating to the mucous lining of the stomach, pylorus, and duodenum.
4. Genetic susceptibility.
5. A combination of the above factors.

Incidence

1. Duodenal ulcer is found most frequently in the 25–40 age group and in males 4 times more than females.
2. Gastric ulcer occurs most frequently in the 40–55 age group and in males 2½ times more often than females.
3. Five to 15% of population in U.S.A. have ulcers; only one half the cases are recognized.
4. Duodenal ulcers occur 10 times more frequently than gastric ulcers (Fig. 10-5).
6. Peptic ulcer occurs 2–2½ times more frequently among siblings with ulcers as among the general population.
7. Duodenal ulcer occurs more frequently in patients with type O blood.

Altered Physiology

(Duodenal Ulcer)
1. Increased mass of gastric mucosa and more parietal and peptic cells
2. Increased sensitivity to gastrin (peptide hormone secreted by gastric antrum stimulates gastric secretion)
3. Increased vagal stimulation, which in turn releases gastrin

4. Increased release of gastrin in response to a meal
5. More rapid gastric emptying
6. Increased acid load to duodenum

Preventive Measures and Health Education

Instruct the patient as follows:
1. Establish regular eating habits.
2. Avoid foods such as alcohol and coffee that strongly stimulate gastric acid.
3. By-pass stress situations, because they stimulate gastric secretion and motility.
4. Avoid irritating drugs, such as aspirin, Alka-Seltzer, and steroids. If it is necessary to administer these medications, have patient ingest milk and crackers between meals and at bedtime for buffering action. Acetaminophen (Tylenol) should be used rather than aspirin.
5. Be aware of high-risk tendency if there is a family history of peptic ulcer.

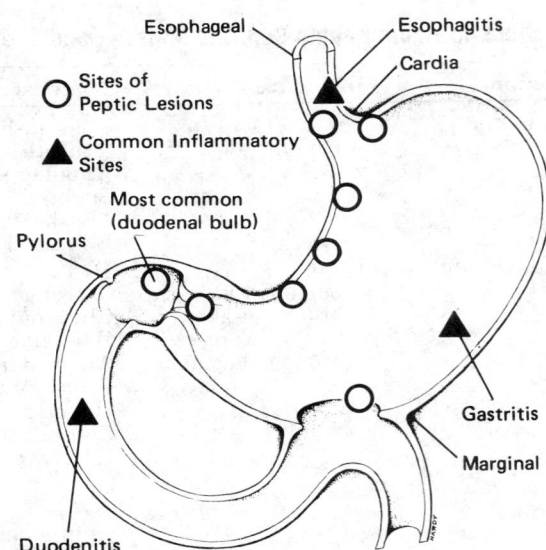

FIGURE 10-5 *"Peptic" lesions may occur in the esophagus (esophagitis), stomach (gastritis), or duodenum (duodenitis). Note peptic ulcer sites and common inflammatory sites.*

Clinical Manifestations

A. *Underlying Observations*

1. Peptic ulcers are more apt to be in the duodenum than in the stomach (ratio of 10 to 1).
2. A peptic ulcer occurs only in the areas of the gastrointestinal tract that are exposed to hydrochloric acid and pepsin (Fig. 10-5).
3. A small percentage of patients will have no symptoms and will first be diagnosed during a bleeding episode (more common in teen-agers).

B. *Pain*

1. Types
   a. Pain or discomfort—quality usually not well described—may be sharply localized in midepigastrium.
   b. Heartburn (substernal burning) is associated with peptic ulcer in many patients.
   c. Pain may radiate to the back if the duodenal ulcer has begun to penetrate the pancreas.
2. Time of occurrence
   a. Pain is worse when stomach is empty—usually ½ to 2 hours after meals; it may waken patient in early A.M. hours (12–3 A.M.).
   b. Pain is seldom present when patient first wakens, because gastric secretion is lowest at this time.
   c. Periodicity occurs in clusters—patient may have trouble for days to weeks, then experience long symptom-free intervals.
3. Relief
   Obtained by food or antacids—if truly effective, this occurs within 5–10 minutes.

C. *Nausea and Vomiting*

Reflex vomiting occurs in 10–20% of patients; it is associated with ulcer pain, also seen with duodenal obstruction in chronic ulcer disease when it usually occurs with or just after evening meal.

D. *Eructation*

Belching is due to increased air swallowing. (This is a nonspecific symptom and is most common in persons with *no* organic gastrointestinal disease.)

E. *Pyrosis (Heartburn)*

This is a burning sensation in lower esophagus and just below the sternum, sometimes with sour eructation.

Diagnostic Evaluation

1. Observation, history, and nursing assessment include the following:
   a. Determine location of pain, whether it is localized, whether it radiates, how long it lasts, and when it occurs.
   b. Find out if pain is relieved by food or alkalies.
   c. Learn if there is a history of tension, problem situations, or anxiety.
   d. Determine whether the patient ingested drug irritants.
   e. Determine whether the patient smokes or consumes alcohol.
2. Fiberoptic panendoscopy, which permits visualization of entire stomach and proximal duodenum, is most accurate.
3. Upper G.I. series (see p. 396).
4. Gastric secretory studies (p. 396) are of value mainly to check for possible Zollinger-Ellison syndrome.

5. Associated diseases
   Associated occasionally with hyperparathyroidism, polycythemia vera, alcoholism, chronic liver disease, chronic respiratory disease, uremia.

Objectives of Treatment and Nursing Management

A. *To promote an atmosphere conducive to physical and mental rest.*

1. Encourage bed rest to reduce physical activity and to separate patient from his usual environment.
2. Offer sedatives or tranquilizers to lessen the response to stimuli and to promote relaxation and sleep.
3. Provide frequent feedings, antacids and other medications given on time.
4. Inform visitors to avoid upsetting conversation.

B. *To relieve pain and discomfort, and to promote healing through the control of gastric acidity by using antacids and antisecretory medications.*

1. Administer antacid medications to neutralize hydrochloric acid and relieve pain.
   a. Liquid antacids are more effective than tablets.
   b. Increasing aluminum in antacids leads to constipation; increasing magnesium leads to diarrhea.
   c. Antacids are given 1 hour after meals, at bedtime, and during the night as required for pain.
   d. Look for antacids that effectively neutralize stomach acid, leave low sodium content, require about 5 ml. to swallow at a time, and are least expensive (Delcid, Maalox therapeutic concentrate).
   e. Antacids with calcium may produce hypercalcemia.
   f. Magaldrate is antacid containing least salt and is useful for patients on restricted salt diet.
2. Administer anticholinergic drugs to suppress gastric secretions and delay gastric emptying. This is most useful at night.
   a. Anticholinergics are contraindicated in patients with glaucoma, urinary retention, gastric retention, and possibly arrhythmia.
   b. Encourage hydration to minimize side effects of anticholinergic medications.
3. If ulcer problems persist after first being treated with antacids, it may be necessary to administer cimetidine (Tagamet).
   a. Cimetidine (Tagamet) owes its effectiveness to its H_2-receptor blocking action in inhibiting gastric acid secretion; to its potency (superior to that of cholinergics); and to its failure to produce acute side effects.
   b. Cimetidine is administered with meals because it is rapidly absorbed and its blood concentration peaks about 75 minutes after ingestion.
   c. Between 60–90% of patients with duodenal ulcers heal within 4 weeks.
   d. About 85% of patients with duodenal ulcers suffer acute episodes which can be effectively managed without surgery.
   e. For short-term therapy, side effects are most unusual.
   f. Symptoms of misuse of Tagamet need to be noted: diarrhea, dizziness, gynecomastia, decreased sperm count, hallucinations, bradycardia.
   g. Cimetidine is effective only in preventing bleeding from starting, not in stopping bleeding once it has started.

C. *To reduce motor and secretory activities of the stomach by means of a therapeutic diet.*

1. Eliminate foods which the patient says cause him pain or distress; otherwise the diet is unrestricted.
2. Offer regular milk since the fat in milk decreases secretion. (Skim milk is usually not given, because the calcium in milk increases secretion.)
3. Give small servings to decrease distention and release of gastrin.
4. Provide frequent feedings to neutralize gastric secretions and to dilute stomach contents.
5. Advise patient to avoid coffee and other caffeinated beverages, and cola drinks.

D. *To assist the patient in understanding how chronic and long-lived his problem is and the very real part he has in controlling it.*

1. Emphasize the need to avoid anxiety-producing situations.
2. Alert him to the irritating nature to the gastric mucosa of certain drugs—especially aspirin and aspirin-containing drugs such as Alka-Seltzer.
3. Review the reasons for smaller meals and midmeal snacks.
4. Suggest that he cut down on smoking; suggest switching from coffee and cola to caffein-free beverages such as ginger ale, 7-Up, and Postum.

Discharge Planning and Health Education

See Objectives of Treatment and Nursing Manage-

Complications

- Hemorrhage ⟶ Shock
- Perforation ⟶ Peritonitis
- Pyloric Obstruction ⟶ Dehydration
- Intractability ⟶ Incapacitation: Surgery

A. *Hemorrhage*

1. Experienced by 15–25% of patients with duodenal ulcer; accounts for 40% of deaths from peptic ulcer.
2. Manifestations
   a. Giddiness, faintness, breathlessness with slight exertion.
   b. Tachycardia, sweating, and coldness of extremities.
   c. Black, tarry stool (melena). (Test for occult blood.)
   d. Vomiting of blood (hematemesis).
3. Medical and Nursing Intervention
   a. Encourage bedrest and check vital signs frequently.
   b. Give medication for restlessness or pain, but be on alert for shock.
   c. Employ nasogastric suction to empty stomach of clots and to monitor rate of bleeding.
   d. Give whole blood and/or plasma to keep circulating blood volume at a safe level. (This is not needed if hematocrit is greater than 30 and vital signs are stable, with no orthostatic drop in blood pressure or rise in pulse.)
   e. Note color, consistency, and volume of stools and vomitus.
   f. Provide treatment if patient goes into oligemic shock (see p. 128).

B. *Perforation*

1. Clinical Manifestations
   a. Severe upper abdominal pain, persisting and increasing in intensity and often spreading from upper to lower abdomen.
   b. Vomiting suddenly
   c. Referring of pain to top of shoulders (phrenic nerve irritation)
   d. Abdomen—extremely tender and rigid
   e. X-ray of abdomen: 50–75% free air visible
   f. Shock, tachypnea
   g. Patient lying still in bed, afraid to move; pain increased by patient's coughing or jostling the bed.
2. Surgical Intervention
   a. Repair fluid deficit (peritoneal "burn").
   b. Close perforation; plication of ulcers is performed (see Postoperative Care, p. 402) if chronic symptoms preceded perforation.

C. *Pyloric Obstruction*

1. Etiology
   Area around pyloric sphincter becomes narrowed from spasm, edema, or scar tissue formed when ulcer alternately heals and breaks down. Inflammation, muscle spasm, or edema may cause a temporary obstruction.
2. Assessment and Major Manifestations
   Nausea, vomiting of retained food, constipation, weight loss, cramping, epigastric pain after meals.
3. Medical and Nursing Intervention
   a. Gastric decompression and intravenous fluids.
   b. Later, test emptying with fluid load and then with solid bolus.
   c. Surgery may follow if clinical course is prolonged and obstruction is unrelieved.

D. *Intractability*

The failure of medical management to accomplish healing of the ulcer—usually a calloused posterior ulcer that penetrates into the pancreas.

1. Manifestations
   Pain continues without adequate relief from milk or antacid.
2. Surgical Intervention
   a. Vagotomy and gastrojejunostomy or pyloroplasty—to abolish cephalic phase of secretion.
   b. Vagotomy and hemigastrectomy—to abolish cephalic and gastric phase of secretion.
   c. Gastric resection—to abolish acid-secreting parietal cells.

Surgical Treatment

Surgery is required in only about 15–20% of ulcer patients; operation is individualized, based on patient's age, ability to withstand procedure, preoperative nutritional status, and particular indications.

OBJECTIVES: to relieve complications
   a. Perforation (described in B, above)
   b. Hemorrhage (described on this page)
   c. Pyloric obstruction (described in C, above)
   d. Intractability (described in D, above)
to treat the tendency to ulcer formation.

A. *Types of Gastric Operations*
A comparison of these may be made for the following: M—mortality rate; UR—ulcer recurrence; PNR—poor nutritional result.

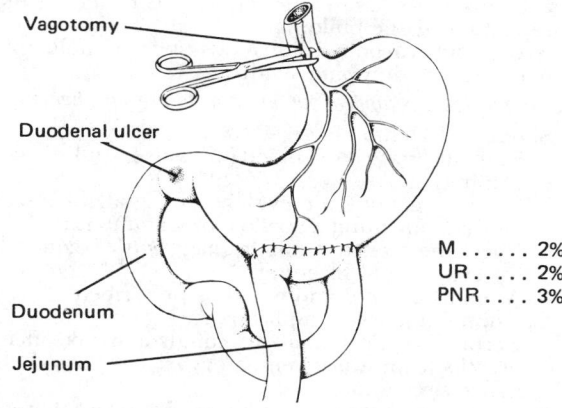

FIGURE 10-6. *Gastrojejunostomy and vagotomy.*

(See Figs. 10-6–10-9 for the incidence of each of these occurrences.)
1. Gastrojejunostomy and Vagotomy (Fig. 10-6)
   The jejunum is anastomosed to the stomach to provide a second outlet of gastric contents. The severed vagus nerve reduces secretions and movements of the stomach (90% good results).
2. Antrectomy and Vagotomy (Fig. 10-7)
   The resected portion includes a small cuff of duodenum, the pylorus, and the antrum (about one-half of the stomach). The stump of the duodenum is closed by suture, and the side of the jejunum is anastomosed to the cut end of the stomach.
3. Subtotal Gastrectomy (Fig. 10-8)
   The resected portion includes a small cuff of the duodenum, the pylorus, and from two-thirds to three-quarters of the stomach. The duodenum or side of the jejunum is anastomosed to the remaining portion of the stomach.
4. Vagotomy and Pyloroplasty (Fig. 10-9)
   A longitudinal incision is made in the pylorus, and it is closed transversely to permit the muscle to relax and to establish an enlarged outlet. This compensates for the impaired gastric emptying produced by vagotomy.

B. *Nursing Management*

(See below, for management of the patient undergoing a gastric resection.)

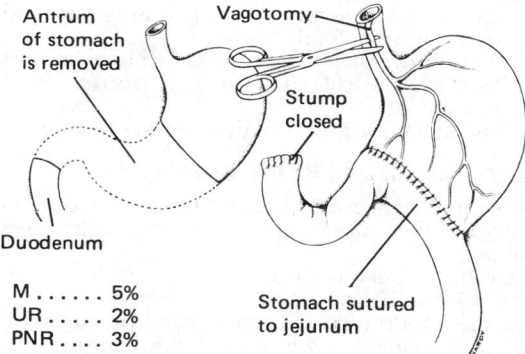

FIGURE 10-7. *Antrectomy and vagotomy.*

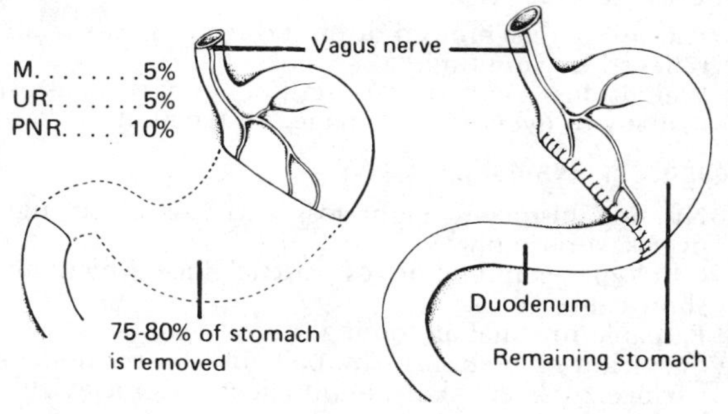

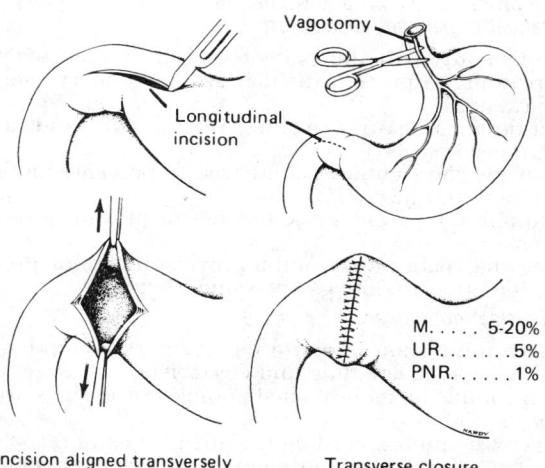

FIGURE 10-8. *Subtotal gastrectomy. It is also possible to do the Billroth II procedure by suturing the gastric stump to the side of the jejunum.*

GASTRIC CANCER

Cancer of the stomach accounts for about 14,000 deaths annually in the United States—usually males of middle age. (See p. 844, Cancer Mortality by Site). There has been a decrease in incidence in U.S.A. over the last 2 decades for unknown reasons.

Clinical Manifestations

A. *Early Manifestations*

(Most often, patient presents with same symptoms as gastric ulcer; later, on evaluation, the lesion is found to be malignant.)
1. Progressive loss of appetite
2. Noticeable change in, or appearance of, gastrointestinal symptoms—gastric fullness (early satiety), dyspepsia of more than 4 weeks duration
3. Blood (usually occult) in the stools
4. Vomiting which may indicate pyloric obstruction or cardiac-orifice obstruction
5. Occasionally, vomiting that has a coffee-ground appearance due to slow leaks of blood from ulceration of the cancer.

FIGURE 10-9. *Vagotomy and pyloroplasty.*

B. *Later Manifestations*

1. Pain is a late symptom often induced by eating and relieved by vomiting.
2. Weight loss, loss of strength, anemia, metastasis (usually to liver), hemorrhage, obstruction.

Diagnostic Evaluation

1. Nursing history—weight loss and loss of strength over several months.
2. Cytologic examination of gastric juice which may show cancer cells.
3. Palpable unusual abdominal mass.
4. Suspicion of metastasis by palpable lymph nodes—surface of liver, skin at umbilicus, supraclavicular nodes, etc.
5. Gastric analysis—absence of acid after maximal stimulation (Histalog, gastrin) indicates ulcer is malignant.
6. Roentgenologic studies, fluoroscopy, and gastroscopy; also cytologic studies and biopsy-fiberoscopy.
7. Stool examination and tests for occult blood may be indicated.
8. Ultrasonography and computed tomography may be required. These are usually reserved for questionable diagnoses since they are more costly tests.

Treatment

1. The only successful treatment of gastric cancer is surgical removal.
2. If tumor is localized to stomach and can be removed, chances are still poor that the patient can be cured.
3. If tumor has spread beyond the area that can be excised surgically, cure cannot be accomplished.
   Palliative surgery such as subtotal gastrectomy with or without gastroenterostomy may be performed to maintain continuity of the gastrointestinal tract. Surgery may be combined with chemotherapy to provide palliation and prolong life.

GASTRIC RESECTION

Gastric resection is the surgical removal of part of the stomach.

Objectives of Treatment and Nursing Management

A. *To promote comfort and wound healing by relieving the patient of pain and discomfort.*

1. Frequently turn the patient and encourage deep breathing to prevent vascular and pulmonary complications.
2. Institute nasogastric suction to remove fluids and gas in the stomach.
3. Provide conscientious mouth care to prevent mouth dryness and ulceration.
4. Administer parenteral antibiotics to prevent infection.
5. See that patient has nothing by mouth until prescribed (to promote gastric wound healing).

B. *To meet nutritional needs of the patient*

1. Give intravenous fluids to prevent shock and to provide adequate fluid and electrolytes.
2. Give fluids by mouth when audible bowel signs are present.
3. Increase fluids according to patient's tolerance.
4. Offer a diet with vitamin supplements when patient's condition permits.

5. Give protein-vitamin supplements to foster wound repair and tissue building.
6. Avoid high carbohydrate foods such as milk that may trigger "dumping syndrome."

C. *To anticipate complications in order to prevent them*

1. Shock and Hemorrhage
   a. Evaluate status of blood pressure, pulse, and respiration.
   b. Observe patient for evidence of apathy, apprehension, air hunger, pallor, or clammy skin.
   c. Check the dressings and drainage bottle frequently for evidence of bleeding.
   d. Administer fluid and blood as prescribed.
2. Cardiopulmonary Complications
   a. Encourage the patient to cough and take deep breaths to produce ventilatory exchange and enhance circulation.
   b. Assist the patient to turn and move, thereby mobilizing secretions.
   c. Promote ambulation as prescribed to increase respiratory exchange.
3. Thrombosis and Embolism
   a. Initiate a plan of self-care activities to promote circulation.
   b. Encourage early ambulation to stimulate circulation.
   c. Prevent venous stasis by use of elastic stockings if indicated.
   d. Check for tight dressings or binder that may restrict circulation.
   e. See also page 340.
4. "Dumping Syndrome"
   This is a complex reaction which may occur because of excessively rapid emptying of gastric contents.
   Manifestations: nausea, weakness, perspiration, palpitation, some syncope, and possibly diarrhea.
   Instruct the patient as follows:
   a. Eat small, frequent meals rather than three large meals.
   b. Avoid meals high in sugars and salt.
   c. Reduce fluids with meals but take them between meals.
   d. Take anticholinergic medication before meals (if prescribed) to lessen gastrointestinal activity.
   e. Relax when eating; eat slowly and regularly.
   f. Take a rest after meals.
5. Phytobezoar Formation (Formation of a gastric concretion composed of vegetable matter)
   a. Avoid fibrous foods such as citrus fruits (skins and seeds), because they tend to form phytobezoars.
      (1) Following a gastric resection, the remaining gastric tissue is not able to disintegrate and digest fibrous foods.
      (2) This undigested fiber congeals to form masses that become coated by mucous secretions of the stomach.
   b. Stress the importance of adequate mastication.

Discharge Planning and Health Education

(Adjustment to self-care and return to the community)
1. Emphasize the importance of coping with stress situations.
2. Review nutritional requirements and regime with patient (Table 10-1).
3. Stress the importance of vitamin B_{12} supplements.
4. Encourage follow-up visits with the physician.
5. Recommend annual blood studies and medical

TABLE 10-1. DIET GUIDELINES FOLLOWING GASTRIC SURGERY

Foods Usually Well Tolerated
Meat, fish, poultry, eggs, cheese, refined breads and cereals (unsweetened)
Unsweetened canned fruits and juices
Cooked mild vegetables, including potatoes
Fats and oils

Foods to Add as Tolerance Improves
Sweetened canned fruits*
Whole grains

Foods Frequently Poorly Tolerated*
Sugar, candy, syrup, sweetened desserts (cake, cookies, pie, pudding, ice cream)

Foods and Beverages to Avoid
Cold high carbohydrate items such as milkshakes, slush, fruit ice
Coffee and tea (unless allowed by physician)

Special Considerations
Begin with *very* small portions; eat 5 to 6 times daily
Take most liquids between rather than with meals
Milk: include in early stages unless poorly tolerated
Fresh fruits and vegetables: gradually include after 2 to 3 wk; chew thoroughly

* Add *gradually* to diet if desired unless bothered by symptoms of dumping.
(From: Behm V, Murchie G and King DR. Nutritional care of the patient following gastric surgery. Dietetic Currents 1974 Mar/Apr; 1(1). Courtesy of Ross Laboratories, Columbus, Ohio)

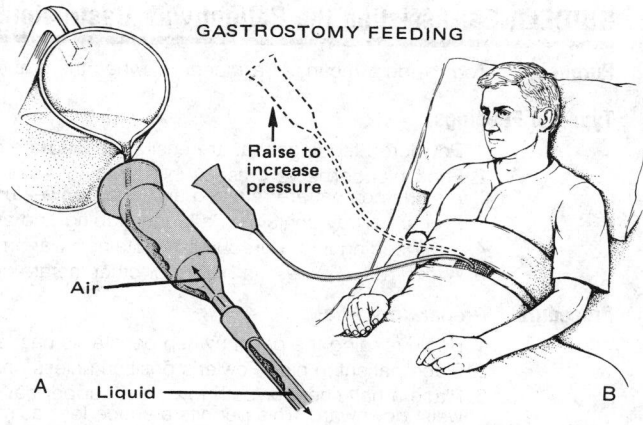

check-ups for any evidence of pernicious anemia or other problems.
6. See above, C-4 "Dumping Syndrome."

GASTROSTOMY

A *gastrostomy* is an opening into the stomach performed for the purpose of administering food and fluids when a complete obstruction of the esophagus exists. The obstruction may be due to scar-tissue contracture such as may result from a lye burn or a carcinomatous growth. A gastrostomy may also be done occasionally in the unconscious or debilitated patient for prolonged nutrition.

Preoperative Patient Care

1. Explain the nature of the problem to the patient and the recommended treatment; use simple line drawings for clarification.
2. Achieve adequate fluid, electrolyte, and nutritional balance by administering the required foods and fluids.
3. Immediate preoperative care is similar to that described on page 88.

Surgery

1. Frequently performed under local anesthesia.
2. The anterior gastric wall is incised through a left rectus incision.
3. A tube is inserted and held in place in the stomach wall with several purse-string sutures. The tube may be a rubber tube or a Foley catheter inflated with 5 to 8 ml. of water or air and pulled taut to the abdominal wall (Fig. 10-10).
4. The skin is closed close to the tube to prevent leakage.
5. The tube is clamped at all times except for feedings.

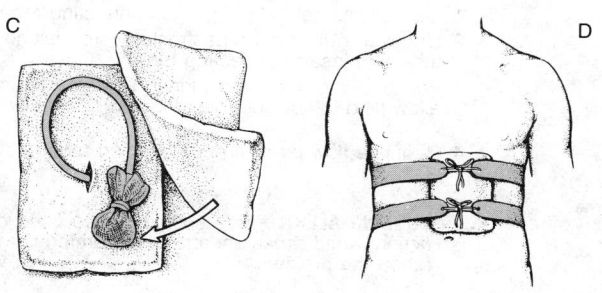

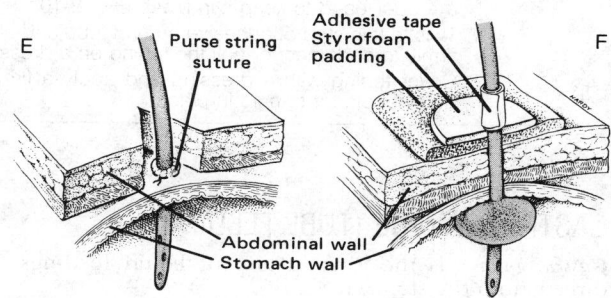

FIGURE 10-10. A. *The receiving receptacle is tilted so that feeding can be poured to allow air bubbles to escape. B. Liquid feeding is poured and permitted to flow into the stomach by gravity. Raising the funnel can increase pressure; lowering it can decrease pressure. At the end of the feeding, flush tubing with water. C. Following the feeding, disconnect catheter and cover the outlet with a sterile gauze square; fasten with a rubber band. Coil tubing on dressing and cover with another dressing or abdominal pad. D. Secure dressing or abdominal pad with Montgomery straps. E. A gastrostomy tube may be a rubber perforated tube; the stomach may be pulled upward and fastened with sutures to prevent leakage. F. Another method is to use a Foley catheter as the gastrostomy tube. It is inflated with 5 ml. of water or air and pulled snugly against upper gastric wall. This tube is anchored in place with tape which rests on a cushion of styrofoam or padding. The nurse recognizes the extra precaution required in handling this latter type of gastrostomy.*

GUIDELINES: Assisting the Patient with Gastrostomy Feedings

Purpose   To provide a means of alimentation when the oral route is inaccessible.

Types of Feedings

1. Powdered feedings that are easily liquefied are commercially available.
2. Food blender is very useful in preparing a normal diet; physiologically it is more acceptable, since fiber and residue content are retained and good bowel function is promoted.
3. Prepare a tray containing a funnel, tubing and adapter plus water at room temperature.
4. Pour feeding into a graduated container; warm to 37.8° C. (100° F) in a basin of water.
5. Avoid milk in excess in blacks or other lactate-deficient patients.

Procedure   **Preparatory Phase**

1. Begin feeding the patient when peristalsis has returned.
2. Place patient in high Fowler's position unless contraindicated.
3. Place a half-sheet or bath towel over upper half of patient; fold top bedding down to cover the patient from the waist downward. This permits a space for gastrostomy tube exposure.

NURSING ACTION (Fig. 10-10)	**RATIONALE/AMPLIFICATION**
Performance Phase	
1. Connect funnel to tubing and connecting tube.	
2. Uncover opening of gastrostomy (or jejunostomy) tube and insert connecting tube.	2. Provides a receptacle for feeding that will lead into gastrostomy tube.
3. Pour feeding into tilted funnel, unclamp tubing and allow fluid to flow into the stomach by gravity.	3. Tilting the funnel allows air bubbles to escape; when tubing is unclamped, air bubbles will not enter stomach.
4. Regulate flow by raising or lowering receptacle.	4. Raising inceases pressure; lowering decreases pressure.

> **NURSING ALERT:** Force should not be used nor should feeding be given directly from the refrigerator; such action would cause abdominal discomfort to the patient. If there appears to be an obstruction, stop feeding and report the problem.

5. After each feeding, the tube should be irrigated with water (room temperature) and clamped.	5. A water flush will prevent the tube from clogging and will assist in keeping it clean.
6. Apply a small dressing over the tube opening, using a rubber band to keep it in place (Fig. 8-10).	6. This will keep the tube opening clean for the next feeding.
7. Twist a thin strip of adhesive around tube and attach firmly to abdomen, or coil the tubing on a dressing.	7. Prevents the tubing from being accidentally pulled out of the stomach.
8. Cover tubing with a dressing and apply a firm abdominal binder to hold in place.	8. Provides maximum mobility for the patient.

GASTRIC GAVAGE (TUBE FEEDING)

Gastric gavage is the introduction of liquid feedings directly into the stomach.

Purpose

1. Effective in persons who have difficulty swallowing (dysphagia), prolonged unconsciousness, or anorexia.
2. Useful when there is oral or esophageal obstruction or trauma.
3. Life-saving in one who is debilitated or who has had surgery on some part of the gastrointestinal tract that does not permit normal ingestion of food.

Avenues (Fig. 10-11)

These vary with the patient and circumstances.
1. Nasogastric—orogastric—see Guidelines, page 392
2. Esophagotomy—a stoma (temporary or permanent) may be created at one of several sites along the esophagus.
   a. The feeding tube is introduced through the skin directly into the esophagus.
   b. The tube is usually removed between meals, making this method easy to manage.
3. Gastrostomy—see p. 403 and Guidelines p. 403
4. Jejunostomy—an abdominal stoma is constructed providing direct access to the jejunum.
   a. This is advantageous when the stomach must be bypassed.
   b. Disadvantages are the high incidence of diarrhea and dumping syndrome.

Feeding Methods

1. Gravity—a funnel or Asepto syringe (minus bulb) (Fig. 10-10) is used as the receptacle for feedings. The rate of flow is affected by raising or lowering receptacle.
2. Drip-regulated
   a. A Murphy drip is connected by tubing to a

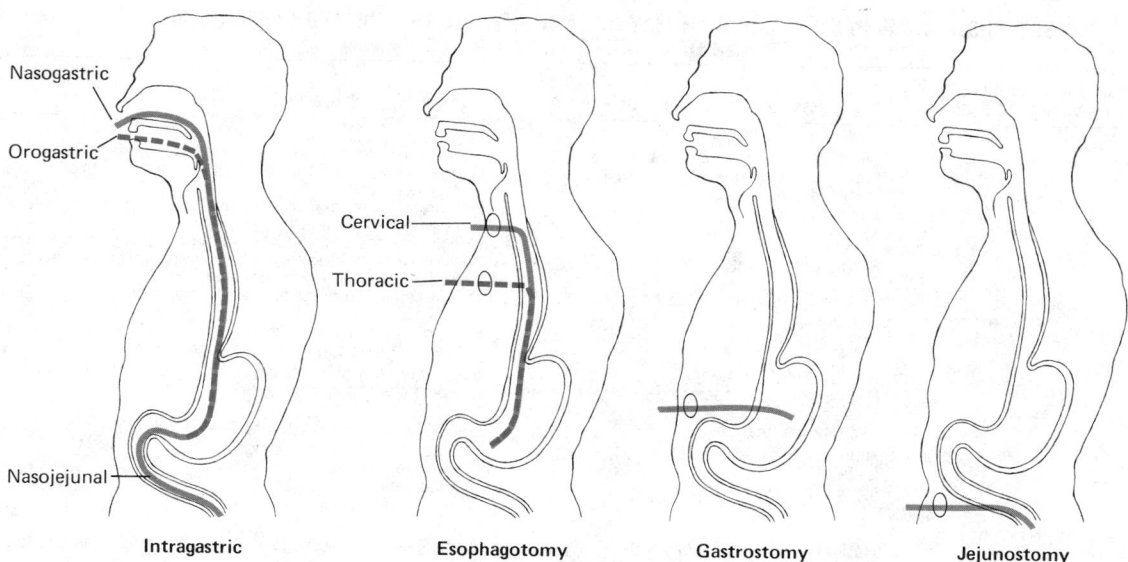

FIGURE 10-11. *Types and sites of gastric feeding.*
Intragastric (nasogastric, NG): *A tube is passed through the nose or mouth into the stomach and secured in place. (A tube passed through the mouth is more correctly called an orogastric tube. An orogastric tube is ordinarily inserted at mealtime and removed following the meal.) Intragastric tube preferred for short-term gavage feeding; easily inserted by physician or nurse, remains in place between feedings. (Some clients are taught to insert their own tube; they may remove the tube between meals.) Variations include nasopharyngeal and nasojejunal feeding tubes.*
Esophagotomy: *A temporary or permanent opening (stoma) is constructed at one of several sites to allow a tube to be introduced through the skin into the esophagus. Feeding tube is usually removed between meals. Advantages: dependable for long term feeding, allows concealment of apparatus, easy to handle.*
Gastrostomy: *A temporary or permanent stoma is constructed allowing food to be introduced through the skin directly into the stomach. Preferred for long-term gavage feeding of children and for long-term feeding of adults when use of esophagus is contraindicated. Disadvantages: partial undressing necessary at mealtime; skin care may pose problems.*
Jejunostomy: *A stoma is constructed which gives direct access to the jejunum. This method of feeding may be used when the stomach must be bypassed. Disadvantages: high incidence of dumping syndrome and diarrhea; adequate nutrient intake difficult to maintain. (Suitor CW and Hunter MF. Nutrition: Principles and Application in Health Promotion, p. 367. Philadelphia JB Lippincott Co., 1980)*

receptacle (Kelly flask) which hangs on an I.V. pole.
  b. From the other end of the Murphy drip, tubing is connected to the feeding tube.
  c. The rate of flow of liquid can be adjusted.
  d. Requires thorough cleaning or may be disposable. Consider cost.
3. Motor pump—feeding is delivered at a pre-set rate.

Continuous Nursing Assessment

1. Recognize that even though some nutritional deficits are corrected, other problems may arise, such as fluid deficit, electrolyte imbalance, diarrhea, esophageal reflux.
2. Cleanse all containers and tubing thoroughly; formulae and feedings make excellent media for bacterial growth.
3. Aspirate the tubing prior to feeding to verify that the tube is in the patient's stomach.
4. Avoid air bubbles in the system (Fig. 10-10 A) which could cause distention.
5. Provide oral and nasal hygiene before and after orogastric and nasogastric feedings for comfort and to prevent infection.
6. Follow last amount of each feeding with water to

flush tubing for cleansing, and to promote fluid balance.
7. Monitor patient for signs of fluid and electroylte imbalance.
8. Record amount of feeding and water; indicate patient's participation and acceptance.
9. See Table 10-2 regarding problems which may be encountered and examples of corrective measures.

Patient Education

1. Since the tube should be changed every 2 or 3 days, the patient may be taught how to do it. (The tube should be clean but not necessarily sterile.)
2. The patient should learn how to feed himself. (He can learn what foods may be taken.)
3. Skin requires special care.
  a. It can be irritated by action of gastric juices that leak out.
  b. Daily dressing of wound averts skin maceration.
  c. Bland ointment, such as zinc oxide or petrolatum, can be applied to area around the tube.
4. After several weeks, the tube may be removed and inserted only for feedings.
5. For problems that may be encountered in tube-fed clients and corrective measures, see Table 10-2.

TABLE 10-2. SOME PROBLEMS WHICH MAY BE ENCOUNTERED IN TUBE-FED CLIENTS AND EXAMPLES OF CORRECTIVE MEASURES

Factors to Assess to Determine How Individual is Tolerating the Feeding	Possible Causes of Problems	Corrective Measures

1. Gastrointestinal function
  a. Vomiting
	Feeding too soon after intubation
	Improper location of tip of feeding tube
	Rapid rate of infusion
	Excessive volume
	  1) Air
	  2) Formula
	Position of patient
		Allow patient time to relax and rest after tube is inserted
		Repositioning of tube by qualifed health professional
		Administer slowly
		Be sure tube feeding container does not run dry before feeding is completed
		Check with doctor regarding number and size of feedings
		Position on right side for ½ hr following feeding—reverse Trendelenburg or semi-Fowlers

Applies to
      both vomiting
      and diarrhea
	{ Food poisoning or
	    infection
	Anxiety
		Check sanitation of formula and equipment
		
		Explain procedures. Provide reassurance and other needed types of support. Provide privacy.

b. Diarrhea	Rapid rate of infusion High osmolarity of formula or high concentration of formula Lactose intolerance	Administer slowly—very slowly if formula is cold Adapt patient to formula gradually Contact physician regarding change of formula
c. Constipation	High content of milk in formula Lack of fiber Inadequate fluid intake	Contact physician regarding: 1) change in formula 2) laxatives 3) increasing fluid
2. Fluid and electrolyte balance a. Dehydration	Rapid infusion of carbohydrate → hyperglycemia → osmotic diuresis → dehydration Excess protein and electrolytes in formula Inadequate fluid intake	Administer slowly. Exogenous insulin sometimes needed Change formula and/or increase fluid according to physician's orders
b. Edema	Excessive sodium in formula	Check with physician about change in formula
3. Nutritional adequacy a. Undernutrition (gradual weight loss)	Inadequate number of calories to meet energy requirements	Check to see if patient is receiving prescribed amount of formula. Estimate client's caloric intake Check with physician regarding increasing the volume, concentration or number of feedings given
b. Overnutrition (gradual gain of undesirable weight)	Excessive caloric intake	Check with physician regarding decreasing the volume, concentration, or number of feedings given
c. Undernutrition (inadequate intake of protein and/or micronutrients leading to biochemical or clinical signs of deficiency)	Amount of standard formula needed to maintain weight is too low to meet requirements for essential nutrients	Check with physician regarding providing appropriate nutrient supplements

(Suitor CW and Hunter MF. Nutrition: Principles and Application in Health Promotion, Phila., J. B. Lippincott Co., 1980, p. 371)

GUIDELINES: Total Parenteral Nutrition (TPN) Hyperalimentation

Total parenteral nutrition (TPN), formerly referred to as "parenteral hyperalimentation," is a means of providing body nutrients by way of the intravenous route when it is impossible or inadvisable to use the normal digestive routes.

Physiological Basis

1. The intravenous route has heretofore not provided adequate nutrition; caloric and nitrogen deficiencies occurred.
2. Because of nutritional deficiencies, the process of *gluconeogenesis* takes place; this is the body's conversion of protein to carbohydrate.
3. Approximately 1500 calories/day are required by the average adult postoperative patient to prevent body protein from being utilized.
4. Body needs are increased when the patient has a hypermetabolic disease, a fever, or injury; these needs may require up to 10,000 calories daily.
5. To meet the fluid volume necessary to provide so many additional calories would exceed fluid tolerance and lead to pulmonary edema or congestive heart failure.
6. This process (TPN) provides desired calories in concentration directly into the intravenous system which rapidly dilutes incoming nutrients to satisfactory levels of body tolerance.
   a. Hypertonic glucose → fulfills caloric requirement → permits amino acids to be released for protein synthesis (not energy).
   b. Potassium → provides proper electrolyte balance → transports glucose and amino acids across cell membranes.
   c. Calcium, magnesium, and sodium chloride → meet cell requirements as determined by serum electrolyte needs.
   d. Other trace elements whose function is not known may be deficient in TPN, since they are not included.

Clinical Indications

1. As a substitute for oral or nasogastric intubation when these are not effective, desirable or even hazardous. Use TPN under the following conditions:
   a. Chronic vomiting
   b. Cancer, chemotherapy, or radiotherapy
   c. Cerebrovascular accident
   d. Anorexia nervosa
2. As a supplement for patients demonstrating large nitrogen losses, e.g., burn patients, those with metastatic cancer, and those who are receiving radiation and chemotherapy.
3. As a means of putting the gastrointestinal tract at rest.
   a. When there is evidence of gastrointestinal fistula
   b. With severe and extensive inflammatory bowel disease
   c. Following major intestinal resection
   d. Instances of intestinal obstruction

Equipment Skin detergent germicide
Sterile drapes and gloves
20-ml. syringe
No. 14 (5 cm.) needle
16 gauge 20-cm. radiopaque catheter
Connecting tubing and adapters
250-ml. flask, 50% D/W
3 x 3 dressings—adhesive for occlusive dressing
Suture material
Antimicrobial ointment
Tincture of benzoin spray

Procedure (Fig. 10-12)

(for subclavian vein catheterization)

NURSING ACTION	RATIONALE/AMPLIFICATION
Preparatory Phase	
1. Explain the procedure to the patient and why it is important for him not to touch the area where the catheter is inserted.	1. To provide reassurance; to prevent dislodging and contaminating catheter.
2. Tell the patient he will probably be ambulatory during the extended time of therapy.	2. In the absence of other conditions requiring bed rest, ambulation is possible.
3. Place patient in head-low position.	3. This position permits dilatation of neck and shoulder vessels, which makes catheter entry easier and prevents air embolus.
4. Suggest that the patient turn his face away from the area selected.	4. To prevent contamination of TPN site.
5. Support patient in proper position to permit hyperextension of shoulder.	5. This position can be facilitated by placing a rolled sheet or towel vertically along spinal column.
6. Shave area if necessary, remove surface oils with acetone or ether, and prepare skin with a detergent-germicide.	6. To reduce probability of contamination to the barest minimum.
7. Instruct patient to be still during insertion of catheter.	7. To prevent the possibility of dislodging of catheter and perforation of subclavian vein.
Performance Phase (by physician)	
1. Clean and drape area for catheter insertion (Fig. 10-12).	1. To prevent infection.
2. Inject local anesthesia to skin and underlying tissues.	2. To promote comfort of patient and prevent patient movement.
3. Using a No. 14 (5 cm.) needle with syringe, insert needle beneath the clavicle and into subclavian vein.	3. Suclavian vein is selected because it leads into the superior vena cava, which has a large volume of blood flow that provides rapid dilution of hypertonic solution.
4. Instruct patient to perform Valsalva maneuver.	4. By the patient's bearing down with mouth closed, positive pressure is produced when syringe and needle are replaced by catheter.
5. Detach syringe and insert a 16-gauge 20 cm. radiopaque catheter through the needle into the vein; withdraw needle.	5. This permits the more flexible catheter to remain in position during subsequent feedings.
6. Attach Intracath to tubing from a flask of 5% dextrose in water.	6. To keep tube patent between other feedings and to provide calories.
7. Prepare patient for x-ray.	7. To insure that tip of catheter is in proper location.

GUIDELINES: Total Parenteral Nutrition (TPN) Hyperalimentation (cont.)

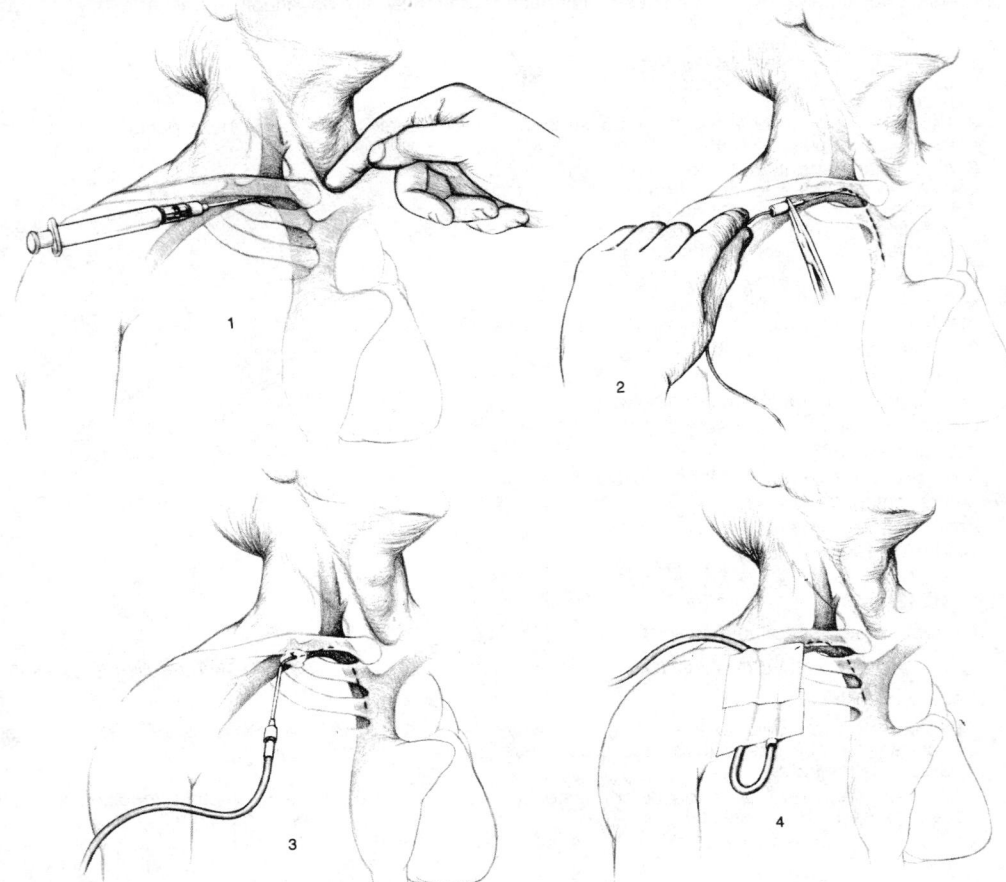

FIGURE 10-12. *Subclavian catheterization for IV feeding is achieved under controlled hospital conditions in these stages:*
1. *Syringe with intracath needle inserted at clavicular curve parallel to patient's chest, advanced under clavicle and over first rib until entire beveled tip enters vein (demonstrated by aspirated blood).*
2. *Syringe detached, needle held by hemostat, catheter threaded into superior vena cava.*
3. *Needle withdrawn, x-ray confirms correct catheter placement in middle portion of superior vena cava.*
4. *Catheter sutured to chest skin, attached to standard IV tubing, adhesive dressing applied, infusion started.*

Solutions may be delivered by gravity flow or propulsion pump. (From Patient Care, Jan 15, 1975.

Procedure (cont.)

NURSING ALERT AND PRIORITIES OF CARE
Patients receiving hyperalimentation are particularly susceptible to catheter-related infections. To minimize this complication:
1. Solutions are to be prepared under a laminar flow hood.
2. Solutions are prepared fresh daily and refrigerated until used.
Maintain sterility during entire TPN procedure to prevent sepsis.
Maintain consistent infusion rate which is calculated on a 24-hour basis.
Monitor patient carefully—including vital signs.
Record data accurately.
Provide emotional support to patient.

Follow-up Phase

1. Remind patient not to touch dressings.

1. Permit him to turn in bed or to ambulate, but caution patient against handling dressings which would cause contamination.

Procedure (cont.)	NURSING ACTION	RATIONALE/AMPLIFICATION
	2. Check infusion rate every 30 minutes. Adjust infusion rate to not more than 10% of the original rate if too fast or too slow.	2. If too rapid → hypermolar diuresis occurs → excess sugar is excreted → intractable seizures occur → coma → death. If too slow → inadequate nutritional intake.
	3. Weigh patient daily and keep accurate intake and output records.	3. Accurate comparison of daily change is noted.
	4. Check vital signs every 4 hours.	4. Note temperature rise, which could signify a complication.
	5. Change dressings every 48–72 hours and as required.	5. Strict aseptic technique must be followed.
	6. I.V. tubing and filters must be changed daily.	6. Procedure is done by a nurse especially taught to do this.
	7. Encourage diversional therapy and activity during extended therapy.	

GUIDELINES: Intravenous Fat Emulsion

Intravenous fat emulsion is a form of essential fatty acids that can be administered to the patient intravenously when these essential nutrients are needed and cannot be acquired in any other way.

Chief Advantage

A concentrated amount of essential fatty acids and calories can be supplied in a relatively small volume of liquid.

Availability

Intralipid 10% (soybean emulsion)—Cutter Laboratories
Liposyn 10% (safflower emulsion)—Abbott Laboratories
Liposyn 20%* (safflower emulsion)—Abbott Laboratories

Clinical Indications

Treatment or prevention of essential fatty acid deficiencies which may be due to:
1. Malignancies, burns, ulcerative colitis, severe renal disorders, nonfunctional gastrointestinal tracts
2. Severe nutritional disorders and inability to take nourishment by mouth
3. Extended semiconsciousness or unconsciousness
4. Specific preoperative and postoperative patients in whom it is necessary to increase caloric intake
5. Essential fatty acid deficiencies: characterized by sparse hair growth, eczematous scaly skin lesions, thrombocytopenia, and poor wound healing

Action

1. Lipid emulsion is introduced into the blood; protein in the blood acts as emulsifier (lipid–protein complex).
2. The lipid–protein complex carries nutrients to the liver, adipose tissue, etc., where they are degraded, synthesized, stored, mobilized, and oxidized for energy.
3. It is delivered with amino acid dextrose solution in order not to deplete patient's protein resources.

Equipment

1. Prepackaged in 500 ml. flasks (1.1 calories per ml.)
   Intralipid 10%—refrigerate until ½ hour before using
   Liposyn 10%—does not require refrigeration
2. Intravenous tubing with Y-connection (Fig. 10-13)
   "Cutter Saftiset"—use with Intralipid (if pump is used, prime the tubing by gravity)
   "Abbot Venoset 78" (macrodrip)—use with Liposyn

NURSING ALERT: Use the administration set as recommended by the manufacturer, since some plastics in combination with lipids cause leaching of diethylhexyl phthalate (DEHP).

Procedure	NURSING ACTION	RATIONALE/AMPLIFICATION
	Preparatory Phase:	
	1. Do not shake emulsion flask.	1. Agitation of emulsion may cause fat globules to aggregate.
	2. Inspect flask of fat emulsion.	2. Look for signs of altered stability: a. Inconsistency in texture and color b. Separation of oil

* 20% solution will provide 2 cal/1 ml. Rate may not exceed 60 ml/1 hour after first 30 minutes of slow infusion.

GUIDELINES: Intravenous Fat Emulsion (cont.)

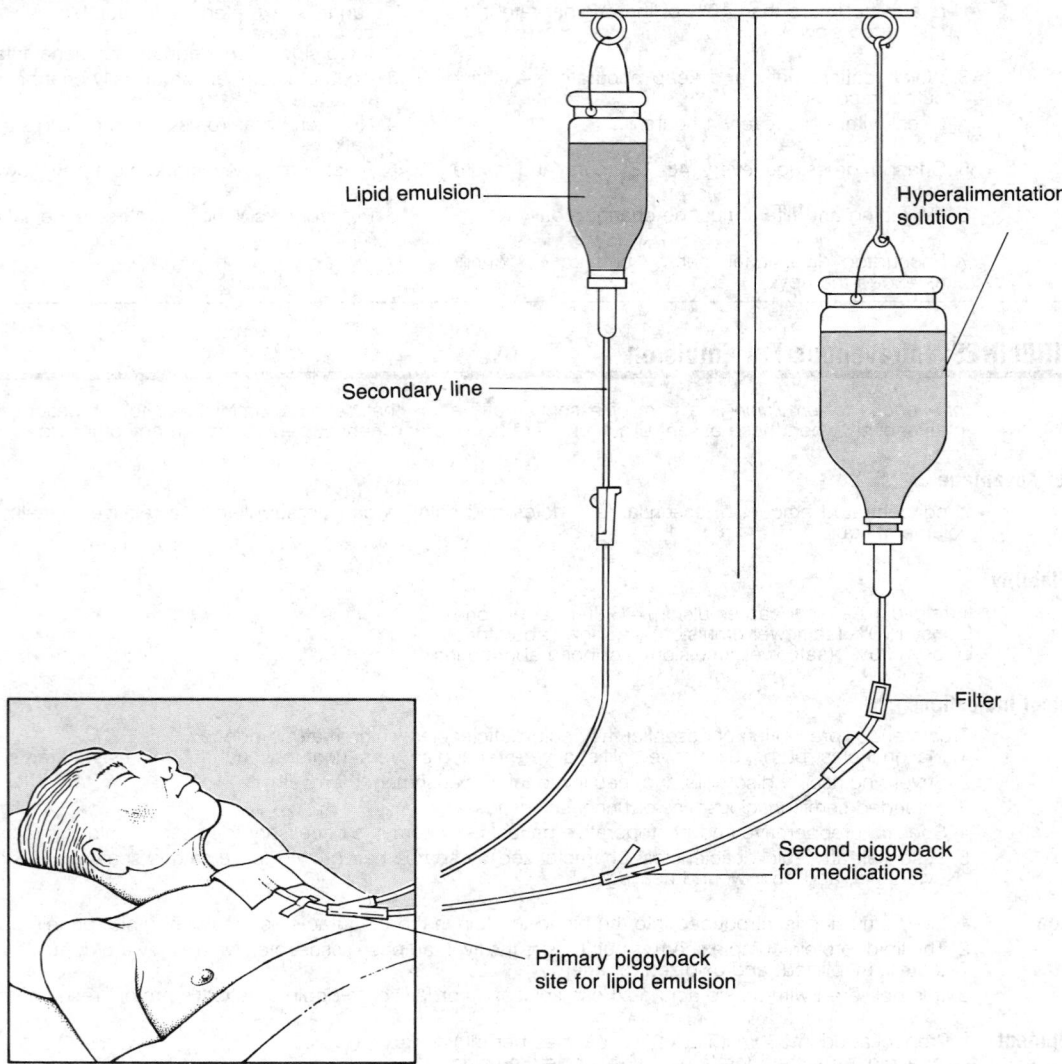

Lipid emulsion

Hyperalimentation
solution

Secondary line

Filter

Second piggyback
for medications

Primary piggyback
site for lipid emulsion

FIGURE 10-13. *Administration of fat emulsion. Note that the flask of fat (lipid) emulsion is higher than the amino acid and dextrose (hyperalimentation) fluid. The reason is that if both were at the same level, backflow and failure to infuse would result because of differences in specific gravity. Primary line is for amino acid and dextrose solution; secondary line is for lipid emulsion.*

Procedure (cont.)

NURSING ACTION	RATIONALE/AMPLIFICATION
3. Connect tubing to emulsion flask and clear tubing of all air (do not use the pump to prime tubing but use gravity only).	3. Air in system may cause an air embolus in patient.
4. Connect I.V. tubing to Y-tube connection which is closest to insertion site; insert tubing primed with I.V. fat emulsion directly into this site.	4. This reduces length of time emulsion comes in contact with substances that may affect its stability.
5. Do not use in-line filters.	5. Particles are too large to go through a filter.
6. If infusion is to be administered by gravity drip, hang fat emulsion flask higher than flask of amino acid solution.	6. This will prevent backflow of fat emulsion (less density) into other amino acid flask (higher density).

Procedure (cont.)

NURSING ACTION	RATIONALE/AMPLIFICATION
7. Explain procedure to patient; tell him that the milk-white solution is unlike other solutions he has received intravenously. Remind him that he is not to leave the unit while this emulsion is running.	7. Patient will have a better understanding of the reason for more frequent vital signs and other observations.
8. Document patient's vital signs.	8. These will be used as a baseline comparison for later evaluation.

Performance Phase:

NURSING ACTION	RATIONALE/AMPLIFICATION
1. Start flow rate at 1 ml./min. for first 30 minutes, monitor vital signs every 10 minutes during this time.	1. Provides opportunity to assess patient for chills, fever, headache, dizziness, sleepiness, allergic reactions, back pain, chest pain, nausea, vomiting, pressure over eyes, etc.
2. If untoward signs occur, stop infusion and notify physician.	
3. If problems occur, physician may prescribe heparin.	3. Heparin will hasten clearing of lipids from patient's plasma.
4. If no complications occur, infusion rate may be increased: a good gauge is to administer 500 ml. in 4–6 hours.	4. Continue constant observation; monitor vital signs hourly.
5. At conclusion of infusion, detach emulsion flask and attach 150 ml. flask of 5% dextrose as per physician request.	5. Dextrose flushes out remaining fat emulsion from tubing.

Follow-up Phase.

NURSING ACTION	RATIONALE/AMPLIFICATION
1. When dextrose has run in, clamp tubing securely until next lipid emulsion is to be given. If this is final treatment, disconnect as with any I.V.	
2. Continue to be alert for delayed adverse reactions.	2. Fat overload syndrome manifestations: headache, low grade fever, nausea, abdominal pain, irritability*
3. Record the nature of lipid emulsion given, amount, time, patient reactions, time of termination of procedure.	3. Include documentation of vital signs.
4. Request periodic serum triglyceride levels and liver function studies.	4. These will provide indicators regarding patient's ability to metabolize and clear the emulsion from the blood stream.
5. Monitor patient for effectiveness of this treatment. Observe for changes in his clinical status.	5. This would determine effectiveness in treating an EFA (essential fatty acid) deficiency.

* This may be indicative of splenomegaly, hepatomegaly, hyperlipemia, thrombocytopenia, jaundice, gastroduodenal ulcer.

GUIDELINES: Duodenal Drainage

Purposes
1. To detect abnormal constituents of bile, pancreatic juice, or duodenal fluid.
2. To assist in diagnosis of cholelithiasis (gallstones), choledocholithiasis (common duct stones), pancreatitis, and pancreatic carcinoma.
3. To assist in diagnosing gallbladder problems when x-rays prove inadequate.
4. To assist in parasitologic studies, especially in detection of *Giardia intestinalis*.

Equipment
Rehfuss' tube (metal tip) with markings: 45, 60, 65, 70, and 90 cm.
    (or rubber tubing with mercury weighted bag), or Abbott-Rawson tube with mercury-weighted tip
Clamp for tubing
Towel and emesis basin
Glass of water; straw
Container for specimen
30 grams of magnesium sulfate in 50 ml. of water
Optional: clear plastic tubing (7.5 cm.) to use as a sleeve over rubber tubing; this can be slipped over tubing and
    kept near teeth to prevent biting of rubber tubing

Procedure   *Preparatory Phase*

1. Explain procedure to patient and tell him how mouth-breathing and swallowing can help in passing the tube.
2. Have patient in a chair or high Fowler's position in bed with neck flexed; place a towel across his chest.
3. Determine with the patient what sign he might use, such as raising his index finger, to indicate "wait a few moments" because of gagging or discomfort.
4. Remove dentures.

GUIDELINES: DUODENAL DRAINAGE (cont.)

Procedure (cont.)

ACTION	RATIONALE/AMPLIFICATION
Performance Phase (by the physician)	
1. Ask the patient to open his mouth and breathe through it.	1. Mouth breathing facilitates the relaxation process.
2. Place the tube's metal tip or the tubing with the mercury bag on the back of the tongue.	2. Proper positioning of the tip encourages and promotes swallowing.
3. Ask patient to close his mouth (without biting the tubing) and swallow.	
4. Permit patient to drink water through a straw as he swallows tubing until the 45 cm. mark is reached. It is even better to have him suck on ice chips.	4. Water aids in lubricating and swallowing. However, avoid administering more than 100 ml. in volume.
5. Instruct patient to sit in chair or on edge of bed and to lean forward with elbows on his knees. The tube is slowly advanced to the 60-cm. mark.	5. These are all maneuvers that have been found helpful in permitting the tube to pass through.
6. Next have the patient curl up on his *right* side with hips on a pillow and shoulders low. Advance tube to the 70-cm. mark.	6. The tube tip should be in the second portion of the duodenum (Fig. 10-14). Check to see if bile can be aspirated and if the pH is greater than 7.0.
7. The patient is then rolled over on his back for 5 minutes.	
8. Drainage procedure may now take place with patient in right lateral position. Following are the ways of testing to see if tube is in duodenum:	
a. Aspirate gently—inspect fluid; instill 30 ml. water.	a. Record color, amount, and consistency of bile as well as duration of flow (normal: clear, golden brown).
b. Instill 30 ml. air rapidly and aspirate immediately; if as much as 5 ml. can be recovered, the tip is probably in the stomach.	b. Usually no air can be recovered from the duodenum.
c. Use a stethoscope to locate tube's tip as air is slowly injected through tubing by syringe.	c. A bubbling sound is substantially louder than elsewhere. The spot should be small and well to the right of the midline. If bubbling can be heard over an area as large as the hand, the tip is in the stomach.
d. To be absolutely sure of position of tube, check position fluoroscopically.	
9. Anchor tube by using plastic guard.	9. To prevent patient's biting rubber tube.
10. Collect specimens as directed by gravity drainage or by low-pressure intermittent suction with container on floor. If the tube is determined to be in the duodenum, an appropriate stimulant is injected and collection begins.	
a. Administer magnesium sulfate solution to stimulate relaxation of sphincter of Oddi and contraction of gallbladder.	a. If gallbladder function is to be evaluated.
b. Administer secretin or secretin-CCK to stimulate pancreatic secretion. Measure volume, bicarbonate concentration, and amylase content.	b. If pancreatic function is to be evaluated.
Follow-up Phase	
1. At conclusion of test, slowly withdraw tubing.	1. Rapid withdrawal may be injurious to mucous lining because of metal tip; teeth also may be injured by metal tip.
2. As tube emerges from the patient's mouth, cover it immediately with a towel.	2. Covering the mouth will help prevent the urge to vomit.
3. Offer toothbrush and paste or mouthwash.	3. To freshen mouth.
4. Record test and patient's reaction.	

INTESTINAL CONDITIONS AND TREATMENT

DIAGNOSTIC STUDIES

Stool Specimen

1. The stool is examined for its amount, consistency, and color; a screening test for occult blood is also done. Normal color varies from light to dark brown.

Special tests may be made for fecal urobilinogen, fat, nitrogen, parasites, food residue, and other substances.

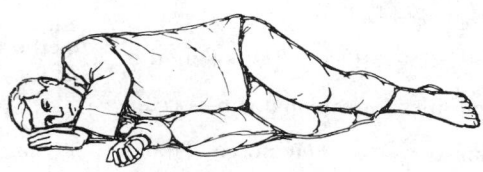

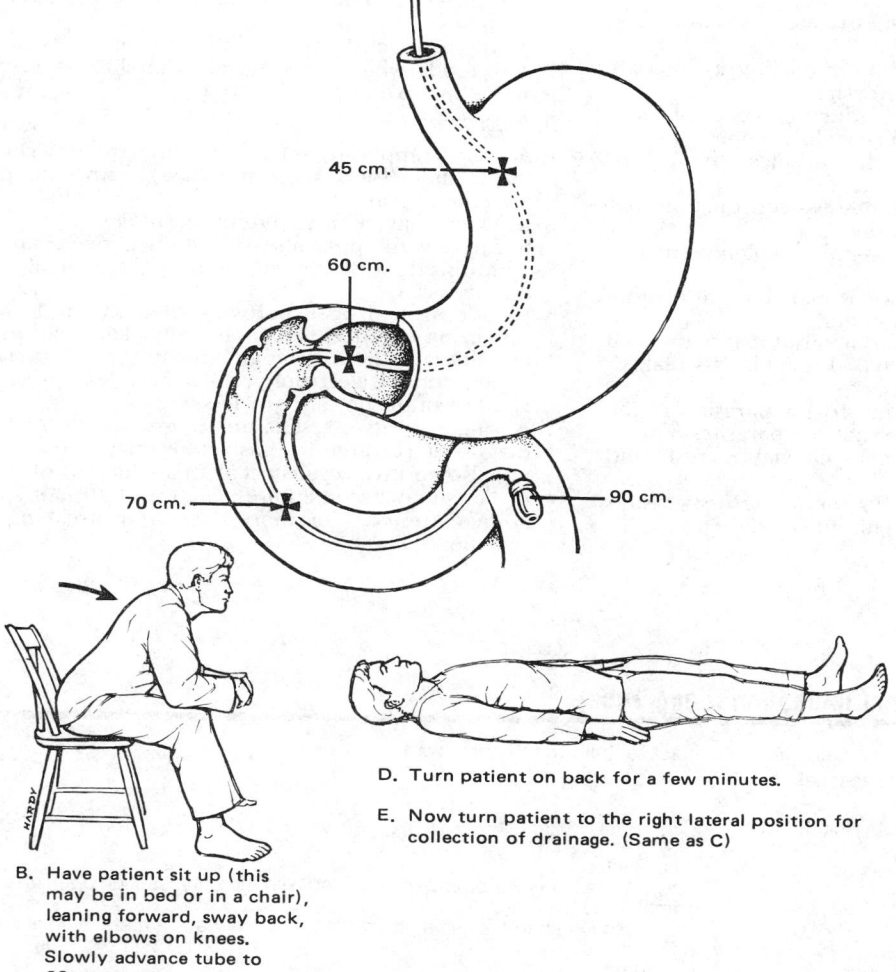

A. With patient in sitting position pass tube to 45 cm. mark.

C. Then have patient curl up on right side with hips on a pillow and shoulder low. Tube is advanced to 70 cm. mark.

45 cm.

60 cm.

70 cm.

90 cm.

B. Have patient sit up (this may be in bed or in a chair), leaning forward, sway back, with elbows on knees. Slowly advance tube to 60 cm. mark.

D. Turn patient on back for a few minutes.

E. Now turn patient to the right lateral position for collection of drainage. (Same as C)

FIGURE 10-14. *Positions to be assumed by the patient in passing a duodenal drainage tube. Note on the central diagram how the tubing is advanced by each position change.*

2. Various foods affect stool color.
   a. Meat protein—dark brown
   b. Spinach—green
   c. Beets—red
   d. Cocoa—dark red or brown
   e. Licorice—black

3. Various medications affect stool color.
   a. Phenylbutazone (Butazolidin, Azolid)—black
   b. Oxyphenbutazone (Tandearil, Oxalid)—black
      Phenazopyridine (Pyridium)—orange-black
   c. Aluminum hydroxide—gray-white
   d. Pyrvinium pamoate (Povan)—red-orange

e. Bismuth compounds—black
f. Senna laxatives—yellow-green
g. Hematinics (iron salts)—black
h. Barium—white
4. Hemoglobin and bleeding affect the stool in the following way:
   a. Considerable quantities of hemoglobin—occult blood
      (not visible to naked eye); use "Hemoccult Stool" testing packet
   b. Upper G.I. bleeding—tarry black (melena)
   c. Lower G.I. bleeding—bright red blood
   d. Lower rectal or anal bleeding—blood streaking on surface of stool or on toilet paper
5. Characteristic clinical entities related to characteristics of stool:
   a. Bulky, greasy, foamy, foul in odor, gray in color with silvery sheen—steatorrhea
   b. Light gray "clay-colored" (due to absence of "acholic" bile pigments)—biliary obstruction
   c. Mucus or pus visible—chronic ulcerative colitis, shigellosis
   d. Small, dry, rocky-hard masses—constipation, obstipation, fecal obstruction
   e. Marble sized stool pellets—spastic colon syndrome

Nursing Management
1. Use a tongue blade to place a small amount of stool in a disposable waxed container.
2. Save a sample of any fecal material if it is unusual in appearance, worms, blood or blood-streaked, unusual color, much mucus.
3. Send specimen to be examined for parasites to the laboratory immediately so that the parasites may be observed under microscope while viable, fresh, and warm.
4. Test for occult blood or to confirm grossly visible melena or blood—hemoccult guaiac slide test.

Hemoccult Guaiac Slide Test

Commercially available guaiac-impregnated slides present a simple, inexpensive, and esthetically acceptable method of testing feces for blood.

A. *Patient Preparation*

(Preparation varies, therefore check with physician.) Common practices are:
1. Diet should be high-residue during preceding 48–72 hours before specimen is collected.
2. Similar diet is followed for next 3 days:
   a. Vegetables—particularly lettuce, spinach, and corn; cooked and raw
   b. Fruits—particularly prunes, grapes, plums, and apples
   c. Any product that is "all bran" for daily cereal
3. Any foods which cause severe diarrhea or severe abdominal pain are to be avoided.

B. *Procedure*
1. A wooden applicator is used to apply a stool specimen to the slide (for 3 successive days). Three samples are taken because:
   a. There may be intermittent bleeding.
   b. There is the possibility of false-negative results.
2. Slides inside a packet can be brought or mailed to the physician.
3. By adding hydrogen peroxide (denatured alcohol-stabilizing mixture) to samples, any blood cells present liberate their hemoglobin, and a bluish ring appears on the electrophoretic paper. Read precisely *at* 30 seconds, no more or less.
4. A single positive test is an indication for further diagnostic research for gastrointestinal lesions.
   a. False-positive results occur in about 10% of tests.
   b. Tests may become false-negative in 10% of specimens tested 4 or more days after streaking on paper.

GUIDELINES: Nasointestinal Intubation (Long Tube)

Purposes
1. To remove fluid and flatus from the intestinal tract (decompression).
2. To assess gastrointestinal bleeding.

Equipment (Choice made by physician)
1. Type of Tube
   Single-lumen tube: Harris, Cantor
   Distal end has a small rubber bag weighted with mercury; suction openings are proximal to bag.
   Some single-lumen tubes use air to inflate balloon or have a metal bulb at distal end.
   Double-lumen tube: Miller-Abbott
   a. One outlet is for drainage.
   b. The other outlet is for filling the small rubber bag near the distal end.
2. Tube Selection
   a. Miller-Abbott tube is used in presence of mechanical bowel obstruction with hyperactive bowel sounds.
   b. Other tubes are used for adynamic ileus (absent bowel sounds).

Procedure *Preparatory and Performance Phases*

NURSING ALERT: All tubes and endoscopes should be routinely pretested for patency and function *before* passage.

Procedure (cont.)

PHYSICIAN ACTION; NURSE ASSISTED	RATIONALE/AMPLIFICATION
1. Similar to passing a short nasogastric tube (p. 392). Exception: *Miller–Abbott.* Carry out the procedure as follows:	
a. Pretest the bag volume; the proper amount of air will fill the bag to just less than fully distended (slightly compressible).	a. This will assure that the bag is not leaky.
b. Place 1 ml. mercury in the bag after it is in the stomach.	b. This helps to pass tubing through the pylorus.
c. After duodenum has been entered, instill 20–50 ml. air in bag according to pretested volume; place other opening on suction.	c. This position checked by x-ray. Air-filled bag acts as a bolus and is carried distally by peristaltic action as suction evacuates retained air and fluid just ahead of bag.
2. After the tubing enters the stomach it passes by peristalsis and gravity into the small intestine.	
a. Change position from Fowler's to a position which has patient leaning forward.	a. This will assist in advancing the tubing to and through the pylorus; tilting to the right is helpful.
3. Upon x-ray confirmation that the tubing is past the pylorus, permit patient to ambulate.	3. Passing the tube through the pylorus and into the duodenum under fluoroscopic guidance allows the entire procedure to be completed in less than 15 minutes with little patient discomfort.
Nursing Action	
4. At specified time intervals, advance tubing 5 to 10 cm. (2–4 inches).	4. Physician may prescribe or suggest these times.
5. Tubing may be taped to the face, and suction may be applied when the tubing tip has reached its destination.	
6. Measure drainage; record its characteristics every 8 hours.	

> **NURSING ALERT:** If drainage is clear and up to 3000 ml. obtained/day, there is complete intestinal obstruction. If drainage is yellow with a fecal odor, the patient may have a small intestinal obstruction.

Follow-up Phase

1. Similar to short nasogastric tube.	1. See page 394.
2. Exception: in removing tubing, patient may feel tube resistance and become nauseated.	2. Due to action of sphincters through which the tube is withdrawn.
3. As tubing is drawn through posterior nasopharynx, have patient open his mouth so that balloon or bag can be grasped with a clamp. Withdraw remaining tubing through the nose.	3. This permits balloon or bag to be removed through the mouth.
4. If tubing has advanced beyond the ileocecal valve, the physician may release it so that it can pass through the gastrointestinal tract. Peristalsis aids in passing the tubing.	4. After distal tube has been retrieved at the rectum, the proximal end can be released at the nose.

Roentgenography of the Colon: Barium Enema

The fasting patient receives a rectal instillation of a barium sulfate suspension which is viewed in the fluoroscope and then filmed. If patient is adequately prepared, fluoroscope will reveal:
  a. Colon—contour of entire colon is visible.
  b. Cecum and appendix—contour and motility observed.
NOTE: Air may be induced to give air contrast studies.
Nursing Management and Patient Instruction
1. Explain to the patient:
  a. What the x-ray procedure involves
  b. That proper preparation provides a more accurate view of the tract
  c. That it is important to retain the barium so that all surfaces of the tract are coated with opaque solution.
2. Two days before the examination, the patient may be given a minimal residue diet.

3. The day before the examination, some physicians restrict food intake to liquids; others advise liquids for the evening meal only.
4. The day before the examination, a cathartic may be prescribed.
5. The evening before and on the morning of the examination, a cleansing enema may be given. Food and fluids are restricted for the examination.
6. The above preparation varies, but the objective remains the same: to have the large intestine as clear of fecal material as possible.

> **NURSING ALERT:** Use nursing judgment regarding the administration of cathartics or enemata in the presence of acute abdominal pain or obstruction. For the patient with ulcerative colitis, cathartics or cleansing enemas may be too rigorous, and can possibly cause bleeding.

7. Administer an oil-retention enema or a cathartic following the barium enema to completely evacuate the barium.
8. Permit patient to eat following the examination, since he has been fasting and is undoubtedly hungry.

Visualization Measures

1. Two visualization measures are sigmoidoscopy and colonoscopy.
2. The details of these two procedures are presented in the following Guidelines.

GUIDELINES: Sigmoidoscopy

A *sigmoidoscopy* is the viewing of the lumen of the sigmoid and rectum by means of a sigmoidoscope, a tubular instrument that can be illuminated.

Equipment
Fleet-type enema—used at least 1 hour before the sigmoidoscopy
Water-soluble lubricant
Sigmoidoscope—a 2-part instrument (obturator and cannula)
—a long, thin metal tube with light bulb at one end
Glass eyepiece to fit on scope during insufflation of air
Inflation bulb
Long applicator sticks (cotton)
Disposable gloves for preliminary digital examination

Procedure **Preparatory Phase**

1. An hour before the sigmoidoscopy, a Fleet enema may be administered by the nurse (or by the patient himself).
2. The enema is retained for 5 minutes before being evacuated.
3. Some physicians request the patient to be on a light diet the evening before and the breakfast before the examination. Others prefer a cathartic the evening prior to the examination.

NURSING ACTION	RATIONALE/AMPLIFICATION
Performance Phase	
1. Have the patient assume the knee-chest or Sims' lateral position.	1. The position used depends upon physician preference, patient condition, and nature of examining table (or bed).

a. Knee/chest position
    (1) Knees are spread comfortably apart.
    (2) Thighs are perpendicular to table.
    (3) Feet are extended over the edge.
    (4) Head is turned sideways to right (head shares pillow with chest).
    (5) Left arm is flexed to side of chest.
    (6) Right arm may rest above head.
	a. This position permits the sigmoid to hang forward, diminishing the angle at the rectosigmoid junction.

b. Sims' lateral position
    (1) Place patient on left side with left leg partially flexed at hip and knees; right leg should be fully flexed.
    (2) Pelvis to be perpendicular to table.
	b. Used for elderly, ill, or arthritic patients or those who are reluctant to assume the knee-chest position.

2. Drape the patient so that only the perineum is visible.	2. A disposable large sheet with a circular opening is practical.
3. Check scope lights after connecting cord to battery.	
4. Physician first examines anal and perianal region. Digital examination indicates the direction of the anal canal, its patency, and the presence of any abnormality.	4. The purpose is to note inflammation, fistula, and ulceration. Digital examination also promotes anal relaxation and helps to lubricate orifice.
5. Warm sigmoidoscope in tap water or sterilizer to slightly above body temperature; lubricate tip of scope.	5. A cold scope would cause discomfort and promote contraction rather than relaxation of perianal muscles. Water-soluble lubricant permits easier passage of scope.
6. Physician spreads buttocks and anal margins with left hand and inserts instrument with right hand (or vice versa).	6. Keep instrument out of view of patient.
7. Nurse encourages relaxation and explains each step in advance.	7. Reassuring patient promotes relaxation.
8. Physician may use a glass eyepiece over viewing end of scope; an insufflation bulb and tubing are attached. He may proceed to pump a small quantity of air into the bowel.	8. The purpose of inflating lower bowel with air is to expand the area viewed so that vision is not obstructed by mucosal folds.

Procedure (cont.)

NURSING ACTION	RATIONALE/AMPLIFICATION
9. The nurse should relay to the physician expressions or complaints of pain by the patient.	9. Tenderness and pain may be experienced by the patient with a history of abdominal surgery; procedure may have to be terminated in order not to risk perforation.
10. As the scope advances, it may be necessary to attach suction to remove secretions, exudate, blood, or excreta.	10. Connect tubing to suction equipment and turn to lowest degree at first.

Follow-up Phase

1. Upon withdrawal of scope, assist patient in gradually assuming a relaxed position.	1. Wipe the perineal area to prevent soilage of garments and to promote comfort.
2. If disposable scope is used, rinse scope and discard in proper receptacle. Reusable scopes are thoroughly cleaned in soap and water.	2. Sterilizable parts are sterilized before scope is stored.
3. Record the procedure and the reaction of the patient.	

GUIDELINES: Colonoscopy

Colonoscopy is the direct visual inspection of the large intestine by means of the colonoscope.

Purposes
1. As a diagnostic aid to view and assess the status of the large intestine (Fig. 10-15).
2. As an operative instrument to remove polyps, to obtain tissue for biopsy, and to remove foreign bodies.

Equipment
Complete colonoscope, possibly with sidearm second observer scope
Water-soluble lubricant
Suction apparatus
Air-insufflating equipment
Snares
Drapes
Fluoroscope

The Colonoscope
The colonoscope is an instrument consisting of a flexible 4-mm. glass bundle (containing about 250,000 glass fibers).

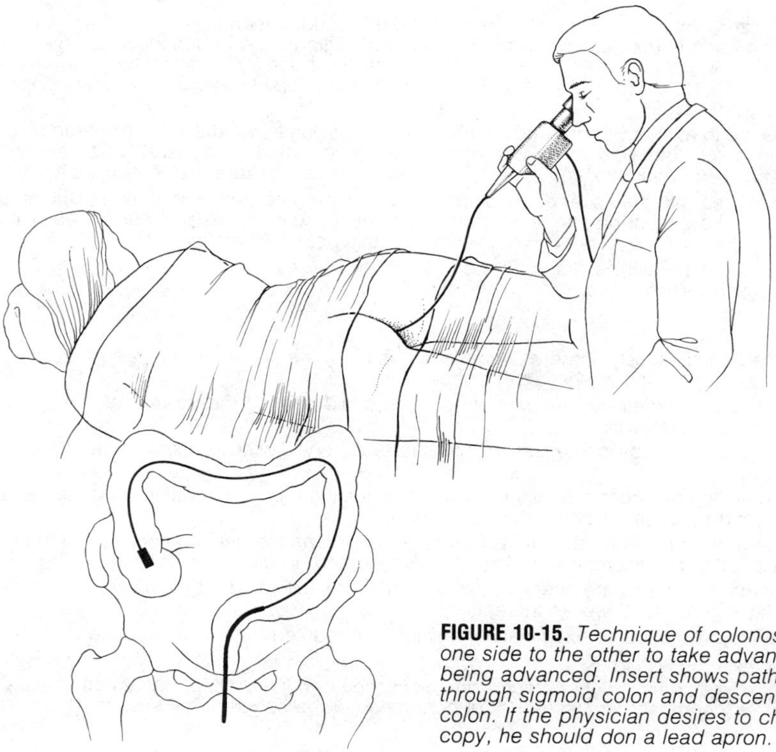

FIGURE 10-15. *Technique of colonoscopy. The patient is turned from one side to the other to take advantage of gravity as the scope is being advanced. Insert shows path of flexible scope from rectum through sigmoid colon and descending, transverse, and ascending colon. If the physician desires to check scope position with fluoroscopy, he should don a lead apron.*

GUIDELINES: Colonoscopy (cont.)

Equipment (cont.)

1. There is a lens at both ends equipped to focus and magnify.
2. Light is transmitted from an external source by way of a fiberoptic bundle to the tip of the scope; an image is transmitted regardless of the looping or twisting of the flexible bundle.
3. Accessory channels provide for
   a. Suction of fluid, blood, and mucus
   b. Insufflation of air or water
   c. Biopsy
4. There are two kinds of colonoscopes:
   a. To visualize left side of colon—105 cm.
   b. To visualize entire colon—165–185 cm.

Procedure

Preparatory Phase

1. Explain procedure to patient; his understanding and cooperation will promote his relaxation and facilitate his comfort during examination.
2. Limit the patient's intake to liquids for 24–48 hours prior to the procedure (as directed by the endoscopist).
3. Serve the patient a cathartic as prescribed, in the evening for 2 days before the examination.
4. Give tap water or saline enemas approximately 3 hours prior to the colonoscopy until the returns are clear.
5. Administer sedative or analgesic as prescribed; sedation is desirable, but the patient must be sensitive to any pain during the examination so that his response can be relayed to the endoscopist.
6. Preferably, this procedure is performed where fluoroscopy is available.

NURSING ACTION (AS ASSISTANT)	RATIONALE/AMPLIFiCATION
Performance Phase (by endoscopist)	
1. Place patient in the left lateral position.	1. This position is assumed to follow the location of the sigmoid-rectum anatomically.
2. The lubricated scope is inserted and passed through the rectum.	2. This procedure is done under direct visualization; valvulae are prominent throughout the colon.
3. At apex of rectosigmoid area, there is a red "blur-out".	3. Blur-out occurs because the tip of the colonscope touches the sigmoid colon wall.
4. The instrument is steadily inserted, rotated, and flexed.	4. This will promote the sliding of the tip along the greater curvature of any loops in the sigmoid colon.
5. If mucosa does not appear red, but seems to blanch or become white, the scope is withdrawn until red mucosa appears.	5. Whitening or blanching is indicative of compression of bowel wall with danger of perforation.
6. The endoscopist utilizes "maneuvers" to straighten difficult curves. A fluoroscope can also be used.	6. By various maneuvers, such as "alpha," "hooking," or "lifting," the endoscopist is able to continue with the insertion and examination of the walls of the colon. Fluoroscopy assists in monitoring position and direction.
7. Maneuvers are resorted to at sharp turns such as the sigmoid-descending colon, the splenic flexure, the transverse colon, and the hepatic flexure.	7. Occasional withdrawal, appearance of a triangular configuration, or a bluish color are techniques and observations to assist in advancing the scope.
8. As the scope is advanced into the ascending colon, the nurse can position the patient on his back or on his right side.	8. This permits the maneuvering of the colonoscope into the cecum. It takes about 20–45 minutes to reach this point in the examination.
9. Observation and close inspection is accomplished during insertion and withdrawal of scope.	

Polypectomy and Postcare

1. Prepare intestinal tract meticulously; if there is any fecal matter in the field near the polyp, the procedure will be postponed and bowel preparation will have to be repeated.
2. Skill is required to remove the optimum amount of polyp, to avoid burning the bowel wall, and to prevent cutting the base too close to the bowel wall.
3. When the tissue has been cut by cauterization, the snare-cautery device is removed and the polyp tissue is withdrawn by suction.
4. Following polypectomy, the colonoscope may be reinserted, the inner bowel insufflated with air, and the operated area carefully examined for possible hemorrhage.
5. Postpolypectomy care depends upon size of the polyps removed and the general condition of the patient. Usually the ambulatory patient can be discharged with no medication and no dietary restriction.
6. For in-hospital patients, vital signs are checked for several hours, full liquid diet is given the day of surgery, and soft, low-residue diet is given for 2 weeks thereafter.
7. Follow-up by complete colonoscopic examination usually is scheduled for 6–8 weeks later.

NURSING ALERT: If polypectomy is done through sigmoidoscope or colonoscope, barium enema should not be done until 7–10 days thereafter because of risk of perforation at the polypectomy site.

MEDICAL AND NURSING MANAGEMENT OF THE PATIENT UNDERGOING MAJOR INTESTINAL SURGERY

Preoperative Objectives

A. *To ensure that the general physical condition of the patient is the best possible.*

1. Administer parenteral therapy to correct fluid and electrolyte imbalance.
2. Correct nutritional deficiencies: protein supplements, between-meal feedings.
3. Provide blood replacement to overcome losses sustained by bleeding, infection, and neoplasm.
4. Assist with diagnostic studies as they relate to the evaluation of the cardiopulmonary, hepatorenal bodily functions.
5. Give the patient psychological support as he encounters the stresses of accepting the diagnosis, surgery, and possibly a colostomy.
6. Insert an indwelling urinary catheter immediately prior to the patient's going to the operating room.
7. Oversee general personal cleanliness to minimize skin and wound infection postoperatively.

B. *To reduce bacteria in the intestinal tract to prevent postoperative infection.*

1. Administer antibiotic agents to suppress aerobic colon microflora.
   Combinations of kanamycin or neomycin with tetracycline, erythromycin, or lincomycin.

NOTE: Evidence that these are preferable to a good intestinal cleansing is lacking.

2. Reduce content of colon.
   a. Give low-residue diet and, when required, change to liquid diet.
   b. Offer laxatives as prescribed. Saline catharsis may be preferred.
   c. Administer enemas or colonic irrigations.
3. Decompress gastrointestinal tract by means of indwelling gastrointestinal tube to control distention and vomiting, if necessary.
   Miller-Abbott or Cantor tube (see p. 414).

Postoperative Objectives

A. *To meet nutritional needs by administering fluids, electrolytes, and nutrients.*

1. Utilize intravenous catheter if intravenous therapy is to continue several days.
   Observe tissue for infiltration of fluid.
2. Maintain meticulous mouth hygiene while patient is on parenteral therapy.

B. *To promote proper functioning of nasogastric decompression and patient comfort.*

1. Observe and record quality and quantity of aspirated material.
2. Lubricate nostrils with water-soluble lubricant.
3. Humidify room to prevent dryness of mucous membranes.
4. Turn patient frequently to minimize discomfort.
5. Remove tube (when required) upon re-establishment of peristalsis (determined by auscultation, passage of flatus rectally).

C. *To alleviate psychosocial concerns of patient.*

1. Encourage patient to express concerns and questions. (See Colostomy and Ileostomy Management if these are pertinent, pp. 438 and 426.)

2. Administer analgesics according to needs.
3. Promote restfulness with appropriate nursing measures prior to giving sedation or hypnotics.

D. *To prevent complications by recognizing early signs.*

1. Evaluate vital signs and recognize patterns of development that may suggest hemorrhage, infection, shock, obstruction, etc.
2. Stress preventive measures, such as turning frequently, maintaining fluid balance, encouraging coughing, emphasizing cleanliness and movement of legs.

E. *To prepare a plan for convalescence and follow-up care.*

1. Encourage ambulation and self-care activities.
2. Stimulate appetite by promoting those measures that will make patient want to eat what he should eat.
3. Help patient set goals toward which he can progress.
4. Emphasize the importance of follow-up visits to evaluate healing process, general physical and psychological adjustment.

APPENDICITIS

Acute appendicitis is an inflammation of the appendix due to an infection. It is almost always a surgical problem.

Incidence

1. Occurs most frequently in young adults but may occur in any age group.
2. Incidence of appendicitis in U.S. has been decreasing during the past decade.

Clinical Manifestations

1. Begins with a progressively severe abdominal pain, beginning in midabdomen (periumbilical) and moving to right lower quadrant after 6–12 hours.
2. An effective early assessment of the patient for acute appendicitis is to have him rise on his toes and then drop down on his heels with a thump or to have him cough. If he has an acute inflammation, he will feel localized pain in the inflamed area.
3. Within a few hours, the acute tenderness becomes localized in the right lower quadrant (McBurney's point).
4. Anorexia, slight or moderate temperature elevation, mild change in bowel habit (usually constipation), and perhaps nausea and vomiting occur.

NOTE: If these clinical manifestations occur in any person, encourage him to see a physician immediately. There is a tendency in the aging person to ignore aches and pains and to delay seeing a physician. Consequently, mortality in elderly persons with inflammatory bowel lesions is as high as 20%.

Diagnostic Evaluation

1. Physical examination noting especially location and localization of pain, rebound tenderness, etc.
2. Blood studies with particular attention to white count; urinalysis.
   A white blood count reveals a moderate leukocytosis.
3. Careful history to rule out other possibilities.
4. In some clinics, when appendicitis is difficult to diagnose, laparoscopy may be utilized.

Treatment and Nursing Management

A. *Palliative Preoperative Care*

1. Place patient in comfortable position to relieve abdominal pain and tension—usually Fowler's position.
2. See that patient takes nothing by mouth—to decrease peristalsis and to allow stomach to empty preparatory to surgery. Note time and nature of last meal.
3. Place ice bag to right lower quadrant—NEVER HEAT because of the possibility of causing a rupture of appendix and peritonitis.
4. Do not administer cathartics for the same reason as preceding precaution concerning heat.
5. Frequently evaluate vital signs—to assess progression of infection.
6. When diagnosis of acute appendicitis is made, administer chemotherapy and/or antibiotics.

NOTE: If there is evidence that perforation has occurred recently and a generalized peritonitis has developed, operative urgency is increased (see below).

B. *Operative*

1. If diagnosis of acute appendicitis is established, a simple appendectomy is performed.
2. Because patient will obtain relief from pain, he usually accepts surgery very willingly, which affords a smooth recovery.
3. Anesthetic may be general or spinal.
4. Incision may be McBurney, muscle-splitting or gridiron, or right rectus.

C. *Postoperative Care* (see also p. 89).

1. Without drainage
   a. Following recovery from anesthetic, Fowler's position is maintained, analgesic is given every 3 or 4 hours as needed, and fluids and food are given as tolerated.
   b. Stitches removed between 5th and 7th day (usually in physician's office).
2. With drainage
   Treat same as for peritonitis (see below).

PERITONITIS

Peritonitis is an inflammation of the peritoneal cavity.

Etiology

Peritonitis indicates transgression of peritoneum by trauma (blunt or penetrating) or inflammatory or neoplastic disease. The point of origin may be the gastrointestinal tract, the ovaries, the uterus or extraperitoneal organs (i.e., inflammation of the kidney).

A. *Primary peritonitis*—acute, diffuse

1. Occurs primarily in young females; often due to pathogenic bacteria (streptococci, pneumococci, gonococci) introduced through Fallopian tubes or through hematogenous spread.
2. In patients with nephrosis or cirrhosis, the offending organism is most often *E. coli.*

B. *Secondary peritonitis*

1. Commonly seen in surgical patients; caused by appendicitis, peptic ulceration, biliary tract disease, colonic inflammation.
2. May occur following gunshot wound, stab wounds, and motor vehicle accidents.

C. *Postoperative*

1. Theoretically preventable.
2. Noted following poor preoperative preparation—inadequate nutrition, fluid and blood replacement, and technical problems.
3. May occur in compromised patients who are diabetic, or have malignancy, or are taking steroids.

Altered Physiology

1. Any irritant such as blood, bile or pancreatic enzymes causes an exudation of plasmalike, protein-rich fluid—"internal burn."
2. Secondary peritonitis often presents a mixed flora which include *E. coli* as well as the enterococci, *Clostridium, Klebsiella, Pseudomonas,* and *Bacteroides.*
3. If there is failure to seal the source of contamination, i.e., perforation along gastrointestinal tract, peritonitis will become progressively worse.
4. When offended, the surface of the peritoneal cavity begins to exude a plasmalike fluid. This process can account for losses of as much as 5 liters/day.
5. Paralytic ileus is usual, with fluid loss into dilated intestinal loops and stomach.
6. Individual is compromised because of fluid loss, abdominal distention with respiratory embarrassment; nutrients are not absorbed, leading to progressive rapid catabolism.

Clinical Features and Initial Physical Assessment

(Dependent upon location and extension of inflammation)
1. Initially local type of abdominal pain tends to become constant, diffuse, and more intense.
2. Abdomen becomes extremely tender and muscles become rigid; rebound tenderness and ileus may be present; patient lies very still, usually with legs drawn up.
3. Often nausea and vomiting occur; peristalsis diminishes; anorexia is present.
4. Elevation of temperature and pulse as well as leukocyte count.
5. Fever and thirst occur.
6. Percussion—resonance and tympany due to paralytic ileus; loss of liver dullness may indicate free air in abdomen.
7. Auscultation—decreased bowel sounds.

Diagnostic Evaluation

1. Blood studies—to show leukocytosis (leukopenia, if severe).
2. Urinalysis—may indicate urinary tract problems as primary source.
3. Peritoneal aspiration—to demonstrate blood, pus, bile, bacteria (Gram stain), amylase.
4. X-ray of abdomen—may indicate free air in abdomen under diaphragm; of thorax—to rule out unexpected pneumonia.

Objectives of Treatment and Nursing Management

A. *To prevent the cause of peritonitis.*

1. Encourage the individual who has early signs and symptoms of appendicitis to see his physician.
2. Instruct patient to avoid taking a laxative or applying heat to abdomen when abdominal pain of unknown cause is experienced.
3. Practice meticulous aseptic technique during abdominal surgery.

B. *To monitor the patient so that the eventual goal of normal hemoglobin and oxygenation, urine output of 30–50 ml./hr., and normal vital signs are realized.*

1. Monitor for central venous pressure (see p. 271).
2. Record urinary output hourly.
3. Note and record blood pressure every other hour.
4. Check vital signs frequently.
5. Obtain baseline and take frequent analyses of hematocrit, blood gases, and electrolytes.

C. *To remove cause of the infection.*

1. If localized:
   a. If acutely inflamed appendix—an appendectomy is called for.
   b. If ruptured duodenal ulcer—ulcer closed or plicated.
   c. Resection of diseased bowel; decompression (gastrostomy, colostomy, ileostomy).
2. If not localized, patient is acutely ill and surgery is not performed until after distention as well as electrolyte and fluid problems are treated.

D. *To combat infection and promote patient comfort.*

1. Give nothing by mouth—to reduce peristalsis; ensure meticulous oral hygiene.
2. Provide fluids by vein to establish adequate fluid level and to promote adequate urinary output.
3. Record accurately intake and output including the measurement of vomitus.
4. Administer antibiotics as prescribed.
5. Observe and describe symptoms accurately: pain and tenderness have a tendency to shift and must be reported precisely.
6. Reassure the patient and establish his confidence, because he usually realizes the seriousness of his condition.

E. *To promote recovery and reduce the possibility of complications.*

1. Following recovery from anesthetic, place patient in Fowler's position to facilitate drainage.
2. Administer fluids by vein, since nothing is given by mouth initially.
3. Prevent nausea, vomiting, and distention by use of nasogastric suction; institute proper nursing measures for nasal and oral comfort.
4. Reduce parenteral fluids and give oral food and fluids when the following occur:
   a. Temperature and pulse rate come down.
   b. Abdomen becomes soft.
   c. Peristaltic sounds return (determined by abdominal auscultation).
   d. Flatus is passed and patient has bowel movements.
5. Be alert for possibility of complications: Report immediately
   a. Wound evisceration—"It feels as if something just gave way."
   b. Abscess formation—an area of abdomen is tender or painful and fever increases.

ABDOMINAL HERNIA

A *hernia* is a protrusion of viscus through the wall of the cavity in which it is normally contained. It is often called a "rupture."

Incidence

1. Occurs 3 times more frequently in men than women; may occur at any age.

2. Results from congenital or acquired weakness of the abdominal wall.
3. Tends to increase in size and occurrence with increase of intra-abdominal pressure brought about by coughing, straining, or pressure from a nearby tumor.

Classification

A. *According to Area*

1. Inguinal
   a. In male—due to weakness in abdominal wall where spermatic cord emerges; enters inguinal canal and then scrotum.
   b. In female—due to weakness in abdominal wall where round ligament is located; enters inguinal canal and then labia.
      (1) Direct inguinal
          Medial-to-deep epigastric artery
          Majority are acquired
      (2) Indirect inguinal
          Lateral-to-deep epigastric artery
          Majority are congenital
2. Femoral
   a. Occurs most often in women.
   b. Located below Poupart's ligament (below groin).
3. Umbilical
   a. Results from failure of umbilical orifice to close.
   b. Occurs most often in obese women and children and in patients with cirrhosis and ascites.
4. Ventral or incisional
   a. Due to weakness in abdominal wall.
   b. May occur following impaired healing of incision because of drainage, infection, etc.

B. *According to Severity*

1. Reducible—the protruding mass can be replaced in abdomen.
2. Irreducible—the protruding mass cannot be moved back into abdomen.
3. Incarcerated—an irreducible hernia in which the intestinal flow is completely obstructed.
4. Strangulated—an irreducible hernia in which the blood and intestinal flow are completely obstructed. Symptoms—pain, vomiting, swelling of hernial sac, fever, lower abdominal signs of peritoneal irritation.

Treatment

A. *Mechanical*

(reducible hernia only)

A *truss* is an appliance having a pad that is held snugly in the hernial orifice.

1. Does not cure a hernia—it prevents abdominal contents from entering hernial sac.
2. May be used in treatment of hernia in adults when, because of disease or age, it is inadvisable to perform surgery. In general, surgical treatment is preferred.

B. *Surgical*

Surgical treatment is recommended to correct the hernia before a strangulation occurs, which then becomes an emergency situation.

1. Hernial sac is dissected free.
2. Contents of sac are replaced in abdominal cavity.
3. Neck of sac is ligated.
4. Muscle and fascial layers are sewed together firmly to prevent a recurrence. If this is not possible, synthetic mesh may be sutured over area.
5. Strangulated hernia requires resection of ischemic bowel in addition to hernia repair.

Nursing Management

A. *Preoperative*

1. If hernia is strangulated, emergency conditions prevail. (See p. 434, *Intestinal Obstruction.*)
2. If surgery is elective, patient is usually in good physical condition.
3. Shave suprapubic region and anterior surface of upper thigh.
4. Observe for upper respiratory infection—if present, surgery will be postponed because coughing or sneezing postoperatively may break the sutures.

B. *Postoperative*

1. Ambulate patient in a day or two.
2. Take following measures for scrotal edema or swelling.
   a. Bed rest
   b. Ice pack, scrotal suspensory for support
3. Observe for urinary retention.

C. *Patient Education*

1. Athletics and extremes of exertion are not permitted for 8-12 weeks postoperatively.

ULCERATIVE COLITIS

Ulcerative colitis is an inflammatory disease of the mucosa and less frequently, the submucosa, of the colon and rectum. Occasionally it involves the distal ileum as well.

Etiology and Incidence

1. Unknown (idiopathic); however, there are several unproven possibilities:
   a. Emotional response alters blood supply to colon mucosa, but there is question as to whether stress is a cause or effect of the disease process.
   b. Unidentifiable organisms cause pathology.
   c. A combination of causative factors: infection, stress, allergy, autoimmunity.
2. Most common in young adulthood and middle life; almost equal between sexes (slightly more in females); more prevalent among Jews; highest in 3rd and 4th decades, familial incidence.

Clinical Manifestations

1. Diarrhea (may be bloody), tenesmus (painful straining), sense of urgency, and cramping.
2. Multiple crypt abscesses of intestinal mucosa that may become necrotic and lead to ulceration.
3. There often is weight loss, fever, dehydration, hypokalemia, anorexia, nausea and vomiting, iron-deficiency anemia, and cachexia.

NOTE: See differences between Regional Enteritis and Ulcerative Colitis, p. 425.

Clinical Features

1. Involvement extends proximally from rectum and is mainly of left colon.
2. The disease usually begins in the rectum and sigmoid and spreads upward, eventually involving the entire colon.
3. There is a tendency for patient to experience remissions and exacerbations.
4. Very high frequency of secondary and often multiple colon cancer.
5. It is a serious disease accompanied by systemic complications (see below) and high mortality rate.

Diagnostic Evaluation

1. Stool examination to rule out bacillary or amebic dysentery.
2. Sigmoidoscopy; proctoscopy to reveal petechiae, hyperemia, and ulcerations.
3. Barium enema x-ray.

> **NURSING ALERT:** If disease is in acute stage, cathartic may be contraindicated because it may cause exacerbation and lead to toxic megacolon.

4. Review of nursing history for patterns of fatigue and overwork, tension, family problems.
5. Assessment of behavioral manifestations indicative of emotional concerns.
6. Assessment of food habits that may have a bearing on triggering symptoms (milk intake may be a problem).
7. Careful clinical assessment to rule out diverticulitis, cancer, etc.
8. Complete blood studies if they appear to be warranted.
9. Fecal analysis if blood and mucus are evident.

Complications

1. Skin ulcers
2. Arthritis
3. Malnutrition
4. Anemia
5. Abscess formation
6. Stricture, anal fistula
7. Erythema nodosum
8. Amyloidosis
9. Electrolyte imbalance
10. Malignancy (colonic cancer)
11. Toxic megacolon
12. Ankylosing spondylitis

Objectives of Treatment and Nursing Management

NOTE: There is no cure for ulcerative colitis because the cause is unknown; the *chief objective* of treatment is to control the disease to achieve patient comfort and improve the quality of life.

This can be done by:
1. Initiating early, effective management of exacerbations.
2. Prolonging remissions with appropriate therapy.
3. Subjecting the patient to surgery only when judiciously necessary.

A. *To promote rest and relaxation of the intestinal tract.*

1. It may be necessary to reduce or eliminate food and fluid and then to resort to parenteral feeding or to low-residue diets.
2. Give sedatives and tranquilizers not only to provide general rest but also to allow peristalsis to slow down and afford rest to the inflamed bowel.
3. Be aware of the possibility of pressures sores in this patient because of malnourishment and enforced inactivity, especially if he is thin.
   a. Cleanse the skin gently after each (or every other) bowel movement. Apply a protective emollient such as petroleum jelly, karaya gel, A&D ointment, Desitin, or a similar agent.
4. Administer tincture of belladonna, atropine, or Lomotil, as prescribed, to lessen intestinal motility. Sulfasalazine (Azulfidine) is effective for antidiarrheal

effect even though it is an antibiotic. Some patients experience side effects (epigastric distress, headache, dizziness); discontinue medication for 2–3 days and gradually introduce it again.

5. Relieve painful rectal spasms (produced by frequent diarrheal stools) with anodyne suppositories.
6. Report any evidence of sudden abdominal distention, since it may indicate toxic megacolon.
7. Reduce physical activity to a minimum or provide frequent rest periods.
8. Provide commode or bathroom next to bed, since urgency of movements may be a problem.

B. *To combat infection and toxic state.*

1. Give sulfa drugs as prescribed: nonabsorbable sulfasalazine (Azulfidine) may be prescribed as an oral medication.
2. Administer corticosteroids as prescribed: the type depends upon the condition of patient—mode of administration may be oral, intravenous, or rectal. Rectal administration may be in the form of hydrocortisone-retention enemas.
3. Provide conscientious skin care because excoriation is common following severe diarrhea.

4. For severe proctitis, nightly instillations of steroids as prescribed (dissolved in tap water, or as suppositories) may produce a remission of symptoms. Belladonna suppositories also may help.

C. *To meet nutritional and fluid needs of the body.*

1. If patient is acutely ill, maintain him on parenteral replacement of vitamins, fluids, and electrolytes (potassium is very important).
2. When resuming oral fluids and foods, select those which are nonirritating to the mucosa (mechanically, thermally, and chemically). If this fails, an elemental diet (such as Precision LR) may be prescribed; the purpose of this diet is to provide low residue which can rest the lower intestinal tract.
3. Consider a milk-free diet, since studies have shown that fewer relapses occur on a milk-free diet; the incidence of lactase deficiency is more frequent in patients having attacks than in those in remission.
4. Provide a well-balanced, low-residue, high-protein diet to correct malnutrition (Table 10-3).
5. Determine which foods agree with this patient and which do not. Modify diet plan accordingly.

TABLE 10-3. LOW RESIDUE (LOW FIBER) DIET (WITH ADAPTATIONS FOR MINIMAL RESIDUE DIET OF NORMAL FOODS)*

Food Group	Amount Allowed	Choices
Milk	Up to 490 ml (2 c) fluid milk†, including that used in cooking In moderation	Whole†, lowfat†, or skim† (fresh, evaporated, or dry); chocolate flavored† Plain yogurt† Cottage cheese (creamed or dry), mild American cheese, cream cheese, Neufchatel
Meat	2–3 servings daily	Lean, very tender beef, ham, lamb, pork, veal, and liver or other organ meats Tender poultry (without skin) Fish or eggs (Prepared by broiling, roasting, baking, or simmering, steaming, pressure cooking, or microwave)
Fruits and vegetables	Up to 4 servings daily, if tolerated	Fruit and vegetable juices† (avoid prune juice), preferably strained Canned or cooked fruit *without* seeds or skin†: apples, apricots, cherries, peaches, pears Potatoes and sweet potatoes (without skin): baked, boiled, creamed, escalloped, mashed Tender cooked asparagus tips and carrots† Strained cooked vegetables†: green or wax beans, peas, spinach, squash (may be eaten as a vegetable or used in soups or gelatin salads)
Grains	At least 4 servings daily	Refined, enriched breads and cereals without seeds, added fruit, or nuts (Examples: white enriched bread, plain rolls, soda crackers, saltines, rusk, melba toast, plain matzo, zwieback) Cooked cornmeal, farina, Malt-o-Meal, strained oatmeal Ready-to-eat rice, corn, and oat flour cereals Cooked white enriched rice and plain pasta
Other Fats	As tolerated	Butter, margarine, cream, vegetable oil
Soups	As desired	Homemade strained vegetable soups† using allowed ingredients, clear broth or broth with noodles or white rice
Desserts and sweets	As calories allow	Plain pudding using milk allowance†, plain ice cream†, sherbet, gelatin, fruit ice, popsicles Angel or sponge cake, meringue Other cakes and cookies (if fat is tolerated) Sugar, honey, syrup, jelly, hard candy
Seasonings	In moderation	Avoid pepper
Beverages	As tolerated	Fruit drinks, noncarbonated soft drinks Stay within milk allowance Avoidance of coffee and carbonated beverages may be helpful in controlling diarrhea

* Minimal residue diet of normal foods resulting in a small volume of stool which may be difficult to pass. Minimal residue *formula* diets result in a small volume of more liquid stool which is easier to pass. The latter type of diet may be advantageous in some circumstances, e.g., when a "clean" bowel is desired prior to gastrointestinal surgery.
† May be omitted from *minimal* residue diets.
(Suitor CW and Hunter MF. Nutrition: Principles and Application in Health Promotion, Phila., J. B. Lippincott Co. 1980, p. 445)

6. Bolster with supplemental vitamin therapy, including vitamin C, B complex, and K.
7. Avoid cold fluids because they increase intestinal motility.
8. Administer proper electrolytes which have been lost in diarrheal bouts, especially potassium.
9. Administer dephenoxylate (Lomotil) as prescribed for symptomatic relief of diarrhea.
10. Prohibit smoking because it also increases intestinal motility.

NURSING ALERT: Since opiates may precipitate toxic megacolon, use only for brief periods, if at all, in acutely ill patients.

11. Administer blood transfusions and iron to correct existing anemia.
12. Carefully note fluid intake and output and character of bowel movements.
13. Weigh the patient frequently and record weight; rapid increase or decrease may relate to fluids.

D. *To cope with and correct psychological disturbances.*
1. Offer psychological support.
2. Educate the patient to accept and learn to live with this chronic disease. This is done on a long-range basis, and the patient should participate in the evaluation and planning of his care.
3. Plan all aspects of patient's care in conference so that a team effort promotes the nursing process and ensures continuity of care, communication, and periodic evaluation.
4. Indicate by actions and expressions that you, the nurse, are responsible for and care for him. Good nurse-patient relationship enables him to satisfy his dependency needs.
5. Solicit the assistance of the family in helping to understand the patient; assist the family in understanding the patient.
6. If patient is to have an ileostomy, before surgery it is helpful to have patient visited by someone who has had a similar operation and has made a good adjustment. After surgery, these persons can also help with management problems (Ostomy Clubs exist in most major cities).

NOTE: Impotence occurs in males rather frequently after a colectomy because of damage to pudendal nerves.

E. *To prevent complications.*
1. Observe for signs of colonic perforation and hemorrhage.
2. Assess carefully the behavior of the patient and all his complaints.

Surgical Treatment and Nursing Management

A. *Indications and Contemplated Surgery.*
1. Approximately 20% of patients with ulcerative colitis in the United States require surgical intervention.
2. Recommended when no improvement occurs through conservative means: evidenced by impending perforation, actual perforation, deteriorating clinical course after 24–48 hours of maximum medical regime, severe hemorrhage, or persistent colonic dilation for longer than 1 week.
3. Total proctocolectomy and permanent ileostomy are recommended.

B. *Preoperative Physical and Psychological Preparation*
1. Institute an intensive program of fluid, blood, and protein replacement.
2. Administer chemotherapy and antimicrobials to reduce intestinal organisms.
3. Recognize psychological needs of this patient:
   a. Fear, anxiety, and discouragement accompany diarrhea.
   b. Hypersensitivity may be evident.
   c. Let him know his complaints are understood.
4. Encourage patient to talk; listen to what he says is bothering him.
5. Answer his questions relative to the permanent ileostomy he is about to have.

C. *Postoperative Care Including Ileostomy Management*
(See Management of Patient having Major Intestinal Surgery, p. 419.)
(See Conditions: Caring for a Patient with an Ileostomy, p. 426.)

Health Education

1. It is important to involve the patient in understanding chronic ulcerative colitis and each component of care prescribed; he should be made to feel that he is sharing responsibility for maintaining his health.
2. This patient needs encouragement and support postoperatively even though surgery is considered curative; there may be problems with skin care; there may also be aesthetic difficulties, surgical revisions.
3. When early indications of relapse are noted, such as bleeding or increased diarrhea, the patient should report these findings early so that steroid treatment may be initiated.
4. Monitoring the patient's condition should continue when new symptoms suggest it or on a regular annual basis.
5. Let the patient know that he has a valuable resource person in the enterostomal therapist and that he should not hesitate to call this person about his ileostomy problems.

REGIONAL ENTERITIS (CROHN'S DISEASE, GRANULOMATOUS COLITIS, TRANSMURAL COLITIS)

Regional enteritis is a chronic inflammatory disease of the small intestine usually affecting the terminal ileum at the region just before the ileum joins the colon. The etiology is unknown (Fig. 10-16).

Incidence

1. Affects both sexes equally.
2. Appears more often in Jewish persons of Eastern European origiin.
3. A familial tendency exists.
4. May occur at any age, but occurs mostly between 15 and 35 years of age.

Clinical Features

1. Intestinal tissue thickens first by edema and later by formation of scar tissues and granulomas.
2. At times, "skip lesions" occur with normal intestine in between.
3. This condition interferes with the ability of the intestine to transport the contents of upper intestine

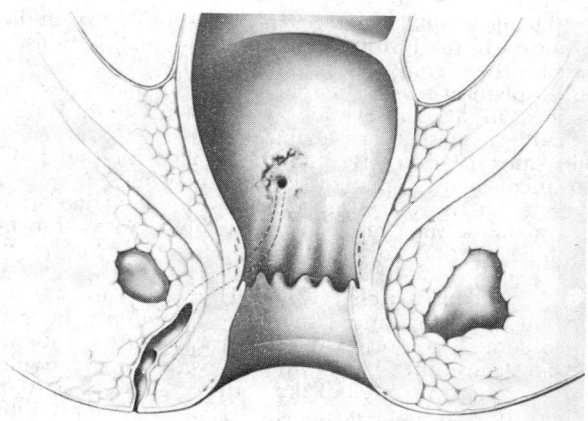

FIGURE 10-16. *Crohn's disease is usually characterized by large, shaggy ulcers, deep abscesses, and unusual fistulas. (Kratzer GL. Manual on the Office Management of Colon and Rectal Diseases. Kenilworth, NJ, Reed and Carnrick).*

through the constricted lumen; this causes crampy pains after meals.
4. Inflammation and ulcers form in the lining membrane, producing a constant irritating discharge.
5. In some patients, the inflamed intestine may perforate and form intraabdominal and anal abscesses.

Clinical Manifestations

These are characterized by exacerbations and remissions—may be abrupt or insidious:
1. Crampy pain after meals; this causes patient to eat in small amounts or even to avoid eating, which then results in malnutrition, weight loss, and possibly anemia (hypochromic or macrocytic).
2. Chronic diarrhea due to irritating discharge may occur; usual consistency is soft or semi-liquid.
3. Milk products and chemically or mechanically irritating food may aggravate the problem.
4. Melena and malabsorption syndrome may occur; occult blood may appear in stool.
5. Low-grade fever occurs if abscesses are present.
6. Lymphadenitis occurs in mesenteric nodes.
7. Abdominal tenderness, especially in right lower quadrant.

Differences Between Regional Enteritis and Ulcerative Colitis

Clinical Complications
1. Stricture and fistulae formation (ischiorectal, perianal—even to bladder or vagina).
2. Hemorrhage, bowel perforation, mechanical intestinal obstruction.
3. Incidence of colorectal cancer is higher in these patients.

Clinical Evaluation
1. Regional enteritis may simulate acute appendicitis.
2. Upper gastrointestinal barium studies—classic "string sign" is noted at terminal ileum that suggests a constriction of a segment of intestine.
3. Barium enema to permit visualization of lesions of large intestine and terminal ileum.
4. Proctosigmoidoscopy to note ulceration.

Medical and Nursing Therapeutic Regimen
OBJECTIVES: to promote patient comfort and maintain adequate hydration and nutrition, and attain remission.
to employ safeguards to prevent transmission of pathogenic organisms from one patient to another—conscientious hand washing as well as proper linen and equipment care.
to transmit feelings of understanding, concern, and helpfulness to this patient who is often dejected, debilitated, embarrassed about frequent and malodorous stools, and even fearful of eating.
1. Administer a diet low in residue, roughage and fat, and high in calories, protein, and carbohydrates, with vitamin supplements (especially vitamin K).
   a. Prepare for hyperalimentation if patient is debilitated.
2. Provide iron medications if anemia is present.
3. Treat pain and diarrhea symptomatically; encourage patient to rest.
4. Consider antimicrobials and sulfonamides such as sulfasalazine (SAS; Azulfidine) for control of inflammatory process.
5. Some clinics treat this patient with sulfasalazine, steroids, and mercaptopurine (Purinethol).
6. If patient does not respond to conservative medical and pharmacotherapy (sulfa drugs, steroids, azo-

	Regional Enteritis	Ulcerative Colitis
Pathology		
Early	Transmural thickening	Mucosal ulceration
Later	Deep, penetrating granulomas	Mucosal minute ulcerations
Clinical Manifestations		
Bleeding	Generally no, but may occur	Common
Perianal disease	Common	Rare
Fistula	Common	Rare
Perforation	Common	Rare
X-ray: Barium Studies		
Stricture	Common	Rare
Distribution	Segmental	Continuous
Associated with malignancy	Not common	Common

thioprine), surgery may be necessary to relieve segmental obstruction. Surgery is determined specifically for each patient. The involved segment may be resected with anastomosis. Bypass procedures may be done. Unfortunately, recurrence of the disease is possible following surgery.

ILEOSTOMY

An *ileostomy* is an opening in the ileum for the purpose of treating intractable granulomatous or ulcerative colitis, of diverting intestinal contents in colon cancer, familial polyposis, congenital defects, or trauma. The opening (*stoma*) is brought out through the abdominal wall, usually the lower right section of the abdomen. This stoma becomes the outlet for discharge of intestinal contents.

Implications for the Patient

(See also Colostomy for Pre- and Postoperative Nursing Management, p. 438)

1. Some patients welcome the ileostomy, since it means the removal of a long-standing incapacitating disease process; in general, however, many patients experience psychological problems that are often overwhelming. Preoperative counseling by the medical and nursing team as well as by a trained visitor from the local chapter of the United Ostomy Association is most helpful.
2. The patient appreciates that now he has the prospect of enjoying a normal diet, as against the low-residue diet to which he was restricted.
3. Patient wears a soft vinyl or rubber pouch with an open-end bottom; a clamp fitted on the bottom of the pouch permits emptying. He empties the pouch 4–5 times a day, usually when he goes to the bathroom to urinate.

4. The ileostomate requires instruction—first from the nurse in the hospital or an enterostomal therapist,* and then from the community nurse.
5. Appliances may be reusable or disposable. They are held in place in several ways—cement, double-faced adhesive discs, karaya rings.
6. Waterproof tape is effective in anchoring the appliance when the patient showers or swims.
7. At first the discharge will be liquid, but later the small intestine will begin to take on its water-absorbing function to permit a more semisolid, pasty discharge.
8. Because the discharge is rich in enzymes, it may cause skin irritation; therefore optimum skin care becomes a top priority consideration for the patient.
   a. Cleanse the skin thoroughly with mild soap and water; rinse well. Take baths or showers as soon after surgery as possible. Dry area thoroughly. For elderly patients, soap may be too drying for the skin; however, oil base soaps may prevent adhesives from adhering.

---

* An *Enterostomal Therapist (E.T.)* is a health care professional with special training in the rehabilitation of persons with ostomies and related problems. Enterostomal therapists are certified by the I.A.E.T. (below).
  The *International Association for Enterostomal Therapy (I.A.E.T.)* is the professional association for enterostomal therapists. Address is 505 N. Tustin, Suite 219, Santa Ana, CA 92705.
  The *Journal of Enterostomal Therapy* is the official publication of the International Association for Enterostomal Therapy and is published six times yearly by AMC Publishers, 2506 Gross Point Road, Evanston, IL 60201
  The *United Ostomy Association (UOA)* is a self-help group for ostomates and other interested persons. The address is 2001 W. Beverly Boulevard, Los Angeles, CA 90057.

GUIDELINES: Changing an Ileostomy Appliance

Purposes
1. To prevent leakage (bag is usually changed every 2–4 days).
2. To permit examination of skin around stoma.
3. To assist in controlling odor if this presents a problem.

Time
1. Early in morning before breakfast or 2–4 hours after a meal when the bowel is least active.
2. Immediately if patient is complaining of burning or itching underneath the disc or has pain around the stoma.

Equipment
Duplicate ileostomy appliance with or without belt (Fig. 10-17); pouch-closing device
Soap, water, and washcloth
Appropriate skin barrier (karaya powder, karaya paste, and/or karaya ring, Stomahesive (Tm), ReliaSeal (Tm), Skin Prep (Tm) or other)
Gauze
Emesis basin
Tape (hypoallergenic)

Procedure

NURSING ACTION	RATIONALE/AMPLIFICATION
Preparatory Phase	
1. Have patient assume a relaxed position. Provide privacy.	1. Encourage patient participation and understanding so that eventually he will be able to change appliance himself.
2. Explain details of this activity to patient.	
3. Expose ileostomy area; remove ileostomy belt (if worn).	
4. Position lamp; wash hands.	

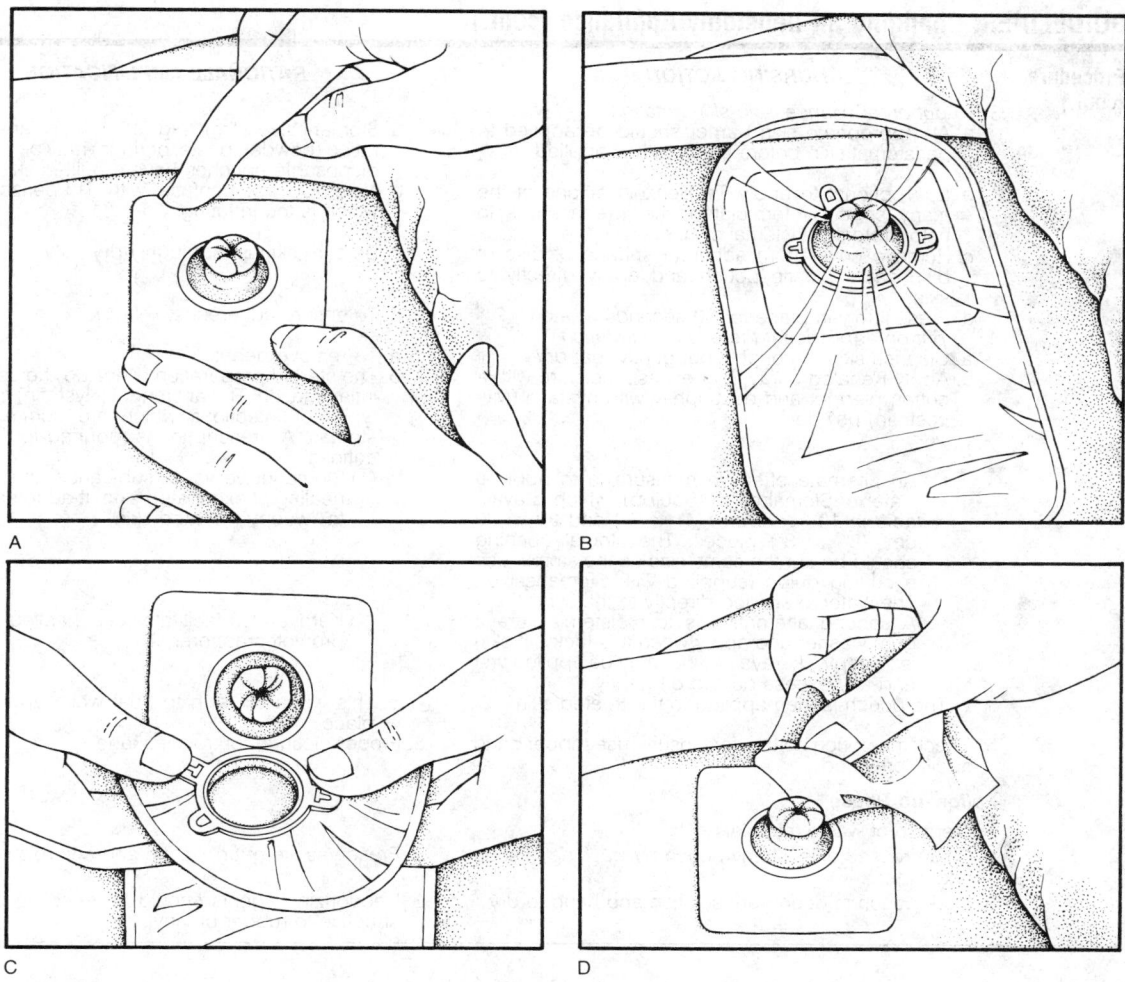

FIGURE 10-17. *Ileostomy Care. A. A Stomahesive wafer with flange (1½", 1¾", 2¼", 2¾") can be applied directly to the peristomal area after it has been thoroughly cleaned and dried. B. An opaque or transparent drainable pouch is positioned at desired angle over stoma. C. Pouch may be removed without removing wafer. D. Stoma may be assessed without removing wafer. (Adapted by permission from ConvaTec, a Division of ER Squibb & Sons, Inc.)*

Procedure (cont.)

NURSING ACTION	RATIONALE/AMPLIFICATION
Performance Phase	
1. *To remove appliance:*	
a. Sit or stand in a comfortable position.	a. Have patient sit on toilet or on a chair facing toilet. If standing, face toilet.
b. Fill a container with prescribed solvent, then fill medicine dropper with solvent; apply a few drops of solvent between disc of appliance and skin. *Do not pull off appliance!*	b. As solvent works, pouch loosens and pulling is unnecessary. Solvent is often unnecessary when skin cement is not used. Pouch can be removed by gently pushing skin away from adhesive.
c. If adhesive residue builds up on skin, use very small amount of adhesive remover on gauze.	c. Do not use acetone, ether, or benzene because they are irritating to skin.
2. *To cleanse skin:*	
a. Remove any excess karaya with dry toilet tissue.	a. During this time, a gauze dressing or pieces of tissue may be used to cover the stoma to absorb excess drainage while skin is being cleaned.
b. Wash skin gently with soft cloth moistened with *tepid* water and mild soap, or bathe before putting on clean appliance.	b. Patient may shower before removing appliance. Micropore or waterproof tape applied to sides of disc will keep it secure while bathing.
c. Rinse and dry skin thoroughly after cleansing.	c. Moisture or soap residue will interfere with appliance adhesion.

GUIDELINES: Changing an Ileostomy Appliance (cont.)

Procedure (cont.)

NURSING ACTION	RATIONALE/AMPLIFICATION
3. *To put on appliance if no skin irritation:*	
a. An appropriate skin barrier should be applied to peristomal skin before the pouch is applied.	a. Stomahesive (Tm) (Fig. 10-17) or karaya preparation (powder, paste, or rings) may be used. Many disposable pouches have a built-in skin barrier.
b. It is optional to apply Tr. Benzoin or one of the many specially formulated skin preparations to help protect peristomal skin.	b. Note: Do not confuse with Tr. benzoin comp., which is too irritating.
c. Remove cover from adherent surface of disc of disposable plastic pouch and apply directly to skin.	c. Be sure skin is thoroughly dry.
d. Press firmly in place for 30 seconds.	d. To ensure adherence.
4. *To put on appliance if there is skin irritation:*	
a. Cleanse skin thoroughly but gently; pat dry.	a. To remove debris.
b. Apply Kenalog spray; blot excess moisture with a cotton pledget and dust lightly with nystatin (Mycostatin) powder.	b. The steroid preparation (Kenalog) helps decrease inflammation. The antifungal (Nystatin) treats those types of infections which are common around stomas. A prescription is required for both medications.
(1) An alternate effective measure is to apply a wafer of Stomahesive (Squibb), which is available in 10 × 10 cm. (4″ × 4″) and 20 × 20 cm. (8″ × 8″) pieces. The stomal opening should be cut the same size as the stoma; use a cutting guide (supplied with Stomahesive). The wafer is applied directly to the skin.	(1) Stomahesive is a substance that facilitates healing of excoriated skin. It adheres well even to "weepy" irritated skin.
(2) A second alternative is to moisten a karaya gum washer and apply when it is tacky. If skin is "weepy," karaya powder may be applied first and any excess dusted off gently.	(2) Karaya also facilitates skin healing. Tackiness promotes adherence.
c. The pouch is then applied to the treated skin.	c. This will allow skin to heal while appliance is in place.
5. Check the pouch bottom for closure; use rubber band or clip provided.	5. Proper closure controls leakage.
Follow-up Phase	
1. Dispose of waste materials.	
2. Clean reusable ileostomy pouch by washing in soap and water.	2. Preserves life of appliance and controls odor.
3. Soak pouch in deodorant solution and hang to dry.	3. Deodorizing agents should be effective but not destructive to rubber or vinyl.

Nutritional Management of the Ileostomate

Nutritional needs of the patient with an ileostomy are similar to those of a healthy individual. With adequate diet, additional vitamins or food supplements are unnecessary. These are the exceptions:

Condition/Problem	Management/Resolution
Negative nutritional balance during or immediately after surgery.	Need for a diet high in calories and protein; also additional vitamin and mineral supplements.
These patients have fewer fluid and electrolyte reserves to tap in case of extra bodily demands: vomiting, diarrhea, excessive perspiration.	Avoid salt tablets, which may act as cathartics. Supplement fluids with athlete beverages (Gatorade, Sportade) which contain electrolytes and glucose.
If a large portion of small intestine has been resected, patient may be unable to absorb adequate amounts of nutrients.	Continue diet high in protein with vitamin and mineral supplements; fat restriction may be necessary. Elemental diets (diet preparations already broken down to simple, easily digested forms) are very helpful until ileum adapts to new shortened length. (e.g., Vivonex (Eaton), Flexical (Mead-Johnson)
Weight gain or loss: If weight loss: patient may be limiting intake to reduce amount of effluent.	Check and record weight daily. Explain to patient that ileostomy will continue to function even if oral intake is limited and that adequate nutritional intake is essential for healing to occur. Dietary supplements are appropriate. Ensure (Ross), Isocal, Sustacal (Mead-Johnson).

Condition/Problem	Management/Resolution
Resection of terminal ileum—this results in loss of specific absorptive site for vitamin B₁₂ and bile salts.	Check blood levels for B_{12}; replacement by injection of Vitamin B_{12} may be necessary. Because bile salt supplementation is not practical, restrict fat, since patient may not be able to digest and absorb fats because of bile salt deficiency. This must be monitored carefully because on a fat-restricted diet patient may lose weight and be unable to absorb fat soluble vitamins: A, D, E, and K. Also, with bile salt deficiency, this patient may be more susceptible to formation of gallstones.
Excessively watery effluent.	Restrict fibrous foods; whole-grain bread and cereals, fresh fruit skins, fresh vegetables, beans, corn, nuts.
Excessively dry effluent.	Increase salt intake. Note: *increased intake of water does not increase effluent because excess water is excreted in urine.*
Stomal obstruction.	Fibrous foods may contribute; be alert to such offenders as celery, cabbage, nuts, corn, and popcorn. Patient should chew all food thoroughly.

Problems Encountered by the Patient with an Ileostomy

Problem	Cause and Assessment	Prevention/Management
Skin excoriation	1. Irritating intestinal effluent. 2. Materials used to hold appliance in place. 3. Allergies 4. Fungal or bacterial growth. 5. Belt applied too tightly. 6. Poor stoma location—peristomal skin folds or scars.	Evaluate for proper fit of appliance. Karaya protects skin—it comes as powder, paste, rings, and sheets. Good substitutes for karaya are Stomahesive (Squibb) or ReliaSeal (Davol). An appropriate skin barrier should always be used between skin and appliance. Avoid products to which patient may be sensitive. Patch test any new or suspect problems on patient's inner arm. If large areas of skin are involved or ulcerated, avoid rubber cement-type adhesive. Severe problems due to poor stoma location necessitate surgical revision.
Minor stomal bleeding	This may occur following wiping the stoma.	Mucosa is friable and easily injured. However, when handled gently, these tissues heal readily because of the rich blood supply.
Prolapsed stoma	This may occur from an oversized opening resulting from 1. excessive bowel shrinkage 2. abdominal pressure due to coughing 3. failure of opposing layers of bowel to adhere in the turnback suture procedure	Remove appliance. Observe bowel for signs of compromised circulation (pale or dark color). Apply cold pads or packs to control edema. Notify surgeon. He will manually replace bowel into abdomen (medical treatment) or suggest surgical correction.
Odor	This may be due to: 1. a reusable appliance that is not changed frequently enough or not cleaned properly. 2. an appliance which is not odor-proof. 3. certain foods: onions, cabbage, eggs, fish.	Be meticulous in cleaning procedure. Alternate reusable pouches; when not in use, allow pouch to hang in fresh air (not sun). If using disposable pouches, select odor-proof materials. Change medications when one is found to be odor-producing.

Problems Encountered by the Patient with an Ileostomy (cont.)

Problem	Cause and Assessment	Prevention/Management
	4. obstruction or dysfunction of ostomy.	Use oral deodorants: chlorophyll derivatives, bismuth subcarbonate, or bismuth subgallate.
	5. certain medications; vitamins, penicillin, estrogens.	Insert deodorizer in appliance: charcoal, Banish (TM-United), or baking soda.
		Foods such as spinach and parsley act on the intestinal tract as deodorizers.
Expulsion of intestinal flatus	This patient has no sphincter control—often feels everyone around him is aware of gas passage.	Limit gas-producing foods such as beans, cabbage, onions, beer.
		Try to avoid air-swallowing which may occur during smoking, talking, eating, emotional upset.
Obstruction	This is suggested by the following signs: 1. abdominal cramping, distention. 2. malodor along with liquid projectile effluent. 3. vomiting. 4. signs of dehydration.	Obstruction or stenosis may be due to edema or lymphatic blockage. More commonly, it is due to food blockage brought about by poor chewing habits and high-cellulose foods. *Nursing Intervention:* 1. Remove appliance. 2. Have patient lie down in bed and apply hot compresses to abdomen, or have patient relax in tub of warm water. 3. Offer hot tea drinks. If this does not help within 2–3 hours, check with physician; it may be necessary to gently irrigate the ileostomy (physician prescribed) with a small volume of saline.
Obstruction due to adhesions or volvulus		This may require surgical correction.
Kidney stones	The incidence is higher in ileostomy patients because of: 1. dehydration—increases formation of urate crystals because of loss of bicarbonate in intestine. 2. increased absorption of oxalates after ileal resection—oxalate stones form	Increase fluid intake of patient. If stones are urate crystals, sodium bicarbonate may be required to alkalinize urine. If stones are calcium, ascorbic acid may be prescribed to acidify urine.
Diarrhea	Observe whether there is an increase in the number of times patient is required to empty pouch. Normal output is about 750 ml./day. Check for food poisoning, mechanical obstruction, stomal stenosis. Assess for signs of dehydration.	Electrolyte imbalance may easily occur. Treat with clear liquids and antidiarrheal medications. Water salts and fluids can be replaced with such commercial preparations as Gatorade, Quick Kick. Another suggestion is to alternate a cup of salted broth and a cup of sweetened tea each hour. Water-absorbing drugs (hydrophilic colloids) such as Metamucil Powder are sometimes effective. If diarrhea does not resolve in 24 hours, patient should seek medical care. I.V. fluids and electrolyic therapy may be necessary.
Medication difficulties	1. Drug action can be affected by the absence of the colon and altered transit time through small intestine.	1. The various functions of the small and large bowel are interrupted or absent.

Problems Encountered by the Patient with an Ileostomy (cont.)

Problem	Cause and Assessment	Prevention/Management
	2. Suggest taking uncoated tablets or liquids for oral medication.	2. Coated tablets may pass undissolved through bowel into ileostomy appliance.
	3. Have patient check effluent to be sure pills are not being passed undissolved.	3. If they do pass undissolved, thereafter crush them and take them with water or applesauce.
	4. Do not use time-release tablets or sustained-release capsules.	4. They may not be absorbed.
	5. Administer Vitamin B_{12} subcutaneously if distal ileum has been removed.	5. The terminal ileum is where absorptive site for B_{12} is located.

Patient Education

Discharge from hospital for patient with ileostomy or colostomy

A. *Clothing*

1. A girdle is permissible—a size larger is recommended to accommodate the pouch.
2. Swim suits (even two-piece) can be worn; men prefer boxer-styled trunks; women may prefer a swim suit with a skirt.
3. For swimming, a rubber belt is preferred to elastic cloth which sometimes loses elasticity when wet.

B. *Medications*

1. The ileostomate should not have laxatives, irrigations, enteric-coated or time-release capsules.

C. *Travel*

1. Travel by plane or any other vehicle is not contraindicated.
2. If traveling by plane, it is suggested that patient carry his ostomy kit with him (in the event that there is a delay in retrieving baggage).
3. Colostomates who irrigate should use only water suitable for drinking.
4. Ileostomates should bring along a suitable antidiarrheal medication.

D. *Sports*

1. All kinds of sports may be participated in, as reported by ostomates: tennis, water surfing, skin diving, water skiing, ice skating, horseback riding.
2. Problems may arise if the ostomate participates in contact sports such as football, ice hockey.

E. *Sexual Intercourse*

1. Approximately 10–20% of male ileostomates experience impaired sexual function; in many individuals this is only temporary.
2. Male colostomates vary from full potency to impotence.
3. Most males who have urinary surgery for malignancy as adults are impotent.
4. In many instances, potency is regained, but this may take up to two years.

F. *Pregnancy*

1. An ostomy is not a contraindication to a successful pregnancy.
2. Careful medical supervision is required for a female ostomate during pregnancy. The ostomy opening may change in size (stretch) as the pregnancy continues; thereafter, changes in the size of the appliance opening may be required. Change in abdominal contour may necessitate the use of a very flexible appliance or faceplate.

G. *Sleeping*

1. Almost any position of comfort can be assumed if the pouch is properly fitted.
2. Sleeping on the stomach is comfortable when a small cushion is placed under the hip on the side of the stoma.

H. *Obstruction or Blockage*

1. Know signs and symptoms; notify enterostomal therapist or physician if necessary.

GUIDELINES: Continent Ileostomy (Kock Pouch)

A *continent ileostomy* is the surgical creation of a pouch of small intestine that can act as an internal receptacle for fecal discharge; a nipple valve is constructed at the outlet to permit drainage from the abdomen. This kind of ileostomy may be done initially for selected patients when they present for an ileostomy, or it may be constructed from the conventional ileostomy (Fig. 10-18).

Preoperative Management

This is essentially the same as for the patient having a traditional ileostomy.

Postoperative Management

1. A catheter will extend from the stoma and be attached to closed suction; drainage will be maintained about 10 days.
2. Catheter irrigation is done usually every 2 hours with a 20–30 ml. saline to ensure patency; return flow is by gravity.
3. Nasogastric suction is used to relieve pressure on suture line by preventing a build-up of gastric contents.
4. Parenteral fluids are administered for 4–5 days; thereafter, clear liquids and diet as tolerated.

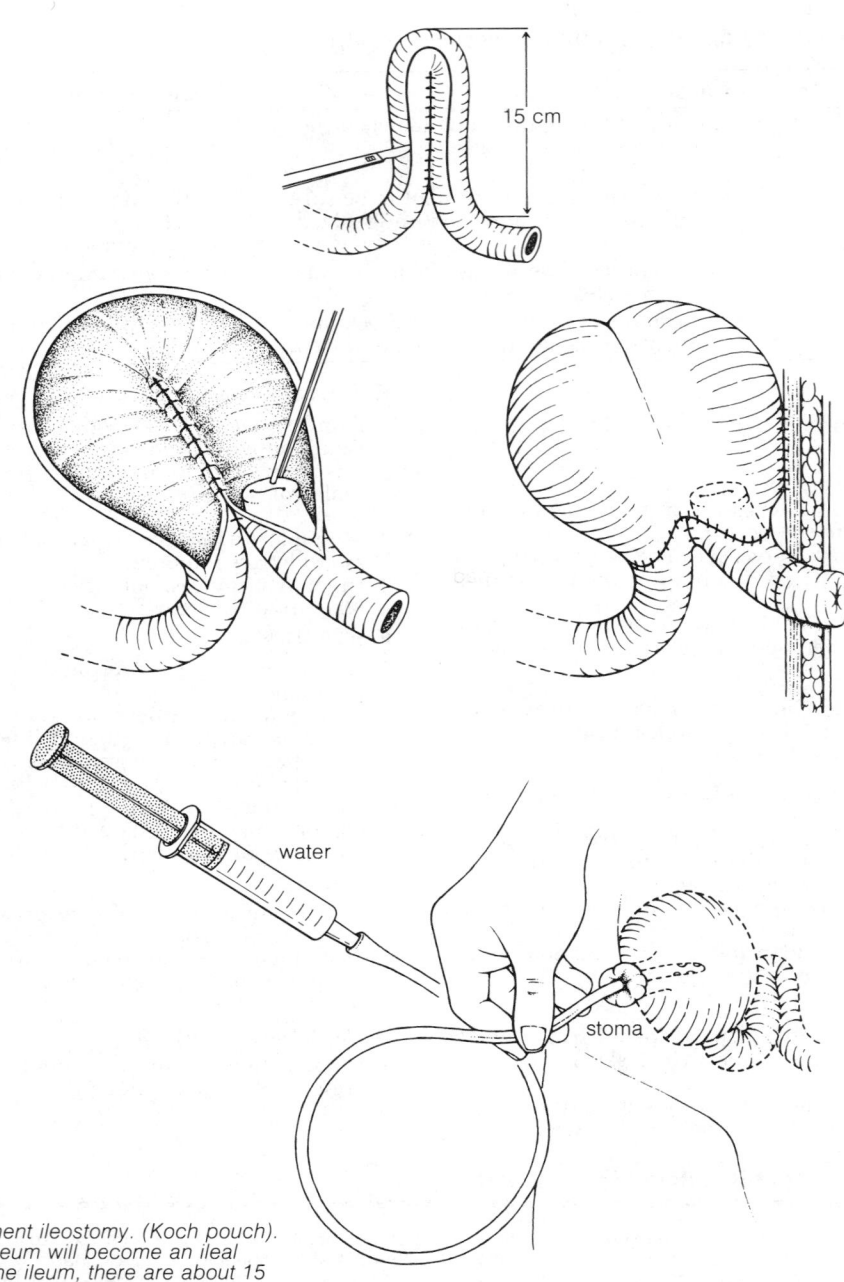

FIGURE 10-18. *Continent ileostomy. (Koch pouch). 1.–About 30 cm of ileum will become an ileal pouch. By looping the ileum, there are about 15 cm on each side as shown. The 2 sides are stitched together in the center. The surgeon then makes a U-shaped incision. 2.–The ileum is opened and the inner section is stitched, much like a seam, to make a smooth inner surface. After this, a valve or "nipple" is constructed on the right between pouch and stoma. Then the top of the ileum is folded to the bottom and stitched closed, as illustrated in part 3. This pouch is stitched to the inner wall for immobilization; likewise, the stoma is fixed to the abdominal wall. In part 4 a lubricated catheter is being gently inserted about 5 cm into the ileal pouch for drainage. (Brunner LS, Suddarth DS. Textbook of Medical and Surgical Nursing. Philadelphia, JB Lippincott Co. 1980)*

GUIDELINES: Continent Ileostomy (Kock Pouch) (cont.)

5. Monitor for nausea and abdominal distention.
6. Pain medication is given as required; early ambulation is encouraged.
7. In about 10–14 days, the catheter is removed from the stoma and the patient participates in the management of his ileostomy.

Equipment
Catheter
Water-soluble lubricant
Gauze squares
Syringe
Irrigating solution in a bowl, emesis or receiving basin.

NURSING ACTION	RATIONALE/AMPLIFICATION
1. Lubricate catheter and gently insert about 5 cm. (2 inches).	1. Resistance may be felt at valve or "nipple."
2. If much resistance, fill syringe with 20 ml. air or water and inject through catheter—gently exert pressure on catheter.	2. This will permit catheter to enter pouch.
3. Place end of catheter in drainage basin (below level of stoma); later this can be done at toilet bowl.	3. Gravity facilitates drainage. Drainage may include flatus as well as effluent.
4. Following drainage, remove catheter. Wash area around stoma; dry and apply absorbent pad. Fasten with hypoallergenic tape.	4. Entire procedure requires about 5–10 minutes. At first, irrigation is done every 2 hours, then gradually extended to 3 times daily. If feces are not too thick, drainage through catheter may occur successfully without irrigation.

DIVERTICULOSIS AND DIVERTICULITIS

A *diverticulum* is a pouch or saccular dilatation leading out from a tube or main cavity (Fig. 10–19).
Diverticulitis is an inflammation of diverticula.
Diverticulosis is the condition in which an individual has multiple diverticula.

Predisposing Factors

1. Probable congenital predisposition
2. Weakening and degeneration of muscular wall of the intestine causing herniation of the lining mucous membrane through a muscle at site of artery penetration
3. Increased mechanical pressure due to abnormal high-pressure contractions of sigmoid colon in response to neurohumoral stimuli
4. Chronic overdistention of the large bowel.

Incidence

1. Usually occurs in individuals over 40 years of age.
2. Diverticula of the large bowel occurs in 5–10% of adults; of these, ⅓ may experience diverticulitis. The condition is most common in sigmoid colon.
3. Small bowel diverticula are unusual but when they occur they are often multiple. They may act as areas of stasis and bacterial overgrowth, leading to malabsorption of fat and vitamin B_{12}.

Altered Physiology

(Colon diverticulosis and diverticulitis)
Constipation from spastic colon syndrome often precedes the development of diverticulosis by many years.
1. Following local inflammation of the diverticula, there may be narrowing of the colon with fibrotic stricture, which then leads to narrowed stools, cramps, and increasing constipation.

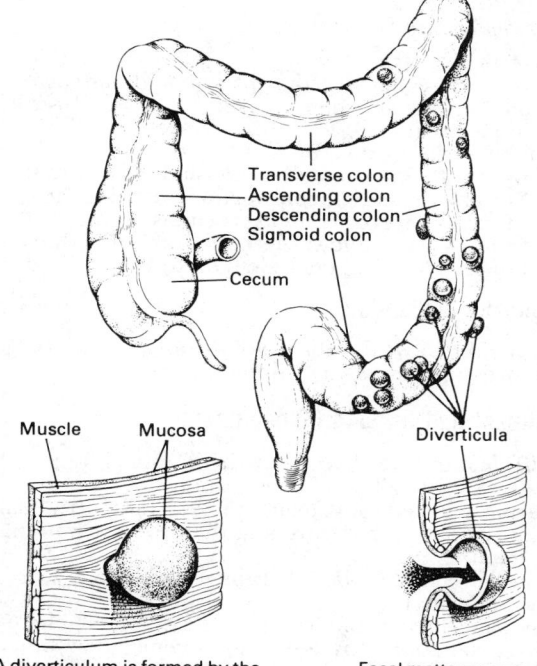

A diverticulum is formed by the herniation of the intestinal mucosa through the weakened muscular wall usually at site of arterial penetration on the mesenteric border of the colon.

Fecal matter accumulates within the diverticulum

FIGURE 10-19. *Diverticula are most common in the sigmoid colon; they diminish in number and size as the colon approaches the cecum. Diverticula are rarely found in the rectum.*

2. With the development of granulation tissue, occult bleeding may occur, producing iron-deficiency anemia; fatigue and weakness are then evident. However, massive bleeding is more common.
3. Abscess development causes a tender palpable mass; fever and leukocytosis also occur.
4. If the diverticulum perforates, local abscess or peritonitis results; peritonitis causes rigidity, abdominal pain, loss of bowel sounds, and eventually shock.
5. Uninflamed or minimally inflamed diverticula may erode adjacent arterial branches, causing acute massive rectal bleeding.

Clinical Manifestations

A. *General Clinical Signs*

1. May occur in acute attacks or may persist as a long, drawn-out smoldering infection.
2. Tends to spread into surrounding bowel wall, increasing the irritability and spasticity of the colon.
3. When infections are severe, perforation of the colon can occur, leading to peritonitis.
4. When infection is less acute but slowly progressive, extensive scarring and abscess formation involving the bowel wall may occur, with the possibility of lower bowel obstruction. Sometimes, fistulae form with the bladder, the adjacent small bowel, the vagina, or even the skin.
5. Sepsis may spread via portal vein to liver, causing liver abscesses.

B. *Specific Clinical Signs*

1. Diverticulosis
   a. Bowel irregularity, constipation, and diarrhea
   b. Sudden massive hemorrhage (occurs in 10–20% of patients)
2. Milder forms of diverticulitis
   a. Bouts of soreness, mild lower abdominal cramps
   b. Bowel irregularity, constipation, and diarrhea
3. Moderately severe acute diverticulitis
   a. Crampy pain in lower left quadrant of abdomen
   b. Low-grade fever, chills, leukocytosis

Diagnostic Evaluation

1. Sigmoidoscopy; possibly colonoscopy
2. Fluoroscopy and x-ray wih barium enema

Treatment and Nursing Management

OBJECTIVES: to provide rest for the intestinal tract and to alleviate constipation.

1. During acute episode, maintain fluid and nutritional requirements with intravenous therapy; give nothing by mouth.
2. Maintain antimicrobial therapy as prescribed to reduce infection.
3. For pain, meperidine (Demerol) is the analgesic of choice because it is less spasmogenic than other analgesics.
4. When indicated, employ stool softeners such as dioctyl sodium or calcium sulfosuccinate (Colace, Bu-Lax, Surfak).
5. Administer bulk additives to counteract tendency toward constipation; a frequently prescribed hydrophilic mucilloid smooth bulk laxative is psyllium (Metamucil).
6. Warm-oil-retention enemas may be used to treat inflammation locally by softening fecal mass.

NOTE: In some patients, an increase in mass results in an increase in symptoms.

7. Check with physician as to type of diet to be followed. Some authorities prefer fiber-content in the diet rather than a low-residue diet. With increased fiber, more bulk is added to give the stool proper consistency. With a low-residue diet, the colon may work harder to propel contents, thereby producing high pressure on the intestinal wall, which in turn promotes diverticula formation.

8. *Surgical*
   a. If there is little response to medical treatment, or if complications such as hemorrhage, obstruction, or perforation occur, surgery is necessary.
   b. Preparation for surgery:
      (1) Low-residue diet or nothing by mouth.
      (2) Antimicrobials, systemic and intestinal surface-acting, to reduce bowel bacterial flora, diminish bulk of stool and soften fecal mass for easier movement.
      (3) Cleansing enemas may be prescribed.
   c. Resection of segment of intestine involved with directicula, reuniting (anastomosing) two ends to maintain continuity.
   d. Temporary colostomy is sometimes performed to divert fecal stream (see p. 428), with continuity restored in later second-stage procedure.

Health Education

OBJECTIVES: to prevent recurrence of diverticular disease.

1. Maintain a diet that is high in soft residue and low in sugar; obtain lists of these foods in order to be familiar with proper dietary control; how well the intestinal tract functions in great measure depends upon proper food intake.
2. Bran products will add bulk to the stool and can be taken with milk or sprinkled over cereal.
3. Establish regular bowel habits to promote regular and complete evacuation; mineral oil can be used nightly if necessary, but dependence on it should be discouraged.
4. Have patient continue periodic medical supervision and follow-up; report problems and untoward symptoms.

INTESTINAL OBSTRUCTION

Intestinal obstruction is an interruption in the normal flow of intestinal contents along the intestinal tract.

The block may occur in the small or large intestine, may be complete or incomplete, may be mechanical or paralytic, and may or may not compromise the vascular supply. Obstruction most frequently occurs in the very young and the very old.

Types of Obstruction

1. Mechanical—a physical block to passage of intestinal contents without disturbing blood supply of bowel
   a. Location
      Extrinsic, e.g., adhesion, hernia, intussusception
      Intrinsic, e.g., hematoma, tumor
      Intraluminal, e.g., foreign body, fecal or barium impaction, polyp
   b. Clinical Pattern
      High small-bowel (jejunal); 80% incidence
      Low small-bowel (ileal); 80% incidence
      Colonic; 20% incidence

2. Paralytic (adynamic, neurogenic) ileus
Peristalsis is ineffective (diminished motor activity perhaps because of toxic or traumatic disturbance of the autonomic nervous system); there is no physical obstruction and no interrupted blood supply.
3. Strangulation
Obstruction also compromises blood supply, leading to gangrene of the intestine.

Causes

1. Mechanical (extramural)
   a. Adhesions—postoperative
   b. Hernia
   c. Malignancy
   d. Volvulus (loop of intestine that has twisted)
2. Mechanical (intramural)
   a. Carcinoma
   b. Hematoma
   c. Intussusception (telescoping of intestine)
   d. Stricture or stenosis (scarring)
3. Paralytic
   a. Spinal cord injuries, vertebral fractures
   b. Postoperatively after any abdominal surgery
   c. Peritonitis, pneumonia
   d. Wound dehiscence (breakdown)
   e. Gastrointestinal tract surgery

NOTE:
1. In postoperative patients, approximately 90% of mechanical obstructions are due to adhesions.
2. In nonsurgical patients, hernia (most often inguinal) is the most common cause of mechanical obstruction.

Altered Physiology

1. Disturbed physiologic responses as a result of mechanical small-intestine obstruction results in increased peristalsis, distention by fluid and gas, and increased bacterial growth proximal to obstruction. The intestine empties distally.
2. Increased secretions into the intestine are associated with diminution in the bowel's absorptive capacity.
3. The accumulation of gases, secretions, and oral intake above the obstruction causes increasing intraluminal pressure.
4. Venous pressure in the affected area increases, and circulatory stasis and edema result.
5. Bowel necrosis may occur because of anoxia and compression of the terminal branches of the mesenteric artery.
6. Bacteria and toxins pass across the intestinal membranes into the abdominal cavity, thereby leading to peritonitis.
7. "Closed-loop" obstruction is a condition in which the intestinal segment is occluded at both ends, preventing either the downward passage or the regurgitation of intestinal contents.

Assessment and Clinical Manfestations

Fever, peritoneal irritation, increased white blood cell count, toxicity and shock may develop with all types of intestinal obstruction.
1. Simple mechanical—high small bowel
Colic (cramps) mid to upper abdomen, some distention, early bilious vomiting, increased bowel sounds (high-pitched tinkling heard at brief intervals), minimal diffuse tenderness
2. Simple mechanical—low small bowel

Significant colic (cramps) midabdominal, considerable distention, vomiting—slight or absent—later feculent, increased bowel sounds and "hush" sounds, minimal diffuse tenderness
3. Simple mechanical—colon
Cramps (mid-to-lower abdomen), later-appearing distention, then vomiting may develop (feculent), increase in bowel sounds, minimal diffuse tenderness
4. Partial chronic mechanical obstruction—may occur with granulomatous bowel (Crohn's) disease.
Symptoms are cramping abdominal pain, mild distention, and diarrhea.
5. Strangulation
Symptoms are initially those of mechanical obstruction but later progress rapidly: Pain is severe, continuous and localized. There is moderate distention, persistent vomiting, usually decreased bowel sounds and marked localized tenderness. Stools or vomitus become melenous or bloody or contan occult blood.
6. Paralytic ileus
Gaseous distention is prominent; abdomen is tense; pain is dull, continuous, and diffuse; obstipation (intractable constipation) is rarely complete, since small amounts of flatus may be passed; peristalsis is usually depressed, and bowel sounds are infrequent or absent; vomiting occurs only after eating (vomiting may later become fecal).

NURSING ALERT: Because of loss of water, sodium, and chloride, signs of dehydration become evident: intense thirst, drowsiness, general malaise, aching; tongue becomes parched, face appears pinched, abdomen becomes distended. Shock may result (pulse increasingly rapid and weak, temperature and blood pressure lowered, skin pale, cold, clammy) ending in death.

Treatment and Nursing Management

OBJECTIVE: to remove the obstruction, treat the fluid and electrolyte imbalance, relieve the distention, and prevent or detect early the complications of shock and peritonitis.

A. *Initial Nursing Assessment and Care*

1. Describe accurately the nature and location of the patient's pain, the presence of distention, the absence of flatus or defecation. The overview of symptoms is important in differentiating intestinal obstruction from other more benign conditions.
2. Elderly patients with poor bowel tonus who often remain in the recumbent position for extended periods are likely to experience air-fluid lock syndrome, which is described below.
   a. Fluid collects in dependent bowel loops.
   b. Peristalsis is too weak to push fluid "uphill."
   c. Obstruction occurs primarily in the large bowel
   d. Management consists simply of alternately turning the patient from supine to prone position every 10 minutes until enough flatus is passed to decompress the abdomen. A rectal tube may help.
3. Monitor and record vital signs (including blood pressure) every 4 hours.

4. Measure and record accurately all intake and output.
5. Save any stool that may be passed; this is to be tested for occult blood.
6. Anticipate physician's request for urinalysis, hemoglobin determination, and blood cell counts.
7. Frequently determine the patient's level of consciousness; decreasing responsiveness may offer a clue to an increasing electrolyte imbalance.
8. Institute long-tube decompression of intestine proximal to block.
9. Recognize the patient's concern and initiate measures to secure his cooperation and confidence in the staff; these measures include ascertaining his specific anxieties and providing him with therapeutic responses.
10. Compare the patient's state of orientation with his admission status; a lessening awareness of his environment may suggest his going into shock.
11. Minimize those factors that would enhance gastric secretions in order to prevent fluid loss (via nasogastric suction); avoid conversation about enticing meals and eliminate meals being served within his range of seeing or smelling.
12. Observe for evidence of postural hypotension as patient is moved from a low Fowler's position to an upright position; this may be suggestive of circulatory insufficiency.
13. Undertake measures to prepare the patient for surgery, since most problems of mechanical obstruction require surgical correction.

B. *Medical, Surgical, and Nursing Management*

1. Relieve distention by introducing a long gastrointestinal tube (p. 414); this can be passed more effectively with the patient lying on his right side; begin decompression to remove gas and fluid.
2. Correct fluid imbalance by initiating
   a. Na+, K+, plasma substitutes
   b. Ringer's lactate to correct interstitial fluid deficit
   c. Dextrose/water to correct intracellular fluid deficit.
3. Administer antimicrobials (neomycin and kanamycin) and possibly a broad spectrum agent to lessen the possibility of infection, particularly peritonitis.
4. Recognize that giving an enema may distort an x-ray picture by introducing gas into the tract distal to the obstruction. An enema may make a partial obstruction worse, hence it is contraindicated.
5. Prevent infarction by carefully assessing status of patient; if pain increases in intensity, localizes, or becomes continuous, it may herald strangulation.
6. Detect early signs of peritonitis, such as rigidity and tenderness, in an effort to minimize this complication.
7. Relieve obstruction by releasing, removing, or repairing the cause of the obstruction; this is done surgically in most instances. Complete small bowel obstruction and colon obstruction requires an operation for relief. When tube suction therapy does not help after 12 hours, surgery is indicated.
   a. *Resection* of obstructing lesion and end-to-end anastomosis is done when no evidence of peritonitis and only minimal edema exist; this requires a proximal colostomy to decompress new anastomosis.
   b. Resection of all necrotic intestine is necessary.
   c. A tube *enterostomy* may be done by introducing a catheter into distended bowel; the other end of

catheter is brought out through the abdominal wall via a separate incision. This is a palliative measure.
   d. A *loop colostomy* is done when relief is sought by drawing a proximal loop or segment of colon up to the skin surface and opening it as a colostomy; the distal portion of colon is treated later.

C. *Postoperative Nursing Care*

1. To meet fluid, electrolyte, and nutritional needs, administer prescribed amounts of fluids; keep accurate intake and output records.
2. For an enterostomy, connect tube to drainage bottle at side of bed; expect considerable amount of fecal drainage during the first 12–15 hours (500–1000 ml.).
   a. Observe frequently the patency of drainage equipment.
   b. If there is difficulty with drainage, it may be necessary to inject 15 ml. of warm saline into the enterostomy tube every 2–4 hours with approval of physician.
   c. Protect skin around enterostomy tube with a skin barrier such as Stomahesive or karaya preparations.
3. Follow additional postoperative management described in Major Intestinal Surgery on page 419.

CANCER OF THE COLON

Incidence

1. Cancer of the colon and rectum will account for over 53,000 deaths annually—the second highest overall death rate in the U.S. for any type of cancer.
2. Males are affected slightly more often than females.
3. The highest incidence occurs in patients about 50 years old.
4. Five-year-survival is 40–50% (best of visceral cancers).

Etiology

1. Familial polyposis (numerous pedunculated growths arising from mucosa and extending into lumen of intestine).
2. Chronic ulcerative colitis—definite risk of colon cancer (up to 20% after 20 years of age with active disease).
3. Diverticulosis and cancer may be found together and simulate each other—no definite evidence that the presence of diverticula is significant in the development of cancer.
4. Cancer of the colon occurs much more frequently in developed countries and rarely in underdeveloped countries. The increased incidence of colon cancer in developed countries is probably related to the relatively lower fiber content of diet in these areas.
5. Unabsorbable fiber deficit appears to be related to intestinal transit time, stool bulk, and consistency.
6. The effect of diet on the colon bacterial flora is a factor possibly contributing to cancer.

Clinical Manifestations

1. Distribution of cancer in the colon is shown in Figure 10–20.
2. Most common symptoms:
   a. Blood in stools (usually occult)—causing anemia.
   b. Partial obstruction—causing constipation alter-

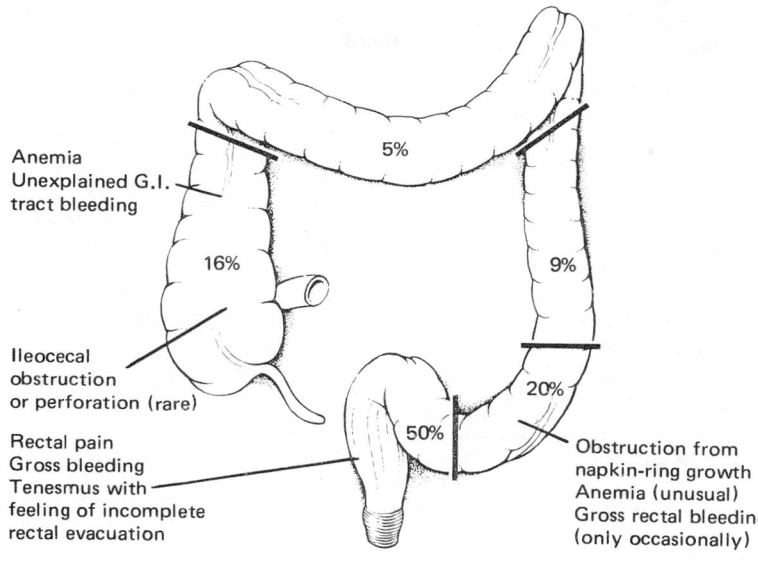

Anemia
Unexplained G.I.
tract bleeding

5%

16%

9%

Ileocecal
obstruction
or perforation (rare)

Rectal pain
Gross bleeding
Tenesmus with
feeling of incomplete
rectal evacuation

50%

20%

Obstruction from
napkin-ring growth
Anemia (unusual)
Gross rectal bleeding
(only occasionally)

FIGURE 10-20. *Distribution of cancer in the colon.*

nating with diarrhea, lower abdominal pains (crampy), distention.
c. Additional signs—progressive weakness, anorexia, weight loss, shortness of breath, anginal pain, anemia.

Diagnostic Evaluation

1. Digital rectal examination—half of all colon and rectal cancers are found this way.
2. Endoscopy (proctosigmoidoscopy/colonoscopy)—⅔ of all colon and rectal cancer can be seen and biopsied via proctoscope alone.
3. Stool examination for blood—often reveals evidence of carcinoma when the patient is otherwise asymptomatic.

NURSING ALERT: Giving a guaiac-impregnated slide kit to individuals over age 40 is an *effective way of screening for colon cancer.* Diet preparation prior to use of 3 slides is optional:
a. Some recommend meat-free, high residue diet with avoidance of peroxidase-producing vegetables (horseradish, turnips, and rutabagas) which produce false-positive results.
b. Some prefer no dietary restriction except retesting those who have a positive test result.

4. Blood-hemoglobin determination for anemia.
5. Barium enema—especially significant in unexplained abdominal mass.
   Napkin-ring-type outline clearly indicates obstruction and possible tumor.
6. Intravenous pyelography and possible cystoscopy may be indicated to assess whether malignancy has spread locally to involve ureter or bladder.

Treatment

A. *Diagnosis confirmed by*

1. Removing rectosigmoid polyps through sigmoidoscope for histologic study.
2. Removing polyps above rectosigmoid by colonoscopy

or laparotomy (if other symptoms are present) to verify diagnosis.

B. *Surgical therapeutic plan*

1. Recommend total colectomy for patient with familial history of polyposis or prolonged, universal, chronically active colitis, even before cancer is confirmed.
2. Most common operative procedures:
   a. Wide segmental resection of colon and mesentery with anastomosis, or
   b. Abdominoperineal resection with colostomy (if lesion is in rectum).
   c. Even more extensive surgery involving removal of other organs if cancer has spread—such as to the bladder, uterus, small intestine, groin, etc.
   d. If cancer is extensive and it may not be in the patient's best interest to do radical surgery, palliative treatment may be done using radon seed implantation (combined surgery and preoperative radiation therapy is being done in several clinics) or local fulguration via colonoscope or proctoscope.

Nursing Management

A. *Preoperative Care* (colostomy not anticipated)

1. Meet nutritional needs of patient by serving a high caloric, low-residue diet for several days prior to surgery if condition permits.
2. Reduce bacterial count of colon by mechanical cleansing and administering antimicrobials as prescribed: erythromycin, neomycin orally; gentamicin and clindamycin systematically. Whatever the choice, it should be effective against the full spectrum of aerobic and anaerobic fecal microbes. The degree of obstruction, acuteness, inflammation—all have a bearing on the nature of antimicrobial administration.
3. Observe and record fluid losses such as may be sustained by vomiting and diarrhea.
4. Record and report any complaints of abdominal pain with a description of nature and location.

5. Assist with and maintain nasogastric suction to minimize postoperative distention.
6. Elicit any concerns or questions patient may have regarding postoperative discomfort, dependency, etc.
7. Prepare patient immediately preoperatively by adequate skin preparation of area. (See page 419 for Care of Patient Having Major Intestinal Surgery.)

B. *Postoperative Care*

See page 419

COLOSTOMY

A *colostomy* is a temporary or permanent opening of the colon through the abdominal wall. The placement of the colostomy will influence the nature of the discharge (Fig. 10-21). The stoma is that part of the colon that is brought above the abdominal wall in a colostomy and becomes the outlet for discharge of intestinal contents.

Purposes

1. It may be part of an abdominoperineal resection for cure or palliation of cancer.
2. It may be palliative when unresectable malignancy is present.
3. It can be a temporary measure to protect an anastomosis, such as after abdominal trauma.
4. It may be temporary to divert fecal stream during radiation or other therapy.

Nursing Management

A. *Preoperative Care*

1. Determine the nature of anticipated surgery; the colostomy must be positioned where the patient can see and care for it (this is determined by the surgeon or enterostomal therapist).
   a. The colostomy should not be placed in the laparotomy incision.
   b. It should be placed where it will not interfere with proper fitting and comfortable wearing of an appliance—away from iliac crest, costal margin, umbilicus, scars, deep folds.
   c. If possible, show patient the intended appliance and have him try it on.
2. Make specific plans for the patient's understanding and acceptance of a colostomy
   a. Collaborate with the surgeon in ascertaining the nature of communication and information exchanged between surgeon and patient, including initial patient contact, in-hospital experience, plans for rehabilitation.
   b. Reinforce the patient's hope for a future that will be manageable and will lead to independent functioning.
   c. Arrange a preoperative visit by a trained visitor from the local chapter of the United Ostomy Association.
   d. Develop a plan with the enterostomal therapist and patient to include short-term and long-term goals. Provide the patient with literature and information according to his level of understanding. Take care not to overwhelm the patient with too much information.
3. Preparation for surgery—follow usual preoperative procedures and modify to meet individual needs.
   a. Follow low-residue diet to limited liquids to nothing by mouth in the prescribed time frame.
   b. Administer antimicrobial agents (neomycin, kanamycin) for bowel disinfection to reduce pathogenic bacterial flora.
   c. Give enemas or lavage for mechanical cleansing of intestinal tract.
   d. Maintain hydration by assisting with intravenous infusion and observing and recording urinary output.
   e. Prepare patient and assist in nasogastric intubation for decompression of intestinal tract.

B. *Postoperative Care*

(Also see p. 419 and below, and Health Education, p. 439.)

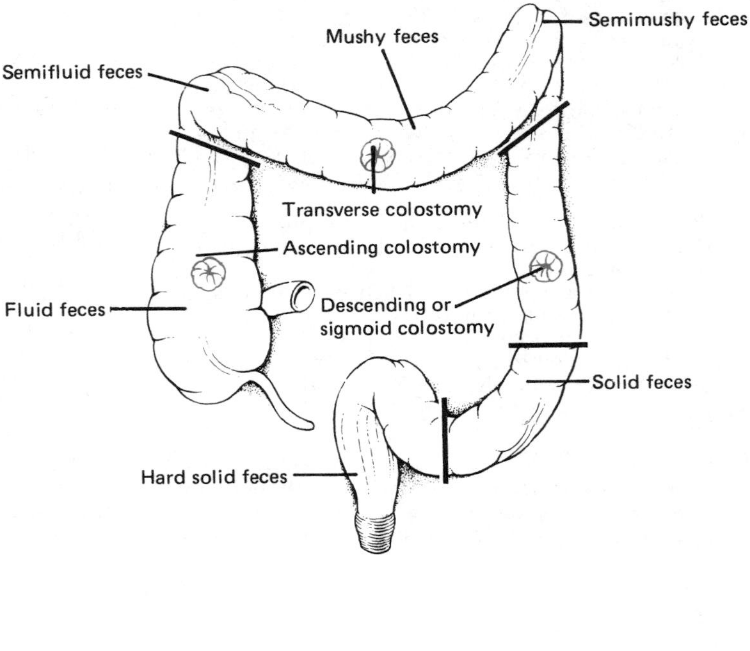

FIGURE 10-21. *A diagrammatic representation of the placement of permanent colostomies and the nature of the discharge at these sites.*

OBJECTIVES: to educate the patient toward gradually learning the care of his colostomy and to carry on with diminishing professional guidance.

Initial Care of the Colostomy

1. Apply a temporary plastic colostomy bag to control odors and soiling.
   a. Tactfully try to have patient look at his colostomy, and encourage him to participate in caring for it. Psychosocial skills and understanding are required. Evaluate learning readiness; never force independence.
2. Begin to irrigate when the immediate postoperative period is past and bowel function has resumed (usually 5th or 6th day) (see Guidelines, p. 440).
3. Utilize the treatment time of irrigating the colostomy as the learning time for the patient to begin to master the art of controlling his colostomy independently.
   a. Recognize that some patients are learning to control their colostomy without irrigation.
4. Although irrigation is widely used, recognize that there are some persons who cannot control the colostomy this way (i.e., the patient with an "irritable" colon, or unpredictable bowel movements). Also, because of the nature of the contents in various parts of the colon (Fig. 10-22), only colostomies in the descending or sigmoid colon can be expected to be controlled by irrigation. Ascending and transverse colostomies have outputs which are too frequent and too liquid to facilitate control.
5. Often the recognition of a bowel movement is when the patient's pouch or dressing is checked; for others, it may be the awareness of the escape of flatus or the contact of stool on the skin.
6. For some there is an awareness of motility which enables them to get to the bathroom in time for discharging stool into the toilet.
7. Frequency and number of movements vary from person to person.
8. Irrigations for most persons are done every other day.
9. The cone-tip is excellent to prevent insertion of a catheter into insensitive mucosa with risk of perforating the bowel wall. The cone-tip is plugged into the stoma for about 2.5 cm and permits irrigation without perforation or leakage.
10. Regulation is enhanced when there is systematic planning, balanced meals eaten at regular intervals, and a regular time for irrigation and evacuation.

Discharge Planning/Health Education

A. *See also Patient Education (Discharge from Hospital), p. 431.*

B. *Irrigation of Colostomy (see p. 440).*

C. *Skin Care*

1. One group of effective skin barriers is made of karaya gum. Karaya is available in powder form, discs, or rings which can be placed on excoriated peristomal skin (i.e., new skin can grow under them). Karaya paste and rings are excellent for preventing skin irritation immediately around the stoma.
2. Hypoallergenic skin shields include Stomahesive (Squibb), ReliaSeal (Davol), and Hollihesive (Hollister). These tend to deteriorate less quickly than the karaya washers and often can be worn in areas where there are creases and wrinkles.
   a. Stomahesive and Hollihesive can be used as 4″ × 4″ sheets or can be cut into washer size. Stomahesive and Hollihesive adhere well on weepy irritated skin and allow healing to occur.
   b. ReliaSeal comes as a round shield (3¾″ in diameter) or as an oval barrier; it is most effective on reddened peristomal skin but not on ulcerated, weepy skin.
3. Coverings over the stoma may be disposable pouch, gauze, facial tissue covered with petrolatum, Saran Wrap, or wax paper over a dressing. Hypoallergenic tape may be used; an Ace bandage is excellent for those allergic to adhesive.
4. For peristomal excoriation, corticosteroid aerosol sprays or nystatin powders are useful when used sparingly.
5. For allergic reactions, try other products until a compatible one is found; antacid suspensions are found practical for some patients.

C. *Odor Control*

1. Avoid foods known to cause odors—for example, onions, members of the cabbage family, eggs, fish, and beans.
2. Note that fecal odors are lessened with yogurt, cranberry juice, and buttermilk.
3. Odors can be controlled by taking one or two tablets of bismuth subcarbonate or bismuth subgallate at mealtimes and bedtime.

D. *Control of Gas*

1. Most gas is due to swallowed air (often taken in while chewing gum), highly spiced foods, and carbonated beverages, including beer.
2. Avoid gas-forming foods: beans, cabbage family, onions, radishes, cucumbers, and highly seasoned foods.

E. *Diet*

1. Avoid overeating and eating irregularly; chew food well.
2. Individualize the diet so that it is balanced and will not cause diarrhea and constipation. A daily diary is effective in determining what foods cause difficulty and can then be eliminated from the diet.
3. Note that fruits, fruit juices, and tomatoes may cause frequent bowel movements. Beer may be a laxative as well as a gas-producer.

F. *Enhanced Life-style*

1. According to the United Ostomy Association, approximately 10–12% of male ostomates suffer impairment of sexual function and potency; fortunately, this impairment is temporary in most cases. Male colostomates vary in degree of potency from full potency to complete impotence. Some patients take up to 2 years to regain potency.
2. An ostomy in a woman does not preclude a successful pregnancy; close medical care is required.
3. There is no contraindication to any form of travel, including horseback riding.
4. Participation in any type of sport is possible.
5. Showering is possible with or without the appliance.
6. Girdles, swim trunks, and pantyhose may all be worn, provided there is neither discomfort nor too much constriction.
7. Promote patient's acceptance of the colostomy by building up self-esteem; encourage the family to assist the patient during the period of adjustment.

8. Contact the community nurse who will serve as a liaison between hospital, physician, and home as a follow-up where the patient continues to adjust to the colostomy at home.
9. Inform the patient of the United Ostomy Association and enroll him in the local group so that he may obtain information and exchange ideas with other ostomates.
10. Provide the patient with literature, addresses, and phone numbers of the following organizations:
    Community Nursing Agencies.
    American Cancer Society.

a. Journal of the Colostomy/Ileostomy Rehabilitation Association, P.O. Box 121, Philadelphia, Pennsylvania 19105.
b. *Ostomy Quarterly.*—Official Publication of the United Ostomy Association. 2001 W. Beverly Boulevard, Los Angeles, CA 90057.
c. The United Ostomy Association also has available many excellent booklets.
d. Many manufacturers of ostomy supplies have free booklets available covering a wide variety of ostomy related topics.

GUIDELINES: Irrigating a Colostomy

Purposes
1. To empty the colon of its contents: fecal, gas, mucus.
2. To cleanse the lower intestinal tract.
3. To establish a regular pattern of evacuation so that normal life activities may be pursued.

Equipment
1. Reservoir for irrigating fluids: enema bag, irrigating can
2. Irrigating fluid: 500–1500 ml. lukewarm tap water or other solution if prescribed by physician
3. Tubing, connecting tubes, and clamp; preferable clamp—one that can be operated with one hand
4. Irrigating tip: soft rubber catheter—No. 22 or No. 24 with some type of shield to prevent backflow of irrigating solution (or soft rubber or plastic cone irrigating tip)
5. Irrigating sleeve or sheath: self-adhering (adhesive) or held in place with a belt (a plastic or rubber sheet can be used as a trough in place of a sheath)
6. Newspaper or plastic bag: to collect soiled dressings and disposable pouch
7. Toilet tissues and water-soluble lubricant

Procedure   *Preparatory Phase*
1. Select a suitable time, preferably after a meal, so that this hour fits into a patient's post-hospital pattern of activity. Irrigation should be done at the same time each day.
2. Hang irrigating reservoir with solution 45–50 cm. (18–20 inches) above stoma (shoulder height with patient seated).
3. Have patient sit in front of toilet commode on chair or on commode itself.
4. Remove dressings or pouch and place in bag.

NURSING ACTION	*RATIONALE/AMPLIFICATION*
IRRIGATION	
1. Apply irrigating sleeve or sheath to stoma. Place end in commode (Fig. 10-22).	1. Helps control odor and splashing. Allows feces and water to flow directly into commode.

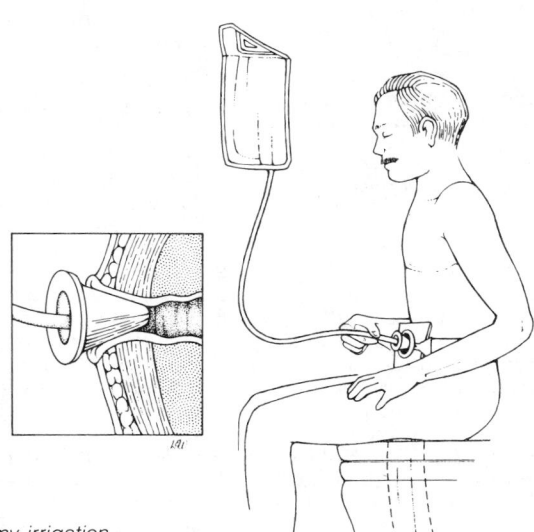

FIGURE 10-22. *Colostomy irrigation.*

	NURSING ACTION	**RATIONALE/AMPLIFICATION**

Procedure (cont.)

2. Allow some of solution to flow through tubing and catheter/cone.

3. Lubricate catheter/cone and gently insert into stoma. Insert catheter no more than 8 cm. (3 inches). Hold shield/cone gently, but firmly, against stoma to prevent backflow of water.

4. If catheter does not advance easily, allow water to flow slowly while advancing catheter. *NEVER FORCE CATHETER!*

5. Allow fluid to enter colon slowly. If cramping occurs, clamp off tubing and allow patient to rest before progressing. Water should flow in over a 5–10 minute period.

6. Hold shield/cone in place 10 seconds after water has been instilled, then gently remove.

7. Allow 10–15 minutes for most of return, then dry bottom of sleeve/sheath and attach it to top, or apply appropriate clamp to bottom of sleeve.

8. Leave sleeve/sheath in place about 20 minutes while patient gets up and moves around.

Follow-up Phase

1. Cleanse area with mild soap and water; pat dry.

2. Apply a karaya preparation or other peristomal skin barrier; replace colostomy dressing or pouch.

3. Clean equipment with soap and water; dry before storing in well-ventilated area.

2. To release air bubbles in the set-up so that air is not introduced into the colon, which would cause crampy pain.

3. These steps are necessary to prevent intestinal perforation.

4. Slow rate of flow helps relax bowel and facilitates passage of catheter.

5. Painful cramps are usually caused by too rapid flow or too much solution. 500 ml. is usually sufficient for initial postoperative irrigation. Volume may be increased with subsequent irrigations to 1000 or 1500 ml. as patient needs for effective results.

7. Most of water, feces, and flatus will be expelled in 10–15 minutes.

8. Ambulation stimulates peristalsis and completion of irrigation return.

1. Cleanliness and dryness will provide patient with hours of comfort.

2. Patient should use pouch until colostomy is sufficiently controlled. Karaya will protect skin from irritation.

3. This will control odor and prolong life of equipment.

ANORECTAL CONDITIONS AND TREATMENTS

PERIANAL ABSCESS; FISTULA IN ANO; FISSURE IN ANO

Condition	**Description**	**Management**
Perianal abscess	Localized infection in fatty tissue near rectum. Condition should raise suspicion of granulomatous bowel disease.	Incision and drainage (see Nursing Management, p. 442).
Fistula in Ano	Abnormal opening from the skin near the anus that winds tortuously into the anal canal. Because it is an infectious area, pus leaks outward. Condition should raise suspicion of granulomatous bowel disease.	1. Surgical identification of the path of a fistula. 2. Cutting fistula open followed by insertion of packing (see Nursing Management, p. 442).
Fissure in Ano	Longitudinal ulcer (a crack that does not heal in the anal canal) frequently associated with constipation, as well as excruciating pain and blood streaking on defecation.	1. Dilatation of anal sphincter. 2. Excision of fissure (see Nursing Management, p. 442).

HEMORRHOIDS

Hemorrhoids are varicose veins of the anal canal; *external* hemorrhoids appear outside the external sphincter, whereas *internal* hemorrhoids appear above the internal sphincter. When blood within the hemorrhoids becomes clotted and infected, the hemorrhoids are referred to as *thrombosed*.

Predisposing Factors

1. Pregnancy
2. Straining at stool
3. Chronic constipation
4. Prolonged sitting
5. Anal infection
6. Hereditary factor
7. Portal hypertension (cirrhosis)

Clinical Manifestations

1. Pruritus (itching)
2. Protrusion
3. Constipation
4. Bleeding during defecation
5. Infection or ulceration
6. Pain noted more in external hemorrhoids

Diagnostic Evaluation

1. History and visualization by external examination and the use of an anoscope or proctoscope.
2. Barium enema also should be performed, since hemorrhoids are often warning signs of more serious colonic lesions, which may be the actual source of observed rectal bleeding.

Treatment and Nursing Intervention

A. *Medical*

1. Patient should adhere to a low-roughage, high fiber diet to keep stool soft. Some authorities suggest a diet that includes 30 gm. miller's bran per day or replacing white bread with whole wheat.
2. Bowel habits should be regulated with nonirritating stool softeners (e.g., mineral oil or milk of magnesia) to keep stools soft.
3. Frequent hot sitz baths.
4. Insertion of soothing anal suppository 2–3 times daily; topical hydrocortisone foam is comforting.
5. Application of witch hazel compresses for comfort.
6. Control of itching by placement of a cotton pledget on folded soft tissue between the buttocks against the anus to absorb moisture.
7. Do not use topical anesthetics chronically on hemorrhoids or fissures as they often produce hypersensitivity (allergic) perianal skin rashes with severe itching.
8. If hemorrhoids are prolapsed and the patient is unable to reduce them himself, the nurse may have to reduce them manually:
   a. Apply cold compresses to anal area.
   b. Gently apply anesthetic ointment with a gloved finger.
   c. Very gently manipulate hemorrhoids back through rectal sphincter.
   d. Apply an anesthetic ointment on a dressing to rectal area.
9. Surgery may be indicated when the following conditions exist:
   a. Prolonged bleeding
   b. Disabling pain
   c. Intolerable itching
   d. General unrelieved discomfort

B. *Surgical*

1. Incision and removal of clot from acutely thrombosed hemorrhoid.
2. Excision of hemorrhoids includes the following procedures:
   a. Dilatation of rectal sphincter
   b. Ligation and excision of hemorrhoid under local or spinal anesthesia
   c. Insertion of drainage tube to permit escape of flatus and blood (Fig. 10-23)
   d. Application of Gelfoam or oxycel gauze to control bleeding if necessary
3. Dilatation—forced dilatation of the anal canal and lower rectum under general anesthesia is another advocated treatment.
   This procedure is not advocated for patients whose main complaints are prolapse or incontinence. It also is not recommended for aging patients with weak sphincters.
4. Cryodestruction—freezing of hemorrhoids.
   It is claimed to be painless; some patients have a foul-smelling discharge for about a week following cryosurgery.
5. Barron ligation with a rubber band is considered "ideal" treatment by many. (Fig. 10-23)
   a. A large anoscope is used; the apex of the internal hemorrhoid is grasped and drawn through a double-sleeved cylinder.
   b. An elastic band is loaded on the inner cylinder and released by a trigger device so that the band encircles the base of the hemorrhoid.
   c. After a period of time, the hemorrhoid sloughs away.

PILONIDAL CYST

A *pilonidal cyst* is a congenital cyst located in the intergluteal cleft on the posterior surface of the lower sacrum; hair frequently protrudes from sinus openings giving the cyst its name—pilonidal (a nest of hair).

Clinical Manifestations

1. Rarely produces symptoms until early adult life when infection produces drainage followed by the development of an abscess.
2. Trauma may be a factor in cyst development.

Treatment

1. Antibiotics are administered.
2. When abscess develops, incision and drainage is indicated.
3. Radical dissection indicated when abscesses recur or secondary sinus infection develops.
4. Healing takes place by granulation, since defect may be too large to heal with suturing.

NURSING OBJECTIVES AND MANAGEMENT IN CARING FOR PATIENTS WITH RECTAL PROBLEMS

Preoperative Care

A. *To recognize the psychosocial concerns of the patient with a rectal problem.*

1. Be an understanding and concerned listener when this patient relates problems of a personal nature.
2. Insure and respect his privacy when attending to personal hygiene, examinations, and treatments.
3. Do not minimize complaints of discomfort.

B. *To assess nature of the rectal problems in order to assist physician in approaching an accurate diagnosis.*

1. Observe the stool for evidence of bleeding. Is stool mixed or coated with blood?

2. Determine presence of pain during and after evacuation. Is there associated abdominal pain? How long does it last?
3. Describe the problem in the patient's words when recording.
4. Note presence of a discharge. Is it purulent, bloody?

Postoperative Care

A. *To promote comfort of patient and healing of wound.*
1. Be gentle in changing dressings, shaving, irrigating or administering perineal care.

2. Use petrolatum gauze in protecting edges of wounds (ex. following incision and drainage of ischiorectal abscess, excision of pilonidal sinus) to prevent crusting and the dressings from sticking to wound.
3. Provide sitz baths when recommended; adjust temperature of solution and provide a comfortable position for the patient.
4. Use caution in applying analgesic or anesthetic ointments since this often leads to secondary skin rashes from allergy.

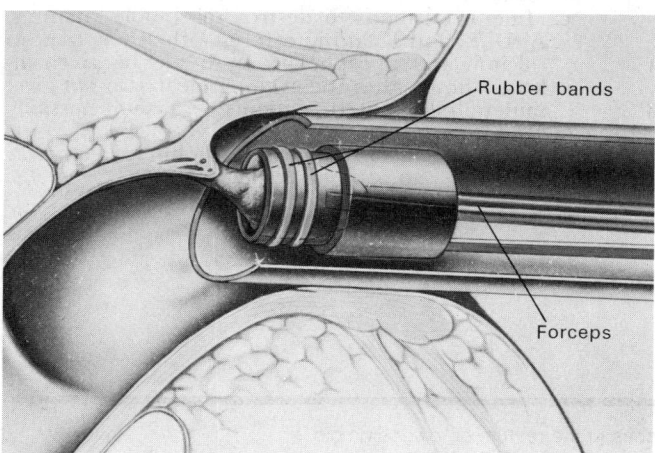

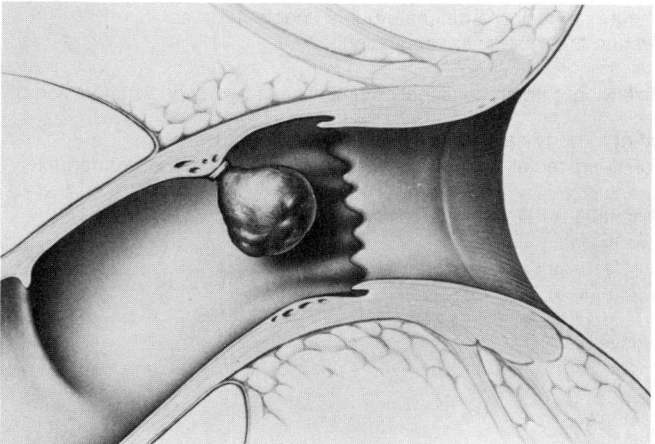

FIGURE 10-23. *Hemorrhoidectomy, using the Barron ligation technique. (Top) The hemorrhoid is grasped with forceps and pulled into a rubber-band-loaded ligator. (Bottom) Elastic ligature is triggered from ligator onto base of internal hemorrhoid. (Kratzer GL. Manual on the Office Management of Colon and Rectal Diseases. Kenilworth, NJ, Reed and Carnrick)*

5. Keep the perineal area clean to minimize or eliminate infection; presence of *E. coli* demands meticulous cleanliness to prevent infection and promote healing.
6. Change patient's position from side to side to prevent added discomfort of pressure areas; use air ring properly inflated—not too full.
7. Prevent constipation by proper attention to diet needs of patient; give mineral oil or mild cathartic only as prescribed; use stool softeners.
8. Encourage voluntary voiding to avoid catheterization; this may be facilitated by getting patient out of bed.
9. Observe vital signs and dressings for evidence of hemorrhage, particularly following hemorrhoidectomy.
10. Daily rectal sphincter dilatation may be needed to relieve pain from spasm, to assure granulation of incisional wounds from bottom out, and to prevent postoperative stricture.

Health Education

(To Prepare Patient for Posthospital Convalescence)
1. Instruct patient on perianal hygiene to minimize the possibility of infection; avoid rubbing area with toilet tissue; instead, pat the area dry.
2. Apply wet dressings (equal parts of witch hazel and water) to relieve edema.
3. Advise patient regarding the effect of diet on stool formation; plant fibers of leafy vegetables and the roughage of bran flakes, whole grains, and whole wheat bread add roughage to the diet to form cellulose. Cellulose absorbs water, swells, and softens stool, thereby stimulating peristalsis and aiding in intestinal elimination. Encourage patient to eat fresh fruits, fruit juice, and fresh vegetables except for seeds, skins, corn, and nuts.
4. Avoid cathartics so that stool is formed rather than being soft or liquid.
5. Recommend hot stiz baths or hot compresses to relieve painful sphincter spasm.
6. Suggest adequate fluid intake and daily exercise to prevent constipation; encourage patient to have a regular time each day for having a bowel movement.
7. Stool softeners are often given until good bowel habits are established.
   a. "Wetting agents" contain dioctyl sodium sulfosuccinate, a substance that penetrates, moistens, and softens hard dry stool.
   b. "Bulk producers" such as psyllium and agar preparations absorb water, add bulk, and add moisture to stool.
   c. Mineral oil tends to destroy oil-soluble vitamins A, D, E, and K and interferes with absorption of calcium and phosphorus. It should be given at least 3 hours after the evening meal. (Do not give mineral oil to elderly patients because of possible aspiration pneumonia.)
8. Administer enemas only when absolutely necessary; rectal suppositories may be helpful.

GUIDELINES: Removal of Fecal Impaction

A *fecal impaction* is the retention of hardened feces in the rectum or lower sigmoid.

Manifestations and Occurrence

1. The patient may say he is constipated; often he has a desire to defecate but is unable to do so.
2. Diarrhea or liquid fecal seepage may occur around the obstructing impaction.
3. The patient may complain of rectal pain.
4. This condition may occur in elderly persons following chronic constipation, insufficient hydration, or ingestion of fibrous foods.
5. Orthopedic patients who have been in traction or in body casts may develop an impaction.
6. Occasionally, impaction occurs in patients following rectal surgery or when barium has not been adequately removed following radiologic examination.
7. Impaction is also common in patients with neurologic or psychotic disorders.

Purpose of Fecal Disimpaction

To remove hardened feces in the rectum or lower sigmoid.

Equipment Clean (not necessarily sterile) rubber or plastic glove
Water-soluble lubricant
Bedpan
Plastic or rubber sheet with cloth protection
Soap, water, washcloth

Procedure

NURSING ACTION	RATIONALE/AMPLIFICATION
Preparatory Phase	
1. Explain procedure to patient.	
2. Position patient on left side with upper knee flexed.	2. To permit access to rectum and lower sigmoid.

Procedure (cont.)

NURSING ACTION	RATIONALE/AMPLIFICATION
3. Drape patient and place protecting pad under buttocks.	3. To prevent chilling and undue exposure.
4. Place bedpan in a convenient place.	4. To serve as receptacle.
5. Put on glove and lubricate index finger generously (some prefer the middle finger because it is longer).	

Performance Phase (Fig. 10-24)

1. Insert gloved finger *gently* into rectum until impaction is felt.	1. This stimulation may increase peristalsis.

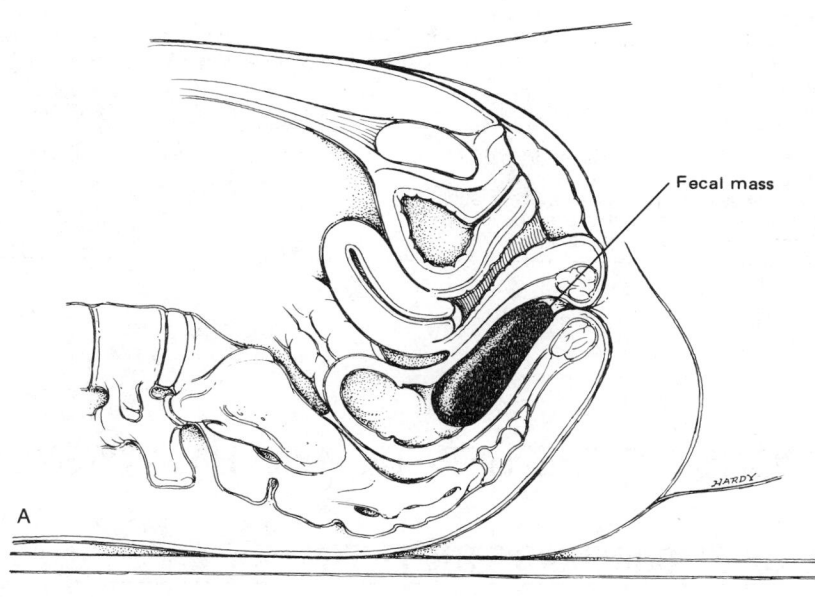

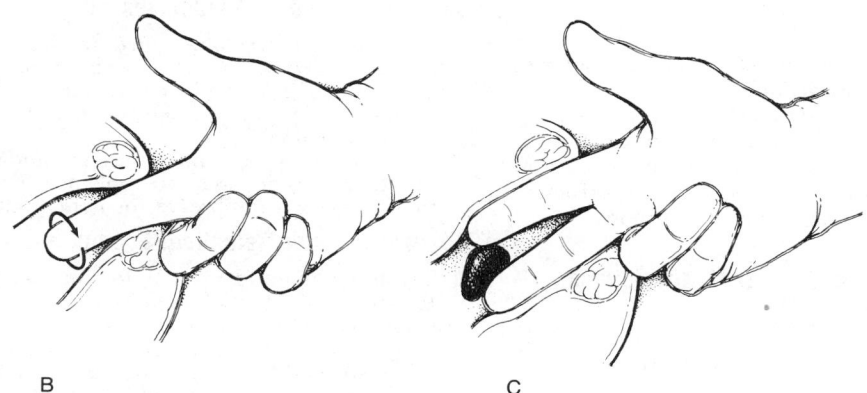

FIGURE 10-24. *Fecal Impaction. A. Note shaded area inside rectal sphincter—this indicates fecal impaction. B. By gently stimulating the rectal wall with a gloved index finger, and using a circular motion, it is possible to loosen fecal material. C. It may be necessary to gently insert 2 fingers in an attempt to crush the fecal mass. A scissor-like motion is used.*

2. *Gently* remove or break fecal material within reach and deposit in bedpan; work finger around and into mass to break it up if possible.	2. The emphasis is on *gentleness*, since this may be painful.
3. Gently stimulate rectal sphincter by making a circular motion once or twice.	3. This may stimulate peristalsis and relax the sphincter.

GUIDELINES: Removal of Fecal Impaction (cont.)

Procedure (cont.)

NURSING ACTION	RATIONALE/AMPLIFICATION
4. If step 3 does not result in removal of the impaction, it may be necessary to *gently* insert the middle and index finger and attempt to break up the mass by a scissorlike movement of the fingers. Repeat steps 2 or 4 until all easily reachable fecal masses are removed.	4. Greater leverage is afforded, and the mass may be more easily broken.
5. Note any bleeding or pain; observe patient for shortness of breath or perspiration.	5. Should any of these responses occur, stop the procedure.

Follow-up Phase

1. Gently wash and dry the rectal area; make the patient comfortable and have him rest.	1. Drying the area prevents skin excoriation and promotes comfort.
2. Note bedpan contents and then empty.	
3. Record color, consistency, and odor of stool.	3. These characteristics may provide clues as to the nature of the problem.
4. Plan health instruction measures in an effort to prevent a recurrence. Explore nutritional and fluid needs of the patient; determine activity level and encourage suitable exercises to promote adequate elimination.	4. Investigate the possibility of using stool softeners; suggest periodic use of Fleet's enema.

3   CONDITIONS OF THE HEPATIC AND BILIARY SYSTEM

MANIFESTATIONS OF DISORDERS OF THE LIVER

Pathophysiology

1. Viral infections and the effects of toxins may lead to hepatocellular dysfunction.
2. Chronic alcohol consumption, along with malnutrition, may cause toxic liver damage (cirrhosis).
3 Impairment of liver function may occur when flow of bile into the intestine is impeded (i.e., obstruction of the biliary tract by gallstones or a tumor).

General Assessment and Clinical Manifestations which may indicate Liver Failure

(Also see p. 37, Physical Assessment of Liver)

Jaundice (Icterus)

The condition of the body when all tissues including the sclerae and skin assume a yellow or greenish-yellow tinge due to an increased concentration of bilirubin. (See p. 449 for types of jaundice.)
1. Normal bilirubin concentration in blood is 0.1–1.0 mg./100 ml. of blood.
2. Over 3.0 mg/100 ml. of blood, jaundice can be detected.

Abnormal Bleeding Tendencies

1. Because of blood coagulation defects, gastrointestinal hemorrhage may occur as well as bleeding gums, blood in urine, rectal bleeding, tarry stool.
2. Minor skin trauma may produce ecchymosis (black and blue marks).
3. Following all types of intramuscular and intravenous injections, it is necessary to apply pressure for longer than usual and to observe for hematoma.

Excessive Water Retention, Edema, and Ascites

1. Tissue edema and intra-abdominal fluid are manifestations of intense sodium and water retention combined with potassium excretion.
2. Hypoproteinemia, iron-decreased hepatic synthesis, and disturbed kidney function are also instrumental in causing fluid retention.

Impairment of Central and Peripheral Nervous System

1. Pyridoxine deficiency can result in nervous irritability and in convulsive seizures in children.
2. Thiamine deficiency may lead to polyneuritis and Wernicke-Korsakoff psychosis.
3. Stupor, somnolence, and confusion from failure to metabolize ammonia arriving from intestine in portal venous system, and from impaired metabolism of sedative drugs.

DIAGNOSTIC EVALUATION OF LIVER DISEASE

LIVER DIAGNOSTIC STUDIES

Test and Purpose	Normal	Clinical and Nursing Significance
Bile Formation and Secretion		
1. *Serum bilirubin (van den Bergh reaction)* Measures bilirubin in the blood; this determines the ability of the liver to take up conjugate and excrete bilirubin. Bilirubin is a product of the breakdown of hemoglobin.		
Direct (conjugated)—soluble in water	0.1–0.2 mg./dl.	Abnormal in biliary and liver disease causing jaundice clinically.
Indirect (unconjugated)—insoluble in water	0.1–0.8 mg./dl.	Abnormal in hemolysis and in functional disorders of uptake or conjugation.
Total serum bilirubin	0.1–1.0 mg./dl.	
2. *Urine bilirubin* Not normally found in urine, but if direct serum bilirubin is elevated, some spills into urine.	None	Mahogany-colored urine; when specimen is shaken, yellow tint to foam can be observed. Confirm with Ictotest tablet or Dipstick. If phenazo-pyridine (Pyridium) is being taken, there may be a false positive bilirubin. (Mark lab slip if this medication is being taken.)
3. *Urobilinogen* Formed in small intestine by action of bacteria on bilirubin. Related to amount of bilirubin excreted into bile.	Urine urobilinogen up to 1–4 mg./ 24 hr. Fecal urobilinogen 40–280 mg./24 hr.	Urine specimen is collected over 2-hr. period after lunch. Place specimen in dark brown container and send it to lab immediately to prevent decomposition. If patient is receiving antimicrobials, mark lab slip to this effect since production of urobilinogen can be falsely reduced.
Protein Studies		
1. *Albumin and globulin measurement* Is of greater significance than total protein measurement.		As one increases, the other decreases; hence,
Albumin—produced by liver cells.	3.5–5.5 gm./dl	Albumin ↓ cirrhosis chronic hepatitis
Globulin—produced in lymph nodes, spleen, and bone marrow and Kupffer cells of liver.	1.5–3.0 gm./dl.	Globulin ↑ cirrhosis chronic obstructive jaundice viral hepatitis.
Total serum protein	6.0–8.0 mg./dl.	
2. *Prothrombin time (PT)* Prothrombin and other clotting factors are manufactured in the liver; its rate is influenced by the supply of vitamin K.	60–100% of control	Prothrombin time may be prolonged in liver disease, in which case it will not return to normal with vitamin K. It may also be prolonged in malabsorption of fat and fat-soluble vitamins, in which case it will not return to normal with vitamin K.
Fat Metabolism		
1. *Cholesterol* It is possible to measure lipid metabolism by determining serum cholesterol levels.	150–270 mg./100 ml. Esters = 60% of total	Serum cholesterol level is decreased in parenchymal liver disease. Serum lipid level is increased in biliary obstruction.

DIAGNOSTIC EVALUATION OF LIVER DISEASE (cont.)

LIVER DIAGNOSTIC STUDIES

Test and Purpose	Normal	Clinical and Nursing Significance
Liver Detoxification *Serum alkaline phosphatase* Since bile disposes this enzyme, any impairment of liver cell excretory function will cause an elevation. In cholestasis or obstruction, increased synthesis of enzyme causes very high levels in blood.	Varies with method: 2–5 Bodansky units, 30–85 I.U./ml.	*Abnormalities:* The level is elevated to more than 3 times normal in obstructive jaundice, intrahepatic cholestasis, liver metastasis or granulomas. Also elevated in osteoblastic diseases, Paget's disease, and hyperparathyroidism.
Enzyme Production Transaminase (SGOT) (Aspartate aminotransferase).	7–40 mU./ml.	An elevation in these enzymes indicates liver cell damage.
Transaminase (SGPT) (Alanine aminotransferase).	10–40 mU./ml.	**NOTE:** Opiates may also cause a rise in SGOT and SGPT. Aspirin may cause an increase or decrease in SGOT and SGPT.

Other "Liver Profile" Tests
GGT (gamma glutamyl transpeptidase), Total Protein, Albumin.
(See Appendix for laboratory values)
Bile acids radioimmunoassay are replacing BSP tests.

GUIDELINES: Assisting with Liver Biopsy

Liver biopsy is the sampling of liver tissue by needle aspiration.

Purpose To establish a diagnosis of liver disease by histologic study of liver tissue.

Equipment Sterile aspiration syringe and biopsy needle (Silverman)
Local anesthetic
Skin antiseptics, sterile fenestrated towel, gloves
Glass slides, specimen bottles containing fixative and/or test tubes

Procedure **Preparatory Phase**

1. Verify that the patient has had prothrombin tests and blood typing by checking the chart.
2. Determine availability of compatible blood inasmuch as these patients often have clotting defects.
3. Determine and record patient's pulse, respiration, arterial pressure and prothrombin time immediately before the biopsy in order to have a base line of comparison with the postbiopsy condition of the patient.
4. Explain the steps of this procedure to the patient to reduce his concerns and gain his cooperation.

NURSING ACTION	RATIONALE/AMPLIFICATION
Performance Phase	
1. Place patient flat in bed with right arm under head and face turned left.	
2. Expose the upper abdomen in readiness for skin disinfection and local anesthetic injection.	2. For optimum exposure and comfort of patient the right hypochondriac region is treated as a surgical area to minimize danger of infection.
3. Determine biopsy site—one interspace below upper border of liver dullness 2 cm. behind anterior axillary line.	
4. Physician anesthetizes the skin, intercostal tissues, and liver capsule with local anesthetic.	4. To promote local comfort.
5. Physician introduces biopsy needle into intercostal tissues but not into liver.	5. To prevent tearing of diaphragm of liver.
6. Instruct patient to inhale and exhale deeply 3 or 4 times, then to exhale and hold his breath.	6. Holding one's breath immobilizes the chest wall and diaphragm; this helps to prevent the needle from tearing the diaphragm or the liver.

Procedure (cont.)	NURSING ACTION	RATIONALE/AMPLIFICATION
	7. The physician rapidly introduces biopsy needle into the liver, aspirates tissue, and withdraws.	
	8. As soon as needle is withdrawn, inform patient to resume normal breathing.	8. Actual insertion and withdrawal of needle takes about 10 seconds.
	Follow-up Phase	
	1. Following biopsy, assist the patient to turn on his right side, place a pillow under his lower rib cage and advise him to remain quiet for several hours.	1. Compressing the liver against the chest wall near the biopsy site, reduces the possibility of bleeding.
	2. Determine and record the patient's pulse and respiratory rates and his blood pressure at frequent intervals until they stabilize.	2. The nurse needs to be aware of the possible complications of liver biopsy; hemorrhage and bile peritonitis. Anticipatory nursing includes early recognition of symptoms.
	3. Recognize that an increasing pulse and decreasing blood pressure may be indicative of hemorrhage; note any indication of pain.	

JAUNDICE

Hemolytic Jaundice

Hemolytic jaundice is attributable to abnormally high concentration of bilirubin in blood exceeding the capacity of normal liver cells to excrete it.
1. Encountered in patients with hemolytic transfusion reactions, hereditary spherocytosis, autoimmune hemolytic anemia, erythroblastosis fetalis, and other hemolytic disorders.
2. Bilirubin in the blood is unconjugated (indirect-reacting).
3. In feces and urine, urobilinogen is increased; urine is free of bilirubin.
4. Prolonged jaundice leads to formation of "pigment stones" in gallbladder. Extremely severe jaundice (unconjugated bilirubin elevated: 20–25 mg./100 ml.) causes brain-stem damage in neonates.

Hepatocellular Jaundice

Hepatocellular jaundice is due to an inability of diseased liver cells to clear the normal amount of bilirubin from the blood.

A. *Causes*

1. Infection—hepatitis A, hepatitis B, hepatitis nonA nonB
2. Drug or chemical toxicity—carbon tetrachloride, chloroform, phosphorus, arsenicals, ethanol, halothane, isoniazid, acetaminophen, mushroom poisoning.

B. *Clinical Manifestations*

1. Mildly or severely ill patient.
2. Lack of appetite, nausea, loss of vigor and strength, weight loss.
3. Elevated transaminase (SGOT) (aspartate aminotransferase) and (SGPT) (alanine aminotransferase)—2 enzymes that are liberated with cellular necrosis
4. Rise in BSP (bromsulphalein) and bilirubin. Alkaline phosphatase mildly elevated.
5. Abnormal serum proteins in prolonged illness; prothrombin time increased.
6. Headache and chills possible in infectious condition.
7. Bile acids radioimmunoassay are replacing BSP tests.

Cholestatic Jaundice

A. *Causes*

1. Extrahepatic obstruction—blockage of bile ducts by gallstone(s), tumor(s), an inflammatory process, or an enlarged pancreas pressing on the duct.
2. Intrahepatic cholestasis—caused by injury to bile canaliculi or blockage of intrahepatic ducts due to tumors or granulomas.
    Certain drugs may cause this, e.g., "cholestatic" agents: phenothiazine derivatives (Thorazine), perphenazine (Trilafon), sulfonamides, tolbutamide (Orinase) and other antidiabetic drugs, thiouracil, and para-aminobenzoic acid (PABA).

B. *Clinical Manifestations*

Due to damming back of bile, it is reabsorbed by blood. The following responses may be noted:
1. Jaundice of skin and sclerae
2. Deep orange-colored urine
3. White or clay-colored stools
4. Itchy skin and dyspepsia due to impaired bile acid excretion
5. SGOT and SGPT rise only moderately.
6. Bilirubin and BSP are increased.
7. Alkaline phosphatase is strikingly elevated.
8. Cholesterol is elevated.

Objectives of Nursing Management

A. *To control pruritus and make the patient more comfortable.*

1. Use starch or baking soda baths, soothing lotions such as calamine.
2. Administer antihistamines, tranquilizers, and sedatives if prescribed.
3. Administer cholestyramine (Cuemid or Questran) to deplete retained acids which cause itching.
4. Assist patient in reducing the strong tendency to scratch his skin:
    a. Resort to activities which can divert his attention.
    b. Keep nails trimmed and clean.
    c. Avoid excessive top bedding.
    d. Give soothing massages particularly at night in preparing patient for sleep since this is an especially likely time to scratch.

e. Provide clean white gloves to use at night if he scratches subconsciously.

B. *To support the patient psychologically.*

1. Instruct staff to avoid remarks or facial expressions which the patient can interpret as referring to his unusual appearance.

2. Notify visitors in a like manner to avoid embarrassing the patient.
3. Encourage patient to talk about his problems; listen to his expressions of concern.
4. Place patient's bed in a position where he cannot look at himself in a mirror.

HEPATITIS

Hepatitis is an inflammation of the liver caused by viruses.

Significance

1. From a community health point of view one is concerned with ease of disease transmission and morbidity.
2. From a socioeconomic point of view one is concerned with prolonged loss of time from school and employment.

Preventive Measures

1. Stress importance of proper public and home sanitation.
2. Recognize merits of conscientious surveillance in the proper and safe preparation and dispensation of food.
3. Promote effective health supervision in schools, dormitories, and camps.
4. Initiate and support health education programs.

Types of Hepatitis

1. Hepatitis A virus; HAV, infectious hepatitis, IH virus, short-incubation hepatitis.
2. Hepatitis B virus; HBV, serum hepatitis, SH virus, homologous serum hepatitis, long-incubation hepatitis.
3. Hepatitis nonA nonB; NANB
   Features of HAV, HBV, and NANB hepatitis are summarized in Table 10-4.

Diagnostic Evaluation

1. By radioimmunoassay test, the presence of hepatitis B antigen (HB_sAg) is detected in individuals who have serum hepatitis.
2. By detection of the presence of HB_sAg, hepatitis can be confirmed before the patient becomes clinically ill.
3. SGPT levels also rise 1–2 weeks before clinical jaundice occurs.

TYPE A HEPATITIS (HAV)

Epidemiology

1. HAV is probably an RNA virus of the enterovirus family.
2. Mode of transmission
   a. Fecal–oral route; respiratory route possible
   b. Poor sanitation; person-to-person (epidemic-type prevalent in camps)
   c. Contaminated food, milk, polluted water, or shellfish
   d. Blood transfusion rarely
3. Incubation: 3–7 weeks; average 4 weeks
4. Occurrence
   a. Worldwide
   b. Usually children and young adults

Assessment and Clinical Manifestations

1. Preicteric phase (prior to period of jaundice)
   a. Most patients are anicteric and symptomless.
   b. Initial symptoms: headache, fatigue, anorexia, fever, flu-like upper respiratory infection.
2. Icteric phase: jaundice, dark urine, vague epigastric symptoms, anorexia, flatulence.
   When jaundice reaches its peak, symptoms tend to subside. Liver is tender and perhaps enlarged.

Nursing Management

1. Provide bed rest and a nutritious dietary regime.
2. Accept the challenge of enticing the patient to eat; although he may resist eating, eventually he will recover his appetite.

TYPE B HEPATITIS (HBV)

Hepatitis B virus is a double-shelled particle containing DNA.

Epidemiology

1. Causative agent—This particle is composed of:
   a. antigenic material in an outer coat—hepatitis B surface antigen (HB_sAg)
   b. antigenic material in an inner coat–hepatitis B core antigen (HB_cAg)
   c. an independent protein circulating in the blood—HB_eAg
2. Antibody—Each antigen elicits its specific antibody:
   a. anti-HB_s (produced early after hepatitis B infection)
   b. anti-HB_c (noted later in convalescence)
   c. anti-HB_e (noted later in convalescence)
3. Significance:
   a. HB_sAg—may be detected transiently in blood of 80–90% of infected persons; may be noted in blood for months and years.
   b. HB_cAg—cannot be detected in blood.
   c. HB_eAg—if absent, patient is an asymptomatic carrier.
   d. HB_eAg—if present, patient may have chronic hepatitis and may be more infectious.
4. Mode of transmission:
   a. Oral–oral via saliva (i.e., mother to child via breast feeding)
   b. Parenterally, or by intimate contact with carriers. Susceptible persons are general surgeons, clinical laboratory workers, oral surgeons, nurses, respiratory therapists.
   c. Male homosexuals
   d. Blood, saliva, semen, vaginal secretions
5. Incubation—2–5 months
6. Occurrence—affects all ages but mostly young adults; worldwide

TABLE 10-4. QUICK SUMMARY OF HEPATITIS

	Hepatitis A Virus (HAV)	Hepatitis B Virus (HBV)	NonA/NonB Hepatitis Virus (NANBH)
Other Names	Type A hepatitis, infectious or epidemic hepatitis; IH virus	Type B hepatitis, serum hepatitis, SH virus, Dane particle	Hepatitis "C", "D"; Type C
Epidemiology			
Cause	Hepatitis A virus	Hepatitis B virus	Another virus
Method of transmission	Fecal-oral; poor sanitation Person-to-person Waterborne, foodborne—shellfish Rarely, if at all, by blood transfusion	Parenterally, or by intimate contact with carriers or those with acute disease; male homosexuals. Vertical transmission from mothers to babies. Contaminated instruments, syringes, needles; renal dialysis*	Transfusion association Personnel in renal transplant and dialysis units Parenteral drug abusers Blood transfusion products Institutions with long-term residents*
Source of virus/antigen	Blood, feces; saliva, occasionally; urine suspected	Blood Saliva Semen, vaginal secretions	Appears to be blood-borne
Distribution by age	Young adults (15–29) and middle-aged who have escaped childhood infection	Affects all ages, but mostly young adults	Same as HBV
Incubation period	3–5 weeks Mean: 30 days	2–5 months Mean: 90 days	Variable: 14–115 days Mean: 50 days
Occurrence	Worldwide	Worldwide	Worldwide Accounts for 20% of sporadic cases
Antibody	Anti-HAV Present in convalescent sera and immune serumglobulin (ISB)	Anti-HB$_c$ (core antigen) Anti-HB$_s$ (surface antigen)	—
Immunity	Homologous	Homologous	—
Severity	Most anicteric and asymptomatic	More severe than HA*	Wide spectrum of severity, resembling HA or HB. Often prolonged illness—months. May progress to chronic hepatitis.*
Nature of Disease			
Signs and Symptoms	May occur with or without symptoms: flulike illness Preicteric phase: Headache, malaise, fatigue, anorexia, lassitude, fever Icteric phase: Dark urine, scleral icterus, jaundice, liver tenderness, and perhaps enlargement	May occur without symptoms 1,000 IU/liter-serum transaminase level May develop antibodies to virus Similar to HAV, but more severe Fever and respiratory symptoms rare, but may have arthralgias, rash	Similar to HBV Less severe and anicteric
Diagnosis and method	Elevated serum transaminase Complement fixation rate Radioimmunoassay	Check serum for HB$_s$Ag, HB$_e$Ag, anti-HB$_c$, in absence of anti-HB$_s$ Elevated serum transaminase Radioimmunoassay—hemagglutination	(Obtainable as a panel)
Severity	Usually mild Fatality rate 0–1%	Variable, may be severe Fatality rate varies: 1–10%	—
Specific treatment	Adequate fluids, rest, nutrition	Same as HAV In research: vaccine antiviral chemotherapy to eliminate chronic HBV carrier state (being tested)	—
Prevention	Good sanitation Proper personal hygiene Effective sterilization procedures Careful screening of food handlers Immune Serum Globulin (ISG) given within a few days of exposure	Specific hepatitis B immune globulin (HBIG) probably useful after exposure by ingestion, inoculation, or splash involving hepatitis B surface antigen (HB$_s$Ag)	Mandatory screening of blood donors: 1) for HB$_s$Ag, 20% 2) for NonA NonB, 80%

* Probably the same, for HBV and NANBH, recent intensive research suggests.

Assessment and Clinical Manifestations

1. Resembles hepatitis A clinically.
2. Symptoms insidious and variable.
3. Arthralgias and rashes may be observed; fever and respiratory symptoms are rare.
4. Jaundice may or may not be present.
5. Anorexia, abdominal pain, generalized ailing, malaise may be noted.

Treatment and Nursing Management

1. Provide adequate fluids, nutrition, and bed rest.
2. Administer alkalies, belladonna, and antiemetics if these agents are required to control dyspepsia and malaise.
3. A newly available gamma globulin with a high titer of anti HB$_s$ seems to reduce severity of hepatitis following needle-stick exposure or contact.

4. Recognize that recovery and convalescence are slow and prolonged, sometimes taking 3–4 months; provide psychosocial stimulation.
5. Hepatitis B vaccine is being tested and should soon become available.

HEPATITIS nonA/nonB

This type of hepatitis is a viral infection that at present does not have an identified agent or antigenic markers.

Epidemiology

1. Over 80% of post-transfusion hepatitis fall into this category
2. Mode of transmission
   a. Associated with blood transfusions
   b. Personnel in renal dialysis units
   c. Parenteral drug abusers
   d. Appears to be blood-borne
3. Incubation—2 months
4. Occurrence—same as Hepatitis B

Assessment and Clinical Manifestations

1. Same as hepatitis B; less severe and anicteric

Treatment and Nursing Management

(Similar to that for Hepatitis B)
1. NonA/nonB hepatitis waxes and wanes over many months. There is probably a chronic carrier state.
2. Gamma globulin significantly reduces incidence of

this hepatitis and reduces the incidence of chronic active liver disease.

Preventive Measures and Health Education

Hepatitis A

Encourage optimum sanitation practices.

Instruct patient to practice good personal hygiene.

Employ proper safeguards to prevent use of blood and its components from infected donors.

Screen food handlers carefully.

Practice safe preparation and serving of food.

Administer Immune Serum Globulin (ISG) intramuscularly within a few days of exposure.

Use disposable needles and syringes; dispose of these carefully.

Wear gloves when handling bedpans and fecal contaminated linens.

Hepatitis B—Hepatitis nonA/nonB

Reject blood donors who have had serum hepatitis.

Instruct patient to maintain a 6-month interval of time since last serving as a donor.

Transfuse a patient only when justified.

Use blood substitutes when feasible.

Use disposable needles and syringes; dispose of these carefully.

Use hyperimmune globulin.

Administer Hepatitis B vaccine.

HEPATIC COMA/HEPATIC ENCEPHALOPATHY

Two Major Types

1. Fulminant—Due to acute massive liver cell necrosis, usually in previously healthy liver. Mortality in adults is 50–60%, but it is lower in younger age groups.
2. Subacute—Due to acute metabolic insult in a cirrhotic patient with borderline compensation of hepatic function. Mortality is only 10–20% and usually reversible if the precipitating cause is withdrawn (see below).

Causes

1. Incomplete metabolism of nitrogenous compounds by the diseased liver—manifestation of profound liver failure.
2. Biochemical abnormalities responsible are not known; however, the accumulation of significant amounts of nitrogenous substances, particularly ammonia, in the blood are believed to be highly suspect.
3. Shunting of portal blood that contains ammonia and other bacterial metabolites of protein around the liver.

Precipitating Factors

1. Progressive hepatocellular diseases are not associated with any acute irritation of the liver.
2. Increased sources of ammonia in the blood; azotemia, high protein diet, gastrointestinal bleeding, following administration of ammonium chloride, thiazides.
3. Infections, paracentesis, acute alcoholism, hypoten-

sion, shock, general anesthesia, minor surgery, hypokalemia, alkalosis, administration of sedatives, or narcotics.
4. Portacaval shunts, especially if protein is not restricted postoperatively in the diet.

Clinical Manifestations

Five stages:
1. Minor mental aberrations—patient slightly confused, untidy, and displaying inappropriate behavior and defective abstract thinking.
2. Motor disturbance—coarse or "flapping" tremor *asterixis* (especially of hands), hyper-reflexia.
3. Progression to gross disturbances of consciousness: somnolence or stupor, hepatic encephalopathy (HE).
4. Complete disorientation to time and place; eventual coma.
5. Decerebrate rigidity, hypoventilation → apnea.

Altered Physiology

A. *Problems*

1. Disruption of enzymatic function in liver cells, muscle, and brain.
2. Failure of liver cells to detoxify the ammonia (by converting it to urea).
3. Accumulation of sympathomimetic amines (false neurotransmitters) from abnormal metabolism of aromatic amino acids.

B. *Sources of Ammonia.* It comes from bloodstream as a result of the following:

1. Its absorption from the *gastrointestinal tract* (largest source)
   Enzymatic and bacterial digestion of ingested protein and of urea passing from blood into the gastrointestinal tract increases blood ammonia
   a. Increases result from
      (1) Gastrointestinal bleeding
      (2) High protein diet
      (3) Ingestion of ammonium salts (diuretic: ammonium chloride)
      (4) Bacterial overgrowth in small bowel (infection)
      (5) Uremia
   b. Decreases result from
      (1) Elimination of protein from diet.
      (2) Intestinal antibiotics—neomycin, kanamycin, chlortetracycline.
2. Its production by metabolizing *kidney* tissue (deamination of various amino acids, especially glutamine)
   a. Increases with
      (1) Diuretics (steroids, chlorothiazide)
      (2) Restriction of dietary sodium (hyponatremia)
      (3) Potassium depletion (hypokalemia)
      (4) Alkalosis
3. Its liberation from contracting *muscle* cells
   Increases during exercise.

Treatment and Nursing Management

1. Evaluate and maintain vital functions
   a. Assess patient's neurologic status (i.e., his ability to perform simple arithmetic calculations and his handwriting). Keep daily record and note differences.
   b. Observe and record the extent and magnitude of characteristic tremor.
   c. Note and record state of consciousness, including: slight drowsiness, slight confusion, drowsy, confused, or disoriented.
   d. Note presence of a "far-away" look.
   e. When patient does not respond, note sucking and grasping abilities; check corneal reflex.

f. Weigh patient daily and keep an accurate intake and output record; record quantity of feces.
g. Correct electrolyte abnormalities, especially hypokalemia.
2. Arrest gastrointestinal bleeding and reduce intraintestinal nitrogen.
   a. If there is upper gastrointestinal bleeding, constant gastric aspiration may be required.
   b. If bleeding has ceased, administer a cathartic or enema to clear blood from intestine.
   c. Cancel requests for ammonium products, sedatives, tranquilizers, and narcotics.
   d. Greatly reduce dietary protein—if patient begins to improve, gradually increase protein intake; provide sufficient calories in absorbable form (i.e., I.V. glucose or lipid emulsion).
   e. Cleanse the intestinal tract of nitrogenous substrates by administering prescribed purgatives such as magnesium citrate or sorbitol, or enemas.
   f. Administer oral lactulose, if prescribed, to reduce intestinal absorption of ammonia.
   g. Give neomycin, a nonabsorbable antibiotic, if prescribed, to suppress urea-splitting enteric bacteria.
3. Reduce and possibly eliminate all sedatives and analgesics. Administer only those specifically prescribed.
4. Prevent complications, if possible; identify and treat complications.
   a. Correct preexisting complicating diseases—cardiovascular, renal, and pulmonary.
   b. Treat any infections, including respiratory infections, since these can become severe in this patient.
   c. Administer antacids to reduce gastric acid and to protect against peptic ulceration. Prophylactic use of intravenous cimetidine to keep gastric pH above 5.0 is helpful.
   d. Monitor blood glucose every 8 hours or whenever level of consciousness deteriorates; administer intravenous glucose.
   e. Monitor status of hydration and correct any electrolyte, acid–base, or fluid imbalance.

HEPATIC CIRRHOSIS

Cirrhosis of the liver is a chronic disease in which there has been diffuse destruction of parenchymal cells followed by liver cell regeneration and an increase in connective tissue. These processes result in disorganization of the lobular architecture and obstruction of the hepatic venous and sinusoidal channels, causing portal hypertension.

Classification of Hepatic Cirrhosis

1. Laennec's cirrhosis of the alcoholic (micronodular)
   a. Fibrosis—mainly around central veins and portal areas
   b. Most commonly due to chronic alcoholism and malnutrition
2. Postnecrotic (macronodular)
   a. Broad bands of scar tissue—due to collapse of necrotic lobules and confluence of portal areas
   b. Due to previous acute viral hepatitis or drug-induced massive hepatic necrosis
3. Biliary
   a. Scarring around bile ducts and lobes of liver

b. Results from chronic biliary obstruction (with or without infection)
c. Much more rare than Laennec's and postnecrotic cirrhosis
4. Posthepatic
   a. Fine bands of scar tissue extend from portal areas whipsawing the lobules
   b. Usually due to chronic viral hepatitis.

Etiology

1. Cirrhosis of the liver is characterized by repeated occurrences of death of the liver cells, replacement with scar tissue, and regeneration of liver cells.
2. Onset is insidious; it may be developing and progressing over many years.
3. Major causes in the U.S. are excessive consumption of alcohol and chronic viral hepatitis.
4. Twice as many men as women are affected; age group most often affected is from 40–60 years.

Altered Physiology: Clinical Manifestations

1. Early in disease—gastrointestinal disturbances, fever and liver enlargement due to cells being loaded with fat; as tissue is replaced, scars contract and become smaller, the surface becomes rough and has a hobnail effect.
2. Anorexia, weight loss, weakness, and fatigability occur; jaundice and fever may be present in the active stage. There are signs of portal hypertension and estrogen-androgen imbalance.
3. Later—chronic failure of liver function and obstruction of portal circulation.
   a. Obstruction of portal circulation, causing portal hypertension with congestion of spleen, pancreas, and gastrointestinal tract.
      (1) Chronic dyspepsia, change in bowel habits—diarrhea, constipation
      (2) Esophageal varices, dilated cutaneous veins around the umbilicus, internal hemorrhoids, ascites, splenomegaly, pancytopenia, and caput medusae
   b. Chronic failure of liver function
      (1) Plasma albumin is reduced, thereby leading to edema and contributing to ascites.
      (2) Weakness increases, leading to depression, wasting, delirium, coma, and eventually death.
      (3) Estrogen-androgen imbalance, causing spider angiomata and palmar erythema, amenorrhea develops in females; testicular and prostatic atrophy, gynecomastia, loss of libido, and impotence develop in males.
      (4) Bleeding tendencies may be evident.

Diagnostic Evaluation

1. Liver biopsy (see p. 448)
2. Esophagoscopy
3. Barium-contrast esophagography (only about 50% accurate) to check for esophageal varices
4. Arteriography or umbilical venous catheterization to visualize portal collaterals; by placement of a catheter in the portal vein via recanalized umbilical vein, direct venous pressure and portovenography can be done in 75% of patients.
5. Radioisotopic liver scans—increased splenic and vertebral uptake of ^{99}Tc (radioactive technetium) sulfur colloid.
6. Paracentesis to examine ascitic fluid, for cell count, for protein content, and for bacterial count.

Treatment

(May be slow and tedious)
1. Prevent further damage to the liver by withdrawing toxic substances, alcohol, and drugs.
2. Offer supportive care of the patient.
3. Maintain adequate nutritional levels.
   a. Provide protein within ability of liver to handle it. Normal nutritious diet with vitamin supplements, especially B, C, and K and folate.
   b. Restrict alcohol consumption.
4. Restrict salt intake when fluid retention occurs.
5. Protect patient from infections and toxic agents.
6. Treat ascites with diuretics gently and only when acute activity of liver damage has subsided.
   a. Portacaval shunt may be tried to control ascites; however, operative mortality is high.
   b. Abdominal paracentesis is to be avoided as long as possible (if necessary, see Procedure, p. 455)

   c. LeVeen peritoneovenous shunt may be tried; this is used only in patients with "intractable" ascites, circulatory failure of cirrhosis, or abdominal hernia with severe ascites.
      (1) Complications:
         (a) Coagulopathy (bleeding); requires monitoring of clotting factors
         (b) Shunt malfunction
7. Treat hepatic coma as necessary (see p. 453)
8. Provide multivitamin supplements and thiamine to compensate for liver's inability to store or activate them.
9. Give folic acid to correct folic acid deficiency anemia.
10. Control or reduce pruritus in patients with liver disease and retention of bile salts.

Nursing Management

1. Instruct and prepare patient for the very many laboratory and x-ray studies needed.
   a. Diagnostic evaluation requires nursing assistance in patient preparation.
   b. Liver studies and nursing significance (see p. 447).
2. Evaluate nutritional status and needs.
   a. Offer small frequent meals rather than 3 large meals.
   b. Consider patient preferences in food.
   c. If patient is severely anorexic or nauseated and eating poorly, tube feeding may be necessary; include milk and starch hydrolysate (Dextri-maltose). Do not increase dietary protein if serum ammonia level is increased.
   d. Give pancreatin (if diarrhea and steatorrhea) to permit better tolerance of diet.
3. Monitor intake and output accurately; weigh carefully.
4. Adjust nutritional offerings if the patient has ascites or edema.
   a. Restrict sodium intake to 200–500 mg. daily (less than 10 mEq. daily).
   b. Maintain caloric and vitamin intake; give protein as tolerated.
   c. Avoid table salt, salty foods, salted margarine, and butter as well as all ordinary frozen and canned foods, mouthwash, baking soda, and all other products containing large quantities of salt.
   d. Use "salt" substitutes such as lemon juice, oregano, thyme to enhance flavor; commercial salt substitute should be approved by physician.
   e. Encourage use of powdered low-sodium milk and milk products.
   f. If water accumulation is not controlled on above regimen, resort to the following:
      (1) Limit sodium allowance to 200 mg. daily.
      (2) Restrict fluids if serum sodium is low.
      (3) Administer oral diuretics: hydrochlorothiazide (HydroDiuril) furosemide (Lasix).
      (4) Administer spironolactone (Aldactone) if prescribed—this is an aldosterone-blocking agent used to reinforce the actions of diuretics and prevent undue potassium loss.
      (5) Promote diuresis slowly to avoid renal failure.
   g. Abdominal paracentesis is to be avoided as long as possible (if necessary, see Procedure, p. 455).
4. Assist the patient in overcoming anorexia, weight loss, and fatigue.
   a. Encourage him to eat all meals and supplementary

feedings by serving them with eye-catching appeal, in small servings, and in small frequent meals.
b. Recognize the effect of esthetic factors—control odors, disturbing conversations, unpleasant situations.
c. Eliminate alcohol but encourage high caloric intake.
d. Give supplementary vitamins (A, B complex, C, and K) and folate.
e. Conserve patient's energy so that total food intake is not expended to replace energy requirements.
f. Provide special mouth care if patient has bleeding from gums.
5. Observe skin and control pruritus.
a. Provide good skin care; bathe without soap; apply soothing lotions.
b. Keep patient's fingernails short to prevent him from scratching his skin.
c. Administer medications as prescribed for pruritus; be alert for side effects of nausea, diarrhea or constipation, and vitamin K depletion, which leads to bleeding.
6. Be cognizant of signs of hematemesis and melena.
a. Assess for anxiety, weakness, restlessness, and epigastric fullness as possibly heralding hemorrhage.
b. Take and record vital signs frequently.
c. Administer vitamin C as prescribed.
d. Observe each stool for color, consistency, and amount. Test for occult blood with Hemoccult.
e. Record nature, amount, and time of vomiting.
f. Note patient's reaction frequently if he receives a blood transfusion.
7. Anticipate manifestations of hemorrhage such as ecchymosis, petechiae, epistaxis, and nose bleeds; initiate preventive measures.
a. Maintain a safe environment to prevent injury.
b. Avoid trauma such as forceful nose blowing, use of hard toothbrush, large gauge needles for injection.

c. Apply pressure to small bleeding sites; record their nature and location.
d. Encourage intake of foods high in vitamin C.
8. Recognize signs of increasing stupor, notify physician, and initiate nursing measures as follows:
a. Be alert for evidences of mental changes, lethargy, hallucinations.
b. Avoid giving patient narcotics and barbiturates.
c. Restrict dietary protein; offer small high caloric feedings frequently.
d. Protect patient by keeping him in bed; pad siderails.
e. Arouse patient at intervals.
f. Limit visitors.
g. Provide constant nursing surveillance and emphasize sensitivity to patient's changes and needs.
h. Provide nasal oxygen when prescribed to oxygenate weakened cells in case more die. Check for adequate fitting of nasal tubings.
9. Treat iron deficiency (from gastrointestinal blood loss) with folate, pyridoxine or pyridoxal phosphate, and iron, if necessary.

Health Education

Instruct patient regarding precautions and regimen to follow upon his discharge from the hospital.
1. Stress the necessity of giving up alcohol completely; urge acceptance of skillful assistance from psychiatrist, Alcoholics Anonymous, or the alcohol treatment unit in the hospital.
2. Provide written dietary instructions, emphasizing the restriction of sodium (and protein, if necessary).
3. Emphasize the significance of rest, a sensible lifestyle, and an adequate, well-balanced diet.
4. Involve the person closest to him (usually spouse) because recovery often is not easy and relapses are common; a close, trusted helper can help patient over the rough spots.
5. See items 4, 5, 7 above, for nutrition, hygiene, and safety aspects.

GUIDELINES: Assisting With Abdominal Paracentesis

Paracentesis (abdominal) is the withdrawal of fluid from the abdominal cavity.

Purposes
1. To remove no more than 1 liter at a time of accumulated fluid from the abdominal cavity to relieve pressure on the following:
a. Diaphragm, which impairs breathing
b. Stomach, which aggravates anorexia
c. Umbilical hernia
2. For diagnostic purposes, especially in patient with unexplained fever, abdominal pain, and change in bowel habits.

Danger and Complications
1. In chronic liver disease, paracentesis may precipitate hepatic coma.
2. Shock and hypovolemia can occur if fluid from general circulation shifts to abdomen to replace withdrawn fluid; this can be minimized if no more than one liter of paracentesis fluid is withdrawn or if lost fluid is replaced in kind by parenteral administration of human albumin (salt poor).

Equipment
Sterile paracentesis tray and gloves
Procaine hydrochloride 1%
Drape or cotton blankets
Scultetus or appropriate abdominal binder
Pail
Skin preparation tray with antiseptic
Specimen bottles and laboratory forms

GUIDELINES: Assisting With Abdominal Paracentesis (cont.)

Procedure NURSING ACTION	RATIONALE/AMPLIFICATION
Preparatory Phase	
1. Have patient void before treatment is begun. See that consent form has been signed.	1. This will lessen the danger of accidentally piercing the bladder with the needle.
2. Position patient in Fowler's position with back, arms and feet supported (sitting on the side of the bed is frequently used position).	2. Patient is more comfortable and a steady position can be maintained.
3. Drape patient with sheet exposing abdomen.	3. Minimizes exposure of patient and keeps him warm.
Performance Phase	
1. Assist physician in preparing skin with antiseptic solution.	1. This is considered a minor surgical procedure requiring aseptic precautions.
2. Open sterile tray and package of sterile gloves; provide anesthetic solution.	
3. Position bucket and be prepared to place end of rubber tubing into bucket.	
4. Assess pulse and respiratory status frequently during procedure; watch for pallor, cyanosis or syncope (faintness).	4. Preliminary indications of shock must be watched for. Keep emergency stimulants available.
5. Physician administers local anesthesia and introduces #20 needle into abdomen through Z-track.	
6. Withdraw fluid by syringe in 50 ml. aliquots, using 3-way stopcock.	6. Fluid withdrawn slowly by needle and syringe. Each aspiration is limited to 1–2 liters to relieve acute symptoms.
7. Apply dressing when needle is withdrawn.	7. Elasticized adhesive patch is effective, serving as waterproof-adhering dressing.
Follow-Up Phase	
1. Assist patient to be comfortable after treatment.	
2. Record amount and kind of fluid removed, number of specimens sent to laboratory, patient's condition through treatment.	
3. Check blood pressure and vital signs every half hour for 2 hours, every hour for 4 hours, and every 4 hours for 24 hours.	3. Close observation will detect poor circulatory adjustment and possible development of shock.
4. Usually a dressing is sufficient; however, if the trocar wound appears large, the physician may close the incision with sutures.	
5. Watch for leakage or scrotal edema after paracentesis.	5. If seen, notify physician at once.

BLEEDING ESOPHAGEAL VARICES

Esophageal varices are dilated tortuous veins found in the submucosa of the lower esophagus; they may extend up in the esophagus and down into the stomach.

Causes

1. Nearly always due to portal hypertension which may result from obstruction of the portal venous circulation and cirrhosis of the liver.
2. Abnormalities of the circulation in splenic vein or superior vena cava.

Altered Physiology and Symptoms

1. Increasing portal vein obstruction—venous blood returning to right atrium from intestinal tract and spleen seeks new pathways, through enlarging collateral esophageal veins.
2. Usually no symptoms are produced by dilated veins unless mucosa becomes ulcerated.
3. Hematemesis and melena plus a history of alcoholism tend to point toward esophageal varices; however, bleeding may result from associated gastritis or duodenal ulcer in 25% of patients with varices.
4. The strain of coughing or vomiting may precipitate variceal rupture, hemorrhage, and death.
5. Irritation of vessels by gastroesophageal reflux may cause esophagitis, esophageal rupture, hemorrhage, and death.

Assessment and Clinical Manifestations

1. Blood loss may be sudden and massive; blood may well up in the throat.
2. Hematemesis, melena, or rectal bleeding (bright red blood)
3. Monitor blood pressure and assess for signs of shock.

Diagnostic Evaluation

1. The patient's history, physical examination, and neurologic examination will assist in identifying any evidence of hepatic encephalopathy.

2. Fiberoptic endoscopy may be used if bleeding is controlled. It is essential to exclude other causes of bleeding.
3. Arteriography may be substituted if bleeding is massive.
4. Splenoportography using diodrast can be effective when studied as a series of x-ray plates or done as a segmental roentgenogram; extensive collateral circulation of esophageal vessels may be indicative of varices.
5. Portal vein pressure above 250 mm. of water is abnormal; this can be measured in the operating room by introducing a needle into spleen or via umbilical vein catheter.
6. Liver function tests include bromsulphalein retention, serum transaminase, bilirubin, serum proteins, alkaline phosphatase.

Treatment and Nursing Management

This patient is critically ill and requires attentive nursing care.
1. Assess for signs of potential hypovolemia:
   a. Monitor blood pressure; CVP monitoring for fluid replacement.
   b. Assess urinary output; indwelling catheter may be required.
   c. Check blood gases to determine oxygenation of blood.
2. Initiate measures to overcome blood loss.
   a. Replace blood with *fresh* whole blood.
      (1) Ammonia content is lower than in stored blood.
      (2) Coagulation effect is greater, particularly if the patient has severe liver disease.
   b. Administer vitamin K intramuscularly.
3. Recognize the importance of controlling hemorrhage.
   a. Purpose
      (1) To lessen transfusion requirements.
      (2) To reduce large amounts of blood in gastrointestinal tract.
      (3) To avoid hepatic coma.
   b. Methods
      (1) Administer Vasopressin systemically to reduce portal pressure and to initiate hemostasis. Intra-arterial infusion into the superior mesenteric artery may be used after angiography, but offers no definitive advantage.
      (2) Ice-water lavage of stomach (gastric hypothermia) may temporarily control bleeding.
      (3) Aspirate blood from the stomach if necessary.
      (4) Esophageal tamponade—pressure is exerted on the cardiac portion of the stomach and against the bleeding varices by a double balloon tamponade (Sengstaken-Blakemore tube). (See below.)
      (5) Treat bleeding by complete rest of the esophagus (parenteral feedings); avoid straining and vomiting and continue gastric suction.
      (6) Initiate vitamin-K therapy; administer multiple blood transfusions.
      (7) Avoid sedation, since it may lead to coma.
      (8) Administer saline cathartic (magnesium citrate) plus enemata to remove blood.

GUIDELINES: Using the Sengstaken-Blakemore Tube to Control Esophageal Bleeding

Purposes
1. To exert pressure on the cardiac portion of the stomach and against bleeding varices by a double balloon tamponade.
2. To reduce transfusion requirements.
3. To prevent blood accumulation in the gastrointestinal tract which could precipitate hepatic coma.

Equipment
Sengstaken-Blakemore tube
Basin with cracked ice
Clamp for tubing
Towel and emesis basin
Glass of water and straw
Flashlight

Procedure (Fig. 10-25)

Preparatory Phase

1. Provide nursing support by reassuring patient that this procedure will help to control his bleeding.
2. Explain procedure to patient and tell him how breathing through the mouth and swallowing can help in passing the tube.
3. Elevate head of bed slightly unless patient is in shock.

NURSING ACTION	RATIONALE/AMPLIFICATION
Performance Phase	
1. Check balloon by trial inflation to detect leaks.	1. This is best done under water because it is easier to see escaping air bubbles.
2. Chill the tube, then lubricate it before physician passes it via mouth or nose (preferable).	2. Chilling will make the tube more firm and lubrication will lessen friction.
3. After the tube has entered the stomach, gavage stomach and aspirate all clots.	

GUIDELINES: Using the Sengstaken-Blakemore Tube to Control Esophageal Bleeding (cont.)

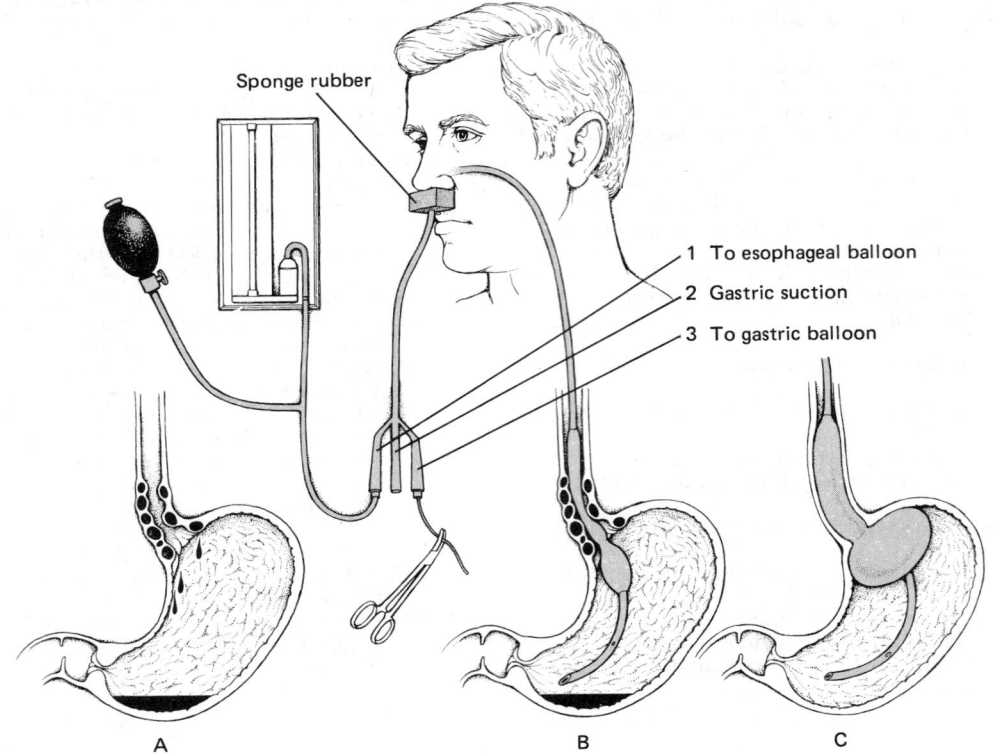

Sponge rubber

1 To esophageal balloon
2 Gastric suction
3 To gastric balloon

A   B   C

FIGURE 10-25. *Diagram showing esophageal varices and their treatment by a compressing balloon tube (Sengstaken-Blakemore). A. Dilated veins of the lower esophagus. B. The tube is in place in the stomach and the lower esophagus but is not inflated. C. Inflation of the tube and compression of the veins which can be obtained by inflation of the balloon. In some instances, it may be necessary to pass an additional tube through the other nostril for the purpose of aspirating secretions.*
Note: The Minnesota four-lumen esophagogastric tamponade tube has an additional outlet for aspiration of the esophagus.

Procedure (cont.)

NURSING ACTION	RATIONALE/AMPLIFICATION
4. After obtaining an x-ray of the lower chest and upper abdomen to check position of the balloon, it is fully inflated (200–250 ml.) of air and then pulled back gently.	4. This is to exert force against cardia. The triple-lumen tube provides 2 channels to inflate each compression bag, one in the stomach and one in the esophagus. Balloons are inflated using a manometer to measure pressure to 25 or 30 mm. Hg.
5. Traction is placed on tubing where it enters the nose of the patient. Then the esophageal bag is inflated to 35–40 mm. Hg. This is tied with double ties to prevent leakage (Fig. 10-26).	5. This keeps balloons in position and assists in exerting proper pressure.
6. Gastric suction may be attached to the 3rd outlet of the catheter.	6. By using suction and irrigating the tubing hourly, it is possible to tell how well the bleeding is controlled by the appearance of the drainage.
7. A second nasogastric (Levin) tube is passed into the lower esophagus.*	7. To aspirate saliva and to check for bleeding *above* the esophageal balloon.
8. Deflate esophageal balloon for 5 minutes at 8- or 12-hour intervals. Do not deflate gastric balloon under traction.	8. To prevent erosion and necrosis of the esophagus or stomach.
9. Pressure on tubes and traction is released in 2–4 days.	9. If bleeding remains controlled, the tubing is removed in 24 hours.

* If the Minnesota four-lumen esophagogastric tube is used, this will not be necessary.

Nursing Responsibilities

1. Maintain *constant* vigilance while balloons are inflated in the patient.
2. Keep balloon pressures at required level to control bleeding. (Hemostats are utilized as clamps.)
3. Observe and record vital signs frequently—bleeding, shock, etc.
4. Be alert for chest pain—may indicate injury or rupture of esophagus.
5. Irrigate suction tube as prescribed; observe and record nature and color of aspirated material.
6. Keep head of bed elevated to avoid gastric regurgitation and to diminish nausea and a sensation of gagging.
7. Maintain nutritional and electrolyte levels parenterally.
8. Maintain nasogastric suction to aspirate saliva through an accessory nasogastric tube.
9. Note nature of breathing: if counterweight pulls the tube into oropharynx, the patient may be asphyxiated.

> **NURSING ALERT:** Keep a pair of scissors taped to the head of the bed. In the event of *acute respiratory distress,* use the scissors to cut across tubing (to deflate both balloons) and remove tubing.

NOTE: This procedure should be reserved for patients who are known without a doubt to be bleeding from esophageal varices, and in whom all forms of conservative therapy have failed.

CHIEF HAZARD: Vomiting with an inflated esophageal balloon tamponade in place, which results in massive pulmonary aspiration. Manage this problem by inserting a nasogastric tube in the free nostril to drain the esophagus above the esophageal balloon, thereby preventing aspiration. The Minnesota four-lumen esophagogastric tamponade tube has the additional outlet for aspiration of the esophagus.

Surgical Intervention

If bleeding of esophageal varices is not controlled by conservative measures, surgical procedures may be employed:

A. *Surgical Procedures*

1. Direct ligation of varices.
2. Surgical by-pass (*portacaval anastomosis*). By shunting portal blood into the vena cava, pressure in the portal system is reduced.
3. Splenorenal shunt. A shunt is made between the splenic vein and the left renal vein; this is done when the portal vein cannot be used because of thrombosis or for other reasons.

B. *Evaluation of Surgery*

1. Varying degrees of success are reported with shunting procedures.
2. The success depends mainly on the condition of the patient; it is used as an emergency procedure following bleeding. Most common use is to prevent recurrence after the patient recovers from an initial variceal bleed.
3. Complications are acute hepatic failure and chronic portal systemic encephalopathy (PSE).
4. Postoperative care is similar to postabdominal surgery complicated by care required for a patient with cirrhotic liver.

DISEASES OF THE BILIARY (GALLBLADDER) SYSTEM

Incidence

1. About 500,000 persons a year in the U.S. are hospitalized for gallbladder disease; ⅔ of these are treated surgically.
2. Women acquire the disease more frequently than men: 4 to 1.
3. Patients are most often past 40, multiparous and overweight; however, the condition is common also in younger patients.
4. Postmenopausal women on estrogen therapy are at greater risk for gallbladder disease; likewise, women on birth control pills are at greater risk than nonusers of pills.

Types of Gallbladder Disease

(Chole—gallbladder)
Cholecystitis—inflammation of the gallbladder
Cholelithiasis—stones in the gallbladder
Choledocholithiasis—stones in the common duct

A. *Chronic Cholecystitis with Cholelithiasis*

1. Assessment and Clinical Manifestations
   a. History of episodic, usually colicky epigastric or right upper quadrant pain often associated with nausea and vomiting
   b. Jaundice due to choledocholithiasis
2. Treatment
   a. Surgery is advised if gallstones are present with typical pain attacks and/or jaundice. Whether asymptomatic stones should be removed surgically is still open to debate.
   b. In the older patient, the risk of surgery must be evaluated in relation to other disease conditions present.
   c. Chenodeoxycholic acid, an investigational drug, can decrease the size of existing stones (dissolve small ones) and prevent new stones from forming.
      (1) The only adverse effects appear to be mild diarrhea and cramps and SGOT elevation; with dose regulation these disappear.
      (2) Stones may recur; therefore, long-term therapy may be required.
      (3) Studies continue to evaluate this drug for its proper place in the management of the patient with cholelithiasis. It is not yet approved by the FDA for routine use outside of controlled trials.

d. Ursodeoxycholic acid (UDCA), is another investigational drug which appears to dissolve gallstones as efficiently as chenodeoxycholic acid but with less diarrhea as a side effect. Not yet available in this country.

B. *Acute Cholecystitis*

1. Clinical Manifestations
   a. RUQ pain, fever, nausea, and vomiting.
   b. The condition may occur at any age, but it is most common in patients over the age of 50.
   c. The chief hazard is perforation with local or generalized peritonitis.
2. Treatment and Nursing Management
   a. Provide hospitalization, bed rest, withholding of oral fluids, and insertion of nasogastric tube with suction.
   b. Administer IV fluids to correct electrolyte imbalance, to maintain adequate urinary output, and to provide nutritional needs.
   c. Administer medication for pain and antimicrobials for infection control.
   d. Prepare patient for laboratory studies, chest x-ray, ECG, and possibly intravenous cholangiogram.
   e. Record vital signs every 4 hours and prepare patient for surgery.

Diagnostic Evaluation of Biliary Conditions

Overall assessment of the patient should include detection of associated disease processes (cardiovascular, pulmonary, and renal); diabetes status; and realization of increased surgical risk if patient is over age 65.

A. *Flat Plate of Abdomen*—used to visualize the 25% of stones that are radiopaque.

B. *Cholecystography*—used to visualize the shape and position of the gallbladder.

NOTE: This test is effective only if the liver cells are functioning properly and are capable of excreting the radiopaque contrast medium into the bile.

1. *Purpose*
   a. To detect gallstones.
   b. To estimate ability of gallbladder to fill, concentrate its contents, contract and empty in a normal manner.
2. *Method*
   a. Because gallstones are usually radiolucent, it is necessary to fill the gallbladder with a radiopaque contrast medium which permits stones to show up as clear areas.
   b. Iodide-containing contrast medium is excreted into bile by the liver and concentrated in the gallbladder. Caution: Prior to administration of iodide, determine whether patient is sensitive to iodine.
      (1) Orally
         (a) Contrast media may be given by mouth (e.g., Telepaque, Priodax, Oragrafin, Teridax, Monophen).
         (b) Iodide preparation is usually given in oral doses of 3.6 gm. approximately 10–12 hours before x-ray. If there is no visualization the next morning, repeat dose of 3.6 gm. the following evening.
         (c) Administer nothing by mouth from the time of iodide administration to the time of x-ray to prevent contraction of gallbladder and expulsion of contrast medium.
      (2) Intravenously
         Intravenous cholecystography involves giving an iodide preparation (e.g., Cholografin) about 10 minutes before x-ray.
3. *Patient Preparation*
   a. At least 1 hour after the evening meal, the patient takes the prescribed tablets or capsules of iodide preparation by mouth.
   b. These tablets are taken one at a time at 3- to 5-minute intervals with at least 8 oz. of water.
   c. From this time to bedtime, nothing is taken by mouth except water; from midnight on, water is also excluded. (If nausea, vomiting, or diarrhea occurs notify physician; test may be postponed.)
   d. No laxatives are given during this time; however, a saline enema may be required on the morning of the x-ray.
   e. Breakfast is withheld and patient goes to x-ray.
   f. Right upper abdominal quadrant is x-rayed.
   g. The patient is fed a fatty meal containing cream, butter or eggs to test contractility of the gallbladder.
   h. X-ray examination is repeated at intervals until gallbladder has expelled contrast medium.

NURSING ALERT: Cholecystography is ineffective in the jaundiced patient, since the liver cells in this situation cannot transport contrast medium to the biliary tract.

C. *Cholangiography*—(contrast medium is injected directly into biliary tree)

1. Advantages
   a. Procedure is best way to visualize biliary tree in patient after cholecystectomy.
   b. All components of the biliary tree can be observed: hepatic ducts within liver, common hepatic duct, and cystic duct, but the gallbladder is often not well visualized.
2. Clinical Usefulness
   a. In differentiating hepatocellular jaundice from jaundice due to biliary obstruction.
   b. In locating stones within bile ducts.
   c. In detecting and diagnosing cancer of the biliary system.
   d. In investigating gastrointestinal symptoms of patients who had cholecystectomy.
3. Patient Preparation
   a. The patient is dehydrated by restricting his fluid intake.
   b. Enema is given early in morning of test.
   c. A sedative is given at least 1 hour before the x-ray.
   d. Contrast medium (e.g., Cholografin Sodium) is injected either intravenously (results not as conclusive) or directly into the common duct.
      (1) Operatively; this can be done during surgery.
      (2) Postoperatively; by injecting contrast medium into the common duct drain.
      (3) Via retrograde endoscopic cannulation of duct via duodenum.
   e. Following the x-ray, regardless of method of contrast medium injection, as much as possible of the contrast medium and bile are aspirated to prevent leakage into the peritoneal cavity, thus avoiding a possible bile peritonitis.

NOTE: Operative cholangiography may be done during gallbladder surgery in the operating room.

D. *Ultrasound Examination (Echogram)*—B scanner and transducer

This test can be used to demonstrate gallbladder distention, bile duct distention, and calculi.

E. *Liver Scan*

1. In the jaundiced patient, this scan may show evidence of hepatocellular disease or metastatic lesions.
2. With radioactive rose bengal, which is excreted by the liver-like gallbladder dyes, obstructive pathology of the biliary tree may be revealed.

F. *Endoscopic Retrograde Cholangiopancreatography (ERCP)*

See Guidelines, p. 462.

Types of Gallbladder Surgery

1. *Cholecystostomy*

Simple opening of gallbladder to remove stones, bile or pus; a tube is then sutured into the gallbladder for drainage.

NOTE: When patient returns to the Recovery Unit, this drainage tube is connected to a drainage bottle.

2. *Cholecystectomy*

Removal of the gallbladder after ligation of the cystic duct and vessels; done in most situations of acute or chronic cholecystitis. A drain (penrose type) may be inserted in the gallbladder bed to permit drainage into dressings.

3. *Choledochostomy*

An opening into the common duct for the purpose of removing obstructing stones; a drainage T-tube is inserted into the duct and is connected to a drainage bottle. Usually a cholecystectomy is done at this time because the gallbladder often contains stones also.

Preoperative Nursing Management

1. Diagnostic evaluation
   a. Gallbladder x-rays (p. 460)
   b. Chest roentgenogram
   c. Examination of urine and stool
   d. Blood studies including liver function tests (p. 447)
2. It may be necessary to administer vitamin K and fresh blood to correct a low prothrombin level.
3. Proper nutritional levels may require supplements of protein hydrolysate to aid in wound healing and to prevent liver damage.
4. Adequate instruction regarding immediate postoperative requirements such as turning, deep breathing and use of incentive spirometry to prevent hypostatic pneumonia, a common postoperative complication.

Postoperative Nursing Objectives and Management

1. To prevent respiratory complications which are common in obese patients and in those having upper abdominal incisions.
   a. Encourage the patient to take 10 deep breaths hourly and to turn frequently.
   b. Administer analgesics as prescribed to permit patient to take deep breaths comfortably (may be painful otherwise).
   c. Place patient in low Fowler's position to facilitate lung expansion
   d. Activate and ambulate as early as permissible; apply a scultetus or appropriate abdominal binder if it will make the patient more comfortable.
   e. Since he may still have a drainage bottle, place it in a below-the-waist pocket or fasten so that it is at a desired level.
2. To promote drainage from T-tube or cholecystostomy tube until normal flow of bile is established.
   a. Place patient in low-Fowler's position and later in semi-Fowler's position as tolerated to facilitate drainage.
   b. Connect drainage tube to drainage bottle at side of bed; observe for kinking, twisting and blockage of tubes.
   c. Check postoperative orders regarding positioning of drainage bottle; often the bottle or tubing is elevated so that bile drains through the apparatus only if pressure develops in the system. This is done purposely to prevent total bile loss and to promote normal bile flow through the common bile duct.
   d. Allow enough tubing leeway to permit the patient to be turned without dislodging tubes.
   e. Observe, describe and record amount and character of drainage frequently.
   f. After 5 or 6 days of drainage, the T-tube may be clamped 1 hour before and after each meal to allow bile to flow into duodenum to aid in digestion. (Done with physician's permission.)
   g. T-tube drain may be removed in 1 to 2 weeks. Cholecystostomy tube is removed in 6 weeks to 6 months. Drainage tube from gallbladder bed may be removed in 5 to 6 days.
3. To maintain fluid and nutritional needs of the postoperative biliary patient.
   a. Intravenous fluids are usually initiated; fluids by mouth are given in 24 hours.
   b. Insert nasogastric tube to relieve distention and promote normal peristalsis.
   c. An enema is usually given after 72 hours after which the patient is offered a soft, low fat diet.
   d. If necessary to feed the patient his own bile (in chronic biliary drainage) it may be best not to tell the patient what the liquid is other than it is to stimulate his appetite; bile may be chilled, strained and diluted with grape or other fruit juice.
   e. Provide diets that are low in fats and high in carbohydrate and proteins (fatty foods are usually avoided because they cause nausea).
   f. It may be necessary to continue to give vitamin K.
4. To observe color changes in skin, sclerae and stool which will indicate whether bile pigment is disappearing from blood and draining again into the duodenum.
   a. Note color and consistency of all stools; chart an accurate description.
   b. Send specimens of urine and stool to the laboratory at frequent intervals for examination of bile pigments.
   c. Observe skin and sclerae for yellowish color which would indicate bile-flow obstruction.
5. To protect skin around incision site due to bile seepage.
   a. Change the outer dressings frequently to provide for absorption of drainage; Montgomery straps may facilitate dressing changes.

b. Apply skin pastes of zinc oxide or petrolatum to prevent the bile drainage from attacking and digesting the skin.

Health Education and Discharge Planning

OBJECTIVE: to stress elements in posthospital care that will assist patient in his convalescence.

1. It is not unusual after cholecystectomy for patient to have "looseness of the bowel," consisting of 1–3 movements a day. This diminishes over a period of a few weeks to several months; within a year, the bowel habit is normal.

2. Usually there are no dietary instructions except to maintain a nutritious diet and to restrict fats for 4–6 weeks. (Otherwise, flatulence may occur.) Thereafter adequate bile will be released into the digestive tract to emulsify fats and permit their digestion.
3. Review medications and their purpose; vitamins, anticholinergics, antispasmodics.
4. Be aware of reportable symptoms: jaundice, dark urine, pale-colored stools, pruritus, pain, or fever.
5. Emphasize the importance of follow-up visits to the physician.

GUIDELINES: Endoscopic Retrograde Cholangiopancreatography (ERCP)

A fiberoptic endoscope (a side-viewing instrument) is placed in the descending duodenum so that the ampulla of Vater can be located and cannulated (Fig. 10-26).

In this examination, both the common and pancreatic ducts may be injected with contrast media to visualize the hepatobiliary tree and pancreatic ducts radiologically.

The clinician is able to diagnose abnormalities of the ductal system, detect disease processes, and obtain direct secretory information as well as cells for cytologic examination.

Indications
1. Biliary disease
2. Pancreatic disease
3. To diagnose:
   Cancer of the papilla
   Obstructive jaundice
   Calculus disease, pre- and postcholecystectomy

   Carcinoma of biliary ducts
   Carcinoma of pancreas
   Pancreatitis

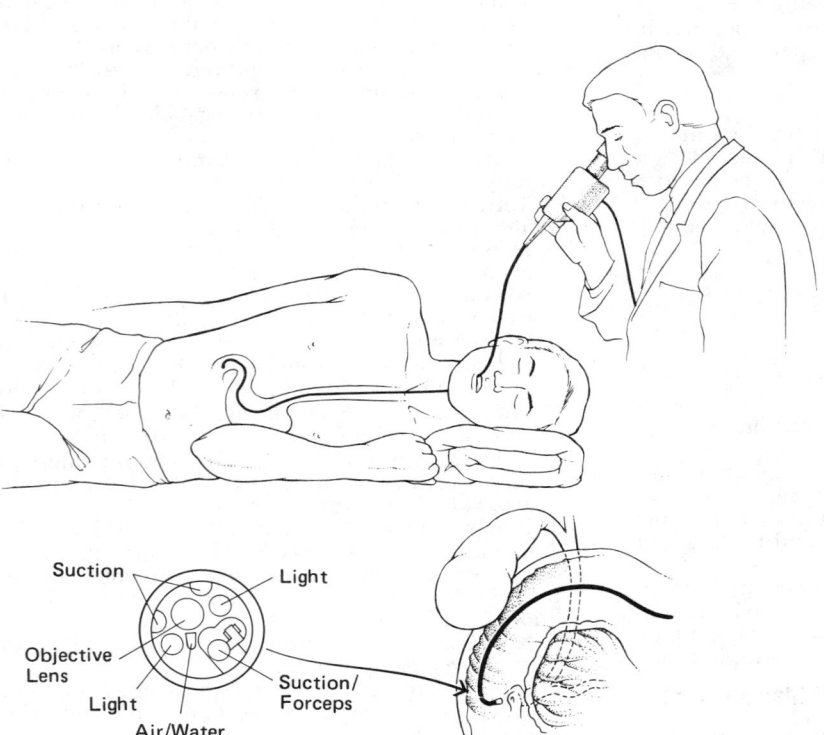

Suction   Light

Objective
Lens
Light

Suction/
Forceps

Air/Water

FIGURE 10-26. *Endoscopic retrograde cholangiopancreatography (ERCP). The patient is moved from left lateral to prone position as the flexible scope is passed. The circle on the left shows the tip of the scope: the objective lens is the viewing section assisted by two side lights. Air or water may be directed to an area and suction is available. If a biopsy is to be taken, a separate channel is available.*

The lower right diagram shows the scope nearing the ampulla of Vater; the scope is in the duodenum; gallbladder is the topmost sac—from which note the biliary and common bile ducts.

Contraindications

1. Acute cardiorespiratory disease
2. Acute recent attack of pancreatitis (within 3 weeks) because of risk of inducing another attack
3. Stricture or obstruction of esophagus or duodenum
4. Acute cholangitis

Equipment

A side-viewing duodenoscope* (to be sterilized after use with suspected infectious patients).
Sterilized cannula.
This duodenoscope is 125 cm. long and 1 cm. in diameter.
Visual fields are oriented 90 degrees to its long axis.
It includes a channel through which a cannula or biopsy forceps can be passed under direct vision.

Considerations

1. ERCP is not a simple endoscopic procedure; it must be done by a skillful, well-trained physician.
2. There are certain risks, described below:
   a. After ERCP a very small percentage of patients develop clinical pancreatitis which may last 1–3 days.
   b. The patient may retain contrast material injected proximal to an obstructed duct; this may result in cholangitis or pancreatitis. Such a patient should be covered with broad-spectrum antibiotics; surgical drainage may be indicated.
   c. A very few patients are sensitive to iodinated compounds.
   d. The more experienced the team in performing ERCP's, the fewer the complications and the better the success rate.

Procedure

NURSING ACTION	PHYSICIAN'S ROLE	RATIONALE/AMPLIFICATION
Preparatory Phase		
1. Remind patient to take nothing by mouth after midnight.	1. Collaborate with nurse in patient preparation.	1. Limited intake produces a basal condition with reduced body secretions; this permits better visualization of tissues.
2. Explain contemplated examination to patient; discuss possibilities of after-effects.		
3. Determine patient's sensitivity to iodine (or fish which contains iodine) or any other medication.		3. A few patients are sensitive to iodine preparations (Hypaque sodium).
4. Take and record vital signs.		4. This information becomes a baseline for later comparison.
5. Offer patient 3 ml. of tetracaine (Pontocaine) to be used as a gargle and swallow.		5. Tetracaine is an oropharyngeal topical anesthetic.
6. (Intravenous infusion may be started by nurse, if qualified.)	6. Start an intravenous infusion with normal saline.	6. This becomes the avenue for direct intravenous medications such as diazepam (Valium) and meperidine (Demerol) to promote relaxation prior to insertion of duodenoscope.
7. Instruct patient to remove dentures; a mouthpiece is inserted.		7. To facilitate insertion of scope.
Performance Phase		
1. Place patient in left lateral position.	1. Scope is passed through patient's mouth into esophagus and stomach.	1. Anatomy is carefully examined as the scope advances.
2. Administer IV medication, which may include Demerol, Valium, atropine, or glucagon.	2. Gently advance tip through pyloric ring into duodenal bulb into descending duodenum.	2. Atropine will produce a hypotonic duodenum and relaxed sphincter at ampulla of Vater; secretion will be reduced.
	3. Minimal air insufflation used to search for the ampulla of Vater.	3. Unless this is obstructed by tumor, it can usually be identified with careful search.
4. Place patient in prone position. (This provides the radiologist with a better position for fluoroscopy and radiography.)	4. Administer glucagon.	4. Glucagon is given to further reduce duodenal motility.

* Olympus Corporation

GUIDELINES: Endoscopic Retrograde Cholangiopancreatography (ERCP) (cont.)

Procedure (cont.)	NURSING ACTION	PHYSICIAN'S ROLE	RATIONALE/AMPLIFICATION
	5. Prepare a special radiopaque Teflon cannulation tube by filling it with contrast medium (to eliminate air).	5. When cannulation tubing is in correct position, contrast medium is slowly injected: 3–5 ml. for pancreatic ductal system; 15–20 ml. for biliary ductal system.	5. Cannulation tube is passed through biopsy channel of scope. Contrast medium is warmed to body temperature. Tube is advanced under fluoroscopy. X-ray pictures are taken while patient is in prone position following injection of contrast media.
	6. Upon completion of film-taking, turn patient to lateral position. Draw blood sample for amylase determination. Use suction to remove oropharyngeal secretions.	6. Keep scope and cannula in place and patient in prone position until films are completed. If films are satisfactory, scope is carefully removed.	6. Await return and reading of films.
	Follow-up Phase		
	1. Check vital signs every 4 hours. Notify family as to when patient will return to his room.		1. Postcannulation patient may experience a temperature rise, chills, abdominal pain. Report these responses to physician.
	2. In the absence of complications, permit the patient to eat in 2–4 hours (light diet); permit a full diet the next day.		2. A mild rise in serum amylase is observed in a high percentage of the patients.
	3. Watch for palpitations related to atropine sulfate injection. Also watch for respiratory depression and transient hypotension.		3. Some patients experience mild to severe epigastric pain, nausea, and vomiting. These discomforts are usually transitory.

4 CONDITIONS OF THE PANCREAS*

ACUTE PANCREATITIS

Acute pancreatitis is an inflammation of the pancreas brought about by the digestion of this organ by enzymes, particularly trypsin, an enzyme it produces.

Etiology

1. Unknown.
2. Associated with excessive intake of alcohol—most common cause in the U.S.
3. Associated with blockage of ampulla of Vater by gallstones, causing activation of pancreatic enzymes.
4. Associated with spasm and edema of ampulla of Vater following duodenitis or after treatment with opiates.
5. May occur as a complication of mumps or bacterial disease.
6. Some congenital hyperlipidemias appear to be related to acute pancreatitis.

Clinical Manifestations

A. *Acute Interstitial Pancreatitis*

1. Pancreatic edema and escape of enzyme into nearby tissues and peritoneal cavity.
2. Fat necrosis of omentum caused by pancreatic lipase.
3. Increase in peritoneal fluid.
4. Abdominal and back pain.
5. Nausea, vomiting; fever

* For discussion of diabetes mellitus see pages 639–650.

6. Tenderness across upper abdomen—often minimal.
7. Elevated blood lipase and amylase.

B. *Acute Hemorrhagic Pancreatitis*

1. A more advanced form of acute pancreatitis.
2. Enzymatic digestion of gland more widespread.
3. Tissue becomes necrotic—blood escapes into pancreas and retroperitoneally.
4. Severe abdominal and back pain; tenderness is often present in epigastrium, but rigidity is often absent.
5. Symptoms similar to acute interstitial pancreatitis, only more severe.
6. Blood lipase and amylase are elevated.
7. Respiratory distress may occur.
8. With severe pancreatitis, there is often psychic disturbance manifested in restlessness, hallucinations, coarse tremor.
9. Severe leakage of exudate from plasma into peritoneum (large 3rd-space loss).
10. Shock, due to activation of kinins.
11. Hypokalemic alkalosis and hypocalcemia usually present.

Diagnostic Evaluation

1. Determination of serum amylase. If serum amylase is elevated, and there is clinical evidence, pancreatitis is likely.
2. An elevated serum lipase may also be present and persists longer than elevation of amylase.

Treatment and Nursing Management

OBJECTIVES: to halt the progress of the illness.
    to treat the hemodynamic abnormality.
    to treat systemic and local complications.

1. Relieve discomfort and pain to control restlessness which increases body metabolism causing stimulation of enzyme secretions.
   a. Give meperidine (Demerol); this is preferred because it depresses the central nervous system. (Opiates on the other hand may produce spasm of biliary-pancreatic ducts.)
   b. Encourage patient to assume position of comfort. Turn frequently to prevent pulmonary-vascular complications.
2. Decrease pancreatic secretions by reducing stimulation.
   a. Give nothing by mouth to eliminate chief stimulus to enzyme secretion.
   b. Offer anticholinergic medications as prescribed to assist in reducing pancreatic secretions by suppressing vagal mechanisms.
   c. Initiate nasogastric suction to remove hydrochloric acid from stomach, thus preventing release of secretin; adynamic ileus is also treated.
      (1) Record color and nature of gastric secretions.
      (2) Measure secretions at periodic intervals.
   d. Maintain the comfort of the intubated patient.
      (1) Assist patient in cleansing and refreshing mouth care.
      (2) Apply lubricant to external nares to prevent irritation of mucous membrane and skin.
      (3) Alternate side-positioning to prevent esophageal and gastric irritation by tube.
      (4) Provide cool mist vapor therapy to increase humidity and control drying of mucous membrane.
3. Monitor blood gases to detect early signs of respiratory failure.
   Administer oxygen therapy if necessary.
4. Provide medications to correct deficiencies and prevent complications.
   a. Give parenteral fluids: electrolytes, blood, and plasma to meet body's nutritional needs, replace losses, and combat shock. Keep accurate intake and output record.
   b. Administer antimicrobials to ward off secondary infection or abscess formation. (Use of antibiotics remains controversial. Some physicians suggest intravenous administration of cephalothin every 6 hours.)
   c. If marked hyperglycemia occurs, give insulin in small doses (crystalline insulin at 6-hour intervals) rather than long-acting insulin.
5. Support cardiopulmonary system in patients with acute hemorrhagic pancreatitis.
   a. Monitor hematocrit (if it rises in first 24–48 hours, volume replacement was inadequate);
      Monitor central venous pressure (keep to 8 to 10 cm. of water above baseline);
      Monitor urinary output (keep to 50–100 ml./hr.).
   b. Provide blood, plasma, and balanced electrolytes to maintain blood volume; limit solutions containing glucose, because this patient is often hyperglycemic.
   c. Maintain surveillance of vital signs.
   d. Monitor blood sugar every 4 hours; administer IV insulin to keep blood sugar levels under 200 mg./100 ml.
   e. Monitor serum calcium; it may be necessary to administer calcium gluconate if calcium falls low enough to produce symptoms.
   f. Keep the body metabolism of the patient low.
      (1) Administer oxygen therapy if breathing is labored.
      (2) Keep patient in bed to control overexertion.
      (3) Turn on air-conditioning to keep body heat under control.
6. Surgical Intervention
   a. There is considerable disagreement about the place of surgery in treating acute pancreatitis. It is considered only if all other therapy has failed.
   b. Laparotomy may reveal an alternate problem which can be corrected:
      (1) Tense gallbadder—cholecystostomy
      (2) Stones in ductal system—establish common duct patency
      (3) Necrotic material and fluid removed by peritoneal lavage.

Health Education and Discharge Planning

Manage recovery phase and offer guidelines to the patient to prevent future attacks of pancreatitis.
1. By the 5th or 6th day, offer the following:
   a. Small amounts of fat-free liquids
   b. Anticholinergics parenterally or orally
   c. Nonabsorbable antacids hourly
2. Instruct the patient as follows:
   a. Gradually resume normal diet.
   b. Interdict alcohol and excessive use of coffee, since they increase pancreatic secretion.
3. Urge follow-up visits with physician. (Biliary tract studies and surveillance may uncover the cause of the pancreatitis.)

CHRONIC PANCREATITIS

Chronic pancreatitis is a chronic fibrosis and calcification of the pancreas with obstruction of its ducts and destruction of its secreting acinar cells.

Incidence

1. Occurs most often in men between 45 and 60.
2. Follows repeated attacks of acute interstitial pancreatitis.
3. Usually occurs in patients having a history of prolonged use of alcohol.
4. Gallstones, hyperparathyroidism, and hyperlipidemia are occasionally associated with chronic pancreatitis.

Clinical Manifestations

1. Recurrent episodes of severe upper abdominal and back pain (morphine often does not relieve pain), vomiting, and low-grade fever. Drug addiction is often a secondary problem.
2. Protein and fat digestion is disturbed because of deficient pancreatic secretion.
3. Steatorrhea; stools that are frequent, frothy, and

foul-smelling with high fat content because of faulty fat digestion.
4. Later formation of calcium stones in the duct as calcification develops.
5. Weight loss.
6. Jaundice may occur because of constriction of common bile duct as it passes through head of pancreas.

Diagostic Evaluation

1. Determine whether levels of serum amylase and lipase are elevated. Levels often are not elevated in chronic creatitis.
2. Examine stool to measure fecal fat and trypsin content.
3. Arteriography and x-ray may show fibrous tissue and calcification.
4. Diabetes or abnormal glucose tolerance may be detectable.

Treatment and Nursing Management

1. Offer patient bland, low-fat diet in 6 feedings daily.
2. Give antacids and anticholinergic medication to reduce acid which would stimulate the release of secretin and enhance pancreatic activity.
4. Pancreatic insufficiency is controlled by giving medication containing amylase, lipase, and trypsin—Pancreatin, Cotazyme, Viokase.
   Medication may need to be administered with antacids or bicarbonates.

NOTE: Steatorrhea should be present before initiating enzyme replacement therapy.

5. Since these patients often develop diabetes, be alert for symptoms such as polydipsia, polyuria, weakness, polyphagia (excessive eating), or weight loss and report these to physician.
6. The use of alcohol should be discouraged, since this will aggravate the pancreatitis; treatment of alcoholism must be done if this is a problem, as it usually is.
7. If hyperparathyroidism or hyperlipemia is diagnosed, these certainly must be treated.
8. Surgical aspects are similar to biliary tract surgery (see p. 461).
9. Nature of surgery is determined by identifying the cause; surgery usually fails if alcoholism or drug addiction persists.
   a. With gallbladder disease—biliary tract surgery to explore common bile duct, choledocholithotomy (removing stones in duct) and cholecystectomy (removing gallbladder).
   b. Sphincteroplasty or sphincterotomy dividing sphincter of Oddi to improve drainage of common bile duct.
      . . . or . . .
   c. Selective or generalized drainage of dilated ducts via pancreaticojejunostomy.
   d. Pancreatectomy may be done when pancreas is severely diseased or when persistent pain is a major problem.

PSEUDOCYSTS AND PANCREATIC ABSCESSES

Pseudocysts of the pancreas are collections of inflammatory fluid walled off by fibrous tissue in the pancreas, usually resulting from local necrosis at the time of acute pancreatitis.

Clinical Manifestations and Diagnosis

1. Cysts may attain considerable size; they develop rapidly or slowly (within 72 hours or over several weeks or months).
2. Because they occur in the posterior peritoneum, they may exert pressure against the stomach or colon, visible on barium studies.
3. Persistent elevation of amylase (serum or urine) is the most common finding. Pain and vomiting may occur.
4. Leukocytosis and fever are common but are usually mild with pseudocysts; these responses are more striking with abscess formation.

5. Sonography has been found useful in confirming the diagnosis.

Treatment
1. Pseudocysts may occasionally subside spontaneously.
2. Symptoms of secondary infection may require surgery for drainage.
3. Drainage may be established into gastrointestinal tract (internal) or through skin surface (external); this latter method is frowned upon, because it presents the risk of the patient's developing pancreatic fistulae.

Nursing Management
1. Should external drainage be done, recognize the irritating qualities of the pancreatic enzyme; meticulous skin care is required.
2. Maintain adequate drainage, avoiding tube dislodgment.

PANCREATIC CANCER

Cancer may arise in the head, body, or tail of the pancreas; insulin-secreting pancreatic islet cells may or may not be involved.

Clinical Manifestations
The "big three" are *weight loss*, *pain*, and *jaundice*.
1. Initial symptoms of cancer of the pancreas are often

vague, thereby accounting for a reported 4–9 months' delay from onset of symptoms to diagnosis.
2. Disease usually occurs in older men; alcoholism may be a contributing cause.
3. Weight loss, anorexia, dyspepsia, nausea, some bowel disturbance, and occasionally chills and fever develop.

4. Intermittent, dull-to-severe, vague, epigastric, or back pain, often aggravated by eating or associated with postcibal fullness and bloating occur.
   a. Right upper quadrant pain suggests involvement of the head of pancreas.
   b. Left upper quadrant pain suggests involvement of the body or tail of pancreas.
   c. Pain often radiates to back or is exclusively in back.
   d. Pain is often worse at night, aggravated in lying-down position and relieved by lying with legs drawn up or by walking bent over.
   e. Fear of eating may take place.
5. The patient may experience depression and loss of ambition combined with a feeling of anxiety and premonition of serious illness.
6. Obstruction of the common bile duct produces jaundice, clay-colored stools, dark urine, and itching (due to cancer of head of pancreas).

   Differentiation must be made between jaundice due to biliary obstruction (due to a stone in the common duct) and jaundice due to hepatic metastases.

Diagnostic Evaluation

1. Blood studies including serum bilirubin, alkaline phosphatase, SGOT, and prothrombin time.
2. Secretin studies and radiologic procedures: UGI series, gallbladder studies, and possibly fiberoptic duodenoscopy with cannulation of papilla and pancreatic ductography, or transhepatic cholangiography.
3. Scanning—^{75}Se-selenomethionine; note that frequent false positive findings occur.
4. Angiography

BIBLIOGRAPHY

Books
General

Abbott MK. Invasive Radiologic Diagnostic Procedures. Philadelphia, F.A. Davis, 1978
Beal VA. Nutrition in the Life Span. Somerset, John Wiley & Sons, 1980
Beeson P, McDermott W and Wyngaarden J. Textbook of Medicine, 15th ed. Philadelphia, WB Saunders, 1979
Brooks FP (ed). Gastrointestinal Pathophysiology. New York, Oxford University Press, 1978
Drain CB and Shipley SB. The Recovery Room: Postoperative Care after Gastrointestinal, Abdominal, and Anorectal Surgery. Philadelphia, WB Saunders, 1979
Fischer J. Total Parenteral Nutrition. Boston, Little, Brown & Co, 1978
Given BA and Simmons SJ. Gastroenterology in Clinical Nursing, 3rd ed. St. Louis, CV Mosby, 1979
Goldberg SM, Gordon PH and Nivatvongs S. Essentials of Anorectal Surgery. Philadelphia, JB Lippincott Co, 1980
Gross L and Bailey Z. Enterostomal Therapy: Developing Institutional and Comunity Programs. Wakefield, Nursing Resources, 1979
Karush A et al. Psychotherapy in Chronic Ulcerative Colitis. Philadelphia, WB Saunders, 1977
Kirsner JB and Shorter RD (eds). Inflammatory Bowel Disease. Philadelphia, Lea & Febiger, 1978
Montgomery WW. Surgery of the Upper Respiratory System, 2nd ed. Philadelpha, Lea & Febiger, 1975
Mullen BD and McGinn KA. The Ostomy Book: Living Comfortably with Colostomies, Ileostomies, and Urostomies. Palo Alto, Bull Publishing Co, 1981

5. Ultrasonography
6. Computed tomography

Treatment

Surgical only: Although surgical cures are possible, 5-year survival is about 25%. Tumor is removed if it has not invaded important surrounding structures.
1. Whipple Resection—removal of head (and sometimes neck) of pancreas; removal of adjacent stomach, distal portion of common duct, and duodenum. Patient has severe malabsorption afterward.
2. If Whipple procedure cannot be done, jaundice should be relieved by diverting bile from gallbladder into jejunum (cholecystojejunostomy). If duodenum is invaded, gastrojejunostomy should be done to bypass duodenal obstruction.
3. For cancer of the body and tail of the pancreas, distal pancreatectomy and splenectomy are the most commonly employed procedures.
4. Total pancreatectomy—en bloc resection of the common bile duct, stomach, duodenum, pancreas, and spleen.

Nursing Management

1. Because of the patient's poor nutritional state, it is a challenge to maintain adequate calorie levels. A bland, low-fat diet is recommended plus whatever he can tolerate without overeating.
2. Medium-chain triglycerides are better tolerated, since they cause less fat excretion.
3. Alcohol to be avoided.
4. Anticholinergics used.
5. See management of the patient undergoing major gastrointestinal surgery (p. 416) and biliary surgery (p. 461).

Nyhus LN and Condon RE (eds). Hernia. Philadelphia, JB Lippincott Co, 1978
Pracy R et al. Ear, Nose and Throat Surgery, New York, John Wiley & Sons, 1977
Sernka T and Jacobson E. Gastrointestinal Physiology. Baltimore, Williams & Wilkins, 1979
Sleisenger M and Fordtran J. Gastrointestinal Disease: Pathophysiology, Diagnosis, Management, 2nd ed. Philadelphia, WB Saunders, 1978
Snow JB Jr (ed). Controversy in Otolaryngology. Philadelphia, WB Saunders, 1980
Suitor CW and Hunter MF. Nutrition: Principles and Application in Health Promotion. Philadelphia, JB Lippincott, 1980
Thorn G et al. Harrison's Principles of Internal Medicine, 9th ed. New York, McGraw-Hill, 1980
Waite DE. Textbook of Practical Oral Surgery. Philadelphia, Lea & Febiger, 1978
Zegarelli EV, Kutscher AH and Human GA. Diagnosis of Diseases of the Mouth and Jaws. Philadelphia, Lea & Febiger, 1978

1 CONDITIONS OF THE MOUTH, NECK, AND ESOPHAGUS

Articles
Mouth

Apfelberg DB et al. Temperomandibular joint disease. Postgrad Med 1979 May; 65(5):167–172
Beck S. Impact of a systematic oral care protocol on stomatitis

after chemotherapy. Cancer Nurs 1979 June; 2(3): 185–199

Bock J. Herpes: Scourge of the seventies. The Canadian Nurse 1980 Jan; 76(1):22–24

Bock MM. Care after dental surgery. Nursing '79, 1979 April; 10(4):94–95

Brown P. TMJ syndrome. Am J Nurs 1980 May; 80(5): 908–910

Daly KM. Everyday concerns. Am J Nurs 1979 Aug; 79(8): 1415–1417

Dupont JB, Guillamondegui OM and Jeese RH. Surgical treatment of advanced carcinoma of the base of the tongue. Am J Surg 1978 Oct; 136(4):501–503

Fann W and Shannon I. A treatment for dry mouth in psychiatric patients. Am J Psychol 1978 Feb; 135(2): 250–252

Gannon EP. Giving your patients meticulous mouth care. Nursing '80 1980 March; 10(3):70–76

Geisler J. Tips for your fractured-jaw patient. RN 1981 May; 44(1):33, 114

Heller KS and Shah JP. Carcinoma of the lip. Am J Surg 1979 Oct; 138(4):600–603

Kempinski C et al. An experience in primary care (Nursing Grand Rounds) (Squamous cell carcinoma—mouth). Nursing '79 1979 Oct; 9(10)45–47

Lee, BC, Hansen EF and Poppell MR. Facial fractures. Nursing '80 1980 Aug; 10(8):43–46

Lieberman ZH, Byrd DL and Davidson TJ. Immobilization of the mandible in oral cancer therapy. Am J Surg 1979 Oct; 138(4):508–511

May M and Hardin WB. Facial Palsy: Interpretation of neurologic findings. Laryngoscope 1978 Aug; 88(8): 1352–1362

Marbach JJ. Arthritis of temperomandibular joint. Am Fam Physician 1979 Feb; 19(2):131–139

McCabe B and Manning R. Physical diagnosis. Ahhh! What the mouth exam can tell you. Patient Care 1978 June 15; 12(11):140–161

Meissner JE. A simple guide for assessing oral health. Nursing '80 1980 April; 10(4):84–85

Osner J. Coping with change. Am J Nurs 1979 Aug; 79(8):1418–1419

Ostchega Y. Preventing . . . and treating . . . cancer chemotherapy's oral complications. Nursing '80 1980 Aug; 10(8):47–52

Potter BE, Yarington CT Jr and Walike JW. Management of intraoral injuries. Am Fam Physician 1978 Nov; 18(5):96–102

Schweiger JL, Lang JW and Schweiger JW. Oral assessment: How to do it. Am J Nurs 1980 April; 80(4):654–657

Van de Heyning J. Levamisole in the treatment of recurrent aphthous stomatitis. Laryngoscope 1978 March; 88(3); 522–527

Vest C, Meinneke JA and Smith R. Herpes zoster oticus. Postgrad Med 1979 April; 65(4):143–150

Yanachek MP. Growing role for the nurse in oral surgery. AORN J 1979 Aug; 30(8):314–326

Dysphagia

Atkinson M. Diseases of the alimentary system-dysphagia. Br J Med 1977 Jan; 1(6053):91–93

Buckley JE, Addicks CL and Maniglia J. Feeding patients with dysphagia. Nurs Forum 1976; 15(1):69–85

Espiritu CR. Swallowing disorders: Clinical features and therapy. Today's Clinician 1978 April; 2(4):27–31

Griffin JW and Tollison JW. Dysphagia. Am Fam Physician 1980 Nov; 22(5):154–160

Martinez LO. Dysphagia: Radiologic aspects of diagnosis. Today's Clinician 1978 April; 2(4):17–23

Head and Neck

Aquilar NV, Olson ML and Shedd DP. Rehabilitation of deglutition problems in patients with head and neck cancer. Am J Surg 1979 Oct; 138(4):501–507

Cornelius J. Screening for head and neck cancers. Nurse Practitioner 1979 Jan; 4(4):15–19

Jesse RH, Ballantyne AJ and Larson D. Radical or modified neck dissection: Therapeutic dilemma. Am J Surg 1978 Oct; 136(4):516–519

Keith CF. Wound management following head and neck surgery. Nurs Clin North Am 1979 Dec; 14(4):761–778

McConnell EA. Radical neck dissection. Nursing '76 1976 Nov; 6(11):58–65

Middleton DB and Ferrante JA. Periorbital and facial cellulitis. Am Fam Physician 1980 Feb; 21(2):97–103

Stuart MS. Skin flaps and grafts after head and neck surgery. Am J Nurs 1978 Aug; 78(8):1368–1374

Esophagus

Gallagher EG, Zumbro GL and Treasure RL. Celestin tube intubation for advanced esophageal carcinoma. Am J Surg 1978 Sept; 136(3):405–407

Israel R and Wood J. Esophagitis related to cromolyn. JAMA 1979 Dec 21; 242(25):2758–2759

Manteuffel SL and McDonough JJ. Esophageal reconstruction with free jejunal grafts. AORN J 1979 Dec; 30(6): 1059–1064

Perro KB, Goetze CM and Monaghan JJ. Esophageal gastric tube airway. Nursing '80 1980 Aug; 10(8):61–63

Rajan RK. Esophageal diverticula. Am Fam Physician 1979 March; 19(3):119–122

Diarrhea and Constipation

Bayless TM. Malabsorption in the elderly. Hosp Pract 1979 Aug; 14(8):57–63

Bertholf CB. Protocol: Acute diarrhea. Nurse Practitioner 1978 May–June; 3(3):17–20

Devroede G. A commonsense approach to overcoming constipation. Drug Therapy 1978 Nov; 8(11):113–117

Devroede G. Evaluation and treatment of chronic constipation. Drug Therapy 1978 Nov; 8(11):61–68

Dhar GJ and Soergel KH. Principles of diarrhea therapy. Am Fam Physician 1979 Jan; 19(1):165–173

Lactulose (Chronulac) for constipation. Med Letter 1980 Jan 11; 22(1):2–3

Matsishe JW and Phillips SF. Chronic diarrhea. Med Clin North Am 1978 Jan; 62(1):141–154

Rodman MJ. Diarrhea: Think twice before giving meds. RN 1980 Oct; 43(10):73–84

Sack DA et al. Prophylactic doxycycline for travelers diarrhea. N Engl J Med 1978 April 6; 298(14):758–763

Summers RW and Christensen J. Acute and chronic diarrhea: Diagnostic and therapeutic considerations. Drug Ther 1978 Nov; 8(11):73–90

2   GASTROINTESTINAL CONDITIONS

Articles

Diagnosis

Baker C and Way LW. Clinical utility of CAT body scans. Am J Surg 1978 July; 136(1):37–44

Bush W, Mullarkey M and Webb RL. Adverse reactions to radiographic contrast material. West J Med 1980 Feb; 132(2):95–98

Endoscopy and upper GI series. Am Fam Physician 1980 Mar; 21(3):182

Exploration needed? 'Go in' with sound. Patient Care 1979 Feb 15; 13(3):53–95

Exploring the abdomen with ultrasound. Patient Care 1979 Feb 15; 13(3):98–154

Harvey CK. Protecting personnel from diagnostic x-ray. AORN J 1979 Oct; 30(4):612

Liebermann TR and Barnes M. Gastrointestinal fiberoptic endoscopy: Diagnostic and therapeutic aspects. Surg Clin North Am 1979 Oct; 59(5):787–786

Sherlock P and Winawer SJ. Differential diagnosis of upper gastrointestinal bleeding and cancer. CA A Cancer Jour Clin 1978 Jan–Feb; 28(1):7–16

Smeltzer C and Urba P. Hemoccult screeing: The nurse's role. Cancer Nurs 1979 Dec; 2(6):475–479

Sterilization or disinfection of flexible fiberoptic endoscopes. AORN J 1979 Aug; 30(2):350–352

X-ray hazards, real and imagined. Harvard Medical School Letter 1978 Nov; 4(1):3–5

Nutrition

Donovan L. Is the doctor starving your patient? RN 1978 July; 41(7):36–40

Martin DS and DuRant RH. A critical analysis of elemental diets. Hosp Formulary 1979 July; 14(7):686–695

Mendeloff AI. Dietary fiber and gastrointestinal diseases. Med Clin North Am 1978 Jan; 62(1):165–171

Mullen JL et al. Implications of malnutrition in the surgical patient. Arch Surg 1979 Feb; 114(2):121–125

Nachlas MN, Crawford DT and Pearl JM. Current status of jejunoileal bypass in the treatment of morbid obesity. Surg Gynecol Obstet 1980 Feb; 150(2):256–270

Zikria BA and King TC. Gastrointestinal function and nutrition in surgical patients. Contemp Surg 1979 June; 14(6):37–41

Intubation

Disposable suction catheters: Product survey. Nursing '79, 1979 May; 9(5):70–75

Giving medication through a nasogastric tube. Nursing '80, 1980 May; 10(5):71–73

Grossman MB. Gastrointestinal endoscopy. Clinical Sym 1980; 32(3):1–36

Hansen BC et al. Nursing intervention in problems of tube feeding, a consortium project. Booklet. Nursing Research, ANA Commission on Nursing Research, pp 8–9, 1979

Hanson RL. New approach to measuring adult nasogastric tubes for insertion. Am J Nurs 1980 July; 80(7):1334–1335

Hanson RL. Predictive criteria for length of nasogastric tube insertion for tube feeding. J Parenteral & Enteral Nutrition 1979 May/June; 3(3):160–163

Hoppe M. The new tube feeding sets or your patients are what you feed them. Nursing '80 1980 March; 10(3):79–85

McConnell EA. Ten problems with nasogastric tubes. Nursing '79 1979 April; 9(4):78–85

Nurse's aid to suction procedures—aspiration—gastrointestinal decompression. Booklet. Gomco Equipment, Chemitron Products, 1979

O'Malley P and Zankofski MA. Disposable suction catheters (A nursing '79 product survey). Nursing '79 1979 April; 9(4):70–75

Ochsner A. The relative merits of temporary gastrostomy and nasogastric suction of the stomach. Am J Surg 1977 June; 133(6):729–732

Oral care for nasogastric tube patients. Nursing '79 1979 May; 9(5):98–99

Persons C. Why risk TPN when tube feeding will do? RN 1981 Jan; 44(1):35–41

Duodenum and Stomach

Atkenson RJ and Nyhus LM. Gastric lavage for hemorrhage in the upper part of the gastrointestinal tract. Surg Gynecol Obstet 1978 May; 146(5):797–798

Babb RR. Cimetidine. Postgrad Med 1980 Dec; 68(6):87–93

Burkle WS. Tagamet. Nursing '80 1980 April; 10(4):86–87

Cimetidine prophylaxis of gastrointestinal bleeding. JAMA 1980 Sept 12; 244(11):126

Dragstedt LR. The pathogenesis of duodenal and gastric ulcers. Am J Surg 1978 Sept; 136(3):286–301

Dyck WP. Cimetidine in the management of peptic ulcer disease. Surg Clin North Am 1979 Oct; 59(5):863–868

Freeman HP and Ganepola GAP. The case for parietal cell vagotomy. Contemp Surg 1978 July; 13(7):11–22

Freund H, Atamian S and Fischer JE. Chromium deficiency during total parenteral nutrition. JAMA 1979 Feb 2; 24(5):496–498

Fujimoto S et al. Carcinoembryonic antigen (CEA) in gastric juice or feces as an aid in the diagnosis of gastrointestinal cancer. Ann Surg 1979 Jan; 189(1):34–38

Gastrointestinal stapling safe. AORN J 1980 Jan; 31(1):62–63

Gordon A Jr. Total parenteral nutrition. Postgrad Med 1979 Jan; 65(1):29

Hall S. Understanding aerophagia. Nursing '79 1979 Nov; 9(11):100–103

Marshall JB and Settles RH. Zollinger–Ellison syndrome. Postgrad Med 1980 July; 68(1):38–50

Morris SJ and Rogers AI. Diarrhea after gastrectomy and vagotomy. Postgrad Med 1979 Jan; 76(1):219–230

Page CP et al. Safe, cost-effective postoperative nutrition. Am J Surg 1979 Dec; 138:939–945

Rodman MJ. The drug interactions we all overlook (antacids). RN 1980 Oct; 43(10):47–49

Singer JA and Rason GR. Gastric ulcer: The importance of follow-up care. Am J Surg 1979 Sept; 136(3):302–305

Parenteral Hyperalimentation

Blackburn GL. Hyperalimentation in the critically ill patient. Heart Lung 1979 Jan–Feb; 8(1):57–70

Colley R and Wilson J. Meeting patients' nutritional needs with hyperalimentation. Nursing '79 1979 May; 9(5):76–83; and 1979 June; 9(6):57–61; and 1979 July; 9(7):50–54; and 1979 Aug; 9(8):56–63; and 1979 Sept; 9(9):62–69

Copeland EM, Daly JM and Dudrick SJ. Intravenous hyperalimentation, bowel rest, and cancer. Crit Care Med 1980 Jan; 8(1):21–28

Driscoll RH and Rosenberg IH. Total parenteral nutrition in inflammatory bowel disease. Med Clin North Am 1978 Jan; 62(1):185–201

Fischer J. Parenteral and enteral nutrition. Disease-a-Month, Chicago, Yearbook Publishers 1978; 24(9):3–84

Freund H, Atamian S and Fischer JE. Chromium deficiency during total parenteral nutrition. JAMA 1979 Feb 2; 24(5):496–498

Gever LN. Parenteral iron supplements. Nursing '80 1980 Aug; 10(8):60

Goodgame JT. A critical assessment of the indications for total parenteral nutrition. Surg Gynecol Obstet 1980 Sept; 151(3):433–441

Gordon A Jr. Total parenteral nutrition. Postgrad Med 1979 Jan; 65(1):29

Hodges RE. Total parenteral nutrition. Postgrad Med 1979 March; 65(3):171–180

Ivey MF. The status of parenteral nutrition. Nurs Clin North Am 1979 June; 14(2):285–303

Kudsk K, Fabri J and Ruberg R. Pyogenic arthritis caused by a total parenteral nutrition line. JAMA 1979 Nov 2; 242(18):1995

Newmark SR. The role of nutritional support in the treatment of gastrointestinal disease. Surg Clin North Am 1979 Oct; 59(5):761–780

Orr G et al. Alternatives to total parenteral nutrition in the critically ill patient. Crit Care Med 1980 Jan; 8(1):29–34

Steiger E and Grundfest S. A review of home hyperalimentation. Contemp Surg 1979 Aug; 15(8):33–40

Articles

Fat Emulsion

Barlow AL (ed). Liposyn Research Conference Proceedings. North Chicago, Abbott Laboratories, 1979

Jacobson NT. how to administer those tricky lipid emulsions. RN 1979 June; 42(6):63–64

Managing I.V. Therapy. Nursing Photobook. Horsham, Intermed Communications, 1980

Appendicitis—Peritonitis—Hernia

Condon RE et al. Symposium. Peritonitis—Part 1. Contemp Surg 1979 Nov; 15(11):65–88; Peritonitis—Part 2. Contemp Surg 1979 Dec; 15(12):51–61

Fine M and Busuttil RW. Acute appendicitis: Efficacy of prophylactic preoperative antibiotics in the reduction of septic morbidity. Am J Surg 1978 Feb; 135(2):210–212

Hiebert CA and O'Mara CS. The Belsey operation for hiatal hernia; A twenty year experience. Am J Surg 1979 Apr; 137(4):532–435

Leape LL and Ramenorsky ML. Laparoscopy for questionable appendicitis. Ann Surg 1980 Apr; 191(4):410–413

Ryan AJ. Validation of appendectomy. Postgrad Med 1979 Jan; 65(1):19–21

Savrin RA. Chronic and recurrent appendicitis. Am J Surg 1979 Mar; 137(3):355–357

Smith DE, Kirchmer NA and Stewart DR. Use of the barium enema in the diagnosis of acute appendicitis and its complications. Am J Surg 1979 Dec; 138(6):829–834

Regional Ileitis (Crohn's Disease)

Bertholf CB. Protocol: Acute diarrhea. Nurse Practitioner 1978 May–June; 3(3):17–20

Dhar GJ and Soergel KH. Principles of diarrhea therapy. Am Fam Physician 1979 Jan; 19(1):165–173

Mendeloff AI and Halberstam MJ. How to tell ulcerative colitis from Crohn's disease—and how to treat both. Mod Med 1980 Dec 15; 48:85–95

Myers S et al. Quality of life after surgery for Crohn's disease: A psychosocial survey. Gastroenterology 1980 Jan; 78(1):1–6

Serebro H, Kay S and Javett S: Sulphasalazine rectal enemas: Topical method of inducing remission of active ulcerative colitis affecting rectum and descending colon. Br Med J 12 Nov 1977; 2:1264

Strauch B et al. Caring enough to give your patient control (Crohn's disease). Nursing '80 1980 Aug; 10(8):54–59

Ileostomy and Colostomy

Bedell K and Kinimaka L. Sexuality in the male following abdominoperineal resection. J Enterost Ther 1980 Mar/Apr; 7(1):14–18

Bille DA. Legal ramifications of the ostomates bill of rights. J Enterost Ther 1980 Jan–Feb; 7(1):12–16

Broadwell DC and Sorrells SL. Loop transverse colostomy. Am J Nurs 1978 June; 78(6):1029–1031

Click C. Chemotherapy and the ostomy patient. J Enterost Ther 1980 Sept–Oct; 7(5):10–12,16

Fowler E, Jeter KF and Schwartz AA. How to cope when your patient has an entero-cutaneous fistula. Am J Nurs 1980 March; 80(3):426–429

Gelernt IM. A step toward the continent colostomy. J Enterost Ther 1977 Summer; 4(3):5–7

Heindel M. How to protect your ostomy patients from post-op skin problems. RN 1978 Jan; 41(1):43–45

Kodner IJ. Colostomy and ileostomy. Ciba Clinical Symp 1978; 30(5):2–36

Lerner J, Harsh J and Eisenstat TE. Why pre-op stoma planning is a must. RN 1980 Aug; 43(8):48–51

Lindensmith S. Body image and the crisis of enterostomy. Canadian Nurse 1977 Nov; 73 (11):24–27

McVay CB et al. Symposium; Abdominal stomas. Contemp Surg 1978 July; 13(7):23–53

Meyers S et al. Quality of life after surgery for Crohn's disease: A psychosocial survey. J Enterost Ther 1980 Sept–Oct; 7(5):25–31

Mahoney JM. What you should know about ostomies. Nursing '78 1978 May; 8(5):74–84

Parlato CD. Tent the tube. Nursing '79 1979 Jan; 9(1):88

Traverso CJ. SOAP noting common stomal problems. J Enterost Ther 1980 Jan–Feb; 7(1):8–11; 1980 Mar–Apr; 7(2):11–12; 1980 May–June; 7(3):8–9

Watt RC. Colostomy irrigation—yes or no? Am J Nurs 1977 March; 77(3):442–444

Wood RY. People with temporary colostomies. Canadian Nurse 1977 Nov; 73(11):28–30

Continent Ileostomy (Kock)

Akwari OE, Kelly KA and Phillips SF. Myoelectric and motor patterns of continent pouch and conventional ileostomy. Surg Gynecol Obstet 1980 March; 150(3):363–371

Cox and Wentworth AA. The ileal pouch procedure. Booklet. Rochester, Minnesota Mayo Comprehensive Cancer Center, 1977

Flake WK et al. Problems encountered with the Kock ileostomy. Am J Surg 1979 Dec; 136(6):851–855

Heyman E et al. The pouch ileostomy. Nursing '77 1977 Sept; 7(9):44–47

Kock NG. A new look at ileostomy. In Nyhus LM. Surg Annu 8:241–256, 1976

MacClelland DC. Kock Pouch: A new type of ileostomy. AORN J 1980 Aug; 32(2):191–201

Shrock TR. Complications of continent ileostomy. Am J Surg 1979 July; 138(1):162–169

Stark KJ. Nursing care of the Kock pouch patient. Aorn J 1980 Aug; 32(2):202–206

Colon

Akwari OE, Kelly KA and Phillips SF. Myoelectric and motor patterns of continent pouch and conventional ileostomy. Surg Gynecol Obstet 1980 Mar; 150(3):363–371

Bell GA. Closure of colostomy following sigmoid colon resection for perforated diverticulitis. Surg Gynecol Obstet 1980 Jan; 150(1):85–90

Berk JE, Colcock BP and McHardy G. New perspectives on diverticulitis. Patient Care 1979 Jan 30; 13(2):152–179

Bland KI, Garrison RN and Knutson CO. Colorectal carcinoma. Postgrad Med 1979 Sept; 66(3):106–115

Check WA. Colorectal cancer: Does extensive surgery help? JAMA 1979 Sept 28; 242(13):1346–1351

Chung RS, Gurll NJ and Berglund E. A controlled clinical trial of whole gut lavage as a method of bowel preparation for colonic operations. 1979 Jan; 137(1):75–81

Devroede G et al. Confirming the elusive colitis diagnosis. Patient Care 1980 June 15; 14(10):38–81

Devroede G et al. Working through history and physical clues to colitis. Patient Care 1980 April 30; 14(8):50–107

Flake WK. Problems encountered with the Kock ileostomy. Am J Surg 1979 Dec; 138(6):851–855

Fonkalsrud EW. Total colectomy and endorectal ileal pull-through with internal ileal reservoir for ulcerative colitis. Surg Gynecol Obstet 1980 Jan; 150(1):1–8

Garnjobst W, Leaverton GH and Sullivan ES. Safety of colostomy closure. Am J Surg 1978 July; 136(1):85–89

Howe HJ. Acute perforations of the sigmoid colon secondary to diverticulitis. Am J Surg 1979 Feb; 137(2):184–197

Kroner K. Are you prepared for your ulcerative colitis patient? Nursing '80 1980 April; 10(4):43–49

Lactose intolerance—milk as a cause of bowel symptoms. Harvard Med School Health Letter 1979 Aug 4; (10):5

Lipkin M. Dietary, environmental, and hereditary factors in the development of colorectal cancer. CA A Cancer Jour Clin 1979 Sept/Oct; 29(5):291–299

Mendenhall MK and Ahlgren EW. Anesthetic considerations in surgery for gastrointestinal disease. Surg Clin North Am 1979 Oct; 59(5):905–918

Miller SF. The detection of asymptomatic colorectal cancer. Am Fam Physician 1978 Sept; 18(3):89–92

Minervini S et al. Comparison of three methods of whole bowel irrigation. Am J Surg 1980 Sept; 140(3):400–402

Nichols RL. Infections following gastrointestinal surgery: Intra-abdominal abscess. Surg Clin North Am 1980 Feb; 60(1):197–212

Nichols RL et al. Intra-abdominal sepsis. Am Fam Physician 1980 April; 21(4):118–126

Rheingold OJ, Barkin JS and Rogers AI. Carcinoma of the colon. Postgrad Med 1979 Nov; 66(5):201–209

Roberts JW. Continent ileostomy. Surg Clin North Am 1979 Oct; 59(5):853–862

Rusch V and Simonowitz DA. Crohn's disease in the older patient. Surg Gynecol Obstet 1980 Feb; 150(2):184–186

Sachar DB and Present DH. Immunotherapy in inflammatory bowel disease. Med Clin North Am 1978 Jan; 62(1):173–183

Sredl D and Wilhite M. The enterostomal therapist—a new breed of nurse. Super Nurse 1980 Jan; 11(1):51–52

Strauch B et al. Caring enough to give your patient control (Crohn's disease). Nursing '80 1980 Aug;; 10(8):54–59

Waye JD. Colitis, cancer, and colonoscopy. Med Clin North Am 1978 Jan; 62(1):211–224

Rectal Conditions

Abcarian H. Anorectal disorders: When is conservative care enough? Mod Med 1980 Jan 15; 48(2):37–52

Amin N. Giardiasis. Postgrad Med 1979 Nov; 66(5):151–156

Eckhauser FE, Lindenauer SM and Morley GW. Pelvic exenteration for advanced rectal carcinoma. Am J Surg 1979 Sept; 138(3):411–414

Fisher SG. Psychosexual adjustment following total pelvic exenteration. Cancer Nurse 1979 June; 2(3):219–225

Green JP et al. Anal carcinoma: Current therapeutic concepts Am J Surg 1980 July; 140(1):151–155

Shambaugh GE III and Major ND. When your patient asks about enemas. Patient Care 1980 March 30; 14(6):129–138

Slawson M. Thirty-three drugs that discolor urine and/or stools. RN Mag 1980 Jan; 43(1):40–41

Agencies

American Celiac Society 45 Gifford Ave, Jersey City NJ 07304

American Dental Association, Bureau of Dental Health Education, 211 E Chicago Ave, Chicago IL 60611

American Dietetic Association, 430 N Michigan Ave, Chicago IL 60611

American Digestive Disease Society, 420 Lexington Ave, New York, New York 10017

National Dairy Council, 6300 N River Road, Rosemont, IL 60018

National Foundation for Ileitis and Colitis, Dept N80, 295 Madison Ave, New York, New York 10017

The Nutrition Foundation, Office of Education and Public Affairs, 888 17th St, NW, Suite 300, Washington, DC 20006

Society for Nutrition Education, 2140 Shattuck Ave, Suite 1110, Berkeley CA 94704

United Ostomy Association, 2001 W Beverly Blvd, Los Angeles, CA 90057

3 CONDITIONS OF THE HEPATIC AND BILIARY SYSTEM

Books

Conn HA and Lieberthal MM. The Hepatic Coma Syndromes and Lactulose. Baltimore, Md, Williams & Wilkins, 1979

Koff RS, Liver Disease in Primary Care Medicine. New York, Appleton-Century-Crofts, 1980

Koff RS. Viral Hepatitis. New York, John Wiley & Sons, 1978

Krugman S and Gocke DJ. Viral Hepatitis, Vol. 15. Major Problems in Internal Medicine. Philadelphia, WB Saunders, 1978

Leevy CM et al. Diseases of the Liver and Biliary Tract. Chicago, Year Book Medical Publishers, 1977

Schiff L. Diseases of the Liver, 4th ed. Philadelphia, JB Lippincott, 1975

Wright R et al. Liver and Biliary Disease. Philadelphia, WB Saunders, 1980

Articles

Liver, General

Babb RB. Diagnosing ascites. Postgrad Med 1978 May; 63(5):219–233

Boyer JL. Exploring disruptions in bile flow. Patient Care 1980 Feb 29; 14(4):58–135

Byrne J. Liver function studies, Part 1: Introduction and bilirubin. Nursing '77 1977 July; (9):12–14

Byrne J. Liver function studies, Part III, Tests that measure protein metabolism. Nursing '77 1977 Oct: 7(10):13

Byrne J. Liver function studies, Part IV. Using metabolism tests to investigate liver function. Nursing '77 1977 Dec; 7(12):14

Byrne J. Liver function studies, Part V. Using enzyme levels to assess liver function. Nursing '78 1978 Jan; 8(1):50–52

Calne RY. Orthotopic liver transplantation. Contemp Surg 1978 Oct; 13(10):21–36

Gaines KC and Sorrell MF. Host resistance in liver disease—its evaluation and therapeutic modification. Med. Clin North Am 1979 May; 63(3):495–505

Hinshaw JR. Cost effectiveness of tests to determine etiology of jaundice. Contemp Surg 1980 July; 17(1):50–52

Kanagasundaram N and Leevy CM. Immunologic aspects of liver disease. Med Clin North Am 1979 May; 63(3):631–642

Kaplowitz N. Cholestatic liver disease. Hosp Pract 1978 Aug; 13(8):83–92

Korobkin M and Goldberg HI. Computed tomography of the hepatobiliary system. Ann Rev Med 1979; 30:181–188

Russell RM. Vitamin and mineral supplements in the management of liver disease. Med Clin North Am 1979 May; 63(3):537–544

Terblanche J, Koep LJ and Starzl TE. Liver transplantation. Med Clin North Am 1979 May; 63(3):507–521

Zimmerman HJ. Drug-induced chronic hepatic disease. Med Clin North Am 1979 May; 63(3):567–582

Zimmons DS, Chang J and Clemett AR. Advances in the management of bile duct obstruction. Med Clin North Am 1979 May; 63(3):593–609

Hepatitis

Aach RD and Kahn RA. Post-transfusion hepatitis: Current perspectives. Ann Intern Med 1980 Feb; 92(4):539–546

Ackley A and Gocke DJ. Viral hepatitis. Am Fam Physician 1980 May; 21(5):156–162

Bauer D. Preventing the spread of hepatitis B in dialysis units. Am J Nurs 1980; 80(2):260–261

Bayer AS. Arthritis associated with hepatitis. Postgrad Med 1980 April; 67(4):175–178

Berman M et al. The chronic sequelae of the Non-A, Non-B hepatitis. Ann Intern Med 1979 July; 91(1):1–6

Bryan JA. Viral hepatitis. 1. Clinical and laboratory aspects and epidemiology. Postgrad Med 1980 Nov; 68(5):66–76; 2. Prevention and Control Postgrad Med 1980 Nov; 68(5):81–86

Dienstag JL. Viral hepatitis: How far have we come, where are we going? Drug Ther 1978 Sept; 8(9):31–33

Favero MS et al. Guidelines for the care of patients hospitalized with viral hepatitis. Ann Intern Med 1979 Oct; 91(4):872–876 (also see—Letters and corrections regarding this article. Ann Intern Med 1980 May; 92(5):706–708)

Herlong HF and Maddrey WC. Viral hepatitis. Primary Care 1979 Sept; 6(3):505–515

Hollinger FB and Graham DY. Viral hepatitis: Types A, B and non-A/nonB. Drug Ther 1978 Sept; 8(9):39–55

Kiernan TW and Ramgopal M. Viral hepatitis: Progress and problems. Med Clin North Am 1979 May; 63(3):611–619

Miller DJ. Seroepidemiology of viral hepatitis. Postgrad Med 1980 Sept; 68(3):137–148

Peterson AN. Acute viral hepatitis. Nurse Practitioner 1979 Jan; 4(4):9–11

Redeker A. When viral hepatitis turns chronic. Patient Care 1979 Nov 15; 13:102–152

Siefkin AD and Bolt RJ. Preoperative evaluation of the patient with gastrointestinal or liver disease. Med Clin North Am 1979 Nov; 63(6):1309–1320

Esophageal Varices

Adamson RJ. Portacaval shunt with portal vein arterioalization. Hosp Pract 1979 Sept; 14(9):88–94

Cirrhosis of the Liver

Ansley JD et al. Effects of peritoneovenous shunting with the LeVeen value on ascites, renal function, and coagulation in six patients with intractable ascites. Surgery 1978 Feb; 83(2):181–187

Babb RR. Diagnosing ascites. Postgrad Med 1978 May; 63(5):214–222

LeVeen HH. Peritoneo-jugular shunt for ascites. Resident Staff Physician 1978 Feb; (2):96–106

Hoyumpa AM Jr. A guide to the treatment of ascites. Drug Ther 1979 Jan; 4(1):33–39

Lund RH and Newkirk JB. Peritoneo-venous shunting system for surgical management of ascites. Contemp Surg 1979 Feb; 14(2):31–45

Seybert PL et al. The LeVeen shunt; new hope for ascites patients. Nursing '79 1979 Jan; 9(1):24–31

Sherman DW et al. Realistic nursing goals in terminal cirrhosis. Nursing '78 1978 June; 8(6):43–46

Steigmann F. Preventing portal systemic encephalopathy in the patient with cirrhosis. Postgrad Med 1979 Feb; 65(2):118–126

Gallbladder

Bell J and Johnson J. Just another patient with gallstones? Don't you believe it. Nursing '79 1979 Oct; 9(10):27–33

Binder SC and Katz B. The benefits of surgery for asymptomatic gallstones. Am Fam Physician 1978 Oct; 18(4):171–173

Feigenberg Z. Routine drainage in cholecystectomy. Am J Surg 1979 March; 137(3):313–316

Ferguson IA et al. Is it gallbaldder disease or isn't it? Patient Care 1980 July 15; 14(13):14–60

Ferguson IA et al. Judging alternatives to cholecystectomy. Patient Care 1980 Sept 15; 14(15):88–133

Ferguson IA et al. When gallbladder disease means surgery. Patient Care 1980 Oct 15; 14(17):120–153

Freeman JB and Olson CM. Refinements in the detection of gallbladder disorders. Contemporary Surg. 1978 Nov; 13(11):9–33

Goldstein F. Tracking and treating gallstones: Sound word on what's new. Mod Med 1979 May 15; 47(9):20–32

Hofmann AF et al. Chenotherapy for gallstone dissolution, induced changes in bile composition and gallstone response. JAMA 1978 March 20; 239(11):1041–1046

Hutcheon DF et al. Postcholecystectomy diarrhea. JAMA 1979 Feb 23; 241(8):823–824

Kurtz K, Kempema J and Birnbaum ML. Coping with acute abdominal crisis and more: multisystem failure (gall bladder). Nursing '78 1978 Nov; 8(11):22–31

McAvoy JM et al. Role of ultrasonography in the primary diagnosis of cholelithiasis. Am J Surg 1978 Sept; 136(3):309–312

Pearlman BJ and Schoenfield LJ. Gallstones, the present and future of medical dissolution. Med Clin North Am 1978 Jan; 62(1):87–105

Redinger RN. Cholelithiasis. Postgrad Med 1979 June; 65(6):56–71

Schoenfield LJ. Chenodeoxycholic acid: Uses and limitations. Hosp Pract 1979 Oct; 14(10):57–65

Tangedahl T. Dissolution of gallstones—when and how? Surg Clin North Am 1979 Oct; 59(5):797–810

Tangedahl TN. Who gets gallstones and why Postgrad Med 1979 Sept; 66(9):175–179

Thistle JL et al. Chenotherapy for gallstone dissolution, 1. Efficacy and safety. JAMA 1978 March 13; 239(11):1041–1046

Thistle JL et al. Chenotherapy for gallstone dissolution. 2. Induced changes in bile composition and gallstone response. JAMA 1978 March 20; 239(12):1138–1144

Thorpe CJ and Caprini JA. Gallbladder disease: Current trends and treatment, Am J Nurs 1980 Dec; 80(12):2181–2185

Tucker L and Bergstrom JF. Identification of gallstone disease. Postgrad Med 1979 Nov; 66(11):163–172

Tucker L and Tangedahl TN. Manifestations of gallstone disease. Postgrad Med 1979 Oct; 66(10):179–184

Watts JM et al. The effect of added bran to the diet on the saturation of bile in people without gallstones. Am J Surg 1978 March; 135:321–324

Pancreas

Development continues on artificial pancreas. AORN J 1979 April; 29(5):925

Kimura T, Zuidema GD and Cameron JL. Acute pancreatitis. Am J Surg 1980 Sept; 140(3):403–408

Macaron C. Primary endocrine-secreting pancreatic tumors. Am Fam Physician 1980 April; 21(4):94–98

Peterson LM and Brooks JR. Lethal pancreatitis: A diagnostic dilemma. Am J Surg 1979 April; 137(4):491–496

Ranson JHC. Acute pancreatitis. Curr Probl Surg 1979 Nov; 16(11):1–84

Reed K, Vose PC and Jarstfer BS. Pancreatic cancer: 30-year review 1947–1977. Am J Surg 1979 Dec; 138(6):929–933

Regan PT and DiMagno EP. Acute pancreatitis: Diagnosis and treatment. Hosp Med 1979 Aug; 15(8):30–41

Skandalakis JE et al. Anatomical complications of pancreatic surgery—Part 1. Contemp Surg 1979 Nov; 15(11):17–40

Skandalakis JE et al. Anatomical complications of pancreatic surgery—Part 2. Contemp Surg 1979 Dec; 15(12):21–50

CONDITIONS OF THE KIDNEYS, URINARY TRACT, AND REPRODUCTIVE SYSTEM

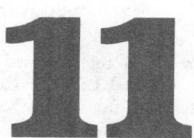

1 RENAL AND GENITOURINARY CONDITIONS

2 GYNECOLOGIC CONDITIONS

1   RENAL AND GENITOURINARY CONDITIONS

CLINICAL MANIFESTATIONS OF URINARY DYSFUNCTION

Pain

1. Genitourinary pain is not always present in renal disease, but is generally seen in the more acute conditions.
2. Pain of renal disease is caused by sudden distention of the renal capsule; severity is related to how quickly the distention develops.
3. Kidney pain—may be felt as a dull ache in costovertebral angle; may spread to umbilicus.
4. Ureteral pain—felt in the back and radiates to the abdomen, upper thighs, testes, or labia.
5. Flank pain (side area between ribs and ilium)—radiates to lower abdomen or epigastrium and often is associated with nausea, vomiting and paralytic ileus; may indicate renal colic.
6. Bladder pain (low abdominal pain or pain over suprapubic area)—may be due to bladder infection or overdistended bladder.
7. Urethral pain from irritation of bladder neck, from foreign body in canal, or from urethritis due to infection or trauma.
8. Pain in scrotal area from inflammatory swelling of epididymis or testis, torsion of testis.
9. Testicular pain due to injury, mumps orchitis, torsion of spermatic cord.
10. Perineal or rectal discomfort from acute prostatitis, prostatic abscess.
11. Back and leg pain from cancer of prostate with metastases to pelvic bones.
12. Pain in glans penis is usually from prostatitis; penile shaft pain is from urethral problems.

Changes in Micturition (Voiding)

1. Hematuria (red blood cells in urine)
   a. Hematuria is considered a serious sign and requires evaluation.
   b. Color of bloody urine dependent upon pH of urine and amount of blood present.
      (1) Acid urine is dark, smoky color.
      (2) Alkaline urine is red color.
   c. Hematuria may be due to systemic cause such as blood dyscrasias, anticoagulant therapy, neoplasms, trauma, extreme exercise.
   d. Painless hematuria may indicate neoplasm in the urinary tract.
   e. Hematuria from renal colic (stones in kidney).
   f. Bloody spotting reveals bleeding from urethra, bladder neoplasms.
   g. Hematuria also seen in renal tuberculosis, polycystic disease of kidneys, septic pyelonephritis, thrombosis and embolism involving renal artery or vein.
2. Proteinuria (albuminuria)
   a. Normal urine does not contain persistent protein in significant quantities.
   b. Proteinuria characteristically seen in all forms of acute and chronic renal disease (more characteristic of glomerulonephritis than pyelonephritis).
      (1) The protein is mainly albumin, but globulin is also present.
      (2) Albumin and globulin escape through damaged glomerular capillaries in a greater amount than can be reabsorbed by the tubules, or damaged tubules fail to reabsorb normal amount filtered.
   c. Proteinura occurs in systemic diseases where there are varying degrees of renal anoxia, as in cardiac decompensation, diabetic glomerulosclerosis.
   d. Mild proteinura may occur from other sources—urethritis, prostatitis, cystitis.
3. Dysuria (painful or difficult voiding)—seen in wide variety of pathological conditions.
4. Frequency—voiding occurs more often than usual, compared to patient's usual pattern (or to a generally accepted norm of once every 3–6 hours).
   a. Determine if habits regarding fluid intake have been altered; it is essential to know normal voiding pattern in order to evaluate frequency.
   b. Increasing frequency can result from a variety of conditions—such as infection and diseases of urinary tract, metabolic disease, hypertension, medications (diuretics).
5. Urgency (strong desire to urinate)—due to inflammatory lesions in bladder, prostate, or urethra, acute bacterial infections, chronic prostatitis in men, and chronic posterior urethrotrigonitis in women.
6. Burning upon urination—as seen in urethral irritation or bladder infections.
7. Enuresis (involuntary voiding during sleep)—may be physiologic to age of 3; after this may be functional or symptomatic of obstructive disease (usually of lower urinary tract).

8. Nocturia (excessive urination at night)—suggests decreased renal concentrating ability or heart failure, diabetes mellitus, poor bladder emptying.
9. Strangury (slow and painful urination); only small amounts of urine voided; blood staining may be noted—seen in severe cystitis.
10. Incontinence (involuntary loss of urine)—may be due to injury to external urinary sphincter, acquired neurogenic disease, severe urgency, etc.
11. Stress incontinence (intermittent leakage of urine due to sudden strain)—indicates weakness of sphincteric mechanism.
12. Polyuria (large volume of urine voided in given time)—demonstrated in diabetes mellitus, diabetes insipidus.
13. Oliguria (small volume of urine; output between 100–500 ml./24 hours)—may result from acute renal failure, shock, dehydration, fluid–ion imbalance.
14. Anuria (absence of urine in the bladder; output less than 50 ml./24 hours)—indicates serious renal dysfunction requiring immediate medical intervention.
15. Pneumaturia (passage of gas in urine during voiding)—caused by fistulous connection between bowel and bladder, rectosigmoid cancer, regional ileitis, sigmoid diverticulitis (most common), and gas-forming urinary tract infections.
16. Hesitancy (undue delay and difficulty in initiating voiding)—may indicate compression of urethra, outlet obstruction, neurogenic bladder.

Gastrointestinal Symptoms Related to Urologic Disease

1. Gastrointestinal symptoms may occur with urological conditions because of:
   a. Renal-intestinal reflexes.
   b. Anatomic relation of right kidney to colon (hepatic flexure), duodenum, head of pancreas, common bile duct, liver, and gallbladder.
   c. Anatomic relation of left kidney to colon (splenic flexure), stomach, pancreas, spleen.
   d. Peritoneal irritation—anterior surface of kidneys covered by peritoneum, which is affected by renal inflammation.
2. Gastrointestinal symptoms related to urologic conditions include nausea, vomiting, diarrhea, abdominal discomfort, paralytic ileus, gastrointestinal hemorrhage with uremia.
3. Appendicitis may present with urinary symptoms.

DIAGNOSTIC EVALUATION FOR UROLOGIC DISEASE

Health History and Assessment

Seek the following information related to urinary and renal function:
1. What is the patient's primary concern? Why is he seeking help?
2. What is the patient's present and past occupation(s)? (Look for occupational hazards related to the urinary tract: contact with chemicals, plastics, pitch, tar, rubber.)
3. What is the past history, especially in relation to urinary problems?
4. Is there any family history of renal disease?
5. What childhood diseases did the patient have?
6. Is there a history of urinary infections?
7. Did enuresis continue beyond the usual age (past 3 years of age)?
8. Are there any voiding disorders?
   a. Dysuria? When does it occur? Where is it felt? Initial or terminal dysuria?
   b. Hesitancy? Straining? Pain during or after urination?
   c. Changes in color of urine? Diminished urine output?
   d. Incontinence? Stress incontinence? Urgency incontinence?
   e. Any history of hematuria?
9. Is pain present?
   Location? Character? Radiation? Duration? Related to voiding? What brings it on? What relieves it?
10. Has the patient had fever? Chills? Passage of stones?
11. Any history of genital lesions or venereal disease?
12. For the female patient:
    What is the number of children? Their ages? Any forceps deliveries? Catheterizations? Any signs of vaginal discharge? Vaginal/vulvar itch or irritation?
13. Does the patient have diabetes mellitus? Hypertension? Allergies?
14. Has the patient ever been hospitalized with a urinary tract infection?
    Urinary tract infection before the age of 12? Ever cystoscoped? Catheterized with an indwelling catheter? Any kidney roentgenologic procedures?

Roentgenography

A. *Roentgenogram*—flat plate, KUB (x-ray of kidney, ureter, bladder) is used to delineate size, shape, and position of kidneys, but includes organs up to the level of symphysis pubis.
1. Gives a baseline reference for subsequent films.
2. Shows the position, number, and size of radiopaque objects suspected of being urinary tract calculi (stones).

B. *Infusion Drip Pyelography*—is an intravenous infusion of a large volume of dilute solution of contrast material to produce opacification of the renal parenchyma and complete filling of urinary tract. Films taken at intervals to demonstrate the filled and distended collecting system.
1. Patient preparation is same as for excretory urography *except that the patient is not dehydrated* (see below).
2. Infusion drip pyelography has almost replaced standard intravenous pyelography; it is used when regular urographic techniques fail to show drainage structures satisfactorily.

C. *Excretory Urography* (intravenous urogram [IVU] or intravenous pyelogram [IVP])—introduction (IV) of a radiopaque contrast medium which concentrates in the urine and thus visualizes the kidneys, ureter, and bladder. The contrast medium is cleared from the bloodstream by renal excretion.

1. Excretory urography is used in:
   a. Initial investigation of any suspected urologic problem, especially in diagnosis of lesions in kidneys and ureters.
   b. To provide a rough estimate of renal function.
2. Patient Preparation
   a. See that patient is not overhydrated—will dilute contrast material and thus cause inadequate visualization (except in patients with myeloma).
   b. Remove obstructing intestinal content, if possible, so as to minimize intestinal gas; enema not usually given, since it may increase gas in the gastrointestinal tract.
   c. It is customary to take no liquids for 8–10 hours before this test, although good films are often obtained in the hydrated patient.

NURSING ALERT: Elderly patients with poor renal reserve or those with multiple myeloma may not tolerate dehydrating procedures and should be given water to drink. Persons with uncontrolled diabetes may be sensitive to fluid restriction.

   d. Give laxative the night before the test to eliminate feces and gas in the intestinal tract.
   e. Ascertain if patient has history of allergies—to find the high-risk patient.
      (1) Evaluate for anaphylactoid reaction (rare) to intravenous dosage of contrast medium. (No contrast medium is completely innocuous.)
      (2) Watch patient during procedure so that reactions are recognized immediately.
         (a) Mild reaction (relatively common)—flushing, metallic taste, nausea, vomiting, faintness, tingling—may be due to osmotic or chemical character of contrast medium.
         (b) Severe reaction—urticaria, edema, asthma, hypotension, convulsions, cyanosis, shock, and cardiac arrest—due to allergic response to contrast medium.
      (3) Have emergency drugs (epinephrine, vasopressors, corticosteroids, etc.), oxygen and tracheostomy equipment ready to restore cardiac activity and maintain adequate respiration and blood pressure. Have equipment available to treat cardiac arrest.

D. *Retrograde Pyelography*—injection of opaque material through ureteral catheters which have been passed up ureters into renal pelvis by means of cystoscopic manipulation. The opaque solution is introduced by gravity or syringe.

1. Retrograde pyelography usually done when nonfunctioning kidney is suspected or if patient is allergic to intravenous contrast material.
2. Performed with decreasing frequency due to improvement of IVP (intravenous pyelogram) techniques.

E. *Cystourethrogram*—visualization of urethra and bladder either by retrograde injection or by voiding of contrast material.

Voiding Cystourethrogram
1. Bladder is filled with radiopaque medium and patient then voids while rapid spot films are taken.
2. With the image intensifier, the presence or absence of vesicoureteric reflux and/or congenital abnormalities

in the lower urinary tract can be demonstrated. Also used to investigate difficulty in bladder emptying and incontinence.

F. *Cystometrogram*—graphic recording of the pressures exerted at varying phases of filling of the urinary bladder. Intermittent filling of the bladder can be recorded and compared with changes in intravesical pressure.

1. Patient is requested to void. Physician observes the time it takes to initiate voiding; size, force, and continuity of urinary stream; degree of straining, hesitancy, intermittency of urination, presence of terminal dribbling.
2. Patient is then placed in lithotomy position and a retention catheter is placed through urethra and into bladder. The residual volume is measured, and the catheter is left in place.
3. The urethral catheter is connected to a water manometer and water is allowed to flow into bladder, usually at the rate of 1 ml. per second.
   a. Patient informs examiner when he feels the first desire to void and again when the bladder feels full. The degree of bladder filling at these points is recorded.
   b. The pressures above the zero level at the symphysis pubis are measured and the pressures and volumes within the bladder are plotted and recorded.

G. *Nephrotomogram*—body section roentgenograms which bring into focus the different layers of the kidney and the diffuse structures in that layer; done also as part of intravenous pyelogram study.

H. *Ultrasonic Scan* (echogram, sonography)—scanning by ultrasound is a noninvasive technique for investigation of renal disease. The kidneys produce a characteristic ultrasonic pattern, making abnormalities readily identifiable. Also used in assessing retroperitoneal disease and in staging malignancies of urinary bladder and prostate. Noninvasive test; no special patient preparation.

I. *Radioisotope Studies of Urinary Tract* (renogram)—delineate structure and function of kidneys without disturbing their normal physiologic processes.

1. Intravenous radioiodine (Hippuran ^{131}I) is given.
2. Sites over both kidneys are monitored with scintillation counters to reveal differences between the 2 kidneys with respect to blood flow, tubular function, and excretion.

J. *Isotopic Localization of Renal Pathology* (renoscan)—delineates the kidney anatomy by external scanning.

1. A radioisotope is given intravenously. A lesion (tumor, infarct) is detected by absence of radioactivity in the involved area and resultant defect in scan.
2. Technetium scan for renal blood flow can be used to show vascular malformations.

K. *Renal Angiography*—visualization of renal arterial supply. Contrast medium is injected through a catheter (which is placed under fluoroscope control) via the femoral or axillary artery into the aorta and/or renal artery.

1. Useful in diagnosing renovascular abnormalities and in differentiating renal masses, primarily renal cyst from renal tumor.
2. *Nursing Responsibilities Before Procedure*
   a. Give cathartic or enema as prescribed to eliminate fecal material and gas from colon and to ensure unobstructed radiographs.

b. Shave proposed injection sites: groin (for femoral approach) or axilla (for axillary approach).

c. Locate and mark peripheral pulses to facilitate postprocedure nursing evaluation.

d. Inform patient what to expect during procedure.
   (1) Procedure is done under local anesthesia; patient will probably be given preoperative medication.
   (2) The procedure may take from 30 minutes to 2 hours.
   (3) There may be a transient feeling of heat along the course of the vessel upon injection of contrast material.

3. *Nursing Responsibilities Following Procedure*
   a. Take vital signs until stabilized; take blood pressure on opposite arm if axillary artery was punctured.
   b. Assess puncture site for swelling and development of hematoma.
   c. Palpate peripheral pulses (radial, femoral, dorsalis pedis).
   d. Note color and temperature of involved extremity, comparing it with the uninvolved extremity.
   e. Apply cold compresses to puncture site—to decrease edema and pain.

L. *Computed Tomography*—provides a cross-sectional view of kidney and urinary tract to detect the presence of and extent of urologic disease; a computer measures small changes in x-ray absorption and magnifies the differences from tissue to tissue so a display can be made and read. No preparation needed; noninvasive.

Urologic Endoscopic Procedures

A. *Cystoscopic Examination*—involves direct visualization of the urethra, prostatic urethra, and bladder by means of a tubular lighted telescopic lens.

1. *Uses*
   a. To inspect bladder wall directly for tumor, stone, ulcer, and to inspect urethra, especially the prostatic urethra prior to surgery.
   b. To allow insertion of catheters into the ureters in order to obtain a separate specimen from each kidney and evaluate renal function separately.
   c. To see configuration and position of ureteral orifices.
   d. To remove calculi from urethra, bladder, and ureter.
   e. To treat lesions of bladder, urethra, and prostate.

2. *Patient Preparation*
   a. Preparation depends on type of anesthesia to be used (general or local).
   b. Give prescribed oral fluids and preoperative medication.

3. *Nursing Support Following Procedure*
   a. Expect patient to have some burning upon voiding, blood-tinged urine, and urinary frequency from trauma to mucous membrane.
   b. Watch patients with prostatic hypertrophy for urinary retention due to edema from instrumentation.
   c. Give warm sitz baths or apply heat to abdomen for pain relief and promotion of muscle relaxation.
   d. Use indwelling catheter if urinary retention persists.

4. *Complications Following Cystoscopy*
   (More apt to occur in patients with obstructive pathology)
   a. Urinary retention
   b. Urinary tract hemorrhage
   c. Infection within prostate or bladder

B. *Renal and Ureteral Brush Biopsy*—introduction of catheter followed by a biopsy brush, which is passed through the catheter; suspected lesion is brushed back and forth to obtain cells and surface tissue fragments for histologic diagnosis.

C. *Renal Endoscopy, Nephroscopy*—introduction of fiberoptic scope into the renal pelvis during an open renal operation (pyelotomy) to view interior of renal pelvis, remove calculi, biopsy small lesions, and diagnose renal hematuria and selected renal tumors.

Needle Biopsy of Kidney

Needle biopsy of the kidney is performed by percutaneous needle biopsy through renal tissue (Fig. 11-1A) or by

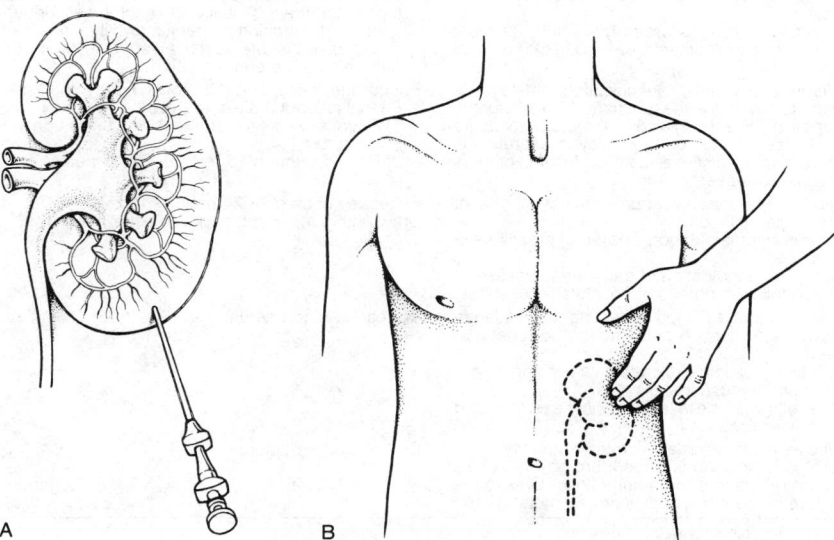

A   B

FIGURE 11–1. A. *Percutaneous needle biopsy of the kidney.* B. *Examining for enlarging hematoma.*

open biopsy through a small flank incision. It is useful in evaluating the course of renal disease.

A. *Prebiopsy Management*

1. Coagulation studies are carried out to identify the patient at risk for postbiopsy bleeding; serum creatinine and urinalysis are done.
2. The patient may be placed on a fasting regimen for 6–8 hours before the test. An IV line may be established.
3. Secure and save a voided specimen before biopsy—for comparsion with postbiopsy specimen.
4. Instruct the patient that he may be asked to hold his breath while the biopsy needle is inserted.

B. *Postbiopsy Nursing Management*

OBJECTIVE: to observe patient for evidences of bleeding.

1. Keep the patient supine as long as directed.
2. Take the vital signs every 5–15 minutes for first hour and then with decreasing frequency if stable to assess for hemorrhage, which is a major complication.
   a. Watch for rise or fall in blood pressure, anorexia, vomiting, or development of a dull, aching discomfort in abdomen.
   b. Assess for flank pain (usually represents bleeding into the muscle) or colicky pain (clot in the ureter).
   c. Assess for backache, shoulder pain, or dysuria.
   d. Persistent bleeding may be suspected when there is an enlarging hematoma which is palpable (Fig. 11-1B).
   e. If perirenal bleeding develops, avoid palpating or manipulating the abdomen after the first examination has determined that a hematoma exists.
3. Measure each voiding and inspect for bleeding. Compare samples with each other and with prebiopsy specimen.
4. Assess for any patient complaints, especially frequency and urgency.

5. Keep the fluid level at 3000 ml. daily if tolerated, unless the patient has renal insufficiency.
6. A hematocrit and hemoglobin study may be done within 8 hours to assess for anemia.
7. Prepare for transfusion and surgical intervention for control of hemorrhage, which may necessitate surgical drainage or nephrectomy (removal of kidney).

C. *Discharge Planning and Patient Education*

Instruct the patient as follows:

1. Avoid strenuous activity, strenuous sports, and heavy lifting for at least 2 weeks.
2. Notify physician if any of the following occur: flank pain, hematuria, light-headedness and fainting, rapid pulse, or any other signs and symptoms of hemorrhage.

TESTS OF RENAL FUNCTION

General Information (Table 11-1)

1. Renal function tests are used to determine the kidneys' excretory functioning effectiveness, to evaluate the severity of kidney disease, and to follow the patient's progress.
2. Renal function may be within normal limits until about 50% of renal function has been lost.

URINE EXAMINATION

Factors Affecting Composition of the Urine

1. Nutritional status
2. Metabolic processes
3. Status of kidney function

TABLE 11-1. TESTS OF RENAL FUNCTION

1. There is no single test of renal function; renal function is variable from time to time.
2. The rate of change of renal function is more important than the result of a single test.

Test	Purpose/Rationale	Test Protocol
Renal Concentration Test Specific gravity Refractive index Osmolality of urine	Evaluates the ability to concentrate solutes in the urine Concentration ability is lost early in kidney disease; hence, this test detects early defects in renal function.	Fluids may be withheld 12 to 24 hours to evaluate the concentrating ability of the tubules under controlled conditions. Specific gravity measurements of urine are taken at specific times to determine urine concentration.
Phenolsulfonphthalein Excretion Test (PSP)	A diagnostic agent (phenolsulfonphthalein) is given to determine the functional capacity of the kidney. (PSP test can also be used as a measure to assess residual urine.) Delayed excretion is seen in renal disease, cardiac failure, primary vascular disease.	Encourage fluids 1 to 1½ hours before the test. Phenolsulfonphthalein is given IV. 1) Record exact time contrast medium is administered. 2) Collect urine in 15 minutes, 30 minutes, and 1 hour.
Creatinine Clearance* (Endogenous creatinine clearance)	Provides a reasonable approximation of rate of glomerular filtration. Measures volume of blood cleared of creatinine in 1 minute. Most sensitive indication of early renal disease. Useful to follow progress of patient's renal status.	Collect all urine over 24-hour period. Draw one sample of blood within the period.
Serum Creatinine	A test of renal function reflecting the balance between production and filtration by renal glomerulus. Amount of creatinine excreted varies and is dependent on muscle mass. Test results may be altered during exercise and in certain diseases.	Do test on blood serum.
Serum Urea Nitrogen (Blood Urea Nitrogen [BUN])	Serves as index of renal excretory capacity. Serum urea nitrogen is dependent on the body's urea production and on urine flow. (Urea is the nitrogenous end-product of protein metabolism.)	Do test on blood serum.

* Clearance is the amount of blood cleansed of a constituent per unit of time. See Appendix, page 1470 for range of values.

Amount

1. 1200–1500 ml./24 hours; less than 500 ml. is considered oliguria.
2. Day volume 2 to 3 times more than night volume.

Appearance

1. Normal urine is clear.
2. Turbid (cloudy) urine is not always pathological. Normal urine may develop turbidity on refrigeration or from standing at room temperature; bacteria ferment urine quickly at room temperature.
3. Abnormally cloudy urine—due to pus, blood, epithelial cells, bacteria, fat, colloidal particles, phosphate, urates.

Odor

1. Normal—faint aromatic odor.
2. Characteristic odors produced by ingestion of asparagus, thymol.
3. Cloudy urine with ammonia odor—urea-splitting bacteria such as *Proteus,* causing urinary tract infections.
4. Offensive odor—bacterial action in presence of pus.

Color

1. Color shows degree of concentration and depends on amount voided.
2. Normal urine is clear yellow or amber due to the pigment urochrome.
3. Color varies with specific gravity:
   a. Dilute urine is straw-colored.
   b. Concentrated urine is highly colored.
4. Abnormally colored urine:
   a. Turbid or smoky colored—may be from hematuria, spermatozoa, prostatic fluid, fat droplets, chyle.
   b. Red or red-brown—is due to blood pigments, porphyria, transfusion reaction, bleeding lesions in urogenital tract, some drugs.
   c. Yellow-brown or green-brown—may reveal obstructive lesion of bile duct system or obstructive jaundice.
   d. Orange-red or orange-brown—from urobilin or from Pyridium, a urinary antiseptic.
   e. Dark brown or black—due to malignant melanoma, leukemia.

Reaction (pH)

1. Reflects the ability of kidney to maintain normal hydrogen ion concentration in plasma and extracellular fluid; indicates *acidity* or *alkalinity* of urine.
2. The pH should be measured in fresh urine since the breakdown of urine to ammonia causes urine to become alkaline.
3. Normal pH is around 6 (acid); may normally vary from 4.6 to 7.5.
4. Urine acidity or alkalinity has relatively little clinical significance unless patient is on special diet or therapeutic program or is being treated for renal calculous disease.
5. Alkaline urine is often cloudy due to phosphate crystals.

Specific Gravity

1. Measure density of particles in urine; reflects concentrating and diluting power of kidneys; may reflect degree of hydration or dehydration.
2. Normal specific gravity ranges from 1.005–1.025.
3. Specific gravity is fixed at 1.010 in chronic renal failure.
4. In a person eating a normal diet, inability to concentrate or dilute urine indicates disease.

Osmolality

1. Osmolality is an indication of the amount of osmotically active particles in urine (specifically, it is the number of particles per unit volume of *water*). It is similar to specific gravity, but is considered a more precise test; it is also easy to do—only 1–2 ml. of urine are required.
2. The unit of osmotic measure is the *osmole*.
   Average values:
   Females: 300–1090 mOsm./kg.
   Males: 390–1090 mOsm./kg.

Abnormal Urine Constituents

1. *Proteinuria* (albuminuria)—characteristically seen in all forms of acute and chronic renal disease.
   a. Normal urine does not have persistent protein in significant quantities.
   b. Proteinuria also occurs in systemic diseases where there are varying degrees of renal anoxia, cardiac decompensation, diabetic glomerulosclerosis, etc.
2. *Glucosuria*—glucose in the urine; seen most frequently in diabetes mellitus.
3. *Ketonuria*—the presence of ketone bodies (acetone, acetoacetic acid, and beta-hydroxybutyric acid). Ketonuria is indicative of incomplete fat metabolism (diabetic ketoacidosis), dehydration, starvation; also seen after aspirin ingestion.
4. *Hematuria*—red blood cells in the urine.
5. *Pyuria*—white blood cells in the urine.
6. *Bacteriuria*—bacteria in the urine.
7. *Crystalluria*—excretion of crystals in the urine.

Dipstick Tests (Reagent Tests)

Strips that have been impregnated with chemicals are dipped quickly in urine and "read" as a means of testing urine.
1. When dipped in urine, the chemicals react with abnormal substances in the urine by changing color.
2. Some dipsticks can test for only 1 substance, whereas others can test several substances simultaneously.

Basic Principles for Collecting Urine Specimens

1. The first morning urine specimen is most concentrated—it reveals sediment abnormalities.
2. Urine should not be left standing at room temperature since it becomes alkaline due to contamination of urea-splitting bacteria from the environment.
3. Microscopic examination should be done within ½ hour after collection—standing causes dissolution of cellular elements and casts and bacterial overgrowth unless obtained under sterile conditions.
4. Urine specimens should be collected from the patient by means of the clean-catch midstream technique (see below) or by careful catheterization.
5. Collection of 24-hour specimen:
   a. Ensure that the patient understands the procedure. *All* urine must be collected within a 24-hour period via clean-catch technique.
   b. Have patient empty the bladder at specified time (Ex. 8:00 A.M.). *Discard urine.*

c. Collect all urine voided during the next 24 hours.

d. Collect last specimen at 8:00 A.M. on following day (or 24 hours after collection was started).

e. Keep collected urine in the refrigerator in a clean bottle; a suitable preservative may be required.

f. Start with an empty bladder and finish with an empty bladder.

GUIDELINES: Technique for Obtaining Clean-catch Midstream Voided Specimen

A *clean-catch midstream specimen* is the best clinically effective method of securing a voided specimen for urinalysis. It is not a simple procedure and requires patient education and active assistance of the female patient.

Equipment

Antiseptic solution or liquid soap solution
Sterile water
4 × 4 sponges
Disposable gloves for nurse assisting female patient
Sterile specimen container

Procedure

NURSING ACTION	RATIONALE/AMPLIFICATION
Male Patient	
1. Instruct the patient to expose glans and cleanse area around meatus. Wash area with mild antiseptic solution or liquid soap. *Rinse thoroughly.*	1. The urethral orifice is colonized by bacteria. Urine readily becomes contaminated during voiding. Rinse antiseptic solution or soap solution thoroughly because these agents can inhibit bacterial growth in a urine culture.
2. Allow the initial urinary flow to escape.	2. The first portion of urine washes out the urethra and contains debris.
3. Collect the midstream urine specimen in a sterile container.	
4. Avoid collecting the last few drops of urine.	4. Prostatic secretions may be introduced into urine at the end of the urinary stream.
5. Send specimen to laboratory immediately.	
Female Patient	
1. Ask the patient to separate her labia to expose the urethral orifice. If no one is available to assist the patient, she may sit backwards on the toilet seat facing the water tank or sit on (straddle) the wide part of the bedpan.	1. Keeping the labia separated prevents labial or vaginal contamination of the urine specimen. By straddling the toilet seat/bedpan, the patient's labia are spread apart for cleansing.
2. Cleanse the area around the urinary meatus with 4 × 4s soaked with antiseptic/soap solution. Rinse thoroughly. a. Wash from front to back. b. Do not use 4 × 4 more than once.	2. The urethral orifice is colonized by bacteria. Urine readily becomes contaminated during voiding.

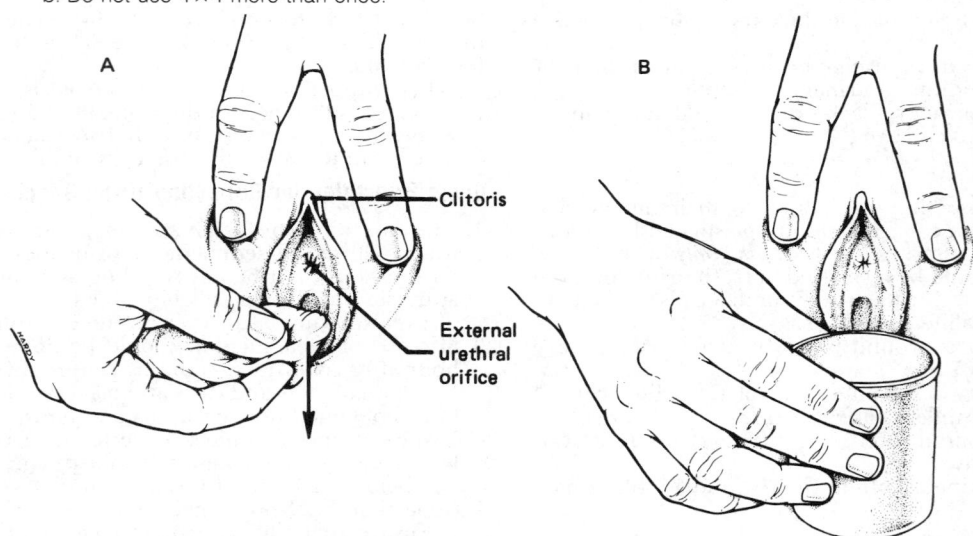

FIGURE 11-2. *Obtaining a clean-catch midstream urine specimen in the female. A. Instruct the patient to hold the labia apart and wash from high up front toward the back with gauze soaked in soap. B. The collection cup is held so that it does not touch the body and the sample is obtained only while the patient is voiding with the labia held apart.*

Procedure (cont.)	**NURSING ACTION**	**RATIONALE/AMPLIFICATION**

NURSING ACTION

3. While the patient keeps the labia separated (Fig. 11-2), instruct her to void forcibly.
4. Allow initial urinary flow to drain into bedpan (toilet) and then catch the midstream specimen in a sterile container, making sure that the container does not come in contact with the genitalia.
5. Send the specimen to the laboratory immediately.

RATIONALE/AMPLIFICATION

3. This helps wash away urethral contaminants.
4. The first portion of urine washes out the urethra. Have the patient remove the container from the stream while she is still voiding.
5. Too long an interval between collection and analysis produces unreliable results.

CATHETERIZATION

GUIDELINES: Catheterization of the Urinary Bladder

Purpose
1. To empty contents of bladder.
2. To obtain a sterile urine specimen.
3. To determine amount of residual urine in bladder after voiding.
4. To allow irrigation of the bladder.
5. To bypass an obstruction.

Equipment   Sterile gloves
Disposable sterile catheter set with water-soluble lubricant for different types of catheters (Fig. 11-3)

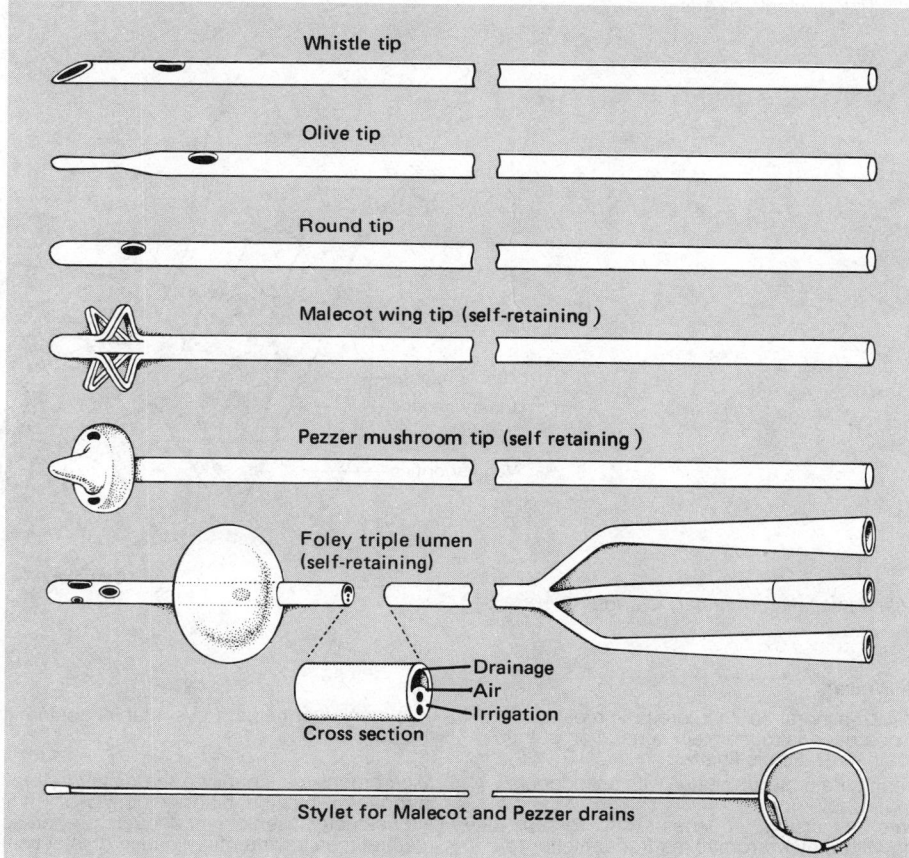

Whistle tip

Olive tip

Round tip

Malecot wing tip (self-retaining)

Pezzer mushroom tip (self retaining)

Foley triple lumen (self-retaining)

Drainage
Air
Irrigation

Cross section

Stylet for Malecot and Pezzer drains

FIGURE 11-3. *Types of catheters.*

GUIDELINES: Catheterization of the Urinary Bladder (cont.)

Procedure

NURSING ACTION

Solution for periurethral cleansing (sterile)
Sterile container for culture
Bath blanket/sheet for draping
Standing lamp (preferred) or flashlight

Selection of Catheter Size

Female: (Adult No. 16 Fr.) (Child No. 8 Fr.)
Male: (Adult No. 16 Fr.) (Child No. 6–8 Fr.)

Procedure for Catheterizing Female Patient

NURSING ACTION

RATIONALE/AMPLIFICATION

Preparatory Phase

1. Place patient at ease.

2. Open catheter tray using aseptic technique. Place waste receptacle in accessible place.
3. Direct light for visualization of genital area.
4. Place patient in a supine position with knees bent, hips flexed, and feet resting on bed about 0.6 m. (2 feet) apart. Drape the patient.
5. Position moisture-proof pad under patient's buttocks.
6. Wash hands. Put on sterile gloves.

RATIONALE/AMPLIFICATION

1. Patient will feel reassured if the procedure is explained and if she is handled gently and considerately.
2. Catheterization requires the same aseptic precautions as a surgical procedure.

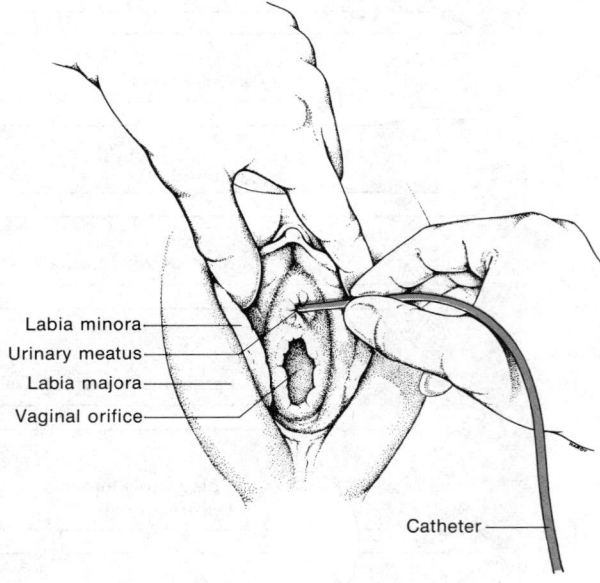

Labia minora
Urinary meatus
Labia majora
Vaginal orifice

Catheter

FIGURE 11-4. *Catheterization of urinary bladder in female.*

Performance Phase

1. Separate labia minora so that urethral meatus is visualized; one hand is to maintain separation of the labia until catheterization is finished.
2. Cleanse around the urethral meatus with an iodophor preparation (Betadine).
   a. Manipulate cleansing sponges with forceps, cleansing with downward strokes from anterior to posterior.
   b. Dispose of cotton sponge after each use.
   c. If patient is sensitive to iodine, benzalkonium chloride or other cleansing agent is used.

1. This maneuver helps prevent labial contamination of the catheter (Fig. 11-4).

2. Microorganisms inhabiting the distal urethra may be introduced into the bladder during or immediately after catheter insertion. Inadequate preparation of the urethral meatus is a major cause of infection.

Procedure (cont.)

NURSING ACTION	**RATIONALE/AMPLIFICATION**

3. Introduce well-lubricated catheter 5–7.5 cm. (2–3 inches) into urethral meatus using strict aseptic technique.
    a. Avoid contaminating surface of catheter.
    b. Ensure that catheter is not too large or too tight at urethral meatus.
4. Pinch off catheter and remove gently when urine ceases to flow.

3. A well-lubricated catheter reduces friction and trauma to the meatus. The female urethra is a relatively short canal measuring 3.0–4 cm. in length.

    b. Too large a catheter may cause painful distention of the meatus.
4. Pinching off the catheter prevents air from entering the bladder as the catheter is removed.

Follow-up Phase

1. Make patient comfortable; dry area.
2. Measure urine and dispose of equipment.
3. Send specimen to lab as indicated.
4. Record time, procedure, amount, and appearance of urine.

Procedure for Catheterizing Male Patient

NURSING ACTION	**RATIONALE/AMPLIFICATION**

1. Carry out all of "preparatory phase" as for female patient except:
2. Place the patient in supine position with legs extended. Place the moisture-proof pad across upper thighs.
3. Position the perineal drape.
4. Lubricate the catheter well.

5. Wash off glans penis around urinary meatus with an iodophor solution (Betadine) using forceps to hold cleansing sponges. Maintain sterility of right hand.
6. Grasp shaft of penis (with left hand) raising it almost straight up (Fig. 11-5). Maintain grasp on penis until procedure is ended.

4. A well-lubricated catheter prevents urethral trauma (decreasing the opportunity for bacterial invasion).
5. Cleanse urethral meatus from tip to foreskin with downward stroke on one side. Discard sponge. Repeat as required.
6. This maneuver straightens the penile urethra and facilitates catheterization. Maintaining a grasp of the penis prevents contamination and retraction of penis.

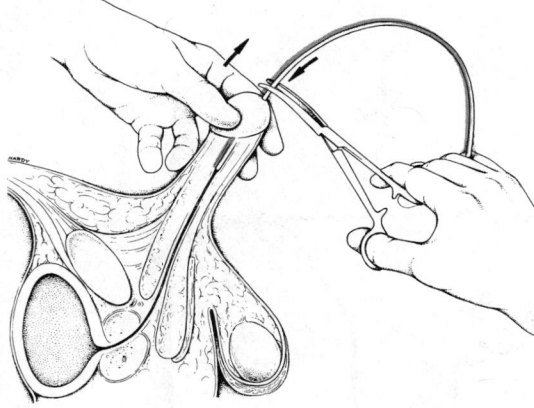

FIGURE 11-5. *Technique for catheterization in male.*

7. Using sterile forceps, insert catheter into the urethra; advance catheter 15–25 cm. (6–10 inches) until urine flows.

8. If resistance is felt at the external sphincter, slightly increase the traction on the penis and apply steady, gentle pressure on the catheter.
    Ask patient to strain gently (as if passing urine) to help relax sphincter.
9. When urine begins to flow, advance the catheter another 2.5 cm. (1 inch).

7. The male urethra is a canal extending from the bladder to the end of the glans penis. The length varies within wide limits; the average length is about 21 cm.
8. Some resistance may be due to spasm of external sphincter. Inability to pass the catheter may mean that a urethral stricture or other forms of urethral pathology exist. The urethra may have to be dilated with sounds by a urologist.
9. Advancing the catheter ensures its position in the bladder.

GUIDELINES: Catheterization of the Urinary Bladder (cont.)

Procedure for Indwelling Catheter

NURSING ACTION	RATIONALE/AMPLIFICATION
1. Advance catheter almost to its bifurcation (for male patient).	1. This prevents the balloon from becoming trapped in the urethra.
2. Inflate the balloon according to manufacture's directions. Be sure catheter is draining properly before inflating balloon.	2. Inadvertent inflation of the balloon within the urethra is painful and causes urethral trauma.

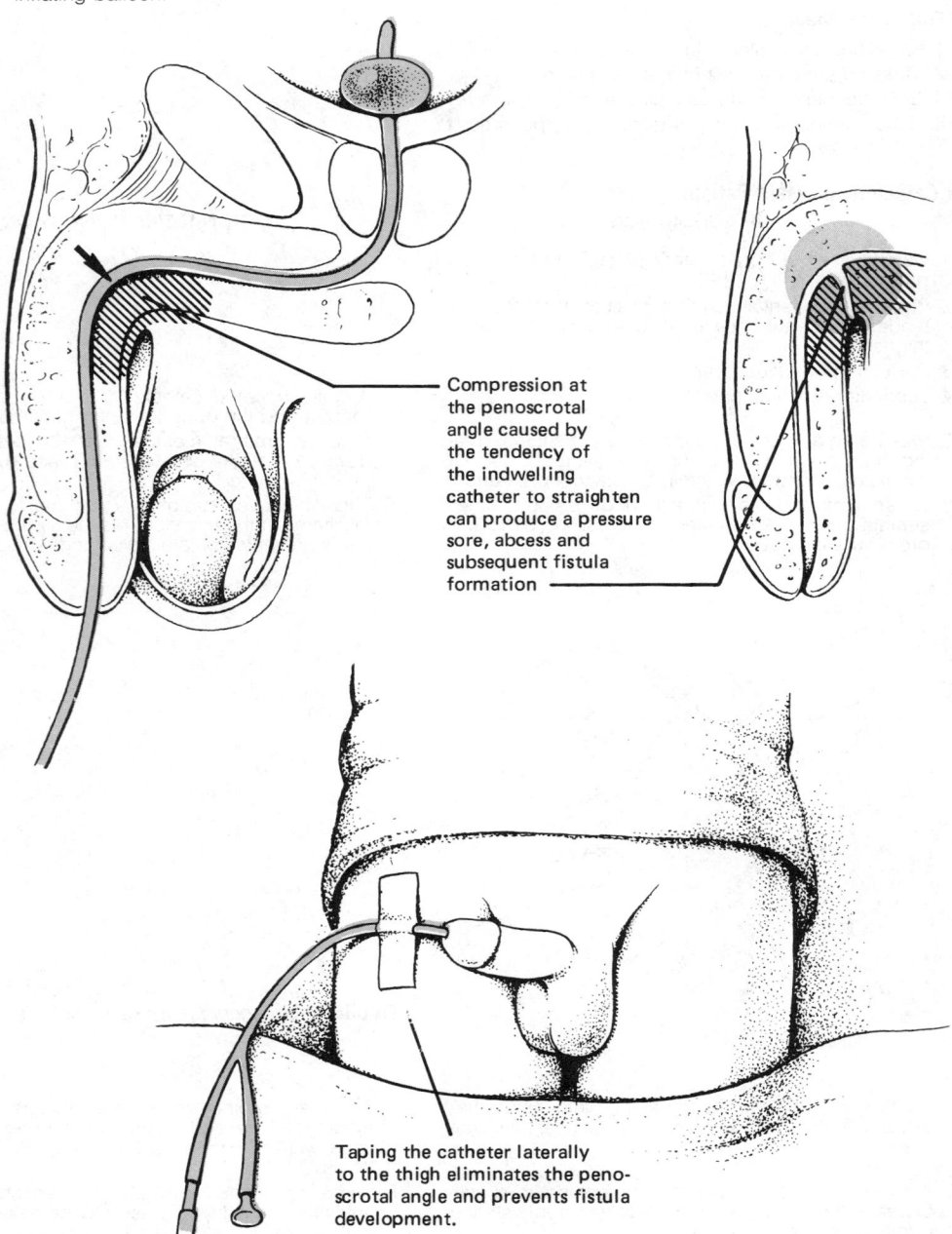

Compression at the penoscrotal angle caused by the tendency of the indwelling catheter to straighten can produce a pressure sore, abcess and subsequent fistula formation

Taping the catheter laterally to the thigh eliminates the penoscrotal angle and prevents fistula development.

FIGURE 11-6. *Tape the penis laterally (or on the abdomen) to smooth out urethral curve and eliminate pressure on the penoscrotal angle which is a source of infection, periurethral abscesses, and urethral fistula formation.*

Procedure (cont.)

NURSING ACTION	RATIONALE/AMPLIFICATION
3. Withdraw catheter slightly and connect to drainage system.	
4. Anchoring the indwelling catheter. Do not pull it tight.	
a. *Female:* Tape the catheter and drainage tubing to the thigh.	a. This prevents traction and tension on the bladder.
b. *Male:* Tape the catheter laterally to the thigh (Fig. 11-6) or on the abdomen.	b. This smooths out urethral curve and eliminates pressure on the urethra at the penoscrotal junction, which can eventually lead to the formation of a urethro-cutaneous fistula.
c. Tape the tubing (not the catheter) to shaved inner aspect of thigh.	c. Taping the tubing to the thigh prevents tension and traction on the bladder.
5. Reduce (or reposition) the foreskin.	5. Paraphimosis (retraction and constriction of the foreskin behind the glans penis), secondary to catheterization, may occur if the foreskin is not reduced.

Follow-up Phase

Same as for female patient.

GUIDELINES: Management of the Patient with an Indwelling (Self-Retaining) Catheter and Closed Drainage System

Purpose
1. To empty urine from the bladder.
2. To clear an obstructed catheter.
3. To rinse the bladder with a continuous solution of an antiseptic or antimicrobial solution to prevent infection (less common use).

Equipment
1. Use a completely closed system (see Fig. 11-7)
2. Catheter tray with triple lumen catheter
3. Drainage solution as prescribed
4. Gauze squares
5. Antibacterial solution for cleansing.

Procedure

NURSING ACTION	RATIONALE/AMPLIFICATION
Performance Phase	
1. Attach the catheter to the drainage apparatus before inserting the catheter into the urethra. Catheterize the patient (p. 481).	1. A closed drainage system is one that is closed to outside air.
2. Prevent introduction of organisms where catheter enters urethral meatus (meatal-catheter junction).	2. Suppurative drainage and encrustation occur at the exit of any tube. Catheter care helps prevent exudate from entering urethra. Encrustations arising from urinary salts may enter bladder when catheter is removed and may serve as nuclei for stone formation. The catheter must be cleansed of blood or pus to maintain antibacterial protection.
a. Cleanse around meatal-catheter junction at least twice daily with an antibacterial solution.	
b. An antimicrobial ointment may be applied at the meatal-catheter junction.	
c. Teach patient how to cleanse around catheter if he/she is able.	
3. Wash the perineal area with soap and water several times daily.	3. Avoid using powders and sprays on the perineal area.
4. *To Secure Urine for Culture:*	4. Avoid separating connecting tube and catheter.
a. Clamp the drainage tubing near the junction of the catheter.	a. The catheter should only be clamped for a brief period.
b. Cleanse the aspiration port or hub of the catheter with alcohol or an iodine-containing solution.	
c. Insert a 25-gauge needle (attached to a syringe) into hub or special port of catheter.	c. Avoid inserting needle into the shaft of the catheter, since this may cause balloon deflation.
d. Aspirate a small volume of urine for culture.	
e. Unclamp the drainage tubing.	
5. *Changing the Catheter:* Change catheter every 2–4 weeks.	
a. Roll the catheter between thumb and finger after removal.	a. This determines the presence of grit or sand along the drainage lumen.
b. If there is calcific deposit present, shorten the interval between catheter changes.	b. The catheter should be relatively free of calcific material.
6. *Principles of Care When Managing a Closed System*	6. Maintain an unobstructed flow at all times. Urine flow must be downhill.

GUIDELINES: Management of the Patient with an Indwelling (Self-Retaining) Catheter and Closed Drainage System (cont.)

Procedure (cont.)

NURSING ACTION	RATIONALE/AMPLIFICATION
a. The drainage bag should not be raised above the level of the patient's bladder.	a. Raising the bag will cause reflux of contaminated urine into the patient's bladder from the bag.
b. Urine should not be allowed to collect in the tubing, since a free flow of urine must be maintained to prevent infection.	b. Improper drainage occurs when the tubing is kinked or twisted, allowing pools of drainage to collect in the loops of tubing.

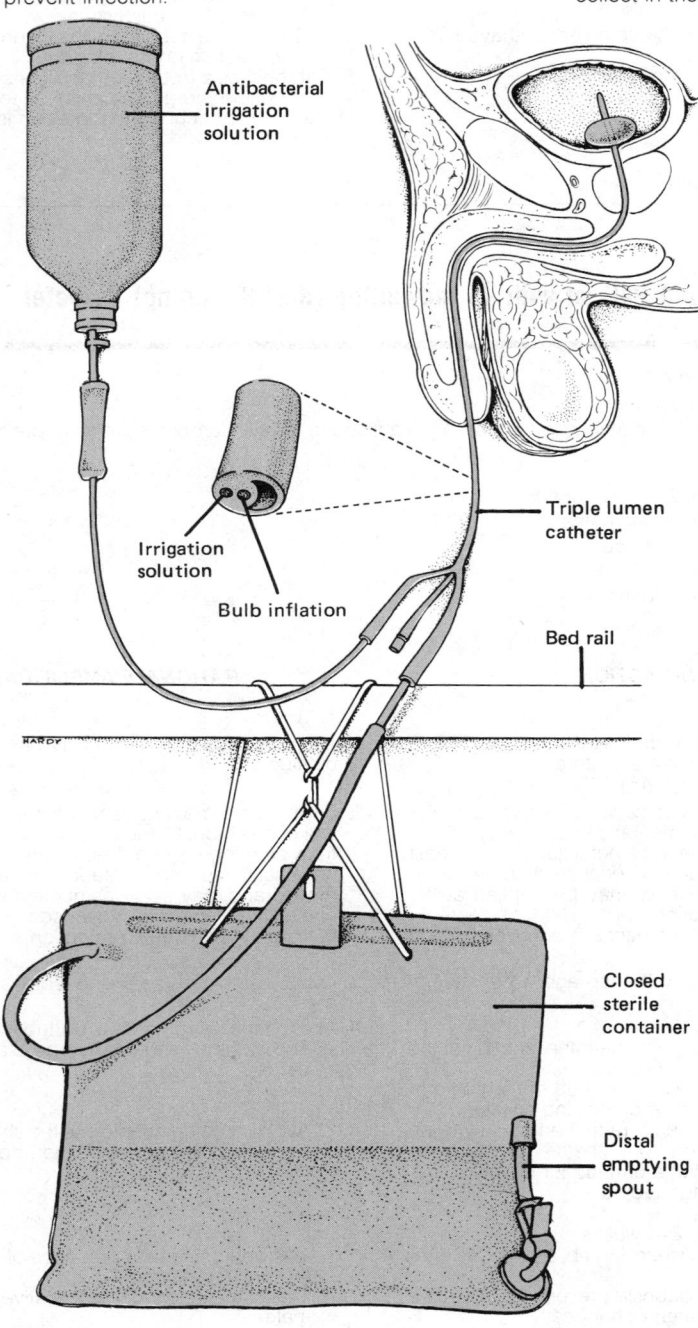

Antibacterial irrigation solution

Irrigation solution

Bulb inflation

Triple lumen catheter

Bed rail

Closed sterile container

Distal emptying spout

FIGURE 11-7. *Closed sterile drainage system.*

Procedure (cont.)	NURSING ACTION	RATIONALE/AMPLIFICATION
	c. The drainage bag should not touch the floor.	c. The bag and tubing should be changed if contamination occurs.
	d. The bag is drained at 8-hour intervals with care taken to see that the drainage tube (valve/spout) is not contaminated.	d. Do not disconnect tubing from drainage bag; use a distal emptying valve to empty the bag. (Fig 11-7)

GUIDELINES: Management of a Continuous Irrigating System

NURSING ACTION	RATIONALE/AMPLIFICATION
1. *Use a 3-way (Triple-Lumen) Catheter (See Fig. 11-3)* a. One lumen—for inflating the balloon holding the catheter in place. b. Second lumen—for outflow of urine and of drainage solution. c. Third lumen—for inflow of irrigating solution (antibacterial rinse) into bladder. 2. *Use of Irrigating Solutions* a. For continuous irrigation (1) If drainage is bright red, allow irrigating solution to run in rapidly until drainage becomes lighter. (2) If drainage is clear, allow irrigating solution to run at rate of 40–60 drops/minute. 3. *Other Measures to Prevent Infection* a. Ensure copious fluid intake. b. Keep the urine acid. (1) Oral intake of ascorbic acid or potassium acid phosphate (2) Acid–ash diet 4. *Measures to Prevent Cross-contamination* a. Wash hands thoroughly between patients. b. Assign only one patient with an indwelling catheter to a room. c. Know the patients at risk.	a. To produce mechanical flushing and dilute urinary elements that cause encrustation. b. To prevent tube obstruction and encrustation by urinary sand and calculous deposits. a. Many urinary tract infections are due to extrinsically acquired organisms transmitted by cross-contamination. b. There appears to be a greater risk of microbial transmission between catheterized patients. c. Female, elderly, debilitated, and critically ill patients are at risk for infection.

GUIDELINES: Assisting the Patient Undergoing Suprapubic Drainage (Cystostomy)

Suprapubic bladder drainage is a method of establishing drainage from the bladder by inserting a catheter or tube through the suprapubic area into the bladder by either a stab incision or puncture with a needle or trocar.

Purpose
1. To drain the bladder via a tube placed in the bladder through the suprapubic area.
2. To divert the flow of urine from the urethra.

Clinical Usefulness
1. When urethral route is impassable—urethral stricture, injuries
2. Following gynecological operations—vaginal hysterectomy; vaginal repair
3. Following bladder surgery
4. Pelvic fractures

Equipment
Sterile suprapubic drainage system package (disposable)
Skin germicide for suprapubic skin preparation
Local anesthetic agent if needed

Procedure	NURSING ACTION	RATIONALE/AMPLIFICATION
	Preparatory Phase 1. Place patient in a supine position with one pillow under head. 2. Expose the abdomen.	

GUIDELINES: Assisting the Patient Undergoing Suprapubic Drainage (Cystostomy) (cont.)

Procedure (cont.)

NURSING ACTION

Performance Phase (by physician)

1. The bladder is distended with 300–500 ml. of sterile saline via an urethral catheter, which is removed. Or the patient is given fluids (oral or IV) before the procedure.

2. The suprapubic area is surgically prepared. After the skin is dried, the needle entry point is located.

3. The procedure may be performed in several ways:
   a. By open operation (incision of the bladder)
   b. By puncture with a trocar/cannula assembly.
   (1) The trocar/cannula is passed in a slightly caudal direction.

   (2) After the bladder has been entered, the trocar is removed, leaving the outer cannula in place.

   (3) The catheter is threaded through the cannula and well into the bladder (Fig. 11-8 *A*).
   (4) The cannula is slowly withdrawn, leaving the catheter in position.
   (5) The catheter is secured with sutures, tape, or a body-seal system (Fig. 11-8 *B*).

RATIONALE/AMPLIFICATION

1. Distention of the bladder makes the bladder easier to locate by the suprapubic route.

2. The needle entry point is approximately 5 cm. (2 inches) above the symphysis.

   (1) Entrance into the bladder is usually felt and can be verified by reflux of urine through a hole in the trocar/cannula.
   (2) Usually a 3-way stopcock is attached to the proximal end of the catheter and connected to a siphon drainage system.

   (5) Aseptic technique is employed in the area around the cystostomy tube.

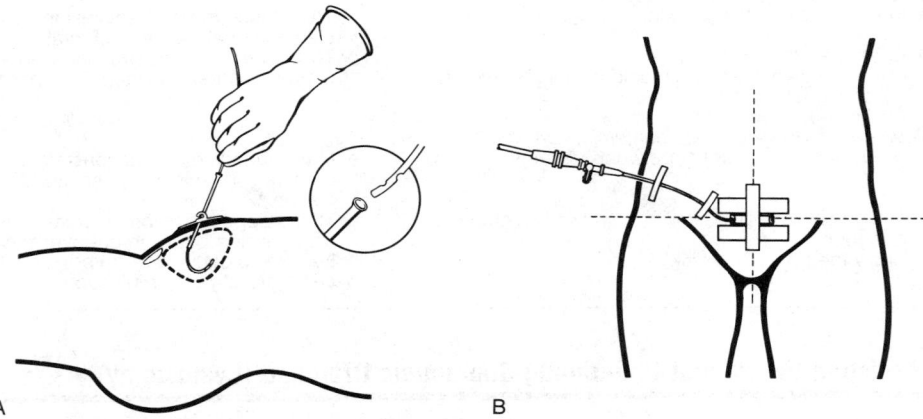

A   B

FIGURE 11-8. (A) Introduction of suprapubic catheter. (B) The body seal and catheter are taped to the abdomen. (Courtesy of Dow Corning Corporation)

   (6) Cover the area around the catheter with a sterile dressing.
   (7) Attach the drainage tubing to a closed sterile system.

4. Secure drainage tubing to lateral abdomen with tape (Fig. 11-8 *B*).

5. If the catheter is not draining properly, withdraw the catheter 2.5 cm. (1 inch) at a time until urine begins to flow. Do not dislodge catheter from bladder.

6. The drainage is maintained continuously for several days.

7. If a "trial of voiding" is requested, the catheter is clamped for 4 hours.
   a. Have the patient attempt to void while the catheter is clamped.
   b. After the patient voids, unclamp the catheter and measure residual urine.
   c. Usually, if the amount of residual urine is less than 100 ml. on 2 separate occasions (A.M. and P.M.), the catheter may be removed.

4. Prevents undue tension on the catheter.

7. Usually, patients will void earlier after surgery with suprapubic drainage than with indwelling catheters.

Procedure (cont.)

	NURSING ACTION	RATIONALE/AMPLIFICATION
	d. If the patient complains of pain or discomfort, or if the residual urine is over the prescribed amount, the catheter is usually left open. 8. The catheter is removed upon request and a sterile dressing is placed over the site.	8. Suprapubic drainage is considered more comfortable than an indwelling urethral catheter; it allows greater patient mobility and there is less risk of bladder infection.

URINE RETENTION

Urinary retention is the inability to urinate despite a desire to do so. Retention may be acute or chronic. Chronic retention will often lead to overflow incontinence or residual urine.

Etiology

Males
1. Benign prostatic hyperplasia
2. Stricture of urethra, calculus or foreign body in urethra, urethritis, tumor
3. Phimosis

Females
1. Urethral obstruction secondary to stricture, stones, vaginal cysts, carcinoma, edema
2. Retroverted gravid uterus

Either Male or Female
1. Following any operation, particularly on anal or perineal region—due to reflex spasm of sphincters
2. Trauma
3. Neurogenic bladder dysfunction—spinal cord tumor, trauma, herniated intervertebral disc, multiple sclerosis
4. Certain drugs (anticholinergics, antihistamines)
5. Fecal impaction
6. Psychogenic urinary retention

Clinical Features (See Figure 11-9)
1. History of no voiding or frequent passing of small amounts of urine without relief.
2. Progressive slowing of urinary stream; hesitancy.
3. Lower abdominal discomfort and distress; severe pain.
   a. Patient may have little or no discomfort if bladder distends slowly.
4. Oval-shaped mass that is palpable over bladder area.
5. Dullness to percussion above symphysis pubis (residual urine below 130 ml. is not usually percussible).
6. Visualization of a rounded swelling arising out of the pelvis.
7. Urine-stained clothing.

Treatment and Nursing Management
OBJECTIVES: to prevent overdistention of the bladder with resultant infection.
to treat underlying cause.
1. Utilize measures to help patient void.
   a. Transport patient to bathroom (or bedside commode) or allow to stand beside bed if possible—many patients are unable to void while lying in bed.
   b. Use warmth to relax sphincters—sitz bath, warm compresses to perineum, warm shower.
   c. Give hot tea to drink.
   d. Have patient listen to sound of running water; place hands in warm water.
   e. Administer bethanechol chloride (Urecholine) only if directed.
   f. Give psychological reassurance and support.
2. Give prescribed analgesic medication postoperatively.
   a. Voiding may be difficult because of pain in incisional area, especially in anterior vaginal operations.
   b. Sphincter spasm is generally present in patients with acute urinary retention.
3. Decompress bladder before overdistention occurs—bladder mucosa which has been stretched from urinary retention is readily infected.
   a. Utilize indwelling catheter and closed drainage.
      (1) It may be advisable to decompress the bladder gradually if patient is elderly or hypertensive or has diminished renal reserve, or if retention of large amounts of urine has persisted for several weeks.
      (2) Call urologist if unable to pass catheter easily; he will use special instruments (or operation may be necessary).
      (3) Blood pressure may fluctuate and renal function decline the first few days after bladder drainage is instituted.
   b. Suprapubic cystostomy may be required if it is impossible to pass urethral catheter (p. 487).
4. Carry out blood urea nitrogen tests and other renal function tests.
5. Assist in carrying out diagnostic tests if obstructive uropathy (pathologic change in urinary tract from obstruction) is suspected.

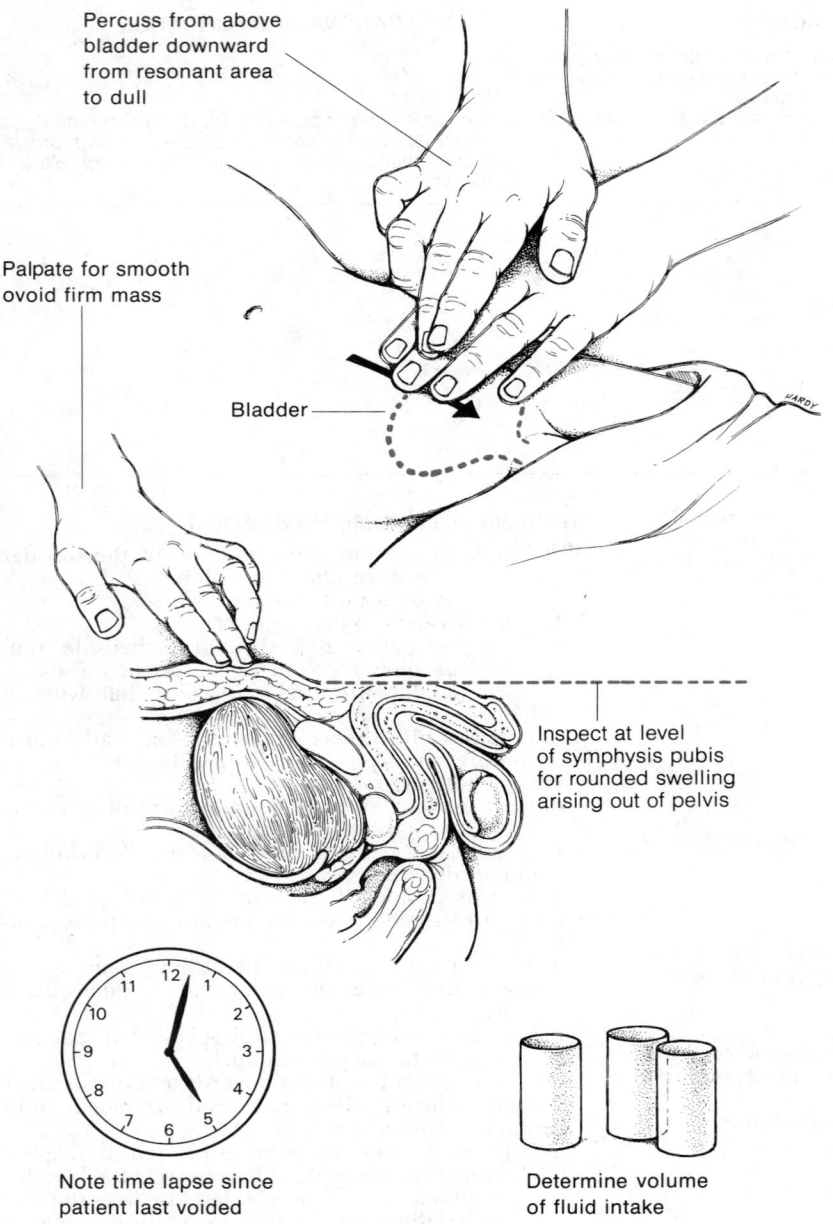

Percuss from above bladder downward from resonant area to dull

Palpate for smooth ovoid firm mass

Bladder

Inspect at level of symphysis pubis for rounded swelling arising out of pelvis

Note time lapse since patient last voided

Determine volume of fluid intake

FIGURE 11-9. *Nursing assessment for urinary retention.*

NURSING ASSESSMENT FOR FLUID AND ELECTROLYTE IMBALANCE

The following signs and symptoms tend to occur in patients with renal disease.

Clinical Manifestations

Signs and Symptoms	Possible Indication
Acute weight loss (in excess of 5%), drop in body temperature, dry skin and mucous membranes, longitudinal wrinkles or furrows of tongue, oliguria or anuria	Volume deficit of extracellular fluid

Signs and Symptoms	Possible Indication
Acute weight gain (in excess of 5%), edema, moist rales in lungs, puffy eyelids, shortness of breath	Volume excess of extracellular fluid
Abdominal cramps, apprehension, convulsions, fingerprinting on sternum, oliguria or anuria	Sodium deficit of extracellular fluid
Dry sticky mucous membranes, flushed skin, oliguria or anuria, thirst, rough and dry tongue	Sodium excess of extracellular fluid
Anorexia, gaseous distention of intestines, silent intestinal ileus, weakness, soft, flabby muscles	Potassium deficit of extracellular fluid
Diarrhea, intestinal colic, irritability, nausea	Potassium excess of extracellular fluid
Abdominal cramps, carpopedal spasm, muscle cramps, tetany, tingling of ends of fingers	Calcium deficit of extracellular fluid
Deep bone pain, flank pain, and muscle hypotonicity	Calcium excess of extracellular fluid
Deep rapid breathing (Kussmaul), shortness of breath on exertion, stupor, weakness	Primary base bicarbonate deficit of extracellular fluid
Depressed respiration, muscle hypertonicity, tetany	Primary base bicarbonate excess of extracellular fluid
Chronic weight loss, emotional depression, pallor, ready fatigue, soft, flabby muscles	Protein deficit of extracellular fluid
Positive Chvostek's sign, convulsions, disorientation, hyperactive deep reflexes, tremor	Magnesium deficit of extracellular fluid

Nursing Responsibilities

1. Observe the clinical course of the patient; record the data collected.
2. Keep an accurate intake and output record.
3. Check the vital signs every 4 hours. Weigh the patient daily.
4. Support the patient having repeated blood examinations for the surveillance of electrolyte balance.

ACUTE RENAL FAILURE

Acute renal failure is a sudden and almost complete loss of kidney function caused by failure of the renal circulation or by glomerular or tubular damage. The substances normally eliminated in the urine accumulate in the body fluids as a result of impaired renal excretion and lead to a disruption in homeostatic, endocrine, and metabolic functions. Renal failure is a disease affecting the entire body.

Precipitating Factors

1. Reduction in renal blood flow—volume depletion, hypotension, shock, trauma, burns, hemorrhage
2. Sepsis
3. Dehydration; trauma
4. Obstructive lesions—vascular lesions, bladder outlet obstruction, calculi
5. Nephrotoxic drugs
6. Multiple blood transfusions and mismatched blood
7. Cardiopulmonary bypass
8. Surgery of aorta, renal vessels, biliary tree
9. Extensive surgery in the elderly

Altered Physiology

Hypotension or nephrotoxins → decrease in renal flow → decreased glomerular filtration rate → renal ischemia → loss of tubular function → oliguria

Preventive Measures

1. Initiate adequate hydration before, during, and after operative procedures.
2. Avoid exposure to various nephrotoxins. Be aware that the majority of drugs or their metabolites are excreted by the kidneys.
3. Prevent and treat shock with blood and fluid replacement. Prevent prolonged periods of hypotension.
4. Monitor urinary output hourly in critically ill patients to detect onset of renal failure at the earliest moment.
5. Schedule diagnostic studies requiring dehydration so that there are "rest days," especially in aged who may not have adequate renal reserve.
6. Avoid infections which may produce progressive renal damage.
7. Pay special attention to draining wounds, burns, etc., which can lead to sepsis.
8. Give meticulous care to patients with indwelling catheters to prevent ascending infections.
9. Take every precaution to ensure that the right person receives the right blood—to avoid severe transfusion reactions, which can precipitate renal complications.

Clinical Phases

1. Period of oliguria (urine volume less than 400–600 ml./24 hours). (However, there can be decrease in renal function with increasing nitrogen retention even when the patient is excreting more than 2–3 liters of urine daily—called high output failure.)
   a. Accompanied by rise in serum concentration of elements usually excreted by kidney (urea, creat-

inine, uric acid, organic acids, and the intracellular cations—potassium and magnesium).
  b. Clinical manifestations—scant, bloody urine, lethargy, nausea.
  c. Lasts about 10–20 days or longer.
2. Period of diuresis—gradually increasing urinary output, which doubles daily until relatively fixed volume is attained—glomerular filtration has started to recover, but renal function is still abnormal. With dialysis, the diuretic phase may not occur.
3. Period of convalescence—improvement of renal function may take 3 months. There may be a permanent loss of some glomerular filtration rate and concentrating ability and a decreased ability to acidify urine.

Objectives of Treatment and Nursing Management

GOAL: to restore the normal homeostatic environment so that repair of renal tissue and restoration of renal function may take place.

A. *To remove the cause of renal failure if possible.*

B. *To prepare for peritoneal dialysis or hemodialysis to prevent metabolic deterioration.* (See pp. 494 and 498.)
1. Dialysis produces a more sustained correction of biochemical abnormalities.
2. Allows for liberalization of fluid, protein, and sodium intake; helps wound healing; diminishes bleeding tendencies and predisposition to infection.

C. *To restore adequate blood flow to the kidneys.*
1. Give intravenous fluids and medications as directed to improve renal blood flow and decrease intrarenal vascular resistance.
2. Restore circulating blood volume.
3. Control shock.
4. Manage local or systemic infections.
5. Debride necrotic tissue.

D. *To maintain fluid and electrolyte balance.*
1. Carry out biochemical studies as prescribed. (Electrolyte administration is guided by serial measurements of central venous pressure, serum and urine electrolyte concentrations, fluid losses, and the clinical status of the patient.)
2. Give only enough fluids to replace current losses during oliguric phase (usually 400–500 ml/24 hours plus measured fluid losses associated with gastrointestinal drainage, fever, surgical drainage, or other routes).
3. Weigh the patient daily to provide an index of fluid balance—expected weight loss 0.2–0.5 kg. (½–1 lb.) daily.
4. Monitor the urinary output and urine specific gravity.
   Measure and record intake and output (include urine, gastric suction, stools, wound drainage, perspiration, etc.).
5. Observe fluid excess by assessing patient's clinical status—dyspnea, tachycardia, distended neck veins, peripheral edema, pulmonary edema.
6. Limit dietary protein during oliguric phase to minimize protein breakdown and to prevent rises in blood urea nitrogen.
   a. Prepare for hyperalimentation with high carbohydrate and amino-acid solutions when adequate nutrition cannot be administered through gastrointestinal tract.

  b. Give high-calorie foods, since carbohydrates have a greater protein-sparing power.
  c. Hard candy usually allowed freely; chewing gum will stimulate saliva flow and lessen thirst.
7. Measure and replace sodium losses, especially if large losses occur from the gastrointestinal tract via suction, vomiting, or diarrhea.
8. Control potassium balance (protein catabolism causes release of cellular potassium into body fluids, resulting in serious potassium intoxication).
   a. Sources of potassium are diet, tissue breakdown, blood in the gastrointestinal tract, blood transfusion, other sources (intravenous infusions, potassium penicillin), and extracellular shift in response to metabolic acidosis.
   b. Evaluate for hyperkalemia (potassium intoxication) by assessment of serum potassium levels correlated with ECG changes and patient evaluation.
   c. Give ion exchange resins—sodium polystyrene sulfonate (Kayexalate); provides for more prolonged correction of elevated potassium.
      (1) Orally (laxative may be given concurrently to avoid fecal impaction), or
      (2) By retention enema since the colon is the principal site for potassium exchange
         (a) Use catheter with balloon to facilitate retention if necessary.
         (b) Assist the patient to retain the resin 30–45 minutes to remove the potassium.
      (3) Sorbitol (induces water loss in G.I. tract) may be given orally or as enema with Kayexalate.
   d. Intravenous glucose and insulin or calcium gluconate sometimes used as emergency (and temporary) measure for potassium intoxication; causes potassium to enter cells.
   e. Give intravenous hypertonic sodium bicarbonate as directed—promotes elevation of plasma pH; when available sodium ions are provided, there is a migration of potassium into the cell and a lowering of potassium in the plasma; this is short-term therapy and is used with other long-term measures.
   f. Be prepared for cardiac arrest since increased potassium elevations lead to acute cardiac arrhythmias.
9. Give IV calcium supplementation if hypocalcemia is present.
10. Assess for an increase in serum phosphate concentrations.
    a. Give phosphate binding antacid (aluminum hydroxide)—to keep phosphate from being absorbed into blood stream and help prevent a continuing rise in serum phosphate levels.
11. Watch for signs of dehydration or hypovolemia during the diuretic phase (reduction in body weight, decreasing skin turgor, dryness of mucous membranes, hypotension, tachycardia).

E. *To prevent infection.*
1. Utilize environmental asepsis.
2. Pay special attention to draining wounds, burns, etc., which may develop sepsis.
3. Avoid use of indwelling urethral catheters if possible.
   a. Give meticulous catheter care to prevent cystitis and ascending pyelonephritis (p. 506). Obstructed catheter may lead to pyelonephritis.
   b. Utilize 3-way closed bladder irrigation system to

decrease incidence of systemic infection if patient has to have indwelling catheter.
4. Turn the patient and encourage him to cough and exercise to prevent pulmonary infections.
5. Be aware of the danger of aspiration of gastric contents in stuporous patients.

F. *To anticipate and forestall complications.*
1. Infection

2. Potassium intoxication
3. Acidosis
4. Circulatory overload (dyspnea, orthopnea, pulmonary congestion, pulmonary edema)
5. Hypertension, hypertensive crisis, convulsions
6. Neurologic complications—abnormalities of mental status.

CHRONIC RENAL FAILURE

Chronic renal failure is a progressive deterioration of renal function which ends fatally in uremia (an excess of urea and other nitrogenous wastes in the blood) and its complications unless hemodialysis or a kidney transplant is performed.

Reversible Causes

1. Urinary tract obstruction and infection
2. Infectious diseases which cause increased catabolism with retention of metabolites and hyperkalemia
3. Hypertension
4. Metabolic disease
5. Nephrotoxic (poisonous to kidney cells) agents
6. Dehydration

Stages of Chronic Renal Failure

Decreased renal reserve → renal insufficiency → renal failure → uremia

Clinical Manifestations

1. Gastrointestinal manifestations—anorexia, nausea, vomiting, hiccoughs, ulceration of gastrointestinal tract, and hemorrhage.
2. Cardiopulmonary manifestations—hypertension, fibrinous pericarditis, pleuritis.
3. Nervous system manifestations—anxiety, delirium, delusions, hallucinations, drowsiness, muscle twitching, convulsions, coma.
4. Anemia
5. Metabolic and endocrine alterations—glucose intolerance, hyperlipidemia, sex hormone disturbances.
6. Personality changes—emotional dullness, lability with impatient, demanding behavior.
7. Skin discoloration (from retained urinary chromogen)
8. Uremic frost on face (late)
9. Ammonia odor on breath

Diagnostic Evaluation

1. Anemia (a characteristic sign)
2. Elevated serum creatinine or BUN
3. Elevated serum phosphorus
4. Decreased serum calcium
5. Low serum proteins, especially albumin
6. Usually low CO_2 and acidosis (low blood pH)

Treatment and Nursing Management

OBJECTIVES: to help the diseased kidneys maintain homeostasis as long as possible.
to make the best possible use of existing renal function.
to preserve the patient's extrarenal health.
to prepare patient for dialysis/transplantation.

1. Detect and treat reversible causes of chronic renal failure (see previous Reversible Causes).
2. Offer diet according to blood chemistry levels and clinical status of the patient.
   a. Restrict protein intake according to impairment of renal function, since metabolites that accumulate in the blood derive almost entirely from protein catabolism.
      (1) Protein should be of high biological value, rich in essential amino acids (dairy products, eggs, meat) so that patient does not rely on tissue catabolism for essential amino acids.
      (2) Low-protein diet may be supplemented with essential amino acids and vitamins.
      (3) As renal function declines, protein intake may be restricted proportionately.
      (4) Protein will be increased if patient is on dialysis program to allow for loss of amino acids occurring on dialysis.
   b. Ensure high calorie intake—essential to spare protein for its own work, to provide energy, and to prevent wasting.
   Encourage intake of hard candy, jelly beans, jellies, flavored carbohydrate powders.
3. Prevent water and electrolyte disturbances.
   a. Weigh patient daily to assess fluid overload or depletion—weight should not increase or decrease over 0.45 kg. (1 lb.) per day.
   b. Treat acidosis if patient is symptomatic; acidosis commonly appears in chronic renal failure.
      (1) Assess patient for stupor, deep, rapid breathing of Kussmaul type, shortness of breath on exertion, weakness, unconsciousness.
      (2) Replace bicarbonate stores by infusion or oral administration of sodium bicarbonate.
   c. Adjust sodium requirements as required (determined by 24-hour urinary sodium excretion and daily weights)—patients with chronic renal diseases cannot tolerate severe restriction or marked excess in sodium intake.
   d. Restrict dietary potassium and administer potassium-binding agents (Kayexalate) if decreasing renal function results in hyperkalemia.
   e. The following measures may or may not be employed:
      (1) Decrease phosphorus intake (restrict meat, milk, legumes, carbonated beverages)—phosphate retention contributes to development of secondary hyperparathyroidism and development of uremic bone disease (renal osteodystrophy).
         (a) Aluminum hydroxide antacids are given because they bind phosphorus in the intestinal tract.

(2) Increase intestinal calcium absorption by dietary and pharmacologic (calcium carbonate or gluconate) means—calcium absorption is usually impaired in renal insufficiency.
f. Give fluids to maintain adequate urinary volume and avoid dehydration.
  (1) Fluid restriction is not usually initiated until renal function is quite low.
  (2) Fluid allowance should be distributed throughout the day.
  (3) Avoid restricting fluids for prolonged periods for laboratory and radiologic examinations since dehydrating procedures are hazardous to those patients who cannot elaborate a concentrated urine.
  (4) Restrict salt and water intake if there is evidence of extracellular excess (congestive heart failure, pulmonary edema, hypertension).
4. Treat associated cardiac conditions with digitalis, diuretics, and antiarrhythmic agents to reverse congestive heart failure and to improve renal hemodynamics.
  a. Patients with chronic renal failure may also have a variety of other conditions—hypertension, neuropathy, bone disease, infection, anemia—that require pharmacologic therapy.
  b. Patients with renal failure have increased sensitivity to drugs due to impaired metabolism and renal excretion.

NURSING ALERT: Patients with impaired renal function may require major adjustments of common therapeutic agents. Give medications with caution.

5. Monitor blood pressure. Hypertension increases rate of renal deterioration and adversely affects the vascular system.
6. Prepare the patient for a chronic intermittent dialysis program and ultimately a kidney transplant (if he is a candidate for this type of therapy).
7. Treat patient's discomforts symptomatically (itching, thirst, etc.).
8. Give attention to "little things" since these chronically ill individuals become weary, discouraged, and despondent.
9. Observe for complications.
  a. Anemia—has many causes and is invariably found in patients with advanced renal failure.
  b. Renal osteodystrophy—uremia is associated with abnormal calcium metabolism causing bone pathology.
  c. Severe resistant hypertension; increasing edema, heart failure.
  d. Infection.
  e. Paresthesias.
  f. Neuromuscular abnormalities.

DIALYSIS

Dialysis refers to the diffusion of solute molecules through a semipermeable membrane, passing from the side of higher concentration to that of lower concentration. The purpose of dialysis is to maintain the life and well-being of the patient until kidney function is restored.

Methods

1. Peritoneal dialysis (see below).
2. Hemodialysis (page 498).

GUIDELINES: Assisting the Patient Undergoing Short-Term Peritoneal Dialysis*

Peritoneal dialysis is a substitute for kidney function during renal failure. The peritoneum is used as a dialyzing membrane.

Purposes
1. To aid in the removal of toxic substances and metabolic wastes.
2. To remove excessive body fluid.
3. To assist in regulating the fluid balance of the body.
4. To control blood pressure.

Equipment
Dialysis administration set (disposable, closed system)
Peritoneal dialysis solution as requested
Supplemental drugs as requested
Local anesthesia
Central venous pressure monitoring equipment
ECG

Suture set
Sterile gloves
Skin antiseptic

* Automated closed-system peritoneal cycling machines are available.

Procedure

NURSING ACTION	RATIONALE/AMPLIFICATION

Preparatory Phase

1. Prepare the patient emotionally and physically for the procedure.

2. See that the consent form has been signed.
3. Weigh the patient before dialysis and every 24 hours thereafter, preferably on an in-bed scale.

4. Take temperature, pulse, respiration, and blood pressure readings prior to dialysis.

5. Have the patient empty his bladder.

6. Assist with insertion of central venous pressure catheter. ECG monitoring may also be employed.

7. Make the patient comfortable in a supine position.

1. Nursing support is offered by explaining procedure mechanics, providing opportunities for the patient to ask questions, allowing him to verbalize his feelings, and giving expert physical care.

3. The weight at the beginning of the procedure serves as a baseline of information. Daily weight is helpful in assessing the state of hydration.
4. A knowledge of vital signs at the beginning of dialysis is necessary for comparing subsequent changes in vital signs.
5. If the bladder is empty there is less likelihood of perforating it when the trocar is introduced into the peritoneum.
6. CVP measurements may be carried out to assess fluid volume changes. Cardiac arrhythmias may occur due to serum potassium changes and vagal stimulation.

Performance Phase (by the physician)

The following is a brief résumé of the method of insertion of the peritoneal catheter (done under strict asepsis).

1. The abdomen is prepared surgically and the skin and subcutaneous tissues are infiltrated with a local anesthetic.
2. A small midline stab wound is made 3–5 cm. below the umbilicus.
3. A thin stylet cannula may be inserted percutaneously, or a trocar is introduced through the incision.
4. The patient is requested to raise his head from the pillow after the stylet/trocar is introduced.

5. When the peritoneum is punctured, the stylet/trocar is directed toward the left side of the pelvis. The stylet is removed, and the catheter is inserted through the trocar and maneuvered into position.
   a. Dialysis fluid is allowed to run through the catheter while it is being positioned.

6. After the trocar is removed, the skin may be closed with a purse-string suture. (This is not always done.) A sterile dressing is placed around the catheter.
7. Flush the tubing with dialysis solution.

8. Attach the catheter connector to the administration set which has been previously connected to the container of dialysis solution (warmed to body temperature, 37° C.)
9. Dry the dialysate bottles before inverting.
10. Drugs (heparin, etc.) are added in advance.

11. Permit the dialyzing solution to flow unrestricted into the peritoneal cavity (usually takes about 10 minutes for completion).

12. Allow the fluid to remain in the peritoneal cavity for the prescribed time period (15–30 minutes). Prepare the next exchange while the fluid is in the peritoneal cavity.

13. Unclamp the outflow tube. Drainage should take approximately 10 minutes or more, although the time varies with each patient.

1. Surgical preparation of the skin minimizes or eliminates surface bacteria and decreases the possibility of wound contamination and infection.
2. The midline area is relatively avascular.

3. Some peritoneal catheters require a surgical approach in the operating room.

4. This maneuver tightens the abdominal muscles and permits easier penetration of the trocar without danger of injury to the intra-abdominal organs.

   a. This prevents the omentum from adhering to the catheter, impeding its advancement or occluding its opening.
6. The catheter is attached to the skin to prevent loss of the catheter in the abdomen.

7. The tubing is flushed to prevent air from entering the peritoneal cavity. Air causes abdominal discomfort and drainage difficulties.
8. The solution is warmed to body temperature for patient comfort and to prevent abdominal pain. Heating also causes dilation of the peritoneal vessels and increases urea clearance.

10. The addition of heparin prevents fibrin clots from occluding the catheter. Potassium chloride may be added on request unless patient has hyperkalemia.
11. The inflow solution should flow in a steady stream. If the fluid flows in too slowly the catheter may need to be repositioned since its tip may be buried in the omentum, or it may be occluded by a blood clot.
12. In order for potassium, urea, and other waste materials to be removed, the solution must remain in the peritoneal cavity for the prescribed time (dwell or equilibration time). The maximum concentration gradient takes place in the first 5–10 minutes and this is the most effective dwell time.
13. The abdomen is drained by a siphon effect through the closed system. Gravity drainage should occur fairly rapidly, and steady streams of fluid should be observed entering the drainage container. The drainage is usually straw-colored.

GUIDELINES: Assisting the Patient Undergoing Short-Term Peritoneal Dialysis* (cont.)

Procedure (cont.)

NURSING ACTION	RATIONALE/AMPLIFICATION
14. If the fluid is not draining properly, move the patient from side to side to facilitate the removal of peritoneal drainage. The head of the bed may also be elevated. Ascertain if the catheter is patent.	14. If the drainage stops, or starts to drip before the dializing fluid has run out, it may indicate that the catheter tip is buried in the omentum. Rotating the patient may be helpful (or it may be necessary for the physician to reposition the catheter).
15. When the outflow drainage ceases to run, clamp off the drainage tube and infuse the next exchange, using strict aseptic technique.	
16. Take blood pressure and pulse every 15 minutes during the first exchange and every hour thereafter. Monitor the heart rate for signs of arrhythmia.	16. A drop in blood pressure may indicate excessive fluid loss from glucose concentrations of the dialyzing solutions. Changes in the vital signs may indicate impending shock or overhydration.
17. Take patient's temperature every 4 hours (especially after catheter removal).	17. An infection is more apt to become evident after dialysis has been discontinued.
18. The procedure is repeated until the blood chemistry levels improve. The usual time for short-term dialysis is 24 hours, using 48 liters of dialysate, depending on the patient's condition.	18. The duration of dialysis depends on the severity of the condition and on the size and weight of the patient. Patients requiring only a few peritoneal dialysis treatments may have a plastic T-shaped button placed in the catheter tract between dialyses to avoid need to repuncture the abdomen for catheter insertion. Patients requiring prolonged peritoneal dialysis have implanted silastic catheters used with closed automated dialysis systems.
19. Keep an exact record of the patient's fluid balance during the treatment. a. Know the status of the patient's loss or gain of fluid at the end of each exchange. b. The fluid balance should be about even or should show slight fluid loss.	19. Complications (circulatory overload, hypertension, congestive heart failure) may occur if most of the fluid is not recovered.
20. Promote patient comfort during dialysis. a. Frequent back care and massage of pressure areas. b. Rotate from side to side. c. Elevate head of bed at intervals. d. Allow patient to sit in chair for brief periods if condition permits.	20. The dialysis period is lengthy, and the patient becomes fatigued.

21. Observe for the following:
a. Respiratory difficulty
  (1) Slow the inflow rate.
  (2) Make sure tubing is not kinked.
  (3) Prevent air from entering peritoneum by keeping drip chamber of tubing three-fourths full of fluid.
  (4) Elevate head of bed; encourage coughing and breathing exercises.
  (5) Turn patient from side to side.
b. Abdominal Pain.
  (1) Encourage patient to move about.
	21. a. This is caused by pressure from the fluid in the peritoneal cavity and the upward displacement of the diaphragm—producing shallow respirations.
	  (3) In severe respiratory difficulty, the fluid from the peritoneal cavity should be drained immediately and the physician notified.
	
	b. Pain may be caused by the dialyzing solution's not being at body temperature, incomplete drainage of the solution, chemical irritation, irritation by the catheter, peritonitis.

c. Leakage
  (1) Change the dressings frequently.
  (2) Use sterile plastic drapes to prevent contamination.
	c. Leakage around the catheter predisposes to peritonitis.

22. Keep accurate records: a. Exact time of beginning and ending of each exchange; starting and finishing time of drainage b. Amount of solution infused and recovered c. Fluid balance d. Number of exchanges e. Medications added to dialyzing solution f. Pre- and postdialysis weight g. Level of responsiveness at beginning, throughout, and at end of treatment h. Assessment of vital signs and patient's condition	
Complications 1. Peritonitis a. Watch for abdominal pain, rebound tenderness, rigidity, cloudy dialysate return. b. Send specimen of dialysate for smear and culture.	1. Peritonitis is the most common complication. Antibiotics may be added to dialysate and also given systematically. Albumin (IV) may be given because of increased loss of protein with peritonitis.

Procedure (cont.)

NURSING ACTION	RATIONALE/AMPLIFICATION
2. Bleeding	2. A small amount of bleeding around the catheter is not significant if it does not persist. During the first few exchanges, blood-tinged fluid from subcutaneous bleeding is not uncommon. Small amounts of heparin may be added to inflow solution to prevent the catheter from becoming clogged.
3. Shock	3. Symptoms of shock may occur due to excessive fluid loss.
4. Protein loss	4. There may be a significant protein loss because most serum proteins pass through the peritoneal membrane during dialysis. Serum albumin determinations are made throughout the treatment.

Continuous Ambulatory Peritoneal Dialysis (Fig. 11–10)

Continuous ambulatory peritoneal dialysis is a practical self-dialysis method that involves almost constant peritoneal contact with a dialysis solution for patients with end-stage renal disease.

1. A permanent indwelling catheter is implanted into the peritoneum.
2. A connecting tube is attached to the external end of the peritoneal catheter, and the distal end of the tube is inserted into a sterile plastic bag of dialysate solution.
3. The dialysate bag is raised to shoulder level and infused by gravity into the peritoneal cavity.
4. Then the plastic bag attached to the connecting tube is folded and placed in a pouch at the waist, under the patient's clothing.
5. At the end of the dwell time (approximately 4 hours) the bag is removed from the pouch, unfolded, and placed near the floor to allow the dialysate to drain by gravity over a 20–25 minute period.
6. After the dialysate is drained, a fresh bag of dialysate solution is attached under aseptic conditions, and the procedure is repeated.
7. The patient performs 4–5 exchanges daily, 7 days per week with an overnight dwell time allowing uninterrupted sleep; most patients become unaware of fluid in the peritoneal cavity.
8. *Advantages*
   a. Physical and psychological freedom
   b. Free dietary intake
   c. Relatively simple and easy to use
   d. Least expensive form of dialysis therapy
   e. Eliminates need for complicated machines/dialyzers
9. *Complications*
   a. Peritonitis (aftereffects may be peritoneal adhesions)
   b. Orthostatic hypotension, hypertriglyceridemia, back pain

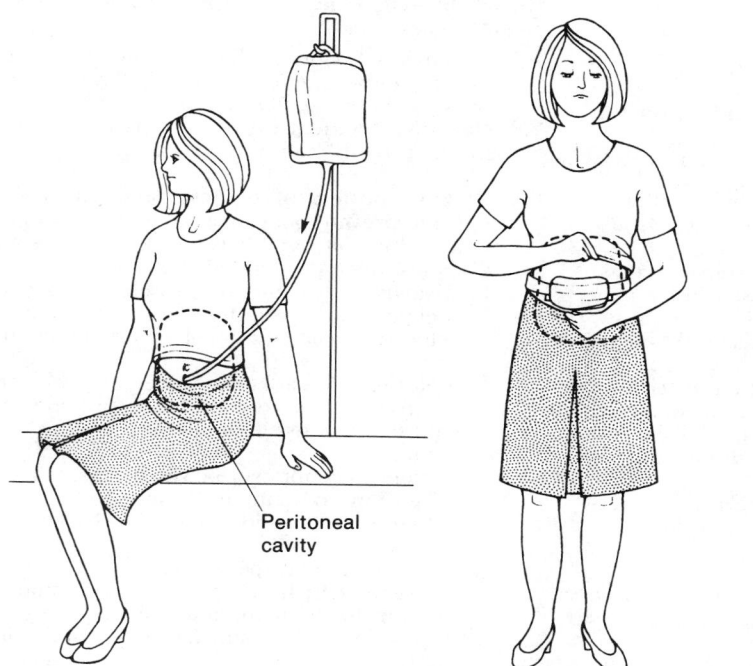
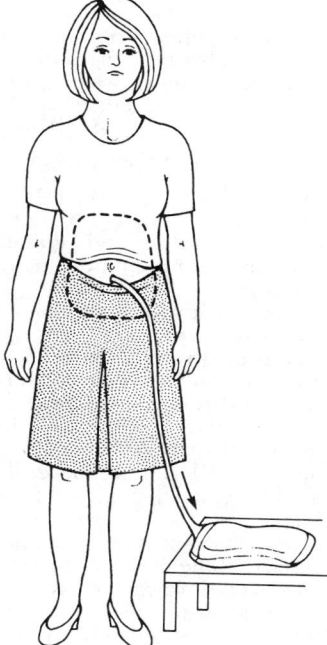

Peritoneal cavity

FIGURE 11-10. *Continuous ambulatory peritoneal dialysis.*

HEMODIALYSIS

Hemodialysis is a process of cleansing the blood of accumulated waste products. It is used for patients with end-stage renal failure or for acutely ill patients who require short-term dialysis.

OBJECTIVES: to extract toxic nitrogenous substances from the blood.
to remove excess water.

Underlying Principles

1. Heparinized blood passes down a concentration gradient through a semipermeable membrane by dialysis to the dialysate fluid.
2. The dialysate is composed of all of the important electrolytes in their ideal extracellular concentrations.
3. Through the process of diffusion, the blood components equilibrate with those in the dialysate. By appropriate adjustment of the dialysate bath composition, noxious substances (urea, creatinine, uric acid, phosphate, and other metabolites) are transferred from the blood into the dialysate so that they can be discarded. Small pores of the membrane hold back desirable blood components.
4. Excess water is removed from the blood (ultrafiltration).
5. The body's buffer system is maintained by the addition and diffusion of acetate from the dialysate into the patient; it is metabolized to form bicarbonate.
6. Purified blood is returned to the body through a vein of the patient.
7. At the end of the treatment the majority of poisonous wastes have been removed, electrolyte and water balances have been restored, and the buffer system has been replenished.

Requirements for Hemodialysis

1. Access to the patient's circulation
2. Dialyzer with semipermeable membrane
3. Appropriate dialysate bath
Time—4–6 hours, 3 times weekly, depending on the type of artificial kidney used.
Place—home (if feasible) or at a dialysis center.

Methods of Access to Patient's Circulation

1. Arteriovenous fistula (AVF)—fistula made surgically by anastomosis of an artery to a vein.
   a. Usually radial artery and cephalic vein are anastomosed in nondominant arm; vessels in leg may also be used.
   b. Following the procedure, the superficial venous system of the arm dilates.
   c. By means of two large-bore needles inserted into the dilated venous system, blood can be obtained and passed through the dialyzer. The arterial end is used for arterial flow and the distal end for reinfusion of dialyzed blood.
   d. Healing of AVF requires several weeks; an external shunt (see below) is used in the interim.
   e. Problems:
      (1) Infection; aneurysm formation
      (2) Disadvantage of being injected with large-bore needles before each dialysis treatment
2. External arteriovenous shunt (cannula)
   a. Teflon-silastic cannula sewn into radial artery and a forearm vein (or placed in leg). The 2 are connected by a teflon bridge.

b. During dialysis, the bridge is removed and the arterial and venous ends are connected to the flow lines of the artificial kidney.
   c. Currently used while AVF is healing.
   d. *Problems*
      (1) Clotting and infection; chronic erosion of the skin
      (2) Limited shunt life—must be surgically revised every few months
      (3) Dislodgement with hemorrhage
      (4) Visible reminder to patient of his disability
3. Biological grafts—bovine carotid graft; autogenous saphenous graft
4. Synthetic grafts—expanded reinforced polytetrafluoroethylene (PTFE) graft
5. Direct cannulation of vessels (femoral vein)

Types of Dialyzers

Many varieties of artificial kidneys have been described, but most conform to one of the following types:
1. Coil dialyzer
2. Flat plate or parallel flow dialyzer
3. Hollow-fiber kidney

Monitoring During Dialysis

The management of the patient on a dialyzer is a complex subject beyond the scope of this discussion. The reader is referred to the written protocol of the machine being used.

NURSING ALERT: Nurses attending patients undergoing hemodialysis are at risk of acquiring hepatitis B.

Dietary Management of Patient on Long-term Hemodialysis

1. The individual patient's dietary regimen is adjusted according to the extent of his residual renal function to avoid wide fluctuation in body chemistry.
2. Dietary management involves restriction or adjustment of protein, sodium, potassium, and/or fluid intake.
   a. Protein—protein of highest biological quality is given to prevent poor protein utilization, to maintain positive nitrogen balance, and replace amino acids lost during each dialysis.
      (1) Usually 1–1.2 gm. of protein per kg. body weight is given; additional supplement given when stress situations (bleeding, infection) occur.
      (2) Calories (35 kcal/kg. body weight) are supplied from carbohydrates and fats to provide energy and to spare tissue breakdown.
   b. Sodium
      (1) Patient may not excrete the necessary amount of sodium to maintain balance.
      (2) Observe for fluid overload—hypertension, edema.
      (3) Or patient may be a "salt loser," unable to conserve salt; he thus loses large amounts of sodium in the urine and will require sodium replacement by pharmacologic and dietary means.
   c. Potassium—potassium is a mineral found in the body cells.

(1) Ability to eliminate excessive amounts of potassium is decreased in chronic renal failure.

(2) Accumulation of potassium in body can be toxic to heart and cause serious arrhythmias.

(3) Potassium is found in practically all foods—fruit juices, salt substitutes, bananas, chocolate, and baked potatoes are rich sources of potassium.

d. Fluid limitations

(1) Fluid is restricted according to output; usually between 500–800 ml. depending on renal function, losses, activity, environmental temperature.

(2) Patient should be able to adjust his fluid intake according to the weight he has gained between dialysis treatments.

(3) "Sourballs" are satisfactory to use as thirst quenchers.

e. Calcium and phosphorus intake may have to be adjusted.

Nutrition: Health Education

Instruct the patient as follows:

1. Avoid eating frequently in places where salt-free cooking cannot be assured.
2. Read food labels carefully; avoid commercially prepared foods that have added sodium.
3. Avoid "salt substitutes"—may contain potassium chloride, which should be avoided.
4. Eat fresh vegetables and fruits within dietary prescription.
5. An excellent dietary guide available for $1.45:
   Jones, W. O.: Diet Guide for Patients on Chronic Dialysis. DHEW Pub. No. (NIH) 76–685, Superintendent of Documents, U.S. Government Printing Office, Washington, D.C. 20402.

Pharmacologic Management

1. Phosphate-binding gels (Amphogel, Aludrox, Basojel)
   a. Phosphorus tends to accumulate, resulting in hyperparathyroidism and osteodystrophy.
   b. These medications bind phosphate in the intestine and may help maintain proper calcium and phosphorus levels in the blood.
2. Potassium-binders (Kayexalate)—binds potassium in intestine to prevent dangerous elevations in blood.
3. Multivitamins—necessary because of significant nutrient losses during dialysis (especially of ascorbic acid and folic acid).

Medical Problems of Patients on Long-term Hemodialysis

Although hemodialysis can prolong life indefinitely, it does not completely control uremia or halt the natural course of the underlying kidney disease. There are various abnormalities, syndromes, and discomforts, and long-term metabolic complications associated with hemodialysis.

1. Arteriosclerotic cardiovascular disease—leading cause of death and major factor limiting long-term survival.
   a. Disturbances of lipid metabolism (hypertriglyceridemia) appear to be accentuated by hemodialysis.
   b. Congestive heart failure, coronary heart disease with anginal pain, stroke, peripheral vascular insufficiency may incapacitate patient.
2. Intercurrent infection—patient has reduced resistance to infection.
   a. Exposure of blood to blood products and foreign material—may cause infection and gram-negative and gram-positive bacteremia
   b. Local infection of shunt site and in fistulas
   c. Hemodialysis-associated hepatitis
3. Anemia and fatigue—may be caused by accelerated red cell loss (from hemolysis and bleeding) and impaired erythropoietin production.
   a. Sleeplessness, fatigue, and malaise may be persistent
   b. Diminution of physical and emotional well-being—lack of energy, drive, loss of interest
4. Intractable pruritus (itching).
5. Bleeding.
   a. Bleeding from heparin rebound
   b. Gastrointestinal bleeding
   c. Subdural hematoma
   d. Hemorrhagic pericarditis
   e. Menorrhagia
6. Hypertension.
7. Bone problems
   a. Renal osteodystrophy (leading to bone pain and fractures)—pathogenesis obscure but excessive parathyroid hormone secretion and vitamin D resistance may be causal factors
   b. Aseptic necrosis of hip
   c. Vascular calcification
8. Chronic ascites—may be due to fluid overload associated with congestive heart failure, malnutrition (hypoalbuminemia), and inadequate dialysis.
9. Disequilibrium syndrome—from rapid fluid and electrolyte changes.
   May produce hypertension, headache, vomiting, convulsions, coma, and psychiatric problems.
10. Dialysis dementia—progressive, irreversible, and fatal neurologic syndrome thought to be due to aluminum intoxication (from aluminum-containing dialysate fluid).

Psychosocial Problems

Long-term hemodialysis has unpredictable and uneven results. The impact of renal disease and the stresses of dialysis can be destructive to the ego and can place its victims under severe mental and emotional stress.

1. Depression—an expected occurrence; most common psychological manifestation seen in patients on hemodialysis
   Depression occurs from multiple causes—losses of bodily functions, working capability, and sexual drive; impotence, other physical complications, chronic illness, feelings of deprivation from diet and fluid restriction, limited capacity to compete, fear of death and dying, unpredictable medical status.
2. Dependence-independence conflict
   a. Although patient is dependent on the machine, personnel, and treatment regimen, he is at the same time encouraged to be independent, work, and lead a "normal" life.
   b. Dependence may create aggressive feelings which cannot be expressed.
   c. May repress hostility toward medical and nursing staff.
   d. Highly dependent patient may "enjoy" hemodialysis.

3. Anxiety—a normal reaction to stress and threat
    a. Patient anxious because of constant changes in his clinical status and unpredictability of his health.
    b. May use denial, fantasy, repression, rejection, etc., as defense mechanisms to deal with anxiety.
    c. Try to clarify the nature of his anxiety before attempts at reassurance.
4. Suicidal behavior—usually an act that stems from depression—suicide rate is more than 100 times that of general population.
    a. Allow patient to express his feelings about self-destruction.
    b. Point out his positive coping mechanisms and emphasize his capabilities.
    c. Psychiatric referral may be necessary.
5. Denial—a common response to a shift in health status
    a. Denial may be protective and useful to a certain extent—may protect patient from emotional decompensation (denial has both adaptive and maladaptive functions).
    b. Failure of this defense may lead to depression.
6. Stress of dietary restrictions—patient may "act out" conflicts by binges of overeating/drinking.
7. Sexual dysfunctions—diminished interest and ability due to biologic, pharmacologic, and psychological reasons.

Impact of Dialysis on Family

1. Altered family life style.
    a. Social activities may be decreased due to large amount of time spent on dialysis.
    b. Close confinement to home (if patient on home dialysis)—may create conflicts, frustration, and depression in some families.
    c. Patient and family may impose unnecessary limitations on their own activities.
2. Decreasing sexual activity—may lead to marital problems.
3. Feelings of resentment (revealed or hidden)—due to personal sacrifices made by family.
4. Feeling that patient is a "marginal" person with limited life expectancy—can be transmitted to patient.
5. Difficulties in communication between patient and spouse—difficult to express anger, negative feelings, and fear of death.
    a. Fear that expressed anger will cause something to happen to patient.
    b. Expressions of anger may be displaced or covered up by anxiety.

Health Education

1. Encourage patient to assume the management and control of his therapeutic regimen.
    a. Determine patient's own value system and ego strengths; use these to help him adapt to a different life style.
    b. Emphasize his capabilities.
    c. Teach patient about his condition and treatment in "small doses."
    d. Deemphasize the patient's image of himself as "sick."
    e. Help him to develop a sense of independence from the machine.
    f. Encourage patient to interact with his surroundings during dialysis.
2. Encourage patient to set realistic goals.
    a. Work activities should be introduced gradually—returning to work may not be a realistic goal for some patients.
    b. Modify attitudes in direction of permissiveness in area of productivity.
3. Encourage patient to express his angry feelings (pain, discomfort, frustration)—helps to reduce level of emotional tension and will help prevent depression.
4. Let family have an opportunity (away from patient) to express their feelings of anger, helplessness, etc.
    a. Help family to accept their negative feelings.
    b. Teach family what is involved in chronic hemodialysis.
5. Organizations helpful to patients on chronic dialysis: National Association of Patients on Hemodialysis and Transplantation, Inc. 505 Northern Boulevard Great Neck, N.Y. 11021

    National Kidney Foundation
    116 East 27th Street
    New York, N.Y. 10016

KIDNEY TRANSPLANTATION

Kidney transplantation is the transplantation of a kidney from a living donor or human cadaver donor to a recipient with end-stage renal failure who requires support from dialysis in order to maintain life.
    Kidney transplants from well-matched related living donors are more successful than those from cadaver donors.

Potential Problems

1. Infection—leading cause of death after transplant.
2. Possibility of recurrence of original disease in the graft
    (Example: rapidly progressive glomerulonephritis)
3. Renal graft failure and renal graft rejection
    Except when the donor is a twin, the immunologic defense of the recipient tends to reject (and destroy) a foreign substance, e.g., the kidney graft.
4. Death from complications

Operative Procedures Done Before Transplantation

Surgical operations on all recipients before transplantation may or may not include:
1. Bilateral nephrectomy—for uncontrolled hypertension (renin variety), for removal of potential source of infection, if present, and for patients with obstructed kidneys or vesicoureteral reflux, rapidly progressive glomerulonephritis, polycystic renal disease.
2. Vagotomy/pyloroplasty—may be done as an acid-reducing gastric procedure for patients with history of gastrointestinal bleeding or duodenal ulcer to lessen potential for postoperative steroid-induced gastrointestinal bleeding.

Surgical Procedure
1. The donor kidney is transplanted retroperitoneally in either iliac fossa.

2. The ureter of the newly transplanted kidney is transplanted into the bladder or anastomosed to the ureter of the recipient.

Preoperative Medical and Nursing Management Before Transplantation

OBJECTIVE: to bring patient's metabolic state as close to normal as possible.

1. Tissue typing done to determine histocompatibility of donor and recipient.
2. Antibody screening for red and white cell antibodies.
3. Immunosuppressive drugs given in order to minimize or overcome body's defense mechanism:
   Azathioprine (Imuran) and prednisone are usually begun 48 hours preoperatively on a scheduled transplant patient.
4. Blood transfusion (if necessary)
5. Blood counts, chemistries, coagulation profiles, liver function tests, required cultures, ECG, state of hydration, blood pressure, TPR and weight are corrected and documented.
6. Hemodialysis (p. 498) is usually done the day before the scheduled transplant.
7. Preoperative skin preparation is meticulous to decrease bacterial count on the skin.
   Preoperative shaving done in O.R.—inadvertent scratches and nicks from shaving serve as nidi for bacterial colonization.
8. Avoid pulmonary complications by:
   a. Cessation of cigarette smoking 2 weeks prior to surgery
   b. Instruction and practice in deep breathing, coughing, and leg and ankle exercises

Postoperative Objectives of Surgical and Nursing Management

GOAL: to maintain homeostasis until kidney transplant is functioning well. (Many facets of care are similar to those of patients having renal and vascular surgery.)

A. *To anticipate at the earliest moment any evidence of threatened rejection.*

1. Watch for signs of rejection—fever, decreased urine output, increased serum creatinine; also assess for increasing blood pressure, weight gain, swelling or tenderness over graft, apprehension.
2. Participate in careful postoperative immunosuppressive management based on immunologic monitoring.
   a. Give combinations of immunosuppressive drugs (Azathioprine [Imuran]), prednisone, or antilymphocyte globulin (ALG), or antithymocyte globulin (ATG), or combination(s) of cyclophosphamide, prednisone, ALG, as directed.
   b. Doses are gradually tapered; therapy is continued indefinitely.
   c. Renal graft failure and rejection may be early (first 24–72 hours), delayed (3–14 days), or late (after 3 weeks).
      (1) Transplanted kidney is removed when rejection is inevitable or when excessive immunosuppression is required to maintain kidney.
      (2) Patient placed back on maintenance dialysis; will require understanding and supportive emotional care.
3. Monitor patient for opportunistic infections—immunosuppression depresses formation of leukocytes, which may produce agranulocytosis; resistance to infection is lowered and lethal sepsis may develop.

B. *To anticipate and avoid all possible complications.*

1. Monitor and protect patient from infection—kidney recipient is susceptible to faulty healing and infection due both to immunosuppressive therapy, which suppresses the immune response, and to complications of renal failure.
   a. Infection may be masked or confused with symptoms of rejection since impaired renal function and fever are evidences of both infection and rejection.
   b. Immunosuppressive drugs render the transplant recipient more vulnerable to infection, permitting opportunistic infections to occur (moniliasis, cytomegalic virus disease, *Pneumocystis carinii* pneumonia.
2. Carry out protective isolation as required; health team members and family may wear masks until immunosuppressive drug dosages are lowered.
3. Give aseptic care to wounds and puncture sites (CVP lines, IV, draining sites, etc.).
   a. Wound healing may be delayed due to effects of renal disease and immunosuppressive drugs.
   b. Change dressings promptly if drainage is present—drainage is an excellent culture medium for bacteria.
   c. Carry out bacteriologic testing of urine and all exit wounds. Catheter and drain tips are cultured on removal.
      (1) Before removing catheter, disinfect skin around entry site of catheter (or drain). Remove.
      (2) Using aseptic technique, cut off tip of catheter or drain and place in sterile container for lab culture.
4. Monitor vascular access to hemodialysis to ensure patency and watch for evidence of infection.
5. Give oral mycostatin mouthwash—to prevent mucosal candidiasis (fungal colonization occurs secondarily to steroid and antibiotic administration).
6. Give regular skin hygiene.

C. *To keep an accurate fluid and electrolyte balance.*

After kidney transplant the following may occur:
1. A few donor kidneys function immediately after grafting.
   a. May produce large quantities of dilute urine (10–15 liters in first 24 hours)—due partly to tubular dysfunction or overhydrated state found in some dialyzed patients.
      Give IV fluid replacement to balance losses.
   b. Cadaver kidney (due to period of ischemia following donor's death) may undergo tubular necrosis and not function for 2–3 weeks.
      Restrict fluid intake—usually approximately 600 ml./24 hours plus amount of fluid losses from drainage, etc.
   c. Or kidney may produce amounts of urine varying from extremes of no urine to large volumes of urine.
2. Monitor central venous pressure, ECG, and skin temperature frequently to guard against occult blood volume depletion and electrolyte imbalance.
   a. CVP readings observed and recorded hourly or more frequently as necessary.
   b. Avoid using dialysis access extremity for IVs, intraarterial monitoring, or restraints.

3. Monitor output from indwelling catheter which has been connected to a closed drainage system.
   a. Measure urine every 30 minutes–1 hour.
   b. Irrigate catheter only on direct request.
   c. Palpate bladder to detect presence of distention.
   d. Instruct patient to void frequently after catheter removal to avoid stressing the bladder closure.
4. Monitor serum and urine electrolytes to determine patient's chemical balance.
   a. Anticipate adjustment of fluid replacement.
   b. Give IV fluids according to urine volume and serum electrolyte levels; serum and urine chemistries are measured at specified intervals.
   c. Notify physician immediately if arrhythmias or other cardiac symptoms develop.
5. Prepare for hemodialysis in postoperative period until transplanted kidney is functioning well.

D. *To be alert for other complications.*

1. Acute renal failure—from ischemia, renal artery thrombosis, hyperacute rejection
2. Gastrointestinal complications
   a. Incidence of GI ulceration and bleeding is high (steroid-induced).
      (1) Steroids mask symptoms of ulceration.
      (2) GI hemorrhage associated with high mortality rate.
      (3) Give antacids frequently as directed until steroid doses are lowered—as a means of protection against GI ulceration.
   b. Fungal colonization of GI tract—occurs secondarily to steroid and antibiotic administration.
   c. Fecal impaction—decrease in colonic motility may occur from steroid effect.
3. Other complications
   a. Infection, diabetes, GI bleeding, thrombosis, osteoporosis, psychosis, disorders of calcium metabolism, cushingoid facies, glaucoma, cataracts, acne—from steroids.
   b. Bone marrow depression—from immunosuppressive therapy
   c. Vascular complications—hemorrhage and thrombosis
   d. Grafted ureter—stricture, fistula (also fistula of bladder)
   e. Viral hepatitis
   f. Hypertension—from renal artery stenosis in allograft, from steroids, from renal–vascular disease.

g. Cancer—persons on long-term immunosuppressive therapy develop cancer more frequently than the general population.

E. *To give continuing psychological support.*

1. Be aware of the stresses associated with renal transplantation—fear of organ rejection, problems associated with immunosuppressants and steroids.
2. Keep the patient informed of his progress, proposed treatment plans, and short- and long-term goals.
3. Observe for changes in behavior, altered thought and feeling processes.
4. See p. 499 for other aspects of psychological support.

Discharge Planning and Health Education

1. The hospitalization period for a kidney transplant may be 6 weeks or longer.
2. The patient receives individualized instruction about the following:
   a. Diet
   b. Medications
      (1) Review medications in detail, including color identification of pills, dose schedules, and the necessity for taking the medication.
   c. Fluids
   d. Daily weight
   e. Daily measurement of urine
   f. Management of intake and output
   g. Prevention of infection
   h. Resumption of activity
3. Instruct patient to report to the physician immediately if any of the following occur:
   a. Decrease in urinary output
   b. Weight gain
   c. Malaise
   d. Changes in blood pressure readings
   e. Fever
   f. Respiratory distress
   g. Tenderness over graft
   h. Anxiety, depression, changes in eating, drinking, or other habit patterns
4. Advise patient to avoid strenuous contact sports after surgery.
5. Patient should know that follow-up care after transplantation is a lifelong necessity.
6. Organization helpful to the patient:
   National Association of Patients on Hemodialysis and Transplantation, Inc.
   505 Northern Boulevard, Great Neck, New York 11021; Publication: NAPHT NEWS.

NURSING MANAGEMENT OF THE PATIENT UNDERGOING RENAL/UROLOGICAL SURGERY

Preoperative Nursing Care

OBJECTIVE: to restore the patient to as normal a physiological state as possible with as little psychological trauma and physical morbidity as possible.

A. *To recognize the fear and anxiety of the patient concerning the threat of impending surgery.*

1. Keep in mind that most patients entering the hospital with urological conditions have pain, fever, hematuria, difficulty in voiding, etc.

2. Encourage the patient to recognize and express his feelings of anxiety.
3. Obtain patient's confidence by establishing a relationship of trust and by giving gentle and considerate care.
4. Increase the patient's understanding of what to expect during the pre-and postoperative periods.
5. Assess for alertness, appetite, and general well-being of the patient.
6. Avoid physical inactivity.
7. Give preoperative medications as prescribed to allay worry and fear.

B. *To assess anatomic and functional status of urinary tract and kidneys.*

1. Complete examination of urinary tract including laboratory evaluation, x-ray studies, renal angiography, etc., as indicated.
2. Give antibacterial agents as indicated before surgery—for infected kidneys, ureters, bladder.

C. *To assess respiratory and cardiovascular function before surgical exposure of the kidney.*

1. Surgical approaches to the kidney predispose the patient to respiratory complications and paralytic ileus.
2. Determine history of patient's ability to engage in physical activity without distress.
   Observe for dyspnea, productive cough, other cardiac symptoms.
3. Do an electrocardiogram on all patients over 50. The preoperative cardiogram also serves as a baseline reference in event of postoperative cardiopulmonary complications.
4. Secure a chest x-ray.
5. Carry out pulmonary function studies and blood gas analysis in patients with impaired respiratory function.
6. Assess status of vascular system of lower extremities (especially varicosities).
   a. Elevate patient's leg and apply elastic stockings to minimize stasis in superficial veins.
   b. Encourage patients to do leg exercises.
7. Inquire if patient has any bleeding tendencies.
8. Teach the patient deep-breathing exercises and an effective cough routine (p. 84).
9. Manage coexisting diseases (diabetes, congestive heart failure).

D. *To discover and correct any abnormalities of fluid and electrolyte balance.*

1. Weigh patient daily to determine status of fluid balance.
2. Assess status of mucous membranes and skin turgor; maintain the hematocrit at optimal level.
3. Measure and record intake and output as an index of hydration.

E. *To determine the drug and allergy history of the patient so that therapeutic corrections can be made if necessary.*

1. Antihypertensives and tranquilizers—predispose to refractory hypotension during general anesthesia.
2. Anticoagulants—depress prothrombin activity; can produce hemorrhagic complications especially in prostatic surgery and operations on retroperitoneal area.
3. Adrenal cortical steroids—may produce adrenal insufficiency during periods of stress.
4. Anticholinergics and antihistamines—may impair emptying of bladder
5. Alcohol—previous overuse may precipitate onset of delirium tremens

Postoperative Nursing Care

OBJECTIVE: to reduce factors that contribute to postoperative complications.

A. *To promote the safety and comfort of the patient.*

1. Employ frequent and close observation of blood pressure, pulse, and respiration in order to recognize symptoms of shock, hemorrhage, and early atelectasis.

2. Give postoperative sedation and pain control on an individual basis to reduce splinting of respiratory movements and to permit coughing, since incision is close to diaphragm; patient will voluntarily tend to splint chest while breathing.
   a. Use narcotics at proper intervals—to help patient perform deep breathing and coughing more effectively.
   b. Use moist heat, massage, and analgesics for muscular aches and pain resulting from position on operating table.
   c. Assess for pain similar to renal colic—caused by passage of clotted blood down the ureter; requires adequate doses of narcotic for relief.
   d. Use incentive spirometer (p. 183) to help maximize lung inflation; encourage coughing after each deep breath to loosen secretions.
3. Be alert for symptoms of postoperative ileus (fairly common following renal surgery).
   a. Assess for abdominal distention, pain, and lack of intestinal peristalsis (determined by stethoscope auscultation).
   b. Avoid oral intake for patient until active bowel sounds are heard (auscultation) or passage of flatus is noted.
   c. Give adequate and appropriate fluid and electrolyte replacement intravenously.
   d. Assist with decompression via nasogastric tube for relief of abdominal distention (p. 392). See page 435 for treatment of paralytic ileus.
4. Monitor fluid intake—by vein and then by mouth when nausea ceases.
   a. Keep accurate intake and output records.
   b. Weigh patient daily to determine status of fluid balance.
5. Make certain that drainage tubes are functioning, since almost all urological patients have drains, tubes, or catheters.
   a. Make sure indwelling catheter is dependent and draining.
      (1) Tape tubing to thigh to relieve traction on bladder. In supine male patient tape catheter to abdomen.
      (2) Give meticulous catheter care.
   b. Change dressings as indicated when patient has profuse drainage.
   c. Employ care with patient with nephrostomy tube drainage (insertion of tube directly into kidney for temporary or permanent urinary diversion). It is attached to closed gravity drainage or to a urostomy appliance. A self-retaining U-tube or loop nephrostomy tube may be used.
      (1) Purpose of nephrostomy drainage:
         (a) To provide drainage from kidney after surgery.
         (b) To conserve and permit physiological restoration of renal tissue that has been traumatized by obstructive disease.
         (c) To provide drainage when ureter is no longer functioning.
      (2) Evaluate for bleeding from nephrostomy site (main complication of nephrostomy).
      (3) Ensure that the nephrostomy tube is draining freely—plugging of the tube causes pain, trauma, bursting of suture lines, and infection.
         (a) Call surgeon *immediately* if tube is inadvertently dislodged.
         (b) Do not clamp the nephrostomy tube.

(c) Irrigate nephrostomy tube only by direct physician request. Use 10 ml. warm sterile saline—to avoid mechanical damage to kidney or infection from pyelorenal backflow.

(d) Encourage adequate fluid intake—to produce effective mechanical flushing and to dilute urinary elements that cause calculous formation.

6. Assess patient with indwelling ureteral catheter or stent (utilized to permit drainage from affected kidney).

a. Ureteral catheters are inserted through a cystoscope and left in place for a period of time; they are taped to indwelling urethral catheter to hold them in place.

b. Tape catheter to thigh to reduce pulling on catheter.

c. Make notation on nursing care plan that catheter is an *ureteral* catheter.

d. Do not irrigate an ureteral catheter; this is done by the urologist.

7. Employ early ambulation techniques as an aid in preventing thromboembolic episodes and improving patient endurance.

a. Ambulation contraindicted in prostatic patients with bleeding and with some types of plastic reconstruction surgery.

b. Encourage patient to do leg exercises in bed

8. See page 523 for management of patient following prostatectomy.

B. *To assess patient constantly for complications.*

1. Hemorrhage (and shock)—chief danger after renal surgery.

a. Watch for pain, blood loss from drain site, mass over flank, shock.

b. Prepare for reoperation; see management of hemorrhage, page 130.

2. Abdominal distention; paralytic ileus (see p. 435).

3. Pneumothorax (p. 216); postoperative atelectasis (p. 131).

4. Infection.

5. Pulmonary embolism (p. 211).

Discharge Planning and Health Education

1. Teach patient/family about care of catheters/tubes and management of dressings if patient is to return home with indwelling tubes.

2. Continue a liberal intake of fluids.

3. Take frequent short rest periods and increase activities gradually.

INFECTIONS OF THE URINARY TRACT

A *urinary tract infection* (UTI) is caused by the presence of pathogenic microorganisms in the urinary tract with or without signs and symptoms. Infection may predominate at the bladder (cystitis), urethra (urethritis), prostate (prostatitis), or kidney (pyelonephritis). Unfortunately, noninfectious conditions may generate symptoms which mimic those of urinary tract infection.

Recurrent urinary tract infections may indicate:

1. Relapse—recurrence of bacteriuria with same infecting microorganism

2. Reinfection—recurrence of bacteriuria with a microorganism different from that of the original infection; i.e., a "new" infection

Bacteriuria refers to the presence of bacteria in the urine. (The normal urinary tract is sterile except near the urethral orifice.)

Colony count of at least 100,000 colonies/ml. of urine on a clean-catch midstream or catheterized specimen implies infection.

> **NURSING ALERT:** Infections in any part of the urinary tract may persist for months or years without symptoms and eventually cause serious kidney damage.

Predisposing Factors

1. Increasing intraluminal pressure or overdistended bladder.

2. Urinary stasis and obstruction (ureteral stenosis, stone, tumor)—slowing of urinary flow causes kidney to be more susceptible to bacterial infection.

3. Reflux

a. urethrovesical reflux—flowing back of urine from urethra into bladder

b. vesicoureteral reflux (ureterovesical reflux)—flowing back of urine from bladder into one or both ureters

4. Fecal soiling of urethral meatus.

5. Instrumentation—catheter, cystoscope.

6. Metabolic disorders (diabetes mellitus) and diseases of blood vessels (arteriosclerosis)—may diminish blood supply to organs of urinary tract.

7. Neurological abnormalities (neurogenic bladder dysfunction).

8. Renal disease—increases susceptibility of kidney to infection.

Pathways of Infection Within Urinary Tract

Bacteria invade and spread within tract by the ascending (most common), bloodstream, and/or lymphatic pathways.

1. Urethra—from ascending bacteria

2. Bladder—from bacteria ascending from urethra (or, less commonly, descending from kidney)

3. Kidney—from ureterovesical reflux (incompetence of ureterovesical valve which allows urine to regurgitate into ureters, usually at time of voiding); bloodborne

4. Prostate—from ascending urethral flora

5. Epididymis—from infected prostate

6. Testis—from bacteria via the bloodstream

CYSTITIS

Cystitis is inflammation of the urinary bladder.

Etiology

1. Ascending infection after entry via the urinary meatus.

a. Women seem to be more apt to develop acute cystitis because of shorter length of urethra, anatomic proximity to vagina, periurethral glands, and rectum (fecal contamination), and the mechanical effect of coitus.

b. Women with recurrent urinary tract infections often have gram-negative organisms at the vaginal introitus; there may be some defect of the mucosa of the urethra, vagina, or external genitalia of these patients that allows enteric organisms to invade the bladder.

c. Poor/abnormal voiding patterns cause decrease in blood supply to bladder.

d. Acute infection in women most often from organisms of patient's own intestinal flora (*Escherichia coli*).

2. In males, obstructive abnormalities (strictures, prostatism)—most frequent cause.
3. Upper urinary tract disease may occasionally cause recurrent bladder infection.

Clinical Manifestations

1. Frequency, urgency, burning, and pain on urination
2. Nocturia
3. Bearing-down sensation in region of bladder; suprapubic pain
4. Changes in composition of urine (bacteria and red blood cells)

Treatment and Nursing Management

OBJECTIVES: to eradicate the causative pathogens.
to prevent recurrences.

1. Obtain uncontaminated urine specimen for smears, culture, and antibiotic sensitivity studies to determine pathogen so that appropriate drug may be selected.
   a. Patient may be treated with single dose therapy or 7–10 day regimen.
   b. Urine culture may be repeated several times during therapy and 7–10 days after completion of treatment to ensure elimination of infection.
   c. Patients with recurring infections should have periodic urine cultures since most recurrences are new infections with different organisms; relapses may occur with same organism.
2. Assist with evaluation studies to determine if infection is secondary to a functional or structural abnormality (x-rays, intravenous urogram, cystoscopy).
   a. Take careful history for previous symptoms of urinary tract disease.
   b. Obtain detailed description of present illness. (Example: frequency)
      (1) How often does patient void?
      (2) How much urine is passed at each voiding?
      (3) How much fluid is taken? What types of fluid?
      (4) Relationship between voiding and other symptoms.
   c. Obtain similar detailed information about dysuria, nocturia, urgency, incontinence, changes in appearance of urine, urinary stream, pain.
   d. Assist with physical examination.
3. Remove the contributing cause(s) and source of obstruction if found (neoplasm of kidney, bladder calculus, prostatism, stricture).
4. Give prescribed antimicrobial medication since urinary infections usually respond to drugs that are excreted in the urine in high concentrations; a potentially effective drug should rapidly sterilize the urine and thus relieve the patient's symptoms.
5. Maintain an appropriate urine pH—efficacy of certain antimicrobial drugs is affected by the reaction

(pH) of the urine. Sodium bicarbonate alkalinizes urine; ascorbic acid acidifies urine.
6. Attempt to enhance body's normal defense mechanism.
   a. Encourage patient to drink sufficient fluids to promote renal blood flow and to flush out bacteria in urinary tract.
   b. Encourage patient to void frequently (every 2–3 hours) and to empty bladder completely, since this enhances bacterial clearance, reduces urine stasis, and prevents reinfection; infrequent voiding overstretches the bladder wall leading to hypoxia of bladder mucosa which is then susceptible to bacterial invasion.
7. Promote patient comfort.
   a. Encourage bed rest during the acute phase.
   b. Give analgesics, antispasmodics, and heat to perineum to relieve pain, spasm, and urgency.

Discharge Planning and Health Education

1. Encourage patient to have follow-up urine studies for at least 2 years or more to determine if asymptomatic infection is present—*there is a marked tendency for infection to recur.*
2. Instruct patients who have had urinary tract infections during pregnancy to have follow-up studies.
3. For women with repeated urinary tract infections, give the following instructions:
   a. Reduce vaginal introital concentration of pathogens by hygienic measures.
      (1) Wash in shower or while standing in bathtub—bacteria in bath water may gain entrance into urethra.
      (2) Cleanse around the perineum and urethral meatus after each bowel movement.
   b. Drink liberal amounts of fluid to flush out bacteria.
   c. Avoid irritants—coffee, tea, alcohol, cola drinks.
   d. Void every 2–3 hours during day and completely empty bladder.
   e. In certain women, sexual intercourse is the initiating event for the development of bacteriuria.
      (1) A single dose of an oral antimicrobial agent may be prescribed following sexual intercourse.
      (2) Void immediately after sexual intercourse.
   f. An antibacterial vaginal suppository may be prescribed to reduce concentration of bacteria in introitus.
   g. Apply antibacterial ointment around urinary meatus as directed.
   h. Patients with persistent bacteria may require long-term antimicrobial therapy to prevent colonization of periurethral area and recurrence of urinary tract infection.
      (1) Take drug the last thing at night after emptying bladder to ensure adequate concentration of drug during overnight period since low rates of urine flow and infrequent bladder emptying predispose to multiplication of bacteria.
      (2) Use dip slides at home to monitor urinary tract infection.
         (a) Wash around urethral meatus several times, using different washcloths.
         (b) Collect midstream specimen.
         (c) Remove slide from its container, dip it into urine sample, and return it to container.
         (d) Incubate slide at room temperature—time according to product directives.

(e) Read the results by comparing slide with colony density chart (comes with the product).

PYELONEPHRITIS

Pyelonephritis is an infection of the renal pelvis, tubules, and interstitial tissue of one or both kidneys with variable manifestations. (Pyelonephritis may be acute or chronic.)

Causes

1. Secondary to ureterovesical reflux (incompetence of ureterovesical valve which allows urine to regurgitate into ureters, usually at time of voiding).
2. Urinary obstruction
3. Enteric bacteria
4. Blood-borne infection
5. Renal disease
6. Trauma
7. Pregnancy
8. Metabolic disorders

Altered Physiology

Swelling of renal parenchyma → patchy distribution of acute infectious processes throughout kidney → swelling and scarring → kidney atrophy → renal failure.

Complications

1. Hypertension
2. Chronic infection (usually silent)
3. Renal insufficiency and renal failure, unilateral or bilateral

Clinical Manifestations

1. Symptoms vary from none to severe.
2. The patient may be asymptomatic for many years although renal damage may be extensive.
3. Scarring of kidneys may follow each acute infection, causing the kidney to become atrophied.

Acute Pyelonephritis
(an active infection)
1. Frequency, dysuria, burning on urination
2. Chills and fever with aching and malaise
3. Dull aching in back or pain and tenderness over costovertebral angle
4. Pyuria and bacteriuria and casts in the urine sediment

Chronic Pyelonephritis
(results from scarring effects of previous bacterial infection; it is a silent disease until it produces renal insufficiency)
1. Fatigue, malaise
2. Headache, anorexia
3. Polyuria, excessive thirst
4. Weight loss
5. Proteinuria; symptoms of chronic renal insufficiency

Diagnostic Evaluation

1. Identification of antibody-coated bacteria (ACB) in urine; bacteria invading kidney induce an antibody response that coats the bacteria—differentiates renal infection from bladder infection.
2. Other radiologic/urinary tests as directed.

Objectives of Treatment and Nursing Management

A. *To determine if obstruction is present and to locate it precisely.*
1. Carry out intravenous urogram and other diagnostic tests—relief of obstructions is essential to save kidney from rapid destruction.

B. *To find and treat conditions known to cause urinary tract infection.*

C. *To obtain permanent eradication of bacteria from urinary tract.*
1. Obtain urine specimen for culture and sensitivity studies (under aseptic conditions) since choice of drug is based on sensitivity studies.
2. Give organism-specific antimicrobial therapy. Antibacterial agent is maintained in urine for a long enough period to prevent reseeding of residual foci of infection.
   a. Acute pyelonephritis usually caused by *E. coli*, which is sensitive to many antimicrobial drugs.
   b. A 10–14 day course of organism-specific antibody therapy is usually given.
3. Obtain urine for repeated cultures to determine patient's response to treatment and to search for secondary organisms.

D. *If patient has chronic or recurring infections:*

OBJECTIVES: to prevent progressive parenchymal damage.
   to preserve renal function.
   to locate and relieve the obstruction causing the infections.
1. Employ continuous treatment with urine-sterilizing agents after initial antibiotic treatment has been employed.
2. Advise patient to keep up this regimen for months to years until (1) there is no evidence of inflammation, (2) causative factors have been treated or controlled and (3) there is evidence of stability of renal function.
3. Emphasize to patient that serial urine cultures and evaluation studies must be done for an indefinite period of time.
4. Encourage patient to have blood counts and serum creatinine determinations if he is on long-term therapy.

E. *For health education, see page 505.*

TUBERCULOSIS OF THE KIDNEY

Tuberculosis of the kidney (and urinary tract) is caused by the organism *Mycobacterium tuberculosis* and is usually disseminated from the lungs via the bloodstream to one or both of the kidneys and to other organs of the genitourinary tract.

Clinical Manifestations

1. Hematuria (microscopic or gross)
2. Bladder irritation—burning on urination, frequency, nocturia
3. Manifestations from infection of prostate and epididymis
4. Slight afternoon fever, loss of weight, anorexia

Diagnostic Evaluation

1. Urine culture for tubercle bacilli (smears of urinary sediment also stained for acid-fast bacilli)
2. Excretory urogram—to reveal renal and ureteral lesions

3. Cystoscopic examination—to determine extent of bladder involvement, for biopsy purposes, and for ureteral catheterization of each kidney to determine if one or both kidneys are affected.
4. Acid urine with persistent symptoms of cystitis and pyuria may yield a negative "routine" culture; it may take special culture media and up to 6 weeks to grow acid-fast bacillus.

> **NURSING ALERT:** A search for tuberculosis elsewhere in the body must be conducted when tuberculosis of the kidney or urinary tract is found.
> Be alert for patient who has had previous contact with tuberculosis.

Treatment

OBJECTIVE: to eradicate the offending organism.
1. Multiple drug regimen appears to delay the emergence of resistant organisms.

2. Combinations of the following drugs usually given—ethambutol, isoniazid, rifampin, and cycloserine.
   All medications may be given together in a single daily dose; certain patients may have to divide cycloserine.
3. General health of patient should be promoted since renal tuberculosis is a manifestation of a systemic disease.
4. Surgical intervention may be necessary to prevent obstructive problems and to remove severely infected organ. However emphasis is on medical treatment.

Discharge Planning and Health Education

Instruct the patient as follows:
1. Follow-up examinations, including periodic urine examinations and excretory urograms are necessary for a prolonged period—to detect reactivation of disease.
2. Report for cystoscopic examination as directed—to detect ureteral stricture formation, which is a complication of genitourinary tuberculosis.
3. For other aspects of health teaching, see page 812.

ACUTE GLOMERULONEPHRITIS

Acute glomerulonephritis refers to a group of kidney diseases in which there is an inflammatory reaction in the glomeruli. It is not an infection of the kidney per se, but rather the result of untoward side effects of the defense mechanisms of the body. It is thought to involve an antigen–antibody reaction, which produces damage to the glomeruli, the filtering bed of the kidney.

Altered Physiology

Cellular proliferation, infiltration of glomerulus by leukocytes → glomerular trapping of circulating immune complexes → thickening of glomerular filtration membrane → scarring and loss of filtering surface → renal failure.

Clinical Manifestations

1. The disease may be so mild that it is discovered accidentally through a routine urinalysis.
2. History of preceding pharyngitis or tonsillitis with fever (2–3 weeks previously)
3. Scant smoky or bloody urine
4. Facial edema and edema of extremities
5. Fatigue and anorexia
6. Hypertension (mild, moderate, or severe)
7. Tenderness over costovertebral angle
8. Anemia—from azotemia (nitrogen retention in blood)

Diagnostic Evaluation

1. Urinalysis—hematuria (microscopic or gross), proteinuria (2+ to 4+), red cell casts, white cells, renal epithelial cells, and various casts in the sediment.
2. Blood—elevated blood urea nitrogen and serum creatinine, low total serum protein level, increased antistreptolysin titre (from reaction to streptococcal organism)
3. Needle biopsy—reveals obstruction of glomerular capillaries from proliferation of endothelial cells.

Clinical Course

1. Diuresis usually starts 1–2 weeks after onset of symptoms.
   a. Renal clearances and blood urea concentration return to normal.
   b. Edema decreases and hypertension lessens.
   c. Microscopic proteinuria or hematuria may persist many months.
2. Recovery is usual in children and young adults; in older person the disease may progress to chronic glomerulonephritis.

Objectives of Treatment and Nursing Management

A. *To protect the poorly functioning kidneys.*

1. Encourage bed rest during the acute phase. (Rest also facilitates diuresis.)
2. Restrict dietary protein moderately if there is oliguria and the BUN is elevated.
   a. Give carbohydrates liberally to provide energy and reduce catabolism of protein.
   b. Restrict protein more drastically if acute renal failure develops (see p. 491).
   c. Restrict sodium intake in presence of edema or signs of congestive heart failure.
3. Measure and record intake and output.
4. Give fluids according to patient's urinary output and daily body weight.

B. *To recognize and treat complications promptly.*

1. Recognize and treat any intercurrent infections promptly.
2. Watch for symptoms of renal failure—nausea, fatigue, vomiting, diminished urinary output (see p. 491).
3. Evaluate patient for:
   a. Hypertensive encephalopathy
   b. Cardiac failure and pulmonary edema
4. Dialysis may be considered if uremia and fluid retention cannot be controlled.

Discharge Planning and Health Education

Instruct the patient as follows:
1. Explain to patient that he must have follow-up evaluations of blood pressure, urinary protein, and BUN concentrations to determine if there is exacerbation of disease activity.
2. Treat any infection promptly.
3. Call physician/clinic if symptoms of renal failure occur.

NEPHROTIC SYNDROME

Nephrotic syndrome is a clinical disorder characterized by (1) marked proteinuria, (2) hypoalbuminemia, (3) edema, and (4) hyperlipidemia as a consequence of excessive leakage of plasma proteins into the urine because of increased permeability of the glomerular capillary membrane to protein.

Etiology

In any condition that seriously damages the glomerular capillary membrane, any of the following etiologies are possible.
1. Chronic glomerulonephritis
2. Diabetes mellitus (intercapillary glomerulosclerosis)
3. Amyloidosis of kidney
4. Systemic lupus erythematosus
5. Renal vein thrombosis
6. Primary lipoid nephrosis in children (see p. 1333)
7. Possible early symptom of malignant disease

Clinical Manifestations

1. Insidious onset of edema; easily pitting edema
2. Marked proteinuria—leads to negative nitrogen balance.
3. Extensive depletion of body proteins (hypoalbuminemia) from extensive urinary protein losses.
4. Hyperlipidemia—may lead to accelerated atherosclerosis.

Diagnostic Evaluation

1. Needle biopsy of kidney—for histologic examination of renal tissue to confirm diagnosis.
2. Serum electrolyte evaluations (protein, albumin, etc.)
3. Triglyceride profile—to evaluate degree of hyperlipidemia
4. Urinary tests—for microscopic hematuria, proteinuria, RBCs, WBCs, casts, fat bodies
5. Renal function tests

Treatment and Nursing Management

OBJECTIVES: to preserve renal function.
1. Keep on bed rest for a few days—to mobilize edema.
2. Utilize dietary treatment—to replace protein losses.
   a. High protein diet—to replenish wasted tissues and restore body proteins.
   b. Mild to moderate sodium restriction—to control severe edema.
   c. High calorie diet (25–50 cal./kg. body weight/day).
3. Give diuretics—if renal insufficiency is not severe.
4. Give steroids (prednisone)—to reduce edema and proteinuria.
5. Immunosuppressive agents may be effective when nephrosis is associated with autoimmune disease.
6. Protect patient from infection—causes exacerbation of symptoms.
7. Evaluate for thromboembolism (renal vein thrombosis, pulmonary emboli, thrombophlebitis)—increased incidence in patients with nephrotic syndrome.
8. See page 507 for nursing the patient with acute glomerulonephritis, and page 493 for care of patient with chronic renal failure.

HYDRONEPHROSIS

Hydronephrosis is dilation of the pelvis and calyces of one or both kidneys with resulting thinning of renal parenchyma due to obstruction of urinary flow. (A partial block may occur at any level in the urinary tract.)

Causes

1. Congenital causes—stenosis of ureteropelvic junction, urethral valves
2. Progressive changes in bladder, ureters, and kidneys from obstruction anywhere in urinary tract.
   a. Obstruction from enlarged prostate
   b. Obstructing calculus
   c. Malignant lesion (cancer of prostate, bladder, or cervix)
   d. Obstruction of ureter—from calculus, stricture, etc.
3. Neurogenic causes
4. Vesicoureteral reflux

Altered Physiology

Interference with passage of urine from kidney → chronic infection → increasing pressure → distention of renal pelvis and calyces → decreased renal blood flow → atrophy of renal parenchyma (as one kidney undergoes gradual destruction, the contralateral kidney gradually enlarges [compensatory hypertrophy]) → impairment of renal function.

Clinical Manifestations

1. Often asymptomatic and insidious onset
2. Aching in flank and back (present with acute obstruction)
3. Bladder irritability—fever and dysuria if infection is present
4. Gastrointestinal disturbances
5. Chills, fever, tenderness, pyuria—from infection
6. Hematuria—hydronephrotic kidney may bleed from congestion
7. Uremia—if condition is bilateral and advanced

Diagnostic Evaluation

Complete urographic survey.

Treatment and Nursing Management

OBJECTIVES: to discover and remove (if possible) the cause of obstruction.
to treat the patient's infection.
to restore and conserve renal function.

1. Relieve obstruction, etc.
   Urine may have to be diverted by nephrostomy or other types of diversion.
   a. Place ureteral catheter to decompress kidney—if patient is having severe flank pain.
   b. See page 503 for care of patient having a nephrostomy.
2. Eradicate infection since residual urine in calyces produces infection and pyelonephritis.
3. Prepare for surgical intervention to correct obstruction. (See p. 502)
   a. Removal of obstructive lesions.
   b. Operations to improve drainage of kidney, such as pyeloplasty—plastic operation to remove and correct results of obstruction at ureteropelvic junction.
   c. Nephrectomy—if one kidney is severely damaged.

UROLITHIASIS

Urolithiasis refers to the presence of stones in the urinary system. Stones are formed in the urinary tract by the deposit of crystalline substances (calcium phosphate, oxalate, uric acid) excreted in the urine. They may be found anywhere in the urinary system from the kidney to the bladder and vary in size from mere granular deposits (called sand or gravel), to bladder stones the size of an orange.

Factors Favoring Stone Formation

1. Obstruction and urinary stasis facilitating precipitation of salts from the urine
2. Infection—particularly of urea-splitting organisms (*Proteus vulgaris*)
3. Dehydration and urine concentration—encourages precipitation of solids
4. Immobilization—produces slowing of renal drainage and altered calcium metabolism
5. Hypercalcemia (abnormally high concentration of blood calcium compounds) and hypercalciuria (abnormally large amounts of calcium in urine)
   a. Hyperparathyroidism
   b. Excessive intake of vitamin D
   c. Excessive intake of milk and alkali
   d. Myeloproliferative disorders (leukemia; polycythemia vera) and patients receiving chemotherapy—excrete increased amounts of uric acid.
6. Excessive excretion of uric acid
7. Vitamin deficiency (especially vitamin A)
8. Foreign bodies in urinary tract
9. High intake of protein, calcium, excessive consumption of tea and fruit juices
10. Small bowel disease or small bowel surgery
11. Heredity—plays a part in calcium oxalate stones (most common type), cystine, and uric acid stones
12. Idiopathic—no cause can be found

Clinical Features

1. The problem occurs predominantly in the 3rd to 5th decade, affecting men more than women.
2. The majority of stones contain calcium or magnesium in combination with phosphorus or oxalate.
3. Infection and obstruction may cause destruction of renal tissue and subsequent loss of a kidney.
4. Most renal stones migrate downward (causing severe, colicky pain) and are discovered in the lower ureter.
5. People who have had 2 stones tend to have recurrences.

Clinical Manifestations

Dependent on presence of obstruction, infection, edema.

1. Stones blocking flow of urine produce symptoms of urinary tract infection—chills, fever, dysuria.
2. Renal stones—produce an increase in hydrostatic pressure and distention of the renal pelvis and proximal ureter, causing:
   a. Pain in renal area—radiates anteriorly and downward toward bladder in female and toward testicle in male.
   b. Renal colic—acute pain with tenderness over loin; nausea and vomiting.
3. Ureteral stones
   a. Acute colicky pain, referring down the thigh and to genitalia (ureteral colic).
   b. Frequent desire to void but little urine is passed.
4. Gastrointestinal symptoms
   a. Due to renal–intestinal reflexes and anatomic relation of kidneys to stomach, pancreas, colon, etc.
   b. Include nausea, vomiting, diarrhea, abdominal discomfort.

Diagnostic Evaluation

1. Laboratory screening studies—CBC, urinalysis/culture, serum chemistry survey; 24-hour urine study for calcium, phosphorus, uric acid, creatinine
2. Intravenous urography

Treatment and Nursing Management

OBJECTIVES: to eradicate the stone.
to determine the stone type.
to control infection.
to relieve any obstruction that may be present.
to prevent nephron destruction.

1. Initiate treatment for renal and ureteral colic; relieve pain until its cause can be removed—morphine or meperidine hydrochloride, hot baths or moist heat to flank areas.
2. Encourage patient to maintain a high round-the-clock fluid intake (250–300 ml. of fluid hourly when awake) to reduce concentration of urinary crystalloids and to ensure a high urinary output; also lowers specific gravity of urine.
3. Strain all urine through gauze for stone analysis—

crystallographic studies and x-ray diffraction are useful in obtaining data about the amount and distribution of chemical components of the stone.
4. Give specific therapy as directed—regimen depends on stone type.
   a. *Calcium stones* (calcium oxalate and calcium phosphate)
     (1) Moderate dietary intake of calcium and phosphorus; restrict oxalate-containing beverages (cola, tea).
     (2) Administer drugs, depending on classification of hypercalciuria—orthophosphates, thiazides, magnesium oxide.
   b. *Uric acid stones* (develop in highly acidic and concentrated urine)
     (1) Alkalinize the urine.
     (2) Limit protein intake; encourage high fluid intake.
     (3) Administer allopurinol—to lower serum and urinary acid levels.
   c. *Cystine stones*
     (1) Increase fluid intake; exclude excess dietary protein.
     (2) Administer D-penicillamine (Cuprimine)—decreases stone formation and sometimes results in stone dissolution.
   d. *Struvite stones* (infection stones)—associated with urinary tract infections with urea-splitting bacteria (*Proteus* species, *Klebsiella*, *Pseudomonas*, *Staphylococcus*).
     (1) Acidify urine.
     (2) Give appropriate antimicrobial therapy.
5. Maintain proper urine reaction (pH); give appropriate drugs to acidify or alkalinize urine (depending on stone type).
   a. Phosphate, oxalate, and carbonate stones form in alkaline urine.
     (1) Drugs used to acidify urine include ammonium chloride and methenamine mandelate (Mandelamine) and vitamine C.
   b. Uric acid, urate, and cystine stones form in acid urine.
     (1) Drugs used for alkalinizing the urine include potassium acetate or citrate, sodium bicarbonate.
6. Employ principles of diet therapy if stone composition is known—to control urine pH, supply proper vitamins, and eliminate stone-forming substances.
7. Treat infection (if present) with appropriate drugs—infection may accelerate stone growth and be difficult to eradicate.
8. Correct obstructive process to prevent impairment of tubular function, atrophy of nephrons, reduced renal blood flow, and increased susceptibility to infection.
9. Treat and correct metabolic problems (hyperparathyroidism, renal tubular acidosis).
10. Prepare for surgical intervention if patient's condition indicates that:
   a. stone is too large to pass, or is
   b. producing obstruction, unremitting pain, infection that does not respond to treatment, or is causing progressive renal damage.

Surgical Procedures

OBJECTIVE: to remove stone with a minimum of trauma to the kidney.
1. Nephrolithotomy—incision into kidney for removal of stone.
2. Nephrectomy—removal of kidney, indicated when kidney is extensively and irreparably damaged and is no longer a functioning organ.
3. Pyelolithotomy—removal of stones from kidney pelvis.
4. Ureterolithotomy—removal of stone in ureter.
5. Cystolithotomy—removal of stone from bladder.
6. See page 502 for management of patient undergoing renal surgery.

Discharge Planning and Health Education

Instruct the patient as follows:
1. Maintain a high fluid intake over a 24-hour period, since stones form more readily in concentrated urine.
   a. Drink at least 3000 ml. daily if you are a stone former.
   b. Drink larger amounts if you perspire freely.
2. Avoid sudden increases in environmental temperatures that may cause a drop in urinary volume.
3. Increase fluid intake when engaging in activities that produce excessive sweating.
4. Avoid prolonged periods of recumbency—slows renal drainage and alters calcium metabolism.
5. Avoid excessive ingestion of vitamins and minerals, especially vitamin D.
6. Test urine pH with a pH indicator if urine pH is a factor in causing particular type of stone.
7. Stay on prescribed diet.

RENAL TUMORS

General Considerations

1. All renal tumors should be considered malignant until proven otherwise.
2. Renal cell carcinoma is the most common malignant renal tumor; occurs more frequently in males and metastasizes early to the lungs, lymph nodes, bones, adrenals, etc.

Clinical Manifestations

1. Many renal tumors produce no symptoms and are discovered on routine physical examinatin as a palpable abdominal mass.
2. Classic triad (late symptoms)
   a. Hematuria (intermittent, microscopic, or gross)—may be initial, terminal, or total depending on location of tumor.
   b. Pain—from distention of renal capsule, invasion of surrounding structures.
   c. Palpable mass in flank.
3. Low-grade fever, anemia, weight loss—systemic effects common to most tumors.
4. Gastrointestinal symptoms—due to reflex action or encroachment on intraperitoneal organs.

Diagnostic Evaluation

1. Plain film of abdomen—often shows kidney enlargement.

2. IVP and IV drip nephrotomogram.
3. Cystoscopic examination—for visualization of tumor by retrograde pyelography.
4. Assessment of urinary lactic dehydrogenase activity; this enzyme may be elevated in carcinoma of the kidney, bladder, prostate, in infection, etc.
5. Ultrasonography—helpful in differentiating renal cyst from renal tumor.
6. Renal angiogram—definitive study.

Treatment

OBJECTIVE: to eradicate the tumor and prevent metastasis.

1. Radical nephrectomy (removal of kidney, the adrenal gland, perinephric fat, most of ureter, and retroperitoneal lymph nodes)—see page 503 for nursing management following renal surgery.
2. Radiation therapy, chemotherapy, hormone therapy, and immunotherapy may be used with varying degrees of success.

Health Education

Have a yearly physical examination and x-ray examination of chest.

INJURIES TO THE KIDNEY

Trauma to abdomen, flank, or back may produce renal injury. Suspicion is high in a patient with multiple injuries.

Types of Injuries

1. Contusions
2. Fissures; lacerations
3. Rupture or renal vascular pedicle injury

Major Problems Following Kidney Trauma

1. Control of hemorrhage—may be persistent or recurring
2. Injuries to other organs
3. Late complications are significant

Clinical Manifestations

1. Hematuria—amount shows no correlation with extent of injury
2. Pain—costovertebral, flank, upper abdomen
3. Nausea, vomiting, abdominal rigidity—from ileus (seen when there is retroperitoneal bleeding)
4. Shock—from severe/multiple injuries

Diagnostic Evaluation

1. History of injury—determine if injury was caused by blunt or penetrating trauma (stab/gunshot wounds)
2. Serial urine studies for hematuria
3. Plain film of abdomen—to determine presence of other fractures (pelvis, ribs, transverse processes of lumbar vertebrae)
4. Excretory urography (IVP)—to define extent of injury to involved kidney and function of contralateral kidney
5. Renal angiography—to assess vascular integrity, outline renal parenchyma

Complications

1. Hemorrhage
2. Infection

NURSING ALERT: Excessive bleeding may occur several days after renal injury. Perirenal abscess or infection may occur 2–4 weeks following injury.

3. Hypertension
4. Stone formation
5. Loss of renal function

Treatment and Nursing Management

OBJECTIVES: to control hemorrhage, pain, and infection.
to preserve and restore renal function.
to maintain urinary drainage.

1. Place patient on bed rest to minimize bleeding.
2. Monitor blood pressure and pulse—to assess for bleeding and impending shock; perirenal hemorrhage may cause rapid exsanguination.
3. Save, inspect, and compare each urine specimen—to follow the course and degree of hematuria.
4. Carry out serial hematocrit and hemoglobin determinations—to assess degree of anemia, since progressive anemia indicates hemorrhage.
5. Evaluate the patient frequently during the first few days following injury.
   a. Assess for flank and abdominal pain, muscle spasm, and swelling over flank—suggests renal hemorrhage and extravasation.
   b. Outline original mass with marking pencil for future comparisons.
   c. Examine renal area for development of bruising and/or swelling.
   d. Watch for any *sudden* change in patient's condition. This may indicate hemorrhage and require surgical intervention.
6. Avoid narcotic analgesia—may mask accompanying abdominal symptoms.
7. Give antibiotics as directed to discourage infection—from perirenal hematoma and/or urinoma (cyst containing urine).
8. Prepare for surgical exploration if patient has increasing pulse rate, hypotension, or shock (see p. 128).

Discharge Planning and Health Education

1. Activity should be restricted for about 1 month following trauma to minimize incidence of delayed/secondary bleeding.
2. Encourage patient to have follow-up examinations after discharge—to detect late-developing complications (post-traumatic hypertension, decreasing renal function).

NEUROGENIC BLADDER

Neurogenic bladder refers to a bladder disturbance due to diseases and disorders of bladder innervation.

Normal Physiology

1. Normal bladder action depends on intact sensory and motor nerve supply.
2. The bladder fills to approximately 300–500 ml.—triggers an emptying reflex.
3. This reflex initiates a contraction of the musculature inside the bladder wall which forces urine out through the urethra until the bladder is empty.

Causes

1. Spinal cord injury; spinal tumor; herniated intervertebral disc
2. Disease—multiple sclerosis, tabes dorsalis, diabetes mellitus, syphilis
3. Certain congenital anomalies (spina bifida, myelomeningocele)
4. Infection

Types of Neurogenic Bladder

A. *Spastic (reflex or automatic)*

1. A bladder disorder caused by any lesion of the cord above the voiding reflex arc (upper motor neuron lesion); most common type.
2. There is loss of conscious sensations and cerebral motor control.
3. Patient has reduced bladder capacity and marked hypertrophy of bladder wall.
4. Bladder behaves in reflex fashion with minimal or no controlling influence to regulate its activity (spontaneous uncontrolled voidings).

B. *Flaccid (atonic, nonreflex or areflexic, or autonomous)*

1. A bladder disorder caused by a lower motor neuron lesion.
2. Bladder continues to fill until it becomes greatly distended—bladder musculature does not contract forcefully at any time.
3. When pressure reaches a breakthrough point, small amounts of urine dribble from urethra as bladder continues to fill (overflow incontinence).
4. Sensory loss may accompany flaccid bladder; patient is not aware of discomfort.
5. Extensive distention causes damage to bladder musculature, infection of stagnant urine, and infection of kidneys by back pressure of urine.

C. *Mixed*

Complications

1. *Infection*—from stasis of urine and subsequent catheterization.
2. *Hydronephrosis*—hypertrophy of bladder wall leads ultimately to vesicoureteral reflux.
3. *Urolithiasis*—from demineralization of bone from bed rest; urinary stasis and infection.
4. *Renal failure*—major cause of death of patients with neurologic impairment of the bladder.

Treatment and Nursing Management

OBJECTIVES: to prevent overdistention of the bladder.
to empty bladder regularly and completely.

to maintain urine sterility with no stone formation.
to maintain adequate bladder capacity without ureterovesical reflux.

A. *Initial Treatment*

Following spinal cord injury, the syndrome of spinal shock is reflected in the bladder; sensation is not perceived and the bladder usually cannot contract and empty itself. The bladder must be decompressed by either intermittent or continuous catheterization.

1. Intermittent catheterization (preferred).
   a. Bladder catheterized at designated intervals (4, 6, or 8 hours) with a small caliber catheter; this intermittent emptying approximates physiological function; circumvents complications usually seen with indwelling catheter.
      (1) Hourly fluid intake and output record is kept to assess individual output patterns.
      (2) Catheterization technique requires strict asepsis and skilled personnel.
      (3) Patients with upper extremity function may be taught to catheterize themselves.
2. Continuous catheterization.
   a. Bladder is catheterized using continuous drainage and irrigation system (p. 487) to avoid overdistention and risk of contracture from being constantly empty.
      (1) Tape catheter to abdomen (male) to remove sharp angulation and pressure at penoscrotal angle (Fig. 11-6).
      (2) Maintain a high fluid intake.
3. Encourage liberal fluid intake—to reduce urinary bacterial count, reduce stasis, decrease the concentration of calcium in urine, and minimize the precipitation of urinary crystals and stone formation.
4. Keep patient as mobile as possible—to reduce incidence of calculosis (presence of calculi).
   a. Turn, move, and exercise patient.
   b. Get patient up on tilt table (p. 70) or in wheelchair as soon as possible.
   c. Give low calcium diet—to prevent calculosis.
5. Evaluation studies (as soon as patient's condition permits)—to assess for bladder and bladder neck problems. Do initial studies to provide a baseline against which later changes can be measured.
   a. Serial studies of BUN, serum creatinine, creatinine clearance—to determine status of renal function
   b. Cystogram—to determine presence of vesicoureteral reflux
   c. Urethrogram—for presence of urethral complications
   d. IV urogram—to outline upper urinary tract
   e. Pressure and flow studies
   f. Cystoscopy—to assess for loss of muscle fibers and elastic tissues; gives opportunity for biopsy

B. *Treatment for Chronic Phase*

Each person with neurogenic bladder disease has a particular type of problem(s); it is difficult to assess what the rehabilitation potential and eventual urological disability may be.

OBJECTIVE: to develop effective spontaneous reflex voiding.

1. Have patient drink a measured amount of fluid from

8 A.M.–8 P.M.; no fluids (except sips) taken after 8 P.M. to avoid bladder overdistention.
2. At specified time, patient attempts to void by using pressure over bladder or stimulates reflex voiding by abdominal tapping or digital stretch of anal sphincter to trigger the bladder.
3. Estimate residual urine by comparing intake and output; palpate and percuss over bladder.
4. Palpate the bladder at repeated intervals to determine if bladder is being emptied (Fig. 11-9).
5. Immediately following voiding attempt, catheterize the patient to determine urine residual.
   a. Measure all urine, voided and catheterized.
   b. Avoid *overdistention* of bladder.
   c. Caution patient to be alert for any sign that his bladder is full—perspiration, coldness of hands or feet, feelings of anxiety, etc.
6. *Intervals between catheterizations.*
   Catheterization intervals are lengthened and program is moved forward as less and less urine is retained; catheterization checks are usually discontinued when the volume of residual urine is at an acceptable level compatible with urine sterility and radiological normalcy of the upper urinary tract.

C. *Treatment for Flaccid Bladder*
1. Patient may be placed on bladder routine (outlined above); the fluid intake and output are adjusted to prevent bladder overdistention.
   Patient may be given orally-administered doses of parasympathomimetic drugs (bethanechol chloride)—to facilitate detrusor contraction.
2. *Or,* if no reflex or only a partial reflex can be induced, the patient is maintained on intermittent catheterization until he develops spontaneous reflex voiding; or surgical intervention may be required.

a. Male patient—may use condom collecting device if bladder empties well and no residual remains.
b. Female patient—may use pads, waterproof pants; or urinary diversion procedure may be required.
3. Surgical intervention may be carried out to correct bladder neck contractures, correct vesicoureteral reflux, or perform urinary diversion procedures (p. 516).
   a. Tubeless cystostomy (continent vesicostomy)—tube formed from bladder wall and brought to abdominal surface; external valve is created by intussusception of the proximal portion of the tube into the bladder; procedure appears useful in patients with neurogenic bladder.
      (1) Bladder emptied by intermittent transabdominal catheterization.
      (2) Urinary collection device not necessary.
      (3) Complications—bladder stone formation, stricture of cutaneous stoma, incontinence (urinary flooding of vesicostomy).
   b. Ileal conduit (See page 516).

Health Education

Instruct the patient to do vaginal and rectal contractions to strengthen periurethral tissue.
1. Tighten the rectum or vaginal vault.
2. Hold the contraction while counting slowly to 6; relax.
3. Continue relaxing and tightening for a 5-minute period.
4. Perform these exercises twice daily for 5 minutes over a 6- to 8-week period—success or failure of exercise program is then evaluated.

GUIDELINES: Intermittent Self-Catheterization: Clean (Nonsterile) Technique

Intermittent self-catheterization is the periodic drainage of urine from the bladder by the patient via catheterization; it is necessitated by temporary or permanent inability to empty the bladder (vesical dysfunction, neurogenic disease, obstructive uropathy, decompensated bladder).

Underlying Considerations

1. Intermittent catheterization is the treatment of choice following spinal cord injury. It is done under aseptic conditions by qualified health professionals until the patient is able to catheterize himself. After discharge from the hospital, the patient may be able to use a "clean" (nonsterile) technique.
2. The patient should be medically followed at regular intervals to prevent complications—reflux, hydronephrosis, external sphincter spasm, infection.
3. Advantages of self-catheterization: Better patient acceptance; promotes independence; fewer complications; permits more normal sexual relations.
4. *Objective:* to decrease morbidity associated with long-term use of indwelling catheter and to achieve a catheter-free status, if possible.

Equipment   No. 14 Fr. catheter (several to be kept in reserve); lubricant
Mirror (female patient)
Shallow pan
Irrigation tip syringe
Clear plastic bag or case—for carrying catheter

Procedure

ACTION (BY PATIENT)	RATIONALE/AMPLIFICATION
1. The patient must understand the importance of frequent catheterization and emptying of bladder at prescribed time regardless of circumstances.	1. An overdistended bladder slows the circulation of blood through the bladder walls and weakens its resistance to infection.
2. Wash hands with soap and water.	2. Do not forgo catheterization if soap and water are not available.

GUIDELINES: Intermittent Self-Catheterization: Clean (Nonsterile) Technique (cont.)

Procedure (cont.)	ACTION (BY PATIENT)	RATIONALE/AMPLIFICATION
	3. Try to void before catheterizing self using reflex triggering mechanisms—pressure on abdomen, thigh stroking, etc.	3. This may help to develop voluntary voiding without catheterization.
	Female	
	1. Position mirror in line of vision with urinary meatus. Assume modified dorsal recumbent position with feet on bed, legs flexed and knees apart; later patient may sit on toilet seat if physical condition permits.	1. This position helps to expose the urethral meatus.
	a. The nurse points out the location of the clitoris, urethral meatus, and vaginal outlet (in the mirror)	a. The patient is taught to confirm the position of the clitoris, urethral meatus, and vaginal outlet by palpation so that eventually a mirror will not be necessary.
	b. Expose the urinary meatus and cleanse.	
	2. Lubricate the catheter with water or water-soluble jelly. Hold the catheter 7.5 cm. (3 inches) from its tip and insert it 5–7.5 cm. (2–3 inches) in a downward and backward direction into the urethra. Allow urine to flow into a shallow pan/toilet or into a disposable plastic urine bag.	
	3. Remove catheter when urine stops flowing.	3. Measure or estimate volume of residual urine.
	Male Patient	
	1. Assume sitting position until technique is learned.	
	2. Lubricate the catheter.	2. A well-lubricated catheter is particularly necessary in the male to avoid traumatic urethritis.
	3. Retract foreskin of penis with one hand; then grasp penis and hold it at right angle to body.	3. This maneuver straightens the urethra and facilitates ease of catheter insertion.
	4. Insert the catheter 15–25 cm. (6–10 inches) until urine begins to flow.	
	5. Then advance catheter about 2.5 cm. (1 more inch) and allow urine to flow into shallow pan/toilet. When urine stops flowing, remove catheter.	5. Measure or estimate volume of residual urine.
	Follow-up Phase	
	1. Wash catheter in warm, soapy water: Rinse.	
	2. Wrap catheter in clean towel/paper towel.	2. The catheter may be carried in a clean plastic bag or case. The emphasis should be on availability and cleanliness.

INJURIES TO THE BLADDER (AND URETHRA)

Types of Bladder Injuries

1. Contusion of bladder
2. Intraperitoneal rupture ⎫
3. Extraperitoneal rupture ⎭ or combination of both
4. Injury to urethra

Types of Urethral Injuries

1. Contusion
2. Partial or complete rupture

Problems Associated with Bladder Injury

1. Injuries to the bladder and urethra are commonly associated with pelvic fractures and multiple trauma. Certain surgical procedures (hysterectomy, surgery of lower colon and rectum) also carry a risk to the bladder.
2. With injury there is a rise in intravesical (within bladder) pressure which produces extravasation of urine into the peritoneal cavity or perivesical space.
3. Rupture of the bladder requires immediate treatment.

Clinical Manifestations

1. Failure to void
2. Hematuria; presence of blood at urinary meatus
3. Shock and hemorrhage—pallor, rapid and increasing pulse rate
4. Suprapubic pain and soreness
5. Rigid abdomen—indicates intraperitoneal rupture

Diagnostic Evaluation

1. Urethrogram—to detect any rupture of urethra. *Do first* (before catheterization)
2. Cystogram—to detect and localize perforation of urinary bladder
3. Plain film of abdomen—may show associated pelvic fracture
4. Excretory urogram—to survey the kidneys for injury

Treatment and Nursing Management

1. Treat for shock and hemorrhage.
2. Carry out retrograde urethrography in suspected injuries involving lower urinary tract.

3. Catheterize patient only after urethrogram is done.
   a. Indwelling catheter serves as a means of continuous urinary drainage.
   b. Catheter also serves as a splint to urethra if urethra has been injured but it may complete a partial rupture if urethral injury is not recognized with a urethrogram.
4. Prepare for surgical intervention if bladder rupture has occurred.
   a. Extravasated blood and urine will be drained and urine diverted with suprapubic cystostomy and indwelling catheter.
   b. Bladder tears will be sutured; urethral repairs may be postponed.
5. Observe drainage systems after surgery.
   a. Suprapubic cystostomy drainage—until healing of bladder is complete.
   b. Indwelling urethral catheter drainage—to divert urine drainage and permit suprapubic incision to heal.
   c. Perivesical areas drained with penrose drain (will be brought out through suprapubic incision).

For Urethral Injury:
1. Assist with cystostomy drainage (p. 487)—to provide urine drainage until reconstructive surgery is done.
2. Treatment modalities determined by level of urethral injury and its effect on bladder continence.

Discharge Planning and Health Education

Urethral stricture, incontinence, and impotence may follow urethral injury.

CANCER OF THE BLADDER

Etiology

It appears that multiple agents are responsible for the development of cancer of the bladder. The specific etiology is unknown.
1. Cigarette smoking
2. Prolonged exposure to aromatic amines or their metabolites—generally dyes manufactured by the chemical industry and used by other industries
3. Causal relationship may exist between excessive coffee drinking and consumption of excessive amounts of analgesics and bladder cancer.
4. Chronic infection and irritation.
5. Bladder schistosomiasis (rare in U.S.).
6. Secondary metastasis from prostate, colon, rectum (males), and lower gynecologic tract (females)

NURSING ALERT: High-risk persons should have annual cytologic examinations of the urine.

Clinical Features

1. Bladder cancer is a highly malignant condition; it occurs 3 times more frequently in males, particularly after the 5th decade.
2. Large numbers of these tumors occur in the lateral and posterior bladder wall and near the trigone.
3. Metastases appear in vesical, hypogastric, common iliac, and lumbar lymph nodes; in liver, lungs, vertebrae, pelvis.
4. Recurrences may occur years after last known tumor is treated.
5. Small bladder tumors are seeded from tumors of renal pelvis.

Clinical Manifestations

1. Painless hematuria, either gross or microscopic—most characteristic sign
2. Dysuria, frequency, urgency—symptoms of bladder irritation
3. Flank pain, chills, fever—from progressive tumor growth, infiltration of bladder wall, ureteral obstruction, and bladder infection
4. Pelvic or back pain—from distant metastasis
5. Leg edema—from invasion of pelvic lymph nodes

Diagnostic Evaluation

1. Intravenous urography (IVU)—to rule out ureteral obstruction or presence of renal pelvic tumor
2. Cystourethroscopy—for visualization and biopsy of lesion
3. Bimanual examination of pelvis—to determine degree of mobility, fixation of tumor, and degree of extravesical extension
4. Retrograde pyelography—to define presence/absence of upper urinary tract pathology
5. Urinalysis (three-glass test)—for blood and bacteria
6. Cytology study of fresh urinary sediment to assess for malignant transitional cells shed from tumor
7. Enzyme studies—urinary lactic dehydrogenase and alkaline phosphatase which may or may not be elevated (a nonspecific test)
8. Chest x-ray and bone survey—to demonstrate distant metastases
9. Bone scan

Treatment

A. *Underlying Rationale*

1. There is no single effective method of treatment. The surgical procedure of choice depends on the characteristics of the tumor and whether or not bladder wall infiltration and local or distant metastasis has occurred. The patient's age and physical, mental, and emotional status are considered.
2. The patient is usually considered incurable if gross extension of the tumor beyond the bladder wall has occurred; in such cases adjuvant modalities such as radiotherapy and chemotherapy may be somewhat palliative.

B. *Modalities of Treatment*

   a. Transurethral endoscopic resection and fulguration.
   b. Partial (segmental) cystectomy.
   c. Cystectomy (removal of bladder) or radical cystectomy for invasive and poorly differentiated tumors.
      (1) Radical cystectomy in male—removal of blad-

der, pelvic peritoneum, prostate, seminal vesicles, and possible regional node dissection and removal of the urethra to the meatus.

(2) Radical cystectomy in female—removal of bladder, pelvic peritoneum, urethra, uterus, broad ligaments, vagina, tubes, and ovaries, and regional lymphadenectomy (iliac and pelvic nodes).

(3) Cystectomy requires diversion of the urinary stream.

(a) Early complications include wound infection (wound dehiscence or evisceration), pneumonitis, ileus, peritonitis, intestinal obstruction, urine leakage, ureterointestinal obstruction, rectal fistula.

(b) Long-term complications include pyelonephritis, calculi, stomal stenosis, conduit fibrosis, progressive loss of renal function.

d. Urinary diversion procedures (see below) to relieve frequency and hemorrhage in patients with inoperable disease.

e. Hydrostatic pressure therapy—placement of water-filled balloon within the bladder to produce tumor necrosis by reducing blood circulation in the bladder wall.

2. Radiation therapy—may be internal or external (see p. 852).

3. Chemotherapy

a. Topical chemotherapy—places a high concentration of drug in contact with neoplastic cells.

b. Systemic chemotherapy.

4. Combinations of surgery, radiation, and chemotherapy.

5. Immunotherapy—BCG given intravesically as well as intradermally to improve immune competence of patient.

URINARY DIVERSION

Urinary diversion refers to diverting the urinary stream from the bladder so that it exits via a new avenue. There are a large number of operative procedures.

Clinical Conditions Requiring Urinary Diversion

1. Malignancy of bladder or ureters; pelvic malignancy
2. Birth defects
3. Stricture and trauma to ureters and urethra
4. Neurogenic bladder
5. Severe ureteral and renal damage due to vesicoureteral reflux or chronic infection
6. Injuries

Methods of Urinary Diversion (Fig. 11-11)

The most common methods of urinary diversion are:

1. *Ileal Conduit*—implantation of the ureters to a section of the terminal ileum or loop of colon which is led out through the abdominal wall. The loop of ileum is a conduit (passageway) for urine from the ureters to the surface.

2. *Ureterosigmoidostomy*—implantation of the ureter(s) into the sigmoid, close to the rectum, thereby allowing urine to flow through the colon and out of the rectum.

3. *Cutaneous ureterostomy*—bringing the detached ureters through the abdominal wall and attaching them to an opening in the skin.

4. *Suprapubic cystostomy* (vesicostomy)—accomplished by inserting special catheter through the abdomen into the bladder either through an incision or by trocar punch technique.

5. *Nephrostomy*—inserting a catheter or silicone loop nephrostomy tube into the renal pelvis percutaneously or via an incision into the flank.

Preoperative Considerations for Patients Having Intestinal Urinary Diversion Procedures (Ileal Conduit and Ureterosigmoidostomy)

1. For patient undergoing renal surgery, see page 502 for general aspects of preoperative care.
2. Pay careful attention to cardiopulmonary status, as the patient is older and undergoing a lengthy, complex procedure.

3. Prepare patient for sigmoidoscopy and barium enema if ureterosigmoidostomy is to be performed.

a. Enemas are given (increasing in amount) to help develop sphincter control.

b. Assess patient's ability to retain enema as a means of evaluating adequacy of rectal sphincter.

4. Prepare the bowel for surgical intervention to minimize fecal stasis and postoperative ileus.

a. Give clear liquids.

b. Administer antimicrobial agents (neomycin, kanamycin)—for bowel disinfection to reduce pathogenic bacterial flora, as bowel contents frequently spill with transection of intestine.

c. Give enemas as directed for mechanical cleansing of lower bowel.

5. Employ adequate hydration procedures including intravenous infusions, to ensure urine flow during surgery.

6. Reinforce the surgeon's explanations of the surgical procedures.

a. The stoma site is planned preoperatively with the patient standing, sitting, and lying—to locate the stoma away from bony prominences, skin creases, and scars, and where the patient can see it.

b. Apply several types of skin adhesives or cement to abdomen preoperatively to determine contact allergies and to facilitate management of ostomy appliance postoperatively.

c. Have patient wear the intended appliance preoperatively.

7. Assist patient undergoing nasogastric intubation before surgery (p. 392); or, temporary gastrostomy may be done during surgery to facilitate gastric decompression.

8. Encourage patient to express his feelings about his situation.

Postoperative Nursing Management

OBJECTIVES: to preserve and maintain renal function.
to assist patient to adapt to his altered body image and to enjoy a full and satisfying life.

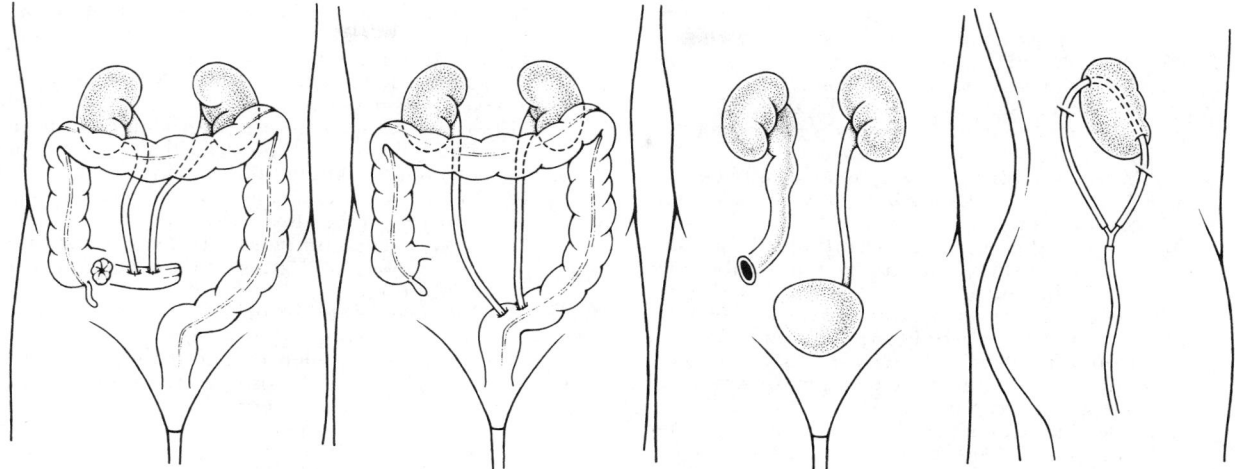

FIGURE 11-11. *Methods of urinary diversion.*

A. *General Considerations*

1. See page 419 for nursing management of patient following intestinal surgery and page 503 for nursing management of patient following urological surgery.
2. Watch for any abnormal signs and symptoms (wound infections, leaking at anastomosis site, peritonitis, paralytic ileus, intestinal obstruction, stenosis of stoma). These operations are extremely taxing, and patients have little or no reserve.
3. Assure adequate circulating volume with blood and plasma.
4. Keep nasogastric tube in place until patient passes gas via rectum.
5. Monitor total parenteral nutrition (p. 406) if patient is unable to return to oral feeding.
6. Accept the depression of the patient which usually follows any surgery that interferes with body integrity.
   a. Accept the patient's irritability and lack of motivation to learn.
   b. Give extra support until he can cope with his situation.

B. *Following Ileal Conduit*

1. Patient wears transparent disposable urinary drainage bags cemented to the abdominal wall until edema subsides and stoma shrinks to normal size. (Some patients prefer using disposable bags permanently.)
2. The patient with an ileal conduit wears a cemented-on appliance day and night. The ileal bladder drains urine constantly (but not feces)
   a. Appliance is connected to a drainage tube and bag; urinary volume is recorded hourly.
   b. Appliance remains in place as long as it is watertight; it is changed as necessary.
3. Inspect stoma for congestion and cyanosis, bleeding and friability of stomal mucosa—during first few postoperative weeks the stoma appears swollen and edematous.
4. Examine skin around stoma for signs of irritation, alkaline encrustation with peristomal dermatitis (from alkaline urine coming in contact with exposed skin), and wound infections.
   a. Alkaline urine is usually a result of bacteria; assess for odorous, cloudy appearing urine.
   b. Keep urine pH below 6.5; test the urine dribbling from the stoma with pH indicator (Nitrazine paper [Squibb]).
   c. Ascorbic acid may be given to acidify urine.
   d. Encourage high fluid intake—to flush ileal conduit and prevent mucus from congealing.
5. *Health Education, Rehabilitation, and Discharge Planning*

OBJECTIVE: to become an expert in the management of stoma and appliance.
   a. The urinary appliance may consist of one or two pieces and may be disposable, semidisposable, or reusable (choice determined by location of stoma, patient activity, body build, and economic status).
      (1) Reusable appliance—has a faceplate that is attached to the body with cement or adhesive.
      (2) Semidisposable appliance—has a reusable faceplate to which disposable pouches are attached.
      (3) Disposable appliance—discarded after each change.
   b. *Determining Stoma Size* (for ordering correct ostomy appliance)
      (1) The stoma will shrink considerably as edema subsides, and the opening is recalibrated every 3–6 weeks for the first few months postoperatively.
      (2) Measure the widest part of the stoma with a ruler. The inside diameter of the faceplate should not be more than one-sixteenth to one-eighth of an inch larger than the diameter of the stoma.
      (3) Patient is taught to dilate stoma himself with a finger in a plastic glove (usually weekly).
   c. *Changing the Appliance* (every 5–7 days)
      (1) Change appliance early in morning—before taking fluids.
      (2) Assemble all equipment needed for the type used.
      (3) Moisten the edge of the faceplate with adhesive solvent or soap and water and gently remove it. Adhesive solvent is not used if skin barriers (ReliaSeal or Stomahesive) are used.
      (4) Instruct the patient to bend over quickly and remain in that position for a minute to allow conduit to empty before the skin is washed and dried.

(5) Clean all cement from the skin with adhesive solvent; use a soft cloth. Wash skin with non-cream-based soap and water. Pat dry. *The skin must be dry or appliance will not adhere.*
   (1) Inspect skin for signs of irritation.
   (2) Keep the skin free from direct contact with urine.
   (3) A gauze or tissue wick may be applied over the stoma to absorb urine while the appliance is being changed.
(6) Prepare the appliance according to the manufacturer's directions; the skin of the abdomen should be taut.
(7) Center the appliance directly over the stoma and apply it carefully. Apply gentle pressure around appliance for secure adherence.
(8) Apply nonallergic tape in a picture-frame effect around the pouch.
(9) The skin under the appliance may be dusted with pure talcum powder and a cotton cover used to absorb perspiration and eliminate warmth from the pouch.
(10) The use of a belt is optional, but follow manufacturer's directions, since an ill-fitting belt can cause abrasion of the stoma.

d. *Odor Control*
   (1) Instruct the patient to avoid foods and medication that produce strong odors.
   (2) Drink liberal amounts of fluids to flush the conduit free of mucus and reduce possibility of urinary infection.
   (3) Introduce a few drops of liquid deodorizer or diluted white vinegar through the drain spout into the bottom of the pouch with a syringe or eye dropper.

e. *Managing the Ostomy Appliance*
   (1) Empty the appliance when it is ⅓–½ full to prevent weight of urine from loosening adhesive seal—urinary ostomy appliances are closed with a drain valve (spigot) for periodic emptying.
   (2) Some patients prefer wearing a leg bag attached with an adapter to the drainage apparatus.
   (3) Attach outlet on appliance to a collecting bottle with plastic tubing for nighttime drainage; have at least 1.5 m. (5 ft.) of tubing to allow patient to turn in bed.
      The tubing may be threaded down the pajama leg to prevent kinking.

f. *Securing a Urine Specimen for Culture from an Ileal Conduit*
   (1) Open catheter set.
   (2) Remove the bag from the stoma. Place a 3 x 4 gauze sponge over the stoma to absorb the urine.
   (3) Don sterile gloves.
   (4) Using a sterile surgical forceps and cotton balls, cleanse the area around the stoma from the center outward.
   (5) Insert a French catheter 5 cm. (2 inches) into the stoma and wait for the urine.

g. *Cleaning and Deodorizing the Appliance*
   (1) Clean faceplate with solvent and remove all adhesive; rinse in clear water.
   (2) Clean appliance with a brush and detergent solution; rinse and soak in white vinegar, washing soda solution, a few drops of Clorox, or any commercial deodorizing solution.

   (3) After soaking (5–10 minutes) hang it up to air-dry.
   (4) Discard equipment that can no longer be cleaned adequately.

h. *General Instructions*
   (1) Urinary stoma care is not difficult or complicated and should be regarded as part of personal grooming and dressing routine.
   (2) The stoma is normally red in color; it may protrude or be flush with the skin. It may bleed if it is bumped or rubbed. Report to your physician if it continues bleeding for several hours.
   (3) Mucus shreds in the urine are normal following an ileal conduit operation.
   (4) Choose an appliance that fits your needs. Successful urinary ostomy requires a well-fitting appliance, meticulous skin care, and control of urinary odor.
   (5) Always carry spare pouches and cement in a small case in handbag or pocket.
   (6) The wearing time of an appliance varies. Experiment with your appliance; usually an appliance may be worn 5–7 days. See page 517 for changing, cleaning, and management of appliance.
   (7) Before changing to a new skin adhesive, apply a test patch to the other side of the abdomen or forearm.
   (8) Wear cotton (rather than nylon) underwear. Avoid a heavy girdle as it may cause chafing of the stoma and leakage from pressure on the pouch.
   (9) Avoid heavy lifting for 6 weeks. Sexual activities, driving the car, returning to work, etc., may be resumed when energy level increases.
   (10) Get in touch with local medical supply distributor or enterostomal therapist or look in *Ostomy Quarterly* (address follows) for manufacturer's advertisements of appliances, deodorizers, skin barriers, and other new products.
   (11) Call your physician for instructions if skin problems develop or if one or more of the following symptoms of kidney complications occur: fever, chills, pain, change in color of urine (cloudy, bloody), diminishing urine output.
   (12) Contact local ostomy association for visits, reassurance, and practical information from ostomy visitor.
   (13) For further information and valuable periodical materials:
      United Ostomy Association, Inc., 2001 W. Beverly Boulevard, Los Angeles, CA 90057.

C. *Following Ureterosigmoidostomy*

1. Patient will have rectal tube (or mushroom catheter) draining urine postoperatively—to ensure drainage and prevent reflux of urine into ureters and kidneys.
  a. Tape the tube to the buttocks.
  b. If the tube must be removed for defecation reinsert the tube approximately 10 cm. (4 inches) into rectum to prevent trauma to site of ureteral anastomosis.
2. Give special skin care around anus to prevent skin erythema and excoriation.
3. Following removal of the tube, the patient voids through his rectum.

a. Encourage patient to empty rectum every 2–3 hours (or more often) to keep rectal pressure low and to minimize the absorption of urinary constituents from the colon.

b. In time the patient will be able to differentiate between the sensation to void and the urge to defecate.

c. Reinsert the tube (catheter) at night (attached to drainage bottle) to permit uninterrupted sleep.

d. Do not give enemas or cathartics.

e. If irrigations are requested, avoid using force because of danger of introducing an infection into newly implanted ureters.

4. Evaluate for electrolyte imbalance and acidosis—potassium and magnesium imbalances may occur from presence of urine in the bowel, which stimulates diarrhea.

a. Maintain fluid and electrolyte balance in immediate postoperative period by serum chemical determinations and intravenous infusions.

b. Low chloride diet supplemented with sodium potassium citrate—to prevent acidosis.

5. *Health Education*

a. Give specific diet instructions when patient can tolerate oral intake.

(1) Avoid gas-forming foods since flatus can cause stress incontinence, socially embarrassing offensive odor, and discomfort.

(2) Watch for air swallowing (chewing gum, smoking, carbonated beverages) to avoid gas.

(3) Reduce salt intake to prevent hyperchloremic acidosis.

(4) Increase potassium intake through medication and foods since potassium may be lost in acidosis.

b. Take prophylactic antimicrobials as directed—pyelonephritis (due to reflux of bacteria from colon) can occur in some patients.

D. *Following Cutaneous Ureterostomy*

1. A urinary appliance is fitted immediately following surgery and is worn at all times.

2. Ureteral dilatation with sterile catheter is performed at regular intervals to assure patency and prevent ureteral stricture.

3. See page 517, nursing considerations for patient having ileal conduit—for general aspects of care.

E. *Following Cystostomy* (temporary or permanent)

1. Usually done on patient with an obstruction below bladder (prostatic obstruction) when it is not possible to insert urethral catheter.

2. Encourage liberal amounts of fluid to avoid encrustation around catheter.

3. See also page 487.

F. *Following Nephrostomy* (temporary or permanent)

1. May be performed rapidly under local anesthesia when other procedures are not technically possible.

2. See page 503 for care of patient.

PROBLEMS AFFECTING THE URETHRA

URETHRITIS

Urethritis is inflammation of the urethra.

Etiology

1. Nonspecific—urethritis not caused by gonococcus. However, a large number of cases are sexually transmitted by:

a. *Chlamydia*—a virus-like intracellular bacterium

b. *Trichomonas vaginalis*

c. *Herpesvirus hominis*, Type 2

d. *Candida*

e. Mycoplasms

f. Unknown organisms

2. Nonsexually transmitted:

a. Bacterial urethritis—may be associated with urinary tract infection

b. From trauma—secondary to passage of urethral sounds, repeated cystoscopy, indwelling catheter

3. Reiter's syndrome—urethritis, conjunctivitis, arthritis of unknown etiology

Clinical Manifestations

1. Itching and burning around area of urethra
2. Dysuria and frequency
3. Urethral discharge; may be scant or profuse; thin, clear, or mucoid; or thick and purulent
4. Penile pain

Diagnostic Evaluation

1. Study of stained urethral smear
2. Culture for gonorrhea
3. Blood test for syphilis

4. History and physical findings (interview to elicit past history of gonorrhea)

Treatment and Nursing Management

1. Give antimicrobial—tetracyclines are effective for *Chlamydia* infection.

a. Give on empty stomach, preferably 1 hour before meals

b. Do not take with milk, antacids, iron supplements—reduce absorption of drug

2. Metronidazole (Flagyl) may be given for *Trichomonas* infection.

3. Treat associated prostatitis (p. 521).

Health Education

1. Advise patient to temporarily discontinue sexual activity and ingestion of alcohol—these activities may prolong the acute phase of urethritis.

2. Urge treatment for sexual partner—in event of treatment failure and recurrence.

3. Support and reassure patient—nonspecific urethritis is usually self-limited and is not a serious health threat.

URETHRITIS FROM GONORRHEA

Etiology

1. *Neisseria gonorrhoeae*—the specific organism.
2. Transmitted through sexual contact.
3. More and more asymptomatic carriers are being recognized.

Clinical Manifestations

Male
1. Inflammation of meatal orifice; burning on urination; *may be asymptomatic*
2. Urethral discharge: scant and serous to thick, yellowish pus (4–10 days or longer after sexual exposure)

Female
1. Purulent urethral discharge
2. Frequency, urgency, nocturia
3. Red, swollen urinary meatus
4. Pelvic infection accompanied by abdominal pain
5. Often is asymptomatic

Complications (local)

1. Male—periurethritis, prostatitis, epididymitis, urethral stricture, sterility due to vasoepididymal duct obstruction
2. Female—pelvic infection, abscess of greater vestibular glands (Bartholin's glands), urethral stricture

Treatment and Health Education

1. See page 808 for treatment of gonorrhea.
2. Instruct the patient to avoid sexual activity with untreated previous sexual partners until they have been treated and examined to prevent reinfection.
3. Emphasize that patient must return in 7–14 days to assess results and determine if there is need for further treatment and tests.
4. Urge patient to have their sexual contacts present themselves for treatment.

URETHRAL STRICTURE

Urethral stricture is a narrowing of the lumen and loss of distensibility of the urethra caused by scar tissue formation and contraction.

Etiology

1. Urethral injury
   a. Urethral instrumentation—transurethral surgical procedures, indwelling catheters, cystoscopic procedures
   b. Straddle injuries, automobile accidents, pelvic fractures, direct trauma to urethra
2. Untreated gonorrheal urethritis
3. Congenital abnormalities.

Clinical Manifestations

1. Diminution in force and size of urinary stream
2. Urinary infection and retention—dysuria and urgency
3. Symptoms of complication from stricture—back pressure produces cystitis, prostatitis, pyelonephritis, etc.

Diagnostic Evaluation

1. Urethrogram and voiding cystogram—to locate site and degree of stricture
2. Elevated WBC, pus and bacteria in urine—if urinary tract infection present
3. Passing of catheter or sounds (bougies)—to determine the diameter and location of urethral narrowings
4. Residual urine measurement

Prevention

1. Treat urethral infections promptly.
2. Utilize utmost care in urethral instrumentation (catheterization, etc.).
3. Avoid prolonged urethral catheter drainage.

Treatment and Nursing Management

1. Dilatation of urethra with urethral sounds.
   a. Sounds of increasing size are used.
   b. Sounds are passed at lengthening intervals (2 weeks, 1 month, 3 months) for an indefinite period depending on how long the strictured lumen is patent.
   c. Hot sitz baths and nonnarcotic analgesics—to control pain after instrumentation.
   d. Antimicrobials may be given several days after dilatation—lessens discomfort and minimizes infectious reaction.
2. Surgical excision, urethroplasty, or suprapubic cystostomy may be necessary for severe strictures.

CONDITIONS OF THE PROSTATE

BENIGN PROSTATIC HYPERPLASIA (HYPERTROPHY)

Benign prostatic hyperplasia is enlargement of the prostate. The etiology is uncertain but is presumably related to endocrine changes associated with aging that initiate hyperplasia of both glandular and cellular tissue of the prostate.

Clinical Manifestations

1. In early or gradual prostatic enlargement there may be no symptoms, since the bladder can compensate for increased peripheral resistance.
2. Obstructive symptoms—hesitancy, diminution in size and force of urinary stream, postvoiding dribbling, sensation of incomplete emptying of the bladder.
3. Symptoms of recurring urinary infection and stasis—frequency, nocturia, chills, fever.
4. Renal symptoms (prolonged obstruction)—ureteral dilatation, hydronephrosis, renal infection, azotemia, uremia.

Diagnostic Evaluation

1. Rectal examination—allows rough estimate of size of gland.
2. Cystourethroscopy—to inspect urethra and bladder and evaluate prostatic size.
3. Catheterization after voiding—to determine amount of residual urine.

4. Excretory urogram—to document upper urinary tract obstruction.
5. Serum creatinine and BUN—to evaluate renal function.

Treatment and Nursing Management

(The plan of treatment depends on the cause, the severity of obstruction, and the condition of the patient.)
1. Conservative treatment if no symptoms of urinary impairment—intermittent catheterization, urethral dilation, prostatic massage—to relieve symptoms of acute obstruction.
2. Prepare patient for surgery (enucleation or removal of hyperplastic prostatic tissue) when obstructive symptoms occur. See page 523 for nursing management of patient having a prostatectomy.
3. Cystostomy drainage of bladder—for poor-risk patient or one acutely ill with retention, uremia, etc.

Health Education

1. Surgical procedures for benign enlargement usually do not result in impotence, but may cause retrograde ejaculation (passing back of semen into the bladder during sexual intercourse).
2. See page 524.

PROSTATITIS

Prostatitis is an inflammation of the prostate gland.

Classification

Acute bacterial prostatitis, chronic bacterial prostatitis, nonbacterial prostatitis, prostatodynia.

Etiology (bacterial prostatitis)

1. Bacterial invasion of prostate
    a. From hematogenous (bloodstream) origin (tonsils, GI tract, GU tract)
    b. From ascent of bacteria from urethra
    c. Secondary to urethritis (p. 519)
2. Descending infection from kidneys

Clinical Manifestations

(from infection and local inflammation)
1. Sudden chills and fever (moderate to high fever)
2. Pain in perineum, rectum, lower back, lower abdomen, and penile head
3. Pain in groin—if seminal vesicles are involved
4. Bladder irritability—frequency, dysuria, urgency, hematuria

Diagnostic Evaluation

1. Culture and sensitivity tests of urethral and prostatic fluid and urine.
    a. The pathogens in each specimen are identified by collection of divided urine specimens and expressed prostatic fluid (obtained by prostatic massage).
    b. The pH of the prostatic fluid is usually elevated.
2. Rectal examination—frequently reveals exquisitely tender, painful, swollen prostate, warm to the touch.

Complications

1. Urinary retention—from swelling of the gland; recurring urinary tract infection
2. Epididymitis, prostatic abscess

3. Bacteremia/septicemia
4. Pyelonephritis

Treatment and Nursing Management

OBJECTIVE: to avoid complications of abscess formation and septicemia

A. *Acute Bacterial Prostatitis*
1. Treat with antimicrobial (trimethoprim-sulfamethoxazole) to which organism causing infection is susceptible.
2. Supportive care:
    a. Bed rest—to relieve perineal and suprapubic pain.
    b. Hot sitz baths—to promote muscular relaxation of pelvic floor and reduce potential for urinary retention.
    c. Antipyretics, analgesics, stool softeners, as necessary.
3. Watch for urinary retention—due to edema of prostatic tissue; suprapubic catheter may be required.

B. *Chronic Bacterial Prostatitis*
1. Give specific therapy (trimethoprim-sulfamethoxazole, minocycline, doxycycline): chronic bacterial prostatitis is difficult to treat because many antibacterial agents diffuse poorly into prostatic fluid.
    a. Continuous suppressive treatment with low-dose antimicrobial drugs may be indicated.
    b. Be alert for relapsing infection.
2. Promote comfort with antispasmodics (relieve bladder irritability), sitz baths, stool softeners.

C. *Nonbacterial Prostatitis*
1. Most common type; etiology obscure.
2. Therapy is directed towards control of symptoms and individualized to meet specific needs; acute symptoms may be controlled with anticholinergic or anti-inflammatory drugs, hot sitz baths, etc.

D. *Prostatodynia*—Patient has symptons of urinary irritation but no evidence of bacteria or inflamed prostatic fluid or tissue. Treatment is symptomatic.

Discharge Planning and Health Education

Instruct the patient as follows:
1. Take antibiotic for the full time period.
2. Use hot sitz baths (10–20 minutes) several times daily.
3. Drink fluids to satisfy thirst, but avoid "forcing fluids," as an effective level of drug must be maintained in the urine.
4. Avoid food and drinks that have diuretic action or increase prostatic secretions (alcohol, coffee, tea, chocolate, cola, spices).
5. Avoid sexual arousal/intercourse during period of acute inflammation; sexual intercourse may be beneficial in the treatment of chronic prostatitis; chronic prostatic infection is *not* sexually transmissible.
6. Be assured that the causative agent of prostatitis is not the type that causes venereal disease. (This may be an unspoken fear.)
7. Avoid sitting for long periods of time.
8. Medical follow-up is necessary for at least 6 months to 1 year since recurrence of prostatitis due to the same or different organisms can occur.

CANCER OF THE PROSTATE

Cancer of the prostate is a malignant tumor of the prostate gland. It arises from the parenchyma of the prostate, usually in the most posterior part; therefore most prostatic cancers are palpable on rectal examination.

Clinical Features

1. Cancer of the prostate is the 2nd leading cause of cancer death among American men.
2. It can spread by local extension, by lymphatics, or via the bloodstream.
3. Prostatic cancer is potentially curable at an early stage; however, the majority of patients present with obstructive symptoms or metastatic lesions.

NURSING ALERT: Annual rectal examination of males over 40 is important for early diagnosis of prostatic cancer.

Clinical Manifestations

1. Symptoms due to obstruction of urinary flow
   a. Hesitancy and straining on voiding, frequency, nocturia
   b. Diminution in size and force of urinary stream
2. Symptoms due to metastases
   a. Pain in lumbosacral area radiating to hips and down legs
   b. Perineal and rectal discomfort
   c. Anemia, weight loss, weakness, nausea, oliguria (from uremia)
   d. Hematuria—from urethral or bladder invasion, or both

Diagnostic Evaluation

1. Digital rectal examination—reveals "stony hard" fixed gland if lesion is advanced (there are indurated lumps without fixation if condition is found earlier)
2. Cystoscopy—helps evaluate local extent of disease
3. Prostatic biopsy
4. Biochemical tests
   Serum acid phosphatase—frequently increased when cancer extends outside prostatic capsule; radioimmunoassay techniques for acid phosphatase may be useful in detecting early lesions
5. Radionuclide bone scan—to detect metastases
6. Skeletal roentgenograms—to reveal osteoblastic metastases
7. Excretory urogram—to demonstrate changes from ureteral obstruction
8. Lymphangiography—to seek evidence of metastases to pelvic and para-aortic lymph nodes
9. Pelvic lymphadenectomy and biopsy—for staging and to determine spread to lymph nodes

Treatment

OBJECTIVES: to control tumor spread.
to draw up a rational plan of treatment.

A. *Curative* (depends on stage)

1. Transurethral resection or open enucleation of prostate—for patients with Stage A disease.
2. Radical prostatectomy—removal of prostate and its capsule, prostatic urethra, and seminal vesicles; may include regional lymphadenectomy
   a. Done by retropubic or perineal approach.

b. Sexual impotence follows radical procedure, but urinary control is usually normal
   c. See page 523 for care of patient undergoing prostatectomy.
3. Radiation therapy—Cobalt ^{60} or high energy x-rays produced by linear accelerator—to region of prostate gland. Some degree of proctitis, diarrhea, and urinary frequency may be seen toward the end of treatment; impotence may occur.
4. Interstitial implantation of ^{125}I radioactive seeds.

B. *Palliative*

OBJECTIVES: to improve quality of life.
to relieve symptoms.

1. *Hormonal manipulation*—the aim of hormonal treatment is to suppress or eliminate the main sources of androgen production (most prostatic cancers are androgen dependent) and thereby to alleviate symptoms and retard progress of disease.
   a. Bilateral orchiectomy (removal of testes)—removes major source of androgen production, since 95% of circulating plasma testosterone originates from testes. Or,
   b. Estrogen therapy (diethylstilbestrol)—thought to inhibit the gonadotropins (responsible for testicular androgenic activity), thus removing androgenic hormone upon which the tumor growth depends.
      (1) Therapy with estrogens has been reported to increase death rate from cardiovascular disease.
      (2) Watch for fluid retention
      (3) Patient may experience soreness and enlargement of breasts (gynecomastia.)
   c. Both orchiectomy and estrogen may be used in treatment.
   d. Chemotherapy (singly or in combination) appears to be beneficial in advanced prostatic cancer.
   e. Radiation therapy for palliation—may also decrease bone pain.
   f. Transurethral resection to remove obstructing tissue.
   g. Suprapubic cystostomy drainage for bladder outlet obstruction when transurethral resection cannot be done.
   h. Transsphenoidal hypophysectomy or adrenalectomy.
   i. See page 851, nursing management of the patient with pain and page 856, care of the patient with late stage cancer.

MANAGEMENT OF THE PATIENT UNDERGOING PROSTATIC SURGERY

Surgical Procedures

A. *Four Approaches for Prostatectomy*

1. Transurethral removal of prostatic tissue by an instrument introduced through urethra.
2. Open surgical removal of prostate (procedures used are named for area of incision).
   a. Perineal
   b. Retropubic
   c. Suprapubic

B. *Factors Influencing Choice of Surgical Approach*

1. Size of gland and severity of obstruction
2. Age and condition of patient
3. Presence of associated disease(s)

Preoperative Objectives of Nursing Management

A. *To establish kidney function at the patient's optimum level.*

1. Maintain adequate bladder drainage via indwelling catheter or suprapubic cystostomy—renal function usually improves with reestablishment of drainage.
   a. Introduce indwelling catheter if patient has continuing retention or if residual urine is more than 75–100 ml. and patient is azotemic.
   b. Utilize cystostomy if patient cannot tolerate urethral catheter.
   c. Give antibiotics (according to culture and sensitivity tests)—to combat and control infection.
   d. Watch patient closely after drainage is instituted—blood pressure fluctuates and renal function may decline first few days after drainage is established.
   e. Ensure adequate hydration—patient is frequently dehydrated from self-limitation of fluids because of frequency.
      (1) Encourage fluid intake of 2500–3000 ml. daily (if cardiac reserve is adequate)—to help in overcoming azotemia.
      (2) Weigh patient daily and monitor fluid intake and output.
      (3) Give intravenous fluids according to need as indicated by clinical status and serum electrolyte determinations.
2. Carry out prescribed renal function studies—to determine if there is renal impairment from prostatic back pressure and to evaluate renal reserve.

B. *To ensure that patient is in best possible condition.* (Older people have diminishing functional reserves of vital organs and may have coexisting disease.)

1. Carry out complete hematologic investigation—to ascertain specific clotting defects since hemorrhage is a major postoperative complication.
2. Correct nutritional deficiencies, hypoproteinemia, vitamin deficiencies and anemia.
3. Give cardiac supporting drugs when indicated—helps alleviate renal symptoms.
4. Prepare patient with pulmonary emphysema with antibacterial agent, tracheobronchial cleansing, and incentive spirometry. Patient should stop smoking at least 2 days before surgery.
5. Teach active leg exercises; apply below-the-knee elastic stockings to prevent deep vein thrombosis.
6. Type and cross match for blood transfusion(s).

Postoperative Objectives of Nursing Management

A. *To evaluate for shock and hemorrhage.*

1. Watch for evidence of hemorrhage in drainage bottle, on dressings, and at incision site.
2. Take blood pressure, pulse, and respiration as frequently as clinical condition indicates. Compare with preoperative vital sign readings to assess degree of hypotension present.
   a. Observe for cold, sweating skin, pallor, restlessness, fall in blood pressure, increasing pulse rate.
   b. Prepare for surgical intervention if bleeding persists (suturing of bleeders or transurethral coagulation of bleeders.)

3. Give blood transfusion as indicated.

B. *To promote adequate drainage of the bladder.*

1. Utilize a closed sterile gravity system of drainage—3-way system is useful in controlling bleeding; irrigating system keeps clots from forming (does not correct the *cause* of bleeding).
2. Watch drainage for evidence of increased bleeding—bright red urine indicates arterial bleeding; dark color suggests venous bleeding.
3. Irrigate bladder (amount and time prescribed by urologist) to avoid clot formation in the bladder.
   a. Frequency of bladder irrigation determined by amount of bleeding.
   b. Irrigation is adjusted to keep urine a light pink to straw color, free of clots, and transparent in appearance.
   c. Avoid overdistending bladder—may produce secondary hemorrhage by stretching the coagulated vessels in the prostatic capsule.
   d. Maintain an input and output record, including the amount of fluid used for irrigation.
4. Explain again to the patient the purpose of the catheter.
   a. Tell him that the urge to void is caused by the presence of the catheter and bladder spasm.
   b. Encourage him to refrain from pulling on catheter—will cause bleeding, clots, plugging of catheter, and distention.
   c. Tape catheter to abdomen or laterally (see Fig. 11-6) to prevent pressure on penoscrotal junction.
   d. Wash urethral meatus adjacent to catheter with soap and water; rinse and apply an antibacterial ointment several times a day as directed.
5. Be alert for blockage of urinary drainage tube by kinking, mucus plugs, and blood clots.
6. Tape the drainage tubing (not the catheter) to shaved inner thigh—to prevent traction on bladder. (However, traction on the catheter by the urologist may control bleeding.)
7. Tape cystostomy catheter to lateral abdomen.
8. Note time and amount of each voiding after removal of catheter.
   a. May be urinary leakage around wound several days after removal of catheter in perineal, suprapubic, and retropubic surgery.
   b. Cystostomy tube may be removed before or after removal of urethral catheter.

C. *To anticipate postoperative complications.*

1. Hemorrhage and shock
2. Urinary infection
3. Epididymitis
4. Pulmonary complications

D. *To promote comfort and rehabilitation of the patient.*

1. Keep patient quiet, and comfortable during *immediate* postoperative period to prevent episodes of bleeding. When a patient experiences pain following prostatectomy, it may cause him to strain (from bladder irritability); this causes pelvic vein engorgement and promotes venous hemorrhage and clot formation.
2. Use tranquilizers, sedatives, antispasmodics, and appropriate analgesics for pain control.
   a. Elderly patients do not usually tolerate barbiturates.
   b. Take blood pressure before administering tranquilizers and analgesics.

3. Give antibiotics as directed—to promote urinary antisepsis.
4. Avoid rectal temperatures, rectal tubes, and enemas following perineal prostatic surgery.
5. Help the patient to ambulate as quickly as possible; avoid sitting for prolonged periods, since this increases intra-abdominal pressure and increases the possibility of bleeding.
6. Promote the comfort of the patient with perineal sutures.
   a. Wash perineum with surgical soap as directed.
   b. Use heat lamp to perineal area (cover scrotum with towel)—to promote healing.
   c. Assist patient with sitz bath as directed—to promote healing.

Discharge Planning and Health Education

The major concerns of the patient usually center on urinary control and sexual competence:
Instruct the patient as follows:

A. *Urinary Control*

1. After the catheter is removed, there may be some burning on urination and/or frequent desire to void. These symptoms will disappear in a few weeks.
2. Expect urinary dribbling for a period of time (especially after catheter removal). Urinary incontinence may follow any type of prostatic surgery.
3. Exercises to gain urinary control.
   a. *Perineal exercises*
      (1) Tense the perineal muscles by pressing the buttocks together. Hold this position as long as possible; relax.
      (2) Perform this exercise 10–20 times each hour.
      (3) Continue with perineal exercises until full urinary control is gained.
   b. *When starting to void*
      (1) Shut off the stream for a few seconds.

(2) Continue with full voiding.
(3) Continue this exercise with each urination until control improves; may take many weeks.
4. Urinate as soon as the first desire to do so is felt.
5. The urine may be cloudy for several weeks after surgery. As the prostate area heals, the cloudiness will disappear.
6. Avoid long automobile trips which increase tendency to bleed.
7. Avoid alcohol which increases urinary burning.
8. Drink adequate fluids (8 glasses/day) since dehydration increases tendency for clot obstruction.
9. Do not take anticholinergics and diuretics unless by direct order of the physician.

B. *Sexual Potency*

1. Prostatectomy does not usually cause impotence.
   a. Total prostatectomy (removal of entire prostatic contents and capsule) results in impotence, since the nerves and muscular tissue surrounding the capsule (which have a function in penile erection) have been severed.
   b. Penile prosthesis (inflatable, semi-rigid and flexible types) may be surgically implanted—used to make the penis rigid for sexual intercourse.
2. In most instances sexual activity may be resumed in 6–8 weeks; this is the time required for healing of the prostatic fossa to take place.
3. Do not be alarmed if no fluid appears on ejaculation; following ejaculation the seminal fluid goes into the bladder and is excreted with the urine. This is not harmful.

C. *Other Considerations*

1. Avoid straining and strenuous exercises.
2. Report to the physician any bleeding or a decrease in the size of the urinary stream.

HYDROCELE

Hydrocele is an abnormal accumulation of fluid within the scrotum around the testicle and within the 2 layers of the tunica vaginalis.

Causes

(Caused by defective or inadequate reabsorption of normally produced hydrocele fluid)
1. Secondary to local injury including hernia operation
2. Secondary to infection
3. Following epididymitis or orchitis; torsion
4. As a complication of tumor of testicle.
5. In edematous states such as congestive heart failure, cirrhosis of the liver
6. Idiopathic

Clinical Manifestations

1. Enlargement of the scrotum
2. Usually painless until fluid accumulation is large enough to cause pressure
3. Transmits light when transilluminated

Treatment

1. No treatment is required unless complications are present.
   a. Circulatory complications involving testicle
   b. Painful large hydrocele which is uncomfortable and cosmetically unacceptable to the patient
2. Surgical intervention—hydrocelectomy (excision of tunica vaginalis of testis) for removal of fluid and control of swelling.
   a. Periodic aspiration of hydrocele fluid in poor-risk patient
   b. Open operation for eversion of hydrocele sac or removal of hydrocele sac
3. See page 525, Treatment and Nursing Management—Varicocele, #3 for postoperative nursing support.

Complications

1. Hemorrhage into scrotal tissues
2. Infection

VARICOCELE

Varicocele is an abnormal dilation of the pampiniform plexus in the scrotum (a network of veins from the testicle and epididymis, constituting part of the spermatic cord).

Clinical Manifestations

1. Subfertility may occur with varicocele—may suppress spermatogenesis due to vascular and temperature changes or more likely to reflux of left adrenal corticosteroids to both testes because of intercommunication of their venous circulations.
2. A dragging sensation in the scrotum is usually the patient's chief complaint.
3. Varicocele on the right may indicate retroperitoneal tumor.

Treatment and Nursing Management

1. Patient wears a scrotal support (or suspensory) to relieve discomfort.
2. Operative intervention—ligation and excision of veins *(varicocelectomy)*.
3. Postoperative nursing support
   a. Apply ice bag to scrotum first few hours postoperatively—relieves edema.
   b. Apply scrotal support for comfort.

TUMORS OF THE TESTICLE

The etiology of testicular tumors is unknown but cryptorchidism (p. 1340), infections, and genetic and endocrine factors appear to play a role in their development.

Clinical Features

1. Tumors of the testicle are usually malignant; they occur primarily in men between the ages of 20 and 40.
2. Most testicular tumors metastasize early to the periaortic and pericaval lymph nodes, lungs, and liver.
3. A patient with a history of 1 testis tumor is more apt to develop another than is the random patient to develop a first testis tumor.
4. Testicular germ-cell tumors are now considered curable.

Clinical Manifestations

1. Mass in scrotum; painless enlargement of the testis accompanied by feeling of heaviness in scrotum.
2. Pain in the testis (if patient has epididymitis or bleeding into tumor).
3. Gynecomastia (enlargement of the breasts) from elaboration of chorionic gonadotropins from testicular tumor.
4. Symptoms of metastases
   a. Left supraclavicular or abdominal mass
   b. Abdominal pain
   c. Cough (lung metastases)

Diagnostic Evaluation

1. Radioimmunoassay of human chorionic gonadotropins (HCG) and alpha-fetoprotein (AFP)—serologic and cellular markers used for diagnosis, detection of early recurrence, staging, and for determining adequacy of treatment.
2. Intravenous urogram to evaluate presence of enlarged lymph nodes as manifested by ureteral displacement
3. Chest film to seek pulmonary or mediastinal metastases
4. Lymphangiography—to assess extent of lymphatic spread of tumor
5. Computed tomography—to identify lesions in retroperitoneum and to follow patient's course during/after treatment.

Treatment and Nursing Management

OBJECTIVE: to eradicate disease and achieve cure.
1. Orchiectomy—removal of testis and its tunica, and spermatic cord—through an inguinal incision. Retroperitoneal lymphadenectomy usually performed after orchiectomy.
   a. Orchiectomy (unilateral) usually has no adverse effects on sexual potency or fertility. Gel-filled prosthesis can be implanted at time of orchiectomy or electively thereafter—to offset absence of one testis.
   b. Possible postoperative complication of loss of ejaculation may occur after retroperitoneal lymphadenectomy; patient will not be fertile, but normal libido and orgasm will be unimpaired. Banking of sperm may be considered preoperatively.
2. Radiation therapy to lymphatic drainage pathways is used in most patients with testicular cancer; treatment of choice for seminoma.
3. Chemotherapy—for patients with recurrent or disseminated nonseminomatous cancer; usually given in combination.
   a. Cyclophosphamide, vinblastine, actinomycin-D, bleomycin, cisplatin—induce a high percentage of durable complete remissions.
   b. These regimens are toxic and require intensive therapeutic support; require high degree of patient commitment and cooperation.
   c. May be used as adjuvant to surgery and/or radiation in advanced disease. See page 843 for nursing management of patient receiving chemotherapy.
4. Provide continuing emotional support, since therapy can cause sexual fears and be a threat to masculinity and self-esteem.

Discharge Planning and Health Education

Instruct the patient as follows:
1. Follow-up evaluation includes chest films, excretory urography and radioimmunoassay of HCG and AFP, examination of lymph nodes—to monitor success of therapy and to detect recurrence of malignancy.
2. Carry out periodic self-examinations of the testes (see Guidelines, p. 526).

GUIDELINES: Self-Examination for Testicular Tumor

1. The testis is easily accessible for self-examination. Most tumors are palpable and can be detected by self-examination.
2. The hormonally-active years (15–35) are the tumor-prone years.

Procedure

ACTION BY PATIENT	EXPLANATION
1. Examine for testicular tumor periodically, preferably while showering/bathing.	
2. Use both hands to palpate (feel). Carefully examine all scrotal contents.	2. A small lump (nodule) can slip away from one hand. You can feel differences in weight between the testicles by using both hands.
3. Locate the epididymis; this is the cord-like structure at the back of the testis.	3. It is important to know what the epididymis feels like so you will not confuse it with an abnormality.
4. The spermatic cord (and vas) extends upward from the epididymis.	
5. Feel each testis between the thumb and first two fingers of each hand.	5. The testes lie freely in the scrotum, are oval shaped, and measure 4–5 cm. in length, 3 cm. in width, and about 2 cm. in thickness.
6. Note size, shape, abnormal tenderness.	6. An abnormality may be felt as a firm area on the front or side of the testicle.
7. Stand in front of mirror and look for changes in size/shape of scrotum.	7. Tumors or cystic masses tend to involve only one side.

EPIDIDYMITIS

Epididymitis is an infection of the epididymis which usually descends from an infected prostate or urinary tract.

Causes

1. Prostatic infection (most common cause); complication of infected urine containing pyogenic bacteria.
2. Trauma.
3. Postoperative epididymitis—complication of prostatectomy and urethral catheterization.
4. Specific causes: gonorrhea, syphilis, tuberculosis, *Chlamydia trachomatis* infection.

Clinical Manifestations

1. Pain and soreness in inguinal region and scrotum
2. Swollen, tender, extremely painful epididymis
3. Edema, redness, and tenderness of scrotum
4. Chills and fever
5. Pyuria and bacteriuria

Diagnostic Evaluation

1. Elevated white blood count (may be as high as 20,000–30,000/cu.ml.)
2. Staining of urethral discharge if preceded by urethritis (either nonspecific or gonorrheal); usually no discharge is present with epididymitis

Treatment and Nursing Management

1. Bed rest during acute phase.
2. Give specific antimicrobial therapy until all evidence of acute inflammatory reaction has subsided.
3. Scrotal support for enlarged testicle—to relieve edema and discomfort and to take the tension off the cord. A cotton-lined athletic supporter may promote comfort.
4. Infiltration of spermatic cord with local anesthetic agent (procaine hydrochloride)—for pain relief if patient is seen within 24 hours after onset.
5. Analgesics for pain relief.
6. Initially, intermittent cold compresses to scrotum—for pain relief.
7. Local heat or sitz bath later—to hasten resolution of inflammatory process.
8. Observe for possible abscess formation.

Discharge Planning and Health Education

Instruct the patient as follows:
1. Avoid straining (lifting, defecation) and sexual excitement until infection is under control.
2. It may take 4 weeks or longer for epididymis to return to normal.
3. Sex partners of patients with chlamydial urethritis or epididymitis should be examined and treated.

VASECTOMY

Vasectomy is the ligation and transection of a section of the vas deferens; a bilateral vasectomy is a sterilization procedure for males.

Clinical Indications

1. Performed as a sterilization procedure.
2. Performed if the patient has recurrent acute epididymitis (see above).

Underlying Considerations

1. A vasectomy interrupts the transportation of the sperm. This procedure has no effect on sexual

potency, erection, ejaculation, or production of male hormones.

2. Seminal fluid is mostly manufactured in the seminal vesicles and prostate which are unaffected by vasectomy.
   a. There will be no noticeable decrease in the amount of ejaculated fluid; the sperm accounts for less than 5% of the volume. The sperm cells are reabsorbed into the body.
   b. Psychological problems have been noted in an occasional patient following this procedure.
3. A vasectomy can be done on an outpatient basis with local anesthesia.
4. A legal consent form must be obtained, usually from patient and his partner.
5. The patient should be advised that he will be sterile but that potency will not be altered following a bilateral vasectomy. Rarely is there a spontaneous reanastomosis resulting in pregnancy.
6. A vasectomy may not be reversible and should be considered permanent; microsurgical techniques are being used for vasectomy reversal (vasovasotomy); success rates are promising.

Postoperative Management

1. Apply ice bags intermittently to the scrotum for several hours after surgery to reduce swelling and relieve discomfort.
2. Reassure patient that discoloration of scrotal skin, swelling, and edema are to be expected.

3. Advise patient to wear suspensory for added comfort and support

Complications

1. Sperm granuloma—due to extravasation of sperm
2. Infection
3. Recanalization of vas deferens (very rare)
4. Bleeding and hematoma

Health Education

Instruct the patient as follows:
1. The primary function of the testicle(s) is the production of hormones and of sperm. A vasectomy will not interfere with these functions but it will interrupt the descent of sperm from the testicle to the ejaculatory ducts.
2. Rest for 48 hours after surgery to prevent discomfort.
3. Avoid strenuous activities for several days
4. Sexual intercourse may be resumed as desired.
5. Contraceptives should be used until the sperm stored distal to the point of interruption of the vas is evacuated; (2 negative semen specimens one month apart). *The patient is still fertile for a variable period of time after vasectomy.*
6. Absence of sperm must be demonstrated microscopically; laboratory tests confirm that no sperm are present in the seminal fluid.
7. A vasectomy does not prevent venereal disease.

CONDITIONS AFFECTING THE PENIS

ULCERATION OF THE GLANS PENIS

Causes

1. Chancre—venereal ulcer caused by *Treponema pallidum*, page 823 Syphilis
2. Cancer
3. Herpes—Small blisters that may produce secondary ulceration
4. Balanitis—inflammation and ulceration produced by a spirochete and a gram-positive bacillus
5. Chancroid—ulceration produced by mixed infection

Clinical Manifestations

Ulceration of the penis should be suspected as being venereal in origin until proved otherwise.

Diagnostic Evaluation

1. Dark field microscopic examination of smear for spirochetes
2. Serological (blood) test for syphilis

Treatment

Varies greatly depending on the cause of ulceration

OTHER CONDITIONS

Gonorrhea.

See page 807.

Phimosis

A condition in which the foreskin is narrowed and cannot be retracted over the glans. The treatment is circumcision.

Paraphimosis

A condition in which the foreskin is retracted behind the glans, and because of narrowness and subsequent edema, cannot be reduced back to its normal position.

Priapism

An uncontrolled persistent erection of the penis occurring from sickle cell thrombosis, chronic irritation, tumor invasion, etc. Treatment includes bed rest, sedation, icepacks, or surgery.

CIRCUMCISION

Circumcision is the excision of the foreskin (prepuce) of the glans penis.

Clinical Indications

1. Usually done in infancy for hygienic purposes
2. Phimosis
3. Paraphimosis
4. Recurrent infections of glans and foreskin
5. Personal desire of patient (or parents if patient is a minor)

Postoperative Nursing Management

1. Watch for bleeding.
2. Change petrolatum (vaseline) gauze dressing as directed.
3. Give analgesia as patient's condition indicates; circumcision can be quite painful in the adult male.
NOTE: *Circumcision is an important preventive measure against carcinoma of the penis.*

2 GYNECOLOGIC CONDITIONS

MENSTRUATION

Menstruation is a physiologic process in the female of childbearing age.
1. If conception does not occur, the ovum dies; tissue lining the endometrial cavity, which has become thickened and congested, becomes hemorrhagic.
2. Tissue lining the uterus, blood cells, and breakdown-products slough off and are discharged through the cervix into the vagina.
3. This cyclic process is called *menstruation* and usually occurs about every 28-30 days.
4. The average flow of blood lasts about 4-5 days and totals 50-150 ml.
   Menarche or onset of menstruation occurs between 11 and 15 years.
   Ovulation refers to the expulsion of an ovum from the ovary—14 days before the onset of the next menstrual period.
   As the endometrium is being shed, the process of repair and regrowth starts again—preparing once more for the reception of a fertilized ovum.

DISTURBANCES OF MENSTRUATION

A relationship with feedback mechanism exists between the hormonal secretions of the ovary, adrenal, thyroid, and pituitary glands. An increase or decrease in the activity of one or more glands can cause a disturbance in menstruation.

Dysmenorrhea

Dysmenorrhea is painful menstruation.

A. *Occurrence*

Common in unmarried women and women who have not borne children.

B. *Types*
1. Primary—due to unknown factors; thought to be intrinsic to uterus; extrinsic pathology such as polyp and fibroids may be a factor.
   May involve emotional and psychological factors.
2. Secondary—due to factors extrinsic to uterus, such as endometriosis, pelvic infection.

C. *Symptoms*
1. Pain may be due to uterine spasm caused by a narrowing of cervical canal (exaggerated uterine contractility).
2. Pain—colicky, cyclic, nagging, dull ache; usually in lower abdomen, may radiate down back of legs. May be severe enough to require bed rest for a day or two.
3. Severe dysmenorrhea may be experienced—with chills, headache, diarrhea, nausea, vomiting, and syncope.

D. *Etiology*
1. Endocrine
   Some investigators believe there is a relation between release of prostaglandin from the endometrium and the symptoms of dysmenorrhea; this has not been proven.
2. Anatomic
   a. Some discomfort results from the passing of a cervical sound or from dilatation of the cervix; a pathological growth could produce the same symptoms.
   b. An infantile or small uterus may contribute to dysmenorrhea but this has not been proven.
3. Constitutional
   Chronic illnesses and general debilitation seem to be associated with a high incidence of dysmenorrhea (anemia, fatigue, diabetes, tuberculosis).
4. Psychogenic
   Most studies indicate that strong underlying psychological factors cause dysmenorrhea. Parental instruction and a healthy emotional environment for the growing young girl, in a setting where realistic family relations are cultivated, almost precludes primary dysmenorrhea.

E. *Treatment and Nursing Management*

Since there is no single treatment for dysmenorrhea, a three-pronged approach seems best to relieve symptoms: Combine therapies as they relate to constitutional, hormonal, and psychological factors.
1. Selective, according to needs of individual and severity of problem.
   a. Proper psychological preparation of girls for menarche.
   b. Good posture; use special exercises to improve posture and correct weak musculature and imbalance.
2. Since emotional makeup may accentuate discomfort, psychotherapy or pharmacotherapy may be necessary.
3. Complete physical examination to rule out other physical abnormalities.
4. Instructions to patient:
   a. Usual activity is possible—should be encouraged.
   b. Mild analgesics for discomfort are permissible.
   c. Avoid use of habit-forming drugs such as narcotics and alcohol.
5. Dysmenorrhea can usually be eliminated by oral contraceptives which block ovulation.
6. Regular exercises (as well as physical activity) are recommended.
7. Administration of a prostaglandin inhibitor such as ibuprofen (Motrin) or mefenamid acid (Ponstel) has recently been recommended and appears to be effective in relieving primary dysmenorrhea.
8. If the above are unsuccessful, surgery may be necessary.
   Presacral and ovarian neurectomy (cutting nerve fibers) may be done.
9. Psychological counseling may also benefit some individuals.

Amenorrhea

Amenorrhea is absence of menstrual flow.

A. *Primary*—when a girl is 16 or 17 and has not menstruated.
1. May be caused by embryonic maldevelopment
2. Treatment is according to etiology

B. *Secondary*—menstruation has begun (initial menarche) but stops.
1. Causes:
   a. Normal pregnancy and lactation
   b. Psychogenic (minor emotional upsets)
      Hypothalamic disturbances (anatomic nervous system) may also be the cause. Example—anorexia nervosa
   c. Constitutional
      Any disturbance of metabolism and nutrition. Examples—diabetes, tuberculosis, obesity
2. Treatment: Directed at cause—constitutional therapy, psychotherapy, hormone therapy, surgery.

Oligomenorrhea

Oligomenorrhea is markedly diminished menstrual flow—nearing amenorrhea.

Menorrhagia

Menorrhagia is excessive bleeding during regular menstruation.

A. *Causes*
1. Endocrine disturbances
2. Inflammatory diseases; benign or malignant pelvic tumors
3. Emotional stress

B. *Treatment*
1. Search for underlying cause.
2. Correct blood deficiency

Metrorrhagia

Metrorrhagia is bleeding from uterus between regular menstrual periods.
   Significant because it is usually a symptom of some disease—often cancer or benign tumors of uterus and adnexa.

Polymenorrhea

Polymenorrhea is frequent menstruation occurring at intervals of less than 3 weeks.

MENOPAUSE

Menopause is the stage of female life when there is physiologic cessation of the menses along with progressive ovarian failure.
   Climacteric is the transition period (perimenopausal period: premenopause, menopause, and postmenopause) during which the woman's reproductive function gradually diminishes and disappears. It usually occurs between the ages of 49 and 55 (mean 51.4).

Clinical Manifestations

1. The monthly menstrual flow becomes smaller in amount, then becomes irregular, and finally ceases.
2. Hot or warm flashes and other vascular disturbances may be in evidence and are of endocrinologic origin.
3. Additional physical signs are:
   a. Manifestations of atrophy: sagging structures, atrophic vaginitis
   b. Evidence of stress incontinence on occasion
   c. Skin dryness; weight gain
   d. Calcium deficiency (which may lead to osteoporotic changes)
4. Psychological manifestations:
   a. Dizziness, weakness, nervousness, insomnia
   b. Headaches; inability to concentrate.
   c. A feeling of being unneeded
   d. Fear of growing old; depression

Treatment and Nursing Management

1. Most women respond favorably to a regimen of education and modification of life style. Adherence to habits that promote good health is desirable.
2. Mild sedatives and tranquilizers may be required by some to relieve nervousness and tension.
3. For persistent or severe hot flashes, it may be necessary to resort to estrogen therapy: diethylstilbestrol, Premarin, or ethinyl estradiol (Estinyl). Close medical supervision is required.
4. Continued use of estrogens to prevent widespread degenerative changes continues to be controversial; however, long-term use of estrogens has been linked with cancer.
   a. Estrogen replacement should not be withheld from women who need it (less than one fourth of menopausal women). Indiscriminate use of estrogens is strongly discouraged.

Health Education

1. "Change of life" is not abnormal nor need it be limiting.
2. Sex life is by no means terminated; in many instances it is enhanced.
3. Avoid overfatigue and stress situations, since these exaggerate minor problems.
4. Encourage a nutritious diet and keep weight under control.
5. Develop outside interests that help to absorb anxieties and lessen tension.
6. Continue to exercise and develop self-fulfilling and enriching activities.
7. Recognize that the expected life span after menopause is 30–35 years.
8. To allay vaginal dryness and pain on intercourse (due to estrogen deficiency), it is safer to use a water-based lubricant (K-Y Jelly or Lubafax) than an estrogen cream.
   Topical estrogens produce systemic effects; therefore, it cannot be assumed that their action has limited local effects.

DIAGNOSTIC STUDIES FOR GYNECOLOGIC CONDITIONS

PELVIC EXAMINATION

A *pelvic examination* is an inspection of the external genitalia for signs of inflammation, swelling, bleeding, discharge, or local skin and epithelial changes. A speculum is inserted to permit the examiner to visualize the vagina and cervix.

(For Guidelines: Vaginal Examination by the Nurse, see p. 531.)

A. *Patient Preparation*

1. Provide psychological support—patient needs reassurance, understanding, and skillful consideration of her emotional as well as physical problems.
2. Instruct patient to avoid douching for 24 hours before examination; cellular deposits might wash away.
3. Encourage patient to go to bathroom before examination—voiding and bowel evacuation before the examination provide more relaxation of perineal tissues.
4. Advise patient to remove sufficient clothing to permit adequate exposure of genitalia and allow for examination of the abdomen.
5. Avoid undue exposure of the patient.

B. *Positioning of Patient* (best done on an examining table but can be achieved on a bed)

1. *Lithotomy*—knees and hips flexed; heels resting on foot rests.
   a. Drape sheet diagonally over patient so that corner may be grasped and pulled upward to expose perineal area.
   b. When examination is done in bed, the patient is positioned across the bed with hips extending slightly over the edge (dorsal supine position); feet are placed on examiner's knees or on 2 chairs placed next to the bed.
2. *Sims' position*—the patient lies on one side, usually the left, with the left arm behind her back. The right (uppermost) thigh and knee are flexed as much as possible; left leg is partially flexed.
3. *Knee-Chest*—Patient kneels on table with feet extending over the end.
   a. Separate knees and maintain thighs at right angles to the table.
   b. Turn patient's head to one side and allow face and chest to rest on a soft pillow.
   c. Patient's arms may grasp sides of table.

C. *Procedure for Examining the Pelvis*

1. A speculum is inserted so that the vaginal tissues and condition of cervix can be visualized.
2. *Cytology Smear* (Papanicolaou) is best made by scraping cervix directly (see Fig. 11-12).

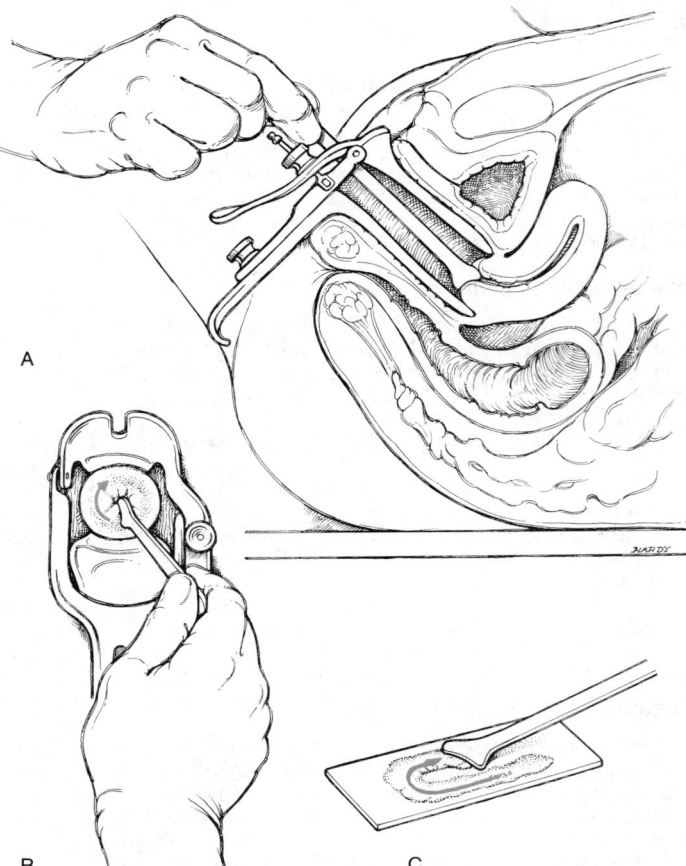

FIGURE 11-12. *A cervical scrape of secretions for cytology is obtained by using a wooden Ayre spatula. A. Shows the speculum in place: the Ayre spatula is inserted so that the longer end is placed snugly in the os. B. A representative sample of secretions is obtained by rotating the spatula. C. Cervical secretions are gently smeared on a glass slide in a single circular motion. The slide is placed in the appropriate fixative. Using a cotton tipped applicator, also obtain a smear from the floor of the vagina below the cervix and preserve in the same manner.*

3. *Bimanual examination*—by inserting 1 or 2 gloved fingers of the left hand in the vagina and palpating the abdomen with the right hand, it is possible to further examine the uterus and adnexa.

4. *Rectal Examination*—to detect abnormalities of contour, motility, and placement of adjacent structures and tissues.

D. *Nursing Intervention and Support*

1. Attend and support the patient by encouraging her to relax, by holding her hand, etc.
2. Focus the light and uncover examining tray with speculum, swabs, cytology necessities, etc.

3. Assist physician by providing gloves, lubricant, etc.
4. At conclusion of examination, wipe discharge from patient before assisting her from the table.
5. Have patient slide up on table before removing feet from stirrups.
6. Allow time for older patient to adjust to sitting position before helping her off the table.
7. Answer any questions patient may have; elaborate on physician's instructions.
8. Assist patient with dressing if necessary.

GUIDELINES: Vaginal Examination by the Nurse

Purposes
1. To inspect the vaginal canal and cervix.
2. To obtain tissue specimen for cervical cytology and other tests.

Equipment

Perineal drape
Vaginal specula
Water soluble lubricant
Sterile gloves

Long swab sticks
Pap smear equipment
Adequate lighting

Procedure   **Preparatory Phase**

1. Have woman void before assistant positions her on examining table.
2. Position woman on examining table (woman's slip may be kept on but other clothing from waist to knees is removed).
   a. Have buttocks at edge of table.
   b. Position feet in stirrups to assume dorsal lithotomy position.
   c. Make patient as comfortable as possible with a small pillow under her head.
   d. Drape patient to permit minimal exposure (but adequate for examiner).
3. Encourage patient to relax; tell her what you are doing and what she may feel.
4. Adjust light for maximum focus.

NURSING ACTION	RATIONALE/AMPLIFICATION
Performance Phase	
1. Be gentle and take your time; don sterile gloves; lubricate fingers.	1. This promotes relaxation of patient, making the procedure easier for both.
2. Observe external genitalia for apparent abnormalities; gently separate labia and continue visual inspection.	2. Note any evidence of irritation, infection, or abnormalities.
3. To encourage relaxation in patient, gently place the tip of 1 or 2 fingers into introitus.	3. Say to patient, "Tighten your muscles and squeeze my fingers—try hard—then relax."
4. Identify cervix manually and depress the perineum downward with your fingers.	4. Downward pressure is away from the more sensitive anterior structures.
5. Gently insert warm speculum horizontally, passing it over your fingers and aiming it toward the cervix.	5. If it is preferred not to initially insert gloved fingers, the speculum is introduced vertically using a downward pressure (after entering the vestibule, the speculum is slowly rotated to the horizontal position).
6. Slowly open the speculum and lock into position. With slow manipulation, the speculum can be turned to permit visualization of the vaginal walls.	6. Walls normally are pink and moist. A pale white secretion may be noted.
7. Inspect the cervix, which should be pink in color. Normally, the os is a dent, unless the women has had children, in which case a slit is noted.	7. If woman is taking oral contraceptive, the cervix may be deep pink to red. A thread coming out of cervix would suggest presence of an IUD.
8. If Pap test is to be done, follow procedure in Fig. 11-12. For a Schiller test, see p. 532.	
9. When removing speculum, hold it open until cervix is cleared; then withdraw speculum and let it close as it will.	9. By the time speculum is completely withdrawn, it will be closed.
10. For palpation (Bimanual Examination) see above	

GUIDELINES: Vaginal Examination by the Nurse (cont.)

Procedure (cont.)	NURSING ACTION	RATIONALE/AMPLIFICATION
	Follow-up Phase	
	1. Gently wipe the perineal area with soft tissue or gauze using firm strokes from the pubic area back to beyond the rectum.	1. This will remove secretions and liquid lubricant.
	2. Instruct assistant in carefully helping patient to remove feet from stirrups.	2. Both feet must be removed at the same time to reduce strain.
	3. Elevate the lower third of examining table to receive legs—permits patient to assume dorsal recumbent position.	3. Keep patient covered with a sheet.
	4. Assist patient in sliding toward head end of table; provide a wide-based stool for her to step on as she gets off table.	4. Do not rush patient as she is getting off the table, since sudden shifting from recumbent to sitting position may cause a feeling of dizziness.
	5. Assist patient in dressing (closing zippers, etc.) if necessary. Answer any queries woman may have.	

OTHER DIAGNOSTIC TESTS

Cytology Test for Cancer (Papanicolaou)

A. *Purpose*—To screen for cervical dysplasia and/or cervical cancer. Occasionally adenocarcinoma of the endometrium will also be discovered.

B. *Procedure*—See Fig. 11-12.

1. Examination and interpretation of cytologic smear is done by the pathologist.
2. Classification of cytologic findings (after Papanicolaou)
   Class 1—Absence of atypical or abnormal cells.
   Class 2—Atypical cytology but no evidence of malignancy.
   Class 3—Cytology suggestive of, but not conclusive for, malignancy.
   Class 4—Cytology strongly suggestive of malignancy.
   Class 5—Cytology conclusive for malignancy.
3. If the patient has an abnormal smear of Class 2, 3, or 4, explain to her that this is not conclusive but requires additional testing such as biopsy and conization.

Schiller Iodine Test

(A simple test to outline unhealthy epithelium.)

A. *Rationale*—Cancer epithelium contains no glycogen whereas normal cervical epithelial cells do contain glycogen; glycogen has the ability to absorb iodine stain.

NOTE: Schiller's test is unreliable for cancer and only suggests some epithelial change.

B. *Procedure*—A long applicator stick is used to paint the cervix with Schiller's 2% iodine solution.

1. *Negative result*—a mahogany brown color covering entire surface indicates a reaction between iodine and glycogen of normal cells.
2. *Positive result*—tissues are not stained brown; this indicates that immature cells are present and suggests the need for a biopsy.

Cervical Biopsy and Cauterization

A. *Purpose*—to remove cervical tissue for laboratory study.

B. *Patient Preparation*

1. To be done preferably at a time when cervix is least vascular (usually a week after the end of the menstrual flow).
2. Explain the nature of the procedure to the patient.
3. Place her in lithotomy position and drape her properly.
4. Explain to her that no anesthesia is required since the cervix does not have pain receptors.

C. *Procedure*

1. After the speculum is positioned in the vagina and the cervix properly exposed, the surgeon, under colposcopic guidance, uses a biopsy forceps to take bits of cervical tissues.
2. Tissue is preserved in 10% formalin, labeled, and sent to the laboratory.
3. If bleeding occurs, suturing and packing may be necessary.

D. *Aftercare of Patient*

1. A brief rest after the procedure is usually necessary before the patient leaves.
2. Discharge instructions/health education:
   Instruct the patient as follows:
   a. Avoid heavy lifting for 24 hours.
   b. Packing will remain in place for 12–24 hours depending on physician's preference.
   c. There may be some bleeding; however, more than that of a normal period must be reported to the physician.
   d. Obtain physician's instructions regarding douching and sexual relations.

Uterotubal Insufflation (Rubin's Test)

Carbon dioxide is injected under pressure through a special cannula into the cervical canal. If one or both tubes are patent, the gas will pass through the fallopian tubes into the peritoneal cavity.

1. The patient is prepared as for a vaginal examination.
2. A Graves speculum is positioned in the vagina.
3. Special cannula is passed through intrauterine canal; cervix is held tightly with a tenaculum against a rubber stopper to prevent gas leakage.
4. Tubing is connected to a machine which measures and records pressure.

Findings

1. Normal—if pressure is below 180 mm. Hg and gas is heard (with a stethoscope) passing through the tubes

2. Partial obstruction—180–200 mm. Hg
3. Complete obstruction—200 mm. Hg and above.

Culdoscopy

A *culdoscopy* is an uncommon operative, diagnostic procedure in which an incision is made into the posterior vaginal cul-de-sac so that a culdoscope can be inserted for the purpose of visualizing the uterus, tubes, broad ligaments, uterosacral ligaments, rectal wall, sigmoid, and even the small intestines.
1. The patient is prepared as for any vaginal operation.
2. Anesthesia may be local, general, or regional.
3. The knee-chest position is best for a culdoscopy.
4. Following the examination, the scope is withdrawn and sutures placed; the patient is returned to her room.

Hysteroscopy

Hysteroscopy—the endoscopic visualization of the uterine cavity by means of a hysteroscope.
1. Earlier attempts were usually unsuccessful because uterine bleeding obscured the view.
2. Today, fiberoptic lighting and the distention of the uterine cavity with dextran solution permits optimum visualization.

A. *Indications*—primarily to complement other diagnostic procedures, chiefly the staging of endometrial cancer.
1. Problem of infertility.
2. When the cause of uterine bleeding is unknown.
3. To view lesions which can be photographed and removed in some instances.
4. To diagnose and manage intrauterine adhesions.
5. For transuterine tubal sterilization.

B. *Contraindications*
1. Pelvic infection.
2. Recurrent upper genital tract infection.
3. Uterine perforation
4. Pregnancy, because of possible disturbance of pregnancy and risk of infection.

C. *Patient Preparation and Examination*
1. Administer the prescribed sedative and mild tranquilizer prior to the examination. Explanation is similar to that for D & C.
2. Place the patient in the lithotomy position as for a D & C.
3. Cleanse the perineum and vagina immediately prior to sterile draping.
4. The examiner performs a bimanual palpation of the uterus.
5. Inject local anesthesia into the cervix, which is positioned with a tenaculum forceps.
6. Insert sounds into the cervical canal for dilatation prior to insertion of endoscope.
7. With endoscope in place, slowly infuse endometrial cavity with a concentrated solution of dextran.
8. Uterine walls are visualized with a 30-degree oblique lens rather than with the 180-degree system.

D. *Follow-up*
1. Following removal of instruments, the patient is returned to bed to rest.
2. She may be discharged later the same day.

X-Ray Studies—Hysterosalpingogram

A *hysterosalpingogram* is an x-ray study of the uterus and fallopian tubes following the injection of a contrast medium.

A. *Purpose*
1. To study sterility problems.
2. To determine extent of tubal patency.
3. To note the presence of pathology in the uterine cavity.

B. *Procedure*
1. Patient is placed in lithotomy position on a fluoroscopic x-ray table.
2. The bivalve speculum is introduced to expose cervix.
3. Contrast medium is injected into uterine cavity.
4. X-rays are taken to determine configuration of pelvic area.

GUIDELINES: Colposcopy

Colposcopy is a stereoscopic examination of the cervix using a binocular instrument with strong light illumination.

Purposes
1. To determine distribution of abnormal squamous epithelium.
2. To pinpoint areas from which biopsy tissue can be taken.

Indications
1. Following atypical vaginal or cervical cytology (in Pap smear).
2. When suspicious cervical lesions are present.
3. Previous treatment for dysplasia or cancer of the cervix.
Advantage: Colposcopy may spare the patient a conization (D & C), which may require hospitalization.

Procedure **Preparatory Phase**
1. Identical to that for preparation of patient having pelvic examination (p. 530).
2. Additional explanation may be required so that the patient will know what to expect.

NURSING ACTION	RATIONALE/AMPLIFICATION
Performance Phase	
1. Use a long cotton applicator stick to dry cervix.	1. This will clear away mucus and other secretions.

GUIDELINES: Colposcopy (cont.)

Procedure (cont.)	NURSING ACTION	RATIONALE/AMPLIFICATION
	2. Swab cervix with saline using long cotton applicator.	2. Moistening of cervical epithelium allows vascular patterns and squamous columnar junction to be visualized.
	3. Examine tissue with colposcope utilizing green filter illuminator.	
	4. Paint cervix with 3% acetic acid.	4. This acts as a mucolytic agent and accentuates epithelial topography.
	5. Note colposcopic patterns—particularly the transformation area (where columnar epithelium is replaced by squamous epithelium).	5. Acetic acid tends to draw moisture from tissues of high nuclear density—this accounts for color changes in the cervical epithelium.
	6. Biopsy (using a fine biopsy forceps) any questionable area; endocervical curettage should also be done.	6. The cervical os has few nerve endings so the patient will experience minimal discomfort.
	7. If bleeding occurs, direct pressure or application of silver nitrate stick will usually stop it. Some clinicians prefer to apply ferric subsulfate (Monsel's solution) via applicator stick for hemostasis.	7. Measures to prevent or control bleeding.
	8. Insert a vaginal tampon following examination.	8. To absorb discharge; may be removed after 5–6 hours.

Follow-up Phase

Similar to that following pelvic examination; see p. 531.

GUIDELINES: Using the Gravlee Jet Washer for Endometrial Cytology

The *Gravlee Jet Washer* is an intrauterine washing device that uses the principle of negative pressure to obtain cytologic and tissue-fragment specimens.

Equipment

Gravlee Jet Washer sterile disposable unit (Upjohn) (Fig. 11-13)
Vaginal specula, tenaculum forceps, sterile uterine probes, water-soluble lubricant, long swab sticks

Sterile gloves for gynecologist   Perineal drape
Antiseptic solution   Pap smear equipment

Procedure

Preparatory Phase

1. Similar to that for a pelvic examination.
   a. Have patient empty bladder immediately before procedure.
   b. Place patient in lithotomy position (legs in stirrups).
2. Explain to the patient that a specimen of tissue lining the uterus will be taken by a flushing-out process that is relatively painless; the patient may experience menstrual-like cramps during the procedure.

NURSING ACTION	RATIONALE/AMPLIFICATION
Performance Phase *(by gynecologist)*	
1. Insert speculum into vagina; perform Papanicolaou smear of cervix and vagina.	1. Cytology studies of tissue from the vagina and cervix can be done.
2. Remove speculum; perform bimanual examination.	2. Size and position of uterus can be noted.
3. Reintroduce speculum. Cleanse vaginal vault and cervix with antiseptic solution.	3. To minimize number of organisms in the area preparatory to entering uterine cavity.
4. Grasp cervix with tenaculum forceps to stabilize the uterus.	4. To reduce the extent of displacement of the uterus.
5. Introduce a sterile probe into cervical canal using extreme caution because of danger of perforating uterine wall.	5. To determine depth and angle of uterine cavity.
6. Prepare cannula from tray by adjusting rubber stopper; bend cannula to conform to curvature of uterine cavity.	6. To indicate length of cannula which can be safely introduced into the uterus and to serve as a water-seal plug at the cervical os.
7. Pour 30 ml. of sterile isotonic saline into reservoir (Fig. 11-13).	
8. Attach cap to receptacle after directing small tube into solution of receptacle; twist receptacle counterclockwise to screw cap in place.	8. To assemble equipment in working order.
9. Introduce cannula into uterine cavity and secure rubber plug into cervical opening.	9. To produce an intact irrigating system.

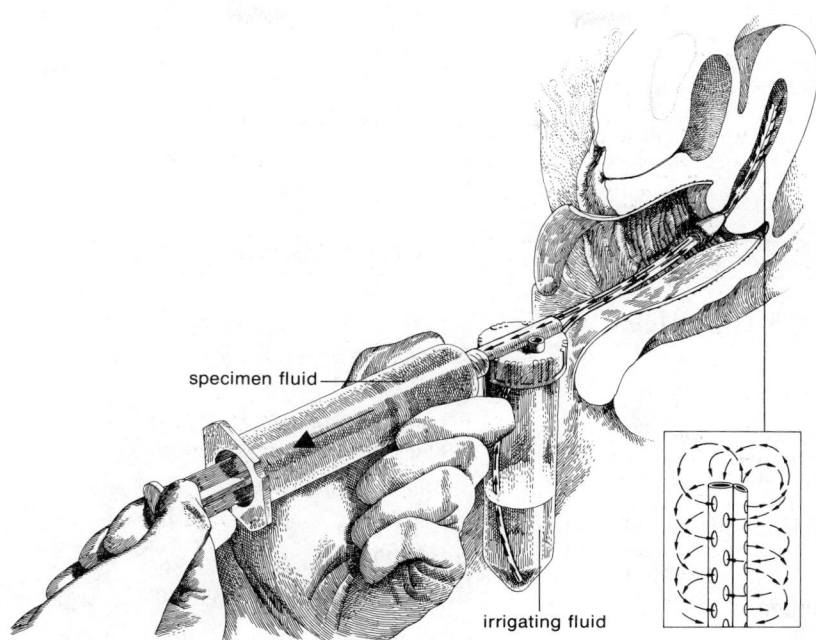

specimen fluid

irrigating fluid

FIGURE 11-13. *Pulling on the plunger of a 30-ml. syringe in the Gravlee Jet Washer creates a negative pressure in the uterine cavity causing sterile saline from the vertical receptacle to be drawn into the uterine cavity for irrigation. Since no more than 1–4 ml. are in this cavity at one time, and since there is negative pressure, fluid does not get out into the fallopian tubes. Note the rubber plug at the cervical os which assists in creating an airtight system. The boxed diagram at the lower right demonstrates how the fluids circulate in the uterine cavity. (Courtesy Upjohn.)*

Procedure (cont.)

NURSING ACTION	RATIONALE/AMPLIFICATION
10. Drawing on the plunger of the syringe causes irrigating fluid to flow into the uterus and out into the barrel of the syringe.	10. Saline bathes the endometrial cavity and dislodges cells and small tissue fragments. This negative-pressure lavage system prevents the possibility of reflux into the fallopian tubes.
11. When the syringe is filled, remove the device from the uterus.	

Follow-up Phase

1. Disconnect syringe, expel its contents into saline reservoir through porthole on top of cap.
2. Expel any tissue collected along cannula into collecting receptacle.
3. Apply unused screw cap, attach identification label, and send to laboratory immediately for block cytology.

1. This forms the handy receptacle which will be sent to the laboratory.

3. If specimen does not go to laboratory immediately, a formalin or alcohol preservative must be added. (5 ml. of 10% buffered formalin or equal parts of ether and 95% ethyl alcohol).

DILATATION AND CURETTAGE (D & C)

Dilatation and curettage is a widening of the cervical canal with a dilator and the scraping of the uterine canal with a curette. The cervix is scraped first without dilatation.

Purposes

1. To secure endometrial and endocervical tissue for tissue study.
2. To control abnormal uterine bleeding.
3. To serve as a therapeutic measure for incomplete abortion.

Nursing Management

A. *Preoperative Care*

1. Inform the patient about the nature of the operation to be done (usually done by a gynecologist).
2. Answer questions patient may have regarding D & C.
3. Ascertain whether patient has been told what to expect with regard to postoperative discomfort, drainage, or incapacity following the D & C.
4. Check with physician regarding perineal shave (some prefer no shave).

5. Prepare bladder and intestinal tract by having patient void and by giving a small enema.

B. *Postoperative Care*

1. Check that perineal pad is in place with a sanitary belt.
2. Replace each perineal pad with a sterile pad as required during the time packing is in place.

3. Report excessive bleeding.
4. Recommend bed rest for the remainder of the day, with bathroom privileges.
5. Offer mild analgesics for low back pain and pelvic discomfort.
6. Offer meals as desired.

CONDITIONS OF THE EXTERNAL GENITALIA AND VAGINA

CONTACT DERMATITIS OF THE VULVA
Nature of the Irritation

1. An inflammation of the vulvar skin is annoying because it causes itching.
2. Itching causes scratching, which presents an open lesion subject to many irritants: vaginal discharge, skin secretions, menstrual discharge, urine, and feces.
3. In addition, there is local irritation caused by close-fitting synthetic-fabric underpants, girdles, panty-hose, and slacks, and by laundry detergents.

Treatment and Health Education

Instruct the patient as follows:
1. Take pharmacotherapeutic agents as prescribed.
2. Carefully cleanse the perineal area with cotton pledgets that have been moistened in a warm bland soap solution.
3. Pat dry with a soft washcloth or dry cotton pledgets.
4. Dust lightly with a nonperfumed powder as an aid in keeping the area dry; cornstarch is very effective.
5. Do not use sprays, perfumed soaps, topical anesthetic agents—they may compound the problem.
6. Replace synthetic-fabric undergarments with loose cotton underclothing.
7. Avoid wearing tight garments over the cotton undergarments.
8. Thoroughly wash and rinse all underclothing (use soap, not detergents).

PRURITUS

Pruritus is an itching of the vulva which often accompanies chronic infections of genital tract such as trichomoniasis, gonorrhea, or yeast infection—particularly in young women.

Clinical Manifestations

1. Itching followed by scratching and a thickening of tissues.
2. Patient often appears nervous.

Treatment

1. Real cause may be difficult to discover.
2. Cleanliness must be scrupulous.
3. Glucosuria and urinary incontinence must be controlled.
4. Temporary relief is obtained from soothing lotions and ointments.

CONDYLOMATA

Condylomata are warty papillary excrescences on the external genitalia.

Cause

1. Irritation and infection.

Types

1. Pointed type associated with gonorrhea.
2. Flat type considered syphilitic.

Clinical Manifestations

Leukorrheal discharge causing irritation.

Treatment

Directed to venereal problem.

KRAUROSIS AND LEUKOPLAKIA

Kraurosis is a disease of the vulva; the skin becomes thin, dry, white and easily fissured.
   Leukoplakia is similar to kraurosis; grayish-white patchy thickening and hardening of vulvar tissues with itching and burning. Treated like kraurosis.

Clinical Manifestations

1. As disease progresses, vulva appears shrunken and leathery.
2. Marked itching.
3. May lead to cancer of the vulva.

Management

1. Ovarian extract, antihistaminics, vitamin A.
2. Advanced problem may require a vulvectomy (p. 537).

VULVITIS AND ABSCESS OF GREATER VESTIBULAR GLAND (BARTHOLIN'S GLAND)

Vulvitis is an inflammation of the vulva; the cause may be infection possibly caused by uncleanliness. Common offending organisms are *Escherichia coli*, staphylococcus, streptococcus, gonococcus, and *Trichomonas vaginalis*.

Clinical Manifestations

1. Burning pain which is worse with intercourse.
2. Red and edematous tissue with profuse purulent exudate.
3. Acute throbbing pain and swelling between labia indicating vulvovaginal abscess (infection of Bartholin's glands).
4. When the acute infection subsides, the problem tends to become chronic.

Treatment and Nursing Management

1. Advise the patient to remain in bed; administer analgesics for the relief of pain.

2. Employ thermotherapy in the form of hot packs and sitz baths for comfort.
3. Administer broad spectrum antibacterial agents to combat infection.
4. Prepare the patient for incision and drainage of the abscess, which will afford immediate relief.
5. Marsupialization (creation of a pouch) with or without biopsy is indicated when there are painful recurrences or obstruction at introitus.
   a. Ice packs are applied intermittently for 24 hours to reduce edema and provide comfort.
   b. Thereafter, warm sitz baths or a perineal heat lamp are comforting.

CANCER OF THE VULVA

Incidence

1. Most common in elderly women; cancer of the vulva represents 3–4% of all malignancies of female reproductive system.
2. Women seem reluctant to seek medical attention in early phases when ulcer is small and on the skin surface; they tend to delay until the ulcer becomes infected and painful.
3. Early radical vulvectomy with complete node dissection is curative. If the lesion is large and treatment late, cures are unlikely.

Clinical Manifestations

1. In orderly progression, symptoms are: severe vulvar pruritus, reddened, pigmented, whitish or slightly elevated lesions with ulceration.
2. Frequent site
   a. Labia majora—mid or anterior portion
   b. Clitoris
   c. Encroachment upon urethra in larger lesions
3. Less frequent sites—fourchette and posterior labial areas.
4. As disease progresses, tissues become edematous and lymphadenopathy is apparent.
5. Secondary infection is responsible for foul-smelling discharge.

Diagnostic Evaluation

1. A biopsy is taken after procaine is injected. The entire lesion, when it is small, may be excised; but final treatment is reserved until laboratory studies are completed.
2. Superficial lymph nodes on both sides are palpated for metastasis.
3. Pelvic examination is necessary to determine the extent of the cancer (clinical stage) and to rule out other pelvic neoplastic disease.

Treatment

This depends on type and extent of malignancy:
1. Basal cell carcinoma requires superficial hemivulvectomy.
2. Carcinoma in situ (noninvasive carcinoma) is treated by simple vulvectomy.
3. Invasive carcinoma calls for a radical vulvectomy and bilateral lymph node resection—often requiring removal of the deep pelvic (retroperitoneal) nodes.

Nursing Management

A. *Preoperative Care*

1. Shave a wide area to include perineal, pubic, and inguinal areas.

2. Encourage the patient to talk about her condition and to ask questions.
   a. Concerns occur regarding fear of mutilation and loss of sexual function.
   b. Possibility of becoming pregnant again may be important to the woman of childbearing age.
   c. The possibility of metastasis, and its effects, cause the cancer patient to be concerned about prognosis, suffering, relation to others in the family, etc.
3. Cleanse the vulva thoroughly 2 or 3 days prior to surgery by using sitz baths twice daily.
4. Evacuate the intestinal tract before surgery to provide the advantage of no bowel movements for 2–3 days postoperatively.

B. *Objectives of Postoperative Care*

1. To maintain proper drainage and compression of tissues, connect drains to suction.
2. To promote comfort, place patient in low Fowler's position with knees slightly elevated with a pillow to lessen tension on sutures.
3. To minimize postoperative complications, mobilize patient on the day of surgery.
4. To prevent infection of wound and bladder, clean the wound daily with warm sterile solutions as prescribed (dilute hydrogen peroxide, saline, antibacterial solution) and follow with a warm water spray. Later, after the stitches are removed, a heat lamp to the vulva for 5 minutes twice a day may be required.
5. To facilitate wound healing, some physicians prefer dry heat such as that provided by a heating lamp until the stitches are removed; this is followed by perineal packs or soaks.
6. To prevent straining on defecation and wound contamination, offer a low residue diet.
7. To prevent bladder infection, give meticulous care to the vagina and urethral orifice.
8. To encourage social adjustment, maintain a relationship conducive to allowing the patient to voice her concerns.
9. To promote tissue repair, sitz baths of pHisoHex solution may be prescribed after the 10th day.
10. To maintain continuity of care upon discharge from the hospital, a follow-up plan is devised to provide for family care, visits by the community nurse, and return visits to the surgeon.

VAGINAL FISTULA

A *fistula* is an abnormal, tortuous opening between 2 internal hollow organs, or between an internal hollow organ and the exterior of the body.

Ureterovaginal fistula is an opening between the ureter and vagina.

Vesicovaginal fistula is an opening between the bladder and vagina.

Rectovaginal fistula is an opening between the rectum and vagina.

Causes

Vaginal fistula may result from
1. Obstetric injury
2. Pelvic surgery (hysterectomy or vaginal reconstructive procedures are most common)
3. Extension of carcinoma or a complication of treatment for carcinoma.

Clinical Manifestations

1. Patient with vesicovaginal fistula will experience continuous trickling of urine into vagina.
2. Patient with rectovaginal fistula will experience fecal incontinence and flatus passed through vagina, a malodorous condition.

Diagnostic Aids in Locating Fistula Site

1. *Methylene Blue Test*
   Following instillation of this dye in the bladder—
   a. Methylene blue appears in vagina in vesicovaginal fistula.
   b. Methylene blue does not appear in vagina in ureterovaginal fistula.
2. *Indigo Carmine Test*—Following a negative methylene blue test, indigo carmine is injected intravenously.
   If dye appears in vagina, this indicates a ureteral fistula.
3. *Intravenous pyelogram*—(see p. 475) is a valuable test for determining presence of hydroureter or hydronephrosis and position or location of the fistula.
4. *Cystoscopy*—performed to determine number and location of fistulas.

Treatment and Nursing Management

In rare cases, a fistula will heal without surgical intervention. The following measures may promote such healing:

1. Maintain cleanliness by encouraging frequent, soothing sitz baths and deodorizing douches.
2. Use perineal pads and plastic or rubber pants if required.
3. Provide optimum skin care to prevent excoriation; bland creams or a light dusting of cornstarch may be soothing.
4. Recognize value of meeting psychosocial needs, such as feminine morale boosters (attractive hairdo, nail polish, perfume, new bed jacket etc.); encourage visitors, diversion, recreation, activities, etc.

A. *Preparation of Patient for Surgery*

1. Fistulas recognized at time of delivery should be corrected immediately.
2. Postoperative fistulas are not treated immediately but delayed, sometimes for 2 or 3 months, to allow for treatment of inflammation.
3. Surgery is recommended if tissues are healthy.
4. Maintain adequate nutrition; increase intake of vitamins and protein content of meals.
5. Promote local cleanliness by vaginal flushing and rectal enemata.
6. Administer chemotherapeutic agents to reduce pathogenic flora in intestine.
7. If the patient is postmenopausal, oral estrogen may be given to promote healthier, more viable tissue in the operative area.

B. *Specific Postoperative Nursing Management*

1. Rectovaginal fistula
   a. Limit bowel activity by keeping patient on clear fluids for several days; progress to a low residue, then a full diet.
   b. Give warm perineal irrigations and perhaps controlled heat lamp treatments to assist the healing process.
   c. Encourage rest because of the high degree of debilitation.
2. Vesicovaginal fistula

a. Maintain proper drainage from indwelling catheter—otherwise, pressure may build up and be exerted against newly sutured tissues.
b. Employ gentleness in administering bladder or vaginal irrigations because of the tenderness of the operative site.
c. Pay particular attention to urinary output.

VAGINAL INFECTIONS

Normal Vaginal Condition

1. The vaginal secretions are acid (pH 3.5–4.5); acidity is produced by the conversion of cellular glycogen to lactic acid by Döderlein's bacilli, which normally inhabit the vagina.
2. When estrogen production is low (before menarche and after menopause) the epithelium is inactive; the cells contain no glycogen, Döderlein's bacilli are absent, and the pH is between 6 and 7.
3. *Leukorrhea* is a whitish vaginal discharge; it is considered normal to have a slight discharge at the time of ovulation or just before menstruation.

Simple Vaginitis

Simple vaginitis is an inflammation of the vagina, with discharge; this may be due to invading organisms, irritation, poor hygiene.

Urethritis often accompanies vaginitis because of the proximity of the urethra to the vagina.

A. *Symptoms*

1. Leukorrheal discharge with itching, redness, burning, and edema.
2. Voiding and defecation aggravate the above symptoms.

B. *Predisposing Factors*

Trichomonas vaginalis, Candida or Monilia, *Haemophilus vaginalis*, pediculosis pubis, contact allergens, excessive perspiration, poor hygiene.

C. *Nursing Assessment* (See Chart, p. 539.)

D. *Objectives of Treatment and Nursing Management*

1. To enhance the natural vaginal flora by administering a weak acid douche, 15 ml. of vinegar to 1000 ml. water (1 T. white vinegar to 1 qt. water).
2. To stimulate the growth of Döderlein's bacilli by administering beta-lactose vaginal suppository; this dissolves with body heat and the sugar then acts.
3. To foster cleanliness by meticulous care after voiding and defecation.
4. To control infection by initiating chemotherapy: Insert medication into vagina via applicator or by using a chemotherapeutic cream locally as prescribed.

Trichomonas Vaginalis

A condition produced by a protozoan which infects the vagina and which is evident as a bubbly, greenish-yellow, irritating leukorrhea and as a red, speckled ("strawberry") cervix.

A. *Characteristics*

1. Caused by a pear-shaped mobile flagellate that thrives in an alkaline medium.
2. *Trichomonas vaginalis* is persistent and resistant.
3. Vulvar edema and hyperemia occur secondary to irritation of discharge.

Nursing Assessment: Simple Vaginitis

Assessment	Rationale
1. Regarding discharge: When was it first noticed? Any other symptoms?	1. May be suggestive of other pelvic difficulty.
2. Menstrual period: Does patient have dysmenorrhea, amenorrhea, dysfunctional bleeding?	2. May be suggestive of other pelvic difficulty. Consider psychogenic problem.
3. Urinary tract: Does she have burning on urination?	3. Suspect cystitis or other urinary difficulties.
4. Type of itching: Is it more prevalent at night?	4. Suspect pinworm.
5. Odor: Is odor offensive?	5. Indicative of poor hygiene, foreign body (lost tampon), or other infection.
6. Husband: Does he have a discharge?	6. Suspect reinfection of each other: *Trichomonas, Candida*, gonoccocus.
7. Use of deodorant spray, strong douche solution, ointment: What products does she use?	7. Suspect sensitivity, overuse of product.
8. Clothing: Is clothing too tight (girdle, pantyhose)?	8. Synthetics and excessive perspiration are irritating.
9. Other disease: Ask if patient has diabetes.	9. This generally is linked to vulvovaginitis.
10. Nature of discharge: Cheese-like . . . . Frothy . . . . Pus-like . . . . Thick and foul-smelling . . . . Whitish-gray, scant, foul odor	Suspect: *Candida* *Trichomonas* Mixed infection Foreign body *Haemophilus vaginalis*

4. Remissions may occur; the organism meanwhile remains inaccessible to treatment in the urinary tract.
5. The male partner may carry the organism in his urogenital tract and reinfect his mate.

B. *Objectives of Treatment and Nursing Management*

1. To destroy infective protozoa give metronidazole (Flagyl) for 10 days (by mouth) If above cannot be tolerated or is contraindicated, insert vaginal suppositories containing trichomonocidal compounds (Tricufuron, Devegan).

NOTE: Flagyl is contraindicated in the first trimester of pregnancy.

2. To counteract alkaline preferred environment of infecting organisms, administer acidic vaginal douches (Massengill, Nylmerate, white vinegar, 15 ml.–1000 ml. (1 T. to 1 qt. of water).
3. To reduce possible vaginal irritants, suggest that the patient avoid scented tampons and vaginal sprays.
4. To prevent reinfection, treat male concurrently with Flagyl.

Monilial Vaginitis

A fungal infection caused by *Candida albicans*.

A. *Incidence*—Six factors have been found to be significantly associated with the incidence of *Candida albicans*.

1. Drug addiction
2. Obesity
3. Pregnancy
4. Antibiotic therapy
5. Diabetes mellitus
6. Birth control pills

B. *Characteristics*

1. *Candida albicans* is a normal inhabitant of the intestinal tract and therefore a frequent contaminant of the vagina.
2. Since this fungus thrives in an environment rich in carbohydrates, it is seen commonly in patients with poorly controlled diabetes.
3. This infection is observed in patients who have been on antibiotic or steroid therapy for a while (reduces natural protective organisms in vagina).

C. *Manifestations*

1. Vaginal discharge is thick and irritating; white, patchy, cheese-like particles adhere to vaginal walls.
2. Itching is common.
3. Appearance of vulva and vagina varies from normal to that of an acute inflammation.

D. *Objectives of Treatment and Nursing Management*

1. To eradicate the fungus, apply miconazole nitrate (Monistat) cream, 1 application daily at bedtime for 14 days, or
   a. Nystatin vaginal tablets twice daily, to be inserted high in the vagina, for 15 days.
   b. Treatment should be continued without interruption even during menstruation.
2. To reduce local irritation and itching apply nystatin, neomycin sulfate, gramicidin, or triamcinolone acetonide (Mycolog) cream to the affected areas twice daily.
3. To treat the symptomatic or uncircumcised partner by applying Mycolog cream to the penis twice a day for a week.
4. To discourage the wearing of clothing that tends to promote moisture and heat in the perineal area since *Candida albicans* thrives best in the presence of moisture and heat.

Atrophic (Postmenopausal) Vaginitis

This is a common postmenopausal occurrence. Because of atrophy of vaginal mucosa, the woman is prone to postmenopausal dyspareunia (painful intercourse due to a tight vagina).
1. Signs and symptoms—vesicovaginal itching, burning, and pain.
2. Treatment
   a. Since this is a manifestation of general body estrogenic depletion, the patient should be treated with oral, water soluble, natural, conjugated estrogen (Premarin).
   b. The condition reverses itself under treatment, which must be maintained.
   c. If infection is also present, this is treated.
   d. Estrogenic or cortisone vaginal cream may be prescribed.

NURSING ALERT: In the postmenopausal woman, if vaginal bleeding occurs, encourage patient to see her physician immediately, because cancer may be suspected.

HERPES VIRUS TYPE 2 INFECTION (Herpes Genitalis, Herpes Simplex Virus [HSV])

Herpes genitalis is a viral infection that causes herpetic lesions on the cervix, vagina, and external genitalia; it is considered to be acquired by venereal transmission.

Clinical Manifestations

1. Herpes genitalis is manifested within three to seven days and is most prevalent in young adults.
2. Multiple vesicles appear on the vulva; surrounding area is inflamed and edematous.
3. Itching may be intense and even painful; scratching may further aggravate the problem.
4. Lesions appear on the vulva, and in most patients, the cervix is also involved; it too may be inflamed and edematous, and bleeds easily when touched.
5. A profuse watery discharge may be present.
6. Fever, malaise, and headache may accompany the acute flare-up.
7. Within 1–4 weeks the sores disappear; however, the virus remains in the body and recurrences are common with leukorrhea, abnormal bleeding, vaginal pain, and dyspareunia.

Implications

1. Babies delivered vaginally may become infected with the virus; there is significant fetal morbidity and mortality. In the early pregnancy, there is increased incidence of spontaneous abortion.
2. Incidence of cervical cancer is higher in women who have had genital herpes.

Treatment and Nursing Management

1. A viral culture is taken as soon as the patient presents for suspected herpes infection.
2. A gel of 2-deoxy-D-glucose or D-glucose in miconazole nitrate (2%) cream or in miconazole alone has been effective in providing relief of pain and dysuria in 12–72 hours. Recurrences seem to be minimized with this treatment.

3. Provide information about the management of the infection; sexual activity should be avoided until the infection is cleared; recognize that this person is a potential transmitter of the disease.
4. Support and understanding are parts of the therapeutic regime.

TOXIC SHOCK SYNDROME (TSS)

Toxic shock syndrome is a condition caused by a bacterial toxin *(staphylococcus aureus)* in the bloodstream; it can be life-threatening. This condition, first identified in 1975, came to public attention in 1980 because of increased incidence. The use of tampons by young women during menstruation has been suspected.

Clinical Manifestations

1. Sudden onset of high fever.
2. Vomiting and profuse watery diarrhea.
3. Rapid progression to hypotension and shock within 48 hours.
4. Sometimes, sore throat, headache, and myalgia are experienced.
5. Rash (similar to sunburn) that is followed by desquamation, particularly of the palms and soles.

Suspected Link

Vaginal tampons used during menstruation are suspected of being one of the causes:
1. It is thought that a tampon dams up the flow of blood, which then acts as a culture medium for *Staphylococcus aureus.*
2. It is suspected that tampons may cause abrasions in the vaginal lining, thereby creating pathways for staphylococci to enter the bloodstream.

Treatment and Nursing Management

1. Antibiotics are administered to control the infection (excluding penicillin).
2. Medications to raise the blood pressure are given.
3. Fluid replacement is instituted to replace fluid and electrolyte deficits.
4. Encourage women who are recovering from TSS not to use tampons until all evidence of the infection is gone.

Health Education

1. Until more definitive research provides answers to this puzzling problem, women are advised to
   a. Alternate use of pads with tampons.
   b. Be alert to the symptoms of TSS.
   c. Change tampons frequently and not wear one longer than 8 hours.
   d. Be careful of vaginal abrasions that can be caused by some applicators.
   e. Avoid using super-absorbent tampons.
2. Since the risk is low (1/1000 over age 30, 4/1000 under age 30), it seems unwarranted to recommend that the use of tampons be discontinued.
3. Cases of toxic shock syndrome are to be reported to State Health departments and to the Center for Disease Control (CDC)* so that additional data can be accumulated.

* Attn: Special Pathogens Branch, Bacterial Diseases Division Bureau of Epidemiology, Atlanta, GA 30333. Phone: (404) 329-3687.

GUIDELINES: Vaginal Irrigation

Purpose   1. To cleanse or disinfect the vagina and adjacent tissues.
               2. To soothe inflamed tissue.

Equipment 1. Sterile reservoir for irrigating fluid—can or bag
               2. Sterile irrigating fluid as prescribed (1000–4000 ml.) at 40.5°–43.3° C. (105°–110° F.)
               3. Tubing, connecting tubes, and clamp (sterile)
               4. Irrigating vaginal nozzle (sterile)
               5. Bedpan or douche pan
               6. Plastic or rubber sheet with cloth protection
               7. Sterile cotton balls, cleansing solution
               8. Sterile disposable gloves

Procedure (Fig. 11–14)

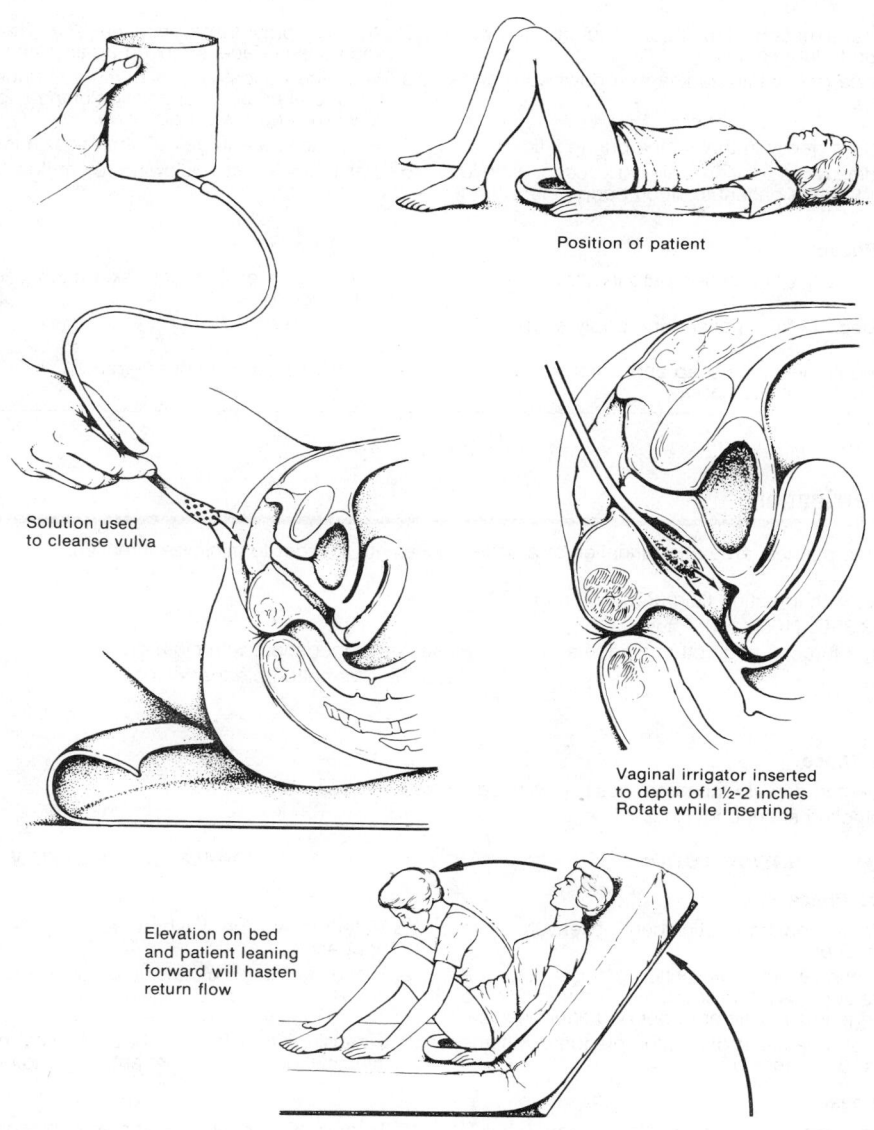

Position of patient

Solution used to cleanse vulva

Vaginal irrigator inserted to depth of 1½-2 inches Rotate while inserting

Elevation on bed and patient leaning forward will hasten return flow

FIGURE 11-14. *Vaginal irrigation.*

GUIDELINES: Vaginal Irrigation (cont.)

Procedure (cont.)

NURSING ACTION	RATIONALE/AMPLIFICATION
Preparatory Phase	
1. Have patient void before beginning irrigation.	1. A full bladder would prevent adequate distention of vagina by solution.
2. Place patient in dorsal recumbent position.	2. To permit gravity to assist in allowing fluid to reach distal areas of vagina.
3. Drape patient.	3. To prevent chilling and undue exposure.
4. Arrange irrigating receptacle at a level just above patient's hips (not more than ⅔ meter, i.e., 2 feet, above hips) so that fluid flows easily but gently.	4. The higher the fluid source, the greater the pressure.
Performance Phase	
1. Cleanse vulva by separating labia and allowing solution to flow over area; if insufficient, use cotton balls saturated in soap solution; cleanse from front toward anal area.	1. Materials found around vaginal meatus may be introduced into vagina and cervix. This is to be avoided.
2. Allow some solution to flow through tubing and out over nozzle to lubricate it.	2. Moisture provides lubrication and less resistance when one surface is moved against another.
3. Insert nozzle gently into vagina in a downward and backward direction.	3. When the patient is in a dorsal recumbent position, the natural anatomical position of the vagina is in the downward-backward direction.
4. Rotate nozzle gently in the vagina during inflow.	4. All surfaces are irrigated when nozzle is rotated.
5. Clamp tubing when solution is almost all used; remove nozzle and permit patient to sit on bedpan for return flow.	5. Gravity will assist in allowing return flow to drain from vaginal tract.
Follow-up Phase	
1. Wipe patient dry using cotton balls in a front-to-back direction.	1. Drying the area prevents skin excoriation and promotes comfort.
2. Remove bedpan from patient and apply sterile perineal pad.	
3. Cleanse equipment with soap and water; dry before storing in well-ventilated area.	3. This will prolong life of equipment.

GUIDELINES: Vulvar Irrigation

Purpose To cleanse the perineal area after urination or a bowel movement in order to minimize infection.

Equipment Sterile pitcher with irrigating fluid (300–500 ml.)
   40.5°–43.3° C. (105°–110° F.)
Sterile sponge forceps and cotton pledgets   Plastic or rubber sheet with cloth protection
Bedpan   Paper bag for cotton pledget disposal

Procedure (Fig. 11–15)

Preparatory Phase
1. Place patient in dorsal recumbent position with legs flexed and separated.
2. Place protecting sheet under patient.

NURSING ACTION	RATIONALE/AMPLIFICATION
Performance Phase	
1. Pour warmed irrigating solution gently over vulva from a sterile pitcher.	1. Materials will be flushed from perineal area into bedpan.
2. Cleanse perineal area with cotton pledget held in a sponge holder; use a top-down direction and discard each sponge in a plastic or paper bag after one use.	2. Friction facilitates cleansing process and the removal of soil.
3. Dry perineal area using dry cotton pledgets in same fashion as for cleansing.	3. Cleansing from front to back assists in preventing intestinal organisms from entering vaginal area.
Follow-up Phase	
1. Apply sterile perineal pad and hold in place with a T-binder.	1. To maintain cleanliness and provide comfort for patient.

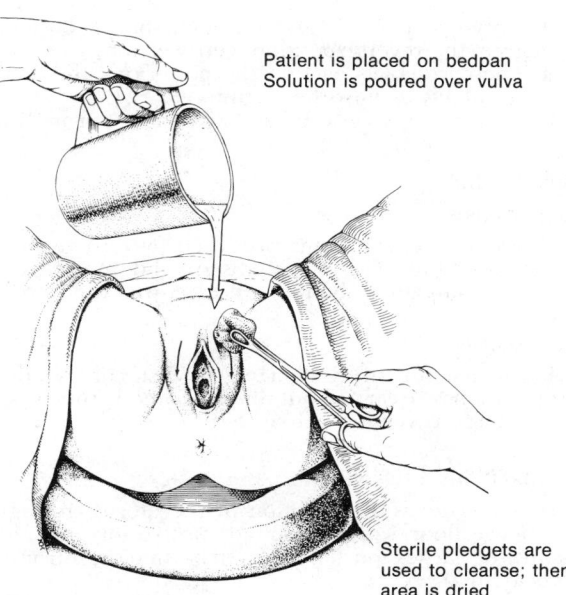

Patient is placed on bedpan
Solution is poured over vulva

Sterile pledgets are
used to cleanse; then
area is dried

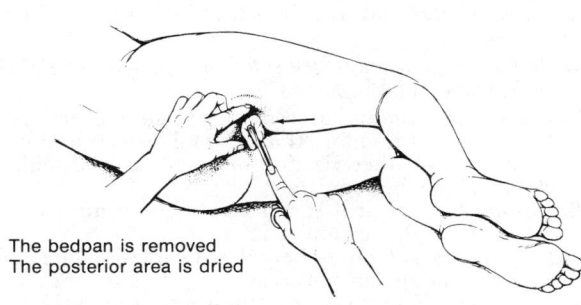

The bedpan is removed
The posterior area is dried

FIGURE 11-15. *Perineal care.*

PROBLEMS RESULTING FROM RELAXED PELVIC MUSCLES

CYSTOCELE

Cystocele is a downward displacement (protrusion) of the bladder into the vagina.

Etiology

1. Associated with obstetrical trauma to fascia, muscle, and ligaments during childbirth (results in poor support).
2. Often becomes apparent years later when genital atrophy associated with aging occurs.

Clinical Manifestations

1. Fatigue and pelvic pressure
2. Urinary symptoms—urgency, frequency, incontinence
3. At times a marked protrusion of anterior wall outside the vulva
4. Interference with coitus (intercourse)
5. Residual urine and urinary infection

Treatment

A. *Medical*
1. Generally, nonsurgical treatment with vaginal pessaries is rarely used.
2. Kegel's pelvic floor exercises are useful and may prove beneficial in some women.
   a. Conscious contraction of the pelvic floor or levator ani muscles.
   b. This can be done many times during the day, as one sits, stands, or lies in bed.

B. *Surgical*
An anterior colpoplasty, usually in conjunction with a vaginal hysterectomy and posterior colpoplasty, is the standard surgical therapy.

RECTOCELE

Rectocele is displacement (protrusion) of the rectum into the vagina.

Etiology

Similar to cystocele; however, posterior vaginal wall is weakened in a rectocele.

Clinical Manifestations

1. Disturbance of bowel function: constipation.
2. A "bearing down" feeling—as though the "pelvic organs were going to fall out."
3. Difficulty in fecal evacuation; some patients state that "they must put their fingers in the vagina to push the mass up" so that defecation can take place.
4. Symptoms disappear in the recumbent position.
5. Incontinence of gas and feces (in patients with a complete tear between rectum and vagina).

Treatment

Posterior colpoplasty (perineorrhaphy)—repair of posterior vaginal wall

Objectives of Nursing Management

A. *To encourage women who have problems resulting from relaxed pelvic muscles to see a gynecologist. Patient may tend to:*

1. Procrastinate and feel embarrassed.
2. Expect that time will take care of it.
3. Be resigned to the fact that this is a normal result of child-bearing.

B. *To enable the patient to relax during preoperative preparation phase*

1. Promote rest particularly in a patient who has been working hard.
2. Suggest low Fowler's position in bed to lessen edema and congestion.
3. Recognize that this problem often occurs in older women.
4. Prepare intestinal tract by administering a cathartic and enema.

C. *To prevent pressure on the suture line postoperatively, and to prevent infection*

1. Encourage voiding to reduce pressure every 4–8 hours, so that no more than 150 ml. will accumulate in bladder—catheterization or use of an indwelling catheter may be required.
2. Administer perineal care to the patient after each voiding and defecation.
3. Employ a heat lamp to help dry the incision line and enhance the healing process.
4. Utilize available sprays for anesthetic and antiseptic effects.
5. Apply an ice pack locally to relieve congestion and discomfort.

D. *To recognize the special care required by patients following operations for a complete perineal laceration*

1. Encourage voiding (catheterization if necessary) to prevent pressure on suture line due to a full bladder.
2. Avoid the use of enemas or a rectal tube for several days to permit wound healing.
3. Provide liquid diet (no milk) for several days to prevent necessity of a bowel movement.
4. Give tincture of opium (paregoric) to reduce peristalsis and inhibit bowel function.
5. Administer mineral oil by about the 6th day and follow with an oil retention enema at sign of a possible bowel movement.

DISPLACEMENT OF THE UTERUS

Considerations

1. Normally the cervix lies in the axis of the vagina with the corpus uteri inclined forward on the bladder.

2. Twenty-five percent of all women have, to some degree, the reverse position (retroversion).
   a. The corpus lies back in the posterior cul-de-sac, essentially against the rectum.
   b. This is in no sense pathological; it is normal for such women.

Retroversion

A. *Symptoms*

There are no symptoms produced by retroversion. Its association with salpingitis or endometriosis is due to complaints about the disease—not the retroversion.

B. *Treatment*

Retroversion is surgically treated when conservative operations are carried out for associated pathology—not the retroversion per se.

Prolapse and Procidentia

Uterine prolapse is a herniation of the uterus through the pelvic floor with a resultant protrusion into the vagina (prolapse) and at times even beyond the introitus (procidentia).

Prolapse

1st degree—cervix, without straining or traction, is at the introitus (spread the labia and it is visible).
2nd degree—the cervix extends over the perineum (Fig. 11–16).
3rd degree—the entire uterus (or most of it) protrudes (Fig. 11–16).

Procidentia

The uterus, vaginal vault, rectum, and bladder (and in some cases the posterior cul-de-sac) protrude.

A. *Factors Aggravating the Condition*

1. Obstetrical trauma
2. Overstretching of the musculofascial supports
3. Standing, straining, coughing, lfting a heavy object

B. *Treatment*

Surgical correction is recommended treatment.
1. Vaginal hysterectomy—combined with anterior and posterior repair.
2. Colpocleisis (Le Fort)—used as a last resort but effective in elderly persons since it involves closing or near closing of the vagina.

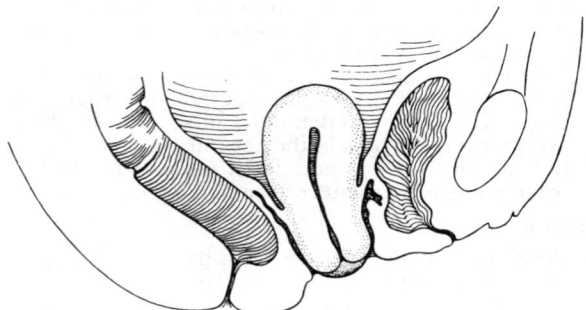 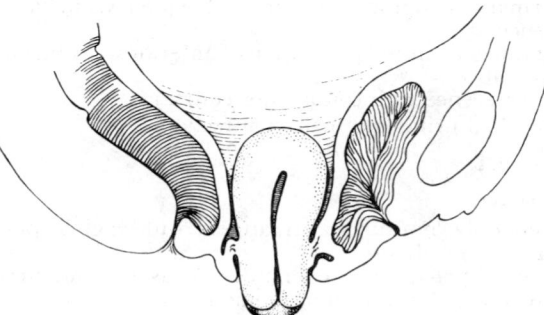

FIGURE 11-16. *Prolapse of the uterus. (Left) Shows second degree prolapse of the uterus. Note that cervix extends over perineum. (Right) Shows third degree prolapse—entire or most of the uterus protrudes. (From Gray LA. Postgrad Med, 30:208–209)*

TUMORS OF THE UTERUS

Incidence and the Importance of Patient Education

1. In the U.S., malignant tumors of the uterus (cervix and endometrium) rank 4th highest among cancers in women (breast, colon-rectum, lung, uterine).
2. The death rate for uterine cancer has been showing a steady decline; this is attributed to the unremitting education of women, which stresses the importance of annual checkups, including the cytology smear.
3. Nurses need to seek out the reasons why millions of women have not had Pap tests—lack of information, no transportation, inconvenient schedules of clinics, fear of results, and general lack of motivation.

CANCER OF THE CERVIX

Etiology

1. It is most common between the ages of 35 and 55, but it can occur at any age.
2. Early cancer of the cervix is usually asymptomatic; it is almost always curable in its preinvasive stage.
3. Early sexual activity and multiple sexual partners appear to be related to the incidence of this cancer.
4. Viral and chronic infections as well as erosions of the cervix appear to be significant in the development of cancer.
5. Incidence of cancer of the cervix is higher in groups with low socioeconomic status; occurs more often in black women than in white.

Clinical Manifestations

1. There are no symptoms of early cervical carcinoma.
2. Initial symptoms of carcinoma of the cervix.
   a. Posttraumatic bleeding (coitus).
   b. Irregular vaginal bleeding or spotting—between periods (metrorrhagia) or after the menopause; at first it may be very slight, but as disease progresses, bleeding becomes more constant.
   c. Leukorrhea—increases in amount, becomes dark and foul-smelling because of necrosis and infection of tumor mass.
3. With advanced cancer there is excruciating pain in back and legs relieved only by large doses of narcotics.
4. Later, extreme emaciation and anemia; occasionally there is irregular fever due to secondary infection, peritonitis, and abscesses in ulcerating mass.

Diagnostic Evaluation

1. Physical and gynecological examination plus a complete history are done initially.
2. Laboratory studies include cytology smear, routine blood examinations plus fasting blood sugar to detect diabetes, total plasma proteins for nutritional status evaluation, and bleeding and clotting time.
3. Colposcopy, Schiller's test, biopsy (cone and punch), and proctoscopic examination are essential diagnostic aids.
4. Roentgen studies should include chest x-ray, intravenous pyelogram, barium enema, and bone studies.
5. Electrocardiogram.

Treatment and Nursing Management

1. Carcinoma in Situ
   a. Hysterectomy is usually recommended, with preservation of the ovaries.
   b. Cervical amputation, wide conization, cryosurgery are alternatives to hysterectomy but there is less assurance of complete removal of the lesion.
2. Invasive Carcinoma
   a. Treatment is individualized, depending on the stage of the disease, age of patient, and general physical condition.
   b. Most often invasive carcinoma is treated by radiation; radical operations (exenteration) are performed on some patients.

Health Education and Follow-up Emphasis

Regardless of the treatment, the nurse must emphasize the necessity of follow-up visits for this patient, since they will be required for the rest of her life:
1. To determine patient's response to treatment
2. To detect spread of cancer (metastasis)
3. To maintain the best health possible
4. To take regular cytologic smears

CANCER OF THE CORPUS UTERI

Incidence

1. Carcinoma of the cervix and carcinoma of the body of the uterus occurred in the ratio of 4:1 a few years ago; at present the ratio is 2:1.
2. Endometrial cancer is most common in women past 40 (peaks at age 55).
3. Seventy-five percent of women with cancer of the corpus uteri are postmenopausal.
4. Often this malignancy occurs when the patient is also affected by obesity, hypertensive cardiovascular disease, and diabetes.
5. Forty years of statistical and laboratory experimentation have failed to show a definite relationship between estrogen and cancer.

Clinical Manifestations

1. The first evidence is usually a serous, malodorous leukorrhea—often this is disregarded by the patient.
2. This is followed by a bloody discharge—it may be spotty or it may be steady.
3. Pain is not a symptom until the late stages.
4. Anemia may result if there is considerable bleeding.

Diagnostic Evaluation

1. Determine source of bleeding; even if it is coming from the cervical canal, it could be caused by other than carcinoma.
   (If tampon is inserted in the vagina overnight, the place where blood is noted on the dressing may offer a clue to bleeding source; i.e., near the string could suggest bladder source, but near the tip of the tampon would suggest cervix as source.)
2. Endometrial biopsy: Positive indicates cancer, whereas negative does not necessarily exclude carcinoma.
3. Fractional curettage is the most effective and accurate diagnostic aid.
4. Gravlee Jet Wash (see p. 534) is used as a screening procedure by some gynecologists.

Treatment

1. Hysterectomy (p. 547)—depending on stage of lesion.

2. Radiation therapy (p. 852)—depending on stage of lesion.

MYOMA OF THE UTERUS

Myomas are benign tumors of the uterus; (they are also called fibromyomas, "fibroids," and leiomyomas).

Incidence and Characteristics

1. Such tumors occur in about 20% of women past age 30.
2. Myomas rarely develop after menopause; tumors which developed earlier may regress slightly after menopause—but the significant ones do not disappear.
3. Incidence is higher in black women than in white.
4. These tumors tend to be of dense musculofibrous structure; they are encapsulated and tend to form small or large nodules.

Clinical Manifestations

1. Small myomas do not cause symptoms.
2. After myomas (or myomata) grow, the first indication of the presence of a tumor is a palpable mass.
3. Excessive or prolonged menstruation is usually the chief symptom (with little or no change in the menstrual interval); intermenstrual or postmenopausal bleeding may also occur.
4. Pain comes with degeneration of the growth and from pressure on adjacent organs. As myomas grow there may be sensation of weight—a heavy feeling.
5. Secondary symptoms may be a feeling of lassitude, general weakness, anemia, and lower abdominal discomfort.

Diagnostic Measures

1. These are done primarily to rule out cancer: cytology, dilatation and curettage, cervical biopsy.
2. Diagnosis is made by abdominal and bimanual palpation.

Treatment

1. If patient is of childbearing age and desires children, treatment is conservative.
   a. If small tumor—myomectomy
   b. If large tumor—hysterectomy
   c. Ovaries are preserved
   d. If tumor is large with excessive bleeding—hysteromyomectomy (tumor and uterus removed)
2. For medical and nursing management, see page 548.

NURSING CARE OF THE PATIENT RECEIVING RADIATION THERAPY OF THE UTERUS

Radiation Therapy (see also p. 852)

1. Radium, cesium-137, or radioactive cobalt is introduced into the endocervical canal and vagina for a prescribed time; radium (or cesium) is placed in tubes designed to filter out most alpha and beta rays while allowing gamma rays to penetrate into the tumor.
2. Such therapy may be supplemented by external radiation (supervoltage x-ray, telecobalt, or linear accelerator sources) directed over the pelvis in an effort to eliminate cancer spread via lymphatic system; energy may be delivered via anterior or posterior portals over lower abdomen or back, or by means of rotational therapy permitting more uniform exposure of pelvis.
3. Therapy is individualized according to stage of disease and patient's response to and tolerance of radiation.
4. A popular method of treatment involves using radiation therapy externally, then shifting to radium application, and then returning to radiation therapy. Total treatment time is 5–6 weeks.

Patient Preparation for Radium (Cesium) Implantation

1. Physician explains to the patient the reason why such therapy is advocated; nurse can amplify or answer any questions patient may later raise.
2. Prepare the patient for various preliminary tests (may be done on an outpatient basis)—blood studies, biopsies (endometrial and cervical), chest x-ray, electrocardiogram, cystoscopy.
3. Be available for questions and conversation with the patient regarding any phase of the preliminary studies or treatment.
4. Following admission to the hospital, prepare the patient for surgery and, in addition, prepare the intestinal tract by enemata and the vaginal tract by a cleansing douche.
5. Cesium-137 has tended recently to supplant radium because it is less expensive.

Radium Application

After-loading Technique Using an Applicator such as a Fletcher-Suit
1. In surgery, the tandem and ovoids are positioned (without radium or cesium).
2. Upon recovery from anesthesia, x-rays are taken in various positions in the x-ray department.
3. Therapeutic radiologist then inserts radium (cesium) into prepositioned apparatus.

Nursing Management

> **NURSING ALERT:** It is imperative to keep the radiation applicator in the uterine canal and to prevent a change of position. Adjust all nursing measures to meet this objective.

A. *While Radium Is in Place*
1. Maintain patient on a low residue diet to prevent bowel movements which might dislodge apparatus.
2. Inspect catheter frequently to insure straight drainage—a distended bladder may cause severe radiation burns.
3. Observe for symptoms of radiation sickness—nausea, vomiting, elevated temperature.
4. Encourage patient to eat by offering a variety of small rather than large servings and present meals attractively to offset poor appetite.
5. Offer citrus fruit juices because vitamin C is valuable in tissue repair.
6. Patient must lie on back; head of bed may be elevated 30 degrees.
7. Provide back care but spend a minimum amount of time at the bedside.

8. Relieve patient of anxiety and fear by utilizing wisely the contact time with the patient—engage in profitable conversation about her medical and nursing problems.

B. *Radium Removal*
1. Notify surgeon when it is time to remove radium (or cesium).
2. Provide sterile gloves, long forceps, and a large waste basin.
3. Note on the chart the number of tubes applied so that this number is accounted for on removal.
4. Practice radium precautions in handling and returning radium (cesium) to the radiotherapy department.
5. Administer a cleansing enema before the patient gets out of bed.

C. *Postirradiation Patient Care*
1. Keep the patient's skin (exposed to radiation) dry; avoid use of soap since it irritates.
2. Apply a soothing powder such as cornstarch to relieve itching and discomfort.
3. For erythematous areas, apply a bland ointment such as A & D ointment to relieve irritation.
4. Nausea or vomiting may occur with large doses of radiation.

> **NURSING ALERT:** Do not tell the patient nausea and vomiting may occur, since the power of suggestion may initiate these symptoms.

5. Observe for any symptoms which might suggest radiation injury to the intestine—diarrhea, tenesmus; report these if they occur.
6. Tell the patient the importance of monthly follow-up visits to her physician for the first 6 months—to assess effects of radiation on tumor.
   a. Cytological smears are taken; if positive, treatment was not successful. This may mean surgery will be required.
   b. If cytology smear is negative and tissue looks satisfactory, follow-up visits after 6 months may be further apart (on a semiannual basis).

> **NURSING ALERT:** Recognize that 5–8% of women who are followed for the treatment of a particular cancer may develop other primary cancers. Therefore, such follow-up visits are essential even though the woman is symptomless.

HYSTERECTOMY

Hysterectomy is the surgical removal of the uterus.

Possible Indications
1. Malignant and nonmalignant growth on uterus, cervix, and adnexa that should be removed
2. Severe (life-threatening) pelvic infection
3. Control of uterine bleeding and/or hemorrhage
4. Correction of problems associated with pelvic floor relaxation: cystocele, rectocele
5. Treatment of endometriosis when conservative measures have failed
6. Irreparable rupture or perforation of uterus

Qualifying Considerations
1. Woman's age
2. Woman's desire to have children
3. Possible effectiveness of alternative treatment
4. Degree of dysfunction
5. Woman's willingness to endure dysfunction in order to retain her uterus

Elective Indications
1. Voluntary sterilization
2. Prophylaxis when there is a significant history of uterine disease

Types of Abdominal Hysterectomy
(Approximately 70% done abdominally)
1. *Subtotal hysterectomy*—corpus of uterus is removed but cervical stump remains.
2. *Total hysterectomy*—entire uterus is removed, including cervix; tubes and ovaries remain.
3. *Total hysterectomy with bilateral salpingo-oophorectomy*—entire uterus, tubes, and ovaries are removed.

Vaginal Hysterectomy
Preferred approach for
1. Repair of pelvic relaxation (uterine descensus, urinary stress incontinence, cystocele/rectocele) is more easily managed vaginally than abdominally.
2. High risk patients, very obese patients, or those unable to withstand prolonged anesthesia.

Advantages
1. Less likelihood of paralytic ileus, postoperative pain, and intestinal adhesions
2. Less chance of pulmonary complications and thrombophlebitis
3. Wound dehiscence possibility is less; shorter hospitalization
4. No abdominal scar

Disadvantages
1. More limited surgical field; inability to examine intrapelvic and intra-abdominal organs
2. May be increased risk of bleeding and postoperative infection

Psychosocial Considerations
1. Patient may have deep-seated fears that cancer or venereal disease may be discovered.
2. There may be a conflict between recommended medical treatment and her personal religious beliefs.
3. Concerns may be raised regarding the possibility that all phases of her reproductive process may be distrubed.
4. She may be disappointed particularly if she never had children.
5. The patient may feel that she will no longer be able to fulfill her role and needs as a woman.
6. Depression and heightened emotional sensitivity to people and situations may have to be assessed.
7. The complexity of problems which are a mixture of physical, emotional, and social factors needs to be considered by the nurse as she assists this patient.

8. Questions arise about how a hysterectomy will affect her participation in sexual relations.
9. The relationship of this woman to her mate and family should be determined.

Postoperative Objectives of Nursing Management—Abdominal Hysterectomy

See Postoperative Nursing Management, p. 89 (surgical section). In addition, note the following specific objectives:

A. *To reduce the possibility of bladder problems (which may occur due to the proximity of the bladder to the surgical site).*

1. Monitor and record intake and output; administer parenteral fluids as prescribed.
2. Insert an indwelling catheter, if prescribed, because edema or nerve trauma may cause temporary bladder atony. A suprapubic catheter may be used (see p. 487).
3. Remove catheter as soon as feasible (as directed).
4. Catheterize patient if no catheter is in place and the patient has not voided after 8 hours, or is uncomfortable.
5. Determine whether there is pooling of residual urine; catheterize patient after each voiding; otherwise, bladder infection may develop.

B. *To relieve the discomfort of abdominal distention.*

1. A nasogastric tube may be inserted while the patient is in the operating room.
2. Fluids and food may be restricted until peristalsis has resumed.
3. Auscultate abdomen for bowel sounds to determine onset of peristalsis.
   a. Apply heat to the abdomen and insert a rectal tube to relieve abdominal flatus.
   b. Permit the patient to sit on edge of bed with feet supported and to get out of bed and walk.
   c. Serve additional fluids and soft diet as peristalsis returns.

C. *To prevent respiratory and cardiovascular disorders*

1. Assist patient in turning every 2 hours and encourage her to take deep breaths.
2. Avoid high Fowler's position and pressure under the knees which might cause stasis and pooling of the blood.
3. Assess dressings or vaginal pad for amount and nature of discharge.
   a. Color of stain; wetness or dryness
   b. Size of stain—record in centimeters; note odor or its absence.
   c. Document observation as well as time of assessment so that differences can be noted at the next observation.
4. Measure amount of blood loss by weighing each pad when removed (before evaporation takes place); compare weight of saturated pad with that of a dry pad (the difference will be weight of blood loss).
5. Evaluate legs for positive Homan's sign (tenderness, pain in calf upon dorsiflexion of foot).
6. Observe legs for the presence of varicosities; promote circulation with special leg exercises.
7. Apply antiembolic stockings as a precautionary measure to promote peripheral circulation.

D. *To counteract effects resulting from removal of a large tumor or unusual blood loss.*

1. Administer high protein diet with iron supplement to combat anemia.
2. Recommend a girdle or apply an abdominal binder following removal of a large tumor to provide support for relaxed abdominal muscles.

Discharge Planning/Health Education

1. A total hysterectomy produces a surgical menopause (if the adnexa were also removed).
2. Explain to patient the importance of hormonal replacement (prescribed) if she has had a total hysterectomy with oophorectomy/salpingectomy.
3. Advise her against sitting too long at one time, as in driving long distances, because of the possibility of pooling of blood in the pelvis and of thromboembolism.
4. Suggest that patient delay driving a car until the 3rd week postoperative, since even pressing the brake pedal may initiate slight discomfort in the lower abdomen.
5. Tell her to expect a "tired feeling" for the first few days at home and, therefore, not to plan too many activities for the first week.
6. Have her plan an adjustment schedule in keeping with the expectation that she will be able to perform most of her usual household activities in a month; in 2 months she will feel her "normal" self.
7. Stress that she should assume employment outside the home only when her physician indicates; this will depend on the type of work, need for it, etc.
8. Tell her not to feel discouraged if at times during convalescence she experiences depression, feels like crying, and seems unusually nervous. This is common, but will not last.
9. Remind her to ask her physician regarding resumption of various preferred physical activities; note that some of the most strenuous tasks are hanging clothes on a line and using the vacuum cleaner. These tasks should be delayed for several weeks. The patient should not lift heavy objects for a month to 6 weeks, at least.
10. Determine what the physician has told the patient regarding resumption of intercourse; reinforce this and explain that too-enthusiastic genital sex may injure the incision site and produce bleeding. In other words, she is to "go easy" at first. Suggest coital position variation.
    a. Usually sexual relations, douching, or use of tampons is discouraged for 4–6 weeks unless otherwise specified by the physician.
11. Showers are permitted but tub bathing is deferred until the physician indicates that tissues are sufficiently healed.
12. Emphasize the importance of follow-up physical and gynecological examinations not only for peace of mind but also to detect any beginning pathology.
    a. Temperature elevation over 37.8° C (100° F), heavy vaginal bleeding, drainage, and foul odor of discharge are reportable.

ENDOMETRIOSIS

Endometriosis is a disease characterized by displaced groups of cells (resembling the cells that line the uterus) growing aberrantly in the pelvic cavity outside of the uterus.

Incidence

1. Frequency of occurrence is about 25—30% in white women.
2. It is rarely encountered in women of the black race.

Characteristics

1. Pelvic endometriosis attacks many areas. Order of frequency is—the ovary, ureterosacral ligaments, the cul-de-sac, ureterovesical peritoneum, cervix, umbilicus, laparotomy scars, hernial sacs and appendix.
2. Misplaced endometrium responds to ovarian hormonal stimulation and even depends on this for survival.
   a. When uterus goes through the process of menstruation, this misplaced tissue also bleeds; because there is no outlet for accumulated blood, pain and adhesions result.
   b. At surgery, concealed bleeding is in evidence because lesions are brown or blue-black.
   c. Ovarian cysts in which such bleeding has occurred are referred to as "chocolate cysts," but all such cysts are not indicative of endometriosis.

Etiology

1. Embryonic tissue remnants may cover pelvic peritoneum and ovaries and may differentiate as a result of hormonal stimulation.
2. Such tissue may be spread via lymphatic or venous channels.
3. Endometrial tissue, during surgery, may accidentally be transferred by way of instruments (uncommon).

Clinical Manifestations

1. Persistent infertility in an otherwise healthy married woman.
2. Lower abdominal and pelvic pain or discomfort, rectal pain, increasing dyspareunia (painful intercourse), and abnormal uterine bleeding.
3. Symptoms are more acute during menstruation and subside after menstruation.
4. When a cyst ruptures, symptoms mimic acute appendicitis or ruptured ectopic pregnancy—an acute abdomen is apparent.

Diagnostic Evaluation

1. Manual rectal and pelvic examinations reveal fixed, tender nodular structures, ovarian abnormalities, and uterus fixed by restraining adhesions.
2. X-ray studies, such as barium enema, may demonstrate constrictions suggestive of endometriosis.
3. Laparoscopy is an effective diagnostic aid because tissue can be visualized.

Treatment and Nursing Management

1. It is necessary for the patient to be included in treatment plans so that she knows why a particular method of treatment has been selected and how her role is a vital one in the success of the team effort.
2. Encourage the patient to express her concerns; often false ideas emerge—such as "perhaps I have endometriosis because I used tampons."
3. The use of estrogen-progestogen "pseudopregnancy"—this therapy changes functioning endometriosis into decidua with subsequent necrosis and healing of lesions.
4. Menopause also improves or cures endometriosis; this is only of value to the older patient.
5. Danazol (Danocrine) is occasionally used to treat endometriosis by producing a temporary menopausal state. It appears successful, and later, when the drug is discontinued, patients are able to become pregnant.
6. Surgery, when indicated, is directed toward resection of cysts and lysis of adhesions.
7. Radical surgery may be necessary in the woman with extensive disease both within and outside the pelvis.

OVARIAN CANCER

Ovarian cancer is high risk cancer of the ovary.

Incidence

1. Barber states that ovarian cancer accounts for about 25% of all gynecologic cancers; it also accounts for about 47% of all genital cancer deaths.
2. Cancer of the ovary is the leading cause of death from gynecological cancer; it is the third most frequent gynecological cancer.

Clinical Manifestations

1. Advanced cancer: Abdominal swelling, pain, and a mass in the abdomen
2. Earliest manifestations—insidious and vague:
   a. Some abdominal discomfort
   b. Indigestion
   c. Flatulence
   d. Slight anorexia
3. These gastrointestinal symptoms may be due to an acid reaction of the peritoneal fluid in ovarian cancer.

Diagnostic Evaluation

1. Because of the high risk nature of ovarian cancer, it is important that every effort be made to diagnose the condition early.
2. The nurse should recognize those conditions in a woman which collectively place her in a high-risk category. High risk individuals include women who are
   a. Infertile
   b. Anovulatory
   c. Nulliparous
   d. Habitual aborters
3. If only *one* of the above conditions is present, along with *three* of the following symptoms, the patient should be labeled as "High Risk."
   a. Increasing premenstrual tension
   b. Irregular menses
   c. Menorrhagia with breast tenderness
   d. An early menopause

4. Semiannual gynecological examination and cervical cytology.
5. Investigate any ovarian enlargement by laparoscopy or laparotomy.
   This is particularly true of postmenopausal women whose ovaries should not be palpable.

Treatment

1. Surgical removal of diseased area—extensiveness depends upon the malignancy.

2. Treatment may be ovariectomy, hysterectomy, bilateral salpingo-oophorectomy, omentectomy, appendectomy.
3. Modalities may be surgery first, radiation and chemotherapy, and finally immunotherapy.
4. Cisplatin (Platinol) is a new intravenous drug which may be combined with doxorubicin (Adriamycin) to treat ovarian cancer.

PELVIC INFECTION

All structures in the pelvic cavity can become infected. Two types can be roughly distinguished according to the site of the infection and its spread.

Etiology

Nongonococcal Infections

Chlamydia trachomatis is a genital tract infection in women which is similar to gonorrhea; the incidence is increasing.
1. This condition may occur with or without a gonorrheal infection.
2. It may be mild enough to be ignored or severe enough to cause symptoms:
   a. Mucopurulent cervical exudate with erythema, edema, and congestion; in addition there may be friability (easily crumbled) of the cervix.

Gonoccocal and Mixed Infection

1. Gonococcal infection originates in the urethra, cervix, and/or rectum.
2. If reinfection does occur following proper treatment, the disease is self-limiting.
3. Most frequently, women are reinfected, and the secondary invaders (streptococcus, staphylococcus, *Escherichia coli,* etc.) take over. Accordingly, as a rule, what started as a self-limiting salpingitis becomes a chronic process. The disease is spread by way of the uterine canal into the tube and through the fimbria.
4. As a rule, the endometritis resulting from gonorrhea is shortlived.
5. The largest group of infections are created by pelvic cellulitis—i.e., endometritis from a complication of pregnancy or an intrauterine device.
6. Here all the cervical and vaginal pathogens are offenders. They spread by way of the lymphatics and blood vessels.
7. Cellulitis tends to be unilateral whereas gonorrhea is a bilateral process.
8. Tuberculous endometritis—uncommon in the United States and common in Israel—is a likely cause of infertility.

Clinical Manifestations

1. Abdominal pain, nausea and vomiting, temperature elevation, malaise
2. Leukocytosis
3. Malodorous, purulent vaginal discharge

Treatment and Nursing Management

OBJECTIVES: to control the spread of infection within the patient.
   to prevent the spread of infection to others, including the nurse.
1. Place patient in a semi-Fowler's position to facilitate drainage.
2. Avoid the use of tampons; catheterization is contraindicated in order to minimize spread of infection.
3. Support patient nutritionally with attractive, well-balanced meals.
4. Administer appropriate antibiotics and chemotherapeutic agents as prescribed.
   a. Nongonococcal (Chlamydiae)—tetracycline regime
   b. Gonococcal—Penicillin G, ampicillin, spectinomycin
5. Control spread of infection by the following safeguards:
   a. Handle perineal pads with extreme precautions:
      (1) Use an instrument or gloves.
      (2) Deposit pad in paper bag for proper disposal.
   b. Wash hands carefully before and after patient contacts.
   c. Disinfect utensils, bedpans, toilet seats, and linen. Adopt procedure appropriate for specific organism.
   d. Instruct patient to protect herself from reinfection and to prevent spread to others.
6. Apply heat to the abdomen externally and hot douches vaginally as prescribed, to improve circulation.
7. Record vital signs, patient responses (physical and mental) to therapy, and nature and amount of vaginal discharge.
8. Recognize the depressing nature of the disease and that the patient needs support and understanding, particularly when she has discomfort and vague symptoms.

Complications from Untreated or Recurrent Infection

1. Chronic pelvic discomfort; disease becomes rampant.
2. Sterility occurs because of closing of fallopian tubes with scar tissue.
3. Ectopic pregnancy is possible if fertilized egg is unable to pass stricture.
4. Inflammatory masses may develop, eventually requiring removal of uterus, tubes, and ovaries.

FERTILITY CONTROL

Basic Principles

1. The nurse should be familiar with the application, advantages and disadvantages of the various methods of contraception available.
2. The most effective method is the one a woman selects for herself and will use consistently.
3. Women are entitled to contraceptive advice as part of good medical care without the burden of moral judgment.

Contraceptive Methods

NOTE: Failure Rate (Pregnancy) is determined by the experience of 100 women for 1 year and is expressed as *pregnancies per 100 woman years.*

A. *Coitus Interruptus*

This is the withdrawal of the penis from the vagina when ejaculation is imminent.
1. Indications—Effective when mechanical devices are unavailable.
2. Contraindications
   a. When male is not able to exert self-control.
   b. Ineffective when premature ejaculation occurs—this is true of almost 50% of males.
3. Undesirable Effects
   a. Failure rate is between 35—40%.
   b. Psychological ill effects for both male and female.
   c. Subsequent prostatitis has been substantiated.

B. *Condom*

Application of a rubber sheath worn over the penis by the male during coitus.
1. Procedure for Use and Precautions
   a. Place condom over erect penis.
   b. Leave a dead space at the tip of the condom (from which air has been expelled) to allow room for ejaculate.
   c. Lubricate (spermicidal) exterior of condom—as an added precaution.
   d. Avoid leaving condom in vagina during withdrawal; this is facilitated by grasping ring around top of condom at time of withdrawal.
2. Advantages
   a. Inexpensive and easy to use; available without a prescription.
   b. Protects against pregnancy and offers some protection against venereal disease.
   c. May lessen premature ejaculation.
   d. Assures males involvement in the contraceptive process.
3. Disadvantages
   a. May dull sensation somewhat for male and fe male.
   b. Requires an erect penis for application.
   c. Condom may tear or rupture and thus be ineffective.
   d. May cause a contact dermatitis
4. Failure Rate (Pregnancy)
   Varies from 15 to 35 (various authorities) undesired pregnancies per 100 woman years.

NOTE: If condom ruptures, the female should see her gynecologist immediately to obtain "morning after pill" (high estrogen) for pregnancy interception.

C. *Diaphragm*

A rubber dome-shaped device with a flexible wire rim which is inserted in the vagina to fit snugly behind the pubic bone and over the cervix into the posterior fornix. It is used to prevent sperm from reaching the cervical os. Spermicidal jelly is often used on both sides of the diaphragm.
1. Indications—preferred by women who
   a. Object to a device in utero.
   b. Object to hormonal or chemical contraceptives.
   c. Do not object to insertion of the diaphragm immediately prior to intercourse.
2. Procedure for Insertion and Follow-up
   a. Bimanual pelvic examination and cytology smear are preliminary to measurement for a diaphragm.
   b. Measure depth of vagina; select largest diaphragm that can be retained comfortably; it too small, the device will be displaced during intercourse.
   c. Teach the patient how to insert diaphragm behind lower edge of pubic bone; use spermicidal jelly or cream for additional contraceptive action.
   d. Instruct her to retain diaphragm for 6-8 hours after intercourse.
   e. Remind patient of annual gynecological examination.
   f. Inform patient that a larger diaphragm may be necessary after a pregnancy.
3. Failure Rate (Pregnancy)
   15 undesired pregnancies per 100 woman years of using diaphragm.

D. *Vaginal Foam*

This is a spermicidal cushioning foam that is available in cream, jel, aerosol, or tablet form. All except the tablet are effective immediately—tablets require 5-10 minutes to dissolve.
1. Advantages
   a. Requires little instruction; a favorite method with lower socioeconomic groups.
   b. May be used to advantage with coitus interruptus.
2. Disadvantage
   Higher failure rate than other contraceptive methods.
3. Failure Rate (Pregnancy)
   Somewhere between 35 and 45 per 100 woman years.

E. *Intrauterine Device (IUD)*

The IUD is a device made of metal or plastic that fits inside the uterus; it may be in the shape of a spiral, loop, shield, or ring.

NURSING ALERT: It is now apparent that the IUD is more dangerous than ever anticipated. Endometritis, ovarian abscesses, ruptured uteri, and their consequences have left a trail of pelvic surgery and permanent crippling that cannot be ignored.

1. Indications
   a. When hormonal medications appear to be contraindicated.

b. When motivation and other resources are lacking, as a last resort.
2. Contraindications
   a. Inflammation or infection of cervix, uterus, or uterine tubes.
   b. Objections on the part of the woman to a foreign device in her uterus.
   c. Severe dysmenorrhea.
3. *Advantages*
   a. Effectiveness listed as 97%–99%
   b. Convenient; permits spontaneity of intercourse
   Disadvantages
   a. Increased dysmenorrhea and amount of menstrual flow
   b. Some discomfort with insertion of IUD
   c. Increased risk of pelvic inflammatory disease
   d. In prolonged use (over three years without IUD having been removed) there is increasing risk of pelvic actinomycosis
4. Procedure for Insertion
   a. Nursing history is obtained to determine contraceptive history and pertinent health information such as:
      abnormal vaginal bleeding, pelvic infections, past surgery on reproductive organs, pregnancy history, nature of menses, presence of other diseases.
   b. Client is counseled as recommended by the US Food and Drug Administration:
      (1) Preinsertion
         What you should know about the IUD
         Use-effectiveness
         What you should tell your physician: adverse reactions
      (2) Postinsertion
         Description of the IUD
         Directions for use
         Side effects
         Warnings
         Special warning about pregnancy with an IUD in place
   c. A pelvic examination and a (Pap) cytology smear is done.
   d. Calibre of interior of the uterus is determined by means of sounding.
   e. Insertion of IUD with the aid of a plastic inserter at time of menstruation is done by a physician (or one specifically trained). Menstruation ensures dilation of cervix and that the patient is not pregnant.
   f. A nylon string attached to the IUD dangles from the cervix and can be detected during vaginal examination.

NURSING ALERT: If the patient is pregnant when an IUD is inserted, she may suffer septic abortion and possibly fatal septicemic shock; hence the wisdom of having the device inserted during menstruation.

5. Patient Education
   a. Inform client how to check for IUD nylon string.
   b. Instruct her to avoid intercourse for 5 days (time to permit IUD to induce endometrial changes).
   c. Recommend follow-up visits as directed.

d. Suggest that she promptly seek assistance if any of the following occurs:
   (1) Unusually heavy or long bleeding
   (2) Bleeding between periods
   (3) Pain; unusual vaginal discharge
   (4) Infection signs—chills/fever
   (5) Inability to locate string
   (6) Signs of pregnancy
   (7) Suspected or obvious expulsion of IUD
e. Provide her with a wallet card showing IUD insertion date, clinic and emergency phone numbers.
f. Suggest that the woman check with her physician as to how long her particular IUD can be worn before being removed. It should be removed and replaced every two to three years.

F. *Oral Fertility Control—the "Pill"*
1. Basis of Operation of Oral Contraceptives
   Oral synthetic preparations of estrogens and progesterone are used. It is believed that in the presence of sufficient amounts of these synthetic compounds, the hypothalamus fails to secrete the usual LH releasing factor and its stimulating product LH which normally occurs about 12-14 days after the onset of the monthly menstrual cycle and is essential to ovulation.
2. Indications
   a. For those desirous of a highly effective contraceptive with no special preparation immediately before intercourse.
   b. For women who will conscientiously adhere to a daily plan of pill-taking.
3. Contraindications
   a. A complete physical examination is required prior to taking the "pill" and 12-month checkups thereafter.
   b. Contraindications are debatable and often not substantiated by hard, reliable data.
4. Methods
   a. Combined steroid therapy
      A pill with an estrogen and progestogen usually taken 20 days during each month beginning on the 5th day after the onset of menstruation.
   b. Microprogestational therapy
      Low dosage of progestational drug given continuously:
         Androgens—19-carbon compounds
         Progesterone—21-carbon compounds
         Estrogens—Menstranol and ethrynyl estradiol

NURSING ALERT: Cigarette smoking increases risk of serious cardiovascular side effects from oral contraceptives. Women who use the pill should be strongly advised not to smoke.

5. Risk Factors and Contraindications
   a. Past history of cardiovascular disease
   b. Known or suspected breast carcinoma
   c. Known or suspected estrogen-dependent neoplasia of uterus (endometrium or cervix)
   d. Liver disease or impaired liver function
   e. Known or suspected pregnancy
   f. Genital bleeding—undiagnosed

6. Risk Factors and Possible Contraindications
   a. Women over 40 years of age
   b. History of migraine, hypertension, epilepsy
   c. Leiomyomas of the uterus
7. Disadvantages
   a. Because oral contraceptives are potent drugs there may be side effects: increased incidence of thromboembolic disease, essential hypertension, disturbance of carbohydrate metabolism—diabetes, acceleration of the process of arteriosclerosis in those with a predisposition.
   b. They require close supervision by a physician.
   c. Interference with laboratory diagnostic procedures: sedimentation rate, thyroid test for protein-bound iodine or thyroxine, cervical smears and biopsy, and even the "Pap" test.
8. Side effects—occur in approximately 1–3% of women on low-dose pill.
9. Failure Rate (Pregnancy)
   Combined—less than 1 pregnancy per hundred woman years.

G. *Topical Spermicide*—chemically active substance which incapacitates spermatazoa; when used properly it is estimated to be 95% effective and even when used improperly, it is considered about 85% effective.

Action
This product consists of two parts:
1. Relatively basic material which
   a. blocks passage of spermatazoa
   b. serves as a vehicle for
2. Spermicide; this incapacitates sperm before it reaches the ovum

Advantages
1. Safe—no proven systemic side effects or serious local reaction
2. Available—no prescription required
3. Convenient and acceptable; simple to use
4. Provides a measure of protection against venereal disease.

H. *Abortion* (See p. 1051.)

Sterilization Procedures
A. *Indications*
1. The patient's desire
   a. Socioeconomic reasons
   b. Therapeutic or eugenic reasons to prevent a pregnancy that might endanger the mother's life
2. Legal considerations
   a. Laws much less rigid than those governing therapeutic abortion.
   b. Written consent required from a legally responsible and informed person.

   c. Must be compatible with state laws.
3. Incidence and indications
   a. Increasing numbers are performed annually in U.S.
   b. Done for multiparity, 2 or more previous cesarean sections, hypertensive cardiovascular disease.
   c. Done for other reasons: vaginal plastic procedures, for inheritable life-threatening disease.

B. *Tubal Sterilization*
1. Types:
   a. Tubal ligation with or without resection
   b. Tubal ligation with or without crushing
   c. Tubal transection and burying of stumps
   d. Cornual resection
   e. Cornual occlusion utilizing cautery
2. Approaches
   a. Abdominal
   b. After a cesarean section
   c. Vaginally
3. Evaluation
   a. There are advantages and disadvantages to each of the above—the individual situation must be considered.
   b. Reversible methods of tubal occlusion or semi-permanent sterilization using metal clips or chemical injections are still experimental.
4. Laparoscopy:
   a. A relatively new procedure in which coagulation and transection of the isthmic tubal segments is done through a laparoscope (an electrical current is passed for 3–5 seconds to cut and coagulate tube).
   b. The procedure is considered rapid, safe, and effective.
   c. The patient is discharged from the hospital about 3 hours postoperatively with minimal discomfort; procedure can be done on an outpatient basis.
   d. Effectiveness
      (1) Hysterosalpingography done 12 weeks postoperatively confirms tubal occlusion in 98% of patients.
      (2) No adverse effects occur in sex relations, menstrual function, or outward bodily appearance.
   e. Hazards:
      (1) Pulmonary embolism, hemorrhage, infection
      (2) Tubal pregnancy
      (3) Some women are disturbed emotionally by procedure; however, 90% of patients who request this have no subsequent regret.

C. *Vasectomy* (See p. 526.) Source of Information:
American Fertility Society, 1801 Ninth Ave., South, Birmingham, Alabama 35205

3   CONDITIONS OF THE BREAST

EARLY DETECTION AND DIAGNOSTIC EVALUATION

A. *Breast Self-examination (BSE)*
1. Clinical value
   a. Experience has verified that more than 90% of breast cancers are found by women themselves.
   b. When women discover lumps in their breasts at

a very early stage, surgery can save 70–80% of proven cases.
2. Health Education
   a. Encourage women to examine their breasts once a month, just after the menstrual period because breasts are less engorged at this time and a tumor

is easier to detect, and at regular monthly intervals after the cessation of menses (Fig. 11-17).

b. The breast can be examined in the sitting or standing position noting in a mirror any contour changes, asymmetry, nipple discharge, or eczematoid scaling around the nipple.

c. Then the breast is examined in the supine position with the breast spread out on the chest wall; use the flattened, more sensitive surface of the fingers

to gently knead breast tissue in the search for abnormalities.

d. Since most of the lesions occur in the upper outer quadrant (see Fig. 11-20B), an effective pattern to follow is to start the examination in the upper outer quadrant, proceed around the breast, and repeat (at the end) the upper outer quadrant. (In this manner, five-fourths of the breast are examined.)

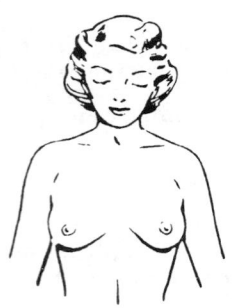
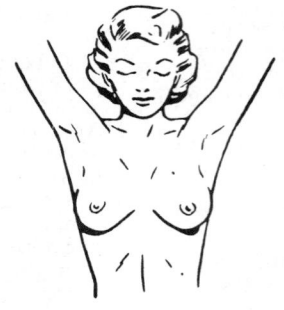
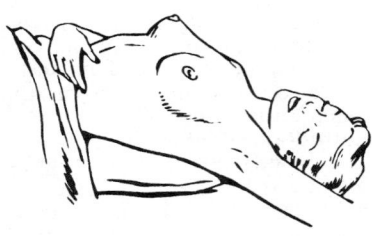

1. Careful examination of the breasts before a mirror for symmetry in size and shape, noting any puckering or dimpling of the skin or retraction of the nipple.

2. Arms raised over head, again studying the breasts in the mirror for the same signs.

3. Reclining on bed with flat pillow or folded bath towel under the shoulder on the same side as breast to be examined.

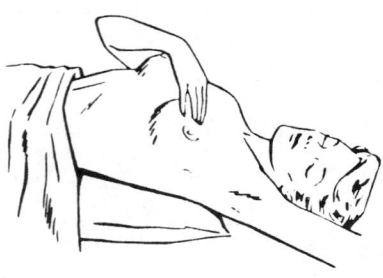
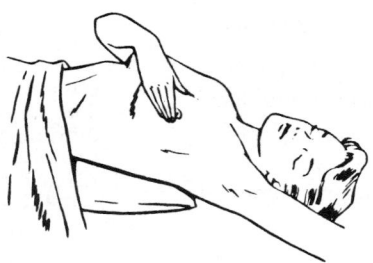
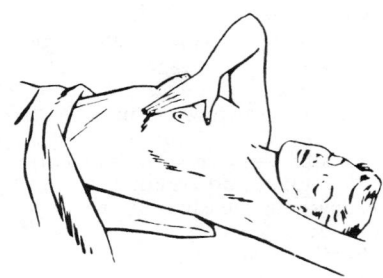

4. To examine the inner half of the breast the arm is raised over the head. Beginning at the breastbone and, in a series of steps, the inner half of the breast is palpated.

5. The area over the nipple is carefully palpated with the flat part of the fingers.

6. Examination of the lower inner half of the breast is completed.

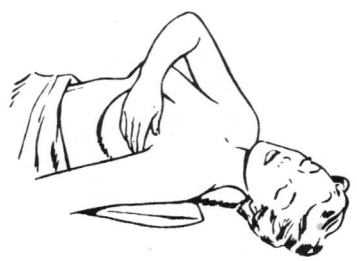
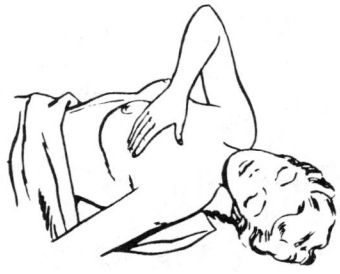
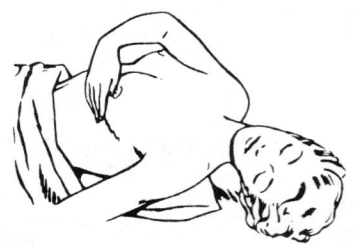

7. With arm down at side self examination of breasts continues by carefully feeling the tissues which extend to the armpit.

8. The upper outer quadrant of the breast is examined with the flat part of the fingers.

9. The lower outer quadrant of the breast is examined in successive stages with flat part of the fingers.

FIGURE 11-17. *Breast self-examination. (Courtesy American Cancer Society.)*

e. When in doubt, compare findings with opposite breast.

3. Suggestions for patients unable to or who are having difficulty doing self-examination:
   a. Determine the problem:
      (1) If patient complains of tenderness, gentle self-examination may be more effective and less painful than examination by someone else.
      (2) For the woman who has cysts or lumps, recommend professional examination annually and instruct her in detecting changes from one month to the next.
      (3) If the patient has large pendulous breasts, encourage her to lie on her back and perform self-examination slowly and in a specific pattern or order.

b. Recommend other diagnostic aids periodically—mammography, thermography, xeroradiography (below) as condition indicates.

4. Community Health Education
   a. Tell women's organizations about the breast self-examination film and advise them to see it.
   b. Arrange for local showings of the film.
   c. Take part in the discussion of the film. Be prepared—know the signs that may mean breast cancer.
   d. Help to create healthy psychological attitudes.
   e. Know the resources within the community where medical help is available, physicians' offices, nearby hospitals, cancer clinics, or cancer hospitals.

GUIDELINES: Examination of the Breast by the Nurse

Purpose
1. To detect abnormalities in the breasts
2. To teach a woman how to perform breast self-examination

Equipment A good lamp and privacy

Procedure

NURSING ACTION	RATIONALE/AMPLIFICATION
Preparatory Phase and Superficial Examination	
1. Have the woman strip to her waist and sit comfortably, facing the examiner.	1. This provides an opportunity to visually observe breasts for lack of symmetry and for gross signs such as redness, irritated nipple, dimpling, orange-peel skin.
2. Wash your hands under warm water and dry them; powder if they feel "sticky."	2. The breast is sensitive to cold.
Examination	
1. Palpate supraclavicular area.	1. Note whether lymph nodes are enlarged, fixed, movable, or difficult to locate.
2. Palpate axillary nodes; hold woman's forearm in your left palm while you check nodes with your right fingertips. Repeat on other side.	2. Same as 1 above.
3. Instruct patient to lie down with her right arm under her head. Place a small pillow under the right shoulder.	3. This will spread breast tissue evenly over chest wall.
4. With the flattened surface of 2 or 3 fingers, gently palpate breast tissue beginning at the upper outer quadrant. a. Proceed in an orderly pattern around the breast and repeat the first quarter examined. b. Repeat procedure for other breast.	4. The sensitive fingers proceeding in a kneading fashion can detect thickened, lumpy, or "buckshot" tissue between the patient's skin and chest wall. Since the majority of breast lesions are in the upper outer quadrant, this segment is double checked.
5. Recognize that there is a prolongation of the axillary extension of normal breast tissue which may extend high into axilla.	5. This is normal if symmetrical; abnormal if asymmetrical.
6. Check the areolar area for crustiness, nipple discharge, signs of infection.	6. Prepare to collect a discharge specimen for cytology if indicated (see Fig. 11-18, p. 557).
7. Record findings and report abnormalities to the physician.	
8. Instruct the patient in performing self-examination on her own (Fig. 11-17). Encourage her to ask any questions; provide her with appropriate literature.	8. 95% of women discover their own abnormalities.

B. *Physical Examination*
1. Annual physical checkup should include breast examination and palpation.
2. Twice-a-year examination recommended for women with a family history of cancer.

C. *Mammography*—roentgenography of breast without injection of contrast medium; 2 views: (1) Caudal, and (2) mediolateral.

Guidelines for use of mammography for breast cancer screening:
1. In women under 35, no mammography.
2. In women 35–39, use only if patient has had a breast cancer.
3. Women in their 40s, use annually if there is a history of breast cancer in immediate family.
   Indications: Greatest value is in detecting suspicious area before a "lump" is felt. Hence,

earlier diagnosis. Other than for cancer screening:

4. Breast disease evident in form of a questionable lump.
5. Lumpy or very large breasts which are difficult to examine.
6. Screening the opposite breast in a woman with a mass on one side.
7. Cancerophobia (fear of cancer).

D. *Thermography*—infrared photography gives a pictorial representation of heat patterns on the surface of the breast which may indicate signs of abnormal circulation (of limited value).

1. Heat sensing equipment is used to detect minute amounts of heat generated in and around areas of increased blood supply.
2. Thermography is a complementary diagnostic tool that may be useful in the evaluation of breast disease when combined with both physical examination under the supervision of a qualified physician and mammography by a trained radiologist.
3. An advantage is that there is no radiation exposure.

E. *Xeroradiography*—a special x-ray technique in which a selenium-coated plate is subjected to an electrical charge; after the x-ray exposure is made, the plate is carefully developed. The xerogram portrays all tissue in bas-relief, like a "positive" film instead of the "negative."

F. *Transillumination*—using a powerful cold light in a completely darkened room, breast tissue can be illuminated and a cyst or neoplasm can easily be demonstrated. The method is not satisfactory in fibrosis because of the density of tissue.

G. *Ultrasound scanning*—a more recent painless noninvasive technique that is still being evaluated.

H. *Biopsy*

1. *Aspiration* (needle)
   Purpose: This is a simple, rapid, and accurate procedure to detect breast cancer.
   a. Tumor or cyst is immobilized between 2 fingers to stabilize it during needle insertion (Fig. 11-18).
   b. Gently create a vacuum in syringe by pulling back and forth on plunger; allow pressure to equalize before withdrawing needle.
   c. Spread needle contents on glass slide; further spread specimen with a 2nd glass slide held at an angle.

NOTE: Positive results are significant. Negative results are ignored; other clinical evaluations must be done.

2. *Incisional* (Surgical)
   A piece of tissue is obtained in the operating room and sent to the laboratory for frozen section, which is then stained and examined under the microscope. It is desirable to allow at least a day or two between the biopsy and definitive treatment.

3. *Excisional*
   Following an incision into the breast, the entire lump is removed for microscopic study.

I. *Estrogen-receptor Assay*—A test of tumor tissue to determine whether or not the cancer cells have estrogen receptor sites. If such sites are present, the patient is more likely to respond to endocrine manipulation.

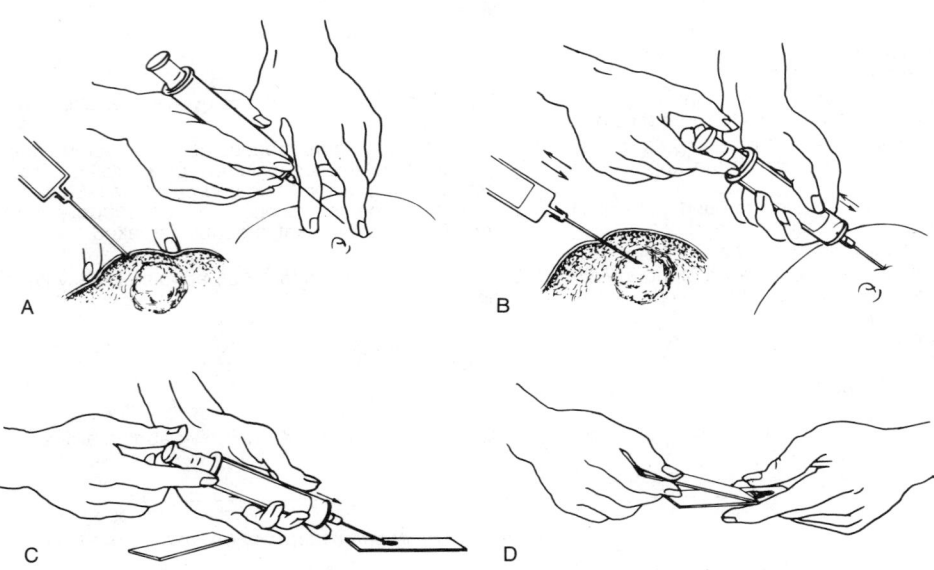

FIGURE 11-18. *Aspiration cytology. A. Tumor is immobilized with two fingers before the needle is inserted. B. A vacuum is created by withdrawing the plunger slowly but forcefully several times. Before the needle is removed, the pressure is allowed to equalize. C. Contents of the needle are placed on a glass slide. D. The smear is spread forward gently with a glass slide inclined at an angle of about 35 degrees, with an up-and-down movement. (Zajdela A. The value of aspiration cytology in the diagnosis of breast cancer. Cancer 35)*

CONDITIONS OF THE NIPPLE

FISSURES AND BLEEDING

	Fissure of Nipple	Bleeding from Nipple

Clinical Manifestations	A *fissure* of the nipple is a longitudinal type of ulcer that occasionally develops in the breast of a nursing mother.
	  a. Nipple appears sore and irritated
	  b. Bleeding from nipple
		Bloody discharge—usually on edge of areola.

Causes	1. Lack of preparation of nipples in prenatal period. 2. Condition aggravated by sucking infant.	1. Most commonly due to wartlike papilloma in one of larger collecting ducts at edge of areola. 2. Occasionally a malignancy is responsible (Fig. 11-19, cytology examination).
Health Teaching	1. Keep nipple clean by washing and drying after each nursing period (see p. 1031). 2. In prenatal period, wash, dry, and lubricate nipples in preparation for nursing.	

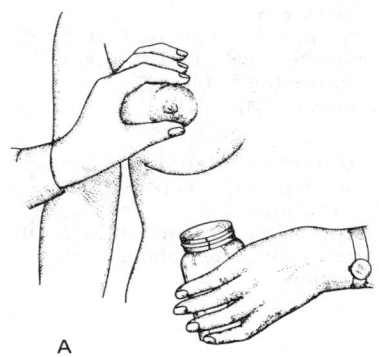

A

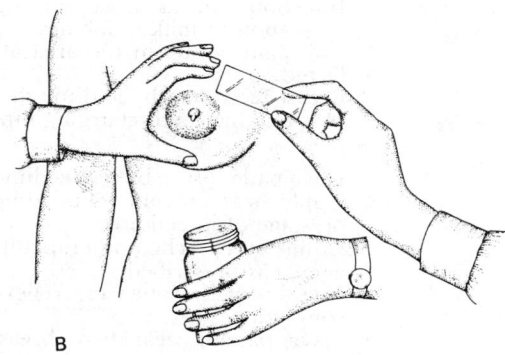

B

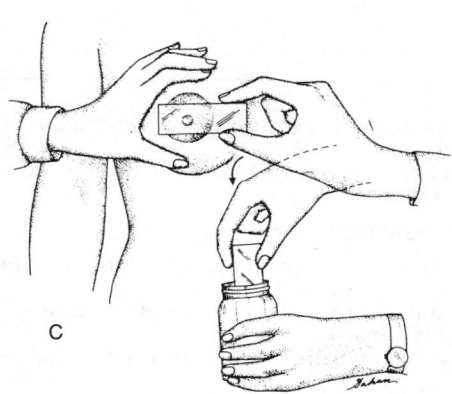

C

FIGURE 11-19. *Obtaining nipple discharge specimen for cytologic examination.*
1. *Wash nipple gently with cotton pledget; pat dry.*
2. *Gently strip duct and express fluid only until a small pea-sized drop appears on nipple.*
3. *Obtain assistance of patient in holding container of fixative solution near breast to receive the prepared slide.*
4. *Stabilize breast with fingers and thumb of one hand (A).*
5. *Gently place one end of slide on nipple (B); rapidly draw slide across nipple and immediately drop into fixative solution (C).*
6. *This may be repeated to secure additional specimens if necessary.*
NOTE: 1. Positive results are significant.
2. Negative results may be "false negatives." This test is never used alone but in conjunction with other diagnostic tests.

	Fissure of Nipple	Bleeding from Nipple

Treatment and Nursing Management	1. Wash nipples with sterile saline solution.
	2. Use artificial nipple for nursing.
	3. If above does not initiate healing process, stop nursing and use breast pump.
		1. Surgery for palpable mass.
		  a. Duct is identified.
		  b. Papilloma is excised (or a wedge of breast from area producing the bleeding is excised if no gross papilloma is identified) through a small peri-areolar incision—send for laboratory analysis.
		  c. Sterile dressings applied.
		2. If no palpable mass, mammography and xerography.

INFLAMMATION OF THE BREAST

ACUTE MASTITIS AND MAMMARY ABSCESS

	Acute Mastitis	Mammary Abscess
Incidence	May occur at beginning or end of lactation.	Often follows acute mastitis.
Source of Infection	1. Hands of patient 2. Personnel caring for patient 3. Infection from baby 4. Blood-borne	Same
Clinical Manifestations	1. Infection attacks duct causing stagnation of milk in lobules. 2. Dull pain occurs in the area affected. 3. Breast feels doughy and tough. 4. May also have a discharging nipple.	1. Area is very sensitive, appears dusky red. 2. Pus may be expressed from nipple. (See Fig. 11-19, nipple discharge for cytology.) 3. Mass is palpable.
Treatment and Nursing Management	1. Have patient stop breast feeding. 2. Apply heat or cold (depending on stage of infection). 3. Administer chemotherapeutic agents as prescribed. 4. Give progesterone to relieve congestion. 5. Have patient wear firm breast support. 6. Encourage patient to practice meticulous personal hygiene.	1. Administer antibiotics and chemotherapy as prescribed. 2. Incise and drain. 3. Apply hot wet dressings to increase drainage and hasten resolution.

FIBROCYSTIC DISEASE

Fibrocystic disease is mammary dysplasia characterized by increased formation of fibrous tissue, hyperplasia of the epithelial cells of the ducts and breast glands, and dilatation of the ducts. It is related to the cyclic stimulation of the breast by estrogen, but represents a departure from the normal stimulation and regression pattern of this process.

Incidence

1. The most common lesion of the female breast; 3 to 4 times more prevalent than cancer.
2. Overgrowth of fibrous tissue around ducts; dilatation of the ducts to form cysts; epithelial hyperplasia in ducts on glands.
3. Occurs usually in women between 30 and 50 and is endocrine related.

Clinical Manifestations

1. Patient complains of an uncomfortable feeling in the breast.
2. Cysts or lumps are usually firm, single or multiple smooth, round masses; bilateral.
3. They are tender on palpation or pressure and slightly mobile.

4. Pain may be of the "shooting" type and may be aggravated by congestion before a menstrual period.

Treatment and Nursing Management

1. Aspiration
   a. Patient is placed in supine position. Under aseptic precautions, skin area is cleaned with a skin antiseptic.
   b. Local anesthesia is given.
   c. The physician immobilizes cyst with thumb and index finger of one hand.
   d. Using a 20 ml. syringe and 16 or 18 gauge needle, the cyst is penetrated and aspirated.
2. Excision

If cyst refills within a week or 2, excisional biopsy is usually performed.
3. The nurse emphasizes the importance of frequent reexaminations.
   a. Individuals with fibrocystic disease have an increased incidence of subsequent malignancy.
   b. Self-examination is difficult in the markedly fibrotic breast.
4. Avoidance of methylxanthines (coffee, tea, cola, and chocolate) tends to resolve these cysts (investigational).

NOTE: The palpable changes of fibrocystic disease may mask an underlying cancer.

TUMORS OF THE BREAST

FIBROADENOMATA

Clinical Manifestations

1. Firm, round, movable, benign tumors of the breast.
2. Appear in breasts of girls in their late teens or early twenties.
3. No pain or tenderness.

Treatment

Removal through a small incision

Prognosis

No malignant potential

CANCER OF THE BREAST

Incidence

1. Breast cancer is the leading cause of cancer incidence and death in black and white women today.
2. One of every 4 women having an initial breast biopsy will have a malignancy.
3. About 110,000 new cases are predicted yearly and it is estimated that there will be 36,000 deaths.
4. Despite all efforts to date, the breast cancer death rate remains high.
5. Over 90% of patients discover their condition themselves through breast self-examination.
6. Survival rates—if cancer has
   a. Spread to axillary lymph nodes: 5-year survival rate is about 55%.
   b. Localized in breast: 5-year survival rate is 80–85%.

Risk Factors in Breast Cancer

A. *Major Risk Factors*

1. Sex—99% occur in females.
2. Age—higher incidence in early 40s; levels off between 45 and 55, then increased evidence in postmenopausal period.
3. Genetics—women whose mothers and sisters have had breast cancer are twice as likely to develop cancer.
4. Parity—decreased risk three to fourfold if first birth is before 18 years of age. Decrease in risk continues, but at a declining rate, up to age 25 for first parity. Increased risks in unmarried women, infertile women, women with fewer than 3 children, and

women who have first child after 34. Lower incidence of breast cancer with early parity.
5. If breast cancer appears in one breast, the likelihood of cancer in the other breast is greater.
6. Benign cystic breast is considered to be a precursor to cancer; likelihood of cancer is about 4 times greater in women who have cystic disease.

B. *Prominent Risk Factors*

1. Prolonged total menstrual activity. Increased incidence under the following circumstances:
   a. When menarche occurs before 12 years of age
   b. In those with 30 or more years menstrual activity
   c. When menopause occurs after 55.
2. Other organ cancers such as ovary, colon, endometrium
3. Wet type cerumen (earwax)—genetic predisposition

C. *Possible Risk Factors*

1. Heavy radiation exposure
2. Immunodeficiency
3. Exogenous estrogen administration
4. Excessive intake of dietary fat.

Clinical Manifestations (Fig. 11-20)

1. Early signs are insidious.
2. A nontender lump appears in the breast, most frequently in the upper outer quadrant; it may be movable and isolated.
3. Pain usually is absent except in the late stages.
   a. A recent study indicated that 13% of patients described pain as a primary symptom; 7% indicated that it was the first clue which led them to probe and examine the breast. Pain was described as a "hurt" or "funny feeling" rather than acute or sharp.
4. Retraction or dimpling of the skin over the mass may be noted.
5. On mirror examination, asymmetry may be observed—the affected breast appears more elevated than the other.
6. Nipple retraction or nipple bleeding may be apparent.
7. Later, the nodule becomes more fixed to the chest wall.
8. Nodular axillary masses may appear.
9. Ulceration appears in late stages.

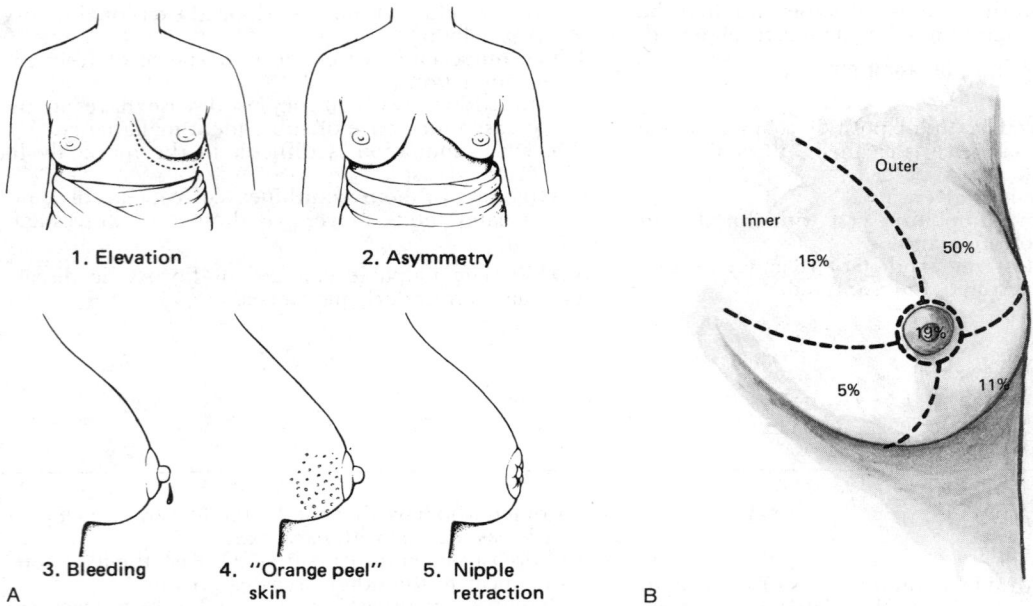

FIGURE 11-20. A. *Signs of cancer of the breast.* B. *Distribution of carcinomas in different areas of breast.*

Classification of Breast Tumors
See Table 11-2.

Treatment and Nursing Management

OBJECTIVES: to preserve the life of the woman.
to achieve permanent local control of the disease.
to minimize the possibility of recurrence.
to provide the best cosmetic result.

These may be accomplished by surgical removal of the cancer. Radiation, chemotherapy, and immunotherapy are other treatment modalities that may be employed independently or in combination with surgery for the purpose of helping to cure, control growth, alleviate pain, and/or prevent recurrence.

Prognosis:
1. When malignancy is confined to breast: 5-year survival—85%
2. When malignancy has spread to axilla: 5-year survival—55%

A. *Seek optimal physical and psychosocial approach in preparing patient for treatment.*
1. Begin emotional support when patient is told that hospitalization and biopsy may be required.
2. Dispel fear by
   a. Listening to patient's concerns and dispelling misconceptions.
   b. Collaborating with physician on a unified approach to informing the patient.
   c. Emphasizing successful program of rehabilitation, use of prosthesis, and possibly reconstruction.
   d. Having a patient who made a satisfactory postoperative adjustment visit present patient.
   e. Soliciting support of the husband and/or significant others.
   f. Providing encouragement and reassurance.

3. Minimize delay before operation.
   a. Determine physical, nutritional, and emotional needs.
   b. If radical surgery is anticipated, have blood replacement available.
   c. Administer hypnotic to minimize concerns of patient.
4. Prepare skin adequately (see p. 85).
   a. Instruct patient to wash operative area with a detergent-germicide for several days before admission.
   b. When skin graft is anticipated, shave and clean donor area (usually anterior aspect of thigh).

B. *Select a surgical approach to remove malignancy, minimize disfigurement, and prevent spread of cancer cells.*

1. *Tylectomy* (lumpectomy, tumorectomy, segmental mastectomy)—removal of lesion with an area of normal tissue surrounding the lesion followed by radiotherapy of the breast and the lymph drainage paths.
   a. Advantages are that cosmetic results are excellent; with negative nodes, follow-up data for 4–5 years are comparable to data for radical mastectomy with negative nodes.
   b. Disadvantages are that cancer may not be completely destroyed and may recur and that later effects of high dose radiotherapy are not yet known.
2. *Simple* or *total mastectomy*—removal of breast without lymph node dissection.
3. Total mastectomy with axillary dissection and preservation of the pectoral muscles (*Modified radical mastectomy*). Results appear to be comparable—better cosmetically and better for an external or internal prosthesis, depending on preference of patient and surgeon.

TABLE 11-2. CLASSIFICATION OF BREAST TUMOR AND PREFERRED METHOD OF TREATMENT

Clinical Anatomic Observation	Treatment
Stage I Breast mass localized; all nodes negative	Variable: Tylectomy (p. 560) Some prefer simple mastectomy plus irradiation. Others prefer simple mastectomy without irradiation. Modified radical mastectomy
Stage II Breast mass localized; axillary nodes positive	Radical mastectomy preferred with or without postoperative irradiation.
Stage III Breast mass locally extensive; axillary, supraclavicular and internal mammary nodes positive	This is considered inoperable for cure. Variable depending on extensiveness: 1. Simple mastectomy with radiation, chemotherapy, and 2. Radiation therapy, chemotherapy, and endocrine manipulation

Stage IV
Distant metastasis
	Variable, depending on location of metastasis (bone, soft tissue, etc.).
	1. Radiation therapy for primary lesion or metastasis
	2. Endocrine manipulation
	  a. Systemic—estrogens, androgens, or steroids
	  b. Ablation—oophorectomy, adrenalectomy, hypophysectomy
	3. Chemotherapy

4. *Classical radical mastectomy (Halsted)*—removal of breast and underlying muscles down to chest wall; also removal of nodules and lymphatics of axilla. This is rapidly being replaced by the modified radical mastectomy.

C. *Initiate postoperative surveillance to minimize complications and hasten recovery.*

1. See Chapter 6 for detailed discussion of postoperative care.
2. Upon patient's return from the recovery room, promote comfort and rest; administer analgesics for pain.
3. Relay any positive verified information related to the successful removal of all tumors, limited spread, etc.; this can accelerate recovery.
4. Encourage fluid and nutritional support as tolerated and desired.
5. Position comfortably in semi-Fowler's position; if arm is free, elevate on a pillow; the most distal part (hand) is placed higher to permit gravity to aid in removal of fluid via lymphatics and venous pathways. Note Fig. 11-21, which describes a practice followed in some clinics.
6. Check dressings for undue constriction, signs of hemorrhage, etc.; ensure that portable suction or other drainage devices are operating properly.
7. Encourage mobility of arm on the affected side as recommended by the surgeon, to prevent such complications as lymphedema and frozen shoulder:
   a. Initiate bed exercises after 24 hours, such as wrist and elbow flexion and extension, hourly.
   b. Encourage patient to use her arm in self-care: washing face, applying lipstick, combing hair.
   c. Table 11-3, page 562, for activities to be resumed eventually
8. Ambulate patient early, as determined by individual patient.
9. Familiarize patient with "Reach to Recovery" program of the American Cancer Society:
   a. Combine this with visits by helpful persons who have had a successful mastectomy rehabilitation.
   b. Acquaint patient with prosthetic possibilities as determined feasible by the surgeon.
   c. Suggest clothing adjustments and possibilities.
   d. Assist patient in addressing psychosocial adjustment problems including sexual problems; include her husband or important others as required.

D. *Be familiar with other treatment modalities and their impact on the patient.*

1. Radiation Therapy
   a. Primary treatment when surgery has been ruled out by advanced age, inoperable condition, other complications.
   b. Adjunct therapy to surgery.
   c. To reduce tumor size; as palliation for pain.
   When radiation therapy is used, follow principles of care, page 852.
2. Chemotherapy—Also see pp. 843–851.

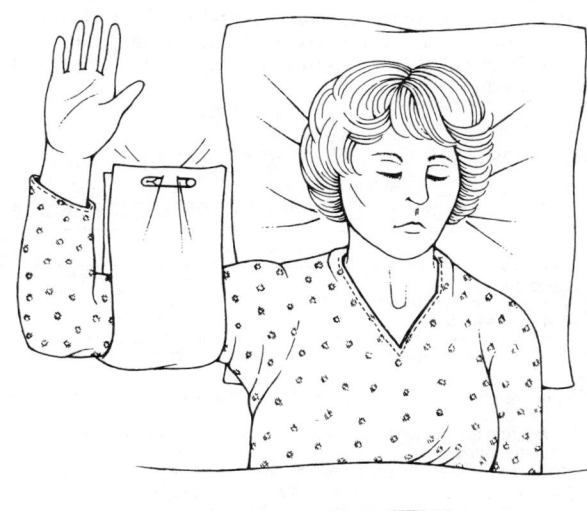

FIGURE 11-21. *One method of intermittent arm elevation. Early in the postoperative period, the arm on the operative side is positioned at right angles to the body. A folded towel (comfortably wide) is placed loosely around the arm to provide support; it is pinned to the bed sheet and underpadding. A pillow may be used to support the forearm to prevent undue extension of the elbow. While awake, the patient is encouraged to rotate her arm, as if reaching for her face. If the patient maintains this position intermittently for 24 to 48 hours, by the time of ambulation she has gained considerable arm movement for adding other exercises. (After Degenshein. Surg Gynecol Obstet 1977 July; 145:77)*

a. Used as adjunct therapy to surgery and/or radiotherapy.

b. Usually various combinations of drugs are preferred.

c. Four major types of drugs are alkylating, antimetabolite, antibiotic, and mitotic inhibitor.

3. Immunotherapy (unproven)

a. Theory is that immunologic response could destroy invading cancer cells while sparing normal cells.

b. Bacille Calmette-Guérin (BCG) and levamisole have shown promise of being able to destroy cancer cells.

4. Prophylactic Mastectomy

Removal of breast tissue (leaving skin and nipple area), followed by insertion of a mammary implant in *carefully selected patients who are in the high-risk group for developing breast cancer.* Implants may be inserted immediately or at a later date.

Postoperative nursing objective: to maintain skin viability and survival over implant area.

a. Keep head of bed elevated about 30° to promote drainage.

b. Instruct patient to keep elbows at her side to prevent stretching of breast skin (3–4 weeks); soft wristlet restraints may be necessary at night.

c. Check dressings and suction drains frequently for evidence of bleeding.

d. Eliminate any pressure on dressings which might restrict circulation.

e. Encourage intake of fluid to prevent dehydration.

f. Advise patient not to turn on her side or abdomen for at least a month to avoid trauma to operated area.

g. Encourage patient to take deep breaths and cough at prescribed intervals to aerate lungs that may otherwise develop complications due to limited movement.

Discharge Planning and Health Education

1. Talk to and listen to patient; encourage questions and provide helpful answers.

2. Prepare the husband for his role in providing the necessary emotional support.

3. Initiate active exercise on the affected side 24 hours postoperatively for hand and elbow. Check with physician on extent of exercise for each individual patient. Exercises will increase daily and the patient will do more of her own activities such as hair combing, teeth brushing, etc. (Table 11-3).

NOTE: Be cautious in exercising the shoulder during the first week after surgery. Excessive abduction of the arm at the shoulder can lift skin flaps from chest wall and increase serous formation.

a. Exercise should not be painful.

b. Bilateral activity is emphasized.

c. Proper posture should be maintained.

d. If the patient has had a skin graft or if the skin was approximated under tension, exercises will be limited.

4. Care of Wound

a. Explain how the wound will gradually change.

b. Note that the newly healed wound may have less sensation due to severed nerves.

c. Bathe gently and blot carefully to dry.

d. Recognize signs of infection—pain, tenderness, redness, swelling; if these are present, report to physician.

e. Massage gently the healed incision with cocoa butter to encourage circulation and increase skin elasticity. This is initiated with physician approval.

5. Use of a prosthesis—sponge rubber, air-filled, or fluid-filled.

a. Type and style are suggested on an individual basis; skilled fitters from reliable companies are most helpful.

TABLE 11-3. EXERCISES FOR THE REHABILITATION OF THE PATIENT FOLLOWING MASTECTOMY

Exercise	Equivalent Daily Activities
1. Stand erect, Lean forward from waist. Allow arms to hang. Swing arms from side to side together; then in opposite direction. Next, swing arms from front to back together; then in opposite direction.	Broom sweeping Vacuum cleaning Mopping floor Pulling out and pushing in drawers Weaving Playing golf
2. Stand erect facing wall with palms of hand flat against wall; arms extended. Relax arms and shoulders and allow upper part of body to lean forward against hand. Push away to original position; repeat.	Pushing self out of bath tub Kneading bread Breast stroke—swimming Sawing or cutting types of crafts
3. Stand erect facing wall with palms of hand flat against wall. Climb the wall with the fingers; descend; repeat.	Raising windows Washing windows Hanging clothes on line Reaching to an upper shelf
4. Stand erect and clasp hands at small of back; raise hands; lower; repeat. Clasp hands back of neck; reach downward; upward; repeat.	Fastening brassiere Buttoning blouse or dress Pulling up a dress zipper Fastening beads Washing the back
5. Toss a rope over the shower curtain rod. Hold the ends of the rope (knotted) in each hand and raise arms sideways. Using a see-saw motion and with arms outstretched, slide the rope up and down over the rod.	Drying the back with a bath towel Raising and lowering a window blind Closing and opening window drapes
6. Flex and extend each finger in turn.	Sewing, knitting, crocheting Typing, painting, playing piano or other musical instrument

b. Observe effect of prosthesis on incision; to prevent irritation, lamb's wool padding may be used.

c. A prosthesis should not be worn unless authorized by the physician.

Complication—Lymphedema of the Arm

Lymphedema is an obstruction to the lymph flow in the arm on the operated side producing a chronic swelling of the part, particularly if it is in a dependent position. Lymphedema is due to lymph node removal and compression of axillary vein by tumor or scar.

A. *Prevention*

See Figure 11-21 and page 335.

1. Exercises indicated in Table 11-3 should be done.
2. The affected arm should be massaged 3 or 4 months postoperatively to increase circulation and lessen edema.
3. The affected arm should be elevated frequently to prevent dependent edema.
4. The arm and operative site should be kept scrupulously clean to prevent infection.
5. Nonconstrictive clothing should be worn to permit adequate circulation.
6. The suggestions in the hand care chart below should be followed diligently.

B. *Treatment*

1. May include a diuretic.
2. An intermittent compression unit with pressurized sleeve may be used to force fluid back into venous system.

Importance of Follow-up Visit

1. Incision healing evaluated
2. Rehabilitative effort assessed
3. Effectiveness of prosthesis determined
4. Patient's psychosocial adjustment evaluated
5. Possible recurrence detected

BREAST MAMMAPLASTY (BREAST RECONSTRUCTION)

Breast mammaplasty is the reconstruction of the breast by using prosthetic implants or fashioning a flap from the patient's own tissues; an areola-nipple reconstruction may also be performed.

A. *Prevalence and Indications:*

1. The possibility of breast reconstruction is receiving more attention for several reasons:
   a. Breast surgery is less radical
   b. Recent advances in plastic surgery
   c. Greater acceptance of cosmetic surgery
2. Reconstruction is performed usually 3 months to a year after a mastectomy; there is no maximum time limit.
3. Reconstruction is not recommended for women under the following circumstances:
   a. Presence of large tumors or extensive nodular involvement; recent history of breast abscess or history of diffuse, painful cystic mastitis
   b. Presence of other diseases which might impair the healing process
   c. Radiation therapy or chest skin grafts
   d. Marked obesity
   e. Advanced age
   f. Previous radical mastectomy

B. *Implants*—flexible plastic sacs filled with silicone gel (greater firmness) or saline (lesser firmness). Some can be subtly adjusted by inflation with air or injection of additional saline (Fig. 11-22).

1. This pouch can be inserted through a small incision at the base-fold area and positioned underneath breast skin.
2. The tightness of the skin often determines the size of the implant; this may require alteration of the remaining breast to match the reconstructed breast.

HAND CARE*

After a radical mastectomy, an arm may swell because lymph nodes and lymph vessels were necessarily removed and the body is therefore less able to combat infection in this extremity.

Make every effort to avoid all cuts, scratches, pin pricks, hangnails, insect bites, burns, and the use of strong detergents as these can lead to serious infection with increased swelling.

Some "DO NOT'S":

DO NOT hold a cigarette in this hand.

DO NOT carry your purse or anything heavy with this arm

DO NOT wear a wristwatch or other jewelry on this arm

DO NOT cut or pick at cuticles or hangnails on this hand

DO NOT work near thorny plants or dig in the garden

DO NOT reach into a hot oven with this arm

DO NOT permit injection in this arm

DO NOT permit blood to be drawn from this arm

DO NOT allow your blood pressure to be taken on this arm

Some "DO'S":

DO wear a loose rubber glove on this hand when washing dishes

DO wear a thimble when sewing

DO apply a good lanolin hand cream several times daily

DO wear your "Life-Guard Medical Aid" tag engraved with "CAUTION—LYMPHEDEMA ARM—NO TESTS—NO HYPOS"

DO contact your doctor if your arm gets red, warm, or unusually hard or swollen

DO return for a check-up and re-measurement for a new sleeve in two months

DO show this Hand Care Sheet to your surgeon

*Reprinted through the courtesy of the CLEVELAND CLINIC Department of Physical Medicine and Rehabilitation.

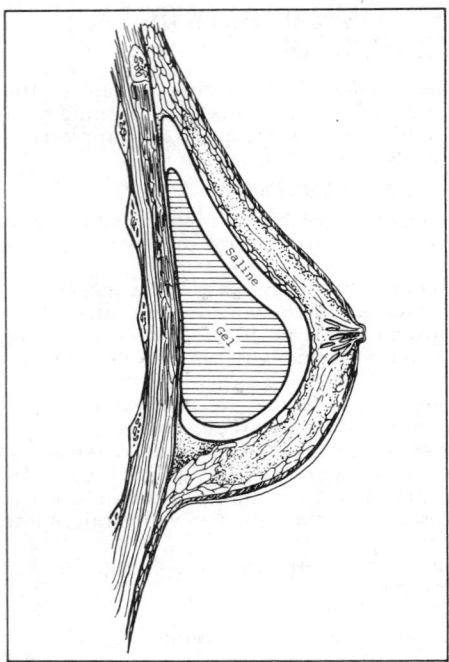

FIGURE 11-22. *The diagrammatic sketch shows the placement of a mammary implant—in this case, one featuring a sealed inner gel implant surrounded by an inflatable outer saline implant (Courtesy American Heyer-Schulte Corporation, Goleta CA 1980)*

Nursing Management and Health Education

1. The woman usually is discharged from the hospital in 2–3 days.
2. She is instructed to keep her elbow close to her side for several days to a week.
3. Full use of her arm is achieved in about a month; however, strenuous arm use in tennis, golf, or swimming may be delayed.
4. A well-fitted brassiere worn day and night for 3 months may assist the breast(s) in taking on the desired shape.
5. Instruct the client to report thinning or discoloration of skin over the implant area.
6. She should be instructed in how to distinguish the prosthesis from normal or abnormal breast tissue during self-examination for breast cancer.

C. *Flap Graft*

This is the transfer of skin from another part of the body, usually in stages, to the mastectomy site. (See Grafts, pp. 593.) This requires several hospitalizations, is costly, and not as cosmetically effective as implants.

D. *Areola-nipple Reconstruction*

The nipple and areola are saved during mastectomy and banked (suturing to a temporary site, usually thigh or abdomen) until the breast reconstruction is done.

1. If banking is not possible, tissue from the other breast, labia, or ear lobe may be grafted.

RECURRENT OR METASTATIC BREAST CANCER

Modalities of Endocrine Manipulation

Theory and Objective: Malignant tumor cells depend on hormonal function in the host; deprivation of hormones reduces tumor's growth. Currently tumor removed at operation is tested for estrogen receptors. If positive, the use of hormonal therapy or ablation can be carried out on a more rational basis than heretofore with an anticipated good response.

A. *Ablative Procedures*

1. Bilateral salpingo-ovariectomy
   a. This is often the initial treatment of choice for premenopausal patients with metastatic breast cancer.
   b. Remission lasts from 3 months to several years (median—1 year).
   c. If signs of reactivation of tumor growth occur, further endocrine therapy may be done (hypophysectomy or adrenalectomy).
2. Hypophysectomy—done microsurgically (transnasal or transsphenoidal)
   a. This is done for postmenopausal patients with metastatic breast cancer.
   b. Remission lasts from 6 months to several years (median—1½ years).
   c. Upon signs of reactivation of tumor growth, cytotoxic chemotherapy is initiated.
3. Adrenalectomy
   a. Bilateral adrenalectomy is usually combined with bilateral salpingo-ovariectomy.
   b. This is often recommended for postmenopausal patients with metastatic breast cancer.
   c. Remission lasts from 6 months to several years (median—1 year).
   d. Women who have had ovariectomy and adrenalectomy and who show signs of recurrence are given cytotoxic chemotherapy.

B. *Hormones*

1. Estrogens
   a. Most commonly used in women who are 5 or more years postmenopausal with recurrent breast carcinoma.
   b. Diethylstilbestrol or ethinyl estradiol are estrogens used.
   c. Remissions last 3 months to several years (median—1 year).
   d. With initial exacerbation of the disease, hormone therapy is immediately terminated.
   e. Recurrence of this disease following remission is treated with hypophysectomy or adrenalectomy.

> **NURSING ALERT:** Observe for fluid retention following estrogen therapy; this can be prevented with dietary sodium restriction and use of diuretics.

2. Progestins (medroxyprogesterone acetate)
   a. Useful in about 30% of postmenopausal women with metastatic carcinoma.
   b. Remission is about 8 months.

c. Failure with progestins suggests a change to other modalities of endocrine therapy.
3. Androgens (fluoxymesterone)
   a. Useful in about 20% of postmenopausal women.
   b. Remissions last about 6 months.
   c. When no longer effective, other kinds of endocrine therapy may be useful.
   d. Side effects:
      (1) fluid retention, which can be prevented by restricting sodium and using diuretics
      (2) virilization (development of secondary male characteristics)
4. Corticosteroids (prednisone, dexamethasone)
   a. Not usually used in primary management of postmenopausal women with metastatic breast cancer because of the possibility of Cushing's syndrome.
   b. Useful as
      (1) an adjunct to radiation therapy in patients with cerebral metastasis
      (2) an adjunct to cytotoxic chemotherapy in pa-

tients with advanced liver and pulmonary metastasis.

C. *Cytotoxic Chemotherapy*

Alkylating agents: 5-fluorouracil, methotrexate, vincristine
1. Remission lasts about 6 months (in 20% of patients).
2. Five-drug combination can boost remission rate to about 9 months (in 65% of patients)—5-fluorouracil, methotrexate, vincristine, cyclophosphamide, prednisone.
3. Recommended for patients who have metastasis to liver or lungs and are poor surgical risks for endocrine ablative surgery.
4. Recommended for premenopausal patients who are not benefitting from ovariectomy or hypophysectomy.
5. Doxorubicin Hydrochloride (Adriamycin) usually used when 5-drug chemotherapy fails.

BIBLIOGRAPHY

1 RENAL AND GENITOURINARY CONDITIONS

Books

Bissada NK and Finkbeiner AE. Lower Urinary Tract Function and Dysfunction. New York, Appleton-Century-Crofts, 1978
Boyarsky S et al. Care of the Patient with Neurogenic Bladder. Boston, Little, Brown, & Co, 1979
Buchsbaum HJ and Schmidt JD. Gynecologic and Obstetric Urology. Philadelphia, WB Saunders, 1978
Chatterjee SN (ed). Renal Transplantation. A Multidisciplinary Approach. New York, Raven Press, 1980
Cockett ATK and Koshiba K. Manual of Urologic Surgery. New York, Springer-Verlag, 1979
Diamond LH and Balow JE. 1980 Nephrology Reviews. New York, John Wiley & Sons, 1980
Hamburger J et al. Nephrology. New York, John Wiley & Sons, 1979
Harrison JH et al. Campbell's Urology, 4th ed, Vols. 1, 2, 3. Philadelphia, WB Saunders, 1979
Jackle M and Rasmussen C. Renal Problems. A Critical Care Nursing Focus. Bowie, Robert J Brady Co, 1980
Javadpour N (ed). Principles and Management of Urologic Cancer. Baltimore, Williams & Wilkins, 1979
Krane RJ and Siroky MB. Clinical Neuro-Urology. Boston, Little, Brown, & Co, 1979
Kunin CM. Detection, Prevention and Management of Urinary Tract Infections, 3rd ed. Philadelphia, Lea & Febiger, 1979
Lancaster LE (ed). The Patient with End Stage Renal Disease. New York, John Wiley & Sons, 1979
Morel A and Wise GJ. Urologic Endoscopic Procedures, 2nd ed. St. Louis, CV Mosby, 1979
Murphy GP (ed). Prostatic Cancer. Littleton, PSG Publishing Co, 1979
Resnick MI and Sanders RC. Ultrasound in Urology. Baltimore, Williams & Wilkins, 1979
Robertson JR. Genitourinary Problems in Women. Springfield, Charles C Thomas, 1978
Silber SJ. Transurethral Resection. New York, Appleton-Century-Crofts, 1977
Smith DR. General Urology, 9th ed. Los Altos, Lange Medical Publications, 1978
Stamey TA. Pathogenesis and Treatment of Urinary Tract Infections. Baltimore, Williams & Wilkins, 1980

Winter CC and Morel A. Nursing Care of Patients with Urologic Disease, 4th ed. St. Louis, C Mosby, 1977

Articles
Assessment and Diagnosis
Colon VF, and Schumann GB. Urine cytology. Part I: Urinary tract cytology. Am Fam Physician 1980 March; 21(3):92–97
McGonigle R and Sharpstone P. Kidney biopsy. Br Med J 1980 Feb; 280(6913):547–549
Schumann GB and Colon VF. Urine cytology. Part II: Renal cytology. Am Fam Physician 1980 April; 21(4):102–106

Dialysis; Transplantation
Abram HS and Buchanan DC. Organ transplantation: Psychological effects on donors and recipients. Med Times 1978 Aug; 106(8):23d–29d
Bauer D. Prevention of the spread of hepatitis B in dialysis units. Am J Nurs 1980 Feb; 80(2):260–261
Denniston DJ and Burns KT. Home peritoneal dialysis. Am J Nurs 1980 Nov; 80(11):2022–2026
Giacchino JL et al. Vascular access: Long-term results, new techniques. Arch Surg 1979 April; 114(4):403–409
Home peritoneal dialysis for end-stage renal disease. Med Lett Drugs Ther 1979 Aug; 21(17):69–70
Irwin BC. Hemodialysis means vascular access . . . . and the right kind of nursing care. Nursing '79 1979 Oct; 9(10):49–53
Kester RC. Arteriovenous grafts for vascular access in haemodialysis. Br J Surg 1979 Jan; 66(1):23–28
Kluthe R et al. Protein requirements in maintenance hemodialysis. Am J Clin Nutr 1978 Oct; 31(10):1812–1820
Lavandero R and Davis V. Caring for the catheter carefully—before, during and after peritoneal dialysis. Nursing '80 1980 Nov; 10(11):73–79
Lemaitre P et al. Polytetrafluorethylene (PTFE) grafts for hemodialysis. Clin Nephrol 1978 July; 10(1):27–31
Levy NB. Psychological problems of the patient on hemodialysis and their treatment. Psychother Psychosom 1979; 31(1–4):260–266
Luke B. Nutrition in renal disease: The adult on dialysis. Am J Nurs 1979 Dec; 79(12):2155–1257
McNamara RM. The bioinstrumentation of hemodialysis. Nurs Clin North Am 1978 Dec; 13(4):611–624
Manis T and Friedman E. Dialytic therapy for irreversible uremia. N Engl J Med 1979 Dec 6; 301(23):1260–1265; Part II, Dec. 13; 301(24):1321–1328

Nose Y. Clinically accepted artificial organs—not a golden rule. Artif Organs 1979 Feb; 3(1):1

Novick AC et al. Current status of renal transplantation at the Cleveland Clinic. J Urol 1979 Oct; 122(4):433–437

Rajapaksa T. Maintenance hemodialysis: How to help patients cope. Med Times 1979 Oct; 107(10):86–88, 91–92

Sorrels AJ. Continuous ambulatory peritoneal dialysis Am J Nurs 1979 Aug; 79(8):1400–1401

Tilney NL et al. Factors contributing to the declining mortality rate in renal transplantation. N Engl J Med 1978 Dec 14; 299(24):1321–1325

Trevino-Becerra A and Boen FST (eds). Today's art of peritoneal dialysis. Contrib Nephrol 1979; 17:1–148

Vaisrub S. Editorial. Dangerous waters. JAMA 1979 Oct 6; 240(15):1630

Wolf JL et al. The transplanted kidney as a source of hepatitis B infection. Ann Intern Med 1979 Sept; 91(3):412–413

Glomerulonephritis

Hirszel P. A new approach to primary glomerulonephritis. Med Times 1979 Oct; 107(10):77–85

Juliana LM. Acute glomerulonephritis. Nursing '79 1979 Sept; 9(9):40–45

Nagar D and Wathen RL. Nephrotic syndrome. Primary Care 1979 Sept; 6(3):541–560

Simon NM and Rosenberg MJ. Medical treatment of glomerular diseases. Med Clin North Am 1978 Nov; 62(6):1157–1181

Infection

Fang LST et al. Urinary tract infections in women. Compr Ther 1979 Sept; 5(9):20–25

Freeman RB. Urinary tract infections. Med Times 1979 Oct; 107(10):40–45

Harding GKM. Prophylaxis of recurrent urinary tract infection in female patients. JAMA 1979 Nov 2; 242(18):1975–1977

Lapides J. Mechanisms of urinary tract infection. Urology 1979 Sept; 14(3):217–225

Mulholland SG. Lower urinary tract antibacterial defense mechanisms. Invest Urol 1979 Sept; 17(2):93–97

Riff LJM. Evaluation and treatment of urinary infection. Med Clin North Am 1978 Nov; 62(6):1183–1199

Roland AR. Treating urinary tract infections in women. Drug Ther 1979 May; 4(5):51–63

Santoro J and Kaye D. Recurrent urinary tract infections. Pathogenesis and management. Med Clin North Am 1978 Sept; 62(5):1005–1020

Wisnia GL et al. Renal function damage in 131 cases of urogenital tuberculosis. Urology 1978 May; 11(5):457–461

Neurogenic Bladder; Urinary Diversion Procedures

Barrett N. Continent vesicostomy: The dry urinary diversion. Am J Nurs 1979 March; 79(3):462–464

Boles DM et al. Two technical aids for intermittent sterile catheterization. Paraplegia 1978 Nov; 16(3):303–305

Editorial. Clean intermittent catheterization. Lancet 1979 Sept 1; 2(8140):448–449

Editorial. The continent urostomy. Br Med J 1978 Aug 19; 2(6136):520–521

Felder L. Neurogenic bladder dysfunction. J Neurosurg Nurs 1979 June; 11(2):94–104

Foster KJ et al. The influence of early post-operative intravenous nutrition upon recovery after total cystectomy. Br J Urol 1978 Aug; 50(55):319–323

Greene WR and Icochea RS. Modifications of nephrostomy tube. Urology 1978 Aug; 12(2):210

Holden S et al. The rationale of urinary diversion in cancer patients. J Urol 1979 June; 121(1):19–21

Link D et al. The use of percutaneous nephrostomy in 42 patients. J Urol 1979 July; 122(1):9–10

Meyer JE et al. Palliative urinary diversion in carcinoma of the cervix. Obstet Gynecol 1980 Jan; 55(1):95–98

Milroy MD et al. Permanent cutaneous ureterostomy: 18 years of experience. J Urol 1978 Dec; 120(6):682–684

Pitts WR Jr and Muecke EC. A 20-year experience with ileal conduits: The fate of the kidneys. J Urol 1979 Aug; 122(2):154–157

Richie JP. Nonrefluxing sigmoid conduit for urinary diversion. Urol Clin North Am 1979 June; 6(2):469–477

Schlesinger RE. The choice of an intestinal segment for a urinary conduit. Surg Gynecol Obstet 1979 Jan; 148(1):45–48

Skinner DG et al. Complications of radical cystectomy for carcinoma of the bladder. J Urol 1980 May; 123(5):640–643

Smith ML. Continent vesicostomy. Obstet Gynecol 1978 Aug; 52(2):247–249

Soloway MS. Rationale for intensive intravesical chemotherapy for superficial bladder cancer. J Urol 1980 April; 123(4):461–466

Renal Failure, Acute and Chronic

Berlyne GM. The place of dietary therapy in the treatment of chronic renal failure. Clin Nephrol 1979 Feb; 11(2):63–65

Blumenkrantz MJ et al. Total parenteral nutrition in the management of acute renal failure. Am J Clin Nutr 1978 Oct; 31(10):1831–1840

Butt KM et al. Kidney transplantation: The ultimate non-dialytic therapy of uremia. Clin Nephrol 1979 March; 11(3):173–176

Fugleberg BB. Management of acute renal failure. Curr Pract Crit Care 1979 1:204–215

Guttman RD. Renal transplantation. N Engl J Med 1979 Nov 8; 301(19):1038–1048

Hogg JE. Neurologic complications of acute and chronic renal failure. Adv Neurol 1978; 19:637–646

Holliday MA et al. Nutritional management of chronic renal disease. Med Clin North Am 1979 Sept; 63(5):945–962

Home peritoneal dialysis for end-stage renal disease. Med Lett Drug Ther 1979 Aug; 21(17):69–70

Kopple JD. Nutritional management of chronic renal failure. Postgrad Med 1978 Nov; 64(5):135–144

Levy NB. The sexual rehabilitation of the hemodialysis patient. Sexuality and Disability 1979 Spring; 2(1):60–65

Luke B. Nutrition in renal disease; the adult on dialysis. Am J Nurs 1979 Dec; 79(12):2155–2157

Marshall JR. Neuropsychiatric aspects of renal failure. J Clin Psychiatry 1979 Feb; 40(2):81–85

Moore MA. Practical management of chronic renal failure. Am Fam Physician 1979 March; 19(3):158–164

Muther RS and Bennett WM. Diagnosis and management of acute renal failure. Compr Ther 1979 Sept; 5(9):12–19

Oestreich SJK. Rational nursing care in chronic renal disease. Am J Nurs 1979 June; 79(6):1096–1099

Oreopoulos DG et al. Continuous ambulatory peritoneal dialysis: a new era in the treatment of chronic renal failure. Clin Nephrol 1979 March; 11(3):125–128

Oreopoulos DG. Peritoneal dialysis is here to stay. Nephron 1979 24; (1):7–9

Schultz BC and Roenigk HH. Uremic pruritus treated with ultraviolet light. JAMA 1980 May 9; 234(18):1836–1837

Shalhoub RJ. The medical management of chronic renal failure. Med Times 1979 Oct; 107(10):23–32

Sorkin MI. Acute renal failure. Med Times 1979 Oct; 107(10):33–39

Watkins YB. Rehabilitation risks of ESRD. J Rehabil 1979 Jan–March; 45(1):30–33

Whelton A. Post-traumatic acute renal failure. Bull NY Acad Med 1979 Feb; 55(2):150–162

Injuries, Surgery, Tumor, Urolithiasis

Bichler K-H. Surgical treatment of urinary calculi. Urol Res 1979 Sept; 7(3):139–142

Bredael JJ et al. Traumatic rupture of the female urethra. J Urol 1979 Oct; 122(4):560–561

Cass AS and Godec CJ. Urethral injury due to external trauma. Urology 1978 June; 11(6):607–611

Editorial. Haematuria after closed trauma. Br Med J 1979 Mar 31; 1(6167):841–842

Evans SC et al. Non-operative management of severe renal lacerations. J Urol 1980 Feb; 123(2):247–249

Finney RP. Experience with new double J ureteral catheter stent. J Urol 1978 Dec; 120(6):678–681

Glass RE et al. Urethral injury and fractured pelvis. Br J Urol 1978 Dec; 50(7):578–582

Karmi SA et al. Classifications of renal injuries as a guide to therapy. Surg Gynecol Obstet 1979 Feb; 148(2):161–167

Kearney GP et al. Useful technique for long-term urinary drainage by inlying ureteral stent. Urology 1979 Aug; 14(2):126–134

Kohler JP et al. Reassessment of circle tube nephrostomy in advanced pelvic malignancy. J Urol 1980 Jan; 123(1):17–18

Moyer JD. Urinary tract injury. Management of renal and bladder trauma. J Kans Med Soc 1978 May; 79(5):189–192

Nanninga JB. Care of the catheter-dependent patient. Urol Clin North Am 1980 Feb; 7(1):41–44

Oliver JA et al. Results of radical nephrectomy in 178 cases of renal cell adenocarcinoma. Can J Surg 1979 Sept; 22(5):409–412

Pak CUC (ed). Symposium on urolithiasis. Kidney Int 1978 May; 13(5):341–426

Peterson NE. Apparent exceptions to the usual patterns of renal trauma. J Urol 1979 April; 121(4):489–496

Peterson NE. The significance of delayed post-traumatic renal hemorrhage. J Urol 1978 April; 119(4):563–565

Pitts GW and Resnick MI. Urinary stone formation: Patient evaluation and management. Urol Clin North Am 1980 Feb; 7(1):45–58

Smith LH et al. Nutrition and urolithiasis. N Engl J Med 1978 Jan 12; 298(2):87–89

Yarnell SK. Intermittent catheterization: Long–term follow-up. Arch Phys Med Rehabil 1978 Nov; 59(11):491–496

Urological Problems (Male)

Abrams PH. Investigation of post prostatectomy problems. Urology 1980 Feb; 15(2):209–212

Belker AM. Urologic microsurgery—current perspectives: 1. Vasovasostomy. Urology 1979 Oct; 14(4):325–329

Blacklock NJ. Prostatitis. Practitioner 1979 Sept; 223 (1335):318–322

Blandy J. Open prostatectomy. Br J Hosp Med 1978 Aug; 20(2):189–197

Blandy JP. Vasectomy. Br J Hosp Med 1979 May; 21(5):520–527

Brosman SA. Benign prostatic hypertrophy—When should you consider prostatectomy for your patient? Geriatrics 1979 April; 34(4):25–29, 33–34

Bruce AW et al. Radiation therapy for adenocarcinoma of the prostate. Can J Surg 1979 Sept; 22(5):421–423

Catalona WJ and Scott WW. Carcinoma of the prostate: A review. J Urol 1978 Jan; 119(1):1–8

Champagne EE and Kane NE. Teaching program for patients receiving radioactive iodine[125] for cancer of the prostate. Oncol Nurs Forum 1980 Winter; 7(1):12–15

Davis JE. Male sterilization. Clin Obstet Gynecol 1979 April; 6(1):97–107

Drach CW. Prostatitis and prostatodynia. Urol Clin North Am 1980 Feb; 7(1):79–88

Early detection of prostatic cancer by radioimmunoassay for prostatic acid phosphatase. Med Lett Drugs Ther 1979 Nov; 21(22):90–91

Editorial. Treatment of advanced prostatic carcinoma. Br Med J 1979 Sept 29; 2(6193):752–753

Fraley EE et al. Germ-cell testicular cancer in adults. N Engl J Med 1979 Dec 27; 301(26):1420–1426

Gorzynski JG and Holland JC. Psychological aspects of testicular cancer. Semin Oncol 1979 March; 6(1):125–129

Javadpour N and Bergman S. Recent advances in testicular cancer. Curr Probl Surg 1978 Feb; 15(2):1–64

Khezri AA et al. Carcinoma of the penis. Br J Urol 1978 June; 50(4):275–279

Klein LA. Prostatic carcinoma. N Engl J Med 1979 Apr 12; 300(15):824–833

Lawson DH and Nixon DW. Modern chemotherapy in the management of testicular tumors. South Med J 1979 Nov; 72:11:1393–1395

Lipshultz LI and Benson GS. Vasectomy—1980. Urol Clin North Am 1980 Feb; 7(1):89–105

Meares EM Jr. Prostatitis: Diagnosis and treatment. Drugs 1978 June; 15(6):412–419

Meares EM. Prostatitis syndromes: New perspectives about old woes. J Urol 1980 Feb; 123(2):141–147

Murphy GP. Prostate cancer. J Urol 1979 Nov; 122(5):644

Pistenma DA and Bagshaw MA. Prostatic adenocarcinoma: Considerations in management. Postgrad Med 1980 April; 67(4):135–145

Romas NA et al. Acid phosphatase: New developments. Hum Pathol 1979 Sept; 10(5):501–512

Slack NH and Murphy GP. Prednimustine for prostate cancer therapy. Compr Ther 1979 Sept; 5(9):54–57

Tobiason SJ. Benign prostatic hypertrophy. Am J Nurs 1979 Feb; 79(2):286–290

Watson RA. Gonorrhea and acute epididymitis. Milit Med 1979 Dec; 144(12):785–787

Yagoda A and Golbey RB (eds). Germ cell tumors. Semin Oncol 1979 March; 6(1):1–138

2 GYNECOLOGIC CONDITIONS

Books

Barber HRK. Manual of Gynecologic Oncology, Philadelphia, JB Lippincott, 1980

Barber HRK. Ovarian Carcinoma. New York, Masson Publishers, 1978

Danforth DN et al. Obstetrics and Gynecology. New York, Harper & Row, 1977

Green TH Jr. Gynecology: Essentials of Clinical Practice, 3rd ed. Boston, Little Brown & Co., 1977

Gwens JR et al. The Infertile Female. Chicago, Year Book Medical Publishers, 1979

Hatcher RA et al. Contraceptive Technology 1978–1979, 9th ed New York, Irvington Publishers, 1978

Hogan R. Human Sexuality: A Nursing Perspective. New York, Appleton-Century-Crofts, 1979

Jackson M et al. Vaginal Contraceptives. Boston, GK Hall & Co, 1980

Kistner RW. Gynecology, 3rd ed. Chicago, Year Book Medical Publishers, 1979

Kjervik DK and Martinson IM (eds). Women in Stress: A Nursing Perspective. New York, Appleton-Century-Crofts, 1979

Martin LL. Health Care of Women. Philadelphia, JB Lippincott, 1978

Quilligan EJ. Current Therapy in Obstetrics and Gynecology. Philadelphia, WB Saunders, 1980

Sloane E. Biology of Women. Somerset, John Wiley & Sons, 1980

Stewart FJ et al. My Body, My Health: The Concerned Woman's Guide to Gynecology. New York, John Wiley & Sons, 1979

Taylor RW and Brush MG. Obstetrics and Gynecology. New York, Macmillan, 1979

Utian WH. Menopause in Modern Perspective: A Guide to Clinical Practice. New York, Appleton-Century-Crofts, 1980

Articles

General

Barber HRK. Fluid, electrolyte and nutritional management of the gynecologic patient. Part II. Curr Probl Obstet Gynecol 1979 Sept; 3(1):1–32

Butts PA. Assessing urinary incontinence in women. Nursing '79 1979 March; 9(3):72–74

Carlson B and Wheeler KA. Group counseling for pre-or-gasmic women. Top Clin Nurs 1980 Jan; 1(4):9–19

Coleman E. The relational cause of sexual dysfunction. Top Clin Nurs 1980 Jan; 1(4):33–37

Goldfarb JM and Little AB. Current concepts: Abnormal vaginal bleeding. N Engl Med J 1980 March 20; 302(12):666–669

Hildebrand BF. Nursing process and chemotherapy for the woman with cancer of the reproductive system. Nurs Clin North Am 1978 June; 13(2):351–368

Hreshchyshyn MM et al: Chemotherapy for gynecologic malignancy. Curr Probl Obstet Gynecol 1979 Feb; 2(6):1–39

Kein MA. The nurse practitioner in ambulatory gynecologic services. Clin Obstet Gynecol 1979 June; 22(2):445–453

McDonough PG and Gambrell RD. The adolescent gynecologic patient and her problems. Clin Obstet Gynecol 1979 June; 22(2):491–507

O'Leary V. Lesbianism. Nursing Dimensions. 1979 Spring; 7(1):78–82

Parker B. Communicating with battered women. Top Clin Nurs 1979 Oct; 1(4):49–53

Richter JM. Physical symptom: A signal of distress in the family system. Top Clin Nurs 1979 Oct; 1(4):31–40

Ruzek SK. Emergent modes of utilization; Gynecological self-help. Nursing Dimensions 1979 Spring; 7(1):73–77

Satterfield SB and Stayton WR. Understanding sexual function and dysfunction. Top Clin Nurs 1980 Jan; 1(4):21–32

Schrader ES. Counseling helps gyn patients handle surgery. AORN J 1979 Aug; 30(2):233–241

Stayton WR. The theory of sexual orientation. The universe as a turn on. Top Clin Nurs 1980 Jan; 1(4):1–7

Watts RJ. Dimensions of sexual health. Am J Nurs 1979 Sept; 79(9):1568–1572

Whipple B and Geck R. A holistic view of sexuality—education for the health professional. Top Clin Nurs 1980; 1(4):91–98

Willson JKV and Young RC. Rising expectations for chemotherapy in gynecologic malignancies. Drug Ther 1980 May; 10(5):47–62

Wilson CL. Beyond the stereotypes: Promoting the personal development of female patients. Top Clin Nurs 1979 Oct; 1(4):21–30

Menstruation

Friedrich EG Jr and Siegesmund KA. Tampon-associated vaginal ulcerations. Obstet Gynecol 1980 Feb; 55(2):149–156

Gever LN. From arthritis pain to dysmenorrhea. Nursing '80 1980 April; 10(4):81

Hann LE et al. Mittelschmerz. Sonographic demonstration. JAMA 1979 June 22; 241(25):2731–2733

Hanna J. Premenstrual syndrome: Defeating the curse of the calendar. Nurs Mirror 1980 Oct 2; 151(14):36–37

Harvey S. New relief for menstrual discomfort. RN 1979 Sept; 42(9):116

Ibuprofen (Motrin) has been approved by the FDA for the relief of dysmenorrhea too. RN 1980 Apr; 43(5):118E

McFarland KF. Amenorrhea. Am Fam Physician 1980 Dec; 22(6):95–101

New hope for dysmenorrhea. The Harvard Med School Health Letter 1979 Nov; 5(1):5

Roberts SJ. Dysmenorrhea. Nurse Pract 1980 July–Aug; 5(4):9–10

Speroff L and Redwine DB. Exercise and menstrual function. The Physic and Sports Medicine 1980 May; 8(5):41–52

Toxic shock syndrome: A tampon tie-in? USPHS, Center for Disease Control, Morbidity Mortality Weekly Rep. 1980 Sept 19; 29(37):229, 242

Menopause, Estrogen Use, and Geriatric Problems

Adlin EV. Postmenopausal estrogen therapy. Ann Intern Med 1979 Sept; 91(3):488–489

DiRaimondo C et al. Gynecomastia from exposure to vaginal estrogen cream. N Engl J Med 1980 May 8; 302(19):1089–1090

Estrogen replacement therapy? Yes! Patient Care 1979 Jan 15; 13(2):23–28

Estrogen use and postmenopausal women. A National Institutes of Health Consensus Development Conference. Ann Intern Med 1979 Dec; 91(6):921–922

Gambrell RD and Greenblatt RB. The menopause: Indications for estrogen therapy. Curr Probl in Obstet Gynecol 1979 Jan; 2(5):1–49

Gruis ML and Wagner NN. Sexuality during the climacteric. Postgrad Med 1979 May; 65(5):197–207

Gynecological exams, a must for older women. Am J Nurs 1979 Nov; 79(11):2004

Hewitt AL et al. Lesions of the geriatric genitalia. Patient Care 1980 Feb 15; 14(3):172–177

Hotchner B. Menopause and sexuality: Gearing up or down? Top in Clin Nurs 1980 Jan; 1(4):45–52

Huffman JW. Counseling the menopausal patient. Postgrad Med 1979 May; 65(6):211–215

Kemmann E. The female climacteric. Am Fam Physician 1979 Nov; 20(5):140–151

Martin P et al. Systemic absorption and sustained effects of vaginal estrogen creams. JAMA 1979 Dec 14; 242(24):2699–2700

Newton M. The problem of postmenopausal bleeding. Consultant 1977 March; 17(3):181–189

Rosenthal MB. Psychological aspects of menopause. Primary Care 1979 June; 6(2):357–364

Udkow GP et al. The safety and efficacy of the estrogen patient package insert. JAMA 1979 Aug 10; 242(6):536–539

Pelvic Examination and Diagnostic Tests

Barber RKB. Pelvic examination: Step-by-step guide. Mod Med 1980 April; 16(4):52–62

Barber RKB. Her first pelvic exam: When and how to do it. Consultant 1979 July; 19(7):33–38

Colon VF and Schumann GB. Gynecologic cytology. Am Fam Physician 1978 Nov; 18(5):135–140

Dunn LJ. Cervical cytologic evaluation. Postgrad Med 1979 March; 65(3):187–192

Knapp RC et al. Put colposcopy to work for you. Patient Care 1979 Aug 15; 13(14):124–137

Newton M. Abnormal Pap smear—What then? Consultant 1979 Nov; 19(11):77–82

Smilkstein G and Coggan PG. Teaching the pelvic examination with a psychosocial format. Fam Med Teacher 1980 May/June; 12(3):8, 18

Infections

An effective treatment for herpes? The Harvard Med School Health Letter 1979 Oct; 4(12):6

Bock J. Herpes: Scourge of the seventies. Can Nurse 1980 Jan; 76(1):22–24

Davis JP et al. Toxic-shock syndrome. N Engl J Med 1980 Dec 18; 303(25):1429, 1439

Drugs for candida infections of the skin and vagina. The Med Letter 1979 May 4; 21(9):39

Eschenbach DA et al. Pathogenesis of acute pelvic inflammatory disease: Role of contraception and other risk factors. Am J Obstet Gynecol 1977 Aug 15; 128(8):838–850

Handsfiedl HH. The latest protocols for sexually transmitted infections. Drug Ther 1979 June; 9(6):43–56

Harrison WO. Trial of minocycline given after exposure to prevent gonorrhea. N Engl J Med 1979 May 10; 300(19):1074–1078

Holmes KK and Stamm WE. Chlamydial genital infections: A growing problem Hosp Pract 1979 Oct; 14(10):105–117

Increasing pelvic infections respond to antibiotics. AORN J 1980 Jan; 31(1):68–70

Ledger WJ. Hospital infections: Gynecologic, obstetric, and perinatal infections. Ann Intern Med 1978 Nov; 89(5):744–776

Lukacs J and Corey L. Genital herpes simplex virus infection: An overview. Nurs Pract 1977 May/June; 2(5):7–9

Management of vaginitis. Am Fam Physician 1979 July; 20(7):143–144

Rosenthal MS. Genital herpes simplex virus infections. Primary Care 1979 Sept; 6(3):517–528

Schachter J. Chlamydia infections. N Engl J Med 1978 Feb 23; 298:428–435; Mar 2; 298:490–495; Mar 9; 540–549

Shands KN et al. Toxic shock syndrome in menstruating women. N Engl J Med 1980 Dec 18 303(25):1429–1439

Skinner G. Herpes simplex virus infections: A cure for some ills. Nurs Mirror 1980 Oct 2; 151(14):38–39

Sulfa vaginal creams. FDS Drug Bulletin 1980 Feb; 10(1):6

Toxic shock syndrome: A tampon tie-in? USPHS, Center for Disease Control, Morbidity Mortality Weekly Rep 1980 Sept 19; 29(37):229, 297

Update on toxic shock syndrome. FDA Drug Bulletin 1980 Nov; 10(3):17–19

Ovary and Uterus

Andrews WC. Medical versus surgical treatment of endometriosis. Clin Obstet Gynecol 1980 Sept; 23(3):917–924

Atunes CMF et al. Endometrial cancer and estrogen use. N Engl J Med 1979 Jan 4; 300(1):9–31

Barber HRK. Ovarian cancer. Part 1, CA 1979 Nov/Dec; 29(6):341–351; Part 2, CA 1980 Jan/Feb; 30(1):2–22

Burchell RC et al: Hysterectomy: For whom, when, how? Patient Care 1980 June 15; 14(11):16–37

Buttram VC and Betts JW. Endometriosis. Curr Probl Obstet Gynecol 1979 July; 2(11):1–58

Butts P. Meeting the special needs of your hysterectomy patient. Nursing '79 1979 Nov; 9(11):40–47

Cisplatin (Platinol) (for ovarian cancer). The Med Letter 1979 April 20: 21(8):33–34

Cohen MR. Laparoscopic diagnosis and pseudomenopause treatment of endometriosis with danazol. Clin Obstet Gynecol 1980 Sept; 23(3):901–915

Gever LN. Cisplatin. Nursing '80 1980 Dec; 10(12):53

Gollober M. Screening for cervical cancer. Nurse Pract 1979 Sept/Oct; 4(5):20–24, 31

Gollober M. Cervical cancer screening. Nurse Pract 1979 Nov/Dec; 4(6):17–21

Hamilton A and Kelley P. An education program for hysterectomy patients. Super Nurse 1979 April; 10(4):19–25

Jick H et al. Replacement estrogens and endometrial cancer. N Engl J Med 1979 Feb 1; 300(5):218–222

Johnson GH. Pelvic mass and diagnosis of carcinoma of ovary. Clin Obstet Gynecol 1979 Dec; 22(4):903–923

Parmley T. Preinvasive cervical cancer. Postgrad Med 1979 Oct; 66(4):169–175

Ramney B. Endometriosis: Pathogenesis, symptoms, and findings. Clin Obstet Gynecol 1980 Sept; 23(3):865–874

Ramney B. Etiology, prevention, and inhibition of endometriosis. Clin Obstet Gynecol 1980 Sept; 23(3):875–883

Segaloff A. The pros and cons of estrogen therapy. Postgrad Med 1979 June; 65(6):106–112

Smith WG. Surgical treatment of ovarian carcinoma. Clin Obstet Gynecol 1979 Dec; 22(4):939–956

Strickler RC. Dysfunctional uterine bleeding. Postgrad Med 1979 Nov; 66(5):135–146.

Weiss NS and Sayvetz TA. Incidence of endometrial cancer in relation to the use of oral contraceptives. N Engl J Med 1980 March 6; 302(10):551–554

Vulva and Vagina

Antonioli D et al. Natural history of diethylstilbestrol-associated genital tract lesions: Cervical ectopy and cervicovaginal hood. Am J Obstet Gynecol 1980 Aug. 1; 137(8):847–853

Blough HA and Guintoli RL. Successful treatment of human genital herpes infections with 2-deoxy-D-glucose. JAMA 1979 June 29; 241(26):2798–2801

Gelms J. Vulvar carcinoma: Pre-, intra-, and post-operative care. Point of View/Ethicon 1980 July 1; 17(3):14–16

Glebatis DM and Janerich DT. A statewide approach to diethylstilbestrol—the New York program. N Engl J Med 1981 Jan 1; 304(1):47–50

Goldfarb JM and Little AB. Current concepts: Abnormal vaginal bleeding. N Engl J Med 1980 March 20; (12):666–669

Herbst AL. DES update. CA 1980 Nov/Dec; 30(6):326–332

Wein AJ et al. Repair of vesicovaginal fistula by a suprapubic transvesical approach. Surg Gynecol Obstet 1980 Jan; 150(1):57–60

Fertility Control

Bartosik D. Oral contraceptives—An update. Am Fam Physician 1979 May; 19(5):149–150

Bressler R and Durand JL. Oral contraceptive risks: A realistic appraisal. Drug Ther 1979 Oct; 9(10):31–94

Cole P. Editorial. Oral contraceptives and endometrial cancer. N Engl J Med 1980 March 6; 302(10):575–576

Connell EB. Update on oral contraceptives. Curr Probl Obstet Gynecol 1979 April; 2(8):1–30

Crabbe P et al. Injectable contraceptive synthesis: An example of international cooperation. Science 1980 Aug; 209(8):992–994

Dawson K. Side effects of oral contraceptives. Nurs Pract 1979; Nov/Dec; 4(6):53–56

Freman WS. When patient "can't" take the pill. Am Fam Physician 1978 Jan; 17(1):143–149

Gambrel D et al. Breast cancer and oral contraceptive therapy in premenopausal women. J Reproduction Med 1979 Dec; 23(12):265–271

Gorline LL. Teaching successful use of the diaphragm. Am J Nurs 1979 Oct; 79(10):1732–1735

Gromko L. Intrauterine devices. Nurs Pract 1980 July/Aug; 5(4):19–26

HEW. FDA issue follow-up report on IUD's. Am Fam Physician 1979 Sept; 20(3):197–200

How to chart your basal body temperature. Patient Care 1979 March 15; 13(5):47–48

Huggins GR. Counseling patients for contraception. Clin Obstet Gynecol 1979 June; 22(2):509–520

IUD's—Update on safety, effectiveness, and research. Population Reports 1979 May; 7(3):B50–B98

Massey KL and Davison MA. Effects of oral contraceptives on nutritional status. Am Fam Physician 1979 Jan; 19(1):119–123

Molitch ME and Reichlin S. Management of post-pill amenorrhea. Drug Ther 1979 Sept; 9(9):93–102

OC (oral contraceptive)—Update on usage, safety, and side effects. Population Reports 1979 Jan; 8(1):A133–A186

Reversing female sterilization. Population Reports 1980 Sept; 8(5):C-97 to C-123

Rioux EJ and Yuzpe AA. Evaluation of female sterilization procedures. Curr Probl Obstet Gynecol 1979 May; 2(9):1–43

Spermicides—Simplicity and safety are major assets. Population Reports 1979 Sept; 8(5):Series H-72 to H-118

Stone SC and Cardinale F. Evaluation of a new vaginal contraceptive. Am J Obstet 1979 Mar 15; 133(6):635–637

Tyler LB. Update on intrauterine devices. Curr Probl Obstet Gynecol 1979 March; 2(7):1–24

Worthington BS. Nutrition during pregnancy, lactation, and oral contraception. Nurs Clin North Am 1979 June; 14(2):269–283

Zimmer JF and Lee TG. Locating a missing IUD by ultrasonography. Am Fam Physician 1979 Dec; 20(6):76–79

Infertility

Alexander NB and Cotanch PH. The endocrine basis of infertility in women. Nurs Clin North Am 1980 Sept; 15(3):511–524

Meeker CI. The infertile patient. Postgrad Med 1980 Dec; 68(6):139–149

Opitz JM et al. Genetic causes and workup of male and female infertility. 1. Prenatal reproductive loss. Postgrad Med 1979 May; 65(5):247–262; 2. Abnormalities presenting between birth and adult life. Postgrad Med 1979 June; 65(6):157–166

Taylor PJ and Cumming DC. Laparoscopy in the infertile female. Curr Prob Obstet Gynecol 1979 June; 2(10):1–59

3 CONDITIONS OF THE BREAST

Books

Brand PC and vanKeep PA. Breast Cancer: Psycho-social Aspects of Early Detection and Treatment. Baltimore, University Press, 1978

Cope O. The Breast: Its Problems—Benign and Malignant—and How to Deal with Them. Boston, Houghton Mifflin, 1977

Donegan WL and Spratt JS. Cancer of the Breast, 2nd ed. Philadelphia, WB Saunders, 1979

Gallagher, HS et al. The Breast. St Louis, C.V. Mosby, 1978

Kushner R. Why me? What every Woman Should Know about Breast Cancer to Save her Life. New York, New American Library, 1977

The Breast Cancer Digest. A Guide to Medical Care, Emotional Support, Educational Programs, and Resources. Bethesda, U.S. Dept. of Health, Education, and Welfare, National Institute of Health, National Cancer Institute, NIH Pub No. 80–1691, Dec 1979

Zalon J and Block JL. I am Whole Again: The Case for Breast Reconstruction after Mastectomy. New York, Random House, 1978

Articles

Albo RJ et al. Immediate breast reconstruction after modified mastectomy for carcinoma of the breast. Am J Surg 1980 July; 140(1):131–136

Bailar JC III. Risks and benefits of mammography. Curr Concepts Oncol 1979 Summer; 1:3–5

Baum G. Ultrasound mammography. Radiology 1977 Jan; 122(1):199–205

Buchanan-Davidson DK. Is breast cancer the same in men and women? Can Nurs 1980 Apr; 3(2):121–130

Degenshein GA. Mobility of the arm following radical mastectomy. Surg Gynecol Obstet 1977 July; 145(1):77

delRegato JA. Cancer of the breast. JAMA 1977 Nov 28; 238(22):2407–2410

Fink R et al. Effects of news events on response to a breast cancer screening program. Public Health Reports 1978 July–Aug; 93:318–327

Finn KL. Augmentation mammoplasty. Nursing '79 1979 Feb; 9(2):60–63

Fleagle JM. Helping the patient with breast cancer adjust to teletherapy. Nursing 80 1980 Apr; 10(4):60–61

Forrest APM. Conservative local treatment of breast cancer. Cancer (Suppl) 1977 June; 39:2813–2821

Foster RS et al. Breast self-examination practices and breast cancer stage. N Engl J Med 1978 Aug 10: 299(6):265–270

Frankl GL. Xeromammography in screening for breast cancer. Postgrad Med 1980 June; 67(6):67–71

Goldwyn RM. Subcutaneous mastectomy. N Engl J Med 1977 Sept 1; 297(9):503–505

Greenwald P et al. Estimated effect of breast self-examination and routine physician examinations on breast cancer mortality. N Engl J Med 1978 Aug 10; 299(6):271–273

Gruber RP. Method to produce better areolae and nipples on reconstructed breasts. Plast Reconst Surg 1977 Oct; 60(4):503–513

Hammond N et al. Predictive value of bone scans in an adjuvant breast cancer program. Cancer 1978 Jan; 41(1):138–142

Henderson IC and Canellos GP. Cancer of the breast, Part I. N Engl J Med 1980 Jan 3; 302(1):17–30

Henderson IC and Canellos GP. Cancer of the breast, Part II. N Engl J Med 1980 Jan 10; 302(1):78–90

Hetter GP. Satisfactions and dissatisfactions of patients with augmentation mammaplasty. Plast Reconst Surg 1979 August; 64(2):151–155

Hicks MJ et al. Sensitivity of mammography and physical examination of the breast for detecting breast cancer. JAMA 1979 Nov 9; 242(19):2080–2083

Hill GJ Jr. Changing concepts in the surgical management of breast cancer. Curr Concepts Oncol 1979 Summer; 1:6–10

If the bra fits. Nursing 80 1980 Feb; 10(2):15

Kirch RLA and Klein M. Prospective evaluation of periodic breast examination programs. Cancer 1978 Feb; 41(2):728–736

Koch SJ. Augmentation mammaplasty. Am J Nurs 1980 Aug; 80(8):1480–1484

Kodlin D and McCarthy N. Reserpine and breast cancer. Cancer 1978 Feb; 41(2):761–768

Lawson NC and Fitzgerald D. Psychological research in cancer—an overview. Cancer Bulletin 1978 Mar/Apr; 30(2):49–51

Levinger GE. Working through recovery after mastectomy. Am J Nurs 1980 June; 80(6):1118–1120

Lippman ME et al. The relation between estrogen receptors and response rate to cytotoxic chemotherapy in metastatic breast cancer. N Engl J Med 1978 June 1; 298(22):1223–1228

Lokich JJ. CEA: A monitor of therapy for breast and colon cancer. Am Fam Physician 1978 April; 17(4):173–176

Mammography may be better than you think. Hosp Pract 1980 Jan; 15(1):26–33

Mammography screening for breast cancer. The Med Letter 1980 June 27; 22(13):53–54

McGuire WL. Steroid receptors and breast cancer. Hosp Pract 1980 Apr; 15(4):83–88

Meyer AC et al. Carcinoma of the breast: A clinical study. Arch Surg 1978 April; 113:364–367

Miller AB. Role of nutrition in the etiology of breast cancer. Cancer (Suppl) 1977; 32:2704–2708

Minton K et al. Responses of fibrocystic disease to caffeine withdrawal and correlation of cyclic nucleotides with breast disease. Am J Obstet Gynecol 1979 Sept 1; 135, 157–158

Moore FD. Breast self-examination. N Engl J Med 1978 Aug 10; 299(6):304–305

Moskowitz M. How can we decrease breast cancer mortality? CA 1980 Sept/Oct; 30(5):272–277

National panel rejects radical mastectomy. AORN J 1979 Nov; 30(5):942–946

NIH breast cancer report controversial. AORN J 1980 Jan; 31(1):128–133

Nursing researchers study breast cancer. Surgical Rounds 1980 May; 15(5):28

Schwartz MK. Hormone receptor assay. Am J Nurs 1977 Sept; 77(9):1445–1446

Snyderman RK. Plastic and reconstructive breast surgery. Am Fam Physician 1979 Oct; 20(4):146–151

Soteropoulos GC et al. Localization with xeromammography. Am Fam Physician 1979 Sept; 20(3):120–123

Todd A. Prophylactic mastectomy. Am J Nurs 1977 Sept; 77(9):1447–1449

Townsend CM. Breast lumps. Clin Symp 1980; 32(2):3–32

Trotta P. Breast self-examination: Factors influencing compliance. Oncol Nurs Forum 1980 Summer; 7(3):13–17

Turnbull EM. Effect of basic preventive health practices and mass media on the practice of breast self-examination. Nurs Res 1978 Mar/Apr; 27(2):98–102

Vaccarino JM. Consent, informed consent, and the consent form. N Engl J Med 1978 Feb 23; 298(8):455

Wolf LE and Biggs TM. Breast reconstruction after mastectomy. Am J Surg 1979 Dec; 138(6):777–782

Wynder EL et al. The epidemiology of breast cancer in 785 United States Caucasian women. Cancer 1978 June; 41:2341–2354

SKIN DISORDERS

12

1 DERMATOLOGY

1 DERMATOLOGY

NURSING PATIENTS WITH DERMATOLOGIC CONDITIONS

Psychological Insights

1. Patients with dermatological problems can see and feel their problems and are more disturbed by their complaints than many patients with other conditions.
2. Skin eruptions evoke feelings of shame, disgust, avoidance, withdrawal, and anger that compound the problems of management of patients with skin conditions.

Touching the patient reduces his sense of isolation.
3. Irritation is a constant feature of skin disease and produces loss of sleep, anxiety, and depression, which in turn reinforce discomfort and fatigue.
4. Cosmetic needs constitute the underlying motive that brings the patient to treatment.
5. Nursing support requires understanding, unending patience, and continuing encouragement for these patients.

Nursing Assessment

Be aware that many systemic conditions may be accompanied by dermatologic manifestations.

A. *History*

1. Obtain a dermatologic history.
   a. How long has the patient had the skin condition?
   b. Has it occurred previously?
   c. Were there any other symptoms besides the rash?
   d. What site was first affected?
   e. What did the rash/lesion look like when it first appeared?
   f. How did it spread?
   g. Are there itching, burning, tingling, or crawling sensations? Loss of sensation?
   h. Is it worse at a particular time?
   i. Does the patient have any idea how it started?
   j. Is there history of hay fever, asthma, urticaria? eczema? allergies?
   k. Was the appearance of the eruption related to the intake of food?
   l. Was there a relationship between a specific event and the outbreak of the rash/lesion?
   m. What medications is the patient taking? What medications (salves, ointments, cream) have been applied to the lesion?
   n. What is the patient's occupation?
   o. What is in his immediate environment (plants, animals) that might be precipitating the problem?
   p. Ask if there is anything else he wishes to talk about in regard to this problem.

B. *Examination of the Skin*

1. Ask the patient to undress; the entire skin must be examined.
2. Have good lighting available. Use a hand magnifying lens to inspect for fine detail (altered skin markings, loss of skin lines, etc.).
3. Inspect the skin in an orderly sequence: hair, scalp, nails, buccal mucosa, skin surface.
4. Look at the distribution, arrangement, and grouping of the rash/lesions.
5. Note the shape, border, color, texture, and surface of the lesion.
6. Palpate the shape, border, texture and surface of the lesion.

C. *Assessment of Patients with Dark or Black Skin*

1. Healthy dark skin has a reddish undertone; buccal mucosa, tongue, lips, and nails normally appear pink.
2. Lightening, darkening, or blotching of the skin are very noticeable and can cause emotional distress.
   a. Hyperpigmentation of the mouth is normal in some individuals.
   b. Some blacks have pigmented streaks on nails; usually normal.
3. Certain procedures (freezing, topical peeling and drying agents or diseases) can cause hypopigmentation (loss or decrease in skin color) or hyperpigmentation (increase in color). These changes are more apparent in dark-skinned patients.

D. *Examination of Black Skin*

1. Have good lighting; look in mouth and nail beds as well as entire skin area.
2. Palpate all suspicious areas.

3. *For rash:*
   a. Ask the patient if he has an area of itching.
   b. Stretch the skin gently to decrease the reddish tone and make the rash stand out.
   c. Palpate by running fingertips lightly over the skin—to feel the differences in skin temperature and to feel the borders of the rash.
   d. Palpate the lymph nodes; take the patient's temperature.
4. *For erythema:*
   a. Inspect for a purplish-grayish cast of skin.
   b. Palpate for increase in warmth and for signs of smoothness (edema) or hardness—to detect possible infection.
5. *For cyanosis:*
   a. Look for a gray cast of the skin.
   b. Inspect areas around the mouth, lips, over cheek bones and ear lobes.
   c. Evaluate for the usual signs of shock. (See p. 128.)
6. Describe and document the dermatosis (abnormal condition of the skin) clearly and in detail.
   a. What is (are) the color(s) of the lesion?
   b. Is there redness, heat, pain, or swelling?
   c. How large an area is involved; where is it?
   d. Is the eruption macular, papular, scaling, oozing, discrete, confluent?
   e. What is the distribution of the lesion—symmetrical, linear, circular?

Description of Skin Lesions

A. *Primary Lesions* (initial lesions)

1. Macule—nonelevated discoloration of the skin; of various sizes, shapes, and colors
2. Papule—a solid, elevated lesion less than 1 cm (0.4 inch) in diameter
3. Nodule—a raised lesion that is larger and deeper than a papule
4. Vesicle—a small elevation of the skin that is filled with clear fluid less than 0.5 cm in diameter
5. Bulla—a large vesicle or blister larger than 1 cm (0.4 inch) in diameter
6. Pustule—vesicle or bulla that contains pus; may form as a result of purulent changes in a vesicle
7. Wheal—transient elevation of the skin caused by edema of the dermis and surrounding capillary dilatation
8. Plaque—a solid, elevated lesion of the skin or mucous membrane, greater than 1 cm in diameter

B. *Secondary Lesions,* (changes that take place in primary lesions and possibly modify them)

1. Scales—heaped-up horny layer of dead epidermis; may develop as a result of inflammatory changes
2. Crusts—a covering formed by the drying of serum, blood, or pus on the skin
3. Excoriations—linear scratch marks or traumatized area of skin. May be self-produced
4. Fissure—a crack in the skin, usually from marked drying and long-standing inflammation
5. Ulcer—lesion formed by local destruction of the epidermis and part or all of the underlying dermis
6. Lichenification—thickening of skin accompanied by accentuation of skin markings
7. Scar—a fibrotic change in the skin following a destructive process

DERMATOLOGIC THERAPY

OPEN WET DRESSINGS

Open wet dressings are wet compresses applied to skin areas.

Purposes

1. To reduce inflammation by producing vasoconstriction—thus decreasing vasodilatation and the local blood flow present in inflammation.
2. To cleanse skin of exudates, crusts, scales—thus making a cleaner and drier surface.
3. To maintain drainage of infected areas.

Clinical Uses

1. Vesicular, bullous, pustular, and ulcerative disorders
2. Acute inflammatory conditions
3. Erosions
4. Exudative, crusted surfaces

Solution and Material	Desired Effect	Nursing Action
Solution Cool tapwater Physiologic saline Burow's Solution (aluminum acetate solution) Magnesium sulfate *Material* Soft toweling Diapers Soft cotton sheeting Kerlix (Bauer and Black)	Effective in treating oozing dermatosis or swollen, infected dermatitis (furunculitis, cellulitis). Relieves inflammation, burning and itching. Has cooling effect. Useless for removing crusts.	Keep dressing cool or at room temperature. Moisten compress to the point of slight dripping. Compresses may be remoistened using an asepto syringe. Add ice cubes to solution if coolness is desired. Apply for 15 minutes every 2–3 hours unless otherwise indicated. Keep patient warm if extensive areas are to be compressed. Do not treat more than $\frac{1}{3}$ of the body at one time. Discard dressing material daily. CAUTION: Avoid burns.

BATHS (BALNEOTHERAPY)

Baths are useful for applying medications to large areas of the skin, removing crusts, scales, and old medications, and relieving inflammation and itching.

Bath Solution and Medication	Desired Effect	Nursing Action

Water
Saline
Colloidal—Oatmeal or Aveeno
    Powdered milk
    Corn starch
    Baking soda
	Used for weeping, oozing, erythematous eruptions.
	Used for widely disseminated lesions.
	Antipruritic and drying.
	
	Cooling
		Fill the tub half full—94 L. (25 gallons).
		Keep the water at a comfortable temperature; avoid *hot* baths.
		
		Do not allow the water to cool excessively.
		Use a bath mat—*medications may cause tub to be slippery.*

Medicated tars (follow package directions)
    Alma-Tar, Balnetar
Bath oils
    Alpha-Keri, Ar-Ex, Avenol, Domol, Lubath, Lubriderm
	Tar baths are used for psoriasis and chronic eczematous conditions.
	
	Bath oils are used for antipruritic and emollient actions.
	Used for acute and subacute eczematous eruptions.
		Remove loose skin debris and crusts after bath.
		Apply a lubricating agent to wet skin after bath if emollient action is desired—increases hydration.
		Dry by blotting with a towel.
		Keep room warm to minimize temperature fluctuations.
		Encourage patient to wear light, loose cotton clothing after the bath.

TOPICAL MEDICATIONS

Type of Medication	Desired Effect	Nursing Action
Lotions Liquid vehicles for carrying medication; act by evaporation	Lubricate Cool through water evaporation. May be protective, antiparasitic, antifungal, antipruritic; may act as sunscreen.	May be applied with cotton gauze or soft paintbrush.
Ointments and Creams Have greasy, nongreasy, or penetrating base depending on nature of lesion and drug applied.	Lubricate Protect the skin. Serve as vehicle for medications. Retard water loss. Used in chronic or localized skin conditions. Cause vasoconstriction; reduce blood flow to skin.	Ointment and creams are rubbed into the skin by hand. Teach patient to apply his own ointment or cream. Ointments may have to be covered with a dressing to prevent soiling of clothing.
Topical Adrenocorticosteroid Agents (many preparations available)	Have anti-inflammatory action.	Apply to localized area requiring medication. Use only a small amount and rub in thoroughly. Use with occlusive dressing as directed—enhances penetration.
Powders (usually with a talc, zinc oxide, or cornstarch base)	Act as hygroscopic agents (take up moisture). Increase evaporation; absorb perspiration. Reduce friction.	Dispense with shaker top. Avoid accumulating powder in intertriginous areas.
Intralesional Therapy Injection with a tuberculin syringe of sterile suspension of medication (usually suspension of corticosteroid) into or just below a lesion	Has anti-inflammatory action.	Be aware that local atrophy may result if injection is made into subcutaneous fat. Check patient for anaphylactoid reaction which may occur.
Systemic Medications Adrenocorticosteroids Antibiotics Antihistamines Sedatives and tranquilizers Analgesics Antineoplastics		

DRESSINGS FOR SKIN CONDITIONS

A. *Occlusive dressing*—an airtight plastic film is applied to cover medicated skin (usually corticosteroid)
1. Purposes
   a. Enhances absorption of topically applied medication.
   b. Increases penetration of corticosteroids into the skin, thus enhancing anti-inflammatory effect
   c. Produces moisture retention; permits medication from evaporating

> **NURSING ALERT:** Prolonged use of occlusive dressings may cause skin atrophy, striae, telangiectasia, folliculitis, nonhealing ulceration, erythema, or systemic absorption of corticosteroids. Dressings should be removed for 12 out of 24 hours to prevent some of these complications.

2. Plastic surgical tape containing corticosteroid is available and can be cut to size.

B. *Other Dressings*

1. Fingers and toes—gauze or cotton cloth; held in place with small size tubular material (Surgitube, Tubegauze)
2. Hands—disposable polyethylene gloves; sealed at wrists
3. Feet—cotton socks or disposable plastic bags
4. Extremities (arms and legs)—cotton cloth covered with tubular material
5. Groin, perineum—disposable diapers; cotton cloth folded in diaper fashion
6. Axillae—cotton cloth taped in place or held by commercial dress shields
7. Trunk—cotton or light flannel pajamas
8. Scalp—turban or plastic shower cap
9. Face—mask made from gauze with holes cut out for eyes, nose, mouth.

THE PATIENT WITH A DERMATOSIS (ABNORMAL SKIN CONDITION)

Objectives of Treatment, Nursing Management and Health Education

A. *To control itching and relieve pain*

1. Examine area of involvement.
   a. Attempt to discover the cause of discomfort.
   b. Record observations in detail, using descriptive terminology.
2. Advise patient to employ measures that produce vasoconstriction.
   a. Maintain cool environment.
   b. Reduce excess clothing or bedding.
   c. Provide tepid, cooling baths.
   d. Apply cool wet dressings.
3. Treat dryness (xerosis) with lubricating creams or lotions applied after bathing and before drying to enhance hydration.
4. Apply prescribed lotions or ointments.
5. Supply analgesic and antipruritic medications as indicated.
6. Administer tranquilizing agents or sedative drugs, as necessary.
7. Instruct patient to refrain from self-medication with salves or lotions that are commercially advertised.
8. Assist the anxious patient to improve his insight and to identify and cope with his problems.

B. *To treat an inflammatory lesion*

1. Apply continuous or intermittent wet dressings to reduce intensity of inflammation.
2. Remove crusts and scales before applying topical medications.
3. Use topical applications containing corticosteroid drugs, as indicated.

   a. Rub topical medicaments well into skin to enhance penetration.
   b. Observe lesion periodically for changes in response to therapy.

C. *To control oozing and prevent crust formation*

1. Provide tub baths and wet dressings to loosen exudates and scales.
2. Remove medications with mineral oil before re-applying.
3. Use mildly astringent solutions to precipitate proteins and decrease oozing.
4. Supply a high protein diet if oozing is voluminous and serum loss substantial.
5. Administer antibiotics by topical application or by mouth, as indicated.

D. *To avoid damage to skin*

1. Protect healthy skin from maceration when applying wet dressings.
2. Remove moisture from skin by blotting gently and avoiding friction.
3. Guard carefully against risk of thermal trauma from excessively hot wet dressings.
4. Advise patient to use sun-screening agents to prevent actinic damage (chemical changes from ultraviolet light).

E. *To ensure efficacy of topical applications*

1. Use occlusive dressings, as needed, to retain medication in constant contact with affected skin.
2. Elicit the patient's cooperation by having him perform his own dermatologic treatments.
3. Instruct patient clearly and in detail to ensure that treatments are carried out as prescribed.

SEBORRHEIC DERMATOSES

Dermatoses refers to abnormal skin conditions.

Seborrhea is excessive production of sebum (secretion of sebaceous glands) in those areas where glands are normally found in large numbers (face, scalp, scrotum).

Seborrheic dermatitis is a chronic inflammatory disease of the skin with a predilection for areas that are well supplied with sebaceous glands or that lie between folds of skin where the bacterial count is high.

Clinical Features

1. Characteristic lesion (remarkably varied)
   a. Dry, moist, or greasy scales
   b. Crusted pinkish-yellow or yellowish patches of varying shapes and sizes
   c. Possible erythema (redness), fissuring (cracking), and secondary infection
   d. Dry, flaky desquamation on scalp with profuse amount of fine, powdery scales (dandruff); itching may be mild or intense
2. Sites
   Scalp (dandruff), eyebrows, eyelids, nasolabial crease, lips, ears, axillae, under breast, groin, gluteal crease.
3. Seborrheic dermatitis is associated with genetic pre-

disposition and aggrevated by physical or emotional stress.
4. There is a tendency to lifelong recurrences lasting for weeks, months, or years.

Treatment

OBJECTIVE: to control the disorder (no known cure at this time) and allow the skin to repair itself.

1. Advise patient to remove external irritants and avoid excess heat and perspiration—rubbing and scratching will prolong the disorder.
2. Suggest local remedies.
   a. *For Scalp*—to control dandruff
      (1) Give the hair an initial cleansing shampoo to remove accumulated scale.
      (2) Use shampoo with selenium sulfide suspension (Selsun); leave shampoo on scalp 10 minutes; rinse thoroughly.
      (3) Shampoos containing tar are also effective, especially in controlling itching.
      (4) Shampoo daily or once or twice weekly, depending on condition of the scalp.
   CAUTION: Observe precautions on container.

b. *Seborrheic dermatitis of the body and face*
 (1) May respond to a topically applied corticosteroid cream—allays secondary inflammation.
 (2) Use with extreme caution on the eyelids, since it can induce glaucoma in predisposed individuals.
 (3) Prolonged use of fluorinated steroids on face can produce acne. Prolonged use in intertriginous areas can produce striae and atrophy. Therefore, plain hydrocortisone is used.
3. Give systemic corticosteroids for severe and acute seborrheic dermatitis (used only rarely).
4. Use antibacterial measures if exudation and crusting occur.
 a. Systemic antibiotic may be required for a spreading infection.

b. Topical antibiotics (cream or lotion) may be applied.
5. Watch for occurrence of secondary moniliasis (yeast infection) that may occur in body creases or folds.
 a. Advise patient to cleanse intertriginous areas carefully; ensure maximum aeration of skin.
 b. Patient with coincidental moniliasis should be evaluated for diabetes mellitus.

Health Education

1. Advise patient to avoid systemic aggravating factors—overwork, lack of sleep, infection, emotional stress.
2 Sunlight may be beneficial.

ACNE VULGARIS

Acne vulgaris is a common disorder of the sebaceous (oil) glands and their follicles (pilosebaceous follicles) characterized by the presence of comedones (blackheads), milia (whiteheads), papules, pustules, nodules, and cysts. The primary sites are the face, chest, upper back, and shoulders.

Predisposing Factors

1. Genetic predisposition—strong genetic overtones
2. Hormonal changes of adolescence—from androgenic stimulation of sebum production
3. Cutaneous flora—high concentration of *Propionibacterium acnes* found in acne-susceptible individuals
4. External irritants—climate, chemical, mechanical irritants, cosmetics, pharmacologic agents

Altered Physiology

Stimulation of androgenic hormones → increase in amount and thickness of oil secretion → lipids arising in the sebaceous glands → follicular bacteria (*P. acnes*) → obstruction of sebaceous glands by blackheads (comedones) → disruption of the follicular epithelium, allowing discharge of the follicular contents into the dermis → inflammatory reaction → papules → pustules → nodules → cysts.

Treatment

OBJECTIVES: to reduce colonization by *P. acnes* bacteria.
 to prevent follicular obstruction.
 to reduce inflammation and combat secondary infection.
 to minimize scarring.
 to eliminate factors that may predispose to acne.
The therapeutic regimen depends on the type of lesion (comedonal, papular, pustular, or cystic).

A. *Prevent obstruction of the oil glands.*
1. Wash face gently 1–2 times daily with mild soap and water—to remove surface oil.
 Mild abrasive soaps and drying preparations may be used for mild involvement (mainly comedones). Avoid excessive abrasion.
2. Shampoo scalp nightly or twice weekly with medicated shampoo.
3. Use bath brush if back is involved.

B. *Topical agents for more severe involvement.*
OBJECTIVES: to clear keratin plugs from follicular ducts.
 to suppress *Propionibacterium acnes* in the follicles.
1. Topical benzoyl peroxide (PanOxyl, Desquam-X, Benazgel)—exerts antibacterial effects, suppresses *P. acnes*, and reduces concentration of surface free fatty acids.
 a. Apply sparingly to completely dry skin; adjusted to point of tolerance.
 b. Advise patient that he may not see improvement for 1–2 and up to 6 weeks.
2. Topical vitamin A acid, (tretinoin [Retin-A])—speeds up the cellular turnover, which forces out the comedones and prevents occurrence of new comedones.
 Instructions to Patient:
 a. Read the product information brochure.
 b. Apply vitamin A acid to thoroughly dry skin—wet skin enhances penetration and increases the potential for irritation.
 c. Keep medication away from eyes, nasolabial folds, corners of mouth—likely to pool in these areas causing local irritation.
 d. Apply as tolerated; the concentration of the preparation used and the frequency of its application are adjusted according to the reactivity of the skin to vitamin A acid.
 e. Wash hands thoroughly after applying vitamin A acid.
 f. Inform the patient that the symptoms may worsen during the early weeks of treatment due to action of medication on previously unseen comedones; there is possibility of some erythema and peeling. Improvement may take 4–8 weeks.
 g. Be cautious during first few weeks about exposure to sun (including sunlamps)—antikeratinizing effect of tretinoin makes patient more sensitive to sunburn.
 h. Avoid other irritants, such as strong soaps.
3. Topical antibiotic therapy—suppresses growth of *P. acnes* and produces decrease in comedones, papules, and pustules.
 a. Topical tetracycline, clindamycin, and erythromycin are available.
 b. Used alone or in combination with other agents.

C. *Systemic Therapy*

1. *Systemic antibiotics* appear to reduce *P. acnes* in pilosebaceous follicles and inhibit sebum production.
   a. Tetracycline, erythromycin, or minocycline is given and adjusted according to therapeutic response.
   b. Long-term, low-dose antibiotic may be given.
   c. May take several weeks for effect of antibiotics to show.
   d. Instruct the patient to take tetracycline at least 1 hour before or 2 hours after mealtime; avoid taking any dairy products (milk, ice cream) within 2 hours before or after taking medication—tetracycline is poorly absorbed with food.
   e. Side effects of tetracycline include nausea, diarrhea, superinfection, and moniliasis. (Vaginitis in women; cutaneous infection in either sex, but more often in men.)
2. *Estrogen therapy* (usually in form of oral contraceptive)—suppresses the androgenic stimulation of sebum production.
   a. Usually reserved for young women with severe cystic acne; not given to males because of undesirable side effects.

D. *Acne Surgery*

1. Comedo extraction (See following Guidelines.)
2. Incision and drainage of cysts and pustular lesions—may be required in large, fluctuant, nodular-cystic lesions.
3. Intralesional injection of corticosteroids (triamcinolone acetonide)
   Diluted steroid suspension is injected into inflamed lesions—leads to rapid resolution.

4. Cryosurgery (freezing with liquid nitrogen)—for nodular and cystic forms of acne
5. Dermabrasion—surgical planing of skin—to reduce surface configuration of old scars and give smooth appearance.

Health Education

1. Gain the patient's confidence. Outline the therapy—try to relieve unspoken fear and guilt.
   a. Acne is not caused by dirt and cannot be washed away; it is a chemical imbalance that causes the oil in the skin to form blackheads.
   b. Acne is *not* related to sexual activity.
2. Keep hands away from face.
3. Do not squeeze pimples or blackheads—squeezing the skin makes acne worse. The majority of blackheads are pushed down into the skin by squeezing. This may cause the follicle to be ruptured.
4. Eat a healthful diet; eliminate any food that you feel worsens your acne.
5. Keep hair off the face; wash hair daily if necessary.
6. Avoid friction and trauma.
   a. Do not prop your hands against your face.
   b. Avoid overzealous washing of face, rubbing the face, pressure from tight collars/helmets.
   c. Avoid perspiration around the face.
7. Avoid cosmetics (including cleansing creams), shaving creams and lotions—contain chemicals that can aggravate acne.
8. Continue treatment even though your skin clears.
9. Be able to talk over your problems with an understanding person—acne may become a source of power struggle between teenager and parent. Emotional stress may worsen acne in certain individuals.

GUIDELINES: Comedo Extraction*

A *comedo* (blackhead) is a mass composed of lipids, keratin, and entrapped follicular bacteria that forms a solid plug in a dilated follicular opening (pore).

Underlying Considerations

1. Blackheads are approximately 4 mm. deep and cannot be washed away.
2. Comedones are considered end-stage lesions and their removal is only of temporary benefit. However, removal reduces the chance of their evolving into papules, pustules, and cysts.

Equipment

Light
Magnifying loupe
Alcohol and sponges

Instruments:
Comedo extractor
Scalpel blade No. 11
No. 18 gauge needle

Procedure

NURSING ACTION	RATIONALE/AMPLIFICATION
1. Wipe off the site with an alcohol sponge.	1. For antisepsis and to allow visualization of lesions.
2. Nick the comedo with No. 18 gauge sterile needle or scalpel blade.	2. This widens the port and facilitates comedo removal.
3. Place opening of the extractor over the lesion and apply firm downward pressure directly on the lesion.	3. This causes extrusion of the plug through the expressor. Overly vigorous attempts to express comedones may result in an increased inflammatory response.
4. Wipe off the site with a fresh alcohol sponge.	
5. Inform the patient that removal of comedones may leave areas of erythema which may take several weeks to subside.	

* This procedure must be performed with skill by a prepared person.

BACTERIAL INFECTIONS

FURUNCLES

A *furuncle*, or boil, is an acute inflammation arising deep within one or more hair follicles; the causative agent is almost always *Staphylococcus aureus*.
Furunculosis refers to multiple or recurrent lesions.
A *stye* is a furuncle that forms on eyelid margin.

Clinical Features

1. Initial occurrence—usually begins around a hair follicle
2. Sites of predilection—back of neck, axillae, buttocks
3. Causative factors—irritation, pressure, friction, excessive perspiration, shaving of axillae (in persons with lowered resistance)
4. Symptoms—tenderness, pain, and surrounding cellulitis; after furuncle localizes, the center becomes boggy and fluctuant, and a soft yellow or white head appears on the surface.

Treatment and Nursing Management

1. Protect area from irritation, squeezing, and trauma.
2. Apply hot wet compresses—to increase vascularization and hasten resolution.
3. Cleanse surrounding skin with antibacterial soap.
4. Apply antibacterial ointment to surrounding skin— to prevent spillage and seeding of the bacteria when furuncle ruptures or is incised.
5. Prepare for surgical drainage when furuncle has become localized and shows fluctuation (wavelike motion upon palpation); furuncle may rupture spontaneously.
6. Give systemic antibiotic therapy (selected by sensitivity study) if spreading still occurs or if area of involvement poses a risk of complications.

> **NURSING ALERT:** Take special precautions with boil on face, since the skin area drains directly into the cranial venous sinuses.
> 1. Place patient with boils on nose, lip, groin, perineal or perianal region on bed rest.
> 2. Give course of systemic antibiotic therapy as prescribed—to control spread of infection.

Health Education

Instruct the patient as follows:
1. Keep draining lesion covered with a dressing.
2. Wash hands thoroughly after caring for lesion.
3. Wrap soiled dressings in paper and burn.
4. Discard razor blades after each use.
5. Bathe with bacteriostatic soap; change and wash clothing and bed linens daily.

CARBUNCLES

A *carbuncle* is an abscess of the skin and subcutaneous tissues—an extension of a furuncle invading multiple follicles; usually caused by staphylococcal infection.

Clinical Features

1. Seen most frequently within the thick, fibrous, inelastic skin of the back of the neck and upper back.
2. More apt to occur in older and debilitated persons; especially frequent in diabetics.

> **NURSING ALERT:** Every patient past middle age with a carbuncle should be suspected of having diabetes.

3. Symptoms
   a. Fever, leukocytosis, extreme pain, and prostration.
   b. Bacteremia is common because the extensive inflammation makes it difficult to completely wall off the infection, so that absorption of toxins takes place; extension of infection to bloodstream may take place.

Treatment and Nursing Management

1. Administer antibiotic (based on sensitivity studies)— antibiotic is continued until infective process is controlled.
2. Determine whether there is an underlying disease condition (diabetes, hematologic disease, etc.).
3. Prepare for surgical incision and drainage when definite fluctuance occurs. (Local surgical incision is usually necessary.)
4. Use supportive modalities (infusions, fever sponges, etc.) for the toxic patient.

IMPETIGO

Impetigo (impetigo contagiosa) is a superficial infection of the skin caused by streptococci, staphylococci, or multiple bacteria.
Bullous impetigo is a superficial infection of the skin caused by *S. aureus* characterized by the formation of bullae from the original vesicles.

Clinical Features

1. Lesion appears as discrete, thin-walled vesicle that ruptures and becomes covered with a loosely adherent, honey-yellow crust.
2. Crusts are easily removed and reveal smooth, red, moist surface on which new crusts soon develop.
3. Areas affected—exposed parts of body (face, hands, neck, and extremities).
4. Impetigo is a contagious disease. It is seen in all ages, but is particularly common among undernourished children living in poor hygienic conditions.
5. Sources of infection—children's pets, dirty fingernails, other children, adults, barber shops, beauty parlors, swimming pools, contaminated clothing, bedding, towels.
6. May be secondary to pediculosis capitis, scabies, herpes simplex, insect bites, poison ivy, eczema.

Treatment and Nursing Management

1. Give systemic antibiotic (benzathine penicillin, oral penicillin). Glomerulonephritis is a complication of

impetigo, depending on strain of streptococcus found. However, this therapy has not been proved to prevent nephritis.
2. Give penicillinase-resistant penicillin (oxacillin; nafcillin) for staphylococci that may be penicillin-resistant.
3. Wash lesions with bacterial soap or treat with warm, moist compresses to remove the loci of bacterial growth and to give topical antibiotic an opportunity to reach the infected site.
4. Apply a topical antibiotic cream (neomycin, bacitracin, polymyxin B) after crust removal.
5. Wear gloves while treating patient.

Health Education

1. The patient and family should bathe at least once daily with bacteriostatic soap as recommended.
2. The child with impetigo should be observed for at least 7 weeks for signs of acute glomerulonephritis.
3. Keep infected child away from other children.
4. Dispose of tissues and materials that come in contact with lesions.
5. Encourage good hygienic practices to prevent spread of disease from one skin area to another and from one person to another.

FUNGAL INFECTIONS

Fungi are plantlike organisms that feed on organic matter; they are responsible for a variety of common skin infections. Secondary infection with bacteria or *Candida* or both may occur.

TINEA PEDIS (ATHLETE'S FOOT) OR RINGWORM OF THE FEET

Tinea pedis (athlete's foot) is a superficial fungal infection which may manifest itself as an acute, inflammatory, vesicular process or as a chronic rash involving the soles of the feet and the interdigital web spaces.

Clinical Features

1. Tinea pedis is the most common fungal infection
2. Causes intense itching and burning
3. Lymphangitis and cellulitis may occur when bacterial superinfection is present

Diagnostic Evaluation

1. Direct examination of scrapings (skin, nails, hair)
2. Isolation of the organism in culture

Treatment

1. Use soaks (potassium permanganate, Burow's solution, saline) to remove scales, crusts, debris, and residual medications; also for mild anti-inflammatory effect.
2. Apply fungistatic creams or lotions such as tolnaftate (Tinactin), haloprogin (Halotex), miconazole (MicaTin) or clotrimazole (Lotrimin) to involved skin.
3. Continue with topical therapy for several weeks—there is a high rate of recurrence.
4. Give systemic antifungal agent (griseofulvin) if there is extension of the infection or resistance to topical therapy.

Preventive Measures and Health Education

Instruct the patient to keep feet dry—moisture encourages the growth of fungi.
1. Dry carefully between the toes.
2. Alternate shoes—to permit adequate drying of shoes between wearings.
3. Wear cotton socks or stockings with cotton feet—synthetic material does not absorb perspiration as well as cotton.
4. Change socks frequently.
5. Wear perforated shoes if feet perspire excessively—to permit aeration of feet.
6. Apply foot powder twice daily—to keep feet dry.
7. Use small pieces of cotton between toes at night—to absorb moisture.
8. Use clogs in community pools, showers, etc.

TINEA CAPITIS (RINGWORM OF THE SCALP)

Tinea capitis (ringworm of the scalp) is a fungal disease of the scalp. See page 1352.

TINEA CORPORIS OR TINEA CIRCINATA

Tinea corporis or tinea circinata is ringworm of the body.

Clinical Features

1. Appearance—begins as erythematous macule advancing to rings of vesicles with central clearing; lesions appear in clusters.
2. Lesions usually appear on exposed areas of body; may extend to scalp, hair, or nails.
3. An infected pet is a common source of infection.
4. Ringworm of the body causes intense itching.

Treatment

1. Apply topical antifungal medication to small areas (clotrimazole, miconazole, tolnaftate, haloprogin).
2. Griseofulvin may be used in very extensive cases. Side effects include photosensitiy skin rashes, headache, nausea, etc.

Health Education

Instruct the patient as follows:
1. Wear clean cotton clothing next to skin.
2. Use a clean towel daily; dry thoroughly all areas and skin folds that retain moisture, since fungi thrive in a warm, moist environment.

PARASITIC SKIN DISEASES

Three varieties of lice infest man; their itching bites are the cause of many skin problems. Lice bite the skin to obtain blood, which they feed on. They leave their eggs and excrement on the skin; lice are passed from person to person.

PEDICULOSIS CAPITIS

Pediculosis capitis is an infestation of the scalp by the head louse, *Pediculus humanus* var. *capitis*.

Clinical Features

1. Appearance—minute white nits (eggs) attached to hair shaft in series: usually on scalp and hair at back of head and behind ears. Look at hair ¾ to 2 inches away from scalp.
2. Most often found in children and persons wearing long hair.
3. The bite of the insect causes intense itching, and the scratching may lead to complications such as impetigo, furuncles, and enlarged cervical lymph nodes.
4. May be transmitted by direct physical contact or contact with infested combs, brushes, wigs, hats, and bedding.

Treatment and Nursing Management

1. Instruct the patient as follows:
   a. Use a shampoo containing gamma benzene hexachloride (Kwell).
   b. Shampoo the scalp at least 4 minutes with this preparation; rinse thoroughly.
   c. Comb hair with a fine-tooth comb dipped in vinegar—to remove remaining nits.
   d. Disinfect comb and brushes with Kwell shampoo; sterilize all washable fomites.
   e. Put on clean clothing and machine wash clothing and bed linen.
   f. Delouse unwashable clothing by sealing in plastic bag for 10 days.
2. Treat all family members and close contacts who are infested.
3. Treat complications—severe pruritus, pyoderma (pus-forming infection of the skin), and dermatitis—with antipruritics, systemic antibiotics, and topical corticosteroids.

Health Education

1. Head lice infestation may happen to anyone; it is not a sign of being dirty.
2. Treatment should be started immediately, since the condition spreads rapidly.
3. Control of school epidemics may be helped by having all of the students shampoo their hair on the same night.
4. Do not use Kwell on infants and children age 2 years or under; it has been associated with convulsions in some cases. Crotamiton (Eurax) lotion is an alternative treatment.

PEDICULOSIS CORPORIS

Pediculosis corporis is an infestation of the body by the body louse, *Pediculus humanus* var. *corporis*.

Clinical Features

1. The body louse lives chiefly in the seams of undergarments and other clothing, to which it clings.
2. Its bite causes characteristic minute hemorrhagic points.
   a. Widespread excoriations may appear on the back and shoulders.
   b. May produce secondary lesions—hyperemia, parallel linear scratches, and hyperpigmentation in persistent cases.
3. Areas of skin involved are those that come in closest contact with the undergarments (neck, trunk, thighs).
4. The lice and nits may be seen in the seams of clothing. They move to the skin for blood feedings and then return to the clothing.

Treatment and Nursing Management

1. Instruct the patient as follows:
   a. Bathe with soap and water.
   b. Put on clean clothing.
   c. Eliminate parasites and nits from clothing, bedding, and sleeping bags—lice adhere to seams of clothing. Machine wash on "hot cycle" or dry clean and press with hot iron.
2. Examine and treat all family members and contacts.
3. Treat pruritus, secondary bacterial infections, and dermatitis.

> **NURSING ALERT:** Body lice are vectors for rickettsial disease, epidemic typhus, relapsing fever, trench fever. The causative organism may be in the gastrointestinal tract of the insect and excreted on the skin surface.

PEDICULOSIS PUBIS

Pediculosis pubis is an infestation by *Phthirus pubis* (crab louse); it is chiefly transmitted by sexual contact and is generally localized to the genital region.

Clinical Manifestations

1. Chief symptom is itching.
2. Black or rust-colored dots clinging to the base of the hairs.
3. Lice may infest hairs of chest, axillary hair, beard, and eyelashes.
4. Gray-blue macules (1–3 cm. in diameter) may be seen on the trunk, thighs, and axillae as a result of the action of the insects' saliva on bilirubin—converts it to biliverdin.

Management and Health Education

1. Instruct the patient as follows:
   a. Bathe with soap and water.
   b. Apply gamma benzene hexachloride (Kwell) cream or lotion to areas of involvement.
      (1) Leave on for 12 hours. Wash off thoroughly. Put on clean clothing.
      (2) Do not apply Kwell to eyebrows.
         (a) Apply ophthalmic petrolatum to eyelashes and eyebrows—smothers the lice and allows easier removal of nits and lice.
         (b) Remove nits manually from eyelashes and eyebrows with cotton-tipped applicator or toothpick.
   c. Machine wash all clothing and bedding.
2. Treat all sexual contacts and family members.

3. Schedule patient for workup for coexisting sexually transmitted disease.
4. Treat secondary bacterial infection, itching, and dermatitis.

SCABIES

Scabies is an infestation of the skin by *Sarcoptes scabiei* (itch mite). Scabies is transmitted by close personal contact.

Clinical Features

1. *Primary lesion*
   a. Adult female burrows into superficial layer of skin after fertilization has occurred on skin surface; burrows are short, wavy, brownish or blackish thread-like lesions.
   b. She extends the burrow, laying eggs daily for up to 2 months, and then dies; larvae hatch in 2–3 days and migrate to skin surface where they reach maturity in 2–3 weeks.
   c. Male mites die shortly after mating.
2. Ask patient where itch is most severe at the time you are examining him; look for burrows (short, wavy, dirty-appearing lines) with a magnifying glass (may or may not see them). See below for procedure for obtaining skin scrapings for mite.
3. Look for small erythematous papules—scabies can imitate almost all pruritic dermatoses.
4. Sites—between fingers, on flexor surfaces of wrists and palms, around nipples, in axillary folds, under pendulous breasts, in or near groin or gluteal fold, penis, scrotum.
5. Secondary lesions include vesicles, papules, pustules, excoriations, and crusts; bacterial superinfection or eczematization may complicate the picture.
6. Symptoms—intense itching, more pronounced at night; usually occurs 1 month after initial infection.

7. The disease may be found in poor persons living under substandard hygienic conditions, but is also found in very clean individuals.
   a. Promoted by close physical contact.
   b. However, infestations are not dependent on sexual activity; since the mites frequently involve the fingers—hand contact may produce infection.
   c. Infestations with mites may also result from contact with dogs, cats, and small animals. (Animal scabies in humans look different; no burrows, only bites.)

Treatment and Health Education

Instruct patient as follows:
1. Take a hot, soapy bath or shower—to remove scaling debris from the crusts.
2. Apply scabicide such as gamma benzene hexachloride (Kwell cream and lotion, Gamene) or crotamiton (Eurax cream and lotion).
   a. Apply thin layer from neck downward, with particular attention to hairy areas around the groin and perianal region.
   b. Leave medication on for specified time. Then wash thoroughly.
   c. Put on freshly laundered or dry-cleaned clothes. Change bed linens.
   d. A bland ointment may be applied to the skin after completion of treatment.
   e. A second or third application may be made at 7-day intervals as necessary.
3. All family members and close contacts may be treated simultaneously to eliminate the mites. Children 2 years and under should not be treated with Kwell.
4. The animal with scabies should be treated by a veterinarian.
5. Advise patient that he may be uncomfortable for some weeks—the treatment solution is irritating to the skin and pruritus may remain for a time.

GUIDELINES: Skin Scraping for Scabies

Purpose To demonstrate the mite *Sarcoptes scabiei* (or ova or feces) in skin scrapings removed from burrows or papules (Fig. 12-1).

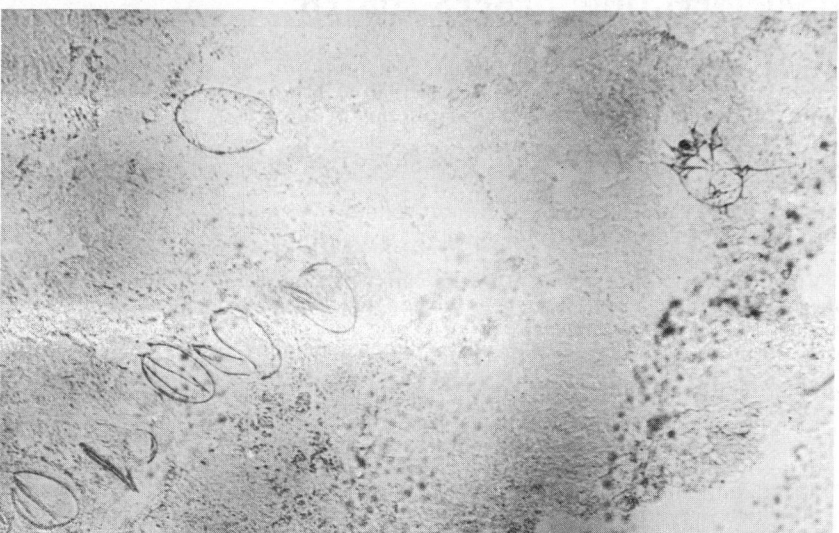

FIGURE 12–1. *Scabies; scraping from a burrow.* (Lower left) *Hatched eggs.* (Upper left) *Intact egg.* (Upper right) *Newly hatched organism.* (Courtesy Mervyn L. Elgart, M.D.)

GUIDELINES: Skin Scraping for Scabies (cont.)

Equipment   Mineral oil in dropper bottle
Scalpel and scalpel blade, No. 15
Glass slide/cover slip
Microscope

Procedure

NURSING ACTION	RATIONALE/AMPLIFICATION
Preparatory Phase	
1. Place a small drop of oil in the middle of a glass slide.	
Performance Phase	
1. Inspect for the burrows of *Sarcoptes scabiei* on lower abdomen, pubic and axillary areas, legs, arms, webs of fingers.	1. The female scabies mite, ova, and fecal deposits may be found in burrows on the skin.
2. Apply a small amount of mineral oil on unexcoriated burrows or papule.	2. The mineral oil causes the mite to float and enhances visualization.
3. Scrape the involved skin with the scapel blade.	
4. Transfer the scrapings to the prepared glass slide. Apply coverslip.	4. To avoid air bubble.
5. Examine the slide with a scanning lens of the microscope.	5. Look for the mites, eggs, and scybala (feces).

BEDBUG INFESTATION

Two species of bedbugs, *Cimex lectularius* and *Cimex hemipterus* invade human habitations. These are nocturnal blood-sucking insects.

Clinical Features

1. Appearance—bites are grouped in a straight line and consist of hemorrhagic spots associated with papular or wheal-like lesions; there may be a tiny red point marking the original site of the bite. New bites appear in the morning.
2. Sites—buttocks, back, and extremities are most frequently bitten—patient experiences itching and burning; urticaria (hives) may accompany the lesions.
3. Secondary infection and pyoderma may occur.

Health Education

1. Direct patient to apply lotions containing menthol and phenol to local areas of bites. Antihistamines may be prescribed for intense itching.
2. Advise patient to eliminate insect by spraying in crevices of furniture, walls, floors, mattresses, and beds.

VIRAL INFECTION: HERPES ZOSTER

Herpes zoster (shingles) is an inflammatory condition in which a virus produces a painful vesicular eruption along the distribution of the nerves from one or more posterior ganglia.

Etiology

Caused by a varicella virus, commonly known as a varicella-zoster virus, which is a member of a group of DNA viruses.

Virus appears to be identical to the causative agent of varicella (chickenpox); herpes zoster may be a reactivation of the latent varicella virus and reflects a lowered immunity.

Clinical Manifestations

1. Eruption usually accompanied or preceded by malaise, itching, tenderness, and pain, which may radiate over entire region supplied by the nerves.
   a. Inflammation is usually unilateral, involving one or two nerve roots in a band-like configuration.
   b. Pain may be burning, lancinating, stabbing, or aching.
2. Vesicles appear in 3–4 days.
   a. Characteristic patches of grouped vesicles on erythematous and edematous skin.
   b. Early vesicles contain serum—they become cloudy (secondary to inflammatory response).
   c. The lesions dry, crust, and clear; scarring may occur.
3. Eruption appears posteriorly and progresses to the anterior and peripheral distribution of the nerves from one or more posterior ganglia.
4. Clinical course varies from 1–3 weeks; healing time varies between 7–26 days.
5. Chickenpox can be acquired through contact with a person who has herpes zoster, particularly if the patient is immunosuppressed, has a malignancy, or has never had varicella.

Treatment and Nursing Management

OBJECTIVES: to reduce or avoid complications.
to make the patient comfortable.
1. The lesions usually clear spontaneously in healthy adults.
2. The following treatment regimen may be given.
   a. Give systemic corticosteroids as directed for pa-

tients with severe and complicated herpes—given for anti-inflammatory effect, relief of pain, and prevention of complications.

b. Vidarabine (Vira-A)—may give rapid pain relief, accelerate clearing of virus from vesicles, halt new vesicle formation.

c. Give analgesics to control pain and antihistamines to control itching.

d. Apply local treatment to skin lesions.
   (1) Apply cool wet dressings to pruritic lesions.
   (2) Apply topical steroid—triamcinolone acetonide (Kenalog) etc.—to give relief and promote healing.
   (3) Do not apply topical steroids if secondary infection is present.

e. Treat secondary bacterial infection of skin lesions—culture and sensitivity studies will indicate appropriate antibiotic.

f. Support the patient undergoing diagnostic studies to investigate the possibility of underlying disease.

> **NURSING ALERT:** Herpes zoster may indicate the presence of serious internal disease, especially in persons past middle age (Hodgkin's disease, lymphosarcoma, malignancy).

3. Watch for complications—higher incidence in patients over 60.
   a. Postherpetic neuralgia—persistent pain of affected nerve following healing.
   b. Ophthalmic herpes zoster—(involvement of ophthalmic branch of trigeminal nerve with keratitis, uveitis, corneal ulceration, and possibly blindness). Patients with ophthalmic herpes zoster should be examined by an ophthalmologist to avoid serious ocular complications.
   c. Facial and acoustic nerve involvement (facial paralysis, vertigo, tinnitus, hearing loss).

CONTACT DERMATITIS

Contact dermatitis (dermatitis venenata) is a common inflammatory, often eczematous, condition caused by a skin reaction due to contact with a variety of irritating or allergenic materials. There is damage to the epidermis by repeated physical and chemical insults.

1. *Primary irritant contact dermatitis* is a nonallergic reaction caused by exposure to an irritating substance.
2. *Allergic contact dermatitis* results from exposure of sensitized individuals to contact allergens.

Causes

1. Poison ivy
2. Cosmetics
3. Soaps, detergents, and scouring compounds
4. Industrial chemicals
5. Hair dye, metals, rubber, chemicals

Predisposing Factors

1. Extremes of heat and cold
2. Frequent immersion in soap and water
3. Preexisting skin disease

Clinical Manifestations

(Skin eruptions begin at point of contact with causative agent.)

1. Itching, burning, erythema, vesiculation, and eczema.
2. Weeping, crusting, drying, fissuring, and peeling.
3. Thickening of skin (lichenification) and pigmentation changes, if repeated reactions occur or if there is continual scratching by patient.
4. Secondary bacterial invasion may occur—prevention of normal sweating produces vesicles, itching, and inflammation.

Treatment and Nursing Management

OBJECTIVE: to protect and rest the involved skin.

1. Inspect the entire body for a distribution pattern—helps differentiate between allergic contact dermatitis and the irritant type.
2. Obtain a detailed history including the *site* of the *initial* eruption.

3. Instruct the patient as follows:
   a. Identify and remove the offending irritant.
      (1) Avoid the use of soap until healing occurs.
      (2) Avoid exposing skin to the causative agent after recovery.
      (3) Wear protective gloves (thin white cotton gloves under rubber gloves) for extended soap and water contact.
   b. *Topical treatment*
      (1) Use bland, unmedicated lotion for small patches of erythema.
      (2) Use cool, wet dressings for small areas of acute, vesicular dermatitis—for soothing and to help stop oozing.
      (3) Cleanse away softened crusts and other debris.
      (4) Apply a thin layer of cream or ointment containing one of the steroids, as directed—usually not as beneficial when blisters are present, although some authorities feel it is helpful in these instances if used more frequently; i.e., at least 5 times daily.
      (5) Use medicated baths at room temperature (p. 573) for larger areas of dermatitis.
4. Give sedatives and antihistamines if necessary to relieve itching and burning.
5. Give systemic antibiotics if secondary bacterial infection is present—purulent exudate and systemic symptoms (fever, lymphadenopathy, etc.).
6. Administer short course of systemic steroids if a more widespread and disabling condition is involved—can shorten the course of a severe disease; allays inflammation.
7. See also the patient with a dermatosis, p. 575.

Health Education

Instruct the patient as follows:

1. Avoid heat, soap, rubbing—all these are external irritants.
2. Avoid topical medications except when specifically prescribed.
3. Wash thoroughly immediately after exposure to antigens.

POISON IVY

Poison ivy grows in the form either of climbing vines or of upright shrubs; the leaves grow in clusters of 3, one at the end of the stalk and the other 2 opposite one another. Poison ivy has a sticky sap that contains an active ingredient known as *urushiol*, an oleoresin (a combination of plant resin and volatile oil). This urushiol can cause an allergic skin reaction (contact dermatitis).

Clinical Manifestations

1. Eruption may develop in hours or days after contact.
   a. Reddened area will be noted, followed by rash and edema.
   b. Eruption occurs in a streak or line; it burns and itches.
   c. Small weeping areas may form (papules, vesicles, blisters)—in more severe cases, large blistered areas with inflammation and swelling may appear.
2. Secondary infection may give lesion the appearance of pyoderma (purulent skin diesease) or plaque of eczema.

Exposure to Urushiol

1. Urushiol must make contact with the skin—contact is usually made by touching the plant leaves or stems.
2. Contact with urushiol may be made indirectly—clothing, tools, or pets touching the plant can pick up the sap and pass it to a person indirectly.
3. Urushiol is present in all parts of the plant, including dead stems and roots.
4. Smoke from burning plants carries droplets containing urushiol which can get on the skin or enter the nose, throat, and lungs.

Treatment

A. *Mild to Moderate Eruption*

1. Apply cold or tepid compresses or use tub baths if rash is diffuse.
2. Apply calamine lotion for soothing effect *or*
3. Apply topical fluorinated corticosteroids in gel base.
   a. If applied before blistering, a gel steroid may stop or ease reaction.
   b. May also be helpful after vesicular stage has resolved to relieve itching, drying, and scaling.

B. *Severe Eruption*

1. Blisters are opened under sterile conditions by physician.
2. Give systemic corticosteroid (prednisone) as directed—to control rash, especially in sensitive patient.
   a. Dosage is adjusted according to severity of reaction and then tapered off gradually.
   b. Buffer the drug with milk or antacid if patient has history of peptic ulcer.

Health Education

1. Advise patient as follows to avoid contact with urushiol (poison ivy, poison oak, or poison sumac).
   a. Do not pull, chop, or burn vines and brush—sap-carrying smoke may produce outbreak in a sensitive person.
   b. Wear protective clothing (long sleeves, gloves, slacks) in heavily wooded areas—to guard against exposure.
   c. Apply protective ointments before working in the vicinity of the plants.
   d. Take off contaminated clothing carefully and wash clothing immediately—urushiol on clothing can cause outbreak of poison ivy.
   e. Wash skin *immediately* with nonirritating soap and rinse well—to remove the sap.

NONINFECTIOUS INFLAMMATORY DERMATOSES

PSORIASIS

Psoriasis is a chronic skin disorder in which there is an abnormally rapid multiplication of the cells of the epidermis. It appears as an eruption of circular patches of all sizes, sharply defined against the normal skin and covered with heavy, dry, silvery scales (Fig. 12-2). In time the patches coalesce, forming extensive irregularly shaped patches.

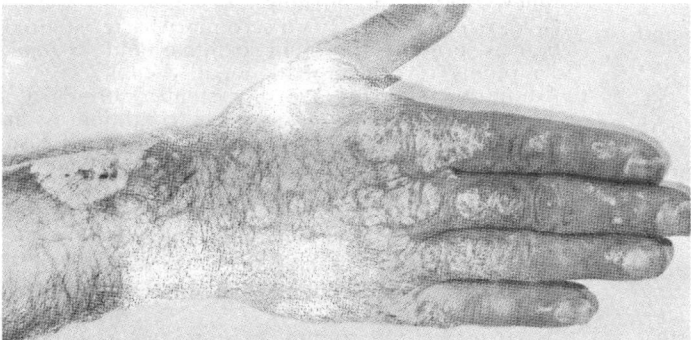

FIGURE 12–2. *Psoriasis. (Sauer G. Manual of Skin Diseases, 4th ed. Philadelphia, JB Lippincott, 1980)*

Clinical Features

1. In psoriasis, the rate of production of the epidermis of the skin is about 9 times faster than normal; this abnormal process does not allow for formation of normal protective layers of skin.
2. There appears to be a loss of normal regulatory mechanisms of cell division.
3. Onset is usually before the age of 20, but all age groups are affected.
4. Psoriasis may be coupled with polyarthritis and cause crippling disability.
5. *Sites* (bilateral symmetry)
   a. Bony prominences (knees, elbows, sacrum), scalp, external ears, genitalia, perianal area, nails and dorsa of hands
   b. Psoriasis of the ears—scaling and dryness
   c. Psoriasis of palms and soles—scaly and pustular pruritic lesions
   d. Psoriasis of nails—thickening, discoloration, crumbling beneath free edges; pitting of nails
   e. Psoriasis between skin folds—smooth, shiny red lesions, easily fissured.
6. The disease may range from a benign cosmetic source of annoyance to a physically disabling and disfiguring affliction with significant morbidity. It may be life-ruining: physically, emotionally, and economically.

Treatment and Nursing Management

OBJECTIVE: to inhibit the rapid proliferation of the epidermis in order to reduce scaling and itching.

1. Instruct patient to take daily tub bath—to help soak off scales.
   a. Gently remove excess scales with a soft brush while bathing.
   b. Apply prescribed ointment after removal of scales.
2. *Topical Therapy* (includes corticosteroids, coal tar, anthralin, salicylic acid, etc.).
   a. Coal tar preparations (ointments/baths)—retard and inhibit the rapid growth of psoriatic tissue
      (1) Coal tar is applied for a period of time; may then be removed; this treatment is followed by carefully graded doses of ultraviolet radiation.
      (2) Begin ultraviolet radiation with low doses (10 seconds) and build up dosage time gradually. Advise patient to wear goggles to protect the eyes.
      (3) Ultraviolet produces mild redness and slight desquamation.
   b. Anthralin preparations (a distillate of crude coal tar)
      (1) Useful for especially thick and resistant psoriatic plaques.
      (2) Instruct patient to apply anthralin medication as directed with a tongue blade or gloved fingers; do not apply to normal skin.
      (3) Wash hands thoroughly after application—medication can produce a chemical conjunctivitis.
      (4) Anthralin stains badly and should be covered in some way (gauze dressings, stockinette, old pajamas).
   c. Topical steroids
      (1) Apply wet dressings to irritated areas of psoriasis.
      (2) Apply corticosteroid preparations—triamcinolone (Kenalog) to skin.
      (3) Hold dressings in place with occlusive film (traps heat and moisture, softens scaly plaques and enhances transepidermal penetration).
         (a) Occlusive dressings over the entire body may be held in place with a large plastic bag with holes cut out for the head and arms; another bag may be used for the legs; extremities (arms) may be wrapped in plastic film.
         Caution the patient not to smoke while wrapped in these dressings.
         (b) In patients being treated at home, a plastic vinyl jogging suit may be used; hands can be wrapped in gloves, the feet in plastic bags, and the head in a shower cap.
3. *Intralesional Therapy* (triamcinolone acetonide)—may be injected directly into psoriatic plaques
4. *Systemic Therapy*
   a. Methotrexate—inhibits DNA synthesis and hence has a marked suppressive effect on the reproduction of rapidly proliferating cells.
   b. Is hepatotoxic and requires pretreatment and follow-up liver biopsies, liver function tests, and blood counts. Birth control measures are necessary.
   c. Patient should avoid alcohol intake while on methotrexate—increases possibility of liver damage.
   d. Hydroxyurea may be used in patients with liver toxicity.
5. *Photochemotherapy (PUVA Therapy)*
   a. Oral psoralen tablets (methoxsalen or 8–MOP, a photosensitizing chemical) followed by exposure to long-wave ultraviolet light (UVA)—in the presence of ultraviolet light, methoxsalen binds to DNA and leads to temporary inhibition of DNA synthesis (inhibits abnormally rapid multiplication of cells).
   b. Considered investigational; long-term concerns include skin cancer, cataracts, aging effect, and systemic effects on other organs.
   c. Methoxsalen capsules taken with milk or food 2 hours before scheduled UVA exposure in a UVA irradiation chamber; exposure is determined by patient's skin type.
   d. An average of 25 treatments given 2–3 times per week is required for clearing; maintenance treatments may be necessary.
   e. *Patient Education*
      (1) Since PUVA treatment produces photosensitization, patient is sensitive to sunlight the entire day of treatment; he must wear protective clothing and use a sunscreen on the face and exposed areas of the body.
      (2) Wraparound gray or green-tinted glasses must be worn throughout treatment period—possibility that some psoralen persists in lens of eye for a longer period of time.
      (3) Initial and follow-up skin biopsies (to determine skin changes), blood tests and urinalysis, eye examinations are required at specified times.
      (4) Birth control measures should be used—effects of methoxsalen on sperm, ovum, or a fetus are unknown.

Health Education

1. The patient must be taught to live with psoriasis; it

is a chronic disease often requiring continuous therapy.
2. Advise the patient that treatment is time-consuming and expensive.
3. If possible, the patient should try to schedule exposure to sunlight on a regular basis. Avoid sunburn, since it can cause a generalized flare.

EXFOLIATIVE DERMATITIS (GENERALIZED ERYTHRODERMA)

Exfoliative dermatitis is a serious condition characterized by progressive inflammation in which erythema and scaling often occur in a more or less generalized distribution. It may be associated with chills, fever, prostration, severe toxicity, and an itchy scaling of the skin.

Clinical Features

A. *Systemic Effects*

Exfoliative dermatitis has a marked effect on the entire body.
1. There is a profound loss of stratum corneum (outermost layer of the skin)—causes capillary leakage, hypoproteinemia, and negative nitrogen balance.
2. Iron loss from the skin produces anemia.

B. *Appearance*

1. Starts acutely as either a patchy or generalized erythematous eruption accompanied by fever, malaise, and occasionally gastrointestinal symptoms.
2. The skin color changes from pink to dark red; then after a week the characteristic exfoliation (scaling) begins, usually in the form of thin flakes which leave the underlying skin smooth and red, new scales forming as the older ones exfoliate (cast off).
3. Hair loss and nail shedding may accompany the disorder.

C. *Multiplicity of Causes*

1. May arise as a primary condition.
2. May follow a previous skin condition (eczema, psoriasis) that had become generalized.
3. May appear as a part of the lymphoma group of diseases and may precede the appearance of lymphoma or leukemia.
4. Also appears as a severe reaction to a wide number of drugs, including penicillin, phenylbutazone, and phenytoin (Dilantin).

Treatment and Nursing Management

OBJECTIVES: to maintain fluid and electrolyte balance.
to prevent intercurrent or cutaneous infection.
1. Discontinue all possibly offending drugs.
2. Hospitalize the patient and place him on bed rest.
Maintain comfortable room temperature—patient does not have normal thermoregulatory control owing to temperature fluctuations from vasodilation and evaporative water loss.
3. Maintain fluid and electrolyte balance—considerable water and protein loss from skin surface.
4. Give systemic corticosteroids as directed—for antiinflammatory action; may be a life-saving procedure.
5. Use compresses, soothing baths, and lubrication—to treat acute extensive dermatitis and give symptomatic relief.

6. Maintain nursing surveillance for intercurrent or cutaneous infection; the erythematous, moist skin is receptive to infection and becomes colonized with pathogenic organisms which produce more inflammation.
Antibiotics are given if infection is present; selected by culture and sensitivity.
7. Watch for symptoms of heart failure (p. 298)—hyperemia and increased cutaneous blood flow can produce a cardiac failure of high-output origin.

Health Education

Advise patient to avoid all irritants, particularly drugs.

PEMPHIGUS

Pemphigus is a serious disease of the skin characterized by the appearance of blisters (bullae) of various sizes on apparently normal skin and mucous membranes (mouth, vagina). See Fig. 12-3.

Clinical Features

1. Appearance
   a. The bullae enlarge and rupture, forming painful raw and denuded areas that eventually become crusted.
   b. The eroded skin heals slowly; eventually, huge areas of the body are involved.
   c. In the mouth, the blisters are usually multiple, of varying size and irregular shape, painful, and persistent.
   d. Bacterial superinfection is common.
2. Available evidence indicates that pemphigus is an autoimmune disease

Treatment and Nursing Management

OBJECTIVES: to bring the disease under control as rapidly as possible.
to prevent loss of serum and development of secondary infection.
to promote re-epithelialization of skin.
1. Administer corticosteroids (prednisone) in large doses, as prescribed—to control the disease.

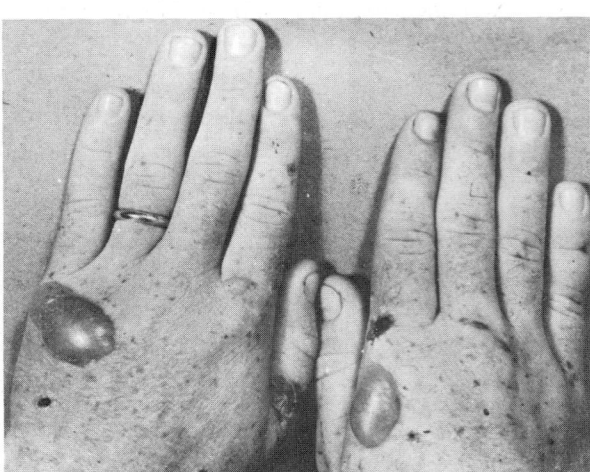

FIGURE 12–3. *Pemphigus; bullous dermatitis of hand (vesicles). (Courtesy Armed Forces Institute of Pathology.)*

a. High dosage level is maintained until remission is apparent.

b. Dosage is reduced to minimum daily maintenance dose as soon as possible.

c. Give medication with or immediately after a meal; may be accompanied by an antacid as prophylaxis against gastric complications.

2. Give immunosuppressive agents (methotrexate; cyclophosphamide, gold) as directed—may be given to help control the disease and reduce the maintenance dose of corticosteroids (steroid-sparing effect).

3. Take fluid measurements of body weight, blood pressure; test urine for glucose. Record fluid balance (input and output).

4. Assess patient for evidence of local and systemic infection—bullae are susceptible to infection, and septicemia may follow. Combinations of steroids and immunosuppressives predispose to severe infection.

5. Evaluate for fluid and electrolyte imbalance—extensive denudation of the skin leads to fluid and electrolyte imbalance.

a. Give soft, high-protein, high-calorie diet—patients with painful oral involvement have difficulty maintaining nutrition.

b. Administer saline infusions as directed—significant loss of tissue fluids and therefore of sodium chloride occur through the skin.

c. Encourage patient to maintain adequate fluid intake.

6. Give blood or component therapy (packed red cells, plasma, etc.) as necessary—large amount of protein and blood lost through denuded skin; nursing management is similar to that of patient with an extensive burn. (See p. 599.)

7. Administer cool wet dressings and/or baths—patients with large areas of blistering have a characteristic odor that is lessened when secondary infection is under control.

a. Potassium permanganate baths help keep areas from becoming infected and to some extent precipitate some of the protein that oozes through open skin.

(1) Dissolve potassium permanganate crystals thoroughly in small container; then pour into bathtub.

(2) Undissolved crystals may be irritating if patient sits on them.

b. Following the bath, dry the patient and cover him with talcum powder as directed—enables patient to move more freely in bed. Fairly large amounts are necessary to keep patient from sticking to sheets.

8. Give meticulous oral hygiene—lesions and painful erosions in the mouth are common.

9. Observe for psychiatric problems caused by high-dose steroids.

ULCERS AND TUMORS OF THE SKIN

ULCERS OF THE SKIN

Ulceration is a superficial loss of surface tissue due to death of cells.

Causes

Ulcers of the skin usually arise from (1) infection or (2) an interference with the blood supply.

1. Infection as cause of skin ulcers.

a. Usually develop from an infection with anaerobic streptococci or from combination of infections (hemolytic streptococci and staphylococci).

b. Tend to progress peripherally—characterized by an overhanging edge.

2. Deficient circulation as cause of skin ulcers—see page 346.

3. Pressure sores (page 64).

TUMORS OF THE SKIN

Cysts

Epidermal cysts are common, slow-growing, firm, elevated tumors consisting of a mass of epidermal cells; frequently found on the back.

Pilar cyst (sebaceous cysts) are cysts which arise from the isthmus (middle) part of the hair follicle. They are common on the face and scalp.

Benign Tumors

A. *Seborrheic keratoses*—tumors are benign wartlike lesions of varying size and color ranging from light tan to black; most common skin tumors in middle-aged and elderly persons.

B. *Verrucae (warts)*—common, benign skin tumors caused by viruses.

1. Many times warts do not need treatment, since they tend to disappear spontaneously.

2. Treatment (remedies are legion)

a. Freezing with liquid nitrogen—liquid nitrogen has a somewhat destructive action, although it tends to spare the epidermis.

b. Area may be treated locally with salicylic acid plasters, electrodesiccation, application of cantharidin, topical fluorouracil, topical vitamin A acid, etc.

C. *Angiomas (birthmarks)*—benign vascular tumors involving the skin and subcutaneous tissues.

1. May occur as flat, violet-red patches (port-wine angiomas) or as raised, bright-red nodular lesions (strawberry angiomas). Strawberry angiomas may involute spontaneously while port-wine angiomas usually persist indefinitely.

2. Most patients use masking cosmetics (Covermark) to camouflage the defect.

D. *Pigmented nevi (moles)*—common skin tumors of various sizes and shapes ranging from yellowish to brown to black.

1. May be flat macular lesions or elevated papules or nodules that occasionally contain hair.

2. Majority of pigmented nevi are harmless; however, in rare cases malignant changes supervene and a melanoma develops at the site of the nevus.

3. Treatment
   a. Nevi at sites subject to repeated irritation from clothing, etc., should be removed—for comfort.
   b. Nevi that show change in size or color, or become symptomatic (itch) should be removed—to determine if malignancy has occurred. This is especially true for nevi with *irregular* borders or variations of blue, red, and/or white color.
   c. Excised nevi should be examined histologically.

E. *Keloids*—benign overgrowths of fibrous tissue at site of scar or trauma in predisposed individuals.

1. More prevalent among black race.
2. Usually asymptomatic—may cause disfigurement and cosmetic concern.
3. Treatment—irradiation or intralesional injection with corticosteroids.

CANCER OF THE SKIN

Clinical Features

1. Skin cancer is the most common malignancy; the number of cases is increasing yearly.
2. There is a 95% cure rate due to early diagnosis, the slow progression of most skin cancers, and the effective methods of treatment available.

Causes

1. Exposure to sun over a period of time. *Sun damage is cumulative.*
2. Persons who do not produce sufficient pigment to protect underlying tissue are susceptible to sun damage—fair, blue-eyed, red-haired persons of Celtic ancestry or those with ruddy or light complexions; those who sunburn and do not tan.
3. Exposure to irradiation (history of x-ray treatment of benign skin lesions).
4. Exposure to certain chemical agents (arsenic, nitrates, tar and pitch, oils and paraffins).
5. Burn scars, areas of chronic osteomyelitis, fistulae of chronic nature.
6. Immunosuppressive therapy.
7. Genetic susceptibility.

Nursing Assessment

Look for:
1. Chronic sunburn
2. Actinic damage—pigment change, splotches, wrinkling, leathery complexion
3. Precancerous lesions (keratosis; leukoplakia)
4. Change in a skin lesion

NURSING ALERT: Any skin lesion that changes in size or color, bleeds, ulcerates, or becomes infected may be skin cancer.

Diagnostic Evaluation

1. Biopsy
2. Histologic evaluation

Types of Skin Cancer

A. *Basal Cell Carcinoma*

1. Most common skin cancer; higher incidence in re-gions where population is subjected to intense and extensive exposure to sun.
2. Lesions are small nodules with a rolled, pearly, translucent border with telangiectasia (dilatation of end blood vessels), crusting, and occasionally ulceration (Fig. 12-4).
3. These tumors may be pigmented, multiple, superficial, or cystic.
   a. Characterized by invasion and erosion of continuous tissues—rarely metastasizes.
   b. Lesions appear most frequently on face, between hairline and upper lip.

B. *Squamous Cell (Epidermoid) Carcinoma*

1. A malignancy that arises on sun-exposed areas of skin and mucous membrane and is considered a truly invasive carcinoma.
2. Appears as solitary rough, thickened, scaly tumor with an inflamed base and an indistinct margin.
3. May be preceded by leukoplakia (premalignant lesion of mucous membrane), actinic keratoses, scarred or ulcerated lesions.
4. Seen most commonly on lower lip, tongue, head, neck, and dorsa of hands.
5. Requires more aggressive approach (wider margin of normal skin included in excision)—greater chance of metastases from squamous cell carcinoma and significantly lower cure rate.

Treatment and Nursing Management

OBJECTIVE: to eradicate the lesion.

1. Method of treatment depends on tumor location; cell type (location and depth); history of previous treatment; and whether or not it is invasive and if metastatic nodes are present.

   Usual modes of treatment are (1) curettage and electrodesiccation and (2) surgical excision.
2. *Curettage followed by electrodesiccation*—usually done on small tumors (less than 1-2 cm.)
   a. Curettage—excision of skin tumor by scraping with a curette; electrodesiccation (alternating high frequency current which results in death of cell) is used to achieve hemostasis and to destroy any

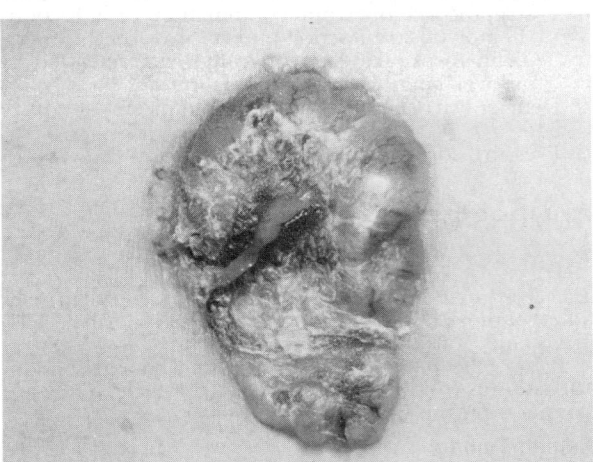

FIGURE 12–4. *Basal cell carcinoma. (Courtesy of Mervyn L. Elgart, M.D.)*

viable malignant cells in margins or in base of wound.

b. This form of treatment takes advantage of fact that the tumor in each instance is softer than surrounding skin and can be outlined by curette, which "feels" the extent of the tumor.

c. Tumor is removed and the base cauterized; process repeated a number of times.

3. *Surgical excision*

a. Wide surgical excision—adequacy of excision verified by microscopic study of sections of the specimen.

b. Histologic study of excised tissue allows determination of whether or not margins are free of tumor.

c. Skin grafting may be necessary

4. *X-ray or irradiation therapy*—usually done for cancer of eyelid, tip of nose, in or near vital structures (facial nerve) where tissue sparing is difficult with other forms of treatment; used for extensive malignancies when goal is palliation or when other medical conditions contraindicate other forms of therapy.

a. Explain to patient that he may experience skin reddening and swelling about the time of the third treatment; may progress to blistering.

b. Apply bland skin ointment as prescribed—to relieve discomfort.

c. Stress importance of follow-up care—there is always the possibility of recurrence or a new primary lesion.

d. Caution the patient against exposure to the sun.

5. *Cryosurgery*—deep freezing to selectively destroy tumor tissue.

a. Liquid nitrogen is applied by cryospray or cryoprobe technique.

b. Site thaws naturally and then becomes gelatinous and heals spontaneously.

6. *Chemosurgery*—combined use of topically applied chemicals and layer by layer surgical excisions to remove tissue; immediate microscopic examination of each specimen is made.

Useful for recurrent skin cancers, since surgical excision is guided by microscopic study.

7. *Topical chemotherapy*—application of topical antitumor agent (fluorouracil) to destroy cancer cells. Only used in very superficial lesions, particularly premalignant actinic keratoses.

Health Education

a. Several days following fluorouracil application, there will be redness, oozing, crusting, and soreness until treatment is completed.

b. Wash hands after each application—fluorouracil can cause conjunctivitis.

c. Do not cover treated area or expose to sunlight.

d. Continue using fluorouracil as long as physician directs. In several weeks the redness should fade and the skin become smooth.

Health Education (Skin Cancer)

Most skin cancer can be prevented by avoidance of and protection from excessive direct exposure to sun. Instruct the patient as follows:

1. Avoid unnecessary exposure to the sun, especially during times when ultraviolet radiation is most intense (10 A.M. to 2 P.M.).

2. Apply a protective sunscreen with recommended sun protection factor if an activity requires a long period of exposure.

a. Sun protection factor (SPF) ranges from 2 (minimal protection) to 15 (ultra or superprotection).

b. Specific SPF number is selected according to skin sensitivity ("burns easily" to "never burns").

c. Sunscreen selected should not come off easily; those which contain 5% para-aminobenzoic acid in 55–70% alcohol do not come off easily.

3. Wear protective clothing (long sleeves, broad-brimmed hat, etc.)—however, damaging radiation to skin still occurs from ground radiation.

4. Have moles removed that are accessible to repeated friction and irritation.

5. Watch for indications of potential malignancy in moles (e.g., change in color, increase in size, ulceration, bleeding, or serous exudation).

6. Have follow-up evaluation throughout lifetime. Watch for development of new lesions.

7. Caution your children and grandchildren, especially those with fair skin, to avoid excessive exposure to the sun so as to prevent later skin cancers.

MALIGNANT MELANOMA

Malignant melanoma is a malignant tumor of the skin melanocytes (pigment cells) that occurs in several forms (see following). It has a higher mortality rate than other forms of skin cancer. The prognosis is related to the depth of dermal invasion of malignant melanocytes in the primary lesion.

Classification

A. *Superficial Spreading Melanoma* (most common)

1. Occurs anywhere on body; usually affects middle-aged persons.

2. Tends to be circular with portion of its outline irregular (either protruding or indenting).

3. Has combination of colors—hues of tan, brown, and black admixed with gray, bluish-black, or white.

4. May be dull pink-rose color in a small area within the lesion.

B. *Nodular Melanoma*

1. Spherical blueberry-like nodule with relatively smooth surface and relatively uniform blue-black, blue-gray or reddish-blue color; occurs commonly on back, head and neck.

2. May be polypoidal, with smooth surface of rose-gray or black color; may be present as elevated, irregular plaque.

3. Least favorable prognosis.

C. *Lentigo-maligna Melanoma*

1. Slowly evolving pigment lesions; occur on exposed skin surfaces of elderly persons.

2. First appears as tan, flat macule—malignant degeneration is manifested by changes in size, color, and topography.

D. *Acral-lentiginous Melanoma*

1. Occurs on palms, soles, subungual areas.

2. Assess for variations in color; may be deeply invasive.

Clinical Features (Fig. 12-5)

1. Signs that suggest malignant change.
    a. *Variegated color*
        (1) Colors that may indicate malignancy in a brown or black lesion are shades of red, white, and blue; shades of blue are considered ominous.
        (2) White areas within a pigmented lesion are suspicious.
        (3) Some malignant melanomas are not variegated but are uniformly colored (bluish-black, bluish-gray, bluish-red).
    b. *Irregular border*—look for angular indentation or notch present in the border of a malignant melanoma.
    c. *Irregular surface*
        (1) Look for uneven elevations of the surface; irregular topography may be palpable or visible; change in the surface (smooth to scaly).
        (2) Some nodular melanomas have a smooth surface.
    d. *Change in size, color; symptoms such as itching, oozing, or bleeding.*
2. Common sites of melanoma—skin of back, legs, between toes, and on feet, face, scalp, fingernails, back of hands.
3. In the black race, melanomas are most apt to occur on less pigmented sites—palms, soles, subungual areas and mucous membranes.
4. Persons at risk: those with light complexion, light-colored eyes, light-colored hair; those who sunburn readily.

Diagnostic Evaluation

1. Appearance of lesion (see above).
2. Biopsy (for histopathologic diagnosis) and micro-staging (determination of level of tumor invasion and thickness).

Treatment

The therapeutic approach depends on the type, level, thickness, and location of the lesion, and the stage of disease.

OBJECTIVE: to improve survival.

1. Wide surgical excision of tumor, sometimes followed by plastic repair or skin grafting. The role of regional node dissection is in dispute.
2. Regional isolation perfusion; specific area is isolated by mechanically controlling its arterial inflow and venous outflow. This allows high concentration of cytotoxic drugs to be delivered to cancer-bearing sites with less systemic toxicity (see page 848).
3. Immunotherapy (BCG)—to stimulate patient's immune system to produce antibodies (investigational).
4. Chemotherapy (dacarbazine [DTIC]—generally used for recurrence of metastasis or as palliation.

Health Education

1. Inform the public that the key factor in development of malignant melanoma is exposure to sunlight. See page 589 for preventive aspects.
2. Educate people to observe their moles and to report moles that *change* colors, enlarge, become raised or thicker, itch, or bleed.
3. Treatment should be initiated immediately.

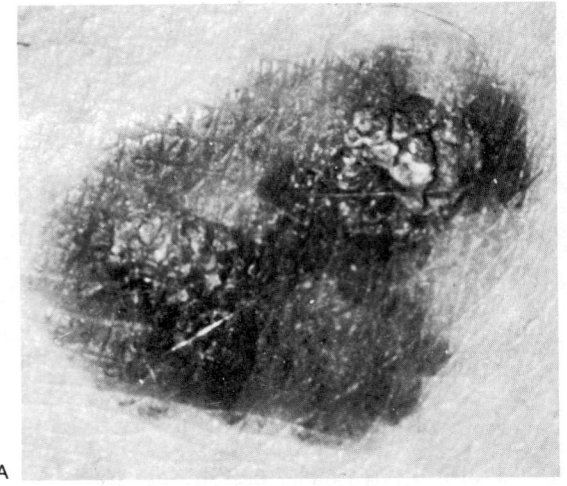

A

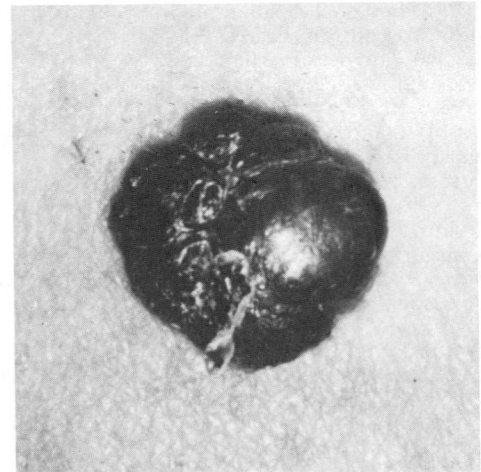

B

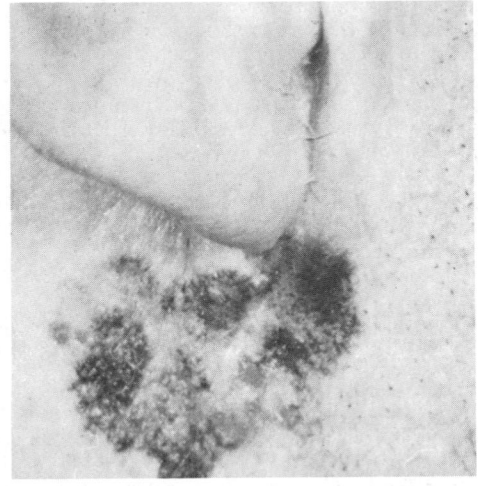

C

FIGURE 12–5. A. *Superficial spreading melanoma; note irregular border.* B. *Nodular melanoma.* C. *Lentigo-maligna melanoma; note irregular pigment pattern. (Courtesy of Arthur J. Sober, M.D.)*

SYSTEMIC DISEASES WITH DERMATOLOGIC MANIFESTATIONS

LUPUS ERYTHEMATOSUS

Systemic lupus erythematosus (SLE) is an autoimmune collagen vascular disease involving multiple organ systems and producing widespread damage to connective tissues, blood vessels, serosal surfaces, and mucous membranes.

Discoid lupus erythematosus is a chronic eruption of the skin which, although often disfiguring, does not pose a threat to life.

Clinical Features

1. Etiology is not understood—evidence indicates that immune, genetic, and viral factors play a role. There is also a drug-induced form of SLE (procainamide; hydralazine; chlorpromazine, etc.).
2. Most frequently found in young women with signs and symptoms referable to the joints and skin.
3. Is characterized by remissions and exacerbations.

Clinical Manifestations

(Multiple organ involvement is explained by the deposit of antigen antibody complexes throughout the body—kidneys, skin, brain, heart, and joints.)
1. Vary greatly, since they can affect every organ system; mimic many other diseases.
2. Arthritis and arthralgia, fever, skin rash, alopecia, and involvement of serosal surfaces (pleurisy and pericarditis).
3. *Skin Manifestations*
   a. Malar rash, alopecia, dermal vasculitis, Raynaud's phenomenon, purpura.
   b. Facial rash with butterfly distribution over bridge of nose and malar bone prominences.
   c. Similar lesions over neck, chest, upper and lower extremities—may become pruritic and scaly.
   d. Brittleness or loss of scalp hair.
   e. Photosensitivity with rashes developing after sun exposure.
4. Generalized lymphadenopathy, anemia, leukopenia, thrombocytopenia.
5. Long-continued low grade fever.
6. Cardiac involvement (pericarditis, myocarditis, pleural effusion).
7. Renal involvement (proteinuria, hematuria, renal insufficiency and failure).
8. Central nervous system involvement (convulsive disorders, abnormalities in mental function and cranial nerves, depression, emotional lability, neurosis, psychosis).

Diagnostic Evaluation

(Many laboratory abnormalities may be found)
1. Clinically documented multisystem disease
2. Documentation of presence of antinuclear antibodies—positive fluorescent antinuclear antibody test (FANA)
3. Tests for complement and antibodies to DNA
4. Blood and renal function tests

Treatment and Nursing Management

(No known cure at this time)
OBJECTIVE: to control the disease by suppressing inflammation and relieving symptoms.

1. Treat intercurrent illness—exacerbations of SLE may follow infection, drug administration, emotional stress, surgical procedures.
2. Other treatment modalities—selection depends on nature and severity of disease.
   a. Corticosteroids (prednisone)—used for suppressing inflammation and thus relieving severe symptoms;
      (1) Observe patient carefully—may be difficult to distinguish between drug effects and those of SLE.
      (2) See page 656 for discussion of side effects of steroids.
   b. Salicylates or nonsteroidal anti-inflammatory agents—for arthritis and arthralgia.
      (1) Patient should take salicylates on a regular schedule so that adequate blood levels are maintained.
      (2) See treatment of arthritis, page 786.
   c. Antimalarials (hydroxychloroquine [Plaquenil])—to control the skin and joint manifestations.
      Patient should be examined by ophthalmologist at least twice yearly—retinal degeneration resulting in visual impairment may be a problem.
   d. Immunosuppressive agents (cyclophosphamide; azathioprine)—to suppress manifestations of SLE.
      (1) Still considered experimental in treatment of SLE.
      (2) Usually reserved for patients who are unresponsive to steroids or who develop unacceptable side effects from steroids.
3. Treat the patient as each problem arises (depending on the organ system involved and its physiological consequences)—nephritis, renal failure, congestive heart failure, central nervous system lupus, etc.
4. Give continuing emotional support. Psychiatric treatment may be indicated for debilitating depression, etc.
5. Be aware that some patients do not react favorably to immunization procedures.
6. Watch for development of complications—uremia, central nervous system disorders, malignancies, infection (namely) "opportunist" bacterial pathogens), acute abdominal catastrophes.

Health Education

1. Obtain physical and emotional rest; fatigue and depression are fairly common.
2. Eat a well-balanced diet.
3. Avoid whatever you know may aggravate the condition.
   a. Avoid sun exposure—sunlight may worsen dermal lesions and precipitate a flare of the disease. Use a sunscreen when exposure to sun is necessary.
   b. Avoid sensitizing drugs (penicillin; sulfa) and avoid using hair sprays and hair coloring agents.
   c. Avoid taking contraceptive pills—anovulatory drugs may precipitate lupus syndrome in susceptible person.
4. Use positive coping mechanisms or seek counseling to deal with stress—emotional turmoil may precipitate a flare-up.
5. The makeup *Covermark®* may conceal facial lesions and scarring (of discoid LE).
6. Report to the physician immediately any worsening

of symptoms—fever, cough, skin rash, increasing joint pain, etc. SLE also compromises the ability to fight infection.
7. See also Health Education, Rheumatoid arthritis, page 788.
8. Support groups:
   Arthritis Foundation,
   3400 Peachtree Road, N.E.,
   Atlanta, Ga. 30326.
   Lupus Foundation of America, Inc.,
   11673 Holly Springs Drive
   St. Louis, Mo. 63141.

POLYARTERITIS (PERIARTERITIS NODOSA)

Polyarteritis (periarteritis nodosa) is a disease of unknown cause characterized by inflammation and necrosis of medium-sized and small vessels, especially arteries, which results in altered function of the organ system in which the arterial supply has been impaired.

Clinical Features

1. The walls of the vessels are involved; spotty inflammation causes changes in circulation and tissue damage.
2. Clinical manifestations vary according to organ(s) involved and amount of necrosis produced by obstructing vascular lesion.
   a. Prolonged fever; myalgia and arthralgia; renal involvement; gastrointestinal manifestations (abdominal pain, nausea, vomiting, diarrhea); cardiovascular manifestations (coronary insufficiency, myocardial infarction); palpable nodules along the arterial trunks—may occur.
   b. Ocular manifestations (retinal exudates and hemorrhages) are fairly common.
   c. Skin lesions are usually in the form of painful nodules that may ulcerate.
      (1) Subcutaneous nodules vary in size and may be located in any part of the body.
      (2) Overlying skin may be reddened or ulcerated.
      (3) Purpuric papules may be present.
3. Periarteritis is apt to run a course of a few years' duration; recovery is unpredictable—death may ensue from renal decompensation, congestive failure, etc.

Treatment

(Treatment is similar to that of systemic lupus erythematosus)

OBJECTIVE: to give the patient symptomatic and supportive care.
1. A search is made for any offending drug that may precipitate the disease.
2. Corticosteroids (prednisone)—given to control symptoms and to prevent progression of disease.
   a. Large doses may be given initially; patient is observed for evidence of disease regression.
   b. See page 656 for management of patient having steroid therapy.
3. Immunosuppressive drugs (cyclophosphamide; azathioprine) may be given in combination with corticosteroids.
4. Watch for and treat intercurrent infections.
5. Advise patient to avoid drugs that may exacerbate symptoms (sulfonamides, iodides, penicillin).

PROGRESSIVE SYSTEMIC SCLEROSIS (SCLERODERMA)

Progressive systemic sclerosis is a disease of unknown etiology characterized by hardening and/or thickening of the skin (scleroderma) and fibrotic, degenerative, and inflammatory changes with vascular insufficiency (Raynaud's phenomenon), resulting in joint changes and dysfunction of certain internal organs (gastrointestinal tract, heart, lungs, kidneys). There are several forms of localized scleroderma.

Clinical Manifestations

1. The disease usually starts insidiously on hands and face:
   a. Painless pitting edema of fingers, hands, feet, legs, face; edema gradually replaced by thickening and tightening of skin, which acquires a tense, wrinkle-free, bound-down appearance.
   b. Wrinkles and lines are obliterated.
   c. Skin is dry—sweat secretion over involved area is suppressed.
   d. Face appears masklike, immobile, and expressionless; mouth becomes rigid.
   e. Condition spreads slowly; extremities become stiff and immobile; the fingers semiflexed, immobile, and useless; the hands clawlike.
2. Detectable clinical changes may occur in the internal organs.
   a. Heart becomes fibrotic—causing congestive heart failure, arrhythmias and conduction disturbances, angina.
   b. Esophagus is hardened, with disruption of normal esophageal peristalsis—gastroesophageal reflux, with heartburn and dysphagia.
   c. Pulmonary fibrosis/pulmonary hypertension.
   d. Intestines become hardened—digestive disturbances.
   e. Progressive renal failure may occur.
   f. Variety of other disturbances develop, including Raynaud's phenomenon and arthritis.

Treatment and Nursing Management

OBJECTIVES: to give symptomatic relief.
　　　　　　　 to preserve muscle strength and mobility.
Treatment modalities may include:
1. Steroid therapy for anti-inflammatory effect.
2. Salicylate therapy—to relieve joint stiffness and maintain joint mobility.
3. Physical therapy—helpful in preventing joint contractures and in maintaining joint mobility.
4. Surgical procedures (as in surgery for arthritis)—for hand deformities.
5. Vasoactive drugs and anti-inflammatory agents—may be helpful for Raynaud's phenomenon.
6. Operative control of gastroesophageal reflux (reconstruction of esophagogastric junction) may be considered for reflux esophagitis.
7. The skin is kept lubricated with topical creams or petrolatum lubricants—to prevent fissuring and ulceration.
8. Cardiac, pulmonary, and renal involvement are treated symptomatically.

Health Education

1. Involve patient and family as co-therapists.
2. Avoid trauma to hands and exposure to cold.

3. Avoid excessive sun exposure—patients burn easily and are prone to heat stroke.
4. Preserve function of hands—warm hand baths, paraffin dips, exercise, reconstructive surgical procedures.
5. For gastrointestinal disturbances:

a. Chew food well and eat slowly to allow esophagus time to empty by gravity, since there is disruption of normal esophageal peristalsis.
b. Elevate head of bed on blocks.
c. Take antacids between meals and before bedtime.

DERMATOLOGIC SURGERY

PLASTIC RECONSTRUCTIVE SURGERY

Reconstructive surgery (plastic surgery) is performed to repair extravisceral defects and malformations, both congenital and acquired, and to restore function as well as prevent further loss of function.

Cosmetic surgery involves reconstruction of the cutaneous tissues around the neck and face; done to restore function, correct defects, and remove the marks of time. (See Table 12-1.)

SKIN GRAFTING

Definitions

1. *Skin graft* (free graft)—a section of skin tissue which is separated from its blood supply and transferred as a free section of tissue to the recipient site.
2. *Skin flap* (pedicle graft)—a section of skin tissue used to cover or fill a defect; it is lifted from its bed but still has partial attachment by a pedicle from which it receives its blood supply until healing takes place in its new location.

   Flaps are used to cover defects in which there is poor vascularity; for reconstruction of eyelids, ears, nose, and cheeks.
3. *Autograft*—transfers or transplants from same person.
4. *Allograft*—transfer or transplants between two individuals of same species.

5. *Isografts*—grafts between identical twins
6. *Xenografts*—grafts between two animals of different species, e.g., rabbit to mouse, baboon to man.
7. *Split-thickness graft* (Thiersch's graft)—graft of approximately one-half the thickness of skin which is removed by a knife or dermatome; deeper layers of dermis are left behind. (Used for coverage and closure of skin defects.)
8. *Full-thickness skin graft*—contains the epidermis and all of the dermis.
   a. Used frequently for reconstruction of facial defects, for it neither contracts nor develops unsightly pigmentation.
   b. Grafts may be further subdivided into thin and thick:
      (1) Thin (0.010–0.015 inch thick)—used to resurface contaminated granulations or recipient sites in which blood supply is jeopardized.
      (2) Thick (0.015–0.020 inch thick)—used where durability is the important factor.
9. *Pinch graft*—a small piece of skin graft obtained by elevating the skin with a needle or forceps and cutting it off with scissors or knife.
10. *Take*—refers to the appearance of the graft between the 3rd and 5th day after transfer, signifying that the vascular connections have developed between the recipient bed and the transplant.

Causes of Graft Failure

1. Fluid beneath the graft

TABLE 12-1. COMMON COSMETIC PLASTIC OPERATIONS

Operation	Purpose	Surgery	Postoperative expectations
Rhinoplasty (Nose)	To improve the shape of the nose in relation to the rest of the face	1–1½ hours. Excess bone or cartilage is removed; nose is re-shaped	Nasal splint; soft intranasal packing; foam rubber dressings
Chin Augmentation	To improve the profile, as is necessary with a receding chin	Incision approach is within the mouth. Inorganic (Silastic) implant is positioned	Healing complete in a week
Rhytidoplasty (Face lift)	To remove excess skin due to elastosis and to tighten remaining skin	Incision is anterior to ear and extended down to nasolabial fold to the mental foramen near the chin and to the midline in the upper neck; the stretched subcutaneous tissues and fascia of the face are folded to provide a basic firmness.	Improvement lasts up to 10 years
Glabellar rhytidoplasty	To remove 2 vertical furrows between eyebrows	Dermabrasion and excision; skin graft may be required	
Otoplasty (Ear)	To correct deformed, flattened, or protruding ears	1–1½ hours. Silicone or plastic implant may be used	Ear bandaged for a week; protection during sleep required for 3 weeks
Blepharoplasty (Eyelid)	To remove wrinkles and bulges caused by herniation of fat, aging, or inheritance	1–1½ hours. Two incisions; one on upper lid and one on lower lid	Neosporin ointment applied around eyes and lids. Individual eye dressings are applied. Swelling and discoloration subside in about 10 days

2. Hematoma—avoid by early inspection and removal of clots
3. Infection

Nursing Management (for Grafting Procedures)

A. *Preoperative Care*
OBJECTIVE: to bring the patient to his optimal physical and emotional level for this procedure.
1. Assess for nutritional status.
   a. Give vitamins and increase protein intake as directed—to facilitate healing.
   b. Note hemoglobin level and clotting time—these levels can affect healing process.
2. Prepare donor and recipient sites for surgical excision.
3. Inform the patient about what to expect postoperatively.
   a. Appearance of the wound—redness, distortion, swelling, and unattractive suture lines are characteristics that will change with time.
   b. Pressure dressings, immobilization devices, etc.
4. Prepare the patient psychologically.
   a. Attempt to establish the reasons why the patient seeks surgery.
      (1) Patient's attitudes toward his disfigurement, his motivations for seeking surgery, and his assessment of how his disfigurement has influenced his life and his psychosocial relationships are taken into consideration before surgery is considered.
      (2) Desirable to have unimpaired body image and realistic acceptance of surgical limitations.
      (3) Poor candidate for cosmetic surgery is one who has delusions concerning his deformity, unhealthy psychological responses, and unrealistic expectations of results.
   b. Explain the limitations of the contemplated procedure, the possibility of complications, and the unpredictability of the result (responsibility of the surgeon).

B. *Postoperative Care*
1. Inspect graft under dressing daily, using a good light—to be sure that edema, blistering, or hematoma has not formed and is not jeopardizing successful graft.
   a. Surgeon carefully teases dressing away from wound—changing dressing may cause avulsion (tearing away) of recent graft around margin of wound.
   b. Surgeon will nick graft to evacuate blood clots.
      (1) Fluid may be rolled out of graft with cotton-tipped applicator or by aspirating with needle and syringe.
      (2) Seromas or hematomas may impede healing.
2. Apply mittens to patient if he is inadvertently scratching the graft during sleep—to protect graft and donor site from subconscious scratching.
3. Apply wet dressings to infected graft as directed.
4. Use prophylactic antibiotic therapy for patient with infected graft.
   Utilize sensitivity testing to identify organism.
5. Elevate grafted extremity for 7–10 days.
   a. Immobilize part—movement of body areas beneath graft may predispose to loss of graft.
   b. Apply cast or immobilizing bandages to restrict all regional movements of the extremity.
   c. Begin ambulation activities very gradually.
6. Inform the patient of the changing hues of the graft—to help him accept his situation.
   a. Free graft is at first pale, then pink and red—it then fades and appears similar to neighboring skin.
   b. Full-thickness grafts may remain deeply red for months.
   c. Anticipate skin scaling in full-thickness grafts.
   d. Teach the patient that the graft is vulnerable to sun; avoid overexposure to the sun.
7. Instruct the patient to apply a thin coating of mineral oil or lanolin on wound after 2nd or 3rd week—to remove superficial crusts, moisten the graft, and stimulate circulation to the wound area.

C. *Care of the Donor Site*
1. The donor site is usually covered with a layer of nonadherent gauze (Xeroform) and held in place with a gauze dressing (Kerlix) without cotton to absorb blood and serum from the wound.
   a. The outer dressings may be removed in 24 hours down to the first layer (Xeroform)
   b. Area may be left exposed after 1st or 2nd postoperative day.
   c. A hair dryer may be employed until dry coagulum is formed.
   d. Xeroform gauze is not disturbed until it separates spontaneously (about 10 days).
2. Prevent area from coming in contact with clothing or bedding—to provide adequate circulation of air to the donor site.
3. Apply wet dressing as directed (silver nitrate solution or acetic acid) if donor site becomes infected.
4. Lubricate donor site with lanolin or cocoa butter after healing—to keep it soft and pliable.
5. Donor sites heal by re-epithelialization; healing should be complete in 2 weeks' time.

Nursing Management (of Patient Undergoing Maxillofacial Surgery)(See p. 374)

A. *Preoperative Care*—See page 82 for nursing support.
B. *Postoperative Care*
1. Maintain an adequate airway.
2. Observe dressings for impairment of circulation and for edema—pressure dressings are frequently used.
   a. Control oral hemorrhage by inserting gauze pad in the mouth and exerting pressure at bleeding point.
   b. Wipe blood from wound—blood under suture line may cause hematoma and infection and spoil the cosmetic result.
3. Watch color of skin flaps—may appear blue and congested due to partial obstruction of the venous circulation.
   a. Surgeon may make small incisions in the flap to relieve the blood congestion and avoid gangrene of the flap.
   b. Moisten flap dressing with warm sterile solution as directed.
4. Relieve pain—expect more pain on operations involving jaw and facial bones.
   a. Apply heat or cold according to direction.
   b. Give analgesics as prescribed.
5. Keep the patient well hydrated and nourished.
   a. Offer cracked ice and water as soon as nausea subsides.
   b. Give soft diet as tolerated.

(1) Provide an adequate quantity and caloric quality to patient on prolonged liquid diet (following jaw surgery, etc.).

(2) Give frequent feedings in order to obtain caloric equivalent of a full diet.

6. Offer appropriate psychological support—numerous operations may be required.

DERMABRASION

Dermabrasion is surgical planing of the superficial portion of the skin.

Clinical Indications

1. Done on selected patients with facial disfigurements from scars due to acne, trauma, nevi, freckles, chickenpox, or smallpox, benign tumors, tattoos.
2. Removal of precancerous lesions (keratosis).
3. To smooth and improve color of transplanted or grafted skin.

Treatment and Nursing Management

Preoperative

1. Wash the part to be treated with pHisoHex for several days before surgery.
2. Administer adequate preoperative sedation as prescribed.

Operative

The epidermis and some superficial dermis are removed, but enough of the dermis is preserved to allow re-epithelialization of the dermabraded areas.

1. The patient is anesthetized.
2. The skin may be sprayed with a topical anesthetic to stabilize and stiffen the skin.
3. The superficial layer of skin is removed by an abrasive machine (Dermabrader) or by sandpapering.
4. Copious saline irrigations are carried out during and after the planing procedure.
5. At the conclusion of surgical planing
   a. The surgeon may apply a layer of Xeroform or Telfa, followed by fluffed gauze and a pressure dressing.
   b. Another method is to apply a thick paste of thrombin (mixture of thrombin powder and saline) to the abraded areas. This controls bleeding and oozing, which dries to form a protective eschar.

Postoperative

1. Mild oozing may be expected for 24 hours. Crusts then form; are shed in 7–10 days. Skin remains pink for 6–12 weeks
2. The patient may be discharged from the hospital the day after surgery. (Some prefer to remain because of their appearance).
3. Techniques vary: some surgeons prefer to leave bulky dressings in place for several days, others prefer the exposure method.
4. When dressings are removed, the patient experiences a "recent sunburn" experience.
5. Caution the patient to avoid exposure to direct sunlight for 3 to 4 months—planed area may become darker or lighter than surrounding skin as a result of exposure.

Health Education

1. In the later stages of healing, Neosporin, bacitracin, or hypoallergenic cold cream may be applied; these aid in the removal of coagulum (crusts). Coagulum should never be forcibly removed because this would injure new epithelium and delay healing.
2. Advise patient to avoid exposure to direct or reflected sunlight.
   Suggest applying an effective sun-screening cream to the affected area; reapply frequently and use for about three months postoperatively.
3. Should hyperpigmentation occur, it regresses in 3 to 18 months. Hypopigmentation occurs occasionally but also regresses. Meanwhile, effective cover-up cosmetics are recommended.

CHEMICAL PLANING

Chemical planing (chemosurgery, chemabrasion, chemical face-lifting) is the application of a cauterant (caustic material) to the skin for the purpose of superficially destroying epidermis and upper levels of dermis.

1. Phenol combined with other agents and trichloracetic acid are the agents commonly used.
2. *Salabrasion* is a combination of chemical and mechanical action occasionally used for tatoo removal.
3. Chemical planing is painful; meticulous care is required over a period of time. It is not corrective surgery but may supplement it. It should be done by a skilled plastic surgeon.

2 BURNS

CARE OF THE BURN PATIENT

Burns are wounds caused by excessive exposure to four categories of agents: thermal, electrical, chemical, and radioactive.

Incidence

1. Over 2 million burn injuries occur annually in the U.S.
2. Approximately 75,000 burn victims require hospitalization each year in this country.
3. Nearly 10,000 persons die from fire and burns each year in the U.S.
4. Most burn accidents occur in the home and are caused primarily by carelessness or ignorance.
5. Authorities estimate that at least 75% of all burns could be prevented.
6. The nurse is in a strategic position for teaching burn prevention and for promoting legislation for safety practices.
7. One-third of burn victims are children.

Surgical Prediction

1. Best survival expectancy occurs in young-adult groups, aged 15–46 years.
2. A burn affecting over 20% of the body endangers life.
3. Prognosis depends on age of patient, depth and extent of burn, past medical history, and current health problems, concomitant injuries, as well as the expertise of the burn management team.
   Sudden drop in WBC and platelets is seen in terminal sepsis—largest killer in burns.
4. Prognosis is largely affected by whether or not a respiratory injury is incurred—respiratory injury (usually reported as pneumonia) is second most frequent cause of death (after infection) in burn victims.

Assessment of Patient's Burn Injury

See Assessment of Burn Injury page 598.

NOTE: This can be done most accurately when wounds are cleaned—otherwise estimate is often erroneous due to presence of soot and debris.

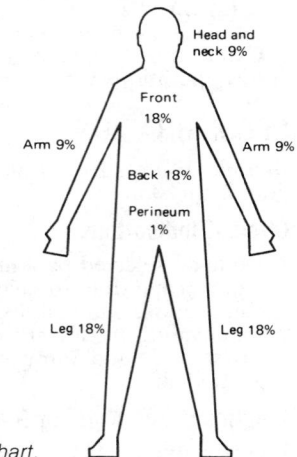

FIGURE 12–6. *"Rule of Nine" chart.*

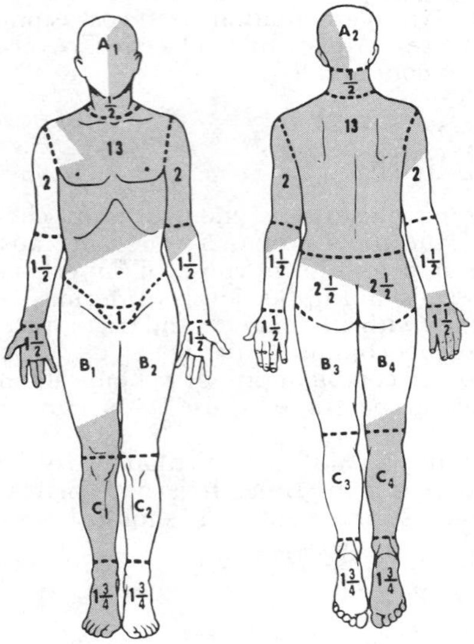

	ANTERIOR		POSTERIOR	
HEAD	A₁	1.5	A₂	1.0
NECK		.5		.5
RT. ARM				1.0
RT. FOREARM		.5		.25
RT. HAND		1.5		1.5
LT. ARM		2.0		2.0
LT. FOREARM		.5		.5
LT. HAND				
TRUNK		10.0		13.0
BUTTOCK	(L)	.5	(R)	1.0
PERINEUM				
RT. THIGH	B₁	1.0	B₄	.75
RT. LEG	C₁	3.5	C₄	3.5
RT. FOOT		1.75		1.75
LT. THIGH	B₂		B₃	
LT. LEG	C₂		C₃	
LT. FOOT				

PERCENT OF AREAS AFFECTED BY GROWTH:

		0	1	5	10	15	ADULT
A = ½	HEAD	9½	8½	6½	5½	4½	3½
B = ½	ONE THIGH	2¾	3¼	4	4¼	4½	4¾
C = ½	ONE LEG	2½	2½	2¾	3	3¼	3½

Mixed ☐ % PARTIAL THICKNESS _____

■ % FULL THICKNESS _____

TOTAL _____ 50%

FIGURE 12–7. *Burn Evaluation Chart—estimation of per cent of body burns. (Crozer-Chester Medical Center).*

A. *Assess extent of body surface burned.*

1. Anatomical location—greater morbidity and mortality for burns affecting hands, feet, face, and perineum requiring specialized care.
2. Determination is based on the use of tables for this purpose, such as the "Rule of Nine" Chart (Fig. 12-6) and the Burn Evaluation Chart (Fig. 12-7). For children, use pediatric evaluation chart, p. 1346. These tables or charts serve as a guide for fluid therapy.
3. Repeat assessment on 2nd and 3rd day inasmuch as demarcation may not be visible until then.

B. *Assess depth of burn: Classification (see Fig. 12-8).*

NOTE: Major burns—Second-degree burns of over 30% of body
Third-degree burns of over 10% of body

Rapid Assessment: Use hair test—if hair can be pulled out easily, there is likelihood of full-thickness injury.
Critical Body Areas: hospitalization usually required
1. Eyes, face, neck
2. Hands
3. Feet
4. Perineum and genitalia

C. *Assess unique contributing factors.*

1. Causative agent: boiling water, chemical, etc.
2. Duration of exposure
3. Thickness of skin
4. Patient's age
5. Preexisting medical complicating factors: heart disease, diabetes, ulcers, alcoholism, epilepsy, psychiatric disorders
6. Prior psychologic status of the patient
7. Circumstances where burn was sustained, e.g., in a closed area—this may cause respiratory damage
8. Chemical, electrical, and radiation burns can cause more damage than appears obvious
9. Concomitant injuries, e.g., patient may have fallen or been thrown in an explosion

D. *Assess the possibility of postburn pulmonary damage.*

1. Look for burns around the mouth or neck.
2. Look for singeing of nasal hairs.
3. Inspect mouth for burns of the oral or pharyngeal mucous membranes.
4. Observe for voice changes or coughing up soot.
5. Determine whether victim sustained burn in a restricted or confined area (forced to inhale hot smoke, etc.).
6. Respiratory status may appear satisfactory initially, but intrinsic and extrinsic edema may cause airway obstruction at any time during first 48 hours postburn. When in doubt, intubate patient to insure an adequate airway until edema subsides several days postburn.

E. *Obtain a brief history.*

1. Previous state of health
2. Allergies
3. Tetanus immunization status
4. Height and weight of patient (pre- and postburn)
5. Vital signs

6. Take a photograph of burned area (with patient's permission) for recording extent of burn
7. Prior treatment: First aid? fluids? drugs? tetanus prophylaxis?
8. Medications currently being taken

Systemic Changes in Major Burn

A. *Fluid Shifts*

1. In addition to changes in the local burned area, there are alterations and disruptions in the vascular and other systems of the body.
2. The water-vapor barrier for the body is the outermost layer of epidermis. When it is rendered nonfunctioning, severe systemic reactions from fluid losses can occur.
3. Blanching of the skin following burn injury is caused by contraction of skin capillaries; redness occurs when arterioles and capillaries dilate.
4. Fluid volume deficit is directly proportional to extent and depth of burn injury.
5. Capillary permeability increases, permitting fluid and protein to move from vascular to interstitial spaces (edema results). Protein-rich fluid is lost in blebs of the burned tissues as well as by weeping of second-degree wounds and surface of full-thickness wounds.
   With reduced vascular volume, the patient will go into shock if untreated.
6. Vascular fluid loss occurs in first 24–48 hours.
7. Capillary permeability returns to normal in about 48 hours—but protein lost in interstitial spaces remains there for 5 days to 2 weeks before returning to the vascular system.
   a. When fluid mobilizes (moves from interstitial spaces back to vascular compartment) patients with good cardiac and renal function will diurese.
   b. Observe carefully for fluid overload and pulmonary edema; patient requires decreased fluid intake, frequent observation of vital signs, CVP, and urine output.
8. Red cell mass is also diminished, due to thrombosis and sludging; as fluid escapes from capillary walls, blood concentrates and the flow is sluggish—hematocrit rises.
9. Capillary stasis may cause ischemia and even necrosis.
10. The body attempts to compensate for losses of plasma volume.
    a. Constriction of vessels
    b. Withdrawal of fluid from undamaged extracellular space
    c. Patient is thirsty. (Oral fluids not given until bowel sounds are heard.)

Fluid Loss

Adult	Amount per Hour per Square Meter of Body Surface
Normal unburned individual	15–20 ml.
Average adult with a flame burn of 40% of his body	100 ml.

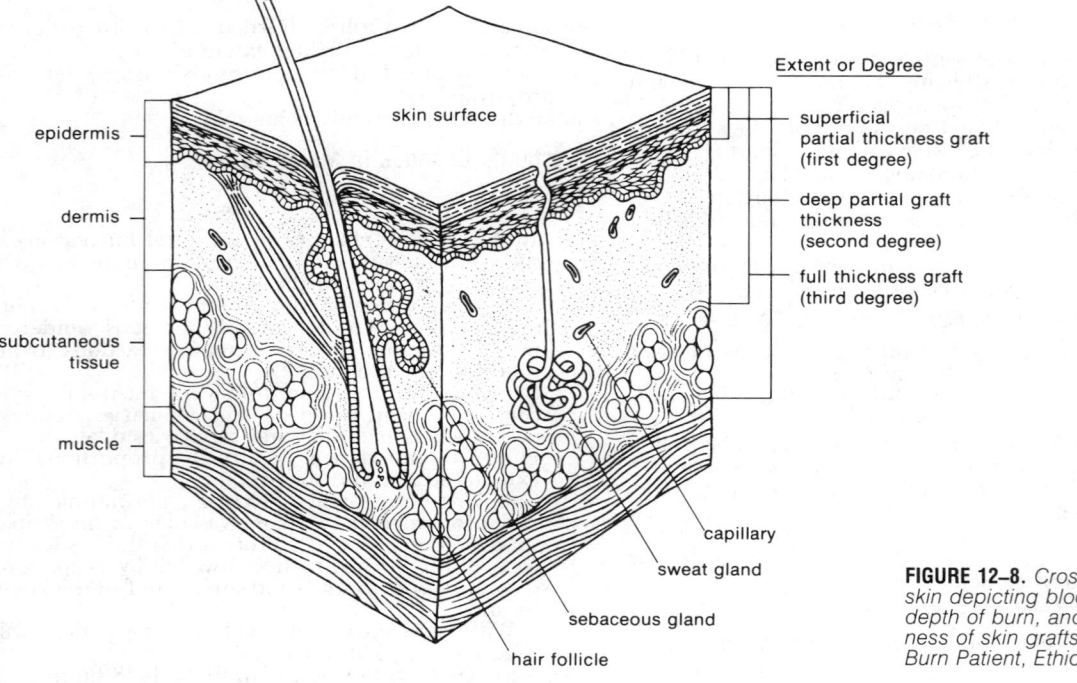

FIGURE 12–8. *Cross section of skin depicting blood supply, depth of burn, and relative thickness of skin grafts. (From The Burn Patient, Ethicon.)*

ASSESSMENT OF BURN INJURY

Extent or Degree	Assessment of Extent	Reparative Process
Superficial Partial Thickness (First degree)	Pink to red; slight edema, which subsides quickly. Pain may last up to 48 hours; relieved by cooling	In about 5 days, epidermis peels, heals spontaneously. Itching and pink skin persist for about a week. No scarring.
Deep Partial Thickness (Second degree)	a. *Superficial:* Pink or red; blisters form (vesicles); weeping, edematous, elastic Superficial layers of skin are destroyed; wound moist and painful.	Heals spontaneously if it does not become infected within 10 days to 2 weeks.
	b. *Deep dermal:* Mottled white and red; edematous reddened areas blanch on pressure. May be yellowish but soft and elastic—may or may not be sensitive to touch; sensitive to cold air Hair does not pull out easily	Takes several weeks to heal. Scarring may occur.
Full Thickness (Third degree)	Destruction of epithelial cells—epidermis and dermis destroyed. Reddened areas do not blanch with pressure	Eschar must be removed. Granulation tissue forms to nearest epithelium from wound margins or support graft. For areas larger than 7–8 cm., grafting is required.
	Not painful; inelastic; coloration varies from waxy white to brown; leathery devitalized tissue is called *eschar.*	Expect scarring and loss of skin function
Fourth degree	Destruction of epithelium, fat, muscles, and bone.	Area requires debridement, formation of granulation tissue, and grafting.

B. *Hemodynamics*

1. Lessened circulating blood volume results in decreased cardiac output initially and increased pulse rate.
2. There is a decreased stroke volume as well as a marked rise in peripheral resistance (due to constriction of arterioles and increased hemo-viscosity.
3. This results in inadequate tissue perfusion, which may in turn cause acidosis, renal failure and irreversible burn shock.
4. A burn injury often upsets the acid-base balance; therefore, careful monitoring of arterial blood gases, serum electrolytes, and urine volume is needed for proper fluid therapy; this will allow one to replace fluid loss and prevent dilatation and paralytic ileus.

C. *Calorie and Nitrogen Losses*

1. Immediately following an extensive burn, there is a breakdown of cells (catabolism) resulting in a marked outpouring of potassium and nitrogen.
2. When adequately treated, an extensively burned patient will probably increase his weight the first 3–4 days, due to collection of fluid in the interstitial spaces; thereafter weight loss will be progressive, at the rate of about 1 pound a day in a young adult, for about a month depending upon nutritional support. *Adequate nutritional therapy* can reduce this loss to no more than 5–10% of pre-burn body weight before weight stabilizes.
3. In spite of all nutritional support, it is almost impossible to counteract a negative nitrogen balance; the sooner a burn wound is closed, the more rapidly a positive nitrogen balance is reached.
4. The postburn adult may require 6000–8000 calories a day; high calories, high protein may be given orally and in some instances by intravenous hyperalimentation or by nasogastric feeding along with normal meals and snacks.

Objectives of Medical and Nursing Management

OBJECTIVES: to prevent burns by initiating and promoting safety practices.

to employ lifesaving measures in the care of the severely burned person.

to provide early specialized and individualized treatment of the burn victim in order to promote tissue repair and to prevent disability and disfigurement.

to recognize that the burn patient is a person with feelings, thoughts, and concerns.

to include the burn patient and his family in the plan of treatment and rehabilitation.

A. *To remove burning agent, alleviate pain, and initiate plan of treatment*

1. Observe for any breathing impairment; prepare for insertion of endotracheal tube if necessary.
2. Remove burned clothing and assess extent of burned area. (This may have to be done in hydrotherapy.) See also detailed assessment, page 598.
3. Make patient as comfortable as possible (morphine intravenously for pain, etc.) while history and physical examination progress; immediately covering burn sites aids in eliminating pain.
4. See also Emergency Management, page 886.

B. *To prevent and treat for burn shock*

1. Prepare for fluid replacement immediately—electrolytes, colloid (plasma or serum protein albumin), and fluid.
   a. Weigh patient on admission if possible (baseline weight) and daily thereafter at the same time each day.
   b. Insert an indwelling catheter; measure hourly output and describe. Maintain urine output in range of 30–50 ml./hr. Check pH, specific gravity, sugar, and acetone.
   c. Assist with cannulization of vein for continuous intravenous therapy.
      (1) A central vein is indicated for large volume replacement. Most physicians recommend 2–4 ml./kg./% (crystalloid) burn surface for first 24 hours.
      (2) Colloids are used for large burns, for children, and after the first 24 hours. After first 24 hours—urine output is best indication of fluid needs, and intravenous infusions are titrated to maintain 0.5ml./kg./hr. (adult) or 1 ml./kg./hr. (children).
   d. Record intake and output conscientiously (Fig. 12-9).
   e. Observe for signs of dehydration or overhydration by use of hematocrit, CVP and urinary output; notify physician if signs occur.
   f. Note any untoward signs indicative of a transfusion reaction (p. 239); if apparent, terminate transfusion and notify physician.
   g. Elevate all burned extremities; check radial and pedal pulses hourly.
      Be alert to decreased circulation in fingers and toes due to circumferential burns (can cause edema to form a tourniquet). Report to physician immediately and prepare for *escharotomy* (an incision through dead eschar to relax constriction).
2. Administer oxygen; it may have to be administered under pressure because of reduced blood volume, in order to saturate plasma.
3. Observe depth and rate of respirations. Circumferential chest burns may constrict chest movement and decrease tidal volume, causing a drop in PO_2 and an increase in PCO_2. Escharotomy may be required to allow adequate chest expansion.

C. *To prepare burn area for assessment and treatment*

1. Cleanse wound gently with bland soap and water or saline; hydrotherapy tub is easiest. See hydrotherapy information, page 600.
2. In some clinics, burn area is prepared by *tangential excision;* a dermatome or knife blade is used to shave burned tissue or devitalized tissue away until normal tissue is reached, since a healthy wound base is more receptive to skin grafts. Area is then usually grafted immediately.

D. *To assess the physical and psychological reaction of the patient to his condition*

1. Take and record vital signs hourly (Fig. 12-10), including CVP; blood pressure may be taken using a "Doppler" to hear pressure if it is inaudible otherwise due to edema. Arterial pressure monitors are available.
2. Draw blood for culture to assess for bacteremia. Note whether blood specimens are taken by the laboratory

Date:	INTAKE						OUTPUT			
	Colloid	Electrolyte	Glucose	Other IV	Oral	Total	Urine	Gastric	Other	Total
7:00 AM										
8:00										
9:00										
10:00										
11:00										
12:00 N										
1:00 PM										
2:00										
8 Hour Summary										

FIGURE 12–9. *Sample 8-hour summary of specific intake and output.*

technician as requested. Also note other methods for bacteriological assessment of the burn wound (Table 12-2)

3. Obtain 24-hour urine specimen if requested. Measure urine output hourly while patient is critical.
4. Talk to patient to determine his concerns; include him in his therapy plan.
5. Observe patient for his reaction to his condition; set goals with him and be consistent in following the therapeutic plan.
6. For the patient who has pain, consider teaching pain intervention techniques such as breathing exercises, relaxation, biofeedback, hypnotherapy response, and other relaxation procedures.

E. *To provide physical comfort and emotional support of the patient.*

1. Administer sedatives and analgesics as prescribed for pain (intravenously, while patient is critical). Some clinics use methadone, which is long-acting and has few side effects.

2. Elevate the burned extremities for comfort and to lessen edema.
3. Place patient in physiological position, keeping in mind the need to prevent contractures. (Position of comfort is the flexed position.)
4. Try to determine what kind of person he is; promote communication links. Allow patient to participate in his own care as much as possible.
5. Provide diversional therapy; allay fear and anxiety.

F. *To meet nutritional needs and control gastrointestinal disturbances.*

When burns exceed 30% of the total body surface, resting and metabolic expenditure may be increased to between 40% and 100% of normal body nutritional needs.

1. Nutritional management must be aggressive to combat acute nutritional deficiency and weight loss; a positive nitrogen balance should be maintained throughout the entire postburn course.
2. Every effort must be exerted to allay pain, fear,

HYDROTHERAPY *Hydrotherapy* ("Tubbing" or "Tanking") is the bathing of the burn patient in a tub or tank of water to facilitate cleansing of the burn area (removal of dead tissue and topical medications).
Advantages:
1. Topical medications, adherent dressings, and eschar are more easily removed.
2. Provides an opportunity for the patient to practice range of motion exercises.
3. Total assessment of the burn area is facilitated; total body cleansing can be achieved.
Disadvantages:
1. Loss of body heat; sodium loss also occurs in tub water.
2. Uncomfortable to the patient and at times painful.
3. Maintenance of IV lines, ventilation care may be difficult during tubbing.
Nursing Plan and Intervention:
1. Describe the procedure to the patient who is experiencing hydrotherapy for the first time.
2. Select the time for future tubbings in collaboration with the patient; administer a pain-control medication, if prescribed, before the treatment so that maximum benefit is realized. Use nursing activities to assist patient with his pain experience. (See D-6, Objectives.)
3. If he has an indwelling catheter, drain and plug it, or maintain a closed system to avoid contamination.
4. Isolation and aseptic technique are adhered to rigidly in preparing the patient for hydrotherapy, during hydrotherapy, and then in redressing wounds and patient following therapy.
5. During hydrotherapy, following cleansing of the wounds, shave and debride as required.
6. Limit therapy to no more than 30 minutes.
7. Never leave the patient unattended in the tub.
8. Respect the patient's feelings and expressions of stress, pain, cold, fatigue.
9. Following treatment, the patient may be weighed before being carefully dressed and returned to his unit.
10. Document significant data, including status of the wound.

	VITAL SIGNS					INTAKE				OUTPUT		
	B.P.	V.P.	T.	P.	R.	TYPE I.V. FLUID & MEDICATION ADDED	READING ON BOTTLE	AMOUNT ABSORBED	ORAL	URINE	SP. GR.	GASTRIC & STOOL
7:00 AM												
8:00												
9:00												
10:00												
11:00												
12:00 N												
1:00 PM												
2:00												
8 Hr.Total												
3:00 PM												
4:00												
5:00												
6:00												
7:00												
8:00												
9:00												
10:00												
8 Hr. Total												
11:00 PM												
12:00 M												
1:00 AM												
2:00												
3:00												
4:00												
5:00												
6:00												
8 Hr. Total												
24 Hr. Totals												

I.V. MEDICATION AND FLUID THERAPY

FIGURE 12–10. *Twenty-four-hour flowsheet for monitoring burn patients during initial treatment. (From The Burn Patient, Ethicon.)*

and anxiety, since they stimulate release of catecholamine stores.

3. Maintaining a warm environmental temperature will help reduce metabolic stress.
4. Initially, patient may be fed by small Silastic nasogastric tube with pump attachment; an antacid such as Maalox, may be given every 2 hours.
5. When caloric requirements cannot be met by enteral feedings, it may be necessary to initiate intravenous fat emulsions intravenously.
6. When bowel sounds return, administer oral fluids *slowly*, so that patient's tolerance can be observed. If no problem, advance diet to regular, as tolerated.
7. If serum potassium levels drop, give fruit juices that contain potassium.
8. After several days, supplement the diet with high protein drinks and vitamins.
9. Offer more solid food after 2–3 days postburn as tolerance for food improves.
   a. Build up daily caloric intake to match daily caloric expenditure.
   b. Provide: 3 gm. protein/kg. body weight; 20% of needed calories in form of fats; remainder in carbohydrates.

10. Imagination and ingenuity may be required to stimulate a sluggish appetite.
11. Encourage patient to feed himself; adapt utensils to his individual needs.
12. Keep record of patient's weight and calorie intake—let him participate in meeting caloric goal by selecting foods he desires.
13. Be alert for evidence of gastric erosion or Curling's ulcer—the incidence is in proportion to the extent of the burn. Hematest gastric aspirate or stools for early signs.

G. *To prevent complications*

1. *Infection*

Burn Wound Sepsis—the proliferation and/or active invasion of the burn wound by microorganisms numbering 100,000 or more per gram of tissue (10^5 per gram of tissue)
   Clinical Manifestation: Elevated temperature, abdominal distention, ileus, disorientation.
   Most common organism—*Pseudomonas*

TABLE 12-2. METHODS FOR BACTERIOLOGICAL ASSESSMENT OF THE BURN WOUND*

Method	Advantage	Disadvantage
Gauze capillarity surface culture	Noninvasive, simple, reproducible, quantitative	Samples surface flora only
Wound biopsy culture (with histologic examination)	Quantitative, samples cross-section of wound	Most expensive, invasive, unsuitable for frequent multiple cultures
Swab culture	Simplest, noninvasive, painless	False negatives, no quantitation, speculation may be incomplete
Rapid slide technique for quantitation of bacteria in specimens	Quantitates specimen bacterial density within a few hours	None if rapid quantitation desirable

* Modified from Edlich RE, Rodeheaver GT, Spengler M, et al.: Practical bacteriologic monitoring of the burn victim. Clin Plast Surg 4:561–569, 1977.

a. Assist in the cleansing and debridement of tissues.
b. Practice rigid asepsis when wound is exposed.
c. Wear mask, cap, and gown in addition to sterile gloves during change of dressings.
d. Obtain wound culture when requested; often, burn-wound biopsy cultures are required every other day until eschar has begun to separate.
e. Keep environment as clean as possible; laminar airflow is used in many burn units.
   (1) Employ good housekeeping practices; do not permit wet mops and dry dust cloths, but utilize wet and dry vacuuming and damp-dusting with a disinfectant.
   (2) Maintain isolation precautions.
   (3) Restrict visitors.
f. Change dressings, once or twice daily, in hydrotherapy; the tank is filled with warm tap water, 37.8°C. (100°F.), to which may be added prescribed amounts of sodium chloride, potassium chloride, calcium hypochlorite, and perhaps a mild soap powder for cleansing purposes.
g. Note any signs of redness at wound edges, purulent drainage, or bad odors; daily wound cultures are done if recommended.
h. Administer antimicrobials as prescribed (usually after first day, since blocked capillaries at burn site will prevent medications from reaching the area); subeschar antibiotic therapy may be initiated for concentration at site of colonization.
i. Recognize changes in vital signs that may indicate infection.
j. Apply topical bacteriostatic substance as directed (silver nitrate, Sulfamylon, Silvadene, etc.).
k. Promote the best personal hygiene for the patient.
   (1) Cleanse unburned areas of the body with antibacterial soap or detergent-germicide; maintain clean nails—hydrotherapy is most effective for this.

(2) Shave hairs from burned areas and adjacent areas; shampoo hair daily.
(3) Provide meticulous mouth care.
(4) Keep all orifices especially clean; give special attention to indwelling catheter and meatus.
l. Administer tetanus toxoid; if patient not immunized previously, also administer tetanus immune globulin and repeat toxoid in 3 weeks.
2. *Impaired circulation to extremities and decreased chest expansion.*
   Assist with escharotomy (incision through tight eschar), particularly if tight eschar is constricting, as in a circumferential burn.
3. *Contractures and deformities*
   a. Maintain proper body alignment, using supports and splints as necessary.
   b. Initiate passive, then active exercises where possible, with physician's permission, on first postburn day.
   c. Turn frequently, encourage deep breathing, and initiate early ambulation as soon as feasible.
   d. Perform range of motion activities in hydrotherapy and at bedside t.i.d. (Fig. 12-11).
   e. Use a footboard to prevent footdrop.
   f. Splint hands at night and even during day when not being used for feeding or other activity.
   g. Have patient feed himself with burned (second-degree) hands as early as first or second postburn day.
   h. Use overhead frame for trapeze and slings to assist with positioning and exercise.
4. *Respiratory difficulty*
   a. Assess respiratory rate, chest movement, and any respiratory stress.
   b. Determine whether patient inhaled smoke, fumes, or flame—whether he has singed nasal hair, red pharynx, hoarse voice, cough, stridor, etc.

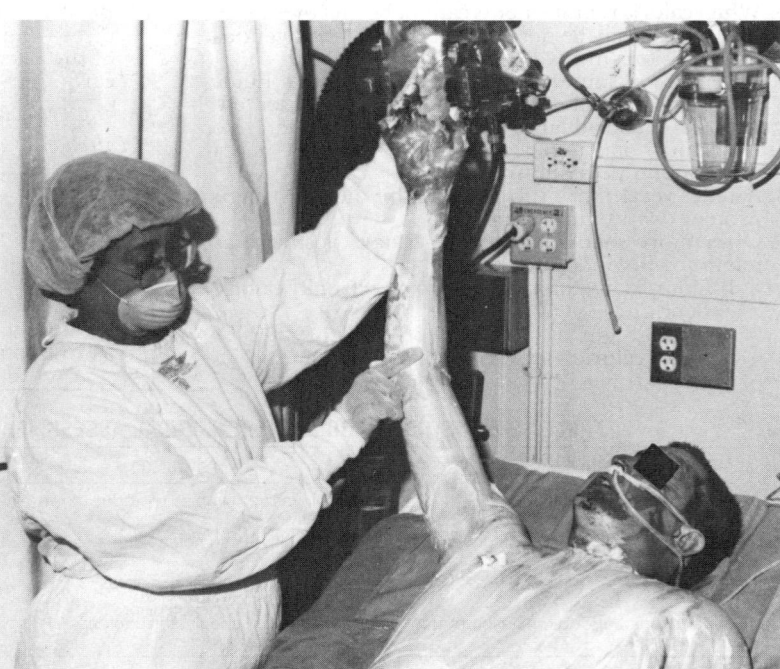

FIGURE 12–11. *The patient is put through full range-of-motion exercises at least twice daily to prevent contractures. (Courtesy of the U.S. Army Institute of Surgical Research, Fort Sam Houston, Texas.)*

c. Have endotracheal tube and oxygen equipment easily accessible.

d. Keep airway free of secretions by frequent oral and nasotracheal suctioning, preferably under sterile conditions.

e. Monitor for signs of pulmonary edema—increased tracheobronchial secretions, rales over both lung fields, blood-tinged expectorations, shortness of breath.

f. Initiate turning, coughing, and deep-breathing regime.

5. *Hazards of immobility*
   a. Prevent pressure sores—use CircOlectric bed to turn if circumferential burns are present.
      (1) Teach patient to change position slightly himself.
      (2) Turn patient and observe possible pressure points every 2 hours.
   b. Prevent pneumonia—provide excellent respiratory hygiene.
   c. Stress conditions may produce Curling's ulcer (see p. 398).

H. *To recognize and treat an inhalation burn injury*

1. Be familiar with the patient's history—note whether he was "overcome with smoke" or in a closed space when injured.

2. Early symptoms are significant and require immediate concern and treatment:
   a. Does he exhibit irrational behavior, have a cough, progressive hoarseness, dyspnea, hemoptysis?
   b. Look for burns in area of head, neck, and chest (circumoral and nasal).
   c. Is there constricting edema of the neck? of chest? May require escharotomy.
   d. Are the nasal hairs singed? (Check with a flashlight).
   e. Auscultate chest for wheezes, rales, and rhonchi—any sign of airway obstruction?
   f. Examine nasal and oral mucosa for soot stains; check sputum for carbon particles.

3. Perform laboratory tests—Serial chest x-rays (first may be normal, but edema and atelectasis may be detected later); serial blood gases (PO_2 and pH decrease, PCO_2 increases); carboxyhemoglobin levels.

NOTE: Initially patient has respiratory alkalosis ($\downarrow pCO_2$) due to hyperventilation from pain and anxiety; with respiratory failure, pCO_2 level may increase.

4. Attempt to determine other related significant factors such as whether patient took alcohol or other drugs, has other medical problems.

5. Initiate therapy:
   a. Maintain adequate airway.
      (1) Insert soft endotracheal tube for 2–3 days while edema persists.

      (2) Employ tracheostomy if patient cannot tolerate intubation, requires continuing ventilatory support, or beyond the 3-day period. (This may be delayed longer—up to 7 days if cuffed endotracheal tube is used.)
   b. Reduce thick and dry secretions to prevent atelectasis by adequate hydration: In addition
      (1) Administer humidified oxygen therapy.
      (2) Encourage the patient to cough; utilize postural drainage and chest percussion if feasible.
      (3) Administer bronchodilators such as aminophylline.
      (4) Promote liquefying of secretions by using such broncholytic agents as parenteral sodium iodide or supersaturated potassium iodide (unnecessary if patient is well hydrated). Hyperventilate intubated patient with Ambu bag hourly, and suction.
   c. Insert nasogastric tube.
      This will aid in preventing gastric dilatation, vomiting, aspiration.
   d. Prevent hypoxemia and maintain acceptable arterial PO_2 levels.
      (1) Administer supplemental oxygen by using a face tent, venti-mask, croup tent, etc.

NURSING ALERT: Nasal cannulae are usually not recommended because air swallowing is likely (would promote gastric dilatation).

Nasal oxygen administration promotes undesirable mucus and drying of bronchi.

      (2) Monitor blood gases and pH every 6 hours.
      (3) Use mechanical ventilator if justified following blood gas determinations.
   e. Prevent pulmonary edema.
      (1) Observe CVP readings.
      (2) Utilize pulmonary capillary wedge pressure readings for accurate observation of left ventricle function.
      (3) Utilize digitalis carefully.
         Monitor serum potassium and diuretics.
   f. Restore blood and fluid volume when appropriate.
   g. Attempt to prevent (or initiate treatment of) pneumonitis.
      (1) Obtain sputum and tracheal aspirate for culture.
      (2) Many authorities recommend broad-spectrum systemic antimicrobial therapy.
      (3) After specific organisms are identified, treat with specific antimicrobials.

INHALATION INJURY

50% to 60% of burn deaths are secondary to inhalation injury.

Mechanism of Occurrence

Carbon monoxide and smoke toxicity are the two major types of pulmonary injury following inhalation.

1. Carbon monoxide (CO) is a colorless, odorless, tasteless, and nonirritating gas produced from incomplete combustion of carbon-containing materials.

2. Affinity of hemoglobin for CO is 200 times greater than for oxygen.

3. Toxicity will depend on concentration of CO in inspired air and the length of time of exposure.

4. Inhalation of hot dry air (148.9° C. [300° F] or higher) appears not to have much effect on lower respiratory tract.
5. From fire in a closed space, most particles of soot are filtered through upper airway, but because they may be superheated, cause direct damage to mucosa.
6. Sulfur dioxide (SO_2) and nitrous oxide (N_2O) (toxic agents) most likely are clinging to soot; in the presence of water they form corrosive acids and alkalies that are extremely toxic.
7. Toxic fumes from burning plastic are more dangerous than smoke; noxious gases include hydrogen cyanide, hydrochloric acid, sulfuric acid, halogens, and perhaps phosgene.
8. Upper airway obstruction may occur during the first 48 hours postburn due to pharyngeal and laryngeal edema resulting from superficial burn of the upper airway. Edema of the neck may also decrease tracheal patency.
9. Restrictive pulmonary complications can occur due to the tourniquet effect of edema seen with circumferential chest burns. Lung compliance and alveolar gas exchange can also be decreased due to pulmonary edema.
10. Evaluate all patients in closed space fires for presence of symptoms of carbon monoxide poisoning: headache, visual changes, confusion, irritability, decreased judgment, nausea, ataxia, collapse.

Assessment

1. If victim was burned in closed area, there should be a high index of suspicion that smoke inhalation has occurred. (Fig. 12-12)
2. Question patient about types of things that burned in this room—type of carpet, vinyl articles, synthetics.
3. Observe for upper body burns, erythema or blistering of lips, buccal mucosa, or pharynx, singed nares hair, soot in oropharynx, dark gray or black sputum.
4. Listen for hoarseness and rales.
5. Obtain blood gases and carboxyhemoglobin levels.
6. Prepare patient for bronchoscopy to confirm presence of mucosal erythema, hemorrhage, ulceration, edema, carbonaceous particles.
7. Obtain chest x-ray for baseline data.
8. See Signs and Symptoms of Toxicity of Reduced Levels of Oxygen Due to Fire Conditions, page 605.

Treatment and Nursing Management

1. Initiate treatment as for any patient with suspected inhalation injury.
   a. Establish airway
   b. Administer 100% oxygen unless patient has known COPD (chronic obstructive pulmonary disease)
   c. Administer 100% oxygen until CO level is re-

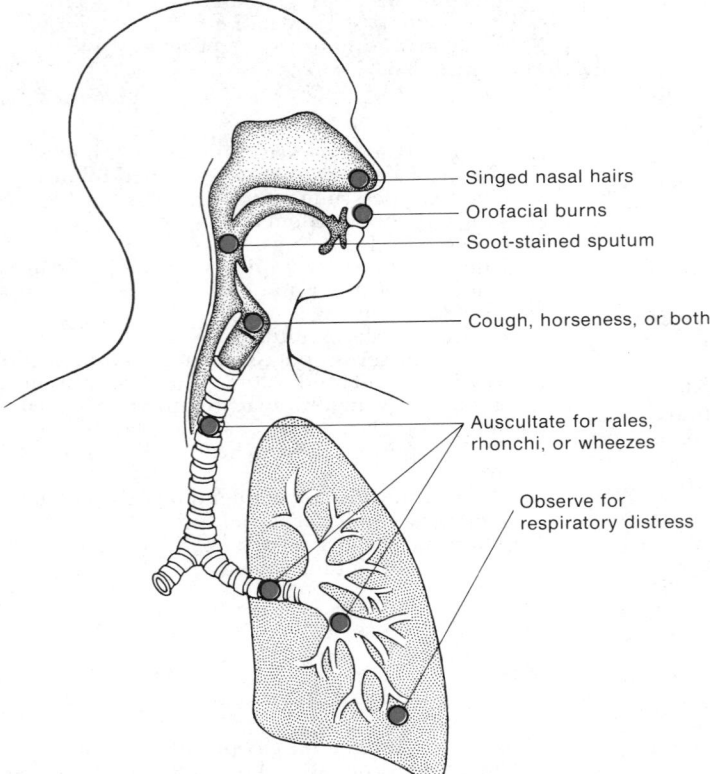

Singed nasal hairs
Orofacial burns
Soot-stained sputum

Cough, horseness, or both

Auscultate for rales, rhonchi, or wheezes

Observe for respiratory distress

FIGURE 12–12. *In the nursing history, determine whether the victim was in a closed area during the fire and whether he lost consciousness. If any of the above physical findings are noted in addition to the nursing history data, the victim should be taken to a health center for further evaluation. Baseline arterial blood gas measurements (hypoxemia) should be taken immediately upon admission.*

Signs and Symptoms of Toxicity of Reduced Levels of Oxygen Due to Fire Conditions*

Percent of Oxygen in Air	Sign or Symptom
20 (or above)	Normal
12 to 15	Muscular coordination for skilled movements is lost
10 to 14	Consciousness continues but judgment is faulty; muscular effort leads to rapid fatigue
6 to 10	Collapse occurs quickly but *rapid treatment would prevent fatal outcome*
6 or below	Death in 6 to 8 minutes

* From Underwriters Laboratories, Inc. Bulletin of Research, No. 53, July 1963, p. 49. Extracted from the January 1952 Quarterly (Vol. 45, No. 3). Copyright © National Fire Protection Association, Boston, Massachusetts. Reprinted by Permission.

ported: even with mild or no burns, CO levels may be high:

  CO levels: 0–10%—normal (high level
       noted in smokers)
       20% —mild
       60% —fatal

2. In mild inhalation injury:
   a. Provide humidification of inspired air.
   b. Encourage coughing and deep breathing.
   c. Prepare for bronchial suctioning.
3. In moderate to severe inhalation injury (also see p. 169):
   a. Initiate more frequent bronchial suctioning.
   b. Monitor urinary output and blood gases.
   c. Administer, judiciously, bronchodilators.
   d. For additional respiratory problems it may be necessary to have patient intubated and placed on mechanical ventilation.
(For additional details, see pp. 186–199.)

Prevention

1. Promote use of smoke detectors: fires often occur at night when persons are sleeping. Common detectors are
   a. Ionizing detectors using a radioactive source to ionize air in detection chambers; since smoke impedes the flow of current, the alarm is sounded.
   b. Photoelectric detectors. Smoke particles scatter the light beam and an alarm is sounded.
2. Reduce number of plastic items in a home (or building); have 2 means of escape from all rooms above first floor.
3. During a fire, move quickly and stay close to the floor where oxygen availability is greatest.
4. Place a damp cloth over nose and mouth if caught in a smoke-filled room. Wear masks even after a fire has been brought under control.
5. If exposed to burning plastic, notify your physician.

METHODS OF TREATING BURNS

OPEN AND CLOSED TREATMENTS

Open Air or Exposure Method

Exposing the burn to the drying effect of air allows the exudate to dry; a hard crust forms in 3 days and then acts as a protection to the wound. This is true of partial thickness wounds; full thickness wounds become hydrated from the edematous tissue beneath, and fluid loss peaks at 15 days postburn.

A. *Advantages and Mode of Action*

1. Effective during disaster, when large numbers of persons must be cared for.
2. Most frequently used to treat burns of face, neck, and perineum, and extensive burns of the trunk.
3. There are no painful dressing changes; therefore, less equipment is used and there is less discomfort for the patient.
4. Infection can be detected earlier.
5. Second-degree burns, beneath crust—regeneration of skin in 2–3 weeks.
6. Third-degree burns, beneath eschar—usually requires grafting.
7. Eschar loosens and must be debrided.

B. *Imperative—Keep Immediate Environment Free of Organisms*

1. Everything that comes in contact with patient must be clean.
   a. Clean, freshly laundered linens on bed. (If sterile, sterility lost rather quickly.)
   b. Masks, sterile gowns, and gloves for persons in contact with patient.
   c. Gowns and masks for visitors—instruct not to touch patient or hand him anything.
   d. "Burn pack" desirable since it contains all linens for patient, and gown and mask for attendant.
2. Room must be kept clean.
   a. Screens on windows.
   b. Dusting and mopping to be done with damp cloth or mop—not dry.
3. Humidity and temperature should be regulated—humidity 40–50%; temperature preferably 24.4° C. (76° F.). (This is warmer than usual but not exactly comfortable for the staff.)
   a. If too warm, patient may lose needed body fluids.
   b. Bed or partial cradle with cover (or a heat shield overhead) can be used to prevent chilling.

C. *Nursing Management*

1. Prevent burn area from sticking to the sheet—use nonadherent disposable sheeting or burn pads to absorb excess exudate.
2. Avoid unnecessary trauma when changing linens by wetting those parts of tissue adhering to linen with sterile saline.
3. Have patient turn frequently to prevent cardiopulmonary complications and contractures.
4. Have patient feed himself if hand burns are not chiefly third degree.
5. Walk patient if complicating fractures are not present.
6. Elevate extremities to prevent edema.

Occlusive (Pressure) Dressings

A. *Advantages*

1. Less pain in first 48 hours postburn.
2. Takes less nursing time.
3. Useful for outpatients who may not have a clean environment or who cannot be relied upon to change dressing with good technique.

B. *Disadvantages*

1. High incidence of burn wound sepsis.
2. Discomfort and pain when changed.
3. If not put in proper position—may encourage development of contractures.

C. *Nursing Management*

1. Observe for signs of infection—temperature elevation, increased pulse, increased pain, perhaps an odor.
2. Change dressings if exudate stain is noted; this may indicate the presence of moisture which may lead to bacterial growth.
3. Elevate extremity to prevent edema.
   See Table 12-3 for further details on open and closed treatments of burns.

TOPICAL ANTIMICROBIALS

Topical medications are used to cover burn areas and to reduce the number of organisms.
1. They are applied directly to the burn area as ointments, creams, or solutions, or they may be incorporated in single-layer dressings that do not stick to the wound but permit drainage. (Fig. 12-13)
2. On top of the fine mesh gauze are placed bulky dry dressings to permit drainage to enter dressing but not come through.
3. Usually these dressings are held in place by a single layer of stretch bandage or by net tube dressings (Surgifix).
4. When the patient is lying in bed, fluffy absorbent dressings or pads are placed on the bed where the burn area will make contact.
5. Desired characteristics in a topical antimicrobial:
   a. Demonstrate action against gram-negative aerobic intestinal bacteria *Pseudomonas aeruginosa* and *Staphylococcus aureus*.
   b. Ability to diffuse through the wound and penetrate the eschar.
   c. Nontoxic and noninjurious to body tissue.
   d. Inexpensive, pleasant to use, odorless, or has pleasant odor; will not stain skin or clothing.
   e. Will not cause resistant strains of pathogenic organisms to develop.
6. To date there is no "ideal" topical antimicrobial.

Silver Sulfadiazine 1% (Silvadene, Flamazine)

In a hydrophilic (readily absorbing moisture) water-soluble cream base.

A. *Advantages and Mode of Action*

1. Chlorides of the body are not readily precipitated, as with silver nitrate. Therefore no electrolyte abnormality occurs and no acidosis develops.
2. Applied as a cream with tongue blades or in impregnated gauze.
3. Little pain experienced with application of cream.
4. Viscous dressings are easily and painlessly removed.
5. Silver sulfadiazine is odorless; absorption of silver is minimal and toxicity is rare.
6. Action occurs by oligodynamic action (active in minute quantities) of silver and is dependent upon chloride and other anions in the wound exudate.
7. It utilizes the special antibacterial action of sulfonamide; it is particularly effective against infections due to gram-negative and gram-positive microorganisms and to *Candida albicans*.
8. It can be bactericidal up to 48 hrs.; however, when wounds are not clean, dressings are changed 2–3 times daily.

B. *Disadvantages*

1. Some patients develop skin rash, probably due to sensitivity to sulfonamides.
2. When dressings are removed, they often have a gray-green appearance—this does not necessarily mean a gross infection.
3. Because sulfa drugs are known to increase possibility of kernicterus, silver sulfadiazine should not be used on infants through the first month of life or on pregnant women near term.
4. If topical proteolytic enzymes are used in debriding, silver sulfadiazine may inactivate them.
5. Lately it has been suggested that with protracted use, gram-negative bacilli, particularly *Enterobacteriaceae*, can become highly resistant.
6. Because isolated incidences of leukopenia have occurred following use of Silvadene, it is suggested that blood counts be carefully monitored.

C. *Mode of Application*

1. Silver sulfadiazine can be applied directly to the burn wound, spread thinly, 2–4 mm., and left exposed; wound should be so covered that no part is visible.

TABLE 12-3. COMPARISON OF CONVENTIONAL OPEN AND CLOSED TREATMENTS OF BURNS*

Open Treatment	Closed Treatment
Advantages	
Ease of examination	Comfort
Delay of sepsis	Transportability
Ease of wound care	Absorption of secretions
Control of temperature	Accelerated debridement
Early physical therapy	Aesthetic considerations
Disadvantages	
Discomfort	Hyperthermia
Delayed eschar separation	Promotion of sepsis
Nontransportability	Difficult examination
Added linen requirement	Odorous dressings
Aesthetically appalling	Delayed physical therapy

* (Peterson HD. Open treatment of the burn wound, *in* Practical Approaches to Burn Management, © 1977 by Flint Laboratories, Division of Travenol Laboratories, Inc., Deerfield, Illinois 60015).

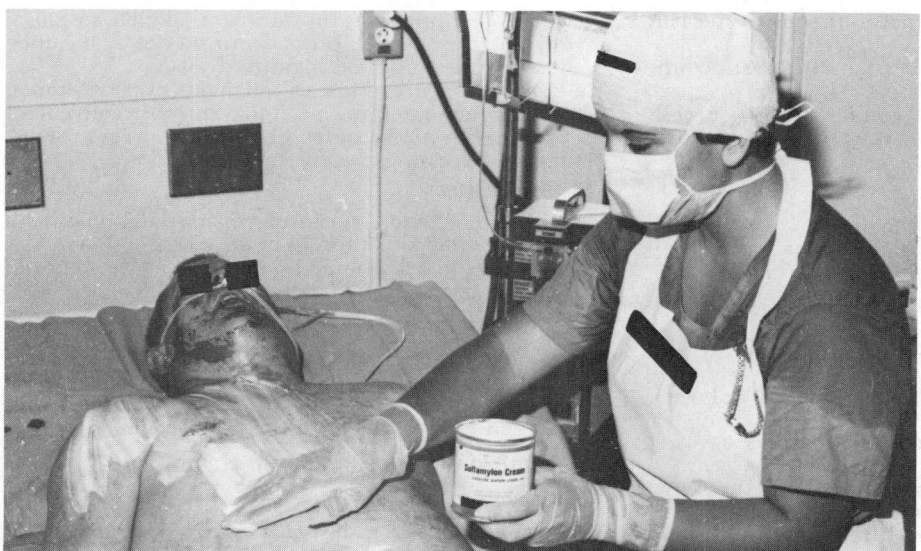

FIGURE 12–13. *Nurse applying a topical agent to protect the patient from infections. The topical agent is applied with sterile gloves. A nasogastric tube is inserted to prevent abdominal distention and for the administration of antacids to prevent Curling's ulcers. (Courtesy of the U.S. Army Institute of Surgical Research, Fort Sam Houston, Texas.)*

2. Some surgeons prefer that after ointment or cream is applied, it should be covered with a single layer of mesh gauze; others apply ointment to gauze and then apply the medicated gauze to the burn. Cover with stockinette or Surgifix.
3. Reapply as it rubs off (remove all old cream before applying new); if occlusive dressings are used, change every 48 hours.

Cerium Nitrate—Silver Sulfadiazine

Modification of silver sulfadiazine with cerium nitrate enhances its clinical effectiveness.

A. *Advantages and Mode of Action*

1. Cerium (a lanthanide element) has a broad antibacterial and antifungal effect.
2. Cerium has low toxicity, is readily available and poorly absorbed from open wounds.
3. Gram-negative bacilli are rarely present when wound is treated by cerium nitrate; however gram-positive bacteria are more effectively treated by silver nitrate or silver sulfadiazine. When combined as cerium nitrate 2.2% with silver sulfadiazine 1% in a cream, results showed promise.
4. Appear to provide more efficient prophylaxis against gram-negative bacteria than other medications did heretofore.

B. *Disadvantage*

1. An occasional methemoglobinemia has occurred.

Silver Nitrate (0.5%) Solution

(Being used less because of its disadvantages)

A. *Advantages and Mode of Action*

1. Silver nitrate is a bacteriostatic chemical and is effective in reducing colonization.
   a. Above 1% produces tissue necrosis.
   b. Below 0.5% solution is ineffective as an antiseptic.

2. Cap, gown, and mask are not required.
3. An effective method for treating large numbers of burns, as during war; is relatively inexpensive.
4. Several layers of 4-ply gauze dressings *must be thoroughly wet every 2–4 hours with silver nitrate solution* to be effective. It is held close to the wound by stretch bandage or net tube dressings.
5. Silver nitrate can be used over grafted areas and donor sites as well as burn surfaces.
6. Bacterial flora with which it is principally effective are gram-negative.

B. *Disadvantages*

1. Since silver nitrate solution only penetrates 1–2 mm. of burn eschar, only surface contaminants can be controlled.
2. The wound must be completely free of oil or grease for silver nitrate solution to be effective.
3. Hyponatremia (loss of sodium ions), hypokalemia (loss of potassium ions) and hypochloremia (loss of chlorine ions) may occur. (For this reason it should not be used for children.)
4. Frequent blood samples are required to determine sodium, potassium, and calcium ion levels.
5. It is necessary to replace electrolytes that are lost.
6. Methemoglobinemia (a modified form of oxyhemoglobin) may be caused due to the reduction of nitrates to nitrites, resulting in cyanosis.
7. Silver nitrate turns black in sunlight.
   a. Clothes, hands, floor, etc. are stained black.
   b. Gloves must be worn by the nurse and assistants.
8. It is a costly agent to use because of the number of dressings required.

Mafenide Acetate (Sulfamylon Acetate)

A. *Mode of Action and Advantages*

1. Accumulated experience with mafenide acetate suggests that use of this agent probably should be limited

to treatment of invasive burn wound sepsis, especially when relatively localized.
2. It will penetrate the eschar (slough) to reduce the number of infecting organisms.
3. In cream form, mafenide acetate diffuses rapidly through the burned skin; this agent must be reapplied at 12-hour intervals.

NURSING ALERT: Careful monitoring of acid-base balance and pulmonary function is essential.

B. *Disadvantages*

1. Causes a burning pain within a half hour following application.
2. Has a tendency to cake; tubbing permits easy removal.
3. Inhibits carbonic anhydrase activity in the renal tubules and may cause metabolic acidosis.
4. Usually not recommended for patients with pulmonary disease, since they cannot use respiratory mechanism sufficiently to maintain acid-base balance in most instances.
5. Some patients are allergic to sulfa drugs.
6. Never use under an occlusive dressing because it will cause severe maceration and contact dermatitis.
7. Appears to inhibit spontaneous epithelial regeneration.
8. Reports of superinfection have been noted, especially by antibiotic resistant *Providencia stuartii;* fungal infections have also been reported.

Povidone-iodine Ointment 10% and Betadine Solution

A. *Advantages:*

1. This agent appears to be effective against a wide variety of gram-negative and gram-positive organisms as well as yeasts, fungi, and viruses.

2. It can be applied as an ointment (similar to Sulfamylon), the solution can be sprayed on, or it can be incorporated into mesh gauze dressings.
3. Usually the dressings are changed every 6 hours, during tubbing; however, it may be more convenient to merely remove outer dressings and rewet inner layer of dressings with Betadine solution.

B. *Disadvantages:*

1. This agent tends to cause crusting—this may be a help in some situations, a hindrance in others.
2. Materials may be stained, but stain can be removed by laundering immediately.
3. Some stinging is noted by patients, but it soon disappears.
4. Some patients are allergic to iodine preparations. Although povidone iodine is recommended for moderate and major burns, more documentation is needed to recommend it for extensive burns.

Gentamicin Sulfate (Garamycin cream) 0.1%

A. *Advantages and Mode of Action*

1. Useful against a wide variety of gram-negative and gram-positive organisms. (Even effective against *Providencia stuartii.)*
2. Application and use are similar to Sulfamylon acetate (See p. 607.)
3. Ointment spreads easily and tends to become invisible.
4. No pain is associated with this cream.
5. It is useful for brief periods when applied to small areas of invasive infection; monitor blood levels of drug carefully.

B. *Disadvantages*

1. Since this drug has a tendency to promote the emergence of gentamicin-resistant organisms that may spread to other patients in the burn unit, it is usually reserved for life-threatening situations.
2. Is nephrotoxic—monitor creatinine levels.
3. With long-term use, superinfection with resistant bacterial strains can occur rapidly.

GUIDELINES: Debridement (Removal of Eschar)

Debridement is the removal of nonviable tissue in preparation for skin grafting. (See p. 593 for skin grafting.)

Effective Methods

1. Surgical primary excision—removing large areas down to fascia.
2. Surgical debridement, (tangential excision)—using a dermatome or scalpel—small areas at a time.
3. Mechanical: Change dry dressings; light anesthesia may be necessary to remove loose tissue. Bathe daily in hydrotherapy—debride small areas daily. Apply wet soaks every 4 hours (saline) using coarse mesh gauze; frequent removal of gauze also facilitates pulling away dead tissue.
4. Enzymatic—using proteolytic enzymes (sutilains ointment [Travase ointment]) with saline to dissolve eschar.

Objectives

1. To prevent bacterial growth which occurs underneath eschar.
2. To debride daily, during each dressing change; this will eliminate less frequent, more fatiguing debridement or the use of anesthesia.
3. To limit the time and stress to the patient by restricting debridement to a maximum area of 10 cm. square (4-inch square) or a maximum time of 20 minutes; this reduces stress as well as limits spread of bacteria.

Equipment

Sterile gloves
Forceps
Scissors

Hemostatic agent (Ex. Oxycel)
4 × 4 gauze squares

Procedure	
NURSING ACTION	**RATIONALE/AMPLIFICATION**
1. Explain to the patient when and why you are going to debride his burn wound.	1. His cooperation makes the procedure proceed more quickly, comfortably, and effectively for him.
2. Using the forceps in one hand, carefully pick up eschar at loosened edge.	2. This gives leverage in cutting the dead tissue.
3. Leave ½ cm (¼ inch) on remaining eschar.	3. To provide a margin of safety in trying to avoid cutting viable tissue.
4. Continue to snip eschar up to limits of time and space.	4. Ten cm. or 20 minutes are acceptable limits for patient comfort.
5. Should bleeding or oozing occur, apply pressure with a gauze square or apply a hemostatic agent (Oxycel).	5. This should control venous and capillary bleeding.
6. Should bleeding continue or spurt and if you have been taught how to clamp and tie vessels, proceed with hemostat and a ligature; otherwise, continue to apply pressure and summon assistance.	6. It is likely that an artery has been nicked. Have available a sterile simple suture set: Hemostat Dressings Suture and ligature Needle and needle holder Scissors Sterile gloves
7. Following debridement, apply topical agent or dressings as prescribed.	
8. Document activity and patient reaction.	

BIOLOGIC DRESSINGS

Biologic dressings are used to cover large denuded surfaces of the body. Usually they are split-thickness grafts harvested either from human cadavers or other mammalian donors such as pigs. Human amnion may also be used.

An *allograft* is a graft of skin taken from a person other than the burn victim and applied to a burn wound temporarily (a cadaver is most common source).

A *xenograft* or *heterograft* is a segment of skin taken from an animal such as a pig or dog. It is useful in preparing debrided area for grafting and is really a biologic dressing. (See p. 593 for Skin Grafting)

Donor Criteria

1. Skin color unimportant since it is only a temporary graft.
2. Donor should be an adult free of infection.

Purpose and Benefits

1. Decreases heat, fluid, and protein losses
2. Reduces bacterial proliferation
3. Closes wound temporarily; enhances production and protection of granulation tissue
4. Protects exposed neurovascular and muscle tissue as well as tendons
5. Reduces pain and facilitates patient comfort
6. Acts as a test-graft to determine when granulating wounds will accept autograft successfully
7. Provides an effective donor-site dressing

Clinical Procedure

1. Porcine skin grafts (xenografts) are the most popular temporary biologic dressings.
2. Devitalized tissue is first removed surgically or enzymatically.
3. Porcine graft is applied directly (epidermis side up) to the denuded area; it may be trimmed to adhere to wound contour. Before applying, it may be dipped in saline solution.
4. Usually grafts are left exposed except when applied to circumferential wounds; stretch gauze (Surgifix) is applied to prevent adherence to as well as to prevent malpositioning by bed sheets.

5. The first xenograft dressing may have to be changed in 24 hours to permit more intimate adherence to granulating wound bed.
6. Thereafter, grafts may be left in place 2 to 5 days between changes; inspect wound daily to detect early signs of suppuration.
7. After good xenograft adherence is achieved, the wound is ready for autografting.

Discharge Planning and Health Education

1. The patient is usually "glad" to be going home (outwardly) but is *frightened* inside. He wonders how others will react to him and whether he can manage his care. He needs to be encouraged to verbalize this. Family should have an opportunity to see the wounds and practice required wound care prior to his discharge.
   a. To overcome this feeling, the nurse must stress the positive, healthy future of the patient. Be hopeful but realistic in helping patient accept a new self-image.
   b. Permit the patient to take brief trips out of the hospital before his discharge—car rides, etc.
   c. Assist patient in exploring feelings of self-worth in light of newly formed self-image.
   d. Prepare family for his coming home—particularly those who haven't seen his changed appearance.
   e. Assist the family in making a transition in their feelings about the patient; they may have expected and adjusted to the fact that the patient was going to die. Now he is coming home to live. They must encourage him to become more and more independent.
2. Develop a plan with the family for helping the patient to become active and interested in an avocation; to prepare to return to work; to make social adjustments. Be alert for need of psychological counseling.
3. Explore the possibility of overcoming scarring and contracture formation by using special formed splints and elastic supports where effective—e.g., for hand and fingers. (Available for whole body.)
4. Explain to the family the gamut of activities the patient can perform, and also inform them of activities for which he will need assistance.

5. Know community resources which will assist with his adjustment; community nursing service agencies may have a physical therapist and medical social worker in the area where the patient lives.
6. Provide written instructions to the patient on skin care, wound care, exercises prescribed, use of elastic garments and splints; what to do for common problems such as blisters, discoloration, itching, flaking of skin.

NOTE: When patients go home, they most often report difficulty sleeping, dreaming about and reliving the burn injury, fearing return to work or other activity that may have been involved with the burn injury. They often become very fire-safety conscious. There may be expressions of boredom (particularly in men who cannot return to work for a while); difficulty resuming sexual activity; feeling out of control, i.e., living from one reconstructive procedure to the next, being unsure when they can resume control and direction of their own lives rather than allowing the health professions to dictate this to them.

BIBLIOGRAPHY

1 DERMATOLOGY

Books

Burton, JL. Essentials of Dermatology. New York, Churchill Livingstone, 1979
Clark WH Jr et al (eds). Human Malignant Melanoma. New York, Grune & Stratton, 1979
Epstein E. Common Skin Disorders: A Manual for Physicians and Patients. Oradell, Medical Economics Book Division, 1979
Epstein E and Epstein E Jr. Techniques in Skin Surgery. Philadelphia, Lea & Febiger, 1979
Fitzpatrick TB et al. Dermatology in General Medicine. New York, McGraw-Hill, 1979
Frank SB (ed). Acne. Update for the Practitioner. New York, Yorke Medical Books, 1979
Gibbs RC. Skin Diseases of the Feet, 2nd ed. St. Louis, Warren H. Green, 1980
Glickman FS. General Dermatology. Littleton, PSG Publishing Co 1979
Helm F. Cancer Dermatology. Philadelphia, Lea & Febiger, 1979
Kopf AW et al. Malignant Melanoma. New York, Masson Publishing USA, 1979
Lazarus GS and Goldsmith LA. Diagnosis of Skin Disease. Philadelphia, FA Davis, 1980
Pillsbury DM and Heaton CL. A Manual of Dermatology, 2nd ed. Philadelphia, WB Saunders, 1980
Sauer G. Manual of Skin Diseases, 4th ed. Philadelphia JB Lippincott, 1980
Sneddon IB and Church RE (eds). Skin Disorders in Clinical Practice. Menlo Park, Addison-Wesley Publishers, 1979

Plastic and Reconstructive Surgery

Chang WHJ (ed). Fundamentals of Plastic and Reconstructive Surgery. Baltimore, Williams & Wilkins, 1980
Cocke W et al. Essentials of Plastic Surgery. Boston, Little, Brown & Co, 1979
Converse JM (ed). Reconstructive Plastic Surgery, 2nd ed. Philadelphia, WB Saunders, 1977
Grabb WC and Smith JW. Plastic Surgery, 3rd ed. Boston, Little, Brown & Co, 1979
Grazer FM and Klingbeil Jr. Body Image: A Surgical Perspective, St. Louis, C.V. Mosby, 1979
McCoy FJ et al. 1980 Year Book of Plastic and Reconstructive Surgery. Chicago, Year Book Medical Publishers, 1980
McDowell F. The Source Book of Plastic Surgery. Baltimore, Williams & Wilkins, 1977
Rees TD. Cosmetic Surgery 2nd ed. Philadelphia, WB Saunders, 1980

Articles

Acne

Bernstein JE and Shalita AR. Topically applied erythromycin in inflammatory acne vulgaris. J Am Acad Dermatol 1980 April; 2(4):318–321
Cahn RL. Current status of acne treatment. Postgrad Med 1980 June; 67(6):117–122
Fisher AA. The safety of topical antibiotics in the treatment of acne vulgaris. Cutis 1980 May; 25(5):474–481
Hurwitz S. Acne vulgaris. Current concepts of pathogenesis and treatment. Am J Dis Child 1979 May; 133(5):536–544
Langer R and Binnick S. Treatment of acne vulgaris. Am Fam Physician 1979 Aug; 20(2):117–118
Melski JW and Arndt KA. Current concepts: Topical therapy for acne. N Engl J Med 1980 Feb 28; 302(9):503–506
Reeves JRT. How I treat acne. Med Times 1980 March; 108(3):82–91
Stoughton RB and Aly R. Topical antibiotic therapy of acne: Laboratory investigation of vehicles, various antibiotics, and stability characteristics. Cutis 1980 Feb; 25(2):216–218, 220
Swinyer LJ et al. Topical agents alone in acne. JAMA 1980 April 25; 243(16):1640–1643

Assessment/Treatment

Feingold DS and Bachta M. Common skin diseases seen by the internist. DM 1979 May; 25(8):5–38
Hazelrigg DE. Scraping for scabies. Am Fam Physician 1978 Jan; 17(1):129
Montgomery BJ. Skin problems in blacks receive scrutiny. JAMA 1979 Dec 21; 242(25):2747–2748
Terezakis NK. Simple treatment for complicated dermatoses. Postgrad Med 1980 June; 67(6):152–163

Herpes Zoster

Becker LE. Herpes zoster: A geriatric disease. Geriatrics 1979 Sept; 34(9):41–47
Koch-Weser J. Antiviral agents. N Engl J Med 1980 April 17; 302 (16):903–907
Nuss DD. Herpes Zoster—the best approach. Med Times 1980 June; 108(6):47–52

Pemphigus

Ahmed R et al. Pemphigus: Current concepts. Ann Intern Med 1980 March; 92(3):396–405
Auerbach R and Bystryn J-C. Plasmapheresis and immunosuppressive therapy. Effect on levels of intercellular antibodies in pemphigus vulgaris. Arch Dermatol 1979 June; 115(6):728–730
Fitzpatrick RE and Newcomer VD. The correlation of disease activity and antibody titers in pemphigus. Arch Dermatol 1980 March; 116(3):285–290

Psoriasis

Arnold V and Rose S. Photochemotherapy for psoriasis. Am J Nurs 1979 March; 79(3):466–468
Cort DH et al. Retrospective analysis of a modified Goeckerman regimen for the treatment of psoriasis. Cutis 1980 Feb; 25(2):201–203; 206–209
Current status of oral PUVA therapy for psoriasis. J Am Acad Dermatol 1979 August; 1(2):106–117

From the NIH: A look at the management of psoriasis. JAMA 1980 April 11; 243(14):1429

Hanno R et al. Methotrexate in psoriasis. J Am Acad Dermatol 1980 Feb; 2(2):171–174

LeVine MJ and Parrish JA. Outpatient phototherapy for psoriasis. Arch Dermatol 1980 May; 116(5):552–554

Saunder DN et al. Suppressor cell function in psoriasis. Arch Dermatol 1980 Jan; 116(1):51–55

Infections/Infestations

Causey WA. Staphylococcal and streptococcal infections of the skin. Primary Care 1979 March; 6(1):127–139

Clayton YM. Dermatophyte infections. Postgrad Med J 1979 Sept; 55(647):605–607

Fisher AA et al. Little lice can make mighty problems. Patient Care 1978 Sept; 12(15):204–224

Lorek M and Maguire H. Specific drugs for superficial fungus infections. Am Fam Physician 1980 Feb; 21(2):164–165

Odom RB. How I treat tinea capitis. Med Times 1980 March; 108(3):46–48

Orkin M and Mailbach, HF. Scabies, a current pandemic. Postgrad Med 1979 July; 66(1):52–65

Pinkus H. Furuncle. J Cutan Pathol 1979 Dec; 6(6):517–518

Skin Cancer; Malignant Melanoma

Briele HA and Das Gupta TK. Natural history of cutaneous malignant melanoma. World J Surg 1979 July; 3(3):255–267

Chanda JJ et al. Malignant melanoma and its therapy: A review. Cutis 1979 June; 23(6):759–783

Mandel MA. Malignant melanoma: An update. Clin Plastic Surg 1980 July; 7(3):379–396

Nathanson L. Immunotherapy of melanoma. J Cutan Pathol 1979 June; 6(3):213–226

Rees RB. How I treat warts. Med Times 1980 March; 108(3):31–35

Robinson JK and Roenigk HH. The big three of skin cancer: Basal cell carcinoma, squamous cell carcinoma and malignant melanoma. Postgrad Med 1980 June; 67(6):92–107

Sober AJ et al. Early recognition of cutaneous melanoma. JAMA 1979 Dec 21; 242(25):2795–2799

Stone SP. Electrodesiccation and fulguration of lesions of the skin. J Fam Pract 1979 Jan; 8(1):171–174

Sullivan BP. Patient responses to BCG therapy for malignant melanoma. Am J Nurs 1979 Feb; 79(2):320–324

Veronesi V and Cascinelli N. Surgical treatment of malignant melanoma of the skin. World J Surg 1979 July; 3(3):279–285

Zimmerman LE and McLean IW. An evaluation of enucleation in the management of uveal melanomas. Am J Ophthalmol 1979 June; 87(6):741–760

Systemic Diseases with Dermatologic Manifestations

Bellows JG. Systemic lupus erythematosus. Compr Ther 1979 July; 5(7):3–4

Black CM. Scleroderma. Br J Hosp Med 1979 July; 22(1):28–37

Cohen RD et al. Clinical features, prognosis, and response to treatment in polyarteritis. Mayo Clin Proc 1980 March; 55(3):146–155

Condemi JJ. SLE: Idiopathic or drug-induced? Geriatrics 1980 March; 35(3):81–88

Decker JL et al. NIH conference. Systemic lupus erythematosus: Evolving concepts. Ann Intern Med 1979 Oct; 91(4):587–604

Farrell JB et al. Role of immune complexes in rheumatoid polyarteritis. Ann Rheum Dis 1979 August; 38(4):390–393

Horwitz DA. Laboratory investigation of systemic lupus erythematosus. Postgrad Med 1980 April; 67(4):193–196; 199–200

Leib ES et al. Immunosuppressive and corticosteroid therapy of polyarteritis nodosa. Am J Med 1979 Dec; 67(6):941–947

Rodman GP (ed). Progressive systemic sclerosis. Clin Rheumatic Diseases 1979 April; 5(1):5–302

Samuelson SJ. Systemic lupus erythematosus. J Am Dent Assoc 1980 April; 100(4):553–557

Travers RL. Polyarteritis nodosa and related disorders. Br J Hosp Med 1979 July; 22(1):38–45

Wasner CK and Fries JF. Treatment decisions in systemic lupus erythematosus. Arthritis Rheum 1980 March; 23(3):283–286

White JF. Teaching patients to manage systemic lupus erythematosus. Nursing '78 1978 Sept; 8(9):26–34

Zurier RB. Systemic lupus erythematosus. Hosp Pract 1979 August; 14(8):45–54

Zweiman B. Editorial. A new therapeutic strategy in systemic vasculitis. N Engl J Med 1979 Aug 2; 301(5):266–267

Plastic and Reconstructive Surgery

Campbell RM. Surgical and chemical planing of the skin. In Converse JM (ed). Reconstructive Plastic Surgery, 2nd ed. Philadelphia, WB Saunders, 1977

Care of cosmetic surgery patients. AORN J 1977 Nov; 26(5):926–928

Chouinard F et al. Vigilant nursing care after reconstructive microsurgery. Nursing 79 1979 June; 9(6):18–25

Finn KL. Rebuilding skin, Part I: A successful graft may be up to you. RN 1977 Oct; 40(10):41–45; Part II: Meeting the challenges of flap care RN 1977 Nov; 40(11):47–52

Hugill JV. Acceleration of healing of skin graft donor sites using scarlet red ointment. Am Surg 1978 June; 44(6):352–355

Johnson CM and Anderson JR. When the patient wants facial cosmetic surgery. Am Fam Physician 1977 Sept; 16(3):170–176

Magil B. Exciting changes in grafting techniques. Contemp Surg 1977 March; 10(3):11–17

More muscles for flaps are emphasis in plastic surgery. AORN J 1980 Jan; 31(1):60–61

Stuart MS. Skin flaps and grafts after head and neck surgery. Am J Nurs 1978 Aug; 78(8):1368–1374

Vasconez LO et al. Musculocutaneous flaps in reconstructive surgery. Contemp Surg 1979 Jan; 14(1):15–26

Wooldridge M and Surveyor JA. Skin grafting for full-thickness burn injury. Am J Nurs 1980 Nov; 80(11):2000–2004

2 BURNS

Books

Artz CP et al. Burns, A Team Approach. Philadelphia, WB Saunders, 1979

Braen GR. Minor Burns, Evaluation and Treatment, American College of Emergency Physicians. Kansas City, Marion Laboratories, 1979

Feller I and Grabb WC. Reconstruction and Rehabilitation of the Burned Patient, Ann Arbor, National Institute for Burn Medicine, 1979

Feller I and Archambeault C. Nursing the Burn Patient. Ann Arbor, National Institute for Burn Medicine, 1973

Feller I et al. Emergent Care of the Burn Victim. Ann Arbor, National Institute for Burn Medicine, 1977

Jacoby FG. Nursing Care of the Patient with Burns, 2nd ed. St. Louis, CV Mosby, 1976

Jones CA and Feller I. Procedures for Nursing the Burned Patient. Ann Arbor, National Institute for Burn Medicine, 1975

Practical Approaches to Burn Management. Deerfield, Flint Laboratories, Division of Travenol Labs, 1977

Articles

Allyn P. Inhalation injuries. Crit Care Q 1978 Dec; 1(3):37–42

Andressen MJC et al. Management of emotional reactions in seriously burned adults. N Engl J Med 1979 Jan 13; 286(2):65–69

Archambeault-Jones C and Feller I. Burn nursing is nursing. Crit Care Q 1978 Dec; 1(3):77–92

Bartlett RH et al. Rehabilitation following burn injury. Surg Clin North Am 1978 Dec; 58(6):1249–1262

Bayley EW and Moore DA. Group meetings for families of burn victims. Top Clin Nurs 1980 July; 2(2):67–76

Brandenburg J. Inhalation injury: Carbon monoxide poisoning. Am J Nurs 1980 Jan; 80(1):98–100

Brown CR. Problems and complications of burn shock resuscitation. Surg Clin North Am 1978 Dec; 58(6): 1313–1322

Christopher KL. The use of a model for hemodynamic balance to describe burn shock. Nurs Clin North Am 1980 Sept; 15(3):617–627

Curreri PW and Luterman A. Nutritional support of the burned patient. Surg Clin North Am 1978 Dec; 58(6): 1151–1156

Dolph JL et al. Amnion; A useful biological dressing. Contemp Surg 1980 Aug; 17(2):65–66

Dyer C. Burn care in the emergent period. J Emergency Nurs 1980 Jan–Feb; (1):9–16

Fitzgerald RT. Prehospital care of burned patients. Crit Care Q 1978 Dec; 1(3):13–24

Fraser G and Beaulieu J. Leukopenia secondary to sulfadiazine silver. JAMA 1979 May 4; 241(18):1928–1929

Gaston SF and Schumann LL. Inhalation injury: Smoke inhalation. Am J Nurs 1980 Jan; 80(1):94–97

Haliurchak DR and Pruitt BA Jr. Use of systemic antibiotics in the burned patient. Surg Clin North Am 1978 Dec; 58(6):1119–1132

Harsperger JE and Dahl LM. Electrical and chemical injuries. Crit Care Q 1978 Dec; 1(3):43–49

Helm PA et al. Burn rehabilitation—a team approach. Surg Clin North Am 1978 Dec; 58(6):1263–1278

Howard RJ. Effect of burn injury, mechanical trauma, and operation on immune defenses. Surg Clin North Am 1979 April; 59(4):199–211

Jackson DL and Beraducci A. Carbon monoxide poisoning—a growing hazard. Med Times 1978 Feb; 106(2):28–37

Jones CA and Feller I. Burns—avoiding and coping with complications before and after grafting. Nursing '77 1977 Nov; 7(1):72–81

Jones CA and Feller I. Burns—the home stretch. Nursing '77 1977 Dec; 7(12):54–57

Kinzie V. What to do for the severely burned. RN 1980 April; 43(4):47–51; 104–110

Leavitt M. Andy was a fighter. Nursing '79 1979 April; 9(4):62–66

MacMillan BG. Closing the burn wound. Surg Clin North Am 1978 Dec; 58(6):1205–1231

MacMillan BG. Infections following burn injury. Surg Clin North Am 1980 Feb; 60(1):185–196

Markley K. Burn care: Infection and smoke inhalation. Ann Intern Med 1979 Feb; 90(2):269–270

Marvin J. Acute care of the burn patient. Crit Care Q 1978 Dec; 1(3):25–35

McHugh ML et al. Family support group in a burn unit. Am J Nurs 1979 Dec; 79(12):2148–2150

Mieszala P. Postburn psychological adaptation: An overview. Crit Care Q 1978 Dec; 1(3):93–111

Monafo WW and Ayvazian VH. Topical therapy. Surg Clin North Am 1978 Dec; 58(6):1157–1171

Morris J and McFadd A. The mental health team on a burn unit: A multidisciplinary approach. J Trauma 1978 Sept; 18(9):658–663

Parks DH et al. Prevention and correction of deformity after severe burns. Surg Clin North Am 1978 Dec; 58(6):1279–1289

Pruit BA Jr. The burn patient, Part 1. Initial Care. Curr Probl Surg 1979 April; 16(4):1–62

Pruit BA Jr. The burn patient, Part 2. Later care and complications of thermal injury. Curr Probl Surg 1979 May; 16(5):1–95

Pruit BA Jr. Fluid and electrolyte replacement in the burned patient. Surg Clin North Am 1978 Dec; 58(6):1291–1312

Pruit BA and McManus WF. Surgical management of burns. Contemp Surg 1980 May; 16(5):11–16

Psychiatric nurse works with burn patients. Am J Nurs 1980 Jan; 80(1):124–125

Schumann L and Gaston S. Commonsense guide to topical burn therapy. Nursing '79 1979 March; 9(3):34–39

Severely burned patients: Anticipating their emotional needs. Nursing '80 1980 Sept; 10(9):47–50

Shuck JM. Outpatient management of the burned patient. Surg Clin North Am 1978 Dec; 58(6):1107–1117

Stoddard JE. Rehabilitation of the burn-injured patient. Crit Care Q 1978 Dec; 1(3):63–76

Trunkey DD. Inhalation injury. Surg Clin North Am 1978 Dec; 58(6):1133–1140

Wooldridge M and Surveyer JA. Skin grafting for full-thickness burn injury. Am J Nurs 1980 Nov; 80(11):2000–2004

Yarborough MF et al. Nutritional management of the severely injured patient (1. Thermal). Contemp Surg 1978 Sept; 13(9):21–28

ALLERGY PROBLEMS

13

THE ALLERGIC REACTION

Definitions

1. *Antigen*—a substance that, when repeatedly in contact with the body, stimulates production of a counteracting substance, a globulin "antibody."
2. *Antibody*—a globulin produced by the lymphoid cells as a result of stimulation of these cells by an antigen; the antibody is capable of combining with the antigen in a very specific manner.
3. *Immunity*—a state of increased resistance to a particular substance.
   a. *Active-acquired immunization*—resistance brought about by the injection of an antigenic substance (e.g., tetanus toxoid).
   b. *Passive-acquired immunization*—resistance brought about by the transfer of antibody-containing serum from an immunized donor to a normal recipient (e.g., tetanus antitoxin).
4. *Allergic reaction*—a manifestation of tissue injury resulting from an interaction between an antigen and an antibody.

Products of Antigen-antibody Union

(Chemical Mediator Products)
1. *Histamine*—released from tissue mast cells by the interaction of an antigen and its corresponding antibody.
   a. Causes contraction of smooth muscle of bronchioles, uterus, intestines.
   b. Dilates and causes increased permeability of capillaries of skin and mucous membrane.
   c. Lowers blood pressure.
   d. Stimulates secretion of nasal, lacrimal, salivary, and gastrointestinal glands.
   e. Produces itching of skin and mucous membrane.
2. *Serotonin*—an amine released at the same time as histamine.
3. *Bradykinin*—acts chiefly by increasing capillary permeability and contractility of smooth muscle.
4. *Acetylcholine*—acts to stimulate autonomic nervous system.
5. *SRS-A*—slow-reacting substance of anaphylaxis.

Antibody-antigen Reaction

1. Consists of:
   a. Those that are protective and beneficial to the body (immunogen).
   b. Those that are not always protective and beneficial to the body (allergen).
      (1) May cause tissue damage.
      (2) May produce discomfort to the patient.
2. Under certain circumstances, an antibody is produced that reacts not only to a noxious agent but also to another harmless agent of similar chemical composition.

Hypersensitivity Phenomena

1. "Sensitivity" is said to exist when the body reacts against substances in the environment which elicit no response from most persons.
2. Some authorities consider that
   a. "Immunity" is produced when antigen and antibody are beneficial to the individual.
   b. "Allergy" is produced when antigen and antibody are harmful to the individual.
3. Inhaled allergens
   a. Plant pollens—ragweed, grasses, tree pollens
   b. Molds, fungi, spores, animal danders, house dust
4. Ingested allergens—cow's milk, egg white, fish, nuts, chocolate, certain fruits
5. Contact allergens—contact dermatitis (see p. 583)
6. Sensitivity reactions
   a. Local or systemic
   b. Mediated by sensitized cells, not circulating globulins
   c. Mediated by circulating immunoglobulin E (IgE) (See Immunoglobulins)

Delayed Hypersensitivity

1. Term for a reaction that reaches its peak 24–48 hours after an antigen is brought into contact with the skin surface of a sensitized individual.
2. The reaction usually consists of erythema and induration.

613

3. Delayed hypersensitivity is mediated by sensitized "T" (thymus-dependent) lymphocytes (not by immunoglobulins).
4. Example: tuberculin skin test, contact dermatitis such as poison ivy.

Immunoglobulins

Antibodies that are formed by lymphocytes and plasma cells in response to an immunogenic stimulus comprise a group of serum proteins called *immunoglobulins*.
1. The abbreviation for immunoglobulin is "Ig."
2. Antibodies combine with antigens in very special ways (lock and key style).
3. There are 5 classes of immunoglobulins:

a. IgM (gamma-M")—largest molecule; tends to stay in bloodstream and is primarily engaged in defense in intravascular compartment.
b. IgG (gamma-G")—most abundant and one of the smallest; readily diffuses into tissue spaces to assist in combating tissue infection.
c. IgA (gamma-A")—circulates in the blood, but its role here is uncertain; it is produced in external secretions (saliva, tears) where it provides a primary defense mechanism.
d. IgD—function has not yet been determined.
e. IgE (gamma-E")—responsible for most of the immediate types of allergic reactions; has property of attaching to human epithelial cells.

PATIENT ASSESSMENT: ALLERGY SURVEY

(Use Allergy Survey Sheet, below.)

Allergy Survey Sheet*

Name _____ Age _____ Sex _____ Date _____

   I. Chief complaint:

  II. Present illness:

 III. Collateral allergic symptoms:

Eyes:	Pruritus _____	Burning _____	Lacrimation _____
	Swelling _____	Injection _____	Discharge _____
Ears:	Pruritus _____	Fullness _____	Popping _____
	Frequent infections _____		
Nose:	Sneezing _____	Rhinorrhea _____	Obstruction _____
	Pruritus _____	Mouth breathing _____	
	Purulent discharge _____		
Throat:	Soreness _____	Post-nasal discharge ____	
	Palatal pruritus _____	Mucus in the morning ____	
Chest:	Cough _____	Pain _____	Wheezing _____
	Sputum _____	Dyspnea _____	
	Color _____	Rest _____	
	Amount _____	Exertion _____	
Skin:	Dermatitis _____	Eczema _____	Urticaria _____

 IV. Family Allergies:

  V. Previous allergic treatment or testing:

Prior skin testing:

Drugs:	Antihistamines	Improved _____	Unimproved _____
	Bronchodilators	Improved _____	Unimproved _____
	Nose drops	Improved _____	Unimproved _____
	Hyposensitization	Improved _____	Unimproved _____
	Duration _____		
	Antigens _____		
	Reactions _____		
	Antibiotics	Improved _____	Unimproved _____
	Steroids	Improved _____	Unimproved _____

Allergy Survey Sheet (cont.)

VI. Physical agents and habits:

Bothered by:

Tobacco for _____ years
Cigarettes _____ packs/day
Cigars _____ per day
Pipe _____ per day
Never smoked _____
Bothered by smoke _____

Alcohol _____   Air cond. _____
Heat _____   Muggy weather _____
Cold _____   Weather changes _____
Perfumes _____   Chemicals _____
Paints _____   Hair spray _____
Insecticides _____   Newspapers _____
Cosmetics _____

VII. When symptoms occur:
Time and circumstances of 1st episode:
Prior health:
Course of illness over decades: Progressing _____   regressing _____
Time of year:
   Perennial _____
   Seasonal _____
   Seasonally exacerbated _____
Monthly variations (menses, occupation):
Time of week (weekends vs weekdays):
Time of day or night:
After insect stings:

VIII. Where symptoms occur:
Living where at onset:
Living where since onset:
Effect of vacation or major geographic change:
Symptoms better indoors or outdoors:
Effect of school or work:
Effect of staying elsewhere nearby:
Effect of hospitalization:
Effect of specific environments:
Do symptoms occur around:
old leaves _____ hay _____ lakeside _____ barns _____
summer homes _____ damp basement _____ dry attic _____
lawnmowing _____ animals _____ other _____
Do symptoms occur after eating:
cheese _____ mushrooms _____ beer _____ melons _____
bananas _____ fish _____ nuts _____ citrus fruits _____
other foods (list) _____
Home: city _____   rural _____
             house _____   age _____
             apartment _____ basement _____ damp _____ dry _____
             heating system _____
             pets (how long) _____ dog _____ cat _____ other _____

Bedroom:	Type	Age	*Living Room:*	Type	Age
Pillow	____	____	Rug	____	____
Mattress	____	____	Matting	____	____
Blankets	____	____	Furniture	____	____
Quilts	____	____			
Furniture	____	____			

Anywhere in home symptoms are worse: _____

IX. What does patient think makes him worse: _____

X. Under what circumstances is he free of symptoms: _____

XI. Summary and additional comments: _____

* From Patterson R. Allergic Diseases, 2nd ed. Philadelphia, JB Lippincott, 1980.

SENSITIVITY TESTS AND IMMUNOTHERAPY (HYPOSENSITIZATION)

Immunotherapy is a procedure designed to increase a person's resistance to offending antigens by administration of small, gradually increasing amounts of a specific antigen over a period of time.

Immunotherapy is preceded by skin testing.

GUIDELINES: Skin Testing

Skin testing is the introduction of an antigen (bacterial, fungal, chemical) to the skin surface or directly beneath the skin to determine body sensitivity and reaction to the antigen.

Purpose
1. Diagnosis
2. Desensitization
3. Immunization

Methods
1. *Patch test*—application of test material either directly to skin or to skin immediately covered with a small gauze dressing (or gauze part of a Band-Aid).
2. *Scratch (prick or tine)*—Antigen is applied to a superficial scratch that penetrates the outer layer of skin.
3. *Intradermal*—Injection of a small amount of antigen into the superficial layers of skin.

Reactions
1. *Positive*
   a. Indicates antibody response to previous contact with the antigen.
   b. Does not prove presence of active infection.
2. *Negative*
   a. Indicates antibodies have been formed against the antigen.
   b. In presence of active infection, it means that not enough time has lapsed to build antibodies.
   c. May mean that antigen has been injected too deeply.
   d. Patient may be anergic (abnormal inactivity).
3. *Suppressed Reaction*—may occur if the patient
   a. Is on corticosteroids.
   b. Is on immunosuppressive drugs.
   c. Is on antihistaminics.
   d. Has received (within 3 weeks) live virus immunizations, e.g., smallpox, measles.
   e. Feels faint or is cold.

Sites
1. Volar or anterior surface of the upper third of the forearm or upper arm (over muscle belly).
2. Back, below top of scapula (Fig. 13-1). (Useful for scratch or tine test.)
3. Anterior thigh (scratch or tine test).

1. Approx. 10 cm. (4 inches) below bend of elbow or 10 cm. above bend of elbow.
2. Avoid spine.

Side Effects

SYMPTOM	TREATMENT
1. Itching, discomfort, pain.	1. Apply cold packs. Apply topical steroids.
2. Vesiculation, ulceration.	2. Keep dry—expose to air.

3. Bleeding
  a. Wheal type—bleeding is of no consequence.
  b. Tine test—bleeding can wash away antigen.
	3. Apply pressure if bleeding is excessive.
	
	  b. Apply pressure if bleeding is excessive. Repeat test in another area.

4. Allergic reaction to preservatives or stabilizers.	4. Discontinue use.
5. Anaphylactic shock.	5. Administer adrenalin (see p. 619).

Procedure
1. Place tests approx. 10 cm. (2 inches) apart.

2. Avoid hairy area.
3. Avoid areas near bone or tendons or areas without adequate subcutaneous tissue.

1. To prevent results of one test from coalescing with those of another.
2. Will interfere with reading.

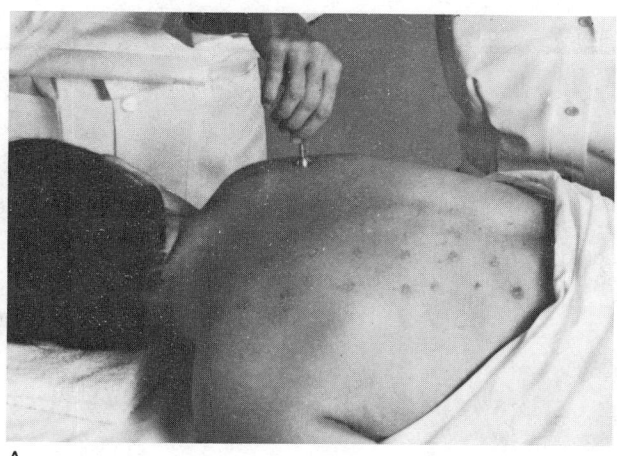
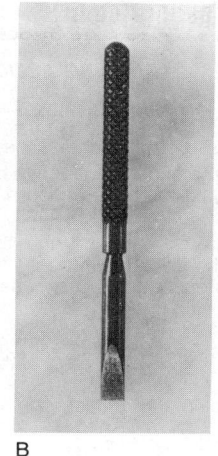
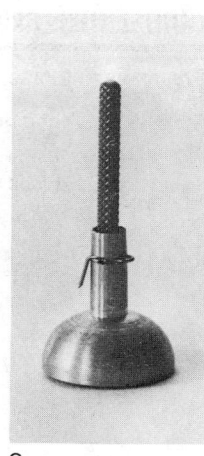

A   B   C

FIGURE 13-1. A. *This shows skin testing from the top of the scapula to the lower rib cage and from the posterior axillary line to 5 or 10 cm. (2 or 4 inches) from the spine. Most scarifications should be at least 5 cm. (2 inches) apart; however, pollen tests should be as much as 10 cm. (4 inches) apart to prevent one reaction from overlapping another. B. Von Pirquet scarifier. C. Robinson bell scarifier. These are small instruments used to scratch the skin preparatory to applying allergen for skin testing. The Von Pirquet scarifier is a small steel chisel which is pressed against the skin and twirled between the thumb and first finger to abrade the outer layer of skin. The Robinson bell is placed on the test site and twirled by the handle. (Courtesy of Hollister-Stier)*

Preparation of Patient

1. Explain to patient what is being done and why.
2. Provide adequate lighting.
3. Thoroughly cleanse testing area with alcohol or ether and allow the area to dry.

PATCH TEST

Advantage:
    Effective in cases involving contact hypersensitivity to topically applied substance.
Disadvantage:
    Not as accurate as other methods.

NURSING ACTION	RATIONALE/AMPLIFICATION
Technique	
1. Apply test material directly to skin for purpose of producing a small area of allergic dermatitis; e.g., plant oils, hair tonic, shaving cream.	1. Leave area exposed, OR Cover with a small gauze dressing and adhesive or use a "Band-Aid."
Reaction	
1. Remove patch after 48 hours.	1. Usually site itches.
2. Wait for 20–30 min. to allow any unrelated reaction to subside.	2. A true allergic reaction persists for several days.

3. Observe reaction and describe:
   + erythema
  ++ erythema, papules
 +++ erythema, papules, vesicles
++++ erythema, papules, vesicles, and severe edema
	3. Positive patch test reactions often show an increase in severity in next 24 hours. Reexamine in 72 hours.

4. Record nature of sensitizers and reactions.	

SCRATCH TEST (PRICK OR TINE)

Equipment:
    Sterile "darning" needle, 4-prong tine scarifier, such as Von Pirquet, Robinson (Fig. 13-1B, C)
    (A needle pricks the skin through a drop of antigen.)
Advantage:
    Relatively little risk of a general constitutional reaction.
Disadvantage:
    May not be sufficiently sensitive unless a very strong antigen is used.

GUIDELINES: Skin Testing (cont.)

Preparation of Patient (cont.)

Technique

NURSING ACTION	RATIONALE/AMPLIFICATION
1. Place a drop of glycerine-saline solution on the skin.	1. This serves as a control.
2. Place a drop of each antigen to be tested on the skin; drops should be spaced about 4 cm. (2 inches) apart.	2. Spacing is required to prevent the coalescing of one reaction with another. Skin-marking pencil may be used to number each antigen.
3. Scratch the skin about 2 mm. through each drop of antigen; the skin should be lightly abraded. If a 4-prong tine is used, grasp forearm firmly and stretch skin tightly.	3. A sterile darning needle or commercially available scarifying instrument may be used. This is to prevent undue movement of the arm when the tine is applied; if the arm moves, a larger scratch results.
4. Apply tine with pressure; hold 1 second.	4. Pressure is applied to produce 4 puncture sites. (A circular depression made by the disc, is also visible.)
5. Remove disc and release skin; discard disc.	5. Discs are never reused.

> **NURSING ALERT:** Do not wipe the skin following a scratch or tine test since this may remove the antigen.

6. Record site, type of antigen, and time when it is to be read.	6. Read in about 30–40 minutes.

INTRADERMAL TEST

Limit number of intradermal tests to no more than 20.
Advantage:
  More dilute solutions of antigen are required.
Disadvantage:
  There is risk of systemic reaction unless this test follows a scratch test.
Equipment:
1. Use sterile tuberculin syringe with gradations of 1/100 of a ml.
2. Use an intradermal needle or No. 26 or No. 27 gauge ¾ or ½ inch needle.
3. Use a separate syringe and needle (preferably disposable) for each antigen.

NURSING ACTION	RATIONALE/AMPLIFICATION
Technique	
1. Eject all air from syringe and needle.	1. Air injected will affect reading.
2. Hold forearm with one hand and use thumb to stretch skin.	2. Left hand can be used if syringe is to be held in right hand (or vice versa).
3. Hold syringe between thumb and forefinger and place plunger against heel of hand.	3. If necessary, air can be expelled by contracting thumb and forefinger.
4. Position bevel upward and place needle and syringe almost parallel along long axis of arm.	4. With bevel upward, needle can penetrate superficial layer of skin and sensitizer can be deposited directly under skin surface.
5. Depress needle into arm and advance until bevel just disappears into corium.	
6. Contract hand and advance plunger, injecting amount needed to raise a bleb of 1 cm. (¾ inch, or 10 mm.)	
7. Remove needle.	7. Transient bleeding is of no significance.
8. Repeat for additional testing.	
9. Record what was given, where it was given, and time when it is to be read.	9. Draw pattern on chart. Usually read in 30–40 minutes.
10. Grading of reactions from negative to positive (intracutaneous tests)* (Fig. 13-2)	

  − no reaction
  + erythema smaller than a nickel in diameter
  + + erythema larger than a nickel in diameter (21 mm.)
  + + + erythema and a wheal without pseudopod formation
  + + + + erythema and a wheal with pseudopod formation

* Patterson R. Allergic Diseases, Philadelphia, JB Lippincott, 1980.

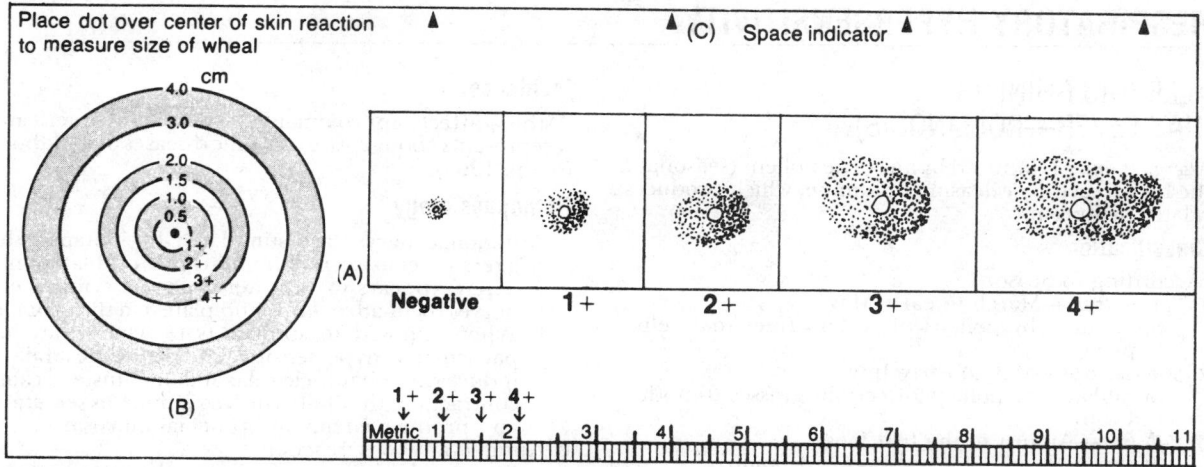

FIGURE 13-2. (A) *These series of reactions indicate the sizes of wheals when the allergist refers to them as 1+, 2+, etc. A negative reaction is shown at the left.* (B) *The target wheal guide can be traced on a transparent sheet (acetate or x-ray film) and then placed over the wheal to measure the size in centimeters or according to plus-size. The relationship between the two is indicated on the lower metric scale.* (C) *Showing placement of test sites spaced uniformly. (Patient Care: Sept. 15, 1973, Copyright © 1973, Patient Care Publications, Inc.; Darien, Conn. All rights reserved)*

RAST *(radioallergosorbent test)* is a technique for laboratory determination of IgE antibodies in serum. It is useful in corroborating skin test findings in questionable situations. It is also a useful substitute when skin testing is contraindicated, e.g., patient objection, generalized dermatitis.

ANAPHYLAXIS

Anaphylaxis is an unusual systemic allergic reaction (hypersensitivity) to a foreign protein or other substance. It is usually precipitated by the injection of a medication or by an insect sting. The reaction occurs rapidly and may cause death because of respiratory obstruction or vascular collapse.

> **NURSING ALERT:** With injection of allergenic extracts, the risk of systemic reaction is always present.
> Skin testing, usually of the intradermal type, has resulted in systemic reactions to pollen, penicillin, and food antigens.

Early Manifestations

1. Feeling of uneasiness or apprehension, weakness, perspiration, sneezing, or nasal pruritus
2. Generalized pruritus, urticaria, angioedema
3. Dyspnea, wheezing, dysphagia, vomiting, abdominal pain
4. Pulse—may be rapid, weak, irregular, or unobtainable
5. Syncope or shock—may follow rapidly

6. Possible urgency, fecal and urinary incontinence, convulsions, and coma

Treatment

Administer epinephrine—the pharmacologic antagonist of the action of chemical mediators on smooth muscle and other effector cells.

A. *Immediate:*

(Anticipate physician's need of the following.)
1. Inject 0.3–0.5 ml. of 1:1000 aqueous epinephrine IM into upper arm; massage.
2. Apply tourniquet above site of antigen injection (allergy injection, insect sting, etc.).
3. Inject 0.3 ml. of 1:1000 aqueous epinephrine into site of previous antigen injection.

B. *If reaction is not reversed by epinephrine:*

(Physician administration)
1. Diphenhydramine chloride is given IV to help prevent development of laryngeal edema.
2. Bronchospasm: aminophylline IV, intravenous fluids.
3. Hypotension: vasopressors, volume repletion, isoproterenol.
4. Laryngeal obstruction: tracheostomy and oxygen.
5. Cardiac arrest: CPR, sodium bicarbonate.
6. Corticosteroids may be helpful for laryngeal edema and hypotension; however, it must be emphasized that steroids are not helpful in immediate anaphylaxis, since they take at least one and probably several hours to act even if given intravenously.

C. *Ongoing monitoring:*

1. Evaluate patient reaction.
2. Repeat aqueous epinephrine, if necessary.
3. Remove tourniquet if reaction seems to be under control.
4. Monitor vital signs as required.
5. Assess for hypotension and respiratory distress.

RESPIRATORY HYPERSENSITIVITY

ALLERGIC RHINITIS (HAY FEVER—POLLINOSIS)

Allergic rhinitis is induced by airborne pollens (seasonal); the body reacts by releasing histamine, which produces related symptoms.

Classification

(According to Season)
1. *Spring types*—March to early May
    Stimulated by pollens of certain trees (oak, elm, poplar)
2. *Summer type*—May to early July
    Stimulated by pollens of certain grasses (timothy, red top)
3. *Fall type*—August to the first frost
    Stimulated by pollens of ragweed family

Clinical Manifestations

1. Rhinitis—leading to edematous, closed nostrils
2. Nasal mucous membranes—itch, burn, and secrete thin, irritating discharge
3. Sneezing—violent paroxysms
4. Eyes—red, burning, lacrimating

Diagnostic Evaluation

Sensitivity Tests
Skin tests confirm patient's hypersensitivity to pollens.

Treatment

1. Advise patient to move to an area where pollen count is low; this, however, is often impractical.
2. Use antihistamines; this will not only control symptoms in 4 out of 5 patients but will also have an atropine-like drying effect.
    a. Be alert for individual reactions to antihistamines, since they are variable: sedation, depression, somnolence, incoordination.
3. If nasal obstruction is a persistent problem, a sympathomimetic may be given (effective for short-term but not long-term therapy).
    Ex. Pseudoephedrine hydrochloride (Sudafed), ephedrine sulfate, phenylpropanolamine (Propadrine), also combination products: Actifed, Dimetapp Extentabs
4. Treat sinusitis and other otolaryngologic infections during symptom-free seasons.
5. Administer prophylactic injections of extract of pollens (specific for the individual); begin several months before the attacks and administer once a week throughout the peak season.
6. Resort to oral corticosteroids when antihistamines are not effective; these act by reducing the responsiveness of mucous membranes to histamine.

BRONCHIAL ASTHMA

Bronchial Asthma is a condition which manifests itself clinically by intermittent episodes of wheezing and dyspnea; it is generally associated with a hyper-responsive state of the bronchi which may be antigen-mediated (allergic).
  The main characteristic differentiating bronchial asthma from other pulmonary conditions is that the former is reversible.

Incidence

Asthma affects approximately 6–8 million Americans; it represents about 25% of chronic diseases of childhood (see p. 1263).

Pathophysiology

1. Autonomic nerves are stimulated by irritants; this triggers mucous secretion and capillary dilatation.
    a. There appears to be a defect in the sympathetic nerves (beta-adrenergic end plates) in the bronchi.
    b. When exposed to stimulants to which they are particularly hypersensitive, these nerves fail to induce smooth muscle relaxation but instead cause contraction; they fail to decrease mucous secretion, and produce edema of bronchial mucosa.
2. Antigen-antibody reaction
    a. Susceptible individuals form abnormally large amounts of IgE when exposed to certain allergens.
    b. This immunoglobulin (IgE) fixes itself to the mast cells of the bronchial mucosa.
    c. When the individual is exposed to certain allergens, the resulting antigen combines with the cell-bound IgE molecules, causing the mast cell to degranulate and release chemical mediators.
    d. These chemical mediators, primarily histamine and slow reacting substance of anaphylaxis (SRS-A) are known to produce bronchospasm.
3. Other factors can precipitate an asthmatic attack. (Also see Fig. 13-3)
    a. Respiratory tract infection
    b. Intolerance to certain drugs, such as aspirin, indomethacin
    c. Cold and sudden barometric changes
    d. Exercise
    e. Emotional upset
    f. Air pollutants—industrial chemicals

Clinical Manifestations

1. There are symptom-free intervals.
2. During an attack of asthma, the amount of airway obstruction determines the degree of severity of symptoms.
    a. During early or mild episodes—cough or mild chest tightness
    b. As asthmatic episode becomes more severe—wheezing, coughing, shortness of breath, which may be stimulated by
        Cold air, air pollutants, psychic factors, varying degrees of exertion.
    c. Dyspnea may become apparent; inspiratory wheezing and use of accessory respiratory muscles
    d. As severity of attack increases, the patient becomes more anxious, restless, and apprehensive.
    e. A fatigue state may follow—respirations are less labored and there is less audible wheezing.
    f. This may lead to respiratory failure with hypercapnia, respiratory acidosis, and hypoxemia.
3. Determine how long the wheezing attack lasts.

NOTE: Instead of wheezing, there may be chest tightness. If attack persists for several days, hospitalization may be required.

4. Can patient talk using long sentences? Does he speak in short phrases as he tries to get his breath?

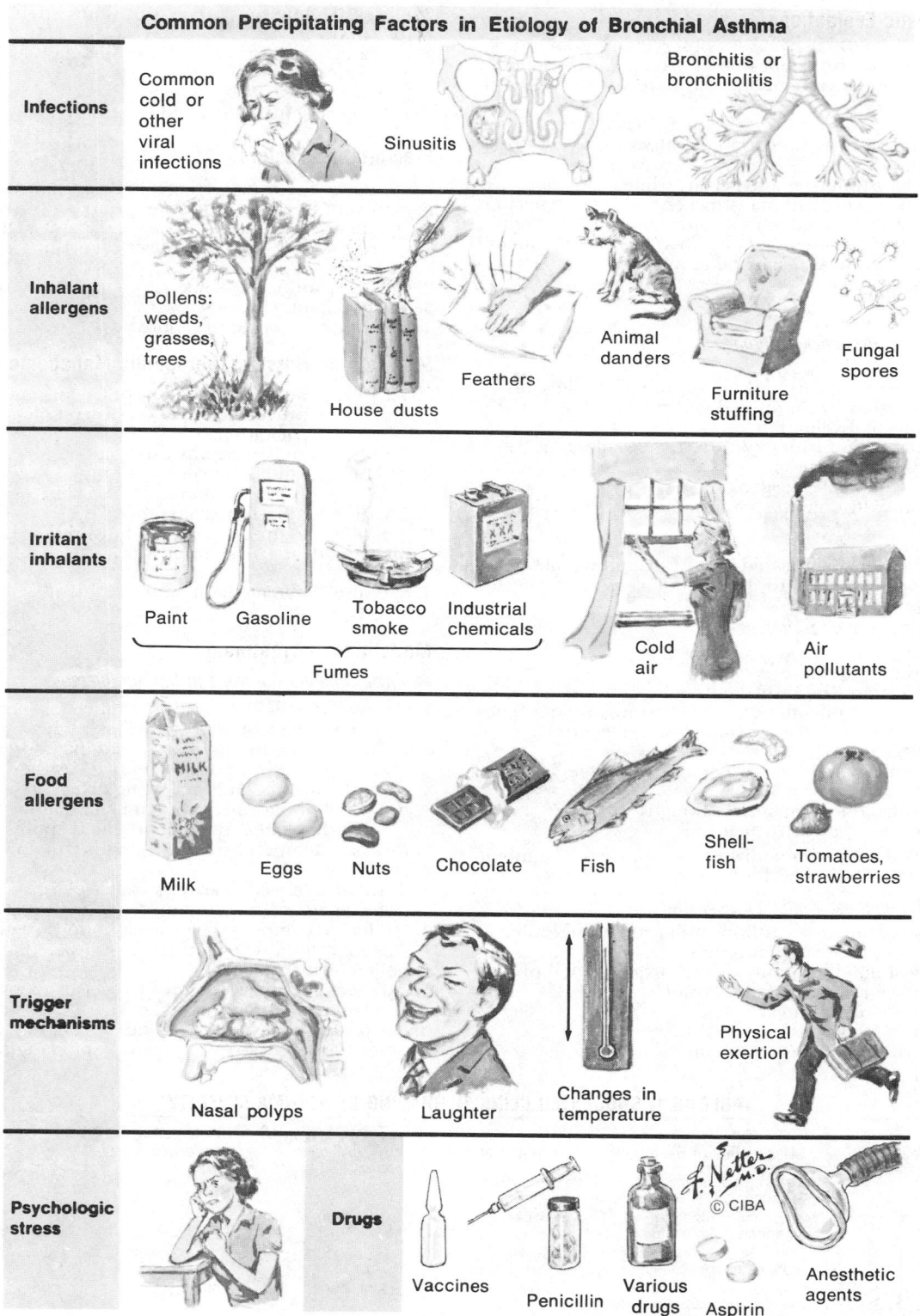

Common Precipitating Factors in Etiology of Bronchial Asthma

Infections — Common cold or other viral infections · Sinusitis · Bronchitis or bronchiolitis

Inhalant allergens — Pollens: weeds, grasses, trees · House dusts · Feathers · Animal danders · Furniture stuffing · Fungal spores

Irritant inhalants — Paint · Gasoline · Tobacco smoke · Industrial chemicals (Fumes) · Cold air · Air pollutants

Food allergens — Milk · Eggs · Nuts · Chocolate · Fish · Shellfish · Tomatoes, strawberries

Trigger mechanisms — Nasal polyps · Laughter · Changes in temperature · Physical exertion

Psychologic stress — Drugs: Vaccines · Penicillin · Various drugs · Aspirin · Anesthetic agents

FIGURE 13-3. (Copyright © 1975 CIBA Pharmaceutical Co., Division of CIBA-Geigy Corp. Reproduced with permission from CLINICAL SYMPOSIA, illustrated by Frank H. Netter, M.D. All rights reserved.)

Diagnostic Evaluation

1. None in particular except observation of an attack.
2. Pulmonary function studies usually show marked improvement after administration of a bronchodilator.
3. Bronchoprovocation techniques may be performed in a pulmonary function laboratory.
4. Sputum tests
   a. Mild asthma—foamy, clear, white
   b. More severe asthma—thicker and more tenacious
   c. Asthma with infection—purulent greenish, yellow
5. To establish baseline data, blood gas evaluation and simple spirometry may be required.

Classification

(Also see Table 13-1)

A. *Extrinsic Bronchial Asthma*

1. Cause
   a. Hypersensitivity reaction to inhalant allergens
   b. Mediated by immunoglobulin E (IgE-mediated)
2. Diagnostic Evaluation
   a. Correlation with exposure to aeroallergens
   b. Positive skin tests
3. Major inhalant allergens
   House dust, mold spores, pollens, feathers, animal danders
4. Prognosis
   Favorable, with avoidance of offending allergens; good response to bronchodilators and specific therapy

B. *Intrinsic Bronchial Asthma*

1. Cause
   a. Nothing definite
   b. Infection—often present
   c. Skin tests of common inhalant antigens and foods are usually negative (non IgE-mediated)
2. Occurrence
   Primary onset before age 5 or after age 35
3. Prognosis
   a. Remission of intrinsic asthma is variable
   b. Control may be difficult

C. *Mixed Asthma*—immediate type appears to combine allergic reaction and infection

D. *Aspirin-induced Asthma* (ASA Sensitive)

(A type of intrinsic asthma induced by ingestion of aspirin and related compounds.)

1. Clinical manifestations spread over a period of time have been described as a "triad":
   a. Bronchial asthma
   b. Nasal polyposis
   c. Severe reactions to aspirin

2. Onset of symptoms after aspirin ingestion (20 min. to 2 hrs)
   a. Watery rhinorrhea, followed by marked flushing of upper part of body
   b. Nausea, vomiting
   c. Wheezing, dyspnea, and cyanosis

Precipitating Factors

Any one of these may trigger an asthmatic attack in person with intrinsic bronchial asthma.

1. Strong odors (fumes): turpentine, paints, chemicals, sprays, heavily scented flowers, perfumes, tobacco smoke
2. Cold air; sudden barometric changes
3. Air pollutants
4. Emotion-triggering situations

Medical and Nursing Therapeutic Management

OBJECTIVE: to achieve sufficient control of symptoms to prevent physical and psychological incapacitation.

1. Treatment must be individualized.
2. Therapy includes concern not only for the physical condition of the person but also for his psychosocial situation and his environment.
3. There is no cure for asthma, but present-day treatment modalities can improve and control the condition.
4. See also "Management of the Patient with an Allergy."

Modalities of Treatment

A. *Environmental Control and Immunotherapy*

1. Control the environment as much as possible to reduce number of allergens (Fig. 13-4).
   a. Particularly in bedroom—eliminate dust (loose carpeting, draperies); remove feather pillows, wool blankets, dust collecting articles.
   b. Exclude house pets, to eliminate dander.
   c. Exclude plants, to eliminate mold spores
2. Regulate temperature and humidity to comfortable levels.
3. Treat any related diseases such as allergic rhinitis to alleviate asthmatic symptoms.
4. Undergo complete hyposensitization regimen involving offending agents such as ragweed, dust, tree pollen, grass.
5. Advise susceptible person to receive hyposensitization to insect stings (wasps, hornets, bees).
6. Discourage moving from one seasonal area to another that has more year-round pollination.

TABLE 13-1. SUGGESTED CLINICAL GRADING OF ASTHMA SEVERITY*

Class	Description of Symptoms	Number of Attacks	Total Duration of Attacks	Restricted Activity or Work-loss Days	Bed Disability Days
Minimal	Annoying, but no marked discomfort	1–2/month	4 hours	1–2/month	0
Moderate	Marked discomfort, but not interfering with usual activities	2/week	4–10 hours	2/week	0
Severe	Some interference with sleep, but not incapacitating	Daily	11–20 hours	3 or more/week	Occasional
Severe (Refractory)	Intolerable; diet and fluid restriction; unable to perform ordinary daily activities	Daily	Continuous	Total	2 or more/week

* Bernstein IL. Asthma in Adults, in Conn HF (ed): Current Therapy, p 584. Philadelphia, WB Saunders, 1980

GUIDE TO "DESENSITIZING" A ROOM

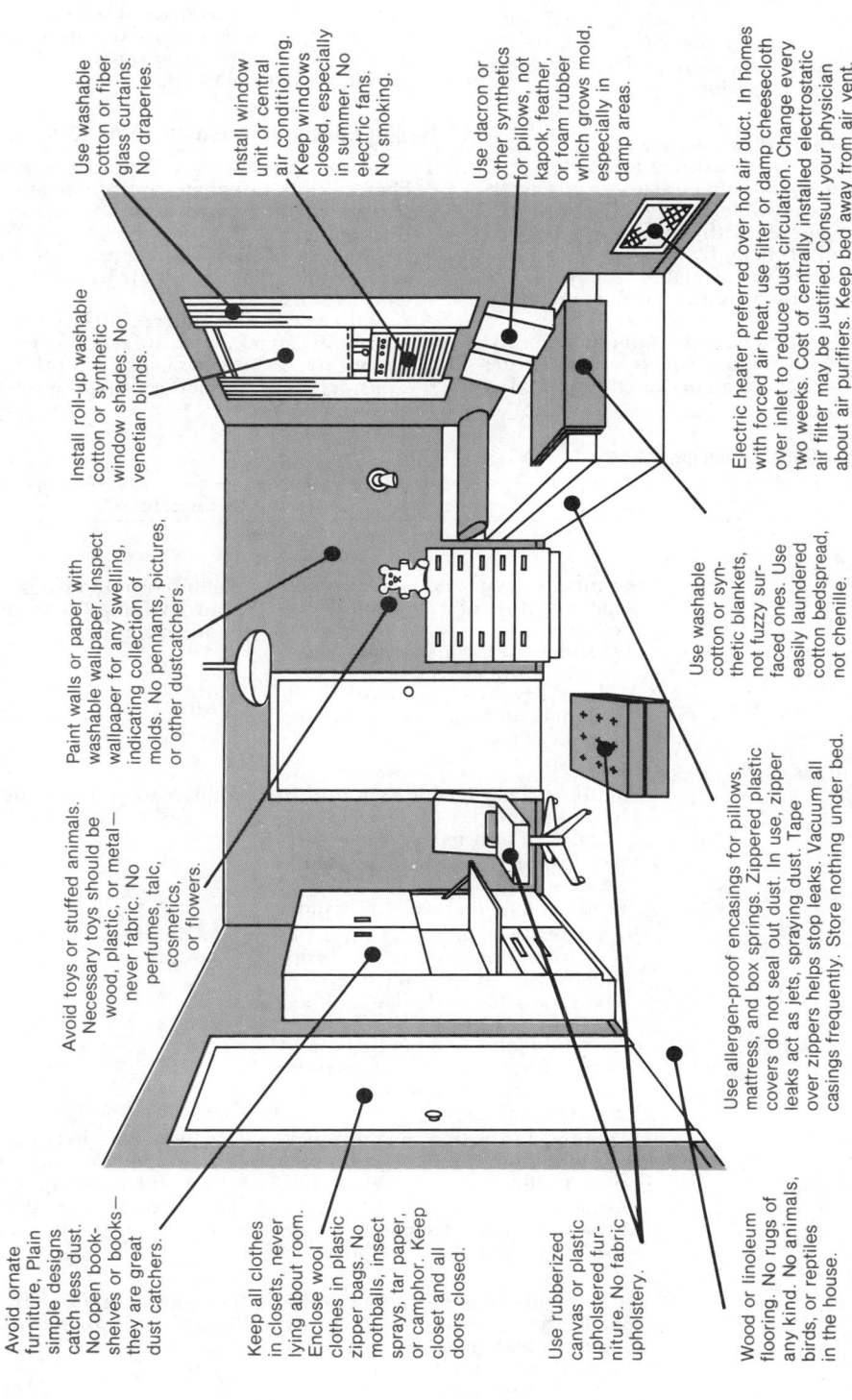

Avoid ornate furniture. Plain simple designs catch less dust. No open bookshelves or books—they are great dust catchers.

Avoid toys or stuffed animals. Necessary toys should be wood, plastic, or metal—never fabric. No perfumes, talc, cosmetics, or flowers.

Use washable cotton or fiber glass curtains. No draperies.

Install window unit or central air conditioning. Keep windows closed, especially in summer. No electric fans. No smoking.

Install roll-up washable cotton or synthetic window shades. No venetian blinds.

Use dacron or other synthetics for pillows, not kapok, feather, or foam rubber which grows mold, especially in damp areas.

Paint walls or paper with washable wallpaper. Inspect wallpaper for any swelling, indicating collection of molds. No pennants, pictures, or other dustcatchers.

Electric heater preferred over hot air duct. In homes with forced air heat, use filter or damp cheesecloth over inlet to reduce dust circulation. Change every two weeks. Cost of centrally installed electrostatic air filter may be justified. Consult your physician about air purifiers. Keep bed away from air vent.

Keep all clothes in closets, never lying about room. Enclose wool clothes in plastic zipper bags. No mothballs, insect sprays, tar paper, or camphor. Keep closet and all doors closed.

Use allergen-proof encasings for pillows, mattress, and box springs. Zippered plastic covers do not seal out dust. In use, zipper leaks act as jets, spraying dust. Tape over zippers helps stop leaks. Vacuum all casings frequently. Store nothing under bed.

Use washable cotton or synthetic blankets, not fuzzy surfaced ones. Use easily laundered cotton bedspread, not chenille.

Use rubberized canvas or plastic upholstered furniture. No fabric upholstery.

Wood or linoleum flooring. No rugs of any kind. No animals, birds, or reptiles in the house.

Cleaning Tips: Wet-dust room twice daily. Damp-mop floor with solution containing disinfectant to prevent growth of mold spores. Oil-mop baseboards.

Vacuum only if followed by airing of room. Use tank-type cleaner, vacuumed itself before using. Attach a second hose to outlet, placing end outside window or in hall to prevent redistributing allergens.

FIGURE 13-4. *Controlling the environment of a room. (Courtesy of A.H. Robins Company)*

B. *Pharmacotherapy*

This phase of management should be integrated with environmental control and immunotherapy; medications are administered in a stepwise approach—one drug is added at a time, and dosage is adjusted to achieve maximum benefit. (See Commonly Used Medications: Bronchial Asthma, below.)

General Considerations:
1. Bronchodilators are used as follows:
   a. Short-term use to reverse asthmatic attacks.
   b. Long-term use to maintain ventilatory capacity as close to normal as possible.
2. The majority of patients with asthma will be well controlled with oral bronchodilators.
3. Sympathomimetics that are available as aerosols are epinephrine (least active), isoproterenol, metaproterenol.
4. There is limited use for sympathomimetic aerosols; they are used primarily to abort an attack or provide some breathing time before an oral medication takes effect (½–2 hours).

5. Subcutaneous and/or intravenous bronchodilators may be indicated for severe asthmatic attacks. Epinephrine and terbutaline are equally effective.
6. The great hazard associated with these medications is that they may be overused; this leads to excessive drying of the tracheobronchial tree and serious cardiac arrhythmias.

Health Education (Also see Fig. 13-5)

1. Promote optimum health practices: good nutrition, liberal fluids, adequate rest, sleep, and exercise.
2. Provide adequate hydration to keep secretions from thickening.
3. Avoid factors that will trigger an asthmatic attack; remove allergenic materials to which patient is specifically sensitive.
4. Avoid crowds and sources of infection, which may initiate an attack; if an infection occurs, encourage patient to see his physician promptly.
5. Consider immunotherapy (hyposensitization) when applicable.

Commonly Used Medications: Bronchial Asthma

Drug	Action	Side Effects
1. Adrenergics		
A. Catecholamines		
Epinephrine (Adrenalin)	Stimulates alpha- and beta-adrenergic receptors of autonomic nervous system: alpha—vasoconstriction beta—bronchodilation A drug of choice because of its potent bronchodilating effect and rapidity of action	Pallor, tremulousness, tachycardia, arrhythmia, headache, nausea and vomiting
B. Noncatecholamines		
Isoproterenol (Isuprel)	Stimulates beta receptors found in smooth muscles of heart, bronchial wall and its capillaries—relaxes muscles and dilates blood vessels Duration of action is relatively short	Similar to epinephrine
Ephedrine	Stimulates beta receptors found in smooth muscles of heart, bronchial wall and its capillaries—relaxes muscles and dilates blood vessels Less potent than epinephrine and isoproterenol but can be given by mouth; also, duration of action is longer (3–6 hours)	Similar to epinephrine and isoproterenol
Metaproterenol (Metaprel) (Alupent)	A potent, fast-acting beta-adrenergic stimulator Given orally or via metered dose inhaler Less active than terbutaline but superior to ephedrine as bronchodilator	Tachycardia, hypertension, palpitation, nervousness, tremor, nausea and vomiting, bad taste Less likely to cause peripheral muscle tremor than terbutaline.
Terbutaline sulfate (Brethine) (Brican) (Bricanyl)	Of sympathomimetic amines, this drug has the least B_1 (cardiogenic) and most B_2 (bronchial smooth muscle) receptor action (oral therapy use) Bronchodilation is provided for 4–6 hours	Peripheral muscle tremor; tachycardia, decreased diastolic blood pressure.

Drug	Action	Side Effects
2. Methylxanthines		
Theophylline	Relaxes bronchial smooth muscles May be given orally or rectally	Nausea, vomiting, headache, epigastric pain, palpitation; agitation, insomnia, seizures
Aminophylline	Relaxes bronchial smooth muscles May be administered orally, rectally, or intravenously	Nausea, vomiting, epigastric distress

NURSING ALERT: New guidelines for initiation and subsequent levels of aminophylline (theophylline products) have been set by FDA (April 1978). Check drug package inserts. (Selected patients are monitored by measurement of serum theophylline concentration.)

3. Cromolyn sodium (Aarane, Intal)	Inhibits allergic reaction if inhaled *before* challenged by antigen. *Ineffective for acute bronchial asthmatic attacks.* Appears to act directly on mast cell and hinders release of chemical mediators (bronchoconstriction). Has no bronchodilator, anti-inflammatory, or anti-histamine action.	Cough, hoarseness, rash, hypersensitivity pneumonitis
4. Corticosteroids—*Use with caution* Oral, parenteral (Prednisone)	Indicated for severe symptoms with full therapy Effective inhibitor of asthmatic reaction	Fluid retention, weight gain, acne, hypertension, cushingoid state, gastritis, gastric ulcers, adrenal suppression, hypokalemia, psychosis.
Inhalation Beclomethasone dipropionate (Beclovent, Vanceril)	Only small proportion is systemically absorbed	Local irritation from spray—Short-term: Occasionally growth of yeast organisms (*Monilia*) in mouth and pharynx. Rinsing or gargling with water or half-strength hydrogen peroxide after inhalation usually prevents this. If unsuccessful, try topical nystatin. Long-term: Same side effects as listed above for oral administration.

STATUS ASTHMATICUS

Status asthmaticus is that state of severe bronchial asthma in which there is no response to conventional therapy (epinephrine, theophylline).
1. Alveolar hypoventilation has progressed to ventilatory failure—arterial pCO_2 is greater than 44 mm.Hg.
2. This is a medical emergency and requires extraordinary therapeutic measures.

Contributing Factors
1. CO_2 retention, followed by acidosis
2. Infection
3. Dehydration
4. Overuse of sedation

Clinical Manifestations
1. Hypoxia causes changes in the central nervous system:
   Fatigue, headache, irritability, dizziness, impaired mental functioning
2. With continued carbon dioxide retention:
   Muscle twitching, somnolence, asterixis (intermittent lapse of an assumed posture—flapping tremor) diaphoresis
3. Tachycardia, elevated blood pressure
4. At very low oxygen levels and high carbon dioxide levels, sudden hypotension may occur
5. Pulmonary vasoconstriction → heart failure, death from suffocation

General Management Principles for the Asthmatic Patient

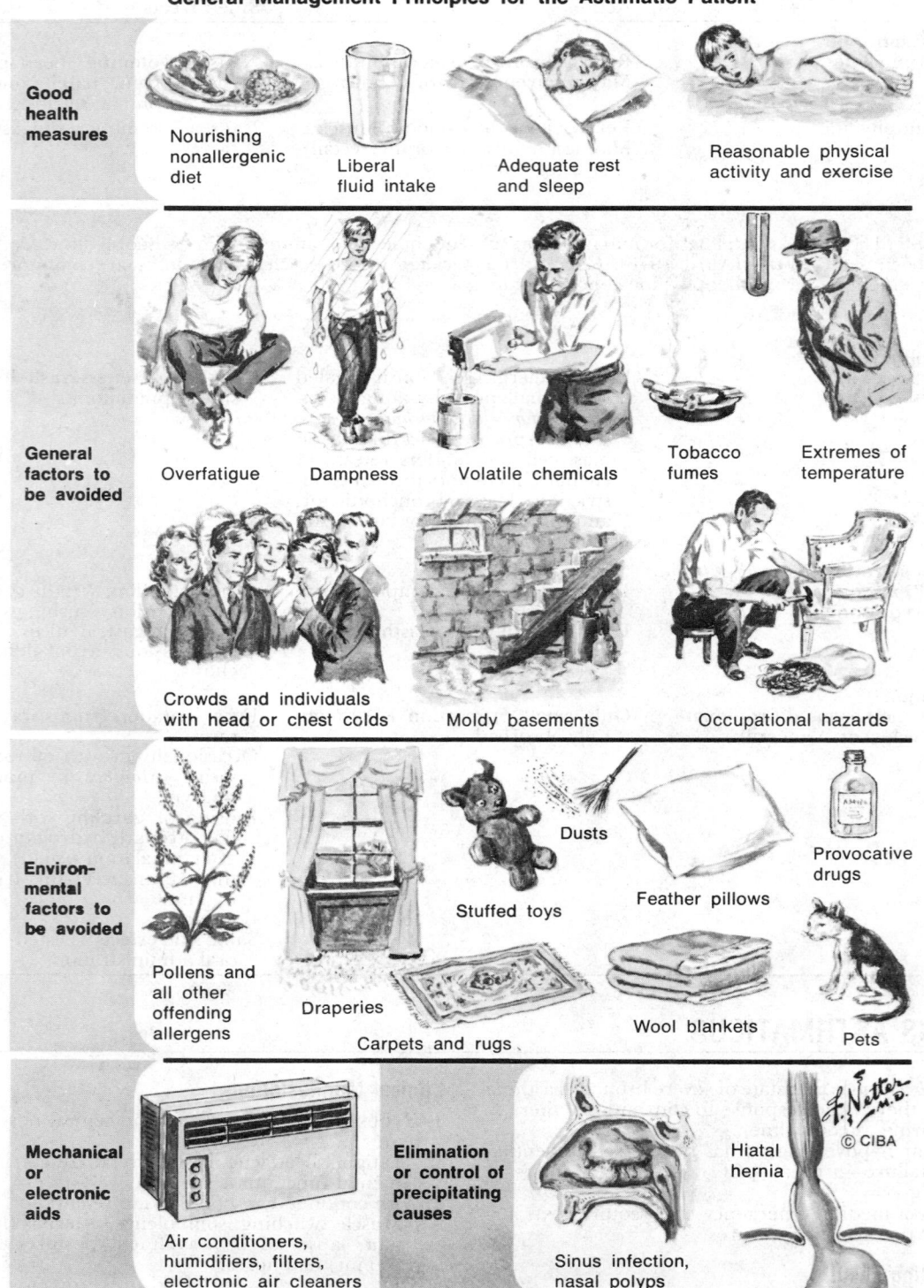

Good health measures

Nourishing nonallergenic diet

Liberal fluid intake

Adequate rest and sleep

Reasonable physical activity and exercise

General factors to be avoided

Overfatigue

Dampness

Volatile chemicals

Tobacco fumes

Extremes of temperature

Crowds and individuals with head or chest colds

Moldy basements

Occupational hazards

Environmental factors to be avoided

Pollens and all other offending allergens

Draperies

Stuffed toys

Dusts

Feather pillows

Provocative drugs

Carpets and rugs

Wool blankets

Pets

Mechanical or electronic aids

Air conditioners, humidifiers, filters, electronic air cleaners

Elimination or control of precipitating causes

Sinus infection, nasal polyps

Hiatal hernia

FIGURE 13-5. *(Copyright © 1975 CIBA Pharmaceutical Co., Division of CIBA-Geigy Corp. Reproduced with permission from CLINICAL SYMPOSIA, illustrated by Frank H. Netter, M.D. All rights reserved.)*

Treatment and Nursing Management

Requires team effort—including allergist, chest physician, anesthesiologist, and respiratory intensive care nurse.

1. Careful monitoring of pH, pCO_2, pO_2, in order to evaluate serially the changes in gas exchange and the patient's response to therapy.

NOTE: In early status asthmaticus, low pO_2 is followed by increased respiratory effort; this leads to low pCO_2 (hyperventilation). Then follow fatigue, reduced ventilation, and increasing pCO_2.

> **NURSING ALERT:** In status asthmaticus, the return to a normal or increasing pCO_2 does not necessarily mean that the asthmatic patient is improving—it may indicate a fatigue state which develops just before the patient slips into respiratory failure.

2. Correction of derangement of blood gases (hypoxemia) and hemoconcentration.
3. Rapid mobilization and removal of bronchial and bronchiolar secretions.
   a. Provide adequate hydration orally and intravenously (humidified oxygen)
   b. Administer expectorant and mucolytic drugs
   c. Remove secretions by coughing, suctioning, or bronchoscopy and lavage.
4. Alleviate patient's anxiety and fear with reassurance and the proper use of adequate doses of tranquilizers.
5. When intravenous fluids are administered, aminophylline may be prescribed and administered by constant infusion; the clinician must be constantly alert for signs of theophylline toxicity.
6. Many physicians administer corticosteroids, and since these act slowly, their beneficial effects may not be apparent for several hours.

MANAGEMENT OF THE PERSON WITH AN ALLERGY

Objectives

1. To encourage the person with an allergy to find out to which antigens he is sensitive.
2. To assist the patient in recognizing the importance of avoiding offending antigens whenever possible.
3. To seek relief for the patient when he has been exposed to an offending antigen.
4. To direct the patient to seek assistance in increasing his resistance to the offending antigen.

Measures to Control the Environment

A. Respiratory Allergies

1. Encourage the patient to modify his environment as much as he can, but not to the point of developing such a rigid regimen that his activities are unduly restricted.
2. *In the Hospital Unit*
   a. Restrict flowers and plants in patient's room, since they introduce antigens or irritating vapors to which he is sensitive.
   b. Avoid dry-dusting and mopping while the patient is in the room.
   c. Do not flourish sheets or plump pillows excessively during bed-making.
   d. Recommend cake face powder rather than loose powder; limit the use of talcums.
   e. Replace feather pillows with dacron or hypoallergenic-filled pillows.
   f. Attempt to find acceptable replacements for items removed from the patient's environment so that his surroundings will still be psychologically therapeutic.
3. *In the Home* (primarily the bedroom)
   Advise the patient as follows:
   a. Use nonallergenic materials for bedding (blankets, comforters, bedpad, pillows).
   b. Enclose the mattress and box springs in plastic airtight covers.
   c. Avoid keeping the window open at night if allergy is due to sensitivity to pollens and grasses.
   d. Replace carpeting with washable throw rugs; heavy draperies with easily laundered light curtains.
   e. Limit the number of dust-catching articles in the room (see Fig. 13-4).
4. *Room Air*
   Advise the patient as follows:
   a. Utilize a system of heating or cooling that can both humidify and filter the air.
   b. Avoid rapid changes in room temperature or variations in humidity that can aggravate or stimulate allergy symptoms.
   c. Weigh the benefits of air conditioning:
      (1) If it tends to circulate dust, it may be a source of irritation.
      (2) If it causes a marked change in temperature when the person moves from one part of the room to another, then it may be undesirable.
      (3) If it provides evenness of temperature, humidity, etc., it may be most desirable.
5. *Smoking*
   Encourage the patient as follows:
   a. Avoid smoking, since smoker is exposed to pollutants likely to aggravate the respiratory passages.
   b. Make an effort to avoid areas where others are smoking.

B. Dietary Allergies

Advise the patient as follows:

1. Recognize the difficulties in trying to determine which foods cause allergic reactions.
2. Develop a pattern of eliminating a certain food for a period of time.
   a. Keep a diary, indicating when food was eliminated from the diet.
   b. Record any allergic reactions or the fact that none occurred.
3. Begin with those foods commonly found to cause reactions—nuts, chocolate, milk, strawberries, eggs, etc.
4. Remember to note contents of prepared foods, canned foods, etc. for the specific ingredients one may wish to avoid.

5. In a restaurant, order those foods which are certain not to include the offending ingredients.

NOTE: Foods are considered a very rare cause of respiratory allergic symptoms.

C. *Contact Allergies*
Instruct patient as follows:
1. Exert extra effort to avoid household items likely to bring on allergic reactions.
   a. Use gloves to avoid skin contact with detergents, fabric dyes, strong soap powders, etc.
   b. Use liquid soaps rather than granules that might permeate the air breathed.
2. Avoid cosmetics unless they are known to be hypoallergenic.
3. Do not rub or scratch itchy skin. (Mild doses of barbiturate or tranquilizers may be necessary if this will assist the patient in such control.)
4. Eliminate items of wearing apparel that irritate the skin, such as those made of wool or nylon. Note that permanent press cottons may be a cause of dermatitis.
5. Avoid overexertion, which causes perspiration and itchiness.

Administration of Medications
1. Warn the patient that it may be dangerous for him to drive during the first few days of antihistaminic therapy, since these medications may cause drowsiness.
2. Advise patient to keep antihistamines out of reach of children—may cause serious accidental poisoning.
3. Utilize corticosteroids with caution because of side effects when administered over a long period of time.
   a. For short-term use, apply drops or ointment form of eye medication effective in relieving conjunctivitis and swollen eyelids.
   b. Avoid long-term use of eye corticosteroids because they may cause an increase in intraocular pressure.
4. When instilling nosedrops, have the patient lie on his back across the bed with his head hanging down; instill drops and have him remain in this position for 1 or 2 minutes; then have the patient turn over for another minute or 2 as though he were trying to look under the bed.
5. Caution the patient about the possibility of recurrent congestion when decongestants are used repeatedly; in such a situation, topical decongestants should be stopped.

BIBLIOGRAPHY

Books
Breneman JC. Basics of Food Allergy. Springfield, Charles C Thomas, 1978
Gershwin ME and Nagy SM Jr. Evaluation and Management of Allergic and Asthmatic Diseases. New York, Grune & Stratton, 1979
Middleton E Jr et al (eds). Allergy, Principles and Practice. St. Louis, CV Mosby, 1978
Parcel GS et al. Teaching Myself about Asthma. St. Louis, CV Mosby, 1979
Patterson R. Allergic Diseases 2nd ed. Philadelphia, JB Lippincott, 1980
Saunders NA and McFadden ER Jr. Asthma—an update: Disease-a-Month. Chicago, Yearbook Medical Publishers, 1978

Articles
General
Atarax (Hydroxyzine) for itching. Med Lett 1980 Jan; 22:4
Harmon AL and Harmon DC. Anaphylaxis—sudden death anytime. Nursing '80 1980 Oct; 10(10):40–43
Hill JS. Urticaria and angioedema. Postgrad Med 1979 April; 65(4):83–90
Hudgel DW and Madsen LA. Acute and chronic asthma: A guide to intervention. Am J Nurs 1980 Oct; 80(10):1791–1795
Mullarkey MF. Allergic and non-allergic rhinitis. Postgrad Med 1979 April; 65(4):97–107
Nalebuff DJ and Fadal RG. IgE screening for allergy. Res & Staff Physician 1980 June; (6):61–67
Parker C. Food allergies. Am J Nurs 1980 Feb; 80(2):262–265
Settipane GA et al. Adverse reactions to cromolyn. JAMA 1979 Feb 23; 241(8):811–813
Slavin RG. Diagnostic tests in clinical allergy. Postgrad Med 1980 March; 67(3):72–81
Webb DR. Drug allergy in clinical practice. Postgrad Med 1979 April; 65(4):62–72
Webber-Jones JE and Brant MK. Over-the-counter bronchodilators. Nursing '80 1980 Jan; 10(1):34–39

Asthma
Al-Bazzaz. Practical management of asthma in adults. Drug Ther 1980 April; 60(4):61–73

Bateman JRM and Clarke SW. Sudden death in asthma. Thorax 1979 Feb; 34(1):40–44
Caplin I. Choosing the right drugs for bronchial asthma. Mod Med 1979 June 15–30; 47(10):70–81
Chodoch A. Rational management of bronchial asthma. Arch Intern Med 1978 Sept; 138(9):1394–1397
Gerhard H and Schachter EN. Exercise-induced asthma. Postgrad Med 1980 March; 67(3):91–102
Golbert TM. Current concepts in food allergy. Am Fam Physician 1980 Aug; 22(2):95–96
Grieco MH et al. Clinical effect of aerosol triamcinolone acetonide in bronchial asthma. Arch Intern Med 1978 Sept; 138(9):1337–1341
I.V. dosage guidelines for theophylline products. FDA Drug Bulletin 1980 Feb; 10(1):4–6
Kriz RJ. Aerosol corticosteroids in the treatment of bronchial asthma. Arch Intern Med 1978 Sept; 138(9):1333
Middleton E Jr. A rational approach to asthma therapy. Postgrad Med 1980 March; 67(3):107–122
Norman PS. Asthma. Drug Therapy 1980 Jan; 10(1):127–138
Pence HL. Stinging insect allergy. Primary Care 1979 Sept; 6(3):587–596
Rands D. Anaphylactic reaction to desensitisation for allergic rhinitis and asthma. Br Med J 1980 Sept 27; 281(2):854
Rodman MJ. The drug interactions we all overlook (antiasthmatic). RN 1980 Nov; 43(11):41–43
Settipane GA et al. Adverse reactions to cromolyn. JAMA 1979 Feb 23; 241(8):811–813
Shim CS and Williams MH Jr. Evaluation of the severity of asthma: Patients versus physician. Am J Med 1980 Jan; 68(1):11–13
Tanphaichitr K. D-penicillamine-induced bronchial spasm. South Med J 1980 June; 73(6):788–790
Toogood J. Steroids in asthma. Lancet 1979 Dec 1; 2(8153):1185–1186
Vogt F. The incidence of oral candidiasis with use of inhaled corticosteroids. Ann Allergy 1979 Oct; 43(4):205–210

Agencies
Allergy Information Association, 3 Powburn Pl, Weston, Ontario, M9R2C5 Canada
Asthma and Allergy Foundation of America, 19 W 44th Street, New York, N.Y. 10036
National Institute of Allergy and Infectious Diseases, National Institute of Health, Bethesda, Md 20205

METABOLIC AND ENDOCRINE DISORDERS

14

1 DISORDERS OF THE THYROID GLAND

2 DISORDERS OF THE PARATHYROID GLANDS

3 DIABETES MELLITUS (PANCREATIC DISORDERS)

4 DISORDERS OF THE ADRENAL GLANDS

5 DISORDERS OF THE PITUITARY GLAND

6 DISORDERS OF PURINE METABOLISM

1 DISORDERS OF THE THYROID GLAND

THE THYROID GLAND AND TESTS OF THYROID FUNCTION

Physiology

1. The thyroid gland affects the rate at which all tissues metabolize.
   a. Speed of chemical reactions
   b. Volume of oxygen consumed
   c. Amount of heat produced

2. The stimulating effect is through the production and distribution of 2 hormones:
   a. Levothyroxine (T_4)—contains 4 iodine atoms; maintains body's metabolism in a steady state; it is believed that T_1 serves as a precursor of T_3.
   b. Triiodothyronine (T_3)—contains 3 iodine atoms; is approximately 5 times as potent as thyroxine;

629

has a more rapid metabolic action and utilization than thyroxine. Most conversion of T_4 to T_3 occurs at the cellular level in the periphery. Some T_3 is produced in the thyroid gland.

Diagnostic Evaluation

See also Physical Assessment, p. 27

A. *Radioiodine (^{131}I) (^{99m}Tc)*

1. ^{131}I *Uptake*
   a. A solution of sodium iodide-131 is administered orally to the fasting patient.
   b. After a prescribed interval (anywhere from 2 to 48 hours, but frequently by 24 hours), measurements are taken with a scintillator of radioactive counts per minute that are detected above the isthmus of the thyroid gland.
   c. Normal thyroid will remove 15–50% of the iodine from the bloodstream.
   d. Hyperthyroidism may result in the removal of as much as 90% of the iodine from the bloodstream.
2. *Thyroidal Iodide Clearance*
   a. Radioiodine clearance test measures the amount of circulating blood that is completely cleared of iodide per unit of time.
   b. Radioiodine is injected intravenously; radioactivity over the thyroid gland is measured continuously for 30–60 minutes—total amount of ^{131}I concentrated in the gland per minute is computed.
   c. Also, plasma ^{131}I content is measured in samples of blood collected 45–70 minutes after injection; these values are averaged.
   d. Thyroid ^{131}I divided by the mean plasma ^{131}I equals thyroid clearance, i.e., ml. of plasma cleared of iodide per minute.
   e. Normal   25 ml./min.
      Hyperthyroidism   250 ml./min.
      Hypothyroidism   1.6 ml./min.
3. ^{131}I *Excretion*
   a. Urinary output of radioiodine is measured during 6 hour and 24-hour periods after ingestion.
   b. Normal   40–80% of ingested
                                    iodine in 24 hours
      Hyperthyroidism   less than 40%
      Hypothyroidism   greater than 80%
4. *Thyroid "Scan"* ^{131}I
   a. Patient ingests sodium iodide-131 and is scanned the next day; if medium is given intravenously, patient may be scanned within ½ to 1 hour.
   b. Patient is supine; the detector head of the scintillation camera with a pinhole collimeter is centered over the patient's neck.
   c. The thyroid images from the oscilloscope of the camera are recorded on film; color adds dimension.
   d. A decrease in ^{131}I uptake in a particular area of the thyroid is considered suggestive of malignancy.
5. *Thyroid "Scan"* ^{99m}Tc
   a. Patient is given an intravenous injection of sodium pertechnetate.
   b. A scintillator electromechanically maps the activity in the scanned area to produce a scintogram.
   c. This simple procedure facilitates the diagnosis of goiterous changes, cold and hot nodules, cystic degeneration, and thyroid malignancy.
6. *Triiodothyronine (T_3) Suppression Test*
   a. Measure 24-hour radioactive iodine uptake.
   b. Place patient on T_3 for 7 days.
   c. Again measure 24-hour radioactive iodine uptake.
   d. Normal: Suppression to a radioactive iodine up-

take below 20% at 24 hours (half original value).
   Graves disease: No suppression.

B. *Serum Thyroxine (T_4)*
1. Normal values 4.5–11.5 µ g/dl.
2. Elevated values found with estrogens and pregnancy.
3. T_4 is bound mainly to thyroxine-binding globulin and prealbumin.

C. T_3 *Resin Uptake*
1. Is an indirect measure of thyroid function based on the available protein-binding sites in a serum sample which can bind to radioactive T_3.
2. The radioactive triiodothyronine is added to the serum sample in the test tube.
3. The effect of estrogen and pregnancy is to produce an increase in binding sites, causing a lowered percentage of binding by the available thyroid hormones.
4. Rates
   a. Normal binding: 25–35%
   b. High T_3 is associated with hyperthyroidism
   c. Low T_3 is associated with hypothyroidism
5. This test is often used in conjunction with B. Serum Thyroxine (T_4).
6. Results may be altered if this patient has been taking estrogens, androgens, salicylates, or phenytoin.

D. *Thyrotropin Radioimmunoassay (TSH)*
1. This is done in conjunction with the RAI test.
2. In patients with primary hypothyroidism, TSH levels are elevated.
3. In patients with hyperthyroidism, TSH levels are low.

E. *Thyrotropin-releasing Hormone (TRH)*
1. Have patient fast overnight.
2. Fifteen minutes prior to TRH injection, draw a blood specimen.
3. Physician injects into arterial system 500 mcg. synthetic TRH; draw blood specimen for TSH (thyroid-stimulating hormone).
4. Draw blood specimens at 15, 30, 45, 60, 90, and 120 minutes.

F. *Protein-bound (PBI)*—A conjugated molecule formed when thyroxine becomes attached to certain plasma-protein fractions.

1. A reasonably accurate index of thyroid function is the concentration of PBI in the blood.
2. Normal values: 3.5–8.0 µg. (0.0035–0.0080 mg./100 ml. of plasma).
   a. Over 8.0—thyroid overactivity
   b. Under 3.5—hypothyroidism

> **NURSING ALERT:** Certain factors impair the PBI test:
> 1. Use of iodine skin antiseptic at venipuncture site
> 2. Ingestion of drugs or administration of dyes containing iodine, such as:
>   a. Expectorants, cough syrups, etc.
>   b. Dyes used in arteriogram, bronchogram, etc.
> 3. Mercurial diuretics, estrogens, sulfonamides, steroids, phenylbutazone, thiocyanates
> 4. Pregnancy

3. In many health-care facilities, this test has been replaced by tests for serum T_3 and serum T_4.

HYPOTHYROIDISM

Hypothyroidism may be classified as primary, secondary, or tertiary. *Primary hypothyroidism* is a condition resulting from the inability of the thyroid gland to secrete a sufficient amount of hormone. *Secondary hypothyroidism* is caused by a failure of the pituitary gland to secrete an adequate amount of TSH (thyroid-stimulating hormone). *Tertiary hypothyroidism* results from failure of the hypothalamus to release thyroid-releasing hormone (TRH).

Cretinism is a condition in which a person is born with a thyroid deficiency. The mother may have a similar deficiency.

Causes

(Primary Hypothyroidism)
1. Prior surgery or radioactive iodine therapy
2. Idiopathic
3. Hashimoto's thyroiditis

Clinical Manifestations

1. Temperature and pulse become subnormal, wants heat turned up in house.
2. Patient begins to gain weight.
3. Skin becomes thickened and dry.
4. The hair thins and falls out.
5. Menorrhagia may develop.
6. Blood pressure is low; feet are cold.
7. Facial expression becomes stolid and mask-like; later, facial bloating and pallor develop.
8. Complaint of fatigue is most common.
9. Mental processes become dulled.
10. Neurological signs are manifested (polyneuropathy, cerebellar ataxia); muscle aches or weakness, clumsiness.
11. Lethargy, poor memory.
12. Severe constipation.
13. There may be a tendency to rapid development of arteriosclerosis.

Diagnostic Evaluation

1. Total serum thyroxine level; low levels are indicative of hypothyroidism.
2. T_3 (radioactive triiodothyronine uptake); low value suggests hypothyroidism.
3. Thyroid-stimulating hormone; elevated level suggests hypothyroidism.
4. Slow reflex return suggests hypothyroidism.
5. Elevation of serum cholesterol.
6. ECG—sinus bradycardia, low-voltage of QRS complexes, and flat or inverted T waves.
7. Check patient's history for previous treatment with radioactive iodine—some of these patients become hypothyroid after such treatment.
8. Complete physical examination.

Treatment and Nursing Management

OBJECTIVE: to restore a normal metabolic state (euthyroid) as rapidly, safely, and inexpensively as possible.
1. Administer thyroid hormone: levothyroxine (Synthroid, Levothroid), thyroglobulin (Proloid), liotrix (Euthyroid, Thyrolar). Give once a day.
2. Monitor patient carefully to anticipate such effects of treatment as:
   a. Diuresis, decreased puffiness

b. Improved reflexes and muscle tone
   c. Accelerated pulse rate
   d. A slightly higher level of total serum thyroxine

ADVANCED HYPOTHYROIDISM

A. *Effects*
1. May lead to *myxedema coma,* often preceded by hypothermia.
2. Causes increased susceptibility to all hypnotic and sedative drugs.
3. Survival rate is 50%.

B. *Clinical Manifestations*
   Hypotension, unresponsiveness, bradycardia, hypoventilation, hyponatremia, possible convulsions, hypothermia (cerebral hypoxia)

C. *Objectives of Treatment and Nursing Management*
1. *To maintain vital functions with supportive therapy.*
   a. Measure arterial blood gases to determine CO_2 retention.
   b. Provide assisted ventilation if needed to combat hypoventilation.
   c. Even though hypothermia exists, do not apply external heat, since the resulting increased oxygen requirements and decreased peripheral vascular tone may compound the existing cardiac failure.
   d. Administer fluids cautiously even though hyponatremia is present.
   e. Give glucose in concentrated amounts to prevent fluid overload if hypoglycemia is in evidence.
2. *To replace thyroid hormone in order to assist in achieving a euthyroid state.*
   a. Because triiodothyronine acts more quickly than thyroxine, give this initially; if patient is unconscious, give via stomach tube.
   b. Administer sodium levothyroxine (Synthroid) parenterally (until consciousness is restored) to restore thyroxine level; continue daily.
   c. Later, continue patient on oral thyroid hormone therapy.
   d. Recognize that with rapid administration of thyroid hormone, plasma thyroxine levels may initiate adrenal insufficiency—hence, steroid therapy may be initiated.
3. *To recognize precipitating factors and avoid them so that further cardiovascular damage is prevented.*
   a. Treat initiating factors such as infection, stress from trauma.
   b. Prevent chilling to avoid increasing metabolic rate, which in turn places strain on the heart.
      Provide bed socks, bed jacket, warm environment.
   c. Recognize sensitivity of patient to hypnotics and tranquilizers; use in small doses and provide effective observation.
   d. Note that patient is usually disturbed by his mental and physical changes; be alert for signs of depression. Be compassionate and understanding.
4. *To initiate comfort measures and promote good care.*
   a. Apply lubricant to the skin since it is usually dry and scaly.
   b. Observe for pressure areas and initiate measures to stimulate circulation to these areas.
   c. Arrange furniture to prevent patient's bumping

into it, since he bruises easily because of increased capillary fragility.
5. *To encourage proper fluid and nutritional intake.*
   a. Offer fluids frequently and include dietary roughage to prevent constipation.

b. Administer stool softeners if necessary.
c. Discourage straining at stool because of increased strain on the heart.
d. Serve attractive low calorie meals; this patient is usually overweight, although his appetite is poor.

HYPERTHYROIDISM

Hyperthyroidism (diffuse toxic goiter) is excessive activity of the thyroid gland.

Incidence

More common in women than in men; occurs in about 2% of the female population.

Types

1. Graves' disease (most prevalent)—diffuse hyperfunction of the thyroid gland associated with ophthalmopathy; most common in younger women; may subside spontaneously.
2. Toxic nodular goiter (single or multiple)—more common in older females with preexisting goiter; will continue to be overactive unless eradicated or kept under suppressive therapy.

Etiology

1. Unknown; immunologic overtones
2. Possible causes
   a. Thyroid-stimulating antibody (TSAb)(formerly LATS—long-acting thyroid stimulator) correlates very closely with the clinical course of Graves' disease.
   b. TSAb, an immunoglobulin found in the blood of patients with Graves' disease, is capable of reacting with the receptor for TSH on the thyroid plasma membrane and stimulating glandular function.
   c. May appear after an emotional shock, infection, or emotional stress
   d. Genetic predisposition, female sex
   e. B and T lymphocytes (immunologic factors)

Clinical Manifestations

1. Single or multiple adenomas
2. Nervousness, emotional hyperexcitability, irritability, apprehension
3. Difficulty in sitting quietly
4. Rapid pulse, at rest as well as on exertion (ranges between 90 and 160); palpitation is evident
5. Low heat tolerance; profuse perspiration; flushed skin (e.g., hands may be warm, soft, moist)
6. Fine tremor of hands; change in bowel habits—constipation or diarrhea
7. Bulging eyes (exophthalmos)—startled expression
8. Increased appetite-progressive weight loss
9. Muscle fatigability and weakness; amenorrhea
10. Atrial fibrillation possible (Cardiac decompensation is common in elderly patients.)

Diagnostic Evaluation

1. PBI
2. Serum thyronine ⎫ if elevated—hyperthyroidism is suspected
3. T$_3$ resin uptake ⎭

Clinical Course

1. Mild, characterized by remissions and exacerbations.
2. In rare instances, it may progress relentlessly—leading to emaciation, extreme nervousness, delirium, disorientation, and eventual death.

Immediate Treatment

1. Hospitalize patient only if "thyroid storm" (see p. 634) or other complications, such as heart failure, are impending.
2. Administer sedatives such as phenobarbital or tranquilizers such as chlordiazepoxide (Librium) to combat nervousness, hyperactivity, and irritability.
3. Give vitamin supplements to offset demands of appetite which may continue after hyperthyroidism is controlled.
4. Administer digitalis if heart failure or atrial fibrillation occurs.
5. Give propranolol for sinus tachycardia and other supraventricular arrhythmias.

Other Modalities of Treatment

1. General Considerations
   a. Types of treatment—pharmacology, radiation, and surgery.
   b. Treatment depends on causes, age of patient, severity of disease, and complications.
2. *According to Causes*
   a. Remission of hyperthyroidism (Graves' Disease) occurs spontaneously within 1–2 years; however, relapse can be expected in half of the patients. All 3 forms of therapy are appropriate.
   b. Nodular toxic goiter—excessive amounts of thyroid hormone secreted. Surgery or radioiodine is preferred.
   c. Thyroid carcinoma. Surgery or radiation.
3. *According to Age of Patient*
   a. Radioiodine therapy may be used in all patients, regardless of age, when other forms of therapy are contraindicated.
   b. Use radioiodine in older patients for whom surgery is contraindicated.
4. *According to Severity* Administer drug therapy before proceeding with radioiodine or surgery.
5. *According to Patient Preference*
   a. Radioiodine or surgery is suggested to patient who does not take medication regularly.
   b. Surgery is recommended to those who prefer it.

Pharmacotherapy—Drugs That Inhibit Hormone Formation

OBJECTIVE: to bring the metabolic rate to normal as soon as possible and maintain it at this level.

Anticipated Results
1. Diagnosis can be confirmed if patient responds to antithyroid therapy.
2. Autonomic nervous system is brought into balance and patient is more comfortable.

3. Opportunity is provided for getting to know the patient.

A. *Thionamides*

1. Preparations
   a. Propylthiouracil
   b. Methimazole (Tapazole)
      (1) Carbimazole—a derivative of methimazole used in Europe.
2. Action.
   a. Depresses the synthesis of thyroid hormone by inhibiting peroxidase.
   b. It has been standard practice to give these medications in divided daily doses (every 8 hours); experimental evidence appears to indicate that once-a-day dosage is effective for 24 hours or longer. Patient compliance is better with this latter medication schedule.
3. Assessment and duration of treatment determined by clinical criteria
   a. Observe clinical course—thyroid gland usually gets smaller.
   b. Measure T_4 and T_3 uptake to determine adequacy of dose.
   c. Continue treatment until patient becomes clinically euthyroid; this varies from 3 months to 1 to 2 years; if euthyroidism cannot be maintained without therapy, then another form of therapy (i.e., RAI or surgery) should be recommended.
   d. Gradually withdraw therapy to prevent exacerbation.
   e. For relapses, recommend radioiodine or surgery.
4. Toxicity
   a. Agranulocytosis is a most serious toxic condition, occurring with a sudden onset—therefore, patient should be apprized of this possibility and urged to report any signs of infection such as fever, sore throat, upper respiratory infection.
   b. Skin rashes, fever, urticaria, granulopenia, inflammation of the salivary glands are other possible side effects.
   c. Substitute an alternate drug if there are toxic manifestations.

Pharmacotherapy—Drugs That Control Peripheral Manifestations of Hyperthyroidism

Propranolol (Inderal)

1. Acts as a beta-adrenergic blocking agent
2. Abolishes tachycardia, tremor, excess sweating, nervousness
3. Controls hyperthyroid symptoms until antithyroid drugs or radioiodine can take effect

Radioactive Iodine

1. Action
   a. Limits secretion of thyroid hormone by damaging and destroying thyroid tissue.
   b. Control dosage so that hypothyroidism does not occur.
2. Advantages and Disadvantages
   a. Chief advantage of radioiodine over thionamides is that a lasting remission can be achieved.
   b. Chief disadvantage is that permanent hypothyroidism can be produced in patients treated with radioiodine.
3. Considerations in Use
   a. Radiation thyroiditis, a transient exacerbation of hyperthyroidism, may occur as a result of leakage of thyroid hormone into the circulation from damaged follicles.
   b. Iodide should not be given prior to radioiodine, since it interferes with the uptake of ^{131}I.
   c. Vigilance is required during treatment to detect occurrence of hypothyroidism.

Psychotherapy

1. Greater emphasis is being placed on the effect that psychogenic factors have on the severity of this disease.
2. A determination needs to be made in caring for each patient about whether psychotherapy would be of value in preventing exacerbations.

Surgery

This modality has become progressively less popular in treating hyperthyroidism because:
1. It is expensive.
2. It requires hospitalization and loss of time from work.
3. It carries risk of hypoparathyroidism and recurrent laryngeal nerve paralysis.

Surgery is an effective treatment modality in selected patients; those with very large goiters, or those for whom the use of radioiodine or thionamides is contraindicated.

A. *Subtotal Thyroidectomy*

Effective in treating hyperthyroidism; involves removal of most of the thyroid gland.

B. *Preparation for Surgery*

1. Patient must be euthyroid at time of surgery.
2. Administer thionamides to control hyperthyroidism.
3. Give iodide to increase firmness of thyroid gland and reduce its vascularity.

> **NURSING ALERT:** Observe patient for evidence of iodine toxicity—swelling of buccal mucosa, excessive salivation, coryza, skin eruptions. If these occur, discontinue iodides.

C. *Complications*

1. Damage to recurrent laryngeal nerve may occur (1–4%).
   a. Unilateral damage—results in minimal voice change.
   b. Bilateral damage—serious airway obstruction develops.
2. Hypothyroidism
   Occurs in 5% of patients in first postoperative year; increases at rate of 2–3%/year
3. Hypoparathyroidism
   a. About 4% occurrence.
   b. Usually is mild and transient.
   c. Requires calcium supplements intravenously and orally when more severe.

D. *Nursing Management*—see page 634.

OPHTHALMOPATHY IN HYPERTHYROIDISM

Exophthalmos is abnormal protrusion of the eyeball, probably due to an autoimmune phenomenon.

Proptosis—a forward bulging (displacement) of the eye.

Ophthalmoplegia—paralysis of the eye muscle.

OBJECTIVE: to protect eyes from irritation.

A. *Mild*

1. Recommend wearing sunglasses.
2. Instill methylcellulose eyedrops 0.5–1% (Tearisol) for comfort; relief from pain and burning.
3. Advise the patient to elevate his head while sleeping to improve drainage.

B. *Rapidly Progressive or Severe* (chemosis, conjunctivitis, proptosis, visual impairment)

1. Tarsorrhaphy (suturing eyelids together) may be required to extend lid when proptosis is so marked that lid does not close during sleep. Operation will prevent corneal ulceration.
2. Administer corticosteroids in high doses to help arrest rapid progression of exophthalmos; with improvement, reduce dose.

C. *Muscle Surgery*

1. Correction of imbalance of extraocular muscles.
2. Lysis of adhesions.

D. *Orbital Decompression Procedures*

Performed only if vision is threatened.

1. Decompression of orbit into ethmoid sinus and maxillary antrum (Ogura procedure).
2. Removal of lateral orbital wall (Krönleim operation).
3. Decompression of orbit into cranial cavity (Naffziger operation).

THYROTOXICOSIS LEADING TO THYROID STORM

Thyroid storm (also called thyroid crisis) is characterized by tachycardia, vasomotor activity, agitation, and, at times, delirium and heart failure. It is assumed to result from a marked increase in beta-adrenergic effect.

Predisposing Factors

1. Decompensation of hyperthyroid state occurs spontaneously.
2. May be precipitated by infection (pneumonia, appendicitis, pharyngitis, cystitis); surgical procedures (thyroidectomy, cesarean section, appendectomy); minor procedures (dental extractions, forceps delivery); insulin reaction; pulmonary embolism; palpation of thyroid gland; and even fear.
3. Crisis may also be precipitated by inadequate surgical preoperative preparation (unrecognized hyperthyroidism).

Clinical Manifestations

1. Hyperpyrexia, diarrhea, dehydration, tachycardia, arrhythmias (Fig. 14-1)
2. Extreme irritation; delirium
3. Coma, leading to shock and death

Objectives of Treatment and Nursing Management

A. *To control synthesis and release of thyroid hormone.*

1. Administer sodium iodide intravenously—inhibits release of hormone from thyroid.
2. Give methimazole or propylthiouracil orally or by nasogastric tube to prevent accumulation of hormone stores.

B. *To diminish metabolic effects of thyroid agents and to reverse peripheral effects of hyperthyroidism.*

Administer propranolol, reserpine, or guanethidine.

C. *To restore and maintain vital functions.*

1. Give steroids because of possibility of a relative adrenal insufficiency state.
2. Administer fluids, electrolytes, and vasopressor agents to treat dehydration, electrolyte imbalance, and hypotension.
3. Control agitation with intravenous barbiturates.
4. Lower the temperature with hypothermia blanket or cooling mattress and salicylates.
5. Try phenothiazines in large doses for hyperpyrexia, but watch for hypotension.
6. Sustain nutritional requirements with glucose intravenously; administer vitamin B.
7. Guard against infection; treat if infection is likely.

MEDICAL AND NURSING MANAGEMENT OF THE PATIENT UNDERGOING THYROIDECTOMY

Preoperative Objectives

A. *To provide a restful and therapeutic environment.*

1. Place the patient in a unit which is away from disturbing sights, very ill patients, and noisy elevators or kitchens.
2. Provide, if possible, a pleasant window view.
3. Suggest radio music programs rather than exciting soap operas or movies.
4. Restrict visitors who may upset the patient with disturbing conversation or boisterous tendencies.
5. Administer soothing back massage at prescribed rest times during the day; draw the blinds for nap times.
6. Be selective in placing a suitable roommate with the patient (preferably one who is convalescing).
7. Gain the confidence of the patient and attempt to uncover anything that might cause aggravation or unhappiness; if a disturbance exists, it could thwart treatment efforts.

B. *To regulate his nutritional intake.*

1. Order an ample diet of carbohydrate and protein foods.
2. Recognize this patient's physiological need for a daily caloric intake of 4000–5000 calories—because of increased metabolic activity and rapid depletion of glycogen reserves.
3. Provide supplementary vitamins, particularly thiamine chloride and ascorbic acid.
4. Avoid tea or coffee because of their stimulating effects.

C. *To study the exact nature of the endocrine problem by supporting the patient undergoing various diagnostic tests.*

1. Explain the purpose and requirements of each prescribed test.
2. Inform the patient and visitors of safeguards required during radioisotope tests.
3. Remind the patient that he must remain in his room until tests are completed.

D. *To prepare the patient for surgery.*

1. Shave the upper chest, neck (bedline to bedline), up to chin edge.
2. Make a special effort to ensure that this patient has a good night's rest preceding surgery.
3. Explain to the patient that speaking is to be minimized immediately postoperatively and that oxygen may be administered to facilitate breathing.

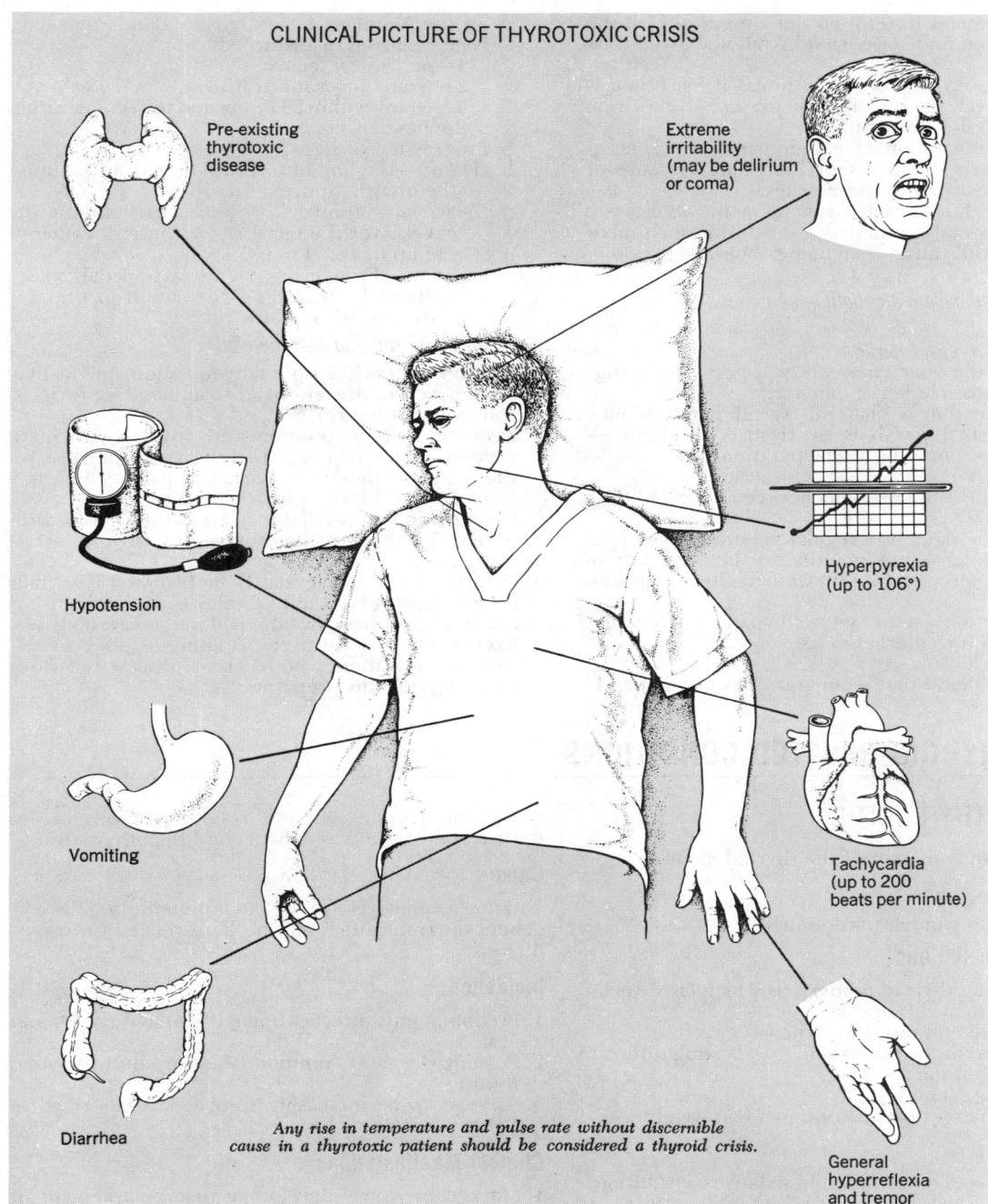

CLINICAL PICTURE OF THYROTOXIC CRISIS

Pre-existing thyrotoxic disease

Extreme irritability (may be delirium or coma)

Hypotension

Hyperpyrexia (up to 106°)

Vomiting

Tachycardia (up to 200 beats per minute)

Diarrhea

Any rise in temperature and pulse rate without discernible cause in a thyrotoxic patient should be considered a thyroid crisis.

General hyperreflexia and tremor

FIGURE 14-1. *Thyrotoxic crisis. (From Hospital Medicine 3, No. 1:39, by permission; © Hospital Publications, Inc.)*

4. Tell the patient that postoperatively, fluids may be given intravenously to maintain fluid, electrolyte, and nutritional needs; glucose may also be given intravenously in the hours before the administration of anesthesia.

5. Proceed with usual preoperative preparation (see p. 80).

Postoperative Objectives

A. *To provide optimum immediate postoperative care in order to avoid complications.*

1. Move the patient carefully; provide adequate support to the head, so that no tension is placed on the sutures.

2. Place the patient in semi-Fowler's position with the head elevated and supported by pillows; avoid flexion of neck.
3. Administer oxygen for a few hours if breathing is labored; check the infusion for prescribed flow rate and smooth flow into patient.
4. Avoid administration of epinephrine, norepinephrine, cholinergic depressants (atropine) because of patient's sensitivity to these drugs.
5. Discontinue antithyroid drugs as a metabolic rate closer to normal is attained (to continue such medication might cause a hypometabolism—hypothyroidism).

B. *To assess the patient's condition as he emerges from anesthesia.*
1. *Damage of laryngeal nerve*
   a. Observe for hoarseness or "whispery" voice suggesting possible nerve damage.
   b. Recognize that a bilateral flaccid paralysis may lead to cord paralysis → closure of glottis → suffocation, months after operation.
2. *Hemorrhage*
   a. Be alert for this possibility between 12 to 24 hours postoperatively.
   b. Watch for signs of irregular breathing, swelling, and choking—signs pointing to the possibility of hemorrhage (see p. 130) and tracheal compression.
   c. Keep a tracheostomy set in the patient's room for 48 hours for emergency use.
3. *Tetany*
   a. The likelihood that tetany may develop depends on the number of parathyroid glands that have been removed or disturbed:
      1—no clinical tetany
      2—tetany mild and transient
      4—tetany within 24 hours and worsening within the next 24 hours
   b. Progression of signs.
      (1) *First*—tingling of toes and fingers and around the mouth; apprehension
      (2) *Second*—positive Chvostek's sign (tapping the cheek over the facial nerve causes a twitch of the lip or facial muscles)
      (3) *Third*—Trousseau's sign (carpopedal spasm induced by occluding circulation in the arm with a blood pressure cuff)

C. *Medical and Nursing Management*
1. Position patient for optimal ventilation; pillow may be removed to prevent head from bending forward and compressing trachea.
2. Keep siderails in position and position patient to prevent injury if a seizure occurs; do not use restraints since they only aggravate patient and may result in muscle strain or fractures.
3. Have equipment available to treat respiratory difficulties; provide tracheostomy and cardiac arrest equipment.
4. Determine calcium levels: If in 48 hours level falls below 7½ mg./100 ml. (3mEq.), replacement of calcium (gluconate, lactate) is done intravenously.
5. Exert caution in intravenous administration of calcium to the patient who has renal disease or who is receiving digitalis preparations.

OTHER THYROID-RELATED CONDITIONS

SUBACUTE THYROIDITIS

Thyroiditis is inflammation of the thyroid gland.

Incidence

Affects younger women predominantly.

Clinical Manifestations

1. Pain, swelling, thyroid tenderness which lasts weeks or months, then disappears
2. Temperature elevation, sore throat
3. Pain referred to the ear, making swallowing difficult and uncomfortable
4. Fever, malaise, chills
5. Irritability, nervousness, insomnia, and weight loss

Management

1. Administer analgesics and mild sedatives; encourage activities that will promote psychosocial comfort.
2. Patient may be placed on thyroid medications to maintain a normal level of circulating thyroid hormone.
3. Steroids may be administered in active inflammatory stage.

LYMPHOCYTIC THYROIDITIS (HASHIMOTO'S THYROIDITIS)

Lymphocytic thyroiditis (Hashimoto's thyroiditis) is a progressive disease of the thyroid gland caused by infiltration of lymphocytes and resulting in progressive destruction of the parenchyma and hypothyroidism.

Cause

Unknown. Believed to be an autoimmune disease, genetically transmitted and perhaps related to Graves' disease.

Incidence

1. Predominantly affects women (95%) in their 40s and 50s.
2. Possibly the most common cause of adult hypothyroidism.
3. Appears to be increasing since it was described in 1912.

Clinical Manifestations

1. Marked by slowly developing firm enlargement of the thyroid gland.
2. Usually no gross nodules.
3. Basal metabolic rate usually low.
4. Normal or high concentration of protein-bound iodine.

Diagnostic Testing

1. 24-hour radioactive iodine (RAI) uptake
2. Thyroid scan
3. Resin T_3 uptake determination
4. Thyroid needle biopsy

Treatment and Nursing Management

1. Patient should be placed on thyroid medications to maintain a normal level of circulating thyroid hormone; this is done to suppress production of thyrotropin, to prevent enlargement of the thyroid and/or to maintain a euthyroid state.
2. Propranolol is often prescribed to control symptoms until thyrotoxicosis remits.
3. Firm nodular thyroid enlargement may at times be associated with tracheal compression, cough, hoarseness. Resection of isthmus can produce relief of symptoms.

CANCER OF THE THYROID

Incidence

1. It has been estimated that of the thyroid lumps which occur in 40,000 out of 1,000,000 persons in any one year, only 25 will be cancerous; this is a relatively rare disease.
2. It occurs twice as frequently in females as in males and more frequently in whites than in blacks; incidence increases with age.
3. It appears well established that an association exists between external radiation to the head and neck in infancy and childhood and subsequent development of thyroid carcinoma. (Between 1949–1960 radiation therapy was often given to shrink enlarged tonsil and adenoid tissue, to treat acne, or to reduce an enlarged thymus.)
    The American Thyroid Association emphasizes that these individuals should:
    a. Consult a physician
    b. Request an isotope thyroid scan as part of the evaluation
    c. Submit to surgical thyroidectomy or take thyroid hormones if abnormalities of the gland are present
    d. Continue with annual checkups if all is normal

Types

1. Papillary and well-differentiated adenocarcinoma (most common)
    a. Growth is slow and spread is confined to lymph nodes that surround thyroid area.
    b. Cure rate is excellent after removal of involved areas.
2. Follicular (rapidly growing, widely metastasizing type)
    a. Occurs predominantly in middle-aged and elderly persons.
    b. Brief encouraging response may occur with x-ray irradiation.
    c. Progression of disease is rapid; high mortality rate.
3. Parafollicular: Medullary thyroid carcinoma (MTC)
    a. Rare, inheritable type of thyroid malignancy which can be detected early by a radioimmunoassay for the hormone, calcitonin.
    b. Screening of familial MTC suspects is done by measuring circulating plasma calcitonin levels.

Diagnosis

1. History and physical examination are important.
2. If a scan is to be done, ^{99m}Technetium pertechnetate is preferred since it delivers a much lower radiation than ^{131}I.
3. ^{123}Iodine, when purified (and when it becomes available), will probably be preferred over ^{131}I and ^{99m}Tc because of even lower radiation.
4. Needle biopsy is recommended only for the very skilled performer and for the experienced pathologist.
5. Surgical exploration.

Treatment

1. Surgical removal is extensive, as required.
2. Thyroid replacement.
    a. Thyroid hormone is administered to suppress secretion of TSH.
    b. Such treatment is continued indefinitely and requires annual checkups.
3. For unresectable cancer, patient is referred to a thyroid specialist for consideration of treatment with ^{131}I, chemotherapy, or radiation therapy.

2   DISORDERS OF THE PARATHYROID GLANDS

THE PARATHYROID GLANDS

The *parathyroid glands* are small, bean-sized structures embedded in the posterior section of the thyroid gland.

Functions

1. Produce, store and secrete parathormone
2. Increase plasma calcium ions by acting on:
    a. The kidney—to decrease elimination of calcium ions in the urine
    b. The gastrointestinal tract—to increase absorption of calcium ions from chyme
    c. Bone—to increase its contributions of calcium ions to the plasma

HYPERPARATHYROIDISM

Hyperparathyroidism is overactivity of the parathyroids.

Cause

An overgrowth of parathyroid glands.

Clinical Manifestations

1. Decalcification of bones
    a. Skeletal pain, backache, pain on weight-bearing,

pathologic fractures, deformities, formation of bony cysts
b. Formation of bone tumors—overgrowth of osteoclasts
2. Formation of calcium-containing stones in the kidneys
3. Depression of neuromuscular apparatus
a. The patient may trip, drop objects, show general fatigue, and experience blurring of the mind
b. Cardiac standstill may result

Diagnostic Evaluation

1. Persistently elevated serum calcium (11 mg./100 ml.); test must be taken 3 times to determine consistency of results
2. Exclusion of all other causes of hypercalcemia—malignancy, vitamin D excess, multiple myeloma, sarcoidosis, milk-alkali syndrome, drugs such as thiazides, Cushing's disease, hyperthyroidism
3. Skeletal changes—revealed by x-ray
4. Diagnosis often extremely difficult (complications may occur before this condition is diagnosed).
5. Cineradiography will disclose parathyroid tumors more readily then x-ray

Complications

1. Kidney disturbances
a. Formation of renal stones
b. Calcification of kidney parenchyma
c. Renal shutdown
2. Gastrointestinal complications
Ulceration of upper gastrointestinal tract (stomach, duodenum) leading to hemorrhage and perforation
3. Skeletal problems
a. Simple demineralization
b. Cysts and fibrosis of marrow—leading to fractures
c. Collapse of vertebral bodies and fractures of the ribs

Objectives of Treatment and Nursing Management

A. *To offset the likelihood of impending complications.*

1. Provide adequate hydration—administer water, glucose, and electrolytes by mouth or intravenously.

NURSING ALERT: A low specific gravity for urine does not necessarily mean adequate hydration.

2. Avoid calcium and alkalies in the diet to prevent stone formation and renal calcification. Obtain daily serum calcium and BUN determinations.
3. Administer diuretic—furosemide (Lasix).

NURSING ALERT: Thiazide diuretics should not be used in the patient with hyperparathyroidism since they decrease the renal excretion of calcium, thereby causing hypercalcemia.

4. Administer phosphate therapy as prescribed to control hypercalcemia.

Obtain daily serum calcium and BUN determinations.
5. Limit operative procedures until primary metabolic disorder is treated.
a. A rising serum calcium level may indicate increasing dehydration—impending crisis.
b. A falling serum calcium indicates dehydration is being corrected.

B. *To treat complications as they arise.*

1. For ureteral stone—cystoscopic manipulation
2. For urinary tract infection—antimicrobials, high fluid input
3. For upper gastrointestinal ulceration—aluminum hydroxide and proteins other than milk
4. For ulcer hemorrhage not stopped by conservative measures—surgical plication
5. For fractures—treatment for vertebral body fractures (see p. 772)
—strapping for broken ribs
—fixation of other long bones
—continued hydration of patient
—earliest mobilization of fracture areas

C. *To operate and remove parathyroid tissue.*

This is resorted to when diagnosis is established and clinical condition warrants definitive treatment.

D. *To develop priorities of care in the postoperative phase that will control possible concomitant complications.*

1. Assess fluid input and output.
2. Recognize that the patient will retain some fluid.
a. This will be manifested by a low urinary output.
b. Therefore, avoid overhydration for first day or two.
3. Avoid giving calcium until nature of the patient's calcium level is determined.
a. To verify success of operation.
b. To observe level to which calcium falls and the rate at which it falls.
(1) If calcium level fails to fall, surgery was inadequate.
(2) If calcium level falls somewhat but not to normal and then rises, surgery was inadequate.
c. To determine patient's skeletal deficit and need for additional calcium.
4. Evaluate signs and symptoms which may lead to tetany.
a. Observe calcium levels—if well below normal and if decline continues into the 2nd week, the skeletal system is absorbing calcium.
If some involvement was noted preoperatively (elevated alkaline phosphatase level), calcium should be administered.
b. Administer calcium—usually lactate or gluconate. When gastrointestinal tract cannot absorb large amount, administer intramuscularly as gluconate, or intravenously in emergency situation.
c. Give vitamin D to increase absorption of calcium.
5. Reassure patient about skeletal recovery.
a. Bone pain diminishes fairly quickly.
b. Cysts, bone tumors, and osteoporosis resolve themselves.
c. Fractures are cared for by usual orthopedic procedures.

HYPOPARATHYROIDISM

Hypoparathyroidism is a condition brought about by a diminution or absence of the secretion of the parathyroid glands.

Cause

1. Decrease in gland function (idiopathic hypoparathyroidism)
2. Surgical or radiation trauma to parathyroid glands
3. Malignancy or metastasis from a cancer to the parathyroid glands
4. Resistance to parathyroid hormone action

Altered Physiology

1. Blood calcium falls to a low level—causing symptoms of muscular hyperirritability, uncontrolled spasms, and hypocalcemic tetany.
2. Blood phosphate level is elevated. Phosphate excretion by renal tubules is decreased.

Clinical Manifestations

1. Due to deficiency of parathormone
   a. Accumulation of phosphorus in blood
   b. Decrease in amount of blood calcium
2. Tetany
   a. General muscular hypertonia; attempts at voluntary movement result in tremors and spasmodic or uncoordinated movements; fingers assume classic position
   b. Chvostek sign—a spasm of facial muscles that occurs when muscles or branches of facial nerve are tapped
   c. Trousseau sign—carpopedal spasm induced by occluding circulation in the arm with a blood pressure cuff
   d. Reduced blood calcium level—to a low level (7.5 mg./100 ml. or less)
   e. Laryngeal spasm
3. Anxiety and apprehension are very marked.
4. Renal colic is often present if the patient has had stones; preexisting stones loosen and migrate into the ureter.

Treatment and Nursing Management

1. Administer calcium.
   a. A syringe and an ampule of a calcium solution are to be kept at the bedside at all times.
   b. Most rapidly effective calcium solution is ionized calcium chloride (10%).
   c. For rapid use to relieve severe tetany, infuse every 10 minutes.
      (1) Administer ionized calcium chloride (10%) slowly. It is highly irritating, stings, and causes thrombosis; patient experiences unpleasant burning flush of skin and, more particularly, of the tongue. Too rapid calcium administration may cause cardiac arrest.
      (2) Give calcium intravenously; calcium carbohydrate combination may also be used—gluconate or heptonate (10%) are not irritating.
   d. Continue a slow drip of intravenous saline containing calcium gluconate until control of tetany is assured; then switch to intramuscular or oral administration of calcium.
   e. Later, add vitamin D to calcium intake—increases absorption of calcium and also induces a high level of calcium in the bloodstream.
2. Control anxiety.
   a. It is difficult to reassure this patient since he has a strong feeling of impending disaster.
   b. Administration of intravenous calcium seems to bring about rapid relief of anxiety.
3. Relieve renal colic.
   Stone may have to be removed cystoscopically or by surgery.
4. Monitor for hypercalciuria. Recommend periodic 24-hour urinary calcium determinations.
5. Monitor blood calcium periodically; variations in vitamin D may affect calcium levels.
6. Inform patient about symptoms of hypocalcemia and hypercalcemia; should these occur, he is to notify his physician.

3 DIABETES MELLITUS (PANCREATIC DISORDERS)

DIABETES MELLITUS*

Diabetes mellitus is a syndrome characterized by persistent hyperglycemia (abnormally high blood glucose). There may be either a deficiency of insulin or a resistance to its action. There are several types of diabetes with different causes, different clinical courses, and different treatment regimens; the common denominator is hyperglycemia.

Altered Physiology

1. In diabetes mellitus there is excessive output of glucose from the liver and inadequate utilization of glucose by muscle and fat cells. Triglycerides are transported from the fat cells to the liver where they

---

* See page 1356 for diabetes mellitus in children and page 1407 for diabetes during pregnancy.

are converted into ketones that can be utilized by the muscles for energy.
2. Insulin is a hormone secreted, when blood glucose rises, by the beta cells of the islets of Langerhans located in the pancreas.
   a. Insulin increases glycogen storage in the liver and the transport of glucose through the cell membrane of muscle and fat cells. Glucose passes into endothelial and nerve cells without the aid of insulin.
   b. The increased secretion of insulin following meals helps maintain the blood glucose at a normal level.
   c. The decreased secretion of insulin between meals facilitates the conversion of glycogen, amino acids, and triglycerides into glucose in the liver (gluconeogenesis).

3. In insulin-dependent diabetes mellitus (IDDM—juvenile or ketotic diabetes) little or no insulin is secreted. In non-insulin dependent diabetes mellitus (NIDDM—maturity-onset diabetes) there is an insensitivity of the glucose-sensing mechanism of the beta cells, and in obese patients with NIDDM there is a decrease in the number of insulin receptors on the cell membrane of muscle and fat cells. Obese patients secrete an excessive amount of insulin, but it is ineffective because of the decreased number of receptors.
4. When blood glucose is sufficiently high, the renal tubules are unable to reabsorb all of the glucose in the glomerulo-filtrate, and glucosuria occurs. This causes an osmotic diuresis accompanied by the loss of water, sodium, chloride, potassium, and phosphate.
5. Diabetic ketoacidosis is due to an absence of effective insulin. The ketone bodies are organic acids and cause acidemia. The patient compensates by hyperventilating and by excreting more water and salt in the urine.
6. Decompensated diabetes mellitus causes loss of fat stores, liver glycogen, cellular protein, electrolytes, and water, eventually resulting in death from ketoacidosis.
7. The sequelae of long-term poorly controlled diabetes (persistent hyperglycemia) are accelerated atherosclerosis in the larger arteries, thickened capillary basement membranes throughout the body, and degenerative changes in the peripheral nerves. These may lead to such complications as coronary thrombosis, stroke, gangrene of the feet, blindness, renal failure, and neuropathy.

Classification of Diabetes

A. *Insulin-dependent diabetes mellitus (IDDM)*

1. These patients are unable to produce endogenous insulin. They require injections of insulin to prevent ketoacidosis and to stay alive.
2. Only 5–10% of all diabetic patients have IDDM. There may be a weak hereditary predisposition to this disease, but sudden onset is apparently caused by a viral infection in predisposed people. It may occur at any age but is most commonly seen in young people.

B. *Non-insulin-dependent diabetes mellitus (NIDDM)*

1. There may be a defect in insulin release from the beta cells of the islets of Langerhans, but most commonly there is resistance to the action of insulin in the peripheral tissues.
2. This type usually develops after age 40 but may be seen in obese children.
3. Most of these individuals are or have been obese.
4. This type is inherited as a dominant trait, but the onset may be prevented or postponed by calorie restriction and weight loss.

C. *Diabetes associated with other conditions*

1. When the pancreas is damaged by inflammation or degeneration it may be unable to produce sufficient insulin.
2. Several drugs, chemicals, hormones, and genetic syndromes are associated with decreased insulin activity and hyperglycemia.

Clinical Manifestations

A. *Insulin-dependent diabetes mellitus (IDDM)*

1. The onset is usually abrupt, with polyuria (excessive urine), polydipsia (excessive thirst), and polyphagia (excessive ingestion of food), followed by weight loss, weakness, and fatigue.
2. The insulin deficiency causes hyperglycemia, which in turn causes glucosuria, osmotic diuresis, and the loss of water and electrolytes.
3. Increased gluconeogenesis from the mobilization of protein and fat stores results in weight loss and muscle wasting.
4. Excess ketogenesis leads to ketonemia and acidosis. Excessive diuresis leads to dehydration and hypovolemia (decreased blood volume).

B. *Non-insulin-dependent diabetes mellitus (NIDDM)*

1. In the early stages there are no symptoms. Pruritus vulvae due to candida infection is the most common presenting complaint. Most often the diagnosis is made by routine screening tests.
2. With increased severity the patient may have polyuria, polydipsia, drowsiness, fatigue, blurred vision, weight loss, muscle cramps, and persistent skin infections.

Diagnostic Evaluation

1. In the presence of classical symptoms (polydipsia, polyuria, polyphagia, and weight loss) a random glucose over 200 mg./dl. is sufficient for diagnosis.
2. Fasting plasma glucose over 140 mg./dl. on two occasions.
3. Fasting plasma glucose under 140 mg./dl. and a two-hour plasma glucose over 200 mg./dl. with one intervening value over 200 mg./dl. following a 75 gm. glucose load (oral glucose tolerance test—OGTT).
4. Impaired glucose tolerance
   a. Fasting plasma glucose under 140 mg./dl. and two-hour plasma glucose between 140 mg./dl. and 200 mg./dl. with one intervening value over 200 mg./dl. following a 75 gm. glucose load.
5. When unsuspected glucosuria is found, the plasma glucose should be determined immediately.
6. Glucose tolerance test is rarely needed for diagnosis and is not accurate unless it is done properly:
   a. Patient should be on an unrestricted high carbohydrate diet and participate in unrestricted physical activity for three days.
   b. The test is done in the morning after a 10- to 14-hour fast.
   c. A 75 gm. glucose load is given in adults; 100 gm. glucose load is given in pregnant women.
   d. The patient should remain seated and not smoke during the test; he should take no medication which affects blood glucose.
   e. Blood is drawn before the glucose is administered and every thirty minutes afterwards for two hours.

Treatment and Nursing Management

OBJECTIVE: to help the patient live a long, comfortable, and useful life by maintaining the plasma glucose as close to normal as possible.
This will correct biochemical and metabolic abnormalities, attain and maintain the ideal body weight, and postpone the progression of the complications of diabetes. *Every new patient requires intensive and extensive*

education in order to learn to eat properly, take prescribed insulin, test urine, and exercise adequately. Reinforcement of diabetic education at every opportunity is an important part of the nursing management of the patient with diabetes mellitus.

A. Dietary Management

OBJECTIVE: to obtain and maintain ideal body weight and ensure normal growth.

1. The diet is planned to contain adequate calories, protein, vitamins, and minerals. Most adults require 30 calories per kg. of ideal body weight.
   a. This may be increased to 35 or 40 calories kg. for children or adults who are extremely active.
   b. This may be reduced to 15 to 25 calories kg. for obese patients and sedentary adults.
2. For most patients the diet is calculated to give protein 0.5 to 1.2 gm. per kg. (15–20% total calories) and carbohydrates 2–4 gm. per kg. (40–60% of total calories).
   a. An effort is made to use high fiber foods that contain complex carbohydrates in contrast to those with rapidly absorbed simple carbohydrates.
3. Fat is added to make up the difference and varies from 0.5 to 1.5 gm. per kg. to give 20–40% of the total calories. Saturated fats are decreased and polysaturated fats increased as much as possible.
4. The menu should be varied according to the patient's ethnic and cultural background, life style, food preferences, exercise routine, and eating habits. The emphasis should be on what is allowed rather than on what is forbidden.
5. When insulin is taken, special consideration must be given to ensure adequate carbohydrate intake to correspond to the time when insulin is most effective and less carbohydrate when insulin is least effective.
6. Obese diabetics should be on a strict weight control program. Many will have a normal plasma glucose after they lose weight. (Remember that obese patients have an excessive amount of circulating insulin but are insulin resistant because of obesity).
7. The American Diabetes Association and American Dietetic Association have prepared exchange lists which reflect these recommendations.
   EXCHANGE LISTS FOR MEAL PLANNING:
   American Diabetes Association, Inc,
   2 Park Ave,
   New York, NY 10016

   American Dietetic Association
   430 North Michigan Ave
   Chicago Ill 60611

8. Each individual patient must be taught how to measure the correct portions at each meal and how to exchange one item for another on the list.
9. Routine urine testing for sugar before each meal and at bedtime is necessary during initial control, in unstable patients, and during illness. Well-controlled, stablized patients may be followed with one test daily. (See page 649).
10. Intensive nutritional counseling by a professional diet counselor should be done initially and repeated several times with every patient.

B. Exercise

Exercise promotes the utilization of carbohydrates and enhances the action of insulin.

1. Insulin-treated patients may develop hypoglycemia after exercise unless they take extra carbohydrate beforehand.
2. Patients should be encouraged to exercise on a regular basis each day.
3. Because insulin is absorbed more quickly from an exercised limb, many patients are more stable when injections are given in the abdomen.

C. Insulin Therapy

1. When the patient cannot produce an adequate amount of insulin, it is necessary to give it by injection.
2. Insulin lowers the blood glucose by decreasing the release of glucose from the liver and increasing the utilization of glucose by muscle and fat cells.
3. One or more insulin injections each day is required for patients with insulin-dependent diabetes.
4. Patients with non-insulin-dependent diabetes may require insulin during an acute illness, infection, stress, or pregnancy.
5. Obese patients can usually achieve a normal blood glucose by calorie restriction.

Insulin Preparations

1. Insulin is extracted from the pancreas of slaughtered pigs and cows.
2. The available preparations vary in onset of action, time of peak effect, and duration of action (Table 14-1). It is important to know the action curve for each type of insulin in order to properly treat the patient.
3. Insulin is prescribed in units. U-100 insulin contains 100 units per milliliter.

Insulin Syringes and Needles

1. The insulin syringe is calibrated according to units. (Example: U100 insulin should be given with a U100 syringe.)

TABLE 14-1. CHARACTERISTICS OF INSULINS AVAILABLE IN THE UNITED STATES

Type of Insulin	Appearance	Protein added	Buffer	Peak action (hrs.)	Duration (hrs.)
Rapid acting					
Regular (CZI)	Clear	None	None	1–2	5–7
Semilente	Turbid	None	Acetate	1–2	12–16
Intermediate acting					
Globin	Clear	Globin	None	2–4	12–18
NPH	Turbid	Protamine	Phosphate	2–8	18–24
Lente	Turbid	None	Acetate	2–8	18–24
Slow acting					
Protamine zinc	Turbid	Protamine	Phosphate	8–12	24–36
Ultralente	Turbid	None	Acetate	8–14	24–36

From Podolsky S. *Clinical Diabetes: Modern Management.* New York, Appleton-Century-Crofts, 1980

2. Needles are numbered according to diameter; the higher the number the thinner the needle.
3. No. 25 or No. 26 needles are usually used; 1.2 to 2.5 cm. (½ to 1 inch).

Regulation of Insulin Doses

1. The dose of insulin is adjusted to maintain the blood glucose within normal range (65–130 mg./dl.) before each meal and at bedtime. Urine sugar tests obtained at this time give an estimate of the blood glucose.
2. Insulin activity curves vary from patient to patient and with the site of injection.
   a. Insulin acts more quickly when injected in the upper extremities than in the lower extremities.
   b. Insulin acts more quickly when injected intramuscularly than when injected subcutaneously.
   c. Insulin acts more quickly if there is vigorous exercise of the extremity which received the injection.
3. New patients with IDDM may be started on 20 units of Lente or NPH given before breakfast.
   a. The dose is increased each day until the blood glucose and urine glucose are normal.
   b. When insulin requirements are changing rapidly, supplemental injections of regular insulin (crystalline zinc insulin) are given before each meal.

NURSING ALERT: There is a narrow margin between the amount of insulin needed to make the blood glucose normal and the amount that will cause hypoglycemia. Exercise and delayed meals decrease the need for insulin, whereas illness and emotional stress increase the need for insulin.

   c. The nurse should know when hypoglycemia is most likely to occur with the type of insulin that is being used.
4. Patients are instructed to test urine for sugar before each meal and at bedtime. In some cases it is helpful to test a second specimen obtained a half hour after the first specimen in order to avoid the hyperglycemia and glucosuria that follow meals.
5. The patient should keep a record of the urine tests and note on this record any changes in insulin dose, diet, or activities.

Insulin Administration

See page 648.

Hypoglycemic Reactions to Insulin

1. *Hypoglycemia* is an abnormally low blood glucose (usually below 50 mg./dl.).
2. Hypoglycemia results from too much insulin, not enough food, and/or excessive physical activity.
3. Hypoglycemia may occur 1–3 hours after regular (crystalline zinc) insulin, 4–18 hours after NPH or Lente insulin, or 18–30 hours after Protamine Zinc or Ultra-lente insulin.
4. Hypoglycemia may occur at any time but it is most commonly seen before meals.

Evaluation of Signs and Symptoms of Hypoglycemia

1. Sweating, tremor, pallor, tachycardia, palpitation, nervousness—from release of adrenalin from the central nervous system when the blood glucose falls rapidly.

2. Headache, lightheadedness, confusion, emotional changes, memory lapses, numbness of lips and tongue, slurred speech, lack of coordination, staggering gait, double vision, drowsiness, convulsions, coma—from depression of the central nervous system when the blood glucose falls slowly.

NURSING ALERT: Patients with long-standing diabetes complicated by autonomic neuropathy may develop hypoglycemia without warning. Severe and prolonged hypoglycemia may cause brain damage. Any abnormal behavior in a patient taking insulin should be considered as resulting from hypoglycemia until proven otherwise.

Management of Hypoglycemia

1. Give some form of sugar orally if the patient is conscious—orange juice, candy, lump sugar, or corn syrup.
2. Give glucagon (subcutaneously or IM) if patient cannot take sugar by mouth—this causes glycogenolysis in the liver if adequate glycogen stores are present.
3. As soon as the patient regains consciousness he should be given carbohydrate by mouth.
4. If the patient does not respond to the above measures, he is given 50 ml. of 50% glucose intravenously or 1000 ml. of 5%–10% glucose in water IV. The recovery will be slow in patients who have had severe and prolonged hypoglycemia.

Preventing Hypoglycemic Reactions Due to Insulin

Instruct the patient as follows:
1. Hypoglycemia may be prevented by maintaining a regular schedule of diet, insulin, and exercise.
2. The early symptoms of hypoglycemia should be recognized and treated.
3. Some form of simple carbohydrate should be carried at all times and taken at the first symptom of hypoglycemia.
4. Between-meal and bedtime snacks may be necessary to keep a normal glucose level.
5. Extra food should be taken before unusual physical exertion.
6. Frequent urine tests are necessary.
7. An identification card or bracelet should be worn.
   a. The card may be obtained from the American Diabetes Association, 2 Park Ave., New York, NY 10016.
   b. Identification bracelet—Medic-Alert Foundation, International, 1000 North Palm, Turlock, CA 95380.

Somogyi Phenomenon

Hypoglycemia is followed by compensatory rebound hyperglycemia that lasts 12–72 hours, and is usually caused by an excessive dose of insulin.
1. The patient will have transient hypoglycemia, but most urine specimens will contain glucose.
2. Gradual reduction of the insulin dose and increase of the diet at the time of the hypoglycemia will help to stabilize the patient.

Local Allergic Reactions to Insulin

A. *Local reactions*

Cause redness, stinging, and induration at the injection site.

1. The reaction may occur within 1 hour but may be delayed for 24 hours.
2. The reaction is usually seen in the early stages of therapy and disappears after a few weeks.
3. If local reactions persist, changing to purified pork insulin will usually correct this problem.
4. A few patients have insulin resistance due to insulin allergy. These should be referred to a medical center for antibody testing.

B. *Insulin lipodystrophy*

Causes either lipoatrophy (a loss of fat) or lipohypertrophy (an indurated fatty tumor) to appear at the site of insulin injection.

1. Insulin lipoatrophy causes pitting at the site of injection. It previously occurred in 25% of the women and children taking insulin but now occurs in only 2% of those who use the new highly purified U-100 insulin.
2. Lipohypertrophy can be prevented by changing the site of injection every day.

C. *Insulin edema*

Results from fluid retention after the sudden correction of prolonged hyperglycemia.

D. *Insulin resistant*

Term applied to patients whose requirements exceed 200 units of insulin each day. This condition is rarely seen.

Oral Hypoglycemic Agents (Table 14-2)

1. Oral hypoglycemic agents may be effective for older, non-insulin-dependent (NIDDM), nonketotic patients who are normal in weight and have persistent hyperglycemia after treatment by only diet adjustment.
2. In the United States, 4 sulfonylurea drugs are available as oral hypoglycemic agents. The initial effect of these drugs is to increase insulin release from the pancreas. There is a long-term effect of increasing the number of insulin receptors. (See package information for side effects and drug interactions.)
3. Patients usually are treated by diet alone before oral hypoglycemic drugs are used.
4. Insulin is required when ketosis or severe infection is present.

TABLE 14-2. ORAL HYPOGLYCEMIC AGENTS SULFONYLUREA COMPOUNDS

Agent	Duration of action (hrs.)	How given
Tolbutamide (Orinase)	6–10 hrs.	Divided doses
Chlorpropamide (Diabinese)	36–60 hrs.	Single dose
Acetohexamide (Dymelor)	10–20 hrs.	Single or divided doses
Tolazamide (Tolinase)	12–24 hrs.	Single or divided doses

ACUTE COMPLICATIONS OF DIABETES

The diabetic may become comatose because of hypoglycemia (see p. 642), diabetic ketoacidosis, and hyperosmolar-nonketotic coma, in addition to all of the conditions that can produce coma in the nondiabetic.

DIABETIC KETOACIDOSIS

Diabetic ketoacidosis results from the absence of effective insulin which causes hyperglycemia, ketonuria, dehydration, and acidosis. Glucose no longer enters muscle cells, and fat is metabolized to produce energy. Free fatty acids are converted to ketone bodies in the liver. The ketone bodies are organic acids that cause metabolic acidosis.

Precipitating Causes

1. Failure to take an adequate amount of insulin
2. Failure to increase the dose of insulin in the presence of acute infection
3. Failure to increase insulin to compensate for pregnancy, injury, surgery, or emotional stress

Clinical Manifestations

A. *Early Manifestations*

1. Polyuria, polydipsia, fatigue, malaise, drowsiness
2. Anorexia, headache, abdominal pains
3. Muscle cramps, nausea, vomiting, constipation

B. *Later Manifestations*

1. Kussmaul breathing—very deep respiratory movements
2. Sweetish odor of the breath due to ketonemia
3. Hypotension and weak thready pulse
4. Stupor and coma

Laboratory Evaluation

A. *Blood*

1. Glucose elevated, bicarbonate decreased, arterial pH decreased, strongly positive plasma ketone

B. *Urine*

1. Strongly positive for sugar and ketone, and moderately positive for protein

Treatment and Nursing Management

OBJECTIVES: to restore normal metabolism.
   to correct hypovolemia.
   to reduce hyperglycemia and correct electrolyte imbalance.

1. Obtain blood and urine samples immediately:
   a. Test blood for glucose, ketone, BUN, electrolytes, complete blood count, arterial pH, PO_2, and PCO_2.
   b. Obtain urine specimen at prescribed time and measure sugar, acetone, and volume. Catheterize only if a voided specimen cannot be obtained.
   c. Start a flow chart which includes vital signs, clinical manifestations, laboratory data, and therapy arranged in a chronological manner.
2. Carry out a rapid physical examination to look for infection, myocardial infarction, stroke, etc.

a. Record vital signs, state of hydration, and mental status.
3. Start intravenous infusion of isotonic saline at a rate of about 500 ml. per hour to rehydrate the patient. Later the type of fluid and rate of administration are changed.
4. Give insulin as directed—to increase glucose utilization and decrease lipolysis. Insulin may be given by:
    a. Continuous infusion low-dose therapy. An infusion pump may be used, or insulin may be put into the bottle containing the intravenous solution. Because ⅓ of the solution sticks to the bottle and tubing, it is necessary to increase the dose as directed.
    b. Deep intramuscular injections of regular insulin into the deltoid may be used instead.
5. As the serum glucose falls, glucose is added to the infusion, and the insulin dose is reduced as directed.
6. Determinations of serum glucose, ketone, bicarbonate, and potassium are done every 3–6 hours.
7. One or more ECG tracings may be needed to rule out silent myocardial infarction, and to monitor intracellular potassium levels.
8. The rapid utilization of glucose under the influence of insulin causes potassium to migrate into the cells, and results in hypokalemia after 4–8 hours of treatment.
    a. This is corrected by administering buffered potassium phosphate (or chloride) at a rate of no more than 20 mEqs. per hour. This is usually added to the infusion after 3 or 4 hours.
9. Hypotension will usually respond to adequate saline infusion.
10. If the patient is given nothing by mouth for 3 hours while rehydration takes place, nausea usually subsides and the patient can usually be given clear liquids.
11. The recurrence of diabetic ketoacidosis can be prevented by adequate patient education. The patient should increase the dose of insulin when there is glucosuria and ketonuria, and seek medical advice when there are symptoms of diabetic ketoacidosis.

NONKETOTIC HYPEROSMOLAR COMA

Nonketotic hyperosmolar coma is characterized by hyperglycemia, hyperosmolarity, severe dehydration, and stupor or coma, but there is no ketonemia or acidosis.

Altered Physiology

1. There is some, but not enough, insulin present. This condition occurs in older people who do not have diabetes but who have been given excessive carbohydrate without adequate fluid administration.
2. Hyperglycemia causes osmotic diuresis resulting in severe loss of water and electrolytes.
3. Water shifts from the intracellular to the extracellular fluid and causes intracellular dehydration.

Clinical Manifestations

1. History of precipitating event: Severe burns, pancreatitis, hemodialysis, hyperalimentation, and excessive use of diuretics may be factors.

2. Severe hyperglycemia with a negative serum acetone and a normal serum bicarbonate.
3. Severe dehydration with poor skin turgor, hypotension, fever, and decreased brain activity. Seizures may occur.
4. Serum osmolarity is greatly elevated.

Treatment and Nursing Management

OBJECTIVE: to correct the volume depletion and hyperosmolar state.
1. Isotonic saline and low dose insulin infusion is the primary treatment.
2. Potassium and glucose are added later as indicated by the blood chemistry tests.
3. As soon as the patient regains consciousness, oral liquids are given.

INFECTIONS

Underlying Considerations

Infections are more protracted and serious in diabetics for the following reasons:
1. Hyperglycemia causes decreased leukocyte phagocytosis. Ketonemia causes decreased leukocyte migration.
2. Diabetes becomes more severe in the presence of infection.
3. Ketoacidosis may be precipitated by infection and inadequate insulin.

Types of Infection

1. Infections of the urinary tract may follow incomplete emptying of the bladder due to diabetic neuropathy or urethral obstruction. Bladder infections may spread to the kidney and cause pyelonephritis.
2. Infections of the extremities due to local injury may occur in patients with diabetic neuropathy who cannot recognize pain. If the skin is dry and cracked, bacteria may penetrate the protective envelope and cause infection.
    a. Inflammation due to infection causes edema of the tissue, decreased blood supply, and decreased resistance to infection.
    b. Atherosclerosis may also cause ischemic injury to the tissue.
3. Dermatologic infections:
    a. Infections of the skin and vagina frequently found in poorly controlled diabetes.
    b. Furuncles and carbuncles due to staphylococcus.
    c. Gas forming infections under the skin and in the genitourinary tract.
4. Tuberculosis occurs with increased frequency in persons with poorly controlled diabetes.

Treatment and Nursing Management

1. The dose of insulin is increased enough to correct the ketonemia and hyperglycemia.
2. The urine is tested frequently for sugar and acetone in order to adjust the insulin dose.
3. Cultures of blood, urine, sputum, and pus are essential for determining the responsible organism and for selecting the correct antibiotic.

LONG-TERM COMPLICATIONS OF DIABETES

Underlying Considerations

1. Diabetes is the most common cause of new blindness and new cases of end-stage renal disease in the United States. Accelerated atherosclerosis causes an increased incidence of myocardial infarction, stroke, and gangrene.
2. Because diabetics are living longer, these complications are becoming more common.

Vascular Complications

1. The specific pathological lesion (microangiopathy) of long-standing diabetes is thickening of the capillary basement membrane in every organ.
2. The prevalence of microangiopathy parallels the duration and severity of hyperglycemia.
3. Intercapillary glomerulosclerosis (Kimmelstiel–Wilson Syndrome), the specific renal disease of diabetes, results from the thickening of the capillary basement membrane in the glomeruli.
4. Microangiopathy of the vessels supplying the skin, peripheral nerves, and walls of large arteries may be a factor in skin diseases, neuropathy, and atherosclerosis.
5. Major vessel occlusion (macroangiopathy) resulting from atherosclerosis causes stroke, myocardial infarction, intermittent claudication, and gangrene. The progress of atherosclerosis is accelerated in diabetics.

DIABETIC RETINOPATHY

Diabetic retinopathy is a progressive impairment of retinal circulation that causes vitreous hemorrhage and loss of vision.

1. Incidence and severity of retinopathy is related to the duration and degree of control of diabetes; half of the patients who have had diabetes for more than 10 years have some evidence of retinopathy.
2. Impaired vision and blindness are caused by hemorrhage into the vitreous with the formation of scar tissue and detachment of the retina.
3. *Treatment*
   a. Photocoagulation—produced when a narrow, intensive beam of light is directed into the eye and focused on the retina; the absorption of light produces heat which coagulates the treated vessel and prevents it from bleeding.
      (1) Used when there are areas of newly formed blood vessels and proliferative retinopathy.
      (2) Photocoagulation must be done when proliferative changes first occur so that bleeding can be prevented.
   b. Vitrectomy—removal of blood and fibrous tissue through a small opening on the side of the eye and replacement with clear fluid that maintains the shape of the eye; may be tried for patients whose blindness is due to vitreous hemorrhage.
4. *Health Education*
   a. All diabetic patients should have yearly examinations of the fundus of the eye; those patients who show changes should be checked more frequently.
   b. Smoking is associated with a two-fold increase in proliferative retinopathy and should be discouraged.

DIABETIC NEUROPATHY

Diabetic neuropathy affects the peripheral and autonomic nervous system and produces a wide variety of syndromes.

1. *Clinical Manifestations*
   a. Peripheral neuropathy—pain (dull, aching, burning, lancinating, or crushing), paresthesia (sensations of tingling or burning or coldness and numbness).
   b. Involvement of autonomic nervous system—orthostatic hypotension, sexual impotency, retrograde ejaculation, pupillary changes, abnormal sweating, bladder paralysis, nocturnal diarrhea.
2. *Assessment of the Feet of Diabetic Patients*
   (The complications of neuropathy and vascular disease are most evident in the feet. Most amputations, other than those occurring from trauma, occur in diabetics.)
   a. Watch for lesions of the feet that do not heal.
   b. Compare the skin color of both feet and ankles. A blue–gray color is caused by diminution of the blood supply.
   c. Change the position of the extremity and note the color change. Pallor on elevation and dusky cyanosis on dependency indicate vascular insufficiency.
   d. Feel the temperature of the skin with the back of your hand and notice decreased temperature.
   e. Examine the toenails. Thick, ridged nails suggest circulatory impairment or fungus infection.
   f. Look for athlete's foot between the toes (epidermophytosis), and fungus infection of the nails (onychomycosis). Fungal infection is more serious in the diabetic and requires treatment.
   g. Look for calluses, corns, blisters, cracks, and abrasions; look between the toes and on the soles of the feet.
   h. Palpate the dorsalis pedis and posterior tibial arterial pulses; absence of a discernible pulse or diminution of the pulses indicate atherosclerosis.

MANAGEMENT OF THE DIABETIC PATIENT UNDERGOING SURGERY

Underlying Considerations

The diabetic patient must be followed closely at the time of surgery because stress, infection, and missed meals change insulin requirements.

1. The trauma of surgery causes hyperglycemia.
2. Infection causes the insulin requirements to rise.
3. Anesthesia may cause hyperglycemia and ketosis.
4. The patient's normal schedule of food intake is usually interrupted.

Treatment and Nursing Management

OBJECTIVE: to achieve the best nutritional balance and best possible metabolic control of the diabetes preoperatively.

A. *Preoperative Preparation*

1. Essential preoperative evaluation studies are urinalysis, blood glucose, BUN, electrolyte, and CBC.
2. The usual diet is given, but the insulin dose may be reduced the day before surgery.

B. *Day of Surgery*

1. A fasting blood glucose is drawn and an intravenous infusion of 1000 ml. of 5% glucose may be given over a 4-hour period for each meal that is missed.
2. The patient is usually given ½ to ¾ his usual dose of insulin.

C. *Postoperative management*

1. Maintain nutrition with intravenous glucose until patient is able to tolerate food by mouth.
2. Give insulin as directed. The usual dose of intermediate acting insulin is started the day after surgery and supplemental regular insulin may be given on a sliding scale according to blood and urine tests.

PRINCIPLES OF HEALTH EDUCATION: MANAGING SELF-CARE

The person with diabetes mellitus must accept a major role in the management of his disease. His education must be amplified, reinforced, and updated continuously, since diabetes is a life-long disease.

OBJECTIVE: to maintain the best possible control of diabetes.

Patient's Objectives

A. *To become familiar with diabetes and how it affects the body*

1. Visit the physician on a regular basis.
2. Study and review available literature from reputable sources.
3. Secure booklets and pamphlets from the American Diabetes Association, Inc, 2 Park Ave, New York, N.Y. 10016
4. Attend available classes.

B. *To maintain health at an optimal level*

1. Maintain a consistent daily routine.
2. Get adequate rest and sleep.
3. Exercise regularly and consistently.
   a. Avoid "spurts" of arduous exercise before meals.
   b. Exercise 1½ hours after meals.
   c. Keep some form of carbohydrate (sugar, candy, orange juice) available during exercise periods.
4. Seek employment with regular hours.
5. Have an annual test for tuberculosis.

C. *To follow the prescribed dietary regimen*

1. Eat 3 or more measured meals each day. Plan ahead for prescribed meals and snacks.
2. Become thoroughly familiar with the food exchange lists.
3. Learn how to follow a calculated diet.
4. Know the caloric value of foods frequently eaten.
5. Use household measures or a gram scale until serving sizes can be judged accurately.
6. Avoid concentrated carbohydrates.
7. Avoid periods of fasting and feasting.
8. Keep weight at optimal level; normalize body weight.
   a. Weigh weekly.
   b. Keep a weight record.
9. If taking insulin, eat extra calories when unusual physical activity is anticipated.
10. Eat a bedtime snack when taking insulin (if permissible).

D. *To be aware of the degree of diabetic control*

1. Test urine for both sugar and acetone at each testing.
2. Test urine before each meal and at bedtime while control is being attained or during periods of illness.
3. Test urine at least once daily.
4. Keep a daily record of urine sugar tests (date, hour, color reaction).
5. Test only freshly voided urine, using the second specimen (voided one half hour after the first specimen).
6. Take the record of urine tests to physician at appointed times.
7. Know that acetone in the urine indicates need for *more insulin* and more food.
8. Protect all urine testing equipment from light, moisture, and heat (to prevent false interpretation due to deterioration of test materials).
9. Monitor blood glucose with Dextrostix when insulin requirements vary and during illness.
   a. Capillary blood is obtained from finger puncture and spread on enzyme strip.
   b. Reaction is quantitated with a reflectance colorimeter.

E. *To become familiar with all aspects of insulin usage (see p. 648 for guidelines for teaching self-injection of insulin).*

1. Know when the prescribed insulin is having its peak action.
2. Adjust insulin dosage according to urine sugar tests as prescribed.
3. Rotate the sites of insulin injections in a systematic manner.

4. Keep the syringe and needle in one particular place.
5. Keep a reserve supply of insulin in the refrigerator.
   a. Keep bottle in current use at *room temperature*.
   b. Avoid injecting cold insulin because it may contribute to tissue reaction.
6. Have an extra insulin syringe available.
7. Know the conditions that produce insulin reactions.
   a. Omission of a meal
   b. Unaccustomed or strenuous exercise
   c. Too much insulin
8. Know the symptoms of an insulin reaction.
   a. Any unfamiliar or peculiar sensation
   b. Hunger, perspiration, palpitation, tachycardia, weakness, tremor, pallor
9. Know how to combat an impending insulin reaction.
   a. Eat carbohydrates (orange juice, sugar, candy) when symptoms first occur.
   b. Test urine.
   c. Carry extra carbohydrate at all times (sugar lumps, candy).
   d. Eat extra carbohydrate before strenuous exercise and during periods of prolonged exercise, or reduce insulin dosage.
   e. Eat a snack at bedtime.
10. Keep a check-off system to ensure taking insulin.
11. Carry diabetic identification card or wear identification bracelet.
12. When traveling, carry diabetic supplies in hand luggage.
    a. Have letter from physician stating that you are a diabetic.
    b. Keep your watch at the time of departure point until arrival at destination; do not change diabetic regimen en route.

F. *To take prescribed oral hypoglycemic medication.*

1. Adhere faithfully to the prescribed diet.
2. Test urine daily.
3. Take the medication exactly as directed.

G. *To appreciate the importance of proper foot care to prevent infection, ischemia, and neuropathy which may lead to amputation and death.*

1. Inspect the feet carefully and routinely for calluses, corns, blisters, abrasions, redness, and nail abnormalities.
   a. Use a small mirror to check bottom of each foot.
   b. Use a magnifying glass under good light if eyesight is poor, or have someone else check feet.
2. Bathe the feet daily in warm (never hot) water.
   a. Do not soak the feet for prolonged periods. (Soaking is defatting.)
   b. Dry feet carefully, especially between the toes.
3. Massage the feet with an absorbable agent (vegetable oil, lanolin, Nivea cream) except between the toes—autonomically denervated foot loses its ability to sweat, and dries and cracks easily.
4. Prevent moisture between the toes to prevent maceration of the skin.
   a. Insert lamb's wool between overlapping toes.
   b. Use powder in the web spaces, especially if feet perspire.
5. Wear well-fitting, noncompressive shoes and socks—long enough, wide enough, soft, supple, and low-heeled.
   a. Buy shoes in the afternoon—feet are larger in the afternoon than in the morning.
   b. Have each foot measured before buying shoes—feet enlarge with age.
   c. Have the measurement taken while standing, since foot is larger in the standing position.
   d. Do not "break in" shoes all at one time.
   e. Avoid rubber- or plastic-soled shoes, which cause the feet to perspire and aggravate fungal infections.
   f. Avoid working in bedroom slippers or other casual footwear.
6. Go to a podiatrist on a regular basis if corns, calluses, and ingrown toenails are present.
   a. Cut toenails straight across to prevent ingrown toenails.
   b. See page 836 for instructions for cutting toenails.
7. Avoid heat, chemicals, and injuries to the feet—do not go barefoot or expose feet to hot water bottles, heating pads, caustic solutions, etc. Heat increases demand for blood which cannot be met because of the reduction of vascular reserve. Diabetic neuropathy causes loss of cutaneous sensation, so that the patient may suffer burns or pressure lesions without being aware of them.
   a. Switch off electric blanket before going to bed; wear socks at night to keep feet warm if necessary.
   b. Avoid overheated baths and sitting too close to a fire.
8. Inspect inside of shoes for foreign objects, etc.
9. If an injury occurs to the foot:
   a. Wash the area with mild soap and water.
   b. Cover with a dry sterile dressing *without* adhesive.
   c. Wear white cotton socks; dye in colored socks and wool may serve as irritants when skin is already irritated.
   d. Call the physician.

H. *To maintain diabetic control during periods of illness or stress.*

1. Call physician immediately when any unusual symptoms become evident; *do not allow diabetes to get out of control.*
2. Make dietary adjustments during illness according to physician's directions.
3. Continue taking insulin; physician may increase dosage during illness.
4. Test urine for sugar and acetone more frequently; keep records.
5. Monitor blood glucose with Dextrostix.
6. Know the conditions that bring about diabetic acidosis.
   a. Nausea and vomiting
   b. Failure to increase insulin when urine sugar is increasing
   c. Failure to take insulin
   d. Stress
   e. Infections
7. Know how to combat impending diabetic acidosis.
   a. Examine urine for sugar and acetone and report results to physician.
   b. Take additional insulin as advised by physician.
   c. Go to bed and keep warm.
   d. Alert someone to be in attendance.
   e. Drink a glass of liquid hourly if possible.

I. *To follow other health directives.*

1. Avoid tobacco—nicotine constricts blood vessels, causing reduction in blood flow to feet.
2. Take only medications prescribed by physician—many drugs enhance effect of insulin and oral antidiabetic agents.

GUIDELINES: Teaching Self-Injection of Insulin

Underlying Considerations

1. Insulin injection should be taught as soon as the need for insulin treatment has been established.
2. A member of the patient's family should also be taught how to administer insulin.
3. An optimistic approach will offer the patient encouragement.
4. Teach insulin injection *first,* since this is the patient's major concern; then teach loading the syringe.

Equipment
Prescribed bottle of insulin
Disposable insulin syringe and needles
Absorbent cotton and alcohol

Procedure

TEACHING ACTION	RATIONALE/AMPLICATION
1. Give the patient the prepared syringe containing the prescribed dose of insulin.	
2. Have patient wipe the skin with alcohol.	
3. Instruct the patient to hold the syringe as he would a pencil.	
4. Show the patient how to spread the skin taut on the anterior thigh (Fig. 14-2A). or Form a skin fold by picking up subcutaneous tissue between the thumb and forefinger if the patient is thin (Fig. 14-2B).	4. Either of the techniques ensures that the needle tip is inserted into subcutaneous tissue and outside the muscle. Avoid pressing the skin *tightly* between the fingers since this is a common cause of local induration and infection.
5. Select areas of upper arms, thighs, flanks and upper buttocks for injection after patient becomes proficient with needle insertion (Fig. 14-2A).	5. The skin is loose and there is more subcutaneous fat in these areas.
6. Assist the patient to insert needle with a quick thrust to the hub at a right angle to the skin surface (Fig. 14-2B).	6. The insulin is injected into deep subcutaneous tissue.
7. Instruct the patient to release the skin fold and pull back on the plunger. If no blood is seen, push in the plunger. (Fig. 14-2C).	7. Pulling back on the plunger and checking for blood ensures that the needle is not in a blood vessel.

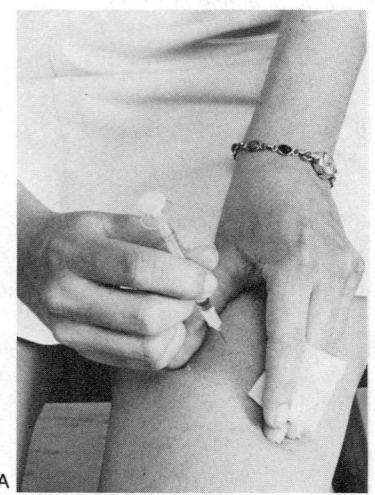 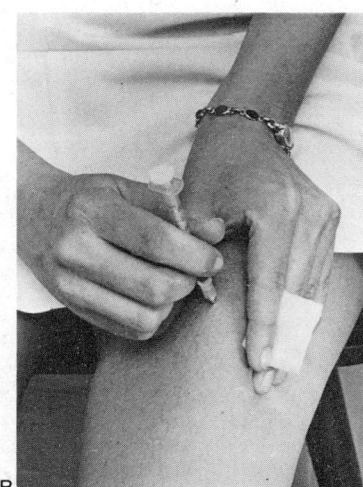 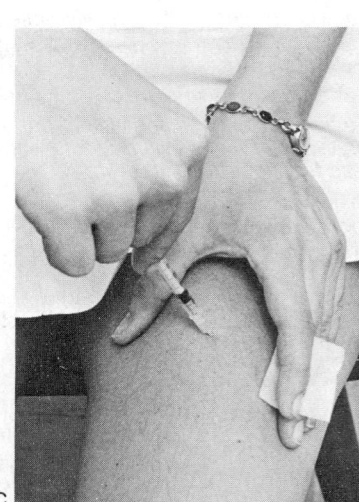

A   B   C

FIGURE 14-2. *Self-injection of insulin. A. The insulin syringe is held perpendicular to the stretched skin before the needle is thrust into the subcutaneous tissues. B. Alternate method: If the patient has only a thin layer of subcutaneous fat, a fold of skin is pinched between the fingers to keep the needle from penetrating into the muscle. C. The patient exerts slight traction on the plunger before the insulin is injected.*

8. Hold the alcohol sponge against the needle and gently withdraw the needle. Wipe area with alcohol sponge.	8. This maneuver prevents painful pulling of the skin as the needle is withdrawn.
9. Develop a systematic plan for insulin administration; e.g., rotation of sites in a clockwise fashion (Fig. 14-3).	9. Systematic rotation of sites will keep the skin supple, will favor uniform absorption of insulin, and will prevent scar formation.

FIGURE 14-3. *Setting up a rotation circle. The sketch shows that the right arm is marked A, the right side of the abdomen is B, and the right thigh is C. The left side of the body going upward is marked D, E, and F, counterclockwise.*

Each of these areas can be marked as a rectangle and divided into 8 squares more than 1 inch on each side. These squares are numbered starting from the upper and outside corner (number 1) to the lowest corner (number 8). All even numbers are toward the body.

If you take the number 1 square and inject into it at each of the 6 areas through F, it will take you 6 days to reach area A again. Then you take square number 2 and inject each time on the squares so numbered in the areas A through F. And so on.

This provides 48 different places for an injection (6 × 8). (From ADA Forecast—the Diabetics' Own Magazine. Jan 1951, Vol. 4, No. 1. Courtesy, Becton, Dickinson.)

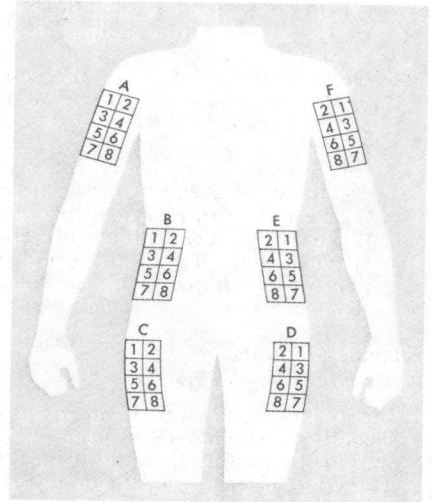

Procedure (cont.)	**TEACHING ACTION**	**RATIONALE/AMPLIFICATION**

To Load the Syringe:

1. Roll the bottle of insulin (Protamine Zinc, NPH and Lente) between the palms of the hands.

1. The rolling action mixes the insulin.

2. Wipe off the top of the insulin vial with an alcohol sponge.

3. Inject approximately the same volume of air into the insulin vial as the volume of insulin to be withdrawn.

3. Air is injected into the vial to keep its contents under slight positive pressure and to make it easier to withdraw the insulin.

To Fill a Syringe with Long- and Short-Acting Insulin Mixture:

1. Wipe off the vial tops with an alcohol swab.
2. Inject air into long-acting insulin first; withdraw needle.
3. Inject air into short-acting insulin bottle and withdraw prescribed amount of insulin.
4. Then withdraw prescribed amount of insulin from long-acting insulin bottle.

RAPID METHODS OF URINE TESTING FOR GLUCOSE (SUGAR) AND KETONES (ACETONE)

Underlying Considerations

1. Sugar appears in the urine when the glucose in the blood rises over 170 mg./dl. In older people, the renal threshold rises above this level.
2. Urinary sugar (glucosuria) may appear when:
   a. More insulin or sulfonylurea is needed.
   b. Patient is eating more than he should.
   c. Exercise is inadequate.
   d. Infection is present.
3. Incorrect tests occur because:
   a. Deteriorated reagent tablets are used.
   b. The directions are not followed accurately.
   c. The patient is taking medication that gives false positive or negative results.

Instructions to the Patient

1. Void and discard the first urine passed after each meal.
2. Collect a second specimen 15–45 minutes later—this recently produced urine will reflect the blood sugar level more accurately.

Tests for Glucose (Sugar)

Copper Reduction Test

A. *Clinitest**—uses a reagent tablet

1. *Two-drop method*—allows estimation of concentration of sugar up to 5%
   a. Hold dropper vertically and place 2 drops (0.1 ml.) of urine in test tube.
   b. Rinse dropper. Add 10 drops (0.5 ml.) of water to test tube.
   c. Add 1 Clinitest reagent tablet. *Do not shake test tube.*
   d. Wait 15 seconds after boiling stops and shake test tube gently to mix contents.
   e. Compare color of urine with appropriate color chart. (Use only the 2-drop method color scale which has 7 colors ranging in value from 0–5%.)
2. *Five-drop method*
   a. Hold dropper vertically and place 5 drops of urine in test tube.
   b. Rinse dropper. Add 10 drops of water to test tube.
   c. Put 1 Clinitest tablet in test tube.
      (1) Watch while reaction takes place.

* Clinitest, Diastix, Acetest, Ketostix, and Keto-Diastix are products of Ames Company, Division of Miles Laboratories, Inc., Elkhart, Indiana 46514.

(2) Do not shake test tube during reaction or for 15 seconds after boiling inside test tube has stopped.
d. Observe the solution in the test tube *while the reaction takes place and during the 15-second waiting period to detect pass-through color changes caused by glucosuria over 2%.*
   (1) If the solution passes through orange and dark shades of green-brown it indicates more than 2% (4+) urine sugar is present.
   (2) Record as such without reference to color scale.
e. After 15-second waiting period, shake test tube gently and compare with the color scale.
f. Record results.

Enzyme Methods

B. *Diastix**—reagent strip
1. Dip reagent end of strip in urine specimen for 2 seconds and remove (or wet end of strip for 2 seconds by passing through urine stream).
2. Tap edge of strip against side of urine container or sink to remove excess urine.
3. Exactly 30 seconds after removing from urine, compare reagent side of strip to closest matching color block on package label.

C. *Tes-Tape***—reagent tape
1. Dip part of the Tes-Tape into the urine.
2. Expose to air 60 seconds—the enzyme requires oxygen for color development.

* Clinitest, Diastix, Acetest, Ketostix, and Keto-Diastix are products of Ames Company, Division of Miles Laboratories, Inc., Elkhart, Indiana 46514.
** Tes-Tape is a product of Eli Lilly and Company, Indianapolis, Indiana 46225.

3. Compare the darkest area with the color chart. If tape indicates ½% or higher, wait 1 additional minute and make final comparison.

Tests for Acetone (Ketone bodies)

A. *Acetest**—reagent tablets
1. Use freshly voided specimen—prolonged standing of urine specimen encourages bacterial growth which can decrease the number of ketone bodies.
2. Place tablet on a piece of white paper.
3. Place 1 drop of urine on tablet.
4. Compare urine ketone test results to color chart at 30 seconds after application of specimen.
5. Acetest* may also give semi-quantitative determinations of ketones in serum, plasma, or whole blood.

B. *Ketostix**—reagent strips
1. Dip test strip in freshly voided specimen or pass it briefly through the urinary stream.
2. Remove immediately. Draw edge of strip against urine container to remove excess urine.
3. Wait 15 seconds. Compare color of test strip with the color chart.
4. See package directions for testing serum and plasma.

Combined (Ketone-Glucose) Reagent Strip

Keto-Diastix*—combined ketone-glucose reagent strip
1. Dip reagent end of strip in urine specimen and remove immediately.
2. Tap edge of strip against side of container to remove excess urine.
3. Compare reagent side of test areas with corresponding color charts at the time specified on the charts. (Glucose is read exactly at 30 seconds, and ketone is read at exactly 15 seconds.)

4 DISORDERS OF THE ADRENAL GLANDS

THE ADRENAL GLANDS

Composition

A. *Medulla*
1. Is not necessary to maintain life but enables a person to cope with stress
2. Secretes 2 hormones:
   a. Epinephrine (adrenalin)
      (1) Acts on alpha and beta receptors
      (2) Increases contractility and excitability of heart muscle, leading to increased cardiac output
      (3) Facilitates blood flow to muscles, brain, and viscera
      (4) Enhances blood sugar—by stimulating conversion of glycogen to glucose in liver
      (5) Inhibits smooth muscle contraction
   b. Norepinephrine (noradrenalin, arterenol)
      (1) Acts primarily on alpha receptors
      (2) Increases peripheral vascular resistance leading to increases in diastolic and systolic blood pressure

B. *Cortex*
1. Is essential to life
2. Secretes adrenocortical hormones—synthesized from cholesterol
   a. Glucocorticoids; cortisone and hydrocortisone
      (1) Enhance protein catabolism and inhibit protein synthesis
      (2) Antagonize action of insulin
      (3) Increase synthesis of glucose by liver
      (4) Influence defense mechanism of body and its reaction to stress
      (5) Influence emotional reaction
   b. Mineralocorticoids
      (1) Aldosterone—supplied by adrenal cortex
      (2) Desoxycorticosterone—usually not present in significant amounts
      (3) Regulate reabsorption of sodium cation
      (4) Regulate excretion of potassium cation by renal tubules
   c. Adrenosterones (adrenal androgens)

ADRENAL HYPERFUNCTION

PHEOCHROMOCYTOMA

Pheochromocytoma is a catecholamine-secreting neoplasm associated with hyperfunction of the adrenal medulla. It may appear wherever chromaffin cells are located; however, most are found in the adrenal medulla. Pheochromocytoma occurs more commonly in early to mid-adult life; it is uncommon in individuals over age 65.

Clinical Manifestations

1. Variable symptoms depend upon whether the tumor secretes epinephrine or norepinephrine.
   Symptoms are often triggered by allergic reactions, physical exertion, emotional upset; they can also occur without identifiable stimulus.
2. Hypertension may be paroxysmal or chronic.
   Chronic form may be difficult to differentiate from "essential hypertension"; however, drugs effective for essential hypertension are not effective in this patient.
3. Tachycardia, excessive perspiration, tremor, pallor or face flushing, nervousness and hyperglycemia.
4. Polyuria, nausea, vomiting, diarrhea and abdominal pain, paresthesia in extremities.

Diagnostic Evaluation

1. If there is sympathetic overactivity along with marked elevation of blood pressure, pheochromocytoma is strongly suspected.
2. Administration of certain drugs produces certain changes in arterial pressure.
   a. Provocative drugs—stimulate a sharp rise in arterial pressure: (histamine, tyramine, tetraethylammonium chloride.
   b. Adrenergic blocking drugs—produce a sharp fall in arterial pressure—phentolamine (Regitine).
3. Intravenous pyelogram (IVP) or x-ray examination may help in identifying the location of tumor.
4. Tests:
   a. Vanillylmandelic acid (VMA) and metanephrine determinations in urine.
   b. Determinations of catecholamines in urine and blood offer an effective test for overactivity of adrenal medulla.
   c. Normal urinary values: VMA 0.7–6.8 mg./24 hrs. Metanephrines: Less than 1.3 mg./24 hrs. Catecholamines: 0–275 µg/24 hrs.
5. Plasma volume is determined, since these patients are very sensitive to blood loss and therefore may benefit from preoperative volume expansion.
6. Adequate hydration is desirable.

Treatment and Nursing Management

OBJECTIVE: to diagnose the condition accurately, and then to remove the cause surgically.

A. *Preoperative Preparation*

1. This requires effective control of blood pressure and blood volume. Often may take 1 or 2 weeks.
2. To accomplish blood pressure control, administer alpha-adrenergic blocking agents such as phentolamine (Regitine) or phenoxybenzamine hydrochloride (Dibenzylene) to inhibit the effects of catecholamines.
3. Catecholamines synthesis inhibitors may also be used; metyrosine (Demser).
4. Propranolol is helpful in controlling cardiac arrhythmias, if present.
5. Localization of tumor(s) is done by computed tomography, ultrasonography, and selective adrenal arteriography.
6. For long-term maintenance of patients with inoperable tumors, metyrosine may be given.
   a. Moderate to severe sedation is a side effect when therapy is initiated; patients are cautioned against driving or participating in activities requiring alertness.
   b. Avoid concurrent use of alcohol or other CNS depressants.
   c. Maintain fluid intake as a precaution against crystalluria; maintain daily urinary output of at least 2000 ml.

B. *Postoperative Care* (see p. 654)

Of particular concern is the evaluation and documentation of 24-hour urine specimens. The patient is considered surgically cured when 24-hour urine specimens are evaluated as "normal" when tested for catecholamines or catecholamine metabolites.

C. *Familial pheochromocytoma.*

Evaluation of the patient's family for pheochromocytoma and medullary carcinoma of the thyroid (p. 637) should be done.

PRIMARY ALDOSTERONISM

Primary aldosteronism is a disorder caused by hypersecretion of the adrenal cortex.

Diagnostic Evaluation and Clinical Manifestations

1. A profound decline in blood levels of potassium (hypokalemia) and hydrogen ions (alkalosis)—results in muscle weakness and inability of kidneys to acidify or concentrate urine, leading to excess volume of urine (polyuria)
   a. Increase in pH
   b. Increase in CO_2-combining power
2. A decline in hydrogen ions (alkalosis)—results in tetany, paresthesias
3. An elevation in blood sodium (hypernatremia)—results in excessive thirst (polydipsia) and arterial hypertension
4. Hypertension

Treatment

Removal of adrenal tumor—adrenalectomy (see p. 654).

CUSHING'S SYNDROME

Cushing's syndrome is a condition in which the plasma cortisol levels are elevated, causing signs and symptoms of hypercortisolism.

Hypercortisolism is characterized by the clinical manifestations listed below. As diagnostic tools have become more sophisticated, hypercortisolism can now be classified in the following 3 categories:

1. Pituitary Cushing's syndrome (Cushing's disease)—

65% of all patients with Cushing's; mostly women in childbearing-age range
2. Adrenal Cushing's syndrome—associated with tumors of the adrenal cortex
3. Ectopic—results from autonomous ACTH secretion by extrapituitary neoplasms

Etiology

1. Cushing's syndrome results mainly from the hypersecretion of cortisol and corticosterone.
2. The disorder may be caused by:
   a. A neoplasm of the adrenal cortex: adenoma or carcinoma
   b. Hyperplasia of both glands due to overstimulation of the adrenal cortex by ACTH
   c. Pituitary tumors
   d. Tumors elsewhere in body producing excess ACTH (e.g., excessive pituitary ACTH secretion)

Diagnostic Evaluation

1. Excessive plasma cortisol levels
2. An increase in blood sugar—diabetes
3. A decrease in concentration of potassium in the blood
4. A reduction in the number of blood eosinophils
5. Elevation in the urine level of 17-hydroxycorticoids and 17-ketogenic steroids
6. Elevation of plasma ACTH in patients with pituitary tumors
7. Very low plasma ACTH levels in a patient with hypercortisolism are characteristic of an adrenal tumor.

Clinical Manifestations

A. *In children*

1. Precocious puberty
2. Affected growth rate

B. *Females* (Cushing's syndrome occurs 10 times more frequently in females than in males.)

1. "Virilism" or masculinization
   a. Hirsutism—excessive growth of hair on the face and midline of trunk
   b. Breasts—atrophy
   c. Clitoris—enlarges
   d. Voice—masculine
2. In utero—possible hermaphrodite

C. *Adult* ("central type obesity")
1. "Buffalo hump" in neck and supraclavicular area
2. Heavy trunk; thin extremities
3. Skin—fragile and thin; striae and ecchymosis, acne
4. Face—rounded, plethoric, oily
5. Muscles—wasted due to excessive catabolism
6. Osteoporosis—characteristic kyphosis, backache
7. Mental disturbances—mood changes, psychosis
8. Increased susceptibility to infections
9. Hypertension, edema

Objectives of Treatment and Nursing Management

A. *To establish the diagnosis*

1. Overnight dexamethasone suppression test.
   a. Dexamethasone is administered the night before in the amount equivalent to amount of cortisol normally produced by the patient in a day.
   b. Dexamethasone will normally suppress ACTH secretion and stop cortisol production.
   c. The next day, blood studies will be done; patients

with Cushing's syndrome will not show suppression below a certain level.
2. If above test does not rule out the possibility of Cushing's syndrome, specific urinary excretion tests are performed with dexamethasone suppression.
3. Additional tests are done to determine whether the problem is due to hyperplasia or adrenocortical tumor.
4. Explain to the patient the necessity for the many blood and urine studies.
5. Recognize the need for accurately recording intake of food and fluid as well as output of urine.
6. Record all pertinent observations that may assist the physician in making the diagnosis.
7. Expect the physician to request tests such as computerized tomography and ultrasonography to determine the exact tumor location.

B. *To consider medical treatment in patients unable to face surgery (e.g., myocardial infarction)*

Expect the physician to:
1. Consider mitotane, an agent toxic to the adrenal cortex (DDT derivative)—"medical adrenalectomy" Serious side effects accompany this drug.
2. Try metyrapone (Metopirone) to inhibit steroid biosynthesis; this is used for temporary control.

C. *To encourage the patient to eat the prescribed diet*

Explain to the patient that his diet (low sodium and high potassium) is as significant to his treatment as his medications.
   a. Foods high in potassium—meats, glandular meats, fish, most vegetables and fruits, legumes
   b. Foods low in sodium—cereal, fruits, squash, potatoes, lettuce, honey, unsalted butter

D. *To be aware of the psychological manifestations of this syndrome*

1. Identify those situations which are disturbing to the patient; record these on the nursing care plan as situations to be avoided.
2. Be alert for evidence of depression; in some instances this has progressed to suicide; therefore, mood changes are most important.
3. Report when depression continues after surgery.
4. Understand the emotional stress in female patients who manifest masculinization tendencies.
5. Reassure the patient who has benign adenoma or hyperplasia that, with proper treatment, evidence of masculinization can be reversed.
6. Note that weakness is a frustrating experience in a patient who heretofore has been active.

E. *To recognize the therapeutic options available when the precise type of Cushing's syndrome is diagnosed*

(See Table 14-3)

F. *To remove the causative factor surgically.*

1. Tumor (adrenal or pituitary)—should be removed or treated with irradiation.
   a. The most recent development in the management of pituitary Cushing's syndrome in adults is transsphenoidal adenomectomy (microsurgery). Obviously this procedure requires skilled neurosurgical and radiological teams.
2. Hyperplasia of adrenals—calls for an adrenalectomy

G. *To administer replacement therapy postoperatively.*

1. Adrenalectomy patients require life-long replacement therapy with the following:

TABLE 14-3. CURRENT THERAPEUTIC OPTIONS FOR THREE DISTINCT ETIOLOGIES OF CUSHING'S SYNDROME*

Treatment	Indication	Prognosis
Surgery		
Transsphenoidal (microresection)	Pituitary Cushing's syndrome	90%–95% remission rates after removal of pituitary microadenoma. Temporary cortisol replacement may be required.
Transfrontal (hypophysectomy)	Pituitary Cushing's syndrome	Panhypopituitarism: permanent replacement therapy
Adrenalectomy	Adrenal Cushing's syndrome	Temporary cortisol replacement therapy required if unilateral; lifelong if bilateral
	Pituitary Cushing's syndrome	Mortality 4%–10%; recurrent hypercortisolism 10%; Nelson's syndrome 10%–20%; lifelong adrenal hormone replacement required if bilateral
Irradiation		
External high-voltage x-ray (cobalt-60)	Pituitary Cushing's syndrome	80% remission in patients under 20 years of age; 20% remission in adults
Cyclotron (α-particle, proton beam)	Pituitary Cushing's syndrome	60% remission in adults; morbidity 7%–8%
Internal yttrium-90, gold-198 (implants)	Pituitary Cushing's syndrome	Requires transsphenoidal surgery; seldom used in U.S.
Drugs		
CNS-active cyproheptadine (24 mg/day orally in 3–4 divided doses	Pituitary Cushing's syndrome	Remission in 60% to 65% after 6–8 week of cyproheptadine; relapse if treatment is discontinued
CNS-active bromocriptine (10 mg/day orally)		
Adrenal-active o,p′-DDD (mitotane) (6.0 gm/day)	Ectopic Cushing's syndrome; inoperable adrenal Cushing's syndrome; pituitary Cushing's syndrome treated with irradiation	Remission of hypercortisolism in up to 90%; adrenocorticolytic; may require gluco- and minealocorticoid replacement
Metyrapone (1.0 gm/day) Aminoglutethimide (1.0 gm/day) Trilostane (0.5 gm/day)	Same as for o,p′-DDD (above); preoperative buildup of patients who are poor surgical risks because of metabolic effects of hypercortisolism	Not adrenocorticolytic; minor side effects; may require cortisol replacement during therapy; relapse if discontinued.

*From Gold EM. Cushing's syndrome: A tripartite entity. *Hospital Practice* 1979 June 14:72

a. A glucocorticoid—cortisone
b. A mineralocorticoid—fludrocortisone (Florinef)
c. Extra salt
2. Following pituitary irradiation or hypophysectomy, patients may require adrenal replacement plus thyroid and gonadal replacement therapy.

3. Following transsphenoidal adenomectomy, patients require hydrocortisone replacement therapy for periods of 12–18 months.
4. Protein anabolic steroids may facilitate protein replacement; potassium stores are usually depleted rapidly and may require replacement.

ADRENAL HYPOFUNCTION

ADRENOCORTICAL INSUFFICIENCY

Primary adrenocortical insufficiency—Caused by bilateral hypofunction of the adrenal cortex (Addison's disease) resulting in deficient production of adrenal steroids:
a. Glucocorticoids (principally cortisol)
b. Mineralocorticoids (principally aldosterone)
Secondary adrenocortical insufficiency—Caused by ACTH deficiency resulting from
a. pituitary disease
b. suppression of hypothalamic–pituitary axis by corticosteroids (used in treating nonendocrine disorders)

ADDISON'S DISEASE

Addison's disease—see primary adrenocortical insufficiency

Cause

A deficiency of cortical hormones due to:
1. Destruction of adrenal cortex
2. Atrophy—following prolonged steroid therapy or secondary to pituitary hypofunction

Clinical Manifestations

Due to (1) disturbance of sodium and potassium metabolism, and (2) depletion of sodium and water—urine loss, severe chronic dehydration.
1. Muscular weakness, fatigue, weight loss
2. Gastrointestinal problems—anorexia, nausea, vomiting, diarrhea, constipation, abdominal pain
3. Low blood pressure, low blood sugar, low BMR, low blood sodium
4. High potassium
5. After a while, symptoms worsen and the patient is forced to go to bed.
   a. Skin color changes to tan, bronze, or brown—diffuse or patchy, freckling.
   b. Mucous membranes also discolor—bluish black or gray.
   c. Mental changes occur—depression, irritability, anxiety, apprehension.
6. Normal responses to stress are lacking.

Diagnostic Evaluation

A. *Blood Studies*
1. Hypoglycemia—decrease in sugar concentration
2. Hyponatremia—decrease in sodium concentration

3. Hyperkalemia—increase in potassium concentration
4. Lymphoid hyperplasia
5. Low fasting plasma cortisol levels

B. *Urine Studies*

24-hour specimen for 17-ketosteroids, 17-hydroxy-corticoids, and 17-ketogenic steroids—all values decreased

C. *Injection of a Potent Pituitary Adrenocorticotropic Hormone to Artificially Stimulate Adrenals*

1. Normal response—normal rise in plasma cortisol and urinary 17-ketosteroids
2. In Addison's disease
   a. Decrease in circulating eosinophils
   b. Increase in uric acid excretion in about 4 hours
   c. No rise in plasma cortisol and urinary 17-ketosteroids

Treatment and Nursing Management

1. Attempt to restore normal electrolyte balance.
   a. Administer high sodium, low potassium diet and fluids.
   b. Treat glucocorticoid deficiency with cortisone, cortisol, or prednisone. Treat mineralocorticoid deficiency with fludrocortisone.
      (1) Overtreatment may be manifested by hypertension, edema from sodium and water retention, weakness due to sodium loss.
2. Detect early signs of *Addisonian crisis.*
   a. Nausea, vomiting, cyanosis
   b. Sudden drop in blood pressure
   c. Very high temperature
3. Recognize that circulatory collapse may result from the following:
   a. Overexertion
   b. Exposure to cold
   c. Acute infection
   d. Decrease in salt intake
   e. Excessive diarrhea
4. Be on guard for later signs of Addisonian crisis.
   a. Fall in systolic pressure to 40–50 mm.Hg
   b. Weak pulse and cold clammy skin
5. Initiate treatment immediately
   a. Administer blood transfusions to replace blood volume.
   b. Start intravenous flow of sodium chloride solution to replace sodium ions.
   c. Give hydrocortisone.
   d. Inject circulatory stimulants.

6. Assess vital signs frequently for deviation.
   a. Monitor vital signs and blood pressure; a drop in blood pressure may suggest impending crisis.
   b. Record the temperature hourly since an elevation may easily be precipitated.
7. Observe carefully the emotional status of the patient.
   a. Promote rest periods to avoid overexertion.
   b. Control the temperature of the room to avoid sharp deviations in patient's temperature.
   c. Maintain a quiet, peaceful environment; avoid loud talking and noisy radios.
8. Record conscientiously the salt intake and urine output.
   Inform the patient's family as well as all nursing personnel who come in contact with this patient that all urine must be saved for a 24-hour urine specimen.
9. Administer optimum physical nursing care.
   a. Do not allow the patient who is in adrenal crisis to do anything for himself.
   b. Assist him in moving and turning, in feeding, and in providing mouth care.
   c. Limit conversation to what is essential to his care.
10. Protect the patient from infection.
    a. Control his contacts so that infectious organisms are not transmitted.
    b. Protect him from drafts, dampness, etc.
11. Be familiar with the nature of hormonal replacement required by the individual patient.
    a. Some require cortisol.
    b. Other patients require additional electrolyte-type medications to maintain homeostasis.
    c. Determine the method of administration of drug for the particular patient: most are taken by mouth, but some are administered intramuscularly.
    d. Note whether there is an effect on fluid retention—weigh patient frequently and record weight.
12. Inform the patient of the nature of long-term therapy for adrenocortical insufficiency.
    a. Inform the patient that therapy must be continued for the rest of his life.
    b. Emphasize the importance of taking more hormones when he is under stress.
    c. Suggest that he carry an identification card on which are indicated the type of medication he is receiving and the phone number of his physician.

MANAGEMENT OF THE PATIENT HAVING AN ADRENALECTOMY

Preoperative

1. Correct hyperglycemia by proper diet and insulin.
2. Administer high protein diet to correct protein deficiency.
3. See page 80—Care of patient is similar to that for general surgery of abdomen.

Postoperative

1. Similar to that for an abdominal operation (see p. 89).
2. Will require administration of hydrocortisone or similar compounds in large amounts; this should begin prior to surgery. If bilateral adrenalectomy is performed, lifetime replacement is necessary.

3. For removal of pheochromocytoma:
   a. Because of manipulation of tumor during surgery, there may be extreme fluctuations of blood pressure.
   b. Upon ligation of vessels from tumor, an abrupt fall of blood pressure may result. Administer large amounts of epinephrine intravenously.

NURSING ALERT: Be prepared to monitor blood pressure frequently for 24 to 48 hours and to regulate vasopressor intravenous medications in order to stabilize the blood pressure.

4. Monitor vital signs, including blood pressure and central venous pressure, up to 48 hours—to detect early changes which may lead to cardiovascular collapse.

5. Anticipate stressful situations for the patient and avoid them; provide rest periods, anticipate his needs, provide comfort measures.

STEROID THERAPY*

Classification of Steroids

(by major metabolic effects on body)
1. Mineralocorticoids
   a. Concerned with sodium and water retention and potassium excretion.
   b. Example—aldosterone and 11-desoxycorticosterone
2. Glucocorticoids
   a. Concerned with metabolic effects, including carbohydrate metabolism
   b. Example—cortisol
3. Sex Hormones
   a. Important when secreted in large amounts or when the growth of hormone-sensitive cancers is stimulated
   b. Examples:
      Androgens—dehydroepiandrosterone, testosterone
      Estrogens—estradiol
      Progestins—progesterone

Effects of Glucocorticoids (corticosteroids, steroids)

1. Antagonize action of insulin—promote gluconeogenesis, which provides glucose.
2. Increase breakdown of protein (inhibit protein synthesis).
3. Increase breakdown of fatty acids.
4. Suppress inflammation, inhibit scar formation, block allergic responses.
5. Decrease number of circulating eosinophils and leukocytes; decrease size of lymphatic tissue.
6. Exert a permissive action (allow full expression of effects of another hormone) on all effects caused by catecholamines.
7. Exert a permissive action on functioning of central nervous system.
8. Inhibit release of adrenocorticotropin.
   IN SUMMARY: Glucocorticoids give an organism the capacity to resist all types of noxious stimuli and environmental change.

Uses of Steroids

1. Physiologically—to correct deficiencies or malfunction of a particular endocrine organ or system, e.g., Addison's disease.
2. Diagnostically—to determine proper functioning of the endocrine system.
3. Pharmacologically—to treat the following:
   a. Rheumatoid arthritis
   b. Acute rheumatic fever
   c. Blood conditions

* Source acknowledgement: Melick ME. Nursing intervention for patients receiving corticosteroid therapy. In Kintzel: Advanced Concepts in Nursing, 2nd ed. Philadelphia, JB Lippincott, 1977

      (1) Idiopathic thrombocytopenic purpura
      (2) Leukemia
      (3) Hemolytic anemia
   d. Allergic conditions—bronchial asthma, allergic rhinitis
   e. Dermatologic problems—drug rashes, giant hives, atopic dermatitis
   f. Ocular diseases—conjunctivitis, uveitis
   g. Collagen diseases—lupus erythematosus, periarteritis nodosa
   h. Gastrointestinal problems—ulcerative colitis
   i. Organ-transplant recipients—as an immunosuppressive
   j. Neurological—cerebral edema
   k. Other conditions—gout, multiple sclerosis
4. Emergency conditions
   a. Status asthmaticus
   b. Acute adrenal insufficiency
   c. Anaphylactic reaction (only after epinephrine has been given)

Preparing the Patient to Receive Steroid Therapy

1. Require a thorough physical examination and medical history.
2. Determine contraindications for such therapy.
   a. Peptic ulcer
   b. Diabetes mellitus
   c. Viral infections
3. Take a tuberculin test to determine need for anti-tuberculin drugs.
   If this is not done prior to steroid therapy, the patient's hypersensitivity to tuberculin may be suppressed.
4. Assess the patient's own level of steroid secretion, if possible.
5. Explain the nature of the therapy, what is required of the patient, how long he is to be on steroid medications, what adverse signs to watch for, and answer any of his questions.

Choice of Steroid and Method of Administration

(See Table 14-4)
1. Determined on an individual basis by physician.
2. May be given for local effects or systemic effects.
3. May be given by a wide variety of methods: orally, parenterally, sublingually, rectally, by inhalation, or by direct application to skin or mucous membrane.
4. Combinations of steroids with other drugs should be avoided.
5. To help avoid steroid side effects, alternate-day therapy should be used if at all possible; this is not always feasible.
6. Sometimes steroids are given in extremely high doses, then sharply reduced; if patient has been taking steroids for a while, doses must be tapered gradually.

TABLE 14-4. CHARACTERISTICS OF PHARMACEUTICAL DERIVATIVES OF ADRENOCORTICOSTEROIDS

Oral Preparations

USP Name	Trade Name(s)	Anti-inflammatory Relative Potency (Cortisol = 1)	Mineralocorticoid Relative Potency (D.O.C. = 1)	Anti-inflammatory / Mineralocorticoid
Dexamethasone	Decadron, Deronil, Dexameth, Gammacorten, Hexadrol	30.0	Mild natriuretic	∞
Betamethasone	Celestone	30.0	Mild natriuretic	∞
Triamcinolone	Aristocort, Kenacort	5.0	0	∞
Methylprednisolone	Medrol	6.0	0.02	300
Prednisone	Deltasone, Deltra, Meticorten, Paracort	4.0	0.04	100
Cortisone	Cortigen, Cortone	0.8	0.03	27
Hydrocortisone (cortisol)	Cortef, Cortifan, Cortril, Hycortole, Hydrocortone	1.0	0.03	33
Fludrocortisone (9α-fluorocortisol)	Cortef-F, Florinef	10.0	4.2	2.4
Desoxycorticosterone (deoxycorticosterone)	Cortate, Decortin, Decosterone, Doca	0	1.0	0
Aldosterone	Not available	0.1	20	0.005

Intravenous Preparations		Topical Preparations*		Slow-release Preparations	
USP Name	Trade Name	USP Name	Trade Name	USP Name	Trade Name
Hydrocortisone hemisuccinate	Solu-Cortef	Triamcinolone acetonide	Aristoderm (Kenalog)	Hydrocortisone acetate	Cortef Acetate
Hydrocortisone phosphate	Hydrocortone Phosphate	Fluocinolone acetonide	Synalar	Methylprednisolone acetate	Depo-Medrol
Methylprednisolone hemisuccinate	Solu-Medrol	Fluorometholone	Oxylone	Deoxycorticosterone trimethylacetate	Percorten
Dexamethasone phosphate	Decadron Phosphate				
Prednisolone phosphate	Hydeltrasol				

* In addition to these topical preparations, most of the anti-inflammatory steroids are supplied in the form of creams, aerosols, eye-drops, etc., for special topical use.
From Bondy PK and Rosenberg LE. Metabolic Control and Disease, 8th ed, p 1450. Philadelphia, WB Saunders, 1980.

Potential Side Effects of Steroid Therapy

See Chart, page 657.

A. *Classification*

1. Mineralocorticoid
   a. Sodium and water retention
      Edema, weight gain, elevated blood pressure
   b. Potassium depletion
      Weakness, tiredness, alkalosis
2. Glucocorticoid
   a. Masking of infections
   b. Osteoporosis
   c. Steroid diabetes
   d. Exacerbation of tuberculosis.

B. *Control or Avoidance of Side Effects*

1. Mineralocorticoid
   Use triamcinolone or newer synthetic steroids. (Some of the newer synthetics cause less sodium retention but have other side effects.)
2. Glucocorticoid
   Difficult to separate anti-inflammatory effects from sodium-retaining effects.

Nursing Management of Patients Receiving Steroid Therapy

1. Know the routes by which steroids are given.
   a. Ascertain advantages of the method chosen for the particular patient.
   b. Determine what is expected of the medication in a particular situation.
   c. Be informed about side effects and untoward manifestations.

   d. NOTE:
   (1) Local application of steroid medications to the skin (to a large area, over a prolonged period, using occlusive dressings) leads to adrenal suppression.
   (2) Local administration to the eye over a prolonged period leads to increased eye pressure, corneal ulceration.
   (3) Long-term systemic cortocosteroid therapy may cause generalized skin atrophy, impaired wound healing, and development of petechiae and ecchymoses in the extremities.
   e. Recognize that it is necessary to understand pharmacologic action of a particular steroid before planning the scheduled doses. Be aware of the following:
   (1) How frequently it can be given.
   (2) How late in the day it may be administered.
   (3) Whether every other day is sufficient, etc.
      Patients on intermittent therapy have few side effects.
2. Be aware of the problems encountered during periods when steroids are being withdrawn or lowered in dosage.
   a. Associate symptoms of tiredness, muscular weakness, and lethargy with drug withdrawal.
   b. Report any stress situations during this time, such as surgery, a family crisis, etc.
   c. Instruct the patient why it may be necessary to save all urine for 24 hours (for determination of 11-hydroxycorticosteroid level).
3. Monitor carefully the patient who is on intravenous corticosteroid therapy.

THE PATIENT ON STEROID THERAPY

Acceptable and Expected Side Effects

Nature of Effect	Action
Facial mooning (Cushing's Syndrome)	May be minimized by restricted calorie intake.
Weight gain	Restrict calorie intake; may require a change in steroid medication; may require a diuretic.
Edema	May require diuretics and potassium
Potassium loss	Prescribe diuretics and potassium.
	May require addition of a fluorinated synthetic.
	Administer potassium supplement.
Acne	Treat with topical medications.
Increase frequency and nocturia	Check for evidence of genitourinary infection or diabetes mellitus; urinalysis.
Insomnia, headache, fatigue, euphoria	Treat symptomatically.
Glycosuria, leukocytosis	

Undesirable and Unacceptable Side Effects

Nature of Effect	Action (Report to Physician)
Allergic reaction to ACTH or steroid	Withdraw drug promptly. Substitute steroid or synthetic ACTH.
Cardiovascular system effects:	
Hypertension	Suggest reduction in dosage of steroids.
Thromboembolic complications	
Arteritis	
Infection	Suggest antimicrobial medications as indicated.
Eye complications:	
Glaucoma	Refer to ophthalmologist.
Corneal lesions	
Subcapsular cataract	
Musculoskeletal effects:	
Osteoporosis	Suggest sex hormones—synthetic estrogens and/or androgens.
Pathologic fractures	
Growth suppression	Suggest calcium supplement.
Myopathies	
Central nervous system:	
Seizures	Refer to neurologist.
Neuritis	
Psychotic reactions	
Adrenal insufficiency (after steroid withdrawal) manifested by peripheral circulatory collapse—in upright position.	Administer hydrocortisone promptly (intravenously). The following day give steroid replacement.

Advice and Admonitions for Patients on Long-term Steroids

1. Recognize that steroids are valuable and useful medications but if taken longer than 2 weeks, they may produce certain side effects.
2. "Acceptable" side effects may include weight gain (perhaps due to water retention), acne, headaches, fatigue, and increased urinary frequency (see above).
3. "Unacceptable" side effects which are to be reported to the physician: dizziness when rising from chair or bed (postural hypotension indicative of adrenal insufficiency), nausea, vomiting, thirst, abdominal pain, or pain of any type (see above).
4. Additional side effects which are reportable are: convulsive seizures, feelings of depression or nervousness, or development of an infection (see above).
5. If the patient has a fall or is in an auto accident, his condition may precipitate adrenal failure. He requires an immediate injection of hydrocortisone phosphate. (Long-term patients should wear a Medic Alert tag and carry a kit with hydrocortisone.)
6. See physician on a regular follow-up basis.

a. Determine the flow rate of fluids necessary to give a precise amount of medication.
b. Observe the tissues, catheter site, flow rate, fluid

level, and patient's response at frequent intervals to be sure the system is functioning well.
c. Note signs and symptoms indicative of adrenal

crisis—restlessness, weakness, headache, nausea, vomiting, diarrhea, and falling blood pressure.

Health Education

1. Be sure the patient or a responsible member of his family knows that he is taking a steroid medication; explain why he is receiving it and what effects are desired.
2. The patient must also know what complications can occur, how to prevent them, and what to do should they occur.
3. Inform patient of the need for him to tell any physician, dentist, or nurse in his future contacts that he is on steroid therapy.
4. Be sure he knows that steroids are unique drugs prescribed in a dosage specific for him and that no one else should use his medications.

GUIDELINES: The Patient Receiving Steroid Therapy— Clinical Assessment, Surveillance, and Health Education

OBJECTIVE: to detect early signs of side effects from steroid therapy.

NURSING ACTION	RATIONALE
Infection Control	
1. Encourage patient to avoid crowds and the possibility of exposure to infection.	Because steroids may affect the circulating blood—resulting in decreased eosinophils and lymphocytes, increased red cells, and increased incidence of thrombophlebitis and infection.
2. Utilize exercise schedules to prevent stasis.	
3. Be aware that cardinal symptoms of inflammation may be masked.	
4. Instruct all personnel coming in contact with this patient to wash hands thoroughly and practice meticulous asepsis.	
Diet and Metabolism Considerations	
1. Determine whether the patient needs assistance in dietary control.	1. Because steroids may cause weight gain and an increase in appetite.
2. Administer a high protein, high carbohydrate diet.	2. Because steroids affect protein metabolism, there may be negative nitrogen balance.
3. Encourage patient to take steroids with milk or food.	3. Because steroids cause an increase in secretion of gastric hydrochloric acid and have an inhibiting effect on secretion of mucus in the stomach, they may aggravate an existing peptic ulcer.
4. Be on guard for early evidence of gastric hemorrhage such as melena, blood in vomitus.	
5. Check urine for evidence of glucose.	5. Because steroids precipitate gluconeogenesis and insulin antagonism, which results in hyperglycemia, glucosuria, decreased carbohydrate tolerance.
Possible Bone Complications	
1. Be on the alert for the possibility of pathologic fractures. Stress safety measures to prevent injury	Because steroids affect the musculoskeletal system, causing potassium depletion and muscular weakness. (Steroids cause increased output of calcium and phosphorus, which may lead to osteoporosis.)
2. Administer a diet high in calcium and protein.	
3. Recommend a program of activities of daily living; normal range of motion for the bedridden.	
Electrolyte Disturbance	
1. Restrict sodium intake and increase potassium intake. a. Lemon juice is high in potassium and low in sodium. b. Avoid saline as a diluent in preparing injectable medications.	Because mineralocorticoid differs from other steroids, resulting in sodium retention and potassium depletion: edema, weight gain.
2. Check blood pressure frequently and weigh patient daily.	
3. Observe for evidence of edema.	
Behavioral Reactions	
1. Watch for convulsive seizures (especially in children).	Because steroids may alter behavior patterns, increase excitability, and affect the central nervous system.
2. Avoid overstimulating situations.	
3. Recognize and report any mood deviating from the usual behavior patterns.	
4. Report unusual behavior, haunting dreams, withdrawal, or suicidal tendencies.	
Stress Reactions	
1. Recommend that the patient carry at all times an identification card indicating that he is on steroid therapy and including the name of his physician and instructions for emergency care.	Because steroids affect the hypothalmic-pituitary-adrenal system, this in turn affects the individual's ability to respond to stress.

2. Advise the patient to avoid extremes of temperature, as well as infections and upsetting situations.

Safety Measures

1. Admonish the patient to avoid injury; stress safety precautions.
2. Observe daily the healing process of wounds, particularly surgical wounds, in order to recognize the potential for wound dehiscence.

Because steroids interfere with fibroblasts and granulation tissue, there is altered response to injury, resulting in impaired growth and delayed healing.

5 DISORDERS OF THE PITUITARY GLAND

DIABETES INSIPIDUS

Diabetes insipidus is a disorder of water metabolism caused by deficiency of vasopressin, the antidiuretic hormone (ADH) secreted by the posterior pituitary.

Etiology

1. Primary: idiopathic, rarely familial
2. Secondary: head trauma (particularly basal skull fracture), brain neoplasm, neurosurgery, irradiation of pituitary

Clinical Manifestations

1. Marked polyuria—daily output of 5–20 liters of very dilute urine; appearance of urine like that of water, with a specific gravity of 1.001–1.005 corresponding to a urine osmolality of 50–200 mOsm./kg.
2. Polydipsia (intense thirst); 4–40 liters of fluid daily; patient has a craving for cold water.

Diagnostic Evaluation

1. Fluid Deprivation Test
OBJECTIVE: to restrict water intake and observe changes in urine volume and concentration.
   a. Fluids withheld for 8–12 hours or until 3% of body weight is lost.
   b. Plasma and urine osmolality studies are determined at beginning and end of test—inability to increase specific gravity and osmolality of urine is characteristic of diabetes insipidus.
   c. Patient is weighed frequently while fluid is withheld.

2. Measurement of urinary ADH by radioimmunoassay.

Treatment and Nursing Management

OBJECTIVES: to replace vasopressin (usually a lifelong therapeutic program)
to search for and correct underlying intracranial pathology

1. Administer antidiuretic hormone (ADH) or its derivative, the principal hormone controlling water balance. Available ADH preparations include:
   a. Vasopressin tannate (Pitressin tannate in oil)—effective for 24–72 hours.
      (1) Administered by IM injection.
      (2) Warm vial and shake vigorously before administering—to ensure uniform dispersion, since active component settles at bottom of vial.
   b. Lypressin (Diapid nasal spray)—drug absorbed through nasal mucosa into blood.
      (1) Duration of action only a few hours.
      (2) May cause chronic nasal irritation.
   c. Desmopressin acetate (DDAVP)—a synthetic vasopressin derivative administered into nose through a soft, flexible nasal tube.
2. For patients who have some residual hypothalamic vasopressin:
   a. Chlorpropamide (Diabinese)—potentiates action of vasopressin on renal-concentrating mechanism.
   b. Clofibrate (Atromid S.)—probably acts by augmenting ADH secretion from neurohypophysis.
   c. Carbamazepine (Tegretol)—stimulates endogenous ADH release.

PITUITARY TUMORS

Types of Pituitary Tumors

1. *Chromophobe Adenoma*—tumor of the anterior pituitary gland of adults.
   a. Most common pituitary tumor; does not secrete clinically significant amounts of hormones but can destroy rest of pituitary gland.
   b. Produces failing vision, optic atrophy, bitemporal hemianopsia, enlargement of sella turcica, and endocrine disturbances.

2. *Eosinophilic Adenoma*—endocrine secretion of tumor produces gigantism in children and acromegaly in adults.
3. *Basophilic Adenoma*—gives rise to so-called Cushing's syndrome with features largely attributable to hyperadrenalism—masculinization and amenorrhea in females, girdle obesity, hypertension, osteoporosis, and polycythemia.

HYPOPHYSECTOMY

Hypophysectomy is removal of the pituitary gland.

Indications

1. Primary neoplasms (tumors) of the pituitary gland
2. Diabetic retinopathy
   a. Used to halt progress of hemorrhagic diabetic retinopathy and to prevent blindness
   b. Also reduces insulin requirements
3. Palliative measure for relief of bone pain secondary to metastasis of malignant lesions of breast and prostate; alters hormonal milieu of body to create a hormonal environment hostile to continued growth of neoplasm

Methods of Pituitary Ablation (Removal)

1. Extirpative hypophysectomy—done by transfrontal, subcranial, or oronasal-transsphenoidal approaches
2. Hypophyseal stalk section
3. Radiation x-ray
4. Destruction with stereotaxic radio frequency (heat) or cryosurgery (freezing)

Management

The absence of the pituitary gland alters the function of many parts of the body.

1. The patient may need substitution therapy with adrenal steroids (hydrocortisone) and thyroid hormone.
2. Menstruation ceases and infertility occurs almost always after total or nearly total ablation.
3. See page 659 for treatment of diabetes insipidus; transient or permanent diabetes insipidus may follow surgery of pituitary gland.
4. See page 715 for nursing management of the patient undergoing cranial surgery.

6 DISORDER OF PURINE METABOLISM

GOUT

Gout is a disease manifested by an acute inflammation of a joint; it is caused by the deposit of uric acid crystals in joints and connective tissues.

1. *Uric acid*—end product of purine metabolism derived from both dietary sources and endogenous synthesis.
2. *Hyperuricemia*—persistent elevation of urates in the blood usually found in gout patients. It is caused by overproduction or underexcretion of uric acid.
3. *Tophi*—deposits of urates in the tissues about the joints or on the ear; development of tophi related to duration of disease, degree of hyperuricemia, and renal function status

Types of Gout

1. *Primary gout*—may be due to a genetic defect of purine metabolism or a renal defect resulting in decreased excretion of uric acid.
2. *Secondary gout* (an acquired disease)—hyperuricemia occurs in conditions in which there is an increase in cell turnover (leukemia, multiple myeloma, psoriasis) and in cell breakdown, or because of impaired renal excretion of uric acid.
   May be precipitated by prolonged ingestion of diuretic agents, aspirin, trauma, treatment of myeloproliferative diseases.

Clinical Manifestations

1. Sudden onset of severe pain in one or more peripheral joints—may be accompanied by intense inflammation, swelling, and tenderness.
   a. First joint of great toe is susceptible; later, other joints of foot are affected.
   b. Joints of feet, ankles, knees, wrist, and elbow commonly affected.
2. Fever 38.3–39.4° C. (101–103° F.)
3. Attacks involving the same joints tend to recur; variable lengths of time between attacks.

Diagnostic Evaluation

1. Clinical history
2. Therapeutic response to colchicine
3. Elevation of serum uric acid levels
4. Identification of uric acid crystals in synovial fluid—obtained by arthrocentesis (aspiration of fluid from a joint cavity)

Treatment and Nursing Management

OBJECTIVES: to relieve acute pain and inflammation. to prevent the development of chronic gouty arthritis, renal calculi, and renal damage.

A. *Acute Attack of Gout*

1. Give colchicine *early* in attack—suppresses inflammatory manifestations of acute gout; useful in establishing diagnosis since it gives dramatic relief if patient has gout.
   a. An initial dose of colchicine is given and is followed by doses every 1–2 hours until the pain disappears and gastrointestinal symptoms develop (nausea, vomiting, abdominal cramping, diarrhea).
   b. Colchicine produces diarrhea—stop drug temporarily until diarrhea subsides. Drug may be given intravenously.
   c. A maintenance dose of colchicine is given as soon as diarrhea stops; it is given as a prophylactic agent against recurrent gouty arthritis.
   d. Colchicine may be given before and after surgery to patients with gout—reduces the incidence of acute attacks of gouty arthritis precipitated by operative procedures.
2. Alternative forms of therapy.
   a. Phenylbutazone (Butazolidin) or oxyphenbutazone or indomethacin (Indocin) are other drugs given during the acute stage of gout—these drugs

reduce the fever and have an anti-inflammatory effect.
   b. Fenoprofen, naproxen, ibuprofen (nonsteroidal anti-inflammatory agents)—also effective in acute gout.
3. Give analgesic for severe pain until specific drug is effective.
4. Immobilize and elevate the affected joint; encourage patient to rest since early ambulation may precipitate a recurrence.
5. Encourage large fluid intake to maintain a high 24-hour urinary volume—urinary urate excretion increases 24 hours after introduction of uricosuric drugs and may lead to stone formation.

B. Chronic Gouty Arthritis
OBJECTIVE: to lower serum uric acid levels to a normal range.
1. Give drug (uricosuric agent for urate-lowering therapy)—acts on renal tubule to inhibit urate reabsorption and thereby increases urinary excretion of urate and lowers the serum urate level; prevents formation of new tophi and reduces size of those already present. Drug selection depends on the mechanism of hyperuricemia.
   a. Probenecid (Benemid)
      Side effects—headache, gastrointestinal disturbances, skin rash.
   b. Sulfinpyrazone (Anturane)
      Side effects—gastrointestinal disturbances (including peptic ulcer), skin rash, hematologic side effects.
   c. Give after meals or with antacids if there are gastric side effects.
2. Or give allopurinol (Zyloprim), a xanthine oxidase inhibitor—interferes with final stages of conversion

of the products of purine metabolism to uric acid (inhibits formation of uric acid).
   Dosage based on serum urate determinations.
3. Encourage large fluid intake to maintain a high 24-hour urinary volume—urinary urate excretion increases 24 hours after introduction of uricosuric drugs and may lead to stone formation and renal complications.
   a. Maintain an alkaline urine in patients with a history of stone formation.
   b. Give sodium bicarbonate or citrate solutions.

Health Education
Instruct the patient as follows:
1. Take colchicine as prescribed as a prophylactic measure against acute gouty attack.
2. Take uricosuric agent (see above) or allopurinol—to prevent further deposition of uric acid in joints.
3. Avoid aspirin since it counteracts uricosuric effect.
4. Avoid foods rich in purine content—glandular meats, liver, shellfish, anchovies, sardines; avoid any food known to precipitate an acute attack. Avoid excessive alcohol intake.
5. Maintain a high fluid intake to sustain high urinary volume—minimizes urate precipitation in urinary tract.
6. Avoid fasting (to lose weight or when on alcoholic spree)—fasting has been found to increase the serum uric acid level.
7. Avoid crash diets—rapid reduction of weight may increase the serum uric acid level; slow weight reduction reduces the serum urate level without inducing an acute attack.
8. Recognize the warnings of an impending attack. Start therapy promptly.

BIBLIOGRAPHY

1   DISORDERS OF THE THYROID GLAND

Books
Alsever RN and Gotkin RW. Handbook of Endocrine Tests in Adults and Children, 2nd ed. Chicago, Year Book Medical Publishers, 1978
Ashkar FS. Thyroid and Endocrine System. Investigations with Radionuclides and Radioassays. New York, Masson Publishers, 1979
Bondy PK and Rosenberg LE. Metabolic Control and Disease. Philadelphia, WB Saunders, 1980
Brown BR Jr. Anesthesia and the Patient with Endocrine Disorders. Philadelphia, FA Davis, 1980
DeGroot LJ. Endocrinology. New York, Grune & Stratton, 1979
Dillon RS. Handbook of Endocrinology. 2nd ed. Philadelphia, Lea & Febiger 1980
Hamburger JI. Clinical Exercises in Internal Medicine, Vol. 1 Thyroid Disease, Philadelphia, WB Saunders, 1978
Hershman JM and Bray GA. The Thyroid. Elmsford, Pergamon Press, 1979
Ryan WG. Endocrine Disorders, 2nd ed. Chicago, Year Book Medical Publishers, 1980
Stanbury JB. Endemic Goiter and Endemic Cretinism. New York, John Wiley & Sons, 1980
Werner S and Ingbar S. The Thyroid, 4th ed. Hagerstown, Harper & Row, 1978
Williams RH. Textbook of Endocrinology, 6th ed. Philadelphia, WB Saunders, 1980

Articles
Ali AS and Akavaram NR. Neuromuscular disorders in thyrotoxicosis. Am Fam Physician 1980 Sept; 22(3):97–102
Bains J and Walfish PG. The assessment of thyroid function and structure. Otolaryngol Clin North Am 1978 June; 11(6):419–443
Clark OH et al. Hashimoto's thyroiditis and thyroid cancer: Indications for operation. Am J Surg 1980 July; 140(1):65–71
Feek CM et al. Combination of potassium iodide and propranolol in preparation of patients with Graves' disease for thyroid surgery. N Engl J Med 1980 April 17; 302(16):883–885
Greenfield LD et al. Radiation safety precautions with [131]iodine therapy. Cancer Nurs 1978 Oct; 1(5):379–384
Guimond JH and Wilson SG. Postirradiation thyroid disorders. Am J Nurs 1980 July; 80(7):1256–1258
Holm L et al. Malignant thyroid tumors after iodine-131 therapy. N Engl J Med 1980 July 24; 303(4):188–191
Jenkins EH. Living with thyrotoxicosis. Am J Nurs 1980 May; 80(5):956–958
Katz AD and Bronson D. Total thyroidectomy. Am J Surg 1978 Oct; 136(4):450–454
Kinderlehrer DA. Thyroid function tests. Am Fam Physician 1980 May; 21(5):116–120
Klementschitsch P et al. Reemergence of thyroidectomy as treatment for Graves' disease. Surg Clin N Amer 1979 Feb; 59(1):35–44

Lowhagen T et al. Aspiration biopsy cytology (ABC) in nodules of the thyroid gland suspected to be malignant. Surg Clin North Am 1979 Feb; 59(1):3–18

Miller JM. Hamburger JI and Kini S. Diagnosis of thyroid nodules. JAMA 1979 Feb 2; 241(5):481–484

Oppenheimer JH (ed). Thyroid Today. A leaflet available almost monthly by Travenol Laboratories. Deerfield, Flint Laboratories.

Palmer ED. Gastrointestinal repercussions of thyroid disease. Am Fam Physician 1979 May; 19(5):131–132

Rees-Jones R et al. Hormonal content of thyroid replacement preparations. JAMA 1980 Feb 8; 243(6):549–550

Saxe AW. Thyroid scans and the diagnosis of carcinoma of the thyroid. Surg Gynecol Obstet 1979 Nov; 149(11):729–730

Schottenfeld D and Gershman ST. Epidemiology of thyroid cancer. CA—A Cancer Jour for Clinicians 1978 March/April; 28(28):66–86

Syed AMN and Greenfield LD. The role of interstitial irradiation in the treatment of thyroid cancer. Contemp Surg 1980 Sept; 17(3):36–50

Wake MM and Brensinger JF. The nurse's role in hypothyroidism. Nurs Clin North Am 1980 Sept; 15(3):453–467

White VA and Kumagai LF. Preoperative endocrine and metabolic considerations. Med Clin North Am 1979 Nov; 63(6):1321–1334

2 DISORDERS OF THE PARATHYROID GLANDS

Articles

Coe FL and Fairis MJ. Does mild, asymptomatic hyperparathyroidism require surgery? N Engl J Med 1980 Jan 24; 302(4):224–225

Edis AJ. Prevention and management of complications associated with thyroid and parathyroid surgery. Surg Clin North Am 1979 Feb; 59(1):83–92

Edis AJ and Beart RW Jr. Parathyroid autotransplantation: An innovative approach. Hosp Pract 1979 Jan; 14(1):78–84

Esselstyn CB Jr. Parathyroid surgery. Surg Clin North Am 1979 Feb; 59(1):77–81

Heath H III et al. Primary hyperparathyroidism. N Eng J Med 1980 Jan 24; 302(4):189–193

Hoffmann JTT and Newly TB. Hypercalcemia in primary hyperparathyroidism. Nurs Clin North Am 1980 Sept; 15(3):469–480

Peskin GE et al. Expanding indications for early parathyroidectomy in the elderly female. Am J Surg 1978 July; 136(1):45–48

3 DIABETES MELLITUS (PANCREATIC DISORDERS)

Books

Drury MI. Diabetes Mellitus. Oxford, Blackwell Scientific Publications, 1979

Grave GD (ed). Early Detection of Potential Diabetics: The Problems and the Promise. New York, Raven Press, 1979

Podolosky S (ed). Clinical Diabetes: Modern Management. New York, Appleton-Century-Crofts, 1980

Rakow R. Podiatric Management of the Diabetic Foot. Mt Kisco, Futura Publishers, 1979

Rifkin H and Raskin P (eds). Diabetes Mellitus. Bowie, Robert J Brady, 1981

Sims DF (ed). Diabetes: Reach for Health and Freedom. St. Louis, CV Mosby, 1980

Articles

Management of Diabetes Mellitus

American Diabetes Association. Principles of nutrition and dietary recommendations for individuals with diabetes mellitus: 1979. Diabetes 1979 Nov; 28(11):1027–1031

Anderson JW et al. Fiber and diabetes. Diabetes Care 1979 July–Aug; 2(4):369–379

Bauer JK and Horwitz DL. New trends in diabetic diets. Compr Ther 1979 Dec; 5(12):12–18

Bernstein RK. Blood glucose-self-monitoring by diabetic patients: Refinements of procedural technique. Diabetes Care 1979 March–April; 2(2):233–236

Burke MD. Diabetes mellitus: Test strategies for diagnosis and management. Postgrad Med 1979 Nov; 66(5):213–220

Ellenberg M et al. Symposium on sex amd diabetes. Diabetes Care 1979 Jan–Feb; 2(1):4–30

From the NIH. Diabetes research is greatly expanding. JAMA 1980 Aug 8; 244(6):549–550

Gonzalez ER. Exercise therapy 'rediscovered' for diabetes; but what does it do? JAMA 1979 Oct 12; 242(15):1591–1592

Guthrie D. Helping the diabetic manage his self-care. Nursing '80 1980 Feb; 10(2):57–64

Hodge RH et al. Multiple use of disposable insulin syringe-needle units. JAMA 1980 July 18; 244(3):266–267

Jenkins DJA et al. Diabetic diets: High carbohydrate combined with high fiber. Am J Clin Nutr 1980 Aug; 33(8):1729–1733

Johnson DG. The pathogenesis of diabetes mellitus. Ariz Med 1979 Oct; 36(10):766–770

Karam JH. Diabetes mellitus: Therapeutic guidelines based on a functional classification. Compr Ther 1980 Aug; 6(8):50–55

Khachadurian AK et al. Management of noninsulin-dependent diabetes mellitus. Am Fam Physician 1980 Feb; 21(2):154–160

Maurer AC. The therapy of diabetes. Am Sci 1979 July–Aug; 67(4):422–431

National Diabetes Data Group. Classification and diagnosis of diabetes mellitus and other categories of glucose intolerance. Diabetes 1979 Dec; 28(12):1039–1057

Podolsky S (ed). Symposium on diabetes mellitus. Med Clin North Am 1978 July; 62(4):625–866

Principles of nutrition and dietary recommendations for individuals with diabetes mellitus: 1979. J Am Diet Assoc 1979 Nov; 75(5):527–530

Programmed instruction: Controlling diabetes mellitus. Am J Nurs 1980 Oct; 80(10):1827–1850

Reaven GM et al. Nutritional management of diabetes. Med Clin North Am 1979 Sept; 63(5):927–943

Shuman CR. When—and how—to use an oral agent. Med Times 1980 May; 108(5):77–86

Turkington RW et al. Diabetes. Compr Ther 1979 April; 5(4):9–74

Watlington CO. The oral glucose tolerance test. J Fam Pract 1979 Nov; 9(5):915–919

Complications of Diabetes

Alberti KGM and Nattrass M. Severe diabetic ketoacidosis. Med Clin North Am 1978 July; 62(4):799–814

Bellows JG. Prevention of diabetic retinopathy. Compr Ther 1980 May; 6(5):3–4

Bradley WE (ed). Aspects of diabetic autonomic neuropathy. Ann Intern Med 1980 Feb; 92(2):289–342

Bruce RA and Letson AD. Ocular manifestations of diabetes mellitus. Postgrad Med 1980 Oct; 68(4):143–157

Cavalier JP. Crucial decisions in diabetic emergencies. RN 1980 Nov; 43(11):32–37

Edwards JE Jr et al. Infection and diabetes mellitus. West J Med 1979 June; 130(6):515–521

Ellenberg M. Chronic complications of diabetes mellitus. NY State J Med 1979 Dec; 79(13):2005–2014

Fisher JN. Management of diabetic ketoacidosis. Compr Ther 1979 April; 5(4):43–48

Garofano CD. Helping diabetics live with their neuropathies. Nursing '80 1980 June; 10(6):42–44

Johnson EW et al. Management of the diabetic neurotrophic foot. Instructional Course Lectures 1979; 28:118–165

Kiser D. The Somogyi effect. Am J Nurs 1980 Feb; 80(2):236–238

Levine ME et al. Prevention and treatment of diabetic complications. Arch Intern Med 1980 May; 140(5):691–696

Lippmann HI and Farrar R. Prevention of amputation in diabetics. Angiology 1979 Oct; 30(10):649–658

Perrin ED. Laser therapy for diabetic retinopathy. Am J Nurs 1980 April; 80(4):664–665

Riley TL and Massey EW. Managing the patient with peripheral neuropathy. Postgrad Med 1980 Oct; 68(4):103–109

Smith IM. Common infections in the elderly diabetic. Geriatrics 1980 Aug; 35(8):55–58

Taylor AL. Diabetic ketoacidosis. Postgrad Med 1980 Oct; 68(4):161–175

Whitehouse FW (ed). Key problems in diabetes. Med Times 1980 May; 108(5):31–118

Williamson JR and Kilo C. Vascular complications in diabetes mellitus. N Engl J Med 1980 Feb 14; 302(7):399–400

Wolbarsht ML and Landers MB. The rationale of photocoagulation therapy for proliferative diabetic retinopathy: a review and a model. Ophthalmic Surg 1980 April; 11(4):235–245

Management of Diabetic Undergoing Surgery

Bessman AN. Management of the diabetic surgical patient. Compr Ther 1979 April; 5(4):57–64

White VA and Kumagai LF. Preoperative endocrine and metabolic considerations. Med Clin North Am 1979 Nov; 63(6):1321–1334

Woodruff RE et al. Avoidance of surgical hyperglycemia in diabetic patients. JAMA 1980 July 11; 244(2):166–168

4 DISORDERS OF THE ADRENAL GLANDS

Articles

Bissada NK. Surgical diseases of the adrenal gland. Am Fam Physician 1977 June; 15(6):130–135

Burke MD. Hypertension: Strategies for laboratory diagnosis. Postgrad Med 1980 June; 67(6):77–85

Byyny RL. Preventing adrenal insufficiency during surgery. Postgrad Med 1980 May; 67(5):219–225

Daughday WH. New criteria for evaluation of acromegaly (editorial). N Engl J Med 1979 Nov 22; 301(21):1175–1176

Garofano CD. Frank's condition—is it serious? Nursing '80 1980 April; 10(4):30–31

Gold EM. Cushing's syndrome: A tripartite entity. Hosp Pract 1979 June; 14(6):67–75

Gold EM. The Cushing syndromes: Changing views of diagnosis and treatment. Ann Intern Med 1979 May; 90(5):829–844

Javadpour N. et al. Adrenal neoplasms. Curr Probl Surg 1980 Jan; 17(1):1–52

Prinz RA et al. Cushing's disease: The role of adrenalectomy and autotransplantation. Surg Clin North Am 1979 Feb; 59(1):159–165

Rincon J et al. 'Not Cushing's Syndrome.' Am Fam Physician 1979 May; 19(5):77–86

Sanford SJ. Dysfunction of the adrenal gland: Physiologic considerations and nursing problems. Nurs Clin North Am 1980 Sept; 15(3):481–498

Schteingart DE. Cushing's disease: An update. Drug Ther 1978 Feb; 8(2):125–135

Tepley JF and Lawrence GH. Pheochromocytoma. Am J Surg 1980 July; 140(1):107–111

Tzagournis M. Acute adrenal insufficiency. Heart Lung 1978 July–Aug; 7(4):603–609

Wilson CB et al. Cushing's disease revisited. Am J Surg 1979 July; 138(1):77–79

Steroids

Blechman WJ et al. Update on anti-inflammatory agents. Patient Care 1978 Feb 15; 12(3):174–181

Dismukes W et al. Disseminated histoplasmosis in corticosteroid-treated patients. JAMA 1978 Sept 29; 240(14):1495–1498

Dixon R and Christy N. On the various forms of corticosteroid withdrawal syndrome. Am J Med 1980 Feb; 68(2):224–230

Gever LN. Reducing the side effects of steroid therapy. Nursing '80 1980 Sept; 10(9):59

Gotch PM. Teaching patients about adrenal corticosteroids. Am J Nurs 1981 Jan; 81(1):78–81

Gottlieb N and Penneys N. Spontaneous skin tearing during systemic corticosteroid treatment. JAMA 1980 March 28; 243(12):1260–1261

Hartley B. Now you're on cortisone. Can Nurs 1978 Feb; 74(2):21–27

Leyden JJ and Kligman AM. Efficacy of steroid-antibiotic combination. Drug Ther 1978 Feb; 8(2):114–120

Newton DW et al. You can minimize the hazards of corticosteroids. Nursing '77 1977 June; 7(6):26–33

One more topical corticosteroid (diflorasone diacetate—Florone). Met Lett Drugs Ther 1978 Dec 15; 20(25):112

Rose LI and Saccar C. Choosing corticosteroid preparations. Am Fam Physician 1978 March; 17(3):198–204

Segaloff A. The status of steroid therapy. Drug Ther 1978 Feb; 8(2):106–113

Toward safer use of topical steroids. Emergency Med 1980 May 30; 12(10):65

White SJ and Williamson K. What to watch for with synthetic adrenocortical steroids. RN 1980 Aug; 43(8):37–39

5 DISORDERS OF THE PITUITARY GLAND

Articles

Diabetes Insipidus

Hau T-H. Current management of diabetes insipidus. Compr Ther 1980 Aug; 6(8):22–25

Moens J. Coping with diabetes insipidus. Can Nurse 1979 April; 75(4):18–20

Oliver RE and Jamison RL. Diabetes insipidus: A physiologic approach to diagnosis. Postgrad Med 1980 Dec; 68(6):120–131

Ross JL and Shenkman L. Diabetes insipidus. Compr Ther 1979 April; 5(4):30–35

Pituitary Tumors

Camunas CE. Transsphenoidal hypophysectomy. Am J Nurs 1980 Oct; 80(10):1820–1823

Herbert P and Breeding P. Self-care after hypophysectomy. J Neurosurg Nurs 1979 June; 11(2):118–120

Morrow LB. Clinical evaluation of pituitary adenomas. Postgrad Med 1980 Dec; 68(6):155–164

6 DISORDERS OF PURINE METABOLISM

Articles

Gout

Boss GR and Seegmiller JE. Hyperuricemia and gout. Classification, complications and management. N Engl J Med 1979 June 28; 300(26):1459–1468

Mangin RJ. Pathogenesis and clinical management of hyperuricemia and gout. J Maine Med Assoc 1979 March; 70(3):118–120;122–127

EYE PROBLEMS

EYE CARE SPECIALISTS*

Definitions

1. An *ophthalmologist* or *oculist* is a physician (M.D.) who specializes in diagnosis and treatment of defects and diseases of the eye, performing surgery when necessary or prescribing other types of treatment, including glasses.
2. An *optometrist,* a licensed, nonmedical practitioner, measures refractive errors (irregularities in the size

or shape of the eyeball or surface of the cornea) and eye muscle disturbances. In his treatment the optometrist uses glasses, prisms, and exercises only.
3. An *optician* grinds lenses, fits them into frames, and adjusts the frames to the wearer and/or teaches patient to use contact lens.

    * Definitions from U.S. Dept. of Health, Education, and Welfare.

NORMAL VISION AND REFRACTIVE ERRORS

Vision

Vision is the passage of rays of light from an object through the cornea, aqueous humor, lens, and vitreous humor to the retina and its appreciation in the cerebral cortex.

A. *Normal*—emmetropia

    Rays coming from an object at a distance of 6 meters (20 feet) or more are brought to a focus on the retina by the lens.

B. *Abnormal*—ametropia

1. Nearsightedness (myopia)
   a. Rays of light coming from an object at a distance of 6 meters (20 feet) or more are brought to a focus in front of the retina.
   b. Correction—concave lens.

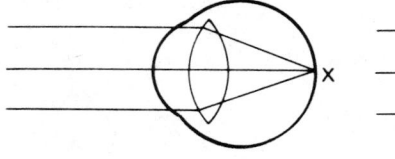

Normal

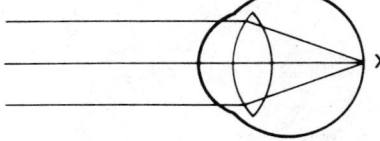

No correction necessary

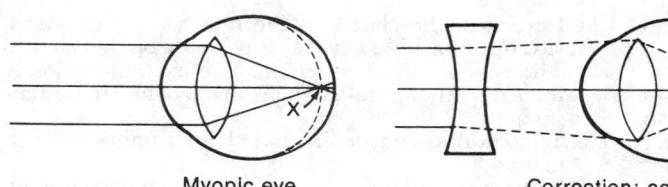

Myopic eye   Correction: concave lens

2. Farsightedness (hyperopia)
   a. Rays of light coming from an object at a distance of 6 meters (20 feet) or more are brought to a focus in back of the retina.
   b. Correction—convex lens.

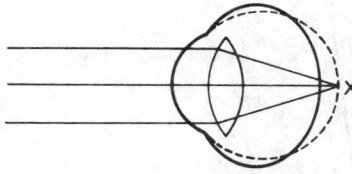

Hypermetropic eye

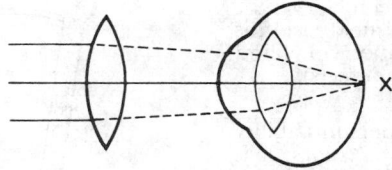

Correction: convex lens

Accommodation

In *accommodation*, the focusing apparatus of the eye adjusts to objects at different distances by means of increasing the convexity of the lens (brought about by contraction of ciliary muscles).

Presbyopia—the elasticity of the lens decreases with increasing age; an emmetropic person with presbyopia will read a paper at arm's length and requires prescription lenses to correct the problem.

Curvature of Cornea

A. *Normal*—equal curvature of cornea

B. *Abnormal*—astigmatism
1. Uneven curvature of the cornea, causing the patient to be unable to focus horizontal and vertical rays on the retina at the same time
2. Correction—cylinder lenses

EXAMINATION AND DIAGNOSTIC PROCEDURES

(For history, physical examination, and assessment see page 21.)

External Examination

Includes examination of eye and adnexa without the aid of special apparatus.

A. *Visual Acuity*

Snellen Chart and other methods.
1. Each eye is tested separately, with and without glasses.
2. Letters or objects are of a size that can be seen by the normal eye at a distance of 6 meters (20 feet) from the chart.
3. Letters appear in rows and are arranged so that the normal eye can see them at distances of 9, 12, 15 meters (30, 40, 50 feet), etc.
4. When a person can identify letters of the size 6 at 6 meters (20 at 20 feet), his eye is said to have 6/6 (20/20) vision.
5. Additionally, if vision is less than 6/60 (20/200), test may be recorded as follows:

Counting fingers at _____meters (feet):	C.F.
Hand motion—ability to detect hand movement at a certain distance:	H.M.
Light perception:	L.P.

	meters	feet
Visual Acuity	6/6	20/20
	6/9	20/30
	6/12	20/40
	6/15	20/50
	6/21	20/70
	6/30	20/100
	6/60	20/200
Then:	C.F.@ _____	meters (feet)
	H.M.	Hand motion
	L.P. & P.	Light perception and projection
	L.P.	Light perception only
	N.L.P.	No light perception

B. *Visual Fields*

To determine function of retina, optic nerve, and optic pathways.
1. Equipment—perimeter, tangent screen, light source, and test objects.
2. Fields
   a. *Peripheral*—useful in detecting disorders that cause

constriction of peripheral vision in one or both eyes.
(1) Patient is seated at a "perimeter."
(2) The left eye is covered while the patient focuses with right eye on a spot in the central portion of the perimeter (0.33 meters from the eye).
(3) A test object (white) is brought in from the side at 15-degree intervals, through 360 degrees.
(4) The patient is asked to signal when he sees the test object.
(5) The object is passed along the same meridian from the seeing to the nonseeing segment and the patient is asked to signal when it disappears.
b. *Central*
(1) Patient is seated 1–2 meters from a 2–3 meter (6–8 foot) black felt tangent screen.
(2) Each eye is covered and central field vision is tested—including a determination of blind spots and scotomas (visual field defects).

C. *Color Vision Tests*

These tests are done to determine the person's ability to perceive primary colors and shades of colors; it is particularly significant for individuals whose occupation requires color perception: transportation workers, surgeons, nurses, artists, interior decorators.
1. Equipment
   a. Polychromatic plates; these are dots of primary colors printed on a background of similar dots in a confusion of colors.
   b. Individual colored discs; each disc is matched to its next closest color.
2. Procedure
   a. Various polychromatic plates are presented to the patient under specified illumination.
   b. The patterns may be letters or numbers which the normal eye can perceive instantly, but which are confusing to the person with a perception defect.
3. Outcome
   a. Color-blindness—person is unable to perceive the figures
   b. Red-green blindness—8.0% of males; 0.4% of females
   c. Blue-yellow blindness—extremely rare

D. *Refraction*

Refraction is a clinical measurement of the error of focus in an eye.
1. Usually this is accomplished by instilling a cyclopegic (atropine or cyclopentolate) into the conjunctival sac.
2. The ciliary muscle is relaxed.
3. Accommodative power is lowered (cycloplegia).
4. The pupil is dilated (mydriasis), which facilitates the examination.
5. The refractive state of the eye can be determined as follows:
   a. Objectively—via retinoscopy
   b. Subjectively—trial of lenses to arrive at the best visual image.

NOTE: *Auto-Refractor*—in eye clinic centers, this device provides automatic refraction of an individual's eyes as he sits in front of the special instrument. Findings are transferred by computer directly onto a printout sheet.

Internal Examination

A. *Ophthalmoscopic Examination*

The interior of the eye is examined when a beam of light is reflected through the pupil while the examiner looks through an ophthalmoscope.

a. Defects in the clarity of the media (e.g., cataracts, vitreous opacities, corneal scars) may be detected.
b. The retinal blood vessels may be examined closely for the pathological changes of diabetes, hypertension, etc.
c. The choroid can be examined for tumors, inflammation.
d. The retina can be examined for retinal detachment, scars, diabetes, etc.

B. *Gonioscopy*

Direct visualization of the junction of the iris and cornea (angle of anterior chamber).

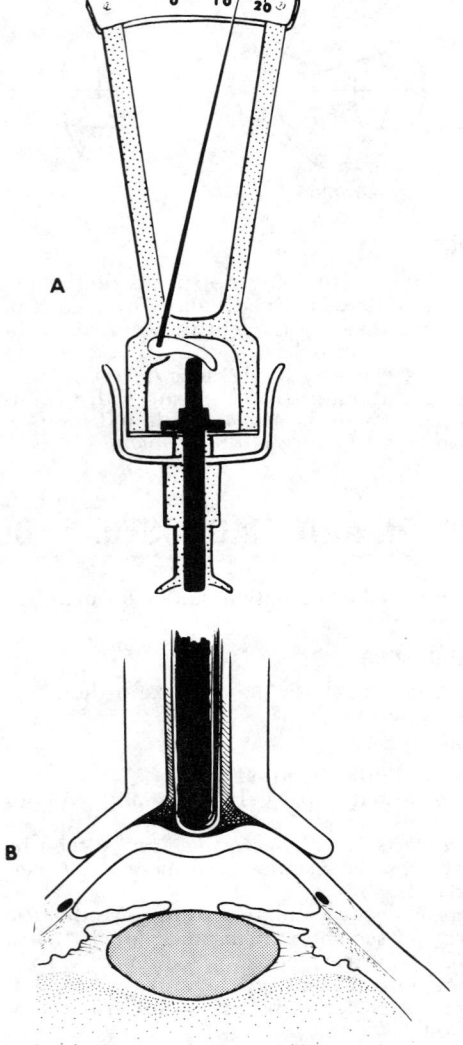

FIGURE 15-1. (A), *Schiøtz tonometer in which the plunger, in black, measures the ease of indentation of cornea. (B), Indentation of the anesthetized cornea by the plunger of the tonometer in order to measure ocular tension. From Newell, Frank W.: Ophthalmology: Principles and Concepts, ed. 4. St. Louis, The C. V. Mosby Co.*

1. *Equipment*—Local anesthetic solutions, goniolens, biomicroscope (Slit lamp)
2. Procedure
   a. A local anesthetic is instilled into the eye.
   b. The goniolens is placed over the cornea; sterile methylcellulose solution is injected between the cornea and the lens.
   c. The patient fixes his gaze as the examiner views the anterior chamber, through the biomicroscope, through a circumference of 360 degrees.

C. *Tonometry*

Measurement of intraocular tension or pressure.
1. Schiøtz tonometry
   a. After instillation of topical anesthesia, the Schiøtz tonometer is gently rested on the eyeball (Fig. 15-1).
   b. The indicator measures the ocular tension in mm.Hg.
   c. Normal tension is approximately 11–22 mm. Hg.
2. Applanation tonometry
   a. This is the most effective measuring method for determining intraocular pressure, however it requires a biomicroscope and a trained interpreter.
   b. After instillation of topical anesthesia, the cornea is flattened by a known amount (3.14 mm.).
   c. The pressure necessary to produce this flattening is equal to the intraocular pressure, counterbalancing the tonometer.
3. Air applanation tonometry
   This requires no topical anesthesia and measures tension by sensing deformation of the cornea in reaction to a puff of pressurized air.

GUIDELINES: Assisting the Patient Undergoing Tonometry

Tonometry is the measurement of intraocular pressure by means of placing a sensitive instrument (tonometer, Fig. 15-2) directly on the partially anesthetized eyeball. Normal reading: 11–22 mm. Hg.

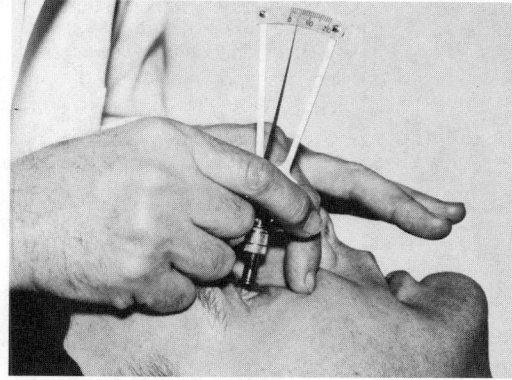

FIGURE 15-2. *The Schiøtz tonometer measures the ocular tension in mm. Hg. (Courtesy, F. H. Roy, M.D.)*

Purpose   To measure one of the diagnostic criteria of glaucoma

Procedure   *Preparatory Phase*
1. The patient is placed in a tilt-type chair, tilted back and instructed to look upward.

ACTION	RATIONALE/AMPLIFICATION
Performance Phase	
1. Physician:	
a. Instills a drop of Proparacaine 0.5% in each eye.	a. This will produce corneal anesthesia within a minute.
b. Places a sterile tonometer gently on the center of the cornea for a few seconds.	b. Pressure from the eyeball will be transferred to the sensitive measuring indicator.
c. Repeats for second eye.	
2. Nurse:	
a. Offers the patient an absorbent tissue.	
b. Instructs patient to pat the *closed* eyes dry.	
c. Cautions the patient against rubbing his eyes.	c. The cornea is still anesthetized; painful abrasions can result from the natural tendency to rub the eyes because of the unusual numb sensation.

Follow-up Phase
1. Remind patient to have an eye-pressure check at least every 2 years if his pressure is normal.

GUIDELINES: Instillation of Eyedrops

Purposes   1. To dilate or contract the pupil.
2. To relieve pain and discomfort.
3. To act as an antiseptic in cleansing the eye.
4. To combat infection; to relieve inflammation.

Equipment   Sterile solution or medication
2 × 2 gauze squares or cotton balls
Sterile eyedropper (Most medications come in plastic bottles with built-in dropper.)

GUIDELINES: Instillation of Eyedrops (cont.)

Procedure   *Preparatory Phase*

1. Inform the patient of the need and reason for instilling eyedrops.
2. Allow him to sit with head tilted slightly backward or to lie in the dorsal recumbent position.
3. Check visual acuity and record: This can be used as a base line to determine subsequent change in condition.

NURSING ACTION	RATIONALE/AMPLIFICATION
Performance Phase	
1. Check patient's name.	1. For proper patient identification.
2. Check orders and bottle or vial for correct medication and correct concentration.	2. To avoid medication error.
3. Check orders designating which eye requires medication: O.D. (oculis dexter)—right eye O.S. (oculis sinister)—left eye O.U. (oculis uterque)—both eyes	
4. Wash hands prior to instilling medication.	4. Good hygiene.
5. Check glass eyedropper for defects. If plastic disposable dropper is used, squeeze plastic to allow medication to come to the tip.	5. Provides an effective and safe vehicle for transmission of medication.
6. Prevent medication from flowing back into bulb end.	6. Loose particles of rubber may slip into medication.
7. Using forefinger, pull lower lid down gently.	7. To expose inner surface of lid and cul-de-sac.
8. Instruct patient to look upward (Fig. 15-3).	8. Prevents medication from hitting sensitive cornea.

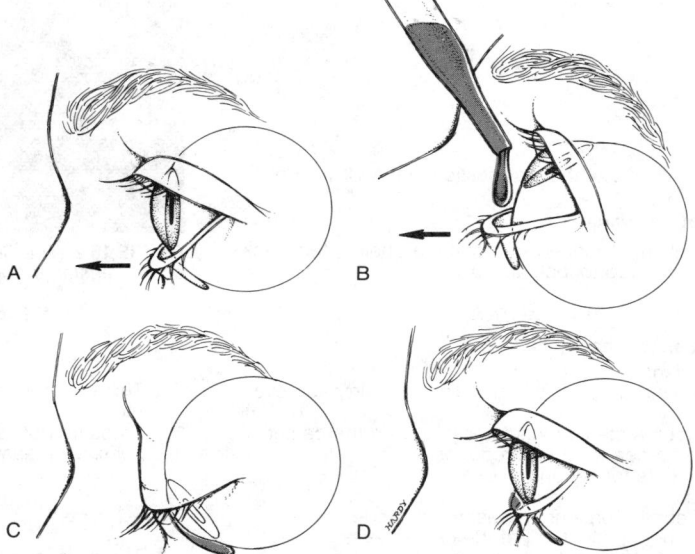

FIGURE 15-3. *Administering eyedrops. A. Pull lower eyelid away (at right angles) from eye to form a pouch—note arrow. B. Drop of medication is dropped into pouch. C. Ask patient to look down as he gently closes his eye; keep eye closed for a minute or two. Medication is trapped next to eye. D. Normally the eye can retain only a fraction of the average eyedrop.*

9. Drop medication into center of lower lid (cul-de-sac).	
10. Instruct patient to close eyes slowly but not to squeeze them.	10. Squeezing would express medication; closing allows medication to be distributed evenly over eye.
11. Wipe off excess solution with a gauze square.	11. Instruct patient not to rub his eye.
12. Wash hands after instilling medication.	12. To prevent transferring microorganisms to self or other patients.

NOTE: Eye ointments are frequently used—procedure is similar to instillation of eyedrops. Ointment from tube is gently squeezed as a ribbon of medication along inner lower lid with care taken not to touch eye with end of tube.

Follow-up Phase

Record time; type, strength, and amount of medication; and the eye into which medication was instilled.

GUIDELINES: Irrigating the Eye (Conjunctival Irrigation)

Purposes
1. To remove secretions from the conjunctival sac.
2. To treat infections, using a prescribed solution.
3. To relieve itching.
4. To provide moisture on the surface of the eyes of an unconscious patient.
5. To irrigate chemicals or foreign bodies from the eye.

Equipment
1. For small amount of solution—an eyedropper
2. For larger amount of solution—asepto bulb syringe or plastic bottle with prescribed solution
3. For copious use (chemical burns)—IV set with sterile normal saline

Procedure **Preparatory Phase**

1. Verify that you have the right patient; check chart, address patient by name.
2. The patient may sit or lie in the dorsal recumbent (supine) position.
3. Have patient tilt head toward the side of the affected eye.

NURSING ACTION	RATIONALE/AMPLIFICATION
Performance Phase	
1. Wash eyelashes and lids with prescribed solution at room temperature; place a curved basin on the affected side of the face to catch the outflow.	1. Any materials on the lids or lashes can be washed off before exposing conjunctiva.
2. Evert the lower conjunctival sac. (If feasible, have patient pull down lower lid with his index finger.)	2. The inner part of the lower lid is less sensitive than the cornea. (This involves the patient and gives him a sense of control.)
3. Instruct patient to look up; avoid touching eye with dropper.	3. To prevent eye injury—never touch cornea.
4. Allow irrigating fluid to flow from the inner canthus to the outer canthus along the conjunctival sac.	4. This prevents the solution from flowing toward the lacrimal sac, duct, and nose (which would aid in transmitting the infection).
5. Use only enough force to flush secretions from conjunctiva. (Allow patient to hold towel or sponges near the eye to catch fluid.)	5. Too much force may be injurious to eye tissues. (Involve patient in his treatment.)
6. Occasionally have patient close his eyes.	6. This allows upper lid to meet lower lid with the possibility of dislodging additional particles.
Follow-up Phase	
1. Pat eye dry and dry patient's face with gauze or cotton ball.	1. Makes patient comfortable.
2. Record kind and amount of fluid used as well as its effect on the patient.	

GUIDELINES: Application of an Eye Patch, Eye Shield, and Pressure Dressings to the Eye

Purposes
1. To keep an eye at rest, thereby promoting healing (patch).
2. To prevent the patient from touching his eye (patch, shield, dressings).
3. To absorb secretions (patch and pressure dressing).
4. To protect the eye (patch, shield, dressing).
5. To control or lessen edema (pressure dressing).

Procedure NURSING ACTION	RATIONALE/AMPLIFICATION
Eye Patch (Fig. 15-4 A, B, C)	
1. Instruct patient to close both eyes.	1. It is too difficult to close only the affected eye.
2. Place patch over the affected eye.	
3. Secure the patch with 3 or more strips of special transparent tape; tape from mid-forehead to below ear.	3. Adhesive tape (Scotch) is easy to remove—use hypoallergenic type if patient is allergic to tape.
4. For the unconscious patient, moisten the eye patch.	4. Dry patch can irritate cornea.
Eye Shield (Plastic or Metal, Fig. 15-4D)	
1. Apply over dressings or directly over the eye (without dressings).	1. Used primarily to protect the eye. Place tab or irregular extension toward the patient's ear.

GUIDELINES: Application of an Eye Patch, Eye Shield, and Pressure Dressings to the Eye (cont.)

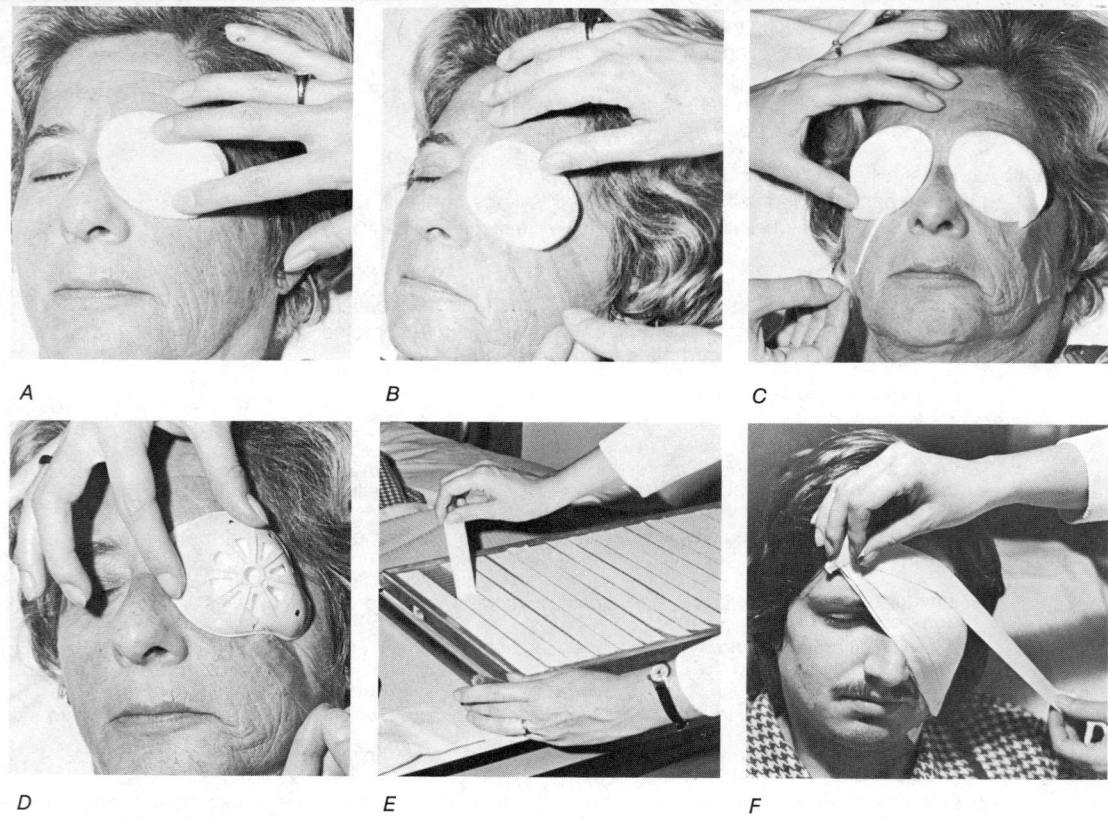

A   *B*   *C*

D   *E*   *F*

FIGURE 15-4. *Application of an eye patch, eye shield, and pressure dressings to the eye. (From Nursing '75, June 1975, pp 54–55.)*

Procedure (cont.)

2. Fasten with special transparent tape; use 2 strips.
3. For metal eye shields, a guard can be placed around flanged edges before use:
   a. Cut 1.2–2.5 cm. (½″ × 1″) piece of latex rubber from a glove finger.
   b. Stretch it around perimeter of shield.

   a. This eliminates the need for adhesive tape around edge.
   b. Two such pieces will add cushioning and provide comfort to the patient.

Pressure Dressings (Fig. 15-4E, F)

1. Prepare 8–10 adhesive strips by cutting 2.5 cm. (1 inch) adhesive tape in 35 cm. (9 inch) lengths. Stretch tape (3M) may also be used.
2. Paint forehead and cheeks with tincture of benzoin compound.
3. Apply two eye patches to the affected eye.
4. Apply strips from forehead over unpatched eye across dressings to the cheek bone (maxillary prominence).

1. Use of a warming tray for strips will improve their adhesiveness.
2. To promote adherence of tape and prevent excoriation of skin.
3. For pressure dressing bulk.
4. This is a secure dressing which accomplishes its purpose while permitting freedom of movement of the head.

EYE INJURIES

Assumptions

1. Recognize that all ocular injuries are potentially serious.
2. Protect the integrity of the visual system and prevent further damage to the injured part.
3. Evaluate the extent of injury; either refer the patient to an ophthalmologist or provide immediate treatment that will not extend damage.
4. Suspect a penetrating ocular injury with every eye wound until suspicion is proved incorrect.
5. Record visual acuity as soon as possible on every eye patient; this is a reflection of the basic integrity of the eye.

NURSING ALERT: All eye emergency patients should have visual acuity checked in each eye, both with and without glasses, as a part of history-taking and preliminary examination and *prior to any* form of treatment.

Emergency Management

A. *Corneal abrasion*
Injury to the cornea which goes no deeper than the epithelium.
1. Instill tetracaine (Pontocaine) solution as requested—to relieve pain and facilitate eye examination. Some ophthalmologists prefer systemic analgesics only.
2. Stain the cornea with fluorescein—to detect existence of an abrasion and its extent.
   a. Gently touch conjunctiva of lower lid with edge of fluorescein paper strip.
   b. The exposed (damaged) layers of epithelium will take the stain and turn green; undamaged areas remain unstained.
   c. Following use of fluorescein, flush the eye well since some patients react to fluorescein as an allergen.
3. Apply pressure bandage firmly but gently over eye—to put eye at rest and to prevent movement of the eyelid, with resultant irritation of abraded corneal area.
4. Give oral analgesic as necessary—abrasions of the cornea are painful.
5. Advise patient to rest his eyes for 24 hours for greater comfort; the corneal epithelium usually heals in 24–48 hours.
6. Instruct the patient to return to ophthalmologist the following day for dressing change and inspection of eye for evidence of infection or ulcer formation.
7. Corneal ulcer is a complication to be guarded against. (See p. 675).

B. *Contusion*
Black eye; hemorrhage into the orbit from trauma.
1. Contusions usually clear slowly and without treatment.
   a. Apply cold compresses intermittently for first 24 hours to control pain and swelling.
   b. Apply warm compresses (after 24 hours) intermittently.
2. Place patient on bed rest with both eyes bandaged for hyphema.
3. To rule out orbital fracture or hyphema (hemorrhage into anterior chamber of eye), consult an ophthalmologist if hemorrhage is severe or if pain and double vision are noted.

C. *Foreign bodies lodged in cornea*
Treatment by ophthalmologist or emergency department physician.
1. Instill sterile anesthetic into the conjunctival sac—to facilitate examination.
2. Ophthalmologist will remove superficial particles with a moist cotton-tipped applicator; foreign body removed with a spud or similar instrument using a slit lamp for magnification.
3. Apply eye patch and reinforce instruction to return to ophthalmologist the following day to determine if healing is underway.

D. *Penetrating injuries to the eye*
1. Cover eye with sterile dressing and call ophthalmologist.
   a. Intraocular foreign bodies should be removed as soon as possible; they cause damage by disintegration or become encapsulated by fibrous tissue.
   b. Apply eye patch lightly—pressure of pad may cause further penetration.
2. Give sedative-analgesic combination as directed; have patient lie quietly until ophthalmologist arrives.
3. Give tetanus prophylaxis for any penetrating eye injury.
4. Give oral antimicrobials in high doses as directed—blood aqueous barrier resists penetration.

E. *Burns of the eye*
Cause drying of the cornea with resulting chronic conjunctivitis and corneal ulceration.
1. *Thermal burns* (associated with face or body burns).
   a. Call ophthalmologist.
   b. Thermal burns are treated in the same way as burns of skin structures.
2. *Actinic Trauma*
   a. Excessive sunlight (or other strong light such as a sun lamp, bright sun on snow) can cause ultra-violet-ray damage to cornea.
   b. Damage may be superficial and resolve in 48 hours; however, punctate keratitis may develop.
   c. An ophthalmologist should be consulted immediately.
   d. Treatment
      (1) Reassure patient.
      (2) Patch both eyes.
      (3) Report to an ophthalmologist.
      (4) Instill anesthetic drops.
      (5) Instill mydriatic–cycloplegic to relax ciliary muscles and iris sphincter spasm.
      (6) Instill emollient antibiotic ointment.
3. *Chemical burns*—may be either acid or alkali in nature. Both cause intense pain and inflammation.
   a. *Irrigate eye with copious amounts of water*—holding the patient's eye directly under running water with lids retracted by gauze flats is the best way to irrigate the eye when immediate irrigation is required.
   b. Irrigate for 20–30 minutes.
   c. Repeat irrigation every 15–20 minutes (using regular eye irrigation equipment) until patient is seen by ophthalmologist.
   d. Control severe pain thereafter with systemic analgesics as prescribed.
   e. Patient may be hospitalized for treatment to enhance healing.

Health Education and Preventive Measures
1. Appropriate glasses should be used for protection against very bright light, sun shining on snow, fumes of sprays or chemicals, etc.
2. Goggles should be worn if there is danger of flying gravel (power-mower lawn cutting), flying wood chips (while chopping wood), flying metal or glass bits (in a machine factory).
3. Children should be reminded of dangers of sling shots, BB guns, "sparklers," darts, arrows, etc.
4. Eyeglasses and sunglasses should have impact-resistant lenses.
5. Many states have school eye safety laws that require all students to use industrial-quality safety eyewear in shops and laboratories.

6. Anhydrous ammonia used as agricultural fertilizer is a very destructive agent. Goggles must be worn when handling this chemical. Sufficient water for irrigation should always be present.

7. Protective lenses or goggles should be worn when using a hammer, mowing the lawn, etc. They are also highly recommended in various sports—hockey, tennis, handball, racket ball, hunting, etc.

GUIDELINES: Removing a Particle from the Eye

Equipment
Local anesthesia
Hand lens
Fluorescein strips
Cotton applicator sticks or tongue depressor
Saline (Irrigating)
Antibiotic solution

Procedure

NURSING ACTION	*RATIONALE/AMPLIFICATION*
1. As patient looks upward, evert lower lid to expose the conjunctival sac. (See *A* in following illustration.)	1. Dust particles are often washed downward by the upper lid.
2. With small cotton applicator dipped in saline, gently remove particle.	2. Wipe gently across lid—inner to outer. Use hand magnifying lens if necessary.
3. If offending particle is not found, proceed to examine upper lid.	
4. Have patient look downward while you stand in front of him.	4. Serves as a safety measure since cornea is away from area of activity. Looking downward relaxes the levator muscle, which is attached to the upper border of the tarsal plate.
5. Encourage patient to relax; move slowly and reassure him that you will not hurt him.	5. This will prevent squeezing the lids shut, a maneuver which contracts the obicularis muscle, making eversion of lid impossible.
6. Place cotton applicator stick or tongue blade horizontally on outer surface of upper lid. Apply pressure about 1 cm. above lid margin. (See *B* in following illustration.)	6. Since the upper tarsal plate extends 10–12 mm. above the lid margin, pressure must be applied at least 1 cm. above lid margin for easy eversion of lid.
7. Grasp upper eyelashes with fingers of other hand and pull the upper lid outward and upward over cotton stick.	7. Particles may be washed under the lid; visual exposure assists in detection. Eyelid will remain everted by itself.
8. With a cotton applicator moistened with saline, gently remove particle. (See *C* in following illustration.)	

NURSING ALERT: It is very important to take a history. Determine what the nature of the particle is—wood? (Fungus infection may result.) Metal? What kind—magnetic? copper? Was it projectile?

If particle cannot be removed by the method described above, it may have become imbedded in lens or vitreous, in which case an ophthalmologist is required.

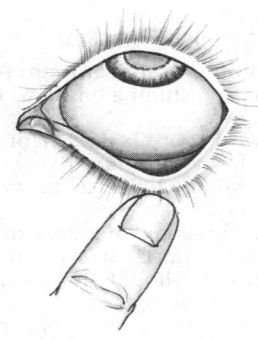

A

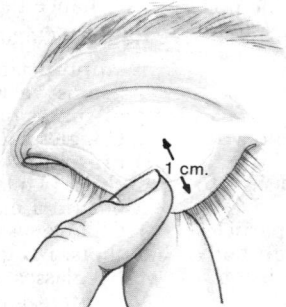

1 cm.

B

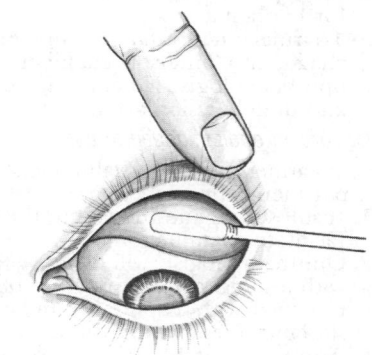

C

GUIDELINES: Removing Contact Lenses

Purpose   Since contact lenses are designed to be worn while awake, if a person is injured and incapacitated due to accident, sickness, or other cause, the lenses should be removed.

> **NURSING ALERT:**
> 1. If the injured person is unconscious or unable to remove his lenses, an optometrist or ophthalmologist should be called.
> 2. If professional help is not available and the lenses must be removed:
>   a. Determine the type of lens.
>   (1) Small *corneal lenses* are most widely used. The diameter is less than the colored part of the eye (smaller than a dime).
>   (2) Larger *scleral lenses* are worn by a few. These cover all the colored part of the eye and some of the sclera (about the size of a quarter).
>   b. *When Not to Remove Lenses:* If the colored part of the eye is not visible upon opening the eyelids, await the arrival of an optometrist or ophthalmologist.

Procedure   *Preparatory Phase*

1. Since the patient will undoubtedly be in the recumbent position, it is acceptable to remove the lens while he is in this position.
2. Wash your hands thoroughly.

NURSING ACTION	*RATIONALE/AMPLIFICATION*

Performance Phase

Corneal Lens (Hard Type)

If an eye suction cup is available (as in Emergency Room) simply separate eyelids to expose lens fully; then place cup over lens and apply slight pressure to cup. The suction produced will permit cup to lift lens from cornea.

1. For right eye, stand on right side of patient so hands will have easier access to eye.
2. Lightly place left thumb on upper eyelid; right thumb on lower eyelid close to the edge and parallel with lids (Fig. 15-5A). Thumbs are placed in a leverage position on the eyelids.
3. Gently pull lids apart and observe if contact lens is visible (Fig. 15-5B). If contact lens is not visible wait for an experienced practitioner.
4. If lens is visible, it should slide with the movement of the eyelids while thumbs are still kept at the edges of the eyelids.
5. Gently open the lids wider beyond the edge of the lens and maintain this position.
6. Press gently downward with right thumb on eyeball (Fig. 15-5C). This should cause the contact lens to tip up on one edge.
7. Then slide the eyelids and thumbs together gently (Fig. 15-5D). The lens should slide out between the lids where it can be taken off.
8. FORCE SHOULD NOT BE USED!
   Cornea may be irreparably damaged.
9. If lens can be seen but cannot be removed, gently slide it to the white sclera.
10. For left eye, move to left side of patient and repeat.

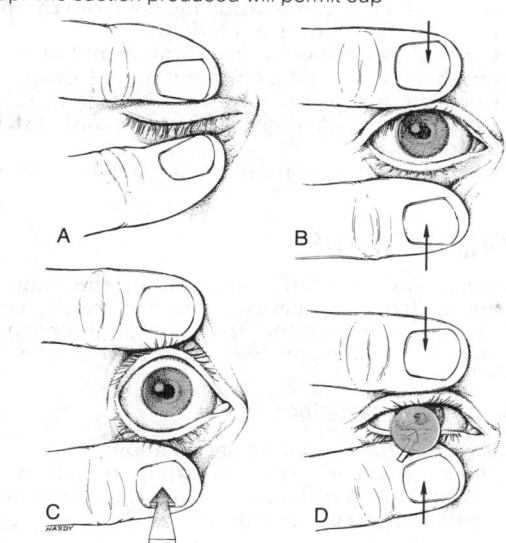

FIGURE 15-5. *Removing corneal contact lens.*

Scleral Lens

1. For right eye, stand on right side of patient.
2. Place left index finger parallel with and at the edge of the lower eyelid (Fig. 15-6A).
3. Press the lid downward and backward until the edge of the scleral lens becomes visible (Fig. 15-6B).
4. Maintain pressure but pull finger with lower lid toward the patient's right ear (Fig. 15-6C). This should cause the lid to slide under the lens. Avoid force.
5. Grasp scleral lens with right finger and thumb.

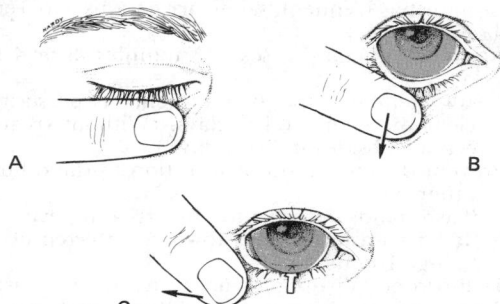

FIGURE 15-6. *Removing scleral contact lens.*

GUIDELINES: Removing Contact Lenses (cont.)

Procedure (cont.)

Soft Contact Lenses
May be removed by gently grasping and pinching lens between thumb and forefinger. This is rarely necessary, since soft contact lens may remain on the eye for many hours without harm. An ophthalmologist can be called to remove lenses if the patient is unable to do so. Also note: if the contact lens cannot be removed with relative ease, discontinue efforts and wait for the ophthalmologist to remove them.

Disposition of Lenses

1. When lenses are found and removed, place in a case or bottle; label "right" and "left."

2. Soft lenses must be kept moist.

1. Since right and left lenses are often different, storing them with proper labels will be appreciated by the patient.

2. Store in normal saline to prevent drying.

INFLAMMATION OF THE EYE

SUPERFICIAL LID INFECTIONS

Blepharitis—infection of eyelids, with crusting, redness, and irritation
Hordeolum (sty)—infection of eyelash follicle
Chalazion—infection of the meibomian gland

Treatment

1. Cleanse lid margins by applying hot moist compresses for 5 minutes 3 or 4 times daily.
2. Carefully wipe loose crusts away from lashes; apply ophthalmic antibiotic ointment and/or drops.
3. Continue for several days until infection clears.
4. Keep patient's hands away from eyes and wash hands after eye care.
5. Chronic chalazion may require incision and curettage.

CONJUNCTIVITIS

Conjunctivitis is an inflammation of the conjunctiva resulting from an allergy, from a bacterial, viral, or rickettsial infection, or from physical or chemical trauma. The infection is often referred to as "pinkeye."

Clinical Manifestations

1. Redness, pain, swelling, lacrimation
2. Discharge according to offending organisms
   Abundant purulence indicates infection caused by pneumococcus or gonococcus.

Treatment and Nursing Management

1. Administer frequent saline irrigations—to remove discharge.
2. Apply warm compresses—15 minutes, 3 or 4 times a day.
3. Instill chemotherapeutic ointments as prescribed—to clear infection in 1–3 days. (Without treatment infection subsides in 7–10 days.)
4. Prevent dissemination of infection to the other eye or other persons.
   a. Wash hands before and after treating eye.
   b. Restrict washcloth and towel to infected eye and change frequently.
5. Trifluridine (Viroptic) is an antiviral agent used in the treatment of keratoconjunctivitis and recurrent epithelial keratitis due to herpes simplex virus.

UVEITIS

Uveitis is an inflammation of the uveal tract (iris, ciliary body, choroid).

Classification

1. Location
   a. Anterior uveitis → iritis, iridocyclitis
   b. Posterior uveitis → choroiditis, chorioretinitis
   c. Panuveitis → entire uveal tract
2. Granulomatous or nongranulomatous
   a. *Granulomatous*

Location:	Any portion, mostly posterior
Onset:	Insidious
Pain:	None or minimal
Circum corneal flush:	Minimal
Course:	Chronic
Prognosis:	Fair to poor

   b. *Nongranulomatous*

Location:	Anterior
Onset:	Acute
Pain:	Marked
Circum corneal flush:	Present
Course:	Acute
Prognosis:	Good

Complications

1. Anterior uveitis—adhesions impede aqueous outflow, leading to glaucoma. May cause cataracts.
2. Posterior uveitis—adhesions impede aqueous flow from posterior to anterior uvea, causing metabolic disturbances of the lens and leading to cataracts.
3. Retinal detachment may result from traction exerted on retina by vitreous strands.

Treatment

1. Directed to specific type of uveitis.
2. Atropine—to reduce likelihood of adhesion formation between iris and lens.
3. Steroids, locally—for anti-inflammatory and anti-allergic action.
   Steroids, systemically, occasionally.
4. Analgesic—for pain.

SYMPATHETIC OPHTHALMIA

Sympathetic ophthalmia is a severe granulomatous bilateral uveitis that may occur after any surgical or traumatic perforation involving the uveal tract. Rare, but severe.

Clinical Manifestations

Photophobia, blurring vision, and injection ("bloodshot") in sympathizing eye.

Treatment

1. Administer corticosteroids, locally and systemically, to reduce the amount of intraocular scarring.

2. Instill atropine (mydriatic) locally to prevent adhesions between the iris and lens.
3. Possibility of preventive enucleation of originally injured eye before sympathetic ophthalmia occurs.

Nursing Management

1. Understand the patient's condition and the objectives desired for him.
2. Recognize the difficult decision facing the patient if enucleation approach is suggested.
3. Assess the psychosocial implications of the individual situation, offer sustaining support, and collaborate in planning immediate and long-term goals.

CORNEAL ULCER

Keratitis is an inflammation of the cornea, which when combined with a loss of substance results in *corneal ulcer.*

Clinical Manifestations

1. Pain, marked photophobia, and increased lacrimation
2. Injected ("bloodshot") eye
3. When a corneal ulcer progresses deeper to involve the iris, iritis develops; pus forms in the anterior chamber and collects as a white or yellow deposit (hypopyon) behind the cornea.
4. If corneal ulcer perforates, iris may prolapse through cornea.

Treatment and Nursing Management

1. Prevention is much easier than treatment.
   a. Foreign bodies must be removed quickly.
   b. Corneal abrasions must be treated promptly.

2. Suggest the wearing of dark glasses to relieve photophobia.
3. Explain to patient that physician may administer mydriatics preparatory to examining the eye and will instill topical anesthetic to relieve pain and fluorescein to outline ulcer.
4. Administer antibiotic or chemotherapeutic agent as prescribed for specific type of infection.
5. Apply warm compresses for comfort as prescribed.
6. Administer systemic antibiotics when prescribed.

NURSING ALERT: Always question patient about allergies to medications, whether topical or systemic, prior to institution of therapy.

EYE CONDITIONS POSSIBLY REQUIRING SURGERY

CARING FOR THE PATIENT HAVING EYE SURGERY

Nursing Objectives and Management

A. *To understand the psychological effect of an eye problem on a patient.*

1. Recognize that dependence on sight is exaggerated when one faces a possible diminution or loss of sight.
2. Observe that the concern of the patient may be manifested as fear, depression, tension, resentment, anger, and even rejection.
3. Encourage the patient to express his feelings in order to determine the underlying problems.
4. Provide diversional and occupational therapy to keep patient occupied mentally within the limits of his decreased vision so as not to accentuate his feelings of depression or despair over loss of vision.
5. Demonstrate interest, empathy, and understanding, but try not to be oversolicitous.
6. Recognize individual differences which affect the method of dealing with patient anxiety.
7. Assure the patient that rehabilitative programs and

personnel are available if his condition requires them.

B. *To assess the physical needs which have to be met while maintaining the highest level of self-sufficiency.*

1. Always orient the new patient who has diminished vision to his surroundings—his room and the people in his immediate environment.
2. Encourage patient to care for himself so that he will be self-sufficient and not feel that he is a burden.
3. Supervise him as he attempts to feed himself so that he does not become discouraged.
4. Promote proper elimination by an adequate diet, laxatives, or an enema as required.
5. Provide a rest period daily if patient is ambulatory.
6. For safety reasons, discourage his reading, smoking, or shaving (done by members of the health team).
7. Caution him against rubbing his eyes or wiping them with a soiled tissue or handkerchief.
8. Instruct him to wear dark glasses if he has had atropine instilled.
9. Maintain a safe environment that is free of obstacles such as footstools or loose rugs.
10. Doors should be completely open or closed.

C. *To assist in the immediate preoperative preparation of the patient.*

1. In preparation for general anesthesia, evacuate lower bowel (enema) in the morning of the day of surgery; offer liquid diet only after this. (This is unnecessary for local anesthesia.)
2. Arrange long hair of female patients (braiding) so that it will be conveniently out of the way.
3. Cut eyelashes of the affected eye, using small, curved, blunt scissors covered with petrolatum so that lashes will adhere to it and not drop into the patient's eye. This is done to reduce the possibility of infection. Lashes will grow back in about 3 weeks.
4. Check local hospital policy regarding preoperative skin preparation; in many hospitals, this is done in the operating room.
5. Remove dentures or artificial eye before patient goes to the operating room.
6. Caution patient to hold his head still during surgery if the operation is to be done under local anesthesia.
7. Instruct patient regarding postoperative restrictions—no reading, no showers, tub baths, or shampoos; no bending from the waist or lifting of heavy objects, no sleeping on operated side. Tell him he will have a patch and shield on eye when he returns from the O.R.
8. Make sure the eye specified on the operative permit and eye to be operated upon are the same.
9. Instill proper preoperative medications in the proper eye.

D. *To provide optimum care for the patient immediately following eye surgery.*

1. Place patient in the dorsal recumbent position with a small pillow under his head, or permit him to lie on unoperated side.
2. Position bed rails so as to offer the patient a sense of security.
3. Place a call bell within reach of the patient; have him call the nurse rather than risk stress or strain in an attempt to be self-sufficient.
4. Direct anyone who enters his room to announce himself; also, let patient know when you are leaving the room. Otherwise he may be left talking to himself.
5. Avoid disturbing the head with such activities as combing the hair; delay combing the hair until patient is allowed out of bed.

E. *To provide a relaxing convalescence.*

1. Consult ophthalmologist before recommending diversional or recreational therapy that is not fatiguing to the eyes—no reading; television in moderation; radio.
2. Recognize the soothing and relaxing effect of soft pastels for the wall and ceiling colors.
3. Regulate lights so that they are not too bright and do not produce a glare.
4. Inform patient before he leaves hospital regarding medications, eye glasses, follow-up visits, type of work he can do and when he can do it.
5. Instruct the patient or family as follows on instillation of eye medications and proper cleansing of eyes:
   a. Wash hands before and after treating eyes.
   b. To clean around the eye, use sterile wet gauze and wipe gently across lid from inner corner to outer corner.
   c. To apply eye medications, pull down lower lid and place eye drop in cul-de-sac, place ribbon of ointment along the entire length of the conjunctiva of lower lid.
   d. Apply protective shield over the operated eye at bedtime.
6. Inform patient of "Talking Book" records, machines, and tapes that are available from most public libraries without charge.
7. Initiate follow-up visits with ophthalmologist. The nurse can make the first appointment for the patient.

Health Education and Discharge Planning

1. Measures listed above are pertinent for transfer teaching and learning for the patient, so that he may practice these habits at home.
2. Upon discharge from the hospital, check the following:
   a. Does patient have a return appointment date with physician confirmed?
   b. Does he have his medication properly identified and labeled? Does he (or a responsible member of the family) know how to use his prescribed medications?
   c. Does the patient understand the restrictions placed upon him and the reasons for them?

CORNEAL TRANSPLANTATION (KERATOPLASTY)

Keratoplasty is the transplantation of a donor cornea to repair a corneal scar, burn, or deformed cornea, as in keratoconus.

Types of Grafts

1. Full thickness (6.5–8 mm.)—most common
2. Partial thickness—lamellar

Cryopreservation

The care and handling of corneal graft by freezing to retain its transparency

1. Because an intact endothelium is required for ultimate transparency of the corneal graft, it is necessary in the preservation process to properly freeze, defrost, and quickly use the graft to reduce the likelihood of damage to the graft.
2. Eye Bank laboratories* cut the cornea from the enucleated eye and place it in several solutions before freezing.
3. During defrosting, the cornea is gently rotated in a glass tube at a certain temperature for a certain period of time. When only a small ice ball adheres to the cornea, it is allowed to melt without shaking the vial.
4. Fluid from the vial is decanted and is replaced with fresh, diluted human albumin for several prescribed minutes before using immediately.
5. The technique described above requires trained skill.
6. Fresh corneas are still preferred and are used within 48 to 72 hours after donation, without cryopreservation.

* Function of Eye Banks:
1. Inform public of need of eye donations.
2. Procure eyes donated to the bank.
3. Assist in the optimum use of the tissue; either retain for local use or arrange for its transportation to the nearest Eye Bank with the greatest need.

Objectives of Treatment and Nursing Management

A. *To recognize and alleviate the concerns of the patient preoperatively.*

1. Psychological preparation for surgery is simplified because the patient is usually optimistic about the imminent transplant.
2. If cultural and spiritual concerns need to be voiced by the patient, the nurse, and possibly the hospital chaplain, should be available so that the patient faces surgery in the best frame of mind possible.

B. *To keep intraocular and external pressure on the operated eye at a safe level.*

This is to protect the eye from loss of aqueous humor or from injury because of the possibility of dislocating the newly transplanted cornea.

1. Prevent sudden turning of the head.
2. Minimize those activities or sources of irritants which may cause sneezing (dusting or sweeping, heavily scented flowers, sprays). (No pepper on trays.)
3. Avoid conversation which annoys or disturbs the patient; caution visitors not to upset the patient since emotional disturbances may increase his intraocular pressure.
4. Instruct patient not to sleep on operated side.

C. *To provide rest for the operated eye in order to enhance the healing process.*

1. Cover both eyes even though only 1 is involved; if 1 eye is left uncovered, both would move because of twin-like movements.
2. Recognize that healing is slow, due to the avascularity of the cornea.

D. *To utilize measures that will prevent infection of the eye.*

1. Assist physician in practicing meticulous aseptic technique during dressing change to reduce the possibility of infection.
2. Discourage the patient from touching the dressings.

E. *To recognize the differences between care requirements of the patient having a full-thickness (penetrating) corneal transplant and those of the patient having a lamellar transplant.*

1. Full-thickness (penetrating) type
   a. Emphasize the need for longer bed rest.
   b. Restrict the patient's activities according to physician's specifications: the patient may be fed, bathed, and provided with bedpan service.
   c. Allow patient to raise his head slightly toward unoperated side.
   d. Initiate passive range of motion activities and deep breathing exercises to prevent circulatory and pulmonary complications.
2. Lamellar type
   a. With physician's sanction, help the patient out of bed and into a chair for short periods of time.
   b. Keep the patient's eyes bandaged, perhaps double patched, according to physician's request.

F. *To implement care that will prevent complications.*

1. Avoid urinary retention by providing adequate fluids.
2. Prevent constipation or straining on defecation by avoiding constipating foods and maintaining adequate hydration.
3. Administer analgesics as necessary to relieve pain.
4. Report unrelieved pain since it may indicate that dressings are too tight, that graft has slipped, or that hemorrhage is occurring—or possible early infection, inflammation, or postoperative glaucoma.
5. Introduce additional activities gradually each day, but continue to avoid those which will require straining.
6. Emphasize the importance of follow-up visits to the ophthalmologist.

> **NURSING ALERT:** For eye patients requiring extensive bed rest (e.g., following keratoplasty, injury, retinal detachment surgery) measures should be taken to prevent pulmonary and/or circulatory complications. This may include passive range of motion activities, antiembolism stockings, special positioning, etc.

RADIAL KERATOTOMY AND KERATOPHAKIA

Radial keratotomy (investigational surgery) is an operation designed to provide correction of myopia (nearsightedness) by making a number of incisions on the outside of the cornea in order to flatten it. This permits images to fall on the retina instead of in front of it.

Keratophakia (investigational surgery) is an operation designed to provide correction of hyperopia (farsightedness) by (1) temporarily removing a segment of cornea; (2) shaping a donor cornea to required shape; and (3) reinserting both pieces in an attempt to steepen or build up corneal curvature. This permits images to fall on the retina instead of in back of it.

DETACHED RETINA

Retinal detachment is the detachment of the sensory retina from the pigment epithelium of the retina.

Altered Physiology

1. The retina perceives light and transmits impulses from its nerve cells to the optic nerve.
2. Tears or holes in the retina may result rapidly from trauma or slowly from the aging process.
3. A tear in the retina allows vitreous humor and transudate from choroid vessels to seep behind the retina and separate it from the pigment epithelium.

Clinical Manifestations

1. Patient complains of flashes of light or blurred, "sooty" vision due to stimulation of the retina by vitreous pull.
2. He notes sensation of particles moving in his line of vision (normally most individuals can see floating filaments when looking at a light background).
3. Delineated areas of vision may be blank (a relative scotoma); there is no perception of pain.
4. A sensation of a veil-like coating coming down, coming up, or sideways in front of the eye may be present.
   a. This veil-like coating, or shadow, is often misinterpreted as a drooping eyelid or elevated cheek.
   b. Straight ahead vision may remain good in early stages.
5. Unless the retinal holes are sealed, the retina will

progressively detach and ultimately there is a loss of central vision as well as peripheral vision.
6. Retinal detachments do not cure themselves; they must be corrected surgically.

Treatment and Nursing Management

A. *Preoperative Nursing Management*

1. Instruct the patient to remain in bed to prevent further detachment of the retina. Both eyes may be bandaged (according to physician's request).
2. Physician will determine proper position to be maintained, according to the area of detachment; such an area must be in a dependent position if adherence is to take place.
3. Since patient will not be permitted to wash his hair for a week following surgery, he may wish to do this the day before the operation.
4. Explain what is to be expected before and after the operation. Tell patient that:
   a. The circumorbital area may be black and blue but this will gradually fade away in a few weeks.
   b. The patient will have a patch on his eye/s after the operation.
5. Have patient wash his face preoperatively with a detergent–germicide to reduce possibility of eye infection; administer sedation and tranquilizing medications for comfort and relief of anxiety.

B. *Surgical Intervention*

OBJECTIVE: to seal the retinal hole, thereby ensuring that the retina will adhere to the retinal pigment epithelium.

Types of Surgery:
   a. *Electrodiathermy*—the passing of an electrode needle through the sclera to allow subretinal fluid to escape. An exudate forms from the pigment epithelium and adheres to the retina.
   b. *Cryosurgery* or *retinal cryopexy*—a supercooled probe is touched to the sclera, causing minimal damage; as a result of scarring, the pigment epithelium adheres to the retina.
   c. *Photocoagulation*—a light beam (either laser or xenon arc) is passed through the dilated pupil, causing a small burn and producing an exudate between the pigment epithelium and retina.
   d. *Scleral buckling*—a technique whereby the sclera is shortened to allow a buckling to occur which forces the pigment epithelium closer to the retina.

C. *Postoperative Nursing Management*

1. Proper positioning in bed is important after the operation and is prescribed according to individual need. Usually patient is permitted out of bed on the 2nd day.
2. Take precautions to avoid bumping the patient's head thus causing the retina to detach further.
3. Following general anesthesia, patient is encouraged to breathe deeply but not to cough since this will increase eye pressure. Vomiting must be avoided.
4. Allow additional activity as type of treatment permits; for example, scleral buckling is less confining than diathermy.
5. Provide for diversional therapy, since this patient often becomes depressed.
   a. Moderate television viewing.
   b. No handwork or reading until physician's permission is obtained.
   c. "Talking books," radio, and visitors permitted.

6. If local anesthesia is used, patient is ambulatory postoperatively if condition permits (age, vision in other eye, other medical or physical problems).
7. Hospitalization ranges from 5-10 days.

D. *Prognosis*

1. Untreated retinal detachment progresses to complete retinal detachment and legal blindness in that eye.
2. Surgical reattachment by scleral buckling, cryotherapy, or diathermy is successful in approximately 90–95% of cases. Secondary operations may be required.
3. Return of visual acuity with a reattached retina depends upon:
   a. Amount of retina detached prior to surgery
   b. Whether the macula was detached
   c. Length of time the retina was detached
   d. Amount of external distortion caused by the scleral buckle
   e. Possible macular damage as a result of diathermy or cryocoagulation
4. Retinal tears that may lead to retinal detachment may be present in the other eye. These may require surgical treatment by cryocoagulation, photocoagulation, or scleral buckling.
5. Two possible complications to watch for and guard against are glaucoma and infection.

Health Education and Discharge Planning

1. When he goes home, the patient is able to care for himself; he may care for all bodily needs in an unhurried manner, being careful to avoid falls, jerks, and bumps.
2. It is advisable to stay home for the first several weeks to avoid accidental injury.
3. Watching television, looking at friends, and using eyes in straight line vision is harmless, but rapid eye movement, as in reading, should be avoided for several weeks.
4. For comfort of the eyes and eyelids, the use of a clean wash cloth, wrung out of hot water is most relaxing and soothing when applied several times during the day for 10 minutes.
5. Avoid straining and bending head below waist; driving is restricted.
6. Use meticulous cleanliness in giving eye medications.
7. The first follow-up visit to the ophthalmologist should take place in 2 weeks and other visits at longer intervals thereafter.
8. Within 3 weeks, light activities may be pursued; in 6 weeks, athletic and heavier activities are usually possible.
9. Acquaint the patient with the symptoms that indicate a recurrence of the detachment; floating spots, flashing light, progressive shadow.
   If they occur, recommend that patient contact his physician.

CATARACTS

A *cataract* is an opacity of the crystalline lens or its capsule; it is the leading cause of blindness in the United States.

Predisposing Factors

1. A cataract may occur at birth (congenital cataract).
2. Occasionally a cataract occurs in young individuals as a result of disease or trauma.

3. Most commonly, cataract occurs in adults past middle age (senile cataract) as a result of the aging process.
4. Recent research indicates that users of hair dye or eyelash dye containing aniline dye para-phenylene-diamine (para-diaminobenzene) may suffer from long-term damage to the lens as a result of its use.

Altered Physiology

1. Normally, the lens is a semisolid body of clear, gelatinous protein encased in a capsule lying behind the iris; the lens possesses great refractive powers (approximately 1/3 of the total).
2. Chemical change in the lens protein may cause coagulation; as a result, the lens loses its pristine transparency and gradually becomes opaque.
3. Physical changes result in a swelling of the fibers which in turn causes a distortion of the image.
4. Metabolic changes that reduce vitamin C and B_{12} in the lens may be instrumental in forming opacities.
5. Although cataract may be readily diagnosed, the basic cause of senile cataract is unknown.

Clinical Mainifestations

1. Alterations in vision are noted
   a. Objects seem distorted and blurred
   b. Glare annoys the patient when there are bright lights
   c. Visual loss is gradual, but eventually the opacity becomes complete
2. The pupil, usually black, becomes gray and later milky-white

Management

1. Surgical removal of the lens is indicated.
2. Proper time for cataract removal is determined by the patient's eyesight, occupation, general health, and convenience.
3. Usually a patient with 1 cataract can manage without surgery.
4. If cataract occurs in both eyes, he need not suffer blindness before he can be helped by surgery.
5. Following surgery and the healing process, the patient is fitted with appropriate eyeglasses or contact lenses.
6. Intraocular lens implants may be implanted at the time of cataract extraction or as an independent procedure.

Traditional Surgical Procedures

A. *Extracapsular Extraction*

1. This surgery is conservative; it is simple to perform and is usually done under local anesthesia.
2. The lens capsule is incised and the cataract is withdrawn.
3. Usually it is performed for congenital and traumatic cataract.
4. The posterior capsule is left in place. This may interfere with vision, and a second operation (a capsulotomy) may be required to produce a clear pupil.
5. A standard sized incision (18-20 mm.) is used.

B. *Intracapsular Extraction*

1. In this surgery, the lens as well as the capsule is removed through an 18 mm. incision.
2. Cryosurgery may be used as the technique for this operation; a pencil-like instrument with a metal probe is cooled to about $-35°$ C; when the lens capsule is available after dissection, the cryosurgical instrument touches the lens and freezes to it so that the lens is easily pulled out.
3. Approximately 5–7 days of hospitalization are required, although this figure is being reduced considerably and varies depending on the surgeon's preference, on the number and size of sutures used, and on the patient's occupation and reliability.

Objectives of Treatment and Nursing Management

A. *Preoperative Care*

1. To make the patient comfortable in his new surroundings.
   a. Explain the plan of care.
   b. Escort the patient as he walks around the unit.
   c. Provide bed rails if he is elderly.
2. To allay his concerns, if he has any, regarding surgery.
   a. Determine how he feels about his operation.
   b. Assess his knowledge level regarding the purpose of surgery and his expectations afterward.
   c. Encourage his questions and provide the answers.
3. To reduce the conjunctival bacterial count to minimize the chance of postoperative infection.
   a. Obtain a conjunctival culture if requested.
   b. Administer local antibiotics as prescribed.
   c. Employ aseptic technique in any eye treatment or procedure.
   d. Instruct patient not to touch his eyes.
4. To introduce rehabilitative measures that the patient will practice postoperatively.
   a. Following general anesthesia, instruct patient to take deep breaths, move extremities, and perform quadriceps muscle setting without moving his head.
   b. Point out the hazard of squeezing the eyelids shut: Teach him how to close his eyes slowly.
5. Determine whether a properly identified and executed operative permit has been obtained. There should be no discrepancies between the patient's understanding of the surgery and the informed consent for surgery.
6. To prepare the eye to be operated upon in the immediate preoperative period.
   a. Instill mydriatic if prescribed.
   b. Note whether pupil dilates after instillation of mydriatic.
7. Administration of the preoperative medications.
   a. Sedatives—barbiturates or chloral hydrate
   b. Anti-emetics—compazine, Vistaril
   c. Narcotics—meperidine for pain relief
   d. Ocular hypotensive agents:
      (1) Cholinesterase inhibitors—acetazolamide
      (2) Osmotic hypotensives.
         Oral—glycerine
         Intravenous—mannitol

B. *Postoperative Care*

1. To prevent pressure build-up within the eye (intraocular) which may exert a stress on the fresh sutures.
   a. Admonish patient to refrain from coughing or sneezing.
   b. Advise patient to avoid rapid movement, but allow him to turn to the unoperated side or remain in the dorsal recumbent position.
   c. Admonish patient not to bend from the waist.
2. To promote comfort of the patient and reorient him to surroundings.

a. Allow patient to turn on unoperated side to relieve back stress; give back rubs.
b. Offer analgesics as prescribed to control pain; report severe pain to physician.
c. Instruct those who enter room to announce themselves and to inform patient when leaving room.
d. Provide a quiet environment to promote patient's relaxation.
e. Allow patient to be ambulatory as permitted by physician.
3. To control symptoms that may lead to serious complication.
a. Sudden pain in the eye may be due to a ruptured vessel or suture and may lead to hemorrhage—notify physician immediately.
b. Restlessness and increasing pulse rate may be indicative of hemorrhage.
c. Nausea may lead to vomiting and increase intraocular pressure—administer antiemetic drugs as prescribed.

New Surgical Procedures

A. *Phacoemulsification (ultrasonic)* (Fig. 15–7)
1. Overview of this type of surgery
   Phacoemulsification is the mechanical breaking up (emulsifying) of the lens by a hollow needle vibrating at 40,000 cycles per second.
   a. The needle tip moves forward and backward (action similar to that of a jackhammer).

b. It is powered by an ultrasound generator to produce the frequency necessary to emulsify the cataract.
c. This action is coupled with simultaneous irrigation and aspiration of the emulsified particles from the anterior chamber through the needle tip.
d. Only a 2–3 mm. incision is required, and the actual procedure takes from 20–30 minutes. (Performed by a specially trained ophthalmic surgeon.)
e. Hospitalization of 1 day is usually required.
f. Normal activities may be resumed the day after surgery.
g. Contact lenses can be used in about 3–6 weeks.
h. Effective in management of soft cataracts in children and young adults.
2. Criteria to be met for this operation.
a. Pupil must be able to dilate fully.
b. Anterior chamber must be deep enough to accommodate the manipulation of the probe-aspirator.
c. Cornea should be healthy.
d. The highly sophisticated phacoemulsifier utilizes expensive materials which are resupplied for each use.
3. Preoperative Nursing Management
a. Take advantage of the opportunity to discuss fears, concerns, and any questions patient may have regarding his surgery since this patient is usually admitted the day before surgery.
b. Acquaint the patient with his surroundings and

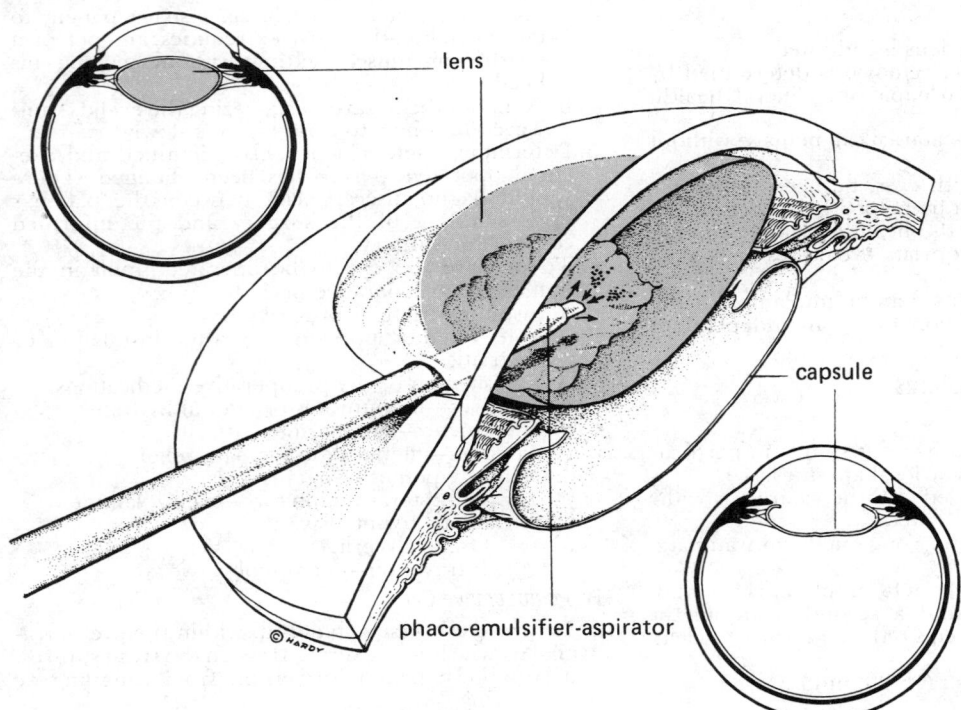

lens

capsule

phaco-emulsifier-aspirator

FIGURE 15-7. *Cataract is shown in orb at upper left. Kelman ultrasonic needle (Cavitron Corp.) is inserted through 2 to 3 mm. incision at corneal-scleral junction to emulsify lens cortex and nucleus and aspirate them. Drawing at right shows cataract removed and posterior capsule intact. Cataract surgery requires a 19–20 mm. incision. (Copyright June 1975, the American Journal of Nursing Co. Reproduced with permission from American Journal of Nursing, Vol. 75, No. 6.)*

his plan of care; if his condition permits, provide him with information regarding postoperative care since this is more flexible and liberal than for other kinds of cataract surgery.

   c. Prepare the patient to receive oral glycerine and intravenous mannitol on the day of surgery; this is to decrease intraocular pressure.

     (1) Monitor vital signs and cardiovascular status.

     (2) Stop the intravenous infusion if untoward signs develop (shortness of breath, chest pain, etc.).

   d. Administer prescribed eye drops to dilate the pupil and to paralyze the muscles of accommodation.

   e. Administer sedation, antiemetics, and/or narcotics as in intracapsular cataract extraction.

4. Postoperative Nursing Management

   a. Remove eye patch and permit patient to get out of bed only when he has fully recovered from anesthesia.

   b. Administer eye medications as prescribed; these may be to prevent infection and to keep posterior capsule in place.

   c. Offer an analgesic if he has any discomfort.

   d. Remind the patient to use his eye medications upon discharge from the hospital, usually the 1st or 2nd day postoperatively.

   e. Explain the time plan for his permanent lenses and describe the need and use of temporary lenses.

5. Considerations and Possible Disadvantages

   a. The posterior lens capsule may later opacify; a percentage of these patients (25%–30%) may require additional surgery (capsulotomy—perforation of capsule).

   b. The cornea may be affected by high frequency vibrations which may later cause degeneration of the cornea.

   c. Possible complications include infection, hemorrhage, and fluid leakage from the eye.

B. *Intraocular Lens* (Fig. 15–8)

1. Basic Concepts

   a. This is the implantation of a synthetic lens—designed for distance vision; the patient wears prescribed glasses for reading and near vision.

   b. Intraocular lens implant is an alternative to sight correction with glasses or contact lenses for the aphakic patient.

   c. Sophisticated calculations are required to determine the power or prescription for lens:

     (1) Corneal curvature

     (2) Depth of anterior chamber

     (3) Axial length of eyeball (by diagnostic ultrasound)

   d. *Unilateral cataract:* Objective is to leave patient slightly myopic (nearsighted)

     (1) Operated eye is used for reading.

     (2) Unoperated eye is used for distance vision.

   e. *Bilateral cataract:* Objective is to leave patient emmetropic (all rays of light focus perfectly on retina).

     (1) Vision is good for distance.

     (2) Glasses required for reading.

   f. Hyperopia (farsightedness) is avoided in implanting a lens because the image would be magnified and cause visual difficulty.

   g. Astigmatism is corrected with eyeglasses.

2. Insertion of intraocular lens.

   a. There are a number of types of intraocular lens available.

   b. Polymethyl methacrylate is a common durable compound from which such lenses are made. Designs and material change as new developments occur. Extended-wear contact lenses may replace intraocular lens.

   c. Various methods of fixation are being used, including (1) fastening by sutures or clips; (2) holding in place in the way that a hub cap is fitted to the rim of a tire; and (3) sealing within the anterior and posterior capsule after extracapsular extraction (capsular fixation). The second method (no sutures) usually requires a miotic (pilocarpine) to keep the iris from dilating too widely—thereby causing displacement of the implant.

3. Advantages of intraocular lens.

   a. Provides an alternative to individuals who cannot wear cataract glasses or contact lenses.

   b. Cannot be lost or misplaced like conventional glasses; does not need to be replaced.

   c. Provides a permanent form of near normal vision.

4. Complications (specific to implantation)

   a. Iritis or vitritis—can be controlled with steriods.

   b. Rosy vision, due to keeping pupil from full constriction; excessive light enters pupil, causing a dazzling of macula.

   c. Degeneration of cornea, chronic uveitis (see p. 674).

   d. Malpositioning or dislocation of lens.

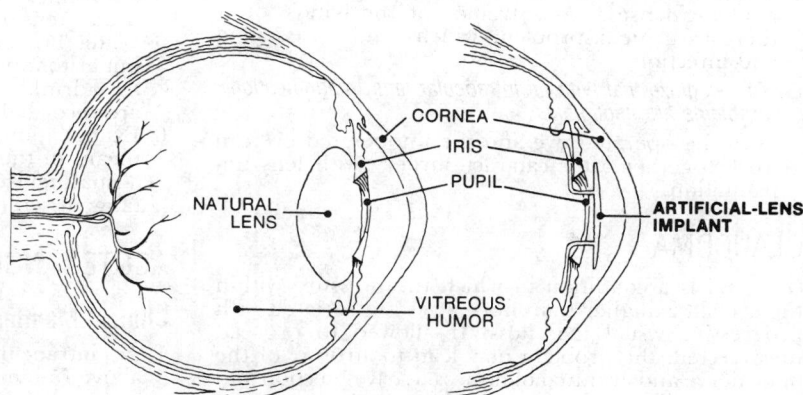

FIGURE 15-8. *Illustration at left indicates position of natural lens; drawing on right shows artificial-lens implant following removal of cataract. (Newsweek—Ib Ohlsson)*

Health Education

During rehabilitative phase of cataract extraction

A. *To encourage the patient to be independent.*

1. Assist patient in getting around his room, locating needed personal items, using bathroom facilities.
2. Gradually increase his activities each day.

B. *To demonstrate to the patient and a responsible member of his family how to administer eye medications.*

C. *To promote patient's interest in diversional activities as he recuperates.*

Try to prevent his becoming bored.

D. *To acquaint patient with the step-by-step requirements of a healthy convalescence.*

1. The use of dark glasses after the eye dressings are removed.
2. Hospitalization—usually 6–10 days following intracapsular extraction.
3. Fitting for temporary corrective lenses for the first 6 weeks, if prescribed.
4. Application of metal or plastic shield over the eye at night to avoid accidental injury during sleep.
5. Prescription for permanent lenses 6–8 weeks after surgery for intracapsular extraction.
6. Prescription for contact lenses about 3–6 weeks after phacoemulsification.

E. *To assist patient in adjusting to the eyeglasses.*

1. If spectacles are to be worn, they will be quite thick, causing the perceived image to be about ⅓ larger than that seen by the patient before cataract formation; peripheral vision is markedly distorted.
2. It is necessary to relearn space judgment—walking, using stairs, reaching for articles on the table, such as cup of coffee.
3. If only one eye is operated for cataract, the patient can use only one eye at a time, with spectacle (glasses) lenses, since the operated eye has a 30% increase in image size and the unoperated eye still has "normal" sized images, which cannot be superimposed.

F. *To familiarize patient with contact lenses, if this is his choice.*

1. With contact lenses, magnification is only about 8%–10%; peripheral vision is not distorted.
2. Since the image size difference between an aphakic eye with a contact lens and the unoperated eye is only 8%–10%, both eyes can be used together.
3. Space judgment presents little difficulty.
4. There may be problems if the patient has difficulty applying lenses, has a tremor of the hands, or if there are hygienic problems which could cause soiling and infection.

G. *To recognize that with an intraocular lens, magnification problems are negligible.*

Both the operated eye and the unoperated eye can work together after cataract surgery with lens implantation.

GLAUCOMA

Glaucoma is a condition in which the pressure within the eyeball is higher than normal; it is associated with progressive visual field loss. If allowed to proceed uncorrected, the problem may lead to atrophy of the optic nerve and eventual blindness. Early detection and treatment will prevent loss of eyesight.

Incidence

1. It is estimated that 1 million Americans have undiagnosed glaucoma.
2. Glaucoma is the cause of blindness in 1 of 10 persons who become blind.
3. Glaucoma is estimated to occur in 1.0 to 2.5% of Americans aged 35 and over.
4. Persons with family history of glaucoma are more susceptible than others.

Altered Physiology

1. Pressure within the eye is determined by the rate of input of aqueous humor as produced by the ciliary body and the resistance to outflow of aqueous humor.
2. Inflow of aqueous humor is through the pupil; outflow is at the meshwork located at juncture of iris and cornea. Clogging at the meshwork by blood, fibrin, or inflammatory cells accounts for the buildup of pressure which produces secondary glaucoma.
3. Thickening of the meshwork appears spontaneously in those older individuals who appear to have a hereditary predisposition; chronic simple glaucoma results and is the most common type.
4. When the iris is abnormally anterior and exerts pressure against the meshwork, acute glaucoma results; this is the least frequent type.

Classification

1. Angle-closure (narrow angle)—acute or chronic
2. Open-angle (wide angle)—chronic
3. Congenital
   Within these classifications, principal contributing factors may be *primary* or *secondary*
   Primary—genetically based
   Secondary—result of ocular disease, injury, neoplasia, or surgery.

Diagnostic Evaluation

1. Because of the relative ease of developing glaucoma, unless a person past 40 has a complete physical examination periodically, including measurement of eye pressure (tonometry), the disease may not be discovered until it is considerably advanced (chronic simple type).
2. Tonometry (see Figs. 15-1, 15-2)
   A reading of 24–32 mm. Hg suggests glaucoma.
3. Gonioscopy—an examination to differentiate angle-closure glaucoma from open-angle type.
4. Tonography—application of tonometer, usually electronic, with a special device that records intraocular tension over a 4-minute period.
5. Water Provocative Test—Breakfast is withheld and initial tonometer reading is recorded. The patient then drinks 1 liter of water, and intraocular pressures are recorded after 30, 45, and 60 minutes.
6. Examination of optic nerve and blood vessels by means of the ophthalmoscope.
7. Visual field examination—with either perimeter or tangent screen.

ACUTE (ANGLE-CLOSURE) GLAUCOMA

Clinical Manifestations

1. As intraocular pressure increases rapidly (often above 75 mm. Hg), severe pain occurs in and around eye.

2. Artificial lights appear to have a rainbow of colors around them.
3. Vision becomes cloudy and blurred.
4. Pupils dilate; nausea and vomiting may occur.
5. Although onset may be insidious, severity of symptoms may progress within hours to include disturbances suggestive of gastrointestinal, sinus, neurological, and dental problems as well as eye pain.
6. If untreated, irreversible blindness may result.

Pharmacotherapy

This will be initiated to control eye pressure before surgery. Medications listed below are prescribed at the discretion of the ophthalmologist according to the patient's condition and needs.

A. *Parasympathomimetic Drugs Used as Miotic Drugs.*

Given as eye drops

1. Drug action—pupil contracts, iris is drawn away from cornea; aqueous humor may drain through lymph spaces (meshwork) into canal of Schlemm.
2. Types: (see chart below).

B. *Sympathomimetic Drugs*

Given as eyedrops (see chart below).

C. *Carbonic Anhydrase Inhibitor*

Given orally or intravenously

1. Drug action—restricts action of enzyme which is necessary to produce aqueous humor.
2. Kind frequently used (see chart below).

D. *Beta-blocker—nonselective*

Given as eyedrops (see chart, p. 684).

E. *Hyperosmotic Agents*

(See chart, p. 684.)

Medication	Action	Effect and Precautions
Parasympathomimetic Drugs		
Pilocarpine hydrochloride	Acts directly on myoneural junction	Action lasts 6-8 hours; may cause ciliary spasm (eye becomes more myopic).
Carbachol (Doryl)	Acts directly on myoneural junction	Used if pilocarpine is ineffective; prolongs pupillary constriction.
Physostigmine salicylate (eserine)	Cholinesterase inhibitor	Action lasts 6-8 hours; allergenic, unstable, short in action.
Echothiophate iodide (Phospholine Iodide)	Cholinesterase inhibitor	Water-soluble; produces less local irritation. Action lasts 24 hours. After instillation, apply finger pressure to tear duct to prevent drainage into nose and throat.
Isofluorophate (DFP) (Floropryl) (ophthalmic solution)	Cholinesterase inhibitor	Oil-soluble miotic. *Caution*: side effects—vomiting, diarrhea, tenesmus.

NOTE: DFP and phospholine iodide are contraindicated in angle-closure glaucoma.

Sympathomimetic Drugs		
Epinephrine	Decreases aqueous humor production rate	Contraindicated prior to iridectomy (may precipitate acute attack of glaucoma). Keep medication refrigerated to maintain effectiveness.

Carbonic Anhydrase Inhibitor		
Acetazolamide (Diamox) Methazolamide (Neptazane) Ethoxzolamide (Cardrase, Ethamide) Dichlorphenamide (Daranide, Oratrol)	Carbonic anhydrase inhibitor	Decreases production of aqueous humor. *Caution*: side effects—gastric distress, shortness of breath, dermatitis, tingling of extremities, general malaise, acidosis, ureteral stones.
		Stress importance of continuing with medications even if side effects occur.
		If diuresis occurs, supplement patient's diet with potassium-containing foods.

Medication	Action	Effect and Precautions
Beta-blocker-nonselective		
Timolol (Timoptic)	Effectively lowers intraocular pressure in glaucoma with a minimum of side effects	May reduce production of aqueous humor. May facilitate outflow of aqueous humor.
	Mechanism of action not completely established	Use cautiously in patients who have bronchial asthma, congestive heart failure, or myasthenia gravis.
	No anesthetic action; has pH similar to that of eye (6.5–7.5)	Check pulse; do not administer if pulse is below 50 beats per minute.
Hyperosmotic Agents		
Intravenous (systemic) Mannitol Urea	Reduces intraocular pressure by increasing blood osmolality	Useful in treatment of acute attacks of pressure and preoperatively.
		May cause agitation and disorientation.
		Keep airway at bedside; use side rails; monitor fluids and vital signs.
Oral Glycerin (Osmoglyn, Glyrol) Isosorbide (Hydronol, Isonol)		Safer than intravenous medication for cardiac patients
		May cause nausea, vomiting, headache; instruct patient to lie down; bed in a flat position.
		Administer medication over cracked ice flavored with citrus juice to avoid nausea.

Surgical Management

1. *Iridectomy*—an incision through cornea so that a portion of the iris may be drawn out and excised—peripheral or sector (keyhole).
   Result—Iris is prevented from bulging forward and causing the angle at cornea and iris to be crowded. Consequently, drainage is facilitated and intraocular tension is reduced and there is relief of pupillary block.
2. *Iridencleisis*—an opening is created between anterior chamber and space beneath the conjunctiva; this bypasses the blocked meshwork, and aqueous fluid is absorbed into conjunctival tissues.
3. *Thermosclerectomy*—thermal cautery of posterior lip of corneoscleral wound combined with iridectomy.
4. *Trabeculectomy*—partial thickness scleral resection with 2-3 mm. removal of trabecular meshwork and iridectomy.

CHRONIC (OPEN-ANGLE) GLAUCOMA

Majority of patients with glaucoma have this type.

Clinical Manifestations

1. Insidious—mild discomfort (tired feeling in eye).
2. Slowly developing impairment of peripheral vision.
3. Possible halos around lights.
4. Progressive loss of visual field.

Pharmacotherapy

1. Often treated with a combination of miotic and carbonic anhydrase inhibitors (p. 683).
2. Remission may occur; however patient should continue to see physician at 3- to 6-month intervals.
3. If medical treatment is not successful, surgery may be required.

Surgery

OBJECTIVE: to provide filtering of fluid in order to decrease intraocular tension.
1. Corneoscleral Trephine—making a permanent opening at the junction of the cornea and sclera through the anterior chamber so that aqueous humor can drain.
2. Iridencleisis—see above.
3. Sclerectomy—similar to trephining iridectomy except that a punch is used instead of a trephine.
4. Cyclocryotherapy—used when other methods fail. A 3 mm. cryoprobe is applied to the eye surface over the ciliary body; this freezes ciliary body and decreases its secretory function.

Postsurgical Nursing Management

1. Patient usually not detained in the recovery room following local anesthesia.
   Operated eye will be covered by an eye patch.
2. Administer eye drops, analgesic, or narcotic as prescribed and required.

3. Assist the patient in getting out of bed the first time following surgery; usually the patient is ambulatory following local anesthesia.
4. Following general anesthesia, patient remains in recovery room until vital signs are stable and he is oriented to time and place; bathroom privileges usually permissible day of surgery.
5. Provide a liquid diet to eliminate straining on defecation. Change to regular diet as condition justifies.
6. Remind patient of periodic eye check-up since pressure changes may occur.

Health Education

1. Even though glaucoma cannot be cured, it can be controlled.
2. Circumstances that may increase intraocular pressure are to be avoided, if possible.
   a. Emotional upsets—worry, fear, excitement, anger
   b. Constricting clothing such as tight collar, belt, or girdle.
   c. Exertion such as snow shoveling, pushing, heavy lifting
   d. Upper respiratory infections
3. Recommended activities
   a. Exercise in moderation to maintain general well-being
   b. Moderate use of eyes for reading and watching television
   c. Maintenance of regular bowel habits (straining on defecation causes increased intraocular pressure.)
   d. Continuous daily use of eye medications as prescribed (unless long-lasting Ocusert is used)
   e. Normal intake of fluids is not restricted even for alcohol or coffee unless these are known to increase eye pressure in the particular patient.
   f. Check-ups with ophthalmologist in order to keep condition under control
   g. Wearing a medical identification tag indicating patient has glaucoma

MONOCULAR VISION*

Each year over 50,000 persons become "one-eyed" because of accidents, disease, or tumors. In addition to the usual postoperative care, the person with monocular vision will need specialized care in adjusting to his condition.

Psychological Adaptations

There are psychological "lows" intermingled with "highs." The support and understanding of family, friends, loved ones, and members of the health team are very important.

Physiological Adjustments

1. Depth perception is impaired and needs readjustment.
   a. Retinal disparity—each eye sees a slightly different image; to make one clear image, the brain notes the size and distance of each object and computes its position.
   b. Convergence—2 images are merged on the retina; this is useful only for objects at a distance of 7.6 m. (25 feet) or less.
   c. Accommodation—only effective in judging distances up to 1.8 m. (6 feet).

NOTE: All sighted persons are effectively one-eyed for distances greater than 6 m. (20 feet).

2. The horizontal field of vision is narrow because of the position of the nose (Fig. 15-9).

Guidelines For Making Necessary Adjustments and Adaptions

1. Relative motion:
   a. By making a quick side movement of the head, one can get 2 slightly different views of an object. Retinal disparity can be overcome by this simple maneuver, and simulation of binocular vision can be created to give a sense of perspective, especially at close range.

* Adapted from Brady FB. A Singular View: The Art of Seeing With One Eye (revised edition). Oradell, Medical Economics, 1979

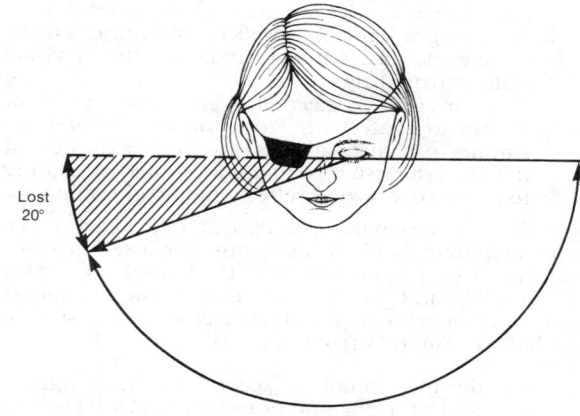

FIGURE 15-9. *The normal field of vision for two eyes is 180 degrees. If a person's vision is limited to one eye, his field of vision encompasses up to 160 degrees, depending on the size of his nose.*

Lost 20°

Visible 160°

2. Perspective:
   a. Note that objects in the foreground are larger than similar objects at a distance (diminishing perspective).
   b. Colors are bolder and brighter in foreground (color perspective).
   c. Close objects are more clearly defined (vanishing perspective).
   d. If a distant object "just grows" in size but does not move, it is on a collision course with the viewer.
3. Coping with activities encountered daily:
   a. In reaching for an object (*e.g.,* door knob or hand in a handshake), move hand in a direct line and keep moving hand until contact is made.
   b. When pouring, actually *touch* the receiving vessel with the one from which the liquid is being poured.

c. Before making a turn to the deficient side, take a good look around by turning the head as far as possible.

d. When dining, choose a place at the table that favors the good eye and is on the same side as the dinner partner; watch out for waiters serving on the sightless side.

e. Watch the *last step* when going up or down steps; feel ahead with the toe and keep one hand on the handrail.

f. In stepping off a curb, keep seeing eye on the edge of the curb so that one can observe its position relative to the backdrop of the street's surface (retinal disparity).

g. Look both ways at the *very last moment* when crossing a street, especially to the side of limited vision.

h. When participating in sports, motion that takes place in two dimensions (bowling, shuffleboard) rather than three dimensions (tennis, basketball) will be easier to master.

i. Swimming is an attractive sport because the swimmer is virtually unaffected by the limits of monocular vision.

j. In fishing, when casting, wear protective glasses with high-impact, shatter-resistant lenses to protect against accidental injury to the good eye.

k. Bouncing a ball off a wall or playing catch (or tossing a frisbee) with a friend can improve visual skills enormously.

l. If an eyeglass is needed, wear impact-resistant glasses to protect the surviving eye. Wear thin-rimmed or rimless glasses, since heavy frames cut down on the visual field; use nonreflective coating to reduce distracting reflections and ghost images.

NOTE: To make emergency "glasses" to read a number in a telephone book when reading glasses are not available: Use a small piece of "cardboard" (size of a calling card), and punch a tiny hole in the cardboard with a pin or bent paper clip. Place eye against hole and hold 15 cm. (6") from page: read.

m. For driving, obtain a second external mirror mounted on right side of car; use curb feelers to assist in parking.

n. Remember that *loss of visual perception* is compensated for by an *increase in degree of alertness.*

o. A "swivel head" also compensates for limited vision.

p. Suggested reading: Brady, Frank B. *A Singular View: The Art of Seeing With One Eye*, revised edition. Oradell, Medical Economics, 1979

Nursing Care of the Non-Seeing Patient

1. Upon entering the room of a non-seeing patient, address him by his name; use a clear, natural voice.
   a. Tell him your name and that you are a nurse.
   b. Indicate why you are there; do not touch him before he knows you are there.
   c. Inform his family and visitors of this procedure when entering the room of the patient, so that he is not startled.

2. Acquaint the patient with his surroundings if he is in a room new to him.
   a. If he is in bed
      (1) Take his hand and show him how to find the call bell and how to use it.

      (2) Help him in using his wash basin, soap, and towel; tell him you have drawn the curtains when he should have privacy.
   b. If he is out of bed
      Assist him to acquaint himself with the room, chairs, bed, doors, bedside table, and place where his personal things are kept.

3. Guide him when walking.
   a. First, remember not to direct the visually handicapped person by steering him from behind—he may bump into things.
   b. Walk ahead of him and have him place his hand in the space at the bend of your elbow; walk normally, at an unhurried pace.
   c. Describe where you are walking and inform him when you are going through a narrow passage or are approaching a curb, steps, or an incline.
   d. Inform him that you are leading him to the bed, chair, or toilet and permit him to feel the front of the object with his knee or hands.

NURSING ALERT: Never permit a non-seeing patient to smoke in bed unattended. If he insists on smoking, have some responsible person remain with him until the cigar or cigarette is extinguished.

4. Provide side rails in the "up" position for the sightless person who has both eyes bandaged for eye treatment or postoperatively.
   a. Hold the patient's hand as you direct him to feel the side rails.
   b. Tell him the side rails are there to remind him not to attempt to get out of bed unassisted.
   c. Place the bell cord within easy reach and inform the patient that someone will answer his bell when he signals. If call light is multipurpose, place a piece of tape over the nurse signal area so that the patient can feel the proper switch.

5. Assist the patient so that he can enjoy his meals.
   a. Read the proposed menu and have him make his selections within his dietary prescription.
   b. Help him to assume a comfortable position when the tray arrives.
   c. Guide his hand to show him where the utensils, plate, cup, etc. are located. Describe food placement on the tray in terms of the face of a clock. If feeding the patient, describe the food: hot, cold, color, flavor.
   d. Plan to have the various items of food always arranged in the same pattern on the tray, so that he will know where the salad, coffee, and bread are. On his plate, the servings should be placed in a specific arrangement so that he knows the meat is in a certain place, etc.
   e. Assist him by cutting the meat into bite-size pieces, buttering the bread, adding sugar and cream to the coffee. Permit him to do as much for himself as he can without embarrassing himself by spilling or knocking food onto the floor.
   f. Provide pleasant conversation or radio music to make mealtime a satisfying time.

6. Solicit his cooperation when he is taking medications.
   a. Tell him you have his medication ready for him; indicate how many pills there are and that they are in a tiny medication cup.
   b. Offer him ½ glass of water to assist in swallowing the tablets.

c. Tell him what the medication is for, if he asks.
d. Prepare him for an injection so that he is not frightened by a "shot."
7. Attend to the psychological and sociological needs of the person with no vision.
  a. Recognize that time does not pass as rapidly when one is inactive.

b. When giving care, mention day of week, date, and time. Radio and television are helpful here.
c. Plan for him to have diversions that interest him—radio, braille books, talking books, visitors, television.
d. Take time to stop and converse with him.

BIBLIOGRAPHY

Books

Bellows JG. Glaucoma: Contemporary International Concepts. New York, Masson Publishers, 1980
Brady FB. A Singular View: The Art of Seeing with One Eye, rev ed. Oradell, Medical Economics Co, 1979
Brockhurst RJ et al. Controversy in Ophthalmology. Philadelphia, WB Saunders, 1977
Chandler PA and Grant WM. Glaucoma, 2nd ed. Philadelphia, Lea & Febiger, 1979
Emery JM and Paton D. Current Concepts in Cataract Surgery. St Louis, CV Mosby, 1980
Fraunfelder FT and Roy FH. Current Ocular Therapy. Philadelphia, WB Saunders, 1980
Hughes WF (ed). 1980 Year Book of Ophthalmology. Chicago, Year Book Medical Publishers, 1980
King JH and Wadsworth J. An Atlas of Ophthalmic Surgery, 3rd ed. Philadelphia, JB Lippincott, 1980
Newell FW. Ophthalmology, 4th ed., St Louis, CV Mosby, 1978
Peyman GA and Sanders DR. Principles and Practice of Ophthalmology. Philadelphia, WB Saunders, 1980
Roth HW and Roth-Witting M. Contact Lenses. Hagerstown, Harper & Row, 1980
Saunders WH et al. Nursing Care in Eye, Ear, Nose and Throat Disorders, 4th ed. St Louis, CV Mosby, 1979
Scheie HG and Albert DM. Textbook of Ophthalmology, 9th ed. Philadelphia, WB Saunders, 1977
Smith JF and Nachazel DP Jr. Ophthalmologic Nursing. Boston, Little, Brown & Co, 1980
Vaughan D and Asbury T. General Ophthalmology, 9th ed. Los Altos, Lange Medical Publications, 1980

Articles

General

Boyd-Monk H. Examining the external eye, Part 1. Nursing '80 1980 May; 10(5):58–63; Part 2 Nursing '80 1980 June; 10(6):58–63
Bresnick GH and Myers FL. Vitrectomy surgery for diabetic retinopathy Annu Rev Med 1979; 300(10):331–338
Cohen KL and Hyndirek RA. Ocular emergencies. Am Fam Physician 1978 Oct; 18(4):178–184
Contact lenses. The Harvard Med School Health Letter 1980 Jan; 5(3):3–4
Dupont J. EENT emergencies. Nursing '79 1979 Nov; 9(11):65–70
Eiferman RA. A primer of conjunctivitis. Primary Care 1979 Sept; 6(3):561–568
Jones M and Tippett T. Assessment of the red eye. Nurs Pract 1980 Jan/Feb; 5(1):10–15
MacFadyen JS. Caring for the patient with a primary retinal detachment. Am J Nurs 1980 May; 80(5):920–921
Pitts RE and Krachmer JH. Evaluation of soft contact lens disinfection in the home environment. Arch Ophthalmol 1979 May; 97(20):470–472
Radical keratotomy—an operation for myopia. The Med Letter 1980 Nov 14; 22(23):97–98
Records RE. Primary care of ocular emergencies. 1. Traumatic injuries. Postgrad Med 1979 May; 65(5):143–152
Records RE. Primary care of ocular emergencies. 2. Thermal, chemical, and nontraumatic eye injuries. Postgrad Med 1979 May; 65(5):157–163
Schrader ES. Perioperative nurses reassure ophthalmologic patients. AORN J 1979 Dec; 30(6):1067–1077
Schumann GB et al. Eye cytology. Am Fam Physician 1980 Dec; 22(6):120–124
Stern EJ. Helping the person with low vision. Am J Nurs 1980 Oct; 80(10)1788–1790

Strickbine-VanReet P et al. Sudden blindness—transient and permanent. Heart Lung 1980 Sept–Oct; 9(5):898–904
Trifluridine (Viroptic) for herpetic keratitis. Med Letter 1980 May 30; 22(11):46–47
Trobe J. The emergent eye. Emergency Med 1978 Sept; 10(9):24–44

Cataract

Boyd-Monk H. Cataract surgery. Nursing '77 1977 June; 7(6):56–61
Jain I etal. Cataractogenous effect of hair dyes: A clinical and experimental study. Ann Ophthalmol 1979 Nov; 11(11):1681–1686
Kolata GD. Lens biophysics and cataract formation. Science 1980 Aug; 209(29):1007–1008
Recommendations made for lens implant use. AORN J 1980 Jan; 31(1):33
Smith JF. Focusing your care for the patient with an intraocular lens implant. RN 1978; 41(3):46, 87

Glaucoma

Boyd-Monk H. Screening for glaucoma. Nursing '79 1979 Aug; 9(8):42–45
Britman N. Cardiac effects of topical timolol. N Engl J Med 1979 March 8; 300(10):566
Katz IM and Soll DB. Beta blockers and glaucoma. Am Fam Physician 1980 April; 2(4):150–151
Quail C and Waddleton C. Treating the glaucomas. Nurses' Drug Alert 1980 Sept; Special Report; 4(12):93–96
Shaivitz S. Timolol and myasthenia gravis. JAMA 1979 Oct 12; 242(15):1611–1612
Zimmerman TJ. Beta blockade; A new approach to glaucoma. Drug Ther 1979 July; 9(7):87–94

Agencies

American Association of Ophthalmology, 1100 17th St, NW Washington, DC 20036
American Council of the Blind, 501 N Douglas Ave, Oklahoma City, Oklahoma 73106
American Foundation for the Blind, 15 W 16th St, New York, NY 10011
American Optometric Association, 7000 Chippewa St, St. Louis, MO 63119
Better Vision Institute Inc, 230 Park Ave, New York, NY 10017
Contact Lens Society of America, 301 First National Bldg, Lexington, KY 40507
Eye-Bank Association of America, 3195 Maplewood Ave, Winston-Salem, NC 27103
Eye-Bank for Sight Restoration, 210 E 64th St, New York, NY 10021
John Milton Society for the Blind, 366 Fifth Ave, Rm 503, New York, NY 10001
Large Print Ltd, 505 Pearl St, Buffalo, NY 14204
Leader Dogs for the Blind, 1039 Rochester Rd, Rochester, Mich 48063
National Braille Press, 88 & Stephen Sts, Boston, MA 02115
National Federation of the Blind, 218 Randolph Hotel Bldg, Des Moines, Iowa 50309
National Society for the Prevention of Blindness, 79 Madison Ave, New York, NY 10016
Recording for the Blind, 215 East 58th St, New York, NY 10022
The New York Times, Large Type Weekly Dept 0229, 220 West 43rd St, New York, NY 10036
The Seeing Eye, Morristown, NJ 07960

EAR DISORDERS

TERMINOLOGY

Ear Care Specialists

1. *Otologist*—a physician who specializes in the diagnosis and treatment of problems of the ear.
2. *Otolaryngologist*—a physician who specializes in problems related to the ear, nose, and throat.
3. *Audiologist*—an individual who specializes in nonmedical evaluation and rehabilitation of hearing disorders (usually not a physician).

Classification of Hearing Loss

1. *Conductive loss*—a hearing loss due to an impairment of the outer or middle ear or both. If causative problem cannot be corrected, a hearing aid may help.
2. *Sensorineural (perceptive) loss*—a hearing loss due to disease of the inner ear or nerve pathways; sensitivity to and discrimination of sounds are impaired. Hearing aids usually are helpful.
3. *Combined hearing loss*—a combination of the above.
4. *Psychogenic hearing loss*—usually a manifestation of an emotional disturbance and unrelated to evident structural changes in the hearing mechanisms. Loss is often total, but without physical basis; thus patient may suddenly recover.

EXAMINATIONS AND DIAGNOSTIC PROCEDURES

NURSING ALERT: In patients with ear pain, suggest examining the good ear first:
1. Otherwise, if sensitive ear is hurt during examination, examiner risks not getting a good look at it or the good ear.
2. If gentleness is demonstrated during examination of good ear, patient is more likely to submit to examination of painful ear.
3. Infection could be transmitted from painful ear to good ear.

MECHANICAL TESTS

See below for assessment procedures: tuning fork (Weber and Rinne Tests). Also see page 24.

NOTE: Tuning fork tests are used only for screening or confirmatory purposes.

AUDIOLOGIC ASSESSMENT

Types

1. Nursing history designed to reveal status of adult hearing (Fig. 16-1).

Ear Condition	Weber Test	Rinne Test
Normal, no hearing loss	No shifting of sounds laterally	Sound perceived longer by *air* conduction
Conductive loss	Shifting of sounds to poorer ear	Sound perceived as long or longer by *bone* conduction
Sensorineural loss	Shifting of sounds to better ear	Sound perceived longer by *air* conduction

A. CHECK, (✓) RIGHT, LEFT, OR BOTH, AND GIVE DURATION (Weeks, Months, Years)

	Right	Left	Both	Duration
Hearing loss?				
Ringing, roaring, or buzzing in ear?				
Fullness or pressure in ear?				
Pain or discomfort in ear?				
Itching in ear?				
Discharge or drainage from ear?				
Do you wear a hearing aid?				

B. ANSWER NO OR YES AND GIVE DATES AND DETAILS

	No	Yes	Dates and Details
Have you had dizzy spells, loss of balance or lightheadedness?			
Have you had any ear operations?			
Have you had tonsil, adenoid, or other nose or throat surgery?			
Have you consulted an ear specialist?			
Are you taking any medication?			
Are you allergic or sensitive to any drugs?			Which ones?
Have you ever taken large doses of aspirin, Anacin, Bufferin, Empirin, or quinine?			
Have you ever received antibiotic injections? (Coly-mycin, streptomycin, Kanamycin, or gentamicin?)			
Do you drink coffee and/or tea?			How much?
Do you smoke?			How much?
Have you been exposed to loud noises? (machinery, gunfire, rock music)			
Is there a history of hearing difficulties in your immediate family?			
Is your general health good?			

FIGURE 16-1. *Status of adult hearing can be determined by a nursing history. (Goodhill V. Ear Diseases, Deafness, and Dizziness, p 99. Hagerstown, Harper & Row 1979)*

2. Pure-tone audiometry.
   a. Sound stimulus consists of a pure (musical) tone.
   b. The louder the tone required before patient hears it, the greater the hearing loss.
   c. *Decibel*—unit of measuring loudness or intensity of sound.
3. Speech audiometry.
   a. Speech Reception Threshold (SRT), with masking* when appropriate.
   b. Speech Discrimination Score (SDS), with masking when appropriate.
   c. Acoustic impedance evaluation.

Pure-Tone Testing—Audiometric Examination

A. *Preliminary Requirements and Procedure*

1. Air conduction and bone conduction pure-tone capabilities.
2. A masking generator.
3. A speech circuit to deliver speech materials (e.g., live voice, taped, or phonographic recording).
4. Acoustically shielded booth (soundproof).
5. Noise level controlled.
6. Patient seated so that he cannot watch hand movement of audiologist during testing.
7. Qualified audiologist, preferably certified in clinical competence by the American Speech and Hearing Association.
8. Patient is instructed to put on earphones and to signal (1) when he hears the tone, and (2) when the tone disappears.
9. *Air conduction* is measured by applying tone directly to external auditory opening.
10. *Nerve conduction* is measured when stimulus is applied directly to the mastoid process.

B. *Audiogram*

1. The vertical lines represent the frequencies at which each ear is tested (25–8,000 Hz or cps) (Fig. 16-2).
2. The horizontal lines represent the degree of deviation from the norm in decibels.
3. Air conduction (AC) levels are plotted (obtained through pure-tone testing).
4. Bone conduction (BC) levels are plotted (obtained through vibrating oscillator placed in back of ear).

C. *Examples of Impairment on an Audiogram:*

1. *Conductive Hearing Loss*
   A problem in the outer and middle ear may result in reduced sensitivity to tones received by air conduction. If the inner ear is unimpaired, bone conduction will be within normal range (see Fig. 16-2).
2. *Sensorineural Hearing Loss*
   A weakening of sound produced in some portion of the sensorineural mechanism (e.g., inner ear) results in reduced thresholds for air conduction. Usually it also causes a reduction in bone conduction (see Fig. 16-3).
3. *Mixed Hearing Loss*
   As mentioned above, weakening of sound in some portion of the sensorineural mechanism results in reduced bone conduction and air conduction. When there is also a lesion in the external auditory canal or middle ear, there will be additional weakening in thresholds for air conduction (see Fig. 16-4).

   * *Masking* is the introduction of noise into the non-tested ear to aid in the elimination of assistance from the good ear (cross-hearing or interaural attenuation).

D. *Evaluation*

1. Normal human ear perception—20 cycles per second (cps) or 20 Herz (Hz) to 20,000.
2. Frequencies significant for speech range—500 to 2000 Hz.

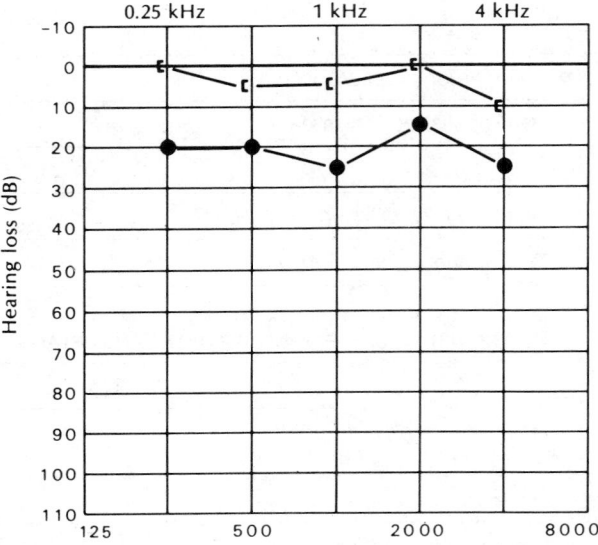

FIGURE 16-2. *An audiogram with reduced air conduction (AC) levels (at least 15 decibels (DB) poorer than bone conduction (BC) levels) and essentially normal bone conduction levels is said to represent a* conductive *hearing loss.*
AC ●——● *unmasked RE (right ear)*
BC [——[*masked RE*

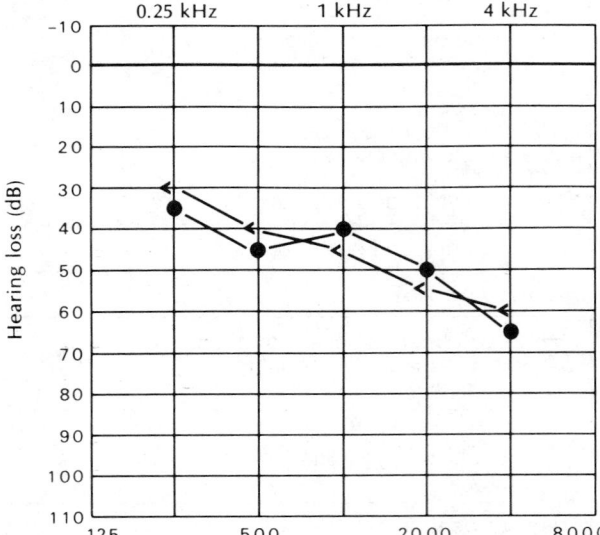

FIGURE 16-3. *When AC = BC ± 10 db, the audiogram is reported to represent a* sensorineural *hearing loss.*
AC ●——● *unmasked RE (right ear)*
BC <——< *unmasked RE*

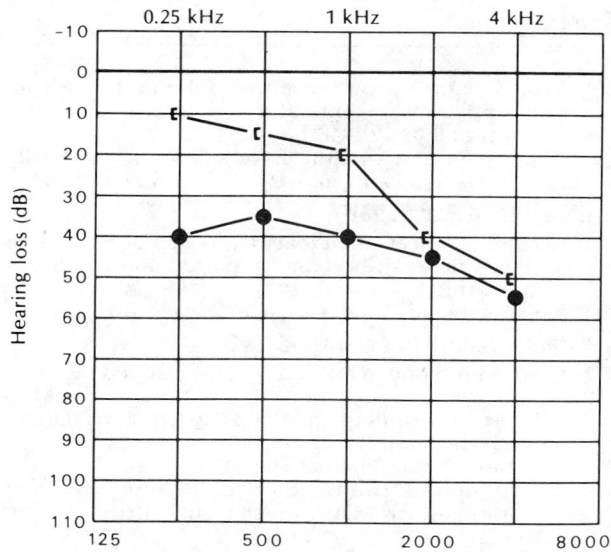

FIGURE 16-4. *When air conduction and bone conduction levels are reduced from normal and the reduction for air conduction is greater than that for bone conduction, the audiogram is said to represent a mixed hearing loss.*
AC •——• *unmasked RE*
BC [——[*unmasked RE*

(Figures 16-2, 16-3, 16-4: Goodhill V. Ear Diseases, Deafness, and Dizziness, pp 143–144. Hagerstown, Harper & Row, 1979)

Speech Audiometry

A. *Speech Reception Threshold (SRT)*

1. This is the softest hearing threshold level at which a person can correctly repeat approximately 50% of very familiar two-syllable words. This is not a test for discrimination but does provide a gross estimate of the patient's ability to recognize and respond to speech.

B. *Speech Discrimination Score (SDS)*

1. This is a supra-threshold measure of speech discrimination.
2. The tester presents phonetically balanced monosyllabic words which the patient is asked to repeat. The percentage of correct responses is the SDS.

C. *Acoustic Impedance Evaluation*

1. An objective measurement (does not require direct patient response) relating to the function of the peripheral auditory mechanism:
   a. Tympanic membrane mobility
   b. Middle ear pressure
   c. Eustachian tube function
   d. Continuity and compliance of ossicular chain
   e. Abnormalities or functional hearing loss
2. The battery of acoustic impedance testing includes:
   a. Measurement of acoustic impedance (static compliance), hindrance, or resistance to passage of sound
   b. Tympanometry
   c. Measurement of acoustic reflex threshold

EAR HYGIENE

Hygienic Measures

1. Avoid putting bobby pins, matches, toothpicks, etc. into the external auditory canal (danger of possible infection and damage to the eardrum). Many physicians even object to the use of Q-tips.
2. If it becomes necessary to remove wax deposits, instill 3 or 4 drops of Debrox twice a day for 3 or 4 days; after the 4th day, irrigate gently with warm water.
3. During an upper respiratory infection, avoid vigorous blowing of the nose, since middle ear infection can result.
4. In the presence of an ear infection, take precautions when swimming—either avoid this sport or insert a lamb's wool plug into the ear canal. It is preferable not to get the head wet.

Noise

1. Excessive noise is detrimental to health and decreases work efficiency; conversely, elimination of noise or substitution of pleasant soft music increases work efficiency.
2. The *decibel* (db) is the unit of measurement of sound intensity.
   a. Leaves rustling in a breeze—10 decibels
   b. Ordinary conversation—50 decibels
   c. Noisy subway—80 decibels
   d. Jet plane (100 feet away)—140 decibels
3. *Frequency*—Number of sound waves emanating from a source per second. This is described as cycles per second (cps or Hz).
4. *Pitch* is related to frequency.
   a. For example—100 cps or Hz is low pitch
   10,000 cps or Hz is high pitch
   b. A healthy young adult can distinguish frequencies from 16 cps to 20,000 cps.
5. Health Implications
   a. Individuals react differently to noise.
   b. The noise level in the home should not exceed 35–40 decibels.
   c. Very loud electrical music can damage hearing.
   d. Protective muffs are recommended in work areas where the noise level exceeds 80–85 decibels.

PROBLEMS AFFECTING THE EXTERNAL EAR

Otitis Externa

Otitis externa is an infection of the external ear canal that may occur 2–3 days after swimming and diving (swimmer's ear).

A. *Prevention*

1. Prevent or minimize by drying the ear canals after diving.
2. Shaking the head vigorously or jumping with head tilted to one side may be effective in removing trapped water in ear canal.
3. Fanning the ear may have a drying effect; a hair dryer held at a comfortable distance from the ear may be helpful.

> **NURSING ALERT:** Use of cotton-tipped applicators to dry the canal or remove ear wax should be avoided because:
> a. cerumen may be forced against tympanic membrane.
> b. the canal lining may be abraded, making it more susceptible to infection.
> c. cerumen that coats and protects the canal may be removed.

4. Use of ear drops after swimming will assist in preventing swimmer's ear. Usually these medications contain several ingredients:
   a. alcohol and glycerol to reduce moisture.
   b. boric acid or acetic acid (vinegar) to limit growth of microorganisms and maintain normal acidity of the ear canal.

B. *Treatment*

1. Alcohol (dries moisture), acetic acid (restores acidity), and antibiotics (curb infection).
2. If canal is swollen and tender, insert cotton wick soaked with Burow's solution (aluminum acetate solution); wick is kept saturated until swelling recedes, usually in 24–48 hours.
3. When pain and swelling have subsided, a specially trained person can remove debris from ear canal.

Cerumen in Ear Canal

1. Accumulated cerumen (earwax) does not have to be removed unless it becomes impacted and interferes with hearing.
2. To irrigate ear canal, see *Guidelines,* below.

Foreign Bodies in External Canal

1. Inserted by young children or handicapped persons.
2. Insects
   Treat by instilling oil drops to smother insect, which then will float out.
3. Vegetable foreign bodies (peas)
   a. Irrigation is contraindicated because vegetable matter absorbs water, which would further wedge foreign body in ear canal.
   b. Unskilled persons should not attempt to remove foreign body because:
      (1) It may be forced into bony portion of the canal.
      (2) The canal skin may be perforated.
      (3) The eardrum may be perforated.
   c. Removal should be done skillfully with instruments; if the victim is very young, general anesthesia is required.

Auricle Cancer

1. This is the most common (70%) ear malignancy; helix and postauricular regions are primary sites.
2. Basal cell cancer (40%) and malignant melanoma (30%) are the most common types.
3. Four-fifths of all patients are male.

Management
Local excision and possibly radiation and/or chemotherapy.

GUIDELINES: Irrigating the External Auditory Canal

Purposes
1. To remove discharge from the canal.
2. To facilitate removal of cerumen or foreign bodies.
3. To apply heat to the tissues of the ear canal.

> **NURSING ALERT:** Ask the patient if he has a history of draining ears, or if he has ever had a perforation or other complications from a previous ear irrigation. If the reply is affirmative, check with the physician before proceeding with the irrigation.

Equipment and Solutions

Kind and amount of solution desired
Tray containing:
Protective towels
Cotton balls and cotton applicators
Solution bowl and emesis basin
Ear syringe or irrigating container with tubing, clamp and irrigating catheter
Paper bag for disposable cotton

Procedure   *Preparatory Phase*

1. After explaining procedure to patient, place him in appropriate position, i.e., sitting or lying with head tilted toward affected ear.
2. Place protective toweling.

NURSING ACTION	RATIONALE/AMPLIFICATION

Performance Phase

1. Use a cotton applicator to remove any discharge on outer ear.
2. Place emesis basin close to the patient's head and under the ear.
3. Test temperature of solution by allowing some to run on inner aspect of wrist. Should be 35 to 40.6° C. (95–105° F.).
4. Ascertain whether impaction is due to a foreign hygroscopic (attracts or absorbs moisture) body before proceeding.
5. Gently pull the outer ear upward and backward (adult); downward and backward (child).
6. Place tip of syringe or irrigating catheter at opening of ear; gently direct stream of fluid against sides of canal (Fig. 16-5).
7. If an irrigating container is used, elevate not more than 15 cm. (6 inches).

8. Observe for signs of pain or dizziness.
9. If irrigating does not dislodge the wax, instill several drops of glycerin, Debrox, or saturated solution of sodium bicarbonate, 2–3 times daily for 2–3 days.

1. To prevent carrying discharge deeper into canal.

2. To provide a receptacle to receive irrigating solution.

3. More comfortable for patient; solutions that are hot or cold are most uncomfortable and may initiate a feeling of dizziness.
4. If water contacts such a substance, it may cause it to swell and produce intense pain.

5. To straighten ear canal.

6. To permit direction for inflow and outflow; if stream is directed forcefully against eardrum, it is possible to rupture it.
7. To provide safe and effective pressure of fluid; if height is more than 6 inches, pressure will be too great and may damage tissue.
8. If they occur, discontinue treatment.
9. To soften and loosen impaction.

Follow-up Phase

1. Dry external ear with cotton pledgets.
2. Remove soiled towels, etc. and make patient comfortable.
3. Record: Time of irrigation, kind and amount of solution used, nature of return flow, effect of treatment.

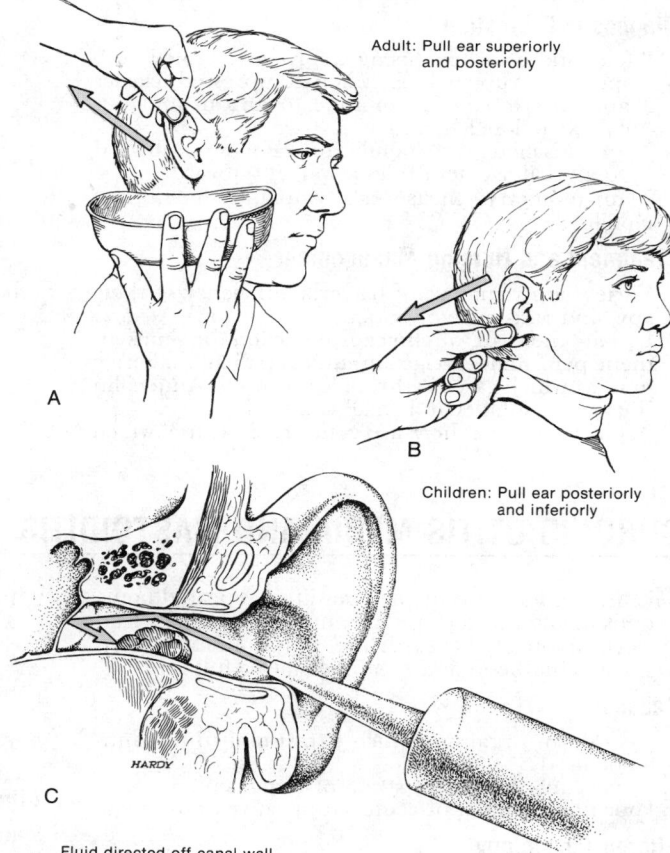

Adult: Pull ear superiorly and posteriorly

Children: Pull ear posteriorly and inferiorly

Fluid directed off canal wall behind cerumen

FIGURE 16-5. *Ear irrigation. A. The external auditory canal in the adult can best be exposed by pulling the earlobe upward and backward. B. The same exposure can be achieved in the child by gently pulling the auricle of the ear downward and backward. C. An enlarged diagram showing the direction of irrigating fluid against the side of the canal. NOTE: This is more effective in dislodging cerumen than if the flow of solution were directed straight into the canal.*

ACUTE OTITIS MEDIA

Acute otitis media is an inflammation of the middle ear caused by the entrance of pathogenic organisms. Normally the middle ear is sterile in its environs.

Etiology

Hemolytic streptococcus, pneumococcus, staphylococcus, influenza bacillus.

Mode of Entry

1. Auditory canal—if drum is perforated.
2. Eustachian tube—during indiscriminate use of nasal drops or nasal douching, or as a result of forcibly sneezing or blowing the nose.
3. Rarely, following a fracture of the skull.

Clinical Manifestations

1. Variable—may be mild or severe.
2. Pain is usually the first symptom—may be in and about the ear and it may be intense.
   May be relieved by spontaneous perforation of the drum or by myringotomy.
3. Fever—may be caused by a virus; in some patients temperature may rise to 40.0°–40.6° C. (104°–105° F.).
4. Headache, difficulty hearing, ear and head noises, anorexia, nausea, and vomiting.

Diagnostic Evaluation

1. Pneumatic otoscopy (using a properly sealed otoscope)—the rubber bulb, when compressed, causes a normal tympanic membrane to flap in and out (total excursion 1–2 mm.).
   In otitis media, the membrane often moves inward to a greater extent than it moves outward.
2. Tympanometry—measures tympanic membrane mobility.

Treatment and Nursing Management

1. Varies with virulence of bacteria, efficiency of therapy, and resistance of patient.
2. Usually the drug of choice is penicillin (or semisynthetic penicillin—cyclacillin) unless patient is allergic to it, in which case erythromycin is used. Ampicillin is used for infants and small children.
3. Aspirin and local heat are comfort measures which may permit patient to rest more comfortably if pain is a problem. (Sedation is usually avoided, for it may interfere with the early detection of intracranial complications.)
4. Some physicians believe the most effective therapy is to administer decongestants along with self-inflation of the ear by the Valsalva maneuver.
   a. This is accomplished by having the patient try to exhale forcefully while holding his nose and mouth tightly—this forces air along the eustachian tube into middle ear.
   b. When successful, the patient will experience a "pop" and an immediate (perhaps temporary) improvement.
   c. It should be performed 10–12 times daily.
5. Employ wide-spectrum antibiotic therapy.

NURSING ALERT:
1. With wide-spectrum antibiotic therapy, acute otitis media may become subacute with continued purulent discharge.
2. Healing may take place, but the patient may be left with a residual deafness.
3. Recognize that such symptoms as headache, slow pulse, vomiting, and vertigo are significant and should be reported.
4. Secondary complications may involve the mastoid or even the brain, producing meningitis or brain abscess.

6. *Myringotomy*—an incision made into the posterior inferior aspect of the tympanic membrane for draining purposes (to relieve pressure and drain pus from middle ear infection).
   a. The incision heals rapidly.
   b. Hearing is not adversely affected.
   c. This procedure is done less frequently now because antimicrobial therapy usually makes it unnecessary. However, it may be done because of failure to respond to antimicrobial therapy, for severe persistent pain, and for persistent conductive hearing loss.

CHRONIC OTITIS MEDIA AND MASTOIDITIS

Chronic otitis media occurs as a result of repeated bouts of otitis media which cause inflammation and may lead to perforation of the eardrum. This condition often begins in childhood and continues into adult life.

Causes

1. A strain of organism which is resistant to the antibiotic used
2. A particularly virulent strain of organism
3. Poor management of acute suppurative otitis media

Altered Physiology

1. Marginal perforation of drum membrane
2. Presence of cholesteatoma (soft ball of dead skin) which erodes vital structures
   a. Caused by an ingrowth of skin from the perforated drum
   b. Fills area in the mastoid and middle ear; bacterial infection frequently develops
   c. May encroach upon vital structures—facial nerve, labyrinth, and brain

Clinical Manifestations

Symptoms are minimal: mild hearing loss, otorrhea (foul-smelling discharge); pain frequently means a CNS complication has occurred.

Diagnostic Evaluation

1. Presence of above symptoms
2. X-rays to note mastoid pathology
3. Pneumatic otoscopy, tuning fork testing, audiometry

Treatment and Nursing Management

OBJECTIVES: to eradicate disease.
to improve hearing.

A. *Medical Therapy*

1. Antibiotic and steroid eardrops may control infection and inflammation.
2. Frequent removal of epithelial debris and purulent drainage.
3. If advanced chronic ear disease is left untreated, inner-ear and life-threatening CNS complications may develop because of erosion of surrounding structures.

B. *Surgery*

1. Indicated when cholesteatoma is present.
2. Indicated when there is pain or complications—profound deafness, dizziness, sudden facial paralysis, stiff neck (may lead to meningitis or brain abscess).
3. *Simple Mastoidectomy*—removal of mastoid cells—indicated when there is persistent tenderness, fever, discharge from ear, or headache.
4. *Radical Mastoidectomy*—removal of all diseased tissue from mastoid area and middle ear.
5. *Posteroanterior Mastoidectomy*—combines simple mastoidectomy with tympanoplasty.

C. *Nursing Concern*

1. Shaving depends upon nature of the incision.
   a. Postaural—(incision behind the ear). Clip hair and shave scalp for 3–4 cm. around ear (only if desired by surgeon).
   b. Endaural—(incision through the ear canal). Shave is unnecessary.
2. Provide for relief of pain preoperatively.
   a. Give aspirin or codeine sulfate.
   b. Apply ice cap to area.
3. Postoperatively, administer sedatives for pain and restlessness.
4. Assist with dressing change since area is packed with gauze for drainage; this may be done daily or every other day—packing is removed on 3rd or 4th day.
5. Observe for possible complications:
   a. Facial paralysis may be indicative of facial nerve injury.
      (1) Immobility on side of face affected
      (2) Eye cannot close, mouth droops
      (3) Patient unable to whistle
      (4) Patient unable to drink without dripping from mouth
      (5) When patient speaks or smiles, immobility of affected side is noticeable
      (6) Administer cortisone preparation as prescribed to assist in restoration of nerve function. (Not used if paralysis is caused surgically.)
   b. Infection
      (1) Observe for clinical signs of inflammation.
      (2) Administer antibiotics.
   c. Vertigo—may be apparent following radical mastoidectomy due to inner ear disturbance.
   d. Spread of infection to brain.
      Unusual rise in temperature, chills, stiff neck, nausea and vomiting.
6. Note status of hearing
   a. If stapes has been removed or dislodged, then hearing is lost.
   b. If stapes or cochlea have not been removed or disturbed, then hearing is regained; a hearing aid may be required.

PERFORATION OF EARDRUM

Etiology and Altered Physiology

1. Infection is the most frequent cause of permanent perforation of the tympanic membrane; often this is due to acute or chronic suppurative otitis media.
2. Trauma is the next cause of permanent perforation; may be due to:
   a. A severe blow on the ear
   b. Blast effect of high explosives
   c. Foreign objects
   d. Force of a stream of water
   e. Burns of face and head
   f. Postmyringotomy defects

Treatment

A. *Medical*

1. Most accidental perforations of the eardrum heal spontaneously.
2. Cauterization of the perforation with trichloroacetic acid at frequent intervals and application of a prosthesis will produce a healed membrane with scar tissue.

B. *Surgical*

Tympanoplasty, Type I—myringoplasty—(simple patching of drum). See below.

TYMPANOPLASTY

Tympanoplasty is a reconstructive operation on the diseased or deformed components of the middle ear.
1. Objective is to improve or preserve the conductive mechanisms in an effort to salvage or improve hearing
2. Impetus for tympanoplasty has been aided by:
   a. Illuminated binocular microscope
   b. Use of antibiotics to prevent or control infection

Physiological Principles of Hearing

Why an intact drum is needed to hear.
1. Sound waves are transformed from airborne vibrations to mechanical stimulation of endolymphatic lymph; this is accomplished by the conductive ability of the eardrum and ossicles.
2. The ratio of the small oval window to the large tympanic membrane is 1:22; this, combined with the vibratory action of the ossicles, means a great increase in force from the air to the inner ear fluids.
3. When there is a disturbance in the above relationships, the result is a loss of hearing.
4. From the oval window, bordered by the annular ligament, impulses are received by the stapes footplate from the incus, malleus, and drum membrane.

5. A lag phase is normal after sound waves stimulate the oval window and before the final effect of the stimulus reaches the round window.

Altered Physiology

1. When there is a perforation of the eardrum, the lag phase (described above) disappears, with the result that sound waves hit the oval and round windows at the same time, causing diminished effect of labyrinth fluid motility → lessened stimulation of hair cells in the organ of Corti → diminished hearing.
2. Infections often produce fibrosis or necrosis of all or part of the ossicular chain.
3. Granuloma, polyps, and fibrous or bony plaques may resist normal function of the oval and round windows.
4. In addition to sequelae from otitis media, otosclerosis may exist.
5. Obstruction of tympanic orifice of the eustachian tube may produce dysfunction.

Types of Tympanoplasty (Table 16-1)

A. *Type I (Myringoplasty)*
1. *Purpose*—to close perforation by placing a graft over it in order to create a closed middle ear section which in turn will improve hearing.
2. *Indications*
    To avoid risk of contamination when patient bathes, swims, or dives—this in turn prevents recurrence of chronic otitis media or mastoiditis.
3. *Contraindications*
    a. Ossicular involvement
        Prediction of surgical results can be made preoperatively by testing for improvement of hearing levels by placing a temporary patch over the defect. If no improvement noticed in audiometric testing, the ossicular chain may be involved.
    b. Presence of active infection
    c. Presence of chronic middle ear infection, impairing or preventing drainage via eustachian tube
    d. Sinusitis or allergy which produces a chronic infectious discharge via nasopharynx
    e. History of acute exacerbations of otitis media
4. *Surgical Repair*
    Perforation is closed using one of the following:
    a. Fascia from temporal muscle (in almost all cases)
    b. Vein grafts from hand or forearm (occasionally)

5. *Postoperative Management*
    a. Administer antibiotics for several days postoperatively to ensure freedom from infection.
    b. Reinforce external dressings if they become soiled; otherwise leave dressings intact.
    c. Remove gauze packing in canal at end of week; do not apply suction or probe canal.
    d. Gentle capillary suction may be attempted by end of 2nd week to remove debris and crusts (Gelfoam remains).
    e. Gently inflate canal to test efficiency of eardrums closed by new graft.
    f. Do not use ear drops, because of danger of loosening graft.
    g. Dust lightly with antibiotic powder (Neosporin).
6. *Patient Education*
    a. Avoid shampooing or showering, which could cause contamination of ear canal, until permission is obtained from physician.
    b. Continue with antibiotics beyond first week if there is evidence of infection.
    c. Use antihistamine with an ephedrine derivative for at least 1 month postoperatively.
    d. Continue using an antihistamine if the patient experiences rhinologic allergy.

B. *Types II to V*
1. *Purpose* (see Table 16-1). These procedures are modifications used to correct various middle ear problems.
2. *Preoperative and Operative Treatment*
    a. Topical and systemic antibiotics are administered when infection is present.
    b. Suitable replacement (polyethylene, stainless steel wire, bone, cartilage) is used to maintain continuity of conduction sound pathway.
    c. The necessity of a 2-stage procedure should be determined.
        (1) First stage—eradication of all diseased tissues; area is cleaned out to achieve a dry, healed middle ear.
        (2) Second stage—(performed 2–3 months after 1st stage) reconstruction, using grafts.
3. *Postoperative Nursing Management*
    a. Reinforce outer dressings as necessary but keep inner dressings intact.
    b. Assist patient in getting out of bed for the first time because he may become dizzy.

TABLE 16-1. TYPES OF TYMPANOPLASTY

Type	Middle Ear Damage		Repair Process
	Tympanic Membrane	*Ossicles*	
I	Perforated	Normal	Close-perforation-myringoplasty.
II	Perforated	Erosion of malleus and/or incus.	Close perforation; graft against incus or whatever remains of malleus.
III	Tympanic membrane destroyed or widely perforated.	Rest of ossicular chain destroyed BUT stapes are intact and mobile.	Grafts implanted to contact the normal stapes. Tympanostapedopexy
IV	Tympanic membrane destroyed or widely perforated.	Ossicular chain destroyed. Head, neck, and crura of stapes destroyed. Stapes footplate mobile.	Expose mobile stapes footplate—graft implanted. Air pocket between graft and round window provides protection. The Cavum minor operation
V	Tympanic membrane destroyed or widely perforated.	Ossicular chain destroyed. Head, neck, and crura of stapes destroyed. Stapes footplate fixed.	Make opening in horizontal semicircular canal; graft seals off middle ear to give sound protection for round window. Tympanoplasty and fenestration of lateral semi-circular canal

c. Notify physician of any dizziness; medication will be prescribed as needed for vertigo and nausea.
d. Caution patient not to blow his nose with force and to avoid wetting dressings during bathing.

e. Note that hearing improvement is achieved in inverse proportion to the amount of surgery required; the simpler the surgery, the better the chance for hearing to improve.

OTOSCLEROSIS

Otosclerosis is a form of deafness caused by the formation of new spongy bone in the labyrinth, fixation of the stapes, and prevention of sound transmission through the ossicles to the inner fluids.

Incidence and Clinical Manifestations

1. Cause is unknown
2. Occurs more commonly in women than men; rare in the black race
3. Has a hereditary basis
4. Patient presents a history of slow, progressive hearing loss with no middle ear infection
5. A frequent complaint is buzzing or ringing noises in the ears; both ears are usually affected equally

Diagnostic Evaluation

1. Audiometry findings substantiate hearing loss.
2. Bone conduction is much better than air condition. Reduced tuning fork transmission by air, whereas there is intensification of bone conduction sound when tuning fork handle is placed over the mastoid bone.

Treatment

1. No known medical treatment for this form of deafness, but amplification with a hearing aid may be helpful.
2. Surgical treatment—stapedectomy (often recommended); see below.

STAPEDECTOMY

A *stapedectomy* involves removal of otosclerotic lesions at the footplate of stapes and the creation of a tissue implant with prosthesis to maintain suitable conduction. To perform such delicate surgery, the otologic binocular microscope is used.

Types of Prostheses

1. Steel wire and fat implant
2. Gelfoam and stainless steel wire
3. Metal or Teflon "piston"
4. Vein graft and polyethylene tubing (least frequent)

Nursing Management

1. Observe for unusual symptoms, such as:

a. Fever—may indicate infection, external otitis, otitis media
b. Headache—may indicate infection, nerve encroachment
c. Vertigo—may indicate labyrinthitis or inner ear reaction
d. Ear pain—may indicate infection or irritation of auditory nerve

2. Position patient postoperatively as desired by physician.
a. Some surgeons prefer that the patient be positioned with operated ear uppermost to maintain position of graft and stability
b. Others prefer that patient be lying on operated ear to permit drainage
c. Still others advocate that the patient assume the most comfortable position

3. Administer antimotion medications and sedatives if patient experiences vertigo, nystagmus, or nausea.
4. Assist patient when he first tries to walk; he may feel dizzy for the first few days.
5. Instruct patient not to blow his nose for a week; air may be forced up the eustachian tube and disturb the operative site.
6. Encourage a restricted head position if the surgeon fears a misplacement of the prosthesis.
7. Replace soiled (bloody) cotton pledget in ear canal as necessary.
8. Administer meperidine or prescribed pain medication for first several hours.
9. Advise patient that it may be weeks before full effect of surgery is determined as far as hearing is concerned. At first, hearing may be impaired because of tissue edema, packing, etc.
10. Note that while patient may be ready for discharge in 4 or 5 days, packing is not removed until the 6th or 7th day, in the physician's office.
11. Instruct patient as follows:
a. Do not smoke.
b. Do not blow nose.
c. Protect ears when going outdoors for the first week.
d. Avoid crowds or exposure to colds so that upper respiratory infection is prevented.

MÉNIÈRE'S DISEASE (ENDOLYMPHATIC HYDROPS)

Ménière's disease involves the inner ear and causes a triad of symptoms: vertigo, hearing loss, and tinnitus.

Etiology

1. Ménière's syndrome stems from labyrinthine dysfunction

2. Suggested theories as to the cause of this syndrome:
a. Increase in pressure of endolymph
b. Emotional or endocrine disturbance
c. Vasomotor changes causing a spasm of the internal auditory artery
d. Allergic manifestation

e. Adrenal pituitary insufficiency
f. Congenital or acquired syphilis

Clinical Manifestations

A. *During Attack*

1. Dizziness, tinnitus, and reduced hearing occur on involved side.
2. Patient complains somewhat of headache, nausea, vomiting, incoordination.
3. Sudden attacks occur in which patient complains that room appears to spin around.
4. Sudden motion of the head may precipitate vomiting.
5. Patient often presents a history of ear trouble, vasomotor rhinitis, and allergies.
6. The most comfortable position for the patient is lying down.
7. Personality changes manifest themselves in irritability, depression, withdrawal, and refusal to eat.
8. Vertigo attacks may last several hours or all day.

B. *After or Between Attacks*

1. Patient behaves normally; may continue his work.
2. Only complaint may be tinnitus or impaired hearing

Diagnostic Evaluation

1. Audiogram for pure tones and speech discrimination.
2. Caloric Test/Electronystagmography.
   a. Useful in differentiating Ménière's syndrome from intracranial lesion.
   b. Fluid, which is above or below body temperature, is instilled into auditory canal.
   c. Reactions
      (1) Normal patient—complains of dizziness
      (2) Patient with acoustic neuroma—no reaction
      (3) Patient with Ménière's syndrome—severe attack (as described above)
   d. Nursing management
      (1) Anticipate possibility of patient vomiting; have emesis basin and protective draping.
      (2) Support patient as he walks after the test, since he may be dizzy.
3. Thyroid function tests, allergy history, and glucose tolerance tests are other diagnostic aids.

Medical Management

Conservative management has included:

1. Psychotherapy, allergic hyposensitization, diuretics, low sodium diet, antihistamines, vasodilators, steroids.
2. Administration of "vertigo sedatives" such as dimenhydrinate, meclizine, droperidol, fentanyl.
3. Administration of aminoglycosides, gentamicin sulfate may control vertigo in many patients.

Surgical Management

1. Conservative
   a. Simple sac decompression, vascular and muscular grafts to the sac, sac "shunts," sac obliteration (all conservative procedures but widely used).
   b. Ultrasound—semicircular canal reached through a mastoid incision; ultrasonic energy applied directly via a probe to the bone in the canal (may cause transient facial paralysis).
2. Destructive Surgery
   a. Labyrinthectomy—recommended if the patient experiences progressive hearing loss and severe vertigo attacks so that he cannot perform normal tasks.
   b. Vestibular nerve section—neurosurgical suboccipital approach to the cerebellopontine angle for intracranial vestibular nerve neurectomy.
   c. Translabyrinthine or middle cranial fossa approach to Scarpa's ganglion.

Nursing Management

1. Recognize the need for encouragement and understanding; this is particularly true when the patient experiences subjective symptoms of a subjective nature.
2. Remind the patient to slow down his bodily movements since jerking or making sudden movement may precipitate an attack.
3. Protect the patient who has an attack by placing him in a bed with side rails in position; if he is standing, help lower him to the floor to avoid injury.
4. Postoperatively, patient may experience vertigo; therefore, he may be more comfortable in bed for the first 2 days.
5. Assist patient when he gets out of bed since he may be unsteady; remind him to change his movements easily.
6. Inform him that dizziness may persist as long as 4–6 weeks.
7. Note that a possible complication is Bell's palsy (a peripheral facial weakness with noticeable pain near the angle of the jaw or behind the ear; see p. 717. This will clear up eventually.

Patient Education

1. Eliminate smoking, and the intake of coffee, tea, stimulating drugs.
2. Control environmental factors and personal habits that may cause stress or fatigue.
3. If there is a tendency to allergic reactions to foods, eliminate those that aggravate these responses (e.g. milk, eggs, chocolate, corn, pork, nuts).
4. Adhere to periodic use of diuretics, as prescribed, to relieve feeling of fullness in the ear, vertigo, and tinnitus.

HEARING IMPAIRMENT

Presbycusis

A progressive bilaterally symmetrical perceptive loss of hearing in the older individual that occurs with the aging process.

Treatment
There is no effective medical or surgical treatment.

Nursing Management

1. Hearing aids are usually unnecessary and may only serve to confuse and upset the patient. When indicated, the patient should be advised by an otologist in collaboration with an audiologist.
2. Helpful aids should be considered, such as a telephone amplifier, radio and television earphone attachments, buzzers instead of a door bell.

TABLE 16-2. DEGREE OF HEARING LOSS AND RELATIONSHIP TO COMMUNICATIVE SEQUELAE

Pure-tone Average of the Better Ear	Effect of Hearing Loss on Communicative Skills	Aural Rehabilitation Requirements
27 to 40 db† (slight)	May only have difficulty with hearing faint speech	May benefit from a hearing aid when loss approaches 40 db Needs preferential seating and lighting May need lip-reading instructions
41 to 44 db (mild)	Understands conversational speech when face to face May miss as much as 50 per cent if voices are faint May exhibit anomalies in language and speech	Individual hearing aid evaluation and training in its use Needs preferential seating Attention to language skills Lip-reading instruction Speech conservation and correction Child should be referred to special education
56 to 70 db (marked)	Will only understand loud conversation Is likely to have defective speech Child is likely to be deficient in language usage and comprehension Will have limited vocabulary	Individual hearing aid evaluation and auditory training Lip-reading instruction Speech conservation and correction Special help in language development Child should be referred to special education
71 or more db (severe)	Will hear only very loud voices May be able to identify some loud environment sounds May be able to discriminate vowels but not all consonants Relies on vision rather than hearing as primary avenue for communication Speech and language defective and likely to deteriorate	Individual hearing aid evaluation Auditory training Child should be referred to full-time special program for deaf children, with emphasis on all language skills, concept development, lip-reading, and speech Continuous appraisal of needs in regard to oral and manual communication

Harrison RJ. Current concepts in the management of hearing loss. Reprinted from January, 1979 issue of American Family Physician, published by the American Academy of Family Physicians.
†All decibel ranges according to American National Standards Institute, 1969 norm.

3. Understanding and help from family members is important.
4. "Cupping" the hand in back of the ear may help funnel sound toward the ear canal. See also Communicating with a Person who has Hearing Impairment (below).

COMMUNICATING WITH A PERSON WHO HAS A HEARING IMPAIRMENT

(See Table 16-2, Degree of Hearing Loss and Relationship to Communicative Sequelae)

When the Person Is Able to Lip-Read

1. Face the person as directly as possible when speaking.
2. Place yourself in good light so that he can see your mouth.
3. Do not chew, smoke, or have anything in your mouth when speaking.
4. Speak slowly and enunciate distinctly.
5. Provide contextual clues that will assist him in following your speech. For example, point to a tray if you are talking about the food on it.
6. To verify that he understands your message, write it for him to read. (That is, if you doubt that he is understanding you.)

When It Is Difficult to Understand the Person When He Speaks

1. Pay attention when the person speaks; his facial and physical gestures may help you understand what he is saying.
2. Exchange conversation with him where it is possible to anticipate his replies—this is particularly helpful in your initial contact with him and may help you become familiar with his speech peculiarities.
3. Anticipate context of his speech to assist in interpreting what he is saying.
4. If unable to understand him, resort to writing or include in your conversation someone who does understand him; request that he repeat that which is not understood.

BIBLIOGRAPHY

Books

Adams GL et al. Boie's Fundamentals of Otolaryngology, 5th ed. Philadelphia, WB Saunders, 1978
Ballantyne J. Deafness, 3rd ed. New York, Churchill Livingstone, 1977
Balltype J. and Groves J (eds). Scott Brown's Diseases of the Ear, Nose and Throat, 4th ed., Vol 2. London, Butterworth & Co, 1979
Bradford LJ and Hardy WG. Hearing and Hearing Impairment. New York, Grune & Stratton, 1979
Gerber SE and Mencher GT. Early Diagnosis of Hearing Loss. New York, Grune & Stratton, 1978
Goodhill V. Ear Diseases, Deafness, and Dizziness. Hagerstown, Harper & Row, 1979
Maurer JF and Rupp RR. Hearing and Aging: Tactics for Intervention. New York, Grune & Stratton, 1979
Saunders WH et al. Nursing Care in Eye, Ear, Nose and Throat Disorders. 4th ed. St. Louis, CV Mosby, 1979

Articles
General

Black FO et al. Easing proneness to motion sickness. Patient Care 1980 March 30; 14(6):114–128
Duvall AJ and Lowell SH. The "chronic" ear: How to manage mild to severe otitis. Postgrad Med 1979 Aug; 66(2):94–101
Meade RH III. Complications of earache. Hosp Pract 1979 Aug; 14(8):78–81
Miller RR. Deafness due to plain and long-acting aspirin tablets. J Clin Pharmacol 1978 Oct; 18 (10):468–471
Newman RK and Johnson JT. Unresponsive unilateral serous otitis. Postgrad Med 1980 March; 67(3):143–149
Schwartz RH. New concepts in otitis media. Am Fam Physician 1979 May; 19(5):91–98
Schwartz RH. Myringotomy: A neglected office procedure. Am Fam Physician 1979 Dec; 20(6):102–108

Stewart TW. Common otolaryngologic problems of flying. Am Fam Physician 1979 Feb; 19(2):113–119

Strauss MB et al. Swimmer's ear. Physic Sports Med 1979 June; 7(8):101–105

Treating Meniere's disease nonsurgically. Am Fam Physician 1980 Dec; 22(6):136

Hearing Loss

Curry JL. The hearing-impaired patient; Stranger in a strange land. Ethicon Point of View 1980; 17(4):18–20

Harrison RJ. Current concepts in the management of hearing loss. Am Fam Physician 1979 Jan; 19(1):135–142

LeBuffe FP and LeBuffe LA. Psychiatric aspects of deafness. Primary Care 1979 June; 6(2):295–310

Pamphlet (# PE 261). Services for special needs. American Bell Telephone Co, 1979

Raafat JR and Adams CT. American sign language. Maryland Nurse 1980 Aug; 37

Schiff M and Cohen IJ. What every otolaryngologist should know about hearing aids. Laryngoscope 1978 June; 88(6):932–948

Weber HJ and Pirkey WP. Selection of hearing aids. Otolaryngol Clin North Am 1978 Feb; 11(1):173–186

Agencies

American Speech–Language–Hearing Association, 10810 Rockville Pike, Rockville, Maryland 20852

American Academy of Otolaryngology, Head and Neck Surgery, American Medical Association, 535 Dearborn St, Chicago, Illinois 60610

Alexander Graham Bell Association for the Deaf, 3417 Volta Place NW, Washington, DC 20007

National Association of Hearing and Speech Agencies, 814 Thayer Ave, Silver Spring, Maryland 20910

National Association of the Deaf, 814 Thayer Ave, Silver Spring, Maryland 20910

National Hearing Aid Society, 24261 Grand River, Detroit, Michigan 49219

Toll-free aid for hearing impaired: 1-800-521-5247 (usable in all states except Michigan) 9 A.M. to 4 P.M. E.S.T. Monday through Friday. Hearing Aid Helpline sponsored by National Hearing Aid Society

17

CONDITIONS OF THE NEUROLOGIC SYSTEM

DIAGNOSTIC EVALUATION OF NEUROLOGIC DISEASE

The neurological examination involves history-taking, an assessment of the patient's mental status, speech, memory, and reasoning ability as well as a physical examination in which special attention is given to examination of the nervous system. This involves testing at each cranial nerve in the manner specified on page 703.

Radiologic Procedures

A. *Skull X-ray*—reveals configuration, density, vascular markings, and intracranial calcification and tumor.

B. *Computed Tomography (CT)* (computerized axial tomography) is an imaging method in which the head is scanned in successive layers by a narrow beam of x-ray. It provides a cross-sectional view of the brain and distinguishes differences in the densities of various brain tissues. A computer printout is obtained of the absorption values of the tissues in the plane that is being scanned. The data are transformed into an image through a series of complex equations. The image is displayed on an oscilloscope or TV monitor and photographed.

1. Lesions are seen as variations in tissue density differing from the surrounding normal brain tissue.
2. Abnormalities of tissue density indicate possible tumor masses, brain infarction, ventricular displacement; useful in patients with head trauma, suspected brain tumor, hydrocephalus. CT also used for diseases of the spinal column and spinal cord.
3. May be done with IV contrast medium enhancement to more accurately define boundaries of certain

lesions and indicate presence of otherwise undetectable lesions.
4. *Patient Preparation*
   a. Inquire about allergies and any previous adverse reaction to contrast agent.
   b. See that a consent form has been signed.
   c. No special preparation is required; this is a non-invasive technique that can be done on an outpatient basis.
   d. Instruct the patient that he must lie perfectly still while the test is being carried out; he cannot talk or move his face as this distorts the picture.

C. *Air Studies*—a gaseous replacement of the fluid within the ventricles and subarachnoid systems serves as a contrast medium because air is less dense than fluid to roentgen rays.

1. *Pneumoencephalogram*—withdrawal of cerebrospinal fluid and injection of air or other gas by means of a lumbar puncture.
   a. Demonstrates ventricular system and subarachnoid space overlying the hemispheres and basal cisterns.
   b. Useful in diagnosing degenerative cerebral atrophy and in detecting mass lesions at the base of the brain.
2. *Fractional pneumoencephalogram*—withdrawal of small amounts of fluid and injection of small amounts of air to visualize the ventricular system.
3. *Ventriculogram*—withdrawal of cerebrospinal fluid and injection of air or gas directly into the lateral ventricles through openings in the skull.

a. Trephines (burr holes) are made through a scalp incision; ventricles are punctured by a special needle.

b. The cerebrospinal fluid is replaced with air, the cannulae are withdrawn, and the scalp wounds are closed.

c. If a lesion is present, there is a change in the size, shape, or position of the ventricular, subarachnoid, or cisternal spaces.

4. *Nursing management following pneumoencephalogram or ventriculogram*

a. Watch the patient for increasing intracranial pressure. (See p. 709.)

(1) Disturbances of intracranial pressure may cause serious complications.

(2) Prepare for ventricular tap and prompt decompression.

b. Take vital signs as frequently as clinical condition indicates and until stabilized.

c. Make frequent neurologic checks, especially of level of responsiveness.

d. Assess for complaints of headache, fever, and for signs of shock.

(1) Place ice cap on head intermittently.

(2) Give analgesics as directed—duration of headache depends on the speed with which the intracranial air is absorbed.

(3) Nausea and vomiting may follow air studies.

(4) Parenteral fluids may be necessary for first 24 hours

D. *Isotope Cisternography*—use of radioactive tracer injected into lumbar subarachnoid space. Useful in studying cerebrospinal fluid circulation, to locate cerebrospinal fluid leak, and to evaluate hydrocephalus, etc.

E. *Cerebral Angiography*—the x-ray study of the cerebral circulation following the injection of contrast material into a selected artery.

1. Contrast material may be injected into common carotid, vertebral, or subclavian artery, or arch of the aorta. Selective catheterization may be done via a femoral artery.

2. After injection of selected artery, x-rays are made of arterial and venous phases of circulation through brain and head.

3. Useful in demonstrating position of arteries, intracranial aneurysms, presence or absence of abnormal vasculature, hematomas, tumors.

4. Nursing Support

a. *Before angiogram*

(1) Withhold meal preceding test.

(2) Patient may be given sedative before going to x-ray department—may help minimize intensity of burning sensation felt along course of injected vessel.

(3) Instruct the patient:

(a) Try to lie quietly during injection.

(b) A burning sensation, lasting for a few seconds, may possibly be felt behind the eyes, or in jaw, teeth, tongue, and lips.

b. *Following angiogram*

(1) Make repeated observations for neurologic sequelae—motor or sensory deterioration, alterations in level of responsiveness, weakness on one side, speech disturbances, arrhythmias, blood pressure fluctuation.

(2) Observe injection site for hematoma formation; apply an ice cap intermittently—to relieve swelling and discomfort.

(3) Evaluate peripheral pulses—changes may develop if there is hematoma formation at puncture site or embolization to a distant artery.

(4) Note color and temperature of involved extremity—to detect possible embolism.

F. *Myelography*—the injection of contrast medium into the spinal subarachnoid space by spinal puncture for radiologic examination; outlines the spinal subarachnoid space and shows distortion of the spinal cord or dural sac by tumors, cysts, herniated intervertebral discs, or other lesions.

1. After injection of the contrast medium, the head of the table is tilted down and the course of the contrast medium is observed radioscopically.

2. Contast material may be removed after test completion by syringe and needle aspiration; patient may complain of sharp pain down leg during aspiration if a nerve root has been aspirated against a needle point—needle point is rotated or an adjustment in needle depth is made.

With newer water soluble contrast agents a smaller needle can be used (less likely to produce headache); material is reabsorbed and need not be removed.

3. *Nursing Responsibilities*

a. *Before test*

(1) Reinforce physician's explanation of procedure; explain that it is usually not painful and that the x-ray table will be tilted in varying positions during the study.

(2) Omit the meal preceding myelography.

(3) Patient may be given light sedative prior to test to help him cope.

b. *Post-test*

(1) Instruct the patient to lie in prone position for several hours; he may be kept in bed in supine position (turning from side to side) for 12–24 hours.

If a water soluble medium (Metrizamide [Amipaque]) has been used, the patient lies with head of bed elevated 15–30 degrees—to reduce rate of upward displacement of the medium.

(2) Encourage patient to drink liberal quantities of fluid—for rehydration and replacement of cerebrospinal fluid and to decrease incidence of postlumbar puncture headache (thought to be due to escape of spinal fluid).

(3) Assess neurologic and vital signs; note motor and sensory deviations from normal.

(4) Check on patient's ability to void.

(5) Watch for fever, stiff neck, photophobia, or other signs of chemical or bacterial meningitis.

G. *Lumbar Epidural Venography*—percutaneous insertion of a catheter into the femoral vein; catheter is guided into ascending lumbar vein and/or internal iliac veins. Contrast medium is injected to opacify epidural venous plexus (fills epidural veins overlying disc spaces).

May reveal deviation or compression of the epidural veins due to herniated disc or tumor.

H. *Discography*—injection of radiopaque substance directly into the intervertebral disc. This study can be used in patients suspected of having herniated disc disease but is infrequently done.

Other Neurologic Investigations

A. *Electroencephalography (EEG)*

Records, by means of electrodes applied on the scalp surface (or by microelectrodes placed within brain tissue), the electrical activity which is generated in the brain.

1. Provides physiologic assessment of cerebral activity; useful in diagnosis of the epilepsies and as a screening procedure for coma and organic brain syndrome; also used as an indicator of brain death.
2. Electrodes are arranged on the scalp to permit the recording of activity in various head regions; the amplified activity of the neurons is recorded on a continuously moving paper sheet.
   a. For baseline recording, the patient lies quietly with his eyes closed.
   b. For activation procedures (done to elicit abnormal electrical discharges, especially seizure potentials), patient may be asked to hyperventilate for 3–4 minutes, look at a bright flashing light, or receive an injection of medication (Metrazol).
   c. EEG may also be made during sleep and upon awakening—some abnormal brain waves are seen only when patient is asleep.
3. Pharyngeal (electrode inserted through nose; rests on mucosa of pharyngeal roof) and sphenoidal (inserted transcutaneously with tips resting on sphenoid bone near foramen ovale) electrodes are used when epileptogenic area is inaccessible to conventional scalp preparation.
4. Patient preparation for routine recording.
   a. Antiepileptic medication and tranquilizers may be withheld 24–48 hours before EEG—may alter EEG wave patterns.
   b. Omit coffee, tea, or cola drinks in meal before test; do not omit meal.
   c. Shampoo hair night before tests; omit hair sprays and hair dressings.
   d. Reassure patient that he will not receive an electrical shock, that the EEG takes approximately 45–60 minutes (more for a sleep EEG), and that the EEG is *not* a form of treatment or a test of intelligence or insanity.

B. *Electromyography (EMG)*

The introduction of needle electrodes into the skeletal muscles to study changes in electric potential of muscles and nerves leading to them. These are shown on an oscilloscope and amplified by a loudspeaker for simultaneous visual and auditory analysis and comparison.

1. Useful in determining the presence of a neuromuscular disorder; helps distinguish weakness due to neuropathy from that due to other causes. Useful in evaluation and follow-up of peripheral nerve injuries.
2. *Nursing Responsibilities*
   a. No special patient preparation is required.
   b. Explain to the patient that he will experience a sensation similar to that of an IM injection as the needle is inserted into the muscle; muscles examined may ache slightly for a short time.

C. *Radioisotope Brain Scanning*—following intake (IV) of radiopharmaceutical, the radioactivity subsequently transmitted through the skull is scanned by a rectilinear scanner which prints out a picture based on the number of counts received from the brain as it scans; (or a gamma camera, which prints out image without actually scanning, may be used; this is a more recent imaging device).

1. This test is based on the principle that a radiopharmaceutical may diffuse through a disrupted blood-brain barrier into the abnormal cerebral tissue or areas where there is new vascularization. (Normal brain tissue is relatively impermeable.) There is an increased uptake of radioactive material at the site of pathology.
2. Brain scanning is useful in early detection and evaluation of intracranial neoplasms, stroke, abscess, follow-up of surgical or radiation therapy of brain.
3. *Nursing Responsibility*
   a. Explain to patient that he will be expected to lie quietly during the procedure.
   b. This is a noninvasive procedure.

D. *Echoencephalography*—the recording of echoes from the deep structures within the skull (generated by the transmission of ultrasound [high frequency] waves) to determine the position of midline structures of the brain and the distance from the midline to the lateral ventricular wall or the third ventricular wall.

1. Useful for detecting a shift of the cerebral midline structures caused by subdural hematoma, intracerebral hemorrhage, massive cerebral infarction, and neoplasms; can display dilation of ventricles; useful in evaluation of hydrocephalus.
2. Ultrasonic transducers are positioned over specified areas of the head; the echoes are imaged and stored on the oscilloscope.
3. *Nursing Responsibilities*
   a. There is no special patient preparation.
   b. Explain that this is a noninvasive test and that some type of liquid (mineral oil) may be used to eliminate the air gap between the transducer and the head.

Tests of Cranial Nerve Function

Nerve	Equipment	Clinical Examination
1. Olfactory	Four small bottles of volatile oils, such as (1) turpentine, (2) oil of cloves, (3) oil of wintergreen, (4) vanilla	Instruct the patient to sniff and to identify the odors. Each nostril is tested separately. The patient is asked if he perceives the smell and if he can identify it.

Tests of Cranial Nerve Function (cont.)

Nerve	Equipment	Clinical Examination
2. Optic	Ophthalmoscope	In darkened room the patient is asked to look straight ahead at a distant object while the examiner looks for choked disc, optic atrophy, and retinal and vascular lesions. Special equipment is used for examination of visual fields. Eye chart is used to check visual acuity.
3. Oculomotor 4. Trochlear 5. Abducens	Flashlight	Because of close association, these nerves are examined collectively. They innervate pupil and upper eyelid and are responsible for extraocular muscle movements.
6. Trigeminal	Test tube of hot water Test tube of ice water Cotton wisp from cotton applicator stick Pin	*Sensory branch*—Vertex to chin tested for sensations of pain, touch, and temperature. This includes reflex reaction of cornea to wisp of cotton. *Motor branch*—Ability to bite is tested.
7. Facial	Four small bottles with solutions which are salty, sweet, sour, and bitter (Four wet cotton applicators)	Observe symmetry of face and ability to contract facial muscles. Instruct patient to taste and to identify substance used. He should rinse his mouth well between each drop of solution. This is a test for the anterior ⅔ of tongue.
8. Acoustic	Tuning fork	Tests for hearing, air and bone conduction.
9. Glossopharyngeal	Cotton applicator stick	Test posterior ⅓ of tongue for taste and also check for gag reflex.
10. Vagus	Tongue depressor	Checking voice sounds, observing symmetry of soft palate will give suggestion of function of vagus.
11. Spinal Accessory		Since this innervates the sternocleidomastoid and the trapezius muscles, the patient will be instructed to turn and to move his head and to elevate shoulders with and without resistance.
12. Hypoglossal		Observe tongue movements.

GUIDELINES: Assisting the Patient Undergoing a Lumbar Puncture

Lumbar Puncture   Insertion of a needle into lumbar subarachnoid space and withdrawal of cerebrospinal fluid for diagnostic and therapeutic purposes.

Purposes
1. To obtain cerebrospinal fluid for examination (microbiologic, serologic, cytologic, or chemical analysis).*
2. To measure and relieve cerebrospinal pressure.
3. To determine the presence or absence of blood in the spinal fluid.
4. To detect spinal subarachnoid block.
5. To administer antibiotics intrathecally in certain cases of infection.
6. To administer anticancer drugs.

Equipment   Sterile lumbar puncture set   Skin antiseptic
Sterile gloves   Band-Aid
Xylocaine 1–2%

* See Appendix for characteristics of normal cerebrospinal fluid.

Procedure

NURSING ACTION	RATIONALE/AMPLIFICATION

Preparatory Phase

1. Give a step-by-step résumé of the procedure.

For Lying Position: (Fig. 17-1)

2. Position the patient on his side with a pillow under his head and a pillow between his legs. He should be lying on a firm surface.

3. Instruct the patient to arch the lumbar segment of his back and draw his knees up to his abdomen, clasping his knees with his hands.

4. Assist the patient in maintaining this position by supporting him behind the knees and neck. Assist the patient to maintain the posture throughout the examination.

For Sitting Position:

5. Have the patient straddle a straight-back chair (facing the back) and rest his head against his arms, which are folded on the back of the chair.

Performance Phase *(by the physician)*

1. The skin is prepared with antiseptic solution and the skin and subcutaneous spaces are infiltrated with local anesthetic agent.

1. Reassures patient and gains his cooperation.

2. The spine is maintained in a horizontal position. The pillow between the legs prevents the upper leg from rolling forward.

3. This posture offers maximal widening of the interspinous spaces and affords easier entry into the subarachnoid space.

4. Supporting the patient helps prevent sudden movements which can produce a traumatic (bloody) tap and thus impede correct diagnosis.

5. In obese patients and those who have difficulty in assuming an arched side-lying position, this posture may allow more accurate identification of the spinous processes and interspaces.

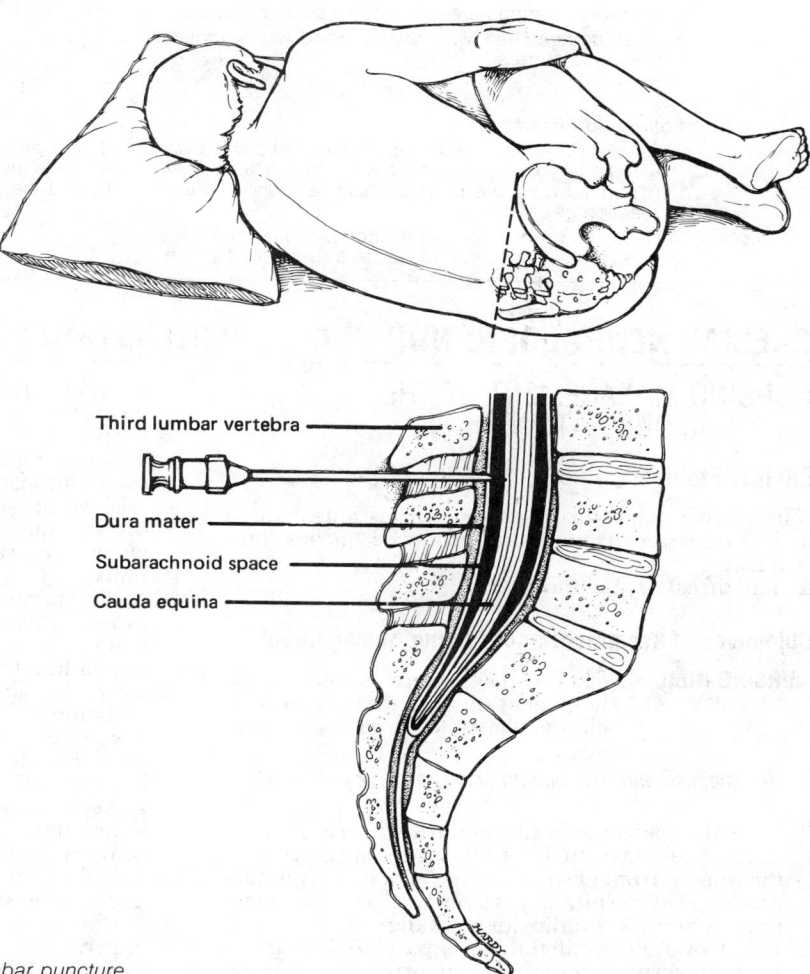

Third lumbar vertebra

Dura mater

Subarachnoid space

Cauda equina

FIGURE 17-1. *Technique of lumbar puncture.*

GUIDELINES: Assisting the Patient Undergoing a Lumbar Puncture (cont.)

Procedure (cont.)

NURSING ACTION	RATIONALE/AMPLIFICATION
2. A spinal puncture needle is introduced between L3–L4 interspace. The needle is advanced until the "give" of the ligamentum flavum is felt and the needle enters the subarachnoid space. The manometer is attached to the spinal puncture needle.	2. L3–L4 interspace is *below* the level of the spinal cord.
3. After the needle enters the subarachnoid space, help the patient to slowly straighten his legs.	3. This maneuver prevents a false increase in intraspinal pressure. Muscle tension and compression of the abdomen give falsely high pressures.
4. Instruct the patient to breathe quietly (not to hold his breath or strain) and not to talk.	4. Hyperventilation may lower a truly elevated pressure. Talking can elevate CSF pressure.
5. The initial pressure reading is obtained by measuring the level of the fluid column after it comes to rest.	5. With respiration there is normally some fluctuation of spinal fluid in the manometer. Normal range of spinal fluid pressure with patient in the lateral position is 70–180 mm. H_2O.
6. About 2–3 ml. of spinal fluid is placed in each of 3 test tubes for observation, comparison, and laboratory analysis.	6. Spinal fluid should be clear and colorless. Bloody spinal fluid may indicate cerebral contusion, laceration, subarachnoid hemorrhage, or a traumatic tap.
Lumbar Manometric Test (Queckenstedt Test) 1. A blood pressure cuff is placed around the patient's neck and inflated to a pressure of 20 mm. Hg (or an assistant compresses jugular vein or veins for 10 seconds). 2. Pressure readings are made at 10-second intervals. 3. After the needle is withdrawn, a Band-Aid is applied to the puncture site.	This test is made when a spinal subarachnoid block is suspected (tumor; vertebral fracture or dislocation). In normal persons there is a rapid rise in pressure of cerebrospinal fluid in response to jugular compression with rapid return to normal when the compression is released. If the pressure fails to rise or rises and falls slowly, there is evidence of a block due to a lesion's compressing the spinal subarachnoid pathways. This test is not done if an intracranial lesion is suspected.
Follow-up Phase 1. Record (a) procedure, (b) appearance of spinal fluid, (c) whether or not specimens were sent to laboratory, (d) spinal pressure readings and (e) condition and reaction of patient. 2. Keep the patient horizontal (prone, supine, or on his side) for 6–12 hours. Encourage a liberal fluid intake.	Some patients suffer from post-puncture headache which is thought to be caused by the leakage of spinal fluid at the puncture site.

SPECIAL NEUROLOGIC NURSING CONSIDERATIONS

NURSING MANAGEMENT OF THE UNCONSCIOUS PATIENT

Clinical Problems

There are 2 major threats to the unconscious patient:
1. The disease or trauma that produced unconsciousness.
2. The threat of the unconscious state.

Objectives of Treatment and Nursing Management

NURSING GOAL: to assume the protective reflexes for the patient until he is aware of himself and can function in his environment.

A. *To establish and maintain an adequate airway* (Fig. 17-2).
1. Place the patient in a three-fourths prone or semi-prone position with his face dependent—prevents the tongue from obstructing the airway, encourages drainage of respiratory secretions, and promotes oxygen and carbon dioxide exchange.
2. Insert oral airway if tongue is paralyzed or is obstructing airway—an obstructed airway increases intracranial pressure. This is considered a short term measure.
3. Prepare for insertion of cuffed endotracheal tube if patient's condition requires (see p. 186)—endotracheal intubation is more effective in permitting positive pressure ventilation. The cuffed tube seals off the digestive tract, preventing aspiration and allowing efficient removal of tracheobronchial secretions.
4. Utilize humidified oxygen therapy, positive pressure assisted breathing techniques, or mechanical ventilation with a ventilator when there is indication of impending respiratory failure (see p. 169).
5. Keep the airway free of secretions with efficient suctioning—in the absence of the cough and swallowing reflexes, secretions rapidly accumulate in the posterior pharynx and upper trachea and can pave the way to fatal respiratory complications.
   a. Keep one end of Y-tube open while inserting the catheter.
   b. When catheter is at desired level close the open end of Y with finger.
   c. Turn the suction on and slowly withdraw catheter with a twisting motion of the thumb and forefinger.
   d. See p. 192 for tracheal suctioning.

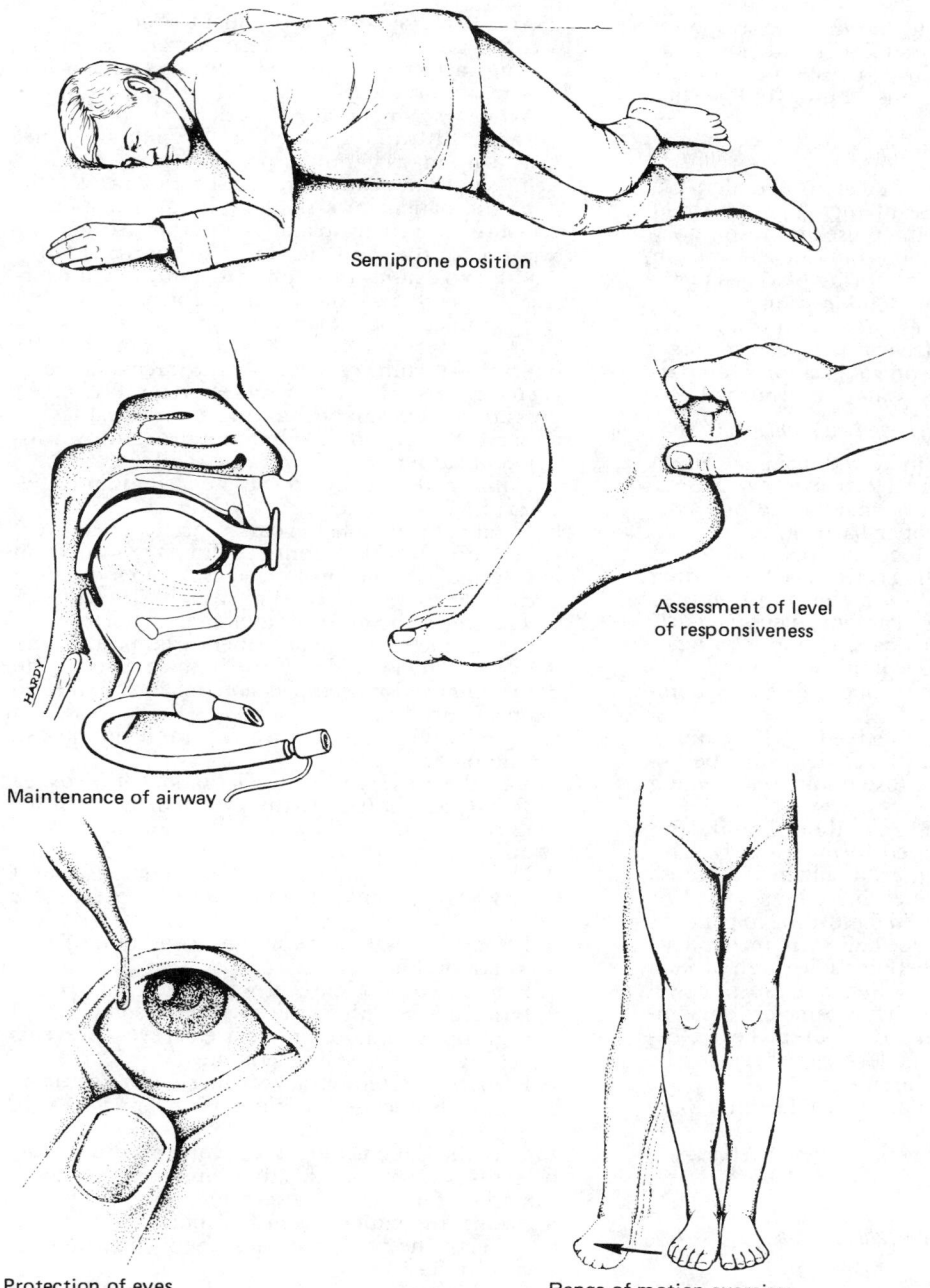

Semiprone position

Maintenance of airway

Assessment of level of responsiveness

Protection of eyes

Range of motion exercises

FIGURE 17-2 *Nursing priorities in the care of the unconscious patient.*

6. Carry out periodic determinations of arterial PO_2 and PCO_2 to determine adequacy of treatment.
7. Prepare for tracheostomy if coma is deepening and there are evidences of inadequate respiratory exchange. (See pp. 188–192 for nursing management of patient with tracheostomy.)
8. Maintain circulation.

B. *To assess the level of responsiveness.*

1. Carry out neurologic examination.

2. Maintain a constant assessment of the patient's level of consciousness and changes in responsiveness—the level of consciousness is the most important measure of the patient's condition. Unconscious patients may deteriorate rapidly from numerous clinical causes.
3. Record the patient's *exact reactions*, eye opening, verbal response, movements, and quality of speech.
   a. Request the patient to speak.
   b. Ask the patient to perform some activity (raise arm, extend tongue, etc.).

c. Apply painful stimuli if there is no response (pinching skin of arms or thighs) and assess patient's perception of pain. No response or a delayed or unequal response is an unfavorable clinical sign.

C. *To evaluate the progression of vital signs.*

1. Know the patient's baseline vital signs and alert the physician if there are significant fluctuations of blood pressure and instability of the pulse and respiratory cycle—fluctuations of vital signs indicate a change in intracranial homeostasis; monitoring of vital signs is also essential to alert for hidden bleeding.
2. Take blood pressure readings, pulse and respiratory rates and temperature at frequently specified intervals until there is evidence of stabilization—temperature-regulating mechanisms may be disturbed.

D. *To maintain fluid and electrolyte and nutritional balance.*

1. Give intravenous fluids as indicated, using a vein in the hand—serial laboratory electrolyte evaluations are made when the patient is maintained on intravenous fluids to ensure proper balance.
2. Or use hyperalimentation feedings, page 406.
3. Or initiate nasogastric feedings (see p. 404)—feeding through a gastric tube ensures better nutrition than does intravenous feeding. Paralytic ileus is fairly frequent in the unconscious patient, and a nasogastric tube assists in gastric decompression.
   a. Insert small gastric tube through nose into stomach.
   b. Aspirate stomach before each feeding. If aspirated residual exceeds 50 ml., the patient may be developing an ileus. Gastric distention and vomiting may result.
   c. Elevate patient's head and thorax and give 100–150 ml. of blenderized formula slowly. Give small amount at first and gradually increase until 400–500 ml. are given at each feeding.
   d. Give 2000–2500 ml. of fluid (according to patient's condition) through the tube daily. An unconscious patient requires adequate fluids since high protein feedings can produce a solute diuresis that will produce dehydration and hyperosmolar coma unless adequate fluid intake is ensured. Fever, excessive sweating, or fluid loss elsewhere in the body increases fluid requirements.
   e. Rinse the tube with water after each feeding. Keep tube feeding refrigerated.
   f. Prepare for gastrostomy if patient's condition indicates.
   g. Measure urinary output.

E. *To give nursing support as the patient's changing condition indicates.*

1. Be aware of the varying phases of restlessness—a certain degree of restlessness may be favorable, since it may indicate the patient is regaining consciousness. However, restlessness is quite common in cerebral anoxia or when there is a partially obstructed airway, distended bladder, overlooked bleeding, or fracture; it may be a manifestation of brain injury.
   a. Have adequate lighting in the room to prevent hallucinations as the patient regains consciousness.
   b. Pad side rails, apply mitts or boxing gloves on hands, or use other devices to protect patient.
   c. Avoid oversedating the patient—Sedatives/narcotics depress level of responsiveness; certain drugs affect pupillary size and reaction, which is an important sign.
   d. Avoid restraints if at all possible.
   e. Speak softly to the patient, calling him by name.
   f. Touch him as gently as possible.
2. Keep the skin clean, dry, and free of pressure—comatose patients are susceptible to formation of pressure sores. Clip patient's nails to prevent excoriation of the skin. (See p. 64 for prevention.)
3. Put all extremities through range of motion exercises 4 times daily—contracture deformities develop early in unconscious patients.
4. Turn the patient from side to side at regular intervals—turning relieves pressure areas and helps keep lungs clear by mobilizing secretions. Prolonged pressure on extremities produces nerve palsies.
5. Observe the patient for indication of an overdistended bladder.
   a. Utilize external sheath catheter (condom catheter) for male patient.
   b. If patient is unable to void, insert 3-way indwelling catheter with continuous drainage—infection invariably follows prolonged use of an indwelling catheter that is attached to straight drainage.
   c. Tape the catheter on the abdomen or horizontally to the side of the male patient (see p. 484) and to the inner thigh of the female patient—to prevent urethral compression (male) and traction on the urethra.
6. Carry out oral care (water, ice chips, and mouthwash solution).
7. Protect the eyes from corneal irritation—the cornea functions as a shield. If the eyes remain open for long periods, corneal drying, irritation, and ulceration are apt to result.
   a. Make sure patient's eye is not rubbing against bedding if blinking and corneal reflexes are absent.
   b. Inspect the size of pupils and condition of eyes with a flashlight.
   c. Remove contact lenses if worn. (See page 673.)
   d. Irrigate eyes with sterile prescribed solution and instill ophthalmic ointment in each eye—prevents glazing and corneal ulceration.
   e. Prepare for temporary tarsorrhaphy (suturing of eyelids in closed position) if unconscious state is prolonged.
8. Protect the patient during convulsive seizures (see below)—patient with head trauma is a potential candidate for convulsive seizures.
   a. Protect the patient from self-injury.
   b. Observe the patient during the seizure and record observations.
   c. Give prescribed anticonvulsant medications through the nasogastric tube.
9. Be alert for the development of complications.
   a. Respiratory complications (infections, aspiration, obstruction, atelectasis)
   b. Fluid and electrolyte imbalance
   c. Infection (urinary, pressure sores, central nervous system)
   d. Bladder and gastrointestinal distention
   e. Convulsive seizures
10. Be aware that the patient will feel uneasy concerning his period of unconsciousness when he gains awareness of what has happened.

a. Give an explanation of what has happened during period of unconsciousness.
b. Permit patient to ask questions and talk about the experience of unconsciousness.

NURSING MANAGEMENT OF THE PATIENT WITH INCREASING INTRACRANIAL PRESSURE

Intracranial pressure is the pressure within the ventriculosubarachnoid space.

Causes

Head injury/hematoma
Cerebral edema; cerebrovascular accident
Abscess, infection
Hemorrhage
Brain tumor
Cranial surgery

NURSING ALERT: As intracranial pressure increases, the brain substance is compressed. A sudden increase may produce an emergency situation in a few minutes. This condition may lead rapidly to death or result in a vegetative existence for the patient.

Clinical Manifestations

1. Change in level of responsiveness (consciousness)
   a. *The level of responsiveness is the most important measure of the patient's condition.*
   b. Look for lethargy, delay in response to verbal suggestions, slowing of speech.
   c. Watch for sudden changes in condition—quietness to restlessness, orientation to confusion, increasing drowsiness, stupor, coma.
   d. *Progressive deterioration is a serious sign* that may require immediate surgical intervention.
2. Subtle changes—restlessness, headache, forced breathing, purposeless movements, and mental cloudiness.
3. Changes in vital signs
   a. Pulse changes—slowing rate to 60 or below; increasing rate to 100 or above.
   b. Respiratory irregularities; slowing of rate with lengthening periods of apnea; Cheyne-Stokes or Kussmaul breathing.
   c. Rising blood pressure or widening pulse pressure (the difference between systolic and diastolic blood pressure).
   d. Moderately elevated temperature.
4. Headache—constant, increasing in intensity; aggravated by movement/straining.
5. Vomiting—recurrent; may be projectile.
6. Papilledema.
7. Pupillary changes—increasing pressure or an expanding clot can displace the brain against the oculomotor or optic nerve, producing pupillary changes.
   a. Inspect the pupils with a flashlight to evaluate size, configuration, and reaction to light. Compare both eyes for similarities/differences.

b. Evaluate gaze to determine if it is conjugate (paired, working together) or if eye movements are abnormal.
c. Evaluate ability of eyes to abduct and adduct.
d. Inspect the retina and optic nerve for hemorrhage and papilledema.

Treatment and Nursing Management

OBJECTIVE: to reduce intracranial pressure rapidly to prevent irreversible brain damage.
1. Provide *continuing* assessment of patient's level of responsiveness.
   a. Response to commands:
      (1) Answers questions readily and correctly
      (2) Can perform a complex maneuver
      (3) Responds to simple command
      (4) Gives delayed or unequal response
      (5) Reacts only to loud voice
      (6) Does not respond
   b. Assessment of spinal motor reflexes (pinch Achilles tendon, arm, or other body site):
      (1) Prompt, purposeful withdrawal
      (2) Sluggish or nonpurposeful movement of extremities
      (3) Facial grimace
      (4) Involuntary voiding
      (5) No response
   c. Observation of patient's spontaneous activity:
      (1) Verbal or other communication
      (2) Changes in posture (frequency)
      (3) Breathing pattern
      (4) Retching, vomiting
      (5) Restlessness, twitching, tremors, convulsions
2. Keep a Neurologic Observation Record (see Table 17-1, p. 710).
   Purpose: To provide a continuing assessment of the patient so that a *change* in condition can be noted immediately. All observations should be compared with and evaluated according to the *baseline* (initial) condition of the patient.
   a. Know the patient's baseline condition.
   b. Carry out *repeated* nursing assessments—to determine clinical improvement or deterioration.
   c. The Glasgow Coma Scale (Fig. 17-3), developed at the University of Glasgow, is a tool for describing objectively the patient's level of responsiveness/consciousness.
3. Use intracranial pressure monitoring system when available (p. 710).
   a. Catheter is inserted into lateral ventricle, or a subarachnoid screw is inserted into dome of skull and attached to pressure transducer; recordings are then made.
   b. Sustained elevations of ICP over 20 mm. Hg should be investigated promptly.
   c. A change in the position of the head (e.g., flattening of bed to give care), endotracheal aspiration, hyperventilation, or compression of jugular veins (head falling to one side) may markedly increase intracranial pressure.
4. Administer pharmacologic agents as prescribed to reduce intracranial pressure.
   a. Hyperosmotic agents (mannitol, urea, glycerol solution)—lower cerebrospinal fluid pressure by reducing the volume of intracranial contents and rate of cerebrospinal fluid formation. Insert indwelling catheter, since hyperosmolar solutions cause diuresis.

TABLE 17-1. NEUROLOGIC ASSESSMENT RECORD*

	Time 7/14 9:30 am	10:00 am		
Spontaneous behavior	Quiet; lies in bed; little activity; complains of headache	No spontaneous activity		
Level of responsiveness to stimulation	Drowsy; can be aroused Responds to voice	Less response; more difficult to arouse but does respond to deep pain (Supra-orbital pressure)		
Orientation (time/place)	Oriented to place, knows year but not day or month			
Movements: Rt. and left arm Rt. and left leg	Moves all 4 extremities left less than right	Moves right side in response to pain; left side gives decerebrate response		
Pupil size (draw) Rt. Left reaction	Rt. ◯ Left ◦ Rt. reacts sluggishly to light	Rt. ◯ Left ◦ Fixed Slight reaction		
Speech Clear Rambling Incoherent Aphasic	Slightly slurred	No speech		
Vital Signs — Blood pressure	150/160	200/60		
Pulse	60	48		
Respirations	18	12		
Temperature	37°C (98.6°)	37°C		

* Based on following patient study: Mr. Elliott Smith, a 36-year-old computer-programmer, sought the services of an ophthalmologist because he had been having generalized headaches for a period of "several months." Moderate papilledema and a left hemianopia field defect (loss of vision in one-half of the visual field of one or both eyes) was noted upon examination. He was admitted immediately to the hospital with a possible brain tumor and increasing intracranial pressure. These nursing observations were part of a continuing assessment record and were made 36 hours after admission.

  b. Steroids (dexamethasone).
  c. Barbiturates—reduce ICP; reduce brain metabolism and systemic blood pressure.
5. Monitor patient's temperature.
  a. Avoid elevation of temperature, since fever increases cerebral metabolism and the rate of cerebral edema formation.
  b. Monitor cardiac output with Swan-Ganz catheter if measures are taken to reduce patient's temperature.
6. Employ passive hyperventilation with volume ventilator when necessary—hyperventilation leads to respiratory alkalosis, which causes cerebral vasoconstriction, decreased cerebral blood volume, and lowered intracranial pressure.
7. Avoid certain positions and activities that produce a rise in intracranial pressure. Avoid the prone position, flexion of the neck, extreme hip flexion, the Valsalva maneuver, isometric muscle contractions, coughing, and straining.
8. Prepare for surgical intervention if patient's condition deteriorates.

CONTINUOUS INTRACRANIAL PRESSURE MONITORING

Intracranial pressure monitoring is the recording of the pressure exerted within the skull by the brain, cerebral blood, and cerebrospinal fluid.

Purpose

1. To provide immediate information for early detection and treatment of intracranial pressure.
2. To guide therapy for control of intracranial pressure.
3. To have access to cerebrospinal fluid for sampling and drainage.

Underlying Principles

1. Intracranial pressure is not in a steady state, but fluctuates; fluctuations are indicated by waves of high pressure and troughs of relatively normal pressure. These waves have been classified as A waves (plateau waves), B waves, and C waves.
2. The plateau (A) waves have clinical significance:

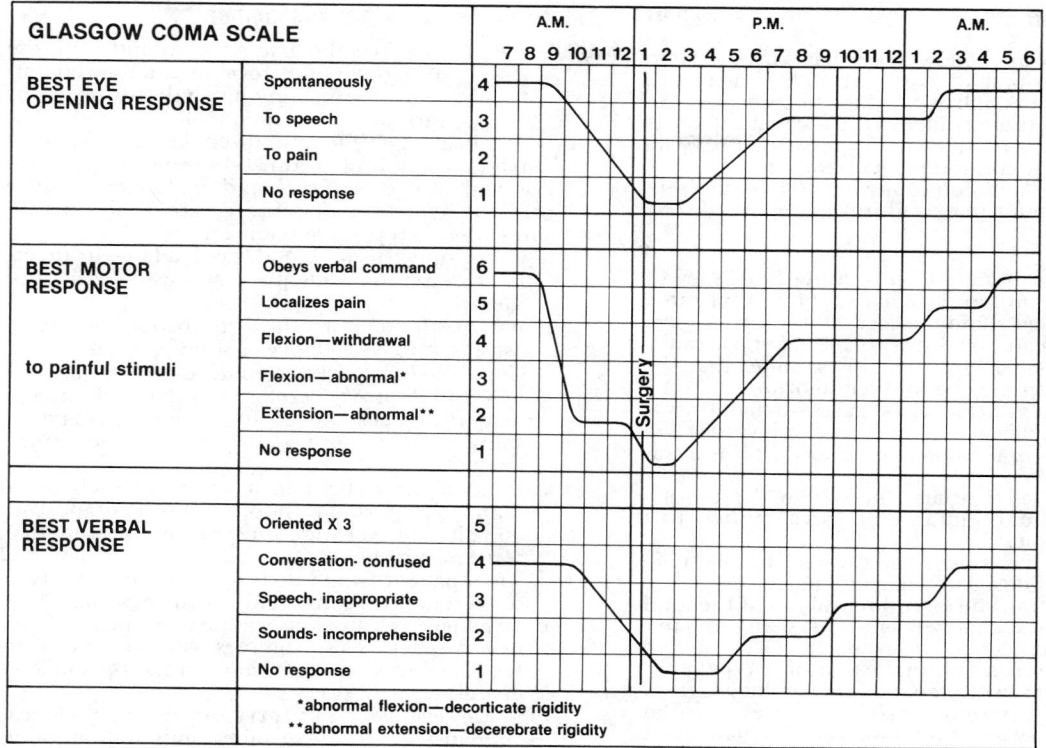

FIGURE 17-3. *Glasgow Coma Scale. How to Score Responses of the Glasgow Coma.*
Scoring of Eye Opening; **4** = *if the patient opens his eyes spontaneously when the nurse approaches;* **3** = *if the patient opens his eyes in response to speech (spoken or shouted);* **2** = *if the patient opens his eyes only in response to painful stimuli such as digital squeezing around nail beds of fingers;* **1** = *if the patient does not open his eyes in response to painful stimuli.*
Scoring of Best Motor Response: **6** = *if the patient can obey a simple command such as "Lift your left hand off the bed.";* **5** = *if the patient moves a limb to locate the painful stimuli applied to the head or trunk and attempts to remove the source;* **4** = *if the patient attempts to withdraw from the source of pain;* **3** = *if the patient flexes only his arms at the elbows and wrist in response to painful stimuli to the nail beds (decorticate rigidity);* **2** = *if the patient extends his arms (straightens his elbows) in response to painful stimuli (decerebrate rigidity);* **1** = *if the patient has no motor response to pain on any limb.*
Scoring of Best Verbal Response: **5** = *if the patient is oriented to time, place, and person;* **4** = *if the patient is able to converse although not oriented to time, place, or person (e.g., "Where am I?");* **3** = *if the patient speaks only in words or phrases that make little or no sense (e.g., "B—H,N—K.");* **2** = *if the patient responds with incomprehensible sounds such as groans;* **1** = *if the patient does not respond verbally at all.*
From Hickey J: The Clinical Practice of Neurological and Neurosurgical Nursing. Philadelphia, JB Lippincott, 1981

a. They are characterized by rapid increases and decreases of pressure with recurring elevations of intracranial pressure that may last from 5 to 20 minutes and range in amplitude between 50–100 mm. Hg.
b. Plateau waves are usually related to cerebral dysfunction and caused by brain shift or distortion.
c. They may be accompanied by transient symptoms—headache, nausea, disturbances of consciousness.
3. B waves are of shorter duration (½–2 minutes) with smaller amplitude (up to 50 mm. Hg). They have less clinical significance and appear to be related to Cheyne-Stokes respiration.
4. C waves are small rhythmic oscillations with frequencies of approximately 6 per minute at amplitudes up to 20 mm. Hg. They appear to be related to rhythmic variations of the systemic arterial blood pressure (Traube-Hering-Mayer waves).

Techniques for Measuring Intracranial Pressure*

1. *Intraventricular catheter*—placement of a catheter into the frontal horn of the lateral ventricle via a burr hole or twist drill hole; the intraventricular catheter is connected to an external pressure transducer by means of tubing filled with normal saline. The output

* The direct measurement of intracranial pressure may be accomplished by a number of monitoring techniques that require complex sensors, transducers, recording devices, etc. The nurse needs a working knowledge of the system being used and its limitations.

from the pressure transducer is displayed on a chart recorder.

2. *Subarachnoid screw*—hollow screw that is inserted into the calvarium (dome of skull) through a small twist drill hole in the skull; it is attached to a pressure transducer via tubing filled with normal saline. A numerical pressure value and a pressure wave form are recorded for continuous monitoring.

3. *Extradural*—implantation of miniature pressure sensor and transmitter in extradural space.

Nursing Management

1. Watch for developing and increasing frequency of plateau waves; no more than 25% of readings in a 30-minute period should exceed 30 mm. Hg.
   Start immediate measures to reduce intracranial pressure (page 709), since this signifies that the brain function may be in disequilibrium.

2. Monitor patient's arterial blood gases—a high $PaCO_2$ will cause vasodilation of the cerebral vessels, an increase in cerebral blood flow, and a rise in intracranial pressure.

3. Keep connections tight and the system closed—any leakage of the fluid column produces a gradual drift from the baseline.
   a. Recalibrate the system according to manufacturer's directions at regular intervals.
   b. Realign the transducer and recalibrate if the level of the bed is changed—most systems require careful referencing of transducers.

4. Avoid excessive rotation or flexion of the patient's head—interferes with the outflow of blood from cranial cavity; temporary occlusion causes a rise in intracranial pressure. Avoid the Valsalva maneuver.

5. Support the patient physically and emotionally—some monitoring systems limit patient mobility.
   a. Monitor site for infection—redness, swelling, leakage.
   b. Change dressing as prescribed.

6. Watch for complications—infection, blocked catheter, equipment malfunction.

NURSING MANAGEMENT OF THE PATIENT WITH A HEAD INJURY

Clinical Manifestations

Unconsciousness or disturbance in consciousness
Headache
Vertigo
Confusion or delirium
Restlessness
Changes in body temperature
Respiratory irregularities
Pupillary abnormalities

Immediate Management in the Emergency Department

See page 880.

NURSING ALERT: Regard every patient who has a head injury as having a potential spinal cord injury. A significant number of patients are under the influence of alcohol at the time of injury, which may mask the nature and severity of the injury.

Treatment and Nursing Management*

OBJECTIVE: to observe the patient constantly for the development of focal or generalized deficits of function that indicate need for surgical intervention.

1. Maintain an open airway and ventilation and ensure maximum respiratory function—oxygen deprivation and an excess of carbon dioxide may produce cerebral hypoxia and cause cerebral edema with subsequent irreparable damage.
   a. Carry out arterial blood gas studies—to determine respiratory adequacy and assess effects of therapy.
   b. Prepare for endotracheal intubation or tracheostomy and ventilatory assistance if indicated. Controlled hyperventilation increases arterial PO_2 and improves cerebral oxygenation. Manipulation of neck during intubation can damage spinal cord if there is associated cervical spine injury.
   c. Position the patient in a lateral recumbent or semiprone position—improves oxygen and carbon dioxide exchange and prevents aspiration of secretions or blood.
   d. Turn patient from side to side—to prevent stasis of secretions in lungs and pressure on skin.
   e. If patient is conscious, elevate the head of the bed 30 degrees—promotes venous return to head, reduces jugular venous pressure, and lowers intracranial pressure.

2. Observe, evaluate, and carry out repeated clinical examinations to determine minute-to-minute, hour-to-hour changes in patient's status—pathologic events occurring as a result of head injury include (1) intracranial hemorrhage (extradural, subdural, intracerebral), which causes elevation of intracranial pressure, (2) edema, and (3) sepsis.

NURSING ALERT: A change in the level of responsiveness is the most sensitive indicator of improvement or deterioration. The level of responsiveness may change from minute to minute.

   a. Make specific documentation of clinical findings including state of responsiveness (consciousness), quality of breathing, changes in respiratory rate and pattern, size and reaction of pupils, motor responses. (See Neurologic Flow Record, p. 710).
   b. Start intracranial pressure (ICP) monitoring for patients with severe injuries, especially those with no eye opening, no verbal response, and nonpurposeful motor responses.
   c. See p. 709, The Patient with Increasing Intracranial Pressure.

3. Obtain computed tomography (CT) scan or angiogram as directed—to determine intracranial pathology.

4. Give fluids and electrolytes in physiologic proportions—to ensure fluid balance and an adequate urinary output.

* See also nursing management of the unconscious patient, p. 706.

a. Do not give fluids by mouth to an unconscious patient.

b. Weigh daily and keep records of intake and output and urinary specific gravity—to determine fluid loss and dehydration and to monitor for development of diabetes insipidus (especially in patients with hypothalamic involvement, craniofacial trauma, basilar skull fracture).

c. Give intravenous solutions fairly slowly—overhydration may lead to cerebral edema.

d. Restrict fluid intake in patients with severe cerebral contusion—to avoid increase in volume of extracellular space.

e. Carry out serial blood and urine electrolyte and osmolality studies—head injuries may be accompanied by disorders of sodium regulation, water retention, and decreased serum potassium levels; assess for apathy, headache, anorexia, nausea, vomiting, and in some instances, coma and convulsions.

f. Give nasogastric feedings (or gastrostomy feedings) if patient is unable to swallow after several days, to maintain homeostasis.

g. Insert indwelling catheter if patient is unconscious—for assessment of urinary volume and to prevent restlessness from distended bladder.

5. Use intensive therapy to keep intracranial pressure at acceptable level.

a. Osmotherapy (mannitol)—to dehydrate brain and reduce cerebral edema.

b. Steroids (dexamethasone)—to reduce brain edema; (controversial) may have *rebound effect.* Give antacid solution through nasogastric tube—gastrointestinal hemorrhage is a common complication in head-injured patients on high doses of steroids.

c. Barbiturates (pentobarbital)—to reduce cerebral metabolism and lower ICP.

d. Muscle relaxants—to prevent coughing and straining while on ventilator, which raises ICP.

e. Hyperventilation—increases arterial PO$_2$ and potentially improves cerebral oxygenation.

6. Control rising temperature with hypothermia blanket, fever sponges—to lower metabolic requirements of the brain.

7. Observe orifices for leakage of spinal fluid through the nose (rhinorrhea) or through the ear (otorrhea)—serious complication of head injury which carries risk of meningitis.

NURSING ALERT: Cerebrospinal fluid leakage may mask the usual clinical signs of an expanding intracranial hematoma without evidence of increased intracranial pressure, changes in vital signs, or alternations in state of consciousness.

a. Tape sterile cotton pad under nose or loosely against ear to collect drainage.

b. Elevate head of bed approximately 20–30 degrees as directed—to reduce intracranial pressure and promote spontaneous closure of leak. (Some neurosurgeons prefer that the bed be kept flat.)

c. Discourage patient from blowing nose, sneezing or straining.

d. Persistence of spinal fluid otorrhea or rhinorrhea usually requires surgical intervention.

8. Treat for shock—from associated injuries of chest, abdomen, pelvis, fractures.

a. Give IV fluids, plasma, or dextran until transfusions can be started.

b. Hourly urinary volume measurements (per indwelling catheter) indicate adequacy of organ perfusion.

9. Support the patient during episodes of restlessness.

a. Avoid restraints if at all possible; straining increases intracranial pressure.

b. Give small doses of chloral hydrate, paraldehyde, or tranquilizing drugs; do not give narcotics and sedatives since these mask the level of responsiveness.

c. Maintain as quiet an environment as possible.

d. Be aware that restlessness may be caused by extradural hematoma, cerebral hypoxia, respiratory obstruction, pain from fractured extremities, tight cast or bandages, or distended bladder.

10. Give phenytoin (Dilantin) or phenobarbital as requested—for control of seizures.

11. Protect the eyes from corneal irritation.

12. Watch for gastrointestinal complications—gastric acid hypersecretion is common in patients with head injuries and may result in ulceration and hemorrhage of stomach and upper intestinal tract (Cushing's ulcer—a potentially perforating ulcer of stomach or duodenum).

13. Carry out rehabilitation techniques.

a. Position the patient correctly to prevent contractures.

b. Put all extremities through range of motion exercises.

c. Begin a program of graded exercises—exercise restores fitness and flagging motivation and assists in elevating the patient's mood to one of optimism.

d. Keep the skin dry, clean, and free of pressure—to prevent pressure sores.

e. Gradually increase physical and mental activity (including resumption of increasingly difficult mental tasks).

14. Be aware of aftereffects of head injury—usually directly related to the severity of the injury.

a. Post-traumatic syndrome
   (1) Headache
   (2) Dizziness and vertigo
   (3) Emotional instability or irritability, inability to concentrate, impaired memory

b. Brain damage

c. Post-traumatic epilepsy

d. Post-traumatic hydrocephalus

e. Post-traumatic neuroses and psychoses

Discharge Planning and Health Education

1. Encourage patient to continue his rehabilitation program following discharge; improvement in status may continue up to 3 or more years following injury.

2. Lessening of headache may be the most reliable guide to recovery; use a second pillow/backrest at night.

3. Encourage patient to return gradually to usual activities.

4. Family may need help in setting limits for injured patient's impulses (anger, emotional lability, etc.) and in realistically evaluating his capabilities. Family may

have difficulty in understanding and accepting alterations in patient's behavior.

5. If patient is discharged from hospital in a relatively short time, tell the family to bring him to the Emergency Department *immediately* if the following signs occur: difficulty in awakening, difficulty in speaking, confusion, severe headache, vomiting, development of unequal pupils, or weakness of one side of body.

GUIDELINES: Administering a Fever Sponge

Fever is an abnormal elevation of body temperature.

A *fever sponge* is the bathing of the body with tepid water (or alcohol and water) for a period of time to reduce fever. It is particularly effective in neurological conditions in which there is a disturbance of the temperature-regulating center. Fever increases both intracranial pressure and the rate of development of cerebral edema.

Causes
1. Infection
2. Disturbance of temperature-regulating center (trauma, central nervous system hemorrhage)
3. Tumors; diseases of blood-forming organs
4. Heat stroke
5. Drug toxicity; allergens
6. Delirium tremens

Purpose To reduce body temperature when fever in itself may be deleterious.

Equipment
Basin of tepid water 21.1–29.1° C. (70–85° F.)
  or
Basin of alcohol (25% saturated with tepid water)
Bath blanket/plastic sheet

Hot water bottle with cover
Ice bag with cover
Towels
7 washcloths or wash mitts

NURSING ALERT: Make certain that the patient is adequately hydrated; unrecognized dehydration can result in decreased circulating blood volume, causing peripheral vasoconstriction which prevents heat loss.

Procedure

NURSING ACTION	RATIONALE/AMPLIFICATION
Preparatory Phase 1. Place plastic sheet under patient and bath blanket over patient. 2. Remove top bedding.	
Performance Phrase 1. Take temperature, pulse, and respiration before starting sponge.	1. This serves as a baseline for determining effectiveness of treatment.
2. Give antipyretic medication as directed 15–20 minutes before starting sponge.	2. There is a more rapid reduction of fever when sponging is combined with administration of antipyretic medication.
a. Aspirin OR	a. Has an anti-inflammatory, antipyretic, or analgesic action.

b. Acetaminophen
   c. Chlorpromazine
	b. Has antipyretic and analgesic action
	   c. Controls shivering

3. Apply ice bag to head.	3. Relieves headache and promotes patient comfort.
4. Apply hot-water bottle to feet.	4. Aids in combating chilliness and shivering.
5. Use the same sequence for sponging as for giving a bed bath.	
6. Place a cold wet compress (washcloth) on neck and in each groin and axilla.	6. The application of cold over superficial large blood vessels aids in lowering body temperature.
7. Expose the body area to be sponged. Place a towel under area.	
8. Using 2 washcloths or mitts alternately, wet in water or alcohol and water solution; pat each area so that solution is uniform over skin surface.	8. Vaporization of water removes heat from the surface of the skin. Alcohol vaporizes at a lower temperature and removes heat from the skin more rapidly. Tepid water and alcohol are highly effective in producing vasodilation and evaporation of heat from skin.
9. If the patient's skin feels cold to the touch, apply skin friction to bring the blood to the surface.	

Procedure (cont.)	NURSING ACTION	RATIONALE/AMPLIFICATION
	10. Bathe each extremity 5 minutes; bathe entire back and buttocks 5–10 minutes; bathe trunk and abdomen 5 minutes.	10. The fever sponge should not exceed 30 minutes.
	11. Allow a fan to blow over the patient while sponging him if fever is high.	11. Increased air movement augments heat loss.
	12. Watch for extreme shivering. Cover the patient and wait a few minutes before proceeding with sponge.	12. Shivering may raise heat production.
	13. Stop sponge if cyanosis, mottling, chilling do not stop when friction (rubbing) is applied to the skin.	13. These symptoms indicate a change in vasomotor tone.

Follow-up Phase

1. Remove bath blanket and plastic sheet. Place a dry gown on patient.
2. Record T.P.R. 30 minutes after sponge is finished.   2. Postsponge temperature indicates whether or not treatment has been effective.

NURSING MANAGEMENT OF THE PATIENT HAVING A SEIZURE

A *seizure* is an involuntary contraction, or a series of contractions, of muscles resulting from abnormal cerebral stimulation.

Nursing Management

OBJECTIVE: to prevent injury to the patient.
1. Observe and record the progression of symptoms during the seizure.
   a. State whether or not the beginning of the attack was observed.
   b. Note the following:
      (1) The first thing the patient does in an attack—where the movements or stiffness starts; position of eyeballs and head
      (2) The type of movements of the part involved
      (3) The parts involved (turn back covers and expose patient)
      (4) Size of both pupils
      (5) Incontinence of urine and feces
      (6) Duration of each phase of the attack
      (7) Unconsciousness, if present, and its duration
      (8) Any obvious paralysis or weakness of arms or legs after the attack
      (9) Inability to speak after the attack
      (10) Whether or not the patient sleeps afterward.
2. Support the patient during the seizure.
   a. Ensure an adequate airway.
      (1) When jaws are clenched in spasm do not attempt to pry open to insert a mouth gag.
      (2) If aura preceded seizure, insert a folded handkerchief between the teeth—to reduce possibility of tongue or cheek being bitten.
      (3) When respiration returns following the seizure and the patient becomes flaccid, turn his head to the side to facilitate drainage of mucus and saliva and prevent aspiration.
      (4) Try to hold the lower jaw forward when the patient is in flaccid stage.
   b. Try to protect the patient from injuring himself.
      (1) Protect his head with a folded blanket/pad to prevent head injury.
      (2) Loosen constrictive clothing.
      (3) Push aside any furniture that the patient may strike during the seizure.
   c. Give the patient privacy and protect him from curious onlookers.
   d. Stay with patient until he is fully conscious.
   e. Reorient him to his environment when he awakens.
   f. Handle the patient with calm persuasion and gentle restraint when seizures are characterized by disturbed behavior.

Family Health Education

Instruct the family as follows:
1. Summon medical assistance if a second seizure follows before consciousness is regained. There is a risk of status epilepticus developing.
2. If the patient has severe postictal (following seizure) excitement, it may be necessary to bring him to the Emergency Department.

NURSING MANAGEMENT OF THE PATIENT UNDERGOING INTRACRANIAL SURGERY

Craniotomy is the surgical opening of the skull to gain access to intracranial structures, remove a tumor, relieve intracranial pressure, evacuate a blood clot, or stop hemorrhage (Fig. 17-4).

Craniectomy is excision of a portion of the skull.

Cranioplasty is repair of a cranial defect by means of a plastic or metal plate.

Treatment and Nursing Management

A. *Preoperative Management*

OBJECTIVE: to determine the precise location of the lesion (clot, tumor, aneurysm).
1. Assist the patient undergoing diagnostic tests and frequent neurologic examinations.
2. Evaluate and record patient's symptoms and signs (paralysis, aphasia) preoperatively in order to make postoperative comparisons.
3. Support the patient with neurologic motor and sensory defects.
   a. Position paralyzed extremities to prevent contracture deformities (see p. 53).
   b. Familiarize the blind patient with his environment.
      (1) Personnel entering room should announce themselves—helps patient understand incoming stimuli.
      (2) Help patient to assume an active role in his care.
   c. Assist the aphasic patient to communicate by means of picture cards, writing materials, gestures, etc.
   d. Protect the confused patient.
      (1) Remove disturbing environmental stimuli.

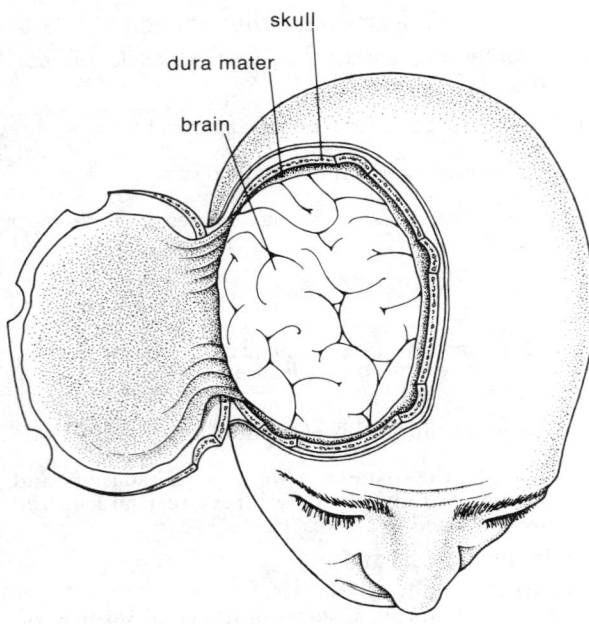

skull

dura mater

brain

FIGURE 17-4. *Craniotomy.*

(2) Keep patient oriented to time and place; place wall calendar and clock where patient can see them.

e. Instruct and encourage the patient and family about the impending surgery—to relieve anxiety and tension.

4. Prepare the patient physically for surgery.
   a. Clip and shampoo the hair with bacteriostatic shampoo; shaving of the area of operation is usually done immediately prior to the surgery. Save the hair.
   b. Report any evidences of scalp infection.
   c. Give enemas only as directed—straining upon defecation raises intracranial pressure.
   d. Give medications and treatments as indicated.
      (1) Steroids—to decrease brain edema.
      (2) Anticonvulsants—to prevent seizures.
      (3) Indwelling spinal catheter connected to a stopcock—to decrease brain edema. Lumbar drainage can be stopped and started as required during procedure.
      (4) Indwelling urethral catheter—to assess urinary volume during dehydrating operative period.
      (5) Parietal burr holes may be made immediately prior to posterior fossa surgery—to facilitate ventricular cannulation if cerebrospinal fluid drainage is necessary.

B. *Postoperative Management*

OBJECTIVES: to watch for life-threatening complications, namely increasing intracranial pressure from edema and bleeding.
to improve the functional status of the patient.

1. Establish proper respiratory exchange—to eliminate systemic hypercarbia and anoxia which increase cerebral edema.
   a. Keep the patient in a lateral or a semiprone position—to facilitate respiratory exchange.

b. Employ tracheopharyngeal aspiration carefully—to remove secretions; suctioning can raise intracranial pressure.
   c. Carry out arterial blood gas studies—to determine respiratory adequacy.
   d. Employ hyperventilation when prescribed—to reduce cerebral blood flow and intracranial pressure.
   e. Elevate the head of the bed 30 cm. (12 inches) after patient is conscious—to aid venous drainage of the brain.
   f. See that the patient has nothing by mouth until an active coughing and swallowing reflex is demonstrated.

2. Assess patient's level of responsiveness.
   a. Response to commands:
      (1) Answers questions readily and correctly
      (2) Can perform a complex maneuver
      (3) Responds to simple command
      (4) Gives delayed or unequal response
      (5) Reacts only to loud voice
      (6) Does not respond
   b. Spinal motor reflexes (pinch Achilles tendon, arm, or other body site):
      (1) Prompt, purposeful withdrawal
      (2) Sluggish or nonpurposeful movement of extremities
      (3) Facial grimace
      (4) Involuntary voiding
      (5) No response
   c. Spontaneous activity:
      (1) Verbal or other communication
      (2) Changes in posture (frequency)
      (3) Breathing pattern
      (4) Retching, vomiting
      (5) Restlessness, twitching, tremors, convulsions
   d. Eye opening (spontaneous, to sound, to pain), reaction of pupils to light.

3. Keep the patient normothermic during the postoperative period—temperature control may be lost in certain neurologic states; a higher temperature increases the metabolic demands of the brain.
   a. Take rectal temperature at specified intervals.
      Extremities may be cold and dry due to paralysis of heat-losing mechanisms (vasodilation and sweating).
   b. Employ measures to reduce excessive fever when present.
      (1) Remove blankets; place loin cloth over patient.
      (2) Give aspirin if indicated. (High fever of central origin is less responsive to aspirin.)
      (3) Apply ice bags to axilla and groin—application of cold over large superficial vessel helps lower body temperature.
      (4) Give tepid water or alcohol sponge (see p. 714).
      (5) Use a fan blowing on patient—to increase surface cooling.
      (6) Use hypothermia blanket.
      (7) Give chlorpromazine (IM)—prevents excessive shivering.
      (8) Utilize ECG monitoring to detect arrhythmias during hypothermia procedures.

4. Evaluate for signs and symptoms of increasing intracranial pressure.
   a. Assess patient (minute by minute, hour by hour) for:
      (1) Diminished response to stimuli
      (2) Fluctuations of vital signs

(3) Restlessness
(4) Weakness and paralysis of extremities
(5) Increasing headache
(6) Changes or disturbances of vision; pupillary changes
b. Control postoperative cerebral edema.
  (1) Give steroids, osmotic dehydrating agents, and glycerol, when prescribed, in post-operative period to reduce brain swelling.
  (2) Keep patient *slightly* underhydrated—to combat cerebral edema.
  (3) Record urinary specific gravity at intervals—especially indicated for surgery of the pituitary and hypothalamus.
  (4) Evaluate electrolyte status:
    (a) Early postoperative weight gain indicates fluid retention; a greater than estimated loss of weight indicates negative water balance.
    (b) Loss of sodium and chlorides will produce weakness, lethargy, and coma.
    (c) Low potassium will cause confusion and lower level of responsiveness.
  (5) Institute hypothermia procedures (see above) to decrease brain metabolism.
  (6) Elevate head of bed 20–30 degrees to reduce intracranial pressure and to facilitate respiration.
5. Perform supportive measures until the patient is able to care for himself.
a. Change position frequently since pain and pressure responses are variable.
b. Give analgesics that do not mask level of responsiveness—codeine, aspirin.
c. Support the patient if convulsive seizures occur (see p. 715).
d. Relieve signs of periocular edema.
  (1) Lubricate eyelids and area around eyes with petrolatum.
  (2) Apply light compresses in pliofilm (taped over eye) at specified intervals.
  (3) Watch for signs of keratitis if cornea has no sensation.
e. Put extremities through range of motion exercises.
f. Use aseptic measures in management of indwelling 3-way urethral catheter (see p. 485).
g. Evaluate and support patient during episodes of restlessness.
  (1) Evaluate for airway obstruction, distended bladder, meningeal irritation from bloody cerebrospinal fluid.

  (2) Pad patient's hands and bed rails—to protect patient from injury.
h. Watch for leakage of cerebrospinal fluid since there is ever present danger of meningitis.
  (1) Differentiate between cerebrospinal fluid (CSF) and mucus.
    (a) Collect fluid on Dextrostix—if CSF is present, indicator will have positive reaction since cerebrospinal fluid contains sugar.
    (b) Assess for moderate elevation of temperature and mild neck rigidity.
  (2) Keep cerebrospinal pressure low.
    (a) Periodic lumbar punctures—to reduce cerebrospinal fluid pressure and decrease its force against the wound.
    (b) Ventricular catheters may be inserted in patient undergoing surgery of posterior fossa (ventriculostomy); catheter(s) connected to a closed reservoir system.
      Patency of the catheter can be noted by the pulsations of the fluid in the tubing.
    (c) Elevate head of bed.
    (d) Give antibiotics as indicated.
i. Reinforce bloodstained dressings with sterile dressing; blood-soaked dressings act as a culture medium for bacteria.
j. Evaluate patient with hypophysectomy (surgery on pituitary) for diabetes insipidus.
  (1) Weigh daily.
  (2) Keep input and output record.
6. Assess for complications.
a. Intracranial hemorrhage. (Postoperative bleeding may be intraventricular, intracerebral, intracerebellar, subdural, or extradural.)
  (1) Watch for progressive impairment of state of responsiveness, signs of increasing intracranial pressure.
  (2) Prepare patient for cerebral angiography; CT scan.
  (3) Prepare patient for reoperation and evacuation of hematoma.
b. Brain edema.
c. Postoperative meningitis.
d. Wound infections (scalp, bone flap)—wound may have to be reopened.
e. Pulmonary complications.
f. Epilepsy.
  (1) Give anticonvulsants on a long-term basis.
  (2) Watch for status epilepticus which may occur after any intracranial operation.
g. Gastrointestinal ulceration (signs and symptoms of hemorrhage and perforation or both).

CRANIAL NERVE INVOLVEMENT

BELL'S PALSY

Bell's palsy (facial paralysis) is due to peripheral involvement of the 7th cranial nerve on one side, producing weakness or paralysis of the facial muscles.

Clinical Manifestations

1. Distortion of face—from paralysis of facial muscles
2. Numbness of face and tongue
3. Eye problems:

a. Epiphora (overflow of tears down the cheek)—from keratitis caused by drying of cornea and lack of blink reflex; laxity of lower eyelid may alter proper drainage of tears.
b. Decreased tear production—may lead to a dry eye which is predisposed to infection.
4. Painful sensations in face, behind ear, and in the eye.
5. Speech difficulties—from facial paralysis.

Clinical Features

1. The etiology of Bell's palsy is unknown. The three theories of possible etiologic causes (and combinations thereof) are vascular ischemia, viral infection, and autoimmune disease.
2. The majority of patients have a viral prodome (upper respiratory infection) 1–3 weeks before onset of symptoms.
3. Bell's palsy can produce grotesque disfigurement with accompanying physical and emotional stress.

Diagnostic Evaluation

1. History of acute onset
2. Tests of cranial nerve function
3. Tests for lacrimation (Schirmer test)—measures the wetting of strip of filter paper placed in lower conjunctival fornix for 5 minutes.
4. Electrodiagnostic study of facial muscles through electromyography—electrodes placed over branches of facial nerve; facial muscles observed for movement

Complications

1. Corneal ulceration; blindness
2. Facial weakness
3. Facial spasm with contracture and synkinesis (unintentional movement)

Treatment and Nursing Management

OBJECTIVES: to maintain muscle tone of the face.
to prevent or minimize denervation.

1. Protect the involved eye—facial paralysis may abolish the blinking reflex; eye is vulnerable to dust and foreign particles.

> **NURSING ALERT:** Keratitis is a major threat to a patient with Bell's palsy.

   a. Protect the cornea with preparation of artificial tears.
   b. Apply tape to upper and lower lid to reduce the amount of ocular exposure.
   c. Use eye ointment at bedtime—helps to keep eyes closed during sleep by sticking the lashes together.
   d. Increase environmental humidity.
   e. Teach patient to close his eye lids frequently with his residually functioning eye musculature or manually.
   f. See that patient wears a protective patch, particularly at night.
      (1) Patch may eventually abrade cornea, as paretic (incompletely paralyzed) eyelids are difficult to keep closed.
      (2) Eyelids may have to be sutured together.
   g. Instruct patient to use protective glasses (wraparound sunglasses or goggles) to decrease normal evaporation from eye.
2. Give steroid therapy (prednisone)—may be helpful in reducing inflammation and edema, which reduces vascular compression and permits restoration of blood circulation in the nerve; early administration appears to diminish severity of disease and mitigate pain.
3. Promote pain relief with aspirin or codeine and by applying heat to involved side of face.
4. Start facial massage (if no nerve tenderness present) as prescribed—to help maintain muscle tone.
5. Prepare for surgical intervention if necessary.
   a. Surgical decompression of facial nerve to decrease edema—may prevent or arrest degeneration.
   b. Surgical procedures to correct eyelid deformities and protect the eye.

Health Education

1. Reassure patient that spontaneous recovery occurs in majority of patients; recovery usually takes place in 3–5 weeks.
2. Reinforce teaching concerning eye care (see above).
3. Keep the face warm and free from drafts.
4. Teach facial exercises—if prescribed—to prevent facial muscle atrophy and to improve strength of remaining innervated muscles. Do the following while looking in a mirror:
   a. Wrinkle forehead
   b. Close eyes
   c. Purse lips
   d. Move mouth from side to side
   e. Blow out cheeks
   f. Whistle

TRIGEMINAL NEURALGIA (TIC DOULOUREUX)

Trigeminal neuralgia (tic douloureux) is a condition of the 5th cranial nerve, characterized by sudden paroxysms of lancinating or burning pain (alternating with periods of complete comfort) in the distribution of one or more branches of the trigeminal nerve.

Etiology

Unknown

Clinical Manifestations

1. Sudden and severe pain appearing without warning—in distribution of one or more branches of trigeminal nerve (Fig. 17-5).
2. Numerous individual flashes of pain, ending abruptly; usually on one side.
3. Attacks predicted by pressure on a trigger point, the terminals of the affected branches. (Movement of the face, talking, chewing, yawning, swallowing, shaving, cold wind, may precipitate an agonizing attack.)

Treatment and Nursing Management

OBJECTIVE: to give pain relief without loss of function.

1. Instruct patient to avoid exposing affected cheek to sudden cold if this is known to trigger the nerve—iced drinks, cold wind, swimming in cold water.
2. Drug Therapy: (antiepileptic drugs)
   a. Carbamazepine (Tegretol) or phenytoin (Dilantin)—relieves and prevents pain in some patients.
   b. Serum levels of drug monitored to avoid drug toxicity.
   c. Observe for evidences of hematologic, hepatic, renal, and skin reactions.
3. Surgical Interruption of Trigeminal System—wide range of surgical procedures used after medical treatment fails to give relief.

OBJECTIVE: to provide optimum pain relief with minimum impairment.

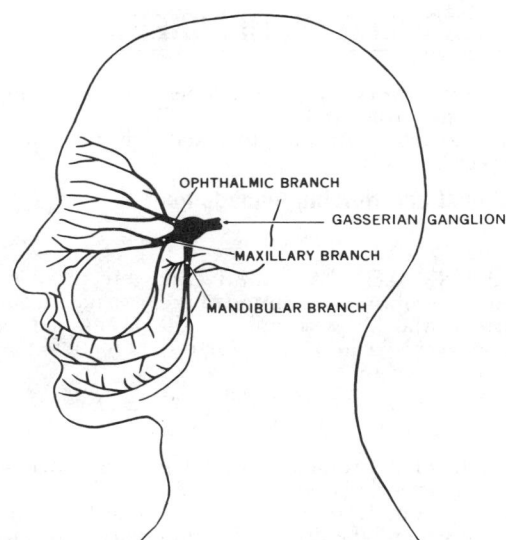

FIGURE 17-5. *The main divisions of the trigeminal nerve are ophthalmic, maxillary, and mandibular. Sensory root fibers arise in the Gasserian ganglion.*

  a. Alcohol injection of ganglion of peripheral branches produces temporary chemical destruction of affected nerves.
    (1) Usually produces complete anesthesia.
    (2) Pain returns after nerve regeneration.

  b. Percutaneous radiofrequency trigeminal gangliolysis (Thermoneurolysis)—introduction of needle electrode through foramen ovale to the desired position of the trigeminal root; low voltage stimulation applied to electrode and a lesion is made. Carefully controlled electrical currents destroy enough of sensory portion of nerve to relieve pain without damaging touch sensation or motor function of face.
    (1) Root selection is made by conscious patient's response to electrical stimulation.
    (2) Permanent relief expected in most patients.
  c. Microvascular decompression of trigeminal nerve—an intracranial approach (retromastoid craniectomy) using an operating microscope to decompress trigeminal nerve; postoperative management is the same as for any intracranial operation. (See page 716.)
  d. Peripheral neurectomy (excision of part of a nerve)
  e. Open surgical retrogasserian rhizotomy (destruction of retrogasserian rootlets)
    (1) Gasserian ganglion lies in the middle fossa and may be reached by a subtemporal, intradural, or extradural route.
    (2) Following operation, patient has a complete loss of sensation in the distribution of the divided nerve fibers.
    (3) See nursing management following craniotomy, p. 716.
    (4) Complications: (burning, stinging, numbness, discomfort in and around eye, herpetic lesions of the face, keratitis, and corneal ulceration).

CEREBROVASCULAR DISEASE

Cerebrovascular disease refers to any functional abnormality of the central nervous system caused by interference with normal blood supply to the brain. The pathology may involve an artery, a vein, or both, when the cerebral circulation becomes impaired as a result of partial or complete occlusion of a blood vessel or hemorrhage resulting from a tear in the vessel wall.

Cerebrovascular Disease from Impairment of Cerebral Circulation

1. *Transient ischemic attacks* (TIA)—transient episodes of cerebral dysfunction commonly manifested by a sudden loss of motor, sensory, or visual function, lasting minutes or up to an hour or more but no longer than 24 hours.
  a. Causes—temporary impairment of blood flow to the brain from atherosclerosis of vessels supplying the brain, or obstruction of cerebral microcirculation by small embolus.
  b. Therapy
    (1) Antiplatelet aggregation drugs (aspirin)—when problem is related to platelet agglutination.
    (2) Anticoagulant therapy (heparin; warfarin).
    (3) Surgical intervention—
      (a) Carotid endarterectomy (p. 720) or
      (b) Extracranial/intracranial bypass grafting—provides revascularization of brain and decreases incidence of further strokes. (See p. 715 for care of patient undergoing intracranial surgery.)
2. *Cerebral thrombosis* (from cerebral arteriosclerosis and slowing of cerebral circulation)—usually produces transient loss of speech, visual disturbance, hemiplegia, or paresthesia in one-half of the body which may precede onset of severe paralysis. (See nursing management of the patient with a stroke.)
3. *Cerebral embolism*—caused by heart disease (infective endocarditis, rheumatic heart disease, prosthetic heart valves, myocardial infarction), pulmonary emboli, arteriosclerotic plaque in carotid artery.
  a. Embolism usually lodges in middle cerebral artery or its branches where it disrupts circulation.
  b. Symptoms—sudden onset of hemiparesis or hemiplegia.
  c. See the nursing management of the patient with a stroke, in the discussion on page 721.

Cerebrovascular Disease from Hemorrhage

1. *Extradural hemorrhage*—hemorrhage occurring outside the dura mater
  a. This is considered a life-threatening emergency.
  b. See care of the patient with head injury for principles of immediate care (p. 712).
2. *Subdural hemorrhage*—hemorrhage occurring beneath the dura mater
  See care of the patient with a head injury (p. 712).
3. *Subarachnoid hemorrhage*—hemorrhage occurring in the subarachnoid space—may result from leaking aneurysm, congenital arteriovenous malformation, hypertension, tumor, or trauma. See treatment of subarachnoid hemorrhage, page 727.
4. *Intracerebral hemorrhage*—hemorrhage occurring within the brain substance—usually from hypertension, cerebral atherosclerosis, aneurysm, etc.

CAROTID ENDARTERECTOMY FOR CEREBROVASCULAR INSUFFICIENCY

Carotid endarterectomy is the removal of atherosclerotic plaque(s) or thrombus from the carotid artery to prevent a stroke and/or bring relief of symptoms.

Clinical Manifestations of Carotid Occlusive Disease

1. Headache, dizziness, blackout spells
2. Memory loss; mental deterioration
3. Transient monocular blindness or homonymous visual field defects
4. Numbness, weakness of extremities
5. Bruit-heard over carotid artery
6. Absent/diminished carotid pulsation in neck

Diagnostic Evaluation

1. Carotid phonoangiography—auscultation, direct visualization, and photographic recording of carotid bruits.
2. Oculoplethysmography (OPG)—measures pulsation in blood flow through ophthalmic artery; gives comparative timing of simultaneously recorded ocular pulse wave forms (by corneal suction cups); light opacity sensors on the ear lobes provide timing of external carotid pulses (Fig. 17-6).
3. Carotid arteriography—to visualize intracranial and cervical vessels.

Treatment and Nursing Management

NURSING ALERT: A carotid endarterectomy requires temporary clamping of the internal carotid artery; the blood supply of the brain may be compromised and neurologic dysfunction may result.

1. Watch for neurologic dysfunction and deficits—result of cerebral ischemia; emboli.
   a. Carry out frequent neurologic checks including assessment of equality, size, and reaction of pupils; handgrip; motor responses; speech; chewing;

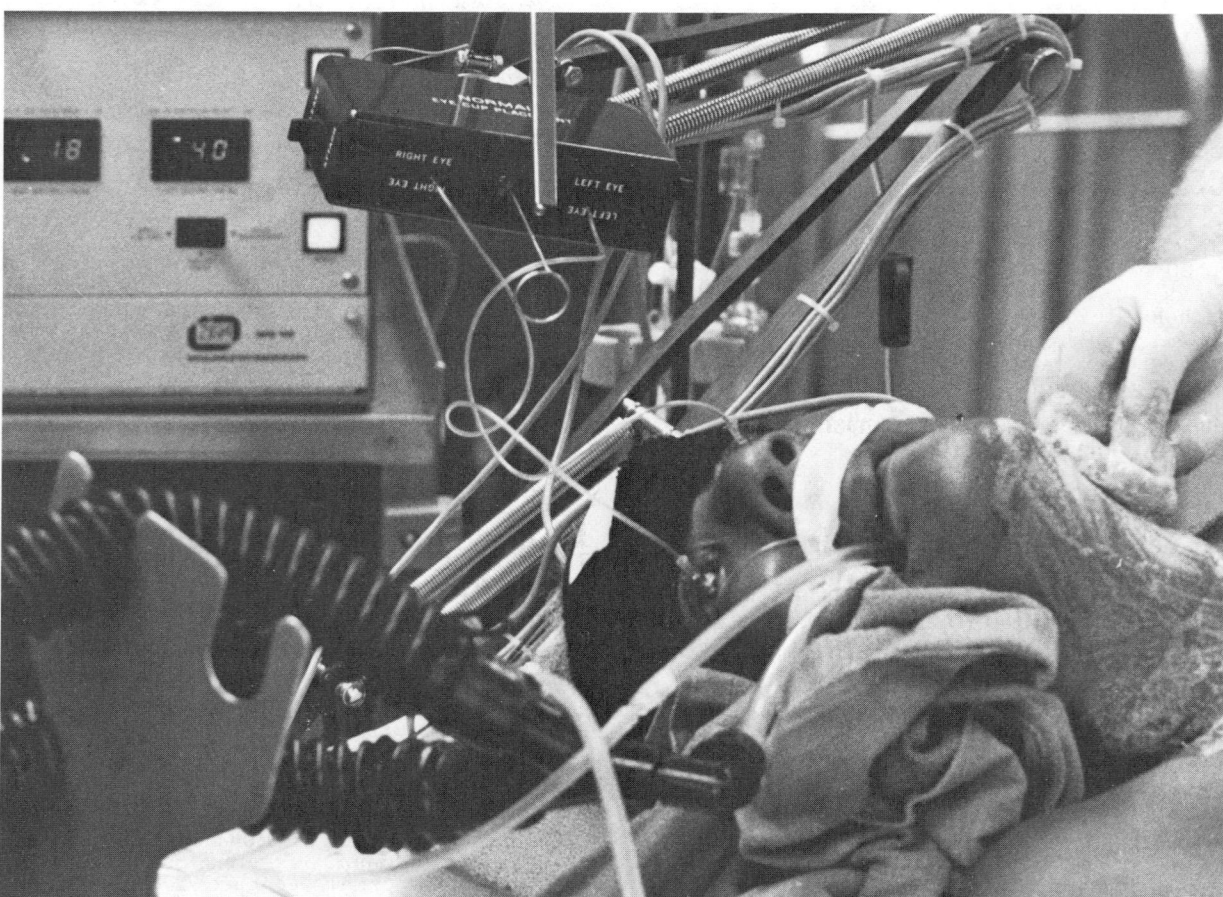

FIGURE 17-6. *Oculoplethysmograph provides continuous monitoring during carotid endarterectomy. (Courtesy of American Journal of Surgery, Vol. 138, No. 5, Nov 1979, and Henry J. Pearce, M.D.)*

swallowing; intellectual capacity; and symmetry of face.
  b. Compare with preoperative status.
  c. Prepare for immediate reoperation if stroke occurs.
2. Watch for respiratory insufficiency—resulting from edema due to operative manipulation or hematoma at operative site.
3. Maintain adequate blood pressure levels in immediate postoperative period—with lactated Ringer's solution and vasopressor agents when necessary.
  a. Avoid hypotension—to prevent cerebral ischemia and thrombosis.

  b. Avoid excessive hypertension by using rapid-acting antihypertensive drugs (trimethaphan [Arfonad]) when necessary—hypertension may precipitate a cerebral hemorrhage. Edema, hemorrhage in operative wound, or disruption of arterial reconstruction may also result from excessive hypertension.
4. Watch carefully for complications—neurologic deficits (stroke), infection/hematoma of wound, carotid artery disruption.
  Long-term complications—myocardial infarction; recurrent cerebrovascular disease.

STROKE OR CEREBRAL VASCULAR ACCIDENT (CVA)

A stroke (*cerebral vascular accident*) is the onset of neurologic dysfunction resulting from disruption of the blood supply to the brain. It is brought on by: (1) thrombosis (blood clot within a blood vessel of the brain or neck); (2) cerebral embolism; (3) stenosis of an artery supplying the brain; and (4) cerebral hemorrhage (rupture of a cerebral blood vessel with bleeding or pressure into the brain substance).

Clinical Manifestations

(depend on size and site of lesion)
1. Motor loss (hemiplegia—paralysis on one side of body)
2. Communication loss
3. Visual loss (homonymous hemianopia—loss of half of the visual field)
4. Sensory loss
5. Bladder impairment
6. Impairment of mental activity and psychological effects

Risk Factors

1. Hypertension
2. Previous transient ischemic attacks
3. Cardiac disease (atherosclerotic/valvular heart disease, arrhythmias)
4. Advanced age
5. Diabetes
6. Oral contraceptives

Treatment and Nursing Management

A. *Acute Phase: The Unconscious Patient*

OBJECTIVES: to keep the patient alive.
to minimize cerebral damage by providing adequately oxygenated blood to the brain.
1. *See Nursing Management of the Unconscious Patient* (p. 706).
2. Carry out a nursing assessment of the following: (Keep neurologic flow sheet.)
  a. A change in the level of responsiveness as evidenced by movement, resistance to changes of position, and response to stimulation.
  b. Presence or absence of voluntary or involuntary movements of the extremities; tone of the muscles; body posture and the position of the head.
  c. Stiffness or flaccidity of the neck.
  d. Comparison of pupils: size, reaction to light, and ocular position.

  e. Color of the face and extremities; temperature and moisture of the skin.
  f. Quality and rates of pulse and respiration; body temperature and arterial pressure.
  g. Ability to speak.
  h. Volume of fluids ingested or administered and volume of urine excreted each 24 hours.
  i. Serial arterial blood gas measurements.
3. Assure an adequate perfusion pressure so that oxygenated blood can reach the brain.
  a. Maintain blood pressure and cardiac output—to sustain cerebral blood flow.
  b. Watch for evidence of myocardial infarction, arrhythmias, and congestive heart failure; arrhythmia may reduce cerebral blood flow and produce cardiac arrest.
  c. Ensure hydration; rehydration may reduce blood viscosity and thereby improve cerebral blood flow.
4. Use endotracheal intubation and mechanical ventilation for patient with massive stroke; respiratory arrest is usually the life-threatening factor in this condition.
5. Reorient the patient when he begins to regain consciousness.
  a. Expect some aphasia if patient has right-sided hemiplegia.
  b. Reassure patient that he has not lost his mind and that he will receive help with communication (speech pathologist or therapist).
  c. *Talk* to the patient while caring for him.
  d. Make every effort to understand the patient.
  e. Maintain a calm and accepting manner during periods of emotional lability.
6. Remove indwelling catheter as soon as patient is conscious.
  a. Offer bedpan or urinal at scheduled short intervals.
  b. Lengthen time intervals as more bladder control is gained.
7. Prepare for surgical intervention if necessary—to halt potential occlusive lesions and restore circulation.

B. *Rehabilitation Phase*

OBJECTIVES: to prevent deformities and loss of range of motion.
to retrain the affected arm and leg.
to help the patient gain independence in self-care.
to help patient adapt and adjust to his residual function.

1. Position the patient in bed correctly—to prevent contractures, relieve pressure, and maintain good body alignment. (These principles of positioning are also carried out during the unconscious phase.) See Figure 17-7A.
   a. Place a board under the mattress—to give the body firm support.
   b. Encourage patient to remain flat in bed except when engaged in activities of daily living—to prevent hip flexion deformities.
   c. Use a footboard at intervals to keep the feet dorsiflexed—prevents footdrop, heel cord shortening, and plantar flexion.
      (1) Some therapists feel that continuous use of a footboard will stimulate plantar flexion.
      (2) Do not allow top bedding to pull affected foot into plantar flexion.
   d. Use a padded posterior splint at night and keep the knee in a fully extended position; secure the posterior splint with an elastic compression bandage.
   e. Apply a trochanter roll from the crest of the ilium to the midthigh (Fig. 17-7B—to prevent external rotation of the hip joint when the patient is in a dorsal position.
   f. Place a pillow in the axilla of the affected side—to keep arm away from the chest and prevent adduction of the affected shoulder (Fig. 17-7A).
   g. Place the affected arm (slightly flexed) on pillow supports with each joint positioned higher than the preceding one—to prevent edema and resultant fibrosis.

FIGURE 17-7. *Positioning for a patient following a stroke. (Dark side of pajamas represents affected or hemiplegic side.)*

A. A pillow is placed in the axilla to prevent adduction of the affected shoulder. Pillows are placed under the arm, which is in a slightly flexed position with each joint positioned higher than the preceding one.

   h. Place the hand in slight supination with fingers slightly flexed; if upper extremity is flaccid, use a volar resting splint to support the wrist and hand in a functional position (Fig. 17-7C). If the upper extremity is spastic, use a dorsal splint to prevent pressure on the palm.
   i. Place the patient in a prone position for 15 minutes to ½ hour daily (Fig. 17-7E)—to prevent knee and hip flexion contractions.
2. Exercise the affected extremities passively and carry out range of motion exercises 4–5 times daily—to prevent contracture development in the paralyzed extremity, to prevent further deterioration of neuromuscular system, to stretch soft tissues, and to enhance circulation.
   a. Involve family in exercise program since care of a stroke patient requires time and effort.
   b. Remind the patient to exercise unaffected extremities regularly at intervals throughout the day—to prevent contracture development in the normal extremities.
   c. Teach patient to put his unaffected leg under the affected one in order to move and turn himself (Fig. 17-8).
   d. Instruct the patient to move his affected arm (and hand) with his good hand (Fig. 17-9).
   e. Teach quadriceps muscle setting and gluteal exercises (5 times daily for 10 minutes)—to improve the muscle strength needed for walking.
      (1) *Quadriceps Setting* (to each extremity)
         Instruct the patient as follows:
         (a) Contract the quadriceps muscle (anterior

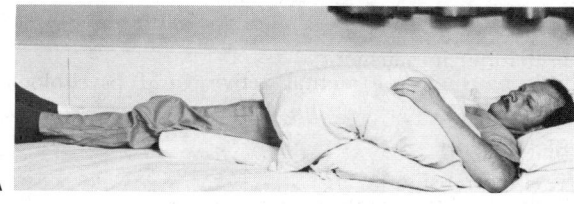

A

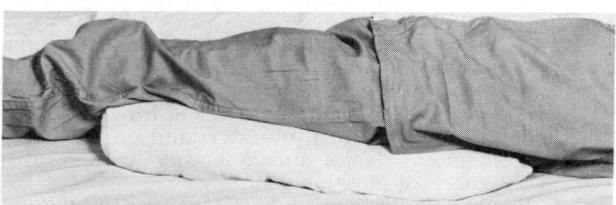

B

B. The trochanter roll should extend from the crest of the ilium to the midthigh, since the hip joint lies between these 2 points. The trochanter roll acts as a mechanical wedge under the projection of the greater trochanter and prevents the femur from rolling.

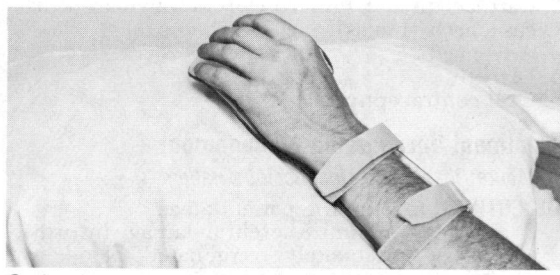

C

C. A volar resting splint may be used to support the wrist and hand if the upper extremity is flaccid.

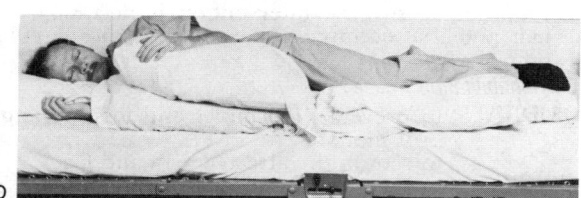

D

D. Lateral or side-lying position. The patient should be turned on his unaffected side. The upper thigh should not be acutely flexed.

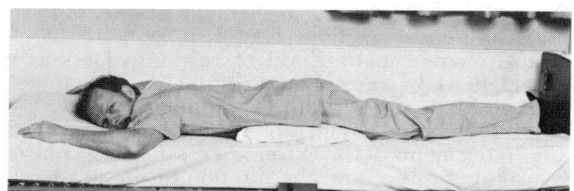

E

E. Prone position. A pillow is placed under the pelvis to help promote hyperextension of the hip joints, which is essential for normal gait. Note position of arms.

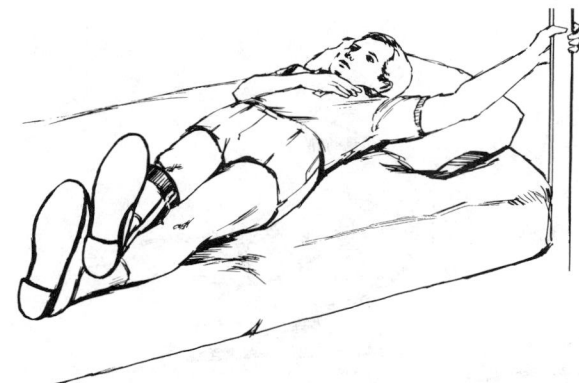

FIGURE 17-8. *Bed exercise for the patient with hemiplegia: moving the legs over the side of the bed. The paralyzed leg is carried by the uninvolved leg. (From Hirschberg G, Lewis L and Vaughan P. Rehabilitation. 2nd ed. Philadelphia, JB Lippincott, 1976)*

portion of thighs) while raising the heel and attempting to push the popliteal space against the mattress.

    (b) Hold the muscle contraction for the count of 5.

    (c) Relax for the count of 5. Repeat.

  (2) *Gluteal Setting*

Instruct the patient as follows:

    (a) Contract or "pinch" the buttocks together for the count of 5.

    (b) Relax for the count of 5. Repeat.

f. Biofeedback may be used to help patient relearn control of activity of lower extremity muscles during early recovery period.

3. Adjust nursing approach to the patient's condition.

  a. Test for hemianopia (defective vision in half of the visual field).

    (1) Show patient an object placed to one side and ask if he can identify it.

    (2) Hemianopia is evident if patient fails to see the object on the correct side, but responds by looking towards it on the other side. (Visual field is likely to be limited on the right if patient has right hemiplegia.)

  b. Place call light, bedside table, etc. on the side of his awareness.

  c. Approach the bed from the uninvolved side.

  d. Encourage the patient to turn his head from side to side to obtain the full view of a normal visual field.

  e. Have patient wear his eyeglasses.

  f. For patient with dysarthria (difficult speech) and dysphagia (difficulty in swallowing)

    (1) Give food and fluids from uninvolved side (if patient has droop of mouth).

    (2) Remind patient to chew on unaffected side.

    (3) Inspect patient's mouth for food collecting between cheek and gums on involved side; frequent oral hygiene is necessary.

    (4) Give nasogastric tube feeding if indicated.

  g. See page 726 for nursing management of patient with aphasia.

4. Maintain bladder and bowel program (see p. 76).

5. Assist the patient in getting out of bed as soon as permitted. Check his blood pressure first.

a. *To Develop Sitting Balance*

  (1) Raise the bed to a sitting position; instruct patient to hold the bedrail with his good hand—helps to regain sense of balance.

  (2) To sit on edge of bed

    (a) Adjust the bed to the low position.

    (b) Instruct the patient to place the strong leg beneath the weak leg and lift it toward the side of the bed.

    (c) Instruct the patient to press the strong elbow (which is flexed to a 90-degree angle) into the mattress and come to a sitting position by transferring weight to the forearm and then to the hand, while lifting the uninvolved leg with the strong leg over the edge of the bed. The force of gravity, set in motion by pushing against the hand and moving the legs, is sufficient to pivot the patient's torso on the buttocks.

    (d) Extend the patient's strong arm with his hand flat on the bed behind him to assist in balancing.

    (e) Stand in front of the patient to observe and, if necessary, help him to maintain this posture.

    (f) A change in color, shortness of breath, increasing pulse rate, or profuse perspiration is an indication that the patient should be placed in bed again. The sitting time is increased as rapidly as the patient's condition permits.

b. *To Develop Standing Balance* (Fig. 17-10)

  (1) Put walking shoes with strong shank on patient for all ambulation activities.

  (2) Seat the patient on edge of bed and place a straight-back chair on each side of him.

    (a) Tie affected hand to the chair if patient lacks grasp strength.

    (b) Assist the patient to a standing position by supporting his lower back with your hands and positioning your knees on the outside of the patient's knees.

  (3) Assess patient for dizziness, pallor, and increasing pulse rate. Have patient practice standing and shifting weight from one leg to the other.

  (4) Assist patient to achieve standing balance at frequent intervals throughout the day.

  (5) Help the patient begin walking as soon as standing balance is achieved (using parallel bars). Stand behind patient and stabilize him at waist level.

  (6) Encourage patient to look at his feet occasionally—proprioceptive loss may accompany hemiplegia.

6. Encourage patient to perform his self-care activities as soon as possible.

  a. Set realistic goals and add a new task daily if possible.

  b. Have the patient immediately transfer all self-care activities to the unaffected side. Teach one-handed methods.

  c. Encourage him to brush his teeth, comb his hair, and bathe and feed himself.

  d. Be sure that the patient does not neglect his affected side.

  e. Encourage the patient to dress himself for ambulatory activities.

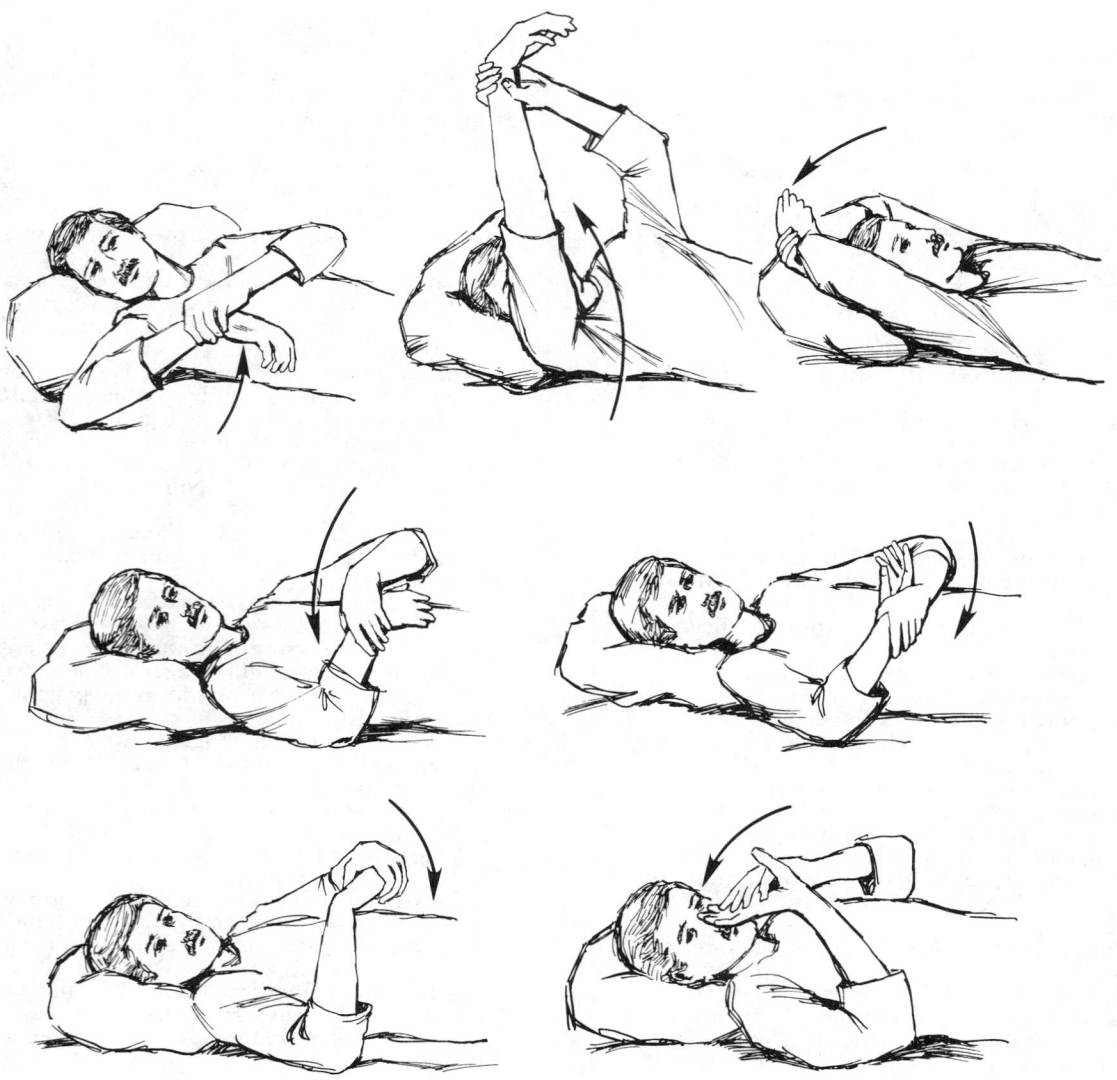

FIGURE 17-9. A. *Exercise to maintain range of motion of the involved shoulder and the elbow in hemiplegia. B. Exercise to maintain range of motion of pronation and supination in affected hand. C. Exercise to maintain range of motion of the wrist and the finger in hemiplegia. (From Hirschberg G, Lewis L and Vaughan P. Rehabilitation, 2nd ed. Philadelphia, JB Lippincott, 1976)*

(1) Instruct family to bring clothing that is one size larger than usually worn.

(2) Have patient dress himself (with assistance if necessary) while seated—to achieve better balance.

(3) Use clothing with front fasteners; stretch fabrics are preferable.

(4) Teach only one activity at a time.

7. Assist in securing supportive devices if needed—most patients develop spasticity of lower extremity and will lack motor control.

a. Secure posterior knee splint if patient has a weakened or absent quadriceps muscle—gives better balance and helps prevent loss of position sense.

b. Secure an adjustable aluminum cane (with 3-prong support if necessary) when patient is able to walk alone.

8. Use a sling on the paralyzed arm when patient is in upright position, if arm is flaccid, or if patient complains of arm pain and heaviness.

a. Remove sling frequently and exercise arm.

b. Instruct patient to interlace his fingers, placing the palms together. With elbows extended, lift

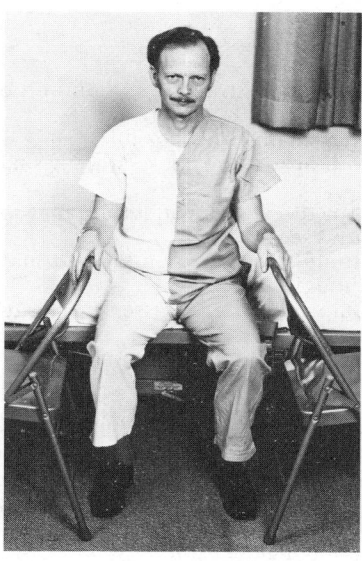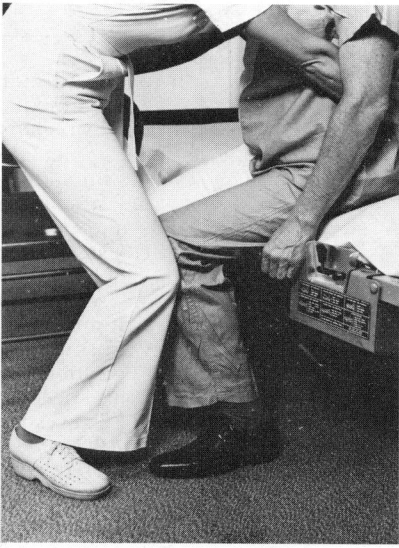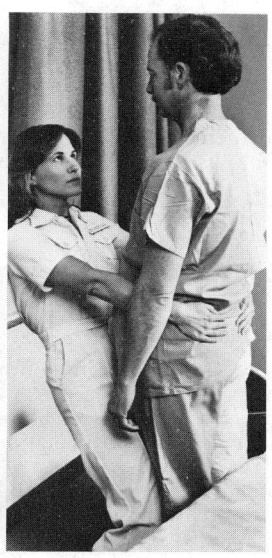

FIGURE 17-10. *Getting the patient out of bed following a stroke. (left) Place the bed in the low position so that the feet are resting on the floor. Observe the patient's reaction and increase the sitting time as rapidly as the patient's condition permits. (center) Getting ready to arise to a standing position. Positioning the nurse's knees on the outside of the patient's knees will prevent the patient's knees from buckling. (right) Stabilizing the patient as he assumes a standing position. Note that the nurse is (1) stabilizing the patient's lower back and knees and (2) assessing his reaction to standing. (Courtesy Washington Adventist Hospital; Glenn Dalby, photographer)*

both arms above head repeatedly throughout day.

c. When seated, keep the affected arm and hand elevated with a pillow.

d. Instruct patient to flex and extend his wrist and fingers with unaffected hand at frequent intervals.

e. Watch for shoulder-hand syndrome—painful shoulder and generalized swelling and pain of hand—can cause atrophy of subcutaneous tissues and contractures.

9. Secure a wheelchair of the correct size with brakes that the patient can manage if he is unable to ambulate.

a. Place wheelchair on patient's unaffected side; allows him to see wheelchair and lead with the stronger leg.

b. Lock wheelchair brake and lift pedals out of the way. To transfer from a chair to wheelchair, instruct the patient as follows:

(1) Move forward in chair, placing weight over strong leg. Push up with strong arm and foot.

(2) Place most of the weight on the strong leg while keeping weak knee locked.

(3) Pivot in the direction of the stronger leg; bring weak leg over to stronger leg. Maintain standing position a few moments.

(4) Lower body into chair gradually, using strong arm and leg.

(5) Push wheelchair by combined action of one hand and one foot.

10. Provide some type of counseling and support system for family—need direction and support in coping with personality and intellectual impairment and psychiatric symptoms.

11. Prepare the patient for discharge to home, rehabilitation center, or extended care facility.

Family Health Education

Instruct the family as follows:

1. Expect some emotional lability and some degree of brain damage if the patient has had a more severe stroke.

a. Patient may have episodes of inappropriate crying/laughing and temper outbursts; change the subject; ask patient to perform a motor act.

b. Hemiplegic patients may be easily confused, forgetful, discouraged, hostile, uncooperative, withdrawn, and dependent.

c. Support him psychologically; hemiplegia has a tremendous psychological impact on the patient (and his family).

2. Avoid doing those things for the patient that he can do for himself.

3. Be supportive and optimistic but firm and direct.

4. Install handrails by the toilet and tub or shower and put safety rails on the bed.

5. Obtain self-help devices to assist in activities of daily living; modify and adapt devices and "gadgets" to encourage independence (see pp. 67–68).

6. See that patient has scheduled rest periods.

7. Encourage patient to keep active and adhere to exercise program, and to remain as self-sufficient as possible.

8. Set realistic goals.

9. Have patient medically evaluated from time to time.

10. Take advantage of community service agencies and the local or regional branch of the State Office of Vocational Rehabilitation.

APHASIA

Aphasia is a disturbance of language function resulting from injury or disease of the brain centers. It may involve impairment of the ability to read and write as well as to speak, listen and comprehend.

Causes

1. Stroke
2. Head injury
3. Brain tumor

Aphasic Syndromes

A. *Fluent Aphasias*—difficulty in comprehension of language

Wernicke's aphasia—patient speaks readily but speech lacks clear content, information, and direction; jargon frequently used.

Anomic or amnesic aphasia—speech is almost normal, but marred by word-finding difficulty.

Conduction aphasia—patient's comprehension of language is good, but he has difficulty repeating spoken material.

B. *Nonfluent Aphasia (motor aphasia, Broca's aphasia)*—difficulty in production of language characterized by sparse verbal output produced with effort; patient usually can comprehend spoken/written word.

C. *Global Aphasia*—fluent and nonfluent aphasia occur together, but one type may predominate; the predominant manifestation may be inability to speak, comprehend speech, repeat, or name; it results from injury to both Broca's and Wernicke's areas.

Medical and Nursing Management

PRINCIPLE: There are a variety of symptoms and disorders underlying aphasia. Therefore, the treatment is individualized.

OBJECTIVE: to stimulate attempts at communication.

1. Determine the communication abilities of the patient—usually done by speech-language pathologist in cooperation with the neurologist.
2. Give the patient as much psychological security as possible.
3. Give the patient plenty of *time* to speak and respond; he cannot sort out incoming messages and formulate a response under pressure.
   a. Speak slowly while making eye contact with the patient.
   b. Face the patient.
   c. Avoid talking too fast, too loudly, or too much.
   d. Use short sentences; pause; see if he indicates that he understands.
   e. Supplement speech with gestures when indicated.
   f. Talk to him while caring for him. Know his former interests.
   g. Be consistent—by using the same wording each time instructions are given and questions are asked.
4. Keep the environment relaxed and permissive.
5. Keep distractions at a minimum—damaged input

pathways cannot sort out distracting stimuli in the environment.

6. Use as many sensory channels as possible.
   a. Supplement auditory stimulation with visual stimulation.
   b. Use visual aids (pictures); ask patient to point to and name what he sees.
   c. Use games to stimulate the patient's mind and help organize thoughts.
   d. Use television, tape recorders, cassettes, etc. to stimulate his interest.
   e. Encourage patient to use any form of communication—gestures, writing, drawing, etc., until his speech begins to return.
   f. Elicit responses from patient . . . e.g., "Please nod your head if you understand." Reinforce every correct response.
7. Give support by assuring the patient that there is nothing wrong with his intelligence.
   a. Treat him as an intelligent adult.
   b. Accept the patient as he is now; avoid artificial praise.
   c. Avoid forcing speech.
8. Maintain a calm, accepting, and deliberate manner, especially during periods of emotional lability.
9. Encourage the patient to socialize with his family and friends.
   a. Seek the help of other people to read aloud, play games, do puzzles.
   b. Have his grandchildren visit and talk with him.
   c. Keep him in the social world.
   d. Be aware of support groups (Stroke clubs) in the community.
10. Watch the patient for clues and gestures if his speech is unintelligible or jargon-like.
    a. Continue to listen to him.
    b. Nod and make neutral statements occasionally.
    c. Shift the topic when appropriate to provide another point of interest and frame of reference.
11. Observe the patient during the course of his daily schedule for clues to evaluate and assess his progress.

Family Health Education

1. See items 1–11, above.
2. The patient's ability to speak may vary from day to day. Fatigue has an adverse effect on speech.
3. The patient is likely to become terribly frustrated by his inability to communicate; ignore swearing and abusive language.
4. Aphasia can also involve the patient's understanding. Some persons cannot express themselves but can comprehend the spoken or written word; others can speak but do not understand; while some who do neither may respond to gesture and actions.
5. Seek information about aphasia:
   American Speech-Language-Hearing Association, 10810 Rockville Pike, Rockville, Md. 20852.
6. Counsel family to continue life of their own and to seek counseling if necessary for dealing with frustration and pressures.

RUPTURE OF INTRACRANIAL ANEURYSM WITH SUBARACHNOID HEMORRHAGE

An *intracranial aneurysm* is a dilation of the walls of a cerebral artery.

Etiology

1. Atherosclerosis—reflects an acquired defect in vessel wall with subsequent weakness of wall
2. Congenital defect of vessel wall
3. Hypertensive vascular disease
4. Head trauma
5. Advanced age

Clinical Manifestations

1. Due to compression of cranial nerves or brain substance
2. Due to leakage from or rupture of aneurysm causing subarachnoid hemorrhage
   a. Headache or head pain, often associated with pain in eye—usually unilateral, frontal, recurrent, and severe; disturbances of consciousness
   b. Pain and rigidity in back of neck and spine—from meningeal irritation
   c. Visual disturbances—visual loss, diplopia (double vision), ptosis (drooping of upper eyelid)—when aneurysm is adjacent to oculomotor (III) nerve
   d. Tinnitus (ringing in the ears)
   e. Dizziness; nausea and vomiting
   f. Hemiparesis (muscular weakness affecting one side of body) or hemiplegia (paralysis of one side of body)
   g. Fever—due to meningeal or hypothalamic irritation

Underlying Principles

1. Early recognition of warning signs should prompt early surgical intervention before major hemorrhage develops.
2. Rupture of an intracranial aneurysm leads to subarachnoid hemorrhage. Other causes of subarachnoid hemorrhage include arteriovenous malformation, tumors, trauma, blood dyscrasia.
3. The mortality rate corresponds to the level of consciousness and neurologic deficit. Many patients ultimately succumb to recurrence of bleeding.

Treatment and Nursing Management

OBJECTIVES: to save the patient's life in the period following subarachnoid hemorrhage.
to prevent recurrent bleeding.

NURSING ALERT: There is a significant incidence of recurrent aneurysmal bleeding with a high mortality rate.

1. Place patient on immediate and absolute bed rest in a quiet, nonstressful setting—activity, pain, stress may elevate blood pressure and potentiate bleeding.
   a. Restrict visitors except family.
   b. Elevate head of bed 30°–35°—to facilitate venous drainage from brain.
   c. Avoid any activity that increases blood pressure or obstructs venous return (Valsalva maneuver, straining, sneezing, pulling up in bed, acute flexion/rotation of head and neck, [compromises jugular veins], cigarette smoking).
   d. Instruct patient to exhale through mouth during voiding/defecation to decrease strain.
2. Monitor patient continually to recognize neurologic deterioration (from recurrent bleeding, increasing intracranial pressure, vasospasm) and to determine optimum time for surgical intervention.
   a. Keep neurologic flow record; check blood pressure, pulse, and level of responsiveness hourly.
   b. Use intracranial pressure monitoring (p. 710) for patients who are unconscious or showing progressive neurologic deterioration.
   c. Angiogram is done when patient is stable—to determine source of bleeding.
   d. See Care of Unconscious Patient, page 706.
3. Use measures to maintain systemic blood pressure at a stable level and prevent rebleeding.
   a. Drugs
      (1) Sedatives (phenobarbital; diazepam)—for sedative and anticonvulsive effects.
      (2) Analgesics (codeine; acetaminophen)—for head and neck pain.
      (3) Antifibrinolytic agents (aminocaproic acid [Amicar])—to inhibit clot lysis and reduce likelihood of recurrent bleeding.
      (4) Stool softeners—to prevent straining.
      (5) Antihypertensive therapy (propranolol; hydralazine; methyldopa)—for elevated blood pressure. Avoid precipitous drop in blood pressure, which can produce brain ischemia.
      (6) Steroids (dexamethasone; methylprednisolone)—to combat cerebral edema (controversial). See also patient with increased intracranial pressure, page 709.
4. Monitor for fluid and electrolyte disturbances—results from inappropriate secretion of antidiuretic hormone (common after subarachnoid hemorrhage).
5. Monitor for cerebral vasospasm (narrowing of cerebral blood vessels which reduces brain blood flow leading to ischemia and cerebral infarction).
   a. Usually occurs 4th–10th day following initial hemorrhage.
   b. May be treated by expanding patient's blood volume and increasing blood pressure to increase perfusion through spastic cerebral vessels.
6. Monitor for other complications—hematoma (intracerebral and subdural), hydrocephalus (from blood in basal cisterns), brain edema, pituitary insufficiency.
7. Prepare for surgical intervention when patient is in suitable condition and his brain's reaction to hemorrhage subsides.
   a. Obliteration of aneurysm by clipping or ligation
   b. Encasement or reinforcement techniques by wrapping aneurysm with plastic, muscle, muslin, or other material or applying a coating substance.
   c. Extracranial-intracranial arterial bypass—to establish collateral blood supply in order to allow surgery on aneurysm.
   d. Postoperative complications

(1) Cerebral vasospasms—produce cerebral ischemia and stroke
(2) Psychological symptoms—disorientation, amnesia, Korsakoff's syndrome
(3) Motor disturbances, aphasia, water and electrolyte disturbances, gastrointestinal bleeding

BRAIN ABSCESS

A *brain abscess* is a localized collection of pus within the brain substance.

Etiology

1. By direct invasion of the brain (intracranial trauma or surgery)
2. By spread of infection from nearby sites (ear, sinus, mastoid)
3. By spread of infection from other organs (remote from the brain) by hematogenous or metastatic spread (lung infections; infective endocarditis)

NURSING ALERT: Have a high degree of suspicion of brain abscess when neurological signs and symptoms develop in a person with a recent history of sinus or ear infection or lung abscess.

Clinical Manifestations

Caused by major alterations of intracranial mass dynamics (edema, brain shift), by infection, or by location of the abscess.
1. Headache—may be from increased intracranial pressure; worse in A.M.
2. Focal neurologic signs (depending on site of abscess)—weakness of arm or leg, visual impairment, focal epileptic seizures, papilledema.
3. Fever and leukocytosis; temperature may be subnormal when there is a thick-walled abscess.
4. Change in patient's mental alertness.

Treatment and Nursing Management

OBJECTIVE: to eliminate the abscess.
1. Give antimicrobial therapy—to reduce the virulence of or to eliminate the organism. Large doses of the appropriate antimicrobial are given to penetrate the abscess cavity.

2. Observe patient for increased intracranial pressure (p. 709)—cerebral edema surrounds an acute brain abscess and may produce sudden increase of intracranial pressure.
   a. Secondary midbrain and brain stem compression can lead to rapid coma and death.
   b. Patient may be given dexamethasone for cerebral edema.
   c. Keep neurological assessment record.
3. Assist in diagnostic studies for determining accurate localization of abscess; nursing assessments, laboratory studies, computed tomography, brain scanning, angiography, and repeated neurological examinations.
4. Give anticonvulsants (phenytoin) as prescribed—risk of epilepsy is high during acute phase and as a complication.
5. Prepare for surgical intervention (the definitive treatment).
   a. Drainage of abscess through burr holes and instillation of appropriate antibiotics.
   b. Craniotomy with elevation of bone flap and radical excision of abscess. (See nursing management of patient undergoing intracranial surgery, p. 715.)
6. Support the patient during repeated computerized tomographic (CT) brain scanning—used to diagnose and localize abscess, determine optimum timing of surgery, and diagnose postoperative complications.
   a. Relapse is common with high overall mortality and morbidity.
   b. Neurologic defects following treatment of brain abscess include hemiparesis, seizures, visual defects, cranial nerve palsies, and learning problems in children.

Health Education

1. It is important that the anticonvulsant medication be taken on a daily basis as prescribed.
2. *Prevention:* Treat otitis media, mastoiditis, sinusitis, and other systemic infections to prevent brain abscess.

Discharge Planning and Health Education

The patient who survives the initial hemorrhage and who does not have surgical repair is at risk for a second hemorrhage. Operative treatment of the aneurysm is necessary unless there are medical contraindications.

BRAIN TUMOR

A *brain tumor* is a localized intracranial lesion which occupies space within the skull and tends to cause a rise in intracranial pressure.

Incidence

1. Tumors of the brain originate in the brain (including the roots of the cranial nerves and the meninges) in about 95% of all patients with this problem.
2. Tumors may be benign or malignant; however any mass within the closed cranial vault may be lethal.
3. The greatest incidence of brain tumors occurs between the ages of 30 and 50 years.

Classification

A. Tumors Originating in the Brain Tissue

Gliomas; infiltrating tumors that may invade any portion of the brain; most common type of brain tumor

Astrocytoma (Grades I–IV)
Ependymoma
Medulloblastoma
Oligodendroglioma
Mixed

} Subclassified according to cell type

B. Tumors Arising from the Covering of the Brain

Meningioma; encapsulated, well-defined, growing outside the brain tissue; compresses rather than invades brain

C. Tumors Developing in or on the Cranial Nerves

1. Acoustic neuroma; derived from sheath of acoustic nerve
2. Optic nerve spongioblastoma polare

D. Metastatic Lesions (most commonly from lung and breast)

E. Tumors of the Ductless Glands

1. Pituitary
2. Pineal

F. Blood Vessel Tumors

1. Hemangioblastoma
2. Angioma

G. Congenital Tumors

Clinical Manifestations

A. General Symptoms

1. Brain tumor is usually characterized by a *progressive* course of symptoms over a period of time.
2. Brain tumors manifest themselves by:
   a. *Symptoms due to increased intracranial pressure*
      (1) Headache—intensified by activity that increases intracranial pressure (stooping, straining); most common in morning
      (2) Vomiting, unrelated to food intake—usually due to irritation of vagal centers in medulla
      (3) Papilledema (choked disc)—edema of optic nerve
      (4) Mental clouding, lethargy
   b. *Localizing symptoms due to local effects of tumor's interference with specific regions of the brain*
      (1) Motor abnormalities—rigidity, lack of coordination, weakness, convulsive seizures
      (2) Sensory abnormalities—aberrations in smell, vision, hearing, and touch

B. Manifestations According to Site

1. *Frontal lobe tumor*
   a. Mental changes (memory loss, euphoria, personality changes, loss of interest, moral laxity)
   b. Headache
   c. Focal seizures
   d. Hemiparesis or aphasia
   e. Failing or blurring vision
   f. Impairment of sphincter control
2. *Temporal lobe* (may be relatively silent)
   a. Focal epileptic seizures
   b. Dysphasia or aphasia
   c. Papilledema
   d. Headache
   e. Behavior disorders

3. *Parietal lobe tumors*
   a. Motor seizures
   b. Sensory loss or visual impairment
   c. Jacksonian convulsions
4. *Occipital tumors*
   a. Visual impairment and visual hallucinations
   b. Focal seizures
5. *Cerebellar tumors* (common brain tumors of childhood)
   a. Disturbances of equilibrium and coordination
   b. Early development of increasing intracranial pressure and papilledema
6. *Tumors of brain stem*
   Symptoms of cranial nerve palsies (dysphagia, dysphonia, nystagmus, ataxia in extremities)
7. *Tumors of the 3rd ventricle*
   Symptoms arise from increasing intracranial pressure

Diagnostic Evaluation

OBJECTIVE: to determine the precise location of the tumor.

1. Clinical assessment of signs and symptoms
2. Computed tomography, specialized cerebral angiography, radionuclide scanning, electroencephalography, pneumoencephalography

Treatment

OBJECTIVES: to eradicate the tumor and cure the patient (if possible).
to achieve palliation by partial tumor removal and by decompression, radiation, or chemotherapy, or combinations of these.

A. Problems Affecting Treatment

1. Effectiveness of treatment depends on type and site of tumor; many tumors are in vital or inaccessible areas (brain stem tumors); even biopsies in such locations can produce unacceptable disabilities.
2. Nonencapsulated and infiltrating tumors make complete removal almost impossible; resulting neurologic defects (blindness, paralysis) would be too severe.
3. Cures may be obtained in certain tumors (meningiomas, acoustic neuromas, cystic astrocytomas of cerebellum, etc.) if treated early; complete removal of infiltrating gliomas not possible.

B. Principles of Treatment

1. Brain tumors require different therapeutic approaches, depending on cell type, tumor location, degree of invasiveness, and association with vital structures; and age and condition of the patient. Each patient (and his lesion) is evaluated individually and the therapeutic program designed accordingly.
2. Treatment usually involves a multidisciplinary approach including surgery, radiation, and chemotherapy, or a combination of the three.
3. Surgical approaches include total tumor excision, decompression, cerebrospinal fluid-vascular shunt. (See p. 715 for nursing management of patient undergoing intracranial surgery.)
4. Support the patient undergoing radiotherapy.
   a. Give steroids (dexamethasone) or osmotic dehydrating agents (urea) as directed—to reduce cerebral edema associated with brain tumors; may be introduced prior to therapy and withdrawn gradually as soon as definitive local treatment (surgery/radiation) has demonstrated clinical results.

b. Total brain irradiation is usually carried out; suprafractionation (more than 1 dose of radiation therapy per day is being investigated).

c. Repeat CT scanning may be used to increase accuracy and safety of radiotherapy.

d. Radiosensitive drugs may be given to increase radiosensitivity of neoplastic tissue.

e. Loss of hair may be expected; regrowth may be expected after several weeks.

f. See page 853 for nursing management of patient undergoing radiation therapy.

5. Encourage the patient undergoing chemotherapy.

a. Chemotherapeutic drugs may be given singly or in combination (BCNU, CCNU, VM-26, procarbazine).

b. Dosages of chemotherapeutic drugs may be limited by their toxicity.

c. See page 849 for nursing management of patient undergoing chemotherapy.

d. See page 842 for nursing management of patient with cancer.

6. Management of patient with brain metastases from systemic cancer (lung, breast, malignant melanoma, leukemia)

a. Patients with systemic tumors may function well until tumor metastasizes to nervous system and rapidly produces frightening and disabling symptoms (motor loss, cranial neuropathies, intellectual impairment, convulsive seizures).

b. Metastases to brain are commonly multiple and often unresectable.

c. Therapeutic approach includes surgery, radiation, and chemotherapy; palliation more effective if treatment is started before major neurologic deficits develop.

d. See page 842 for nursing management of patient with cancer.

THE EPILEPSIES

The *epilepsies* are a symptom-complex of several disorders of brain function characterized by recurrent seizures. There may be associated changes in behavior, mentation, and motor or sensory activity. The basic problem is thought to be an electrical disturbance (dysrhythmia) in the nerve cells in one section of the brain that causes them to give off abnormal, recurrent, uncontrolled electrical discharges.

Causes

The underlying disorder of the brain may be structural, chemical, or physiological or a combination of all three.
1. Genetic tendency
2. Trauma—head/brain
3. Brain tumor
4. Circulatory disorder (stroke, arteriovenous malformation)
5. Metabolic disorder (hypoglycemia, hypocalcemia, anoxia)
6. Toxicity (drugs and alcohol)
7. Infection (encephalitis, meningitis, abscess)

Clinical Manifestations

1. Loss of consciousness
2. Disturbances of the mind
3. Excess or loss of muscle tone or movement
4. Disorders of sensation or special senses
5. Disturbances of the autonomic functions of the body

Diagnostic Evaluation

1. History of seizures (as noted by patient and observers)
2. Electroencephalograph (EEG)—finds and measures brain electrical discharge pattern; useful in locating the site where epileptic discharge begins, its spread, intensity, duration; helps classify seizure type (Fig. 17-11).
3. EEG and television monitoring of patients–split screen techniques show the patient during a seizure with simultaneous EEG tracing (Fig. 17-11).
4. Telemetering computer equipment—patient wears a device which holds electrodes on scalp and which houses a small radio transmitter; EEG signals are picked up by receiver and tape-recorded; helps identify seizure patterns before and after they occur.

Classification of Seizures*

There are wide variations in the types, frequency, and severity of seizures. The most common types of seizures are:
1. *Generalized tonic-clonic (grand mal)*—the "typical" seizures, in which the patient may have jerky and strong muscle contractions and lose consciousness: stupor or brief sleep may follow.
2. *Absence (petit mal)*—brief "blank spells," especially prevalent in childhood and often occurring dozens of times a day.
3. *Complex-partial (psychomotor, temporal lobe)*—different forms of seizure activity, often appearing as irrational or odd behavior which lasts only a few minutes and is not remembered. Electroencephalogram (EEG) discharges frequently come from one or both of the brain's temporal lobes.
4. *Simple-partial (Jacksonian)*—seizures may start in the toes of one foot or the fingers of one hand, moving upward as more neurons are affected and crossing to the other side of the body. Early signs may be followed by grand mal type seizures.

Treatment and Nursing Management

OBJECTIVES: to determine and treat (if possible) the primary underlying cause of the seizures.
to prevent a recurrence of seizures and therefore allow the patient to live a normal life.
to gain an understanding of the patient and his relationship to his environment.

1. Emphasize the importance of *regularity* in taking the prescribed antiepileptic medication to reduce number and/or severity of seizures.

a. Objective of drug therapy: to suppress seizure activity with minimum dosage of medication and without side effects.

* Adapted from the NINCDS Research Program. Epilepsy 1980

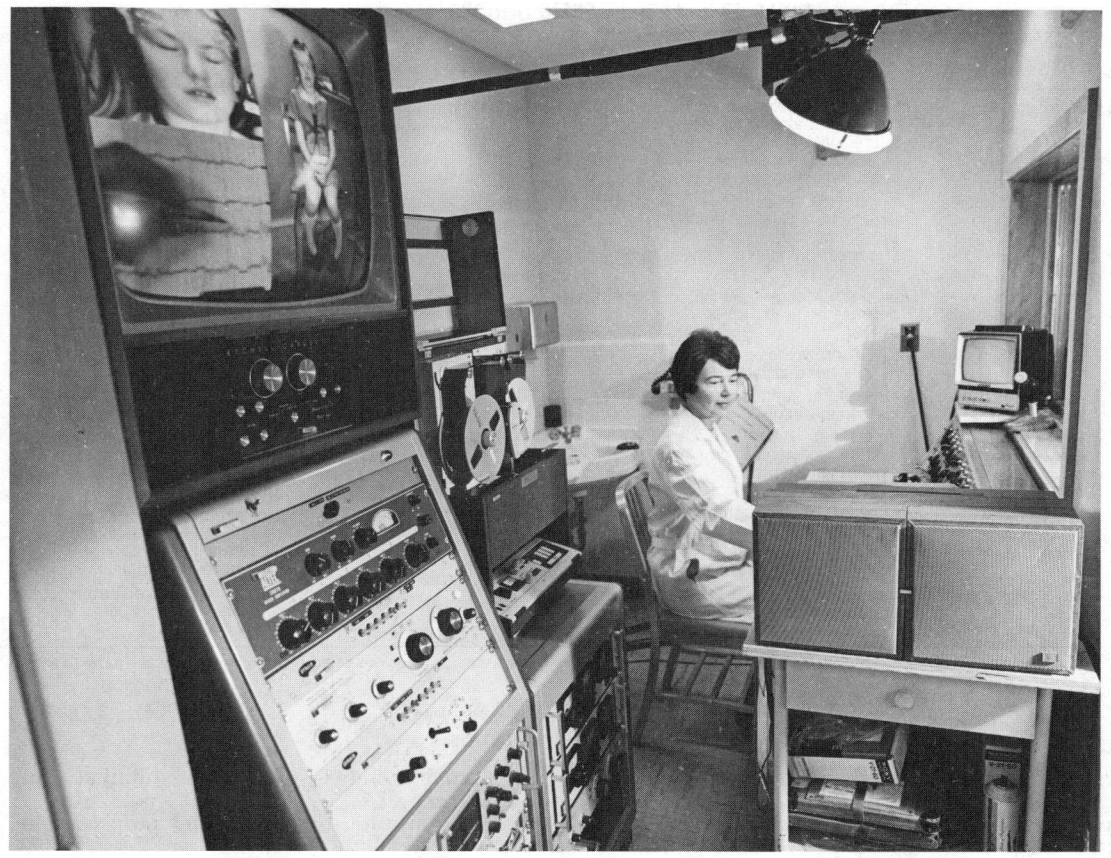

FIGURE 17-11. *Technician videotapes three-way split-screen television presentation of seizures induced by hyperventilation. Two cameras see the patient full body and close-up while the third camera shows EEG tracing. (Courtesy, National Institute of Neurological and Communicative Disorders and Stroke.)*

b. Drug therapy is regarded as a form of control; not a cure.
  (1) The choice of drug(s) is selected by the type of seizure.
  (2) Treatment is usually started with one drug; the dosage is adjusted until seizures are controlled and effective blood concentration of the drug is achieved and maintained or toxic symptoms develop; a second drug may be added if there is partial improvement.
  (3) See Table 17-2 for list of drugs in current use.
c. Instruct the patient to keep a record of events surrounding his seizures (number, duration, time of occurrence, sleep/eating patterns)—to help determine proper therapy/patient compliance.

> **NURSING ALERT:** The patient should not stop taking his antiepileptic medication without medical supervision, since sudden wtihdrawal can cause an increase in seizure frequency or precipitate the development of status epilepticus.

d. Patient should watch for toxic effects of antiepileptic medication—drowsiness, gingival hyperplasia, nervousness, visual difficulties, motor incoordination, staggering ataxia, bone marrow depression leading to blood dyscrasias.
  (1) Advise patient to avoid taking medication on an empty stomach; gastritis is apt to occur, especially with phenytoin (Dilantin).
  (2) Instruct patient to brush teeth frequently and massage gums to prevent gingival infection.
e. Encourage patient to have periodic blood evaluations when taking antiepileptic drugs that may depress hemopoiesis.
2. See nursing management of patient with seizures, page 715).
3. Use a multidisciplinary approach to cope with social, emotional and vocational pressures on the person with epilepsy. See Health Education, page 732.
4. Biofeedback training, in which the patient is taught to control his brain wave activity, holds promise.
5. Neurosurgical management of the Epilepsies: Surgical procedures are performed when epilepsy results from intracranial tumors, abscess, cysts, vascular abnormalities, or when the patient has intractable seizures not responding to drug therapy. If the seizures originate in a reasonably well circumscribed area of the brain that can be excised without pro-

TABLE 17-2. ANTIEPILEPTIC DRUGS*†

Generic Name	Trade Name	Side Effects	Generic Name	Trade Name	Side Effects
carbamazepine	Tegretol	Dizziness, drowsiness, eye muscle imbalance causing blurred vision and nystagmus, nausea, vomiting, headache, skin rashes, blood dyscrasias	paramethadione	Paradione	Nausea, anorexia, insomnia, diplopia, skin rash, bleeding gums, blood dyscrasias
clonazepam	Clonopin	Drowsiness, ataxia, neurologic symptoms, behavior changes, palpitations, hair loss, anorexia	phenacemide	Phenurone	Gastrointestinal disturbances, anorexia, drowsiness, insomnia, paresthesias, psychic changes, hepatitis, blood dyscrasias, skin rash, nephritis
diazepam	Valium	Drowsiness, fatigue, ataxia, depression, headache, tremor	phenobarbital	Luminal	Drowsiness, nystagmus, ataxia
			phensuximide	Milontin	Nausea, ataxia, dizziness, drowsiness, skin eruptions, blood dyscrasias, hematuria
ethosuximide	Zarontin	Nausea, drowsiness, lethargy, headache, dizziness	phenytoin	Dilantin	Ataxia, slurred speech, nystagmus, mental confusion, motor twitching, nausea, rash, gingival hyperplasia, hirsutism
ethotoin	Peganone	Dizziness, fatigue, skin rash, insomnia, diplopia			
mephenytoin	Mesantoin	Nervousness, ataxia, nystagmus, pancytopenia, exfoliative dermatitis, drowsiness	primidone	Mysoline	Ataxia, vertigo, anorexia, fatigue, hyperirritability, drowsiness
mephobarbital	Mebaral	Dizziness, headache, nausea, facial edema, skin rash	trimethadione	Tridione	Bone marrow depression, pancytopenia, exfoliative dermatitis, photophobia, nephrosis, hepatitis
metharbital	Gemonil	Drowsiness, dizziness, gastric distress, irritability, skin rash			
methsuximide	Celontin	Nausea, vomiting, anorexia, ataxia, rash, drowsiness, dizziness, blood dyscrasias	valproate sodium	Depakene	Gastrointestinal disturbance, altered bleeding time, liver toxicity

* Side effects and sensitivity to antiepileptic drugs vary among patients and at different times in the same patient. The dose for each patient is based on the patient's clinical response (free of seizures and side effects) and the monitoring of plasma concentrations.
† Adapted from Official Names of Antiepileptic Drugs. *Epilepsia, 18*:123, 1977.

ducing significant neurologic deficits, the removal of the focus generating the seizures seems to give long-term control and improvement. See page 716 for postoperative care.

Discharge Planning and Health Education

1. Encourage the patient to study himself and his environment to determine what specific factors precipitate his seizures—illness, emotional stress, physical stress, hyperventilation, altered sleep patterns, photosensitivity, or other sensory stimuli, menses, etc.
2. The medication must be taken daily to prevent seizures; medication may have to be adjusted due to recurrent illness, weight gain, increase in stress, etc.
3. Practice *regularity* and *moderation* in daily activities; diet, exercise, rest, avoidance of certain stimulating stresses.
   a. Have regular hours for sleep.
   b. Avoid emotional overstimulation (watching late TV, etc.). or photic stimulation (flickering light).
   c. Eat a well-balanced diet—long-term antiepileptic therapy can cause deficiencies, particularly of vitamin D.
   d. Avoid alcohol when seizures are known to follow alcoholic intake.
   e. Avoid swimming alone or engaging in sports, jobs, or hobbies involving serious risks.
   f. Seek help and counseling (if necessary) during periods of crisis—death in family, divorce, etc.).
4. Report any changes in health status—easy bruising, purpura, bleeding gums, jaundice, fever, recurrent infections or dermatosis.
5. Have follow-up urinalysis and blood studies.
6. Stress the importance of activity, both physical and mental. Activity tends to inhibit, not stimulate, epileptic seizures.
7. Reorient the attitude of patient and family to the disease.
   a. Help the family to understand that the patient has experienced rejection, anxiety (due to unpredictable seizure activity), feelings of being "different."
   b. Encourage patient or family to discuss feelings and attitudes about epilepsy.
   c. Help patient/family towards self-acceptance; reinforce areas of strength.
   d. Epilepsy can be *controlled;* it is not insanity or a supernatural condition.
8. Have a wallet card and wear a medical-alert bracelet indicating that the wearer has epilepsy.
9. Learn of the services and publications of: Epilepsy Foundation of America, 1828 L Street, N.W., Washington, D.C. 20036.

STATUS EPILEPTICUS

Status epilepticus (acute prolonged repetitive seizure activity) is a series of generalized seizures without return to consciousness between attacks. The term has been broadened to include continuous clinical and/or electrical seizures lasting at least 30 minutes even without impairment of consciousness.

Underlying Considerations

1. Status epilepticus is considered a serious neurologic emergency. It has a high mortality and morbidity rate (subsequent mental retardation or neurologic defects).
2. Common factors that precipitate status epilepticus

include withdrawal of antiepileptic medication, fever, and intercurrent infection.
3. Convulsive status epilepticus may be brought on by other conditions (cerebrovascular disease, head trauma, anoxic factors, metabolic abnormalities).

Medical and Nursing Treatment

OBJECTIVES: to stop the seizures as quickly as possible to prevent permanent brain damage and death.
to ensure adequate cardiorespiratory function and brain oxygenation.
to maintain the patient in a seizure-free state.
1. Establish an airway.
2. Ensure adequate oxygenation and monitor blood gases—there is some respiratory arrest at height of each seizure which produces venous congestion and hypoxia of the brain.

3. Give diazepam (Valium) IV slowly—to halt seizures immediately.
   a. Effects of diazepam may be of short duration (30–60 minutes).
   b. Other antiepileptic drugs (phenytoin, phenobarbital) are given after diazepam administration—to maintain seizure-free state.
4. Establish an intravenous route and monitor electrolytes, blood urea, and glucose—to monitor for metabolic abnormalities and as a guide for maintenance of biochemical homeostasis.
5. Employ electroencephalographic monitoring—to determine nature of epileptogenic activity.
6. Monitor vital and neurological signs on a continuing basis.
7. Assist with neurological workup and metabolic screening tests for causative factors.

PARKINSON'S DISEASE

Parkinson's disease is a progressive neurologic disorder affecting the brain centers responsible for control of movement. It is characterized by bradykinesia (slowness of movement), tremor, and muscle stiffness or rigidity.

Pathophysiology

The major lesion appears to be loss of pigment and of neurons in the substantia nigra of the brain.

Etiology

1. Unknown.
2. Viruses, encephalitis, cerebrovascular disease, and poisoning or toxicity (manganese, carbon monoxide) have been suspected.
3. Theory advanced that there is an imbalance of 2 neurochemical systems, cholinergic and dopaminergic, and that the symptoms of parkinsonism are caused by overactivity or underactivity of one or the other of these systems.
4. Genetic susceptibility (positive family history).

Clinical Manifestations

1. Bradykinesia (dyskinesia, hypokinesia)—usually becomes the most disabling symptom
2. Tremor—tends to decrease or disappear on purposeful movement
3. Rigidity, particularly of large joints
4. Muscle weakness—affecting eating, chewing, swallowing, speaking, writing
5. Mask-like facial expression; unblinking eyes
6. Depression
7. Dementia

Treatment and Nursing Management

Treatment is based on a combination of drug therapy, physical therapy and rehabilitation techniques, and patient and family education.

OBJECTIVE: to keep the patient functionally useful and productive as long as possible.

A. *Drug Therapy* (regimen changes as disease progresses)
1. *Antihistamines* (diphenhydramine [Benadryl])—thought to help patients with tremor because of their anticholinergic properties.

2. *Anticholinergics* (block the action of acetylcholine)—given to relieve tremor and augment levodopa therapy.
   a. Frequently used anticholinergics include trihexyphenidyl (Artane and others); benztropine mesylate (Cogentin); ethopropazine (Parsidol); orphenadrine (Disipal).
   b. Assess for side effects of anticholinergic agents—dryness of mouth, blurred vision, urinary retention, constipation, mental confusion.
3. *Tricyclic antidepressants* (amitriptyline [Elavil])—to control depression associated with parkinsonism.
4. *Amantadine* (Symmetrel)—an antiviral drug that may increase release of dopamine in the brain.
5. *Levodopa* (Larodopa, Bendopa, Dopar)
   a. Levodopa (an amino acid which is depleted in the substance of the brain involved in nerve transmission in patients with parkinsonism) is given in increasing doses until patient's tolerance is reached; it relieves rigidity in majority of patients and usually improves tremor for a period of time.
   b. Dosage is increased gradually until maximum therapeutic effect is achieved and side effects appear—nausea, vomiting, anorexia, postural hypotension, mental changes (confusion, agitation, mood alterations), cardiac arrhythmias, twitching.
   c. Beneficial effects most pronounced in first few years of treatment; adverse effects may increase with continued use.
      (1) Abnormal involuntary movements (dyskinesia)—typically choreoathetoid in nature, affecting face and mouth initially, and then involving body and extremities.
      (2) On-off phenomena—sudden episodes of immobility ("off effect") lasting minutes to hours, followed by sudden return of effectiveness ("on effect").
      (3) Psychiatric reactions—confusion, memory impairment, hallucinations, delusions.
6. *Combination of levodopa and a decarboxylase inhibitor*—carbidopa, a decarboxylase inhibitor, slows down the peripheral metabolism of dopa.
   Sinemet (combination of carbidopa and levodopa)—potentiates therapeutic effects of levo-

dopa; appears to achieve a therapeutic effect with much lower dose of levodopa and thus reduces incidence of side effects.

7. *Dopamine Agonists*
   a. *Bromocriptine* (Parlodel)—crosses blood brain barrier and stimulates dopaminergic receptors.
      (1) Given when patient has intractable symptoms despite therapy with levodopa.
      (2) Adverse effects—confusion, delusions, hallucinations, gastrointestinal upset, abnormal involuntary movements.

B. *Exercise and Physical Therapy*

1. Encourage patient to continue on an exercise and physical therapy program to increase muscle strength, improve coordination and dexterity, treat muscular rigidity, prevent contractures, and compensate for lack of automatic movements.
2. Emphasize the importance of a *daily* exercise program (walk, ride stationary bike, swim, garden)—to maintain joint mobility.
   Instruct patient to:
   a. Exercise each joint daily
   b. Lengthen stride when walking; swing arms while walking—loosens arms and shoulders and lessens fatigue.
   c. Practice breathing exercises—to mobilize rib cage.
3. Advise patient to do stretching exercises (stretch-hold-relax) to loosen the joint structures.
4. Teach postural exercises and walking techniques to offset shuffling gait and tendency to lean forward:
   a. Use a broad-based gait (feet wide apart).
   b. Make a conscious effort to swing arms, raise the feet while walking, use a heel-toe, heel-toe gait, and increase the width of the stride.
5. Encourage patient to take warm baths, massage, and passive and active exercises—to help relax muscles and relieve painful muscle spasms that accompany rigidity.
6. Advise patient to have frequent rest periods—patient becomes fatigued and frustrated by his symptoms.
7. Try to have patient seen by a physical therapist on a regular basis—reinforces his program; introduces new program of exercises.

C. *Psychological Support*

1. Help patient establish achievable goals (improvement of health and mobility, lessening of tremors).

2. Encourage patient to be an *active* participant in his therapy and in social and recreational events—parkinsonism tends to lead to depression and withdrawal.
3. Have a planned program of activity throughout day—prevents daytime sleeping, disinterest, and apathy.
4. Reemphasize that disability can be prevented or delayed; offer realistic reassurance.
5. Try to dispel anxiety and fears of patient that may be as disabling to him as his disease.

Health Education

1. See A through C, pages 733–734.
2. Try the following routine when feet and legs seem to be "glued" to the floor.
   a. Raise head.
   b. Raise toes (eliminates muscle spasm).
   c. Rock from side to side while bending knees slightly.
   d. Or raise arms in a sudden, short motion.
3. Attempt to get out of a chair quickly, placing feet well apart, to overcome pull of gravity.
   For the patient who has difficulty rising up from a chair:
   a. Hold his hand and push forward (gently but firmly) on his head with the other hand.
   b. Choose straight-back wood chairs with armrests (captain's chair); raise rear legs of chair 2 inches to give chair a slight forward tilt.
4. Establish a regular bowel routine, consciously increase fluid intake, and eat foods with a moderate fiber content—patients with parkinsonism have trouble with constipation because of muscle weakness, lack of exercise, inadequate fluid intake, and drug effects.
5. Eat a well-balanced diet—nutritional problems develop from slowness of movement, difficulties in chewing and swallowing, and dry mouth from medications.
6. Avoid over-the-counter sedatives.
7. Learn all one can about Parkinson's disease. The American Parkinson Disease Foundation, 147 East 50th Street, New York, N.Y. 10022, has illustrated booklets and a newsletter for patient education.

MULTIPLE SCLEROSIS

Multiple sclerosis (MS) is a chronic, frequently progressive disease of the central nervous system characterized by the occurrence of small patches of demyelination in the brain and spinal cord. Demyelination results in disordered transmission of nerve impulses. (*Demyelination* refers to the destruction of myelin, the fatty and protein material that ensheathes certain nerve fibers in the brain and spinal cord.) There are numerous hypotheses concerning the etiology of MS; namely, infection by a slow virus, altered immunologic status, hereditary factors, epidemiologic factors, etc.

Clinical Manifestations

The signs and symptoms reflect the location and areas of demyelinization within the central nervous system. Patients with MS have a wide range of clinical symptoms; there is great variability in the course of the disease, with many remissions and exacerbations.

1. Weakness and sensory disturbances
2. Abnormal reflexes, either absent or hyper
3. Visual disturbances; impaired vision, diplopia
4. Tremor, ataxia, incoordination
5. Paresthesias
6. Sphincter impairment
7. Impaired vibration and position sense
8. Slurring, scanning speech (dysarthria)
9. Emotional lability; euphoria, depression

Incidence

Multiple sclerosis can be one of the most disabling of the neurologic diseases that strike young adults during their most productive years (20 to 40 years of age). It maximizes the medical, psychologic, social, and economic problems encountered by the patient and his family. However, a number of these patients have little or no disability for many years after diagnosis.

Objectives of Treatment and Nursing Management

OBJECTIVES: to keep the patient as active and functional as possible in order to lead a purposeful life.

to relieve the patient's symptoms and provide him with continuing support.

A. *To strengthen muscles and to prevent and treat muscle spasticity—spasticity interferes with normal function.*

1. Patient should do muscle stretching exercises daily—to minimize joint contractures.
   a. Give particular emphasis to hamstrings, gastrocnemius, hip adductors, biceps, wrist and finger flexors.
   b. Teach patient's family passive exercises and range of motion exercises for patients with severe spasticity.
   c. Teach the stretch-hold-relax routine and encourage patient to do it throughout the day for relaxation.
   d. Spasticity may also be treated with baclofen (Lioresal)
2. Advise patient to avoid muscle fatigue; stop physical activity just short of fatigue and take frequent short rest periods, preferably lying down.
3. Patient should do general body-strengthening exercises for correcting/preventing specific muscle weakness of disuse and for balance and coordination.
4. Prevent muscle contractures and loss of muscle power from lack of use—diminishing motor power is a significant problem in multiple sclerosis.
5. Encourage patient to sleep prone—to minimize flexor spasm at knees and hips.
6. Advise patient to participate in walking exercises—to improve gait affected by loss of position sense in legs.
7. Give muscle relaxants (diazepam) as directed.
8. Utilize braces, canes, crutches, walker when necessary—to keep patient ambulatory.
9. Prepare patients with severe spasticity and contractures for surgical intervention—to prevent further contractures and disability.

B. *To avoid skin pressure and immobility—since there is usually sensory loss, pressure sores accompany severe spasticity in an immobile patient.*

1. Relieve pressure.
   a. Change position at least every 2 hours if patient is in bed.
   b. Change position every 30 minutes if in wheelchair.
   c. Use flotation pad, sheepskin, alternating air pressure mattress, and other modalities to distribute pressure away from bony points and over a wider area.
   d. Teach patient to inspect pressure areas (using a long-handled mirror for posterior sites) for evidences of redness and heat.
2. Avoid skin trauma, heat, cold, and pressure.
3. Give careful attention to sacral and perineal hygiene.
4. See page 64 for discussion of prevention and treatment of pressure sores.

C. *To assist patient to overcome effects of incoordination—caused by motor dysfunction.*

1. Teach patient to walk with feet wider apart—to widen his base of support and increase his walking stability.
2. Have patient use a cane or walker.
3. Utilize weighted bracelets, wrist cuffs, eating utensils—to help overcome incoordination of upper extremities.

D. *To support the patient with bladder disturbances—bladder dysfunction may lead to progressive renal failure.*

1. See page 512 for management of patient with a neurogenic bladder.
2. Assess for urinary retention.
   a. Catheterize patient; insert indwelling catheter only if absolutely necessary.
   b. Give urinary antiseptics—to reduce incidence of bacteriuria.
3. Ensure adequate fluid intake (3–5 liters daily)—to reduce urinary bacterial count, minimize precipitation of urinary crystals and stone formation and encrustation of the lumen of the indwelling urethral catheter.
4. Support the patient who has urinary incontinence (or frequency and urgency).
   Female Patient
   a. Set up a voiding time schedule; every 1½ to 2 hours initially with lengthening time intervals if regimen is successful.
   b. Encourage the patient to drink a measured amount of fluid every 2 hours.
   c. Have the patient try to void 30 minutes after drinking.
   d. Use low fracture bedpan at night; set alarm clock for patient with diminished warning sensation.
   e. For permanent urinary incontinence, urine may have to be diverted by means of ileal conduit (see p. 516).
   Male Patient
   a. See a, b, c, under Female Patient, above.
   b. Use urinal at night.
   c. For permanent incontinence, patient may wear external sheath or condom appliance for urine collection.

E. *To place the patient on a bowel program if he has bowel incontinence.*

1. Establish a program of *regularity.*
   a. Have patient eat regularly scheduled meals; include high fiber foods.
   b. Establish bowel evacuation at *same time each day.*
2. Encourage patient to drink 120 ml. (4 ounces) of prune juice at bedtime (same time each night).
3. Insert a glycerin or Dulcolax suppository into the rectum 30 minutes before scheduled bowel evacuation time—*after* eating a meal (preferably after breakfast).
4. Advise patient to attempt to have a bowel movement within 30 minutes of eating, using as normal a position for defecation as possible.
   a. Instruct patient to bear down and contract abdominal muscles.
   b. Teach patient to apply pressure to abdomen with his hands—to assist with defecation.
5. After this routine is established, mechanical stimulation with a suppository may not be necessary.

F. *To treat the patient with appropriate therapy during periods of exacerbation—the residual effects of the disease may increase with each exacerbation.*

1. Give ACTH for short periods during acute exacer-

bations—may reduce severity of episode by reducing edema and inflammation.

2. Corticosteroids and cytotoxic agents may be prescribed for short treatment in chronic progressive MS patients to produce immunosuppression.
3. Encourage bed rest for a few days during acute exacerbation—continued activity appears to worsen attack.
4. Try to have patient avoid any known factor that causes exacerbation—allergy, infection, cold, etc.
5. Aim to prevent permanent damage; continue with range of motion exercises, specific muscle exercises, etc., as physical strength permits.
6. Take corrective action for each new problem as it arises.
7. Invent, adapt, and modify equipment that can be used for self-help devices so that patient will not regress.

G. *To help patient with optic and speech defects—cranial nerves affecting sight and speech are affected by multiple sclerosis.*

1. Utilize eye patch, frosted lens—to block visual impulses of one eye when patient has diplopia (double vision).
2. Secure services of speech pathologist or therapist—to strength the muscles of speech.
3. Prism glasses may be useful for bedridden person.
4. For person who has impaired eyesight or who is unable to hold book, turn pages, or read regular print, secure books and magazines recorded on discs, tape cassettes, and open reel magnetic tape provided free of charge by: Division for the Blind and Physically Handicapped, Library of Congress, Washington, D.C. 20542.

H. *To train patient in activities of daily living—to keep patient as independent as possible.*

1. Teach transfer activities (see p. 71).
2. Secure services of a knowledgeable wheelchair dealer to select correct wheelchair.
3. Use assistive and self-help devices.
   a. Toilet facilities—raised toilet seat or bedside commode
   b. Bathing facilities—use stool in shower or tub and hand rails
   c. Self-care aids—prism glasses, telephone modifications, long-handled combs, tongs, modified clothing.

Discharge Planning and Health Education

1. Review A through H, pages 735–736.
2. Help the family (and patient) understand the stresses imposed by multiple sclerosis.
   a. There are embarrassing and humiliating symptoms to which the person may respond "inappropriately."
   b. Patient may have brain damage with resultant denial of his disease, euphoria, or depressive and paranoid behavior.
   c. MS patients are often forgetful and easily distracted.
3. Understand that patients adapt to illness in many ways—frustration, anger, denial, depression, withdrawal, inactivity, resentment, etc.
4. Patient may have feelings of alienation from family, others, work, and social life; he feels that his personal worth is lessened.
   a. Try to keep him in the mainstream of life as much as possible.
   b. Contact local chapter of the National Multiple Sclerosis Society* for services, publications, and contact with other MS patients.
   c. Encourage patient to keep up social interests and activities.
5. Try to keep up the activities (physical, social, etc.) that patient is able to do; once lost, certain abilities are almost impossible to regain.
   a. Physical abilities may vary from day to day.
   b. Devise modifications that will allow continuance of certain activities; obtain gadgets and adaptive devices for self-help (mail-order gift companies, medical supply catalogs, rehabilitation literature).
6. Try to avoid physical and emotional stresses—may worsen symptoms and impair performance.
   a. Avoid exposure to heat/cold—appears to increase fatigue
   b. Avoid fatigue—lessens motor power
7. Assist the patient to accept his new identity as a handicapped person and cope with the disruption in his life.
8. Keep channels of communication open.
9. Offer meaningful and realistic short-term goals—to achieve a sense of purpose.

* National Multiple Sclerosis Society, 205 E. 42nd St., New York, N.Y. 10017.

MYASTHENIA GRAVIS

Myasthenia gravis is a disorder affecting the neuromuscular transmission of impulses in the voluntary muscles of the body; it is characterized by excessive fatigability of muscle function. Myasthenia gravis is considered to be an autoimmune disease in which acetylcholine receptor (AChR) antibodies are the principal factors interfering with neuromuscular transmission.

Altered Physiology

Defect in transmission of impulses from nerve to muscle cells due to loss of available or normal receptors on the postsynaptic side of neuromuscular junction.

Clinical Manifestations

1. Diplopia (double vision), ptosis (drooping of one or both eyelids)—from involvement of ocular muscles
2. Abnormal muscle weakness characteristically worse after effort and improved by rest; may involve any striated muscle
3. Sleepy, masklike expression—from involvement of facial muscles
4. Speech weakness, difficulty in swallowing, choking, aspiration of food—from weakness of laryngeal and pharyngeal muscles

Diagnostic Evaluation

1. Pharmacological tests:
   a. Edrophonium (Tensilon) test—intravenous injection of edrophonium may relieve weakness markedly in 30 seconds; useful for patients with ocular, facial, or oroparygeal weakness
   b. Neostigmine methylsulfate (Prostigmin) test—given to evaluate extremity strength; positive result evidenced by increase in muscular strength about 30 minutes after injection; permits measurement of changes in strength of all muscles
2. Electromyographic testing (EMG) to measure electrical potential of muscle cells
3. Chest x-ray—to rule out thymoma (tumor of the thymus)

Treatment and Nursing Management

OBJECTIVE: to increase muscle strength.

A. *Primary Drug Therapy.*

1. Anticholinesterase drugs—will increase response of muscles to nerve impulses and improve strength; by temporarily inhibiting acetylcholinesterase at the neuromuscular junction, they enhance the action of acetylcholine there.
   a. Pyridostigmine bromide (Mestinon)
   b. Ambenonium chloride (Mytelase)
   c. Neostigmine bromide (Prostigmin)
2. Drug given exactly on time to control symptoms; a delay in drug administration may result in patient's losing his ability to swallow.
3. Toxicity and side effects of anticholinesterase:
   a. Gastrointestinal—abdominal cramps, nausea, vomiting, diarrhea.
      (1) Drug may be taken with small amount of milk, crackers, or other buffering substance or after meals.
      (2) Side effects may be ameliorated or prevented by addition of atropine or atropine-like drugs to regimen.
      (3) Give diphenoxylate hydrochloride (Lomotil) for diarrhea.
   b. Skeletal—fasciculations (fine twitching), spasm, weakness.
   c. Central nervous system—irritability, anxiety, insomnia, headache, dysarthria, syncope, coma, convulsions.
   d. Other—increased salivation and lacrimation, increased bronchial secretions, moist skin.

> **NURSING ALERT:** Watch for increase in muscle weakness within one hour after taking anticholinesterase drug; be alert for signs of respiratory embarrassment.

4. After initial medication adjustment has been made, patient learns to take his medication according to his needs. Individual doses may vary with physical or emotional stress, intercurrent infection, etc.
5. Anticholinesterase drugs are not to be taken with morphine, ether, quinine (commerical cold preparations), procainamide, and certain antibiotics.
6. Sedatives and tranquilizing drugs are given with caution; may aggravate hypoxia and hypercapnia and cause respiratory and cardiac depression.

7. Steroid therapy—may be of great benefit to patient with severe generalized myasthenia.

B. *Surgical Intervention (Thymectomy)*—may give improvement or remission of the disease, especially in patients with tumor or hyperplasia of the thymus gland.

1. May be carried out by transcervical or sternal-splitting procedure.
2. Preoperative evaluation includes assessment of respiratory status (tidal volume, vital capacity), muscular strength, and patient's chewing, swallowing, and ocular movements.
3. Postoperative nursing management (in intensive care unit) includes:
   a. Monitoring and caring for patient on mechanical ventilator, if needed.
   b. Continuing assessment of ventilatory function
   c. Temporary cessation of anticholinesterase medications

C. *Plasmapheresis (plasma exchange)*—removal of the plasma containing acetylcholine receptor antibodies to improve muscle strength temporarily in patients with severe symptoms who do not respond to other treatment.

D. *Crises in Myasthenia Gravis—sudden exacerbation of weakness that may endanger life.*

1. Sudden respiratory distress combined with varying signs of dysphagia (difficulty in swallowing), dysarthria (difficulty in speaking), eyelid ptosis, and diplopia are indications of impending crisis.
2. Types of crises in myasthenia gravis.
   a. Myasthenic crisis—may result from natural deterioration of disease, emotional upset, upper respiratory infection, surgery, or trauma; or may be brought about by ACTH therapy.
      Patient may be temporarily resistant to anticholinesterase drugs or may need increased dosage.
   b. Cholinergic crisis—from overmedication with anticholinergic drugs.
   c. Brittle crisis—occurs when the receptors at the neuromuscular junction become insensitive to anticholinesterase medication; not controlled by increasing or decreasing anticholinesterase therapy.
3. Nursing and Medical Management During Crisis.
   a. Place patient in intensive care unit for constant monitoring—myasthenia gravis is a disease of rapidly fluctuating intensity and patient is on verge of respiratory arrest.
   b. Provide ventilatory assistance when muscles of respiration and swallowing become involved; endotracheal intubation and mechanical ventilation may be needed.
      (1) Suction patient as indicated—*aspiration is a common problem*
      (2) See Chapter 7 for management of patient requiring ventilatory support.
   c. Determine the time of onset of symptoms in relation to the last dose of anticholinesterase—may show whether patient is undermedicated or having a cholinergic reaction.
      Tensilon may be given to differentiate type of crisis; Tensilon (IV) improves patient in myasthenic crisis, temporarily worsens patient in cholinergic crisis, and is unpredictable in brittle crisis.

d. Give appropriate drugs as determined by patient's status:
   (1) For myasthenic crisis: Neostigmin methylsulfate (Prostigmin) administered parenterally if patient is in true myasthenic crisis.
   (2) For cholinergic crisis: all anticholinesterase drugs are withdrawn. Atropine may be given to reduce excessive secretions.
e. Administer fluids, medication, and food via nasogastric tube if patient is unable to swallow.
f. Avoid giving enemas—may cause sudden collapse.
g. Develop a communication system for patient on ventilator (or if he is too weak to speak).
   (1) Try to read lips of patient.
   (2) Use picture cards, hand signals, etc.
   (3) Give hand bell to patient.
h. Give continuing psychological support since patient is usually alert and anxious. Reassure him that the crisis will pass and that he will not be left alone.

Health Education

Instruct the patient as follows:
1. Know the basic facts about anticholinergic drugs: action, reason for and importance of timing, dosage adjustment, symptoms of overdose, and toxic effects. Know the drugs that interact with anticholinesterase drugs.
2. Have mealtimes coincide with peak of anticholinesterase effect (when swallowing ability is best); have standby suction available in home if swallowing difficulties occur. (Use a blender when necessary.)
3. Wear an identification bracelet signifying that you have myasthenia gravis.
4. Try to prevent factors (emotional upset, infections) which may increase weakness and precipitate myasthenic crisis.
5. Wear an eyepatch over one eye (alternating from side to side) if diplopia occurs.
6. Avoid vigorous physical activity and other factors leading to fatigue.
7. Avoid contracting colds and influenza—respiratory infections are extremely dangerous to the myasthenic individual.
8. Avoid excessive heat and cold (hot baths, sun bathing); weak spells may follow long exposure to excessive heat/cold.
9. Advise the dentist that you are myasthenic, since Novocain is usually not well tolerated.
10. Rest before fatigue sets in; do not force yourself to continue with an activity.
11. Use adaptive and self-help devices to handle motion impairment problems.
12. Learn all you can about the condition; with good management the patient should be able to live a relatively full life. The Myasthenia Gravis Foundation, Inc., 230 Park Avenue, New York, N.Y. 10007.

AMYOTROPHIC LATERAL SCLEROSIS (ALS, LOU GEHRIG'S DISEASE)

Amyotrophic lateral sclerosis is a progressively incapacitating and fatal disease of unknown cause in which there is loss of motor neurons (nerve cells controlling muscles) in the anterior horns of the spinal cord and the motor nuclei of the lower brain stem. There is usually progressive paralysis with death occurring within 3–5 years after onset.

Clinical Manifestations

(Depends on location of affected motor neurons, since specific neurons activate specific muscle fibers.)
1. Progressive weakness and atrophy of muscles of arms, trunk, or legs—from loss of neurons of the spinal cord
2. Progressive difficulty in speaking and swallowing; nasal and unintelligible speech—when bulbar muscles are affected

Treatment and Nursing Management

OBJECTIVE: to support the patient and improve quality of life.
1. Teach patient active exercises and range of motion exercises—to strengthen uninvolved muscles that can substitute for impaired ones; to prevent disuse weakness.
2. Instruct the patient to use energy conservation and work simplification methods; use self-help and assistive devices.
3. Use orthoses (braces) (p. 75) to help patient function as long as possible.
   a. Ankle-foot orthoses for weak dorsiflexors—help keep patient mobile.
   b. Hand splints—for optimal joint position and to provide a stronger grip.
4. Help family to secure equipment to assist with care—hospital bed, mechanical lift, wheelchair, catapult spring seats.
   a. Teach family positioning, turning, and transfer techniques.
   b. Teach pressure sore prevention. See Rehabilitation Nursing Chapter, page 64.
5. Watch for symptoms of respiratory failure—occurs late in the disease. See page 169 for management.
6. Use techniques to assist patient with bulbar symptoms (choking, difficulty in swallowing and speaking).
   a. Have standby suction available—*aspiration* is a constant danger.
   b. Drink and eat in an upright position with neck flexed.
   c. Use a soft cervical collar if patient has difficulty holding his head up.
   d. Give semi-soft foods; avoid easily aspirated pureed foods and mucus-producing foods (milk).
   e. Consider nasogastric or gastrostomy feeding.
   f. Understand that patient may have outbursts of laughing/crying.
   g. Develop some form of a communication system when speech is lost—eye movement and eye blinks may be patient's only means of communication.
   h. Remember that the patient is alert and retains vision, ocular movement, intelligence, and consciousness even though he is paralyzed and cannot speak/swallow.
7. Give the patient and family compassionate and caring support.
   a. Allow expressions of feelings and frustrations about losses and eventual outcome.
   b. Depression is normal and expected.

8. Advise patient/family of helping services of ALS Society of America, 15300 Ventura Blvd., Suite 315, Sherman Oaks, Calif. 91403 (pamphlets, newsletter, patient care tips), and Muscular Dystrophy Association, 810 Seventh Ave., New York, N.Y. 10019 (services and equipment).

POLYRADICULITIS (GUILLAIN-BARRÉ SYNDROME; INFECTIOUS POLYNEURITIS)

Polyradiculitis is a clinical syndrome of unknown cause involving the peripheral nervous system and cranial nerves; it is characterized by paresthesias of the extremities and by muscle weakness or paralysis. It may be due to an allergic or immunologic reaction and is frequently preceded by an infection.

Clinical Manifestations

1. Paresthesia (tingling and numbness) of lower extremities
2. Muscle weakness of legs—may progress to rapidly ascending paralysis involving the trunk, upper extremities, and facial muscles (complete paralysis)
3. Difficulty in chewing, swallowing, and talking—from cranial nerve involvement
4. Loss of sensation and sphincter disturbances of bladder and rectum
5. Absence of deep tendon reflexes

Treatment and Nursing Management

OBJECTIVE: to support respiration when rapidly ascending paralysis develops.
1. Monitor vital capacity, since respiratory failure is a common cause of death.
   a. Watch for breathlessness while talking, shallow and irregular breathing, increasing pulse rate, and *change* in the respiratory pattern.
   b. Place patient on mechanical ventilator when he shows signs of respiratory insufficiency (p. 193)—may require prolonged controlled mechanical ventilation.
2. Monitor for dysphagia resulting from respiratory paralysis—patient cannot cough normally and is at risk of choking to death; use nasogastric tube for feeding.
3. Monitor for cardiac arrhythmias—cardiac arrest may occur if vagus nerve becomes affected.
4. Watch for urinary retention—thought to be due to involvement of autonomic fibers passing through the sacral nerve roots.
5. Give corticosteroids; may be of value if given early in course of disease.
6. Put extremities through range of motion; use nursing support to prevent contractures, pressure sores. (See Rehabilitation Nursing Chapter, p. 53.)
7. Establish some form of communication (eye blinking, lip reading)—patient is unable to talk, laugh, or cry because of paralysis, tracheostomy, intubation.

Health Education

There may be a rather lengthy convalescence; patients usually recover in 3 to 6 months; a few have sequelae lasting up to several years.

SPINAL CORD INJURY

Spinal cord injury may vary from a mild cord concussion with transient numbness to immediate and permanent quadriplegia. The most common sites are the cervical areas C-5, C-6, and C-7 and the junction of the thoracic and lumbar vertebrae (T-12, L-1). Traumatic injury of the spinal cord may result in loss of function (paralysis) below the level of cord injury. There is usually a high frequency of associated injuries and medical complications.

Causes

1. Trauma—automobile and motorcycle accidents, falls, diving and surfing injuries, gunshot wounds, hard contact sports—may cause compression, contusion, or laceration of the cord, hemorrhage into its substance, or compression of its vascular supply.

Clinical Manifestations

1. Total sensory loss and motor paralysis below level of injury
2. Loss of bowel and bladder control; usually urinary retention and bladder distention
3. Loss of sweating and vasomotor tone below level of cord lesion
4. Marked reduction of blood pressure—from loss of peripheral and vascular resistance
5. Neck pain; back pain
6. Priapism—persistent erection of penis

Pathogenesis of Spinal Cord Injury

1. Damage to the spinal cord ranges from transient concussion to contusion, laceration, and compression (either alone or in combination), to complete transection of the cord.
2. The cord's response to injury is ischemia, edema, and hemorrhage that lead to an irreversible cycle of progressive destruction unless there is appropriate intervention.

Treatment and Nursing Management

OBJECTIVES: to reduce the fracture dislocation and obtain immobilization of the spine as soon as possible to prevent cord damage. to observe for symptoms of progressive neurologic damage.
1. See page 881 for moving the patient from the scene of the accident on a transfer board.
2. Transfer the patient to a Stryker frame. (If none is available, place on a firm mattress with a bedboard under the mattress.)
   a. Keep patient in an extended position—do not allow body to be twisted or turned.

b. Place patient (who is strapped to a transfer board) directly on the posterior frame of a Stryker frame.

c. Place a blanket roll between the patient's legs.

d. Place anterior frame in position. Secure frame straps.

e. Turn the patient to the prone position.

f. Remove frame straps, head bandage, and posterior frame. Remove transfer board.

3. Assess the breathing pattern and maintain airway—patients with injuries at high levels are at risk for respiratory failure.

a. Assess strength of cough.

b. Measure vital capacity—a guide to respiratory insufficiency.

c. Intubate patient with extreme care; do not flex the neck—can result in extension of cord injury.

4. Evaluate the patient constantly for motor and sensory changes—motor and sensory loss occurs from cord edema, hemorrhage, etc., which may further compromise cord function. Document findings carefully.

a. Test motor ability by requesting the patient to spread his fingers, squeeze examiner's hand, move toes, etc.

b. Test sensation by pinching the skin, starting at shoulder level and progressing down the sides of all extremities. Ascertain when patient feels pinching sensation.

c. Note presence/absence of level of sweating.

5. Report immediately any decrease in neurologic function.

a. Keep a neurologic assessment record (flow sheet).

b. Observe for symptoms of progressive neurologic damage—symptoms of cord compression depend on level at which compression occurs. Clinical symptoms of cord compression are indistinguishable from those of cord edema.

(1) Loss of sensation

(2) Inability to move extremities

6. Prepare for laminectomy if progressive symptoms of cord compression occur—permits direct exploration and decompression of cord (p. 743).

7. Evaluate for presence of spinal shock—spinal shock represents a sudden loss of continuity between spinal cord and higher nerve centers. There is a complete loss of all reflex, motor, sensory, and autonomic activity below the level of the lesion.

a. Falling blood pressure

b. Paralysis and lack of sensation below level of cord injury

c. Bladder distention—from paralysis of bladder

d. Bowel distention—caused by depression of reflexes; retroperitoneal hemorrhage may occur with fracture of low back, producing paralytic ileus

8. Maintain the patient's body defenses until shock remits and the system has recovered from the traumatic insult. (Spinal shock is temporary, but may last several weeks.)

a. Support the airway, especially in cervical cord injury.

b. Support circulation—give blood transfusions as indicated.

c. Avoid overdistention of bladder—after spinal injury, the bladder may lack functional nerve supply; overstretching of bladder may produce permanent damage. (Urinary tract infection is common cause of death after spinal injury.)

(1) Utilize intermittent catheterization early in acute phase if possible, or insert indwelling catheter.

(2) See page 512 for management of neurogenic bladder.

d. Treat for acute gastric dilatation and ileus.

(1) Observe for abdominal distention and listen with stethoscope for presence or absence of peristaltic sounds.

(2) Initiate gastric suction to reduce distention and prevent vomiting and aspiration.

(3) Give neostigmine methylsulfate—for severe bowel distention.

(4) Administer rectal tube to relieve gaseous distention.

(5) Give intravenous infusions for fluid replacement; avoid overloading the labile cardiovascular system.

(6) Place patient on bowel training regimen as required (see p. 76).

Definitive Management of Patient With Cervical Spinal Injury

To manage a cervical spine injury there must be immediate immobilization, early reduction and stabilization.

1. To reduce the fracture dislocation and maintain alignment of the cervical spine, some form of skeletal traction with skull calipers or tongs is applied, or the halo-cast or halo-vest technique is used. OR the patient may require open reduction (surgery); measures will still be required to maintain reduction.

Skeletal Tongs

a. A variety of skeletal tongs in use—Crutchfield, Barton, and Vinke tongs, all of which are inserted into the skull through holes made with a special drill under local anesthesia. The Gardner-Wells tongs require no predrilled holes; pins are tightened by hand.

b. Traction is applied to the tongs by weights (4.5 to 9 kg.—10–20 lbs.) or more, depending on the patient's size.

c. The traction is gradually increased by addition of weights—as the amount of traction is increased, the spaces between the intervertebral discs widen and the vertebrae slip back into position. Reduction will take place after correct alignment has been regained.

d. X-rays are taken after each addition of weight until reduction is obtained; monitor patient carefully as weights are added.

e. When reduction is obtained, the weights are gradually removed until the amount of weight needed to maintain the alignment is obtained.

f. Keep traction tongs several inches from top of bed and allow weights to hang free—to prevent interference with traction.

2. Watch for signs of infection, including drainage around the tongs.

3. Check back of head periodically for signs of pressure; massage back of head periodically.

4. Give back care by pressing down on the mattress with one hand and washing and massaging with the other.

5. Duration of cervical traction depends on severity and mechanism of injury; usually a minimum of 6 weeks.

6. Fitted molded collar usually applied when patient is mobilized after traction is removed.

Halo Traction

a. Halo traction devices consist of a stainless steel "halo ring" which fits around the head and is attached to the skull by four skull pins inserted through threaded holes in the ring. It can be connected to a plaster body cast or to a plaster halo vest or girdle which suspends the weight of the unit circumferentially around the chest.
   (1) Patient may be intially distressed by bizarre appearance of halo; usually adapts readily to device.
   (2) Anticipate some inflammation and drainage around the pin sites; patient may experience a slight headache or minor pain around the skull pins for several days following application.
   (3) Cleanse around the pin sites daily and shorten patient's hair periodically.
   (4) Have torque screwdriver readily available in the event that the screws on the frame need tightening.

Other Aspects of Management

1. Prevent pressure sores—inadequate peripheral circulation from spinal shock can cause pressure ulcer to develop within 6 hours.
   a. Patients with initial vasovagal instability as well as associated injury may not be able to tolerate positional changes because of episodes of cardiopulmonary arrest.
   b. Pressure on the denervated skin will sooner or later result in tissue breakdown. Spasticity, friction, and poor nutrition are contributing factors.
   c. *Objective:* to avoid ischemia of the skin.
      (1) Turn every 2 hours, using turning frame, if patient can be turned. Inspect vulnerable skin areas.
      (2) See page 64 for prevention and treatment.
2. Maintain patient in proper alignment to prevent contracture deformities.

Dorsal or Supine Position

a. Position feet against padded footboard—to prevent footdrop.
b. Be sure there is a space between end of mattress and foot of bed—to allow for free suspension of the heels.
c. Apply trochanter rolls from crest of ilium to midthigh of both extremities—to prevent external rotation of the hip joints.
d. Initiate passive range of motion exercises for affected extremities within 48–72 hours *upon order*—to preserve joint motion.
e. Ambulate only upon physician's request—if patient has partial cord function, activity may produce further cord injury.
3. Assess for complications.
   a. Vein thrombosis or pulmonary embolism—from immobilization, muscular and vaso-motor paralysis, factors affecting blood coagulation (hypoproteinemia, infection, etc.).
   b. Hyperthermia—during period of spinal shock, patient does not perspire on the paralyzed portions of his body since sympathetic activity is blocked.

c. Autonomic dysreflexia (autonomic hyperreflexia)—syndrome occurring in patients with spinal cord lesions at or above T_6. Characterized by exaggerated autonomic responses to stimuli: distended bladder or bowel, stimulation of skin (tactile, pain, thermal stimuli), distention or contraction of visceral organs; may be accompanied by immediate and dangerous elevation of arterial blood pressure.
   (1) Syndrome characterized by pounding headache, profuse sweating, nasal congestion, piloerection (goose flesh), bradycardia, severe hypertension.
   (2) Treatment

> **NURSING ALERT:** Autonomic dysreflexia (autonomic hyperreflexia) is considered an emergency.

OBJECTIVE: to remove the triggering stimulus and avoid possible serious complications.
   (a) Place patient in sitting position—to help lower the blood pressure.
   (b) Drain the bladder via catheter. (Do not irrigate catheter with more than 30 ml. of irrigating solution.)
   (c) Insert Nupercainal ointment in rectum if fecal mass is present. (Mass is removed manually *after* symptoms subside.)
   (d) Remove any other stimuli that may be triggering episodes; cold air, object on skin, etc.
   (e) Give ganglionic blocking agent slowly IV, if elevated blood pressure does not respond immediately to above measures. Monitor blood pressure.
   (f) Tag patient's chart with an "Allergic" marker; patient is apt to have another episode of hyperreflexia.
d. Contractures.
e. Kidney and bladder infections.
f. Depression.
g. Endocrine, nutritional, metabolic diseases.
h. Stress ulcers.
4. See Paraplegia for psychological support, page 744 and page 745 for sexual counseling.
5. Employ active rehabilitation procedures when patient's spine is stable enough to assume upright position or following surgery involving stabilizing procedures.
   a. Program is designed according to neurological deficit.
   b. *Objective:* to strengthen muscles still innervated or when return of function is evident.
      (1) An exercise conditioning regimen is started early.
      (2) Muscle strengthening exercises for shoulder depressors, maintenance of sitting balance, getting up and down from wheelchair, or whatever is possible for individual patient.
      (3) Period of immobilization determined by patient's condition (usually 6 weeks on a turning frame and 6 weeks of gradual mobilization with brace or cast, depending on level of lesion, etc.).

HERNIATION OF INTERVERTEBRAL DISC (RUPTURED DISC)

Herniation of the intervertebral disc is a protrusion of the nucleus of the disc into the annulus (fibrous ring around the disc), with subsequent nerve compression. The herniation may occur in any portion of the spine.

Types of Disc Herniation

1. Cervical
2. Lumbar
3. Thoracic (rare)

Causes

1. Degeneration
2. Trauma (accidents, strain, repeated minor stresses)
3. Congenital predisposition

Clinical Manifestations

Depend on location, size, rate of development (acute or chronic), and effect on surrounding structures

A. *Cervical Disc*

1. Pain and stiffness in neck, top of shoulders, and in region of scapulae
2. Pain in upper extremities and head
3. Paresthesia and numbness of upper extremities

B. *Lumbar Disc*

1. Low back pain accompanied by varying degrees of sensory and motor impairment
2. Pain in buttock and thigh radiating to calf and ankle—aggravated by actions that increase intraspinal pressure (sneezing, straining, lifting)
3. Postural deformity of lumbar spine
4. Pain induced by stretching sciatic nerve
   a. Place patient on his back with his knees straight.
   b. Raise the unflexed leg (one at a time).
   c. This maneuver causes stretching of sciatic nerve that is transmitted to nerve roots, producing pain that radiates into the leg.
   d. Patient will experience little or no pain if leg is raised while bent at the knee since this relaxes tension on sciatic nerve.
   e. Lasègue's sign—pain with straight-leg raising and absence of pain with bent-leg raising.
5. Muscle weakness
6. Alterations in tendon reflexes
7. Sensory loss

Diagnostic Evaluation

1. X-ray of spine—to rule out other lesions that cause similar signs and symptoms
2. Computed tomography
3. Myelogram—demonstrates area of pressure and localizes herniation of disc; disc protrusion is seen as indentation of contrast medium
4. Electromyography—localizes specific spinal nerve involved
5. Lumbar venogram

Treatment and Nursing Management

A. *Cervical Disc;* usually occurs at C5–6 or C6–7.

OBJECTIVES: to rest and immobilize the cervical spine to allow for healing of soft tissues.
to reduce inflammation in supporting tissues and affected nerve roots in the cervical spine.

1. Immobilize and rest the cervical spine by one of the following methods:
   a. Cervical collar—allows maximal opening of intervertebral foramina.
      (1) Collar should hold the head in a neutral or slightly flexed position.
      (2) Inspect under the collar at intervals for skin rash.
      (3) In acute herniation the collar may have to be worn night and day until pain subsides (2–3 weeks).
      (4) Cervical isometric exercises are started when patient is pain-free—to strengthen neck musculature in preparation for "weaning" from collar.
   b. Cervical traction (accomplished by head halter attached to a pulley and a weight)—increases vertebral separation and thus relieves pressure on the nerve roots.
      (1) Cervical traction should be comfortable.
      (2) Keep head of bed elevated and make sure that traction is in alignment.
      (3) Inspect for skin burns from cervical halter; pad under the halter as necessary.
      (4) Encourage male patient not to shave since beard offers a form of padding; shaving may cause irritation.
   c. Bed rest—reduces inflammation and edema in soft tissues around disc, relieving pressure on nerve roots; relieves cervical spine of supporting weight of head.
   d. Brace
2. Give muscle relaxant—to interrupt cycle of muscle spasm and allow for patient comfort; to increase range of motion of cervical spine.
3. Administer anti-inflammatory medications, e.g., aspirin, phenylbutazone (Butazolidin), oxyphenbutazone (Tandearil), or steroids—to treat inflammatory response.
   a. Give food or antacid with anti-inflammatory agents—to prevent gastrointestinal irritation.
   b. Take periodic blood counts—to watch for development of blood dyscrasias.
4. Give analgesics and sedatives—to control discomfort and anxiety often associated with cervical disc disease.
5. Apply moist hot compresses (10–20 minutes, several times daily) to back of neck—to increase blood flow to muscles and help relax patient and spastic muscles.
6. Prepare for surgical intervention if significant neurologic deficit from nerve root compression occurs, for unremitting and recurrent pain, or for signs of cord compression.
7. *Discharge Planning and Health Education* (cervical disc) It may take 6 weeks to recuperate from significant disc herniation.
   Instruct the patient as follows:
   a. Avoid extreme flexion, extension, and rotation of the neck while working.
   b. Keep head in a neutral position while sleeping.
      (1) Pillow should be filled with feathers or down.
      (2) Sleep on side or back; do not sleep prone.
      (3) Avoid excessive neck flexion—do not prop up in bed with several pillows.
   c. Avoid excessive automobile riding during acute phase—vibration has adverse effect on spine.

B. *Lumbar Disc*—majority of herniations occur at L4—L5 or L5—S1 interspace.

OBJECTIVES: to relieve the pain and slow the progress of the disease.

to increase the functional ability of the patient.

1. Encourage the patient to remain on bed rest—disc is freed from stress when the patient is horizontal.
   a. Place patient in position of comfort—usually semi-Fowler's with moderate hip and knee flexion.
   b. Place hinged bedboard under mattress—to limit spinal flexion.
   c. Help patient to ambulate (usually after 2 weeks bed rest) when inflammatory reaction and edema from disc herniation have subsided.
   d. Use corset or brace if necessary to mobilize patient (for obese patient with poor abdominal musculature).
2. Use appropriate drug therapy and physical therapy.
   a. Muscle relaxants—muscle spasm is prominent in acute phase.
   b. Anti-inflammatory drugs—to counter inflammation occurring in supporting tissues and nerve roots.
   c. Analgesic agents—to relieve patient's acute pain.
   d. Utilize heat and massage—to relax muscle spasm; also provides analgesia.
3. Watch for development of neurologic deficit.
   a. Muscle weakness and atrophy
   b. Loss of sensory and motor function
   c. Unrelieved acute pain
4. Have the patient increase activities gradually if his symptoms abate.
5. Prepare for surgical intervention when indicated (hemilaminectomy with removal of ruptured disc). Indications for operative intervention include compression of cauda equina (motor and sensory paresis, loss of sphincter control), nerve root compression, and lack of response to conservative therapy.
   a. Patients with multilevel involvement may have recurrences of pain and disability and may require reoperation(s).
   b. Spinal fusion may be required on reoperation.
6. Chemonucleolysis—injection of chymopapain into diseased disc; has a proteolytic action that dissolves the nucleus pulposus, reducing the pressure on the adjacent nerve roots (investigational).
7. *Discharge Planning and Health Education*
   a. Encourage patient to do exercises after acute symptoms subside: (1) exercises to strengthen abdominal muscles and (2) gentle stretching exercises to improve the suppleness and elasticity of the paraspinal muscles and ligaments.
      (1) Start exercises gently and gradually.
      (2) Discontinue exercises if pain worsens.
   b. Advise patient to sleep on side with knees and hips flexed (pillow between knees).
      (1) Do not sleep in prone position—hyperextends the spine.
      (2) Pick up loads correctly (bend knees, keep back straight, avoid lifting anything above the elbows) and keep load close to body.
      (3) Avoid lifting while back is in a flexed or rotated position.
   c. Encourage proper posture while standing, sitting, walking, and working.
   d. A lumbar sacral support (corset) may be necessary for persons with poor abdominal musculature—serves to pull in abdomen and alter lumbar-sacral curve, which relieves strain on ligaments.
   e. Carry out weight control program—obese patient with protruding abdomen and lordotic posture has chronic back strain.
   f. See also health education, low back pain, page 784

MANAGEMENT OF THE PATIENT FOLLOWING DISC SURGERY

Surgical excision of a herniated disc is done when there is evidence of a progressive neurologic deficit (muscle weakness and atrophy, loss of sensory and motor function, loss of sphincter control), and continuing pain and sciatica. Microsurgical techniques are now making it possible to remove a herniated nucleus pulposus through a small incision without a laminectomy.

Diskectomy—removal of herniated disc tissue and related matter.

Laminectomy—removal of the lamina to expose the neural elements in the spinal canal. It allows inspection of the spinal canal and identification and removal of pathology and compression from the cord and roots.

Laminotomy—division of the lamina of a vertebra.

Spinal fusion—bone graft is used to fuse the vertebral spinous processes; the object of spinal fusion is to bridge over the defective disc so as to stabilize the spine.

Postoperative Nursing Management

OBJECTIVE: to relieve pressure on nerve root in order to relieve pain.

(See also the postoperative principles for patient undergoing orthopedic surgery, p. 775).

A. *Cervical Disc*

1. Check neurologic and vital signs at frequent intervals—there is always the possibility of respiratory difficulty, and hoarseness from recurrent laryngeal nerve injury, resulting in the inability to cough effectively and eliminate respiratory secretions.
2. Be aware that a sore throat will be a major complaint.
   a. Give throat spray (Chloraseptic spray) as directed to relieve pain.
   b. Do not give any spray or throat lozenges that numb the throat, since this may cause choking.
   c. Observe for pulmonary secretions since patient may be afraid to cough because of pain from sore throat.

B. *Lumbar Disc*

1. Check vital signs and inspect wound for evidence of hemorrhage—vascular injury is a complication of disc surgery.
2. Assess sensation, motor power, color and temperature of lower extremities—postoperative neurologic deficits may result from nerve root injury.

3. Assess for signs of urinary retention.
4. Position the patient effectively.
   a. Use pillow under head and elevate the knee rest slightly—slight knee flexion relaxes muscles of the back.
   b. Encourage the patient to move and turn from side to side to relieve pressure.
      (1) Turn patient as a unit (log rolling); place pillow between his legs while turning.
      (2) Place pillow between legs when patient is lying on his side.
      (3) Avoid extreme knee flexion when patient is on side.
5. Encourage early ambulation as soon as patient is able. To get the patient out of bed:
   a. Raise head of bed as patient lies on his side.
   b. Support patient's head and shoulders while he pushes up to a sitting position while another person eases his legs over the side of the bed.
   c. Advise him to move from sitting to standing position in one smooth motion.
6. Give narcotics and sedatives to relieve pain and anxiety; discomfort in immediate post-operative period may vary from mild to severe pain.
7. Explain to the patient that there may be varying degrees of pain and sensory mainfestations in the legs (sciatica type pain) due to temporary inflammatory changes, edema, and swelling of compressed nerve.

Discharge Planning and Health Education

1. It may take 6 weeks for ligamentous attachments of the muscles and skin to heal.
2. Instruct the patient as follows:
   a. Increase activities as tolerated—move up to the point of individual tolerance.
   b. Avoid activities that produce flexion strain on the spine—stair climbing, automobile riding.
   c. Have scheduled rest periods.
   d. Apply heat to back when indicated—helps absorb exudates in the tissues; tub bathing is helpful.
   e. Avoid heavy work for 2–3 months after surgery.
   f. Resume exercises to strengthen abdominal and erector spinae muscles as directed.
   g. A brace or corset may have to be worn if back pain persists.
3. See health teaching for herniation of intervertebral disc, page 743, and management of low back pain, page 783.

PARAPLEGIA

Paraplegia is loss of motion and sensation in the lower extremities.

Quadriplegia is loss of motion and sensation involving both upper and lower extremities.

Causes
1. Trauma—accidents, gunshot wounds
2. Spinal cord lesions (intervertebral disc, tumor, vascular lesions)
3. Multiple sclerosis
4. Infections and abscesses of spinal cord
5. Congenital defects

Nursing Management
1. See nursing management of the patient with spinal cord injuries for immediate management principles, page 739.
2. Understand the psychological significance of the disability.
   a. Support the patient through his stages of adjustment to injury—shock and disbelief, denial, depression, grief, acknowledgement, and adaptation.
   b. Allow the patient to work through his feelings about his disability at his own pace (unless his responses continue to be exaggerated or maladaptive).
      (1) Realization of the finality of paraplegia or quadriplegia may prolong the grief process.
      (2) Patient experiences a loss of self-esteem in areas of self-identity, sexual identity, and social and emotional roles.
   c. Be aware that the patient may take 1 of 2 courses:
      (1) Acceptance of disability leading to development of realistic goals for the future.
      (2) Rejection of disability—may exhibit self-destructive neglect, noncompliance with therapeutic program.

Patient and family may require supportive psychotherapy and additional recreational therapy to prevent social and intellectual isolation.
3. Prepare for weight-bearing activities—patient with complete cord severance should start early weight bearing to decrease osteoporotic changes in long bones and to reduce incidence of urinary infections and the formation of renal calculi.
   a. Apply elastic hose from toes to thigh or a Jobst counterpressure leotard—to prevent pooling of blood in abdominal area; a patient with spinal cord paralysis lacks vasomotor tone in the lower extremities and will become hypotensive in the upright position.
   b. Use tilt table—to help patient overcome vasomotor instability and tolerate upright posture (p. 70).
      (1) Start with elevation of 45 degrees and gradually increase angle of elevation over a period of days.
      (2) Take blood pressure immediately before and as soon as patient is positioned on tilt table.
      (3) Observe for nausea and excessive perspiration, pallor, dizziness, or syncope.
   c. *Or* use high-back reclining wheelchair with extension leg rests; raise backrest slowly and lower leg rest gradually over a period of 7–10 days.
4. Initiate bladder training program. See neurogenic bladder, page 512.
5. Start bowel training program.
   a. Objective is to obtain reflex bowel evacuation by conditioning.
   b. See page 76 for bowel training process.
6. Build the unaffected part of body to optimal strength, endurance and coordination—to prepare for transfer and mobilization activities.

a. Weight lifting, manual resistance, etc., are employed.
b. Encourage patient to continue with muscle strengthening exercises for hands, arms, shoulders, chest, spine, abdomen, and neck—patient must bear full weight on these muscles.
   (1) Do push-ups in prone position.
   (2) Do sit-ups in sitting position.
   (3) Extend and flex arms while holding weights.
   (4) Squeeze rubberball to promote hand strength.
c. Graded therapeutic exercises are supervised by physical therapist.
7. Prevent the complications of paraplegic disorders.
a. Infection of urinary tract; urinary calculi; urethrocutaneous fistula (see neurogenic bladder, p. 512).
   (1) Prevent overdistention of the bladder.
   (2) Do frequent urinalyses.
   (3) Encourage fluid intake of at least 4000 ml./24 hours; urinary output should be 2000 ml./24 hours.
   (4) Prevent periurethral abscess formation and urethrocutaneous fistula from catheter—in male patient tape the penis horizontally to the side to prevent pressure and kinking of the urethra on the catheter at the penoscrotal angle (Fig. 11-6).
b. Development of pressure sores
   (1) See page 64 for prevention.
c. Fecal impaction.
   (1) Ensure total evacuation of fecal material from lower bowel every day.
     (a) Employ regular digital examination of rectum—to determine presence of impacted fecal material.
     (b) Keep patient on bowel training program (see p. 76).

d. Ankylosis of joints; contractures; spasticity
   (1) Start passive exercises and range of motion early in course of treatment.
   (2) Position patient in functional positions (see p. 53).
   (3) Use muscle stretching exercises for spasticity.
   (4) Use splints and supports for spastic joints as indicated by patient's condition.
e. Autonomic dysreflexia (see p. 741).
8. Support the counseling services provided for the patient and family.
a. Rehabilitation engineering services—provide a greater range of self-help and mobility devices
b. Occupational therapy—selects and utilizes devices which can aid patient in mealtime, dressing, and other activities
c. Vocational assessment and rehabilitation counseling
d. Sexual counseling
   (1) Most cord-injured persons can have some form of meaningful sexual expression and relationship, but some modifications will have to be made to cope with anxiety.
   (2) Implanatation of penile prosthesis may be considered.
   (3) Female patient may experience little sensation during intercourse, but fertility and ability to bear children are usually not affected.
   (4) Counseling and small group meetings provide an opportunity to share feelings, sexual concerns, give and receive information, and develop positive attitudes and adjustment.
   (5) See sexuality of the disabled, page 53.
e. Family may require counseling and social services to help them cope with burden of spinal cord injury on their life-style and socioeconomic status.

NEUROSURGICAL MANAGEMENT OF INTRACTABLE PAIN

Intractable pain is pain that causes incapacitation of function and that cannot be relieved satisfactorily by drugs short of drug addiction or incapacitating sedation.

Causes

1. Malignant disease (especially of cervix, bladder, prostate, lower bowel)
2. Trigeminal neuralgia; spinal cord arachnoiditis
3. Uncontrollable ischemia or other forms of tissue destruction

Neurosurgical Procedures for Management of Intractable Pain

OBJECTIVE: to interrupt the pathways by which the painful sensations are perceived.

A. *Rhizotomy*

1. *Posterior or spinal rhizotomy*—surgical interruption of selected posterior spinal nerve roots between the ganglion and the cord. This results in permanent loss of sensation and may be done at any spinal level. *Clinical uses*—pain relief of lung cancer, head and neck malignancies.
2. *Percutaneous rhizotomy*—radio frequency current is used to deliver heat selectively to coagulate small pain fibers; the fibers concerned with touch and proprioception are preserved.
3. *Chemical rhizotomy*—injection of alcohol (phenol or mixture of drugs) into the subarachnoid space; medication is maneuvered over affected nerve roots by tilting the patient to achieve desired level. The patient's perception of pain is absent but motor nerve root sensations are not.

B. *Cordotomy*—surgical interruption of the anterolateral quadrant of the spinal cord for the relief of intractable pain.

1. Obliterates pain and temperature sense but leaves motor function intact.
2. May be done by percutaneous needle insertion. An electrode is introduced through the spinal needle and a lesion produced by a radio frequency current at the desired level. This is useful for patient who cannot tolerate a laminectomy; or by open operation (via laminectomy). Cordotomy is helpful for patients with unilateral pain of malignant origin, especially of thorax, abdomen, or lower extremities.
Nursing Management Following Cordotomy
a. Watch for complications:
   (1) Respiratory
     (a) Observe for fatigue and weakening of voice.

(b) Monitor arterial blood gases. Patients with reduced oxygen levels may require oxygen at night until blood gas levels return to normal. (Patient may ventilate adequately while awake but may experience progressive hypercarbia and hypoxia while asleep.)

(c) Assisted mechanical ventilation may be required.

(2) Urinary retention (usually transient)

(3) Ipsilateral (on the same side) leg weakness—usually disappears in a few days

(4) Hemorrhage—may produce motor and sensory loss; immediate surgical intervention is indicated

Test motion, strength, and sensation of each extremity every few hours during the first 48 hours.

b. See management of the patient following disc surgery, page 743, for principles of care also relevant to these operations.

c. Keep the patient flat as prescribed—less tension on incision.

d. For cervical incision, keep the neck in a neutral position.

e. Feel patient's skin temperature at intervals to ascertain skin temperature changes.

f. Watch for development of pressure sores.

(1) Teach patient to inspect his skin using a hand mirror to view hard-to-see areas.

(2) Place patient on bladder training program (p. 76) if high cervical procedure has caused loss of bladder control.

3. *Family and Patient Health Education*

a. Proctect patient against external temperature changes and extremes of weather; he may not be aware of sunburn/frostbite; watch for skin lacerations due to unnoticed injury.

b. Test bath water before getting in tub.

c. Avoid constricting clothing that impairs circulation.

d. Sexual function is usually impaired in males.

C. *Sympathectomy*—interruption of afferent pathways in the sympathetic division of the autonomic nervous system; used to control pain from causalgia and peripheral vascular disorders (eliminates vasospasm and improves peripheral blood supply).

D. *Psychosurgical Approaches*—procedures altering patient's response to pain

1. *Thalamotomy*—destruction (unilaterally or bilaterally) of specific cell groups within thalamus. It is accomplished through burr holes—a lesion is produced by radio frequency current, cryosurgery, etc. This technique is useful for pain of central origin.

2. *Cingulumotomy*—unilateral or bilateral interruption of the anterior cingulate bundle in the frontal lobe of the brain.

a. Accomplished by either open or stereotaxic approach.

b. Tends to modify the patient's affective reaction to pain.

E. *Suppression of pain by electrical stimulation* (neuromodulation)

Neuromodulation is a method of suppressing pain by applying an electronic device that stimulates the different parts of the nervous system for pain relief. It is accomplished by (1) transcutaneous electrical nerve stimulation or (2) dorsal column stimulation.

1. *Underlying Principles*

a. This therapy is based on the theory (gate control theory) that nondestructive stimuli can interfere with the transmission of pain within the central nervous system. It is thought to relieve pain by preventing pain messages from reaching the brain. The exact mechanics are not yet fully known.

b. It is nondestructive in nature and does not carry the potential risks of weakness, numbness, dysesthesia, bladder/bowel incontinence, impotence, or irreversibility as do destructive surgical procedures for pain relief.

c. The system consists of a pulse generator (containing the power source and electronics of the system), a pair of electric cables, and 2 flexible electrodes which transfer the stimulating signal.

d. *Objective:* to help the patient live with his pain without permitting it to affect his life adversely.

2. *Transcutaneous electrical nerve stimulation*—passage of small electrical currents through the skin for the purpose of controlling pain.

a. Electrodes, are placed over or around patient's pain area or on any peripheral nerve pathway.

b. Procedure:

(1) The skin is washed with mild soap and water and dried thoroughly to reduce skin resistance.

(2) Electrode gel is applied to the electrodes, which are then placed over the nerves that serve the painful area. Electrodes are secured with nonallergenic tape.

(3) The patient operates the amplitude control until stimulation is felt (buzzing or tingling sensation). The amplitude is increased until the sensation is strong but not uncomfortable.

(4) The patient is taught to control the amplitude, frequency, and duration of stimulation.

c. *Health Education*

(1) Give the patient the instruction booklet provided by the manufacturing company.

(2) Batteries must be replaced whenever levels of stimulation cannot be achieved.

(3) The electrodes are washed with alcohol and water after each use. The pulse generator and cables are wiped clean with a damp cloth moistened with alcohol/water solution.

(4) Apply talcum powder to the cables periodically to prevent tangling.

(5) Avoid getting the pulse generator wet; avoid pulling or kinking of the cable wire.

3. *Dorsal column stimulation*—is a method for the relief of chronic intractable pain that uses a surgically implanted device that allows the patient to apply pulsed electrical stimulation to the dorsal aspect of the spinal cord to block pain impulses.

a. The unit consists of a radio-frequency stimulation transmitter, a transmitter antenna, a radio-frequency receiver, and a stimulation electrode.

b. The battery-powered transmitter and antenna are worn externally, and the receiver and electrode are implanted.

(1) A laminectomy is performed above the highest level of pain input and the electrode is placed in the epidural space over the posterior column of the spinal cord. (Placement of stimulating systems is varied.) A small subcutaneous pocket is constructed over the clavicular area (site may vary) for placement of receiver. The 2 are connected by a subcutaneous tunnel.

c. A careful preoperative evaluation is performed to select patient who will benefit from dorsal column stimulation—history, physical examination, pain questionnaire, examination to determine areas of pain involvement, psychological and psychiatric evaluation, and a trial of transcutaneous stimulation.
  (1) Trial of transcutaneous stimulation (see above) gives opportunity for patient to receive stimulation sensation—to test his tolerance of the sensation, his ability to operate the system, and the efficiency of the system.
  (2) It is essential that the patient understand that the stimulator will replace drugs and that it is installed for a lifetime.
d. Postoperative nursing management
  (1) See page 743 for the nursing management following disc surgery.
  (2) Assess for paraplegia, quadriplegia, and urinary incontinence.
  (3) Evaluate extremities for leg movement hourly. Report any decrease in movement immediately.
  (4) Look for leakage of cerebrospinal fluid at operative site—dura is opened in surgery.
  (5) Give medication as prescribed for relief of incisional pain.
  (6) Withdraw narcotics as rapidly as possible.
  (7) Help patient to become independently involved with his activities of daily living as rapidly as possible—inactivity serves to compound his problems.
  (8) Look for signs of infection at implantation site—dorsal column stimulator is a foreign body within the patient.
  (9) The dorsal column stimulating system may be tested when the patient is fully alert; initial testing may not be accurate because of overlying bandage at receiver site.
e. *Health Education*
  (1) Give patient the manufacturer's instruction booklet to acquaint him with the system.

    (a) The stimulation transmitter has 4 basic controls: 2 for the patient to use during operation of the system and 2 for the physician to use when determining the voltage the patient will receive.
  (2) The patient is taught method of attaching the antenna to the skin (and proper skin care), use of battery pack, and how to make and modify dorsal column stimulation setting.
    (a) Antenna is secured in place by an adhesive disc centered over the implanted receiver. (The antenna site is cleansed daily and the adhesive discs are changed daily.)
    (b) Connect transmitter to antenna and adjust settings slowly to the point at which the patient first feels a definite sensation and the stimulation results in the desired effect.
    (c) Encourage patient to try different stimulation frequencies to determine which frequency gives best pain relief.
    (d) Have the patient keep a record of stimulation use.
    (e) Instruct the patient that postural changes will cause changes in stimulation intensity.
    (f) Warn patient not to adjust physician's controls.
    (g) Instruct patient to keep several batteries in reserve; battery life depends on extent of use. Patient should be instructed in battery changing procedure.
    (h) Clean transmitter and antenna according to the manufacturer's directions.
4. *Percutaneous epidural neurostimulation*—a method of neuromodulation in which electrodes are inserted percutaneously into spinal epidural space. Effective in treating arachnoiditis and postamputation neuroma.
5. *Brain stimulation*—implantation of stimulating electrodes in the periventricular area of posterior third ventricle. Allows self-stimulation of periventricular gray area to produce analgesia.

BIBLIOGRAPHY

Books

American Nurses' Association. Division on Medical–Surgical Nursing Practice and the American Association of Neurosurgical Nurses: Standards of Neurological and Neurosurgical Nursing Practice. Kansas City, American Nurses Association, 1977

Bakay L and Glasauer FE. Head Injury. Boston, Little Brown & Company, 1980

Barrows HS. Guide to Neurological Assessment. Philadelphia, JB Lippincott, 1980

Bucheit WA and Truex RC Jr (eds). Surgery of the Posterior Fossa. New York, Raven Press, 1979

Caillet R. The Shoulder in Hemiplegia. Philadelphia, F.A. Davis, 1980

Cottrell JE and Turndorf H. Anesthesia and Neurosurgery. St. Louis, C.V. Mosby, 1980

Davis JE and Mason CB. Neurologic Critical Care. New York, Van Nostrand Reinhold, 1979

Duvoisin RC. Parkinson's Disease—A Guide for Patient and Family. New York, Raven Press, 1978

Eadie MJ and Tyrer JH. Anticonvulsant Therapy, 2nd ed. New York, Churchill Livingstone, 1980

Freeman SW. The Epileptic in Home, School and Society. Springfield, Charles C Thomas, 1979

Gilroy J and Meyer JS. Medical Neurology, 3rd ed. New York, Macmillan, 1979

Green JR and Thompson RA. Critical Care of Neurologic and Neurosurgical Emergencies. New York, Raven Press, 1980

Harcus AW et al. Pain—New Perspectives in Measurement and Management. New York, Churchill Livingstone, 1977

Jacox AK. Pain: A Source Book for Nurses and Other Health Professionals. Boston, Little, Brown & Co, 1977

Jeffreys E. Disorders of the Cervical Spine. London, Butterworths & Co, 1980

Johns DF (ed). Clinical Management of Neurogenic Communicative Disorders. Boston, Little, Brown & Co, 1978

Kertesz A. Aphasia and Associated Disorders. New York, Grune & Stratton, 1979

Lipton S. Relief of Pain in Clinical Practice. Oxford, Blackwell Scientific Press, 1979

Merritt HH. A Textbook of Neurology, 6th ed. Philadelphia, Lea & Febiger, 1979

Mulder DW (ed). The Diagnosis and Treatment of Amyotrophic Lateral Sclerosis. Boston, Houghton Mifflin, 1980

Newmark ME and Penry JK. Genetics of Epilepsy: A Review. New York, Raven Press, 1980

Pia HH et al (eds). Cerebral Aneurysms: Advances in Diagnosis and Therapy. New York, Springer-Verlag, 1979

Pierce DS and Nickel VH. Total Care of Spinal Cord Injuries. Boston, Little, Brown & Co, 1977

Popp AJ et al. Neural Trauma. New York, Raven Press, 1978

Pryse-Phillips W and Murray TJ. Essential Neurology. Garden City, Medical Examination Publishing Co, 1978

Rasmussen T and Marino R Jr. Functional Neurosurgery. New York, Raven Press, 1979

Rathke FW and Schlegel K-F. Surgery of the Spine. Stuttgart, Georg Thieme Publishers, 1979

Report of the Panel on Communicative Disorders to the National Advisory Neurological and Communicative Disorders and Stroke Council. NIH Publication 79-1914. Washington, DC, U.S. Government Printing Office, 1979

Report of the Panel on Inflammatory, Demyelinating and Degenerative Diseases to the National Advisory Neurological and Communicative Disorders and Stroke Council. NIH Publication 79-1916. Washington, DC, US Government Printing Office, 1979

Report of the Panel on Stroke, Trauma, Regeneration and Neoplasms to the National Advisory Neurological and Communicative Disorders and Stroke Council. NIH Publication 79-1915. Washington, DC, US Government Printing Office, 1979

Roberts AH. Severe Accidental Head Injury. London, Macmillan, 1979

Ross RT. How to Examine the Nervous System. Springfield, Charles C Thomas, 1978

Salcman M (ed). Neurologic Emergencies. New York, Raven Press, 1980

Samuels RR. Manual of Neurologic Therapeutics. Boston, Little, Brown & Co, 1978

Smith RR. Essentials of Neurosurgery. Philadelphia, JB Lippincott, 1980

Smith WL et al. Pain. Meaning and Management. New York, SP Medical and Scientific Books, 1980

Suchenwirth R. Pocket Book of Clinical Neurology. Chicago, Year Book Medical Publishers, 1979

Sullivan MW. Living with Epilepsy. New York, Nellen, 1979

Taylor JW and Ballenger S. Neurological Dysfunctions and Nursing Intervention. New York, McGraw-Hill, 1980

Thompson RA and Green JR. Critical Care of Neurologic and Neurosurgical Emergencies. New York, Raven Press, 1980

Trieschmann RB. Spinal Cord Injuries. New York, Pergamon Press, 1980

Wilson CB and Hoff JT. Current Surgical Management of Neurologic Disease. New York, Churchill Livingstone, 1980

Wolf JK. Practical Clinical Neurology. Garden City, Medical Examination Publishing Co, 1980

Articles

Amyotrophic Lateral Sclerosis

Bartels EJ. Helping the patient with "Lou Gehrig's disease." RN 1979 Dec; 42(12):48–50, 79–82

Blount M et al. Management of the patient with amyotrophic lateral sclerosis. Nurs Clin North Am 1979 March; 14(1):157–171

DeLisa JA et al. Amyotrophic lateral sclerosis: Comprehensive management. Am Fam Physician 1979 March; 19(3): 137–142

Lehner WE et al. Home care utilizing a ventilator in a patient with amyotrophic lateral sclerosis. J Fam Pract 1980 Jan; 10(1):39–42

Plank C. MS: ALS, MS, MD—What's the difference? Am J Nurs 1980 Feb; 80(2):282–283

Rasmussen DJ. Amyotrophic lateral sclerosis. Am J Nurs 1980 Nov; 80(11):2050–2052.

Assessment/Diagnosis

Marsh ML et al. Neurosurgical intensive care. Anesthesiology 1977 Aug; 47(2):149–163

Miller L. Neurological assessment: A practical approach for the critical care nurse. J Neurosurg Nurs 1979 March; 11(1):2–5

Rimel RW and Tyson GW. The neurologic examination in patients with central nervous system trauma. J Neurosurg Nurs 1979 Sept; 11(3):148–155

Ross AJ et al. Neuromuscular diagnostic procedures. Nurs Clin North Am 1979 March; 14(1):107–121

Brain Abscess/Brain Tumor

Burger PC et al. The morphologic effects of radiation administered therapeutically for intracranial gliomas. Cancer 1979 Oct; 44(4):1256–1272

Hirsh LF. Metastatic brain tumors. Postgrad Med 1979 Feb; 65(2):145–151

Legg NJ. Intracerebral abscess. Br J Hosp Med 1979 Dec; 22(6):608–614

Lieberman A and Ransohoff J. Treatment of primary brain tumors. Med Clin North Am 1979 July; 63 (4):835–848

Ransohoff J and Lieberman A. Surgical therapy of primary malignant brain tumors. Clin Neurosurg 1978; 25:403–411

Rosenblum ML et al. Decreased mortality from brain abscesses since advent of computerized tomography. J Neurosurg 1978 Nov; 49(5):658–668

Rosenblum ML et al. Nonoperative treatment of brain abscesses in selected high-risk patients. J Neurosurg 1980 Feb; 52(2):217–225

Snell GE. Sinogenic and otogenic brain abscesses. A review of 63 cases occurring at Toronto General Hospital. J Otolaryngol 1978 Aug; 7(4):289–296

Walker MD. The contemporary role of chemotherapy in the treatment of malignant brain tumor. Clin Neurosurg 1978; 25:388–396

Wilson CB. Current concepts in cancer: Brain tumors. N Engl J Med 1979 June 28; 300(26):1469–1471

Wilson CB and Gutin PH. Therapy of malignant brain tumors: An update on progress. Tex Med 1980 Jan; 76(1):40–43

Cerebral Aneurysms

Caplan LR. Intracerebral hemorrhage: New clues to an old entity. Med Times 1978 Oct; 106(10):55–61.

Crowell RM and Zervas NT. Management of intracranial aneurysm. Med Clin North Am 1979 July; 63(4):695–713

Fox JL et al. Microsurgical treatment of vascular disease. Intracranial aneurysms, intracranial and intraspinal arteriovenous malformations. Neurosurgery 1978 Sept–Oct; 3(2):305–320

Friedberg SR. Treatment of intracranial hemorrhage. Primary Care 1979 Dec; 6(4):805–812

Hirsh LF. Modern treatment of intracranial aneurysms. Postgrad Med 1980 March; 67(3):153–156, 158, 160

Illingworth R. Surgical treatment of ruptured intracranial aneurysms. Am Heart J 1979 Aug; 98(2):269–271

Lee K. Aneurysm precautions: A physiologic basis for minimizing rebleeding. Heart Lung 1980 Mar–Apr; 9(2): 336–343

Peerless SJ. Pre-and postoperative management of cerebral aneurysms. Clin Neurosurg 1979; 26:209–231

Salazar JL. Treatment of ruptured and unruptured internal carotid artery aneurysms. Surg Neurol 1979 June; 11(6):451–455

Tarlov E. Subarachnoid hemorrhage. Primary Care 1979 Dec; 6(4):791–803

Cerebrovascular Disease

Goldstein M et al. Cerebrovascular disorders and stroke. Adv Neurol 1979; 25:1–394

Greer M. Current concepts in managing TIAs and stroke. Geriatrics 1979 Apr; 34(4):53–55, 59

Holland AL. Treatment of aphasia following stroke. Stroke 1979 Jul–Aug; 10(4):475–477

Johnson JH and Cryan M. Homonymous hemianopsia: Assessment and nursing management. Am J Nurs 1979 Dec; 79(12):2131–2135

Jones HR (ed). Stroke: Diagnosis and management. Primary Care 1980 March; 7(1):1–106

Kwaan JHM et al. Successful management of early stroke after carotid endarterectomy. Ann Surg 1979 Nov; 190(5):676–678

McCormick GP and Williams M. Stroke: The double crisis. Am J Nurs 1979 Aug; 79(8):1410–1411

Meador B and White P. The post-op dangers in carotid endarterectomy. RN 1980 April; 43(4):54–57

Norman S. Diagnostic categories for the patient with a right hemisphere lesion. Am J Nurs 1979 Dec; 79(12):2126–2130

Norman S and Baratz R. Understanding aphasia. Am J Nurs 1979 Dec; 79(12):2135–2138

Palmer EP. Language dysfunction in cerebrovascular disease. Primary Care 1979 Dec; 6(4):827–842

Pearce JH et al. Continuous oculoplethysmographic monitoring during carotid endarterectomy. Am J Surg 1979 Nov; 138(5):733–735

Persson AV and Kopreski MS. The surgical management of carotid artery disease. Primary Care 1980 March; 7(1):59–79

Ramirez-Lassepas M. TIAs: The forewarning of stroke. Geriatrics 1980 Apr; 35(4):73–83

Redford JB and Harris JD. Rehabilitation of the elderly stroke patient. Am Fam Physician 1980 Sept; 22(3):153–160

Robertson JJ and Watridge CB. The surgical management of extracranial and intracranial occlusive disease. Med Clin North Am 1979 July; 63(4):681–693

Sherman DG and Easton JD. Cerebral edema in stroke. Postgrad Med 1980 July; 68(1):107–120

Shiavi RG et al. Efficacy of myofeedback therapy in regaining control of lower extremity musculature following stroke. Am J Phys Med 1979 Aug; 58(4):185–194

Spetzler RF. Extracranial–intracranial arterial anastomosis for cerebrovascular disease. Surg Neurol 1979 Mar; 11(3):157–161

Spetzler RF et al. Microsurgery in stroke management. AORN J 1979 Nov; 30(5):885–890

Thompson JE and Talkington CM. Carotid surgery for cerebral ischemia. Surg Clin North Am 1979 Aug; 59(4):539–553

Thompson JE. Complications of carotid endarterectomy and their prevention. World J Surg 1979 July; 3(2):155–165

Wallhagen MI. The split brain: Implications for care and rehabilitation. Am J Nurs 1979 Dec; 79(12):2118–2125

Yared I et al. Carotid endarterectomy under local anesthesia: A retrospective study. Am Surg 1979 Nov; 45(11):709–714

Yatsu FM. For your stroke-prone patients: A guide to drug treatment. Geriatrics 1980 Feb; 35(2):34–47

Zeluff GW et al. Strokes in young people. Heart Lung 1979 Mar–Apr; 8(2):353–360

Cranial Nerve Involvement

Baker D (ed). Symposium on facial paralysis. Clin Plast Surg 1979 July; 6(3):273–486

Bayer DB and Stenger TG. Trigeminal neuralgia: An overview. Oral Surg 1979 Nov; 48(5):393–399

Gregg JM et al. Radiofrequency thermoneurolysis of peripheral nerves for control of trigeminal neuralgia. Pain 1978 Oct; 5(3):231–243

Jannetta PJ and Tew JM. Treatment of trigeminal neuralgia. Neurosurgery 1979 Jan; 4(1):93–94

Jelks GW et al. The evaluation and management of the eye in facial palsy. Clin Plast Surg 1979 July; 6(3):397–419

Shaber EP and Krol AJ. Trigeminal neuralgia—A new treatment concept. Oral Surg 1980 Apr; 49(4):286–293

Smith MFW and Goode RL. Eye protection in the paralyzed face. Laryngoscope 1979 Mar; 89(3):435–442

Epilepsy

Bruni J. Recent advances in drug therapy for epilepsy. Can Med Assoc J 1979 April; 120(7):817–824

Bruni J. Valproic acid. Review of a new antiepileptic drug. Arch Neurol 1979 July; 36(7):393–398

Dreifuss FE. Use of anticonvulsant drugs. JAMA 1979 Feb 9; 241(6):607–609

Drugs for epilepsy. Med Lett Drugs Ther 1979 March 23; 21(6):25–28

Garvin JS. Management of convulsions in surgical patients. Surg Annu 1979; 11:25–32

Gaser GH et al. Antiepileptic drugs: Mechanisms of action. Adv Neurol 1980; 27; entire volume.

Hawken M and Ozuna J. Practical aspects of anticonvulsant therapy. Am J Nurs 1979 June; 79(6):1062–1068

Massey EW et al. Managing the epileptic patient. Postgrad Med 1980 Feb; 67(2):134–143

Morris HH and Bodensteiner JB. Seizure disorders. J Fam Pract 1980 Feb; 10(2):305–315

Penry JK and Porter RJ. Epilepsy: Mechanisms and therapy. Med Clin North Am 1979 July; 63(4):801–812

Penry JK and Newmark ME. The use of antiepileptic drugs. Ann Intern Med 1979 Feb; 90(2):207–218

Guillain-Barré Syndrome

Hogg JE et al. The Guillain–Barré syndrome epidemiologic and clinical features. J Chron Dis 1979; 32(3):227–231

Kennedy RH. Guillain–Barré Syndrome: A 42-year epidemiologic and clinical study. Mayo Clin Proc 1978 Feb; 53(2):93–99

Samonds RJ. Guillain–Barré syndrome: Helping the patient in the acute stage. Nursing '80 1980 Aug; 10(8):34–41

Head Injury/Intracranial Pressure/Intracranial Pressure Monitoring

Burry M. The decerebrate patient. J Neurosurg Nurs 1979 March; 11(1):6–9

Byrnes DP. Head injury and the dilated pupil. Am Surg 1979 March; 45(3):139–143

Cheek WR et al. Device for extradural monitoring of intracranial pressure: Technical note. Neurosurgery 1979 Dec; 5(6):692–694

Darmody W and Tintinalli JE. Head Injuries. JACEP 1979 March; 8(3):118–121

Feiring EH. Management of head injuries. Compr Ther 1979 Jan; 5(1):53–58

Fryer TB et al. Telemetry of intracranial pressure. Biotelem Patient Monit 1978; 5(2):88–112

Igneizi R. Cerebral edema: Present perspectives. Neurosurgery 1979 April; 4(4):338–342

Jennett B. The problem of mild head injury. Practitioner 1978 July; 221(1321):77–82

Jones C. Glasgow coma scale. Am J Nurs 1979 Sept; 79(9):1551–1553

Levin AB et al. Treatment of increased intracranial pressure: A comparison of different hyperosmotic agents and the use of thiopental. Neurosurgery 1979 Nov; 5(5):570–575

Marshall LF et al. The outcome with aggressive treatment in severe head injuries. Part I. The significance of intracranial pressure monitoring. J Neurosurg 1979 Jan; 50(1):20–25

Moss E and McDowall DG. Monitoring intracranial pressure. Int Anesthesiol Clin 1979 Summer–Fall; 17(2–3):375–390

Palmer MA et al. Intracranial pressure monitoring in the acute neurologic assessment of multi-injured patients. J Trauma 1979 July; 19(7):497–501

Rosner MJ and Becker DP. ICP monitoring: Complications and associated factors. Clin Neurosurg 1976; 23:494–519

Sigsbee B and Plum F. The unresponsive patient. Diagnosis and management. Med Clin North Am 1979 July; 63(4):813–834

Stevenson BE. Initial management of the acute head injury. Otolaryngol Clin North Am 1979 May; 12(2):279–291

Teasdale G and Jennett B. Assessment of coma and impaired consciousness. A practical scale. Lancet 1974 July; 2(7872):81–84

Trubuhovich RV. Management of acute intracranial disasters. Int Anesthesiol Clin 1979 Summer–Fall; 17(2,3): entire volume.

White RJ. Intracranial injuries. New methodology in diagnosis and treatment. Surg Annu 1979; 11:295–311

Wright BD and Young B. Automatic intracranial pressure regulation. Crit Care Med 1978 Nov–Dec; 6(6):373–375

Intervertebral Disc/Spinal Cord Injuries

Baxter RT and Linn A. Sex counseling and the SCI patient. Nursing '78 1978 Sept; 8(9):46–52

Berkman AH et al. Sexual adjustment of spinal cord injured veterans living in the community. Arch Phys Med Rehabil 1978 Jan; 59(1):29–33

Chawla JC et al. Techniques for improving the strength and fitness of spinal injured patients. Paraplegia 1979 July; 17(2):185–189

Comarr AE. Urinary bladder disorders from spinal cord injury. Compr Ther 1979 Sept; 5(9):37–46

Dabezies EJ, and Brunet M. Chemonucleolysis vs laminectomy. Orthopedics 1978 Jan–Feb; 1(1):26–29

Frost EAM. The physiopathology of respiration in neurosurgical patients. J Neurosurg 1979 June; 50(6):699–714

Goald HJ. Microsurgical removal of lumbar herniated nucleus pulposus. Surg Gynecol Obstet 1979 Aug; 149(2):247–248

Golji H. Experience with penile prosthesis in spinal cord injury patients. J Urol 1979 Mar; 121(3):288–289

Hudgins WR. The crossed straight leg raising test. A diagnostic sign of herniated disc. JOM 1979 June; 21(6):407–408

Javid MJ. Treatment of herniated lumbar disc syndrome with chymopapain. JAMA 1980 May 23–30; 243(20):2043–2048

Kewalramani LS. Autonomic dysreflexia in traumatic myelopathy. Am J Phys Med 1980 Feb; 59(1):1–21

Lawson NC. Significant events in the rehabilitation process: The spinal cord patient's point of view. Arch Phys Med Rehabil 1978 Dec; 59(12):573– 579

Meyer GA et al. Diagnosis of herniated lumbar disc with computed tomography. N Engl J Med 1979 Nov 22; 301(21):1166–1167

Nursing grand rounds. Family-centered conference for better trauma care. Nursing '78 1978 Oct; 8(10):70–77

Pfaudler M. Care of patients with severe spinal cord injuries. Curr Prac Crit Care 1979; 1:216–228

Rhame FS and Perkash I. Urinary tract infections occurring in recent spinal cord injury patients on intermittent catheterization. J Urol 1979 Nov; 122(5):669–673

Rutecki B and Seligson D. Caring for the patient in a halo apparatus. Nursing '80 1980 Oct; 10(10):73–77

Thomas DG. Genitourinary complications following spinal cord injury. Practitioner 1979 Sept; 223(1335):339–346

Williams AL et al. Computed tomography in the diagnosis of herniated nucleus pulposus. Radiology 1980 April; 155(1):95–99

Wiseley SF. Clinical management of spinal cord injury: Experience in a smaller state rehabilitation unit. Bull NY Acad Med 1979 Oct; 55(9):822–828

Young JS. Spinal cord injury: Associated general trauma and medical complications. Adv Neurol 1979; 22:255–260

Zackin HJ. Management of decubitus ulcers in paraplegic patients. South Med J 1978 May; 71(5):574–576

Pain/Neurosurgery

Frost EAM. The physiopathology of respiration in neurosurgical patients. J Neurosurgery 1979 June; 50(6):699–714

Gersh MR. Postoperative pain and transcutaneous electrical nerve stimulation. Phys Ther 1978 Dec; 58(12):1463–1466

Ghia JN et al. Therapeutic nerve blocks for chronic pain. Am Fam Physician 1979 July; 20(1):74–78

Lamb S. Neuroaugmentation for the chronic pain patient. J Neurosurg Nursing 1979 Dec; 11(4):215–220

Lampe GN. Introduction to the use of transcutaneous electrical nerve stimulation devices. Phys Ther 1978 Dec; 58(12):1450–1454

Mannheimer MA. Electrode placements for transcutaneous electrical nerve stimulation. Phys Ther 1978. Dec; 58(12):1455–1462

McKelvy PL. Clinical report on the use of specific TENS units. Phys Ther 1978 Dec; 58(12):1474–1477

North JB et al. Postoperative epilepsy: A double-blind trial of phenytoin after craniotomy. Lancet 1980 Feb 23; 1(8165):384

Penney MD et al. Hyponatremia in patients with head injury. Intensive Care Med 1979 March; 5(1):23–26

Richardson DE. Thalamic stimulation in the control of pain. South Med J 1980 March; 73(3):283–285

Richardson RR. Spinal epidural neurostimulation for treatment of acute and chronic intractable pain: Initial and long-term results. Neurosurgery 1979 Sept; 5(3):344–348

Tankaku A et al. Postoperative complications in 1000 cases of intracranial aneurysms. Surg Neurol 1979 Aug; 12(2):137–144

Multiple Sclerosis/Myasthenia Gravis/Parkinson's Disease

Blount M et al. Plasma exchange in the management of myasthenia gravis, Nurs Clin North Am 1979 March; 14(1):173–190

Burnfield A and Burnfield P. Common psychological problems in multiple sclerosis. Br Med J 1978 May 6; 1(6121):1193–1194

Calne DB et al. Advances in the neuropharmacology of parkinsonism. Ann Intern Med 1979 Feb; 90(2):219–229

Catanzaro M. Nursing care of the person with MS. Am J Nurs 1980 Feb; 80(2):286–291

Davies GM. The problems of nursing patients with advanced multiple sclerosis at home. J Adv Nurs 1978 Nov; 4(6):635–645

Dolan B. Multiple sclerosis. J Neurosurg Nurs 1979 June; 11(2):83–93

Drugs for parkinsonism. Med Lett Drugs Ther 1979 May 4; 21(9):37–38

Eisler T. Parkinsonism—new drugs and new approaches. DM 1979 Mar; 25(6):1–51

Elias SB and Appel SH. Current concepts of pathogenesis and treatment of myasthenia gravis. Med Clin North Am 1979 July; 63(4):745–757

Fahn S et al. The role of bromocriptine in the treatment of parkinsonism. Neurology 1979 Aug; 29(8):1077–1083

Feldman RG et al. Baclofen for spasticity in multiple sclerosis. Double-blind crossover and three-year study. Neurology 1978 Nov; 28(11):1094–1098

Field EJ and Joyce G. Multiple sclerosis: What can and what cannot be done. Br Med J 1979 Dec 15; 2(6204):1571–1572

Gresh C. Helpful tips you can give your patients with Parkinson's disease. Nursing '80 1980 Jan; 10(1):26–33

Hallpike JF. New treatment for multiple sclerosis. Br J Hosp Med 1980 Jan; 23(1):63–64, 66, 68

Hofmann WW. The treatment of myasthenia gravis. Ration Drug Ther 1979 Feb; 13(2):1–8

Kinley AE. MS: From shock to acceptance. Am J Nurs 1980 Feb; 80(2):274–275

Lesser RP. Analysis of the clinical problems in parkinsonism and complications of long-term levadopa therapy. Neurology 1979 Sept; 29(9PartI):1253–1260

Lieberman A et al. Treatment of Parkinson's disease with dopamine agonists. A review. Am J Med Sci 1979 July–Aug; 278(1):65–76

McDonnell M et al. MS: Problem oriented nursing care plans. Am J Nurs 1980 Feb; 80(2):292–297

Newson-Davis J et al. Long-term effects of repeated plasma exchange in myasthenia gravis. Lancet 1979 March 3; 1(8114):464–468

Parkes JD. Bromocriptine in the treatment of parkinsonism. Drugs 1979 May; 17(5):365–382

Plank NM. Multiple sclerosis: An update and review. J Neurosurg Nurs 1979 Mar; 11(1):44–47

Plasmapheresis for myasthenia gravis. Med Lett Drugs Ther 1979 July 27; 21(15):64

Poser CM. Multiple sclerosis. A critical update. Med Clin North Am 1979 July; 63(4):729–743

Price G. MS: The challenge to the family. Am J Nurs 1980 Feb; 80(2):283–285

Riley TL and Marsey EW. Managing the patient with Parkinson's disease. Postgrad Med 1980 Sept; 68(3):85–92

Slater RJ and Yearwood AC. MS: Facts, faith and hope. Am J Nurs 1980 Feb; 80(2):276–281

Sneddon J. Myasthenia gravis: A study of social, medical and emotional problems in 26 patients. Lancet 1980 March 8; 1(8167):526–528

Winkler LH and Winkler GF. Myasthenia gravis: Pathogenesis, diagnosis and therapy. Postgrad Med 1979 Aug; 66(2):50–56

Yearwood AC. MS: Being disabled doesn't mean being handicapped. Am J Nurs 1980 Feb; 80(2):299–302

18

MUSCULOSKELETAL CONDITIONS

SPECIFIC PROBLEMS ASSOCIATED WITH ORTHOPEDIC CONDITIONS

PAIN

Assessment of Musculoskeletal Discomfort

A. *Types of Pain*

1. Sharp pain—may be from bone infection with muscle spasm or pressure on sensory nerve; fracture pain is sharp and piercing, relieved by rest and immobilization.
2. Soreness and aching—due to muscular pain
3. Increasing pain—due to progression of an infectious process or malignant tumor or to vascular complication
4. Pain increasing with activity—may indicate joint sprain
5. Pain that is worse in bad weather, felt in more than one part of body—may be secondary to arthritis
6. Radiating pain—rupture of intervertebral disc and pressure on the nerve root
7. Bone pain—deep, boring, and intensifying at night

B. *Nursing Assessment*

1. What activities precipitated the pain?
2. Is the body in proper alignment?
3. Is there pressure from traction, splints, cast, other appliances?
4. How does the patient describe the pain? Can he localize it?
5. Does it radiate? Is it continuous? What is the character of the pain? (dull? sharp? etc.)
6. What relieves the pain? makes it worse?

Nursing Management

OBJECTIVES: to alleviate pain and discomfort.
              to prevent deformity or deterioration.

1. Evaluate the effect of any physical, emotional, and social factors that may be present.
2. Position the patient in correct alignment.
3. Support the painful parts under the joints.
   a. Move the patient slowly and steadily.
   b. Avoid bumping the bed.
   c. Use a turning sheet when possible.
   d. Elevate the affected extremity.
4. Apply heat or cold to relieve muscle spasm.
5. Apply cold to relieve pain in inflammatory conditions or postoperatively.
6. Give analgesic, analgesic with sedative, or muscle relaxant as indicated.
7. Evaluate vascular status.
8. Help the patient to become involved in his rehabilitation program—muscle and joint exercises; promote early function, utilization of proper posture and gait.

CONTRACTURE DEFORMITIES

Assessment

A. *Types of Contracture Deformities*

1. Contracture deformities are caused by limitation of motion and disuse.

2. Pain and muscle spasm produce limitation of motion.
3. Inflammation limits joint motion and causes fibrous tissue to form, producing fibrous or bony ankylosis (abnormal rigidity of joint).
4. Deformities may be congenital, developmental, metabolic, infectious, traumatic, or neoplastic.

B. *Nursing Assessment*

1. When was the deformity noted?
2. Was the onset accompanied by injury?
3. Is the deformity increasing? Decreasing?
4. Is there neurological loss (sensory or motor deficit)?
5. Is there hypoesthesia, paresthesia, hyperesthesia?
6. Is there weakness, stiffness, difficulty in walking?
7. Is there paralysis? Time and mode of onset?
8. Are there any disturbances in control of bladder and bowel?

Nursing Management

1. Position the patient in accordance with principles of body mechanics—to prevent muscle contractures and loss of joint function.
2. Place patient on a firm mattress. Secure a trapeze.
3. Avoid semirecumbent position for prolonged periods—promotes flexion deformities of the hip.
4. Place the patient in a prone position several times daily when possible.

5. Encourage and assist patient to perform passive and active exercises—to maintain and improve muscle strength, maintain and restore optimal joint function, prevent deformities, stimulate circulation, and build endurance.

PSYCHOSOCIAL PROBLEMS

Assessment

Watch for reactive behaviors (denial, anger, bargaining, depression, acceptance) exhibited by patient and family following orthopedic injuries.

Nursing Management

1. Clear up any misconceptions about therapeutic program.
2. Develop a supportive relationship. Direct patient towards appropriate expression of feelings.
3. Keep the patient busy—activity absorbs anxiety.
4. Schedule a program of activity to include exercise program and occupational therapy—to promote feelings of independence.
5. Help integrate physical care (physical therapist, occupational therapist, etc.) so that patient's needs are met.

DIAGNOSTIC EVALUATION OF MUSCULOSKELETAL DISORDERS

A. *Patient's History*

B. *Physical Examination*

1. Observation for muscle atrophy or swelling, skin discoloration
2. Observation of gait and posture
3. Examination of joints—shape, alignment, circumference, range of motion, stability, instability, presence of abnormal joint fluid
4. Evaluation of bone—integrity, size, tenderness, masses
5. Palpation for skin temperature, local swelling, tenderness
6. Measurement of muscle strength, length of extremities, circumference of extremities
7. Neurologic evaluation—including cranial nerve testing, motor and sensory nerve testing, reflexes of extremities
8. Vascular assessment—peripheral pulses, nail growth, presence of hair on extremities.

C. *X-ray Studies*

1. Of bone—to determine bone density, texture, erosion, changes in bone relationships
2. Of cortex—to detect any widening, narrowing, irregularity
3. Of medullary cavity—to detect any alteration in density
4. Of involved joint—to show fluid, irregularity, spur formation, narrowing, changes in joint contour

D. *Special X-ray Techniques*

1. *Laminography or tomography*—shows in detail a specific plane of involved bone
2. *Myelography*—injection of radiopaque dye into subarachnoid space at lumbar spine (to determine level of disc herniation or site of tumor)—see page 702.
3. *Arthrography*—injection of radiopaque substance or air into joint cavity—outlines soft tissue structures and contour of joint
4. *Computed tomography*—useful in identifying tumors of the soft tissues or injuries to ligaments or tendons; helpful in identifying the location/extent of fractures in difficult-to-define areas.
5. *Bone scanning*—parenteral injection of bone-seeking radioactive isotope; increased concentration of isotope uptake revealed in primary skeletal disease (osteosarcoma), metastatic bone disease, inflammatory skeletal disease (osteomyelitis)

E. *Other Studies*

1. *Arthrocentesis*—insertion of needle into joint and aspiration of synovial fluid for purposes of examination.
2. *Electromyography*—provides information on the electric potential of the muscles and nerves leading to them.
3. *Thermography*—measures the degree of heat radiating from the skin surface; used to investigate the pathophysiology of inflamed joints and pain patterns, and to assess patient's response to anti-inflammatory drug therapy.
4. *Arthroscopy*—endoscopic procedure which allows direct visualization of a joint, especially the knee. May be combined with arthrography.
   Technique
   a. Under local or general anesthesia, a large bore needle is inserted into the suprapatellar pouch and the joint is distended with saline.
   b. An arthroscope is introduced and the knee joint visualized, including the synovium, articular surfaces, and menisci.
   c. Patient may be advised to limit his activities for several days following the procedure, which is relatively painless.

MUSCULOSKELETAL TRAUMA

CONTUSIONS

A *contusion* is an injury to the soft tissue produced by a blunt force (blow, kick, or fall).

Clinical Manifestations

1. Hemorrhage into injured part (ecchymosis)—from rupture of small blood vessels; also associated with fractures
2. Pain, swelling, and discoloration

Treatment

1. Elevate the affected part.
2. Apply cold compresses for first 8–10 hours (20–30 minutes at a time)—to produce vasoconstriction and decrease edema.
3. Apply heat to affected area after 8–10 hours (for 20–30 minutes)—to promote absorption: may be followed by cold applications to minimize secondary effects of heat.
4. Apply pressure bandage—to reduce hemorrhage and swelling.

> **NURSING ALERT:** Soft tissue injuries and fractures may result in compartment syndrome, with severe pain and loss of sensation or motion. Immediate intervention (fasciotomy) is required.

SPRAINS AND STRAINS

A *sprain* is an injury to ligamentous structures surrounding a joint; it is usually caused by wrenching or twisting.
A *strain* is tearing of the musculotendinous unit caused by excessive force or stretching.

Clinical Manifestations

A. *Sprains*

1. Rapid swelling—due to extravasation of blood within tissues
2. Spasm of muscles that move the joint
3. Pain upon passive movement of joint

B. *Strains*

There is usually hemorrhage into the muscle, swelling, tenderness, and pain with isometric contraction of the muscle.

Treatment and Nursing Management

1. X-ray injured area—to ensure that there is no bone injury.
2. Elevate and rest affected part.
3. Apply cold compresses (or ice bag) for 15–20 minutes intermittently for 12–36 hours—vasoconstricting effects of cold retard extravasation of blood and lymph (edema) and suppress pain.
4. After 24 hours apply mild heat (15–30 minutes, 4 times daily)—to promote absorption.
5. Support injured structure with compressive dressings and splinting.
6. For more severe sprains (tearing of fibers and disruption of ligaments) patient may require surgical repair and/or cast immobilization so that joint will not lose its stability.

TRAUMATIC JOINT DISLOCATION

A *dislocation of a joint* is a condition in which the articular surfaces of the bones forming the joint are no longer in anatomic contact (bones are "out of joint").

Clinical Manifestations

1. Pain
2. Deformity
3. Change in the length of the extremity
4. Loss of normal movement
5. Change in axis of dislocated bones

Treatment

1. Immobilize part while patient is transported to emergency department, x-ray or clinical unit.
2. X-ray affected part—to confirm diagnosis and rule out associated fracture.
3. The dislocation is reduced (displaced parts brought back into normal position) usually under anesthesia.
4. Essentials of nursing management are the same as for reduction of fractures (see p. 756).

FRACTURES

A *fracture* is a break in the continuity of bone. Although the bone is the part most directly affected, other structures may be involved, resulting in soft tissue edema, hemorrhage into muscles and joints, joint dislocations, ruptured tendons, severed nerves, damaged blood vessels, and injury to body organs.

Classification of Fractures (Fig. 18-1)

A. *Types of Fractures*

1. *Complete*—a fracture involving the entire cross section of the bone; usually displaced (removed from normal position)
2. *Incomplete*—a fracture involving only a portion of the cross section of bone; usually undisplaced
3. *Open*—break in the skin and underlying soft tissue leading directly into the fracture or its hematoma
4. *Closed*—the fracture does not communicate with outside area

B. *Specific Types of Fractures* (Fig. 18-1)

1. *Greenstick*—a fracture in which one side of a bone is broken and the other side is bent
2. *Transverse*—the fracture is straight across the bone
3. *Oblique*—a fracture occurring at an angle across the bone (less stable than transverse)
4. *Spiral*—a fracture twisting around the shaft of the bone
5. *Comminuted*—a fracture in which bone has splintered into several fragments
6. *Depressed*—a fracture in which fragment(s) is (are) in-driven (seen frequently in fractures of skull and facial bones)
8. *Compression*—a fracture in which the fractured bone has been compressed by another bone(s) (seen in vertebral fractures)

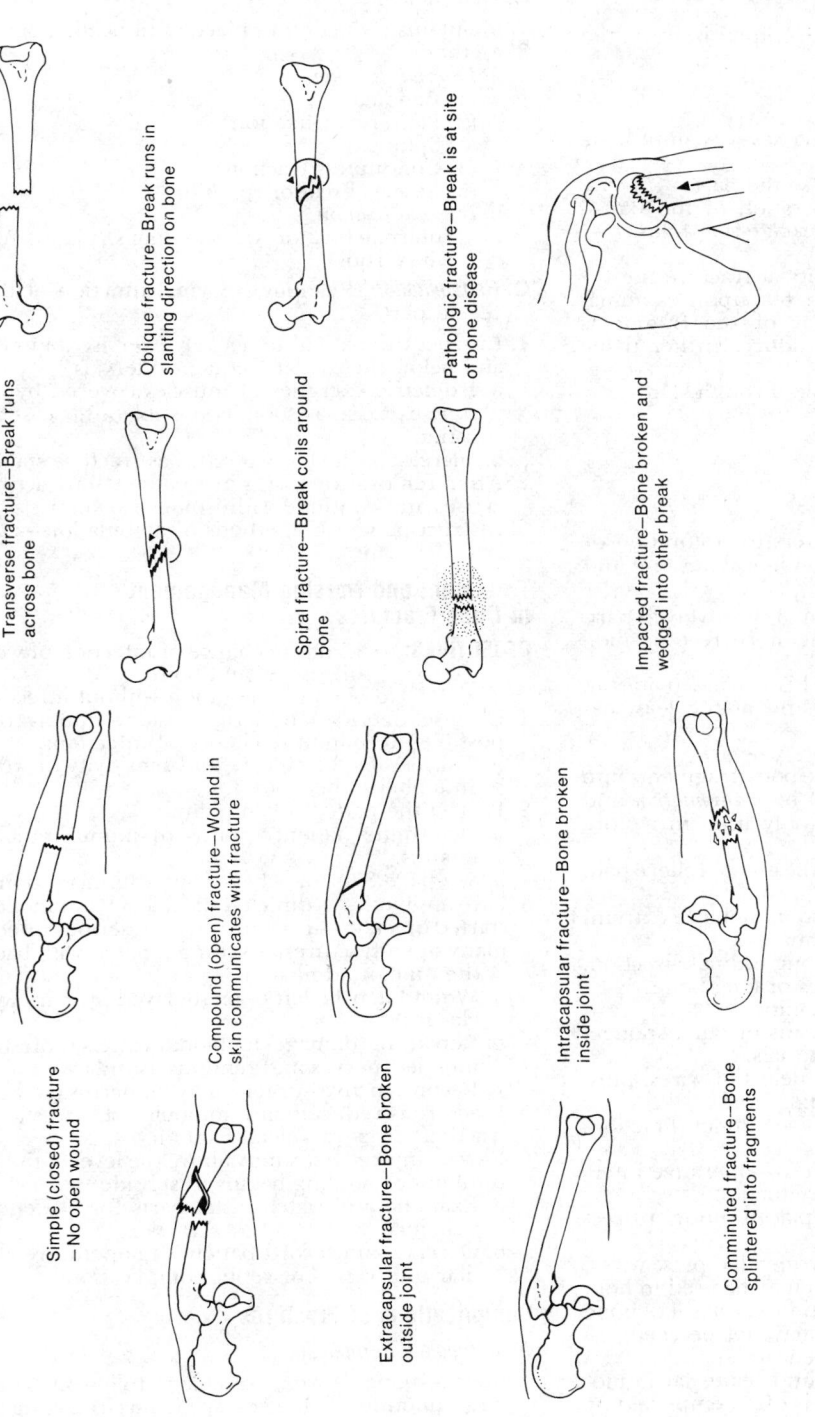

Transverse fracture—Break runs across bone

Oblique fracture—Break runs in slanting direction on bone

Spiral fracture—Break coils around bone

Pathologic fracture—Break is at site of bone disease

Impacted fracture—Bone broken and wedged into other break

Fracture dislocation—Break complicated by bone out of joint

Depressed fracture—Broken skull bone driven inward

Simple (closed) fracture—No open wound

Compound (open) fracture—Wound in skin communicates with fracture

Extracapsular fracture—Bone broken outside joint

Intracapsular fracture—Bone broken inside joint

Comminuted fracture—Bone splintered into fragments

Greenstick fracture—Bone broken, bent but still securely hinged at one side

Longitudinal fracture—Break runs parallel with bone

FIGURE 18-1. *Types of fractures. (From Nursing Care of the Patient in the O.R. Somerville, New Jersey, Ethicon, Inc.)*

9. *Pathologic*—a fracture that occurs through an area of diseased bone (bone cyst, Paget's disease, bony metastasis)
10. *Avulsion*—fragment of bone pulled off by ligament or tendon and its attachment
11. *Epiphyseal*—separation of the epiphysis from the rest of the bone

Clinical Manifestations

1. Pain—continues with increasing severity until bone fragments are immobilized
2. Loss of function; inability to use the part
3. Localized swelling and discoloration of the skin—from trauma and from hemorrhage that follows
4. Deformity (visible or palpable)
5. False motion; abnormal mobility at fracture site
6. Crepitation—grating sensation felt upon examination, due to rubbing together of the fragments (testing for crepitation can produce further tissue damage)
7. In open fracture, bone is visible through skin

Emergency Management

See page 884.

Treatment

A. *Reduction* (setting the bone)—refers to restoration of the fracture fragments into anatomical position and alignment.

OBJECTIVES: to regain the function of the involved part.
to regain and maintain correct position and alignment.
to return patient to his usual activities in the shortest time and at the least expense.

1. Methods
   a. *Closed reduction*—bringing the bony fragments into apposition (ends in contact) by *manipulation* and *manual traction* (most commonly used to restore alignment).
      (1) Usually done under anesthesia—to relieve pain and relax muscles.
      (2) Cast is usually applied—to immobilize extremity and maintain reduction.
   b. *Traction*—force applied in a longitudinal direction.
      (1) May be used for fractures of long bones.
      (2) Traction applied to extremity by:
         (a) Skin traction —by means of tape, sponge, rubber, or plastic materials.
         (b) Skeletal traction—by means of wires, pins, or tongs placed through bone
      (3) For nursing management see under Traction, pages 763–766.
   c. *Open reduction* (open operation)—operative intervention to achieve fracture reduction.
      (1) Bone fragments are replaced under direct visualization.
      (2) Internal fixation devices (metallic pins, wires, screws, plates, nails, rods) may be used to hold bone fragments in position until solid bone healing occurs (may or may not be removed after bony union has taken place)
      (3) After closure of the wound, external immobilization of the fracture is often employed by application of splints or casts.
      (4) For nursing management following open reduction, see Nursing Management of the Patient Undergoing Orthopedic Surgery, pages 775–776.
   d. *Endoprosthetic replacement*

B. *Fracture Immobilization*

1. Maintains reduction in place until healing occurs.
2. Methods
   a. *External fixation*
      (1) Bandages
      (2) Plaster cast fixation
      (3) Splints
      (4) Continuous traction
      (5) External fixator (p. 766)
   b. *Internal fixation*
      Internal fixation devices (nails, plates, screws, wires, rods)

C. *Rehabilitation* (Regaining normal function of the affected part)

1. Instruct the patient to actively exercise joints above and below the cast at frequent intervals.
   a. Isometric exercises of muscles covered by cast—start exercise as soon as possible after cast application.
   b. Increase isometric exercises as fracture stabilizes.
2. After removal of cast, have patient start active exercises and continue with isometric exercises.
3. Instruct patient in methods of ambulation—walker, crutches, cane.

Treatment and Nursing Management of Open Fractures

OBJECTIVES: to minimize chance of infection of wound, soft tissue, and bone.
to obtain bone union without infection.

1. Cleanse, debride, and irrigate the wound as soon as possible—to minimize chance of infection.
   a. Take swabs for culture and sensitivity of wound.
   b. Immobilize the wound.
2. Protect the patient from tetanus.
   a. Determine patient's status of immunization for tetanus.
   b. See page 874 for schedule of administration.
3. Give antibiotics as directed (usually IV antibiotics are started quickly)—to avoid and treat serious infection; many open fractures are contaminated with bacteria at the time of admission.
4. a. Wound may be left open (delayed primary wound closure).
   b. Repair of damage to blood vessels, soft tissue, muscles, nerves and tendons as indicated.
   c. Reconstructive surgery may be necessary.
5. Fracture is reduced and immobilized by cast, splint, traction, or extraskeletal fixation
6. Elevate injured extremity above the level of the heart until initial swelling begins to subside.
   a. Examine and watch distal parts for evidences of ischemia.
   b. Observe and record patient's temperature at regular intervals—for septic complications.

Complications of Fractures

A. *Immediate Complications*

1. Shock—bone is very vascular; following trauma, large amounts of blood escape from circulating blood into soft tissues or through open wounds (especially in femoral and pelvic fractures).
   a. May be fatal within a few hours after injury.

b. Treatment and Nursing Management (see also p. 128)
 (1) Replace the depleted blood volume; maintain arterial blood pressure.
 (2) Relieve the patient's pain.
 (3) Provide adequate splinting.
 (4) Protect the patient from further injury.
2. Hemorrhage (see p. 130).
3. Fat embolism syndrome—embolization of marrow or tissue fat or lipids with platelets and circulating free fatty acids within the pulmonary capillaries; pulmonary capillary leak may result, producing respiratory distress and central nervous system dysfunction.
 a. Onset may occur within 48 hours after injury.

NURSING ALERT: Have a high degree of suspicion of fat embolism syndrome in patients with multiple fractures, and fractures of long bones and pelvis. Hypoxemia is an early manifestation and is detected by arterial blood gas analysis.

 b. Assess patient for:
 (1) Respiratory distress—tachypnea, dyspnea, hypoxemia, rales, wheezing, acute pulmonary edema—lung filters and traps embolic material, producing disturbed ventilation, perfusion and interstitial pneumonitis.
 (2) Mental disturbances—irritability, restlessness, confusion, disorientation, stupor, and coma—effects of systemic embolization and severe hypoxemia (may be first sign).
 (3) Fever.
 (4) Petechiae—in buccal membranes, conjunctival sacs, on the hard palate, retina, chest, and anterior axillary folds—from occlusion of capillaries by fat and fibrin platelet particulate substances.

B. *Treatment and Nursing Management*

OBJECTIVE: to maintain satisfactory pulmonary gas exchange and support the respiratory system.
 (1) Draw arterial blood for gas analysis—arterial hypoxia is present with fat emboli; cannot always be recognized clinically.
 (2) Administer oxygen as indicated by results of blood gas analysis (respiratory failure is the most common cause of death).
 (3) Assist with endotracheal intubation (for airway control); controlled volume ventilation and positive end-expiratory pressure (PEEP)—to obtain maximum aeration of lungs.
 (4) Administer steroids—to block chemical inflammation caused by free fatty acids; decreases endothelial damage (controversial).
 (5) See treatment of respiratory failure and insufficiency, page 169.
4. Thromboembolism (particularly of fractures of lower extremities).
5. Infection—all open fractures are considered contaminated. (See also gas gangrene, p. 819, and tetanus, p. 818).
6. Disseminated intravascular coagulation (DIC)—a group of bleeding states with diverse causes.
 a. Many serious illnesses predispose to DIC, including massive tissue trauma.
 b. Clinical manifestations: unexpected bleeding during or after surgery, ecchymoses, anemia; bleeding from mucous membranes, venipuncture sites, gastrointestinal and urinary tracts.
 c. See page 259 for treatment of DIC.
7. Peripheral nerve injury—bone ends may injure nerves.

C. *Delayed Complications of Fractures*
1. Delayed union—signifies that a specific fracture has not healed in the time considered average for this fracture.
2. Nonunion—failure of the ends of a fractured bone to unite (and union not expected to occur).
3. Avascular necrosis of bone—may occur when the bone loses its blood supply following fracture or dislocation (notably in the hip) or in certain diseases.

CASTS

A *cast* is an immobilizing device made up of layers of plaster bandages or alternatives to plaster (fabric tape impregnated with light sensitive resin, thermoplastic polymer resin, or polyurethane).

Purposes
1. To immobilize and hold bone fragments in reduction
2. To apply uniform compression of soft tissues
3. To permit early mobilization
4. To correct and prevent deformities

Types of Casts (Fig. 18-2)
1. *Short-arm cast*—extends from below the elbow to the proximal palmar crease
2. *Gauntlet cast*—extends from below the elbow to the proximal palmar crease, including the thumb (thumb spica).
3. *Long-arm cast*—extends from upper level of axillary fold to proximal palmar crease; elbow usually immobilized at right angle
4. *Short-leg cast*—extends from below knee to base of toes
5. *Long-leg cast*—extends from upper thigh to the base of toes; foot is at right angle in a neutral position
6. *Spica or body cast*—incorporates the trunk and an extremity
 a. *Shoulder spica cast*—a body jacket that encloses trunk, shoulder and elbow
 b. *Hip spica cast*—encloses trunk and a lower extremity
 (1) Single hip spica—extends from nipple line to include pelvis and one thigh
 (2) Double hip spica—extends from nipple line or upper abdomen to include pelvis and extends to include both thighs and lower legs
 (3) One and a half hip spica—extends from upper abdomen, includes one entire leg, and extends to the knee of the other
7. Cast brace

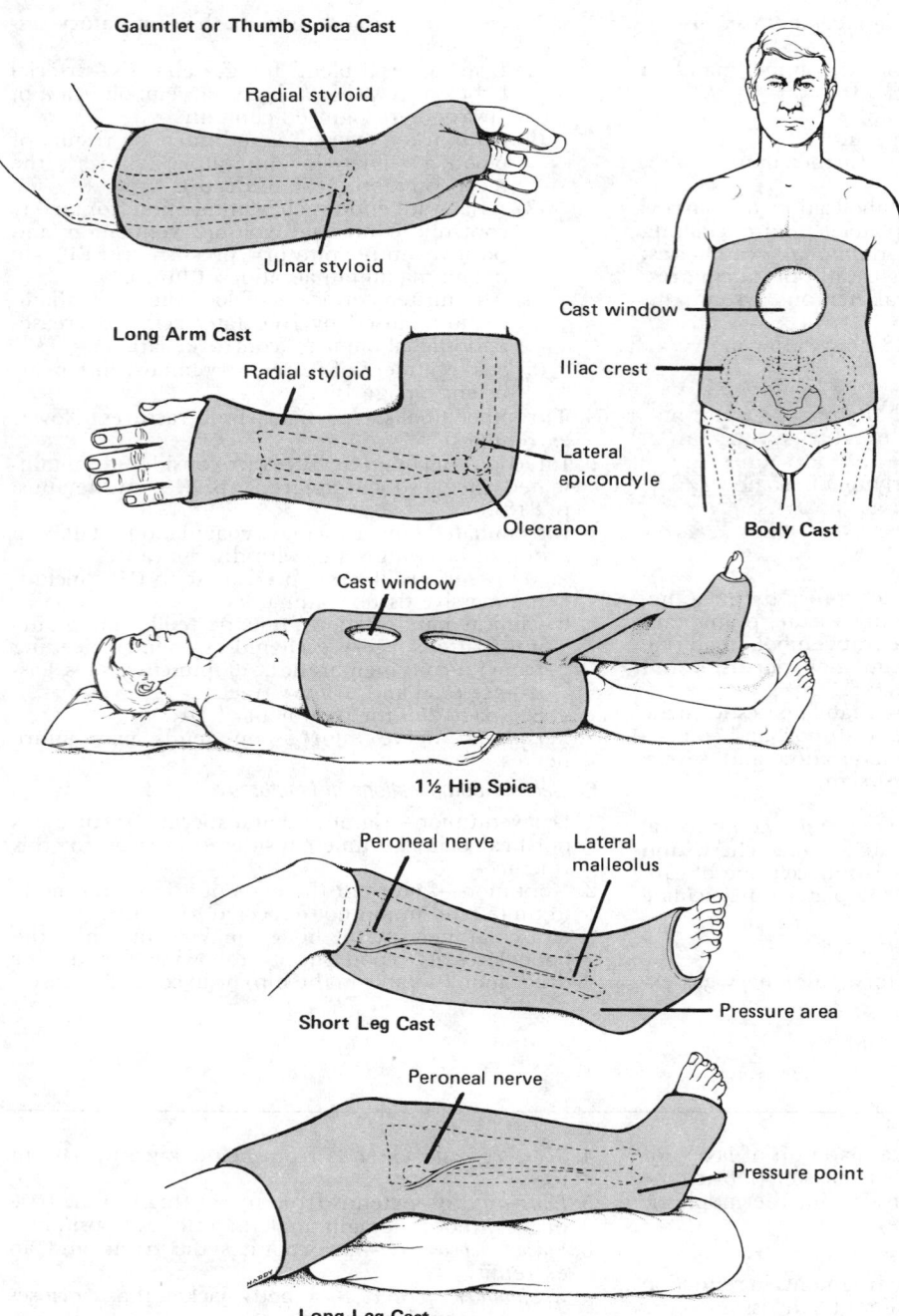

FIGURE 18-2. *Pressure areas in different types of casts.*

Application of Cast

See Guidelines: Application of a Plaster Cast, page 761.

Complications

A. *Constriction of Circulation*

Trauma or surgery affecting an extremity will produce swelling (result of hemorrhage from bone and surrounding tissue and of tissue edema). Vascular insufficiency and nerve compression due to unrelieved swelling can cause a reduction in or obliteration of blood supply and peripheral nerve damage to an extremity.

1. *Symptoms and Signs*
   a. *Unrelieved pain or increasing pain*
   b. Swelling

c. Blanching or discoloration
   (1) Test nail beds and pulp of digits of injured extremity for prompt capillary return. A rapid return of color should appear on release of pressure.
   (2) The color should be pink; blueness suggests venous obstruction.
   (3) Whiteness and cold fingers or toes suggest arterial obstruction.
   (4) Compare uninjured with injured extremity.
d. Tingling or numbness
e. No pulse or diminished pulse
   Compare pulse on uninjured extremity with that of injured extremity.
f. Inability to move fingers or toes; pain on extension of foot or hand may indicate ischemia.
g. Temperature change of skin—cold extremity may indicate ischemia.
2. *Nursing Management*
   a. Bivalve the cast; split cast on each side over its full length into 2 halves.
   b. Cut the underlying padding—blood-soaked padding may shrink and cause constriction of circulation.
   c. Spread cast sufficiently to relieve constriction.

B. *Pressure of Cast on Neurovascular Structures and Bony Parts*

1. Causes necrosis, pressure sores, nerve palsies from prolonged pressure on nerve trunk.
2. *Symptoms*
   Severe initial pain over bony prominences; this is a warning symptom of an impending pressure sore. *Pain decreases when ulceration occurs.*
3. *Pressure Sites*
   a. *Lower extremity*—heel, malleoli, dorsum of foot, head of fibula, anterior surface of patella.
   b. *Upper extremity*—medial epicondyle of humerus, ulnar styloid.
   c. When plaster jackets or body spica casts are used—sacrum, anterior and superior iliac spines, vertebral borders of scapulae.
4. *Nursing Management*
   a. Examine the skin over the area by creating a "window" in the plaster cast at the pain point (over bony prominence).
   b. Or bivalve (split) the cast but do not disturb the alignment; keep extremity in one portion of bivalved cast.

NURSING ALERT: Do not ignore the complaint of pain of the patient in a cast. Suspect circulatory complications or a pressure sore.

Care of Patient While Cast Dries

A. *Extremity Cast*

1. Explain to the patient that he will experience the feeling of heat under the plaster; however, plaster application is not painful.
2. Leave area enclosed in cast *uncovered* until the cast is dry—covers restrict escape of heat, especially in large casts. A fan helps to circulate the air.
3. Elevate the extremity on cloth-covered pillow above the level of the heart *after the cast has cooled* and started to dry. Keep the heel off the mattress.

4. Avoid resting cast on hard surfaces or sharp edges that can cause denting or flattening of the cast and consequent pressure sores.
5. Avoid weight bearing or stress on cast for 24 hours.

B. *Spica or Body Cast*

1. Place a bedboard under the mattress—prevents sagging of bed from pressure of cast.
2. Support the curves of the cast with cloth-covered flexible pillows—prevents cracking and flat spots while cast is drying.
   a. Place three pillows crosswise on bed for body cast.
   b. Place one pillow crosswise at the waist and two pillows lengthwise for affected leg for spica cast. If both legs are involved, use two additional pillows.
3. Handle moist cast with palms of hands.
4. Turn patient every 3 hours while cast dries (see below).

Observation of the Patient in a Cast

1. Listen to the patient's complaints (see complications).
2. Ask the patient to localize the exact site of pain.
3. Avoid giving analgesics for pain. Do not mask the pain until the cause has been determined.
4. Watch for signs of pressure and constriction of circulation.
5. Notify physician if symptoms persist. Cast may have to be removed.

Care of Patient After Cast Dries

A. *Hip Spica Cast* (see Fig. 18-2)

1. Keep the cast level by elevating the lumbar sacral area with a small pillow when the head of the bed is elevated or when the patient is placed on the bedpan.
2. Protect the toes from the pressure of the bedding.
3. Encourage the patient to maintain physiologic position by:
   a. Using the overhead trapeze.
   b. Placing good foot flat on bed and pushing down while lifting himself up on the trapeze.
   c. Avoiding twisting motions.
   d. Avoiding positions that produce pressure on groin, back, chest, and abdomen.
4. Provide hygienic care of the patient.
   a. Cover perineum with a towel and apply spray (lacquer-type) to perineal area of cast. Tuck 10 cm. (4-inch) strips of thin polyethylene sheeting under perineal area of cast and tape to cast exterior. Replace when soiling occurs.
   b. Clean outside of cast with dry cleanser on almost-dry cloth.
   c. Pull stockinette taut, trim, and fasten to cast edges with adhesive.
   d. Inspect skin for signs of irritation:
      (1) Around cast edge.
      (2) Under cast—pull skin taut and inspect under cast, using a flashlight for illumination.
   e. Reach up under cast and massage accessible skin.
   f. Use a fracture bedpan. Roll patient onto bedpan; place pillow in lumbosacral area.
5. Turn the patient.
   a. Move the patient to the side of the bed, using a steady, even, pulling motion.
   b. Place pillows along the other side of the bed; 1 for the chest and 2 (lengthwise) for the legs.
   c. Instruct the patient to place his arms at his side or above his head.

d. Turn the patient as a unit. Avoid twisting the patient in the cast.

e. Turn the patient toward the leg not encased in plaster or toward the unoperated side if both legs are in plaster.

(1) One nurse stands at other side of bed to receive patient's shoulders.

(2) Second nurse supports leg in plaster while the third nurse supports the patient's back as he is turned.

(3) DO NOT GRASP CROSS BAR OF SPICA CAST TO MOVE PATIENT. The purpose of the bar is to strengthen the cast.

f. Turn patient to a prone position twice daily—provides postural drainage of bronchial tree; relieves pressure on back.

6. Encourage patient to drink liberal quantities of fluid—to avoid urinary calculi.

7. Have patient exercise the parts of the body that are not immoblized by the cast at regular and frequent intervals. Also encourage deep breathing exercises and coughing at regular intervals.

NURSING ALERT: Watch for symptoms (*nausea*) of cast syndrome (acute obstruction of duodenum) after spica or body cast is applied. (See intestinal obstruction, p. 434.)

If symptoms occur

1. Place patient prone to relieve pressure symptoms.

2. Remove patient from cast if necessary.

3. Employ nasogastric suction.

4. Maintain normal electrolyte balance by intravenous replacement of fluid.

Surgical intervention (duodenojejunostomy) may be necessary when conservative measures fail to relieve duodenal obstruction.

B. *Leg Cast*

1. Prevent or reduce swelling.

a. Elevate the extremity in the cast above the level of the heart.

b. Apply ice bags (⅓–½ full) to each side of the cast, making sure they do not make indentations in plaster.

c. After patient begins ambulation, encourage him to elevate the cast when he is seated. Encourage patient to lie down several times daily with cast elevated.

2. Prevent irritation at cast edge—pad edges of cast with moleskin or petal the cast edges with strips of adhesive tape.

3. Examine toes and foot for:

a. Blanching or cyanosis

b. Swelling

c. Inability to move toes

4. Ascertain if patient is experiencing sensory disturbances to foot (numbness, tingling, burning, cold)—peroneal nerve injury from pressure at the head of the fibula is a common cause of footdrop; may be initial finding in vascular compromise.

5. *Be alert for evidences of thromboembolic complications.*

High risk individuals (increased age, previous thromboembolism, obese, congestive heart failure, cancer of pancreas or lung, trauma) may require prophylaxis against thromboembolism.

6. Encourage the patient to move about as normally as possible.

a. Do prescribed exercises faithfully.

b. Do not cover a leg cast with plastic or rubber boots since this causes condensation and wetting of the cast. Avoid walking on wet floors or sidewalks.

c. Report to the physician if the cast cracks or breaks; instruct the patient not to try to fix it himself.

C. *Arm Cast*

1. Check neurovascular status. Watch for symptoms of circulatory disturbance in hand (blueness or cyanosis, swelling, inability to move fingers, forearm pain on extension of fingers).

2. Reduce and control swelling.

Elevate arm with each joint positioned higher than preceding joint (i.e., elbow higher than shoulder, hand higher than the elbow).

NURSING ALERT: Guard against Volkmann's contracture—a severe fibrosis with resulting contracture of muscles which have become ischemic by obstruction of the arterial flow to the forearm and hand. This complication is prevented by proper care; if allowed to develop, the results are disastrous.

Health Education

1. Watch for these danger signs (arm or leg cast): blueness or paleness of fingernails or toenails accompanied by pain and tightness, numbness, cold or tingling sensation.

a. Elevate the affected limb above the heart and wiggle fingers/toes.

b. Call the physician if condition persists.

2. Teach the patient to perform isometric exercises—contracting the muscles without moving the joint, to maintain muscle strength and prevent atrophy (performed hourly when awake).

3. Exercise every joint that is not immobilized. Move the rest of the body.

4. Actively exercise joints that do not move bone fragments.

a. Leg-cast—"Push down on the popliteal (knee) space, hold it, relax, repeat." Move toes back and forth; bend toes down, then pull them back.

b. Arm cast—"Make a fist, hold it, relax, repeat." Move shoulders.

5. Avoid getting cast wet, especially padding under cast—causes skin breakdown.

6. Do not place sharp objects under the cast.

7. To clean the cast:

a. Remove surface soil with slightly damp cloth.

b. Rub soiled areas with household scouring powder.

c. Wipe off residual moisture.

8. Report to the physician if cast breaks; do not attempt to fix it yourself.

GUIDELINES: Application of a Plaster Cast

Equipment   Plaster bandages; 5, 7.5, 10, 15, 20 cm. (2, 3, 4, 6, 8 inch) widths
Cast padding (Webril cotton padding)
Stockinette (tubular knitted material)
Plaster splints (for reinforcement)
Cotton, polyester, or polyurethane foam padding for bony prominences
Knives, scissors, indelible pencil
Polyethylene sheeting or newspaper—to protect floor
Disposable gloves—to protect hands of operator
Large plastic-lined pail of water at room temperature—21–24° C. (70–75° F.)

Underlying Considerations

1. The application of a cast requires 2–3 persons; one to apply the plaster (operator), one to dip and hand the plaster bandages to the operator, and a third person to hold the extremity in correct position. (Body spicas may require additional personnel.)
2. Plaster of paris bandages and splints may be fast-setting (5–8 minutes) and extra-fast-setting (2–4 minutes); the technique of application varies somewhat according to the manufacturer.
3. The operator should practice cast application on a model. Plaster sets rapidly and this is a skill that requires experience.
4. There should be no movement of the extremity while the cast is being applied.
5. In general, the joints above and below the involved bone are usually immobilized.

Procedure

ACTION	RATIONALE/AMPLIFICATION
Preparatory Phase	
1. Spread polyethylene sheeting or newspaper on floor.	
2. Explain to the patient that there will be a feeling of warmth as the plaster is applied.	2. Heat is produced by crystallization as plaster sets. The reaction of water with plaster of paris liberates heat.
3. Apply stockinette and roll cast padding on the extremity or part to be immobilized. a. Sheet wadding: Apply as smoothly and snugly as possible so that each turn overlaps the preceding turn by ½ the width of the roll. b. Extra pieces of padding may be placed over bony prominences; olecranon process, malleoli, patella.	3. Padding is used to pad the sharp cast margins for patient comfort and to prevent pressure areas, minimize circulatory problems, and facilitate cast removal. a. & b. Sheet wadding is applied from the distal to the proximal end of the extremity. When too much padding is used, it may roll up and produce pressure under the cast, causing muscle atrophy.
4. While keeping the thumb under the forward edge of the bandage, submerge the plaster bandage vertically in water (room temperature) for a minute or so, or until bubbles cease to rise.	4. Water that is too warm will accelerate setting time, may cause a burn, and may result in excessive plaster loss by loosening the adhesive agents that bond the plaster to the fabric.
5. Expel excess water by squeezing (not wringing) towards the center of the bandage; hand bandage to operator with free end hanging loose.	5. The cast will dry more quickly (and thus will acquire maximum strength sooner) if a well-squeezed bandage is used.
Performance Phase (by operator)	
1. Starting at the distal end, roll the bandage gently and evenly on the extremity, overlapping the preceding turn by ½ the width of the roll.	1. Roll inward towards the patient's body for ease of control.
2. Keep the bandage moving and in constant contact with the surface of the extremity. Smooth and rub down successive layers or turns of each bandage into the layers below with the thumbs and thenar eminences (mound on the palm) in circumferential and longitudinal directions.	2. This keeps the cast uniformly thick. Rubbing the plaster as it is applied will form a smooth, solid and well-fused cast. Avoid indenting the cast with the fingertips since this will produce pressure sores on underlying skin.
3. Take tucks in the lower border of the bandage by lifting the bandage off the surface (without tension) and overlapping it in a V-shaped fashion.	3. Tucking the bandage helps to contour the cast to the changing circumference of the extremity. Do not twist or reverse the bandage to change its direction since this produces sharp cutting edges.
4. Trim the cast to size with a sharp knife.	4. Do not pull too vigorously on the stockinette since this may cause pressure on bony pressure points.
5. Ask the patient if there is any discomfort or pain.	5. If a patient complains of pain, the cast and encircling dressings should be split to avoid constriction, circulatory problems, and pressure sores.
Follow-up Phase	
1. Write the diagnosis and date of injury and cast application with an indelible pencil on the cast.	

GUIDELINES: Application of a Plaster Cast (cont.)

Procedure (cont.)

ACTION	RATIONALE/AMPLIFICATION
2. Support the cast with the palm of the hand while moving the patient. Avoid indentations from tips of fingers.	2. Finger indentation on a fresh cast can produce pressure sores.
3. Expose the cast to warm, circulating dry air. Or blow air over cast with a circulating fan to increase the evaporation of water and consume heat.	3. Avoid covering the cast when it is drying as this delays drying time and causes a rise in temperature. Usually the cast will reach its maximum temperature 5–15 minutes after it is applied and will then cool rapidly. The ultimate cast strength is obtained after the cast is dry (up to 48 hours depending on outside temperature and humidity).
4. Clean plaster from equipment and store ready for use.	

GUIDELINES: Removal of a Cast

Equipment

Cast cutter—an electric saw with circular blade that oscillates through the plaster
Cast spreader
Surgical, linoleum, or plaster knife
Scissors

Procedure

NURSING ACTION	RATIONALE/AMPLIFICATION
Preparatory Phase	
1. Describe to the patient how and where the cast cutter will be used and the expected sensations. Turn on the cutter and allow the patient to hear the motor.	1. Reassures the patient that the cutter produces vibrations but not pain.
2. Determine whether or not the cast is padded.	2. An electric plaster cast cutter should not be used on unpadded casts.
3. Determine where the cut will be made. Mark, with a felt pen, the area to be cut.	3. The line should be in front of the lateral malleolus and behind the medial malleolus on a lower extremity cast. An upper extremity cast is usually split along the ulnar or flexor surface.
4. Dampen the cast along the portion to be cut.	4. Dampening diminishes the cloud of plaster dust.
Performance Phase	
1. Inform the patient that plaster dust may be irritating to his eyes.	
2. Grasp the electric cutter as illustrated (Fig. 18-3A).	
3. Rest the thumb on the plaster.	3. The thumb serves as a depth gauge and acts as a guard in front of the blade.
4. Turn on the electric cutter. Push the blade firmly and gently through the cast while holding the thumb against the cast to steady the blade while cutting through the cast.	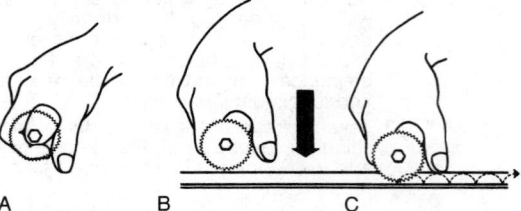
5. As the blade cuts through the plaster, a sudden lack of resistance is felt; plaster will "give" (or "dip") when the cut is completed.	
6. Lift the cutting blade up a degree (but not out of the cutting groove) and advance the blade at a slightly higher or lower level. The cast is cut by a series of alternating pressure and linear movements along the line of the cut (Fig. 18-3B, C).	**FIGURE 18-3.** *Operating a cast cutter. (Courtesy of Stryker Corporation.)*
7. Avoid drawing the cutting blade along the extremity in a single motion.	7. This will cut the skin. If saw blade is in contact with padding too long, patient will feel burning sensation on skin from rapidly oscillating blade.
8. Cut the cast on both sides. Then rock the anterior portion of the cast over the posterior portion.	8. This maneuver allows the operator to determine if the cast is completely cut.

Procedure (cont.)	**NURSING ACTION**	**RATIONALE/AMPLIFICATION**
	9. Insert the blades of the cast spreader in the cut trough. Separate the 2 halves with the spreader at several sites along the cast split. Separate the cast with the hands.	9. Or spread the cast while cutting, to facilitate its removal.
	10. Cut through the padding and stockinette with scissors, keeping the scissor blade that is closest to the skin parallel to the skin.	10. Use bandage scissors; place the flat blade closest to the skin.
	11. Lift the extremity carefully out of the posterior portion of the cast. Support the extremity so that it is maintained in the same position as when in the cast.	11. When the support of the cast has been removed, stresses and strain are placed on parts that have been at rest.
	After Removal of Cast	
	1. Cleanse the skin gently with bland soap and water. Blot dry. Apply a skin cream.	1. Explain to the patient that the skin will be scaly and the extremity will appear "thin" from disuse. Reassure him that it will take a few weeks to regain normal appearance and function.
	2. Emphasize the importance of continuing the prescribed exercises, reporting for physical therapy, etc.	2. Exercises are necessary to redevelop and increase strength and function. Pain and stiffness may be expected after cast removal.

TRACTION

Traction is force applied in a specific direction. To apply the force needed to overcome the natural force or pull of muscle groups, a system of ropes, pulleys, and weights is used. Traction may be applied to the skin or to the skeletal system.

Purposes

1. To reduce and immobilize fracture.
2. To regain normal length and alignment of an injured extremity.
3. To lessen or eliminate muscle spasm.
4. To prevent fracture deformity.
5. To give the patient freedom for "in bed" activities.
6. To reduce pain.

Methods

A. *Skin Traction*—accomplished by a weight that pulls on tape, sponge rubber, or plastic materials attached to the skin or a special device (boots); traction on the skin transmits traction to the musculoskeletal structures.

1. Skin traction is used as a temporary measure in adults; used prior to surgery in treatment of intertrochanteric hip fracture (Buck's extension); Russell's traction is used for applying traction to the femoral shaft with the knee flexed. Skin traction may be used definitively to treat fractures in children.
2. *Application and Nursing Assessment*—see pages 764 and 765.

B. *Skeletal Traction*—is traction applied to bone using wires, pins, or tongs placed through bones; this is the most effective means of traction. It is applied by the orthopedic surgeon under aseptic conditions.

1. Skeletal traction is used most frequently in treating fractures of the femur, humerus (supracondylar fractures), tibia, and cervical spine.
2. *Nursing Assessment and Responsibilities:*
   a. Watch for signs of infection, especially around the pin tract.
      (1) The pin should be immobile in the bone and the skin wound should be dry.
      (2) If infection is suspected, percuss gently over the tibia; this may elicit pain if infection is developing.
      (3) Assess for other signs of infection: heat, redness, fever.
   b. If directed, clean the pin tract with sterile applicators and prescribed medication/ointment—to clear drainage at the entrance of tract and around the pin, since plugging at this site can predispose to bacterial invasion of the tract and bone.
   c. Apply a cork or adhesive over the sharp edges of the pin.
   d. Check traction apparatus at repeated intervals to see that the direction of pull is correct and the ropes are unobstructed; that weights are in proper position; and that patient is comfortable.
   e. See below for nursing management.

C. *Cervical Traction*—see page 740.

D. *Pelvic Traction*—used for treatment of back disorders or injuries.

Nursing Management of Patient in Traction

1. The patient is placed on a firm mattress, often with a hinged bedboard beneath it.
2. The ropes and the pulleys should be in straight alignment.
3. The pull should be in line with the long axis of the bone.
4. Any factor that might reduce the pull or alter its direction must be eliminated.
   a. Weights should hang free.
   b. Ropes should be unobstructed and not in contact with the bed or equipment.
   c. Help the patient to pull himself up in bed at frequent intervals. Traction is *not* accomplished if the knot in the rope or the footplate is touching the pulley or the foot of the bed, or if the weights are resting on the floor.
5. The amount of weight applied in skin traction must not exceed the tolerance of the skin. The condition of the skin must be inspected frequently.

6. There is always the possibility of bone infection when skeletal traction is used. Be alert for odors, signs of local inflammation, or other evidence of infection.
7. The patient's skin should be examined frequently for evidences of pressure or friction over bony prominences.
8. Provision should be made for supplying additional countertraction by increasing the pull in the opposite direction, i.e., by raising the bed in such a manner that the weight of the patient's body tends to oppose the pull of the traction.
9. Active motion of all unaffected joints should be encouraged.
10. *Every complaint of the patient in traction should be investigated immediately.*

Principles of Balanced Suspension Traction

Balanced suspension traction is produced by a counterforce other than the patient's body weight. The extremity balances or floats in the traction apparatus. The line of traction on the extremity remains fairly constant despite changes in the patient's position.

Nursing Management
1. The patient may be elevated, turn slightly, and move as desired.
2. The angle of hip flexion is approximately 20 degrees (the angle between the thigh and the bed).
3. The ropes and the pulleys should be freely movable; the traction should be applied securely to the leg.
4. Observe for skin irritation around the traction bandage.
5. Check the patient for odor and signs of infection.
6. Observe for pressure under the sling at the popliteal space.

7. Provide foot supports to prevent footdrop.
8. The traction must be continuous to be effective.

Principles of Running Traction

Running traction is a form of traction in which the pull is exerted in one plane. It may utilize either skin or skeletal traction, and it may be either unilateral or bilateral. Example: Buck's extension.

A. *Activities Permitted the Patient*
1. The head of the bed may be elevated to the point of countertraction—e.g., if the countertraction is 20 cm. (8 inches), the head of the bed may be elevated 20 cm.
2. The patient may not turn from side to side because the position of the leg on the bed will cause the bony fragments to move against each other.

B. *Nursing Management*
1. The foot should be inspected for circulatory difficulties within a few minutes and then periodically after the elastic bandage has been applied.
2. Special care must be given to the back at regular intervals, because the patient maintains a supine position.
3. Any complaint or burning sensation under the traction bandage should be reported immediately.
4. Observe for wrinkling or slipping of the traction bandage.
5. The patient should have foot supports to prevent footdrop.
6. Check peripheral pulses and the color and temperature of the fingers and toes.
7. Check for calf tenderness and for possible Homan's sign for evidence of thrombophlebitis.

GUIDELINES: Application of Buck's Extension Traction

Buck's extension (unilateral or bilateral skin traction) is a form of traction used as a temporary measure to provide support and comfort to a fractured extremity until definitive treatment is accomplished (Figs. 18-4, 18-5).

Equipment

Traction tape: (Flex-Foam Traction Bandage or adhesive traction bandage) *or* prepadded boots
Elastic bandage, 10 cm. (4 inch)
Cast padding
Spreader block or metal spreader
Pulley, nylon rope, and weights (2.3–3.1 kg. [5–7 lbs] is usual)
   (Amount of weight is prescribed by physician)
Tincture of benzoin (for adhesive traction)
Sheepskin pad
Shock blocks

Procedure

NURSING ACTION	RATIONALE/AMPLIFICATION
Preparatory Phase	
1. Place bedboard under the mattress and shock blocks under the wheels at the foot of the bed if indicated. This depends on the size of the patient and the weight applied.	1. Elevating the foot of the bed (countertraction) helps prevent the patient from sliding down toward the foot of the bed.
2. Question the patient to determine previous skin conditions (contact dermatitis). Inspect skin for evidences of atrophy, abrasions, and circulatory disturbances.	2. The skin must be in healthy condition to tolerate skin traction.
3. Make sure that the skin of the extremity is clean and dry.	3. A clean, dry skin helps traction tape adherence.
4. Document the neurovascular status of the extremity, any evidence of skin problems or varicosities.	

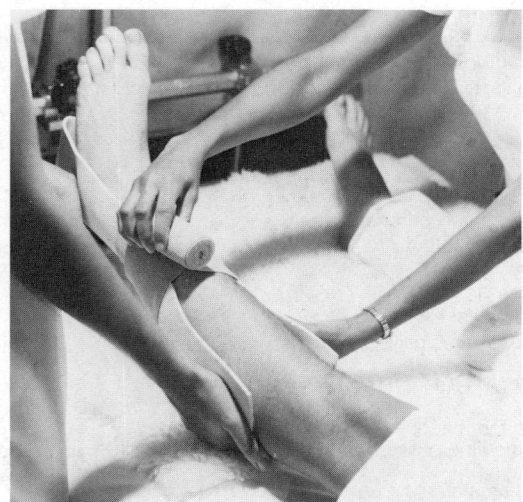

FIGURE 18-4. *Applying elastic bandage for Buck's extension traction.*

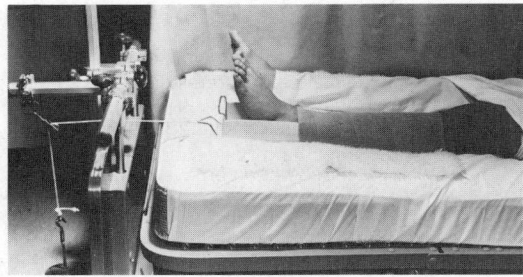

FIGURE 18-5. *Lower extremity in Buck's extension traction.*

Procedure (cont.)

NURSING ACTION	RATIONALE/AMPLIFICATION

Performance Phase

1. For nonadhesive traction bandage:
   a. Pad both malleoli and proximal fibula with cast padding.

   a. Pressure sores and skin necrosis may result from pressure applied directly over malleoli. Pressure over the region of the fibular head and common peroneal nerve may produce peroneal palsy and footdrop.

   b. Apply Flex-Foam (with the foam surface against the skin) on each side of the affected extremity, leaving a loop projecting 10–15 cm. (4–6 inches) beyond the sole of the foot.

   b. Prepadded boots may be used.

2. For adhesive traction bandage:
   a. Pad both malleoli and proximal fibula. Apply tincture of benzoin to the skin.

   a. Adhesive strapping is infrequently used. A skin adhesive, tincture of benzoin, may help protect the skin, although the tape adheres satisfactorily without it.

   b. Gently stroke the tape onto the skin. Apply adhesive skin tape in the same manner as nonadhesive traction bandage.

   b. Stroking the tape onto the skin promotes skin adherence and prevents wrinkles and creases.

   c. Make 0.6–1.2 cm. (¼–½ inch) oblique cuts along each border of the tape if necessary.

   c. Clipping the border of the tape allows it to conform to the contour of the leg. Uneven tension contributes to skin breakdown.

3. Have a second person elevate and support the extremity under the ankle and knee while the elastic bandage is applied (Fig. 18–4). Beginning at the ankle, wrap the elastic bandage snugly over the tape up to the tibial tubercle.

3. The elastic bandage improves adherence of tape to the skin and helps prevent slipping.

4. Attach a spreader block (or metal spreader) to the distal end of the tape. Attach a rope to the spreader block and pass it over a pulley fastened to the end of the bed (Fig. 18–5).

4. The spreader block prevents pressure along the side of the foot. The spreader should not be too narrow (causes pressure sores on ankle) or too wide (pulls traction tape away from the heel).

Follow-up Phase

1. Make sure knots are tied securely. Gently attach the traction weight. Release gradually.

1. The rope should be unobstructed; the weight should hang free of the bed and should not touch the floor.

2. Place a sheepskin pad under the leg (or use a commercial heel protector).

2. Sheepskin is used to reduce friction of the heel against the bed.

3. Assess the patient to ensure he is in proper alignment.

3. The part of the body in traction should be in line with the pull of the weight.

GUIDELINES: Application of Buck's Extension Traction (cont.)

Procedure (cont.)

Nursing Assessment of the Patient following Application of Buck's Extension

1. Palpate over area of traction tapes daily. If area is tender to palpation, suspect skin irritation and report it immediately. The traction bandage may have to be removed.
2. Inspect for skin irritation and pressure on:
   a. Achilles tendon
   b. Peroneal nerve (as it passes around the neck of the fibula just below the knee)
3. Inspect dorsum of foot for loss of sensation, weakness of dorsiflexors of foot and toes, inversion of foot—may be caused by tight traction tape and pressure on the common peroneal nerve.
4. Unwrap the elastic bandage periodically and assess neurovascular status; check for evidence of slipping of traction tape.
5. Assess for complaints of persistent itching and burning.
6. Maintain the extremity in a neutral position. Avoid external rotation.
7. The patient may not turn from side to side because the position of the leg on the bed will cause the bony fragments to move against each other.
8. Inspect and bathe back. To give back care instruct the patient to:
   a. Place hands on overhead trapeze.
   b. Bend the knee of unaffected extremity and place foot flat on bed.
   c. Push down on the uninvolved foot while at the same time pulling up on the trapeze—allows the entire body and trunk to rise off the bed.
      The shoulders, back, and buttocks must move as a single, straight unit.
9. See page 763 for other aspects of nursing management.

EXTERNAL FIXATION FOR COMPLICATED FRACTURES

External fixation is a technique of fracture immobilization in which a series of transfixing pins is inserted through bone and attached to a rigid external metal frame (Fig. 18-6). The method is mainly used in the management of open fractures with severe soft tissue damage.

Advantages

Permits rigid support of severely comminuted open fractures, infected nonunions, and infected unstable joints.

Facilitates wound care (frequent debridements, irrigations, dressing changes) and soft tissue reconstruction (delayed wound closure, muscle flaps, skin grafts).

Allows early function of muscles and joints.

Allows early patient comfort.

Procedure

Under general anesthesia the skin is cleansed and transfixing pins are inserted through small incisions above and below the fracture and drilled through the bony cortex. Following reduction of the fracture, the appliance is tightened by adjusting and tightening the bars connecting the sets of pins.

Nursing Management

OBJECTIVES: to achieve wound and fracture healing.
   to maintain continuing assessment for complications.

1. Reassure patient that the procedure is done under general anesthesia and although the fixator appears clumsy and cumbersome, it should not hurt once it is in place.
2. Following the procedure, the extremity is placed in balanced suspension traction to reduce swelling.
   a. Extremity can be suspended by hanging the fixator directly to the traction frame; support the foot.
   b. See care of the patient in traction, page 763.

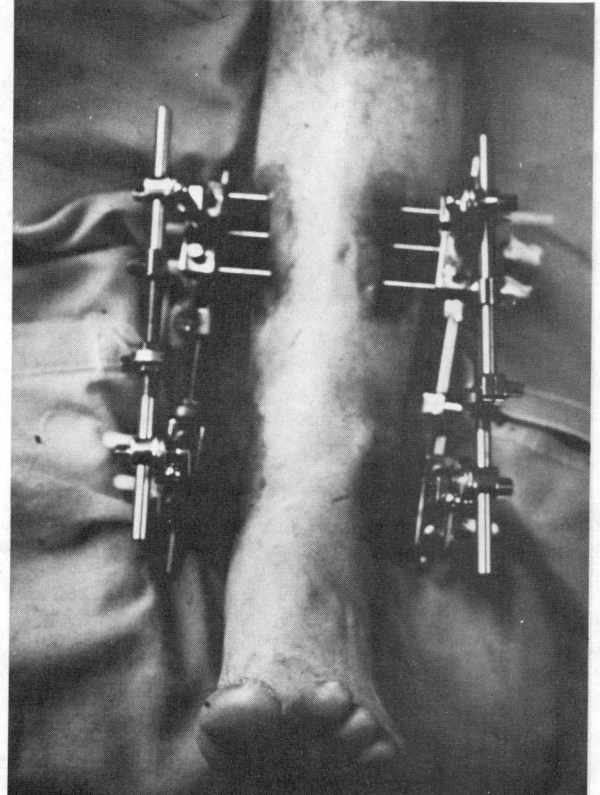

FIGURE 18-6. *External fixation. (Courtesy of University of Texas Health and Science Center at Dallas.)*

3. Pin tract and fixator care:
   a. Inspect each pin site for redness, drainage, tend-erness, pain, and loosening of the pin.
   b. Cleanse pin tract and remove crusts with sterile cotton applicator dipped in hydrogen peroxide or alcohol 1–2 times daily—crusts formed by serous drainage can prevent fluid from draining and cause infection.
   c. Apply nonocclusive antimicrobial agent around pin sites as directed.
   d. Be sure the sharp pin heads are covered with plastic covers or cork or rubber plugs—to protect other extremity and bed linens.
   e. Wipe off fixator with sterile cloth dampened with sterile water.
4. Wound care:
   a. The open wounds at the fracture site are usually treated by daily dressing changes. Allow ample time.
   b. Use sterile technique.
   c. Change dressings around pins first and under-neath fixator rods last.
5. Care of extremity:

a. Quadriceps exercises and range of motion for joints are usually started on first postoperative day.
b. To move the extremity, grasp the frame and assist patient to move. Reassure patient that the fixator can withstand normal movement.
c. Patient ambulates on crutches when soft tissue swelling has diminished; weight-bearing is done only as prescribed.

Health Education

1. Inspect around each pin site daily for signs of infection and loosening of pins. Watch for pain, soft tissue swelling, and drainage.
2. Cleanse around each pin tract daily, using aseptic technique. *Do not touch wound with hands.*
3. Clean fixator regularly—to keep it free of dust and contamination.
4. *Do not tamper with clamps or nuts*—can alter compres-sion and misalign fracture.
5. Showers can be taken when wound has healed; do not swim in chlorinated or sea water—may corrode fixator.

FRACTURES OF SPECIFIC SITES*

There is no one solution in the management of frac-tures. Consideration is given to the severity of the fracture, damage to soft tissues, the age and condition of the patient, and economic factors before a specific form of treatment is selected.

OBJECTIVE: to restore the function of the affected part to as near normal as possible.

Assessment

Watch for neurovascular impairment in all patients with fractures: pain, decreased circulation, decreased sensation, and decreased motor activity.

FRACTURES OF THE UPPER EXTREMITY

Fracture of the Clavicle (Collar Bone)

1. The clavicle helps to hold the shoulder upward, outward, and backward from the thorax.
2. Aim of reduction: to hold the shoulder in the position described above.
3. Most fractures of the clavicle are treated by closed reduction and immobilization accomplished by one of the following methods:
   a. Clavicular strap (Pad axilla to prevent nerve dam-age from pressure.)
   b. Sling
   c. Figure 8 bandage
   d. T-splint.
   { Watch for tingling in hands; too tight a clavicu-lar strap or figure 8 band-age may cause circulatory impairment.
4. Open reduction and internal fixation may be done for marked displacement and angulation of bone ends. Following surgery, the patient's arm is kept in a sling.

* For fracture of the skull see page 712; fracture of the cervical spine, page 740; and rib fractures, page 216.

Health Education

1. Exercise elbow, wrist, and fingers as soon as possible.
2. Do shoulder exercises to obtain full shoulder motion as prescribed. (Fig. 18-7).

Fractures of the Surgical Neck of the Humerus (Fractures of the Proximal Humerus)

1. Most occur from falls in which the outstretched arm strikes the ground (impacted fracture). Osteoporosis is a predisposing factor.
2. Many impacted fractures of the surgical neck of the humerus do not require reduction. The weight of the arm helps to correct displacement.
   a. Place a soft pad under the axilla to prevent skin maceration.
   b. The arm is supported by a sling and swathe or Velpeau bandage for comfort (Fig. 18-8).
   c. Advise the patient that he will sleep more com-fortably when supported in an upright position.
3. Displaced fractures are treated with reduction under x-ray control, open reduction, or replacement of humeral head with prosthesis.
   a. A program of exercises is started after a specified period of immobilization with emphasis on range of motion of the shoulder (Fig. 18-7).
   b. Watch for postoperative infection.

Health Education
OBJECTIVE: to restore shoulder function and prevent adhesions.
1. Start active motion of shoulder joint early—to pre-vent limitation of motion and stiffness of shoulder.
2. Instruct patient to lean forward and allow affected arm to abduct and rotate.

Fractures of the Shaft of the Humerus

1. Fractures of the shaft of the humerus are most frequently caused by direct violence—falls, blow to arm, auto injuries.

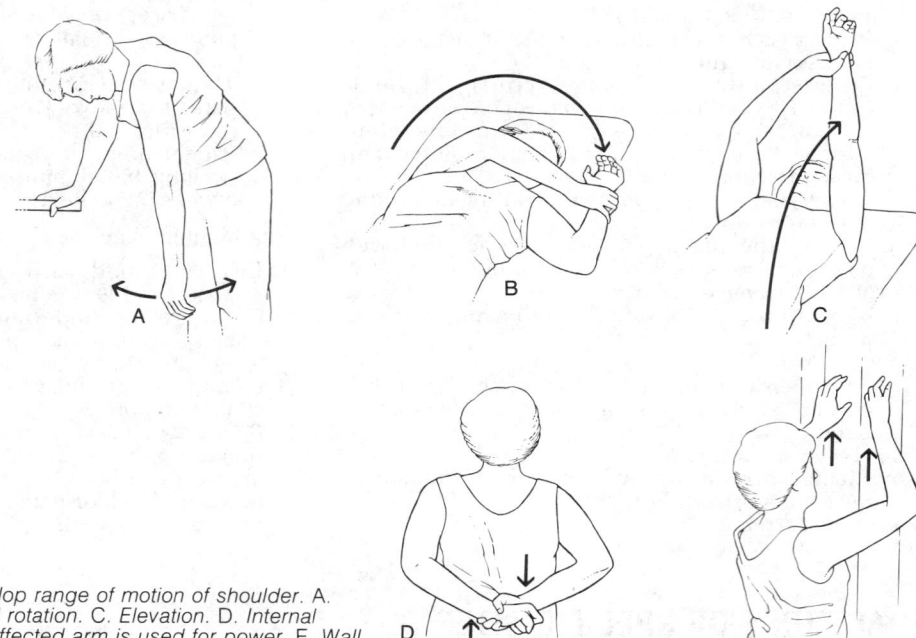

FIGURE 18-7. *Exercises to develop range of motion of shoulder. A. Pendulum exercise. B. External rotation. C. Elevation. D. Internal rotation. In all of these, the unaffected arm is used for power. E. Wall climbing.*

2. The radial nerve may be injured in this fracture because it lies immediately adjacent to the midportion of the humerus in the musculoskeletal groove.
3. Sling and swathe, splints, or hanging casts may be used.
4. Hanging cast is frequently applied to oblique, spiral, and displaced fractures with shortening of humeral shaft—the weight of the arm helps to correct displacement.

> **NURSING ALERT:** A hanging cast for treatment of fracture of the shaft of the humerus must be dependent (remain unsupported) to provide a traction force. Continuous traction on long axis of arm is affected by the weight of the cast. The patient must avoid supporting the elbow in the lap while seated.

5. See that the patient sleeps in a fairly upright position to maintain uninterrupted 24-hour traction.
6. Exercise fingers immediately after the application of the cast.
7. Start pendulum exercises as directed—provides active exercise of shoulder to prevent adhesions of the shoulder joint capsule after cast removal (Fig. 18-7A).
8. Open reduction and internal fixation (usually by compression plate) are performed when satisfactory alignment cannot be obtained with closed treatment, when there is associated vascular injury, and when the fracture is the result of a pathologic (malignant) lesion. Internal fixation is often supplemented by methyl methacrylate (bone cement).

   Following a surgical procedure, the arm is placed in a sling and swathed until bone union has taken place at the fracture site.

Fractures and Dislocations about the Elbow

1. Dislocations or fractures about the elbow usually occur as the result of a fall on the elbow or the outstretched hand, or from a direct blow (sideswipe injury).
2. Each fracture is different, hence specific treatment cannot be described.
3. Treatment may be nonoperative (cast immobilization) or operative (open reduction and internal fixation; orthoplasty).

Nursing Management

1. Watch for signs of impaired circulation in forearm and hand.
   a. Observe hand for swelling, skin color (blueness or blanching of nailbeds), and temperature, comparing it with the unaffected hand.
   b. Evaluate radial pulse; if it weakens or disappears, call orthopedic surgeon *immediately*, since irreversible ischemia may develop.
2. Assess for paresthesias (prickling and burning sensations) in the hand—indicate nerve injury or impending ischemia.
3. Encourage patient to move his fingers frequently.
4. Exercises to increase range of motion are started when prescribed.

Fractures of the Head and Neck of the Radius

1. Usually produced by indirect trauma (fall on outstretched hand) or by direct trauma (blow).
2. *Undisplaced fracture*
   a. Aspiration of hemarthrosis (blood in joint) at the elbow may be done to relieve pain and allow earlier range of motion.
   b. Immobilization by plaster slab or sling.

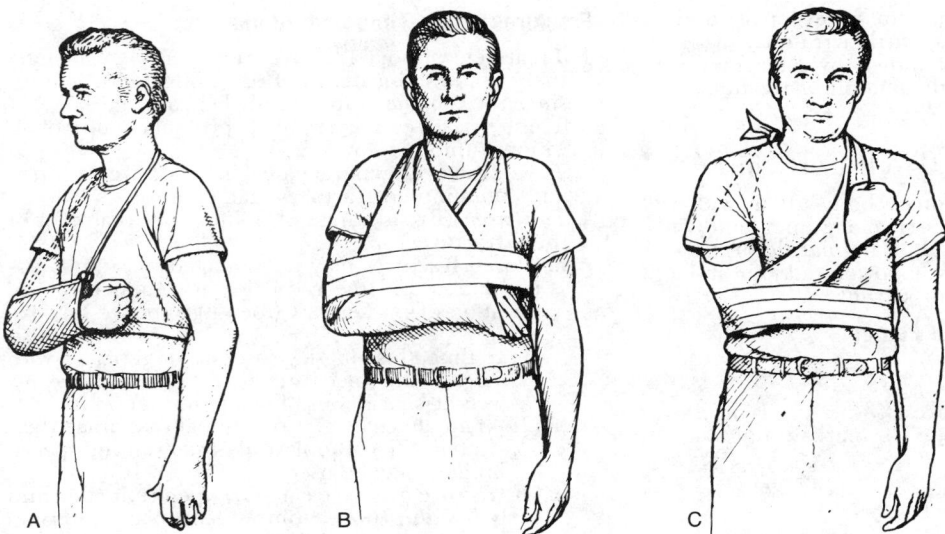

FIGURE 18-8. *The types of immobilizing dressings used for upper humeral fractures. A. A commercial sling and swathe that permits easy removal of the arm for exercises and is comfortable on the neck. B. A conventional sling and swathe. C. A stockinette Velpeau and swathe used when there is an unstable surgical neck component, because this position relaxes the pectoralis major. (From Rockwood, CA and Green DP. Fractures. Philadelphia, JB Lippincott Co.)*

3. *Displaced fracture*—open operation with excision of radial head when indicated.
   a. Postoperatively the arm is immobilized in a posterior plaster splint and sling and elevated.
   b. Early active motion of elbow and forearm is encouraged when prescribed.

Health Education
Encourage patient to continue *daily* program of repetitive, progressive exercises (as prescribed). The exercise program is designed to restore full extension and supination.

Fractures of the Shafts of the Radius and Ulna

1. Objective of treatment is to preserve function of forearm.
2. *Undisplaced fractures*—treated by immobilizing arm in a long-arm cast with elbow flexed 90 degrees.
   a. Watch circulation and function of hand.
   b. Encourage active flexion and extension of fingers at frequent intervals to reduce edema. Encourage shoulder motion.
3. *Displaced fractures*—open operation with internal fixation accomplished by compression plate or some other fixation device.
   a. Postoperatively, a closed drainage system may be used to decrease hematoma and resultant swelling.
   b. The arm is usually immobilized in plaster splints or cast until there is evidence that fracture is healing.

Health Education
Encourage patient to move his fingers and the shoulder of the involved extremity.

Fracture of the Wrist

1. Colles' fracture is a fracture of the radius 1.2–2.5 cm. (½–1 inch) above the wrist with dorsal displacement of the lower fragment.
2. Treatment usually consists of closed reduction and plaster of paris splint or cast support (or by skeletal pins incorporated in plaster).
   a. Elevate arm above level of heart for 48 hours after reduction.
   b. Watch for swelling of fingers—indicates decreased venous and lymphatic return. Check for constricting bandages or cast.

Health Education
Instruct patient to do finger exercises to reduce swelling and prevent stiffness.
1. Hold hand above level of heart.
2. Move fingers from full extension to flexion (fist position). Hold and release.
3. Repeat at least 10 times every half hour when awake—as long as hand has a tendency to swell.

Fractures of the Hand

1. Numerous injuries to the hand require extensive reconstructive surgery which is beyond the scope of this book. The reader is referred to specialized texts on the hand.
2. Objective of treatment is to regain maximum function of the hand.
3. *Undisplaced fracture of the distal phalanx*
   a. Drainage of the hematoma under the fingernail may be necessary.
   b. Finger is splinted (to adjoining finger or by a

dorsal or volar splint)—to relieve pain and to protect finger tip from further trauma.
4. *Open fractures* may be handled by Kirschner wire fixation following debridement and irrigation.

FRACTURES OF THE LOWER EXTREMITY

OBJECTIVES: to obtain adequate bony union with full length and normal alignment and without rotational or angular deformity.
to restore muscle power and joint motion.
to allow weight bearing.

Fracture of the Shaft of the Femur

> **NURSING ALERT:** Fracture of the shaft of the femur may be accompanied by marked concealed blood loss.

1. Closed reduction
   a. Fracture reduced and stabilized by means of balanced skeletal traction, such as Thomas leg splint with a Pearson attachment (Fig. 18-9).
   b. Thomas splint suspends the thigh; Pearson attachment applied to the splint allows knee flexion and supports the leg below the knee. Examine skin under the ring on Thomas splint.
   c. Skeletal traction in long axis of thigh is applied by means of a Kirschner wire or Steinman pin.
   d. May be supplemented with cast brace (for fractures of the shaft of femur—after a period of traction).
2. Open reduction with intramedullary (within the bone) fixation
   a. See nursing management following orthopedic surgery, page 775.
   b. Observe for complications: postoperative infection, chronic osteomyelitis.
   c. A cast-brace may be used in conjunction with internal fixation of fractured femur.
3. See Rehabilitation and Health Education After Fracture of Lower Extremity, page 771.

Fractures of the Tibia and Fibula

1. Treatment of tibial fractures represents a challenge; there is a high incidence of open infected fractures, since the tibia lies superficially beneath the skin.
2. These fractures may require prolonged immobilization—union is slow.
3. Tibial fractures generally heal in 12–16 weeks; open and comminuted fractures take longer.
4. *Treatment:* (Broad range of opinion on treatment of these fractures)
   a. Closed fractures may be managed by simple manipulation and the reduction maintained by application of plaster cast (toe to groin; see Fig. 18-2).
      (1) In time, this long-leg cast may be replaced with a below-the-knee functional cast which permits weight-bearing and knee joint motion.
      (2) As an alternative, a functional cast-brace (fabricated with orthoplast-like material and special hinges) may be used (see Fig. 18-10).
   b. Or fracture may be treated by open reduction and early fixation (plate, compression plate, intermedullary nails, or Hoffman external fixator) as indicated by etiology, type of trauma, and type of fracture.
   c. Pay special attention to ankle joint—may be problem of stiffness.

Nursing Management Following Knee Surgery

Problems of the knee include fractures, disease states (tumors, degenerative processes, neuromuscular disorders), and congenital abnormalities.
1. Elevate extremity; gatch the foot of the bed.
2. Evaluate for effusion of the knee—a common complication following knee surgery which produces marked pain.
   a. Cut pressure dressing and reapply if pain is severe. Call physician.
   b. Support patient undergoing aspiration of fluid from knee joint
3. Encourage quadriceps exercise to prevent atrophy of the thigh muscles; do also on unoperated leg.
4. Progressive exercises (straight leg raising, progressive resistive exercises) usually follow.

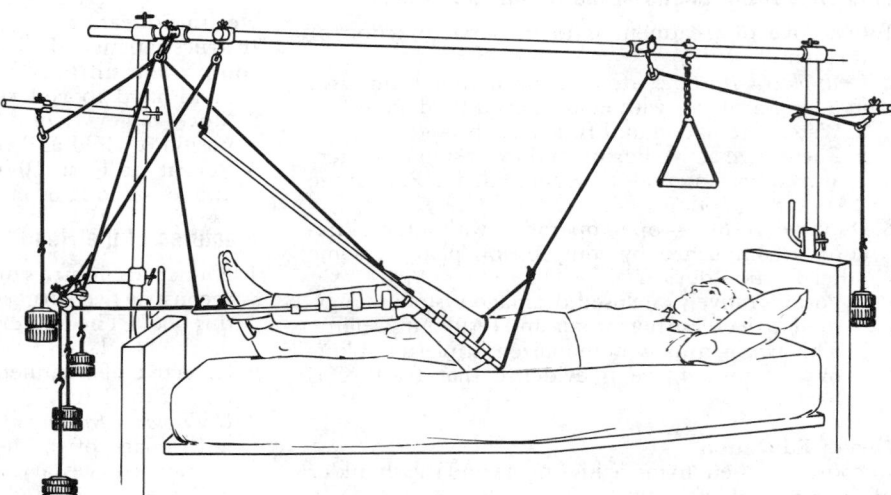

FIGURE 18-9. *Balanced traction with Thomas leg splint with Pearson attachment.*

5. Heat may be used as an adjunct to exercises—loosens muscles and ligaments, relieves discomfort.
6. Intermittent elevation and an elastic knee support to combat knee effusion are used following certain knee injuries.

Rehabilitation and Health Education After Fracture of Lower Extremity

1. Apply elastic stocking to uninvolved leg—maintains pressure on deeper leg veins, helps prevent stasis of blood, edema, and thrombophlebitis.
2. Elevate unaffected leg at intervals throughout day— to promote venous return.
3. Elevate affected extremity to promote venous return and relieve pain.
   a. The early reestablishment of venous return helps absorb blood and tissue fluid (edema from bleeding is a common cause of disability following fractures).
   b. Chronic edema predisposes extremity to fibrosis and ulceration.
   c. *It is desirable to lie down when elevating a leg cast.*
4. Exercise regularly all joints which do not move the bone fragments.
5. Avoid placing extremity in dependent positions for prolonged periods.
6. Mobilize the patient as soon as possible. Instruct in methods of ambulation—walker, crutches, and cane.
7. Physical therapy procedures may be utilized after cast removal (heat, cold, massage, exercise)—to restore joint mobility, increase muscle strength and endurance.
8. Instruct patient to wear elastic bandage or hose after cast is removed to support venous circulation and to reduce edema.
9. Advise patient to move feet up and down in pedaling motion to exercise calf muscles.
10. Recommend that patient start moving affected extremity under water if necessary, since water supports the extremity and provides warmth, which helps promote muscle relaxation.

CAST-BRACE

A *cast-brace* (fracture orthosis) is an external support about a fracture that permits early ambulation. Some cast-braces are constructed with hinges at the hip, elbow, wrist, and ankle (Fig. 18-10).

Rationale

Cast-bracing is based on the concept that some weight bearing is physiologic and will promote the formation of bone and contain fluid within a tight compartment which compresses soft tissues, providing a distribution of forces across the fracture site.

Purposes and Advantages

1. Permits progressive weight bearing
2. Allows motion of joints
3. Allows gradually increasing skeletal stresses and promotes fracture healing by transmission of forces through the bone.
4. Allows early return to mobility and independence.
5. Allows earlier hospital discharge and reduces expenses.
6. Lessens detrimental effect on body physiology by

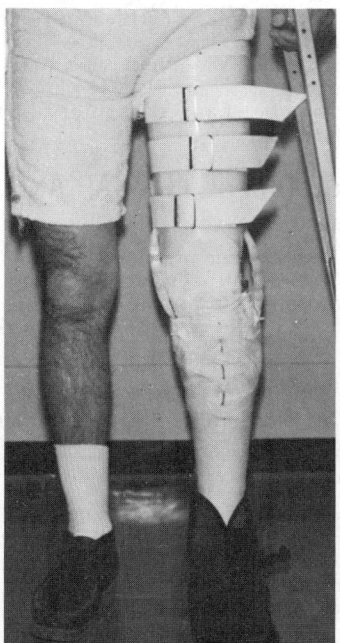

FIGURE 18-10. *Cast-brace provides circumferential support to a segment of a fractured limb while allowing mobility of nearby joints.*

shortening the period of recumbency—earlier return of bladder and bowel function, less chance of renal calculi, muscle atrophy, etc.

Clinical Indications

Fractures of tibia and of femoral shaft; supracondylar fractures of the femur (open or closed)
1. Tibial fracture—functional below-knee walking brace may be applied 2–3 weeks after fracture or earlier.
2. Femoral fracture—long leg cast-brace may be applied 2–6 weeks after patient has been in balanced suspension traction.
3. Cast-brace—applied after initial edema and pain have subsided and there is evidence of fracture stability.

Nursing Management and Health Education

1. The patient is usually permitted to get up 24–48 hours after cast-brace is applied.
   a. As much weight is borne on affected extremity as can be tolerated.
   b. Be sure patient uses proper crutch gait (3-point gait) so that normal gait and rhythm are established.
2. Advise patient that he should be closely monitored.
   a. Angular deformity may occur during first weeks of ambulation.
   b. Standing weight-bearing anteroposterior and lateral x-rays are taken at intervals.
3. Watch for skin breakdown and circulatory problems.
   a. Watch for excessive swelling of exposed area of knee.
   b. Report signs of skin discoloration, numbness, breakdown.

4. Protect cast from soiling (urine and feces)—cast may extend to groin.
5. Elevate extremity when not walking—to promote venous return.
6. The cast may be changed at intervals until clinical union is achieved.

FRACTURES OF THE LUMBAR AND DORSAL SPINE*

Fractures of the vertebrae of the dorsal and lumbar spine may involve the vertebral body, lamina and articulating processes, and spinous processes or transverse processes. (Fractures of the cervical spine are discussed on p. 740).

Clinical Manifestations

Severe pain in back—may radiate down legs or to the abdomen and chest

Clinical Problems

1. Fractures of the vertebral bodies may be compression fractures; they are frequently multiple and comprise the most common types of fractures of the spine.
2. The majority of vertebral fractures seem to be related to osteoporosis or trauma.
3. A spinal cord injury may occur with fracture or dislocation of a vertebra.

Treatment and Nursing Management

OBJECTIVES: to determine if there is injury to the spinal cord.
to assess for complications.
1. Assess and treat the patient for spinal cord injury (see p. 739).
2. Evaluate for paralytic ileus and difficulty in voiding—may occur in the first few days after compression fracture of the lower dorsal or lumbar spine—may be from retroperitoneal hemorrhage.
    a. Assess anal sphincter tone.
    b. Observe for fecal retention.
3. Use measures to prevent risk of thromboembolic complications—elevate foot of bed, apply elastic stockings, encourage active ankle motion, give anticoagulant therapy for high risk patient.

Management
A. *For stable injuries to vertebrae:*
1. Treat symptomatically for pain, and encourage patient to ambulate—or
2. Place patient on a firm mattress and keep on bed rest until pain subsides.
    a. Encourage patient to roll from side to side; patient should not sit up during acute stage.
    b. Give analgesics and muscle relaxants as required, since pain may be severe.
    c. Patient is permitted to ambulate with assistance (wearing shoes) when discomfort subsides.
    d. Encourage patient to do the prescribed back exercises—to increase or maintain the strength of back muscles (2–3 weeks after fracture).
        (1) Exercises are prescribed that strengthen spinal extensor muscles.
        (2) Exercises that encourage spinal flexion are contraindicated.

* See page 740 for fracture of cervical spine.

e. Patient may feel better with a corset-type brace or back support when he is ambulating; remove appliance while in bed.
f. Patient with a more severe injury may require a more substantial back brace or cast.

B. *For unstable fractures/displacement:*
1. The fracture may be reduced by postural positioning, protracted periods of immobilization, or open operation with internal fixation (Harrington rod).
2. The patient may then be placed in a body cast for immobilization. (See nursing management of patient in a cast, page 759.)
3. Mobilize the patient when physical examinations and x-ray evaluations determine there is no displacement or neurologic deficit.
4. Prepare the patient for laminectomy (see p. 743) when indicated.

FRACTURES OF THE PELVIS

Clinical Manifestations

1. Inability to bear weight without discomfort
2. Local swelling and tenderness at site of fracture
3. Symptoms of hemorrhage and shock

Treatment and Nursing Management

OBJECTIVES: to control hemorrhage and shock.
to carry out ongoing nursing assessment for injuries to the bladder, rectum, intestine, and intra-abdominal organs.
1. Control bleeding—hemorrhage is an immediate threat to life.
    a. External compression suit (G-suit) (see Fig. 22-5) allows compression of pelvic area—provides tamponade for bleeding and immobilizes fracture.
    b. Angiographic visualization of pelvic vascular tree—for localization of bleeding points. Bleeding artery may be occluded by an injection of autologous clotted blood deposited proximal to bleeding vessel, by Gelfoam, or by balloon-tip catheter.
2. Determine the extent of internal injuries.
    a. Request patient to void. Urine is examined for blood. A cystourethrogram and intravenous urogram are performed—to detect genitourinary injuries.
    b. Assess and evaluate for intra-abdominal hemorrhage—pelvic fractures may cause death from extraperitoneal and retroperitoneal hemorrhage.
        (1) Peritoneal lavage (p. 875) is carried out to diagnose intraabdominal hemorrhage.
        (2) Monitor stools and urine for blood.
        (3) Palpate peripheral pulses—absence of peripheral pulses may indicate major vessel disruption (torn iliac arteries, veins, etc.).
    c. Look for other injuries—direct force to pelvic girdle may involve intra-abdominal organs; commonly associated with perforation/rupture of bladder, and urethra, vascular injuries, and injuries to liver and spleen.
    d. Evaluate for other complications that are likely to develop as a result of shock, massive soft tissue injury, and multiple fractures—intravascular coagulation, thromboembolic complications, fat emboli, pulmonary complications, infection from large hematomas.
3. Definitive treatment of pelvic fractures
    a. Method of treatment depends on whether the

pelvic ring has been disrupted and whether the fracture involves the weight-bearing portion of the pelvis.
  b. Pelvic fractures may be immobilized and stabilized by
    (1) Bed rest
    (2) Pelvic slings
      (a) Fold sling back over buttocks to enable patient to use the bedpan.
      (b) Reach under sling to give skin care—sheepskin may be used to line sling to prevent pressure sores.
      (c) Loosen the sling only upon physician request.
    (3) Skeletal traction
    (4) Bilateral hip spica cast (p. 759)
    (5) External fixation
    (6) Open reduction with or without internal fixation
  c. Mobilization and weight bearing are determined by x-ray and the patient's reaction to mobility.

HIP FRACTURES (TREATED BY AN INTERNAL FIXATION DEVICE) (Fig. 18-11)

Prevention

Hip fractures are the most frequent cause of death after the age of 75; they occur more frequently in women, often after insignificant injuries. The following preventive measures are advocated to protect against hip fractures:
1. Vigorous physical activity
2. Dietary vitamin D and calcium
3. Exposure to sunlight
4. Use of a cane by the person with osteoporosis

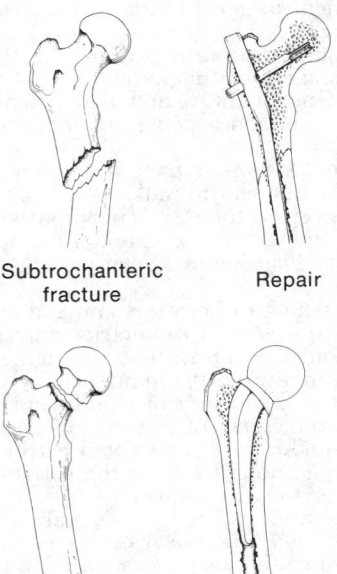

Subtrochanteric fracture   Repair

Femoral neck fracture   Repair

FIGURE 18-11. *Hip fractures and techniques used in their repair.*

Clinical Manifestations

1. Shortening and external rotation of affected leg
2. Pain; usually inability to move extremity

Types of Hip Fractures

Intracapsular—femur is fractured inside the joint (femoral neck fracture)
Extracapsular—femur fractured outside the joint (intertrochanteric fracture)

Treatment and Nursing Management

OBJECTIVES: to prevent physical, psychological, and social dependence.
to restore the ambulatory function of the hip joint (if the patient was ambulatory before the fracture).

A. *Preoperative Nursing Management*
1. Alleviate the pain.
  a. Prepare the bed with a trapeze and flotation mattress.
  b. To transfer patient onto the bed (from Emergency Department):
    (1) Place a pillow between the legs—to keep affected leg in a secure position.
    (2) With two nurses positioned at each side of the bed, use the sheet under the patient and lift the patient off the stretcher onto the bed.
    (3) Turn the patient on the affected side while supporting the shoulder and thigh, and remove the sheet.
    (4) Position the patient supine. Place a pillow under the affected leg from mid-thigh to ankle and a sandbag under the pillow on the side of the patient's affected calf.
    (5) Raise the head of the bed slightly, no higher than 40°.
  c. The patient may be treated with either Buck's extension or pillow positioning.
    (1) Assist with the application of Buck's extension as indicated. Buck's extension is used to afford patient mobilization and to relieve pain until the operative procedure is performed (see p. 764). (Split-Russell's traction may be used.)
    (2) The patient with an intracapsular fracture will assume a flexed and externally rotated position. Support extremity in this position with pillows until surgery is performed.
  d. Handle the affected extremity gently.
  e. Give analgesics as patient's condition indicates.
  f. Keep the skin dry and relieve pressure areas—pressure sores develop rapidly in the preoperative period. (See p. 64 for prevention of pressure sores.)
    (1) Check the neurovascular status of the extremity.
    (2) Inspect the heel *daily*—a patient with a painful hip tends to let weight of leg press the heel against the bed; area loses sensation when blood supply diminishes and nerve endings necrose.
    (3) Support leg with pillow if permitted—distributes pressure more evenly.
    (4) Place a sheepskin pad under the leg.
    (5) Check traction frequently, especially elastic bandages.
2. Ensure that the patient is in as favorable a condition as possible preoperatively.

a. Coordinate studies to assess cardiovascular, pulmonary, renal, and hematologic systems.
b. Correct fluid and electrolyte disturbances. Give intravenous infusions *slowly*—older patients with limited cardiac reserve cannot tolerate additional circulatory loading.
c. Determine if patient is oriented to time, place, and person—mental confusion may be due to underlying systemic illness, particularly to cardiopulmonary disease with inadequate cerebral oxygen transport, stroke, etc.
d. Carry out an ongoing nursing assessment—mental alertness, bright facial expression, and good skin turgor are considered favorable prognostic indications.
3. Use anticipatory nursing assessment and techniques to avoid complications.

NURSING ALERT: Thromboembolism is the most common complication following hip fractures, and it frequently occurs without clinical signs.

a. Prevent thromboembolism with leg exercises, elastic stockings, early ambulation.
b. Warfarin, low-molecular weight dextran, aspirin, or low doses of heparin given subcutaneously may be effective in reducing the incidence of venous thrombi.
c. Elevate foot of bed 25 degrees—to promote venous drainage.
d. Use orienting activities to prevent confusion—clock, calendar, television, explanations and reassurance, same care-giver. (See p. 833 for care of the confused elderly patient.)
e. Teach the use of incentive spirometer, coughing, deep breathing, and exercises, especially quadriceps setting.
f. Notify Social Services Department—to plan postoperative care to avoid unnecessary prolonged hospital care.

B. *Intraoperative Considerations*
1. Surgical procedure is usually carried out as soon as possible after full medical assessment since these patients are usually elderly and prolonged bed rest is detrimental.
2. Stable fractures are usually reduced and fixed with a nail, nail-plate combination, multiple pins, screw, sliding nails, etc, by replacement of the femoral head, or by a total hip procedure.

C. *Postoperative Nursing Management*
1. See Nursing Management of the Patient Undergoing Orthopedic Surgery, page 775.
a. Carry out neurovascular check of affected extremity.
b. Monitor drainage from portable suction.
c. Position affected leg as directed—usually on a pillow with mild abduction.
For patient with femoral head prosthesis, the hip should be kept in abduction, extension, and slight external rotation.
2. Encourage the patient to move by herself as much as possible to decrease the likelihood of complications (thromboembolism, diminished cerebral perfusion, aspiration of secretions and pneumonia, gastrointestinal stasis, urinary problems, increase in bone mineral loss, pressure sores).
a. Teach patient to assist with turning by having her grasp the trapeze or bedrails.
b. Place pillow between legs—to maintain alignment.
c. Using two persons, gently pull patient onto affected side; when lying on unoperated side, keep the affected extremity in position of abduction.
d. Encourage patient to take deep breaths while turning.
3. Get the patient out of bed as soon as possible.
a. Wrap the lower extremities with elastic compression bandages or elastic hose—increases venous velocity in legs and helps minimize dependent edema.
b. Use the tilt table as soon as patient's condition permits (p. 70). With the use of the tilt table the patient becomes accustomed to the upright position, and circulation and respiratory functioning improve.
c. Assist the patient into a wheelchair several times daily as prescribed—helps avoid arterial hypotension, helps maintain strength, aids pulmonary function, and is beneficial psychologically.
  (1) With the aid of the overhead trapeze, encourage the patient to move into the dangle position. (Use a Hi-Low bed.)
  (2) Assist patient to stand on the *unaffected extremity* and transfer to the chair.
  (3) If weight-bearing is permitted, patient may be encouraged to ambulate with walker, applying as much weight to extremity as is comfortable.
  (4) Certain types of fractures must be supported and protected until bone union is secure and displacement of fractures unlikely. If this is the case, the patient may have to be lifted into the chair.
  (5) Allow the patient to get up at her own pace; avoid hurrying.
d. Encourage the patient to participate in activities of daily living (eating, bathing, hair care)—to condition the patient for future ambulation activities and to help maintain a degree of independence.
4. Start active exercises as soon as pain and soreness subside to prepare the patient to walk.
a. Encourage quadriceps setting exercises hourly—the quadriceps femoris muscle extends the leg and is one of the major muscles necessary for ambulation.
b. Do heel-cord stretching of both legs and abdominal and gluteal contractions (isometric contractions). Isometric muscle contractions strengthen the muscle but do not move the joint.
c. Assist the patient to perform arm strengthening exercises (flexion and extension of the arms). The muscles in the shoulder girdle and upper extremities must be strong enough to bear the patient's weight while she is using the walker.
d. Assist the patient to learn to use the walker—ambulating with a nonweight-bearing (or partial weight-bearing depending on the fracture and its fixation) technique.
e. Remind the patient *not* to bear weight on the affected extremity until the orthopedist gives permission and the x-rays reveal sufficient healing. Early weight-bearing before bony union occurs exerts too much stress and may cause bending or

breaking of the pin, crushing of the bone, or loss of fixation due to the device's cutting through the bone.

5. Watch for and prevent complications.
    a. Thromboembolism—most common complication. (See p. 341.)
    b. Pneumonia—have the patient breathe deeply and cough at intervals to clear tracheobronchial tree of secretions. Use incentive spirometer to maximize lung inflation.
    c. Fat embolism—characterized by fever, tachycardia, dyspnea, and cough. (Fat embolism sometimes occurs after fractures of the long bones, particularly in elderly patients.)
    d. Knee contractures
        (1) Maintain the knee in a position of extension while patient is in bed.
        (2) Flex the knee in a 90-degree angle while the patient is in the chair—Avoid extending the knee for long periods when the patient is in a sitting position because extension produces undue strain on the fractured hip.
        (3) Move the knee through assisted range-of-motion exercises.
    e. Urinary tract infection
        (1) Avoid the routine use of an indwelling catheter—infection almost always follows the use of an indwelling catheter. (A urinary tract infection can cause a prolonged period of morbidity, incontinence and confusion in the elderly.)
        (2) Watch the color, odor, and volume of urinary output.
        (3) Maintain a liberal fluid intake (within limits of cardiorenal function).
    f. Pressure sores
        (1) Encourage the patient to move about freely using the overhead trapeze as an assistive device—peripheral arterial insufficiency, poor nutrition, and lack of movement contribute to skin breakdown.
        (2) (See page 64.)
    g. Infection—usually related to intercurrent medical problems, debility, and infection elsewhere in the body.
    h. Nonunion and avascular necrosis.
    i. Dislocation of the prosthesis.
    j. Pain.
    k. Rotation of limb.
    l. Loss of motion.

SPECIAL NURSING CONSIDERATIONS

NURSING MANAGEMENT OF THE PATIENT UNDERGOING ORTHOPEDIC SURGERY

Underlying Consideration

Orthopedic operations usually require a longer period of convalescence and rehabilitation than other surgical procedures.

Nursing Management

A. *Preoperative Care*

1. Assess nutritional status. Assure adequate protein and calorie intake.
2. Question patient to determine whether he has had previous therapy with corticosteroids (especially with patients with arthritis).
    a. Steroid therapy (current or past) may adversely affect patient's response to anesthesia.
    b. Steroids should be administered per request to cover stress of surgery.
3. Have patient practice voiding in bedpan or urinal in recumbent position before surgery. This helps reduce necessity of postoperative catheterization.
4. Acquaint patient with traction apparatus, necessity for splints and cast—to familiarize him with his postoperative environment.
5. Prepare skin according to health agency's policy.

B. *Postoperative Care*

1. Evaluate the blood pressure, pulse, and respiratory rates frequently—rising pulse rate or slowly falling blood pressure indicates persistent bleeding or development of a state of shock.
2. Assess changes in respiratory rate or in patient's color—may indicate obstruction of respiratory exchange or pulmonary or cardiac complications.
3. Elevate affected extremity and apply ice packs as directed.
4. Carry out neurovascular checks (nerve function and circulation) of affected extremity. Watch circulation distal to the part where cast, bandage, or splint has been applied.
    a. Prevent constriction leading to interference with blood or nerve supply.
    b. Watch toes and fingers for healthy color.
    c. Check pulses of affected extremity; compare with unaffected extremity.
    d. Note skin temperature—raised skin temperature may indicate bleeding or infection.

> **NURSING ALERT:** Abnormal coolness of skin, cyanosis, rubor, or pallor indicates interference with circulation.

    e. Notify surgeon and loosen cast or dressing at once.
5. Watch for excessive bleeding—orthopedic wounds have a tendency to ooze more than other surgical wounds. Measure suction drainage if used.
6. Maintain sufficient pulmonary ventilation.
    a. Avoid or give respiratory depressant drugs in minimal doses.
    b. Change position every 2 hours—mobilizes secretions and helps prevent bronchial obstruction.
7. Maintain urinary output.
    a. Maintain adequate fluid intake.
    b. Watch for urinary retention—elderly men with some degree of prostatism may have difficulty in voiding.

Long-term Management

1. Encourage early resumption of activity.
2. Watch for development of pressure sores. See page 74 for prevention and management.
3. Watch for complications due to prolonged disability.
   a. Venous thrombosis. See page 342 for clinical manifestations.
   b. Prevent venous complications.
      (1) Encourage the patient to exercise by himself with a planned program of exercise as soon as possible after surgery.
      (2) Have patient flex his knee, extend the knee with hip still flexed, and then lower the extremity to the bed.
      (3) Encourage patient to move fingers and toes periodically.
      (4) Advise patient to move joints which are not fixed by traction or appliance through their range of motion as fully as possible.
      (5) Suggest muscle-setting exercises (quadriceps setting) if active motion is contraindicated.
      (6) Wrap lower extremities with elastic bandages or apply elastic hose.
      (7) Treatment for venous thrombosis is discussed on page 343.
   c. Give prophylactic anticoagulants as directed (heparin, warfarin, aspirin, etc.).
4. Give a normal balanced diet.
   a. Give supplemental vitamins (B and C) to elderly patients or those with chronic disease.
   b. Avoid giving large amounts of milk to orthopedic patients on bed rest—adds to calcium pool in the body and demands more calcium excretion by the kidneys, predisposing to the formation of urinary calculi.
5. Watch for signs and symptoms of anemia—especially after fracture of long bones.
   a. Hemoglobin determination usually done on 3rd postoperative day or sooner.
   b. Give iron supplements as directed.

LOWER EXTREMITY AMPUTATION

Indications

1. Vascular disease; diabetes mellitus
2. Trauma
3. Malignant tumor
4. Congenital deformities

Treatment and Nursing Management

(Conventional approach)

A. *Preoperative Care*

OBJECTIVE: to have the patient attain his highest physical and emotional level in preparation for wearing a prosthesis (artificial limb) and/or attaining mobility by other means.

1. Assist the patient undergoing hemodynamic evaluation; arterial blood flow evaluated by Doppler pressure measurements and xenon ^{133}flow studies—for accurate and optimum amputation level determination.
   a. Amputation usually not performed until control of gangrene or advancing infection is achieved.
   b. Modern trend is toward selecting most distal amputation level (below knee) consistent with wound healing.
   c. The status of the sound limb is evaluated.
   d. Heart studies are carried out.
   e. Culture and sensitivity tests of draining wounds are often carried out.
2. Support the patient psychologically. Knowing what to expect helps reduce anxiety.
   a. Explain various phases of rehabilitation involved—active participation in rehabilitation is essential for a successful outcome.
   b. Explain to the patient that he will continue to "feel" the foot for a time; this sensation may be helpful for the placement of the prosthetic foot while he is learning to use the prosthesis.
   c. The physician will discuss the possibilities of obtaining and using a prosthesis—not all amputees can benefit from a prosthesis.
      (1) Diabetes mellitus, heart disease, infection, CVA, COPD, peripheral vascular disease, and increasing age are factors limiting full rehabilitation.
      (2) Wound breakdown, infection, and delay in healing of amputation stump are significant limiting factors.
   d. Amputation may be viewed as a surgical reconstructive procedure and as the first step in rehabilitation for the patient who has had prolonged periods of disability from peripheral vascular disease.
   e. Avoid unrealistic and misleading reassurance—management of a prosthesis can be slow and painful.
3. Build up the patient's nutritional status.
4. Have the patient strengthen the muscles of the upper extremity, trunk, and abdomen as a preparation for crutch walking. (Develop arm extensors and shoulder depressors, which are the muscle groups needed for crutch walking.) Instruct the patient as follows:
   a. Flex and extend arms while holding traction weights.
   b. Do push-ups from a prone position.
   c. Do sit-ups from a seated position.
5. Teach the patient to crutch walk preoperatively—prepares for postoperative mobility, maintains mobility and arm function, and instills confidence.

B. *Postoperative Care*

OBJECTIVES: to achieve optimal physical and emotional status in order to minimize problems in fitting and use of prosthesis.
to avoid complications.
to prevent prolonged disability.

> **NURSING ALERT:** Amputation of the lower extremity can be a life-threatening procedure, especially in patients over 60 with peripheral vascular disease. Significant morbidity accompanies above-knee amputations because of associated poor health and disease as well as the complications of sepsis and malnutrition and the physiological insult of amputation.

1. Watch for signs and symptoms of hemorrhage.
   a. Keep tourniquet (in view) attached to end of bed—to apply to residual limb (stump) if excessive bleeding occurs.

b. Raise foot of bed slightly to elevate residual limb. Do not flex patient's hips by elevating stump on pillow since this will produce a hip flexion contracture.

c. Reinforce dressing as required using aseptic technique.

d. Monitor suction drainage.

2. Prevent deformities in the immediate postoperative period. Contracture of the next joint above an amputation is a frequent complication.

a. Deformities include:
   (1) Flexion deformities
   (2) Nonshrinkage of residual limb
   (3) Abduction deformities

b. Encourage patient to turn from side to side.

c. Place patient in prone position twice daily—to stretch the flexor muscles and prevent flexion contracture of the hip.
   (1) Keep patient's legs close together—to prevent abduction deformity.
   (2) Place pillow under abdomen and residual limb while patient is prone.

d. Encourage patient to move residual limb—to avoid contractures.

e. Start range of motion exercises—contracture deformities develop rapidly and cause serious problems in management of prosthesis.

3. Observe and protect the remaining foot from injury.
   a. Examine remaining foot and malleoli daily.
   b. Keep pressure (bedclothes) off foot.

4. Continue with muscle strengthening and balancing exercises—to strengthen muscles, mobilize joints, and increase balance sense.
   Instruct patient as follows (stand behind patient and stabilize him at the waist, if necessary):
   a. Arise from chair and stand.
   b. Stand on toes while holding on to a chair.
   c. Bend the knees while holding on to a chair.
   d. Balance on one leg without support.
   e. Hop on one foot while holding on to a chair.

5. Shrink and shape the residual limb into a conical form—for maximum comfort for subsequent prosthetic application.
   a. Apply elastic stump shrinker or
   b. Use elastic bandages—to prevent edema and shrink residual limb.
      (1) Apply bandage smoothly with no folds;

creases will produce skin abrasion (Fig. 18-12).
   (2) Apply bandages snugly to adductor area to prevent formation of adductor roll. Keep pressure firm enough to maintain the pressure gradient and control fluid contents of residual limb.
   (3) Bandages are worn constantly; rewrap when necessary.
   (4) Prosthesis is measured and fitted when maximum shrinkage occurs.

c. Or—air splint may be applied to residual limb to control edema.

6. Have the patient do residual limb conditioning exercises—to harden the residual limb.
   a. The patient pushes the residual limb against a soft pillow.
   b. Gradually he pushes residual limb against harder surfaces.
   c. Teach the patient to massage the residual limb to soften the scar, decrease tenderness, and improve vascularity.
      (1) Massage is usually started when healing takes place.
      (2) Initially, massage is usually done by physical therapist.

7. Protect the residual limb from infection.
   a. Use plastic material to protect dressing if patient is incontinent.
   b. Wash residual limb with mild soap and water.
   c. Expose residual limb to air and sun.

8. Watch for deterioration of remaining leg—from disuse, poor vascular supply, foot trauma. (Obliterative arteriosclerotic vascular disease may necessitate *bilateral* lower extremity amputation.)

9. Keep the patient active—decreases occurrence of phantom-limb pain.
   a. If patient is not a candidate for prosthesis/ambulation, teach him to participate in self-care activities in a special wheelchair designed for amputees.
   b. Reassure patient that phantom-limb sensation (painful sensation that amputated foot is still there) will soon pass.

10. Accept the frustrations and behavior of the patient.
    a. Patient views amputation as death of part of his body; expect some depression and withdrawal.
    b. The self-image has to be adjusted after ampu-

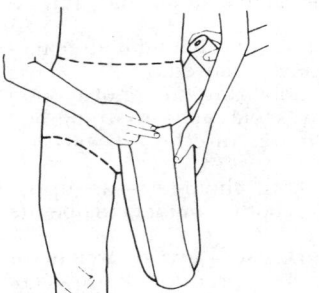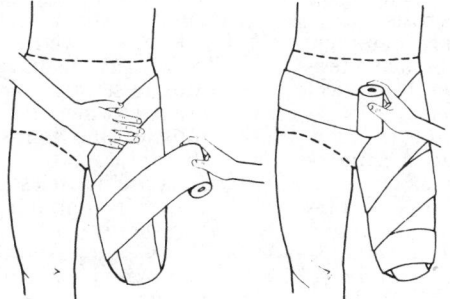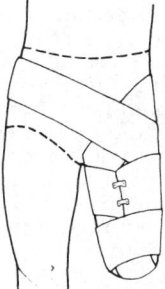

FIGURE 18-12. *Shrinking and shaping the residual limb (stump) in a conical form helps ensure comfort and fit of the prosthetic device. Bandaging supports the soft tissue and minimizes the formation of edema fluid while the residual limb (stump) is in a dependent position. (From Orthopedic and Prosthetic Appliance Journal 1957 June; 11(2):54)*

tation. It will take time for the patient to make this modification.

c. A positive approach combined with physical therapy helps improve patient's outlook on his potential.

Rigid Dressing with Immediate or Early Postoperative Fitting of Prosthesis

Rigid plaster dressing is applied immediately after surgery with provision for the attachment of a prosthetic extension (pylon) and a prosthetic foot immediately or within 10–30 days.

A. *Rationale of Rigid Dressing*

This allows optimum pressure gradients to be exerted on the residual limb—to control edema, support circulation, minimize pain on movement, help shape the residual limb, and promote healing. It allows earlier fitting of the prosthesis, shortens the interval between amputation and walking, and is of tremendous psychological value to the patient.

B. *Modifications of Immediate Prosthetic Technique*

1. Removable below-the-knee rigid dressing now available; allows residual limb observation without need of cast removal and reapplication.
2. Air splint (pneumatic prosthesis)—applied upon completion of amputation and inflated. It provides uniform compression of the residual limb, controls residual limb edema by adjustment of external pressure, gives easy access to residual limb for inspection, and is useful when skilled personnel are not available to apply the rigid cast and pylon prosthesis properly.
3. Unna paste boot

C. *Preoperative Nursing Management*

See page 776.

D. *Postoperative Surgical and Nursing Management*

1. Watch for signs and symptoms of hemorrhage from the residual limb.
2. Make sure that the residual limb remains in the plaster cast socket during the patient's hospitalization; if the socket inadvertently comes off, excessive edema will form very rapidly, causing a delay in rehabilitation.
   a. Rewrap the residual limb immediately with elastic compression bandage (Fig. 18-12).
   b. Prepare for immediate reapplication of cast socket.
3. Control pain.
   Assess for development of complications: increasing residual limb pain, hematoma, odor emanating from cast, infection, residual limb necrosis.
4. Observe and protect the remaining foot from injury.
5. Start patient on standing and ambulation activities.
   a. The timing depends on age, general physical status, condition of remaining foot, etc.
   b. Although the rigid dressing is vital to care, early weight bearing is not always desirable in patients with severe peripheral vascular disease.
   c. The patient may stand by his bed (or on tilt table) within 48 hours postoperatively with the prosthetic foot touching down (no weight-bearing)—helps minimize fear of pain and promotes confidence of patient in his ability to handle himself; allows prosthetist to check length of pylon.
   d. Weight-bearing to tolerance of pain is carried out progressively.
   e. Progressively longer periods of standing and walking in parallel bars or walker are initiated (with protected weight-bearing while prosthesis is in place).
   f. Progressive ambulation following first change of dressing is carried out under the supervision of physical therapist or nurse. Gait training is continued under the direction of physical therapist.
   g. A going-home prosthesis is fitted as soon as possible following surgery. The permanent prosthesis is fitted when the residual limb is fully conditioned.

E. *Health Education*

1. The patient will require rehabilitation services to learn mobility skills, transfers, wheelchair or automobile locomotion, etc.
2. Tube socks (athletic socks without a heel, with elastic band cut off) are sometimes used instead of standard wool stump socks for below-knee amputations.

UPPER EXTREMITY AMPUTATION

Indications

1. Trauma (acute injury, electrical burns, frostbite)
2. Congenital malformations
3. Malignant tumors

Surgical Management and Nursing Care

A. *Preoperative Care* (when time permits)

OBJECTIVE: to optimize the rehabilitation of the patient.

1. Give the patient psychological support to help him adapt to changes in his life style.
   a. Listen to his fears and concerns. Patient will have impaired personal body image, loss of sensory input, and inadequate motor output.
   b. Discuss with him the available prosthetic replacement (by orthotist, physical therapist).
   c. Demonstrate aids to independence (one-handed knife for cutting, elastic shoelaces, one-handed methods of functioning)—usually done in cooperation with occupational therapist.
2. Instruct the patient in postoperative exercises (by physical therapist).

B. *Postoperative Care*

1. When the patient returns from the operating room he will have either a rigid plaster of paris socket with provision for the application of a temporary prosthesis or a conventional compression bandage in place.
2. Monitor the amount and character of the suction drainage—used to eliminate hematoma and approximate the tissues.
3. Encourage active motion of residual limb after mobility restrictions have been removed.
   a. Muscle setting, joint mobilizing, range of motion are performed as soon as tolerated—to strengthen muscles and joints (under direction of physical therapist).
   b. Exercise muscles of both shoulders—an upper extremity amputee uses both shoulders to operate prosthesis.
   c. Carry out postural exercises—loss of weight of amputated extremity may produce postural abnormality.
4. Assist with dressing change and suture removal; wound is inspected and sutures removed in 7–10 days.
   a. Rigid Dressing.

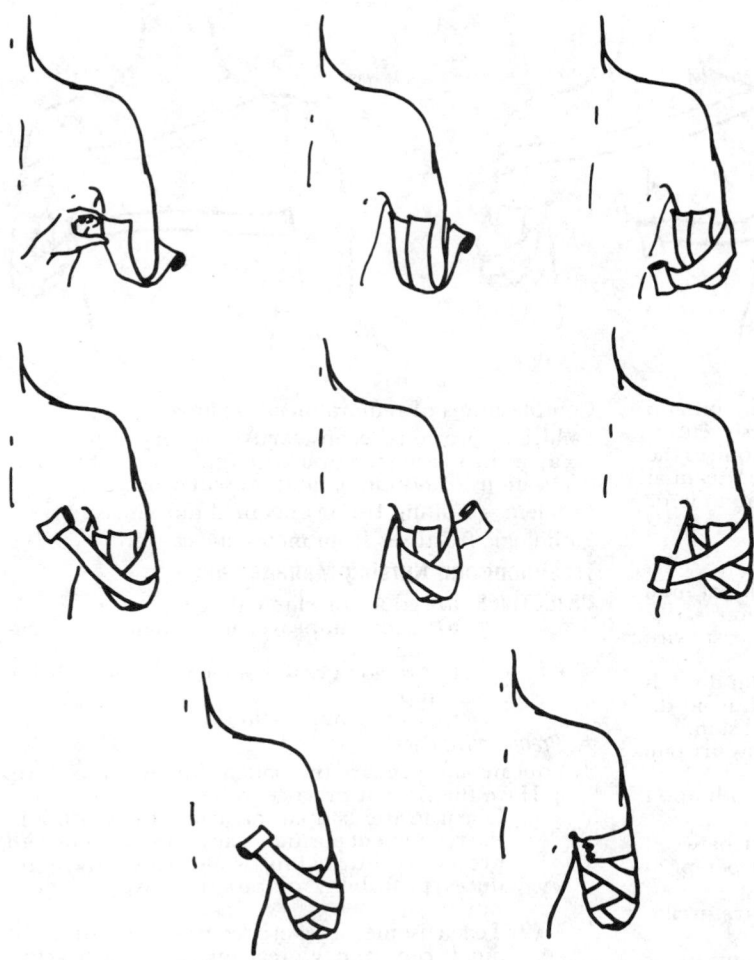

FIGURE 18-13. *Steps in the application of an elastic bandage to a standard or long above-elbow residual limb (stump). (From Bender LF. Prostheses and Rehabilitation after Arm Amputation, 1974. Courtesy of Charles C Thomas, Publisher, Springfield, Illinois.)*

A plaster socket with temporary prosthetic device is applied—increases patient's endurance, allows early prosthetic training and fitting of permanent prosthetic device.

b. Compression Dressing.

(1) Rewrap the residual limb 3–4 times daily—to maintain proper tension in the bandage and to reduce the fluid and shape the residual limb so that a prosthesis may be fitted.

(2) See Figs. 18-13, 18-14 for technique of residual limb wrapping. Make sure that the patient and his family know the correct technique of application since residual limb wrapping will be continued until the permanent prosthesis is fitted (6 weeks to a year).

(3) Keep residual limb snugly wrapped with elastic bandage for 24-hour period except for periods of bathing and exercise.

5. Start patient on one-handed self care activities as soon as possible—to promote independence. Occupational therapist teaches self-feeding, bathing, grooming, etc.

6. Exercises are carried out to prevent contracture, obtain full range of motion, combat muscle atrophy, increase muscle strength, and prepare residual limb for prosthesis.

7. Assess for complications:

a. Neuroma—sensitive tumor of nerve cells growing at end of severed nerve

b. Skin problems—from irritants in prosthetic components, lack of ventilation

c. Residual limb contraction or residual limb contour problems

d. Phantom sensation (feeling that limb is still present)

e. Psychological problems (denial, withdrawal)—responses influenced by support and encouragement of rehabilitation team, by early introduction of one-handed activities, and by discussion of prosthetic options and capabilities.

8. The fitting of the prosthesis depends on the level of amputation, age of patient, and whether or not weakness or limitation of range of motion of joints proximal to amputation site is present.

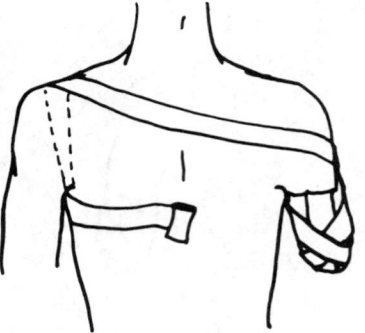
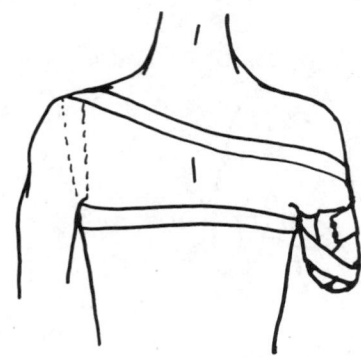

FIGURE 18-14. *An elastic bandage applied to a short above-elbow residual limb (stump) usually must be wrapped one or more times through the normal axilla to hold the stump wrapping in place. (From Bender LF. Prostheses and Rehabilitation after Arm Amputation, 1974. Courtesy of Charles C Thomas, Publisher, Springfield, Illinois.)*

a. Patient will require instruction in putting on and removing prosthesis, control of prosthesis, etc.
b. Ultimate patient rehabilitation ideally requires the services and supervision of rehabilitation team at a comprehensive medical rehabilitation unit or center.

Health Education

Instruct the patient to maintain careful residual limb hygiene to prevent skin irritation and infection.
1. Wash and dry residual limb thoroughly at least twice daily.
2. Wear residual limb sock. Change daily (and wash immediately)—to absorb perspiration and avoid direct contact between prosthetic socket and skin.
3. Avoid wrinkles in residual limb sock—may irritate skin.
4. Wipe the socket of prosthesis with damp cloth upon removal in evening.
5. Wear cotton tee shirt—to prevent contact between skin and shoulder harness and to absorb perspiration. Change daily.
6. Inspect the skin under harness for pressure, irritation, and abrasion.
7. Launder the washable portions of the harness as often as necessary; if practical, have two harnesses so that one can be laundered while the other is worn.
8. Have prosthesis checked periodically.

HIP ARTHROPLASTY (TOTAL HIP REPLACEMENT)

Arthroplasty is an operation to restore motion to a joint and function to the structures (muscles, ligaments, soft tissues) that control it. It may involve either replacement of the joint by a prosthesis or surgical reshaping of the bones of the joint.

Total hip replacement (total joint arthroplasty) is the replacement of a severely damaged hip with an artificial joint. Although a large number of implants are available, most consist of a metal femoral component topped by a spherical ball fitted into a plastic acetabular socket and held in place with bone cement (Fig. 18-15). Total joint arthroplasty is an exacting and meticulous procedure.

Clinical Indications

For patients (over 50) with unremitting pain, irreversibly damaged hip joints
   Primary degenerative arthritis (osteoarthritis)
   Rheumatoid arthritis

Complications of femoral neck fractures
Failure of previous reconstructive surgery (osteotomy, cup arthroplasty, femoral head replacement for complications of nonunion and avascular necrosis)
Problems resulting from congenital hip disease
Pathologic fractures from metastatic cancer

Treatment and Nursing Management

OBJECTIVES: to reduce or eliminate pain.
to restore, improve, or maintain joint function.
to provide greater stability of the arthritic hip.
to avoid complications.

A. *Preoperative Care*
1. Educate and prepare the patient for the procedure.
   a. Have the patient practice in-bed activities:
      (1) Learn to use bedpan or urinal for voiding in the recumbent position—acquaints patient with procedure of voiding while lying down; reduces probability of postoperative catheterization.
      (2) Teach isometric exercises (muscle setting) of quadriceps and gluteal muscles; teach active ankle motion.
      (3) Fit with crutches and instruct patient to walk

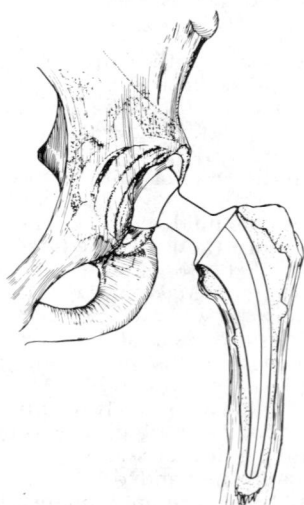

FIGURE 18-15. *An example of total joint arthroplasty, total hip replacement. (Courtesy of Zimmer, U.S.A.)*

without weight-bearing (if prescribed)—to develop crutch walking ability and facilitate patient's postoperative ambulation.

(4) Teach bed-to-wheelchair transfer without going beyond the hip flexion limits (usually 45°).

(5) Demonstrate deep breathing exercises—to assist in complete expansion of the lungs.
  (a) Use incentive spirometer.
  (b) Urge patient to stop smoking in preoperative period.

(6) Show balanced suspension apparatus, abduction splint, overhead traction frame and trapeze—to acquaint patient with postoperative environment.

(7) Educate patient concerning his postoperative regimen; e.g., extended exercise program will be carried out after surgery—atrophied muscles must be reeducated and strengthened.

2. Prevent thromboembolic complications
  a. Prophylactic anticoagulation may be started.
  b. Graded compression anti-embolism stockings are worn—appear to reduce incidence of leg vein thrombosis.

3. Utilize all precautions to avoid infection.
  a. Antimicrobials usually given immediately preoperatively, intraoperatively, and postoperatively to reduce incidence of infection.
  b. Scrupulous assessment made for septic foci—urinary tract, ears, nose, throat; an untreated infection precludes surgery.
  c. Operative area is scrubbed twice daily—microorganisms of the skin are potential cause of infection.
  d. Give "on call" preoperative medication into uninvolved extremity.
  e. Special precautions carried out in OR (impermeable OR attire, clean air system) to reduce particulate matter and bacterial count of air.

B. *Postoperative Care*

OBJECTIVES: to maintain the affected extremity in the desired position.
to prevent and treat complications.

1. The patient is usually positioned flat in bed with the affected extremity held in slight abduction by either an abduction splint or pillows (may or may not be in Buck's extension)—to prevent dislocation of the prosthesis until soft tissue healing has occurred.

NOTE: There are numerous modifications with differing requirements in the postoperative positioning of these patients.

2. Turn the patient (as required by his prosthesis and condition) when indicated by surgeon.
  a. Two nurses lift the patient clear of the bed while a third nurse washes and massages the back.
  b. Two nurses turn patient on unoperated side while supporting operated hip securely in an abducted position; the entire length of leg is supported by two pillows.
    Use pillows to keep the leg abducted; place pillow at back for comfort.
  c. Keep bed flat except during prescribed intervals (meals)—to prevent hip flexion contraction.
    (1) The bed is usually not elevated more than 45 degrees; placing the patient in an upright sitting position puts a strain on the hip joint and may cause dislocation.
    (2) Support the low back with a small pillow or

towel when patient is supine—to relieve strain placed on muscles by the flat position.
  d. As the patient becomes familiar with the turning routine, assist him to change position by using overhead trapeze.
    Patient must not adduct or flex operated hip—may produce dislocation.
  e. To use the fracture bed pan: instruct patient to flex the unoperated hip and knee and pull up on the trapeze to lift buttocks onto pan. Instruct patient *NOT* to bear down on the operated hip in flexion when getting off the pan.

3. Assess neurovascular status of operated extremity—check sensation, pulses, color, and skin temperature and compare with unoperated leg.

4. Monitor blood loss—portable suction is used to decrease incidence of wound hematoma, which is a possible focus of infection.

5. Give narcotics as required the first 24 hours postoperatively and then taper to nonnarcotic analgesia thereafter.

6. Encourage patient to carry out prescribed exercise program, usually under direction of physical therapist.
  a. Pain medication is usually given ½ hour before exercise session as required.
  b. Instruct patient to think about the motion required to contract the appropriate muscles.
  c. Encourage him to breathe deeply while exercising.
  d. Exercise activities depend on procedure and on condition of patient.
    (1) Active motion of affected foot and ankle started first postoperative day.
    (2) Isometric exercise of quadriceps, gluteals, abductors started upon direction of orthopedic surgeon.
    (3) Flexion, extension, abduction, rotation exercises, and ambulation are started upon direction of surgeon.

7. Use an abduction splint or pillows while assisting patient to get out of bed.
  a. Keep the hip at maximum extension.
  b. Instruct patient to pivot on unoperated extremity.
  c. Assess patient for orthostatic hypotension.
  d. When patient is ready to ambulate, teach him to advance the walker and then advance the operated extremity to the walker, bearing most of the weight on the hands.
  e. Patient progresses to use of crutches as directed, to prevent excessive use of hip abductors before healing occurs.

8. Use anticipatory nursing measures to prevent complications.
  a. Thromboembolism (major threat following reconstructive hip operations).
    (1) Continue to exercise ankles and legs—accelerates blood flow and prevents venous stasis.
    (2) Antiembolic stockings for uninvolved extremity—to increase venous velocity; elastic stocking applied to operated extremity when elastic compression dressing is removed.
    (3) Check for calf edema, tenderness, local pain.
    (4) Heparin, warfarin, dextran, aspirin—may be used for thromboembolic prophylaxis.
  b. Infection
    (1) Give antimicrobials as directed.
    (2) Watch for elevation of temperature and inspect wound at intervals.

(3) Infection may not become apparent until months or years after surgery.

(4) Deep infection almost always requires removal of implant.

c. Complicating medical conditions (cardiac, gastrointestinal, genitourinary).

d. Dislocation of prosthesis, fatigue fracture of metal component, avascular necrosis or dead bone caused by loss of blood supply, heterotrophic ossification (formation of bone in periprosthetic space).

Health Education

Instruct the patient as follows:

1. Continue to wear elastic stockings after going home until full activities are resumed.
2. Avoid excessive hip adduction, flexion, and rotation.
   a. Avoid sitting in low chair/toilet seat.
   b. Keep knees apart; do *not* cross legs.
   c. Limit sitting to 30 minutes at a time—to minimize hip flexion and the risk of prosthetic dislocation and to prevent hip stiffness and flexion contracture.
3. Continue quadriceps setting and range of motion as directed.
   a. Have a *daily* program of stretching, exercise, and rest throughout lifetime.
   b. Acquire a stationary bicycle if possible.
   c. Do not participate in any activity placing undue or sudden stress on joint (jogging, jumping, lifting heavy loads, becoming obese, excessive bending and twisting).
   d. Use a cane when taking fairly long walks.
4. Use self-help and energy saving devices.
   a. Handrails by toilet
   b. Raised toilet seat if there is some residual hip flexion problem
   c. Bar-type stool for shower and kitchen work
5. Lie prone twice daily for 30 minutes.
6. Report for follow-up evaluation and testing; supportive equipment (crutches, cane) is modified as needed.
7. Take prophylactic antibiotic if undergoing any procedure known to cause bacteremia (tooth extraction, manipulation of genitourinary tract).

TOTAL KNEE ARTHROPLASTY

A *total knee arthroplasty* is an implant procedure in which tibial, femoral, and patellar joint surfaces are replaced because of destroyed knee joint(s). Different types of implants are used, depending on degree of destruction and stability of joint (Fig. 18-16).

Indications

Disabling pain and loss of stability and function (from degenerative or rheumatoid arthritis of knee).

Preoperative Nursing Management

1. Patient is advised of implant he will receive and what will be expected of him postoperatively.
2. See page 780.

Postoperative Nursing Management

The postoperative nursing management is essentially the same as that for total hip arthroplasty (p. 781) with the exception that balanced suspension traction is not used.

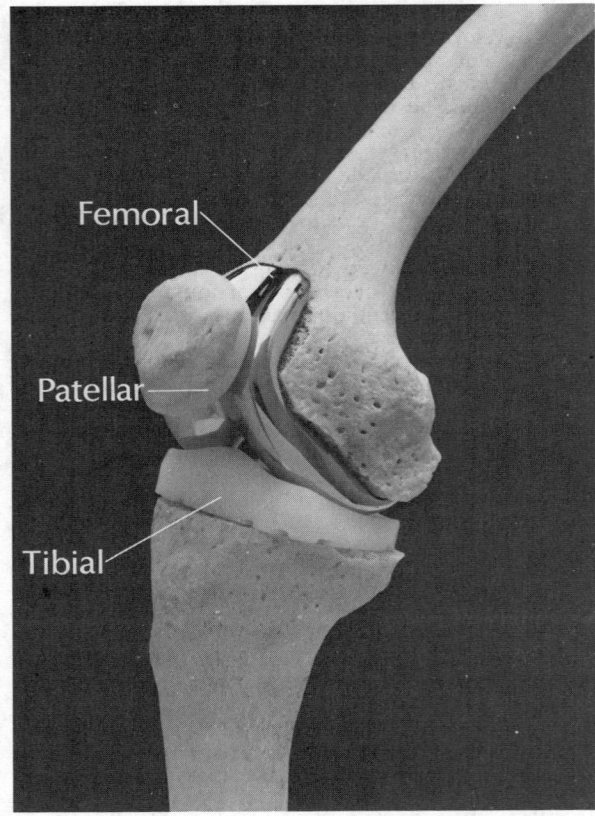

Femoral

Patellar

Tibial

FIGURE 18-16. *Total knee replacement. (Courtesy of Richards Manufacturing Co., Inc.)*

OBJECTIVES: to achieve freedom from pain.
to achieve stability and mobility.

1. The knee may be immobilized in extension with a firm compression dressing and an adjustable soft extension splint or long leg plaster cast.
   a. Leg may be elevated on pillows above the level of patient's heart.
   b. Head of bed not usually elevated except during meals.
2. Quadriceps setting exercises are started preoperatively and resumed on 1st postoperative day—quadriceps muscle is important in achieving full extension of the knee.
3. Suction drainage tubes removed when bloody drainage ceases (usually 24 hours).
4. Gentle knee motion usually started after first dressing is changed.
   a. Give pain medication before exercise period if necessary; cold applications may be beneficial.
   b. Patient assisted in straight leg raising until he is able to lift leg independently.
   c. Patient encouraged to perform active flexion and extension exercises.
   d. Exercises progress to active extension of knee through its fullest arc of motion within the limits of pain.
   e. A pulley and sling setup may be used for assisted hip and knee flexion.

5. Patient may transfer out of bed into wheelchair with extension splint in place; no weight bearing is permitted at this time.
6. Partial weight bearing (with crutches or parallel bars) may be achieved by end of 1 week; patient usually has 70–90 degrees of flexion.
   If knee flexion is less than 70 degrees by 10–14th postoperative day, gentle manipulation is carried out under anesthesia.
7. Use bilateral supportive walking equipment—proper supportive equipment enables patient to walk while bearing weight to tolerance.
   a. Protect wrist and finger joints from extreme stress, especially if patient has rheumatoid arthritis.
   b. Use forearm trough walker, forearm trough cane, axillary crutches, etc.

8. Complications:
   a. Early: Infection, thromboembolic complications, peroneal nerve palsy
   b. Late: Deep infection, loosening of prosthetic components, implant wear and dislocation, fatigue fracture of tibia, fracture of components.

Health Education

Instruct the patient as follows:
1. Use the resting splint at night for 3–4 weeks to maintain knee at full extension.
2. Use stationary bicycle to improve range of motion and strength muscles.
3. Use cane in contralateral hand when walking.
4. See page 782.

LOW BACK PAIN

Low back pain is characterized by an uncomfortable or acute pain in the lumbosacral area associated with severe spasm of the paraspinal muscles, often with radiating pain.
   Muscle spasm is a condition in which muscles are painfully contracted.

Etiology

(multiple causes)
1. Mechanical (joint, muscular, or ligamentous sprain)
2. Congenital disorders
3. Degenerative disc disease; acute herniation of disc(s).
4. Lack of physical activity and exercise; weakness of musculature
5. Arthritic conditions
6. Predisposing endocrine and systemic diseases
7. Diseases of bone (Paget's disease, metastatic carcinoma)
8. Infections of disc spaces or vertebrae
9. Spinal cord tumors
10. Referred pain from other areas

Diagnostic Evaluation

1. History—to determine when, where, and how the pain occurs, aggravating or relieving factors, relationship of pain to specific activities, presence of numbness or paresthesia.
2. Neurologic evaluation—to spot localized weakness of extremities and reflex and sensory loss; to exclude neurogenic disease.
3. Evaluation of muscular system—for changes in strength, tone, and flexibility of key posture muscles.
4. Electromyography—to record changes in electric potential of muscle and of nerve leading to it.
5. X-ray—of lumbar spine (anteroposterior, lateral, and oblique)
6. Myelography; computed tomography

Nursing Management

OBJECTIVES: to relieve muscle spasm.
   to gain normal elasticity of affected muscles.
   to return normal joint motion.
   to correct underlying conditions.

1. Advise the patient to rest in bed in a semi-Fowler's position (hips and knees flexed)—to relieve painful muscle and ligament sprain, heal soft tissue injury, remove stress from lumbar sacral area, relieve tension on sciatic nerves, and open the posterior part of the intervertebral spaces.
   a. Keep pillow between flexed knees while in side-lying position.
   b. Acute spasm should subside in 3–7 days if there is no nerve involvement or other serious underlying disease.
   c. Do prescribed isometric exercises hourly while on bed rest if possible.
2. Use heat or ice to relax muscle spasm and relieve discomfort.
   a. Apply moist warm heat (moist towels, hydrocolator packs).
   b. Follow heat by massage.
3. Use appropriate medications to relieve pain. (Rest in bed may eliminate the need for pain medications.)
   a. Give oral pain medication and muscle relaxants.
   b. Inject painful trigger points with hydrocortisone/xylocaine for pain relief (by physician).
   c. Use parenteral pain medication in acute severe pain syndromes.
   d. Pelvic traction and manipulation may be used.
4. Encourage patient to do prescribed back exercises (Fig. 18-17). Exercise keeps postural muscles strong, helps recondition the back and abdominal musculature, and serves as an outlet for emotional tension.
   Pelvic tilt (small of back is pressed against a flat surface)—decreases lordosis.
5. Advise patient to start activity as soon as possible—activity speeds recovery and helps prevent loss of muscle function.
6. Lumbosacral support may be used—provides abdominal compression and decreases load on lumbar intervertebral discs.
7. Psychiatric intervention may be needed for patient with chronic depression, anxiety, and low back syndrome. Encourage patient to discuss problems which may be contributing to his backache.
   a. Patient may undergo psychological testing (Minnesota Multiphasic Personality Inventory [MMPI])
   b. Psychotropic medication may be used for treatment of depression and anxiety, which potentiate pain.
8. Prepare patient for myelogram if he shows no improvement after 7–10 days of conservative treat-

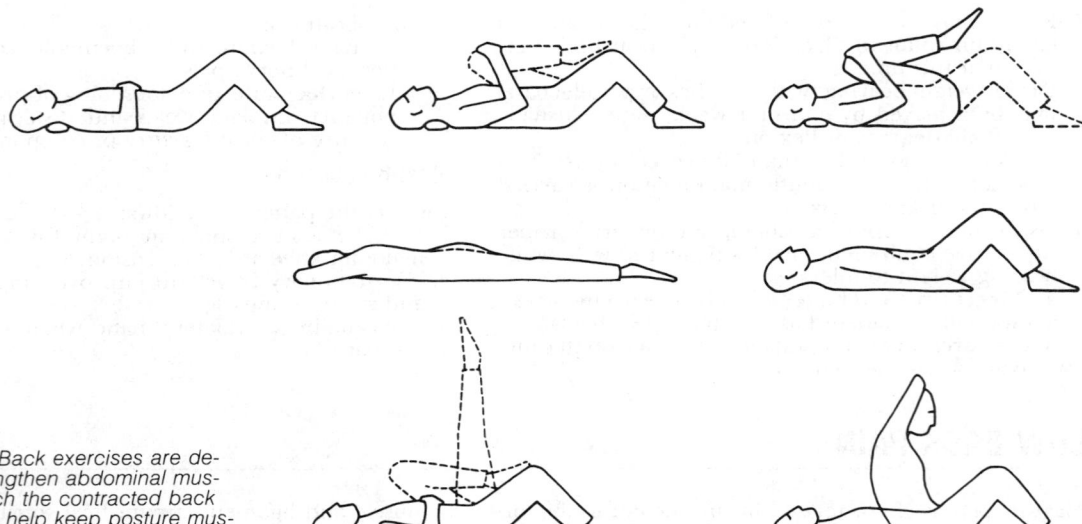

FIGURE 18-17. *Back exercises are designed to strengthen abdominal muscles and stretch the contracted back muscles. They help keep posture muscles strong and flexible.*

ment, when there is a neurologic deficit, intractable pain, loss of bowel or bladder control; operative intervention may be necessary. (See page 742 for treatment of herniated nucleus pulposus.)

Prevention and Health Education

Instruct the patient to avoid recurrences as follows:
1. Standing, sitting, lying, and lifting properly are necessary for a healthy back.
2. Pace yourself. Keep *moving* and *active*, alternating periods of activity with periods of rest.
   a. Avoid prolonged *sitting* (intradiscal pressure in lumbar spine is higher during sitting), standing, and driving.
   b. Avoid assuming tense, cramped positions.
   c. Sit in a straight back, fairly high-seated chair. Sit with the knees higher than the hips. Use a footstool.
   d. Flatten the hollow of the back by sitting with the buttocks "tucked under."
   e. Avoid knee and hip extension. When driving a car, have the seat pushed forward as necessary for comfort. Place a cushion in the small of the back for support.

3. When standing for any length of time, rest one foot on a small stool or wooden box to relieve lumbar lordosis.
4. When lying on the side, place a pillow under the head and one between the legs, which should be flexed at the knees.
   a. Rest at short intervals—fatigue contributes to spasm of the back muscles.
   b. Avoid sleeping in a prone position.
   c. Use a firm mattress.
5. Pick up objects or loads correctly.
   a. Maintain a straight spine.
   b. Flex knees and hips while stooping.
   c. Keep load close to body.
   d. Lift with the legs. Avoid twisting trunk while lifting.
   e. Avoid lifting above waist level and reaching up for any length of time.
6. *Daily exercise is important in the prevention of back problems.*
   a. Do prescribed back exercises twice daily.
   b. Walking outdoors (progressively increasing distance and pace) is recommended.
   c. Reduce weight if necessary.

DEGENERATIVE JOINT DISEASE (OSTEOARTHRITIS)

Osteoarthritis, the most common of all joint diseases, is the degeneration of the articular cartilage in the joints. It is characterized by bony spur formation at the edges of the joint surfaces, thickening of the capsule and the synovial membrane, and thinning of articular cartilage.

Although the exact underlying mechanism is not known, there appears to be a biochemical abnormality of cartilage.

Predisposing Factors

1. Aging of the cartilage
2. Anatomic abnormality; malalignment
3. Trauma (acute or repetitive)
4. Excessive joint use/abuse; obesity
5. Systemic diseases
6. Genetic influences

Clinical Manifestations

1. Pain and swelling in one, two, or more joints
2. Stiffness (morning stiffness; stiffness after sitting)
3. Limitation of joint motion
4. Heberden's nodes—nodular bony enlargements that grow on the distal joints of some or all of the fingers
5. Primary joints involved—hips, knees, vertebrae, and fingers

Objectives of Treatment and Nursing Management

OBJECTIVES: to control joint pain.
to protect the joints from undue strain and trauma.
to improve patient's functional capacity.

A. *To relieve strain on the affected joints.*

1. Give anti-inflammatory agents when synovial inflammation is present (see Table 18-1, p. 787).
2. Give analgesics for pain control.
3. Rest involved joints—excessive use aggravates the symptoms and accelerates degeneration.
   a. Use splints, braces, cervical collars, traction, lumbosacral corsets as necessary.
   b. Have prescribed rest periods in recumbent position.
4. Advise the patient to avoid activities that precipitate pain.
5. Use heat—relieves pain, muscle spasm, and stiffness and allows a more effective follow-up exercise program.
6. Try cold applications if heat is not effective.
7. Support the patient undergoing intra-articular (into the joint) injections of long-acting steroids.
8. Teach the patient to use correct posture and body mechanics.
9. Sleep with a rolled terry towel under the neck—for relief of cervical osteoarthritis.
10. Have patient use crutches, braces, or cane when indicated—to reduce weight-bearing stress on hips and knees.
    Hold cane in hand on opposite side of involved hip/knee.

11. Wear stretch gloves at night—to relieve pain and stiffness of fingers.

B. *To avoid trauma and further degeneration of the weight-bearing joints.*

Instruct the patient as follows:
1. Use postural exercises to correct poor posture.
2. Wear corrective shoes and metatarsal supports for foot disorders—also helps in the treatment of arthritis of the knee.
3. Carry out weight reduction program under nursing and medical supervision—to decrease stress on weight-bearing joints.
4. Avoid engaging in excessive activity and unusual exercise or effort.

C. *To restore function to the maximal extent.*

1. Keep active as much as possible without causing pain; avoid activities that cause pain.
2. Use range of motion exercises to maintain joint mobility and muscle tone for joint support; to prevent capsular and tendon tightening; and to prevent deformities.
3. Avoid flexion and adduction deformities—if deformities are avoided, pain is more apt to disappear.
4. Use isometric exercises and graded exercises to improve muscle strength around the involved joint.
5. Support the patient undergoing orthopedic surgery for unremitting pain and disabling arthritis of joints.
   a. Surgery for joint malalignment to alleviate abnormal joint stiffness
   b. Repair of joint-supporting structures (tendon repairs)
   c. Debridement of loose bodies (cartilage, bone, large spurs)
   d. Osteotomy to redistribute joint forces; arthrodesis (fusion of joint)
   e. Joint replacement (hip, knee, ankle, shoulder, elbow)

Health Education

See A, B, C, above.

RHEUMATOID ARTHRITIS

Rheumatoid arthritis is a chronic systemic disease of unknown cause, characterized most prominently by recurrent inflammation involving the synovium or lining of the joints, leading to destructive changes in the joints. Any or every organ or system may be involved by the rheumatic disease.

Clinical Manifestations

1. Inflammation of the joints characterized by pain, stiffness, swelling, heat, redness, and limitation of function and deformity
2. Subcutaneous nodules over bony prominences, bursae, and tendon sheaths; may appear in myocardium, aorta, and lung
3. Constitutional symptoms (may accompany or precede arthropathy):
   a. Fatigue
   b. Anemia
   c. Weight loss
   d. Fever

Pathophysiology Underlying Joint Destruction

Inflammation of joint (synovitis) → synovial effusion → granulation tissue covering articular cartilage (pannus) → joint capsular and subchondral bone destruction → pain → loss of mobility of joint → muscular weakness about the joint → damage to tendons and ligaments → joint instability and deformity → joint malfunction and disuse → muscular atrophy and contracture deformity.

Diagnostic Evaluation

1. History (onset of symptoms, areas and patterns of involvement, associated constitutional symptoms) and physical examination
2. Laboratory tests
   a. Blood tests—most patients have mild anemia
   b. Erythrocyte sedimentation rate—elevated during periods of active arthritis
   c. Tests for rheumatoid factor in the serum: positive in 70–80% of patients with rheumatoid arthritis

Latex fixation test

Antinuclear antibody test

d. Serum protein electrophoresis—increased globulins (gamma and alpha globulins); decreased albumin

3. Roentgenograms of involved joints—to determine extent, rate of progress, and structural changes within bones; reveals swelling of soft tissue, erosion of bone at articular margins, narrowing of joint space

4. Thermography—pinpoints areas of inflammation and increased metabolic activity in the body by pictorially recording (mapping) the heat emitted from the skin over the affected areas

5. Synovial fluid analysis—to distinguish between inflammatory, traumatic, or degenerative arthritis

6. Arthroscopy—endoscopic examination of knee joint; allows observation of synovial lining, articular cartilage, and minisci; permits examination of knee during passive movements and allows biopsy under direct vision; detects pathology earlier than other methods.

Objectives of Treatment and Nursing Management

OBJECTIVE: to maintain independence and prevent crippling deformities by

1. decreasing or suppressing inflammation
2. maintaining joint mobility and muscle strength and preventing deformities
3. relieving pain and promoting comfort
4. decreasing the activity of the disease
5. educating and helping the patient and family to adjust to a chronic disability
6. repairing damaged tissues

The treatment program includes rest, exercise, drug therapy, and education, and possibly surgical intervention.

A. *To maintain joint mobility and muscle power.*
(Inflammation, scarring, and mechanical damage to joint structures produce pain and disability.)

1. Regular rest at specified periods is needed to relieve pain and control fatigue—arthritis affects the whole body.
   a. Complete bed rest for patients with active widespread inflammatory disease.
   b. Have patient rest in a recumbent position (one pillow under head) on a firm mattress—to take the weight off the joints.
   c. Advise patient to establish one or more daytime rest periods of 30–60 minutes.
   d. Encourage patient to rest in bed 8–9 hours at night.
   e. Instruct patient to lie in prone position twice daily to prevent hip flexion and knee contractures.
   f. Pillows should not be placed under painful joints—promotes flexion contractures.

2. Painful inflamed joints may be rested with splints—to locally decrease synovitis; to reduce pain, stiffness, and swelling (in wrists and fingers); and to rest inflamed joints in optimum position and to prevent/correct deformities (Fig. 18-18).
   a. Use correctly designed splints: a "working" splint (Fig. 18-19) for daytime, to allow continuing function despite a painful joint, and a "resting" splint for nighttime may be indicated.
      (1) A resting splint is used at night to keep knee in extension.
      (2) The wrist is splinted with slight dorsiflexion—

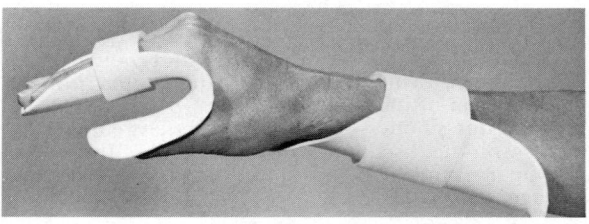

FIGURE 18-18. *Rest splint for hand. Rest of the hand is important when soft tissues are acutely inflamed. Instruct the patient to maintain full range of motion of all joints and maintain tendon excursion while wearing a rest splint to prevent loss of important hand function. (Photo courtesy of The Western Pennsylvania Hospital, Pittsburgh, Pa.)*

useful in patients with carpal tunnel syndrome (compression of median nerve within carpal canal).
   b. Splints may need modifications as joint structures change.
   c. Metatarsal bars or pads (for shoes), inserts, or custom made shoes may be used to decrease pressure on painful arthritic feet.
   d. Cervical collar to prevent cervical motion may help if patient has painful neck.
   e. Exercise is usually prescribed with splinting—to prevent joint deterioration and muscle weakness.

3. Have patient do exercises—to maintain function of all joints, to strengthen muscles that support the joints, to improve circulation, and to promote endurance.
   a. Encourage the patient to follow a prescribed *daily* program of exercise composed of conditioning exercises and specific exercises for particular joint problems (after inflammatory process is controlled).
      (1) Avoid *excessive* exercise.
      (2) Stop exercise before tiring.
      (3) Pain lasting more than $\frac{1}{2}$ hour after activity indicates that exercise is too vigorous; decrease, but do not stop activity.
      (4) Exercise slowly and smoothly in short, frequent bouts.
   b. See that patient performs isometric exercises—to help prevent muscle atrophy which contributes to joint instability.
   c. Have patient move joints through full range of motion 1 to 2 times daily to prevent loss of joint motion.
      (1) Assist patient in performing required joint motion if necessary.
      (2) Avoid grasping painful joints; grasp belly of muscle.
   d. Have patient do progressive resistive exercises—for muscle building, after joint inflammation has been controlled.
   e. Self-help devices can be used to help with daily activities.
      (1) Eating utensils with built-up handles
      (2) Raised chair seats, toilet seats
      (3) Special fastenings on clothing
   f. Crutches or cane held in hand opposite affected knee/hip can be used—to reduce the load on the affected knee/hip.

4. Control pain
   Instruct patient as follows:

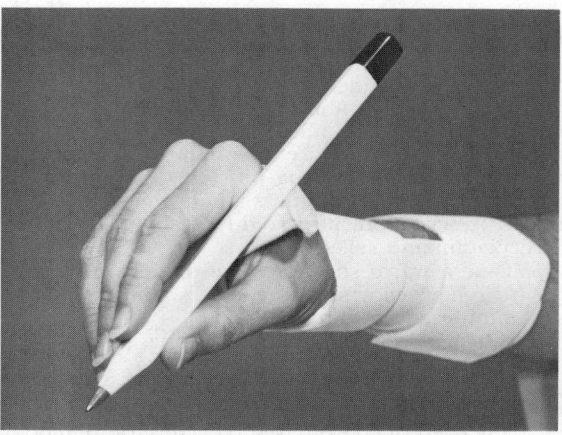
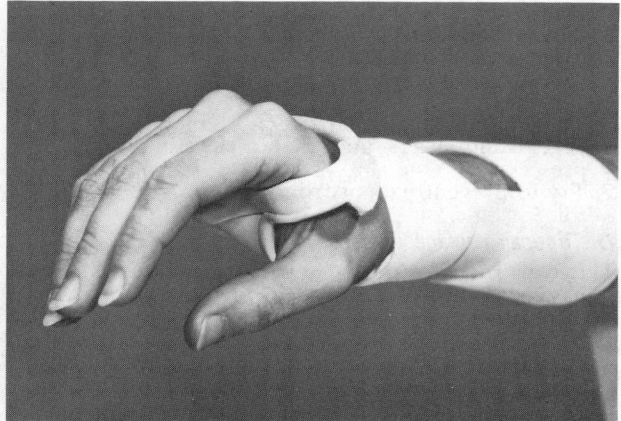

FIGURE 18-19. *Arthritic cock-up splint is a type of working splint that allows continuing function despite a painful joint. (Courtesy of The Western Pennsylvania Hospital.)*

a. Apply moist heat (15–30 minutes) to reduce muscle spasm and post-rest stiffness; provide as much relief from pain as possible so that exercise program can be carried out.
   (1) Take warm tub bath or shower upon arising—shortens period of morning stiffness.
   (2) Use hot paraffin baths for fingers, hands.
b. Use cold packs or ice when indicated for hot, swollen, acutely inflamed joints; heat is sometimes contraindicated when a joint is acutely inflamed. Cold will relieve swelling and pain and help restore function. (Keep commercial cold packs in freezer.)
c. Employ gentle massage to relax muscles.
d. Take joints through range of motion after heat treatments.
e. Advise rest to alleviate pain.
f. Take medication to relieve pain (although the primary function of salicylates in rheumatoid arthritis is anti-inflammatory).
g. Take non-narcotic analgesic if there is pain at night.

B. *To give medications to reduce inflammation and pain in joint tissues and surrounding structures and to suppress the disease process as much as possible, as well as to allow more effective exercise.*

1. Goal is to find drug that gives maximum pain relief with minimum side effects.
2. See Table 18-1 for drug therapy.
3. Patient may respond to all drugs, to only one, or to none.

C. *To support the patient who is depressed and anxious because of the constant, unremitting nature of the disease.*

1. Maintain a supporting relationship—successful management usually requires a long period of treatment.
2. Discuss nature of disease and positive expectations of treatment; encourage patient to set goals.
3. Adopt a positive but realistic attitude.
4. Emphasize that something can and will be done to relieve the patient's pain and mobilize his joints.
   a. Encourage him to express his feelings—patient

TABLE 18-1. DRUG THERAPY IN RHEUMATOID ARTHRITIS

Drug	Dosage (daily)	Adverse Effects	
Salicylates			
Acetylsalicylic acid (Aspirin)	3.0–4.5 g	Salicylism	The salicylates and the nonsteroidol anti-inflammatory drugs are all associated with gastric irritation, even gastrointestinal ulceration and bleeding, in a significant number of patients. Except for the salicylates, headache may be a prominent, often transient, early symptom of drug intolerance. In all, dizziness and tinnitus may occur. Skin rashes and pruritis are infrequent and respond promptly to drug discontinuance
Indole derivates			
Indomethacin (Indocin)	75–150 mg	Psychic change	
Tolmetin (Tolectin)	1200–1800 mg	Fluid retention	
Propionic acid derivatives			
Ibuprofen (Motrin)	900–2400 mg	Fluid retention	
Fenoprofen (Nalfon)	2400–3000 mg	Somnolence	
Naproxen (Naprosyn)	500–750 mg	Fluid retention	
Hydroxychloroquine (Plaquenil)	200 mg	Gastric irritation with anorexia, nausea, and rarely diarrhea; skin rash; rarely, ocular toxicity at this dosage level	
Gold (Myochrysine, Thiomalate)	10 mg initially, increasing to 50 mg weekly; after response, maintenance at 50 mg q 3–4 weeks	Skin rash and rarely an exfoliative dermatitis; stomatitis; depression of granulocytes and platelets; hepatitis; neuritis; proteinuria, rarely nephrotic syndrome	
Penicillamine	250–750 mg	Skin rash; hepatic dysfunction; nephropathy with hematuria and proteinuria; hematologic depression	
Adrenal corticosteroids (Prednisone)	5–15 mg daily or on alternate days	Peptic ulceration, osteoporosis, muscle wasting, capillary purpura, cataracts, ischemic bone necrosis, suppression of adrenal function; cushingoid habitus	

From Harvey AM et al. Principles and Practice of Medicine, 20th ed. New York, Appleton-Century-Crofts, 1980.

becomes hostile and angry because of chronic pain, stiffness, and loss of mobility.
  b. Let the patient know that you are aware of his fears and that his future is important to the health team.
5. Try to modify or adapt to stress-producing situations.
6. Give tranquilizers and mood elevating drugs as prescribed.
7. Try to prevent patient from adopting a dependent role.

D. *To repair damaged tissues*
1. Reconstructive surgery is performed after disease has been optimally controlled when particular structural problems persist.
2. In general, surgery is indicated for progressive synovitis, severe joint deformity, loss of function, constant severe pain, faulty alignment, tendon ruptures, nerve compression, and ankylosis.
3. See total hip arthroplasty, page 780, and total knee arthroplasty, page 782.

Health Education
OBJECTIVE: to maintain function of all joints.
1. Understand the disease, accept the realities of arthritis, and live within the limits imposed by it.
  a. Learn the nature of the disease and its treatment.
  b. Have confidence in your physician and treatment program.
  c. Avoid "miracle cures," dietary fads, drugs not prescribed by your physician, and other forms of "quackery."
  d. Report to the physician or clinic *regularly* for evaluation; have regular medical and functional reevaluation to determine if there is any loss of joint function.
2. Maintain independence.
  a. Rely on your own capabilities.
  b. Participate in as many activities as possible without producing fatigue.
  c. Conserve energy and simplify daily activities using self-help devices, work simplification methods, and energy-saving methods.
  d. Work at an even pace.
  e. Alternate periods of work, exercise, and rest. Avoid overdoing on good days.
  f. Alternate sitting and standing tasks; do not remain seated too long.
3. Take the medication exactly as prescribed, on a regular schedule.
  a. Aspirin is the primary drug (used for its anti-inflammatory effect). It must be taken over a long period and at high doses to achieve desired

response. Long-term use does *not* lead to addiction.
  b. Report ringing in the ears or decreased hearing, as this is a guide in controlling dosage.
  c. Watch for symptoms of gastric irritation.
  d. Take with food (a buffering agent).
  e. Do not substitute acetaminophen (Tylenol), etc. for aspirin—this drug possesses no anti-inflammatory properties but is a pain reliever.
4. Use prescribed heat or cold treatments for muscle relaxation and relief of pain.
  a. Take a warm shower or tub bath upon arising to relieve morning stiffness; rest in bed 20–30 minutes after warm bath.
  b. If heat or cold treatment intensifies pain, discontinue and notify physician.
  c. Try an electric blanket to ascertain its usefulness in relieving morning stiffness.
5. Do the prescribed exercises to preserve joint motion and to gain muscular strength and coordination.
  a. Exercise also in water (pool; bathtub)—water provides buoyancy, support, and relaxation; muscles are exercised while joints are supported by water.
  b. Review publications from The Arthritis Foundation, 3400 Peachtree Road, N.E., Atlanta, Georgia 30326.
6. Wear stretch nylon gloves at night to relieve numbness and tingling fingers.
7. Protect joints from further damage.
  a. Consciously maintain correct posture—pain and swelling cause one to assume a position of deformity, which makes muscles work harder.
  b. Lower yourself gently into a chair, using the sidearms. Collapsing into a chair produces knee and hip joint trauma.
  c. Use an elevated chair if knee and hip joints are affected.
  d. Straighten up before walking.
  e. Avoid tension and stress on fingers and thumb joints.
  f. Avoid obesity, which places greater strain on weight-bearing joints.
  g. Use a cane—to reduce load and impact on diseased joint.
8. Seek sexual counseling (position and techniques) if arthritic involvement is a barrier to sexual performance.
9. Surgical procedures are available for relief of pain and deformity (when recommended by physician).
10. The therapeutic program must be maintained for a lifetime; there is no cure at this time.

GUIDELINES: Paraffin Hand Bath for Rheumatoid Arthritis

Purposes
1. To relieve pain.
2. To decrease duration of morning stiffness of fingers, hand, and wrist.

Equipment
Double boiler or a slow cooker
4 lbs. paraffin to 1 pint of light mineral oil
Plastic wrap
Towel
Candy thermometer

Procedure

NURSING ACTION	RATIONALE/AMPLIFICATION
Preparatory Phase	
1. Melt the paraffin and oil in a double boiler or a slow cooker.	1. The addition of mineral oil lowers the melting point of the wax to 52.0° C. (125.6° F.).

Procedure (cont.)

NURSING ACTION	RATIONALE/AMPLIFICATION
2. Use a candy thermometer to determine exact temperature (52–54° C, or 126–130° F).	
3. Allow mixture to cool until a film forms on top.	
4. Remove jewelry. Wash and dry hands thoroughly.	

Performance Phase

NURSING ACTION	RATIONALE/AMPLIFICATION
1. Dip the hand and wrist in warm paraffin rapidly while keeping the fingers still.	1. The heat is transferred from the paraffin to the skin by conduction.
2. Allow the wax to harden slightly after each immersion.	
3. Immerse the hand in paraffin again; allow the wax to harden, and reimmerse. Repeat 8–10 times.	3. This builds up a glove of warm wax about 0.3-cm. (⅛-inch) thick which also acts as a splint.
4. Wrap hand with plastic and cover with a towel.	4. Wrapping with plastic and a towel helps to retain the heat.
5. Allow paraffin to remain on hand 15–20 minutes or until cool.	
6. Peel off paraffin and replace in double boiler for next application.	
7. Put fingers and wrist through range of motion exercises after paraffin has been removed.	7. Heat relieves the patient's pain and enables him to exercise his fingers and wrists with greater mobility.

MALIGNANT BONE TUMOR

Osteogenic sarcoma is a primary malignant bone tumor usually characterized by early hematogenous dissemination of cancer and the establishment of micrometastases in the lung.

Clinical Manifestations

1. Pain in the involved bone—from effects of tumor (destruction, erosion, and expansion of bone)
2. Swelling
3. Limitation of motion and joint effusion
4. Significant weight loss (an ominous finding)
5. *Physical findings*
   a. Palpable, tender, fixed bony mass
   b. Increase in skin temperature over mass
   c. Superficial veins dilated and prominent
6. *Sites of occurrence*—metaphyseal part of long bones (particularly region of knee)
7. *Sites of metastases*—lung, other bone, local recurrence, brain

Diagnostic Evaluation

1. X-ray will usually reveal bone tumor
2. Bone scan—helpful in detecting initial extent of malignancy, planning therapy, defining level of amputation, and following course of radiation/chemotherapy
3. Serum alkaline phosphatase—usually increased
4. Biopsy of bone—to confirm suspected diagnosis
5. Intravenous urogram and creatine clearance—to evaluate renal function
6. Chest x-ray and lung scan—to determine if metastases are present
7. Arteriography—to assess soft tissue involvement

Treatment and Nursing Management

OBJECTIVE: to destroy or remove malignant lesion by the most effective method possible.

Assumption: The treatment of osteogenic sarcoma requires a multidisciplinary approach, preferably in a cancer treatment center.

1. Surgical ablation of the tumor (may require amputation or disarticulation of affected extremity). See nursing management following amputation, page 776.
   a. Some centers are performing limb-salvaging procedures (resection of affected bone and surrounding normal muscle tissue and reconstruction using metallic prostheses or allografts for bone/joint replacement).
   b. Prophylactic lung irradiation may be carried out—to suppress metastases.
   c. Thoracotomy (pulmonary resection)—for treatment of pulmonary metastases.
2. Chemotherapy—to eradicate micrometastatic lesions.
   a. Chemotherapy used in combination to achieve a greater patient response at a lower toxicity rate and to minimize potential problems of drug resistance.
   b. Chemotherapy may be administered before and after surgery.
   c. Combinations of chemotherapeutic agents may be given in varying courses separated by rest periods.
   (1) Vincristine, high dose methotrexate with citrovorum factor, doxorubicin and cyclophosphamide in various combinations.
      (a) Vincristine—given IV before methotrexate infusion—may promote methotrexate uptake by tumor cells
      (b) High-dose methotrexate—given by infusion to destroy malignant cells
      (c) Citrovorum factor—"rescue" of the patient from methotrexate by allowing larger doses of methotrexate; prevents excess toxicity
   (2) Doxorubicin (antitumor antibiotic) given in high doses; may be given alone or in combination with other agents.
   (3) Chemotherapy may be used in combination with radiation therapy.
   (4) Or immunotherapeutic approach may be selected.

3. See nursing management of patient undergoing chemotherapy (p. 849).
   a. Encourage patient who has to cope with discomfort from disagreeable toxic effects, alopecia, and uncertain outcome of disease.
   b. Oropharyngeal mucositis of oral membranes is a frequent severe manifestation of gastrointestinal toxicity of methotrexate.
      (1) Instruct patient to cleanse oral mucous membranes with a Waterpik®, using a solution containing hydrogen peroxide, water, and mouthwash. Cleanse mouth after eating and at bedtime.
      (2) Stomatitis with superinfection of oral membranes with *Candida albicans*—may be controlled with oral nystatin.
      (3) Bone marrow depression (leukopenia and thrombocytopenia)—may require platelet transfusion.

OSTEOPOROSIS

Osteoporosis is a condition in which there is a reduction in the amount of normal bony material in the skeleton. It is characterized by generalized loss of density and tensile strength throughout the skeleton. The bones become progressively more porous and fragile, eventually leading to fractures, collapse of vertebral bodies, and skeletal deformity.

Causes

1. Postmenopausal or "senile" osteoporosis—there is a relationship between bone loss and reduction of estrogen levels after menopause
2. Immobilization from injury or inactivity
3. Low calcium intake, lack of vitamin D, inadequate supply of protein, vitamins, minerals, malabsorption syndrome
4. Conditions that accelerate bone loss—hyperthyroidism, hyperparathyroidism, large doses of steroids

Clinical Manifestations

Majority of patients have no symptoms.
1. Back pain
   a. Dull ache in lower thoracic/lumbar region
   b. Sharp, severe pain aggravated by motion—usually due to vertebral fracture
2. Tendency to kyphosis; loss of stature—postmenopausal women may lose 2–15 cm. (1–6 inches) in height from vertebral compression
3. Tendency to fractures—vertebral bodies, hip, Colles' fracture of forearm

NURSING ALERT: Osteoporotic bone fragility leads to vertebral collapse and hip fractures. It is the principal cause of fractures in the aged (as a result of minimal or questionable trauma).

Diagnostic Evaluation

1. Roentgenograms—show increased radiolucency of bones
2. Bone scan—to rule out tumor
3. Bone biopsy—may be necessary to rule out malignant disease
4. Laboratory studies

Treatment and Nursing Management

OBJECTIVES: to keep the patient active.
to provide optimal nutrition and induce calcium retention.
to prevent fractures.

1. Administer estrogen therapy as directed—appears to slow progression of bone loss, relieve osteoporotic pain, and stimulate positive calcium-phosphorus balance.
   a. Estrogen may produce breast and endometrial hyperplasia and increase risk of stroke, myocardial infarction, etc.
   b. Instruct patient to have pelvic, cytologic, and breast examination twice yearly.
2. Instruct patient to take prescribed calcium preparation (calcium carbonate)—to increase the amount of calcium absorbed and reduce urinary hydroxyproline excretion. Vitamin D supplementation (necessary for calcium absorption) may be added.
3. Provide dietary counseling—in general, a diet high in calcium, protein, and vitamin D is prescribed to slow rate of bone loss.
4. Insure daily exercise (walking) to prevent bone demineralization.
5. For vertebral compression fractures from osteoporosis.
   a. Give analgesics as required.
   b. Provide bracing and support when needed—to allow as much activity as possible as early as possible.

Health Education

Instruct the patient as follows:
1. Sleep on a firm mattress.
2. Make environment safe to prevent falls.
3. Increase muscle tone of trunk flexors and extensors by isometric exercises.
4. Keep physically active (walking, swimming) to strengthen muscles and prevent disuse atrophy and further bone demineralization.
5. Weigh periodically—indicates whether or not disease is stabilized.
6. Avoid lifting and carrying heavy weights or bending over a great deal—to avoid compression fractures of vertebral bodies.
7. Have daily outdoor activity—to provide Vitamin D (sunlight) and stimulate osteoblastic cells.
8. Estrogen replacement therapy should be considered for women with premature menopause (surgical or spontaneous)—to arrest or prevent bone loss.

PAGET'S DISEASE OF THE BONE (OSTEITIS DEFORMANS)

Osteitis deformans is a bone disease of unknown cause marked by excessive bone resorption (bone loss) and disordered formation of bone. Increased bone turnover and loss of normal bone architecture causes distortion of normal bone anatomy, e.g., enlarged and deformed bones with increasing vascularity. In time the involved bone becomes sclerotic and brittle.

General Features

1. Bony overgrowth and deformities occur and sometimes cause pressure on soft tissue structures.
2. May develop in any part of the skeleton—usually the skull, vertebral column, pelvis, or long bones.
3. Eventually produces marked hypertrophy and bowing of the long bones and irregular deformities of the flat bones.
4. Increased blood flow to affected bone(s) may lead to increased cardiac output and high-output cardiac failure.

NURSING ALERT: Osteitis deformans predisposes to spontaneous fractures and malignant bone tumors.

Clinical Manifestations

(Majority of patients do not complain of symptoms.)
1. Bone pain; tenderness on pressure; increased skin temperature overlying bone
2. Bone deformity:
   a. Bowing of femur and tibia
   b. Kyphosis or lordosis—producing a decrease in height
3. Enlargement of the skull
4. Hearing loss—from pronounced thickening of skull and bony overgrowth which impinges on vital structures

Diagnostic Evaluation

1. Skeletal roentgenograms—involved bones appear to be expanded and have greater than normal density
2. Serum alkaline phosphatase (serves as index of bone resorption)—markedly elevated
3. 24 hour urinary hydroxyproline excretion—used to assess skeletal metabolic activity; reflects increased bone resorption
4. Bone scan—to evaluate location and activity of disease and reveal early lesions

Treatment and Nursing Management

OBJECTIVE: to relieve symptoms and prevent progression of disease.

1. No particular treatment is recommended in patient without symptoms.
2. Therapeutic regimens used to suppress bone resorption:
   a. Calcitonin—a polypeptide hormone comprising 32 amino acids—retards bone resorption by decreasing the number and activity of osteoclasts.
      (1) Calcitonin-salmon (Calcimar) given by injection—patient may be taught to give his own injection.
      (2) Improves or relieves bone pain and produces a fall in serum alkaline phosphatase and urinary hydroxyproline excretion (showing its effect on osteoclasts); halts progression of bone lesions.
      (3) Side effects include transient feeling of warmth, nausea, and tingling sensation in extremities and pharynx.
   b. Diphosphonate therapy
      (1) Etidronate disodium (Didronel)—slows rate of bone turnover; reduces levels of both total urinary hydroxyproline and serum alkaline phosphatase; produces remission of clinical symptoms.
      (2) Can be taken orally; mild nausea and diarrhea are main side effects.
   c. Mithramycin (Mithracin)—cytotoxic antibotic that appears to have a hypocalcemic effect; reduces urinary calcium and hydroxyproline levels; gives symptomatic improvement (relief of bone pain and headaches).
      (1) Hepatic, renal, and hemorrhagic toxicity associated with this drug.
      (2) Usually reserved for patients with severe or extensive disease.
3. Supportive and symptomatic treatment:
   a. Give aspirin and other nonsteroidal anti-inflammatory agents—for pain relief and/or anti-inflammatory effects.
   b. Surgical intervention—to relieve joint pain and stress across adjacent joints, spinal cord compression, etc.
   c. Watch for occurrence of fractures—stress fractures occur with minimal trauma.
      (1) Fractures usually treated with internal fixation.
      (2) Avoid immobilization—increases hazard of hypercalciuria and stone formation.
      (3) For temporary immobilization due to fracture, limit calcium intake and provide high fluid intake—to avoid serious hypercalcemia and the development of kidney stones.
   d. Watch for evidences of bone sarcoma (see p. 789).

BIBLIOGRAPHY

Books

Adams JC. Standard Orthopaedic Operations, 2nd ed. New York, Churchill Livingstone, 1980
Barzel US. Osteoporosis, 2nd ed. New York, Grune & Stratton, 1978
Benjamin A and Helal B. Surgical Repair and Reconstruction in Rheumatoid Disease. NY, John Wiley & Sons, 1980

Brashear HR and Raney RB. Shands' Handbook of Orthopaedic Surgery, 9th ed. St. Louis, C.V. Mosby, 1978
Brooker AF and Edwards CC. External Fixation. The Current State of the Art. Baltimore, Williams & Wilkins, 1979
Brooker AF and Schmeisser G. Orthopaedic Traction Manual. Baltimore, Williams & Wilkins, 1980
Carini GK and Birmingham JJ. Traction Made Manageable. New York, McGraw-Hill, 1980

Cogburn NE and Cogburn SB. Manual of Orthopedics. St. Louis, C.V. Mosby, 1980

Dahlin DC. Bone Tumors, 3rd ed. Springfield, Charles C. Thomas, 1978

Devas M (ed). Geriatric Orthopaedics. New York, Academic Press, 1977

Edmonson AS and Crenshaw HH (eds). Campbell's Operative Orthopaedics, 6th ed. St. Louis, C.V. Mosby, 1980

Ehrlich GE. Rehabilitation Management of Rheumatic Conditions. Baltimore, Williams & Wilkins, 1980

Engleman EP and Silverman M. The Arthritis Handbook. A Guide for Patients and Their Families. Sausalito, Painter Hopkins Publishers, 1979

Fisk JW. A Practical Guide to Management of the Painful Neck and Back. Springfield, Charles C. Thomas, 1977

Fries JF. Arthritis: A Comprehensive Guide. Reading, Mass., Addison-Wesley Publishing Co, 1979

Gartland JJ. Fundamentals of Orthopaedics, 3rd ed. Philadelphia, WB Saunders, 1979

Ghista DN and Roaf R. Orthopaedic Mechanics: Procedures and Devices. New York, Academic Press, 1978

Golding DN. Concise Management of the Common Rheumatic Disorders. Bristol, John Wright & Sons, 1979

Hartman JT. Fracture Management. A Practical Approach. Philadelphia Lea & Febiger, 1978

Heppenstall RB. Fracture Treatment and Healing. Philadelphia, WB Saunders, 1980

Hollingsworth JW. Management of Rheumatoid Arthritis and Its Complications. Chicago, Year Book Medical Publishers, 1978

Huvos AG. Bone Tumors. Diagnosis, Treatment and Prognosis. Philadelphia, WB Saunders, 1979

Iversen LD and Clawson DK. Manual of Acute Orthopaedic Therapeutics. Boston, Little, Brown & Co, 1977

Kelly WN et al. Textbook of Rheumatology. Philadelphia, WB Saunders, 1981

Kerr A. Orthopedic Nursing Procedures, 3rd ed. New York, Springer Pub. Co., 1978

McCarty DJ. Arthritis and Allied Conditions. Philadelphia, Lea & Febiger, 1979

Mears DC. Materials in Orthopaedic Surgery. Baltimore, Williams & Wilkins, 1979

Mercier LR and Pettid FJ. Practical Orthopedics. Chicago, Year Book Medical Publishers, 1980

Mirra JM et al. Bone Tumors: Diagnosis and Treatment. Philadelphia, JB Lippincott, 1980

Mourad L. Nursing Care of Adults with Orthopedic Conditions. New York, John Wiley & Sons, 1980

Müller ME et al. Manual of Internal Fixation. New York, Springer-Verlag, 1979

Roaf R and Hodkinson LJ. Textbook of Orthopaedic Nursing, 3rd ed. Oxford, Blackwell Scientific Publications, 1980

Rockwood CA and Green DP. Fractures, Vols 1 and 2. Philadelphia, JB Lippincott, 1975

Rosenbaum EE. Rheumatology: New Directions in Therapy. Garden City, Medical Examination Publications, 1979

Roth SH. New Directions in Arthritis Therapy. Littleton, PSG Publications, 1980

Uhthoff HK and Stahl E. (eds). Current Concepts of Internal Fixation of Fractures. New York, Springer-Verlag, 1980

Wallace R et al. Staff Manual for Teaching Patients About Rheumatoid Arthritis. Chicago, American Hosp Association, 1979

Vitali M et al. Amputations and Prostheses. London, Baillière Tindall, 1978

Zauder HL. Anesthesia for Orthopaedic Surgery. Philadelphia, F.A. Davis, 1980

Articles

Amputation

Eyre NC. Rehabilitation of the upper limb amputee. Physiotherapy 1979 Jan; 65(1):9–12

Hudson CC. Morbid implications of above-knee amputations. Report of a series and review of the literature. Arch Surg 1980 Feb; 115(2):165–167

Lee BY et al. Noninvasive hemodynamic evaluation in selection of amputation level. Surg Gynecol Obstet 1979 Aug; 149(2):241–244

Malone JM et al. Therapeutic and economic impact of a modern amputation program. Ann Surg 1979 June; 189(6):798–802

Meador R. Learning to live with a new leg. Am J Nurs 1979 Aug; 79(8):1393–1395

Potts JR et al. Lower extremity amputation. Review of 110 cases. Am J Surg 1979 Dec; 138(6):924–928

Steinbach T-V. Upper limb amputation. Prog Surg 1979; 16:224–248

Towne NB and Condon RE. Lower extremity amputations for ischemic disease. Adv Surg 1979; 13:199–227.

Wu Y et al. An innovative removable rigid dressing technique for below-the-knee amputation. J Bone Joint Surg 1979 July; 61A(5):724–729

Arthritis/Joint Anthroplasty

Bain LS. The management of rheumatoid arthritis. Practitioner 1980 Jan; 224(1339):29–33

Barnes RW et al. Efficacy of graded compression antiembolism stockings in patients undergoing total hip arthroplasty. Clin Orthop 1978 May; 132:61–67

Bennett RM. Management of rheumatoid arthritis. Compr Ther 1979 Aug; 5(8):23–35

Brown JM et al. Helping the family withstand the stress of disease. Nursing '79 1979 Sept; 9(9):50–55

Brown-Skeers V. How the nurse practitioner manages the rheumatoid arthritis patient. Nursing '79 1979 June; 9(6):26–35

Cabanela ME et al. Total joint arthroplasty. The hip. Mayo Clin Proc 1979 Sept; 54(9):559–563

Calin A. Rheumatoid arthritis. Am Fam Physician 1978 July; 18(1):89–94

Dunn AW. Replacement and resurfacing of joints. Postgrad Med 1980 March; 67(3):225–237

Edmonds J. The management of rheumatoid arthritis. Aust Fam Physician 1978 Aug; 7(8):925–935

Ehrlich GE. Pathogenesis and treatment of osteoarthritis. Compr Ther 1979 Aug; 5(8):36–40

Fries JF. The approach to the rheumatic disease patient. Compr Ther 1979 Aug; 5(8):8–15

Gever LN. Penicillamine: Newest weapon against rheumatoid arthritis. Nursing '80 1980 Feb; 10(2):65

Golding DN. Osteoarthrosis. Practitioner 1980 Jan; 224 (1339):19–25

Huskisson EC. Osteoarthritis. Changing concepts in pathogenesis and treatment. Postgrad Med 1979 March; 65(3):97–104

Jergesen HE et al. Bilateral total hip and knee replacement in adults with rheumatoid arthritis: An evaluation. Clin Orth 1978 Nov–Dec; 137:120–128

Laskin RS. Total knee replacement. Orthop Clin North Am 1979 Jan; 10(1):223–247

McBeath AA. Late complications of total hip replacement and their prevention. Curr Pract Orthop Surg 1979; 8:58–76

Nelson CL et al. Results of infected total hip replacement arthroplasty. Clin Orthop 1980; 147:258–261

Nonsteroidal anti-inflammatory drugs for rheumatoid arthritis. Med Lett Drugs Ther 1980 April 4; 22(7):29–31

Peterson LFA et al. Total joint arthoplasty. The knee. Mayo Clin Proc 1979 Sept; 54(9):564–569

Pollard JP. Antibiotic prophylaxis in total hip replacement. Br Med J 1979 March 17; 1(6165):707–709

Ritter MA and Stringer EA. Predictive range of motion after total knee replacement. Clin Orthop 1979 Sept; 143:115–119

Spruck M. Gold therapy for rheumatoid arthritis. Am J Nurs 1979 July; 79(7):1246–1248

Weaver JK. Activity expectations and limitations following total joint replacement. Clin Orthop 1978 Nov–Dec; 137:55–61

Fractures

Ahstrom JP Jr. Rehabilitation of the knee. Curr Pract Orthop Surg 1979; 8:77–85

Alho A. Clinical manifestations of fat embolism syndrome. Arch Orthop Trauma Surg 1978 Aug; 92(2-3):153–158

Anderson CE. Keeping up with the best in casting. Patient Care 1979 July 15; 13(3):24–97

Anderson LB. Treatment of open fractures: A review. Va Med 1978 Sept; 105(9):648–657

Carlson RE. The fat emboli syndrome. Med Times 1979 May; 107(5):8d–10d, 15d–18d

Chapman MW and Mahoney M. The role of early internal fixation in the management of open fractures. Clin Orthop 1979 Jan–Feb; 138:120–131

Clancey GJ and Hansen ST. Open fractures of the tibia: A review of one hundred and two cases. J Bone Joint Surg 1978 Jan; 60(1):118–122

Cohen S and Viellion G. Programmed Instruction: Nursing care of a patient in traction. Am J Nurs 1979 Oct; 79(10):1771–1798

Colyer RA. Compression external fixation after biplane femoral trochanteric osteotomy for severed slipped capital femoral epiphysis. J Bone Joint Surg 1980 June; 62(4):557–560

Cooney WP et al. External pin fixation for unstable Colles' fractures. J Bone Joint Surg 1979 Sept; 61(6A):840–845

Crossland S and Deyerle WM. Compartmental syndrome. Nursing '80 1980 Nov; 10(11):51–53

Crow I. Fractures of the hip. A self study. ONA J 1978 Aug; 5(8):12–30

Dunnery E. Fractured hip: How to position and mobilize patients—without undoing their surgery. RN 1979 June; 42(6):44–57

Edwards CC et al. Management of compound tibial fractures using external fixation. Am Surg 1979 March; 45(3):190–203

Farrell J. Casts, your patients and you. Part 1. A review of basic procedures. Nursing '78 1978 Oct; 8(10):65–69

Farrell J. Casts, your patients and you. Part 2. A review of arm and leg cast procedures. Nursing '78 1978 Nov; 8(11):57–61

Farrell J. Casts, your patients and you. Part 3. A review of hip-spica procedures. Nursing '78 1978 Dec; 8(12):53–57

Fleming LL et al. Clinical experience with a new casting tape. South Med J 1980 May; 73(5):569–571

Flint LM et al. Definitive control of bleeding from severe pelvic fractures. Ann Surg 1979 June; 189(6):709–716

Gossling HR and Donohue TA. The fat embolism syndrome. JAMA 1979 June 22; 241(25):2740–2742

Gustilo RB. Use of antimicrobials in the management of open fractures. Arch Surg 1979 July; 114(7):805–808

Hielema FJ. Epidemiology of hip fracture. A review with implications for the physical therapist. Phys Ther 1979 Oct; 59(10):1221–1225

Jackson RP et al. External skeletal fixation in severe limb trauma. J Trauma 1978 March; 18(3):201–205

Jacobs RR et al. Internal fixation of intertrochanteric hip fractures: A clinical and biomechanical study. Clin Orthop 1980 Jan–Feb; 146:62–70

Kryschyshen PL and Fischer DA. External fixation for complicated fractures. Am J Nurs 1980 Feb; 80(2):256–259

Lamb K. Effect of positioning of postoperative fractured-hip patients as related to comfort. Nurs Res 1979 Sept–Oct; 28(5):291–294

Laskin RS et al. Intertrochanteric fractures of the hip in the elderly: A retrospective analysis of 236 cases. Clin Orthop 1979 June; 141:188–195

Lupien AE. Head off compartment syndrome before it's too late. RN 1980 Dec; 43(12):38–41, 114

Martin DW et al. Conservative management of rheumatoid arthritis. West J Med 1978 Aug; 129(2):121–125

Matalon TS et al. Hemorrhage with pelvic fractures: Efficacy of transcatheter embolization. AJR 1979 Nov; 133(5):859–864

Maxwell GP and Hoopes JE. Management of compound injuries of the lower extremity. Plast Reconstr Surg 1979 Feb; 63(2):176–185

McAvoy JM and Cook JH. A treatment plan for rapid assessment of the patient with massive blood loss and pelvic fractures. Arch Surg 1978 Aug; 113(8):986–990

Meredith S. Formidable: That's the only word for the external fixation device—and for the care it demands. RN 1979 Dec; 42(12):19–24

Meredith S. Preparing your patient to live with his cast. RN 1979 July; 42(7):34–43

Mikhail SF et al. Optimism in the management of hip fracture in elderly patients. J Am Geriatr Soc 1978 Jan; 26(1):39–42

Miller CW. Survival and ambulation following hip fracture. J Bone Joint Surg 1978 Oct; 60(7):930–934

Morris GK and Mitchell JRA. Editorial. Can death from venous thromboembolism be prevented in elderly patients with hip fractures? Am Heart J 1978 Feb; 95(2):139–140

Moskovitz PA et al. Low-dose heparin for prevention of venous thromboembolism in total hip arthroplasty and surgical repair of hip fractures. J Bone Joint Surg 1978 Dec; 60(8):1065–1070

Oh WH and Mital MA. Fat embolism: Current concepts of pathogenesis, diagnosis and treatment. Orthoped Clin North Am 1978 July; 9(3):769–779

Putnam N and Yager J. Traction intolerance syndrome: a psychiatric complication of femoral fractures. Int J Psychiatry Med 1977–1978; 8(2):133–143

Spiegel PG (ed). Symposium on problems and solutions in the management of fractures. Orthop Clin North Am 1980 July; 11(3):379–679

Stoltenberg JJ and Gustilo RR. The use of methylprednisolone and hypertonic glucose in the prophylaxis of fat embolism syndrome. Clin Orthop 1979 Sept; 143:211–221

Stone JP et al. The management of open and complex fractures of the tibia. Bull NY Acad Med 1980 April; 56(3):323–340

Uhthoff HK. Current concepts of internal fixation of fractures. Can J Surg 1980 May; 23(3):213–214

Williams MA et al. Nursing activities and acute confusional states in elderly hip-fractured patients. Nurs Res 1979 Jan–Feb; 28(1):25–35

Zickel RE. Fractures of the adult femur excluding the femoral head and neck. Clin Orthop 1980 March–April; 147:93–114

Low Back Pain

Boyd RJ. Low back pain—Assessment and management. Curr Pract Orthop Surg 1979; 8:1–11

Brewer BJ. Low back pain. Am Fam Physician 1979 June; 19(6):114–118

Donovan L. Low back pain. Where care is the key to recovery. RN 1978 Oct; 41(10):70–73

Gilbertson B. Low back pain. What to look for—what to do. RN 1978 Oct; 41(10):74–77

Hitch M. Nursing assessment of a patient with low back pain. ONA J 1979 Dec; 6(12):484–488

Mooney V. Surgery and postsurgical management of the patient with low back pain. Phys Ther 1979 Aug; 59(8):1000–1006

White AH et al. Epidural injections for the diagnosis and treatment of low-back pain. Spine 1980 Jan–Feb; 5(1):78–86

Osteoporosis

Drugs for postmenopausal osteoporosis. Med Lett Drugs Ther 1980 May 30; 22(11):45–46

Nachtigall LE et al. Estrogen replacement therapy I: A 10 year study in the relationship to osteoporosis. Obstet Gynecol 1979 March; 53(3):277–281

Nordin BEC. Treatment of postmenopausal osteoporosis. Drugs 1979 Dec; 18(6):484–492

Skillman TG. Can osteoporosis be prevented? Geriatrics 1980 Feb; 35(2):95–102

Wallach S. Management of osteoporosis. Hospital Pract 1978 Dec; 13(12):91–98

Bone Tumor—Paget's Disease of Bone

Breur K and van der Schueren E. Adjuvant therapy in the management of osteosarcoma: Need for critical reassessment. Recent Results Cancer Res 1978; 68:5–15

Ibbertson HK et al. Paget's disease of bone: Assessment and management. Drugs 1979 July; 18(1):33–47

Lukert BP. Paget's disease of bone. J Kans Med Soc 1979 June; 90(6):345–348

Sim FH. Total joint arthroplasty. Applications in the management of bone tumors. Mayo Clin Proc 1979 Sept; 54(9):583–589

Simons RM. Paget's disease in the head and neck. Gerontology 1980 26(3):155–159

Siris ES et al. Paget's disease of bone. Bull NY Acad Med 1980 April; 56(3):285–304

Taylor WF et al. Trends and variability in survival from osteosarcoma. Mayo Clin Proc 1978 Nov; 53(11):695–700

THE INFECTION PROCESS

Causative Agent

Type: Bacterium, virus, fungus, parasite, rickettsia, chlamydia, etc.
1. Pathogenicity (ability to cause disease)
2. Virulence (disease severity) and invasiveness (ability to enter and move through tissue)
3. Infective dose (number of organisms needed to initiate infection)
4. Organism specificity (host preference), antigenic variations
5. Elaboration of toxins

Reservoir

(the environment in which the agent is found)
1. Human—man is the reservoir of diseases that are more dangerous to humans than to other species
2. Animal—responsible for infestations with trophozoites, worms, etc.
3. Nonanimal—street dust, garden soil, lint from bedding

Mode of Escape from Reservoir

1. Respiratory tract (most common in man)
2. Gastrointestinal tract
3. Genitourinary tract
4. Open lesions
5. Mechanical escape (includes bites of insects)
6. Blood

Mode of Transmission (to the next host)

1. *By Contact Route*
   a. Direct contact (person to person)
   b. Indirect contact (usually an inanimate object)
   c. Droplet spread
2. *By Vehicle Route*
   a. Contaminated food—salmonellosis
   b. Water—shigellosis
   c. Drugs—pseudomonas infections from contaminated ophthalmic ointment
   d. Blood—hepatitis
3. *Airborne*
   a. Residue of evaporated droplets that remain suspended in air
   b. Dust particles
   c. Skin squames
4. *Vector borne*
      Mosquito—malaria

Mode of Entry of Organisms into Human Body

1. Respiratory tract
2. Gastrointestinal tract
3. Genitourinary tract
4. Direct infection of mucous membranes/skin

Host Factors

Illness following entrance of infection into the body depends on:

1. Age, sex, genetic constitution of host
2. Nutritional status, fitness, environmental factors
3. General physical, mental, and emotional health
4. Absent or abnormal immunoglobulins
5. Status of hematopoietic system; efficacy of reticulo-endothelial system
6. Presence of underlying disease
7. Steroids, radiation, antibiotics—may influence response of host to infection

Epidemiology, Therapy, and Control of Communicable Infections

See Table 19-1, page 796.

Emerging Problems in Infectious Diseases

1. Increase in number of different organisms that are developing resistance to increasing numbers of available antimicrobials.
2. Increasing number of persons in state of immunosuppression. These persons, who would formerly have died from cancer, leukemia, etc., are now surviving but are susceptible to invasion by any type of organism, including those usually considered nonpathogenic.

CONTROL AND MANAGEMENT OF INFECTIOUS DISEASES

Nursing Objectives and Management

A. *To assist in identifying the etiologic agent and in establishing the diagnosis*

1. Obtain specimens of blood, urine, stools, sputum, throat swabbings, nasal secretions, and pyogenic exudates for bacteriologic study.
2. Secure or assist in securing smears of blood and other materials for microscopic examination.
3. Assist with aspirations of spinal fluid, bone marrow, and other body fluids or tissues for cytologic, serologic, and bacteriologic tests.
4. Carry out appropriate skin tests for specific diagnostic reactions as directed.

B. *To control the infection in the patient*

1. Administer the appropriate antimicrobial agents as directed.
2. Assist in administering specific immune therapy, if available, employing immune antiserum, gamma globulin, antitoxin, toxoid, vaccine, or an appropriate mixture of antigen and antibody, depending on the circumstances.
3. Observe patient carefully for evidences of drug or serum sensitivity.

C. *To prevent spread of the infection to others*

1. *Wash hands immediately after contact with each patient and after every contact with material that may be contaminated and potentially infectious.*
   a. Use paper towel to turn off faucet if sink is not equipped with foot-, knee-, or elbow-operated faucets.
   b. Use individualized soap tissues.
2. Carry out isolation techniques as required by disease (see p. 788).
3. Observe asepsis as indicated.
4. Use mask technique effectively. (Masks are not currently being used as much as in the past.)
   a. Change mask frequently—moisture increases the mask's permeability, promoting bacterial growth.
   b. Refrain from handling mask while in use.
5. Use gown as required by patient's disease (see p. 798).
   a. Use gown once and discard in appropriate receptacle.
   b. Collect linen in water-soluble bags; double-bag and mark "Isolation."
6. Use gloves when indicated by patient's condition (see p. 798).
   a. Disposable single-use gloves are preferable.
   b. Use once and discard in appropriate container.
7. Handle needles and syringes with *extreme* care.
   Rinse nondisposable needles and syringes in cold water and wrap using double-bag technique—place in clean bag in contaminated area and then place in a second clean bag outside the patient's room.
8. Disinfect and handle wastes with all due precautions.
9. Handle bed linens and fomites with care.
10. Carry out concurrent disinfection of fomites.
11. Control dissemination of infectious droplets.
    a. Encourage patient to cover nose and mouth when coughing or sneezing.
    b. Wrap contaminated tissues and articles in paper before disposal.
12. Control dust.
    a. Avoid creating aerosols—e.g., shaking bedlinens.
    b. Require damp dusting of furniture and wet vacuum cleaning of floors.
    c. Maintain cleanliness of surroundings; wash soil from walls as soon as it appears.
    d. Reduce to a minimum the activity of personnel in the patient's room.
13. Ventilate the patient's room properly with a system that directs room air to the outside.
    Keep the door to the room closed.

D. *To protect the patient who is immunosuppressed or immune-incompetent (organ transplant, leukemia, etc.)*

1. Use meticulous hand-washing technique.
2. Use protective isolation units—life islands, laminar airflow units with high efficiency filters (controversial).
3. Remember that every item in the room is potentially dangerous to the patient.
4. Some authorities suggest that flowers, plants, and water sources be removed from patient's environment when advisable to decrease patient's contacts with bacteria and fungi that are associated with these items.

E. *To provide physiologic support of the patient*

1. Ensure adequate hydration in the event of excessive fluid loss through vomiting, diarrhea, or excessive sweating.
   a. Encourage liberal fluid intake.
   b. Prepare for the administration of intravenous fluids as required.

TABLE 19-1. EPIDEMIOLOGY, THERAPY, AND CONTROL OF COMMUNICABLE INFECTIONS

Disease	Infective Organism	Infectious Sources	Entry Site	Method of Spread
Amebiasis	*Entamoeba histolytica*	Contaminated water and food	Gastrointestinal tract	Patients and carriers; fecal-oral route
Bacillary Dysentery	*Shigella* group	Contaminated water and food	Gastrointestinal tract	Patients and carriers; fecal-oral route
Brucellosis	*Brucella melitensis* and related organisms	Milk, meat, tissues, blood, absorbed fetuses and placentas from infected cattle, goats, horses, pigs	Gastrointestinal tract	Ingestion of or contact with infective material
Chancroid	Ducrey bacillus	Human cases and carriers	Genitalia	Direct sexual contact
Chickenpox (Varicella)	Virus	Human cases	Probably nasopharynx	Probably respiratory droplets
Diphtheria	*Corynebacterium diphtheriae*	Human cases and carriers; fomites; raw milk	Nasopharynx	Nasal and oral secretions; respiratory droplets
Encephalitis, epidemic (eastern and western equine)	Viruses	Chicken and wildbird mites; horses; hibernating garter snakes	Skin	Mosquitoes
Gonorrhea	*Neisseria gonorrhoeae*	Urethral and vaginal secretions	Urethral or vaginal mucosa; pharynx; rectum	Sexual activity
Granuloma Inguinale	Donovan body (bacillus)	Infectious exudate	External genitalia; cervix	Sexual intercourse
Type A Hepatitis (HAV)	Hepatitis A virus	Person-to-person contact; contaminated food or water; feces; blood; urine	Gastrointestinal tract; skin	Fecal-oral route; ingestion of or parenteral inoculation with infected blood or blood products, sexual contact
Type B Hepatitis (HAB)	Hepatitis B virus	Infected blood donor; contaminated injection equipment	Skin	Parenteral injection of human blood, plasma, thrombin, fibrinogen, packed cells, and other blood products from an infected person; contaminated needles and syringes; venereal contact
Infectious Mononucleosis	E-B virus	Human cases and carriers	Mouth	Probably oropharyngeal route; via blood transfusion in susceptible recipients
Influenza	Virus (types A and B)	Human cases; animal reservoir	Respiratory tract	Respiratory
Lymphogranuloma Venereum	*Chlamydia trachomatis*	Human cases	External genitalia; urethral or vaginal mucosa	Sexual intercourse; indirect contact with contaminated articles/clothing
Malaria	*Plasmodium vivax, falciparum, malariae,* and *ovale*	Human cases	Skin	Mosquitoes (Anopheles)
Measles	Virus	Human cases	Respiratory mucosa	Nasopharyngeal secretions
Meningococcal Meningitis	*Neisseria meningitidis*	Human cases and carriers	Nasopharynx; tonsils	Respiratory droplets
Mumps	Virus	Human cases (early)	Upper respiratory tract	Respiratory droplets
Paratyphoid Fever	*Salmonella paratyphi A* and *B* and related organisms	Contaminated food, milk, water; rectal tubes; barium enemas	Gastrointestinal tract	Infected urine and feces
Pneumococcal Pneumonia	*Streptococcus pneumoniae*	Human carriers; patient's own pharynx	Respiratory mucosa	Respiratory droplets
Poliomyelitis	Poliovirus (Types I, II, III)	Human cases and carriers	Gastrointestinal tract	Infected feces; pharyngeal secretions
Rocky Mountain Spotted Fever	*Rickettsia rickettsii*	Infected wild rodents, dogs, wood ticks, dog ticks	Skin	Tick bites
Rubella (German Measles)	Virus	Human case	Respiratory mucosa	Nasopharyngeal secretions
Scarlet Fever	*Group A Streptococcus*	Human cases; infected food	Pharynx	Nasal and oral secretions

* Research developments produce changes in drug therapy. The reader is referred to drug brochures and digests to keep abreast of changing dosages and uses.

Incubation Period	Chemotherapy*	Prevention and Control
Variable	Metronidazole; emetine; chloroquine; iodoquinol; chlortetracycline	Detection of carriers and their removal from food handling; plumbing safeguards
24–48 hours	Ampicillin; chloramphenicol; tetracycline; sulfa-trimethoprim	Detection and control of carriers; inspection of food handlers; decontamination of water supplies
6–14 days	Tetracycline, streptomycin, or chloramphenicol	Milk pasteurization; control of infection in animals
2–5 days	Sulfonamides; streptomycin; tetracycline	Effective case-finding and treatment of infection
14–16 days	None	Varicella-zoster immune globulin (VZIG) (an investigational drug) used in high-risk susceptible children exposed to varicella zoster within 72 hours
2–5 days	Diphtheria antitoxin; penicillin; erythromycin	Active immunization with diphtheria toxoid
Variable	None	Eastern equine encephalitis vaccine, dried (available from Center for Disease Control)
2–9 days	Aqueous procaine pencillin G preceded by probenecid or alternative regimens outlined by U.S.P.H.S.	Examination; culture; treatment of sexual partners
Unknown, presumably 8–80 days	Tetracyclines; erythromycin	Chemotherapy of carriers and contacts; case-finding and treatment of patients
15–45 days	None	Enteric and blood precautions for infected cases; immune serum globulin (ISG)—offers protection against clinical manifestations if given early in incubation period
60–180 days	None	Screening of blood donors; avoidance of unnecessary use of blood and blood derivatives; Hepatitis B immune globulin (HBIG) to exposed patient
2–6 weeks	None	None
24–72 hours	Amantadine	Specific virus vaccine
5–21 days	Tetracyclines	Case-finding and treatment of infection
Variable, depending on strain	Chloroquine; primaquine; amodiaquine; quinine; proguanil	Coordinated measures for wide-scale mosquito control; prompt detection and effective treatment of cases; suppressive drugs in malarious areas
8–13 days	None	Measles vaccine
2–10 days	Penicillin; chloramphenicol	Meningococcal polysaccharide vaccine to persons at risk; rifampin for carriers or contacts
12–26 (aver. 18) days	None	Live mumps vaccine
7–24 days	Chloramphenicol; ampicillin; sulfa-trimethoprim	Control of public water sources, food vendors, food handlers; treatment of carriers
Variable	Penicillin	Polyvalent pneumococcal vaccine; control of upper respiratory infections; avoidance of alcoholic intoxication
7–12 days	None	Oral polio vaccine (OPV), the live attenuated vaccine containing all 3 strains of poliovirus—produces long-lasting immunity in most recipients
3–10 days	Tetracyclines; chloramphenicol	Avoidance of tick-infected areas, or wearing of protective clothing in such areas; frequent search for and prompt removal of ticks from body; specific vaccination of exposed persons
14–21 days	None	Rubella virus vaccine; immune serum globulin (human) given to contacts of rubella. Pregnant women should *not* be given rubella vaccine. Rubella in early stages of pregnancy legally recognized as indication for abortion
3–5 days	Penicillin	Isolation; prophylactic chemotherapy with penicillin; asepsis during obstetrical procedures; specific chemoprophylaxis for persons with rheumatic fever, endocarditis

(continued on next page)

TABLE 19-1. EPIDEMIOLOGY, THERAPY, AND CONTROL OF COMMUNICABLE INFECTIONS (Continued)

Disease	Infective Organism	Infectious Sources	Entry Site	Method of Spread
Syphilis	*Treponema pallidum*	Infected exudate or blood	External genitalia; cervix; mucosal surfaces; placenta	Sexual activity; contact with open lesions; blood transfusion; transplacental inoculation
Tetanus	*Clostridium tetani*	Contaminated soil	Penetrating and crush wounds	Horse and cattle feces
Trichinosis	*Trichinella spiralis*	Infected pigs	Gastrointestinal tract	Ingestion of infected pork, undercooked
Tuberculosis	*Mycobacterium tuberculosis*	Sputum from human cases; milk from infected cows (rare in U.S.)	Respiratory mucosa	Sputum; respiratory droplets
Tularemia	*Francisella tularensis*	Wild rodents and rabbits	Eyes; skin; gastrointestinal tract	Handling infected animals; ingestion of undercooked infected meat; drinking contaminated water; bites from infected flies, ticks
Typhoid Fever	*Salmonella typhi*	Contaminated food and water	Gastrointestinal tract	Infected urine and feces
Typhus, endemic	*Rickettsia typhi (mooseri)*	Infected rodents	Skin	Flea bites
Whooping Cough (Pertussis)	*Bordetella pertussis*	Human cases	Respiratory tract	Infected bronchial secretions

2. Reduce the fever when indicated (it is often important to watch temperature curve).
   a. Administer antipyretic drugs as prescribed.
   b. Employ cool sponges cautiously as indicated (see p. 714).
3. Measure and record body temperature, pulse, and respiratory rates frequently.
4. Measure arterial pressure at regular intervals if patient exhibits a tendency to vascular collapse.
5. Weigh patient periodically, preferably at same hour of the day, on the same scale.

F. *To provide symptomatic relief*

1. Combat generalized aching and malaise.
   a. Utilize warm applications and massage as indicated.
   b. Apply cold compresses for headache.
   c. Administer analgesic medications as prescribed.
   d. Attend to oral hygiene.
   e. Limit physical activity.
2. Relieve cough.
   a. Humidify inspired air.
   b. Administer hot gargles and throat irrigations.
   c. Supply expectorants or cough depressants as indicated and prescribed.
3. Relieve anxiety and depression.
   a. Employ a nonjudgmental approach to the patient with sexually transmitted disease.
   b. Recognize loneliness of the isolated patient.
   c. Lend encouragement to patient faced with prospect of prolonged convalescence.

G. *To protect exposed individuals and the public at large against infectious illness*

1. Make available, facilitate, or perform whatever vaccination procedures are known to be effective and are indicated for the stimulation of active immunity in exposed and susceptible individuals (see p. 801).
2. Furnish specific immune serum (heterologous or human convalescent) or human gamma globulin if indicated, to provide passive immunity and temporary protection to contacts who are particularly vulnerable.
3. Isolate patients with communicable infections, as well as known carriers and contacts, when required.
4. Educate the public with respect to:
   a. Availability and importance of prophylactic immunization
   b. Manner in which infectious illnesses are spread and methods of avoiding spread
   c. Importance of seeking medical advice in the event of a febrile illness or skin eruption
   d. Importance of environmental cleanliness and personal hygiene
   e. Importance of adequate housing and nutrition
   f. Means of preventing the contamination of food and water supplies:
      (1) Discipline, cleanliness, and inspection of food handlers
      (2) Dangers of "perishable" foods; the identity of foods that tend to promote bacterial growth; and methods of food preservation
      (3) Significance of milk pasteurization
      (4) Indications for and methods of sterilizing food by means of heat
      (5) Importance of meat inspection
   g. Knowledge of insect, rodent, and other animal vectors and reservoirs of human infections and the importance of eliminating them.

CLASSIFICATION OF INFECTIOUS DISEASES REQUIRING ISOLATION OR PRECAUTIONS*

Strict Isolation

Private room—*necessary*; door must be kept closed.

Gowns—must be worn by all persons entering room.

* From *Isolation Techniques for Use in Hospitals*, 2nd ed., U.S. Department of Health, Education and Welfare, Center for Disease Control, 1975.

Incubation Period	Chemotherapy*	Prevention and Control
10–70 days	Penicillin; erythromycin; tetracycline	Case-finding by means of routine serologic testing and other methods; adequate treatment of infected individuals
4–21 days (aver. 10 days)	Tetanus immune globulin (human) [TIG] and penicillin	Wound debridement; toxoid booster injections for patients previously immunized; tetanus toxoid and tetanus immune globulin (separate sites and separate syringes) for nonimmune persons
2–28 days	Steroids; thiabendazole	Regulation of hog breeders; adequate meat inspection; thorough cooking of pork
Variable	Isoniazid; ethambutol; rifampin; streptomycin	Early discovery and adequate treatment of active cases; milk pasteurization
1–10 days	Streptomycin; tetracyclines; chloramphenicol	Use of rubber gloves when skinning/handling potentially infectious wild animals; avoidance of contact with potentially infected rodents; adequate cooking of wild rabbit dishes; vaccination of hunters, butchers, laboratory workers risking heavy exposure
1–3 weeks	Chloramphenicol; ampicillin; sulfa-trimethoprim	Decontamination of water sources; milk pasteurization; individual vaccination of high risk persons; control of carriers
1–2 weeks	Tetracyclines; chloramphenicol	Delousing procedures; case quarantine
Commonly 7 days	Erythromycin; ampicillin	Active immunization with vaccine; case isolation

Masks—must be worn by all persons entering room.
Hands—must be washed on entering and leaving room.
Gloves—must be worn by all persons entering room.
Articles—must be discarded or wrapped before being sent to Central Supply for disinfection or sterilization.

Diseases Requiring Strict Isolation*
1. Anthrax, inhalation
2. Burn wounds (major) infected with *Staphylococcus aureus* or group A streptococcus
3. Congenital rubella syndrome
4. Diphtheria (pharyngeal or cutaneous)
5. Disseminated neonatal *Herpesvirus hominis* infection (herpes simplex)
6. Herpes zoster, disseminated
7. Lassa fever
8. Marburg virus disease
9. Plague, pneumonic
10. Pneumonia, *Staphylococcus aureus* or group A streptococcus
11. Rabies
12. Skin infection (major) infected with *Staphylococcus aureus* or group A streptococcus
13. Smallpox
14. Vaccinia (generalized and progressive, and eczema vaccinatum)
15. Varicella (chickenpox)

Respiratory Isolation
Private Room—*necessary*; door must be kept closed.
Gowns—not necessary.
Masks—must be worn by any person entering room unless that person is not susceptible to the disease.
Hands—must be washed on entering and leaving room.
Gloves—not necessary.

   * See *Isolation Techniques for Use in Hospitals* for details and recommended duration of isolation.

Articles—those contaminated with secretions must be disinfected.

Diseases Requiring Respiratory Isolation*
1. Measles (rubeola)
2. Meningococcal meningitis
3. Meningococcemia
4. Mumps
5. Pertussis (whooping cough)
6. Rubella (German measles)
7. Tuberculosis, pulmonary—including tuberculosis of the respiratory tract, suspected or sputum-positive (smear)

Protective Isolation
Private room—*necessary*; door must be kept closed.
Gowns—must be worn by all persons entering room.
Masks—must be worn by all persons entering room.
Hands—must be washed on entering and leaving room.
Gloves—must be worn by all persons having direct contact with patient.
Articles—See *Isolation Techniques for Use in Hospitals*.

Conditions That May Require Protective Isolation†
1. Agranulocytosis
2. Dermatitis; noninfected vesicular, bullous, or eczematous disease, when severe and extensive
3. Extensive, noninfected burns in certain patients
4. Lymphomas and leukemia in certain patients (especially in the late stages of Hodgkin's disease and acute leukemia)

Enteric Precautions
Private room—*necessary for children only.*
Gowns—must be worn by all persons having direct contact with patient.
Masks—not necessary.
Hands—must be washed on entering and leaving room.

Gloves—must be worn by all persons having direct contact with patient or with articles contaminated with fecal material.

Articles—special precautions necessary for articles contaminated with urine and feces. Articles must be disinfected or discarded.

Diseases Requiring Enteric Precautions*
1. Cholera
2. Diarrhea, acute illness with suspected infectious etiology
3. Enterocolitis, staphylococcal
4. Gastroenteritis caused by:
   Enteropathogenic or enterotoxic *Escherichia coli*
   Salmonella species
   Shigella species
   Yersinia enterocolitica
5. Hepatitis, viral, type A, B, or unspecified
6. Typhoid fever *(Salmonella typhi)*

Wound and Skin Precautions

Private room—desirable.

Gowns—must be worn by all persons having direct contact with patient.

Masks—not necessary except during dressing changes.

Hands—must be washed on entering and leaving room.

Gloves—must be worn by all persons having direct contact with infected area.

Articles—special precautions necessary for instruments, dressings, and linen.

Diseases Requiring Wound and Skin Precautions*
1. Burns that are infected, except those infected with *Staphylococcus aureus* or group A streptococcus that are not covered or not adequately contained by dressings (see Strict Isolation)
2. Gas gangrene (due to *Clostridium perfringens*)
3. Herpes zoster, localized
4. Melioidosis, extrapulmonary with draining sinuses
5. Plague, bubonic
6. Puerperal sepsis—group A streptococcus, vaginal discharge
7. Wound and skin infections that are not covered by dressings or that have copious purulent drainage that is not contained by dressings, except those infected with *Staphylococcus aureus* or group A streptococcus, which require strict isolation
8. Wound and skin infections that are covered by dressings so that the discharge is adequately contained, including those infected with *Staphylococcus aureus* or group A streptococcus; minor wound infections, such as stitch abscesses, need only secretion precautions

Discharge Precautions

A. *Secretion Precautions—Lesions*
1. Use a "no-touch" dressing technique (do not touch the wound or dressings with the hands) when changing dressings on these lesions.
2. Employ proper handwashing procedures.
3. Wash hands before and after patient contact; use sterile equipment when changing dressings; double-bag soiled dressings and equipment.
4. These precautions apply only with lesions from which there is a discharge.

* See *Isolation Techniques for Use in Hospitals* for details and recommended duration of isolation.

Diseases; Duration of Precautions
1. Actinomycosis, draining lesions—for duration of drainage
2. Anthrax, cutaneous—until culture-negative
3. Brucellosis, draining lesions—for duration of drainage
4. Burn, skin, and wound infections, minor—for duration of drainage
5. Candidiasis, mucocutaneous—for duration of illness
6. Coccidioidomycosis, draining lesion—for duration of drainage
7. Conjunctivitis, acute bacterial (including gonococcal)—until 24 hours after start of effective therapy
8. Conjunctivitis, viral—for duration of illness
9. Gonococcal ophthalmia neonatorum—until 24 hours after start of effective therapy
10. Gonorrhea—until 24 hours after start of effective therapy
11. Granuloma inguinale—for duration of illness
12. *Herpesvirus hominis* (herpes simplex), except disseminated neonatal disease—for duration of illness. For disseminated neonatal disease, see Strict Isolation; for oral *H. hominis* disease, see Secretion Precautions, Oral.
13. Keratoconjunctivitis, infectious—for duration of illness
14. Listeriosis—for duration of illness
15. Lymphogranuloma venereum—for duration of illness
16. Nocardiosis, draining lesions—for duration of illness
17. Orf—for duration of illness
18. Syphilis, mucocutaneous—until 24 hours after start of effective therapy
19. Trachoma, acute—for duration of illness
20. Tuberculosis, extrapulmonary draining lesion—for duration of drainage
21. Tularemia, draining lesion—for duration of drainage

B. *Secretion Precautions—Oral*
1. The diseases listed in this section can be spread to susceptible persons by contact with oral secretions.
2. Attention should be given to the proper disposal of oral secretions to prevent spread of infection.
3. Instruct the patient to cough or spit into disposable tissues held close to the mouth; discard tissues in an impervious (impenetrable) bag at the bedside.
4. If the patient has nasotracheal suction or tracheostomy, the suction catheter and gloves should be placed in an impervious bag for disposal.
5. Seal the bag before discarding in the trash.

Diseases; Duration of Precautions
1. Herpangina—for duration of hospitalization
2. Herpes oralis—for duration of illness
3. Infectious mononucleosis—for duration of illness
4. Melioidosis, pulmonary—for duration of illness
5. Mycoplasma pneumonia—for duration of illness
6. Pneumonia, bacterial, if not covered elsewhere—for duration of illness
7. Psittacosis—for duration of illness. (It may be desirable to place patient with acute psittacosis who is coughing and raising sputum in respiratory isolation.)
8. Q fever—for duration of illness
9. Respiratory infectious disease, acute (if not covered elsewhere)—for duration of illness
10. Scarlet fever—until 24 hours after start of effective therapy
11. Streptococcal pharyngitis—until 24 hours after start of effective therapy

C. *Excretion Precautions*
1. The diseases listed in this section can be spread to susceptible persons through the oral route by contact with fecal excretions from a person infected with the organism.
2. Strict attention should be paid to careful handwashing following any patient contact and especially following contact with excretions.
3. Instruct the patient on the necessity of careful handwashing after defecating.
4. Make sure there is proper sanitary disposal of excretions; a standard sewage system is adequate.

Diseases; Duration of Precautions
1. Amebiasis—for duration of illness
2. *Clostridium perfringens (C. welchii)* food poisoning—for duration of illness
3. Enterobiasis—for duration of illness
4. Giardiasis—for duration of illness
5. Hand, foot, and mouth disease—for duration of hospitalization
6. Herpangina—for duration of hospitalization
7. Infectious lymphocytosis—for duration of hospitalization
8. Leptospirosis (urine only)—for duration of hospitalization
9. Meningitis, aseptic—for duration of hospitalization
10. Pleurodynia—for duration of hospitalization
11. Poliomyelitis—for duration of hospitalization
12. Staphylococcal food poisoning—for duration of symptoms
13. Tapeworm disease (only with *Hymenolepsis nana* and *Taenia solium* [pork])—for duration of illness
14. Viral diseases, other (ECHO or Coxsackie gastroenteritis, pericarditis, myocarditis, meningitis)—for duration of hospitalization

D. *Blood Precautions*
1. The diseases in this category are associated with circulation of the etiologic agent in blood; be aware of the route of transmission.
2. Blood precautions should be taken for the duration of clinical disease or for as long as the etiologic agent can be demonstrated in the blood. Blood precautions should be taken with anyone who is HB_s Ag-positive.
3. Disposable needles and syringe should be used for patients in isolation. They must not be reused.
4. Used needles need not be recapped; they should be placed in a prominently labeled, impervious, puncture-resistant container designated for this purpose. Needles should not be purposefully bent, because accidental needle puncture may occur.
5. Used syringes should be placed in an impervious bag. Both needle and syringe bags should be incinerated or autoclaved before discarding.
6. Rinse reusable needles and syringes thoroughly in cold water after use; place the needle in a puncture-resistant rigid container; wrap syringes and needles using double-bag technique and return to proper department for decontamination and sterilization.
7. These specifications pertain to needle and syringe

precautions and to labeling of blood specimens. Label blood specimens with patient's diagnosis (so that necessary precautions will be taken).

Diseases; Duration of Precautions
1. Arthropod-borne viral fever (dengue, etc.)—for duration of hospitalization
2. Hepatitis, viral, type A, B, or unspecified (also listed under Enteric Precautions)—for duration of hospitalization
3. Malaria—for duration of hospitalization

IMMUNIZATION

Immunity is the resistance that an individual has against disease.
1. Specific immunity to a particular organism implies that an individual has either generated the appropriate antibody in his own body or received ready-made antibodies from another source.
2. Immunization may be natural (not acquired through previous contact with the infectious agent) or acquired.
3. Acquired immunity may be *passive* or *active*.

Passive Immunity

Passive immunity to a disease is a state of relative temporary protection produced by the injection of serum containing antibodies which have formed in another host.

There are 3 types of preparations:
1. Human immune serum globulin (for general use)
2. Human immune serum globulin with a known antibody content (for specific illnesses)
3. Animal antiserum or antitoxins

Active Immunization

Active immunization is immunization that has been produced by natural or acquired stimulation so that the body produces its own antibodies.
1. It may be produced by clinical or subclinical infection (the person gets the disease); by vaccination with live or killed microorganisms or their antigens; or by inactivated vaccines and toxoids.
2. The organisms have been treated by heating or by chemical inactivation to destroy their harmful properties without destroying their ability to stimulate antibody protection.
3. Active immunizations that are available for adults include tetanus and diphtheria toxoid, adult-type tetanus toxoid, influenza virus vaccine, and rubella virus vaccine.
4. Vaccines are also available for pneumococcal pneumonia, cholera, plague, rabies, typhoid, typhus, yellow fever, Rocky Mountain spotted fever, and smallpox.
5. Current recommendations for the use of vaccines and other biologicals are available from the Public Health Service Advisory Committee on Immunization Practices, Center for Disease Control, Atlanta, Georgia 30333.

SEXUALLY TRANSMITTED DISEASES (STD)

Sexually transmitted diseases are transmitted by sexual activity and include venereal diseases as well as nonspecific urethral and genital infections, enteric infections, and parasitic infestations (Table 19-2).
1. Sexually transmitted diseases are the most common infections in the United States; patients present with physical symptoms, urethral/vaginal discharge, le-

sions, and rashes. Gonorrhea (p. 807) and syphilis (p. 823) are the most important STD because their prevalence constitutes a world-wide health problem.
2. Persons at high risk are those who frequently change partners and homosexuals with multiple sex partners.

TABLE 19-2. SEXUALLY TRANSMITTED DISEASES SUMMARY*

	Etiology	Prevalence	Clinical Presentation
Gonorrhea	*Neisseria gonorrhoeae* A non-motile, gram negative diplococcus. 0.6 μ to 1.0 μ in diameter.	1,013,436 (468.3/100,000) cases reported in 1978. Highest reported case rates are in age groups 20-24 and 15-19.	Men have dysuria, frequency, and urethral discharge that is usually purulent and often more severe in the morning. Women experience vaginal discharge and cystitis. 5-20% of men and about 60% of women have no symptoms.
Syphilis	*Treponema pallidum* A motile spirochete with 6-14 spirals and ends pointed with finely spiral terminal filaments. 6-15 μ in length.	21,656 (10/100,000) infectious cases reported in 1978. Highest reported case rates are in age groups 20-24 and 25-29.	*Primary syphilis:* Classical chancre is a painless, eroded papule with a raised, indurated border. Atypical lesions are common; multiple lesions may occur. Extragenital chancres may appear on any part of body. Unilateral or bilateral lymphadenopathy may accompany. *Secondary syphilis:* Various cutaneous and mucous membrane lesions, alopecia, generalized lymphadenopathy, mild constitutional symptoms.
Nongonococcal Urethritis (NGU)	1) *Chlamydia trachomatis*—estimated to cause NGU in about 50% of cases. An obligate intracellular parasite. Diameter 250-500 nm. 2) *Ureaplasma urealyticum*—estimated by some workers to cause NGU in about 30% of cases. A mycoplasma of the T strain, less than 150 nm in diameter. 3) *Other Etiologic Agents*—estimated to cause NGU in 10-20% of cases. *Trichomonas vaginalis* *Candida albicans* Herpes simplex Coliform bacteria	Age distribution of nongonococcal urethritis parallels that of other sexually transmitted diseases, notably gonorrhea. Recurrences are very common.	Urethral discharge varies from profusely purulent to slightly mucoid. Dysuria may or may not be present. In half of the cases, the incubation period appears to exceed 10 days. Some men may have asymptomatic infection.
Trichomoniasis	*Trichomonas vaginalis* A motile protozoan with 4 anterior flagella and a short, undulating membrane. 5-15 μm in length.	Prevalence ranges from as low as 5% of private gynecologic patients to as high as 50-75% of prostitutes. Colonization rates are higher among women than men.	From no signs or symptoms to erythema and edema of external genitalia and frothy greenish-gray vaginal discharge. Granular vaginitis may include punctuate hemorrhages and may involve the cervix. Most men are asymptomatic, though some may present with urethritis.
Genital Herpes Infection	Herpes virus—Type 2 A spherical DNA virus, enveloped, with cubic symmetry. 150 nm.	Prevalent among adolescents, young adults, and the sexually active.	Vesicular lesions on vulva, perineum, vagina, and cervix in women; lesions on penile shaft, prepuce, glans penis, and (less frequently) scrotum and perineum in men. Recurrent infections. Tender adenopathy, dysuria, and constitutional signs more common with primary infections than those recurring.
Vulvovaginal Candidiasis	*Candida albicans* A dimorphic gram positive fungus that appears as oval, budding yeast cells, has hyphae and pseudohyphae. 3 × 6 μm.	Saprophytic in the oropharyngeal and gastrointestinal tracts in 50% of the population and in the vagina in 20% of nonpregnant women.	Vulva is usually erythematous and edematous. Vaginal discharge, when present, may be thick and white, resembling cottage cheese. Occasionally discharge is thin and watery. Satellite lesions may spread to the groin. Many women have no symptoms. Sexual partners may develop balanitis or cutaneous lesions on penis.
Corynebacterium Vaginale Vaginitis or Hemophilus Vaginalis Vaginitis	*Corynebacterium vaginale* Or *Hemophilus vaginalis* Gram negative pleomorphic coccobacillus, precise taxonomy not decided. Measures 1-3 μm × 0.4-0.7 μm.	Cultured from 23-96% of women with vaginitis. Recovered from 0-52% of asymptomatic women.	Homogenous, relatively thin, occasionally frothy vaginal discharge, usually gray-white. Punctate hemorrhages and vulvar irritation are occasionally seen. Between 10% and 40% of culture-positive patients have no symptoms.

* U.S. Department of Health and Human Services.

Diagnosis	Therapy	Complications
Presumptive identification— Microscopic identification of typical gram negative, intracellular diplococci on smear of urethral exudate from men or endocervical material from women OR Positive oxidase reaction of typical colonies from specimen obtained from anterior urethra, endocervix or anal canal, and inoculated on Modified Thayer Martin Medium.	Aqueous procaine penicillin G, 4.8 million units IM at 2 sites with 1 g of probenecid orally OR Tetracycline HCl, 0.5 g orally q.i.d. for 5 days, 10 g total OR Ampicillin, 3.5 g or amoxicillin, 3 g, either with 1 g of probenecid orally.	Epididymitis Pharyngitis Meningitis Septicemia Arthritis Endocarditis Conjunctivitis in Newborn Pelvic Inflammatory Disease (PID)
Demonstration of *T. pallidum* from exudate of primary or secondary lesions by darkfield microscopy. Typical lesions, reactive reagin test for syphilis (VDRL or RPR), and FAT/ABS will confirm except in early primary cases.	Benzathine penicillin G, 2.4 million units IM at 1 visit OR Aqueous procaine penicillin G, 4.8 million units total: 600,000 units IM daily for 8 days OR Tetracycline HCl, 500 mg orally q.i.d. for 15 days.	Late syphilis Congenital syphilis
Clinical picture of dysuria and/or urethral discharge; discharge on examination; polymorphonuclear leukocytes or urethral smear negative for *Neisseria gonorrhoeae* and negative culture for gonorrhea on Modified Thayer-Martin Medium.	Tetracycline, 500 mg q.i.d. for 7-21 days. Many clinicians recommend similar therapy for sexual consorts.	Epididymitis Prostatitis Proctitis Cervicitis Salpingitis Reiter's Disease Ophthalmia neonatorum
Microscopic examination of wet mount of vaginal discharge. Papanicolaou smears may show the parasite. Culture methods are available.	Oral metronidazole 2 g p.o. STAT OR 250 mg t.i.d. for 7 days. Advise patient against consuming alcohol. Treat steady sex partners.	Rare Epididymitis Prostatitis
Clinical appearance of herpetic lesions. Papanicolaou smears from lesions, stained to show multinucleated giant cells with intranuclear inclusion bodies. Tissue culture.	No specific therapy is available. Symptoms may be relieved by warm baths.	Keratitis Encephalitis Neonatal Herpes Infection
Microscopic examination of gram-stained smears of introital or vaginal wall scrapings. Microscopic examination of wet mount of vaginal discharge. Culture on Sabouraud's modified agar.	Nystatin vaginal suppositories b.i.d. for 7 to 14 days OR Miconazole vaginal cream qd. for 7 days. Discuss with patient predisposing factors and means of avoiding a recurrence.	Nil
Clinical picture, microscopic examination, and culture. Gram stain of vaginal exudate may show tiny, gram negative coccobacilli ("clue cells") adhering to vaginal epithelial cells, though specificity of this finding is low. Wet mount far less sensitive than gram stain.	Oral ampicillin 500 mg q.i.d. for 7-10 days (Examine patient for syphilis or gonorrhea before prescribing this regimen, as ampicillin may mask symptoms) OR Oral metronidazole 250 mg t.i.d. for 7 days.	Nil

(continued on next page)

TABLE 19-2. SEXUALLY TRANSMITTED DISEASES SUMMARY* (Continued)

	Etiology	Prevalence	Clinical Presentation
Pediculosis Pubis	*Phthirus pubis* Pubic louse, an oval, grayish insect which becomes reddish-brown when engorged with blood. 1-4 mm in length.	Age group of patients affected by pubic lice parallels that of patients with gonorrhea. Transmitted during sexual intercourse, very rarely by bedding or clothing.	Erythematous, itching papules. Nits or adult lice adhering to pubic hair or hair around the anus, abdomen, and thighs.
Scabies	*Scarcoptes scabiei* The adult female mite is 300-400 μm long and has 4 pairs of short legs. Posterior legs end in long bristles. Male is 100-200 μm in length.	Transmitted via close bodily contact, often incidental to coitus, infested bedding and clothing.	Linear burrows 1 to 10 mm in length, often with a red papule which contains the mite. Scratching may produce excoriation. Most common sites are finger webs, wrists, elbows, ankles, penis. Nighttime itching is characteristic.
Genital Warts (*Condyloma acuminata*)	Human papillomavirus A small DNA virus, icosahedral, of the papovavirus group.	Age distribution of venereal papillomatous lesions parallels that of patients with gonorrhea.	Flesh-colored to pinkish papillary or sessile growths which occur around the vulva, introitus, vagina, cervix, perineum, anus, anal canal, urethra, and glans penis.
Chancroid	*Hemophilus ducreyi* A coccobacillus that is non-motile, non-acid-fast, gram negative. Size 1-1.5 μm × 0.6 μm.	May occur in conjunction with other genital infections, particularly genital herpes and syphilis.	A ragged, tender ulcer that is not indurated ("soft chancre"), its base covered with gray or yellow necrotic exudate. May be multiple ulcers. Tender inguinal adenopathy, usually unilateral. Women contacts are usually asymptomatic.
Lymphogranuloma Venereum	*Chlamydia trachomatis* An obligate intracellular parasite. Diameter 250-500 nm.	Occurs frequently in tropical and semi-tropical regions, although 348 cases (0.2 per 100,000) were reported in the U.S. in 1977.	Primary lesion is an evanescent, painless vesicle or superficial non-indurated ulcer on the genitalia. Adenopathy of the regional lymph nodes is common. A frank purulent proctocolitis may signal rectal involvement. Rare.
Granuloma Inguinale	*Calymmatobacterium granulomatis* A non-motile coccobacillus that is gram negative. Size 2 μm × 0.8 μm.	Though fairly common in a few underdeveloped nations, frequency has declined from a high of 2611 cases reported in 1949 to 75 in 1977 in the U.S. More common among men than women, and in Southern States.	Single or multiple subcutaneous nodules may erode through the skin, producing clean granulomatous, beefy-red lesions (usually painless).
Hepatitis B Infection	Hepatitis Virus—Type B A virus of probable DNA nucleic acid content, 26 μm or less.	Common among homosexuals and prostitutes.	Onset is usually insidious, with vague abdominal discomfort, anorexia, nausea, arthralgia, which often progresses to jaundice. Fever may be absent or mild. Asymptomatic, anicteric hepatitis may occur.

BACTERIAL INFECTIONS

NOSOCOMIAL (HOSPITAL ACQUIRED) INFECTIONS

Nosocomial infections are infections acquired in a health care facility during hospitalization; infection is neither present nor incubating at the time of admission unless it is related to a previous hospitalization. The major cause of hospital-acquired infections in the United States is gram-negative bacteria.

Gram-negative Infections

Gram-negative infections are bacterial infections caused most frequently by *Escherichia coli, Enterobacter* species, *Klebsiellae, Pseudomonas aeruginosa, Proteus* species, and *Serratia marcescens.*

Related Terms

Septic shock—circulatory shock occurring as a complication of a severe infection (usually by gram-negative enteric bacilli, although gram-positive cocci can cause bacterial shock)

Bacteremia—bacterial invasion of the bloodstream

Predisposing Events

1. Most gram-negative bacilli are not invasive in normal hosts; they are opportunistic bacteria that become invasive in persons with diminishing defense mechanisms.
2. Diagnostic and treatment procedures (tubes, catheters, etc.) result in disruption of usual protective barriers normally provided by the skin and mucous membranes.
3. The advent of potent immunosuppressive drugs, cytotoxic drugs, steroids, radiation therapy, and previous splenectomy contribute to diminishing the defense mechanisms of the patient.
4. Neonates and the elderly are susceptible to infection.
5. The following contribute to the development of gram-negative infections:
   a. Genitourinary tract—indwelling catheters, instrumentation, urinary obstruction
   b. Gastrointestinal tract—from obstruction, perforation, neoplasia, abscesses, diverticuli
   c. Biliary tract—cholangitis, obstruction (stones), surgical procedures

Diagnosis	Therapy	Complications
Clinical observation of lice OR microscopically, by identification of nits at base of hair.	1% Y-benzene hexachloride lotion 25% benzyl benzoate lotion. Combine with appropriate antimicrobials if secondary infection is noted.	Rare Impetigo Furunculosis Pustular eczema
Identifying the burrows and microscopic identification of the mites.	25% benzyl benzoate emulsion. Y-benzene hexachloride crotomiton. Combine with appropriate antimicrobials if secondary infection is noted. Trace and treat family, domestic, and sex contacts.	Impetigo Pustular eczema
Clinical appearance. Histology. Electron microscopy.	Podophylin 10-25% in tincture of benzoin, applied weekly. Electrocautery. Curettage. Cryotherapy.	Rare Malignant change
Clinical appearance. Exclude possibility of syphilis through absence of indurated lesions and negative darkfield. Gram stained exudate from lesion or aspirates from nodes may reveal short, gram negative rods, OR culture on blood agar or media with blood derivatives.	Sulfasoxazole 1 gm orally q.i.d. OR Tetracycline 500 mg q.i.d. for 10-14 days OR Kanamycin 500 mg IM b.i.d. for 10-14 days, or Streptomycin 500 mg IM b.i.d. for 10-14 days. Fluctuating gland masses will call for aspiration.	Chronic fistulas of gland masses in groin.
Clinical picture. Complement Fixation Test (CFT), significantly positive with a titer of 1:16 or higher in more than 80% of cases. Material for Frei Skin Test is no longer available.	Tetracycline 500 mg orally q.i.d. for 2-3 weeks OR Sulfasoxazole 4 g orally, followed by 500 mg q.i.d. for 3 weeks. Fluctuating gland masses indicate a need for aspiration.	Rare Elephantiasis Rectal strictures producing tenesmus, pain, and constipation. Men: Ulcerative and fistular lesions of urethra, penis, scrotum Women: Ulcerative genital lesions
Clinical picture. Intracytoplasmic rods ("Donovan's bodies") in large mononuclear cell from biopsy material stained with Giemsa or Wright's stain.	Tetracycline 500 mg orally q.i.d. for 2-3 weeks OR Gentamicin 40 mg IM b.i.d. for 2 weeks.	Rare Elephantiasis Urethral, vaginal, or rectal stricture from cicatrix following healing. Massed pelvic glands; occasional bony involvement.
Detection of hepatitis B surface antigen (HBsAg) in blood by radioimmunoassay, passive hemagglutination, or other techniques.	Symptomatic	Death Carriers (Rare) Cirrhosis (Late & Rare)

d. Reproductive system—abortion, instrumentation, postpartum period
e. Vascular system—venous cutdowns, intravenous catheters, intracardiac pacemakers, prosthetic heart valves, total parenteral nutrition, pressure-monitoring devices, surgical procedures
f. Skin—wound infections, burns, pressure sores
g. Respiratory tract—tracheostomy, mechanical ventilation, aspiration

Prevention

1. Handwashing by personnel and patient—fundamental to the control of all infections
2. Protective isolation (p. 799) for patients receiving large doses of immunosuppressive drugs.
3. Strict aseptic technique for all diagnostic/therapeutic procedures—wounds, tracheostomies, tube drainage, catheters, intravenous therapy, cardiac pacing, ventilatory equipment
   a. Avoid prolonged IV therapy.
   b. Anchor IV catheter securely to prevent movement in vein.
4. Use of nursing surveillance to prevent cross-infection
5. Monitoring of sterilization procedures and cleaning practices
6. Obtaining environmental and patient cultures as indicated.

7. Try to avoid housing 2 patients with indwelling catheters in the same room
   a. Use closed urinary drainage system if an indwelling catheter is required
   b. Regard outside of catheter and drainage bag as highly contaminated.

Clinical Manifestations

1. Shaking chill and rapid rise in temperature
2. Warm, dry skin (during early stage)
3. Alteration in personality (inappropriate behavior)—due to reduction in cerebral blood flow
4. *Hypotension and shock*
   a. Tachycardia/tachypnea
   b. Cool, clammy skin
   c. Peripheral cyanosis
   d. Oliguria
   e. Vascular collapse—death may occur as a result of vascular collapse
5. Intravascular coagulation

Treatment and Nursing Management

OBJECTIVES: to recognize and treat the development of bacteremia.
to improve perfusion to the vital organs.
1. Examine patient carefully to identify source of sepsis.
   a. Assist with collection of blood culture—to identify

etiologic agent and for sensitivity testing.
b. Obtain other smears and cultures as indicated.
2. Administer appropriate antimicrobial agent—give promptly when patient is too ill to await result of culture.
   a. Most severe infections leading to septic shock are caused by a relatively small number of organisms. Therapy is usually started before bacteriological diagnosis is made because of seriousness of illness.
   b. Drugs in common use in the treatment of gram-negative infections include cephalosporins, aminoglycosides (gentamicin, tobramycin, amikacin) chloramphenicol, carbenicillin, and ticarcillin.
3. Remove any foreign source of possible infection (when possible)—venous or bladder catheters.
4. Assist with surgical drainage of localized infection.
5. Prevent and treat shock and other complications.
   a. Monitor the state of responsiveness; skin temperature, moisture, color, turgor; appearance of mucous membranes and nails; pulse and respiration; input and output; blood pressure.
   b. Administer adequate volume of fluid and blood.
      (1) Insert 2 or 3 large IV catheters—for rapid fluid and blood replacement, to ensure perfusion of vital organs.
      (2) Administer blood, plasma, low molecular weight dextran, or saline as directed for volume expansion and to combat vascular collapse.
      (3) Follow central venous pressure measurements—provides gauge for restoration of volume replacement (rate and amount)
      (4) Follow measurements of left ventricular filling pressures (Swan-Ganz—see p. 268).
   c. Administer oxygen to keep arterial PO_2 at desired level.
      (1) Follow blood gas and pH measurements (p. 158) to assess patient's need for assisted ventilation. Inadequate respiratory exchange is a frequent cause of death in gram-negative shock.
      (2) Patient is usually hypoxic from increased AV shunting and from hypermetabolism from high fever.
   d. Monitor serum electrolytes every several hours.
   e. Administer sodium bicarbonate if severe acidosis exists.
   f. Administer isoproterenol or dopamine, digitalis, diuretics, and other pharmacologic agents as directed.
   g. Treat disseminated intravascular coagulation (p. 259).

STAPHYLOCOCCAL INFECTIONS

Staphylococci are responsible for a wide variety of infections. They cause most superficial infections, but they also produce serious infections of the lungs, pleural space, bones, kidneys, and surgical wounds.

Examples of Staphylococcal Disease

1. *Skin and soft tissue infections*—furuncles (boils), impetigo, carbuncles, cellulitis, abscesses, infected lacerations
2. *Invasion of lymphatics*—axillary, cervical, mediastinal, retroperitoneal, and subdiaphragmatic abscesses
3. *Invasion of bloodstream*—endocarditis, pneumonitis, empyema, perinephritic abscess, hepatic abscess, splenic abscess, staphyloccocal enteritis, septic ar-

thritis, meningitis, osteomyelitis, generalized septicemia

Infectious Agent

Various strains of coagulase-positive staphylococci (*Staphylococcus aureus*)

Modes of Transmission

Direct hand transfer

Ingestion of food

Nasal secretions, draining wound, asymptomatic nasal carrier

Aerosolization during dressing changes

Intravenous needles (drug abusers)

Hospital Staphylococcal Infections

(Include all of the above infections)

A. *Susceptible Hospital Patients*

1. Chronically ill or debilitated patients
2. Patients receiving systemic steroids or cancer chemotherapy
3. Patients undergoing major or prolonged surgery
4. Infants in the nursery
5. Patients with impairment of skin integrity (dermatoses, burns, abrasions)

B. *Prevention and Control*

1. All hospitals and extended care facilities should enforce aseptic techniques supervised by infection control committee of the individual health agency.
2. Personnel with staphylococcal lesions should not work in the health agency until healing has occurred or cultures have become negative after treatment.
3. Patients with staphylococcal infections should be placed under strict isolation precautions until antibiotic treatment has rendered cultures negative for staphylococci.
4. Reduce cross traffic between hospital areas housing infected patients and those in which noninfected patients are quartered.

Specific Therapy for Staphylococcal Infections (Systemic)

1. Penicillinase-resistant penicillins (methicillin, nafcillin) and cephalosporins (cephalothin); vancomycin; clindamycin, etc.; selected according to sensitivity study
   a. Intravenous administration is usually selected because of large doses of drug required.
   b. Serious staphylococcal infections may require 4–6 weeks of treatment.
2. Provide supportive care—surgical measures, pain relief, treatment of fever, etc.

Nursing Isolation Procedures Required for Staphylococcal Disease (*S. aureus*)

1. Burns—strict isolation, wound and skin precautions or secretion precautions, depending on extent of infection, for duration of illness; (wounds or lesions: until they stop draining)
2. Enterocolitis—enteric precautions until patient is off antibiotics and is culture-negative
3. Gastroenteritis—excretion precautions for duration of illness
4. Lung abscess, draining—strict isolation for duration of illness (until drainage stops)

5. Pneumonia—strict isolation for duration of illness
6. Skin infection—strict isolation, wound and skin precautions, or secretion precautions for duration of illness (depending on extent of infection)
7. Wound infection—strict isolation, wound and skin precautions, or secretion precautions (depending on extent of infection) for duration of illness

Preventive Measures and Health Education

1. Public should be educated concerning personal hygiene.
2. Persons with draining lesions should be isolated from their group and treated.

STREPTOCOCCAL INFECTIONS

Most *streptococcal infections* in humans are caused by group A hemolytic streptococci. Beta hemolytic streptococci gain entrance to the body primarily through the upper respiratory tract or skin; transmission is by persons with streptococcal infections or by asymptomatic carriers.

Beta Hemolytic Streptococcal Infections

1. Streptococcal sore throat ("strep" pharyngitis, p. 142).
2. Scarlet fever (streptococcal throat with a rash which occurs if infectious agent produces erythrogenic toxin to which patient is not immune)
3. Sinusitis, otitis media, mastoiditis, peritonsillar abscess
4. Pericarditis, arthritis, peritonitis, meningitis
5. Pneumonia and empyema
6. Wound and skin infections—impetigo, puerperal infections, cellulitis, erysipelas

Poststreptococcal Diseases (sequelae of Hemolytic Streptococci)

1. Rheumatic fever
2. Acute glomerulonephritis

Diagnostic Evaluation

1. Throat culture and sensitivity test
2. Culture from wounds

Treatment

1. Penicillin is the drug of choice in streptococcal infections (except enterococcal streptococci group D infections).
   a. Therapy should be continued for at least 10 days—to eliminate the organism, reduce frequency of suppurative complications, prevent the majority of cases of rheumatic fever (and to a lesser extent acute glomerulonephritis) and help prevent further spread of streptococci.
   b. Cephalosporins, erythromycin, or clindamycin may be used for penicillin-sensitive patients.
2. Make sure the patient understands the importance of *completing* the course of antimicrobial treatment.

Nursing Isolation Procedures

Streptococcal disease (group A)
1. Burns—strict isolation, wound and skin precautions or secretion precautions (depending on extent of infection) until wounds or lesions stop draining
2. Endometritis (puerperal sepsis)—wound and skin precautions until 24 hours after initiation of effective therapy
3. Pharyngitis—secretion precautions until 24 hours after initiation of effective therapy
4. Pneumonia—strict isolation until 24 hours after initiation of effective therapy
5. Scarlet fever—secretion precautions until 24 hours after initiation of effective therapy
6. Skin infection—strict isolation, wound and skin precautions or secretion precautions (depending on extent of infection) until wounds or lesions stop draining
7. Wound infection—strict isolation, wound and skin precautions or secretion precautions (depending on the extent of infection) until wound stops draining
8. Streptococcal disease (not group A) unless covered elsewhere—none

Preventive Measures and Health Education

1. Public should be educated concerning the relationship of streptococcal infections to heart disease and glomerulonephritis
2. Food handlers should be instructed about and monitored for hygienic procedures.
3. Obstetrical patients should be protected from personnel or visitors with respiratory or skin infections.
4. Long-term penicillin prophylaxis may be used for high-risk individuals (rheumatic heart disease)—to prevent a repeat attack.

GONORRHEA

Gonorrhea is an infection involving the mucosal surface of the genitourinary tract, rectum, and pharynx; it is caused by the gonococcus *Neisseria gonorrhoeae*. It is an infectious disease which is transmitted sexually, the exception being gonococcal ophthalmia of the newborn. It may be acquired by sexual intercourse, orogenital, and/or anogenital contacts between members of opposite sexes as well as members of the same sex.

Epidemiology

1. Changes in sexual behavior; liberalization of attitudes
2. Sexual contact at earlier ages
3. Greater personal mobility

Clinical Problems

1. Gonorrhea is the most common reportable communicable disease in the U.S.
2. Gonorrhea has a short incubation period which permits rapid spread; a high percentage of infected females are symptom-free.
3. Syphilis and gonorrhea are frequently observed in the same patient.
4. Gonorrhea is becoming increasingly resistant to penicillin.

Complications

1. Sterility and pelvic infection in women; postgonococcal urethritis in men
2. Secondary foci of infection may develop in any organ system—disseminated gonorrhea, gonococcal arthritis, tenosynovitis, bursitis, endocarditis, pelvic infection, meningitis, lesions of the skin, severe proctitis

Clinical Manifestations

NURSING ALERT: A large number of women who have gonorrhea are asymptomatic and unaware that they are infected. There is a fairly high incidence of asymptomatic males with gonorrhea. Therefore many patients are untreated and remain infectious.

A. *Women (small percentage)*

Vaginal discharge; abnormal uterine bleeding

Urinary frequency and pain

Pelvic infection, when gonococcus spreads through fallopian tubes (salpingitis)

Fever

Nausea and vomiting

Abdominal pain/tenderness

Disseminated gonococcal infection

B. *Men (incubation period 3–5 days or longer)*

Urethritis—purulent discharge followed by painful urination

Spread of infection to posterior urethra, prostate, seminal vesicles, and epididymis

Prostatitis

Pelvic pain and fever

Epididymitis

Severe pain, tenderness, and swelling

Postgonococcal urethritis and urethral stricture become major problems in males

C. *Anorectal Manifestations*

Anal burning, itching, bleeding, mucopurulent discharge or painful defecation; may be asymptomatic

D. *Pharyngeal Manifestations*

Sore throat, but may be asymptomatic

Diagnostic Evaluation

(See Guidelines: Obtaining Culture Specimen for Diagnosis of Gonorrhea, p. 809.)

A. *Women*

Culture specimens obtained from cervix and anal canal and inoculated on selected media such as modified Thayer-Martin (T-M) medium. (T-M medium contains antibiotics to inhibit growth of other bacteria.)

B. *Men*

Smear of urethral exudate for microscopic examination (See Fig. 19-1C)

C. *The pharyngeal and rectal site should be cultured in persons engaging in oral and/or rectal sex.*

Treatment and Nursing Management

OBJECTIVE: to eradicate the organisms.

1. Drug regimens for uncomplicated gonorrheal infection:*
   a. Aqueous procaine penicillin G: 4.8 million units injected at 2 sites with 1.0 gm. of probenecid by mouth; *OR*
   b. Tetracycline hydrochloride: 0.5 gm. by mouth 4 times a day for 5 days; *OR*
   c. Ampicillin or amoxicillin: ampicillin 3.5 gm., or

* Gonorrhea. Center for Disease Control Recommended Treatment Schedules, 1979.

amoxicillin 3.0 gm., either with 1 gm. probenecid by mouth.
   d. Patients who are allergic to the penicillins or probenecid should be treated with oral tetracycline as above. Patients who cannot tolerate tetracycline may be treated with spectinomycin hydrochloride, 2.0 gm., in one intramuscular injection.
2. Treatment of sexual contacts: examined, cultured, and treated with one of the above regimens.
3. Follow-up cultures should be obtained from infected sites in 3–7 days; cultures also obtained 4–6 weeks after treatment to detect reinfection.
4. Secure serologic test for syphilis at time of diagnosis.
5. Patients with gonorrhea who also have syphilis must be given additional treatment depending on stage of syphilis.
6. Treatment of complications of gonorrhea (endocarditis, bacteremia, arthritis, etc.) is individualized.

Nursing Isolation Procedure

Use secretion precautions (p. 800) for duration of illness (until lesions stop draining)

Principles of Control

1. Gonorrhea is a reportable disease; public health authorities are notified so that sexual contacts can be found and treated.
2. Each patient should be interviewed for names of contacts. Conduct interview and record history in nonjudgmental, empathetic manner.
3. Contacts of known gonorrhea cases should be investigated; known contacts should be treated within 10 days.
4. The patient should be instructed to avoid reinfection by sexual activity with untreated previous sexual partners until they have been tested and treated.

Health Education

1. Venereal disease (VD) is acquired by sexual contact (vaginal sexual intercourse, anal intercourse, oral intercourse) and by close and direct contact with an infected person.
2. A person who thinks that he or she may have VD or who has been exposed to someone who might have it should have a checkup. Immediate treatment should be sought if symptoms develop.
3. Anyone who is sexually active with a number of sexual partners should have regular checkups.
4. Washing the sex organs (before and after sexual contact) and the use of a condom may give limited protection against VD.
5. Birth control pills and IUDs give no protection against VD.
6. Gonorrhea and syphilis are different diseases, caused by different germs; they attack the body in different ways but are spread in the same manner. A person may have both gonorrhea and syphilis at the same time.
7. There appears to be no natural or acquired immunity to gonorrhea and syphilis. A person can get gonorrhea and syphilis again and again.
8. Pregnant women may pass infection of syphilis to unborn child. Pregnant women may pass gonorrhea to baby during the birth process.
9. Bacteria from gonorrhea may enter the bloodstream and affect joints, joint linings, heart valves, etc.
10. VD National Hotline: 800-227-8922 or 8923; provides information and referral services for sexually transmitted diseases.

GUIDELINES: Obtaining Culture Specimen for the Diagnosis of Gonorrhea*

Purpose To obtain specimens from the cervix (women), anal canal (men and women), urethral specimen (men) or oropharynx specimen (men and women) for culture for *N. gonorrhoeae*.

Equipment Vaginal speculum
Ring forceps
Cotton balls
Sterile, cotton-tipped swabs
Sterile calcium alginate urethral swabs
Sterile wire loop
Sterile disposable gloves
Selective medium—Martin-Lewis (ML), modified Thayer-Martin (MTM), or New York City (NYC) (for isolation of *N. gonorrhoeae*)

Procedure

NURSING ACTION	RATIONALE/AMPLIFICATION
Preparatory Phase	
1. Place patient in dorsal lithotomy position with adequate draping.	
2. Put on sterile disposable gloves.	
Performance Phase	
FOR FEMALE PATIENT: *Cervical Culture*	
1. Moisten vaginal speculum with warm water. Do not use any other lubricant.	
2. Separate labia. Depress the perineum and posterior vaginal wall with the finger of one hand.	2. This maneuver helps avoid uncomfortable pressure against the more sensitive anteriorly placed structures.
3. Gently insert a bivalve vaginal speculum.	3. The speculum is made self-retaining by adjusting one or more screws. The short blade should be uppermost. The tip of the posterior blade is pushed down into the posterior fornix.
4. Remove excessive cervical mucus with a cotton ball held in ring forceps.	

5. Insert sterile cotton-tipped swab into endocervical canal (Fig. 19-1*A*).
  a. Move from side to side in cervix.
  b. Allow 30 seconds for absorption of organisms by the swab.
	5. The endocervical canal is considered the best culture site. Movement of the cotton swab ensures adequate sampling.

Anal Canal Culture (Rectal Culture)	
1. Obtain anal specimen *after* getting cervical specimen.	1. The anal canal is the most likely site to be positive when the cervix is negative.
2. Insert sterile cotton-tipped swab approximately 2.5 cm. (1 inch) into the anal canal (Fig. 19-1*B*).	2. Use another swab to obtain specimen if swab is inadvertently pushed into feces.
3. Move swab from side to side in anal canal.	3. Movement of the swab in anal canal permits specimen to be secured from anal crypts.
4. Allow 10-30 seconds for absorption of organism by the swab.	
Oropharynx Culture	
1. Swab the posterior pharynx and tonsillar crypts with a cotton-tipped applicator.	1. Oropharyngeal specimens should be obtained from patients suspected of having disseminated gonococcal infection.
FOR MALE PATIENT: *Urethral Culture*	
1. Use sterile bacteriologic wire loop or a sterile calcium alginate urethral swab to obtain a specimen from the anterior urethra by gently scraping the mucosa (Fig 19-1*C*). Do not insert loop or swab more than 2 cm. into urethra.	1. A urethral culture of the male is indicated when the Gram stain of urethral exudate is not positive, in tests-of-cure, or as a test for asymptomatic urethral infection. Avoid using a standard cotton-tipped swab as it is too large.

* Adapted from Criteria and Techniques for the Diagnosis of Gonorrhea, U.S. Public Health Service, Center for Disease Control.

GUIDELINES: Obtaining Culture Specimen for the Diagnosis of Gonorrhea (cont.)

Procedure (cont.)

NURSING ACTION	RATIONALE/AMPLIFICATION
Anal Canal Culture	
(Same as in women)	
Oropharynx Culture	
(Same as in women)	

To Inoculate Selective Medium in Plates:

A. *Candle Jar System*

1. Roll swab in a large "Z" pattern on selective medium (Fig. 19-1*D*). If a second specimen is collected, inoculate on a separate part of medium.

1. This pattern provides adequate exposure of swab to plate for transfer of organisms.

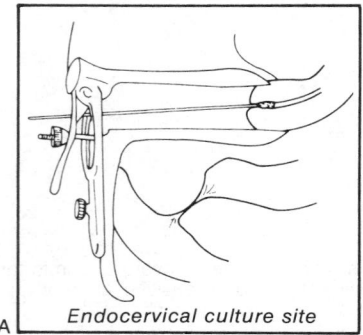

A *Endocervical culture site*

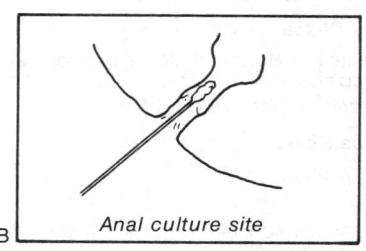

B *Anal culture site*

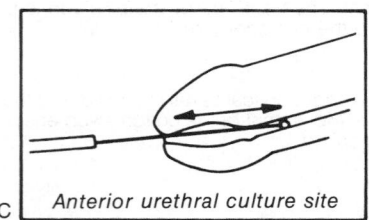

C *Anterior urethral culture site*

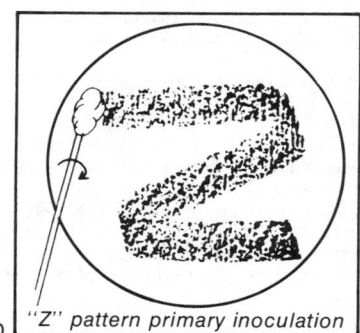

D *"Z" pattern primary inoculation*

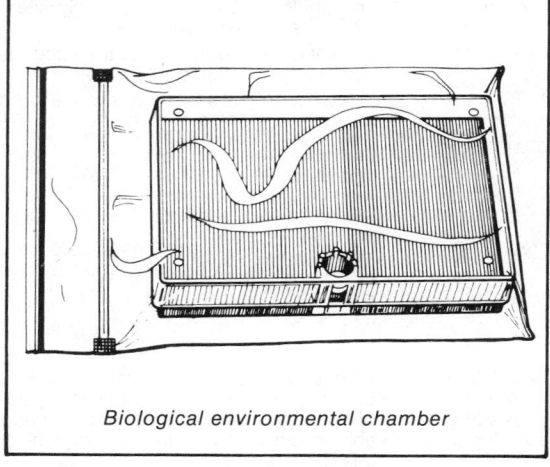

E *Biological environmental chamber*

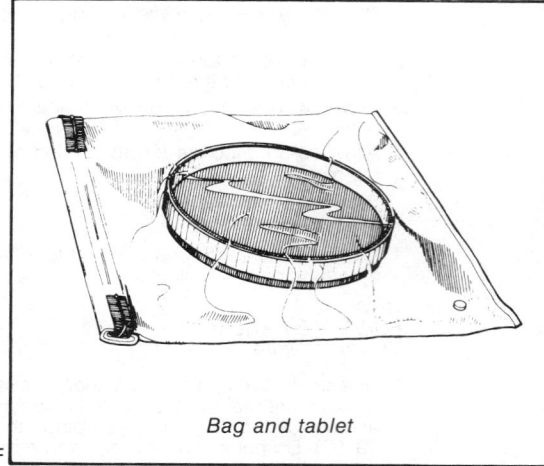

F *Bag and tablet*

FIGURE 19-1. *Obtaining culture for specimen in diagnosis of gonorrhea. From: Criteria and Techniques for the Diagnosis of Gonorrhea. U.S. Public Health Service, Center for Disease Control.*

Procedure (cont.)

NURSING ACTION	RATIONALE/AMPLIFICATION
2. Cross streak immediately with a sterile wire loop or tip of swab (in the clinical facility).	2. Streaking with a wire loop isolates colonies of *N. gonorrhoeae* from the few contaminants that occasionally grow on selective medium.
3. Place the culture plate in a CO_2-enriched atmosphere (candle jar) within 15 minutes of inoculation.	3. Placing the culture plate in a candle jar retards drying and provides an appropriate carbon dioxide environment. Successful recovery of *N. gonorrhoeae* requires an atmosphere enriched with carbon dioxide. The candle must be lit each time the jar is open.
4. Incubate plates within 1–2 hours at 35°–36° C.	
B. *CO_2 Tablet/Plastic Bag System*	
1. After the medium is inoculated, place the CO_2-generating tablet in a special well of the plate (Biological Environmental Chamber), *not* on the medium surface (Fig. 19-1*E*). Use forceps to handle the tablets. Secure the top of the plate tightly.	1. Read the package inserts on the handling and storing of CO_2 tablets.
2. Another method is to drop a CO_2-generating tablet into the plastic bag (Fig. 19-1*F*).	2. The tablet and plastic bag system is easy to use, safe, and economical.
3. Place plate in plastic bag. Expel excess air from the bag and seal it tightly. No portion of the bag is to be left open.	3. Moisture from the medium will activate the CO_2-generating tablet.
4. Incubate plates within 1–2 hours at 35°–36° C. (95°–96.8° F.).	

PULMONARY TUBERCULOSIS

Tuberculosis is an infectious disease caused by the tubercle bacillus, *Mycobacterium tuberculosis*. It usually invades the lungs, but it also involves and sometimes produces gross lesions in other organs and tissues.

Transmission

1. The term *mycobacterium* is descriptive of the organism, which is a bacterium that resembles a fungus. The organisms multiply slowly and are characterized as acid-fast aerobic organisms which can be killed by heat, sunshine, drying, and ultraviolet light.
2. Tuberculosis is an airborne disease transmitted by droplet nuclei, usually from within the respiratory tract of a person with active ulcerative lesions who expels them during coughing, talking, sneezing, or singing.
3. When an uninfected susceptible person inhales the droplet-containing air, the organism is carried into the lung to the pulmonary alveoli.

Pathology

1. Tubercle bacilli infect the lung, forming a tubercle (lesion).
2. The tubercle
   a. May heal, leaving scar tissue.
   b. May continue as a granuloma.
      (1) May heal.
      (2) May be reactivated.
   c. May eventually proceed to necrosis (death), liquefaction, sloughing, and cavitation.
3. The initial lesion may disseminate tubercle bacilli:
   a. By extension to adjacent tissues
   b. Via bloodstream
   c. Via lymphatic system
   d. Through the bronchi

Risk Factors for Activation of Tuberculosis

Persons at risk:
1. Adults whose initial infection was acquired many years previously; these persons harbor live dormant bacilli that at any time may reactivate and spread disease.
2. Persons with silicosis, diabetes mellitus, postgastrectomy state.
3. Patients receiving corticosteroid therapy; patients with chronic renal failure who are undergoing hemodialysis; patients with cancer or organ transplants who are receiving immunosuppressive therapy; patients who have had intestinal bypass surgery for obesity.

Clinical Manifestations

Patient may be asymptomatic or may have insidious symptoms that are ignored.
1. Generalized systemic signs and symptoms
   a. Fatigue, anorexia, weight loss, low grade fever, night sweats, indigestion
   b. Some patients have acute febrile illness, chills, generalized influenza-like symptoms
2. Pulmonary signs and symptoms
   a. Cough (insidious onset) progressing in frequency and producing mucoid or mucopurulent sputum
   b. Hemoptysis; chest pain; dyspnea (indicates extensive involvement)
3. Extrapulmonary tuberculosis: *Mycobacterium* can infect any organ in the body (pleurae, lymph nodes, genitourinary tract, bones/joints, peritoneum, central nervous system)

Diagnostic Evaluation

1. Sputum smear and culture—diagnosis made by finding the acid-fast bacilli in sputum obtained by coughing and expectoration, induced by inhaled aerosols, bronchoscopic aspiration, transtracheal aspiration, gastric aspiration (swallowed sputum in aspirate is cultured).
2. Chest x-ray—to determine presence and extent of disease.
3. Tuberculin skin test—inoculation of tubercle bacillus extract (tuberculin) into the intradermal layer of the inner aspect of the forearm (see p. 814).
4. Screening tests—multiple puncture tests—introduc-

tion of tuberculin into skin by instruments that pierce skin at several points simultaneously.
  a. Used for screening, since there is no way to standardize the amount of tuberculin introduced.
  b. Tests available include Tine, Mono-Vacc, Sterneedle.
  c. See product information sheet for reading and interpretation.

Treatment

OBJECTIVES: to eliminate all viable tubercle bacilli.
to prevent transmission of infection.
to return the patient to his usual life style as quickly as possible.

1. Administer prescribed antituberculosis drugs.
   a. A combination of drugs (to which bacilli are susceptible) is given to destroy viable microbial organisms as rapidly as possible and to minimize the emergence of drug-resistant organisms. *Choice of drugs and length of treatment vary.*
      (1) Isoniazid (INH) and rifampin (RIF) may be used for 9–12 months.
         (a) One or two supplementary drugs may be added in the initial intensive phase of treatment to avert consequences of primary and acquired resistance.
         (b) If resistance is found, revision of the chemotherapy regimen and length of treatment is required.
      (2) See Table 19-3 for most commonly used drugs (first-line and second-line drugs); second-line drugs are used for treatment of recurring tuberculosis or when first-line drugs are not suitable.
2. Majority of patients improve rapidly after antituberculosis therapy is begun; symptoms abate and number of acid-fast bacilli on sputum smear decreases.

Nursing Isolation Procedure

Respiratory isolation (p. 799) until effective therapy begins and there is clinical improvement (sputum smear becomes negative).

Preventive Treatment (Chemoprophylaxis)

Prevention of tuberculosis by prophylactic use of chemotherapeutic agent.

OBJECTIVE: to identify infected persons and give preventive therapy to those at risk of developing disease and becoming transmitters.

Most cases occur in persons known to be positive tuberculin reactors. These patients are the source of infection in 80%–90% of future cases of active tuberculous disease.

Isoniazid Therapy

1. The following high-risk groups are recommended for preventive (isoniazid, [INH]) therapy:*
   a. Household members and other close associates of persons with recently diagnosed tuberculous disease.
   b. Positive tuberculin skin test reactors with findings on the chest roentgenogram consistent with nonprogressive tuberculous disease, in whom there are neither positive bacteriologic findings nor a history of adequate chemotherapy.

   * Joint statement of the American Thoracic Society, American Lung Association, and the Center for Disease Control.

   c. Newly infected persons (recent skin test converters).
   d. Positive tuberculin skin test reactors in special clinical situations. To a varying degree the following situations increase the risk of developing tuberculous disease and may require preventive therapy in the infected: (a) prolonged therapy with adrenocorticoids, (b) immunosuppressive therapy, (c) some hematologic and reticuloendothelial diseases, such as leukemia or Hodgkin's disease, (d) diabetes mellitus, (e) silicosis, and (f) after gastrectomy.
   e. Reactors without special risk factors, under 35 years of age.
2. Complication of isoniazid therapy
   a. Liver dysfunction (hepatitis)
      (1) Question patient who is receiving isoniazid. Do you have loss of appetite? fatigue? joint pain? fever? dark urine?
      (2) Monitor serum transaminase values for persons at risk of developing hepatitis—over 35, daily drinkers, those taking potentially hepatotoxic drugs, history of liver disease.
3. BCG vaccine
   a. BCG vaccine (bacillus Calmette-Guérin)—produces a high level of immunity; may be given to populations with excessive/unavoidable exposure to tuberculosis.
   b. In developing countries, BCG is considered the first line of tuberculosis control.
   c. Only given in U.S. under specific circumstances. (BCG vaccination converts the PPD skin test, making it useless as a screening test for tuberculosis.)

Health Education

1. Educate patient about his disease. He must understand importance of continuing to take his medicine for prescribed time.
2. Secure the booklet *Understanding Tuberculosis Today: A Handbook for Patients* from local Lung Association to give insight into and knowledge of the disease.
3. Review the side effects of the drug therapy with the patient (p. 813); he should report to the clinic if any of these occur.
4. Review possible complications with patient and family: hemorrhage, pleurisy, symptoms of recurrence (persistent cough, fever, or hemoptysis).
5. Train patient to control propagation of secretions while coughing.
   a. Cover mouth and nose with double-ply tissue when coughing/sneezing. Do not sneeze into bare hand.
   b. Wash hands after coughing/sneezing.
6. Encourage patient to eat a nutritious diet.
7. Patients with problems of alcoholism should be referred to an alcoholic clinic or other appropriate health agency.
8. Avoid job-related exposure to excessive amounts of silicone (working in foundry, rock quarry, sand blasting).
9. Encourage patient to report to clinic/physician at specified intervals for sputum smears and chest films.

NURSING ALERT: Patient compliance remains a major problem in eradicating tuberculosis.

TABLE 19-3. TREATMENT OF MYCOBACTERIAL DISEASE IN ADULTS AND CHILDREN

First-Line Drugs	Dosage* Daily	Dosage* Twice Weekly	Most Common Side Effects*	Tests for Side Effects*	Remarks*
Isoniazid	5–10 mg./kg. up to 300 mg. PO or IM	15 mg./kg. PO or IM	Peripheral neuritis, hepatitis, hypersensitivity	SGOT/SGPT (not as a routine)	Bactericidal. Pyridoxine 10 mg as prophylaxis for neuritis; 50–100 mg. as treatment
Ethambutol	15–25 mg./kg. PO	50 mg./kg. PO	Optic neuritis (reversible with discontinuation of drug; very rare at 15 mg./kg.), skin rash	Red-green color discrimination and visual acuity†	Use with caution with renal disease or when eye testing is not feasible
Rifampin	10–20 mg./kg. up to 600 mg. PO	600 mg. PO	Hepatitis, febrile reaction, purpura (rare)	SGOT/SGPT (not as a routine)	Bactericidal. Orange urine color. Negates effect of birth control pills
Streptomycin	15–20 mg./kg. up to 1 gm. IM	25–30 mg./kg.	8th nerve damage, nephrotoxicity	Vestibular function, audiograms;† BUN and creatinine	Use with caution in older patients or those with renal disease
Second-Line Drugs					
Viomycin	15–30 mg./kg. up to 1 gm. IM		Auditory toxicity, nephrotoxicity, vestibular toxicity (rare)	Vestibular function, audiograms;† BUN and creatinine	Use with caution in older patients. Rarely used with renal disease
Capreomycin	15–30 mg./kg. up to 1 gm. IM		8th nerve damage, nephrotoxicity	Vestibular function, audiograms;† BUN and creatinine	Use with caution in older patients. Rarely used with renal disease
Kanamycin	15–30 mg./kg. up to 1 gm. IM		Auditory toxicity, nephrotoxicity, vestibular toxicity (rare)	Vestibular function, audiograms;† BUN and creatinine	Use with caution in older patients. Rarely used with renal disease
Ethionamide	15–30 mg./kg. up to 1 gm PO		GI disturbance, hepatotoxicity, hypersensitivity	SGOT/SGPT	Divided dose may help GI side effects
Pyrazinamide	15–30 mg./kg. up to 2 gm. PO		Hyperuricemia, hepatotoxicity	Uric acid, SGOT/SGPT	Combination with an aminoglycoside is bactericidal
Para-aminosalicylic acid (aminosalicylic acid)	150 mg./kg. up to 12 gm. PO		GI disturbance, hypersensitivity, hepatotoxicity, sodium load	SGOT/SGPT	GI side effects very frequent making cooperation difficult
Cycloserine	10–20 mg./kg. up to 1 gm. PO		Psychosis, personality changes, convulsions, rash	Psychologic testing	Very difficult drug to use. Side effects may be blocked by pyridoxine, ataractic agents or anticonvulsant drugs

* Check product labelling for detailed information on dose, contraindications, drug interaction, adverse reactions, and monitoring.
† Initial levels should be determined on start of treatment.
From American Thoracic Society: Treatment of Mycobacterial Disease. American Review of Respiratory Disease, 1977, 115,185.

GUIDELINES: Tuberculin Skin Test

The *tuberculosis intradermal skin test* is used to detect tuberculosis infection.

Purposes
1. To detect infection, either past or present, with *Mycobacterium* tuberculosis.
2. To serve as a diagnostic procedure in selected patients.

Equipment
PPD (purified protein derivative) tuberculin antigen
Tuberculin syringe
Short 1.25 cm (½ inch) 26 or 27 gauge steel needle
Alcohol sponge

Procedure

NURSING ACTION	RATIONALE/AMPLIFICATION
1. Determine if patient has ever had BCG vaccine, recent viral disease, immunosuppression by disease, drugs, or steroids.	
2. Draw up PPD-tuberculin into tuberculin syringe.	2. Follow the manufacturer's directions. Each 0.1 ml. dose should contain 5 TU (tuberculin units of PPD-tuberculin). Use the antigen immediately to avoid absorption onto the plastic/glass syringe.
3. Cleanse the skin of either the volar (palm side) or dorsal surface of the arm with alcohol. Allow to dry.	
4. Stretch the skin taut.	
5. Hold the tuberculin syringe close to the skin so that the hub of the needle touches it as the needle is introduced, bevel up.	5. This reduces the needle angle at the skin surface.
6. Inject the tuberculin into the superficial layer of the skin to form a wheal 6 mm. to 10 mm. in diameter.	6. If no wheal appears (because the injection was made too deep), inject again at another site at least 5 cm. (2 inches) away.

TO READ THE TEST:

1. Read the test within 48-72 hours.	1. Tuberculin skin tests are tests of *delayed* hypersensitivity.
2. Have a good light available. Flex the forearm slightly at the elbow.	
3. Inspect for the presence of *induration*. Inspect from a side view against the light. Inspect by direct light.	3. Induration refers to hardening or thickening of tissues.
4. Palpate: lightly rub the finger across the injection site from the area of normal skin to the area of induration. Outline the diameter of induration.	4. Erythema (redness) without induration is generally considered to be of no significance.
5. Measure the maximum transverse diameter of induration (not erythema) in millimeters with a flexible ruler.	

INTERPRETATION:

1. *Positive Reaction:* Induration 10 mm. or more.	1. A positive reaction indicates that a patient has had contact with tubercle bacillus. It does not necessarily mean that active disease is present in the lung.
2. *Doubtful Reaction:* Induration of 5–9 mm.	2. Individuals who are in close contact with persons with active tuberculosis and who have reactions in the 5–9 mm. range should be considered positive and receive preventive treatment.
3. *Negative Reaction:* Induration 0–4 mm.	3. This shows either a lack of tuberculin sensitivity or a low-grade sensitivity that most likely is not caused by *M. tuberculosis*. A negative test does not rule out the presence of tuberculosis.

NOTE: A tuberculin converter is a person whose tuberculin reaction changes from less than 10 mm. in diameter to 10 or more mm. in diameter and increases by at least 6 mm. (American Lung Association).

Follow-up Phase

Record:
1. Size of induration.
2. Name of antigen, strength of antigen, lot number, date of testing, date of reading

SALMONELLA INFECTIONS (SALMONELLOSIS)

Salmonellosis is a form of food poisoning characterized by acute gastroenteritis; it is caused by certain species of the genus *Salmonella*. The patient is infected via the oral route by contaminated food or drink.

Infectious agent—1500 known serotypes of salmonella—most common in U.S. are *S. typhimurium, S. enteritidis, S. newport, S. heidelberg, S. infantis,* and *s. st. paul.*

> **NURSING ALERT:** Common food offenders causing salmonella infections include commercially processed meat pies, poultry (especially turkey), sausage (lightly cooked), foods containing egg or egg products, and unpasteurized milk or dairy products.

Clinical Manifestations

(Usually 8–48 hours after ingestion of contaminated food)
1. Diarrhea—sudden onset of frequent, bulky stools followed by profuse, watery diarrhea; may lead to marked dehydration
2. Abdominal pain
3. Nausea and vomiting
4. Fever
5. Other manifestations due to infectious agent localizing in any body tissue—abscesses, cholecystitis, arthritis, endocarditis, meningitis, pericarditis, pneumonia, pyelonephritis

Diagnostic Evaluation

Stool culture

Treatment and Nursing Management

OBJECTIVE: to prevent dehydration and electrolyte imbalance.
Treatment is supportive:
1. Restrict food until nausea and vomiting subside.
2. Offer clear liquids as tolerated.
3. Correct fluid and electrolyte depletion with intravenous infusions.
4. Treatment is similar to that for typhoid fever (p. 816) if patient has focal (abscess) or systemic infection.

Nursing Isolation Procedure

Use enteric precautions for duration of illness (see p. 799).

Preventive Measures and Health Education

1. Food service workers should have training courses and ongoing in-service training in facts about foodborne illnesses, avoidance of food contamination, food storage methods, cleaning of food preparation and service areas, and maintenance of good personal hygiene.
2. Raw eggs or egg drinks should not be eaten, nor should cracked or dirty eggs be used.
3. All foods from animal sources, especially fowl, egg products, and meat dishes, should be thoroughly cooked.
4. Foods should be refrigerated during storage and should be protected against insects/rodents.
5. Any person handling food should be instructed to wash hands after toilet use, before and after food preparation.
6. Chicks, ducklings, and turtles (as well as other domestic animals and pets) are sources of infection.
7. The patient must wash his hands after toilet use, particularly during illness and carrier state (2–4 weeks)—to prevent infection of others.
8. Diarrhea in infants should be investigated immediately, since salmonellae play an important role, particularly in infants less than one year old.

SHIGELLOSIS (BACILLARY DYSENTERY)

Shigellosis, an acute bacterial disease of the intestinal tract, includes a group of enteric infections caused by bacilli of the *Shigella* group of which there are 4 types: *S. dysenteriae, S. flexneri, S. boydii, S. sonnei.* The source of infection is feces from an infected person. The route of spread is fecal-oral. Foodborne outbreaks can almost always be traced to contamination of food by a food handler. Shigellosis may also be of sexual origin.

Clinical Manifestations

1. Fever and headache
2. Abdominal cramps
3. Persistent diarrhea—passage of varying amounts of blood, mucus, and pus

Diagnostic Evaluation

Culture of freshly passed stool

OBJECTIVES: to maintain fluid and electrolyte balance. to prevent the spread of shigellosis to the patient's contacts, i.e., to eliminate the carrier state.
1. Determine the type of shigella—organism is recovered from patient's stool.
2. Do sensitivity testing for selection of antibiotic—multiresistance to antibiotics is common.
3. Give antibiotics which are absorbed from intestinal tract (ampicillin, tetracyclines, chloramphenicol, sulfamethoxazole-trimethoprim)—may shorten duration of illness and carrier state.
4. Maintain fluid and electrolyte balance—to prevent profound dehydration resulting from an excessive loss of salts in the diarrheal stools.
   a. Assess weight loss, skin turgor, dryness of mucous membranes, urinary volume, vital signs.
   b. Weigh daily and measure urinary volume.
5. Offer clear fluids during acute stage of illness; supplementary potassium may be required.
6. Carry out epidemiology studies of every patient in whom the organism is found.
   a. Question patient about travel to underdeveloped countries, exposure to crowded institutions, swimming in contaminated rivers. Inquire about water supplies, food eaten at home/restaurant.
   b. Notify local and state authorities.

Nursing Isolation Procedure

Use enteric precautions (p. 799) until 3 consecutive cultures of feces taken 24 hours apart after cessation of antimicrobial therapy are negative for infecting strain.

Preventive Measures and Health Education

1. See Health Education for typhoid fever, below
2. Program of fly control
3. Surveillance of water sanitation; adequate sewage disposal
4. Detection and treatment of carriers
5. Handwashing after defecation
6. Untreated sexual partners may reinfect patient

TYPHOID FEVER

Typhoid fever is a bacterial infection transmitted by contaminated water, milk, shellfish, or other foods. It is caused by *Salmonella typhi*, which is harbored in human excreta. Today it is spread chiefly by carriers, patients who have recovered from the fever, but whose stools or urine may spread these bacilli for years. The ingestion of infected oysters or shellfish taken from waters contaminated by offshore sewage disposal depots is another common source of infection. The characteristic lesion of typhoid fever consists of ulcers which form in the ileum and colon, and its distinctive clinical features consist of long-continued fever, rose-spot rash, enlarged spleen, slow pulse, and leukopenia.

Altered Physiology

The organism enters the body by the gastrointestinal tract; it invades the walls of the gastrointestinal tract, leading to bacteremia which localizes in mesenteric lymph nodes, in the masses of lymphatic tissue in the mucous membrane of the intestinal wall (Peyer's patches), and in small, solitary lymph follicles in the ileum and colon; ulceration of the intestines may ensue.

Clinical Manifestations

A. *Gradual onset*

1. Severe headache, malaise, muscle pains, nonproductive cough.
2. Chills and fever; temperature rises slowly, reaching highest level in 3–7 days (40–41° C. [104–105° F.])
3. Pulse is full and slow in comparison to height of fever; may have distinct dicrotic wave.
4. Skin eruption—irregularly spaced small rose spots on abdomen, chest, back. Each spot fades over a period of 3–4 days

B. *Second week*

1. Fever remains consistently high.
2. Abdominal distention and tenderness; constipation or diarrhea
3. Delirium in severe infections—from severe toxemia

C. *Third week*

Gradual decline in fever and subsidence of symptoms

Diagnostic Evaluation

1. White blood count—leukopenia is a distinctive hematologic feature but is not always present
2. Blood culture—positive for organism after 1st week
3. Stool culture—positive for organism after 1st week
4. Urine culture—organism may or may not be present
5. Blood serum agglutination test usually becomes positive by end of 2nd week

Treatment and Nursing Mangement

OBJECTIVES: to give supportive care.
to observe for intestinal hemorrhage, perforation, and other complications.

1. Give specific treatment for typhoid.
   a. Chloramphenicol as directed. Monitor blood count to detect chloramphenicol toxicity.
   b. Combination of sulfamethoxazole and trimethoprim may be given for chloramphenicol-resistant strains of typhoid.
   c. Ampicillin or amoxicillin are also in use.
2. Give supportive care—typhoid fever is a nursing challenge.
   a. Support patient during period of toxemia—patient may be drowsy, partially incontinent, or delirious.
   b. Give steroids if prescribed for toxic or delirious patients.
   c. Prepare for blood transfusions if indicated.
   d. Take rectal temperature every 2–4 hours.
      (1) Give fever sponge (p. 714) for temperature of 40° C. (104° F) or more.
      (2) Encourage a high fluid intake.
   e. Watch for bladder distention—patient may lose urge to void during toxic state. Keep input and output record.
   f. Observe for retention of feces.
      (1) Enemas are given under *low* pressure to diminish chance of intestinal perforation.
      (2) Relieve distention with rectal tube, inserted for a short time.
   g. Give a high calorie, low residue diet during febrile stage.
3. Watch for complications which can occur after an apparent clinical cure.
   a. *Intestinal hemorrhage*—from erosion of blood vessel in ulcerated small intestine (occurs in 10% of patients)
      (1) Clinical manifestations
         Apprehension, sweating, pallor
         Weak, rapid pulse; narrowing pulse pressure
         Hypotension
         Bloody or tarry stools
      (2) Treatment
         Withhold food
         Give blood transfusions
   b. *Perforation of intestine*—from erosion of one of the ulcers; most common during 3rd week
      (1) Symptoms
         Sudden, sharp abdominal pain—may stop suddenly
         Abdominal rigidity
         Shock
      (2) Treatment
         Prepare for intestinal decompression procedure (p. 414), intravenous fluids, and surgical intervention if conservative measures do not produce clinical improvement.
   c. Other complications—thrombophlebitis, urinary infections, cholecystitis, anemia, hepatitis.

Isolation Nursing Procedure

Use enteric precautions (p. 799) until 3 successive cultures of feces taken after cessation of antimicrobials are negative for *S. typhi*.

Prevention and Health Education

1. *Prevention:* typhoid vaccine, 1 subcutaneous injection followed by second injection 4 or more weeks later; booster injection every 3 years for selected individuals. (See recommendations of the Public Health Service Advisory Committee on Immunization Practices.)

2. *Maintain environmental hygiene.*
   a. Protect and purify water supplies.
   b. Employ sanitary waste disposal techniques.
   c. Pasteurize milk and dairy products; refrigerate while transporting.
   d. Supervise foods served, especially raw foods.
   e. Ensure that food handlers use handwashing facilities.
3. Patient must be followed with routine stool culture after recovery to detect the development of the carrier state—approximately 2–5% of typhoid patients become permanent carriers, harboring the organism and excreting it in their urine and stools.
   a. Carriers may be given ampicillin or amoxicillin—to attempt to abolish carrier state (there is evidence that treating certain patients with salmonella in their stools may prolong the carrier state).
   b. Positive chronic carrier state—documented evidence of *S. typhi* in stool or urine for a year or more.
   c. Carriers must not become food or milk handlers.

MENINGOCOCCAL INFECTION (MENINGOCOCCAL MENINGITIS)

Meningitis—inflammation of the meninges, or coverings of the brain; may be caused by bacterial, mycobacterial, or viral agents.

Bacterial meningitis is most frequently caused by *Neisseria meningitidis*, *Streptococcus pneumoniae* (in adults), and *Haemophilus influenzae* (in young children). It starts as an infection of the nasopharynx or the tonsils and is followed by meningococcal septicemia, which extends to the meninges of the brain and the upper region of the spinal cord. There are several distinct immunologic strains of the meningococcus, but groups A, B, and C are the most important.

Clinical Manifestations

Symptoms result first from infection and then from increased intracranial pressure.
1. High fever
2. Nausea and vomiting
3. Sudden severe headache, irritability, confusion, delirium, convulsions
4. Neck, shoulder, and back stiffness—from spasms of extensor muscles due to meningeal irritation
5. Appearance of petechiae (usually on trunk and legs); may progress to large ecchymotic or purpuric lesions
6. Resistance to neck flexion
   a. *Positive Kernig's sign*—when lying with the thigh flexed on the abdomen, patient cannot completely extend his leg (a sign of meningeal irritation).
   b. *Positive Brudzinski's sign*—when the patient's neck is flexed on the chest, flexion of the knees and hips is produced. When passive flexion of the lower extremity on one side is made, a similar movement will be seen on the contralateral (opposite) extremity.

Diagnostic Evaluation

Organism usually demonstrated by smear and culture of cerebrospinal fluid and blood.

Clinical Features

1. Human cases and carriers are sources of infection; transmission is by contact or droplet infection.

2. Meningococcus may localize in the brain, skin, or joint synovia.
3. Predisposing factors include otitis media, mastoiditis, sickle cell anemia (or other hemoglobinopathies), recent neurosurgical procedures, head trauma, respiratory infection, immunologic defects.
4. The disease occurs in winter and spring months; epidemics are most apt to occur when people live in crowded quarters.

Treatment and Nursing Management

OBJECTIVE: to observe and treat for vasomotor shock and collapse.
1. Support patient undergoing diagnostic lumbar puncture (p. 704)—cerebrospinal fluid will usually be cloudy with elevated pressure.
2. Give specific drug therapy, depending on culture and sensitivity tests; therapy continued for minimum of 10 days.
   a. Penicillin G (drug of choice); chloramphenicol or ampicillin given in high IV doses—to achieve high blood concentrations.
   b. Most antimicrobials enter cerebrospinal fluid and central nervous system inefficiently.
3. Maintain a clear airway—altered consciousness may lead to airway obstruction.
   a. Carry out arterial blood gas determinations.
   b. Provide oral airway or cuffed endotracheal tube or tracheostomy as patient's condition indicates.
   c. Administer oxygen to maintain arterial PO_2 at desired levels.
4. Provide monitoring procedures and care for patient with fulminating (coming on suddenly, with severity) disease. Death may occur within the first few hours after recognition of the disease.
   a. Assess patient for shock, widespread vasoconstriction, circumoral cyanosis, cold extremities—may lead to coma.
   b. Keep a flow sheet of vital signs, signs and symptoms, medications, number of petechial lesions, etc.
   c. Monitor blood pressure continuously (by Doppler method if available).
   d. Monitor the central venous pressure—to assess for incipient shock (which precedes cardiac or respiratory failure) and to estimate adequacy of fluid therapy.
   e. Monitor input and output.
5. Provide for rapid intravenous replacement of fluids, electrolytes, blood, and plasma.
6. Encourage a liberal fluid intake.
7. Give diazepam (Valium) or phenytoin (Dilantin) to control seizures. See page 715 for care of patient having seizures.
8. Employ measures to reduce temperature in patient with high fever (see p. 714)—to decrease the load on the heart and the oxygen demand of the brain.
9. Give adrenal corticosteroids as prescribed.
10. Be on constant alert for complications—disseminated intravascular coagulation, shock, heart failure, pericarditis, pneumonia.

Nursing Isolation Procedure

Use respiratory isolation precautions (p. 799) until 24 hours after initiation of effective therapy.

Health Education

1. Persons having close contact with patient with the

disease should be considered for antimicrobial prophylaxis—rifampin is given for 2 days.
2. Close contacts should be observed and immediately evaluated if fever or other signs and symptoms of meningococcal meningitis develop.
3. Prevent overcrowding of living quarters.
4. Improve practices of personal hygiene, particularly control of droplet infection.
5. Monovalent A, monovalent C, and bivalent A-C vaccine may be given as an adjunct to antimicrobial prophylaxis for close contacts of patients with meningococcal disease.

TETANUS (LOCKJAW)

Tetanus is an acute disease caused by the tetanus bacillus *Clostridium tetani*, whose spores are introduced into the body when an injury becomes contaminated with soil, street dust, or animal or human feces. The bacillus is an anaerobe (cannot live in presence of oxygen).

Clinical Manifestations

(Caused by potent neurotoxins elaborated by *C. tetani* which have a special affinity for nervous tissue.)
1. Hyperirritability; restlessness, headache, low-grade fever
2. Rigidity of muscles, muscle spasms of both flexor and extensor muscle groups
   a. *Trismus*—painful spasms of masticatory muscles; difficulty in opening the mouth (lockjaw); neck rigidity, stiffness, dysphagia
   b. *Risus sardonicus*—grinning expression produced by spasm of facial muscles
   c. Recurrent painful reflex spasms of almost every muscle group in body—involvement of respiratory muscles may lead to respiratory failure

Treatment of Tetanus

OBJECTIVE: to prevent respiratory and cardiovascular complications.
1. Maintain an adequate airway—tetanic spasm of larynx, pharynx, and respiratory muscles usually occurs during convulsions and may lead to hypoxia, asphyxia, and death.
   a. Place patient in an intensive care unit—requires expert respiratory management with early endotracheal intubation and mechanical ventilation.
   b. See page 193 for management of patient requiring respiratory intensive care.

> **NURSING ALERT:** The hearing of the patient with respiratory paralysis may be acute. Do not make unguarded comments in his presence.

2. Give tetanus immune globulin (human) (TIG) in an effort to neutralize the toxins and to ensure that appropriate circulating levels will be present when the wound is debrided.
3. Carry out effective wound care; debride all necrotic tissue—necrotic tissue favors growth of tetanus bacillus.
4. Give antimicrobials (penicillin)—to eradicate persisting *C. tetani* and other pathogens from the wound and stop the production of new toxin.

5. Support the patient during tetanic spasm and convulsions—caused by the action of toxins in the cells of central nervous system; mortality rate of patients with frequent and severe spasms is high. Give diazepam (Valium) and sedatives to treat muscle rigidity and reflex spasms.
   a. Give neuromuscular blocking agents (metocurine iodide [Metubine]) for reflex spasms and to prevent seizures.
   b. Provide cardiac monitoring—overactivity of sympathetic nervous system may lead to "sympathetic crisis" and death.
      (1) Watch for isolated unexplained tachycardia, temporary hypertension, premature ventricular contractions, sweating.
      (2) Requires aggressive physiologic monitoring and pharmacologic treatment (propranolol to control tachycardia; phentolamine to control hypertensive episodes).
6. Provide for continuing assessment and support of the patient.
   a. Plan nursing management for minimal patient disturbance—tactile stimulation may promote spasms.
      (1) Place patient in a quiet, semidark environment when sedation has maximum effect—to avoid stimulating reflex spasms.
      (2) Avoid sudden stimuli and light—slightest stimulation may trigger paroxysmal spasms.
      (3) Keep vein open—for infusions and in the event of cardiac/respiratory arrest.
      (4) Maintain fluid and electrolyte balance. Parenteral nutrition may be required—aspiration is a constant threat.
      (5) Avoid contractures and pressure sores—from prolonged immobility.
      (6) Watch for urinary retention—occurs when perineal muscles are affected.
      (7) Be alert for the development of fractures of the vertebral bodies which may occur with severe spasm.
   b. See page 715 for management of the patient with convulsive seizures and page 706 for management of the unconscious patient.
7. After recovery, the patient should receive the primary immunization series (for tetanus) plus booster dose every 10 years.

Prevention of Tetanus

1. Consider every break in the skin a potential portal of entry for *C. tetani*.
   a. Tetanus-prone wounds—compound fractures; gunshot injuries; burns; foreign bodies; wounds contaminated with soil or feces; wounds neglected for more than 24 hours; puncture wounds; wounds infected with other microorganisms; wounds from induced abortions; wounds made by dirty hypodermic needles (drug addicts).

> **NURSING ALERT:** Tetanus-prone wounds are those in which there has been an invasion of soil or feces or those involving a severe traumatic injury. Tetanus may develop from an insignificant wound contaminated by soil.

2. All individuals should receive active immunization against tetanus and a booster every 10 years in the absence of injury.
3. When an injury has occurred, treatment depends on the immunization status of the patient, the nature and age of the wound; and the conditions under which it has occurred.
   a. After injury, an additional dose of tetanus toxoid is given if a year has passed since last booster.
   b. For dirty wounds, give tetanus immune globulin (human); clean and debride wound, removing all foreign and devitalized material.
   c. In unimmunized patient with clean, minor wound, give initial immunizing dose of tetanus toxoid; administer again twice at 4-week intervals.
   d. For other wounds in unimmunized patient, give tetanus toxoid (as noted above) and tetanus immune globulin (human) at different sites with separate syringes, surgical debridement of wound, and antimicrobial therapy (tetanus organism is sensitive to penicillin, tetracycline).
   e. Equine or bovine antitoxin is usually *not* given because of high incidence of allergic and anaphylactic reactions. *If used, its administration must be preceded by careful screening for sensitivity according to manufacturer's directions.*

CLOSTRIDIAL MYONECROSIS (GAS GANGRENE)

Gas gangrene is a severe infection of skeletal muscle caused by gram-positive clostridia which may complicate compound fractures and contused or lacerated wounds by producing exotoxins that destroy tissue. Several species of clostridia (*C. welchii, C. perfringens, C. septicum, C. novyi, C. histolyticum, C. sporogenes* and others) may produce gas gangrene. These organisms are anaerobes and spore-formers; they are normally found in the intestinal tract of man and in soil.

Altered Physiology

Injury → bacteria (*Clostridia*) invade devitalized tissue, especially where blood supply is compromised → bacteria multiply and produce toxins → toxins cause hemolysis, vessel thrombosis, and damage to myocardium, liver, and kidneys.

Clinical Manifestations

1. Sudden and severe pain at site of injury—caused by gas and edema in the tissues.
2. Appearance of wound:
   a. Skin is white and tense initially; then progresses to bronze, brown, or black color.
   b. Soft tissue crepitus (crackling)—produced by gas in the tissue.
   c. Vesicles appear; are filled with red, watery fluid.
   d. Muscle is dark red or black and edematous; contains red, watery, foul-smelling fluid.
   e. Gas bubbles seen emanating from tissues—toxins ferment muscle sugar; produce acid and gas, which digest muscle protein. (Obvious gangrene is present.)
3. Rapid, feeble pulse progressing to circulatory collapse—death from toxemia is frequent.
4. Anemia (from hemolysis); prostration; apprehension.
5. Delirium and stupor.

Treatment and Nursing Management

1. Prepare patient for surgical removal and debridement of necrotic tissue—this is preventive as well as curative.
   a. Early excision of all devitalized and infected tissue with wide incisions will render wound unsuitable for growth of clostridium.
   b. Extensive incisions (once infection has developed) in affected part allows air to inhibit growth of anaerobic organisms.
2. Prepare patient for transfer to facility with a hyperbaric oxygen chamber—increases the dissolved oxygen in the arterial system by increasing the partial pressure of the oxygen breathed by the patient; may interrupt toxin formation and microbial replication (reproduction).
3. Give antimicrobial therapy (penicillin; clindamycin; chloramphenicol)—may prevent spread of infection.
4. Support the patient with toxemic manifestations—gas bacillus infection produces an intense toxemia.
   a. Monitor central venous pressure, pulmonary capillary wedge pressure; and urinary output (patient at risk for developing renal failure).
   b. Give IV fluids to support cardiovascular system; maintain fluid and electrolyte balance; give transfusions to maintain adequate hematocrit levels.

Isolation Nursing Procedure

Use wound and skin precautions (p. 800) until the wound stops draining.

BOTULISM*

Botulism is a type of poisoning that affects the central nervous system; it is caused by eating food in which *Clostridium botulinum* has grown and produced toxins. The organism is widely distributed in soil. Human intoxication usually follows ingestion of contaminated foods: home-canned, dried, or smoked foods; or poorly processed foods.

Clinical Manifestations

(Usually begin 12–36 hours after ingestion of contaminated food)

The toxins elaborated by *C. botulinum* are extremely potent and are rapidly absorbed by the G.I. tract; they become bound to neural tissues and produce a neuroparalytic syndrome.
1. Nausea and vomiting
2. Blurred vision; diplopia
3. Dizziness
4. Severe dryness of mouth and throat
5. Difficulty in speaking and swallowing
6. Symmetrical descending weakness and paralysis
7. Progressive respiratory weakness and paralysis with normal mental status

Course

1. Variable; illness may be prolonged with a high risk of superinfection and fatal outcome.
2. Recovery in survivors may be prolonged

* Botulism is an intoxication, not an infection. The Center for Disease Control, Atlanta, Georgia 30333, offers diagnostic consultation and laboratory testing services and support for epidemiological studies of botulism.

Clinical Evaluation

1. Electromyography (p. 703)—to document electro-physiologic abnormalities
2. Mouse-toxin neutralization test—for detection of botulinal toxin; patient's serum sent to laboratory that has capacity for performing this test
3. Examination of fecal samples, serum, gastric contents, incriminated food, for botulinal toxin

Treatment and Nursing Management

OBJECTIVES: to prevent respiratory failure.
to eliminate the toxin and *C. botulinum* from the gastrointestinal tract.

1. Give intensive respiratory support—death is frequently due to onset of respiratory failure.
   a. Prepare for endotracheal intubation; mechanical ventilation.
   b. Carry out blood gas determinations as necessary.
2. Administer trivalent ABE botulinal antitoxin as directed to neutralize any toxin that may be in the circulation.
   a. Determine if there is a history of allergy, asthma, hay fever—high rate of untoward reaction to antitoxin.
   b. Perform a skin test for sensitivity; read package insert.
   c. Have ventilatory equipment and emergency drugs ready in event of life-threatening reaction.
3. Give cathartics, enemas, and gastric lavage (when these can be safely administered)—to eliminate unabsorbed toxin and *C. botulinum* from the gastrointestinal tract.
4. Guanidine hydrochloride may be administered—enhances the release of acetylcholine from the nerve terminals; not as effective in overcoming respiratory paralysis as it is in combating paralysis of extremities and extraocular muscles.
5. Treat superimposed infections with antibiotics if necessary.
6. Provide ECG monitoring—to detect signs of cardiac arrest.

Prevention and Health Education

1. Home canners should be taught how to prevent botulism.
2. Home-canned foods should be inspected before being eaten—foods contaminated with *Clostridium botulinum* may look soft, contain gas bubbles, and give off an odor of decay. However, contaminated food items may have a normal appearance and taste.
3. Canned foods should be heated at temperatures over 80°C (176°F) for 30 minutes or boiled for 10 minutes—toxins are heat-labile and destroyed by proper cooking of foods.
4. Be careful in preparing food for canning at high altitudes since it is difficult to provide a temperature high enough to destroy the spores of *Clostridium botulinum*. Use pressure cooker method of canning at high altitudes.

Nursing Isolation Procedure

No precautions are necessary. Botulism is an intoxication, not an infection.

ACTINOMYCOSIS

Actinomycosis is a chronic, suppurating, granulomatous disease. The usual pathogen in man is an anaerobic gram-positive branching filamentous bacterium, *Actinomyces israelii*, a normal commensal that may be found in the tonsillar crypts, dental caries, and colon of apparently healthy people. Minor trauma, aspiration, or surgical manipulation may initiate the infectious process.

Pathology

1. The characteristic lesions are firmly indurated granulomas which spread slowly to adjacent tissues and break down focally to form multiple sinus tracts which penetrate to the surface.
2. The exudate from the sinus tracts contains the characteristic sulfur granules which are visible masses of the organisms.

Clinical Manifestations

Actinomycosis involves 3 major forms of infection:
1. *Cervicofacial type*—swelling about the teeth, submaxillary region, and neck producing a flat, hard, painless tumor mass which is fixed firmly to the jawbone. Granuloma ultimately breaks down and becomes riddled with abscesses which perforate externally.
2. *Abdominal type*—affects any visceral organ, especially the cecum and appendix, ovaries and tubes. Tumor mass, resembling carcinoma, develops. By extension it may involve the abdominal wall, discharging externally through open sinuses.
3. *Thoracic type*—acute and chronic inflammatory reaction may involve lungs, pleura, mediastinum, chest wall, and pericardium, producing chest pain, fever, cough, and hemoptysis.

Diagnostic Evaluation

Culture and histologic identification of affected tissue.

Treatment

1. Give penicillin (drug of choice)—therapy should be continued for weeks to months to prevent recurrence; alternative antimicrobials are given if patient is allergic to penicillin.
2. Surgical drainage, resection of damaged tissue, and excision of sinuses and fistulous tracts may be required.

Nursing Isolation Procedures

Secretion precautions until wounds or lesions stop draining.

Health Education

1. Encourage good dental hygiene to reduce infection around teeth.
2. There appears to be a relationship between intrauterine device use and colonization or infection of the genital tract with *Actinomyces,* especially when pelvic infection is present.

VIRAL INFECTIONS

INFLUENZA

Influenza is an acute infectious disease caused by an RNA-containing myxovirus. It is characterized by respiratory and constitutional symptoms. Epidemics of influenza develop rapidly; there is a fairly high mortality rate among the elderly and those debilitated by chronic disease.

Etiology

1. The primary factor in the etiology of influenza is a filtrable virus of which 3 major strains have been isolated; designated Types A, B, and C.
2. The numerous variants within a given type are called subtypes.
3. Group A appears to be the most virulent and is responsible for the most recent epidemics.
4. Influenza appears to become epidemic when antibody levels wane or when the antigens of prevalent influenza viruses have changed enough to render the population susceptible.
5. Transmission is by close contact or by droplets from the respiratory tract of an infected person.

Clinical Course

1. The virus is airborne and multiplies in the upper respiratory tract—selected invasion of nasal, tracheal, and bronchial mucosal cells.
2. Influenza virus damages the ciliated epithelium of the tracheobronchial tree, rendering the patient vulnerable to the development of secondary invaders such as pneumococci or staphylococci, *Hemophilus influenzae*, streptococci, and other organisms.

Clinical Manifestations

1. Sudden onset of fever (39–40° C. [102–104° F.]), malaise, sore throat, cough, rhinorrhea, headache, myalgia.
2. Gastrointestinal symptoms—nausea, vomiting, abdominal pain, diarrhea.

Treatment and Nursing Management

OBJECTIVES: to offer the patient supportive therapy. to prevent and treat complications (respiratory, cardiac, neurological).

1. Give aspirin or acetaminophen (Tylenol) every 4 hours for fever, headache, and myalgia—take regularly to avoid marked swings of temperature with sweating and chills.
2. Offer cough syrup for dry, hacking cough.
3. Use a vaporizer—to reduce irritation to respiratory mucosa.
4. Encourage liberal fluid intake.
5. Watch for complications; persons at risk include those over 65, those with chronic pulmonary or cardiac disease, diabetes or other metabolic disorders, chronic renal disease.
   a. Pneumonia—watch for dyspnea early in course of illness.
   b. Neurologic complications—meningoencephalitis, cranial nerve palsies.
   c. Myocarditis, heart block, peripheral vasoconstriction.
6. Antiviral therapy for high-risk persons. (See below.)

Prevention

1. *Vaccination*
   a. Active immunization consists of a single dose of vaccine (influenza virus vaccine, bivalent) for either primary or annual booster vaccination.
   b. Influenza vaccine should be given by mid-November.
2. Annual vaccination is recommended for persons over 65 with chronic conditions such as:
   a. Heart disease of any etiology, particularly with mitral stenosis or cardiac insufficiency
   b. Chronic bronchopulmonary diseases, such as asthma, chronic bronchitis, bronchiectasis, tuberculosis, and emphysema
   c. Chronic renal disease
   d. Diabetes mellitus and other chronic metabolic disorders
3. *Antiviral Therapy*
   a. Amantadine hyrochloride (Symmetrel)—used for *prevention and treatment* of respiratory tract infection caused by influenza A viruses.
      (1) Chemoprophylaxis for unvaccinated high-risk persons exposed to influenza—used immediately after exposure to influenza because virus replication occurs early in disease.
      (2) Treatment for high-risk persons who have influenza (those with chronic heart/lung, metabolic, neuromuscular, immunodeficiency disease; elderly in extended care facilities) may reduce severity and duration of symptoms.
   b. Side effects—dizziness, nervousness, insomnia.

Nursing Isolation Procedures

Usually none. There may be some instances when respiratory isolation of patients with influenza is indicated, especially if the diagnosis can be made on or soon after admission.

Health Education

1. The risk of developing influenza is related to crowding and close contacts of groups of individuals.
2. Restrict visiting privileges within health care facilities during epidemics—to minimize chance of introducing influenza.
3. It appears wise to humidify home and office air and to discourage cigarette smoking for high-risk persons.

INFECTIOUS MONONUCLEOSIS

Infectious mononucleosis ("mono") is an acute infectious disease of the lymphatic system caused by the Epstein-Barr virus (EBV), a member of the herpes group. Cytomegalovirus infection can produce a clinical picture closely resembling that of infectious mononucleosis. Infectious mononucleosis occurs in individuals without antibodies to EBV.

Incidence and Transmission

1. Occurs mainly between ages of 14 and 30; high frequency of occurrence in college students and military population.
2. The virus is excreted in saliva of patients with active disease or of those who are carriers, and is spread

by intimate personal contact. It can also be transmitted by blood transfusion.

Clinical Manifestations

(May be vague and masquerade as those of leukemia, streptococcal sore throat, hepatitis, drug rash)
1. Sore throat, fever, lymphadenopathy (particularly in anterior and posterior cervical lymph nodes, producing neck pain)
2. Periorbital edema, headache, malaise, muscle aches
3. Skin rash, petechiae on hard palate
4. Enlargement of spleen

Diagnostic Evaluation

1. Blood smears—show lymphocytosis and atypical lymphocytes
2. Heterophil antibody agglutination test—increase in titer
3. EBV specific antibody test (positive)
4. Abnormal liver function tests

Treatment and Nursing Management

1. The treatment is symptomatic and supportive.
   a. Encourage patient to obtain additional rest and to tailor activity to individual tolerance.
   b. Give aspirin for headache, muscle pains, and fever.
2. Steroids may be helpful in severe cases; EBV infection can be fatal.
3. Observe for complications—rupture of spleen, Guillain-Barré syndrome (p. 739) causing respiratory failure, glottic edema, hepatic failure, renal failure.

Health Education

1. Fatigue may remain for a period of time.
2. Patient must avoid heavy lifting, strenuous exercise, and competitive sports until recovery is complete—exertion or trauma may cause rupture of spleen.
3. Observe for upper quadrant pain radiating to shoulder with signs of peritoneal irritation—evidence of splenic rupture.

Nursing Isolation Procedures

Secretion precautions for duration of the illness.

RABIES (HYDROPHOBIA)

Rabies is a severe viral infection of the central nervous system that is communicated to humans in the saliva of infected animals, especially wildlife (skunks, raccoons, foxes, squirrels, bats) and cattle. The infection is transmitted by a bite or by contact of the animal's saliva with mucous membrane or an open cut or wound in the skin.

Incubation Period

1. Varies from 18–60 days (occasionally shorter or much longer)
2. Direct relationship between severity and location of bite and length of incubation; may appear in 10 days if head or face is severely bitten.

Clinical Manifestations

A. *Prodromal Stage*

1. Headache and nausea
2. Fever
3. Malaise; loss of appetite; mental depression

4. Sore throat
5. Pain and paresthesia of bitten areas
6. Unusual sensitivity to sound, light, and changes in temperature
7. Dilation of pupils; increased salivation

B. *Acute Neurologic Period*

1. Episodes of irrational excitement alternating with periods of alert calm
2. Convulsions
3. Severe and painful throat spasms when patient attempts to swallow (or even view) liquids (hydrophobia); violent spasms of inspiratory muscles
4. Death usually occurs in this stage from cardiac or respiratory failure

C. *Paralytic Stage*

Fatal progressive paralysis

Diagnostic Evaluation

1. History of exposure and development of characteristic symptoms
2. Demonstration of rabies antibodies in patient's blood
3. Demonstration of characteristic *Negri bodies* in samples of brain tissue of infected animal

Local Treatment of Wound

1. Immediately wash wound and surrounding skin area with soap and water—to remove saliva from area.
2. Provide tetanus prophylaxis and antibacterial therapy as required.

Management of Biting Animal

1. Capture dog or animal that inflicted the bite and keep under veterinary surveillance—this may enable bitten person to avoid undergoing rabies vaccination unnecessarily.
   a. If animal remains healthy for 10 days, it is assumed that it was not infective.
   b. If animal becomes ill or dies, notify local health department; animal is humanely killed and brain examined for characteristic Negri bodies.
2. Kill wild animal that bites a person and send head to health department—brain examined for rabies.
3. If the biting animal escapes or is unknown, determination of the degree of risk is judged by the following factors:
   a. Prevalence of rabies in the area
   b. Species of biting animal
   c. Severity of wound(s)
   d. Whether attack was provoked or unprovoked

Rabies Postexposure Prophylaxis

1. There are two types of immunizing products *which should be used concurrently for rabies postexposure prophylaxis:* vaccine (preferably HDCV) and passively administered antibody (preferably RIG).
   a. *Vaccines*
      (1) Human diploid cell rabies vaccine (HDCV)—preferred; administered in conjunction with RIG.
      (2) Or duck embryo vaccine (DEV).
   b. *Globulins*
      (1) Rabies immune globulin, human (RIG)—preferred.
      (2) Or Antirabies Serum (equine) (ARS).
2. See product information sheets for drug data and schedule.

SPIROCHETAL INFECTIONS

SYPHILIS (LUES)

Syphilis is a chronic infectious multisystem disease caused by *Treponema pallidum* (a spirochete). It is acquired by sexual contact or may be congenital in origin.

Epidemiology

Tracing the source and spread of infections by interviewing known patients for sex contacts.
1. Interviewing and re-interviewing every reported patient with syphilis for sex contacts.
2. Rapid investigation to identify contacts for examination within a minimal time period.
3. Identifying and conducting blood tests of other persons who by definition (suspect or associate) are possibly involved sexually in an infectious chain (cluster procedure).
4. Epidemiologic (preventive or prophylactic) treatment of sexual contacts and infectious syphilis cases.

Clinical Manifestations

Syphilis is capable of destroying tissue in almost any organ in the body; it thus produces a wide variety of clinical manifestations.

Stages of Untreated Syphilis

A. *Incubation period*
1. 10–90 days; average 21 days
2. No symptoms or lesions
3. Spirochetemia is present; patient's blood is infective

B. *Primary (early) Syphilis*
1. Most infectious stage; lasting 1–6 weeks.
2. Manifestations include:
   a. Chancre or primary sore, a painless ulcer with heaped-up firm edges, appears at the site where the treponema enters the body (genitalia, rectum, oral cavity, fingers); generally related to pattern of sexual behavior.
   b. Chancre becomes eroded and heals after 4–6 weeks, leaving a small scar; in some patients, no primary sore can be found.
   c. Enlargement of regional lymph nodes.

> **NURSING ALERT:** Syphilis should be suspected when an indolent, painless ulceration appears on the body.

C. *Secondary Syphilis*
1. Lesion appears 6–8 weeks after onset of primary lesion; may involve any cutaneous or mucosal surface of the body as well as any organ.
2. Skin lesions—generalized maculopapular rash; bilaterally symmetrical in distribution, polymorphous (macular, papular, follicular, pustular)
   a. Moist papules occur most frequently in anogenital region (condylomata) and in mouth.
   b. Lesions of mouth, throat, and cervix (mucous patches) frequently occur in secondary stage; lesions highly infectious.
   c. Generalized patchy hair loss on scalp.
3. Generalized lymphadenopathy

4. Arthritic and bone pain
5. Acute iritis
6. Hoarseness, chronic sore throat

D. *Late Syphilis* (clinically destructive stage after latent period)—manifestations may occur 10–30 years after exposure; recovery unpredictable.
1. Granulomatous lesions appear in skin, bones, liver, cardiovascular system, and central nervous system.
2. Syphilis will mainly affect cardiovascular system (aneurysm of ascending aorta, aortic insufficiency), central nervous system, and skeletal system.

Diagnostic Evaluation

There are 2 types of serologic tests:

A. *Nontreponemal or reagin tests*—screening tests to detect antibody-like substances, called reagin, found in serum of infected patient.
1. Venereal Disease Research Laboratory (VDRL) slide test.
2. Rapid plasma reagin (RPR) card tests.

B. *Treponemal tests*—measure specific antibodies to *Treponema pallidum;* recommended for patients who have reactive reagin tests and atypical signs of primary or secondary syphilis and for diagnosis of late syphilis.
1. Fluorescent treponemal antibody absorption test (FTA-ABS).
2. Microhemagglutination test (MHA-TP).

Treatment and Nursing Management (early syphilis)

1. Give benzathine penicillin G (IM)—drug of choice because it provides effective treatment in a single injection *OR* aqueous procaine penicillin G (IM) daily for 8 days.
   a. Screen for history of previous reaction to penicillin; reaction can occur in patient with negative history.
   b. Patient should be detained 30 minutes after administration of parenteral penicillin in case of development of anaphylactoid reaction.
2. Patients who are allergic to penicillin may be given tetracycline or erythromycin.
3. Post-treatment follow-up is essential—treatment failures do occur and retreatment is required, followed by quantitative VDRL at 1, 3, 6, and 12 months.
4. Jarisch-Herxheimer Reaction—a reaction appearing within hours after initiating treatment of syphilis (particularly in the secondary stage) and subsiding within 24 hours; consists of transient fever and flu-like symptoms of malaise, chills, headache, and myalgia. It may involve release of endotoxin-killed treponemes or from an allergic phenomenon.
   a. Managed by bed rest and aspirin.
   b. Warn patient that this reaction may be expected.

Nursing Isolation Procedures

Secretion precautions for mucocutaneous manifestations until 24 hours after initiation of effective therapy.

Prevention and Health Education

1. Patients who have been exposed to infectious syphilis within the preceding 3 months should be treated as for early syphilis.

2. All patients with early syphilis should return for repeat nontreponemal tests 3, 6, and 12 months after treatment. Patients with syphilis of more than one year's duration should, in addition, have a serologic test 24 months after treatment. (Spinal tap may be necessary.)
3. Instruct the patient to refrain from sexual contact with previous partners who are not under treatment.

4. A program of sex education and epidemiologic screening should be ongoing. Mass screening of special groups with a known high incidence of sexually transmitted disease should be conducted.
5. VD National Hotline: 800-227-8922 or 8923—toll-free telephone numbers; provides information and referral services about sexually transmitted diseases.

RICKETTSIAL INFECTIONS

ROCKY MOUNTAIN SPOTTED FEVER

Rocky Mountain spotted fever (tick-borne typhus fever) is characterized by continuous fever and headache. It is caused by the bite of an infected tick, by crushing an infected tick on the skin, or via conjunctival contamination with infected tick juice.

Etiology

1. The organism responsible for Rocky Mountain spotted fever is *Rickettsia rickettsii.*
2. The infection reservoir includes rabbits, small, wild rodents, and dogs. The wood tick and the American dog tick are the most important vectors of *R. rickettsii* in man.
3. Most prevalent in South Atlantic and South Central states.

Clinical Manifestations

During infection, *R. rickettsii* localize and proliferate in the vascular endothelium of small vessels, producing widespread swelling and degeneration. This generalized vasculitis accounts for the manifestations of the disease and may involve virtually every organ.
1. Severe headache, malaise, anorexia, photophobia, muscle and joint pain
2. High fever—up to 42°C. (107°F.) in severe cases—subsides by lysis
3. Rash—appears in 3–7 days (discrete maculopapular rose lesions appearing on distal parts of body (wrists, ankles, soles, and palms) and spreading to central parts of the body may progress to petechial or purpuric stages; large subcutaneous hemorrhages may appear.
   a. Areas of skin necrosis may appear as a result of endarteritis—necrosis may involve ear lobes, fingers, toes, and scrotum.
   b. Generalized edema—from generalized vascular involvement and resulting escape of serum.
4. Restlessness, insomnia, hyperesthesia, and delirium.
5. Thrombocytopenia.

Diagnostic Evaluation

1. History of exposure to ticks; typical clinical picture
2. Positive Weil-Felix agglutination test and specific complement fixation test

Nursing Management

1. Administer one of the tetracyclines or chloramphenicol as directed—effective if given in the *early* stages of the disease.
2. Give sedatives and analgesics as required for restlessness, insomnia, and pain.
3. Utilize supportive nursing measures for combating fever and promoting patient comfort.

a. Turn frequently and give skin care; position patient carefully—disease can cause vasculitis (inflammation of a vessel) with severe edema and necrosis.
   b. Measure circumference of abdomen, arms, and legs—to determine extent of edema.
   c. Keep input and output records for determination of oliguria—patient may develop renal failure due to poor tissue perfusion from vascular degeneration.
4. Watch for signs and symptoms of disseminated intravascular coagulation, circulatory collapse, hypotension, oliguria, azotemia, hypoproteinemia, myocarditis, and pulmonary complications—Rocky Mountain spotted fever is an infectious vasculitis and can produce marked physiologic disturbances.
   a. Central venous pressure measurements are used to guide fluid and electrolyte replacement because myocarditis is present in some patients and there is a risk of congestive heart failure.
   b. Packed red cells and platelets may be given.
   c. Monitor for thrombocytopenia—patients may succumb from hemorrhagic complications.

Nursing Isolation Procedure

No isolation precautions are required.

Prevention and Health Education

1. Advisory Committee on Immunization Practices recommends vaccine routinely for persons with laboratory exposure to *R. rickettsii* and for those with regular occupational exposure.
2. Clean weeds and cut brush and grass in recreational areas. Spray heavily infested areas (chemical control of recreation sites).
3. Exterminate rodents—serve as hosts for immature ticks.
4. Avoid sitting on grass/logs in infested areas.
5. In a tick-infested area:
   a. Tick repellent should be applied to exposed parts of body and clothing.
   b. Body and clothing should be examined for ticks 2–3 times daily. Ticks must be attached several hours for infection to occur.
   c. Tick should be removed with a pair of forceps; pull gently and firmly without crushing the tick. If forceps are not available, use a bent twig or fingers covered with paper.
   d. Do not crush the tick, thus avoiding contamination of the broken skin with infectious tick secretions.
   e. Hands should be protected with gloves or paper while tick is being removed.
   f. The bite should be disinfected immediately.
   g. Examine household pets for ticks on a regular basis.

PROTOZOAN INFECTIONS

MALARIA

Malaria is an acute infectious disease caused by protozoa that strongly resemble leukocytes. Transmission is by way of an intermediate host (the bite of an infective female *Anopheles* mosquito). Malaria has also been transmitted via blood transfusions and from the use of shared needles and syringes by narcotic addicts.

Etiology

1. Four species of malaria parasites—grouped under genus *Plasmodium,* each causing a different type of malaria: *P. falciparum; P. vivax; P. malariae; P. ovale.*
2. The parasite has a complicated life cycle. Not all patients demonstrate classical cycles of fever and chills.
3. *P. falciparum* is the most serious type of malaria because of the development of high parasitic densities in blood; infected red cells tend to agglutinate and form microemboli.

Clinical Manifestations

1. Paroxysms of shaking chills; rapidly rising fever followed by profuse sweating
2. Headache, muscle aches
3. Splenomegaly, hepatomegaly, orthostatic hypotension, anemia
4. Paroxysms may last about 12 hours, after which the cycle may be repeated daily, every other day, or every third day.

Diagnostic Evaluation

1. Demonstration of malaria parasites in blood films (taken every 6–12 hours throughout the cycle) by microscopic examination—microscopic examination confirms presence, species, and density of parasites
2. Residence in or travel in an endemic area is an important diagnostic clue

Clinical Problems

1. Malaria causes more disability and a heavier economic burden than any other parasitic disease.
2. In parts of Southeast Asia, Africa, South America, Panama, and Oceania, *P. falciparum* infections are increasingly drug-resistant.
3. Mosquitoes evolve resistance against insecticides.

Treatment and Nursing Management

OBJECTIVE: to destroy the blood trophozoites and schizonts of *Plasmodium* that cause the signs and symptoms and the pathologic effects that characterize the disease.

1. Determine the species of parasite infecting the patient (by blood smear). The most favorable time for discovery of the parasite is during and 12–18 hours after a chill.
2. Give specific therapy. The use of antimalarial drugs depends on the stage of the life cycle of the parasite that is involved; malarial parasites can evolve drug-resistant forms.
   a. Chloroquine is given for infections with *P. malariae* or sensitive *P. falciparum.*
   b. The above regimen is followed by primaquine phosphate (to eradicate secondary exoerythrocytic

forms) for *P. ovale* and *P. vivax* infections.
   c. Quinine is given with either pyrimethamine and sulfadiazine or tetracycline for chloroquine-resistant *P. falciparum* strains.
3. Give supportive nursing care.
   a. Have patient under close monitoring and nursing surveillance.
   b. Keep input and output records to prevent pulmonary edema and to evaluate for development of renal failure; dialysis may be lifesaving.
   c. Take a sample of venous blood daily for estimating serum quinine, bilirubin, blood urea nitrogen concentrations, parasite count, and packed red cells.
   d. Determine arterial blood gases and plasma electrolytes if respiratory or renal symptoms occur.
   e. Consider patient with severe falciparum malaria as a medical emergency.
      (1) Administer IV quinine as directed—given in intermittent IV infusions.
      (2) Watch for neurological toxicity (from quinine infusion)—twitching, delirium, confusion, convulsions, and coma.
      (3) Oxygen may be administered—tissue anoxia is thought to be common in this disease.
      (4) Watch for jaundice—related to density of the falciparum parasitemia (presence of malarial parasites in the blood); abnormalities of hepatic function are also common in falciparum malaria.
      (5) Evaluate degree of anemia—related to severity of infection.
      (6) Watch for abnormal bleeding (nose bleeds, oozing of blood from venipuncture sites, passage of blood in the stool)—may be due either to decreased production of clotting factors by a damaged liver or to disseminated intravascular coagulation (DIC).

Nursing Isolation Procedures

1. Blood precautions for duration of hospitalization.
2. Screened rooms in tropical climates.

Preventive Measures and Health Education

1. Control and destroy mosquitoes.
   a. Drain and fill breeding places (pools of stagnant water).
   b. Control mosquitoes in an epidemic area by aerial or ground ultra low-volume application of insecticides.
2. Advise travelers of risk in areas where malaria is endemic—Center for Disease Control (CDC) booklet *Health Information for International Travel* annually updates the current status of malaria in each country.
   a. Limit dusk-to-dawn outdoor exposure, wear protective clothing, live in screened quarters, sleep under mosquito netting, and use topical repellents.
   b. Advise malaria chemoprophylaxis when traveling to areas where malaria is endemic. Varying combinations of chloroquine, primaquine, Sulfadoxine, and pyrimethamine are prescribed.
   c. Advise traveler to seek prompt health care if he develops fever after stopping prophylaxis.
   d. Travelers to malarious areas should not donate blood for up to 3 years.

AMEBIASIS (AMEBIC DYSENTERY)

Amebiasis is a worldwide parasitic disease which is responsible for multiple medical-surgical problems. It is caused by the protozoa *Entamoeba histolytica* and is acquired by ingestion of the cyst stage of *E. histolytica* in food or water contaminated by infected human feces. It is also acquired by person-to-person transmission of enteric pathogens by orogenital, oroanal, or proctogenital sexual activity, particularly among homosexuals.

Incidence

1. Occurs as an endemic infection of man in most regions of the world.
2. In the U.S., found in rural areas or in patients who have lived or traveled in the tropics. Generally limited to warmer regions.

Pathological Insights

1. *E. histolytica* lives in the large intestine and feeds mainly on bacteria.
2. Amebas may be located in the bowel lumen and intestinal wall or outside the gastrointestinal tract.
   a. Trophozoites develop from viable cysts in small intestine.
   b. Trophozoites may erode intestinal mucosa, invade the bloodstream, and travel to the liver via the portal circulation.
   c. Amebas can produce abscesses and other serious complications.

Clinical Manifestations

1. Colicky abdominal pain
2. Diarrhea—watery, foul-smelling stools, often containing blood-streaked mucus

Diagnostic Evaluation

1. Stool specimen for *E. histolytica*. (Trophozoites or cysts may be found in the feces.)
   a. Several stool specimens should be collected daily.
   b. Stool specimen should be examined *immediately* for trophozoites.
2. Positive serological tests (indirect hemagglutination test and indirect fluorescent antibody test.

3. Examination of exudate from liver abscess for trophozoites.

Complications

1. Liver abscess
2. Thoracic complications—secondary to rupture of amebic liver abscess through diaphragm
3. Meningoencephalitis
4. Intestinal obstruction, rupture of colon; peritonitis
5. Ameboma (amebic granuloma found in cecum, rectum, transverse colon, sigmoid)

Treatment and Nursing Management

OBJECTIVES: to give specific therapy.
    to support the patient's general condition.
1. Metronidazole (Flagyl) followed by iodoquinol—produces cessation of diarrhea and eradicates encysted organisms in most patients.
   a. Caution patient not to drink alcohol when taking Flagyl; may cause severe reaction.
   b. Serial follow-up of stools is necessary—relapses are common.
2. Keep patient on bed rest if diarrhea is acute.
3. Give intravenous infusions as indicated to correct fluid and electrolyte imbalance resulting from severe diarrhea.
4. Prepare for aspiration of liver abscess; metronidazole plus chloroquine phosphate may be given for liver abscess.

Nursing Isolation Procedures

Excretion precautions (p. 801) for the duration of illness.

Prevention and Health Education

1. Prevent contamination of food and water with human feces.
2. Carry out health education in personal hygiene—hand washing after defecation, before food preparation and eating.
3. Avoid ground-grown vegetables (lettuce, etc.) and local water supply when traveling in areas where amebiasis is endemic.
4. Examine contacts of recently diagnosed patients.
5. Advise male homosexuals of person-to-person transmission of enteric pathogens by sexual activity.

SYSTEMIC MYCOTIC INFECTIONS (FUNGAL INFECTIONS)

MYCOSES AND HISTOPLASMOSIS

Fungi are primitive organisms that take their nourishment from living plants and animals and from decaying organic material. The 3 main types of mycoses (fungal infections), determined by the tissue level at which the fungus settles, are:
1. Systemic or deep mycoses—primarily involve the internal organs, usually centering in the lungs.
2. Subcutaneous mycoses—involve the skin, subcutaneous tissue, and sometimes the bone
3. Superficial or cutaneous mycoses—grow in outer layer of skin (epidermis), in hair, and in nails
Histoplasmosis is a chronic systemic fungus infection caused by a spore-bearing mold called *Histoplasma capsulatum*. This highly infectious mycosis is transmitted by airborne dust which contains *H. capsulatum spores*. (Partially decayed droppings of pigeons, chickens, birds offer an excellent medium for growth of this fungus.)

Clinical Manifestations

(Fungal infections mimic symptoms of other diseases.)
1. Closely resembles pulmonary tuberculosis, including symptoms of fever, cough, dyspnea, anorexia, and loss of weight and strength.
2. Patient may present findings of malignant lymphoma, including anemia, thrombocytopenia, splenomegaly, hepatomegaly.
3. Other patients may develop ulcerations at mucocutaneous junctions, e.g., lip margins and perianal area.
4. Histoplasmosis may produce bleeding gastrointestinal ulcers and the syndrome of Addison's disease.

Diagnostic Evaluation

1. X-ray—appearance of lesions scattered throughout the lung fields
2. Positive sputum culture of *H. capsulatum*
3. Skin test with histoplasmin—shows hypersensitive reaction; of limited value in endemic areas where most of population is already positive
4. Histoplasma latex agglutination test
5. Complement fixation titers for histoplasma yeast

Treatment

Most patients do not require treatment.
1. Amphotericin B is the mainstay of therapy for disseminated or acute pulmonary disease.
   a. Dosage is controlled by blood level studies. (Patient is assessed for renal toxicity, manifested by rising blood urea nitrogen, decreased creatinine clearance, and other laboratory tests.)
   b. Severe toxic reactions to amphotericin B include nausea and vomiting, chills, fever, diarrhea, hypokalemia, phlebitis; pretreatment with meperidine may control chills.
2. Surgery may be done for persistent lung cavitation.

Nursing Isolation Procedures

None required (no patient-to-patient spread of disease).

Health Education

Avoid stirring up dust around bird-roosting sites (raking and sweeping, etc.).

HELMINTHIC INFESTATIONS

TRICHINOSIS

Trichinosis is infestation by the parasite *Trichinella spiralis,* one of the roundworms. It is acquired by consuming infected meat, usually pork.

Clinical Course

1. Tiny embryos of the parasite *Trichinella spiralis* become encysted in the muscle fibers of an infected pig.
2. These calcified cysts appear in meat (chiefly pork); resemble tiny grains of sand.
3. If insufficiently cooked pork is eaten, the embryos are set free by the gastric juice and develop in the intestine during the following week, becoming adult worms 3–4 mm. long.
4. These worms make their way into the mucous membranes and there produce myriad embryos (larvae) (period of invasion).
5. The larvae, carried by the bloodstream and their own activity, migrate to all parts of the body (period of migration).
6. The larvae gradually become encysted in striated skeletal muscle.

Clinical Manifestations

Intestinal Stage
1. Malaise
2. Gastrointestinal complaints, diarrhea
3. Mild fever—progresses to high and spiking by 3rd week
4. Nausea and vomiting

Muscular Invasion (symptoms derive from inflammatory process developing in the muscles)
1. Edema of the eyelids; scleral hemorrhages; pain on eye motion
2. Generalized pain and soreness in the muscles (myalgia)
3. Cardiac irregularities (occasional)—from trichinae in the heart muscle; may be fatal
4. Difficulty in breathing, masticating, swallowing, speaking

Diagnostic Evaluation

1. Biopsy specimen of muscle—reveals larvae. (Deltoid, biceps, gastrocnemius muscles are sites of biopsy.)
2. Positive serologic tests (precipitin, complement-fixation, bentonite-flocculation, fluorescent-antibody)—demonstrable titers 3–4 weeks after infection.
3. Rising eosinophil count—appears in 2nd week.

Treatment and Nursing Management

The treatment is symptomatic; there is no satisfactory treatment.
1. Thiabendazole (Mintezol)—may produce clinical improvement and prevent or minimize effects of illness.
   Adverse effects—nausea, vertigo, vomiting, rash.
2. Corticosteroid agents may be given to relieve symptoms in the acute stage.
3. Keep the patient on bed rest until he experiences some relief of symptoms.
4. Give analgesics to relieve muscle pain.
5. Carry out ECG evaluations to determine evidence of myocarditis.

Nursing Isolation Procedures

None required.

Prevention and Health Education

1. The public should be educated about the importance of thoroughly cooking all pork and pork products, especially sausage. There should be no trace of pink in cooked pork.
2. Smoking, pickling, seasoning, and spicing do not make pork safe unless it is thoroughly cooked (especially homemade sausage).
3. Beef hamburger may be contaminated by a meat grinder that has been used for pork.
4. Garbage intended for feed for hogs should be cooked.
5. Pork should be inspected to determine if disease is present.

HOOKWORM DISEASE

Hookworm disease (ancylostomiasis; "ground itch") is the result of infestation of the small intestine by one of two quite similar roundworms about 1.2 cm. (½ inch) long. Two species are parasitic in the human intestinal tract:

Necator americanus (predominant species in U.S.)

Ancylostoma duodenale

The infection is usually contracted by penetration of the skin by infected larvae in the soil.

Incidence

1. Southeastern U.S.
2. Endemic in tropical and subtropical countries

Clinical Course

1. Hookworm eggs are passed in human feces onto the ground (indiscriminate defecation habits). Eggs develop into infective larvae.
2. The larvae *bore through the skin of bare feet* ("ground itch") or enter by mouth when food is eaten with dirty hands.
3. After gaining access to the blood or lymph vessels, they are carried via the blood to the lungs, migrate from the pulmonary capillaries into the alveoli, reach the pharynx, and are swallowed, maturing to adult forms in the bowel.

Clinical Manifestations

1. Dermatitis ("ground itch")—occurs at site where larvae penetrate skin
2. *Gastrointestinal symptoms*—maturation of worms in the intestine is usually marked by epigastric/abdominal pain, diarrhea, and other gastrointestinal symptoms.
3. Low-grade fever and malaise.
4. Coryza, pharyngitis, laryngitis, sensation of obstruction in throat, cough—from larval migration to upper respiratory tract.
5. *Severe anemia* and hypoproteinemia—the worms attach to intestinal mucosa and suck blood; a single adult worm can extract 0.05 ml. of blood daily. The patient's iron stores become depleted. A low serum protein often develops (protein malnutrition).

Diagnostic Evaluation

1. History of anemia and malnutrition
2. Recovery and identification of the eggs in feces

Treatment and Nursing Management

1. Mebendazole—specific therapy of choice.
2. Ensure that the patient is eating a nutritious diet—hookworm disease occurs in persons suffering from malnutrition.
   a. Correct anemia prior to therapy for worms in patients with severe anemia.
   b. Give protein and iron supplementation—to aid in correction of anemia.

Nursing Isolation Procedures

None required.

Prevention and Health Education

1. Dispose of excreta in a sanitary manner; this is an important facet of health education.
2. Instruct the patient to wear shoes at all times.
3. Night soil (human excrement used as fertilizer) and sewage affluents should not be used for fertilizer.

ASCARIASIS (ROUNDWORM INFESTATION)

Ascariasis is an infection caused by *Ascaris lumbricoides* (intestinal roundworm). It is characterized by an early pulmonary invasion from larval migration and a later more prolonged intestinal phase.

Incidence

Occurs throughout the world in both temperate and tropical areas, particularly in areas of poor sanitation.

Clinical Course

1. Indiscriminate defecation in streets, fields, and doorways provides a major source of infective eggs.
2. Infection may be contracted from eating raw vegetables when night soil is used for fertilizer; water pollution may cause water transmission.
3. Eggs are swallowed and pass into intestine where they hatch into larvae.
4. Larvae penetrate the intestinal mucosa and enter lymphatics and blood vessels.
5. After reaching the lungs, they pierce the capillary wall, crawl up the trachea, are swallowed, and are returned to the small intestine where they grow, mature, and mate.

Clinical Manifestations

1. *Pulmonary Phase*—cough, fever, and blood-tinged sputum
2. *Intestinal Phase*—masses of worms cause gastrointestinal discomfort, colicky and epigastric pain.

NURSING ALERT: Large masses of worms may migrate into various organs of the body and cause obstruction (to trachea, bronchi, bile duct, appendix, pancreatic duct).

Diagnostic Evaluation

1. Stool specimen—for detection of ova and worms in stool.
2. Patient occasionally vomits a worm.

Treatment

1. Mebendazole or piperazine citrate.
2. Follow-up stool examination should be done 1–2 weeks after treatment.

Nursing Isolation Procedures

None required.

Preventive Measures and Health Education

1. All patients with infestations should be treated.
2. Adequate toilet facilities should be provided.
3. The importance of personal hygiene should be explained.

ENTEROBIASIS (PINWORM DISEASE; OXYURIASIS)

The pinworm or seatworm (*Enterobius vermicularis*) causes the most common form of intestinal roundworm infestation in the U.S. and is most prevalent in children.

Clinical Problems

1. One pinworm may produce 5,000–15,000 eggs.
2. Ingested eggs hatch in the small intestine; embryos reach adulthood in the cecum.
3. The gravid female worm migrates down the large intestine and deposits eggs on the skin of the perianal area.
4. The eggs that survive are ingested and reach maturity in 2–6 weeks in the gastrointestinal tract.
5. Scratching leads to contamination of the hands and nails; hand to mouth contact results in reinfection.
6. Infective eggs may contaminate food and drink, bed linen, dust, etc.

Clinical Manifestations

(Pinworm-infected person may be asymptomatic.)
1. Intense itching (nocturnal) around the anus—from nocturnal migration of gravid females from anus and deposition of eggs in perianal folds of skin.
2. Restlessness; nervousness
3. Vaginitis—from pinworm migration into the vagina

Diagnostic Evaluation

1. Anal impressions on cellophane tape taken in morning before going to toilet or bathing, so that ova deposited during the night will not be removed (Fig. 19-2)
   a. A family member may be taught the method so that the test may be carried out first thing in the morning.
   b. Wash hands thoroughly.
2. Detection (inspection) of characteristic eggs about the anus

Treatment

Mebendazole in a single oral dose usually results in cure.

Prevention of Reinfection; Health Education

1. All members of the family should be treated, or reinfection is apt to occur. Treat on the same day to eliminate cross-infection.
2. To prevent reinfection:

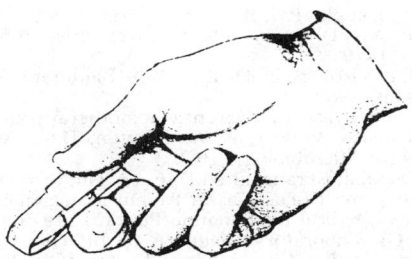

FIGURE 19-2. *Most suitable method of finding eggs in perianal area: Bend cellophane tape back over index finger with sticky part out. (Courtesy of "Forum on Infection")*

a. Cut fingernails short—eggs may be obtained from beneath the nails of infected person.
   (1) Avoid nail biting.
   (2) Wash hands frequently during treatment period.
   (3) Scrub nails with a brush, especially before going to bed.
b. Wash hands with soap and water after using toilet and before meals.
c. Wash around anal area upon arising (after diagnostic test).
d. Apply salve or ointment to anal area—to prevent dispersal of eggs.
e. Infected child should wear snug-fitting cotton pants—to discourage contact of hands with perianal region and contamination of bed linen.
f. See that infected person sleeps alone.
g. Handle bedding and nightwear carefully—there are large numbers of infective eggs in a contaminated house that cause reinfection.
h. Clean sleeping quarters frequently.
i. Reassure mother and family members that pinworms are not a sign of poor hygiene or housekeeping.

Nursing Isolation Procedures

Excretion precaution (p. 801) for duration of illness.

BIBLIOGRAPHY

Books

Barlow D. Sexually Transmitted Diseases. The Facts. New York, Oxford University Press, 1979

Benenson AS. Control of Communicable Diseases in Man. Washington, D.C., The American Public Health Association, 1981

Brooks SM et al. Handbook of Infectious Diseases. Boston, Little, Brown & Co, 1980

Buchanan RE and Gibbons NE. Bergey's Manual of Determinative Bacteriology. Baltimore, Williams & Wilkins, 1974

Caplin M. The Tuberculin Test in Clinical Practice. London, Bailliere Tindall, 1980

Castle M. Hospital Infection Control. New York, John Wiley & Sons, 1980

Chin J and Morrison FR (eds). Guidelines for Analysis of Communicable Disease Control Planning. U.S. Department of Health, Education and Welfare Pub. No. 79–50080, 1979

Dick G (ed). Immunological Aspects of Infectious Diseases. Baltimore, University Park Press, 1979

Eisenberg MD, Furukawa C, Ray CG. Manual of Antimicrobial Therapy and Infectious Diseases. Philadelphia, WB Saunders, 1980

Fuchs PC. Epidemiology of Hospital-Associated Infections. Chicago, Am Soc Clin Pathol, 1979

Galasso GJ, Merigan TC, Buchanan RA. Antiviral Agents and Viral Diseases of Man. New York, Raven Press, 1979

Gantz NM and Gleckman RA. Manual of Clinical Problems in Infectious Disease. Boston, Little, Brown & Co, 1979

Ginsberg M and Tager I. Practical Guide to Antimicrobial Agents. Baltimore, Williams & Wilkins, 1980

Gracey DR and Addington WW. Tuberculosis. Garden City, Medical Examination Pub. Co., 1979

Grieco MH (ed). Infections in the Abnormal Host. New York, Yorke Medical Books, 1980

Kolff CA and Sanchez R. Handbook for Infectious Disease Management. Menlo Park, Addison-Wesley Pub. Co., 1979

Maegraith B. Adams and Maegraith: Clinical Tropical Diseases, 7th ed. Oxford, Blackwell Scientific Publications, 1980

Mandell GL, Douglas RG, Bennett JE. Principles and Practice of Infectious Diseases, Vols. 1–2. New York, John Wiley & Sons, 1979

McLean DM. Virology in Health Care. Baltimore, Williams & Wilkins, 1980

Nelson JD and Grassi C. Current Chemotherapy and Infectious Disease, Vols. 1, 2. Washington, D.C., American Society for Microbiology, 1979

Noble RC. Sexually Transmitted Diseases: Guide to Diagnosis and Therapy: Discussions in Patient Management. Garden City, Medical Examination Pub. Co., 1979

O'Connell CJ. Laboratory Diagnosis of Infectious Disease, 2nd ed. Garden City, Medical Examination Pub. Co., 1980

Rosenthal SR. BCG Vaccine: Tuberculosis–Cancer. Littleton, PSG Pub. Co., 1980

Shulman JA and Schlossberg D. Handbook for Differential Diagnosis of Infectious Diseases. New York, Appleton-Century-Crofts, 1980

Thadepalli H. Infectious Diseases: Focus on Clinical Diagnosis. Garden City, Medical Examination Pub. Co., 1980

Warin JF. Lecture Notes on the Infectious Diseases. Boston, Blackwell Scientific Publications, 1980

Willcox RR. The Management of Sexually Transmitted Diseases. A Guide for the General Practitioner. Copenhagen, World Health Organization, 1979

Youmans GP, Paterson PY, Sommers HM. The Biologic and Clinical Basis of Infectious Diseases. Philadelphia, WB Saunders, 1980

Articles

Control of Infectious Diseases

Dunn JE Jr. The epidemiologic approach. JAMA 1980 Oct 12; 242(15):1658

Fedson DS. Recent developments in immunization. Primary Care 1979 March; 6(1):169–194

Nadolony MD. Infection control in hospitals. What does the infection control nurse do? Am J Nurs 1980 March; 80(3):430–431

Bacterial Infections

Abengowe CU. Comparative clinical trial of amoxycillin and chloramphenicol in the treatment of typhoid in adults. J Int Med Res 1979; 7(3):247–252

Adams B et al. Single or combination therapy of staphylococcal endocarditis in intravenous drug abusers. Ann Intern Med 1979 May; 90(5):789–791

Addington WW. The treatment of pulmonary tuberculosis. Current options. Arch Intern Med 1979 Dec; 139(12):1391–1395

Alfrey DD and Rauscher LA. Tetanus : A review. Crit Care Med 1979 April; 7(4):176–181

Andriole VT. Staphylococci and combination therapy. Arch Intern Med 1979 Oct; 139(10):1090–1091

Banner AS. Tuberculosis. Clinical aspects and diagnosis. Arch Intern Med 1979 Dec; 139(12):1387–1390

Bayer AS and Guze LB. Staphylococcus aureus bacteremic syndromes: Diagnostic and therapeutic update. DM 1979 June; 25(9):7–42

Bosworth DC. Reversible adrenocorticol insufficiency in fulminant meningococcemia. Arch Intern Med 1979 July; 139(7):823–824

Bubrick MP and Hitchcock CR. Necrotizing anorectal and perineal infections. Surgery 1979 Oct; 86(4):655–662

Buchanan JR and Gordon SL. Gas gangrene in a wound treated without skin closure: A case report. Clin Orthop 1980 May; 148:233–236

Cooke DB et al. Gonococcal endocarditis in the antibiotic era. Arch Intern Med 1979 Nov; 139(11):1247–1250

Denny AE et al. Serious staphylococcal infections with strains tolerant to bactericidal antibiotics. Arch Intern Med 1979 Sept; 139(9):1026–1031

Devereux PM and Goldstein EJC. Legionnaires' disease. Finding answers to the riddle. Am J Nurs 1980 Jan; 80(1):81–85

Dutt AK and Stead WW. Short-course treatment regimens for patients with tuberculosis. Arch Intern Med 1980 June; 140(6):827–829

Edmondson RS and Flowers MW. Intensive care in tetanus: Management, complications and mortality in 100 cases. Br Med J 1979 May 26; 1(6175):1401–1404

Felman YM and Nikitas JA. Diagnosis and treatment of sexually transmitted disease. NY State J Med 1980 April; 80(5):781–783

Fiumara NJ. Pharyngeal infection with Neisseria gonorrhoeae. Sex Transm Dis 1979 Oct–Dec; 6(4):264–266

Freeman PB. Gonorrhea. JEN 1980 May; 6(3):17–22

Glassroth J Robins AG, Snider DE Jr. Tuberculosis in the 1980s. N Engl J Med 1980 June 26; 302(26):1441–1450

Goodhart GL, Kramer M, Zaidi AA. Characteristics of defaulters in treatment for infection with Neisseria gonorrhoeae. J infect Dis 1979 Oct; 140(4):649–651

Hager WD et al. Pelvic colonization with Actinomyces in women using intrauterine contraceptive devices. Am J Obstet Gynecol 1979 Nov; 135(5):680–684

Harris AA and Karakusis P. Diagnosis and management of tuberculosis. Primary Care 1979 March; 6(1):43–62

Henderson DK et al. Infectious diseases emergencies: The clostridial syndromes. West J Med 1978 Aug; 129(2):101–120

Holst E and Lund P. Cervico-facial actinomycosis. A retrospective study. Int J Oral Surg 1979 June; 8(3):194–198

Jacobson, JA. Shigellosis in adults. West J Med 1979 Oct; 131(4):349–351

Jara FM, Toledo–Pereyra LH, Magilligan DJ. Surgical implications of pulmonary actinomycosis. J Thorac Cardiovasc Surg 1979 Oct; 78(4):600–604

Jones MC et al. The prevalence of Actinomycetes-like organisms found in cervicovaginal smears of 300 IUD wearers. Acta Cytol (Balt) 1979 July–Aug; 23(4):282–286

Jupa JE. Venereal diseases. Primary Care 1979 Mar; 6(1):113–126

Kaplan JE et al. Botulism, Type A, and treatment with guanidine. Ann Neurol 1979 July; 6(1):69–71

Korzeniowsi OM et al. Evaluation of cefamandole therapy of patients with bacterial meningitis. J Infect Dis (Suppl) 1978 May; 137:S169–S179

Leff A and Geppert EF. Public health and preventive aspects of pulmonary tuberculosis. Arch Intern Med 1979 Dec; 139(12):1405–1410

Licht JH. Penicillinase-resistant penicillin/gentamicin synergism. Effect in patients with Staphylococcus aureus bacteremia. Arch Intern Med 1979 Oct; 139(10):1094–1098

Majmudar B. Actinomycosis and the IUD: Infection under-diagnosed. South Med J 1980 July; 73(7):835–836

McCabe WR. Endotoxin, microbiological, chemical, pathophysiologic and clinical correlates. Semin Infect Dis 1980; 3:38–88

Musher DM, Fainstein V, Young EJ. Treatment of cellulitis with ceforanide. Antimicrob Agents Chemother 1980 Feb; 17(2):254–257

Nolan CM and White PC Jr. Treatment of typhoid carriers with amoxicillin. Correlates of successful therapy. JAMA 1978 June 2; 239(22):2352–2354

Owen WF. Sexually transmitted diseases and traumatic problems in homosexual men. Ann Intern Med 1980 June; 92(6):805–808

Pizzo PA, Ladisch S, Robichaud K. Treatment of gram-positive septicemia in cancer. Cancer 1980 Jan; 45(1):206–207

Portnoy D and Seah S. Typhoid fever: Treatment failure and multiple relapses with trimethoprim-sulfamethoxazole and chloramphenicol therapy. Can Med Assoc J 1979 May; 120(10):1264–1265

Promisloff RA and Johnson RF. Modern management of tuberculosis. Compr Ther 1979 Oct; 5(10):25–37

Puggiari M and Cherington M. Botulism and guanidine. Ten years later. JAMA 1978 Nov 17; 240(21):2276–2277

Recommendations of the Public Health Service Advisory Committee on Immunization Practices. BCG vaccines. MMWR 1979 June; 28(21):241–244

Reichman LB (ed). International Conference on Tuberculosis. Chest (6 Suppl) 1979 Dec; 76:737–817

Ryan JL et al. Enterococcal meningitis: Combined vancomycin

and rifampin therapy. Am J Med 1980 March; 68(3):449–451

Sands M. Treatment of anorectal gonorrhea infections in men. JAMA 1980 March 21; 243(11):1143–1144

Sbarbaro J. Tuberculosis. Med Clin North Am 1980 May; 64(3):417–431

Schumer W. Septic shock. JAMA 1979 Oct 26; 242(17): 1906–1907

Seminar on tuberculosis chemotherapy. Bull Pan Am Health Organ 1979; 13(2):197–200

Skiles MS, Covert GK, Fletcher HS. Gas-producing clostridial and nonclostridial infections. Surg Gynecol Obstet 1978 July; 147(1):65–67

Slack WK. Hyperbaric oxygen therapy in anaerobic infections. Med Times 1978 Oct; 106(10):15d–16d, 21d

Spires R. Tuberculosis today: The siege isn't over yet. RN 1980 Aug; 43(8):42–47

Stead WW and Dutt AK. Tuberculosis. Clin Chest Med 1980 May; 1(2):165–284

Treatment of gonorrhea. Med Lett Drugs Ther 1979 Aug 10; 21(16):66–68

Wajchenberg B et al. The adrenal response to exogenous adrenocorticotrophin in patients with infections due to *Neisseria meningitidis.* J Infect Dis 1978 Sept; 138(3): 387–391

Weissbluth M. Diagnosis and treatment of streptococcal infections. Compr Ther 1980 Jan; 6(1):47–52

Wiesner PJ and Thompson SE. Gonococcal diseases. DM 1980 Feb; 26(5):5–44

Wilson SZ et al. Quantitative nasal cultures from carriers of *Staphylococcus aureus:* Effects of oral therapy with erythromycin, rosamicin, and placebo. Antimicrob Agents Chemother 1979 Mar; 15(3):379–383

Fungal Diseases

Presant CA. Amphotericin B. Arch Intern Med 1980 April; 140(4):469–470

Shaffer PJ, Medoff G, Kobayashi GS. New directions in diagnosis and treatment of fungus infections. Semin Infect Dis 1979; 2:193–216

Yoshikawa TT. Drugs for fungal infections. Am Fam Physician 1980 Oct; 22(4):145–150

Helminthic and Parasitic Infections

Altus P, Blanco R, Chazal R. Trichinosis masquerading as a penicillin allergy. JAMA 1980 Feb 22–29; 243(8):767–768

Bender JL and Huh DC. Trichinosis. IMJ 1979 Dec; 156(6):466–467

Greydanus DE and McAnarney ER. Chlamydia trachomatis: An important sexually transmitted disease in adolescents and young adults. J Fam Pract 1980 April; 10(4):611–615

Miller TA. Hookworm infection in man. Adv Parasitol 1979; 17:315–384

Sitprija V et al. Renal involvement in human trichinosis. Arch Intern Med 1980 April; 140(4):544–546

Tan JS. Common and uncommon parasitic infections in the United States. Med Clin North Am 1978 Sept; 62(5):1059–1081

Wright KA. *Trichinella spiralis:* An intracellular parasite in the intestinal phase. J Parasitol 1979 June; 65(3):441–445

Yoshikawa TT. Antiparasitic drugs. Am Fam Physician 1980 March; 21(3):132–138

Protozoan Infections

Becker GL Jr et al. Amebic abscess of the brain. Neurosurgery 1980 Feb; 6(2):192–194

Bell D. Chemoprophylaxis in malaria. J Antimicrob Chemother 1980 Jan; 6(1):7–9

Committee on Public Health. The New York Academy of Medicine. Statement on amebiasis. Bull NY Acad Med 1980 April; 56(3):341–342

Dritz SK and Goldsmith RS. Sexually transmitted protozoal, bacterial and viral enteric infections. Compr Ther 1980 Jan; 6(1):34–40

Garcia LS and Turner JA. Malaria. Am J Med Technol 1980 Jan; 46(1):17–20

Kang JY, Stiel D, Doe WF. Proctocolitis caused by concurrent amoebiasis and gonococcal infection. The "gay bowel" syndrome. Med J Aust 1979 Nov; 2(9):496–497

Rothrock JF. Primary amebic meningoencephalitis. JAMA 1980 June 13; 243(22):2329–2330

Stek M. Malarial chemoprophylaxis. Postgrad Med 1980 Feb; 67(2):121–131

Teutsch SM. Malaria—An American problem. Int J Dermatol 1979 Sept; 18(7):575–577

Verghese M et al. Management of thoracic amebiasis. J Thorac Cardiovasc Surg 1979 Nov; 78(5):757–760

Rickettsial Infections

Bradford WD. Rocky Mountain spotted fever: A family affair. Clin Pediatr 1979 Oct; 18(10):634–635

Donohue JF. Lower respiratory tract involvement in Rocky Mountain spotted fever. Arch Intern Med 1980 Feb; 140(2):223–227

Raff MJ and Melo JC. A clinical approach to the choice of antimicrobial usage. Case number six: Fever and petechiae. J Ky Med Assoc 1979 June; 77(6):289–290

Walker DH, Paletta CE, Cain BG. Pathogenesis of myocarditis in Rocky Mountain spotted fever. Arch Pathol Lab Med 1980 Apr; 104(4):171–174

Spirochetal Infections

Fiumara NJ. Treatment of primary and secondary syphilis. Serological response. JAMA 1980 June 27; 243(24): 2500–2502

Horwitz CA. Laboratory investigation of syphilis. Postgrad Med 1980 Aug; 68(2):71–79

Syphilis therapy regimens. JAMA 1979 March 9; 241(10):982

Viral Infections

Alexander ER. Human diploid cell rabies vaccine: More protection for less risk. JAMA 1980 Aug 22–29; 244(8):816

Amantadine: Does it have a role in the prevention and treatment of influenza? A National Institute of Health consensus development conference. Ann Intern Med 1980 Feb; 92(2)(Part 1):256–258

Amantadine gains recognition in flu treatment. Am Pharm 1980 Jan; 20(1):46

Anderson LJ and Winkler WG. Aqueous quaternary ammonium compounds and rabies. J Infect Dis 1979 April; 139(4):494–495

Baer GM. Advances in post-exposure rabies vaccination. A review. Am J Clin Pathol (1 Suppl) 1978 July; 70:185–187

Blum A. Fatal mononucelosis? Don't rule it out. JAMA 1980 May 9; 243(18):1793, 1977

Bryson YJ et al. A prospective double-blind study of side effects associated with the administration of amantadine for influenza A virus. J Infect Dis 1980 May; 141(5):543–547

Fry J. Infectious mononucleosis: Some new observations from a 15-year study. J Fam Pract 1980 June; 10(6):1089–1090

Goodman RA et al. Influenza and influenza vaccination. Am Fam Physician 1980 Jan; 21(1):101–105

Recommendations of the Immunization Practice Advisory Committee (ACIP). Rabies prevention. MMWR 1980 June; 29(23):265–280

Seneca H. Influenza: Epidemiology, etiology, immunization and management. J Am Geriatr Soc 1980 June; 28(6):241–250

Sumaya CV, Marx J, Ullis K. Genital infections with herpes simplex virus in a university student population. Sex Trans Dis 1980 Jan–Mar; 7(1):16–20

Ullurich IH and Hoover D. Mononucleosis syndromes. W Va Med J 1980 March; 76(3):54–58

THE AGING PERSON

20

Definitions

Aging—a normal process of time-related changes that occur throughout life; old age is a normal part of human development and is the final phase of the life cycle.

Geriatrics—branch of medical science concerned with the study and treatment of problems and diseases associated with aging.

Gerontology—study of the aging process and its effects on older persons.

HEALTH MAINTENANCE AND PREVENTIVE CARE

OBJECTIVES: to maintain health and function.
to detect disease at an early stage.
to prevent deterioration of an existing condition.

A. *To maintain health and function.*

1. Promote positive feelings about the health of the aged.
2. Educate the older person on ways to conserve his health.
3. Encourage periodic health appraisal and counseling to give attention to health before illness develops and to prevent deterioration of an existing condition. Health assessment techniques utilize automated procedures, computer analysis, and read-out results to obtain baseline health information and determine state of wellness.
4. Promote accident prevention among the elderly and their families.
   a. High incidence of falls due to age, pathological conditions, locomotor disabilities, decline of postural control, environmental risks, and fear of falling.
   b. Maintain physical and mental activities—to improve confidence and mobility.
   c. Rise to an upright posture *slowly* from a supine position.
5. Protect patient against infectious diseases by immunization (especially against influenza).
6. Promote socialization to prevent mental deterioration and depression and to preserve a reason for living.
   a. Encourage the aged to continue to take on intellectual challenges.
   b. Encourage a variety of interests and activities.
   c. See that the patient has sensory input from the outside world.
7. Schedule and coordinate preventive, therapeutic, and restorative health services.

B. *To detect disease at an early stage.*

Explain diagnostic tests available for early detection of problems; provide support and encouragement.
1. Electrocardiogram—to show subtle heart abnormalities.
2. Chest x-ray—for tuberculosis, lung cancer, heart size, changes in large blood vessels and bony structure of the chest.
3. Pulmonary function tests—to rule out chronic bronchitis and emphysema.
4. Tonometer test—to measure intraocular pressure for glaucoma.
5. Blood glucose test—to detect diabetes mellitus.
6. Papanicolaou smear—to detect cancer of the cervix.
7. Blood and urine tests.
8. Hearing and vision tests—sensory deprivation can cause a downhill course.

C. *To prevent deterioration of an existing condition.*

Assess patient's health habits and knowledge of disease.
1. Advise patient to avoid temperature extremes.
2. Encourage him to stop smoking.
3. Educate about proper foot care.
4. Ensure proper nutrition and monitor weight.
5. Educate patient to avoid undesirable effects of drugs.
6. Provide education programs on specific health problems of the elderly.

D. *Community Resources*

1. Every person over 70 who is living alone should be visited regularly by a health visitor (nurse, social worker, volunteer health aid).
2. Use comprehensive services available for elderly: (diagnostic centers, extended care facilities, home care programs, homemaker services, friendly visitors, "Meals on Wheels," daily telephone calls ["buddy system"], day care centers, mental health services, vocational projects, continuing education, foster grandparents).

HEALTH PROBLEMS OF THE AGED

Underlying Considerations

1. Although aging is not synonymous with illness, the aged are vulnerable to disease because of decreased physiologic reserve, less flexible homeostatic processes, and less effective defense mechanisms of the body.
2. Disease in the aged does not always present classic signs and symptoms; the usual clinical manifestations may be absent, attenuated, or diguised; and atypical signs and symptoms may be present.
3. More than one disease may be present.
4. Resistance to stress is diminished—one major illness lowers resistance and allows other illnesses to appear.
5. Illnesses tend to cluster during closing years of the very old person's life—chain reaction of one degenerative process leading to another and finally to death.

DISEASE ASPECTS

Circulatory System Disorders

Diseases of the circulatory system are the most common in this age group.
1. Multiple small thromboses of arteries in the cerebral cortex are responsible for mental deterioration.
2. Arteriosclerosis may cause occlusive vascular disease of lower extremities (p. 347).
3. Atherosclerosis involving coronary arteries produces angina, acute coronary insufficiency, acute myocardial infarction, arrhythmias, and heart failure.
4. Impairment of kidney function may lead to chronic renal failure.

Gastrointestinal Disorders

Gastrointestinal disturbances commonly occur because of neoplastic disease, reduction of blood supply to the GI tract, neuromuscular degenerative changes, alterations of intestinal linings, and loss of secretions.

Respiratory Infections

Respiratory infection in the older person is an acute emergency and requires vigorous treatment; confusion may be the first sign of respiratory infection.

Other Disorders

Other frequently occurring disorders include atrophic and ulcerative lesions of the skin and mucous membranes, enlargement of the prostate with urethral obstruction, etc.

MENTAL HEALTH ASPECTS

Psychological Needs

1. Basic psychological needs of all people include respect, security, self-esteem, and the need to feel appreciated and valued by others.
2. The elderly person is vulnerable to emotional and mental stress from many losses.
   a. Losses through death of spouse, children, other "significant persons."
   b. Loss of social roles and resources—affects status and prestige; person may withdraw and disengage himself from the mainstream of life.

   c. Socioeconomic losses—decreased income; inflation.
      Affect quality of health care, self-esteem, and position in society.
   d. Loss of work role—produces sense of uselessness, feelings of nonparticipation.

Psychiatric and Cognitive Disorders

Incidence increases with age; disorders include depression, senile dementia, and persistent paranoid state.

A. *Depression*—most common emotional disorder of the aged; may result from accumulation of many losses or biochemical, metabolic, or endogenous factors.
1. Patient may complain of physical illness or behavior may mimic dementia.
2. See page 931 for management of depression.

B. *Senile dementia* (senile dementia of the Alzheimer's type)
1. *Dementia*—refers to signs and symptoms of intellectual dysfunction due to differing etiologies and varying pathophysiologic mechanisms. An estimated 5% of the population over 65 suffers from dementia.
2. Neuropathologic changes associated with changes in the patient's cognitive function (attention, learning, memory) may include loss of neurons, neurofibrillary tangles, granulovascular changes, and neuritic (senile) plaques in the brain leading to widespread breakdown of tissues and disintegration of neural pathways.
3. *Clinical Manifestations:* gradual deterioration of memory, gradual impairment of intellectual function and judgment, disorientation, shallow/labile affect, behavioral changes; the individual's ability to carry out self-care activities, relate to others, and cope with environmental situations is affected.
4. *Management of Dementias:*
   a. Keep the patient functioning as long as possible; continue social contacts.
   b. Maintain orderly and rather ritualistic schedule—to promote sense of security.
   c. Use orientation aids (lists of daily activities, labeled items, color-coded bathroom door) to help in day-to-day living.
   d. Give prescribed drug to reduce emotional lability, agitation, and irritability or an antidepressant if depression accompanies the problem.
   e. See Nursing Approach to the "Confused" Older Person.

NURSING APPROACH TO THE "CONFUSED" OLDER PERSON

A. *Confusion may be the first sign of illness in the elderly.*
1. Expect an underlying physical cause in any patient who has *sudden* changes in intellectual functioning.
2. Confusion and disorientation may be the first sign of infection, cardiac failure, coronary occlusion, electrolyte imbalance, stroke, dehydration, anemia, malignancy, or adverse effect of medication.

B. *Aging is not synonymous with senility*—senile dementia is a degenerative disease of the elderly.

C. *Consider when and how the confusion developed.*
1. When was the patient last clear mentally?
   a. Are there any other symptoms? urinary frequency? cough? pain?
   b. What medications are being taken? Ask to see them—drug-induced mental disorders may clear in several days.

D. *Assess the patient.*

Physical Status
1. Observe respiration and pulse; take temperature.
2. Check the state of hydration—tongue, tissue turgor.
3. Examine for peripheral edema.
4. Look for alterations in color.
5. Check for evidence of injury.

Mental Status
1. Where are you now?
2. What is today's date? day of the week? year?
3. How old are you?
4. When is your birthday?
5. Where do you live?

E. *Consider the effect of a new environment*—may bring on confused or "senile" behavior without physiological causes.
1. Be optimistic about this turn of events; act on the assumption that this behavior is temporary.
2. Accept the person as he is, without judgment or criticism.
3. Maintain eye contact.
4. Pay attention to what the patient is saying—often a person who is considered confused is only transiently so and much of what he is saying makes sense.
5. Pick out "meaningful" comments and continue talking with him.
6. Explain the patient's situation to him repeatedly.
7. Make short, frequent contacts.
8. Call the person by name each time a contact is made; touch the patient when you speak to him.
   a. Talk directly to him.
   b. Answer questions in simple, short sentences.
9. Show the person your name tag.
10. Convey a therapeutic attitude—listening, smiling, talking, and touching.

F. *Provide sufficient sensory input that is recognized as friendly.*
1. Keep the patient oriented with respect to time, place, and person (repeatedly).
   a. Remind him of time, date, and place each morning and whenever necessary.
   b. Keep a calendar and clock, both with easily readable numbers, within his range of vision.
   c. Color-code the bathroom door.
2. Encourage family to bring in pictures, family album, etc., since familiar objects promote a sense of continuity, aid memory, and provide security and comfort.
3. Use pictures, music, color, indoor gardens, etc. to enhance the environment.
4. Read newspaper headlines. Discuss current events.
5. Take the patient outdoors.
6. Give the patient something to occupy his hands and mind.
7. Keep the room well-lighted to reduce confusion and fear; use nightlights to reduce risk of "sundowning" (worsening of a condition at night).

8. Maintain a calm environment. Remove unduly stressful stimuli.
9. Arrange for visits from others to counteract isolation.
   a. Have family members sit by bed so that patient can see and touch them.
   b. Utilize services of a volunteer if no family is available.
   c. Work with family toward specific goals.
10. Encourage patient to reminisce; use volunteers when necessary to listen.
11. Treat the person as though he is aware of everything happening around him.

G. *Respect the patient's territorial rights.*
1. Do not move his personal belongings.
2. Avoid changing rooms—difficult for marginally oriented person to cope with change.
3. Have the patient's personal belongings where he can see and use them.

H. *Attempt to deal positively with wandering behavior.*
1. Evaluate for underlying pathology (cardiac decompensation).
2. Ascertain if patient is trying to satisfy a need (hunger, warmth, etc.).
3. Allow the patient mobility without jeopardizing safety.
4. Plan nighttime activities for the nocturnal wanderer; nocturnal agitation is frequently seen in deteriorative diseases of the central nervous system.
5. Allow the nocturnal wanderer to "rest" in an arm chair near the nurse's station.
6. Be aware that boredom and tension may be the basis of wandering.
7. Try restorative and reality orientation programs—may promote well-being and improve sleep patterns.

I. *Encourage the patient to assume a* well *and* active *role.*
1. Encourage him to dress in clean, attractive clothing *daily*—the wearing of nightwear confuses the concept of day and night (suggest up-to-date clothing as gifts).
2. See that he wears shoes—not slippers.
3. Encourage the patient to *walk* and not use the wheelchair, which limits his environment.
4. Encourage the patient to eat at a table and not at the bedside.
5. See that he wears his glasses, hearing aid, dentures, or other prostheses.
6. Be sure that he is drinking adequate fluids.

J. *Attempt to alleviate the patient's anxiety and restlessness.*
1. Try "laying on of hands"—touching, stroking, hugging; many aged persons have no one to touch them.
2. Use warm baths, warm milk, back massage, and also understanding and compassion as therapeutic modalities.
3. Give the patient gentle and constant reassurance.
4. Schedule the patient's daily activities and adhere to the schedule—order and predictability reduce anxiety and promote security.

K. *Avoid endorsing senile behavior.*
1. Do not agree with confused statements.
2. Direct patient back to reality. Avoid letting the patient "ramble."
3. Be consistent. Each member of the health care team should know the nursing objectives and use the same approach.
4. Give "permission" to express grief, anger, and hostility.

APPROACH TO THE AGED PATIENT

ASSESSMENT OF THE ELDERLY PATIENT

In addition to the health history and physical examination, the nursing assessment involves an attempt to determine the functioning ability, assets, and limitations of the patient.

Physiologic Assessment

1. How does the patient describe the activities of a "typical" day?
2. How does he view his health?
3. How effective is the patient at self-care?
4. How much physical capacity does the patient have?
5. How much muscle strength and coordination does he/she have?
6. How well does the patient see and hear?
7. What are the patient's usual eating, sleeping, elimination, and activity patterns? What constitutes a "normal" bowel movement?
8. How does he/she handle his/her sexual feelings?
9. Does he/she have any sexual concerns or problems?
10. Are there any changes in bodily functions?
11. What will the patient have to do to regain or maintain functioning ability?

Socioeconomic Assessment

1. What is the patient's background? early history?
2. How many person-to-person contacts does the patient have in a day?
3. Who is his "significant other"? (Include pet.)
4. Who visits the patient?
5. What is the patient's religion?
6. What are the patient's living arrangements?
7. Is he in proximity to relatives or helping neighbors?
8. Are the patient's activities limited because of transportation problems? high-crime environment?
9. How much independence does the patient possess?
10. What are his feelings about living at home?
11. Does the patient participate in any phase of community life?
12. How can the environment be adjusted to maintain independence?

Psychological Assessment

1. Is the patient alert and optimistic in outlook?
2. What does the patient identify as his major concerns and problems?
3. What are the patient's attitudes toward aging?
4. What are the patient's attitudes toward himself/herself? Is there a feeling of being needed? useful?
5. What psychological defenses does the patient use?
6. What are the patient's activities, interests, and hobbies?
7. What ego strengths and coping skills did the patient use in the past?
8. Are there any disturbances in experiencing pleasure?
9. What are the patient's plans and hopes?

MANAGEMENT OF SPECIAL NEEDS AND PROBLEMS

Nutritional Considerations for the Aged

1. Nutritional requirements of the elderly are similar to those of adults except that calorie intake should be reduced. Older persons need a *variety* of foods.
   a. Energy needs diminish with age—both metabolic rate and activity decrease, so that calorie requirements of the aged are reduced.
   b. The calorie intake is adjusted on an individual basis to maintain normal weight.
   c. Protein requirements are not reduced but protein utilization may be less efficient in old age.
2. Nutritional deficiencies are frequently seen in dietary iron, vitamins A and C, and calcium.
   a. Vitamin C and vitamin K deficiency—ecchymoses due to capillary fragility.
   b. Vitamin A deficiency—fissuring of skin around mouth; reduced visual sensitivity.
   c. Vitamin B deficiency—glossitis, angular stomatitis.
   d. Mineral deficiencies—demineralization of bone.
3. Factors affecting nutritional habits of the elderly.
   a. Food habits of a lifetime.
   b. Social factors (eating alone).
   c. Susceptibilty to food fads.
   d. Dental problems.
   e. Shopping problems.
   f. Reduced income.
   g. Lack of motivation for meal planning and food preparation.
   h. Decreased appeal of food—loss of taste buds; less acute sense of smell.
   i. Drug interference.
4. Assistance programs.
   a. Multipurpose senior centers.
   b. Home-delivered meals; "Meals on Wheels."
   c. Friendly visitor program.
   d. Nutritional counseling.
   e. Food stamps.
   f. Day care for the elderly.
   g. Self-help eating devices.

Drug Therapy and the Aged

A. *Factors Altering Drug Response in Elderly*

1. Absorption, distribution, metabolism, and excretion of many drugs are affected by aging.
   a. *Absorption*—affected by gastric pH, rate of gastric emptying, reduction in intestinal blood flow.
   b. *Distribution*—affected by alterations in body composition, protein binding, tissue permeability.
   c. *Metabolism*—decreased metabolic capacity for detoxifying drugs and decreased number of receptors at which drug may act; diminished cardiac output.
   d. *Excretion*—decreased filtration rate and tubular function.

B. *Nursing Implications*

1. Be aware that drug effect is more pronounced in old persons. The potential for adverse reactions and interactions is greater.
   a. Older persons may not be able to handle multiple medications.
   b. They appear to be more sensitive to digoxin, diuretics, aspirin, oral antidiabetic drugs, sedatives, analgesics, psychotropic agents, etc.
2. Obtain a medical history and drug history.
   a. Check nutritional status.
   b. Find out if patient is taking drugs not currently prescribed.

c. Ask what over-the-counter medications patient is taking (laxatives, antacids, aspirin)—may affect interaction of prescription drugs.
3. Usually the physician will hold the dosage to lowest effective amount; doses may be given further apart.
   a. Reinforce verbal instructions with *written* instructions.
   b. Give instructions also to relative/friend to reinforce patient education.
   c. Write what the drug is used for—e.g., "to thin the blood."
   d. Explain possible side effects.
   e. Be sure that the drug name and instructions for taking it are typed in large letters on the label. Bottles may have color-coded strips.
   f. Arrange drug schedule to coincide with a regular activity (arising, eating, retiring)—helps patient to remember to take drug.
   g. Arrange some sort of check-off system.
4. Carry out periodic drug review.
   a. Ask patient to bring all medication on next visit to physician or clinic.
   b. Assess for patient compliance, response to therapy, possible side effects, drug interactions—rate of noncompliance is high in elderly.
   c. Give patient friendly support.

Hygienic Care

A. *Skin Care*

1. Aging skin is dry, thin, and inelastic; sweat gland and sebaceous gland activity and water binding capacity of skin are decreased.
   a. Avoid bathing in hot water and using detergent soaps—aggravate dryness.
   b. Be sure that soapy water is removed from skin, especially between fingers and toes.
   c. Lubricate skin with ointment that traps moisture.
   d. See page 64 for prevention of pressure sores.

B. *Oral Care*

1. Common oral complaints include loss of teeth, dry mouth, abnormal taste, and burning sensations in mouth.
2. Components of dental/oral care include proper diet, maintaining health of oral and denture-bearing structures, and using available dental services.
   a. Use electric toothbrush and WaterPic® to remove retained food particles between teeth.
   b. Encourage increased fluid intake in persons with decreased salivary flow.

C. *Elimination Problems* (See p. 76.)

D. *Foot Care*

1. Degenerative and systemic diseases, trauma, neglect, and misuse cause foot problems in elderly.
2. Systemic diseases such as diabetes mellitus, arterial insufficiency, and the arthritides often are compounded by loss of sensation, abnormal gait patterns, and impaired vision; thus the assessment made by the nurse is of prime importance.
3. See pages 330, 645 for assessment of feet.

GUIDELINES: Trimming the Toenails (Fig. 20-1)

The nails of elderly persons usually grow very slowly, but they have a tendency to become thickened and deformed from trauma to the nail matrix, vascular insufficiency, and nutritional changes.

Equipment

Foot Care Tray containing
1 sterile nail nippers: 11 cm (4½ inch)
1 sterile tissue nippers: 7.5–10 cm (3–4 inch)
1 sterile curette: 1.5–2 mm.
Suture scissors
Antiseptic
Sterile Kling or adherent gauze

Band-Aids
Towel
Sterile 2 x 2's
Sterile 4 x 4's
Sterile Telfa or nonadherent dressing
Sterile cotton-tipped applicators
Emery boards

Procedure

NURSING ACTION	RATIONALE/AMPLIFICATION
Preparatory Phase	
1. Explain the procedure to the patient.	1. Proper explanation of any procedure reduces apprehension and ensures patient cooperation.
2. Soak the feet in tepid water for 10–15 minutes. An antibacterial skin cleanser may be added to the soak.	2. Soaking softens the nail plate, loosens subungual debris, decreases the possibility of bacterial infection, and relaxes the patient.
3. Dry the feet by blotting instead of wiping.	3. The use of friction may injure delicate, atrophic, and ischemic skin.
Performance Phase	
1. Sit facing the patient. Place his feet on a foot rest or improvised foot rest (hassock).	
2. Observe the nails, skin temperature, texture, and color. Look for breaks in the skin, infection, redness, and edema.	
3. Locate the nail and differentiate the nail from the nail bed. A curette can be used for this.	3. The growth pattern of some nail plates is altered so that it is frequently difficult to differentiate nail plate from nail bed.
4. Apply antiseptic to areas around toenails before debriding or cutting nail plates.	4. This is a precaution which reduces the chance of secondary bacterial infection.

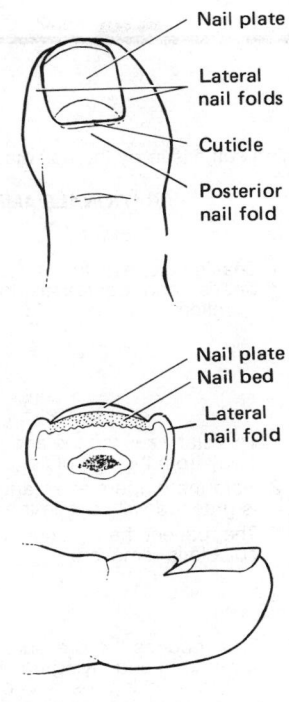

Nail after cutting

FIGURE 20-1. *(Top)* Anterior view. *(Center)* Cross section of toenail. *(Bottom)* After the nail is cut, the nail plate should be long enough so that it rests freely and without pressure on the nail bed.

	NURSING ACTION	RATIONALE/AMPLIFICATION
Procedure (cont.)	5. Thin the nail plate by rubbing the emery board across the nail surface if necessary.	5. The nails may be so thick that thinning is required before cutting is possible.
	6. Using only the tip of the sterile nail nippers, start at one corner and take small bites across the entire nail plate, following the contour of the nail plate. Little or no force should be necessary.	6. The nail should be cut so that it rests freely and without pressure on the nail bed (see Fig. 20-1). It should be cut even with the end of the toe.
	7. Smooth the nail edges with an emery board.	7. This prevents irregular nail edges from irritating adjacent toes and from tearing hose.
	8. Use a curette to carefully debride around and under the nail plate.	8. Debriding removes subungual debris which may be causing discomfort.
	9. Apply antiseptic to nail plates and toes that have been treated.	9. This action helps prevent infection.

NURSING ALERT: Avoid cutting nails if force is required, if a toe is exuding purulent material or is gangrenous, or if a subungual neoplasm is suspected.

GUIDELINES: Ingrown Toenail (Onychocryptosis)

Ingrown toe nail (onychocryptosis) is a condition in which the free edge of a nail plate has penetrated the surrounding skin (ungualabia, or nail lip), either laterally or anteriorly. It may be accompanied by secondary infection and/or granulation tissue.

Causes
1. Improper self-treatment.
2. External pressure—tight shoes or hose.
3. Internal pressure—deformed toes secondary to trauma, growth under nail (melanoma; exostosis).
4. Trauma.
5. Infection (bacterial; mycotic).

GUIDELINES: Ingrown Toenail (Onychocryptosis) (cont.)

Equipment Foot Care Tray (see p. 836).

Objective of Treatment

To relieve pain by decreasing the pressure on the surrounding soft tissue by the nail plate.

Procedure

NURSING ACTION	RATIONALE/AMPLIFICATION

Preparatory Phase

1. Soak the patient's feet in a basin of tepid water containing an antibacterial skin cleanser for 10–15 minutes.
2. Apply an antiseptic to the affected toes.

1. Soaking softens the nail plate, loosens subungual debris, and decreases the possibility of bacterial infection.

Performance Phase

To remove the offending spicule (needle-like piece of nail):
1. Grasp the toe firmly on each side.

2. Insert the tip of the small, sterile nail nippers and split the free edge of the nail on the affected side.
3. Grasp the spicule with the tip of the sterile mosquito forceps and extract it by rotating the forceps away from the nail bed.
4. Carefully check the nail groove and clean with sterile applicator and/or curette.
5. Place a small amount of sterile cotton in the nail groove and under the nail plate on the affected side. Packing can be inserted with a sterile cotton applicator.
6. Apply an antiseptic to affected toe. Apply sterile dry dressing (Band-Aid, Telfa, Kling, etc.).

1. This stabilizes the toe and draws the lateral nail folds away from the nail plate.
2. Hold the nippers at an angle so that the portion that is grasped will contain the offending spicule.
3. The patient has immediate relief as soon as the spicule is removed.

5. This reduces the pressure by keeping the nail plate away from underlying nail bed and nail groove. The packing usually comes out by itself after repeated bathing by the patient.

NURSING ALERT:
1. If the toe is infected or if there is a question about serious pathology, the podiatrist should be notified so that appropriate measures can be taken.
2. When secondary infection is present, appropriate cultures, drainage, soaks, and specific antibiotic therapy may be indicated.
3. A toenail may have to be excised if there is severe infection due to superficial mycosis. Oral antifungal medication may be prescribed.
4. If a neoplasm or gangrene is associated with an ingrown toenail, the patient is immediately hospitalized for appropriate care.

GUIDELINES: Onychogryphosis (Ram's Horn Nail)

Onychogryphosis (Ram's horn nail) is hypertrophy of the nail causing an unusually large and curved nail plate. The nail plate becomes discolored, thick and claw-like (Fig. 20-2, *Left*)

Causes
1. Trauma (most common etiology).
2. Recurrent infection.
3. Fungus infection.
4. Systemic condition (e.g., psoriasis).

Equipment Foot Care Tray (see page 836).

Objective of Treatment

To control the thickness of the nail plate.

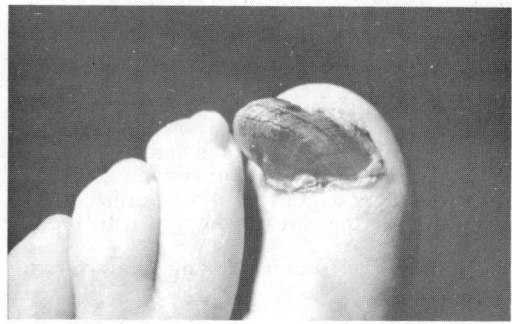 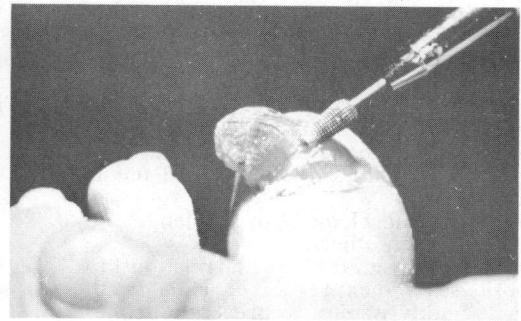

FIGURE 20-2. *(Left)* Ram's horn nail. *(Right)* Treatment of Ram's horn nail by podiatrist.

Procedure	RATIONALE/AMPLIFICATION
NURSING ACTION	

By the Nurse

1. Soak the patient's feet in a basin of tepid water containing an antibacterial skin cleanser.
2. Apply antiseptic to toe.
3. Use straight nail nippers and carefully cut the nail plate from one side to the other, using small bites.
4. When approaching the center of the nail, clip it off carefully.
5. Thin the nail plate by rubbing an emery board crosswise over the nail surface.
6. Remove the subungual debris with a brush or sterile curette.
7. Apply antiseptic and sterile dressing. Apply emollient to the feet.

By the Podiatrist

1. The nail plate may be reduced to normal thickness by the use of a burr attached to a drill (Fig. 20-2, *Right*).
2. The entire nail plate can be removed surgically. Surgical removal is carried out if the nail cannot be salvaged.

RATIONALE/AMPLIFICATION

1. This softens the nail plate. Hypertrophy of nail plate causes pain due to pressure from footgear.

7. This lubricates periungual structures.

SUMMARY OF PRINCIPLES UNDERLYING THE NURSING MANAGEMENT OF THE ELDERLY PATIENT

1. Growth and adaptation continue to occur when the individual's strengths and potential are recognized and reinforced.
2. Nursing care must be individualized, taking into consideration the patient's past experiences, needs, and individual goals.
3. Realistic and attainable goals, which are understood by the patient, are set to help him gain a sense of accomplishment and purpose.
   a. Have an optimistic view of aging and the older person.
   b. Engage in mutual goal-setting when possible.
   c. Keep communicating to the patient and family the planned goals of his care.
   d. Support his belief in his own inner resources.
4. The patient should be an active participant in his own plan of care.
   a. Learn something about him before the initial encounter; find out the patient's strengths.
   b. Consult his preferences.
   c. Concentrate on what the patient can do.
   d. Ask his opinions.
   e. Encourage him to make choices and decisions.
   f. Praise even minimal achievements.
   g. Avoid making decisions for him; this promotes low self-esteem, dependency, and depression.
   h. Support him during his periods of anxiety; allow expression of troubles and difficulties.
   i. Urge him to remain active. Direct attention to gains being made.
5. Nursing activities should be done *with* the patient rather than *for* him.
6. Necessary modifications and compromises imposed by the physiological limits of aging must be made in the medical and nursing management of the patient.
7. The individuality of the patient should be encouraged—to preserve his identity and sense of control.
   a. Encourage him to have and use personal posses-

sions that help bridge the gap between past and present.
b. Respect the right to self-direction.
c. Give the patient *time* to express his feelings.
d. Help him retain the social graces.
e. Help him cope with thoughts of death.
8. Elderly persons should be kept in the mainstream of life to prevent physical, emotional, and mental deterioration.
a. Avoid removing the element of challenge. Encourage contact with others.
b. Give dignity and privacy for personal relationships with opposite sex and expression of sexual needs.
c. Work out a "buddy system" to prevent loneliness and isolation.
d. Stimulate mental acuity and sensory input—minimizes preoccupation with body monitoring.

e. Encourage physical activity.
f. Share your world with the patient.
g. Remember his preferences; accept his idiosyncracies.
h. Provide opportunities for him to do some tasks of daily living (water plants; wash own hose).
i. Provide meaningful diversional activity.
j. Give him something to look forward to.
9. The patient's potentialities should be utilized.
a. Select activities that are in keeping with lifelong interests.
b. Do not attempt to alter lifelong character and behavior patterns.
c. Give the patient time to listen, to learn, and to adapt.
d. Help the patient to learn new ways to maintain independence.

BIBLIOGRAPHY

Books

Atchley RC. The Social Forces in Later Life. Belmont, California, Wadsworth Pub. Co., 1980
Burnside IM (ed). Nursing and the Aged. New York, McGraw-Hill, 1981
Burnside IM, Ebersole P, Monea HE. Psychosocial Caring Throughout the Life Span. New York, McGraw-Hill, 1979
Burnside IM (ed). Psychosocial Nursing Care of the Aged. New York, McGraw-Hill, 1980
Busse EW and Blazer DG. Handbook of Geriatric Psychiatry. New York, Van Nostrand Reinhold, 1980
Carnevali DL and Patrick ML. Nursing Management for the Elderly. Philadelphia, JB Lippincott, 1979
Colavita FB. Sensory Changes in the Elderly. Springfield, Charles C Thomas, 1978
Comfort A. Practice of Geriatric Psychiatry. New York, Elsevier, 1980
Eliopoulos C. Gerontological Nursing Practice. New York, Harper & Row, 1979
Futrell M et al. Primary Health Care of the Older Adult. North Scituate, Duxbury Press, 1980
Gibbs RC. Skin Diseases of the Feet. St. Louis, Warren H. Green, 1980
Glen, AIM and Walley LJ. Alzheimer's Disease. Edinburg, Churchill Livingstone, 1979
Hickey T. Health and Aging. Monterey, Brooks/Cole Pub. Co., 1980
Jackson JJ. Minorities and Aging. Belmont, Wadsworth Pub. Co., 1980
Kart CS, Metress ES, Metress JF. Aging and Health. Menlo Park, Addison–Wesley Pub. Co., 1978
Kohut S Jr, Kohut JJ, Fleishman JJ. Reality Orientation for the Elderly. Oradell, Medical Economics Co., 1979
Landreth GL and Berg RC (eds). Counseling the Elderly. Springfield, Charles C Thomas, 1980
Maurer JF and Rupp RR. Hearing and Aging: Tactics for Intervention. New York, Grune & Stratton, 1979
Mezey MD, Rauckhorst LH, Stokes SA. Health Assessment of the Older Individual. New York, Springer Pub. Co., 1980
Natow AB and Heslin J. Geriatric Nutrition. Boston, CBI Pub. Co., 1980
Pearson LJ and Kotthoff ME. Geriatric Clinical Protocols. Philadelphia, JB Lippincott, 1979
Poe WD and Holloway RA. Drugs and the Aged. New York, McGraw-Hill, 1980
Reichel W (ed). The Geriatric Patient. New York, HP Publishing Co., 1978
Schwartz AN and Peterson JA. Introduction to Gerontology. New York, Holt, Rinehart and Winston, 1979

Seymour E (ed). Psychosocial Needs of the Aged. Los Angeles, University of Southern California Press, 1978
Toga CJ, Nandy K, Chauncey HH. Geriatric Dentistry. Lexington, Lexington Books, 1979
Weber H. Nursing Care of the Elderly. Reston, Reston Pub. Co., 1980
Yale I. Podiatric Medicine. Baltimore, Williams & Wilkins, 1980
Zarit SH. Aging and Mental Disorders. New York, The Free Press, 1980

Articles

Beck C. Mental health and the aged: A value analysis. ANS 1979 April; 1(1–4):79–87
Blumenthal MD. Depressive illness in old age: Getting behind the mask. Geriatrics 1980 April; 35(4):34–43
Bozian MW and Clark HM. Counteracting sensory changes in the aging. Am J Nurs 1980 March; 80(3);473–476
Butler RN et al. Self-care, self-help and the elderly. Int J Aging Hum Dev 1979–1980; 10(1):95–117
Clausen K. When the goal is self-reliance, success depends on you. RN 1978 May; 41(5):50–52
Cummings J, Benson F, LoVerme S. Reversible dementia. JAMA 1980 June 20; 243(23):2434–2439
Dolan MB. Being old is not the same as being ill. Nursing '80 1980 April; 10(4):41–42
Falk G and Falk UA. Sexuality and the aged. Nursing Outlook 1980 Jan; 28(1):51–55
Gasek G. How to handle the crotchety, elderly patient. Nursing '80 1980 March; 10(3):46–48
Gilchrist AK. Common foot problems in the elderly. Geriatrics 1979 Nov; 34(11):67–70
Gioiella EC. Give the older person space. Am J Nurs 1980 May; 80(5):898–899
Grieco MH. Use of antibiotics in the elderly. Bull NY Acad Med 1980 March; 56(2):197–208
Ham R. Alternatives to institutionalization. Am Fam Physician 1980 July; 21(7):95–100
Health care for the aged. Hospitals 1980 May 16; 54(10):61–123
Hellebrandt FA. Aging among the advantaged: A new look at the stereotype of the elderly. Gerontologist 1980 Aug; 20(4):404–417
Hunt TE. Practical considerations in the rehabilitation of the aged. J Am Geriatr Soc 1980 Feb; 28(2):59–64
Kennie DC and Moore JT. Management of senile dementia. Am Fam Physician 1980 Dec; 22(6):105–111
King G and Vaughn S. You may be the aged's only advocate. RN 1978 May; 41(5):48–50

Meissner JE. Assessing a geriatric patient for institutional care. Nursing '80 1980 March; 10(3):86–87

Overstall PW. Prevention of falls in the elderly. J Am Geriatr Soc 1980 Nov; 28(11):481–484

Renshaw D. Sex and the senior citizen. Med Times 1979 Dec; 107(12):27–33

Stead EA Jr and Stead NW. Problems and challenges in the treatment of the aging population. DM 1980 Aug; 26(11):5–41

Stokes SA, Rauckhorst LM, Mezey MD. Health assessment—considerations for the older individual. J Gerontol Nurs 1980 June; 6(6):328–337

Strax TE and Ledebur J. Rehabilitating the geriatric patient: Potential and limitations. Geriatrics 1979 Sept; 34(9):99–101

Task Force Sponsored by the National Institute on Aging. Senility reconsidered. JAMA 1980 July 18; 244(3):259–263

Wahl PR. Therapeutic relationships with the elderly. J Gerontol Nurs 1980 May; 6(5):260–266

Waisman M. A clinical look at the aging skin. Postgrad Med 1979 July; 66(1):87–96

Wister E (ed). Symposium on gerontologic nursing. Nurs Clin North Am 1979 Dec; 14(4):577–664

Witte NS. Why the elderly fall. Am J Nurs 1979 Nov; 79(11):1950–1952

Yesavage J. Dementia: Differential diagnosis and treatment. Geriatrics 1979 Sept; 34(9):51–59

GENERAL CONSIDERATIONS

The Optimistic Side of Cancer

1. One-third of all cancer patients are cured.
2. Improved treatment modalities enable patients with cancer to live longer, more comfortably, and more productively.
3. Most cancer patients spend almost all their time away from hospitals and only come to the hospital intermittently for treatment.
4. More intense efforts at patient rehabilitation are proving effective.
5. Research continues unabated, and, as findings accumulate, prospects for specific cures are encouraging.

Cancer's Warning Signals

C hange in bowel or bladder habits
A sore that does not heal
U nusual bleeding or discharge
T hickening or lump in breast or elsewhere
I ndigestion or difficulty in swallowing
O bvious change in wart or mole
N agging cough or hoarseness

Early Detection of Cancer

Early detection provides a very effective way to reduce the morbidity and mortality of several cancers. Table 21-1 offers recommendations that represent important ways in which an asymptomatic individual can protect his health at greatly reduced risk, cost, and inconvenience.

Benign and Malignant Tumors

	Benign	Malignant
Type of Cell	Adult cell	Young cell
Nature	Closely resembles parent tissue	Tends to be anaplastic (reverting to primitive cells)
Growth	Slow	Rapid, usually
Encapsulated	Often	Never
Effect on surrounding tissue	Never invades	Invades widely
Localization	Remains at original site	Nonlocalized—forms secondary growths by metastasis
Recurrence after removal	Does not tend to recur	Tends to recur

Metastasis

Metastasis is the transfer of disease cells from one organ or part to another not directly connected with it.

1. *Extension and invasion*—because they are not encapsulated, it is easy for cancer cells to invade other tissues and extend themselves rapidly via lymphatic and blood circulatory systems; cancer may also recur in treated areas.
2. *Lymph*—secondary growths of tumor cells are often caught in the lymph filter, the lymph node.
3. *Blood*—by invasion, tumor cells enter the blood vessels and are carried to organs where the venous blood passes through a capillary bed.

Incidence

1. The annual death toll from malignancy in the U.S. is at least 405,000.
2. Cancer ranks second as the leading cause of death in the U.S.
3. About 1 million Americans are under medical care for cancer.
4. Cancer strikes at any age. It affects children as well as adults, but it strikes with increasing frequency with advancing age.
5. There will be about 785,000 new cancer cases this year (diagnosed for the first time).
6. No organ of the body is exempt. (See accompanying charts for cancer death rates by site.)

TABLE 21-1. SUMMARY OF RECOMMENDATIONS OF THE AMERICAN CANCER SOCIETY FOR THE EARLY DETECTION OF CANCER IN ASYMPTOMATIC PERSONS.

Test or Procedure	Population		
	Sex	Age	Frequency
Sigmoidoscopy	M & F	over 50	every 3-5 years; after 2 negative exams 1 year apart
Stool guaiac slide test	M & F	over 50	every year
Digital rectal examination	M & F	over 40	every year
Pap test	F	20-65; under 20, if sexually active	at least every 3 years after 2 negative exams 1 year apart;
Pelvic examination	F	20-40	every 3 years
		over 40	every year
Endometrial tissue sample	F	at menopause women at high risk[1]	at menopause
Breast self-examination	F	over 20	every month
Breast physical examination	F	20-40	every 3 years
		over 40	every year
Mammography	F	between 35-40	baseline
		under 50	consult personal physician
		over 50	every year
Chest x-ray		not recommended	
Sputum cytology		not recommended	
Health counseling and cancer checkup[2]	M & F	over 20	every 3 years
	M & F	over 40	every year

[1] History of infertility, obesity, failure of ovulation, abnormal uterine bleeding, or estrogen therapy.
[2] To include examination for cancers of the thyroid, testicles, prostate, ovaries, lymph nodes, oral region, and skin.
Courtesy of American Cancer Society. From CA-A Cancer Journal for Clinicians. 30(4):231, July-August 1980.

Treatment

1. Modalities of treatment include surgery, radiotherapy, radioactive substances (including radioisotopes), various drugs (pharmaceuticals and hormones), and immunotherapy. (See pp. 855–856.)

2. Method of treatment will depend on the type of malignancy, stage, localization or spread, condition of patient, and the physician; a single method or combination of methods may be required.

SURGERY

Definitions

1. *Biopsy*—surgical removal of a piece of tissue from the questionable area; the tissue sample is sent to the pathology laboratory for diagnostic verification.
2. *Preventive or prophylactic surgery*—removal of lesions which, if left in the body, are apt to develop into cancer. Example: polyps in rectum may lead to cancer of the colon.
3. *Palliative surgery*—a type of surgery which attempts to relieve the complications of cancer, e.g., obstruc-

tion of the gastrointestinal tract, pain produced by tumor extension into surrounding nerves.
4. *Curative surgery*—the removal of the primary site of malignancy and any lymph nodes to which the neoplasm has extended. Such surgery may be all that is required.
5. *Surgery combined with radiation, chemotherapy, or immunotherapy*—combinations of treatment required to halt the spread of a malignancy.

NOTE: Details of surgical treatment are given in the sections relating to specific disease entities.

CHEMOTHERAPY FOR CANCER

Value of Chemotherapy in Treating a Malignancy

1. As yet no drugs are available to cure most malignant tumors. Chemotherapy is used successfully in treating choriocarcinoma and leukemia.
2. Effects of chemotherapy:
   a. May produce a regression of the tumor or of its metastases.
   b. May reduce or slow the appearance of secondary growths.
   c. May relieve pain and other symptoms for a time.
   d. May improve quality of survival.
3. Cancer chemotherapy offers some relief to patients for whom surgery and irradiation are no longer beneficial.

4. Chemotherapeutic agents are useful in treatment of leukemias, Hodgkin's disease, lymphomas, Ewing's tumor, Wilms's tumor, testicular tumors, and retinoblastomas. Can lead to remissions—sometimes for many years.
5. Combinations of chemotherapeutic agents are often more effective and no more toxic than single agents.
6. Recent value of chemotherapy has been demonstrated in the management of patients who have been treated successfully by surgery and/or radiotherapy but in whom the recurrence risk is high.
7. Many chemotherapeutic agents have unpleasant systemic effects in addition to their effect on malignant tissue; therefore, it is imperative that these be recognized by the nurse.

Male Cancer Death Rates by Site
United States, 1930–1977

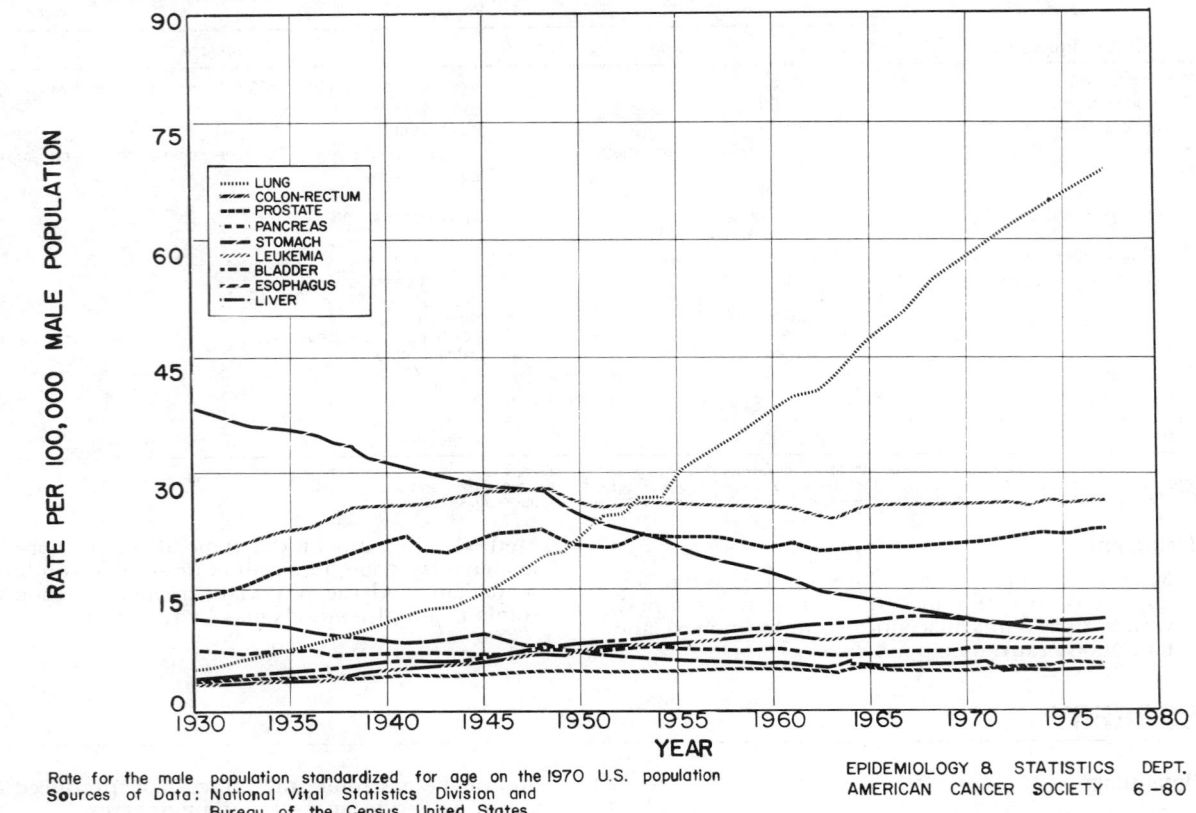

Rate for the male population standardized for age on the 1970 U.S. population
Sources of Data: National Vital Statistics Division and
Bureau of the Census, United States.

EPIDEMIOLOGY & STATISTICS DEPT.
AMERICAN CANCER SOCIETY 6 –80

---

8. Combination with immunotherapy appears promising.
9. Precise scheduling of dosages is necessary to achieve effective results.

Pharmacologic Action (Tables 21-2, 21-3)

1. These drugs are capable of destroying young, rapidly multiplying cells, such as malignant cells.
2. They interfere with manufacture of nucleic acids (inhibit the chain of synthesis or function of DNA and RNA) so that cellular growth and reproduction are inhibited.
3. Since many normal cells in the body also grow rapidly and have short life spans (e.g., bone marrow, gastrointestinal tract lining, hair follicles), many chemotherapeutic agents directly attack these normal cells. Herein lies the challenge.

Method of Administration

Drugs may be given orally, intravenously, intramuscularly, or intra-arterially, depending on the drug.

A. *Intravenous Administration*

1. See page 93 for principles of intravenous therapy. Additional specific concerns related to administration of chemotherapeutic agents include the following:

a. In general, avoid venipuncture in an arm where:
   (1) Dissection of the axillary nodes has been performed
   (2) Radiotherapy has caused marked fibrosis in the axillary area
b. Avoid areas of sclerosis, thrombosis, or scar formation
c. Avoid prolonged tourniquet application when the platelet count falls below 20,000/mm.[3] in order to prevent cutaneous hemorrhage.
2. If a small focal hematoma develops during insertion of needle into a vein, do not use this avenue for administration of toxic chemotherapeutic agents because of the danger of extravasation.
3. Maintain constant supervision during administration of potentially locally toxic chemotherapeutic agents.
4. If any doubt exists regarding vein patency or safety of drug administration, discontinue administration.
5. It is better to prevent *extravasation* than to treat it.
   a. Symptoms
      Pain (severe enough to cause patient to cry out); area may appear red, mottled, and/or swollen— often leading to necrosis.
   b. Treatment
      (1) Apply ice compresses to slow down local tissue metabolism.
      (2) Some individuals recommend local infiltration

Female Cancer Death Rates by Site
United States, 1930–1977

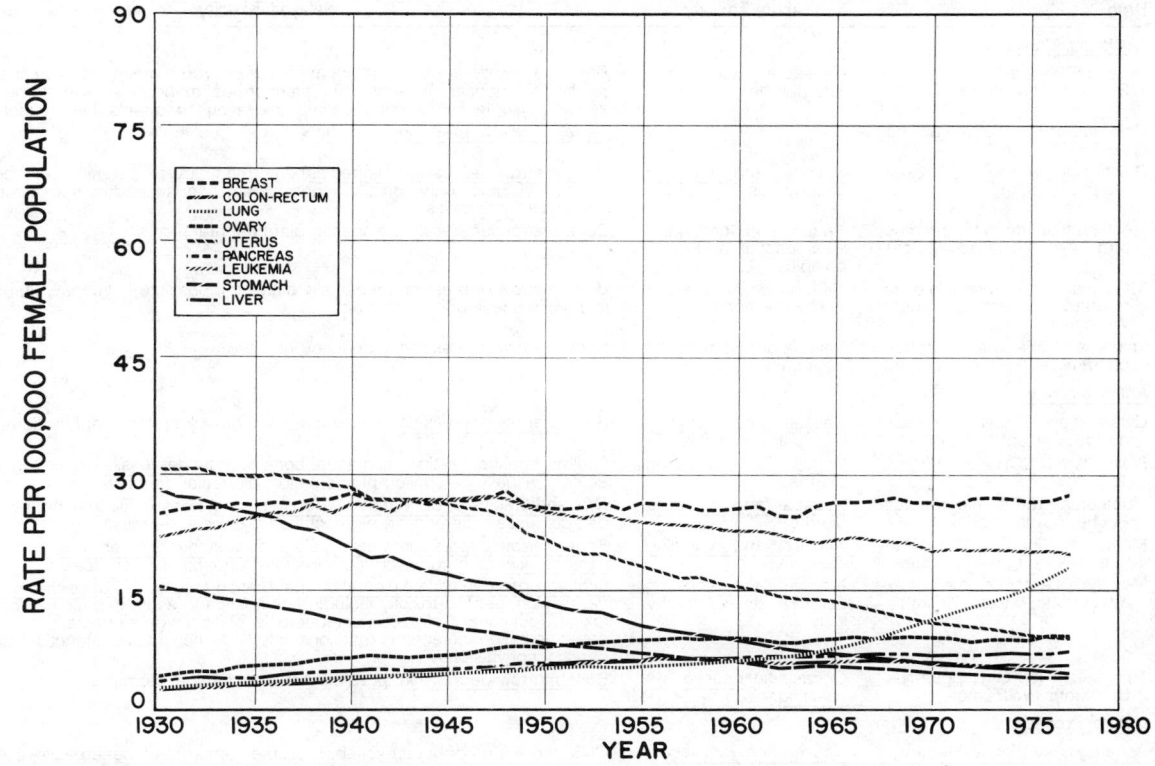

Rate for the female population standardized for age on the 1970 U.S. population
Sources of Data: National Vital Statistics Division and
Bureau of the Census, United States.

EPIDEMIOLOGY & STATISTICS DEPT.
AMERICAN CANCER SOCIETY 6 – 8 0

of the involved area with an anti-inflammatory agent, i.e., hydrocortisone.
(3) Later, warm compresses may be applied; local management as indicated.
c. If only a small amount of drug is extravasated and frank necrosis does not occur, phlebitis may still result, causing pain for several days and/or induration at the site that may last for weeks or months.
d. For one agent, Mustargen, the specific antidote is sodium thiosulfate, which should be injected immediately (subcutaneously or intradermally) into the area of extravasation.
6. Observe for occurrences other than extravasation:
a. Intraluminal
(1) Symptoms
(a) Patient may describe sensations of pain, stretching, or pressure within the vessel, originating near venipuncture site or 7.5–12.5 cm. (3–5 inches) along vein course.
(b) Discoloration—deep blue or purple 5–10 cm. (2–4 inches) proximal to venipuncture site.
(2) Treatment
Wait and observe; change puncture site or discontinue administration of drug.
b. Subcutaneous Tissue

(1) Symptoms
Itching, muscle cramp, pressure within arm, possible urticaria.
(2) Treatment
(a) Wait and observe; change puncture site, or discontinue administration of drug.
(b) Notify physician if systemic effects are observed.
7. Phenomena described above (in 5 and 6) may be associated with:
Daunorubicin; doxorubicin hydrochloride (Adriamycin); dacarbazine (DTIC); mechlorethamine hydrochloride (Mustargen); and BCNU.
B. *Isolation-Perfusion*—administration of large doses of extremely toxic drugs to an isolated extremity, organ, or region of the body (excluding systemic circulation). Usually such a dose cannot be tolerated by the entire body. By this means, short, intensive recirculation of high doses of antineoplastic drugs is used.
1. Areas
a. Lower extremity—iliac, femoral, popliteal arteries and veins
b. Pelvis—abdominal aorta, vena cava
2. Patient Preparation
a. Weigh patient since drug dosage is calculated on basis of kilograms of body weight.

TABLE 21-2. COMMERCIALLY AVAILABLE CANCER CHEMOTHERAPEUTIC DRUGS*
Note: major or dose-limiting effects are underlined

Drug	Acute Toxicity	Delayed Toxicity
Alkylating Agents		
Busulfan (Myleran-Burroughs Wellcome)	Nausea and vomiting; rare diarrhea	Bone marrow depression; pulmonary fibrosis; hyperpigmentation; cutaneous reactions; alopecia; gynecomastia; amenorrhea; menopausal symptoms; sterility; azoospermia; leukemia; chromosome aberrations; cataracts; hyperuricemia
Chlorambucil (Leukeran-Burroughs Wellcome)		Bone marrow depression; pulmonary fibrosis; leukemia
Cyclophosphamide (Cytoxan-Mead Johnson)	Nausea and vomiting; anaphylaxis	Bone marrow depression; alopecia; hemorrhagic cystitis; sterility (may be temporary); pulmonary fibrosis; hyperpigmentation; secondary malignancies; nonspecific dermatitis
Mechlorethamine (nitrogen mustard; HN2; Mustargen-Merck)	Nausea and vomiting; local reaction and phlebitis	Bone marrow depression; alopecia; diarrhea; oral ulcers
Melphalan (1-phenylalanine mustard; Alkeran-Burroughs Wellcome)	Mild nausea; hypersensitivity reactions	Bone marrow depression (especially platelets); possible pulmonary fibrosis; interstitial pneumonitis; leukemia
Thiotepa (triethylenethiophosphoramide; Thiotepa-Lederle)	Nausea and vomiting; local pain	Bone marrow depression; alopecia (one case)
Antimetabolites		
Cytarabine HCl (cytosine arabinoside; Cytosar-U; Upjohn)	Nausea and vomiting; diarrhea; anaphylaxis	Bone marrow depression; megaloblastosis; oral ulceration; hepatic damage
Floxuridine (FUDR-Roche)	Nausea and vomiting; diarrhea	Oral and gastrointestinal ulceration; bone marrow depression; neurological defects, usually cerebellar; pigmentation; alopecia; dermatitis
Fluorouracil (5-FU; Fluorouracil-Roche; Adrucil-Adria)	Nausea and vomiting; diarrhea	Oral and GI ulcers; bone marrow depression; increased lacrimation; neurological defects, usually cerebellar; pigmentation; alopecia; dermatitis
Mercaptopurine (6-MP; Purinethol-Burroughs Wellcome)	Nausea and vomiting; diarrhea	Bone marrow depression; cholestasis and rarely hepatic necrosis; oral and intestinal ulcers; chromosomal aberrations; anorexia; hyperuricemia
Methotrexate (MTX; Methotrexate-Lederle; Mexate-Bristol)	Nausea and vomiting; diarrhea; fever; anaphylaxis	Oral and gastrointestinal ulceration, perforation may occur; bone marrow depression; hepatic toxicity including cirrhosis and acute hepatic necrosis; renal toxicity; pulmonary infiltrates; osteoporosis; chills, fever; alopecia; depigmentation; cutaneous reactions; infertility; menstrual dysfunction; aphasia; paresis; convulsions
Thioguanine (6-TG; Thioguanine-Burroughs Wellcome)	Occasional nausea and vomiting	Bone marrow depression; possible hepatic damage; stomatitis
Natural Products		
Asparaginase (Elspar-Merck)	Nausea and vomiting; fever, chills; headache; hypersensitivity, possible anaphylaxis; abdominal pain; hyperglycemia leading to coma	CNS depression or hyperexcitability; acute hemorrhagic pancreatitis; coagulation defects; renal damage; hepatic damage
Bleomycin (Blenoxane-Bristol)	Nausea and vomiting; fever; anaphylaxis and other allergic reactions	Pneumonitis and pulmonary fibrosis; cutaneous reactions; stomatitis; alopecia; hyperpigmentation; Raynaud's phenomenon
Dactinomycin (actinomycin D; Cosmegen-Merck)	Nausea and vomiting; diarrhea; local reaction and phlebitis	Stomatitis; oral ulceration; bone marrow depression; alopecia; folliculitis
Daunorubicin (Daunomycin; Cerubidine-Ives)	Nausea and vomiting; red urine (not hematuria); severe local tissue damage and necrosis on extravasation; transient ECG changes	Bone marrow depression; cardiotoxicity; alopecia; stomatitis; cutaneous toxicity; hyperuricemia; anorexia; diarrhea; fever and chills
Doxorubicin (Adriamycin-Adria)	Nausea and vomiting; red urine (not hematuria); severe local tissue damage and necrosis on extravasation; diarrhea; transient ECG changes; ventricular arrhythmia; hypertensive encephalopathy; angioneurotic edema	Bone marrow depression; cardiotoxicity (may be irreversible); alopecia; stomatitis; cutaneous toxicity; hyperuricemia; anorexia; diarrhea; fever, chills; urticaria; anaphylaxis; conjunctivitis; lacrimation
Mithramycin (Mithracin-Dome)	Nausea and vomiting; diarrhea; fever	Hemorrhagic diathesis; bone marrow depression (thrombocytopenia); hepatic damage; hypocalcemia and hypokalemia; stomatitis; cutaneous reactions
Mitomycin (Mutamycin-Bristol)	Nausea and vomiting; local reaction if extravasation; fever	Bone marrow depression (cumulative); stomatitis; renal toxicity; alopecia; pulmonary fibrosis; hepatotoxicity at high doses
Vinblastine sulfate (Velban-Lilly)	Nausea and vomiting; local reaction and phlebitis if extravasation	Bone marrow depression; alopecia; stomatitis; loss of deep tendon reflexes; jaw pain; paralytic ileus

* The Medical Letter (Nov. 28, 1980)—56 Harrison St., New Rochelle, NY 10801

Drug	Acute Toxicity	Delayed Toxicity
Vincristine sulfate (Oncovin-Lilly)	Local reaction if extravasation	Peripheral neuropathy (loss of deep tendon reflexes, numbness, tingling and muscle weakness); neuritic pain; alopecia; mild bone marrow depression; constipation leading to paralytic ileus
Other Synthetic Agents		
Carmustine (BCNU; BiCNU-Bristol)	Nausea and vomiting; local phlebitis	Delayed leukopenia and thrombocytopenia (may be prolonged); pulmonary fibrosis (may be irreversible); delayed renal damage; gynecomastia
Cisplatin (Cis-Diammine-dichloroplatinum; Cis-DDP; Platinol-Bristol)	Nausea and vomiting; anaphylactic-like reactions; fever	Renal damage; bone marrow depression; ototoxicity; hemolysis; hypomagnesemia; hyperuricemia; peripheral neuropathy; hypocalcemia; hypokalemia
Dacarbazine (DTIC; DIC; DTIC-Dome)	Nausea and vomiting; anaphylaxis; pain on administration	Bone marrow depression; flu-like syndrome; alopecia; renal impairment; hepatic necrosis; facial flushing, paresthesia; rash; photosensitivity
Hydroxyurea (Hydrea-Squibb)	Nausea and vomiting; allergic reactions to tartrazine dye	Bone marrow depression; hyperkeratosis and hyperpigmentation; stomatitis; dysuria, alopecia, neurological disturbances rare
Lomustine (CCNU; CeeNU-Bristol)	Nausea and vomiting	Delayed (4 to 6 weeks) leukopenia and thrombocytopenia (may be prolonged); stomatitis; alopecia; transient elevation of transaminase activity; neurological reactions
Mitotane (o,p'-DDD; Lysodren-Bristol)	Nausea and vomiting; diarrhea	CNS depression; dermatitis; visual disturbances; adrenal insufficiency; brain damage with long-term high dosage; hematuria, hemorrhagic cystitis, albuminuria; hypertension; orthostatic hypotension
Procarbazine HCl (Matulane-Roche)	Nausea and vomiting; CNS depression	Bone marrow depression; stomatitis; dermatitis; peripheral neuropathy; pneumonitis
Hormones		
Estrogens		
Diethylstilbestrol (DES)	Nausea and vomiting; cramps	Fluid retention; hypercalcemia; feminization; uterine bleeding; if given during pregnancy, may cause vaginal carcinoma in offspring; increased frequency of vascular accidents
Ethinyl estradiol (Estinyl-Schering; others)		Fluid retention; hypercalcemia; feminization; uterine bleeding; increased incidence of vascular accidents
Androgens		
Dromostanolone propionate (Drolban-Lilly)		Fluid retention masculinization; hypercalcemia
Fluoxymesterone (Halotestin-Upjohn)		Fluid retention; masculinization; cholestatic jaundice; hypercalcemia; painful hypertrophy of clitoris; hirsutism
Testolactone (Teslac-Squibb)	Local pain, inflammation at injection site	Hypercalcemia; rare alopecia
Testosterone propionate (Oreton-Schering; others)		Fluid retention; masculinization; hypercalcemia
Progestins		
Hydroxyprogesterone caproate (Delalutin-Squibb)	Local abscess, pain	Hypercalcemia; cholestatic jaundice
Medroxyprogesterone acetate (Provera-Upjohn; others)	Orally: nausea (rare) IM: local pain, abscess at injection site	Fluid retention; hypercalcemia
Megestrol acetate (Megace-Mead Johnson)	Allergic reactions to tartrazine dye	Fluid retention; thromboembolism
Corticosteroids		
Prednisone or prednisolone		Mental aberrations; gastric ulcers; glucose intolerance; osteoporosis; hypertension; cataract formation
Antiestrogen		
Tamoxifen citrate (Nolvadex-Stuart)	Nausea and vomiting; hot flashes; transient increased bone or tumor pain	Vaginal bleeding and discharge; rash; hypercalcemia; retinopathy; corneal changes; decreased visual acuity; peripheral edema; depression; dizziness; headache

b. Obtain blood, urine, and x-ray studies.

c. Explain to the patient the nature of the procedure and the reason for applying tourniquets.

3. Operative Procedure

a. A totally occlusive tourniquet may be applied to an extremity in order to separate this area from systemic circulation.

b. A pump oxygenator is used to circulate patient's blood in a closed system for the involved part of the body.

c. Concentrated doses of the chemotherapeutic agent are injected.

d. Duration of perfusion depends on drug and on extent and location of growth.

e. Oxygenated blood is pumped into the artery; it passes through the extremity affected by the tumor and out through the vein, where the blood is reoxygenated and recirculated.

f. For an abdominal or lower pelvic tumor, a laparotomy may be done.

(1) Blood supply to the tumor area is blocked from systemic circulation by means of pneumatic tourniquets on the legs and special clamps on the inferior mesentery artery and vein.

(2) Catheters are inserted into the major vessels near the tumor site.

(3) The desired drug is injected into the artery; venous blood is conveyed to an oxygenator for

TABLE 21-3. SOME INVESTIGATIONAL DRUGS
Note: major or dose-limiting effects are underlined

Drug	Acute Toxicity*	Delayed Toxicity*
Aclacinomycin A	Anorexia	Bone marrow depression; cardiac toxicity
Aminoglutethimide	Skin rash; lethargy	Hypothyroidism (rare); bone marrow depression; fever, chills; gastrointestinal toxicity
Amsacrine (AMSA; 4'-(9-acridinylamino) methanesulfon m-anisidide)	Nausea and vomiting; diarrhea; pain or phlebitis on infusion	Bone marrow depression; hepatic injury; convulsions; stomatitis; ventricular fibrillation; alopecia
5-Azacytidine	Nausea and vomiting; diarrhea; fever	Leukopenia (may be prolonged); thrombocytopenia; hepatic damage; rash; muscle pain and weakness
Estramustine (estracyt; Emcyt-Roche)	Nausea and vomiting	Mild gynecomastia
Etoposide (VP16-213-Bristol)	Nausea and vomiting; diarrhea; fever	Bone marrow depression; alopecia; peripheral neuropathy
Hexamethylmelamine (HMM)	Nausea and vomiting	Bone marrow depression; CNS depression; peripheral neuritis; visual hallucinations
Ifosfamide (Cyfos-Mead Johnson)	Nausea and vomiting	Bone marrow depression; hemorrhagic cystitis; alopecia; sterility (may be temporary)
Mitobronital (dibromomannitol; myelobromol)	GI disturbances	Bone marrow depression; skin pigmentation; alopecia
Mitolactol (dibromodulcitol)	Mild nausea	Bone marrow depression
Semustine (methyl-CCNU)	Nausea and vomiting	Delayed leukopenia and thrombocytopenia (may be prolonged); pulmonary fibrosis; leukemia; renal failure
Streptozocin (streptozotocin; Zanosar-Upjohn)	Nausea and vomiting; local pain; chills	Renal damage; hyperglycemia
Tegafur (Ftorafur-Mead Johnson)	Nausea and vomiting; CNS symptoms including dizziness and lethargy	Stomatitis; bone marrow depression; pigmentation; alopecia; dermatitis
Teniposide (VM-26-Bristol)	Nausea and vomiting; diarrhea; phlebitis	Bone marrow depression; alopecia; peripheral neuropathy
Vindesine (Eldesine-Lilly)	Local reaction if extravasation; fever; nausea and vomiting; diarrhea	Bone marrow depression; alopecia; peripheral neuropathy; rash

* Information is preliminary; additional or more severe adverse effects may be reported.

oxygenation, and is then pumped back into arterial system.
(4) Upon completion of treatment, fresh blood may be transfused if necessary; clamps and tourniquets are removed and the surgical wound is closed.

C. *Intra-arterial Infusion*—the introduction percutaneously of a catheter into a major artery under fluoroscopic guidance. This does not require major surgery and can be repeated at intervals. The continuous administration of the chemotherapeutic agent into the artery leading to the tumor may last for several days or several weeks.

1. Routes
   Brachial, axillary, carotid, or femoral artery—determined by location of tumors.
2. Uses and Advantages
   a. This method is used preferably when the tumor is completely encompassed by the vessels in question; to check this, fluoroscein may be injected into the catheter and the tumor observed under a special lamp for fluorescence.
   b. Arterial infusion acts on the tumor over a longer period of time than is possible with isolation perfusion.
   c. By increasing regional concentrations and using minimal systemic drug concentrations, systemic toxicity is limited.

D. *Adjunct Chemotherapy*—administration of a chemotherapeutic agent at the time of surgery to kill any tumor cells which may spill into the bloodstream when the tumor is manipulated.

E. *Combined Chemotherapy and Irradiation*—permits drug to enhance the effect of irradiation. This has been particularly effective in treating head and neck lesions.

MEDICAL AND NURSING CARE OF PATIENTS RECEIVING PERFUSION OR ARTERIAL INFUSION

Before Special Treatment

1. The patient needs concerned care; these are procedures (perfusion and arterial infusion) which are tried because the disease is advanced, although limited to an anatomic area.
2. Provide encouragement and enough information to acquaint patient with the possible benefits as well as dangers of the procedure.
3. Give emotional support since the unpleasant side effects of chemotherapy can cause depression.

During Chemotherapy

1. Be familiar with the nature of the chemotherapeutic agent being used (toxic manifestations, etc.).
2. Observe arterial injection site to see that catheter is properly positioned. Guard against hemorrhage, leakage, sepsis, and tissue irritation.
3. Note any signs of malaise, nausea, vomiting, diar-

rhea, temperature elevation, changes in blood pressure and pulse.
4. Report input and output accurately.
5. If necessary, administer fluids intravenously for first 48 hours to maintain general hydration as well as dilution of post-treatment antineoplastic drugs.
6. Record local or systemic changes in detail (e.g., diarrhea or melena).
7. Observe skin tissue in local area for reaction—erythema, blistering, edema, petechiae.
8. Check mucous membranes for signs of tissue breakdown, hemorrhage, or infection.
9. Turn patient frequently because of increased possibility of pressure area breakdown.

Management of Complications

A. *Blood Difficulties*

1. Withdraw drugs if leukocyte or platelet counts fall to dangerous levels.
2. If leukocyte count is below 1200, obtain a culture to assist in determining specific treatment.
3. Practice reverse isolation when leukocyte count falls to low levels, or discharge the patient.
4. Administer packed cells if anemia occurs.
5. Give platelet transfusions if thrombocytopenia (decrease in number of blood platelets) is severe; steroids may also be used.

B. *Other Problems*

Difficulties such as nausea and vomiting, diarrhea, mucositis, infection, alopecia (hair loss) are discussed in the next section: *Nursing Care of the Patient Receiving Chemotherapeutic Agents for Neoplastic Disease.*

NURSING CARE OF THE PATIENT RECEIVING CHEMOTHERAPEUTIC AGENTS FOR NEOPLASTIC DISEASE

1. Recognize *signs of toxicity* due to the chemotherapeutic agent being administered.
   a. Note that signs vary from patient to patient.
   b. Utilize combative measures to offset disturbances, such as antiemetics for nausea.
   c. Anticipate that the patient will experience discomforts, but avoid suggesting to him that they might occur, since psychologically this might hasten their occurrence.
2. Assess status of *oral mucosa* and utilize measures to minimize *mucosal trauma* and *stomatitis*.
   a. Initiate a program of oral hygiene so that mouth does not become a breeding place for bacteria.
   b. Cleanse the mouth with nonabrasive soft materials, such as a very soft toothbrush or finger wrapped with a layer of gauze and dipped in a cleansing solution.
   c. Use mouthwash of 3 parts saline to 1 part hydrogen peroxide (dilute further if this is irritating).
   d. Avoid commercial mouthwashes which may irritate sensitive tissue.
   e. If mouth is sore, avoid spicy, hot, and acid foods; avoid irritating foods and fluids such as toast and citrus fruit juices.
   f. Suggest and serve ice cream, ice milk, and popsicles for a refreshing change.
3. Be alert for evidence of *gastrointestinal tract disturbances: nausea and vomiting.*

   a. Nausea
      (1) Administer antiemetic about ½ hour before or immediately after chemotherapy.
      (2) Offer ice chips or a fruit popsicle at onset of nausea.
      (3) Try giving patient a cup of tea and crackers.
      (4) Have patient eat small meals frequently and chew food thoroughly.
      (5) Encourage good mouth hygiene before and after meals.
      (6) If no stomatitis is present, some patients find lemons or dill pickles enjoyable.
      (7) In situations where antiemetics do not help, some patients have obtained relief from delta-9-tetrahydrocannabinol (THC)—the main active ingredient of marihuana.
      (8) Provide distraction such as television or some diversion.
   b. Vomiting
      (1) Provide emesis basin and tissues; empty and clean basin after use.
      (2) Apply a cool wrung-out washcloth to forehead, face and neck.
      (3) Administer an antiemetic; assess for dehydration.
      (4) Offer items for oral care after vomiting: mouthwash, toothbrush, and toothpaste.
4. Assess for *fluid retention* and *diarrhea*, which are common problems.
   a. Note evidence of superficial edema and signs of congestive heart failure (see p. 298).
   b. Prevent undue pressure on bony prominences since retained fluid stretches and weakens skin; turn patient frequently, massage and lubricate pressure points.
   c. Be alert for signs of hypokalemia and modify diet to increase potassium.
   d. Diarrhea
      (1) Place patient on a diet low in roughage and higher in constipating foods.
      (2) Administer antidiarrheal medication.
      (3) Assess for signs of dehydration; monitor fluids and electrolytes.
5. Maintain adequate *nutritional levels*, recognizing that there may be nausea, vomiting, anorexia, stomatitis, and oral mucositis.
   a. Regulate temperature of fluids and foods coming in contact with the oral mucosa; avoid temperature extremes (too hot or too cold).
   b. Serve high protein and high carbohydrate food; allow patient to choose his foods; guide his selection so that well-balanced diet of nutritionally desirable foods is served.
   c. Present food as attractively as possible and serve it in a pleasant setting.
   d. Ensure that patient is physically comfortable; encourage having friends or family provide company during mealtime if this helps.
   e. Encourage fluids because tissue metabolic rate is elevated and patient needs to clear wastes from his body.
   f. Entice the anorexic patient with refreshing mouth care before serving meals; a bad taste in the mouth discourages eating.
      (1) Try giving patient high-protein, high-calorie foods.
      (2) Monitor weight loss.
   g. Modify chemical and mechanical factors in an

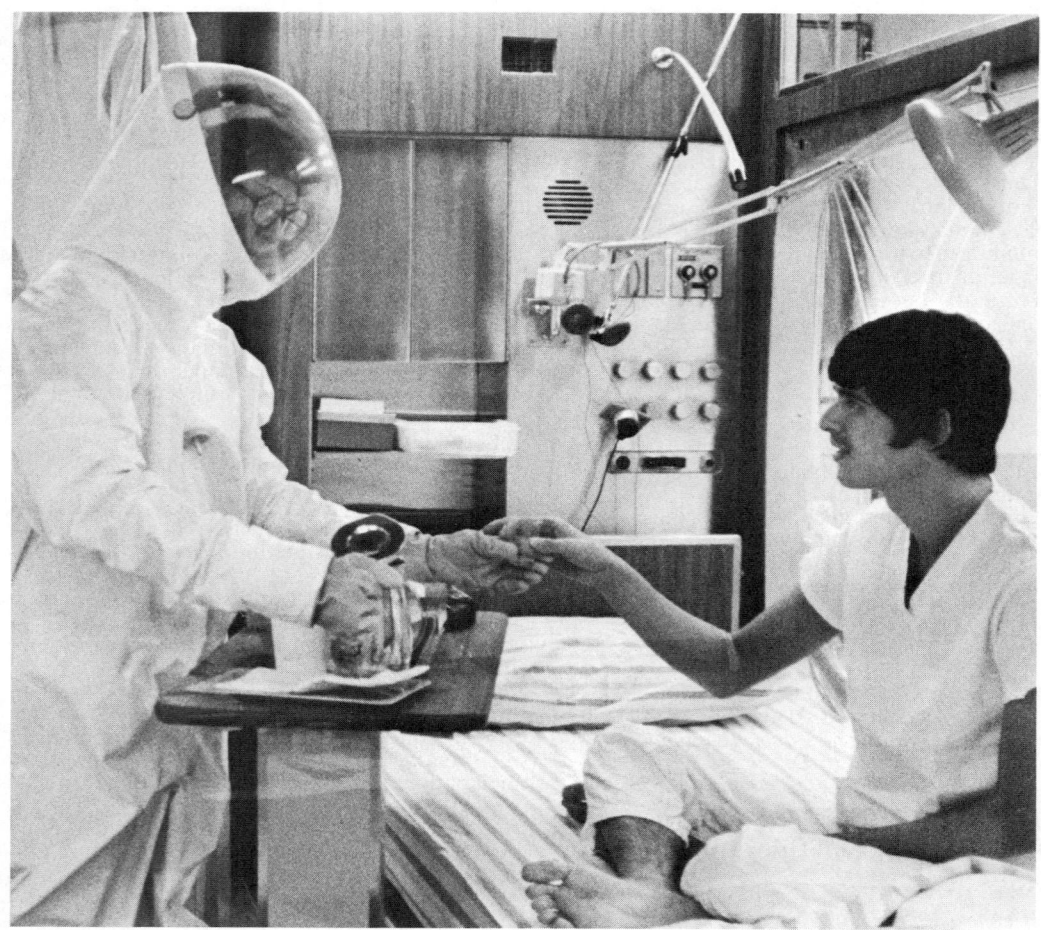

FIGURE 21-1. *A nurse gives nursing care to the patient inside a germ-free unit. All materials in this unit are sterile, and vertical airflow (laminar) prevents cross-contamination from nurse to patient. The nurse wears a special outfit which is attached to a train allowing her to move about freely. (Courtesy of RN Magazine: 35(2).)*

effort to avoid tissue trauma to the mouth—use soft toothbrush and soothing dentifrices and mouthwash; avoid ill-fitting dentures.

h. Avoid highly seasoned foods, even if patient ordinarily thrives on such foods.

i. Discourage smoking and use of alcoholic beverages since these irritate the mucous membranes.

j. Recognize that occasionally cancer and/or treatment may cause an alteration of taste perception, such as a keener taste of bitterness and loss of ability to detect sweet tastes.

6. Note the manifestations of *bone marrow depression.*

a. Check for reduction in number of leukocytes, erythrocytes, and platelets; report abnormal findings.

b. Note any swelling or redness of any body part.

c. Observe for evidence of infection and bleeding tendencies.

d. Explain to the patient that he is susceptible to infection; caution him to guard against exposure to upper respiratory infections and other infections.

e. Instruct patient to avoid cuts, bruises, or trauma; give injections only if absolutely necessary.

f. Apply site pressure (if an injection must be given) to avoid prolonged bleeding.

g. Stress importance of cleanliness and hand washing.

h. Utilize "Life Island" when available, to provide a protected environment. (Fig. 21-1)

7. Anticipate possible signs of *anemia.*

a. Caution patient about physical overexertion, encourage him to rest frequently and to expect a tired feeling.

b. Explain that blood transfusions, if given, are a part of therapy and not necessarily an indication of a setback.

SPECIAL PRECAUTIONS WITH CERTAIN ANTICANCER DRUGS:

Anticancer Drug	Problem	Nursing Action
Actinomycin D (Cosmegen)	Contact with skin	Rinse area with water for 10 minutes Rinse finally with buffered phosphate solution (e.g., Buff)
Methotrexate (MTX)	Contact with skin	Wash skin thoroughly; apply bland ointment to relieve stinging
Actinomycin D Azathioprine (Imuran) Carmustine (BCNU) Lomustine (CeeNU) Melphalan (Alkeran) Nitrogen mustard (Mustargen)	Especially irritating to eyes	Protect eyes well by using goggles or other protective device

c. Observe skin color; monitor laboratory results (HgB, RBC).
8. Inspect body for signs of *nasal infections, eye infections, rectal abscesses.*
   a. Teach patient how to keep these vulnerable areas clean to avoid infection.
   b. Alert him to the importance of avoiding persons who have infections.
   c. Recognize that with an altered blood count, he may be easily fatigued and therefore requires daily rest periods.
9. Promote patient comfort and administer analgesics if he is experiencing *pain.*
   a. Administer Tylenol instead of aspirin for general or local discomfort; aspirin may be irritating to the stomach.
   b. Offer viscous Xylocaine to use as a mouth wash and gargle; this acts as a topical anesthetic agent to relieve pain.
10. Expect that with some chemotherapeutic agents (doxorubicin, cyclophosphamide, vincristine) and with certain methods of administration, there may be *alopecia (hair loss).*
    a. Reassure patient that hair will grow back.
    b. Suggest wearing a turban or head scarf.
    c. Temporary use of a hair piece or wig may be suitable; have wig fitted before chemotherapy is started.
    d. Scalp tourniquet and hypothermia (ice packs) are used to control alopecia; results are variable.
11. Attend to the *psychosocial needs* of the patient receiving chemotherapeutic agents.
    a. When there is hair loss, recognize that this change in physical appearance may result in antisocial behavior and depression (see *10,* above).
    b. Utilize any and all measures that will tend to distract the patient from himself; provide diversional and recreational therapy.
    c. Provide rest periods that are conducive to rest—quiet, relaxing backrubs, soft music, comfortable surroundings.

d. Be honest with the patient about all aspects of his therapy and condition. To promote self-sufficiency and self-esteem, allow him to be a participant in the planning of his care.
    e. Encourage the patient to stay on the therapeutic program.
    f. Provide patient with stimuli to combat sensory deprivation if he is on reverse isolation.

NURSING PRECAUTIONS IN HANDLING CYTOTOXIC ANTICANCER DRUGS

See Special Precautions With Certain Anticancer Drugs, above.
1. Most cytotoxic anticancer drugs are irritating to the skin, eyes, and mucous membranes.
2. If mishandled, these drugs can result in local toxic or allergic reactions.
3. Because research has not yet substantiated cause-and-effect damage as a result of handling these drugs, it would be prudent to employ safeguards:
   a. Wear protective gloves and eye protection in order to avoid direct contact of the drug with skin and eyes.
   b. Wear a face mask when handling such a drug in powder form.
   c. Hold drug ampules away from the face when they are being opened to remove contents.
   d. Wash contaminated skin and surfaces with copious amounts of soap and water.
   e. Dispose of leftover ampule contents by carefully flushing down a drain, using liberal amounts of water.
   f. Wear gloves, a face mask, and eye protection when cleaning up spills of cytotoxic material:
      (1) Wipe up spills with a damp cloth or paper towels.
      (2) Place all of the material in a plastic bag, seal it, place in a second plastic bag, and seal.
      (3) Mark outer bag "Dangerous Material" and send to incinerator.

RADIATION IN DIAGNOSIS AND THERAPY

Radiation is frequently used in diagnosing and treating cancer.

Sources of Radiation

1. Naturally occurring radioactivity—radium, radon
2. Artificially produced radioactivity—radioisotopes
   a. Internal application

Gold	^{198}Au
Phosphorus	^{32}P
Cobalt	^{60}Co
Iodine	^{131}I
Iridium	^{192}Ir

   b. External application

Cobalt teletherapy	^{60}Co
Cesium teletherapy	^{137}Cs

   c. X-ray machines
      30–120 Kev
      250 Kev
      Million volt
      Van de Graaff (2 Mev)
      Betatron (24 Mev)
      Linear accelerator

Definitions

1. *Nuclide*—any atomic entity capable of existing for a measurable lifetime, usually more than 10^{-9} seconds.
2. *Radionuclide* (radioactive nuclide)—one that disintegrates with the emission of particulate or electromagnetic radiations.
3. *Radioactivity*—the disintegration of the atom which gives up energy in the form of rays or particles.
4. *Isotope*—an element whose nucleus contains a fixed number of protons but has a differing number of neutrons, thereby changing its weight.
   a. Optimal ratio between proton and neutron is stable.
   b. By using nuclear reactors, it is possible to bombard a stable isotope with additional free neutrons.
   c. Most radioisotopes emit:
      (1) Particulate radiation—small fragments of the nucleus having mass and size (alpha and beta particles).
      (2) Electromagnetic radiations—rays that have no mass (x-rays).
5. *Radioactive Decay or Disintegration*
   a. The rate of decay varies from isotope to isotope.
   b. "Half-life" or decay rate is the time required to reduce a particular radioactive substance by one-half of its atoms, thereby reducing it to half of its initial activity.
      Example: Radium–225—half-life of over 1600 years.
   c. A radioisotope administered to a patient in unsealed form has a relatively short life and is essentially inactive after therapeutic use has been completed.
      Example: ^{131}Iodine—half-life about 8 days.
   d. Longer lasting isotopes are implanted temporarily in the patient in a sealed container.
      Example: ^{60}Co—half-life about 5 years.
6. *Units of Measurement (Activity)*
   a. Curie (c.)—basic unit for measuring amount of activity in a radioactive sample
   b. Millicurie (mc.)—one thousandth of a curie
   c. Microcurie (μc.)—one millionth of a curie
   d. Picocurie (pc.)—one billionth of a curie

7. *Units for Measuring Radiation Exposure or Absorption*
   a. Roentgen (r.)—a standard unit of exposure (usually applied to x-ray or gamma rays)
   b. Milliroentgen (mr.)—one thousandth of a roentgen
   c. Rad—a unit to measure absorbed dose
      (1 rad = amount of radiation required to deposit 100 ergs of energy per gram of irradiated material)
   d. Rem—a unit of measure of radiation-dose equivalent which relates to biological effectiveness (roentgen equivalent man)
      Standards have been established by the International Committee on Radiation Protection (I.C.R.P.) that the maximum permissible dose (M.P.D.) for radiation workers is 5 rems for persons over age 18.

Biological Aspects and Clinical Application

A. *Nature and Indications for Use*

1. Individualized to produce effective ionization within a tumor while avoiding unnecessary irradiation of normal structures
2. Low voltage—Kev (thousand electron volts)
   Super voltage—Mev (million electron volts)
3. Tissues most likely to respond to radiation exposure—those originating from reticuloendothelial tissues (leukemia, lymphomas) and those from embryonal tissues (teratomas)
4. Tissues least likely to respond—bone and muscle

B. *Factors Affecting the Benefit of Radiation Exposure vs. Risk of Tissue Damage*

1. *Dose rate*—a prescribed dose causes less tissue destruction if given in small amounts over a long period of time rather than given all at once.
2. *Area of Body Exposure*—the larger the area exposed, the greater the effect.
3. *Cell susceptibility*
   Greater susceptibility—rapidly dividing cells with no specialized function (e.g., lymphocytes and germ cells)
   Lesser susceptibility—nondividing cells and highly differentiated cells (e.g., nerve or muscle cells)
4. *Biological variability*—individual differences play a role in human susceptibility.
   Examples:
   a. Healthy person more responsive than malnourished individual.
   b. Skin is especially vulnerable to radiation injury.
   c. Bone marrow is very radiosensitive; therefore, such damage is potentially the most lethal.
   d. Radiation cataracts result from excessive eye exposure.
   e. Lung fibrosis may occur following radiation of chest.

C. *Symptoms of Radiation Syndrome—High Level*

(Major portion of body exposed to large doses of irradiation (*over 100 rems*) in a short period of time.)

1. Prodromal—nausea, vomiting, malaise
2. Latent—symptoms subside
3. Illness—general malaise, epilation (hair loss), hemorrhage (petechiae, nosebleed), pallor, diarrhea, inflammation of mouth and throat, leukopenia
4. Recovery or death

D. *Symptoms of Radiation Syndrome—Low Level*

(Low levels of radiation over a long period of time.)
Examples:
1. Radiologists—may acquire leukemia
2. Clock dial painters—may develop sarcomas (from radium-containing luminizing paint)
3. Gonad exposure to radiation—may affect progeny

E. *Roentgenologic Precautions During Radiography, Fluoroscopy, or Radiotherapy*

1. No one permitted in the room where the patient is undergoing x-ray therapy or roentgenography.
2. Fluoroscopic equipment should not leak radiation.
3. Fluoroscopy room attendants should be protected from scattered radiation by wearing lead aprons and, if necessary, lead-impregnated gloves.
4. Appropriate lead shielding should be available to protect the patient's gonads during radiation exposure.

Nursing Support and Action in Radiation Therapy

A. *Physical and Psychological Preparation of the Patient*

1. Provide psychological support to this patient because radiation therapy is associated with fears:
   a. of being burned
   b. of being disfigured
   c. of dying and death
   d. of inability to perform normal bodily functions
   e. of pain
   f. of sterility and loss of sexual function
2. Recognize systemic responses to fear:
   a. Mouth dryness, pupillary dilatation
   b. Hand tremor, vomiting, severe palpitations
3. If above signs are noted, initiate open discussion, since this often relieves anxiety.
4. Remove all opaque objects such as pins, buttons, and hairpins, and replace clothing with a gown for body x-rays.
5. Have patient remain perfectly still; maintain position with use of sandbags, etc. if required.
6. Tell patient that there will be no sensation or pain accompanying either picture-taking or penetration of x-rays.
7. Advise him that he will be alone in the room for the protection of the technician but that he will be in voice contact.
8. Determine from the physician what he has told the patient about radiotherapy, particularly in the case of the patient with advanced cancer.
9. If a series of treatments is to be given, include the patient in the planning phase.
10. Give special attention to diet and medications; administer antinauseants, analgesics, specific medications for diarrhea, proctitis, and cystitis.

11. Explain the need for routine blood counts.

B. *Skin Manifestations*

1. Inform the patient that some skin reaction can be expected but that it varies from patient to patient. Example: dry erythema, desquamation, moist erythema, healing, epilation, tanning, telangiectasis.
2. Apply no lotions, ointments, cosmetics, etc. to the site of radiation unless prescribed by the physician; avoid talcum powder because it contains heavy metals that can be irritating.
3. Discourage vigorous rubbing, friction, or scratching because it can destroy skin cells; apply a bland ointment (with vitamins A and D).
4. Take precautions against irritation from friction, exposure to sunlight, and extremes in temperature.
5. Do not apply adhesive or scotch tape to the skin.

C. *Mucous Membrane Damage*

1. Oral mucosa
   a. There may be a change in or loss of taste.
   b. There may be various degrees of soreness and inability to swallow.
   c. Avoid irritants such as smoking, spicy food, alcoholic beverages.
   d. Use mild cleansing agents in the mouth.
2. Digestive tract
   a. Diarrhea is a common symptom if large areas are irradiated or if colon is significantly affected.
   b. Treat diarrhea with simple measures such as Kaopectate or opiate-like agents (Lomotil); it may be necessary to suspend radiotherapy for a few days.

D. *Dietary Disturbances*

1. Provide dietary restrictions to relieve symptoms of chronic radiation enteritis:
   Administer diet free of gluten, protein, and lactose to overcome or avoid absorptive problems resulting from atrophy of intestinal villi.
2. Maintain high level of nutrition but eliminate those foods that irritate the mucous membrane; this may preclude the need for nasogastric feeding.
3. Consider parenteral hyperalimentation (p. 406).

E. *Systemic Reactions*

Nausea, vomiting, fever, loss of appetite, malaise.
1. Administer sedatives for greater comfort.
2. Select fluids and foods that will not induce or aggravate nausea.
3. Provide small, frequent meals rather than 3 larger meals.
4. Suggest time for rest and relaxation; avoid noise, confusion.
5. Recognize that the patient needs encouragement and understanding.

RADIOISOTOPE THERAPY

Types of Radioisotope Therapy

A. *Teletherapy*—utilizes gamma rays from a radioactive source which is kept in a shielded unit placed at a distance from the patient.

1. Radioisotope Cobalt-60 (^{60}Co) and Cesium-137 (^{137}Ce) deliver radiation similar to that produced by supervoltage x-ray apparatus.

2. ^{60}Co therapy unit requires extra shielding because rays are being emitted constantly. Because gamma rays cannot be entirely absorbed, personnel are advised to spend minimum time in this room.
3. *Advantages of ^{60}Co over conventional x-ray*
   a. Skin problems are significantly reduced.
   b. Bone or cartilage involvement is lessened.
   c. Electronic circuits are not required.

4. *Disadvantages of* ^{60}Co
   a. Because it has a half-life of 5 years, it is necessary to replace the ^{60}Co.
   b. Radiation energy cannot be varied.
   c. Cost of room shielding is high.

B. *External Molds*—a packaged and screened container in which a radioisotope can be placed and applied directly to the skin surface.

Examples:
1. ^{60}Co can be applied in this manner to small areas, as in the treatment of carcinoma of the lip, larynx, ear, etc.
2. ^{182}Ta (radioactive tantalum) can be applied in a flexible wire mold (e.g., to the external surface of a retinoblastoma involving eyeball and optic nerve).
3. ^{90}Sr (radioactive strontium) and ^{90}Y (yttrium) as in external molds used for shallow irradiation of eye neoplasms.

C. *Intracavitary Isotope Therapy*

Example:
   Liquid radioisotopes:
   —^{198}Au (radioactive colloidal gold)
   — ^{20}Na (radioactive sodium)
   — ^{82}Br (radioactive bromine)
   used in the balloon of a catheter inside the bladder for internal bladder radiation of a few millimeters.

D. *Interstitial Isotope Therapy*

Examples:
1. Radioactive needles, seeds, tubes, or wires can be implanted directly into tumor tissue: Cobalt-60, Cesium-137, Gold-198, Radon-222, Tantalum-182, Iodine-125.
2. Implants may be temporary or permanent; they may be supplementary to surgery or to external beam irradiation.
3. Radioactive solutions may be injected directly into the tumor or surrounding tissue. Colloidal solution of radioactive colloidal gold (^{198}Au) is one of the most commonly used solutions.

E. *Internal Irradiation*

Examples:
1. Oral ingestion of solutions of radioiodine (^{131}I)—administered to patients with hyperthyroidism.
2. Intravenous injection of sodium phosphate (^{32}P)—used in the treatment of polycythemia vera.
Clinical Action
   In above instances, the target tissue has an affinity for the therapeutic agent; the isotope concentrates within the substance.

Nursing Management of Patients Receiving Radioisotopes

A. *Identification of the Patient as a Radiation Source*

1. Have patient wear a wristband with a radioactive symbol.
2. Identify the chart cover, doctor's and nurse's order sheets, and special radiation instruction sheet with the radioactive symbol.
3. For patients receiving the most minute quantities of tracer radioisotopes, such identification (see above) is not necessary.
4. Personnel who may be exposed to penetrating radiation (x-ray or gamma rays) should wear film badges on front of the body.

B. *Radiation Instruction Sheet*

1. Type of radioactivity used
2. Time of insertion
3. Anticipated time of removal
4. Precautions to follow
5. Whom to notify when in doubt or in an emergency

C. *Factors Affecting the Amount of Radiation*

1. *Amount* of radioactivity present, 10mc., 20mc., 30mc., etc.
2. The *distance* of the nurse from the patient

NOTE: The inverse square law applies: doubling the distance from a radiation source cuts intensity received to one-fourth.

3. Amount of *time* spent in actual contact with patient
4. Degree of *shielding* utilized
   Chosen according to type of radiation—alpha, beta, gamma (Fig. 21-2).
5. Amount of *body area exposed* to radiation

> **NURSING ALERT:** During the period of greatest radioactivity (24–72 hours), limit amount of time spent with the patient to that required for essential care. Require patient to remain in his bed or room during course of treatment.

D. *Vital Nursing Measures in Caring for the Patient with Internal Radiation*

1. Be acquainted with the nomenclature describing dissipation of radioisotopes.
   a. *Physical half-life*—a constant rate in which one-half of radioactivity is dissipated in a given time.
   b. *Biologic half-life*—the time it takes for a radioisotope to disappear from the body via normal metabolic processes.
   c. *Effective half-life*—a combination of physical half-life and biologic half-life.
2. Recognize that an isotope that is completely dispersed throughout the body (or a major portion of it) is less hazardous to an organ or tissue than an isotope concentrated by the body into a limited area.
3. Recognize that an isotope that is excreted rapidly is less hazardous than radium, which may be kept in the body for long periods.
4. Take appropriate measures associated with *sealed sources of radiation* implanted within a patient (sealed internal radiation).
   a. Follow directives on precaution sheet which is

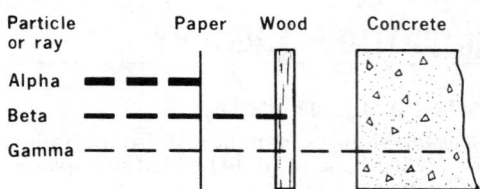

FIGURE 21-2. *Relative penetration of alpha, beta and gamma radiation. (U.S. Atomic Energy Commission.)*

placed on chart of all patients receiving radiotherapy.

b. Do not remain within 1 meter (3 feet) of the patient any longer than required to give essential care.

c. Know that the casing material absorbs all alpha radiation and most beta radiation, but that a hazard concerning gamma radiation may exist.

d. Do not linger longer than necessary in giving patient care, even though all precautions are followed.

e. Be alert for implants that may have become loosened (those inserted in cavities that have access to the exterior), e.g., check the emesis basin following mouth care for a patient with an oral implant.

f. Notify the radiologist of any implant that has moved out of position.

g. Utilize long-handled forceps or tongs and hold at arm's length when picking up any accidentally dislodged radium needle, seeds, tubes, etc., that may appear on dressings, bed, or floor. *Never pick up a radioactive source with your hands.*

h. Do not discard any dressings or linens unless sure that no radioactive source is present.

i. Wash hands with soap and water after caring for a patient who is being treated with a radioisotope. When wearing gloves, wash them with soap and water before removing them.

NOTE: This is not necessary for sealed sources.

j. Encourage patients who are ambulatory to remain in their own rooms.

k. Upon discharge of a patient, it is a good policy for the radiologist to check the room with a radiograph or survey meter to be certain that all radioactive materials have been removed.

l. Continue radiation precautions when a patient has a permanent implant, until the radiologist declares precautions unnecessary. (See p. 853 for nursing care of the patient receiving radiation therapy.)

5. Take appropriate measures associated with *unsealed sources;* radioactivity may be (1) widely spread in the body, (2) localized, or (3) present in any body tissue or fluid.

Examples:

a. *Radioactive iodine*
   (1) Circulates in bloodstream, excreted by kidneys—urine and blood contain radioactive material.
   (2) Can be secreted by sweat glands.
   (3) May be found in vomitus of patient who recently took oral dose.

b. *Radioactive colloidal gold*
   (1) May be noted in wound seepage as pink, red, or purple stain following intracavitary injection.
   (2) May be noted in small amounts in urine.

c. *Radioactive phosphorus solution*
   Be alert for contamination from excreta (urine and feces) and vomitus.

IMMUNOTHERAPY

The *immune system* of the body has the ability to recognize and to defend itself against infection and invasion by foreign cells such as those of cancer. The immune system may be weakened or overwhelmed by the invasion of foreign cells so that it cannot function effectively.

Immunotherapy employs the immune mechanism of the body to combat cancer and overcome it. The immunotherapeutic approach to cancer is based on the fact that most tumors provoke an immune response (such as anti-tumor activity, production of tumor antigens) in the patient (host).

Although it is still considered investigational, significant research in immunotherapy is going on and progress is being made.

Objectives of Immunotherapy

1. To successfully treat the cancer patient.
2. To challenge and to induce mobilization of the patient's immune defenses by utilizing a chemical or microbial agent to which the patient has previously been sensitized.
   a. This produces a delayed hypersensitivity response that can be employed against the cancer.
   b. Once developed in this way, immunocompetence (either alone or in combination with radiation, chemotherapy, or surgery) can fight the cancer.

Various Approaches of Immunotherapy

A. *Active Specific Immunotherapy*

1. Utilization of the patient's own immune mechanisms to reject or control his own malignant cells.

2. To date, active immunization, used alone, appears incapable of boosting the immune mechanism in the patient with advanced disseminated cancer.

B. *Active Nonspecific Immunotherapy*

1. Primarily activates macrophages and enhances delayed hypersensitivity of cellular immunity.
2. Utilization of bacteria or bacterial products as an immunologic adjuvant to enhance the immune response.
   a. *BCG* is a live attenuated strain of tubercle bacillus
   b. *MER* (methanol extraction residue) is a more highly refined, nonviable component of BCG
   c. *C. parvum* is a killed anaerobe
3. These agents are easy to distribute widely, and the responses achieved in patients with melanoma and several other solid tumors, as well as acute leukemia, make them attractive for a large number of therapy protocols.

C. *Passive-Adoptive Immunotherapy*

1. Utilization of the immunity of a competent donor.
2. The use of hyperimmune serum for rubella (passive) or for immunodeficiency diseases (adoptive) appears possible.
   Example: Immune RNA and lymphocyte transfer factor (LTF).
3. Again, further study is needed.

D. *Adjunctive Immunotherapy*

Because the above immunotherapeutic approaches appear inadequate, immunotherapy may be best utilized as an adjunct to other modalities (and even following

curative methods, to eliminate the few remaining malignant cells).
1. *Immunotherapy and Surgery*
   a. Following surgical removal of the bulk of a tumor, immunotherapy may be effective in attacking small foci of cancer cells.
   b. Whereas surgery is directed toward larger primary tumors, immunotherapy can control small foci of metastatic disease at distant sites.
2. *Immunochemotherapy*
   a. Timing is critical in successfully combining immunotherapy with chemotherapy.
   b. Cancer chemotherapeutic drugs are often immunosuppressive, but certain chemotherapeutic

agents actually stimulate the immune response to some antigens.
3. *Immunoradiotherapy*
   a. A problem associated with chemotherapy and radiation therapy is that they attack normal cells as well as cancer cells; because of the selectivity of immunotherapy, it could logically be combined with these other modalities.
   b. If the patient is given tumor-specific antibodies that are attached to isotopes, large doses of radiation could be directed to tumor cells; this would combine the destructive effects of radiation with the specificity of immunotherapy.

CARE OF THE PATIENT WITH ADVANCED CANCER

Objectives of Nursing Management

A. *To halt the spread of the malignant growth.*

1. Prepare the patient for the prescribed modality of treatment: surgery, chemotherapy, or radiation.
2. Assist with diagnostic evaluation in an attempt to determine precise location(s) of involvement or spread.
3. Control local and generalized infections.
4. Promote optimum nutritional, fluid, and electrolyte levels by correcting deficiencies.
5. Provide the patient with psychosociological support.
   a. Listen to his concerns.
   b. Observe and support his reactions where appropriate.
   c. Explain the aspect of treatment that is pertinent at that time.
   d. Empathize with him and offer reassurance where appropriate.
6. Assist with the prescribed forms of therapy.

B. *To encourage the patient to pursue purposeful or diversional activities as long as possible.*

1. Invite him to participate socially, visit with other individuals, take walks, etc.
2. Provide opportunities for communication and mind-occupying activities.
   Accept him as an individual with natural defense mechanisms; encourage him to talk about himself, his concerns, his understanding, his future—even the possibility of dying.
3. Support the patient as he taps his spiritual resources.
4. Understand his behavioral deviations, even when socially unacceptable; when the episode passes, assist in restoring his self-esteem.
5. Empathize with him in an effort to show concern and understanding.
6. Include the patient's family in planning with him meaningful day-to-day activities.

C. *To promote comfort of the patient and relieve his pain.*

1. Assist the patient in bathing and with personal hygiene; personal cleanliness is a comfort measure.
2. Provide warmth when required; in cool seasons the debilitated patient is more sensitive to chilling.
3. Assist him as required in moving, turning, getting out of bed, walking, etc., in an effort to promote maximum activity and minimum amount of pain.
4. Evaluate objectively the nature of his pain (location,

duration, quality) and manner in which the patient tolerates or accepts it.
5. Convey the impression that his pain is understood and that relief is forthcoming.
6. Ascertain pain source—is it carcinoma-related? Is there some other physical source? Is is psychological?
7. Administer medications as specifically required:
   a. Sedative and hypnotics—to induce and promote sleep
      Assist patient in controlling his pain by allowing him a degree of independence in use of pain cocktails, such as Brompton's cocktail.
   b. Local anesthetics—for localized pain
   c. Ataractic drugs—for fear and apprehension
   d. Specific medications—for nausea and vomiting
   e. Muscle relaxant and antispasmodic drugs—to relieve tenseness
   f. Tranquilizers—to promote a sense of well-being
   g. Analgesics—for discomfort or pain
   h. Narcotics—for more intense pain

NURSING ALERT: Recognize that elderly debilitated patients have increased sensitivity: Avoid this cycle: a narcotic → drowsiness → less food and fluid → dehydration → nausea and vomiting → increased pain → more narcotic (and a resumption of the cycle).

8. Prepare the patient for surgical pain-relieving interventions.
   a. Percutaneous procedures: intrathecal alcohol injection, nerve block
   b. Localized radiotherapy
   c. Presacral neurectomy for visceral pain
   d. Sacral rhizotomy
   e. Midline myelotomy
   f. Hypophysectomy—transsphenoidal route
   g. Cordotomy for intractable pain
   h. Neurosurgical nerve interruption

D. *To cope with the annoying and discomforting side effects of radiation therapy.*

1. Radiation sickness
   a. Administer sedatives, antiemetics, and antihistamines as prescribed.

b. Encourage adequate fluid intake.

c. Tempt patient with small, frequent, high calorie, high protein feedings.

d. Record his reactions.

2. Skin reactions

a. Observe skin for dryness, tautness, erythema, desquamation.

b. Apply bland cream or oil to radiation site as directed.

c. Cleanse skin gently with bland soaps (Neutrogena) and lukewarm water.

d. Protect skin from sunlight, heat, trauma, constricting clothing.

e. Note changes such as telangiectasis (small network of dilated arterioles).

f. Offer medicated mouthwashes to soothe oral mucosa.

3. Diarrhea

a. Give antidiarrhea medications as prescribed.

b. Avoid serving foods that aggravate the problem, such as stewed prunes.

c. Provide suppositories as suggested.

d. Keep diet restricted to low residue or bland foods.

4. Blood cell depression

a. Protect the patient from injury and infection.

b. Observe for evidences of bleeding or infection and take measures to correct.

E. *To assist in overcoming bladder and bowel disturbances.*

1. Bladder frequency or incontinence

a. Keep an accurate input and output record.

b. Establish a bladder control program (see p. 76).

c. Maintain perineal cleanliness.

d. Insert an indwelling catheter if other measures fail.

2. Constipation

a. Maintain an adequate fluid level.

b. Omit constipating foods from diet—ensure adequate fruits and vegetables.

c. Administer glycerin suppository or mild laxative as prescribed.

> **NURSING ALERT:** Avoid giving enemas when patient has leukopenia or is taking drugs that irritate the intestinal tract (e.g., 5-fluorouracil).

F. *To maintain an intact skin and prevent tissue breakdown.*

1. Offer regular back and body massages; these can stimulate poor circulation and promote relaxation as well.

2. Ensure wrinkle-free, dry bedding—helps prevent skin breakdown in debilitated patients. Special mattress pads can be used.

3. Control skin breakdown following radiation treatment as indicated on page 853.

4. Maintain an exercise program utilizing range of motion activities.

5. Control edema of extremities by elevating the part as well as supporting it.

6. Initiate measures to prevent pressure sores (see p. 64).

G. *To control odors which tend to emanate from the affected tissues.*

1. Promote an esthetically comfortable environment.

2. Encourage good personal hygiene.

3. Irrigate external wounds with saline and use mechanical cleansers as prescribed (half strength hydrogen peroxide, diluted antiseptic detergents, etc.).

4. Remove soiled dressings promptly and change all soiled linens frequently—wrap dressings in paper and place in covered container immediately.

5. Provide fresh circulating air—use aerosol deodorants when necessary.

6. Change packing or pads frequently, irrigate thoroughly any affected body cavities and shave where hair presents a problem—mouth, nasal area, vagina, rectum.

7. Avoid dressing changes at inopportune times—visiting hours, meal times, etc.

H. *To anticipate and control hemorrhage.*

1. Monitor vital signs to detect increase in pulse rate and respiration and decrease in blood pressure.

2. Apply pressure, if active bleeding occurs, at convenient pressure points between the site and heart.

3. Employ emergency hemorrhage-control measures.

4. Note and record amount and nature of bleeding; notify physician

5. Reassure and comfort patient.

6. Use packing if bleeding involves accessible cavity, e.g., rectum, vagina.

7. Administer platelet or whole-blood transfusion.

8. Prepare patient for cauterization and ligation if necessary.

I. *To keep the patient at the optimum physical and psychological level of which he is capable.*

1. Provide a high calorie and high vitamin diet; cater to his personal food likes.

2. Offer between-meal feedings.

3. Change patient's environment if possible by encouraging him to walk and go outdoors.

4. Promote physical activities as much as possible; encourage rest periods.

5. Allow him to verbalize his feelings, thoughts; provide unhurried time for listening.

6. Maintain an optimistic atmosphere; limit the time plans to hour by hour or day by day (not week by week, month by month, or year by year).

J. *To assist patient as he strives for peace of mind in preparing for death. (See below.)*

PSYCHOSOCIAL SUPPORT OF THE DYING PATIENT

Reactions of the Patient to Dying*

A. *Stage of Denial*

1. Period of denial allows patient to mobilize his defenses.

   * Adapted from Kübler-Ross, E.: On Death and Dying. New York, Macmillan, 1970.

2. Patient will exhibit withdrawal and avoidance of subject of death.

3. Usually a temporary defense to be replaced in time by partial acceptance.

4. Patient may talk of death and then change topic abruptly.

5. Patient may be in a temporary state of shock.

B. *Stage of Anger*

1. Denial may be replaced by anger, rage, envy, and resentment.
2. Anger may be displaced and projected into environment.
   a. Anger frequently directed at hospital staff. (Avoid reacting personally to this anger.)
   b. Try to tolerate rational and irrational anger. Patient may experience considerable relief in expressing anger.

C. *Stage of Bargaining*

Bargaining is an attempt to postpone the inevitable and to extend life.

D. *Stage of Depression*

1. This is a stage in which the patient is preparing himself to accept the loss of everything and everyone he loves.
2. Patient may be undergoing anticipatory grief to prepare himself for the final separation; may mourn the loss of meaningful people in his life.
   a. Allow the patient to express his sorrow—helps make the final acceptance easier.
   b. Sit with the patient.
   c. Use touch therapy if appropriate.

E. *Stage of Acceptance*

1. Patient is neither depressed nor angry about his impending death; he bows to the sentence.
2. May contemplate his demise with quiet acceptance and expectation—detachment may make death easier.
3. During this stage, patient may be almost devoid of feelings—his circle of interest diminishes.
4. Patient will sleep and rest more—does not desire news or visitors from outside world.
5. Patient may just wish someone to hold his hand—reassures him that he is not forgotten.
6. Patient may reach the point where death comes as a relief.
7. Family may require more support during this stage.

Supportive Attitudes and Actions to the Patient, Family, and Health Team

OBJECTIVES: to allow the patient to live as fully as possible.
to relieve his discomfort and distress.
to be attuned to the special needs of the dying.
to help the patient achieve death with dignity.

A. *Physical Support of the Dying Patient*

See page 856.

B. *Emotional Support of the Dying Patient*

1. Make sure the patient has continuing, personal, and caring contacts—gives comfort and reassurance.
   a. Avoid changing personnel.
   b. Be willing to become involved with the patient—personal involvement is necessary if human interaction is to be supportive.
   c. Make sure the nursing approach reflects the mutuality of human interaction.
   d. Take *time* with the patient—gives him the feeling that he is being cared for.
   e. Do not withdraw from the presence of death.
2. Give the patient an opportunity to talk about himself, his illness, and his dying.
   a. Accept the patient as he is now.
   b. Be able to accept the patient's anger—whether overt anger or that expressed as depression.
   c. Encourage him to talk about changes made by his illness.
   d. Demonstrate interest in patient's total life style.
      (1) Learn what supports his ego and self-esteem.
      (2) Be accessible.
3. Allow the patient to act out his feelings without judgment.
   a. Understand that the patient is increasingly overwhelmed by feelings of rage, anger, fear, guilt, futility, despondency, and pain.
      (1) Understand the patient rather than judge him.
      (2) Demonstrate patience, tolerance, and support.
   b. Allow the patient to keep his hold on *hope*—hope is therapeutic and will help maintain the patient through his suffering.
      (1) Maintain hope with the patient.
      (2) Avoid reinforcing hope after the patient has given up (stage of acceptance).
   c. Understand the patient's dread of being deserted.
4. Be alert for behavioral changes—patient may be trying to communicate something.
   Anticipate that the patient's behavior will be altered by his deteriorating physical condition.
      (1) Withdrawal from customary interests
      (2) Impairment of self-esteem
5. Encourage the patient to retain confidence in his health team.
   a. Emphasize to the patient that he and the health team are in the battle together—patient will not be as fearful of loneliness, rejection, deceit.
   b. Reassure him that everything possible will be done for him.
   c. Let the patient know that he is respected and understood; treat him as a fellow human being.
   d. Seek the opinions of the patient—bolsters his self-esteem.
   e. Encourage the patient to take some initiative in his care.
   f. Keep the room neat and confusion at a minimum.
6. Help the patient who must undergo the "business" of dying.
   a. Settling of affairs, settling problems in human relationships, planning future for children, parent, spouse.
   b. Utilize services of chaplain, legal counselor, social worker, etc.
7. Pay attention to the patient's day-to-day complaints.
   a. Recognize the wide variety of symptoms accompanying anxiety—palpitation, nausea, insomnia, diarrhea, irritability.
   b. Be aware of the symptoms of depression—fatigue, lethargy, disturbances of sleep and appetite, inability to concentrate, psychomotor retardation.
   c. Try to alleviate each symptom.
   d. Reassure the patient that his pain will be relieved—helps the patient to cope with his discomfort.
   e. Give appropriate drugs to help the dying patient face death, cope with his anxiety and depression, and alter his sensitivity to pain.
   f. Help make each day as good a day as possible.

C. *Support of the Family of the Dying Patient*

Anticipatory grief—mourning that occurs over an extended period of time before actual death:

Bereavement starts when one realizes that loss is inevitable.

Family experiences awareness of loss and depression.

Family may begin to adapt, physically and psychologically, to the consequences of death.

1. Understand that the family may be undergoing anticipatory mourning and reacting to anticipated loss.
   a. Recognize that various family members behave differently while working out their anticipatory grief.
      (1) Avoid showing disapproval of the behavior of others—may produce feelings of shame, guilt, and inadequacy.
      (2) Understand that family members may feel guilty when they are unable to demonstrate grief—there may be little or no feeling at actual time of death because family members have worked through their grief during the anticipatory period.
      (3) Family may withdraw emotional investment from the patient as they perceive he has no future.
   b. Be alert for untoward reactions to death—family member may need supportive therapy and counseling.
2. Accept the feelings and attitudes of the family— helps avoid mutual hostility and recriminations.
   Feelings include:
      (1) Fear and anxiety
      (2) Sorrow and grief
      (3) Overt or suppressed hostility interwoven with guilt feelings; self blame
      (4) Ambivalent feelings toward dying member
      (5) Overprotective attitude
      (6) Depersonalization
      (7) Projection of guilt to medical personnel
      (8) Submission or excessive courtesy—may mask hostility
3. Realize the problems faced by the family—anticipated separation of loved one, financial problems, disruption of family life, problems of communication.
4. Demonstrate concern for the family.
   a. Inform them of practical help—financial assistance, social worker, other supporting services of local helping agencies.
   b. Reassure family that they will not be left alone.
   c. Provide opportunity for family member to ventilate his conflicts—anger, depression, victimization by illness.

D. *Support of the Health Team*

1. Examine your own attitudes and ability to face terminal illness and death.
   a. Look at possessions and relationships in context of inevitability of death.
   b. Plan for disaster and death.
2. Monitor your own feelings.
   a. Accept the ideas of denial, fear, and guilt.
   b. Assess and correct one's own biases and fears.
   c. Watch emotional responses to challenges of incurable disease and "difficult" families.
3. Do not withdraw from the presence of death.
   a. Face the reality of the dying patient.
   b. Become skilled and sensitive in the art of human interaction.

BIBLIOGRAPHY

Books

Burgess ML and Mangan HM (eds). The Challenge of Cancer Nursing (booklet). U.S. Dept HEW, Pub. No. (NIH) 79–760, 1979

Blumberg B, Flaherty M, Lewis J (eds). Coping with Cancer. A Resource for the Health Professional. U.S. Dept Health and Human Services. NIH Pub No. 80–2080, Sept 1980

Cancer Information Clearinghouse. Coping with Cancer. An annotated Bibliography of Public, Patient, and Professional Information and Education Materials. U.S. Dept HEW, NIH Pub No. 80–2129, May 1980

Carter SK, Bakowski, Hellman K. Chemotherapy of Cancer, 2nd ed. New York, John Wiley & Sons, 1981

Cassileth BR. The Cancer Patient. Philadelphia, Lea & Febiger, 1979

Clark RL and Hickey RC (eds). 1980 Year Book of Cancer. New York, Year Book Medical Publishers, 1980

Cline MJ and Haskel C. Cancer Chemotherapy, 3rd ed. Philadelphia, WB Saunders, 1980

Committee on Hazardous Substances in the Laboratory, National Research Council Assembly of Mathematical and Physical Sciences. Prudent Practices for Handling Hazardous Chemicals in Laboratories. Washington, D.C., National Academy Press, 1981

Cooper JS and Pizzarello DJ. Concepts in Cancer Care. Philadelphia, Lea & Febiger, 1980

Dietz JH. Rehabilitation Oncology. New York, John Wiley & Sons, 1981

Dorr RT and Fritz WL. Cancer Chemotherapy Handbook. New York, Elsevier, 1980

Fletcher GH. Textbook of Radiotherapy, 3rd ed. Philadelphia, Lea & Febiger, 1980

Germain CPH. A Cancer Unit: An Ethnography. Wakefield, Nursing Resources, 1979

Kellogg CJ and Sullivan BP (eds). Current Perspectives in Oncologic Nursing. St. Louis, CV Mosby, 1978

Kopf AW et al. Malignant Melanoma. New York, Masson, 1979

Leahy IM, St. Germain JM, Varricchio CG. The Nurse and Radiotherapy. St. Louis, CV Mosby, 1979

Kokich JJ. Clinical Cancer Medicine. Boston, GK Hall, 1980

Marino LB. Cancer Nursing. St. Louis, CV Mosby, 1980

McCalla J (ed). Laminar Air Flow (Pamphlet—Nursing Dept. Clinical Center). U.S. Dept HEW, Pub. No. (NIH) 79–907, 1979

Outcome Standards for Cancer Nursing Practice (booklet). Oncology Nursing Society and ANA Division on Medical–Surgical Nursing Practice, 1979

Proceedings of the Nursing Mirror International Cancer Nursing Conference. Nursing Mirror. New York, Masson, 1979

Simonton OC, Mathews-Simonton C, Creighton J. Getting Well Again—A Step-by-Step, Self-Help Guide to Overcoming Cancer for Patients and Their Families. Los Angeles, JP Tarcher, 1978

Smith E. A Comprehensive Approach to Rehabilitation of the Cancer Patient. New York, McGraw-Hill, 1976

Smith E. Psychosocial Aspects of Cancer Patient Care. New York, McGraw-Hill, 1976

Tache J, Selye CC, Day SB. Cancer, Stress, and Death. New York, Plenum Medical Books, 1979

Articles

General

Baird SB. Economic realities in the treatment and care of the cancer patient. Top Clin Nurs 1981 Jan; 2(4):67–80

Barber J and Gitelson J. Cancer pain: Psychological management using hypnosis. CA—A Cancer Jour for Clinic 1980 May/June; 30(3):130–142

Beck S. Impact of a systematic oral care protocol on stomatitis after chemotherapy. Cancer Nurs 1979 June; 2(3):185–199

Butler RN and Gastel B. Aging and cancer management. Part II: Research perspectives. CA—A Cancer Jour for Clinic 1979 Dec; 29(6):333–340

Butler JH. Nutrition and cancer: A review of the literature. Cancer Nurs 1980 April; 3(2):131–136

Daeffler R. Oral hygiene measures for patients with cancer. Cancer Nurs 1980 Oct; 3(5):347–356.

Daeffler R. Oral hygiene measures for patients with cancer. Cancer Nurs 1980 Dec; 3(6):427–432

Davis A. Brompton's cocktail: Making good-bye's possible. Am J Nurs 1978 April; 78(4):610–612

Dietz JH. Adaptive rehabilitation in cancer. Postgrad Med 1980 July; 68(1):145–153

Diggory G and Tiffany R. The use of Entonox in the relief of pain. Cancer Nurs 1979 Aug; 2(4):279–282

Epting SP. Coping with stress through peer support. Top Clin Nurs 1981 Jan; 2(4):47–59

Fagan–Dubin L. Causes of cancer. Cancer Nurs 1979 Dec; 2(6):435–441

Friedman BD. Coping with cancer: A guide for health care professionals. Cancer Nurs 1980 April; 3(2):105–110

Frytak S. Is THC an effective antiemetic for cancer patients? CA—A Cancer Jour for Clinic 1980 Sept/Oct; 30(5):278–282

Garfinkel L, Poindexter CE, Silverberg E. Cancer in black Americans. CA—A Cancer Jour for Clinic 1980 Jan/Feb; 30(1):39–44

Gever LN. Brompton's mixture. Nursing '80 1980 May; 10(5):57

Government says cancer rate is increasing? Science 1980 Aug 29; 209:998–1002

Herzoff NE. A therapeutic group for cancer patients and their families. Cancer Nurs 1979 Dec; 2(6):469–474

Holland J. Understanding the cancer patient. CA—A Cancer Jour for Clinic 1980 Mar/Apr; 30(2):103–112

Hunter G and Johnson SH. Physical support systems for the homebound oncology patient. Oncol Nurs Forum 1980 Summer; 7(3):21–23

Jones LS, Miller NH, Wegmann J. Organizing cancer inpatient care: Scattered-bed versus oncology unit approach. Oncol Nurs Forum 1981 Winter; 8(1):31–36

Lewis KP. Pain cocktails. Nurses' Drug Alert 1980 Aug; 4(10):76–77

Lipman AG. Drug therapy in cancer pain. Cancer Nurs 1980 Feb; 3(1):39–46

Manchester PB. The adolescent with cancer; Concerns for care. Top Clin Nurs 1981 Jan; 2(4):31–37

Maxwell MD. How to use methadone for the cancer patient's pain. Am Nurs 1980 Sept; 80(9):1606–1609

Maxwell MD. Cancer and suicide. Cancer Nurs 1980 Feb; 3(1):33–38

McGuire DB. Familial cancer and the role of the nurse. Cancer Nurs 1979 Dec; 2(6):443–452

Megliola B. Multiple myeloma. Cancer Nurs 1980 June; 3(3):209–218

Oleske D. Questions about cancer: Indicator for patient education. Top Clin Nurs 1981 Jan; 2(4):1–8

Peterson BA and Kennedy BJ. Aging and cancer management. Part I, Clinical observations. CA—A Cancer Jour for Clinic 1979 Dec; 29(6):322–332

Public attitudes toward cancer and cancer tests. CA—A Cancer Jour for Clinic 1980 Mar/Apr; 30(2):92–98

Rovinski CA. Nurses and cancer's seven warning signals. Cancer Nurs 1980 Feb; 3(1):53–55

Seipp CA et al. In search of an effective antiemetic (marijuana research). Cancer Nurs 1980 Aug; 3(4):271–276

Silberman H. Hyperalimentation in patients with cancer. Surg Gynecol Obstet 1980 May; 150(5):755–757

Target: Cancer. The Harvard Med School Letter 1980 April, 5(6):1–5

Two professions—two perspectives. Nursing '79 1979 Sept; 9(9):35–38

Welch D. Hi-protein nutritional supplement. Oncol Nurs Forum 1980 Summer; 7(3):24

Cancer Chemotherapy

Adrian RM, Hood AF, Skarin AT. Mucocutaneous reactions to antineoplastic agents. CA—A Cancer Jour for Clinic 1980 May/June; 30(3):143–157

Barlock A, Howair D, Hubbard S. Nursing management of adriamycin extravasation. CA—A Cancer Jour for Clinic 1980 Sept/Oct; 30(5):256–259

Cancer chemotherapy. The Harvard Med School Health Letter 1980 June; 5(8):3–4

Cancer chemotherapy. Patient Care 1979 Oct 15; 13(17):25–123

Fairchild W et al. The incidence of bladder cancer after cyclophosphamide therapy. Urol 1979 Aug; 122(8):163–164

Gever LN. Cisplatin—a break-through for the cancer patient. A nursing challenge for you. Nursing '80 1980 Dec; 10(12):53

Gormican A. Influencing food acceptance in anorexic cancer patients. Postgrad Med 1980 Aug; 68(2):145–152

Gray JC et al. Quick cancer screen. RN 1980 Jan; 43(1):44–50

Hussar DA. New antineoplastic agents. Drug Ther 1979 Nov; 9(11):119–122

Kaempfer SH. The effects of cancer chemotherapy on reproduction: A review of the literature. Oncol Nurs Forum 1981 Winter; 9(1):11–18

Kennedy M et al. Chemotherapy related nausea and vomiting: A survey to identify problems and interventions. Oncol Nurs Forum 1981 Winter; 8(1):19–22

Knowles R and Virden J. Handling of injectable antineoplastic agents. Br Med J 1980 Aug 30; 2:589–591

Law D. Successful chemotherapy: Quality care for the cancer patient. Can Nurse 1980 Feb; 76(2):19–22

Levitt DZ. Cancer chemotherapy. RN 1980 June; 43(6):53–56; 1980 Aug; 43(8):57–60; 1980 Sept; 43(9):51–54; 1980 Dec; 43(12):33–37, 112

Marihuana for nausea and vomiting due to cancer chemotherapy. The Med Letter 1980 May 16; 22(10):41–43

McKusick BC. Prudent practices for handling hazardous chemicals in laboratories. Science 1981 Feb 20; 211(4484):777–780

Ostchega Y. Preventing and treating cancer chemotherapy's oral complications. Nursing '80 1980 Aug; 10(8):47–52

Satterwhite BE. What to do when adriamycin infiltrates. Nursing '80 1980 Feb; 10(2):37

Todres R and Wojtiuk R. The cancer patient's view of chemotherapy. Cancer Nurs 1979 Aug; 2(4):283–286

Immunotherapy

Benjamini E and Rennick DM. Cancer immunotherapy: Facts and fancy. CA—A Cancer Jour for Clinic 1979 Dec; 29(6):362–370

Cox KO and Em M. Immunology. Immunotherapy II. Cancer Nurs 1980 Aug; 3(4):307–321

Em M. Immunity. Basic concepts (Programmed instruction). Cancer Nurs 1980 Feb; 3(1):59–68

Em M. Immunology. Immunotherapy (Programmed instruction). Cancer Nurs 1980 June; 3(3):229–238

Em M. Immunology. Bone marrow transplantation (Programmed instruction). Cancer Nurs 1980 Oct; 3(5):387–400

Koren ME and Herrmann CS. Cancer immunotherapy: What, why, when, how? Nursing '81 1981 Jan; 11(1):37–41

McKhann C. Cancer immunotherapy; A realistic appraisal. CA—A Cancer Jour for Clinic 1980 Sept/Oct; 30(5):286–293

Radiation/Radiotherapy

Champagne EE and Kane NE. Teaching program for patients receiving interstitial radioactive Iodine[125] for cancer of the prostate. Oncol Nurs Forum 1980 Winter; 7(1):12–15

Dietz K. Radiation therapy (Programmed instruction). Cancer Nurs 1979 June; 2(3):233–244

Gillick KM. Radiation therapy. Internal radiation. (Programmed instruction). Cancer Nurs 1979 Aug; 2(4): 313–325

Gunn WB. Radiation therapy for the aging patient. CA—A Cancer Jour for Clinic 1980 Nov/Dec; 30(6):337–347

Haylock PJ and Hart LK. Fatigue in patients receiving localized radiation. Cancer Nurs 1979 Dec; 2(6):461–467

Isler C. Could you cope with a nuclear accident? RN 1979 June; 42(6):66–77

Kelly PP and Tinsley C. Planning care for the patient receiving external radiation. Am J Nurs 1981 Feb; 81(2):338–342

Land CE. Estimating cancer risks from low doses of ionizing radiation. Science 1980 Sept 12; 209:1997–1203

Steinfeld AD. Radiation oncology. Am Fam Physician 1980 April; 21(4):131–138

Varricchio CG. The patient on radiation therapy. Am J Nurs 1981 Feb; 81(2):334–337

Warren S. Effects of radiation on normal tissues. CA—A Cancer Jour for Clinic 1980 Nov/Dec; 30(6):350–355

Welch DA. Assessment of nausea and vomiting in cancer patients undergoing external beam radiotherapy. Cancer Nurs 1980 Oct; 3(5):365–371

ADVANCED CANCER AND DEATH

Books

Cohen KP. Hospice—Prescription for Terminal Care. Germantown, Md, Aspen Systems Corp, 1979

Kübler–Ross E. Death. The Final Stage of Growth. Englewood Cliffs, Prentice–Hall, 1975

McGrail JH. Fighting Back: One Woman's Struggle Against Cancer. New York, Harper & Row, 1979

Ryan C and Ryan KM. A Private Battle. New York, Simon & Schuster, 1979

Stoddard S. The Hospice Movement: A Better Way of Caring for the Dying Patient. New York, Vantage Books, 1979

Articles

Friel M and Tehan CB. Counteracting burn-out for the hospice care-giver. Cancer Nurs 1980 Aug; 3(4):285–293

Liaschenko JM. Assessment of anxiety and depression in the dying patient. Top Clin Nurs 1981 Jan; 2(4):39–45

McGinty C and Weinstein L. Care of the terminally ill. Cancer Nurs 1979 Dec; 2(6):491–492

Wald FS. Terminal care and nursing education. Am J Nurs 1979 Oct; 79(10): 1762–1764

Welch D. Nursing the patient with advanced liver metastasis. Cancer Nurs 1979 Aug; 2(4):297–304

EMERGENCY NURSING

EMERGENCY MANAGEMENT*

Emergency management has traditionally referred to the care given to patients with urgent and critical needs. However, the philosophy of emergency care has broadened to include the concept that an emergency is whatever the patient or his family considers it to be.

Principles of Assessment and Emergency Management

Underlying consideration: Injuries or conditions interfering with vital physiologic function take precedence. Treat the potentially life-threatening problems first.

OBJECTIVES: to preserve life.
  to prevent deterioration before definitive treatment can be given.
  to restore patient to useful living.

---

* This section will deal mainly with emergency management of trauma and other conditions not found elsewhere in this book. Management of acute heart conditions is found on page 263 and management of acute respiratory problems on page 169.

1. Maintain a patent airway, employing resuscitation measures when necessary.
     Assess for chest injuries with subsequent airway obstruction.
2. Control hemorrhage and its consequences.
3. Evaluate and restore cardiac output.
4. Prevent and treat shock; maintain or restore effective circulation.
5. Carry out a rapid and ongoing physical examination; the clinical course of the injured or seriously ill patient is not static.
6. Protect wounds with sterile dressings.
7. Splint suspected fractures, including fractures of cervical spine in patients with head injuries.
8. Check to see if patient has a Medic Alert or similar identification designating allergies, etc.
9. Start a flow sheet of patient's vital signs, blood pressure, etc., to guide decision making.

Obtaining Data (History)

If possible, a brief history of the accident/illness is taken from the patient or the person accompanying him—relative, emergency medical technician.

1. What were the circumstances, forces, location, and time of injury?
2. When did the symptoms appear?
3. How did the patient reach the hospital?
4. What was the health status of the patient before the accident or illness?
5. Is there a past history of illness? of past admissions?
6. Is patient currently taking any medications—especially hormones, insulin, digitalis, anticoagulants?
7. Does he have any allergies?
8. Does he have any bleeding tendencies?
9. Is he under a physician's care? (Name of physician.)
10. When did he eat his last meal? (Important if an anesthetic is to be given.)
11. What was the date of the patient's most recent tetanus immunization?

Psychological Management of Patients and Families in Emergencies

Underlying Consideration: Body trauma is an insult to physiological and psychological homeostasis; it requires both physiologic and psychologic healing.

OBJECTIVE: to prevent psychological incapacity following trauma.

A. *Approach to the Patient*

1. Understand and accept the basic anxieties of the acutely traumatized patient. Be aware of the patient's fear of death, mutilation, and isolation.
   a. Personalize the situation as much as possible—speak, react, and respond in a warm manner.
   b. Give explanations on a level that the patient can grasp—an informed patient can cope with psychologic/physiologic stress in a more positive manner.
   c. Accept the rights of the patient and family to have and display their own feelings.
   d. Maintain a calm and reassuring manner—helps emotionally distressed patient or family to mobilize their psychological resources.
2. Understand and support the patient's feelings concerning his loss of control (emotional, physical, and intellectual).
3. Treat the unconscious patient as if he were conscious—touch him, call him by name, and explain every procedure that is done. Avoid making negative comments about the patient's condition.
   a. Orient patient to person, time, and place as soon as he is conscious; reinforce by repeating this information.
   b. Bring patient back to reality in a calm and reassuring way.
   c. Encourage family, when possible, to orient patient to reality.
4. Be prepared to handle all aspects of acute trauma; know what to expect and what to do—alleviates nurse's anxieties and increases patient's confidence.

B. *Approach to the Family*

1. Inform the family where the patient is and give as much information as possible about the treatment he is receiving.
2. Recognize the anxiety of the family and allow them to talk about their feelings—allow expressions of remorse, anger, guilt, and criticism.
3. Allow the family to relive the events, actions, and feelings preceding admission to the emergency department.
4. Deal with reality as gently and quickly as possible; avoid encouraging and supporting denial.
5. Assist the family to cope with sudden and unexpected death. Some helpful measures include the following:
   a. Take the family to a private place.
   b. Talk to all of the family together—so that they can mourn together.
   c. Assure family that everything possible was done; inform them of the treatment rendered.
   d. Avoid using euphemisms such as "passed on," etc. Show the family that you care by touching, offering coffee, etc.
   e. Allow family to talk about the deceased and what he meant to them—permits ventilation of feelings of loss. Encourage family to talk about events preceding admission to the emergency department. Encourage family to support each other and to express emotions freely: grief, loss, anger, helplessness, tears, disbelief.
   f. Avoid volunteering unnecessary information (patient was drinking, etc.).
   g. Avoid giving sedation to family members—may mask or delay the grieving process which is necessary to achieve emotional equilibrium and prevent prolonged depression.
   h. Encourage family members to view the body if they wish to do so—helps to integrate the loss (cover mutilated areas).
      (1) Go with family to see the body.
      (2) Show acceptance of the body—by touching—to give family "permission" to touch, talk to, etc. the body.
      (3) Spend a few minutes with the family, listening to them.
6. Encourage the emergency department staff to discuss among themselves their reaction to the event—to share intense feelings, for review, and for group support.

CARDIOPULMONARY RESUSCITATION AND AIRWAY MANAGEMENT

Cardiopulmonary resuscitation is described in the Guidelines which follow. Artificial ventilation is also accomplished by a bag-mask unit (p. 180) or tracheal intubation (p. 186). Cricothyroidotomy (p. 869) and esophageal obturator airway (p. 870) are used in certain emergencies for resuscitation. The management of foreign-body obstruction is included on pages 867 and 869. Airway management and artificial ventilation are discussed in detail under Respiratory Insufficiency and Failure, Chapter 7, page 169.

GUIDELINES: Cardiopulmonary Resuscitation for Cardiac or Respiratory Arrest*

Cardiac arrest is a sudden and unexpected cessation of the heartbeat and effective circulation that results in inadequate delivery of oxygenated blood to vital organs.

Causes

1. Cardiac arrest
   Ventricular fibrillation
   Ventricular standstill
   Cardiovascular collapse

2. Respiratory arrest
   Drowning
   Stroke
   Heart attack
   Airway obstruction
   Drug overdose
   Electrocution
   Suffocation
   Accident/Injury
   Head trauma

Signs and Symptoms

1. Absence of palpable carotid or femoral pulse; pulselessness in large arteries
2. Immediate loss of consciousness
3. Absence of breath sounds or air movement through nose or mouth
4. Ashen gray color

Purpose

1. To establish effective circulation and respiration promptly for a victim of cardiac or respiratory arrest through cardiopulmonary resuscitation.
2. To prevent irreversible cerebral anoxic damage.

Equipment

Trained personnel
Arrest board
Oral airway
Bag and mask device

IV setup
Defibrillator
Emergency cardiac drugs
ECG machine

ABCs of CPR* (Fig. 22-1)

1. Airway
   Open the airway
   Determine whether patient is breathing (look, listen, feel)
2. Breathing
   Rescue breathing (mouth to mouth)
   Foreign-body airway obstruction
3. Circulation
   Establish presence or absence of pulse
   Active emergency medical services (EMS)
   Begin chest compression (if pulse absent)

Procedure

NURSING ACTION	RATIONALE/AMPLIFICATION
Performance Phase	
1. Note the time as soon as the cardiac/respiratory arrest is determined. Summon help immediately. Place the patient in a horizontal position on a firm surface.	**NURSING ALERT:** Lack of effective circulation to the central nervous system for more than 3–5 minutes may result in irreversible brain damage.
2. When a monitored patient undergoes cardiac arrest, deliver a precordial thump (a single, sharp blow over the mid-portion of the sternum) using the fleshy part of the fist and striking from a distance of 20.3–30.5 cm. (8–12 inches) above the chest. Then proceed with defibrillation, intubation, etc., as required.	2. The precordial thump is useful when the pulse cannot be detected following a witnessed cardiac arrest or when dealing with a patient who is being monitored or is being paced for a known AV block. The precordial thump should be administered within the first minute after cardiac arrest; it produces a small electrical stimulus.
ARTIFICIAL VENTILATION	
1. Open the airway. Move the lower jaw forward; this is done as follows: a. *Head Tilt* (1) Place one hand on victim's forehead and apply firm, backward pressure with the palm OR	1. Moving the lower jaw forward lifts the tongue off the back wall of the pharynx and opens the airway. (1) This maneuver produces maximal backward tipping of the head.

* Adapted from "Standards and Guidelines for Cardiopulmonary Resuscitation (CPR) and Emergency Cardiac Care (ECC)." JAMA 1980 Aug 1; 244 (5), pp 453–509.

Cardiopulmonary Resuscitation (CPR)

(Basic Life Support—Adult)

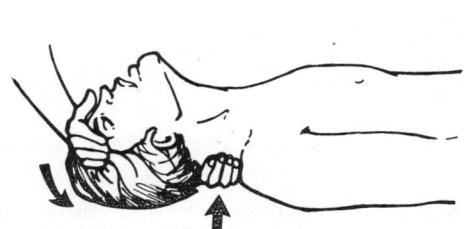 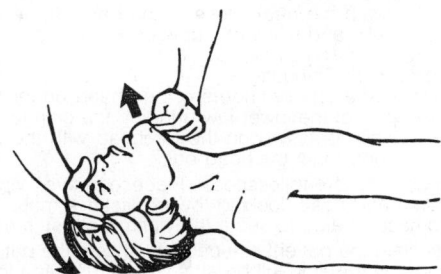

Airway

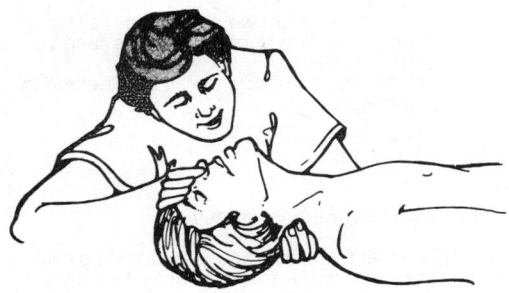 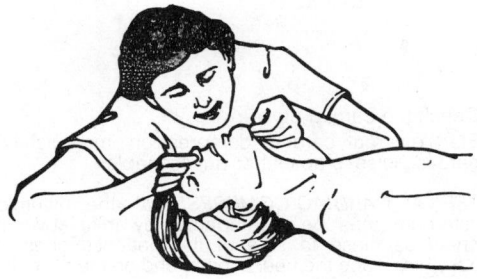

Breathing

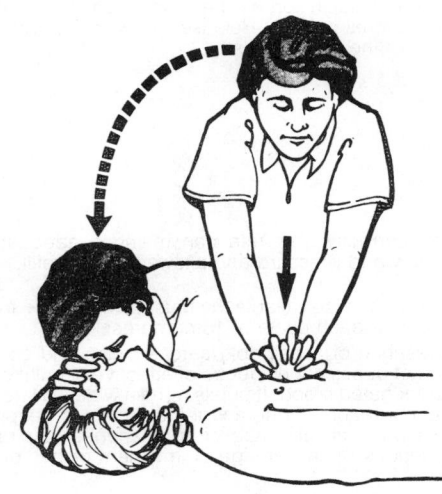 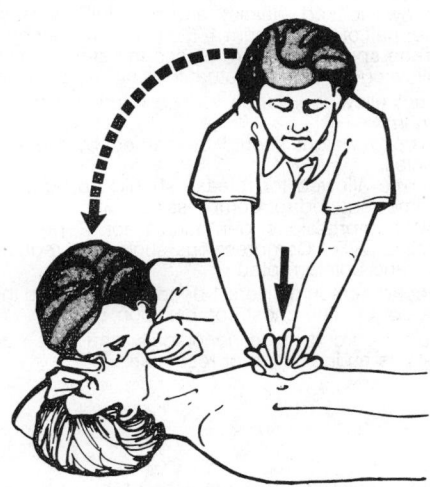

Circulation

FIGURE 22-1. *Cardiopulmonary resuscitation. (Reprinted from the Supplement to Journal of the American Medical Association, August 1, 1980. Copyright 1980, the American Medical Association. Reprinted with permission from the American Heart Association.)*

GUIDELINES: Cardiopulmonary Resuscitation for Cardiac or Respiratory Arrest (cont.)

Procedure (cont.)

NURSING ACTION	RATIONALE/AMPLIFICATION

b. *Head Tilt-Neck Lift*
  (1) Place one hand on victim's forehead (to apply backward pressure) and the other hand beneath the neck close to the back of the head to lift and support it upward.
OR
c. *Head Tilt-Chin Lift*
  (1) Place tips of fingers of one hand under bony part of the lower jaw bringing the chin forward while pressing on the forehead with the other hand to tilt the head back.	

2. Check for breathlessness. Place ear over victim's mouth and nose, looking toward victim's mouth and stomach. Watch to see if the victim's chest is rising.	2. If the chest is rising; the lungs are being ventilated.
3. Ventilate the patient if necessary. Inflate the patient's lungs by 4 quick, full breaths without allowing for full lung deflation between beats.	3. Forceful ventilation helps maintain positive pressure in the airway and helps overcome airway obstruction by increasing the pressure gradient of air movement and dilating the upper airway.
a. Pinch the nostrils closed with the thumb and index finger of the hand that is on the forehead.	a. To prevent air from escaping.

b. Take a deep breath, open mouth wide; and place it outside of the victim's mouth, making a tight seal.	b. Adequate ventilation is determined by:
	  (1) Seeing the chest rise and fall.
	  (2) Feeling in your own airway the resistance and compliance of the victim's lungs as they expand.
	  (3) Hearing and feeling the air escape during exhalation.

4. Check the carotid pulse.	
5. Start external cardiac compression immediately if carotid pulse is absent or questionable.	

EXTERNAL CARDIAC COMPRESSION—the rhythmic application of pressure over the lower half of the sternum (must be accompanied by artificial ventilation.)

NURSING ACTION	RATIONALE/AMPLIFICATION
1. Kneel as close to side of the patient's chest as possible. Place the heel of one hand on the lower half of the sternum 3.8 cm (1½ inches) from the tip of the xiphoid.	1. Proper placement of the hands reduces possible complications of fractured ribs or injury to adjacent abdominal organs. The heart is located to the left of the middle of the chest between the lower sternum and spine.
2. Place the other hand on top of the first one, with the fingers of both hands directed away from the rescuer.	2. The fingers may be either extended or interlaced but should not touch the chest wall.
3. Using your weight while keeping the arms straight and elbows locked, quickly and forcefully depress the lower half of the sternum 4–5 cm. (1½ to 2 inches) toward the spine, and then release the sternal pressure; allowing the chest to return to its normal position.	3. Each compression forces the blood from the heart into the arterial system. Release following compression allows the heart to rest.
a. Do not allow the hands to lose contact with the sternum.	
b. The body weight should be carried by the arm muscles.	
c. The time allowed for release should be equal to the time required for compression.	
4. Use 60 compressions per minute for 2 persons performing CPR.* Compressions should be regular, smooth, and uninterrupted.	4. If done correctly, this rate can maintain adequate blood flow and pressure and allows cardiac refill.
5. The second person delivers 1 deep breath during the upstroke of the fifth chest compression.	5. If only 1 person is available, he must give 2 quick, full breaths after each cycle of 15 compressions.
6. Palpate for carotid pulse periodically and note size of pupils as an indication of response.	6. The presence of a palpable carotid pulse and constriction of pupils are evidence of effective circulation and oxygenated blood. If pupils remain widely dilated and do not react to light, and if the patient is deeply unconscious with absence of spontaneous respirations, serious brain damage is imminent or has occurred.
7. Insert an artificial airway, endotracheal tube, or esophageal airway as soon as possible.	7. This keeps the airway patent and prevents aspiration.

* This procedure is done best by 2 persons. If only 1 person is available, he must perform both artificial ventilation and external cardiac compression, using a 15:2 ratio consisting of 2 quick lung inflations after each 15 chest compressions. The single rescuer must perform each series of chest compressions at a faster rate of 80 compressions per minute because of interruptions for lung inflation.

Procedure (cont.)

NURSING ACTION	RATIONALE/AMPLIFICATION
DEFINITIVE THERAPY	
1. While resuscitation proceeds, simultaneous efforts are made to start an intravenous infusion. Have suction ready and attach ECG electrodes to the patient.	1. An IV line provides access to the circulation for drugs/solutions.
2. Continue to assess status of pulses (palpable carotid pulse/femoral pulse) and spontaneous respiratory movement.	
3. Initiate hemodynamic monitoring.	
4. Monitor ECG. Stabilize rhythm.	
5. Draw arterial blood gases.	5. To determine oxygenation and acid base status.
6. Correct electrolyte and acid base abnormalities.	6. Tissue anoxia from cardiac arrest leads to metabolic acidosis. Sodium bicarbonate (IV) will correct acidosis.
7. The decision to terminate resuscitation is a medical one and takes into consideration the cerebral and cardiac status. Cardiac compression should continue until the patient can maintain blood pressure, etc., or the situation becomes hopeless.	7. If ventricular fibrillation occurs, conversion to a normal sinus rhythm must be effected by electric countershock delivered by a defibrillator.
8. Place the patient in an intensive care unit.	**NURSING ALERT:** The patient who has been resuscitated is at risk for another episode of cardiac arrest.

GUIDELINES: Management of Foreign-Body Airway Obstruction*

Foreign-body obstruction of the airway may be either partial or complete.

Assessment of Clinical Manifestations

Weak, ineffective cough; high-pitched noises on inspiration
Respiratory distress
Inability to speak or breathe
Cyanosis; collapse

Emergency Management

NURSING ACTION	RATIONALE/AMPLIFICATION
1. Carry out a sequence of back blows, manual thrusts, and finger sweeps.	
Back Blows	
a. Administer 4 sharp blows with the heel of the hand over the spine between the shoulder blades while supporting the patient with the other hand on the sternum.	a. Apply the back blows forcefully in rapid succession; they may be administered with the victim sitting, standing or lying.
b. If possible, have patient's head lower than his chest.	
Manual Thrusts	
Abdominal thrust for standing patient:	
a. Stand behind patient and wrap your arms around his waist. The rescuer's arms should be just above the belt line.	a. Manual thrusts to the upper abdomen (abdominal thrust) or lower chest (chest thrust) force air out of the lungs and create an artificial cough intended to remove the foreign body.
b. Make a fist with one hand and grasp the fist with your other hand. Place thumb side of your fist against the patient's abdomen between the waist and the rib cage (Fig. 22-2).	
c. Press your fist 4 times into the patient's abdomen with a quick inward-upward thrust.	c. A combination of back blows and manual thrusts may be effective in removing obstruction.
For lying (unconscious) patient:	
a. Position the patient on his back.	
b. Sit astride the patient's hips, facing his head; with one of your hands on top of the other, place the heel of the bottom hand on the patient's abdomen between the waist and rib cage.	b. Spleen or liver injury may result from sudden increase of abdominal pressure.
c. Press into the abdomen with an inward and upward thrust.	

* Adapted from "Standards and Guidelines for Cardiopulmonary Resuscitation (CPR) and Emergency Cardiac Care (ECC)." JAMA 1980 Aug. 1; 244(5): 464–467.

GUIDELINES: Management of Foreign-Body Airway Obstruction (cont.)

Emergency Management (cont.)

NURSING ACTION

RATIONALE/AMPLIFICATION

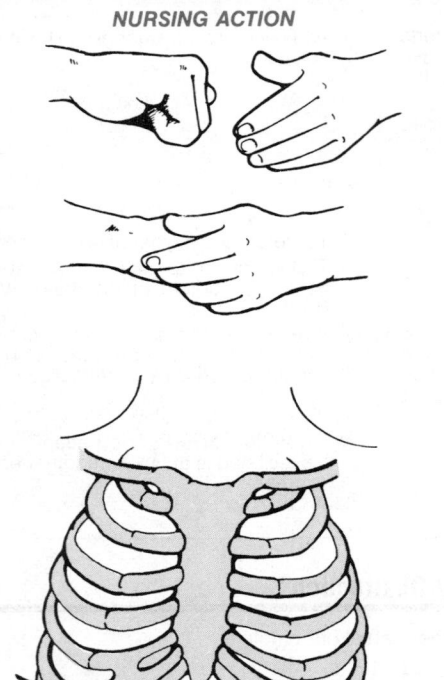

FIGURE 22-2. *Hand placement for abdominal thrusts. (Reprinted from the Supplement to Journal of the American Medical Association, August 1, 1980. Copyright 1980, the American Medical Association. Reprinted with permission from the American Heart Association.)*

Chest Thrust
   a. Stand behind the victim with your arms under his axillae and encircling his chest.
   b. Place the thumb side of your fist on the middle of his breast bone.
   c. Grasp your fist with your other hand and exert four backward thrusts.

2. Apply the finger sweep.
   a. Open patient's mouth by grasping both the tongue and lower jaw between your thumb and fingers and lift the tongue and jaw.
   b. Sweep your index finger inside the patient's mouth using a hooking action to dislodge and remove foreign body.
   c. If patient is still unconscious, attempt to ventilate with mouth-to-mouth ventilation; repeat back blows, manual thrusts, and finger sweep.

a. Chest thrust is an alternate technique.

b. Avoid the xiphoid process and the margins of the rib cage.
c. Each thrust is performed with the intent of relieving the obstruction without having to complete the full series.

a. This maneuver draws the tongue away from the back of the pharynx and the obstructing foreign body.

c. During unconsciousness, muscles relax and these maneuvers may become more effective.

GUIDELINES: Heimlich Maneuver for Upper Airway Obstruction

The *Heimlich maneuver* is a procedure designed to dislodge a food bolus (or other foreign body) located in the base of the throat so that it occludes the airway. Choking on food (café coronary) is the 6th leading cause of accidental death in the U.S.

Clinical Manifestations

(Vary according to cause and *rapidity* of onset)
1. Inability to speak or breathe
2. Paleness—deep cyanosis
3. Collapse—death occurs in 4–5 minutes.

Procedure

NURSING ACTION*	RATIONALE/AMPLIFICATION
1. Stand behind the patient and wrap your arms around his waist.	1. The rescuer's arms should be just above the belt line. The patient's head, arms and upper torso are allowed to hang forward.
2. Make a fist with 1 hand and grasp the fist with your other hand. Place the thumb side of your fist against the patient's abdomen slightly above the navel and below the rib cage.	
3. Press your fist into the patient's abdomen with a quick upward thrust.	3. This action produces a sudden sharp rise in intra-thoracic pressure which will eject the bolus or foreign object that is occluding the airway.
4. This action may be repeated several times.	4. Have a second person prepared to remove the foreign body from the mouth if necessary.
If the patient is sitting:	
1. Stand behind the patient's chair and perform the maneuver in the same manner.	
If the patient is lying on his back:	
1. Sit astride the patient (facing his head) and with one of your hands on top of the other, place the heel of the bottom hand on the patient's abdomen slightly above the navel and below the rib cage.	
2. Press into the patient's abdomen with a quick upward thrust.	2. Place the patient on his side, if he begins to vomit, to prevent aspiration.
3. The patient should be examined by a physician after the emergency maneuver is performed.	

* From Heimlich, H.J.: A life-saving maneuver to prevent food choking. JAMA, 234: 398–401, 27 Oct. 1975.

GUIDELINES: Cricothyroidotomy

Cricothyroidotomy is the puncture or opening of the cricothyroid membrane to establish an emergency airway in certain emergency conditions when endotracheal intubation or tracheostomy is not possible.

Equipment 11-gauge needle

Procedure

NURSING ACTION	RATIONALE/AMPLIFICATION
1. Extend the neck.	1. So that the cricothyroid membrane can be palpated readily.
2. Insert a needle or any sharp instrument at a 10- to 30-degree caudad angle in the midline just above the upper part of the cricoid cartilage.	
3. Listen for air passing back and forth through the needle synchronously with the patient's respirations.	
4. Direct the needle downward and posteriorly.	4. To avoid injury to the vocal cords (located cephalad to the cricothyroid membrane).
5. Tape the needle with adhesive.	5. To prevent laceration or perforation of the posterior tracheal wall.
6. Prepare for endotracheal intubation/tracheostomy.	
7. Potential complications: vocal cord injury, subcutaneous emphysema, bleeding.	

GUIDELINES: Esophageal Obturator Airway (EOA)

The *esophageal obturator airway* is a ventilatory device used in respiratory emergencies for resuscitation. It consists of (1) a face mask—to seal off the nose and mouth and anchor the airway; (2) a flexible tube with openings at the level of the pharynx—to permit ventilation of the lungs; and (3) a balloon on the distal end of the tube—to block the esophagus, thus reducing the possibility of aspirating gastric contents.

Purpose to ventilate an apneic, unconscious patient when endotracheal intubation is not feasible.

Equipment Esophageal obturator airway
50-ml syringe

Lubricant jelly
Bag and mask unit

NURSING ACTION	RATIONALE/AMPLIFICATION
Preparatory Phase	
Lubricate the tube and attach the mask to the tube.	This procedure is contraindicated in conscious or semiconscious patients or in those with corrosive poisoning, esophageal disease, or a foreign body in the trachea.
Performance Phase	
1. Grasp the patient's tongue and lower jaw between the thumb and index finger and lift upward and forward.	
2. Insert the esophageal obturator airway into the mouth, carefully guiding the tube over the tongue and past the pharynx; rotate the tube 180 degrees into the esophagus.	
3. Stop advancing the tube when the mask reaches the face; press the mask firmly against the face.	
4. Ventilate the patient by blowing a few breaths through the tube or by attaching a bag mask to it. If the chest does not rise or no breath sounds are heard, withdraw the tube immediately for reinsertion.	4. *If the tube is in the esophagus, the chest will rise.* Inadvertent tracheal intubation is a complication associated with the use of the EOA.
5. Auscultate over both lung fields to check that *both* lungs are receiving adequate ventilation and that the airway is in the esophagus and *not* in the trachea.	
6. Inflate the cuff (balloon) with approximately 30 ml. of air.	6. Inflating the balloon prevents air from entering the stomach and prevents regurgitation/vomiting.
7. Connect the end of the esophageal obturator to a bag-mask or mechanical ventilator, or continue mouth-to-tube ventilation.	7. Air or oxygen is blown into the sealed mask and exits through the holes at the hypopharynx, passing into the trachea and lungs.
8. One type of EOA unit has a central lumen that allows passage of a nasogastric tube (Fig. 22-3).	8. This allows suctioning and decompression of the stomach.
9. Do not remove the EOA until the patient regains consciousness or has a gag reflex OR until endotracheal intubation has been accomplished.	9. If the tube is taken out prematurely, regurgitation and aspiration are almost inevitable. The EOA tube must be deflated before it is removed.

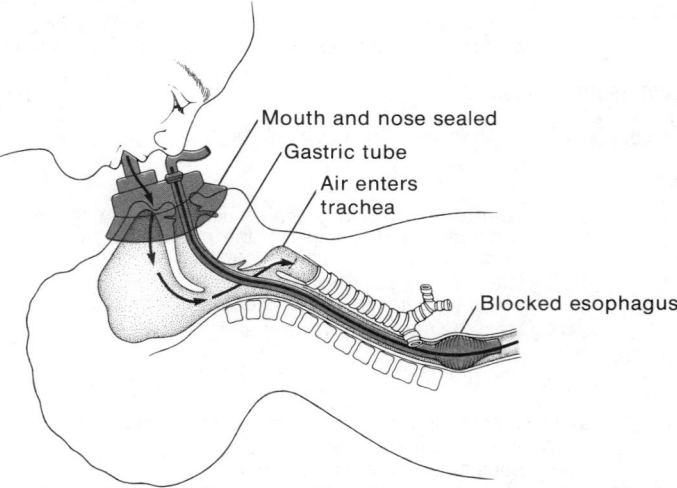

Mouth and nose sealed
Gastric tube
Air enters trachea
Blocked esophagus

FIGURE 22-3. *The Esophageal (Gastric Tube) Airway®. Courtesy of Brunswick Mfg. Co., Inc. (Redrawn)*

HEMORRHAGE

OBJECTIVES: to control bleeding.
to maintain an adequate circulating blood volume for tissue oxygenation.
to prevent shock.

Assessment

(Signs and symptoms of shock occur)

Cool moist skin—from poor peripheral perfusion

Falling blood pressure

Increasing heart rate

Decreasing urine volume

Emergency Management

1. Cut the patient's clothing away quickly and carry out a rapid physical examination.
2. Apply firm pressure over the bleeding area or the artery involved (Fig. 22-4); almost all bleeding can be stopped by direct pressure. Unchecked arterial bleeding produces death.
3. Apply a firm pressure dressing. Elevate the injured part to stop venous and capillary bleeding. Immobilize an injured extremity to control blood loss.

4. Insert intravenous cannula to provide means of blood replacement.
   a. Withdraw blood samples for analysis, typing, and cross-matching.
   b. Give replacement fluids, including isotonic electrolyte solutions, plasma or plasma protein solution, and blood (depending on clinical estimates of type and volume of fluids lost).
      (1) Fresh blood is infused when there is massive blood loss—to prevent loss of platelets and coagulation factors.
      (2) Additional platelets and clotting factors are given when large amounts of blood are needed, since replacement blood is deficient in clotting factors.
      (3) Warm the blood (commercial warmer or basin of warm water)—massive blood replacement has a cooling effect that can cause cardiac arrest.
   c. Rate of infusion depends on severity of blood loss and clinical evidence of hypovolemia.
5. Take the following steps for internal bleeding:
   a. Suspect internal bleeding in patients with hypo-

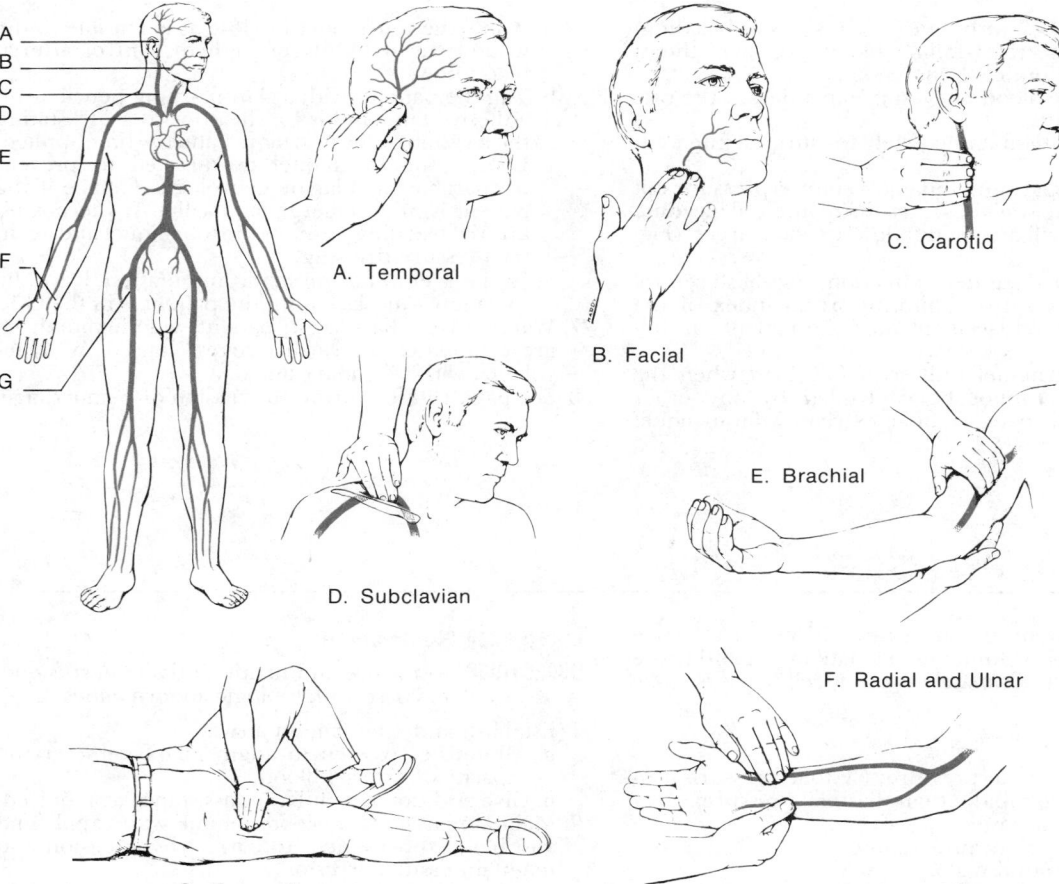

A. Temporal

B. Facial

C. Carotid

D. Subclavian

E. Brachial

F. Radial and Ulnar

G. Femoral

FIGURE 22-4. *Pressure points for control of hemorrhage.*

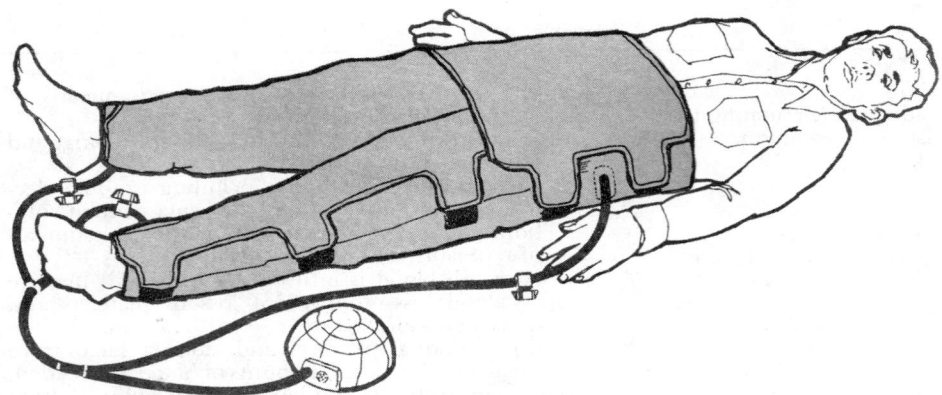

FIGURE 22-5. *The Medical Anti-Shock Trouser (MAST) is a garment designed to correct and counteract internal bleeding conditions and hypovolemia by developing an encircling pressure of up to 2 psi or 104 mm. Hg around both legs and abdomen, thus effectively*
a. slowing or stopping arterial bleeding
b. forcing any available blood from the lower body to the heart, brain and other vital organs in the upper body, and
c. preventing return of available circulating blood volume to the lower extremities.
It should be applied as soon as possible after injury, preferably before patient is transferred to the Emergency Department. (Courtesy of David Clark Co., Inc., 373 Franklin Street, Worcester, Mass. 01604.)

volemic shock with no external signs of bleeding: rising pulse rate; falling blood pressure; thirst; apprehension; cool, moist skin.

b. Give whole blood or plasma expanders at the rate of blood loss.

c. Prepare patient immediately for surgical intervention.

d. Apply wraparound inflatable counterpressure suit ("G" suit) if available—to control internal bleeding and to facilitate blood flow to vital areas (Fig. 22-5).

e. Obtain blood gas determinations; establish central venous pressure monitoring as an index of the amount of replacement fluid the patient can tolerate.

6. Apply a tourniquet only as a *last resort* when the hemorrhage cannot be controlled by any other method. Anticipate loss of an extremity if tourniquet is applied.

a. Apply the tourniquet as close as is feasible to the wound; tie it tightly enough to control arterial blood flow.

b. Tag the patient (with a skin-marking pencil or on adhesive tape on his forehead) with a "T" stating the location of the tourniquet and the time applied.

c. Loosen the tourniquet as directed to prevent irreparable vascular or neurologic damage if the patient is in an emergency facility. If there is no arterial bleeding, remove the tourniquet and again try pressure dressing.

d. In the event of a traumatic amputation, leave the tourniquet in place until the patient is in the O.R.

7. Watch for cardiac arrest; patients who hemorrhage are candidates for cardiac arrest caused by hypovolemia with secondary anoxia.

8. See page 130 for further discussion of hemorrhage.

CONTROL OF HYPOVOLEMIC SHOCK

Shock is a condition in which there is loss of effective circulating blood volume; inadequate organ and tissue perfusion result, ultimately causing cellular metabolic derangements.

Clinical Manifestations

1. Decreasing arterial pressure; (systolic pressure usually falls more rapidly than diastolic pressure)
2. Increasing pulse rate
3. Cold, clammy skin; prostration
4. Pallor; circumoral pallor
5. Thirst
6. Alterations of mental status
7. Suppression of kidney function

Emergency Management

OBJECTIVES: to restore and maintain tissue perfusion.
to correct physiologic abnormalities.

1. Establish and maintain an airway.
   a. Administer oxygen to augment oxygen-carrying capacity of arterial blood.
   b. Give additional ventilatory assistance as required.
2. Maintain circulatory blood volume with rapid fluid and blood replacement to correct hypotension and maintain tissue perfusion.
   a. Insert central venous catheter in or near right atrium (p. 271)—to serve as a guide for fluid replacement. (Continuing CVP reading gives di-

rection and degree of change from baseline reading; also is a vehicle for emergency fluid volume replacement.)

   b. Insert large gauge intravenous needles or catheters into peripheral vein(s); 2 or more catheters may be necessary for rapid replacement in profound shock; the emphasis is on volume replacement.

     (1) Establish IV lines in both upper and lower extremities if there is suspicion that a major vessel in the chest or abdomen has been disrupted.

     (2) Withdraw blood for specimens, arterial blood gases (arterial blood), chemistry studies, typing and cross-matching, and hematocrit.

3. Start intravenous infusion at a rapid rate until CVP rises to a satisfactory level above baseline measurement or until there is improvement in clinical condition.

   a. Infusion of lactated Ringer's solution is useful initially to allow time for whole blood typing and cross-matching and to restore circulation and serve as an adjunct to whole blood.

   b. Start transfusion of blood component therapy, especially when blood loss has been severe or when patient continues to hemorrhage.

   c. Control hemorrhage; hemorrhage will compound the shock state. Carry out serial hematocrit examinations if continued bleeding is suspected.

   d. Maintain the systolic blood pressure at 90–110 mm. Hg by administering fluid and blood.

4. Insert a urinary catheter. Urinary volume reveals adequacy of kidney perfusion.
5. Carry out a rapid physical assessment to determine cause of shock.
6. Maintain ongoing nursing surveillance of *total patient*—blood pressure, heart, and respiratory rates; skin temperature, color; CVP, arterial blood gases, and urinary output—to assess patient response to treatment. Keep a flow sheet of these parameters—trend analysis reveals improvement or deterioration of patient.
7. Elevate the feet slightly to improve cerebral circulation and promote return of venous blood to the heart. (*This position is contraindicated in patients with head injuries.*)
8. Give specific pharmacologic agents (sodium bicarbonate, dopamine, etc.) when indicated by the patient's condition.
9. Support the defense mechanisms of the body.

   a. Reassure and comfort the patient; sedation may be necessary to relieve apprehension.

   b. Relieve pain by *cautious* use of analgesics or narcotics.

   c. Maintain the body temperature.

     (1) Too much heat produces vasodilatation, which counteracts the body's compensatory mechanism of vasoconstriction and also increases fluid loss by perspiration.

     (2) A patient who is in septic shock should be kept cool, since high fever will increase the cellular metabolic effects of shock.

WOUNDS

Wounds (injury to tissues) vary from minor lacerations to severe crushing injuries.

Underlying Considerations

Life-threatening problems such as airway obstruction, hemorrhage, and shock must be dealt with before the wound is treated.

Emergency Management

OBJECTIVES: to avoid complications.
               to promote rapid healing.
               to minimize scarring and prevent deformity.

1. Ask the patient *when* as well as *how* the wound occurred; a delay over 3 hours in treatment increases the risk of infection developing.
2. Inspect the wound using aseptic technique—to determine the extent of damage to underlying structures.

   a. Shave around wound (with exception of eyebrows) only if directed.

   b. Cleanse around wound with antimicrobial agent. Do not allow cleansing solution to get into wound, since it may be injurious to exposed tissues.

   c. Infiltrate with local anesthetic intradermally through the wound margins or by regional block.

3. Cleanse and debride the wound.

   a. Irrigate gently and copiously with isotonic sterile saline—to remove surface dirt.

   b. Remove devitalized tissue and foreign matter—impairs wound's ability to resist infection.

   c. Clamp and tie small bleeding vessels (or achieve hemostasis with a cautery).

4. Suture wound if primary closure is indicated (depends on nature of wound, length of time since injury was sustained, degree of contamination, vascularity of tissues).

   a. Subcutaneous fat is approximated loosely with a few sutures to close off dead space.

   b. Subcuticular layer or dermis is then closed.

   c. Epidermis is closed; sutures placed close to wound edge with skin edges carefully leveled to prevent uneven scar surfaces.

   d. Sterile strips of reinforced microporous tape may be used to close clean superficial wounds.

5. Apply water soluble ointment if directed.
6. Apply dressing—to protect the wound; may serve as a splint and as a reminder to patient that he has sustained an injury.
7. For delayed primary closure:

   a. A thin layer of gauze covered by occlusive dressing (to ensure drainage and prevent pooling of exudate) may be used, or split-thickness cadaver or porcine xenografts may be used to hold the wound apart.

   b. Splint the wound in position of rest—to prevent motion.

   c. Close the wound (with local anesthesia) when there are no signs of suppuration.

8. Give antimicrobial treatment as directed—depends on how injury occurred, age of wound, presence of soil-infection potential, etc.
9. Immobilize the site if wound is contaminated; elevate site to limit accumulation of fluid in wound interstitial spaces.
10. Give tetanus prophylaxis as indicated.

Tetanus Prophylaxis in Wound Management*

Underlying Considerations

1. Available evidence shows that complete primary immunization with tetanus toxoid provides long-lasting protective antitoxin levels.
   a. Additionally, protective antitoxin develops rapidly in response to a booster dose in persons who have previously received at least 2 doses of tetanus-toxoid.
   b. Therefore, passive protection with TIG (Tetanus Immune Globulin) or antitoxin need be considered only when the patient has had less than 2 previous injections of tetanus toxoid or when the wound has been untended for more than 24 hours.
2. The following table is a conservative guide to active and passive tetanus immunization at the time of wound cleansing and debridement. It assumes a reliable knowledge of the patient's immunization history.
3. When tetanus toxoid and TIG are given concurrently, separate syringes and separate sites should be used.

* From Morbidity and Mortality Weekly Report. Vol. 20, No. 43, 1971, page 5.

Guide to Tetanus Prophylaxis in Wound Management*

History of Tetanus Immunization (Doses)	Clean, Minor Wounds		All Other Wounds	
	Td	TIG	Td	TIG
Uncertain	Yes	No	Yes	Yes
0–1	Yes	No	Yes	Yes
2	Yes	No	Yes	No[1]
3 or more	No[2]	No	No[3]	No

[1] Unless wound more than 24 hours old.
[2] Unless more than 10 years since last dose.
[3] Unless more than 5 years since last dose.
NOTE: Td = Tetanus and diphtheria toxoids (adult type)
TIG = Tetanus Immune Globulin, human

4. If TIG is unavailable, equine or bovine antitoxin may be used but there is a risk that serious anaphylactic or serum sickness reactions will follow. *If used, its administration must be preceded by careful screening for sensitivity in accordance with instructions accompanying the antitoxin.*
5. See also page 818.

INTRA-ABDOMINAL INJURIES

Intra-abdominal injuries may be either penetrating or blunt.

PENETRATING ABDOMINAL INJURIES

Persons with *penetrating abdominal injuries* (gunshot wounds, stab wounds, etc.) should be treated like critically ill patients.

High velocity missiles (bullets) create extensive tissue damage; such damage usually requires surgical exploration.

Stab wounds may be managed more conservatively.

Assessment

1. Assess the patient for progression of distention, involuntary guarding, tenderness, pain, muscular rigidity or rebound tenderness, diminished bowel sounds, hypotension, and shock.
2. Auscultate for bowel sounds because the absence of bowel sounds is an early sign of intraperitoneal involvement. If signs of peritoneal irritation are present, an immediate exploratory celiotomy (surgical incision into the abdominal cavity) is usually performed.
3. Record all physical signs as the patient is examined.
4. Look for chest injuries, which frequently accompany intra-abdominal injuries.

Emergency Management

OBJECTIVES: to control the bleeding.
to maintain blood volume.

1. Keep the patient on the stretcher, since movement may fragment a clot in a large vessel and produce massive hemorrhage.
   a. Cut the clothing away from the wound.
   b. Assess respiratory and cardiac status.
   c. Tabulate the number of wounds.
   d. Look for entrance and exit wounds.
2. Assess for signs and symptoms of hemorrhage. Hemorrhage frequently accompanies abdominal injury, especially if the liver and spleen have been traumatized.
3. Control the bleeding and maintain the blood volume until surgery can be performed.
   a. Apply compression to external bleeding wounds.
   b. Insert indwelling intravenous catheter(s) for rapid fluid replacement to restore circulatory dynamics.
   c. Watch for occurrence of shock after an initial positive response to transfusion therapy; this is often the first sign of internal hemorrhage.
4. Aspirate the stomach contents with nasogastric tube—also helps detect gastric wounds and prevents lung complications from aspiration.
5. Cover protruding abdominal viscera with sterile saline dressings to protect viscera from drying.
   a. Flex patient's knees, since this position will prevent further protrusion.
   b. Withhold oral fluids to prevent increased peristalsis and vomiting.
6. Insert indwelling urethral catheter to ascertain the presence of hematuria and to monitor the urinary output.
7. Keep an ongoing flow sheet of the patient's vital signs, urinary output, central venous pressure readings, hematocrit values, and neurologic status.
8. Prepare for paracentesis or peritoneal lavage (see p. 475) when there is uncertainty about intraperitoneal bleeding.
9. For stab wounds, prepare for sinography to determine whether there is peritoneal penetration.

a. Purse string suture is placed around wound.
b. Small rubber catheter or IntraCath is introduced through wound.
c. Contrast medium is introduced through catheter; x-rays are made and will reveal whether peritoneal penetration has taken place.
10. Carry out tetanus prophylaxis as directed.
11. Give broad-spectrum antimicrobial as directed to prevent infection, since bacterial contamination is a frequent complication (depending on history and nature of wound).
12. Prepare for surgery if patient shows evidence of shock, bleeding, wound hemorrhage, free air, evisceration, hematuria, etc.

BLUNT ABDOMINAL TRAUMA

Underlying Considerations

1. Trauma to the abdomen is frequently associated with extra-abdominal injuries—chest, head, and extremities.
2. The incidence of delayed trauma-related complications is greater than that associated with penetrating injuries; this is especially true of blunt injuries involving the liver, spleen, or blood vessels, which can lead to substantial blood loss into the peritoneal cavity.

Clinical Manifestations

1. Pain; pain on movement
2. Exquisite tenderness; rebound rigidity
3. Muscle guarding
4. Diminishing or absent bowel sounds

Emergency Management

1. Take a detailed history (frequently unobtainable, inaccurate, and misleading); obtain all possible data about the following:
   a. Method of injury.
   b. Time of onset of symptoms.
   c. Passenger location (driver frequently sustains spleen/liver rupture).
   d. Time of last food/fluid intake.
   e. Bleeding tendencies.
   f. Concurrent disease.
   g. Immunization history, with attention to tetanus.
   h. Allergies.
2. Carry out ongoing examination (inspection, palpation, auscultation, and percussion of the abdomen).
   a. Avoid moving the patient until initial assessment is done—movement may fragment a clot in a large vessel and produce massive hemorrhage.
   b. Look for chest injuries, especially fracture of lower ribs.
   c. Inspect front, flanks, and back for bluish discoloration, asymmetry, abrasions, contusions.
   d. Evaluate for signs and symptoms of hemorrhage— frequently accompanies abdominal injury, especially if the liver and spleen have been traumatized.
   e. Note tenderness, rebound tenderness, guarding, rigidity, and spasm.
      (1) Press the area of maximal tenderness (let patient point to the area).
      (2) Remove the fingers quickly; pain at suspected point indicates peritoneal irritation.
   f. Look for increasing abdominal distention. Measure abdominal girth at umbilical level upon admission—serves as a baseline from which changes can be determined.
   g. Auscultate for bowel sounds.
   h. Note loss of dullness over solid organs (liver; spleen)—indicates presence of free air; dullness over regions normally containing gas may indicate presence of blood.
   i. Assist with rectal examination/vaginal examination—for diagnosis of injury to pelvis, bladder, and intestinal wall.
3. Avoid giving narcotics during observation period— may mask clinical picture.
4. Monitor vital signs frequently and carefully—may be the only clue to intra-abdominal bleeding.
5. Obtain baseline laboratory studies.
   a. Urinalysis—as a guide to possible urinary tract injury; to monitor urine output.
   b. Serial hemoglobin and hematocrit levels—their trend reflects presence or absence of bleeding.
   c. CBC—white blood cell count may be elevated with rupture of spleen.
   d. Serum amylase—elevation usually indicates pancreatic injury or trauma to bowel.
6. Obtain abdominal and chest x-rays—may reveal free air beneath diaphragm, indicating ruptured hollow viscus.
7. Assist with peritoneal lavage—to test for intraperitoneal bleeding (see below), especially if patient is obtunded.
8. Assist with insertion of nasogastric tube—to prevent vomiting and subsequent aspiration; helpful in decompressing (removing fluid/air) from gastrointestinal tract.
9. Patient may be admitted for observation or exploratory laparotomy.

GUIDELINES: Peritoneal Lavage

Peritoneal lavage is the introduction of solution into the peritoneum for the evaluation of trauma to the abdomen.

Purpose
1. To detect intra-abdominal bleeding.
2. To look for injuries requiring surgical treatment.
3. To test patients with equivocal abdominal findings.
4. To avoid unnecessary operation, especially in patients with altered states of consciousness (from head injuries, drugs, alcohol) and when physical findings are unreliable (spinal cord injuries).

Contraindications

1. Multiple abdominal scars
2. Pregnancy

GUIDELINES: Peritoneal Lavage (cont.)

Equipment   Peritoneal dialysis tray
Sterile solution (lactated Ringer's solution)
IV tubing; IV pole
Peritoneal dialysis catheter (multiple perforations)
Local skin anesthetic; sterile gloves

Procedure

NURSING ACTION	RATIONALE/AMPLIFICATION
Preparatory Phase	
1. Explain the procedure to the patient; see that the consent form has been signed.	
2. Empty the bladder (by catheter if necessary).	2. To prevent puncture of urinary bladder.
3. Shave the lower abdomen from umbilicus to pubic area. Prepare the abdomen as for suurgery.	3. To minimize or eliminate surface bacteria and decrease the possibility of wound contamination and infection.
4. Fill the IV tubing with solution using aseptic technique.	
Performance Phase *(by the physician)*	
1. The skin is infiltrated 2–3 cm. (.7–1.2″) below the umbilicus in the midline with local anesthetic.	1. The midline area is relatively avascular. Epinephrine may be injected with local anesthetic to produce capillary constriction and prevent a false-positive tap.
2. A small vertical incision is made down to the linea alba.	
3. Bleeding vessels are carefully ligated.	3. Ligation of vessels helps avoid a false-positive lavage.
4. The peritoneum is brought upward between 2 hemostats and is punctured under direct vision. The peritoneum is opened and a peritoneal dialysis catheter is directed into the incision and advanced toward the pelvis.	
5. A gauze sponge is packed into the subcutaneous tissue.	5. To absorb minor bleeding.
6. A syringe is attached to the catheter and the peritoneal cavity is aspirated.	6. If nonclotted blood is obtained (or bile or intestinal contents) the tap shows positive findings and the patient is prepared for immediate celiotomy (incision into abdominal cavity).
7. If no blood is present, the catheter is attached to the IV tubing; 500–1000 ml. of solution is infused into the peritoneal cavity through the intravenous tubing attached to the dialysis catheter.	7. If not contraindicated by the patient's condition, he may be turned from side to side to ensure that the solution reaches all parts of the abdominal cavity.
8. Clamp off the IV tubing. Remove the empty IV bottle from the pole and lower the bottle to the floor.	8. Lowering the bottle creates a siphon effect to drain the excess fluid. As much of the fluid as possible is siphoned out of the peritoneal cavity by gravity.
9. Dislodge the air vent from the rubber stopper by removing the IV tubing. Reinsert the IV tubing into the vent hole itself. Unclamp the tubing and allow the fluid to be siphoned from the abdominal cavity.	
10. The fluid recovered from the peritoneal cavity is examined visually and is usually sent to the laboratory for cell counts and microscopic inspection of a spun down sediment.	
INTERPRETATION OF LAVAGE FLUID	
1. *Gross examination (visual)* Inability to read newsprint through the intravenous tubing usually means that the amount of blood is sufficient to indicate a laparotomy.	If the test is positive, a laparotomy is usually done. If the test is negative, the catheter is removed and the wound closed. If the test is questionable, the catheter may be left in place and the lavage repeated.
2. *Laboratory evaluation (positive tests)* RBC greater than 100,000/cu. mm. WBC greater than 500/cu. mm. Bacteria—pathologic when present Bile—pathologic when present Amylase level—greater than 100 Somogyi units/ 100 ml.	If the test is weakly positive, the patient may have echography and arteriography if his condition is stable.
Follow-up Phase	
1. Assess patient for complications.	1. Complications include visceral perforation, wound hematoma, perforated bowel, puncture of bladder, laceration of major vessels, and lack of fluid return.
2. Watch the patient closely for any type of deterioration.	2. Repeated physical examinations of the abdomen should be carried out when intra-abdominal injury is suspected.

CRUSH INJURIES

Crush injuries occur when a person is crushed beneath debris, run over, or compressed by machinery.

Clinical Manifestations

1. Oligemic shock—due to extravasation of blood and plasma into injured tissues after compression has been released.
2. Paralysis of part, erythema and blistering of skin—damaged part (usually an extremity) becomes swollen, tense, hard.
3. Renal dysfunction—prolonged hypotension causes kidney damage and acute renal insufficiency.

Emergency Management

1. Control shock.
2. Observe carefully for acute renal insufficiency (see p. 491)—injury to back may cause severe kidney damage.
3. Splint major soft tissue injuries to control bleeding and pain.
4. Elevate the extremity. Incise fascia if the blood supply is blocked to relieve the pressure of extravasated fluid.
5. Administer medication for pain and anxiety.

CHEST INJURIES

Injuries to the chest are dire emergencies and are potentially life-threatening because of disturbances to cardiorespiratory physiology. See page 215 for a more complete discussion of chest injuries.

Emergency Management (Fig. 22-6)

OBJECTIVE: to restore normal cardiorespiratory function as rapidly as possible.

A. *Airway Assessment*

1. Undress patient completely in order to evaluate respiratory pattern and to look for other injuries; multiple injuries frequently occur with chest injuries.
2. Is the chest wall intact?
3. Are there active respiratory movements and lung expansion?
4. What is the respiratory rate?
5. Is there shortness of breath, inspiratory or expiratory stridor, cyanosis or pain?
6. Determine if the patient is ventilating properly. Auscultate both sides of the chest.
7. Are the neck veins distended?—May indicate cardiac tamponade.
8. Is there swelling of neck and face?—Swelling due to torn bronchus or laceration of lung may cause subcutaneous emphysema.
9. Palpate the abdomen in all thoracic injuries; look for rigidity and tenderness over liver, spleen, kidneys.
10. Look for fracture of the pelvis and long bones since these fractures may cause hemorrhage and shock.
11. *Priorities*
    a. Ensure the airway.
    b. Perform a rapid physical examination to detect associated injuries.
    c. Assist with insertion of a tube into the chest cavity if indicated.
    d. Elevate the head and chest unless the patient is in shock.
    e. Prepare for blood transfusion; patients with severe thoracic injuries need blood to replace that which has been lost in the pleural cavity.

B. *Sucking Wounds*—air passes through hole in the chest wall (from stab or bullet wound, etc.), causing the lungs to collapse and the mediastinum to shift. There is an audible passage of air from the wound during inspiration and expiration.

1. Instruct the patient to exhale.
2. Cover the wound with petrolatum gauze and a pressure bandage applied by circumferential strapping—prevents further shifting of mediastinum and allows for airtight closure of wound; petrolatum gauze dressing helps seal the leak.
3. Insert chest tube connected to a water-seal and controlled suction drainage system—pneumothorax almost invariably accompanies these wounds. (See p. 879.)
    a. The skin is cleansed and infiltrated with a local anesthetic by the physician.
    b. A small incision is made between the 5th and 6th intercostal space in the midaxillary line.
    c. The chest tube is inserted and sutured in place.
    d. Chest tube is attached to a closed water-seal drainage system to evacuate blood and air and to measure blood loss.
4. Continue to assess respiratory status. Treat the patient symptomatically until surgical closure of the chest wall wound can be carried out.

C. *Flail Chest*—usually results from multiple rib fractures, which cause instability of the chest wall and subsequent respiratory impairment.

1. Immobilize the flail portion of the chest by stabilizing it with the hands and then applying a pressure dressing with adhesive strapping (Fig. 22-6).
2. Prepare for tracheostomy or endotracheal intubation plus mechanical ventilation with volume-controlled ventilator to expand the lungs and give adequate oxygenation and to promote stability of the chest wall.
3. Place patient on his injured side; ensure that injury is compressed—by padding or a sandbag.
4. Assist with insertion of tube into the chest cavity.
5. Insert a central venous catheter.
    a. Draw blood for hemoglobin, hematocrit determinations, typing, and cross matching.
    b. Monitor central venous pressure.
    c. Administer intravenous fluids.
6. Draw arterial blood for blood gas analysis to indicate the adequacy of ventilation and the required concentration of inspired oxygen.

EMERGENCY MANAGEMENT OF PATIENT WITH CHEST INJURIES

Objectives: Restore normal cardiopulmonary function
as rapidly as possible
Assess patient to determine physiological status

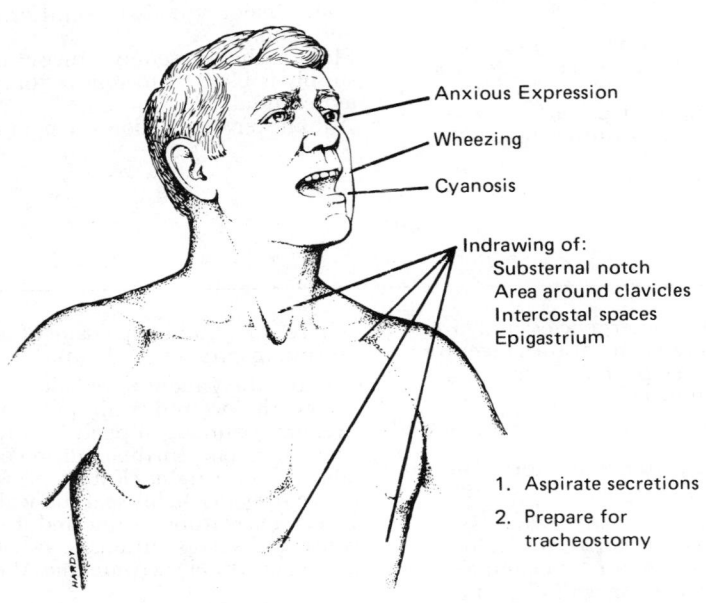

Anxious Expression

Wheezing

Cyanosis

Indrawing of:
Substernal notch
Area around clavicles
Intercostal spaces
Epigastrium

1. Aspirate secretions
2. Prepare for
   tracheostomy

Clinical Assessment

Flail Chest

Dyspnea
Cyanosis

Chest pain

Paradoxical
movement of
involved chest
wall

Emergency Management

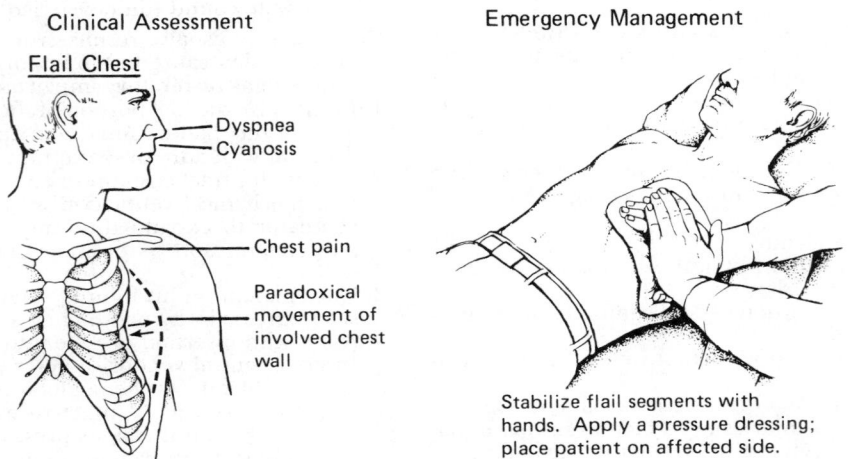

Stabilize flail segments with
hands. Apply a pressure dressing;
place patient on affected side.

FIGURE 22-6. *Emergency management of patient with chest injuries.*

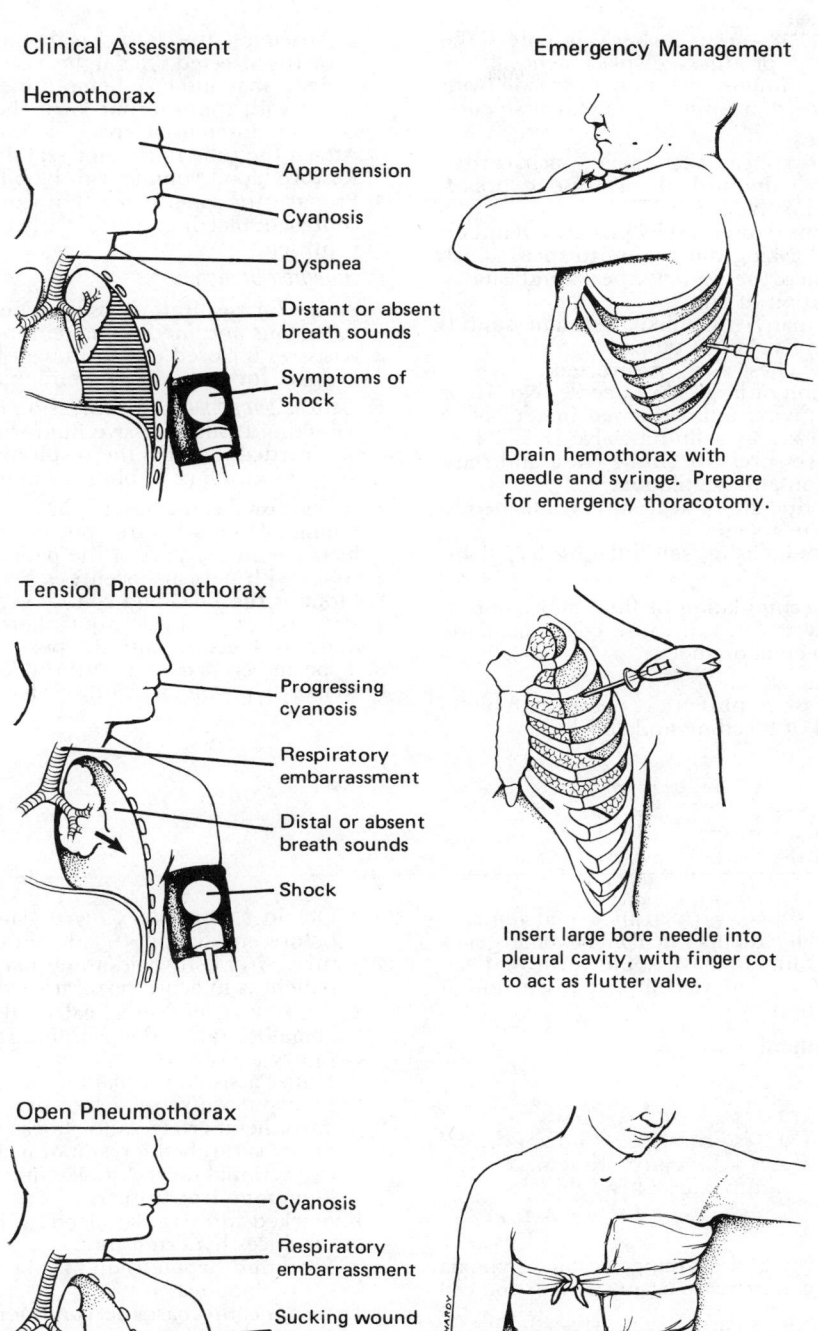

Clinical Assessment

Emergency Management

Hemothorax

- Apprehension
- Cyanosis
- Dyspnea
- Distant or absent breath sounds
- Symptoms of shock

Drain hemothorax with needle and syringe. Prepare for emergency thoracotomy.

Tension Pneumothorax

- Progressing cyanosis
- Respiratory embarrassment
- Distal or absent breath sounds
- Shock

Insert large bore needle into pleural cavity, with finger cot to act as flutter valve.

Open Pneumothorax

- Cyanosis
- Respiratory embarrassment
- Sucking wound of chest
- Shock

Instruct patient to exhale forcefully. Place occlusive dressing firmly in place. Make wound airtight.

FIGURE 22-6. *(Continued)*

D. *Tension Pneumothorax*—occurs when air enters the pleural cavity and produces displacement of the heart and mediastinum to the uninvolved side (with resultant severe cardiorespiratory embarrassment).

1. Assess the patient.
   a. Evaluate for dyspnea, chest pain, tachycardia, tachypnea, and diminished or absent breath sounds on the involved side.
   b. Test for fremitus (vibration) by placing a hand on the thorax and asking the patient to speak. Lack of fremitus when the patient speaks indicates a large accumulation of air.
   c. Listen for tympany (drumlike resonant sound) when the patient's chest is tapped.
   d. Secure portable chest x-ray as directed.
2. Assist with insertion of large bore needle (No. 16 or 18) into pleural cavity; attach incised finger cot to hub of needle to act as a flutter valve (Fig. 22-6). The needle reduces pressure in the chest and reestablishes circulation and ventilation.
3. Assist in the introduction of a chest tube attached to water-seal drainage system.
4. Ventilate the patient using self-inflating bag if indicated.

E. *Hemothorax*—an accumulation of fluid and blood in the pleural cavity which can cause collapse of the lung and hypovolemia or shock.

1. Assess the patient.
   a. Note any increase in pulse rate, decrease in blood pressure, signs of bleeding and shock.

   b. Auscultate the chest. An absence of breath sounds on the affected sides at the base and in the midlung fields may indicate hemothorax.
2. Assist with the insertion of a chest tube at the 5th and 6th intercostal space in the midaxillary line. Attach the tube to a water-seal drainage system.
3. Restore blood volume with blood and fluids.
4. Prepare for emergency thoracotomy for operative control of bleeding, particularly if large hemothorax is present.

F. *Ruptured Bronchus*

1. Assess for respiratory distress, hemoptysis, and subcutaneous and mediastinal emphysema.
2. Assist with closed chest drainage.
3. Prepare for surgical intervention to repair bronchus.

G. *Cardiac tamponade*—compression of the heart resulting from excessive fluid within the pericardial sac. It is the result of intrapericardial injury secondary to blunt or penetrating trauma.

1. Assess for distant heart sounds, *distended neck veins,* falling blood pressure, pulsus paradoxus, and reluctance on the part of the patient to lie down.
2. Assist with pericardiocentesis (p. 274).
3. Monitor the ECG and central venous pressure.
4. Prepare for thoracotomy if there is continuing evidence of bleeding into the pericardium.
5. Type and cross match for possible blood transfusion.
6. Repair hypovolemia with fluids.

HEAD INJURIES

Head injuries are classified as open or closed injuries. About 15 to 20% of all patients who come to emergency departments for treatment have some form of head trauma. (See p. 712 for a more complete discussion of treatment of head injuries.)

Emergency Management

> **NURSING ALERT:** Exercise care when moving the patient's head and neck. Fracture of the cervical spine frequently accompanies a head injury.

1. Maintain the airway and exchange of air—hypoxia and hypercapnia can increase brain swelling and cell damage.
   a. Keep the patient in a lateral recumbent, prone, or semiprone position with head to one side, after making certain that there is no cervical spine injury. Prone position facilitates drainage from the tracheobronchial tree and minimizes aspiration of nasopharyngeal and gastric secretions.
   b. Clear the respiratory passages by means of suctioning.
   c. Ensure adequate oxygenation and humidification. (Hypoxia of the brain, which leads to increased intracranial pressure, is the most frequent cause of death following head injury.)

   d. Obtain a portable x-ray of lateral cervical spine before entubation, to rule out cervical spine fracture. A cricothyroidotomy may be considered if patient is in acute respiratory distress.
   e. Assist with endotracheal intubation if patient is comatose (after determining that a cervical neck injury is not present).
   f. Utilize assisted ventilation if necessary. (The brain is very sensitive to lack of oxygen.)
2. Control hemorrhage and shock.
   a. Shock is rarely the result of head injury—look for extracranial source of bleeding (abdomen, thorax, long bone fracture).
   b. Marked intracranial bleeding in an adult usually produces hypertension.
   c. Profound hypotension may be secondary to acute scalp blood loss.
3. Determine the baseline condition of the patient—serves as a basis for comparison as patient's condition changes.
   a. Assess level of responsiveness (see p. 709). Record exactly what patient does and can do on command and to verbal and painful stimuli.
   b. Determine the presence of headache, double vision, nausea, vomiting, papilledema, retinal hemorrhage.
   c. Evaluate pupil size and reaction to light.
   d. Measure blood pressure, pulse, respirations.
   e. Evaluate for signs of rising intracranial pressure—deterioration in level of responsiveness, slowing

of pulse, rising systolic pressure, increasing pulse pressure, changes in pattern of respiration, dilating, nonreacting pupils.

f. Evaluate motion and strength of extremities.

g. Assess for injuries to other organ systems.

4. Evaluate for changes in patient's condition. *(Change in level of responsiveness is the most sensitive sign of improvement or deterioration.)*

5. Prepare for computed tomography or angiography—to diagnose type of pathology and plan definitive care.

6. Utilize intracranial monitoring (if available)—for recognition of increased intracranial hypertension and to help guide therapy.

7. See page 712 for definitive therapy of head trauma.

SPINAL CORD INJURY

Spinal cord injury may vary from a mild cord concussion with transient numbness to an immediate and permanent quadriplegia.

Any person with a head, neck, or back injury should be suspected of having a potential spinal cord injury until the suspicion is proved groundless.

Clinical Manifestations

1. Intercostal paralysis with diaphragmatic breathing—indicates cervical spinal cord injury.

2. Total sensory loss and motor paralysis below level of injury.

3. Loss of bowel and bladder control; usually urinary retention and bladder distention.

4. Loss of sweating and vasomotor tone below level of cord lesion.

5. Marked reduction of blood pressure—from loss of peripheral and vascular resistance.

6. Neck pain.

7. Priapism—persistent erection of penis.

Emergency Management

1. Immobilize the patient. Keep him on the transfer board or on a hard, flat stretcher.

> **NURSING ALERT:** A spinal cord injury can be made worse during the acute phase of injury. Proper handling is an immediate priority.

a. Keep the head and neck in a straight line with the long axis of the body. Do not move the spine; avoid flexion or rotation of the head and neck or flexing, extending, or twisting the spine.

b. Keep the head and neck in a neutral position while applying a cervical collar to maintain stability.

c. Move the patient on a firm transfer board; at least 4–5 persons are needed to move the patient as one unit to the board.

d. Apply continuous, gentle traction to the head.

e. Transport to a spinal cord center (if available) or special care unit as rapidly as possible.

f. Upon admission to the hospital, carry out radiological studies while patient is on the board.

g. Transfer to a special frame (Stryker) after initial evaluation (p. 739).

2. Evaluate the patient's respiratory exchange—death may occur from respiratory failure in cervical cord victims.

3. Evaluate and examine patient for level of spinal cord injury and associated injuries; the presence of spinal shock (p. 740) may make assessment difficult.

a. Test for strength and motion of extremities.

(1) Request patient to flex and extend elbows and to squeeze fingers of examiner.

(2) Request patient to move hips, knees, ankles, toes.

(3) Observe pattern of respirations—intercostal muscle paralysis causes paradoxical movement of chest and abdomen.

(4) Observe for priapism (persistent erection of penis)—a sign of spinal cord injury.

b. Test for sensory impairment—prick the skin with a pin.

c. Test the biceps, triceps, quadriceps, and Achilles reflexes.

d. Evaluate vital signs.

e. Look for the presence of associated injuries.

4. Continue with repeated neurologic examinations to determine if there is deterioration in the spinal cord lesion.

5. Evaluate the patient's respiratory exchange. Prepare for tracheostomy if there is a high cervical lesion.

6. Introduce nasogastric tube—to prevent and treat adynamic ileus, gastric and intestinal distention.

7. Catheterize the patient—patient with spinal cord injury cannot empty his bladder.

8. Start intravenous infusion.

9. Administer dexamethasone—has been found empirically to help diminish or prevent swelling.

10. See page 739 for definitive management of spinal cord injury.

MULTIPLE INJURIES

Underlying Considerations

1. The patient with multiple injuries requires a team approach with one person responsible for coordinating the treatment.

2. *Evidence* of gross trauma may be slight or may be completely absent. The injury regarded as the least significant may be the most lethal.

3. Any injury interfering with a vital physiologic function is an immediate threat to life and has highest priority for immediate treatment (obstructed airway, hemorrhage).

4. The patient should be completely undressed and a rapid physical examination should be carried out as quickly as possible after the airway has been established.
5. Mortality in patients with multiple injuries is related to the severity of the injuries and the number of systems and organs involved.

Emergency Management (Fig. 22-7)

OBJECTIVES: to determine the extent of injuries.
to establish priorities of treatment.

Carry out a *rapid* physical examination to determine if patient is breathing, bleeding, or in shock; determine the status of his responsiveness and if he has severe wounds or fracture deformities.

1. Establish an open airway.*
    a. Ask conscious patient if he is having difficulty in breathing. Ask if he has chest pain.
    b. Apply suction to clear the trachea and bronchial tree.
    c. Insert oropharyngeal airway—to prevent occlusion by tongue.
    d. Ventilate the patient (bag-mask system) to alleviate hypoxia—see page 180.
    e. Prepare for endotracheal intubation (p. 186) with positive pressure breathing if adequate airway cannot be maintained.
    f. Suspect serious intrathoracic injuries if respiratory distress continues after adequate airway has been established. See pages 215–217 for management of chest injuries.
2. Assess cardiac function and treat cardiac arrest—hypoxia, metabolic acidosis, and chest trauma may precipitate cardiac arrest.*
    a. For cardiac arrest, start closed chest compression and ventilation (p. 864).
    b. If chest wall is unstable (flail chest), emergency thoracotomy and manual compression may be necessary.
    c. Give sodium bicarbonate (IV) to compensate for acidosis if indicated—severely traumatized patients with respiratory and circulatory embarrassment will have some degree of metabolic acidosis.
3. Control hemorrhage.*
    a. Apply pressure over bleeding points if hemorrhage is overt.
    b. Expect significant blood loss in patient with fracture of shaft of femur, with multiple fractures, or with major pelvic trauma.
    c. Use tourniquet(s) for massive arterial bleeding from extremities which cannot be halted with pressure.
    d. Prepare for immediate surgical intervention if patient is bleeding internally.
4. Prevent and treat hypovolemic shock.*
    a. Insert at least 2 (sometimes 4) IV lines, one above diaphragm and one below.
    b. Draw blood for laboratory studies as directed (typing and cross-matching, baseline CBC, electrolytes, blood urea nitrogen, glucose, prothrombin time).
    c. Introduce central venous catheter to monitor patient's response to fluid infusion and to prevent fluid overload.
    d. Start intravenous infusions.

* Imperative lifesaving procedures are performed simultaneously by the emergency team.

(1) Balanced saline solution (lactated Ringer's solution) and sterilized plasma are given for volume replacement until blood is available.
(2) Give blood (contains oxygen-carrying red cells and some clotting factors)—massive transfusions have a cooling effect which can cause cardiac irritability and arrest; blood should be warmed.
    e. Give balanced saline solution rapidly enough to keep central venous pressure readings at 5–15 cm. H_2O (see p. 271); monitor rate and direction of change (important parameters).
    f. Insert indwelling urethral catheter and monitor urinary output. Do not force the catheter—the patient may have a ruptured urethra.
    g. Monitor ECG—to detect changes.
    h. Carry out ongoing clinical evaluation to observe for improvement or deterioration; changes in vital signs, improvement in level of responsiveness, skin warmth, speed of capillary filling, etc., shows reversal of shock state.
    i. Prepare for immediate surgical intervention if patient does not respond to fluids or blood. Inability to restore blood pressure and circulatory volume in patient usually indicates major internal bleeding.
5. Assess for head and neck injuries.
    a. Make definite statements concerning baseline neurologic status of patient (level of responsiveness, size and reactivity of pupils, motor power,
    b. Neck (and chest) films may be taken; apply cervical collar until x-rays preclude possibility of cervical spine injury.
    c. Catheter may be inserted into ventricle of brain (p. 711) to measure intracranial pressure.
6. Administer dexamethasone as directed—corticosteroids appear to protect pulmonary function in patients with multiple injuries and help prevent posttraumatic pulmonary insufficiency. (However, this is considered a controversial issue.)
7. Splint fractures to prevent further trauma to soft tissues and blood vessels and to relieve pain; note presence or absence of pulses in fractured extremities.
8. Assess patient for gastrointestinal injuries.
    a. Examine patient repeatedly for abdominal pain, muscular rigidity, tenderness, rebound tenderness, diminished bowel sounds, hypotension, and shock.
    b. Prepare for peritoneal lavage to assess for intraperitoneal bleeding.
    c. Assist with insertion of nasogastric tube if upper gastrointestinal bleeding is suspected or if gaseous distention of stomach develops—will decrease incidence of vomiting and aspiration.
    d. Prepare for laparotomy if patient shows continuing signs of hemorrhage and deterioration.
9. Continue to monitor urinary output hourly—reflects cardiac output and state of perfusion of visceral organs.
    a. Assess for hematuria and oliguria.
    b. Record measurements on a flow sheet.
10. Evaluate patient for other injuries and institute appropriate treatment including tetanus immunization. (See wound treatment, p. 874).
11. Carry out a more thorough physical examination after resuscitation and management of above priorities.

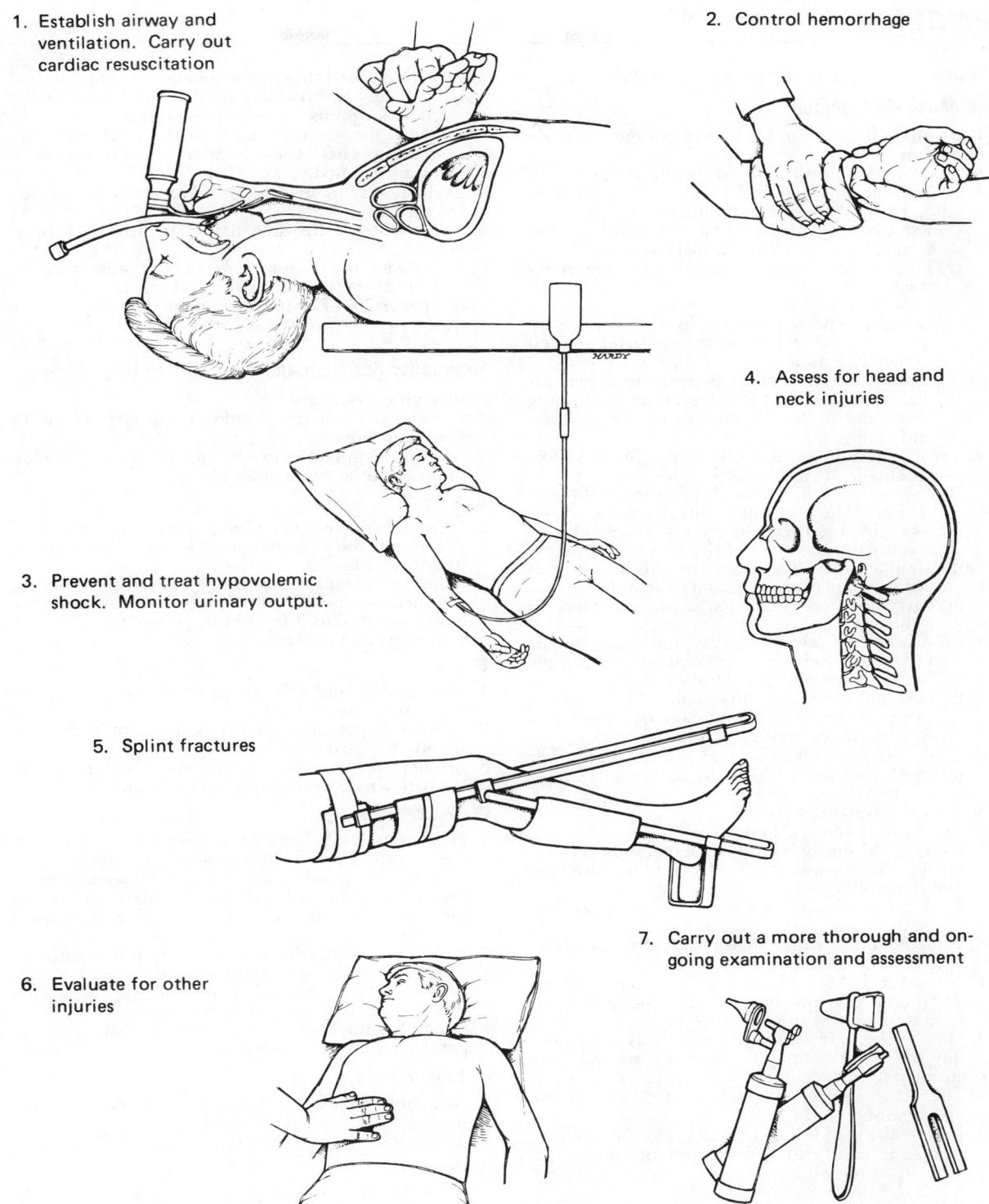

1. Establish airway and ventilation. Carry out cardiac resuscitation

2. Control hemorrhage

3. Prevent and treat hypovolemic shock. Monitor urinary output.

4. Assess for head and neck injuries

5. Splint fractures

6. Evaluate for other injuries

7. Carry out a more thorough and on-going examination and assessment

FIGURE 22-7. *The patient with multiple injuries. Any injury that interferes with vital physiologic function and poses an immediate threat to life takes priority for immediate treatment. Imperative lifesaving procedures are performed simultaneously by the emergency team.*

FRACTURES

A *fracture* is a break in the continuity of the bone.

Emergency Management

1. Give immediate attention to the patient's general condition.
   a. Evaluate for respiratory difficulties—caused by edema due to facial and neck injuries, accumulation of secretions in respiratory tract, etc.
      (1) Examine chest for evidences of sucking chest wounds, pneumothorax, flail chest, etc.
      (2) Prepare for tracheal intubation or emergency tracheostomy.
   b. Control hemorrhage.
      (1) Control venous bleeding by direct pressure along with digital pressure over artery closest to bleeding area.
      (2) Suspect internal hemorrhage (pleural, pericardial, or abdominal) in the event of continuing shock and in the presence of injuries to chest and abdomen.
   c. Treat for shock—usually the result of blood loss in patients with fractures.
      (1) Assess for falling blood pressure, cold and clammy skin, and rapid, thready pulse.
      (2) Keep in mind that heavy loss of blood may accompany fractures of the femur and pelvis.
      (3) Maintain the blood pressure with intravenous infusions, plasma, or plasma expanders.
      (4) Give blood transfusion(s) as soon as blood is available.
      (5) Administer oxygen—cardiopulmonary embarrassment produces decreased oxygen supply to the tissues and circulatory collapse.
      (6) Give analgesic to control pain. (Splinting the extremity and controlling pain are essential in treating shock accompanying fractures.)
   d. Look for evidence of head, chest, and other injuries—patients with multiple fractures may have other serious injuries.
2. Inspect the fractured part(s).
   a. Cut away clothing if necessary.
   b. Observe the entire body using a methodical head-to-toe system—inspect for lacerations, swelling, and deformities.
   c. Look for *angulation* (bending), *shortening*, and *rotation.*
   d. Feel the pulse distal to the extremity fracture. Check all peripheral pulses.
   e. Assess for coolness, blanching, decreased sensation and motor function, diminished or absent pulses—indicate injury to the blood supply.
   f. Handle the part gently and as little as possible.
3. Apply the splint before the patient is moved since splinting relieves pain, improves circulation, prevents further tissue injury, and prevents a closed fracture from becoming an open one.
   a. Immobilize the joint above and below the fracture; place one hand distal to the fracture and apply some traction while placing the other hand beneath the fracture for support.
   b. Extend the splints well beyond the joints adjacent to the fracture.
      (1) Use the patient's clothing for padding (tie, shirt) if nothing else is available.
      (2) Use newspapers, magazines, pillows, tree limbs, and boards for splints if necessary. (Specialized splints and traction are used in the hospital.)
      (3) Splint joints in functional positions.
   c. Check the vascular status of the extremity after splinting; check color, temperature, pulse, blanching of nail bed.
4. Evaluate for neurological deficits caused by the fracture.
5. Apply a sterile dressing if the fracture is an open one.
6. Investigate any complaint of pain or pressure.
7. Transport the patient gently and carefully.
8. See pages 767–775 for a complete discussion of the treatment of fractures at specific sites.

Emergency Splinting and Transporting (Fig. 22-8)

Underlying Concepts
1. A suspected fracture should be splinted before the patient is moved.
2. A splint is applied so that the joints above and below the fracture are immobilized.

A. *Skull*

1. If there is no cervical spine injury, elevate the head slightly on the stretcher, but do not place a pillow under the head.
2. Maintain adequate respiration. Transport patient with head to one side to promote drainage of mucus, blood, or vomitus if level of responsiveness does not permit patient to do so himself.

B. *Jaw*

1. Hold jaw up and in by tying with bandage (if there is no spinal cord injury).
2. Transport patient in a sitting position with head slightly forward.
3. Be alert for possible vomiting—cut bandages immediately to prevent aspiration of vomitus.

C. *Cervical Spine*

1. Place your hands on each side of the head so that the ears are cupped in the hands. (The thumb should be in the temporal region, the 2nd finger just below the zygoma, the 3rd finger along the zygoma, and the 4th finger beneath the mandible, extending traction.)
2. Hold the patient's head, keeping it in line with the body. Slide him onto a rigid surface, flat on his back, face up. The entire body is moved as a unit. Avoid twisting, turning, or pulling the spine.
3. Watch for inadequate respiratory exchange due to paralysis of chest muscles and for neurogenic shock.

D. *Lumbar Spine*

1. Straighten patient carefully and place him on a firm surface such as a long spinal board.
2. Avoid flexion, extension, or rotation of the spine.

E. *Pelvis*

1. Turn the patient carefully on his back.
2. Place padding between the legs and splint them together to prevent unnecessary motion.
3. Immobilize the pelvis by binding a folded blanket around the pelvic area.
4. Transport on a firm stretcher.

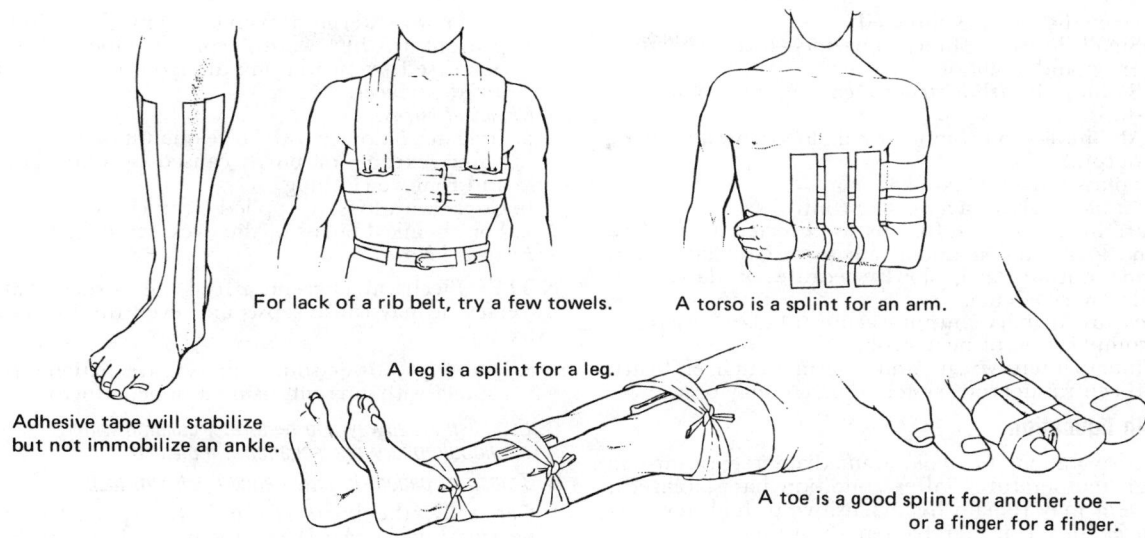

For lack of a rib belt, try a few towels.

A torso is a splint for an arm.

A leg is a splint for a leg.

Adhesive tape will stabilize but not immobilize an ankle.

A toe is a good splint for another toe—or a finger for a finger.

FIGURE 22-8. *Splinting in emergency conditions. (Courtesy of Emergency Medicine.)*

F. *Shoulder, Arm, and Elbow*

1. Place elbow at right angle and apply sling.
2. Bind arm and sling to body with a circular bandage or binder; do not compromise the circulation with bandage in antecubital area.
3. Check radial pulse.
4. If injured elbow is in extension, bandage the extremity to the body in the position in which it was found.

G. *Forearm, Wrist, Hand*

Immobilize with newspaper splint, or with commercial or inflatable air splint, and place in sling with elbow at right angle.

H. *Hip*

1. Splint from axilla to ankle with board, or bind legs together.
2. Use a half-ring traction if available; traction is obtained by means of a hitch around foot and ankle.
3. Transport on stretcher.

I. *Lower extremity*

1. Apply steady, even traction and splint fracture from hip to ankle.
2. Transport on stretcher.

J. *Ankle*

1. Wrap pillow around lower leg, ankle, and foot.
2. Transport on a stretcher.

TEMPERATURE EMERGENCIES

HEAT STROKE

Heat stroke is a medical emergency caused by failure of the heat-regulating mechanisms of the body when the temperature-humidity index is high. The following are particularly vulnerable: persons who (1) are not acclimatized to heat exposure, (2) are at the extremes of age, (3) are engaging in strenuous exercise, and (4) have cardiovascular disease. Heat stroke is a leading cause of death in athletes in this country.

Clinical Manifestations

1. History of exposure to elevated ambient temperature and/or excessive exercise
2. High fever (40.6° C. [105° F.]) and above
3. Central nervous system dysfunction (delirium, psychosis, stupor, convulsions, coma)
4. Weak, rapid, or irregular pulse

Emergency Management

OBJECTIVE: to reduce high temperature as rapidly as possible.

1. Reduce the core (internal) temperature to 39° C. (102° F. rectally) as *rapidly* as possible. Monitor the rectal temperature by a rectal thermistor probe (if available) left in place. One or more of the following temperature-lowering methods may be used.
   a. Immerse patient in ice-water bath.
      (1) Rub extremities continuously during immersion—promotes circulation and maintains cutaneous vasodilation.
   b. Place patient on a hypothermia blanket if available.
   c. Sponge patient continuously with ice water; place electric fan so that it blows on patient, since air movement increases evaporation.
   d. Give chilled saline enemas if temperature does not come down.
2. Monitor patient carefully; vital signs, ECG, CVP, and level of responsiveness change with rapid alterations in body temperature.
3. Administer oxygen to supply tissue needs exaggerated by hypermetabolic condition. Intubate patient with cuffed endotracheal tube and attach to ventilator if necessary to support failing cardiorespiratory systems.

4. Give medications as directed.
   a. Small doses of chlorpromazine—to control shivering and agitation.
   b. Sodium bicarbonate—to correct metabolic acidosis.
   c. Mannitol—to promote renal blood flow and urine output.
   d. Potassium—for hypokalemia.
   e. Anticonvulsant agents—to control seizures.
5. Start intravenous infusions as directed to replace fluid losses and maintain adequate circulation and urine output; give slowly because of danger of pulmonary edema.
6. Measure urinary output—acute tubular necrosis is a complication of heat stroke.
7. Admit to intensive care unit—permanent liver, heart, and central nervous system damage may occur.

Health Education

1. Advise patient to avoid immediate reexposure to high temperatures (after condition has stabilized); patient may remain hypersensitive to high temperatures for a considerable length of time.
2. Have patient maintain adequate fluid and salt intake, wear loose clothing, and rest frequently in hot weather.

BURNS*

Immediate Management

A. *Stop burning process to prevent further tissue destruction.*

1. Remove patient from source of injury.
2. When clothes catch fire, have victim fall to floor or ground and roll him in a carpet or blanket if available; otherwise *stop, drop, roll*, and beat out flames with anything available.
   a. Running would fan flames.
   b. Standing would force victim to breathe flames and smoke, cause his hair to be ignited, or cause facial disfigurement.
3. Remove clothing only if smoldering or hot, or for a scald burn (clothing holds heat).

B. *Initiate immediate treatment.*

1. *Small areas:*
   a. Immerse burn areas in cool water for 10 minutes, or apply cool water compresses (en route to hospital). This limits tissue destruction, relieves pain, prevents edema, and may reduce blister formation.
2. *Large exposed areas:*

> **NURSING ALERT:** Grease, ointment, or antiseptic solutions should *not* be applied to any large burn as an emergency measure.
> Avoid cold or ice water immersion for larger areas because cold may exaggerate vasoconstriction and impair peripheral circulation. Cold thermal injury may cause local tissue necrosis.

   a. Stop the burning process. Allow the wound to cool.

* See also page 595.

b. Cover with sterile dressings or any clean cloth to prevent further wound contamination; pain is decreased by preventing air from contacting injured surfaces.
3. *Chemical burns:*
   a. Irrigate copiously with large quantities of running water (except for burns caused by phosphorus) and remove clothing.
   b. Cover with loosely applied clean cloth.
   c. For chemical burns of the eyes, see page 671.
4. *Electrical burns:*

NOTE: Electrical current affects all tissues that it traverses; it may cause sepsis and even the loss of an extremity.

   a. Interrupt power source or remove patient from contact with current, using a nonconductor.

C. *Establish an airway and restore circulation with cardiopulmonary resuscitation if indicated.*

D. *Transport patient to emergency treatment facility.*

1. Generally, the burn victim is transported to the nearest Emergency Department. A physician there would initiate transfer to a Burn Center unless the ambulance group has standing orders about this.
2. If treatment facility is more than 30 minutes away, Ringer's lactate solution may be started intravenously at scene of accident. If there is difficulty in starting IV, do not lose time but head for the Emergency Treatment Center.
3. It is recommended that morphine not be administered at the scene of the accident because it may depress respirations and interfere with subsequent evaluation of other injuries.

Management of Specific Burns in the Emergency Treatment Center

OBJECTIVES: to maintain ventilation and circulation.
to prevent or treat shock and acute renal failure.
to prevent the depth of injury from increasing.
to complement subsequent burn treatment.
to care for the patient compassionately and make him as comfortable as possible.

A. *General Assessment and Protocol*

1. Assist with evaluation of thermal injury to assess extent of burns and their probable depth (see p. 596).
2. Determine the history: Retain victim's family members or his associates as information sources.
   a. Circumstances of accident
   b. Approximate duration of exposure to heat
   c. Age and *previous health condition* (diabetes, renal disease, etc.)
   d. Time, place, and mechanism of injury
   e. Mental status
   f. Care given patient before coming to Emergency Department.
3. Carry out rapid physical examination.
   a. Assess for hoarseness of voice and respiratory stridor (in patients with head and neck burns).
   b. Look for other injuries, especially in patients burned from automobile accidents or explosions.
4. Use rigid asepsis (cap, mask, gown, sterile gloves) when indicated (when wounds are exposed).

5. Cater to patient as a person; anticipate his needs and concerns.

B. *Initiate Subsequent Management*

1. Maintain adequate airway; provide adequate oxygenation, especially for patients with major burns and for elderly persons; recognize that carbon monoxide poisoning commonly accompanies burn injury, especially if victim was exposed to smoke.
2. Prepare for laryngoscopic, nasotracheal, or endotracheal intubation (tracheostomy is a last resort if intubation is not possible) in the following circumstances:
   a. Patients with deep burns of face, neck, and respiratory tract; injuries from inhalation of gases
   b. Stridor, tachypnea, restlessness, and inadequate respiratory exchange
   c. Patients unable to handle tracheobronchial secretions: drooling, excessive salivation
3. Replace fluids.
   a. Withdraw blood for typing, cross matching and blood gas samples.
   b. Start intravenous fluids; use central line (subclavian).
      (1) Patient loses significant intravascular protein, salt, and water during first few hours after burn; plasma volume is greatly reduced.
      (2) See page 598 for fluid therapy protocol following a burn.
      (3) Start fluid summary record.
4. Combat shock—due to local blood vessel damage with increased capillary permeability and loss of fluid into injured tissues.
   a. Insert indwelling urinary catheter—to assess urine volume, pH, specific gravity, sugar, acetone.
   b. Insert central venous pressure catheter (see p. 271).
   c. Assess patient for fractures, bleeding, head injuries, hemothorax, cardiac tamponade.
   d. Give definitive treatment for shock (p. 129).
5. Assist in care of the burn wound (see p. 599).
   a. Avoid further damage and contamination.
   b. Assist in performance of escharotomy (incision through eschar) since circumferential eschar on chest or extremities will prevent expansion of tissues and will cause compression of the neurovascular bundle.
6. Give analgesic as indicated (intravenously, in small doses).
   a. Patients with extensive superficial burns will complain of pain because of irritated hypersensitive nerve endings.
   b. Patients with deep extensive burns may require no medication during shock phase because of destruction of nerve endings in burned tissue.
7. Start a record of vital signs, treatments, and patient reactions.
8. Give systemic antimicrobial drugs as indicated—for burn wound sepsis.
9. Administer tetanus immune globulin or toxoid for tetanus prophylaxis.
10. Insert nasogastric tube to allow evacuation of air from stomach and prevent gastric dilatation.

C. *Protocol for Patients with Electrical Burns*

1. Initiate cardiopulmonary resuscitation if necessary; most likely to be required for the patient with a high-voltage electric injury.

2. Monitor for cardiac irregularities—death may ensue from ventricular fibrillation.
3. Watch for complications of myoglobinuria—large amounts of myoglobin pigment result from electrical muscle destruction. May need increase in fluids or mannitol to prevent renal tubular blockage.

D. *Disposition of Patient for Next Phase of Treatment*

1. Critically burned person should be moved to a well-equipped burn unit that has a medical and nursing staff experienced in burn care. This includes victims with:
   a. Respiratory tract burns
   b. Partial-thickness burns—more than 30% of body surface
   c. Full-thickness burns—more than 10% of body surface
   d. Burns of face, hands, feet, genitalia
   e. Burns complicated by fractures, major soft tissue injury, electrical injury
   f. Patients at extremes of age (under 2 or over 60) or with chronic disease (COPD, cardiac, diabetic)
2. Moderately burned person may be taken to a community hospital. This includes victims with:
   a. Partial-thickness burns—15–30% of body surface
   b. Full-thickness—less than 10% of body surface
3. Minimally burned person may be treated in a physician's office or hospital outpatient department. This includes victims with:
   a. Partial-thickness burns—less than 10%
   b. Full-thickness—less than 2%

COLD INJURIES TO EXTREMITIES (FROSTBITE)

Underlying Considerations

1. The extent of injury from exposure to cold is not always known when the patient is seen initially. A frozen extremity appears white, yellow-white, or mottled blue-white and is hard, cold, and sensitive to touch.
2. Color changes (purple: cyanosis) after rewarming may be transient *or* they may indicate pressure within the fascial compartment.

Emergency Management

OBJECTIVE: to restore normal body temperature.
1. Do not allow the patient to walk if lower extremities are involved.
2. Remove all constrictive clothing.
3. Rewarm extremity rapidly in warm-water bath 40°–42° C. (104°–108° F.) for 20 minutes or until erythema (flushing) occurs—early thawing appears to give better chance for maximum tissue preservation.
   a. Handle part gently to avoid further mechanical injury.
   b. Protect thawed part; do not rupture blebs.
   c. Administer analgesic for pain if necessary—thawing process may be quite painful.
4. Carry out physical examination—to look for concomitant injury (soft tissue injury, fracture, dehydration, alcoholic coma, fat embolism).
5. Restore electrolyte balance; check for acidosis.
6. Give tetanus prophylaxis if indicated by associated trauma.
7. Use bedside isolation with sterile technique during

bleb stage—to protect patient from contamination. Place sterile gauze/cotton between affected fingers or toes to prevent denudation. Elevate affected extremity.
8. Encourage hourly active motion of affected digits to promote maximum restoration of function.
9. The following measures may be carried out when appropriate.
   a. Whirlpool bath to affected extremity
   b. Escharotomy to prevent constriction
   c. Fasciotomy and sympathectomy—if there is distal ischemia
10. Prohibit use of tobacco because of vasoconstrictive effect.

ACCIDENTAL HYPOTHERMIA

Accidental hypothermia is a condition in which the core (internal) temperature of the body is less than 35° C. (95° F.) as a result of exposure to cold.

Underlying Considerations

1. There is progressive deterioration marked by apathy, poor judgment, ataxia, dysarthria, drowsiness, and eventually coma. Shivering may be suppressed below a temperature of 32.2° C. (90° F.).
2. Below this temperature, the body's self-warming mechanisms become ineffective. The heartbeat and the blood pressure may be so weak that the peripheral pulsations become undetectable. Cardiac irregularities also may occur. Other physiologic abnormalities include hypoxemia and acidosis.

Emergency Management

Management consists of continual monitoring, rewarming, and supportive care.
1. Monitor patient—vital signs, CVP, urinary output, arterial blood gases, electrolytes, glucose, BUN.
   a. Monitor body temperature with esophageal or rectal thermistor probe.
   b. Employ continuous ECG monitoring. Cardiac arrhythmias may occur during rewarming period.
   c. Maintain arterial line for recording blood pressure and to facilitate blood sampling.
2. Rewarm patient rapidly: rewarming methods include active core (internal) rewarming, active external rewarming, and passive or spontaneous rewarming. There are different opinions about which method is best.
3. Supportive care during rewarming includes:
   a. IV fluids (warmed)—to correct hypotension and maintain urinary output
   b. External cardiac massage; electrical cardioversion of ventricular defibrillation
   c. Correction of metabolic acidosis
   d. Mechanical ventilation with volume ventilator and warmed humidified oxygen—to maintain tissue oxygenation

ANAPHYLACTIC REACTION

Anaphylactic reaction is a sudden, generalized systemic (and frequently fatal) reaction occurring within seconds to minutes after exposure to a causative agent, namely, foreign sera, drugs, or insect venoms.

Altered Physiology

1. An anaphylactic reaction is the result of an antigen-antibody interaction in a sensitized individual who, as a consequence of previous exposure, has developed a special type of antibody (immunoglobin) that is specific for this particular allergen.
2. The antibody immunoglobulin IgE is responsible for the great majority of immediate type of human allergic responses—the individual becomes sensitive to a particular antigen after production of IgE to this antigen.

Causes

Penicillin, sera, other drugs, bee and wasp stings, or almost any repeatedly administered parenteral or oral therapeutic agent.

Clinical Manifestations

1. *Respiratory signs* include possible respiratory distress which progresses rapidly (caused by bronchospasm or edema of the larynx), sneezing and coughing, tightness of the chest, and other respiratory difficulties such as wheezing, dyspnea, and cyanosis.
2. *Skin manifestations* appear in the form of flushing with a sense of warmth and diffuse erythema. *Generalized itching over the entire body indicates that a general systemic reaction is developing.* Urticaria (hives) may also appear. When massive facial angioedema develops, upper respiratory edema may occur.
3. *Cardiovascular manifestations* include tachycardia or bradycardia and peripheral vascular collapse, indicated by pallor, imperceptible pulse, falling blood pressure, and circulatory failure leading to coma and death.
4. *Gastrointestinal discomforts,* such as nausea, vomiting, and colicky abdominal pains or diarrhea, may contribute to the general sense of malaise.

Emergency Management

1. Establish an airway while another person administers epinephrine.
   a. Turn patient's face to one side; support angles of mandible.
   b. Insert oropharyngeal or endotracheal tube; apply oropharyngeal suction for excessive secretions.
   c. Employ resuscitative measures (especially for patients with stridor and progressive pulmonary edema).
   d. If glottic edema is present, an incision through the cricothyroid ligament will provide an airway.
   e. Use positive-pressure oxygen therapy by mask and compression bag.
   f. Use closed-chest cardiac massage if necessary.
2. Give epinephrine as directed—to provide rapid relief of hypersensitivity reaction. This should be done while another person is establishing the airway. Use judgment in choosing route of administration for epinephrine.

a. Subcutaneous injection for mild, generalized symptoms.

b. Intramuscular or sublingual injection when reaction is more severe and progressive and when there is concern that vascular collapse will inhibit absorption.

c. Intravenous route (aqueous epinephrine diluted in saline and given *slowly*) for profound hypotension: this method may precipitate cardiac arrhythmias.

3. Start an intravenous infusion of saline for emergency route.

4. Apply tourniquet above injection site if the anaphylactic reaction followed an injection or insect sting—to retard absorption. Infiltrate injection site with epinephrine as directed.

5. Give antihistamine drugs, e.g., diphenhydramine hydrochloride (Benadryl) (IM)—may help block systemic effects of histamine released during anaphylaxis.

6. Give aminophylline IV *slowly* over a period of time for patients with severe bronchospasm and asthmatic symptoms. This is usually not given if patient is responding to epinephrine.

7. Treat prolonged hypotension with plasma or colloids (dextran), vasoconstrictors (metaraminol bitartrate [Aramine]), or levarterenol bitartrate (Levophed); patient with reduced cardiac output may respond to an infusion of isoproterenol or dopamine.

8. Watch for arrhythmias and cardiorespiratory arrest.

9. If the patient is convulsing, give IV injection of short-acting barbiturate or diazepam over a period of several minutes.

10. Administer corticosteroids if the patient is having a prolonged reaction and persistent hypotension or bronchospasm.

Preventive Measures and Health Education

1. Be aware of the danger of anaphylactic reactions.

2. Ask about patient's previous allergies to any medication; if positive, do not give the medication or injection.

3. Question patient before giving a foreign serum or other type of antigenic agent to determine if he has had it at some earlier time.

4. Question patient about previous allergic reactions to food or pollen.

5. Avoid giving drugs to patients with hay fever, asthma, and other allergic disorders unless absolutely necessary.

6. Avoid giving parenteral medications unless absolutely necessary; anaphylactic reactions are more likely to occur when therapeutic agent is given parenterally.

7. Do skin testing before administering foreign serum.

a. Skin testing can precipitate anaphylaxis in highly susceptible individuals.

b. A negative skin test does not always indicate safety.

c. Have epinephrine on hand to control acute untoward reactions.

8. If patient is being treated as an outpatient, keep him in office, hospital, or clinic at least 30 minutes after injection of any agent.

9. Caution patients who are sensitive to stinging insects or other antigens to carry commercial kits equipped with epinephrine.

10. Encourage allergic individual to wear identification tag.

POISONING

Poison is any substance which when ingested, inhaled, absorbed, applied to the skin, injected into or developed within the body, in relatively small amounts, produces injury to the body by its chemical action. (See p. 1451 for prevention of poisoning.)

SWALLOWED POISONS

Objectives of Emergency Management

1. To remove or inactivate the poison before it is absorbed.

2. To give supportive care to maintain vital organ systems.

3. To use the specific antidote to neutralize the poison.

4. To give treatment to hasten the elimination of the absorbed poison.

General Aspects of Management

1. Maintain the airway.

a. Administer oxygen for respiratory depression, unconsciousness, cyanosis, shock.

b. Administer artificial respiration if respiration is depressed; positive expiratory pressure applied to airway may help keep alveoli inflated.

2. Try to discover the nature of the poison (name, manufacturer) and the amount used. Call poison control center in the area if an unknown toxic agent has been taken or if it is necessary to identify an antidote for a known toxic agent.

a. Was ingestion accidental, intentional, or related to drug abuse?

b. Take arterial blood samples to measure pH and blood gas tensions.

c. Insert indwelling catheter to monitor kidney function.

d. Assess for central nervous system depression.

3. Monitor vital signs; try to calm and reassure the patient.

4. Treat shock appropriately.

5. Consider emesis or gastric lavage as the situation dictates—to prevent further absorption of poison.

a. Emesis *is not* indicated when caustic or petroleum distillate products have been ingested or when patient is comatose, convulsing, unresponsive, or without a gag reflex.

b. Intubate with endotracheal tube before gastric lavage to prevent aspiration.

6. Give specific therapy. Administer special chemical antidote (if indicated) or specific pharmacologic antagonists as early as possible.

7. Support the patient having convulsions; many poisons excite the central nervous system; the patient may convulse because of oxygen deprivation.

8. Monitor central venous pressure as indicated.
9. Monitor fluid and electrolyte balance.
10. Reduce elevated temperature.
11. Provide constant nursing surveillance and attention to the patient in a coma (p. 706); coma from poisoning results from interference with brain cell function or metabolism.
12. Give analgesics for pain with caution; severe pain causes vasomotor collapse and reflex inhibition of normal physiologic function.
13. Assist in securing specimens of blood, urine, stomach contents, or vomitus for laboratory analysis and drug screen.
14. Assist with forced diuresis, hemodialysis, or peritoneal dialysis to shorten period of unconsciousness in the event of barbiturate and other hypnotic or tranquilizer poisoning.
15. Refer for psychiatric consultation if suicide attempt or drug abuse is involved.

Corrosive Poisons

A. *Types of Corrosive Poisons*
1. Acid and acid-like substances; sodium acid sulfate (toilet bowl cleaners), acetic acid (glacial), sulfuric acid, nitric acid, oxalic acid, hydrofluoric acid (rust removers), iodine, silver nitrate.
2. Alkali corrosives—most common are sodium hydroxide (lye; drain cleaners), dishwasher detergents, sodium carbonate (washing soda), ammonia water, sodium hypochlorite (household bleach).

B. *Clinical Manifestations*
1. Severe pain; burning sensation in mouth and throat
2. Painful swallowing or inability to swallow
3. Vomiting
4. Destruction of oral mucosa, esophageal burns

C. *Emergency Management*
1. If the patient can swallow after ingestion of a *corrosive poison,* he may be offered milk as an emollient agent (controversial). Do not induce vomiting if patient has consumed a strong acid, alkali, or other corrosive substance.
2. Esophagoscopy may be performed (early) to assess for presence of esophageal stricture.

Noncorrosive Poisons
Emergency Management

1. *Remove poison from patient's stomach immediately by inducing vomiting.*

> **NURSING ALERT:** Do not induce vomiting if victim has consumed a strong acid, alkali, or other corrosive or hydrocarbon solvent. Do not induce vomiting if patient is in a coma, is unconscious, or is having convulsions.

  a. Give 3–4 glassfuls of milk or water to drink—to dilute poison.
  b. Induce vomiting by giving syrup of ipecac or by inserting the index finger or blunt end of a spoon at the back of the patient's throat.
2. Carry out gastric lavage procedure (see below) to remove any unabsorbed poison. This procedure is *not* done if corrosives or hydrocarbon solvents have been ingested. (Example: turpentine, gasoline, kerosene, liquid wax, charcoal fluid lighter, etc.)
  A patient who has ingested hydrocarbons should have a chest film done to evaluate for chemical pneumonia.
3. Instruct family to bring unused poison to hospital for identification.

GUIDELINES: Assisting with Gastric Lavage

Gastric lavage is the aspiration of the stomach contents and washing out of the stomach by means of a gastric tube.

Purposes
1. To remove unabsorbed poison after poison ingestion.
2. To diagnose gastric hemorrhage and for the arrest of hemorrhage.
3. To cleanse the stomach before endoscopic procedures.
4. To remove liquid or small particles of material from the stomach.

> **NURSING ALERT:** Gastric lavage may be dangerous (1) after the ingestion of acids, alkalis, hydrocarbons, or petroleum distillates and (2) in the presence of convulsions. It is dangerous after the ingestion of strong corrosive agents.

Equipment
Stomach tubes (large lumen)
Large irrigating syringe with adapter
Large plastic funnel with adapter to fit stomach tube
Water soluble lubricant
Tap water or appropriate antidote (milk, saline solution, sodium bicarbonate solution, fruit juice, activated charcoal)*
Bucket for aspirate
Mouth gag; nasotracheal or endotracheal tubes with inflatable cuffs
Containers for specimens

* Activated charcoal adsorbs (binds) many drugs in the gastrointestinal tract and prevents their absorption in the bloodstream.

Procedure

NURSING ACTION	**RATIONALE/AMPLIFICATION**
1. Remove dental appliances and inspect oral cavity for loose teeth.	
2. Measure the distance between the bridge of the nose and the xiphoid process. Mark with indelible pencil or tape.	
3. Lubricate the tube with water soluble lubricant.	
4. If the patient is comatose, he is intubated with a cuffed nasotracheal or endotracheal tube.	4. A cuffed endotracheal tube prevents aspiration of gastric contents.
5. Place the patient in a left lateral position with the head, neck, and trunk forming a straight line. After the lavage tube is passed, the head of the table is lowered. Have standby suction available.	5. This position prevents fluid from running into the trachea and keeps reflux vomitus from being aspirated.
6. Pass the tube via the oral (or nasal) route while keeping the head in a neutral position. Pass the tube to the adhesive marking or about 50 cm. (20 inches).	6. The depth of insertion of the tube will vary with the height of the patient. If the tube enters the larynx instead of the esophagus the patient will experience coughing and dyspnea.
7. Submerge free end of tube below water level at the moment of patient's exhalation.	7. If tube is inadvertently in the lungs, the water will bubble with each exhalation.
8. Aspirate the stomach contents with syringe attached to the tube before instilling water or antidote. Save the specimen for analysis.	8. Aspiration is carried out to remove the stomach contents.
9. Remove syringe. Attach funnel to the stomach tube or use 50-ml. syringe to put lavage solution in gastric tube. Volume of fluid placed in the stomach should be small.	9. Overfilling of the stomach may cause regurgitation and aspiration or force the stomach contents through the pylorus.
10. Elevate funnel above the patient's head and pour approximately 120–300 ml. of solution into funnel.	10. If the syringe method is used, the turbulence from the pressure of the syringe will cause the fluid to mix with the stomach contents and assist in washing all of the mucosal surface. It is possible for poison/drugs to be trapped in the rugae of stomach.
11. Lower the funnel and siphon the gastric contents into the bucket.	
12. Save samples of first 2 washings.	12. Keep first washings isolated from other washings for possible analysis.
13. Repeat lavage procedure until the returns are relatively clear.	
14. At the completion of lavage: a. Stomach may be left empty. b. Antidote may be instilled in tube and allowed to remain in stomach. c. Cathartic may be put down tube.	c. To speed elimination of the poison through gastrointestinal tract.
15. Pinch off tube during removal or maintain suction while tube is being withdrawn.	15. Pinching off the tube prevents aspiration and the initiation of the gag reflex. Keeping the patient's head lower than the body also gives this protection.
16. Give the patient a cathartic if prescribed.	16. A cathartic may be given if the poison has no corrosive action on the bowel. The cathartic will help remove unabsorbed material from the intestine.

INHALED POISONS

Carbon Monoxide Poisoning

May occur as an industrial or household accident or as an attempted suicide.

A. *Underlying Principles*

1. The effect of carbon monoxide is to render the hemoglobin useless as an oxygen-carrying chemical, because it unites so firmly with the pigment in place of oxygen. As a result, tissue anoxia occurs.
2. Clinical manifestations:
   a. Patient may appear intoxicated (result of cerebral hypoxia).
   b. Headache, muscular weakness, palpitation, dizziness, mental confusion—may progress rapidly to coma.
   c. Skin may be cherry red or cyanotic and pale—skin color is *not* a reliable sign.
3. History of exposure to carbon monoxide should justify immediate treatment.

B. *Emergency Management*

OBJECTIVES: to reverse cerebral and myocardial hypoxia.
  to hasten carbon monoxide elimination.

1. Give 100% oxygen at atmospheric or hyperbaric pressures to reverse hypoxia and accelerate elimination of carbon monoxide.
2. Observe the patient constantly—psychoses, spastic paralysis, visual disturbances, and deterioration of personality may persist following resuscitation and may be symptoms of permanent central nervous system damage.

SKIN-CONTAMINATION POISONS

Emergency Management

1. Drench skin with water (shower, hose, faucet)—burning continues as long as agent is on the skin.
2. Apply stream of water on skin while removing clothing.
3. Cleanse skin thoroughly with water; rapidity in washing is most important in reducing extent of injury.
   a. Wash with soap if agent is noncaustic.
   b. For phosphorus burns—treat with agents that neutralize offending agent (copper sulfate).

INJECTED POISONS

Stinging Insects

(Bee, yellow jacket, hornet, wasp)

> **NURSING ALERT:** A patient may have an extreme sensitivity to *Hymenoptera* stings (yellow jackets, bees, hornets, wasps). This constitutes an acute emergency. Stings of the head and neck are especially serious, although stings in any area of the body can result in anaphylaxis.

A. *Clinical Manifestations*

Anaphylactic reaction (p. 888)
1. Severe fall in blood pressure
2. Difficult breathing
3. Edema of face, lips
4. Urticaria
5. Itching
6. Bronchial constriction
7. Diarrhea, abdominal cramps

B. *Emergency Management and Health Education*

1. Give epinephrine as requested. Massage the site to hasten absorption.
2. See page 888 for treatment of anaphylactic reaction.
3. Patients known to be sensitive to *Hymenoptera* venom should carry a commercially available emergency kit with epinephrine in prefilled syringes, tourniquet, alcohol swabs, capsule containing antihistamine and ephedrine; available on prescription.*
   a. Instruct the patient to take epinephrine immediately if he is stung.
   b. Flick stinger off with the fingernail, if possible.
   c. Do not squeeze venom sac—may cause additional venom to be injected.
   d. Report to nearest medical facility for observation.
4. Instruct patient to limit exposure to stinging insects by:
   a. Avoiding locales with stinging insects (camp and picnic sites).
   b. Staying away from insect feeding areas—flower beds, ripe fruit orchards, garbage, fields of clover.
   c. Not going barefoot outdoors—yellow jackets may nest on ground.
   d. Avoiding perfumes, scented soaps, bright colors—attract bees.
   e. Keeping car windows closed.

   * Hollister-Stier Laboratories and Nelco Laboratories, Inc. market emergency insect sting kits.

   f. Spraying garbage cans with rapid-acting insecticide.
   g. Securing a professional exterminator to dispose of wasp/hornet nests or bee hives in home area.
5. A person with this allergy should consider undergoing immunotherapy with venom extract.
6. All allergic individuals should wear medical warning bracelets indicating hypersensitivity.

FOOD POISONING*

Food poisoning is a sudden, explosive illness which may occur after the ingestion of food or drink.

Emergency Management

1. Determine the source and type of food poisoning.
   a. Have family bring suspected food to medical facility.
      (1) How soon after eating did the symptoms occur? Immediate onset suggests chemical, plant, or animal poisoning.
      (2) What was eaten in the previous meal? Did the food have any unusual odor or taste? Most foods causing bacterial poisoning do not have unusual odor or taste.
      (3) Did anyone else eating the same food become ill?
      (4) Did vomiting occur? What was the appearance of the vomitus?
      (5) Did diarrhea occur? Diarrhea is usually absent with botulism, or with shell-fish or other fish poisoning.
      (6) Are any neurologic symptoms present? These occur in botulism, chemical, plant, and animal poisoning.
      (7) Does the patient have a fever? Fever is seen in salmonella, favism (ingestion of fava beans), and some fish poisoning.
      (8) What is the patient's appearance?
2. Collect food, gastric contents, vomitus, serum, and feces for examination.
3. Monitor vital signs on a continual basis.
   a. Assess respiration, blood pressure, sensorium, central venous pressure (if indicated), and muscular activity.
   b. Weigh the patient for future comparisons.
4. Support the respiratory system. Death from respiratory paralysis can occur with botulism, fish poisoning, etc.
5. Maintain fluid and electrolyte balance; severe vomiting produces alkalosis; and severe diarrhea produces acidosis; large amounts of electrolytes and water are lost by vomiting and diarrhea.
   a. Watch for oligemic shock from severe fluid and electrolyte losses.
   b. Evaluate for apathy, rapid pulse, fever, oliguria, anuria, hypotension, and delirium.
   c. Carry out blood electrolyte studies.
6. Correct and control hypoglycemia.
7. Control the nausea.
   a. Give antiemetic drug parenterally if patient cannot tolerate fluids or medications by mouth.
   b. Give sips of weak tea, carbonated drinks, and tap water for mild nausea.
   c. Give clear liquids 12 to 24 hours after nausea and vomiting subside.
   d. Graduate to a low-residue, bland diet.

   * Botulism is discussed on pages 819–820, since the treatment differs.

DRUG ABUSE

Drug abuse is the use of drugs for other than legitimate medical purposes. There is a growing tendency among drug users to take a variety of drugs simultaneously, including alcohol, barbiturates, tranquilizers, and sedatives, which may have additive effects. The clinical manifestations may vary with the drug used, but the underlying principles of management are essentially the same.

Emergency Management

OBJECTIVES: to support the respiratory and cardiovascular functions.

to give definitive treatment for drug overdose.

1. Maintain the patient's respirations.
   a. Use a cuffed endotracheal tube and provide assisted ventilation in a severely depressed patient with absent gag or cough reflexes.
   b. Measure arterial blood gases—for hypoxia due to hypoventilation, acid-base derangements, etc.
   c. Administer oxygen.
2. Start intravenous fluids and stabilize the cardiovascular system; this is done simultaneously with airway management.
   a. Begin external cardiac compression and ventilation in the absence of heartbeat.
   b. Start ECG monitoring—to observe arrhythmias and detect electrolyte abnormalities.
3. Give specific drug antagonist if drug is known; naloxone hydrochloride (Narcan) is frequently used.
4. Remove the drug from the stomach as soon as possible (if drug has been ingested).
   a. Induce vomiting if patient is seen *early* after ingestion; save vomitus for toxicologic study.
   b. Use gastric lavage if the patient is unconscious or if there is no way to determine when the drug was ingested; save gastric aspirate.
      (1) In patients with absent gag or cough reflexes, carry out this procedure only after intubation with cuffed endotracheal tube to prevent aspiration of stomach contents.
      (2) Activated charcoal may be a useful adjunct to therapy and is used after emesis or lavage.
5. Save samples of blood, urine, and any other specimens for future laboratory analysis.
6. Try to maintain a free flow of urine since the drug or metabolites are excreted by the kidneys.
7. Consider hemodialysis or peritoneal dialysis for potentially lethal poisoning.
8. Do a thorough physical examination to rule out insulin shock, meningitis, subdural hematoma, stroke, trauma.
   a. Look for needle marks, constricted pupils.
   b. There is a high incidence of infectious hepatitis among drug users which is thought to be the result of communal use of nonsterile needles and syringes.
   c. Keep in mind that many drug users take numerous drugs at one time.
   d. Examine breath for characteristic odor of alcohol, acetone, etc.
9. Try to obtain a history of the drug experiences (from the person accompanying the patient or from the patient himself).

   a. Adopt a supportive, empathetic, and realistic relationship with the patient.
   b. Do not leave the patient alone.
10. Make every effort to enroll the patient in a drug treatment program (detoxification and rehabilitation) to intervene in a life-style that fosters addiction.

NARCOTIC ABUSE

Examples

Heroin (most frequently involved)
Opium or paregoric
Morphine, codeine, synthetic narcotics (methadone)

Clinical Manifestations

1. Pinpoint pupils (may be dilated with severe hypoxia)
2. Depressed vital signs
3. Apnea or slow respirations (2–6/minute)
4. Fresh needle marks along course of any superficial vein

Emergency Management

1. Maintain respiration.
   a. Give mouth-to-mouth resuscitation; then establish intubation and assisted ventilation.
   b. Have second person listen with stethoscope for breath sounds over both lung fields.
   c. Maintain circulation; use external cardiac compression.
2. Give narcotic antagonist (naloxone hydrochloride [Narcan]) to reverse severe respiratory depression and coma.
3. Continue to monitor the level of responsiveness and respirations, pulse, and blood pressure—duration of action of naloxone hydrochloride (Narcan) is shorter than that of heroin, etc., and repeated dose(s) may be necessary.

   Do not leave patient alone—may lapse back into coma rapidly; clinical status may change from minute to minute.
4. Establish an intravenous line—patient may be given a bolus of 50% glucose to eliminate possibility of hypoglycemia.
5. Send urine to laboratory for analysis—opiates can be detected in urine.
6. Secure blood for chemical and toxicologic analysis; also for baseline studies and blood gases.
7. Secure an ECG.
8. Hemodialysis may be indicated for severe drug intoxication.

Heroin Withdrawal Syndrome

A. *Clinical Manifestations*

1. Lethargy; yawning
2. Perspiration, lacrimation, runny nose
3. Dilated pupils, poorly reactive to light
4. Gooseflesh, muscular aches
5. Twitching, anorexia, nausea, vomiting, abdominal pain
6. Chills and fever

B. *Management*

1. Methadone may be prescribed if patient is receiving

treatment at a methadone center, or substitution therapy should be given in a hospital setting.
2. Give intravenous fluids since patient is dehydrated from vomiting; may progress to toxic delirium.
3. Assess for concomitant medical problems (hepatitis, pneumonia, severe diarrhea).
4. Place patient in protected environment under proper medical supervision.
5. Make every effort to enroll patient in a narcotics treatment program—to intervene in a life style that fosters addiction.

HALLUCINOGENS OR PSYCHEDELIC-TYPE DRUGS

Common Forms
1. Lysergic acid diethylamide (LSD)
2. Phencyclidine HCl (PCP); (see Emergency Management, #9)
3. Mescaline, Psilocybin
4. Jimson weed seeds

Clinical Manifestations
1. Marked anxiety bordering on panic
2. Confusion, incoherence, hyperactivity
3. Hallucinations
4. Hazardous behavior (delirium, mania, self-injury)
5. Flashback—recurrence of LSD-like state may occur up to 1 year after drug use.
6. Convulsions, coma, circulatory collapse, death

Emergency Management
1. Determine if patient has ingested hallucinogenic drug or has a toxic psychosis.
2. Try to communicate with the patient—use "vocal anesthesia" to reassure him (except for PCP abusers).
   a. "Talking down" involves understanding the process through which the patient is proceeding and helping him overcome his fears while establishing contact with reality.
   b. Remind the patient that fear is common with this problem.
   c. Reassure the patient that he is not losing his mind; that he is experiencing effect of drugs and that this will wear off.
   d. Instruct the patient to keep his eyes open—reduces intensity of reaction.
   e. Do not leave the patient alone.
3. Sedate the patient if his hyperactivity cannot be controlled—diazepam (Valium) or a barbiturate may be given.
4. Search for evidences of trauma—hallucinogenic users have a tendency to "act out" their hallucinations.
5. Manage convulsions; place patient in Intensive Care Unit.
6. Watch patient closely—his behavior may become hazardous.
7. Monitor for hypertensive crisis if patient has prolonged psychosis due to drug ingestion.
8. Place patient in a protected environment under proper medical supervision to prevent self-inflicted bodily harm.
9. *For phencyclidine intoxication*
   a. Drug effects are unpredictable and prolonged.
   b. Symptoms are likely to exacerbate; patient be-

comes out of control (resembles schizophrenic psychosis)
   c. Management:
      (1) Place patient in calm, supportive environment to minimize stimuli.
      (2) Avoid "talking down." See page 897 for management of combative behavior. Protect from self-injury.
      (3) Treat symptoms as they occur.
      (4) Refer to drug treatment center for evaluation and treatment.

AMPHETAMINE-TYPE DRUGS
(Pep pills, "uppers," "speed")

Examples
Amphetamine (Benzedrine)
Dextroamphetamine (Dexedrine)
Methamphetamine (Desoxyn)

Clinical Manifestations
Abrupt or insidious development of behavioral disturbances
1. Aggressive type of behavior
2. Irritability, insomnia
3. Visual misperceptions; auditory hallucinations
4. Fearful anxiety/depression; cold, distant hostility
5. Hyperactivity, stereotyped activities; rapid speech, euphoria
6. Paranoid suspiciousness
7. Increasing pulse rate and blood pressure
8. Hallucinosis; high temperature
9. Convulsions → coma → death

Emergency Management
1. Try to communicate with patient—amphetamine paranoid psychosis is frequently seen.
   a. Patient may have delusions of persecution, ideas of reference, visual and auditory hallucinations, changes in body image, hyperactivity, excitation.
   b. Maintain tranquil environment.
2. Perform gastric evacuation followed by activated charcoal and saline cathartic.
3. Use specific drug therapy to alleviate agitative state.
   a. Usually within 24 hours after last dose of amphetamine, patient will begin to spend increasing amounts of time sleeping.
   b. Keep patient relatively quiet and reassured; patient may become aggressive/assaultive and reach a state of panic.
4. Carry out urine checks for amphetamines.
5. Place patient in protective environment—observe for suicidal attempts.
   a. Use techniques of dealing with acutely paranoid individuals; do not move close to patient or behind him.
   b. Avoid confined spaces.

BARBITURATES—ACUTE INTOXICATION

Examples
Pentobarbital (Nembutal)
Secobarbital (Seconal)
Amobarbital (Amytal)

Clinical Manifestations

(Barbiturates depress cardiovascular and pulmonary systems)
1. Flushed face
2. Decreased pulse rate
3. Increasing nystagmus
4. Decreasing tendon reflexes
5. Decreasing mental alertness
6. Difficulty in speaking
7. Poor motor coordination
8. Dilated; nonreacting pupils
9. Coma; death

Emergency Management

1. Maintain airway and stimulate depressed respirations.
   Consider endotracheal intubation or tracheostomy if there is any doubt about the adequacy of airway exchange.
2. Support cardiovascular and respiratory functions.
3. Start intravenous infusion through large gauge needle or intravenous catheter to support blood pressure—coma and dehydration result in hypotension and respond to infusion of intravenous fluids with elevation of blood pressure.
   Sodium bicarbonate may be given to alkalinize urine—increases excretion of phenobarbital.
4. Start gastric evacuation; gastric lavage (after endotracheal intubation) may be carried out followed by instillation of activated charcoal through gastric lavage tube.
5. Carry out physical and neurologic examinations.
6. Maintain neurologic and vital sign flow sheet.
7. Patient awakening from overdose may demonstrate hostility; this can stimulate automatic angry responses by health personnel.
8. Refer for psychiatric consultation to assess suicidal intent, drug abuse, etc.

Barbiturate Withdrawal Syndrome

A. *Clinical Manifestations*

1. Shakiness, anxiety, muscular irritability
2. Orthostatic hypotension, tachycardia
3. Seizures; withdrawal psychosis
4. Hyperpyrexia; death

> **NURSING ALERT:** Symptoms of barbiturate withdrawal are serious because abrupt withdrawal from the drug may be life-threatening and may begin when patient is recovering from an overdose.

B. *Emergency Management*

1. Maintain airway and stimulate depressed respiration.
2. Administer phenobarbital according to level of patient's tolerance; gradually reduce dosage of barbiturates until drug-free state is achieved.
3. Give oxygen and intravenous fluids as required.
4. Watch for excessive agitation, confusion, and convulsions.

NONBARBITURATE SEDATIVES

Examples

Glutethimide (Doriden)

Methyprylon (Noludar)
Ethchlorvynol (Placidyl)
Ethinamate (Valmid)
Meprobamate (Miltown, Equanil)
Chlordiazepoxide (Librium)
Diazepam (Valium)

Clinical Manifestations

1. Decreasing mental alertness
2. Confusion
3. Slurred speech
4. Ataxia
5. Pulmonary edema
6. Coma, possible death

Emergency Management

1. Insert endotracheal tube as a precaution; utilize assisted ventilation.
   Watch for sudden apnea and laryngeal spasm (especially in patients habituated to Doriden).
2. Start ECG monitoring.
   Watch for cardiovascular instability with arrhythmia.
3. Assess for hypotension.
   a. Insert indwelling catheter for comatose patient—decreased urinary volume is an index of reduced renal flow associated with reduced intravascular volume or vascular collapse.
   b. Start volume expansion with saline, plasma, or dextrose as required.
4. Assist with gastric lavage followed by activated charcoal.
5. Use hemodialysis therapy if needed.

ASPIRIN AND OTHER SALICYLATE POISONING

Clinical Manifestations

1. Abdominal pain, hematemesis (early)
2. Late signs and symptoms:
   a. Tachypnea
   b. Disturbed acid-base balance
   c. Tinnitus and vertigo
   d. Disorientation
   e. Hyperventilation
   f. Convulsions; coma

Emergency Management

1. Treat respiratory depression.
2. Carry out gastric lavage—will remove significant amounts of salicylates up to 10 hours following ingestion, or give ipecac as directed.
3. Give water, milk, or activated charcoal—to delay absorption of ingested poison after emesis or lavage.
4. Support patient with intravenous infusions to correct electrolyte imbalance and maintain hydration.
5. Correct acid-base disturbances; monitor electrolytes.
6. Administer blood transfusion if indicated.
7. Prepare for peritoneal dialysis (p. 494) or hemodialysis for patients with severe intoxication.
8. Give vitamin K for bleeding—salicylates lower plasma prothrombin by interfering with vitamin K utilization in the liver.

ALCOHOL ABUSE

ACUTE ALCOHOLISM

Clinical Manifestations

(Caused by depressant action of alcohol on nervous system)
1. Drowsiness, incoordination, slurring of speech—or
2. Belligerency, grandiosity, uninhibited behavior
3. Odor of alcohol on breath or clothing
4. Stupor—hypoventilation, hypotension

Emergency Management

1. Approach the patient in a nonjudgmental manner. (Alcoholic patients have a tendency to stimulate rejecting behavior in health care personnel.)
   a. Expect patient to use mechanisms of denial and defensiveness.
   b. Adapt a firm, consistent, accepting, and reasonable attitude.
   c. Speak calmly.
   d. If patient appears drunk, he is probably drunk even though he denies any alcohol intake.
2. Take a blood alcohol test as directed.
3. Allow the drowsy patient to "sleep off" the state of alcoholic intoxication.
   a. Observe for symptoms of CNS depression; keep patient under observation.
   b. Protect the airway.
   c. Undress the patient and cover with a blanket.
4. Sedate the belligerent, noisy patient as directed. Monitor the patient carefully.
5. Examine the patient for injuries and organic disease which can easily be masked by alcoholic intoxication; chronic alcohol abusers suffer more injuries and illnesses than the general population.
   a. Look for symptoms of head injury. Assess the neurologic status of the patient.
   b. Assess for alcoholic coma—a medical emergency.
   c. Evaluate for pneumonia, which is common in alcoholic individuals—due to impaired defense system and tendency toward gastric aspiration.
   d. Watch for hypoglycemia.
6. Hospitalize if necessary, or admit to detoxification center; an effort should be made to examine the problems underlying substance abuse (see p. 942).

DELIRIUM TREMENS (ALCOHOLIC HALLUCINOSIS)

Delirium tremens is an acute toxic state that follows a prolonged bout of steady drinking or the diminution or cessation of alcoholic intake. It may be precipitated by acute injury or infection.

> **NURSING ALERT:** Delirium tremens is a serious complication and poses a threat to the life of the alcoholic patient.

Clinical Manifestations

1. Anxiety; uncontrollable fear
2. Tremulousness, restlessness and agitation, irritability, insomnia
3. Talkativeness; preoccupation
4. Visual, tactile, and auditory hallucinations (usually of a frightening nature)
5. Autonomic overactivity—tachycardia, profuse perspiration, fever

Emergency Management

OBJECTIVE: to give proper sedation and support to enable the patient to rest and recover without the danger of injury or exhaustion.

1. Take the blood pressure since the patient's subsequent medication may depend on his blood pressure readings.
2. Carry out physical examination to identify preexisting or contributing illnesses or injuries (cerebral injury, pneumonia, etc.).
3. Sedate the patient with sufficient dosage of medication to produce adequate sedation—to reduce his agitation, prevent exhaustion, and promote sleep.
   a. A variety of drugs and combinations of drugs are used—chloral hydrate, diazepam (Valium), hydroxyzine (Vistaril), etc.
   b. The dosage may be adjusted according to the patient's symptoms and blood pressure response.
4. Place the patient in a private room where he can be observed closely.
   a. Keep room lighted—to reduce incidence of visual hallucinations.
   b. Close closet and bathroom doors to eliminate shadows.
   c. Keep environment calm and nonstressful; call patient by name.
   d. Observe patient closely—he may become homicidal or suicidal in response to his hallucinations if he is having alcoholic hallucinations.
   e. Have someone stay with the patient as much as possible—presence of another person has a reassuring and quieting effect.
   f. Explain every procedure done to the patient in detail.
   g. Take patient to bathroom if permitted.
   h. Explain visual misinterpretations (illusions)—strengthens link with reality.
   i. Use restraints if patient is not under direct and constant observation.
5. Maintain electrolyte balance and hydration via oral or intravenous route—fluid losses may be extreme because of profuse perspiration and agitation.
6. Record temperature, pulse, respiration, and blood pressure frequently (every 30 minutes in severe forms of delirium)—in anticipation of peripheral circulatory collapse and/or hyperthermia (the 2 most common lethal complications).
7. Administer phenytoin (Dilantin) or other anticonvulsant drugs as prescribed to prevent or control alcoholic or epileptic convulsions.
8. Assess respiratory, hepatic, and cardiovascular status of patient—pneumonia, liver disease, and cardiac failure are complications.
   a. Hypoglycemia may accompany alcoholic withdrawal because alcohol depletes liver glycogen stores and impairs gluconeogenesis; many patients also suffer from malnutrition.

b. Administer parenteral dextrose if liver glycogen is depleted.

c. Give orange juice, Gatorade, or other carbohydrates to stabilize blood sugar and to counteract tremulousness.

9. Give supplemental vitamin therapy and a high protein diet; these patients are usually vitamin deficient.

10. Refer to alcoholic treatment center for subsequent follow-up and rehabilitation.

PSYCHIATRIC EMERGENCY

Psychiatric emergency is an urgent, serious disturbance of behavior, affect, or thought which makes the patient unable to cope with his life situation and interpersonal relationships.

Behavioral Manifestations

A. *Overactive (or violent)*

1. Disturbed, uncooperative, unpredictable paranoid behavior
2. Anxiety and panic-like state
3. Assaultive and destructive impulses and behavior (patient may be noisy or disturbed from acute alcohol or drug intoxication)
4. Crying, depression, intense nervousness

B. *Underactive (or depressed)*

1. Depression
2. Fearfulness, detached attitude
3. Slowing of responses
4. Sad facial expression

C. *Suicidal*

Emergency Management

OBJECTIVE: to maintain the patient's self-esteem (and life, if necessary), while carrying out assessment and intervention.

A. *Overactive Patient*

1. Determine (from family, ambulance driver, etc.) if patient has had past mental illness, hospitalizations, injuries or serious illnesses, uses alcohol or drugs, or has experienced crises in interpersonal relationships or intrapsychic conflicts.
2. Be aware that abnormal thought and behavior may be manifestations of an underlying physical disorder (hypoglycemia, stroke, epilepsy) and drug toxicity, including alcohol toxicity.
3. Try to gain control of the situation.
   a. Approach the patient with a calm, confident, and firm manner—this attitude is therapeutic and will help calm the patient.
   b. Introduce yourself by name to the patient.
   c. Tell him "I am here to help you."
   d. Repeat patient's name from time to time.
   e. Speak in one-thought sentences. Be consistent.
   f. Give the individual space. Let him slow down by himself and allow him to become compliant.
   g. Be interested in and listen to the patient—encourage him to talk of his thoughts and *feelings*.
   h. Offer appropriate explanations. Tell the truth.
4. Give tranquilizer or psychotropic agent for emergency management of functional psychosis. Chlorpromazine (Thorazine) or haloperidol (Haldol) act specifically against psychotic symptoms of thought fragmentation and perceptual and behavioral aberrations.
   a. Initial dosage depends on body weight and severity of symptoms.

b. Observe patient for 1 hour after initial dose to determine degree of change in psychotic behavior.

c. Subsequent dosages depend on patient's reaction.

d. If behavior is caused by hallucinogens (LSD, etc.), psychotropic drugs (exerting an effect on the mind) are not used.

5. Use restraints only as a last resort.
6. Admit to psychiatric unit or arrange for psychiatric outpatient treatment.

B. *Violent Patient*

Violent and aggressive behavior is usually episodic and is a means of expressing feelings of anger, fear, or hopelessness about a situation. Patients who display violent behavior usually fall into one of four diagnostic categories: (1) functional (usually psychotic); (2) organic brain syndrome; (3) toxic psychosis; or (4) drug withdrawal.

Emergency Management:

OBJECTIVES: to protect the patient and staff from harm. to control the violent/disturbed episode.

1. If possible, have 2 persons see the patient initially; a specially designated room should be used, in which no objects that could be used as weapons are in sight.
2. Keep the door of the room open and be in clear view of the staff. Do not block the patient's exit to the door; patient may feel closed in and threatened.
3. Give the patient space. Do not make any sudden movement. If the patient is carrying a weapon, ask him to place it in a neutral area.
4. Adopt a calm, noncritical approach and remain in control of the situation. External calm and structure may help patient to gain control.
5. Talk and listen to the patient.
   a. Crisis intervention is best done with an attitude of interest in the patient's well-being and with an attempt to "tune in" to the patient while at the same time remaining firm.
   b. Acknowledge the patient's state of agitation: "I want to work with you to relieve your distress," etc. Ask if he is thinking of hurting someone.
   c. Give the patient the opportunity to ventilate his anger verbally.
   d. Try to hear what the patient is saying.
   e. Convey to the patient that help is available for him to gain control.
      (1) Let patient know that his behavior is frightening to those around him.
      (2) Describe the help available in crisis situations—clinic, emergency department, mental health facility.
6. Allow the security personnel/police to intervene if the patient does not become calm.
   a. Offer protection of hospitalization—usually welcomed by the patient who fears his loss of control.
   b. Use restraints when necessary but with minimum of force.

(1) Have enough personnel available when applying restraints.
(2) Talk reassuringly to patient while applying restraints.
c. Administer intramuscular medication (haloperidol, diazepam, chlorpromazine) as directed.
d. Refer patient for further mental health treatment after combativeness, agitation, and fear have cooled.

C. Underactive or Depressed Patient

The underactive or depressed patient will be fearful, depressed, and slow to respond, will be plagued by feelings of worthlessness, guilt, ambivalence, and indecision, and will be prone to insomnia, a worsening mood in the morning, sad facial expression, and feelings of isolation.

Emergency Management
1. Listen to the patient in a calm, unhurried manner.
   a. Patient will benefit from ventilation of feelings.
   b. Give patient an opportunity to talk about his problems.
   c. Anticipate that the patient may be suicidal.
   d. Attempt to find out if the patient has thought about or attempted suicide.
      (1) "Have you ever thought about taking your own life?"
      (2) The patient is generally relieved because of the opportunity to discuss his feelings.
   e. Find out if there is an illness, perceived or real.
   f. Assess whether there has been sudden worsening of depression.
   g. Notify relatives about a seriously depressed patient. Do not leave the patient alone since suicide is usually an act committed in solitude.
2. Give antidepressant and antianxiety agents as prescribed.

3. Point out to the patient that depression is treatable.
4. Be aware of crisis and supportive services in the community; telephone counseling and referral, suicide prevention centers, group therapy, marital and family counseling, drug/alcohol counseling, adolescent counseling, befriending programs.
5. Refer patient for psychiatric consultation or to psychiatric unit.

D. Suicidal Patient

Suicide is an act that stems from depression (the loss of a loved one, the loss of body integrity or status, poor self-image) and can be viewed as a cry for help and intervention.

Persons at Risk
Older person, male, unusual loss or stress, unemployed, divorced, living alone, showing significant depression (weight loss, sleep disturbances, somatic complaints, suicidal preoccupation), history of previous suicidal attempts, psychiatric illness.

Emergency Management
1. Treat the consequences of the suicide attempt (gunshot wound, drug overdose, etc.).
2. Prevent further self-injury—a patient who has made a suicidal gesture may do so again.
3. Employ crisis intervention (a form of brief psychotherapy)—to determine suicide potential; discover areas of depression and conflict; find out about the patient's support system; and determine whether hospitalization, psychiatric referral, etc. is warranted.
4. Admit to intensive care unit (if condition warrants), arrange follow-up care, or admit to psychiatric unit, depending on assessment of suicide potential. (See p. 949.)

SEXUAL ASSAULT

Rape is defined as unlawful carnal knowledge of a female by force or the threat of force against her will. The patient should be seen immediately upon entrance into the Emergency Department.

Emergency Management

OBJECTIVES: to provide physical care and emotional support.
to gather available evidence for possible legal proceedings.
to reduce the emotional trauma of the patient.

A. Respect the privacy and sensitivity of the patient; be kind and supportive.

1. The manner in which the patient is received and treated in the Emergency Department is important to the future psychological well-being of the patient. Crisis intervention should begin when the patient enters the health facility.
   a. Emotional trauma may be present for weeks, months, years. Patient may go through phases of psychologic reactions:
      (1) Phase of disorganization—fear, guilt, humiliation, anger, self-blame
      (2) Phase of resolution (putting incident into per-

spective)—may have sleep disturbances, phobias, sexual fears
   b. Reassure patient that anxiety is natural and that appropriate support is available from professional and community resources.
2. Accept the emotional reactions of patient (hysteria, stoicism, overwhelmed feeling, etc.).
3. Do not leave the patient alone.

B. Assist with the physical examination.

1. Secure informed consent from patient (or parent/guardian if patient is a minor) for examination and for the taking of photographs if necessary and for release of findings to police.
2. Take history *only* if patient has not already talked to police officer, social worker, crisis intervention worker, etc. Do not ask the patient to repeat the history.
3. Ask if patient has bathed, douched, brushed teeth, changed clothes, or defecated since attack—may alter interpretation of subsequent findings.
4. Record time of admission, time of examination, date and time of alleged rape, and the general appearance of the patient.
   a. Document any evidence of trauma—discoloration, bruises, lacerations, secretions, torn and bloody clothing.

b. Record emotional state.
5. Assist patient to undress; drape properly.
a. Save clothing; label. Note tears/holes in clothing and indicate on label.
b. Give to appropriate law enforcement authorities.

C. *Assist with pelvic and rectal examinations.*
1. Advise the patient of the nature and necessity of each procedure; give the rationale for each question asked.
a. Use water-moistened vaginal speculum for examination; do not use lubricant.
b. Note color and consistency of any discharge present.
2. Assist with securing laboratory specimens.
a. Collect vaginal aspirate, which is examined for presence or absence of motile/nonmotile sperm.
b. Use sterile swab to draw from vaginal pool for acid phosphatase, blood group antigen of semen, and precipitin test against human sperm and blood.
c. Obtain separate smears from vulva.
d. Obtain culture of body orifices for gonorrhea (see p. 809).
e. Conduct test for pregnancy if there is a possibility that patient may be pregnant.
f. Collect foreign material (leaves, grass, dirt) and place in a clean envelope.
g. Comb the pubic hairs with prepackaged, clean comb; place in separate container.
h. Inspect fingers for broken nails and tissue and foreign materials under nails.
i. Label all specimens with name of patient, date, and initials of personnel handling specimens to preserve chain of evidence; give to pathologist or designated person (forensic laboratory, etc.) and obtain an itemized receipt.

j. Photographs are taken by designated person; film is usually given to police for development and printing.

D. *Treat associated injuries as indicated.*

E. *Give patient option of prophylaxis against venereal disease.*
1. Probenecid orally, followed in 30 minutes by IM penicillin.
2. Patient with allergy to penicillin may receive alternate therapy (p. 808) which may not be effective in treatment of incubating syphilis; patient should have a serology check in 6 weeks.

F. *Offer antipregnancy measures if patient is of childbearing age, is using no contraceptives, and is at high risk in menstrual cycle.*
1. Postcoital contraceptive drugs may be given after pregnancy test—ethinyl estradiol (Estinyl) or conjugated estrogens (Premarin).
2. Antiemetic may be given to decrease discomfort from side effects.
3. Inform patient that if she misses a menstrual period she has the option of having menstrual extraction or abortion.

G. *Offer cleansing douche, mouthwash, and fresh clothing.*

H. *Provide for follow-up services:*
1. Make appointment for follow-up surveillance for pregnancy and venereal disease.
2. Encourage patient to return to previous level of functioning as soon as possible.
3. Inform patient of counseling services to prevent long-term psychologic effects; counseling services should be made available to family.
4. Patient should be accompanied by family/friend when leaving health care facility.

BIBLIOGRAPHY

Books

Barber JM and Budassi SA. Mosby's Manual of Emergency Care. St. Louis, CV Mosby, 1980
Burgess AW and Holmstrom LL. Rape: Crisis and Recovery. Bowie, Robert J Brady, 1979
Cain HD. Flint's Emergency Treatment and Management. Philadelphia, WB Saunders, 1980
Cameron CTM. Public Relations in the Emergency Department. Bowie, Robert J Brady, 1980
Czajka PA and Duffy JP. Poisoning Emergencies. St. Louis, CV Mosby, 1980
Daly BH (ed). Intensive Care Nursing. Garden City, Medical Exam Pub. Co., 1980
D'Arcy PFD and Griffin JP. Drug-induced Emergencies. Bristol, John Wright & Sons, 1980
Dixon SL. Working with People in Crisis. St. Louis, CV Mosby, 1979
Gill W and Long WB. Shock Trauma Manual. Baltimore, Williams & Wilkins, 1979
Grant H and Murray R. Course Planning Guide for Emergency Care, 2nd ed. Bowie, Robert J Brady, 1978
Henderson J. Emergency Medical Guide, 4th ed. New York, McGraw-Hill, 1978
Hill GJ. Outpatient Surgery, 2nd ed. Philadelphia, WB Saunders, 1980
Hunt TK and Dunphy JE. Fundamentals of Wound Management. New York, Appleton–Century–Crofts, 1979
Kaye S. Handbook of Emergency Toxicology, 4th ed. Springfield, Charles C Thomas, 1980
Klippel AP and Anderson CB. Manual of Emergency and Outpatient Techniques. Boston, Little, Brown & Co., 1979
Lanros NE. Assessment and Intervention in Emergency Nursing. Bowie, Robert J Brady, 1978
McFee AS and Franklin ME. Evaluation of the patient with multiple injuries. In Zauder HL. Anesthesia for Orthopaedic Surgery, pp 9–15. Philadelphia, FA Davis, 1980
McCombie SL. The Rape Crisis Intervention Handbook. New York, Plenum Press, 1980
Millar S et al (eds). Methods in Critical Care. Philadelphia, WB Saunders, 1980
Nursing Skillbook. Giving Emergency Care Competently. Horsham, Intermed Communications, 1978
Nursing Skillbook. Nursing Critically Ill Patients Confidently. Horsham, Intermed Communications, 1979
Oaks WW, Bharadwaja K, Hertz L (eds). Emergency Care. New York, Grune & Stratton, 1979
Puryear DA. Helping People in Crisis. San Francisco, Jossey–Bass Publishers, 1979
Rosen P and Sternbach GL. Atlas of Emergency Medicine. Baltimore, Williams & Wilkins, 1979
Rutherford WH et al. Accident and Emergency Medicine. Kent, Pittman Medical, 1980
Schwartz GR et al (eds). Principles and Practice of Emergency Medicine. Vols. 1 and 2. Philadelphia, WB Saunders, 1978
Shires GT. Care of the Trauma Patient, 2nd ed. New York, McGraw-Hill, 1979
Thompson RA and Green JR. Critical Care of Neurologic and Neurosurgical Emergencies. New York, Raven Press, 1980

Warner CG. Rape and Sexual Assault. Germantown, Aspen Systems, 1980

Weiszer I. Allergic emergencies. In Patterson R (ed): Allergic Diseases, 2nd ed, pp 374–394. Philadelphia, JB Lippincott, 1980

Wilkins EW et al (eds). MGH Textbook of Emergency Medicine. Baltimore, Williams & Wilkins, 1978

Zuidema GD, Rutherford RB, Ballinger WF. The Management of Trauma. Philadelphia, WB Saunders, 1979

Articles

Airway Management/CPR

Gann DS. Emergency management of the obstructed airway. JAMA 1980 Mar 21; 243(11):1141–1142

Key GK. Use of the esophageal obturator airway. Postgrad Med 1980 Feb; 67(2):189–194

Linscott MS and Horton WC. Management of upper airway obstruction. Otolaryngol Clin North Am 1979 May; 12(2):351–373

Luce JM et al. New developments in cardiopulmonary resuscitation. JAMA 1980 Sept 19; 244(12):1366–1370

Meislin HW. The esophageal obturator airway: A study of respiratory effectiveness. Ann Emerg Med 1980, Feb; 9(2):54–59

National Conference on Cardiopulmonary Resuscitation and Emergency Cardiac Care. Standards and guidelines for cardiopulmonary resuscitation (CPR) and emergency cardiac care (ECC). JAMA 1980 Aug 1; 244(5):453–509

Perro KB, Goetz MC Monaghan JJ. Making every minute count with an esophageal gastric tube airway. Nursing '80 1980 Aug; 10(8):61–63

Trott A. Recurrent upper airway obstruction. JACEP 1979 Oct; 8(10):407–408

Anaphylaxis, Insect Sting

Bagenstose AH and Tennenbaum JI. Anaphylaxis: A medical emergency. Compr Ther 1980 Apr; 6(4)6–10

Banov CH. Insect allergy revisited. J SC Med Assoc 1979 Oct; 75(10):447–448

Barclay WR. Emergency treatment of insect-sting allergy. JAMA 1978 Dec 15; 240(25):2735

Editorial. Iatrogenic collapse. Br Med J 1979 Aug 18; 2(6187):408

Harmon AL and Harmon DC. Anaphylaxis. Sudden death anytime. Nursing '80 1980 Oct; 10(10):40–43

Lamphier TA. Current diagnosis and treatment of acute anaphylaxis. J SC Med Assoc 1979 Oct; 75(10):449–452

Lichtenstein LM, Valentine MD, Sobotka AK. Insect allergy: The state of the art. J Allergy Clin Immunol 1979 July; 64(1):5–12

Lichtenstein LM et al. Once stung. Twice shy. JAMA 1980 Oct 10; 244(15):1683–1684

Toewe CH. Bug bites and stings. Am Fam Physician 1980 May; 21(5):90–94

Valentine MD. Emergency treatment for insect stings. Ann Intern Med 1979 Jan; 90(1):119–120

Wolf CJ, Nashed MS, Smith RW. Anaphylactoid reaction: The ultimate allergic emergency. J Am Podiatr Assoc 1979 Feb; 69(2):105–109

Approach to Patient and Family

Ballou M. Crisis intervention and the hospital nurse. J Nurse Care 1980 Jan; 13(1):15–19

Breu CS. Behavioral responses of critically ill patients. Curr Pract Crit Care 1979; 1:253–267

Early GL and Redfering DL. Anxiety in ambulatory emergency patients. JACEP 1979 Sept; 8(9):350–352

Rasie SM. Meeting families' needs helps you meet ICU patients' needs. Nursing '80 1980 July; 10(7):32–35

Schultz CA. Sudden death crisis: Pre-hospital and in the emergency department. JEN 1980 May–June; 6(3):46–50

Soreff SM. Sudden death in the emergency department: A comprehensive approach for families, emergency medical technicians and emergency department staff. Crit Care Med 1979 July; 7(7):321–323

Vande Creek L. How to tell the family that the patient has died. Postgrad Med 1980 Oct; 68(4):207–209

Drug and Alcohol Abuse

Beede MS. Phencyclidine intoxication. Insights into a growing problem of drug abuse. Postgrad Med 1980 Nov; 68(5):201–209

Dilts SL, Berns BR, Casper E. The alcohol emergency room in a general hospital. A model for crisis intervention. Hosp Community Psychiatry 1978 Dec; 29(12):795–796

Erb HL. Emergency treatment of drug overdose. Can Nurse 1979 May; 75(5):30–35

Fauman BJ and Fauman MA. Recognition and management of drug abuse emergencies. Compr Ther 1978 May; 4(5):38–43

Rappolt RT. Editorial. Alcohol and the ER. Clin Toxicol 1978 Dec; 13(5):631–632

Rothstein RJ. Emergency management of poisoning and overdose. Compr Ther 1979 Jan; 5(1):7–14

Weiler JM. Health care for chronic alcohol abusers. Can Med Assoc J 1978 Sept; 119(6):633–635

Woolf DS, Vourakis C, Bennett G. Guidelines for management of acute phencyclidine intoxication. Crit Care Update 1980 June; 7(6):16–24

Poisoning

Brandeburg J. Inhalation injury: Carbon monoxide poisoning. Am J Nurs 1980 Jan; 80(1):98–100

Cantrell RW et al. Foreign body and caustic ingestion: Management 1979. Ann Otol Rhinol Laryngol 1979 Nov–Dec; 88(6 pt. 1):872–879

Jackson DL and Menges H. Accidental carbon monoxide poisoning. JAMA 1980 Feb 22–29; 243(8):772–774

Kuhn PJ. "It didn't look quite right, but I ate it anyway." Diagnostic Medicine 1980 May–June; 3(3):46–51

Penner GE: Acid ingestion: Toxicology and treatment. Ann Emerg Med 1980 July; 9(7):374–379

Yarington CT Jr. The treatment of caustic ingestion. Otolaryngol Clin North Am 1979 May; 12(2):343–350

Psychiatric Emergencies

Eggland E. Dealing with tragedy: The aftermath of suicide. J Nurs Care 1978 Dec; 11(12):14–15

Motto JA. New approaches to crisis intervention. Suicide Life Threat Behav 1979 Fall; 9(3):173–184

Pisarcik G et al. Psychiatric nurses in the emergency room. Am J Nurs 1979 July; 79(7):1264–1266

Ruben HL. Managing suicidal behavior. JAMA 1979 Jan 19; 241(3):282–284

Speich PL. Taking a psychosocial stress "pulse." JEN 1979 July–Aug; 5(4):43–47

Weimer SR. Use of physiological monitoring in crisis interviewing: intervention in suicidal states. Gen Hosp Psychiatry 1980 Mar; 2(1):52–55

Whitman J. When a patient attacks: strategies for self-protection when violence looms. RN 1979 Sept; 42(9):3–33, 114

Sexual Assault

Daniels JS. Emergency department management of rape. Ohio State Med J 1979 June; 75(6):351–352

Frazier WH and Moynihan B. The emergency service based rape counseling team. Conn Med 1978 Feb; 42(2):91–94

Josephson GW. The male rape victim: Evaluation and treatment. JACEP 1979 Jan; 8(1):13–15

Moynihan B and Coughlin P. Sexual assault: A comprehensive response to a complex problem. JEN 1978 Nov–Dec; 4(6):22–26

Sredl DR, Klenke C, Rojkind M. Offering the rape victim real help. Nursing '79 1979 July; 9(7):38–43

Temperature Emergencies

Cold facts concerning hypothermia (news). JAMA 1980 Apr 11; 243(14):1403–1404, 1409

DaVee TS and Reineberg EJ. Extreme hypothermia and ventricular fibrillation. Ann Emerg Med 1980 Feb; 9(2):100–102

DeLapp TD. Taking the bite out of frostbite and other cold-weather injuries. Am J Nurs 1980 Jan; 80(1):56–60

Dyer C. Burn care in the emergent period. JEN 1980 Jan–Feb; (1);9–16

Gedrose J. When cold can be a killer. Prevention and treatment of hypothermia and frostbite. Nursing '80 1980 Feb; 10(2):34–36

Ledingham IMA et al. Central rewarming system for treatment of hypothermia. Lancet 1980 May 31; 31(8179): 1168–1169

Luterman A and Curreri PW. Emergency treatment of burn injuries. Hosp Med 1980 Jan; 16(1):66–79

Moncrief JA. Burns. I Assessment. JAMA 1979 July 6; 242(1):72–74

Moncrief JA. Burns. II Initial treatment. JAMA 1979 July 13; 242(2):179–182

Stine RJ. Heat illness. JACEP 1979 Apr; 8(4):154–160

Trauma

Albin MS. Resuscitation of the spinal cord. Crit Care Med 1978 July–Aug; 6(4):270–276

Altemeier WA et al. Symposium on diagnosis and management of abdominal and thoracic trauma. Bull NY Acad Med 1979 Feb; 55(2):123–283

Bruce DA, Gennarelli TA, Langfitt TW. Resuscitation from coma due to head injury. Crit Care Med 1978 July–Aug; 6(4):254–269

Dula DJ. Trauma to the cervical spine. JACEP 1979 Dec; 8(12):504–507

Edlich RF et al. Modern concepts of treatment of traumatic wounds. Adv Surg 1979; 13:169–197

Greer M. Emergency evaluation of head inuries in the elderly. Geriatrics 1979 Oct; 34(10):73–84

Lindsey D. Teaching the initial management of major multiple system trauma. J Trauma 1980 Feb; 20(2):160–162

Lucas CE et al. Impaired pulmonary function after albumin resuscitation from shock. J Trauma 1980 June 20(6): 446–451

McEnany MT. Emergency care of chest injuries. RI Med J 1980 July; 63(7):258–260

Meislin HW (ed). Priorities in multiple trauma. Top Emerg Med 1979 May; 1(1):1–157

Miller ME. Cycle trauma: Nursing's three key roles. Nursing '80 1980 July; 10(7):26–31

Pfaudler M. Care of patients with severe spinal cord injuries. Curr Pract Crit Care 1979; 1:216–228

Schumer W. Hypovolemic shock. JAMA 1979 Feb 9; 241(6):615–616

Shields CB et al. Early management of head injuries. J Ky Med Assoc 1980 Jan; 78(1):9–13

Stevenson BE. Initial management of the acute head injury. Otolaryngol Clin North Am 1979 May; 12(2):279–291

Wilder JR and Kudchadkar A. Stab wounds of the abdomen. JAMA 1980 June 27; 243(24):2503–2505

Yeo JD. First-aid management of spinal-cord injuries. Med J Aust 1979 Nov; 2(10):531–532

PSYCHIATRIC NURSING*

PART 2

* The opinions expressed herein are those of Dr. Gertrude McFarland and Dr. Evelyn Wasli and do not necessarily reflect those of the Division of Nursing, Health Resources Administration, DHHS; or those of Saint Elizabeths Hospital, National Institute of Mental Health, DHHS, respectively.

PSYCHIATRIC NURSING

PART 2

CONCEPTS OF MENTAL HEALTH AND MENTAL ILLNESS

23

Concepts of Mental Health

1. *Medical concept* of mental health is described as freedom from pain, gross pathology, and disability. Disorders are carefully defined.
   See *Diagnostic and Statistical Manual of Mental Disorders* (DSMIII).
2. *Cultural concept* of mental health is described as the capacity to be competent in performance of social roles within a wide range of behaviors.
3. *Statistical concept* of mental health is described as behaviors distributed within a normal curve, with deviant behaviors occurring at both extremes.
4. *Process concept* of mental health is described as the ability to effectively integrate biological, psychological, and social systems as life events are met at progressive stages of growth and development.
5. *Legal concept* of insanity is described as the inability to distinguish right from wrong and to conform behavior to law. Codes to define mental health are being developed by states.
6. Two Theoretical Constructs of Mental Health
   a. Jahoda's Six Cardinal Aspects. These aspects include a positive attitude toward self, presence of growth and development or self-actualization, integration, autonomy and independence from social influences, accurate perception of reality, environmental mastery.
   b. Roger's Process of Self-Actualization. Includes concepts of openness to experience, lack of defensiveness, accuracy in symbolization, congruency, flexibility, self-evaluation, unconditional self-regard, creative adaptation, effective reality testing, harmony with others.

Statistics Regarding Mental Illness

1. About 15% of the population experiences a mental disorder.
2. General health service system and not the specialty mental health services system provides most of the care.
3. Schizophrenia and depression cause people to seek mental health services frequently.
4. Depression is the most common psychiatric disorder in the community.
5. Patient care episodes for 1977 were an estimated 6,894,000 with 70% of the episodes in outpatient

settings, 27% in inpatient settings, and 3% in day treatment.*
6. Number of estimated resident patients in state and county mental hospitals in 1977 was 158,800; the most frequent diagnosis was schizophrenia (49%) and the next most frequent diagnosis was organic brain disorder (18%).†
7. Federally funded community mental health centers reported 1,882,000 people under care during the year 1977. Persons added during the year were diagnosed most frequently as depressive disorder (14%), schizophrenia (12%) and alcohol disorder (11.9%).‡

Causal and Relationship Factors in Mental Illness

1. There is a lack of specific causal factors in mental illness. However, several factors have been shown to have a relationship to the occurrence of mental illness.
2. *Physiological factors* include defective genes, disturbance in neurotransmission, hormone imbalance, abnormal blood factors, malnutrition, vitamin deficiencies, low blood sugar, sensory deprivation, and sleep and dream deprivation.
3. *Psychological factors* include maternal attachment and deprivation, sibling position, parental behavior and child-rearing practices, double-bind process in communication, conflict, stress, and coping styles.
4. *Sociocultural and spiritual factors* include age, sex, race, marital status, occupation, education, economic status, social class, religious beliefs and values, migration, roles, ethnic mores, lack of participation in the community, overcrowding, rapid social change, and availability of and impediments within health care systems.

* From Witkin MJ. Trends in patient care episodes in mental health facilities, 1955–1977. Mental Health Statistical Note No. 154. U.S. Department of Health and Human Services, September 1980, p. 2.
† From Survey and Reports Branch. Additions and resident patients at end of year state and county mental hospitals by age and diagnosis, by state, United States 1977. Unpublished material, Division of Biometry and Epidemiology, NIMH, April 1980, p. 55.
‡ From Survey and Reports Branch. Provisional data on federally funded community mental health centers 1977–1978. Unpublished material, Division of Biometry and Epidemiology, NIMH, May 1980, pp. 16, 38.

Psychodynamic Approach

Emphasizes the influences of intrapsychic forces on observable behavior. *Illness* is defined in terms of behavior disorders that originate in conflicts occurring before age 6 among the id, ego, superego, and/or environment. Anxiety is then experienced as a result of these conflicts. Excessive use of mental defense mechanisms can lead to serious behavioral disturbances.

A. *Theoretical Basis*

1. Freud is recognized as the founder of the psychoanalytic school of thought.
2. Psychic activity is influenced by two drives: sexual and aggressive.
3. Structural aspects of the psyche are:
   a. *Id*—the part containing instinctual drives and impulses. The ego and superego develop from the id.
   b. *Ego*—the part that assists the psyche in relating to the environment through such functions as memory and thinking and in resolving psyche conflicts. One of the more important functions is reality testing (the ego's function in sorting perceptions coming from the id and from the environment). Its primary growth period is 6 months to 3 years of age. It is the "I."
   c. *Superego*—the part that evaluates thought and actions, rewarding the good and punishing the bad.
4. The psyche is divided into levels of consciousness.
   a. *Conscious*—the awareness of self and environment which occurs when a person is awake.
   b. *Preconscious*—contains memories and thoughts that are easily recalled.
   c. *Unconscious*—contains memories and thoughts which ordinarily do not enter consciousness.
5. *Anxiety* is an automatic response occurring when the psyche is flooded with uncontrollable stimulation.
6. *Signal anxiety* is a type of anxiety produced by the ego in anticipation of danger, such as loss of a loved one or disapproval of superego.
7. *Pleasure principle* states that the psyche seeks pleasure and avoids displeasure without regard for consequences.
8. *Reality principle* states that the psyche tends to delay satisfaction by accommodation to situational factors.

B. *Psychosexual Stages of Development*

These stages are crucial for they are periods during which unconscious conflicts among id, ego, and superego develop. Also, fixation, or arrest of development, at any stage may occur as a result of excessive gratification or deprivation.

1. *Oral Stage* (Birth to 1½ years)
   a. The infant obtains relief from biological and psychological tensions through his mouth and lips.
   b. He learns to depend on external objects.
   c. He sucks, swallows, takes in, bites, chews, spits, and cries.
   d. A warm, trusting, and dependent pattern of relating is experienced.
   e. He gratifies his needs and begins to delay their immediate satisfaction.
   f. Ego development begins primarily through the process of identification.
   g. Problems and/or traits related to Oral Stage:
      Over-dependency, clinging behavior, pessimism, optimism, narcissism (self-love), "world-

owes-me-a-living" attitudes, alcoholism, smoking, overeating, drug addiction, refusing to eat, vomiting, gullibility.
2. *Anal Stage* (1½ to 3 years)
   a. The infant achieves control over anal sphincter and gives up some of his control as he experiences toilet training.
   b. He and his parents are involved in issues of control over defecation.
      (1) May give the feces as a gift or keep them or expel them violently.
      (2) May control the time of defecation or do what he wants with the feces.
      (3) May relinquish his control or comply with the control imposed.
   c. The sense of "I" becomes well-developed.
   d. Problems and/or traits related to Anal Stage:
      Compliance, defiance, perfectionism, obsessive-compulsive, antagonistic, negativistic, sadomasochism (pleasure from inflicting pain on others or self), procrastination, miserliness, stuttering, phobias, compulsions, constipation, bed wetting, over-conformity, competitiveness, generosity, creativity, possessiveness.
3. *Phallic Stage* (3 to 6 years)
   a. Child experiences the genitals, particularly the penis, as the main source of pleasurable sensation and interest.
   b. Parents are vital in the process of developing sexual identity.
   c. *Oedipus complex* is term used to describe the emotional attachment of male child for mother and ambivalent feelings toward father. The boy fears retaliation and possible loss of penis (*castration fear*) and he has wishes of killing father.
   d. *Electra complex* is term used to describe a girl's wishes for the penis of the father and hopes to take the place of mother, whom she blames for not having penis.
   e. The complex is resolved by girl or boy in the identification of the child with the parent of the same sex.
   f. The superego is strengthened as the child accepts the standards of the parent.
   g. Problems and/or traits related to Phallic Stage: homosexuality, transsexuality, problems with authority, over-involvement in being sexually attractive.
4. *Latency Stage* (6 to 12 years)
   a. Child experiences a quiet period during which the sexual drive is dormant.
   b. Sexual and aggressive drives are channeled into school activities, play, and work.
   c. Relationships are mostly with peers of same sex.
   d. Problems noted in Latency Stage:
      delinquency, rebelliousness, tics, restlessness, hysteria, anxiety states, anorexia.
5. *Genital Stage* (12 years to adulthood)
   a. Person experiences onset of puberty, renewed interest in sexual activity, and conflicts that were unresolved in past developmental stages.
   b. He learns to develop mature relationships with males and females.
   c. He begins to stop depending on parents.
   d. Problems arising in Genital Stage can include conflicts, character disorders, and other mental disorders.

C. Defense Mechanisms

Unconscious processes used by the ego to reduce anxiety and conflict. Most frequently used ones include:
1. *Repression*—Major response used to keep painful thoughts, feelings and impulses from consciousness.
2. *Denial*—Response acknowledges no awareness of a painful event.
3. *Reaction formation*—Response expresses opposite feelings to those being experienced.
4. *Projection*—Response ascribes to another person or object the unacceptable thoughts and feelings.
5. *Rationalization*—Response justifies behavior by an attempt to logically explain it.
6. *Undoing*—Response cancels the effect of another response just made.
7. *Displacement*—Response is misdirected from original person or object to safer target.
8. *Sublimation*—Response partially substitutes socially acceptable activities for unacceptable impulses.
9. *Regression*—Response in which person deals with anxiety by behaving at a level more appropriate to an earlier age.
10. *Identification*—Response by which the actions and feelings of a person are the same as the significant other.
11. *Introjection*—Response in which an aspect of behavior or thought of another is taken into the ego structure.
12. *Isolation*—Response in which person blocks the feeling associated with unpleasant, threatening situation or thought.
13. *Suppression*—Response which is not unconscious and deliberately forces certain ideas from thought and action.

D. Therapy

1. *Psychoanalysis* is an intense relationship with a psychiatrist for a period of time for the purpose of assisting the person to establish conscious control of affect and behavior.
2. Through dream analysis, free association, interpretation, analysis of resistance and *transference* (ascribing to the psychiatrist the thoughts and feelings associated with parents or other important people), and neutrality, the therapist assists the patient in reducing the anxiety associated with thought.
3. Conflicts are brought into awareness and thus resolved.

Interpersonal Approach

Emphasizes the importance of interpersonal relationships and communication on behavior. *Behavior disorders* are a result of patterns of avoidance, use of substitutive processes, and experiences with significant adults.

A. Theoretical Basis

1. Sullivan is noted for interpersonal theory of psychiatry.
2. *Satisfaction* is achieved through interaction to obtain relief from tension from biological drives or needs of water, food, rest, sleep, shelter, and sex.
3. *Security* is achieved when basic needs are satisfied in relationship to a mothering person without the presence of anxiety.
4. *Self System* refers to all behaviors functioning to avoid or decrease anxiety.
   a. Is developed out of the dynamic interplay of the basic needs and the interpersonal process to achieve satisfaction and security.
   b. Modes of experiencing describe one's perception and thoughts.
      (1) *Prototaxic mode*—Person identifies with whole world; thoughts and responses are undifferentiated.
      (2) *Parataxic mode*—Person recognizes that things go together, but there is no logic. Things are put together only because one event occurs and is followed by another.
      (3) *Syntaxic mode*—Person is able to use logic in explaining events.
   c. Person appraises himself through parents' reactions and organizes the appraisals in terms of:
      (1) Bad me—acts which result in anxiety.
      (2) Good me—acts which are anxiety free.
      (3) Not me—acts which are totally disapproved; severe anxiety is experienced.

B. Stages of Growth and Development

Reflect emphasis of interpersonal approach.
1. Infancy—lasts until the appearance of speech which enables baby to change the environment.
2. Childhood—lasts to emergence of need for peers.
3. Juvenile—lasts to need for close relationship.
4. Preadolescence—lasts to puberty and beginning interest in opposite sex.
5. Early adolescence—lasts to development of relationships with opposite sex.
6. Late adolescence—lasts to the establishment of stable love relationship with another.

C. Anxiety

1. First develops as infant experiences tension or insecurity of mother.
2. Later is experienced whenever a threat of disapproval from a significant person occurs.
3. Avoidance behaviors develop to deal with anxiety.
   a. Physically avoiding the situation.
   b. Changing the interaction in the situation.
   c. Using selective inattention, which is the process the individual uses to not attend to that which causes anxiety.
   d. Using substitutive processes in which person dissociates certain aspects of interpersonal system. The term *security operations* is also used to describe these processes; these are similar to the defense mechanisms of Freud.

D. Therapy

1. Therapist is a participant observer and not a neutral object.
2. *Elucidation* is a principle which states that behavior change can occur when one can identify one's behavior, conceptualize, and evaluate it.
3. Focus of interview is on exploring the avoidance behaviors, anxiety experiences, and the interpersonal context in which the avoidance behaviors and anxiety occur.

Behaviorist Approach

Emphasizes observable and measurable behavioral processes. *Maladaptive behavior* can be classified as behavior excess, behavioral deficit, distortion of reinforcing stimuli, distortion of discrimination stimuli, and aversive behavior.

A. *Theoretical Basis*

1. Pavlov and Skinner contributed to the development of the behaviorist school of thought.
2. All behavior follows learning principles; therefore, behavior may become maladaptive, but is not considered abnormal.
3. *Respondent Conditioning*—Concept that states that a specific stimulus elicits a certain response.
4. *Operant Conditioning*—Concept that states that behavior responses are influenced by what follows the response.
5. *Reinforcement*—A behavior response can be influenced by positive and negative rewards.

B. *Therapy*

1. *Functional Analysis* is analysis of the manifest behavior.
   a. What behaviors are problematic?
   b. Under what conditions does the behavior occur?
   c. What are the positive reinforcers?
   d. What are the negative reinforcers?
   e. What are the effective behaviors that could be used as substitutes or as reinforcers?
2. Techniques frequently used are systematic desensitization, assertive training, sex therapy, progressive relaxation, and operant conditioning.

Developmental Approach

Emphasizes the development of the healthy personality throughout the life span; developed by Erikson. *Illness*—Problems with self, relationships, or society may cause extension of developmental period. Malfunctioning is related to dominance of a mode (e.g., incorporation) or of a zone (e.g., oral).

A. *Theoretical Basis*

1. Human beings progress through a series of eight psychosocial developmental stages.
2. The growth plan is governed by both social experiences and innate capacities, the epigenetic principle.
3. In each developmental stage, the potential exists for the person to develop a new task which serves as a building block for subsequent stages.

   Physical and psychosocial hazards may thwart the person from achieving the task central to a given developmental stage which negatively affects subsequent developmental stages and may lead to maladaptive behavioral patterns.

B. *Erikson's Eight Developmental Stages*

1. *Infancy* (Birth to 18 months)
   a. During this stage, the infant learns to *trust* self and others, provided his needs have been met in a consistent and satisfying manner.
   b. Confidence, realistic trust, hope, optimism, and the ability to form relationships in later life stem from such an attitude of trust.
   c. Subject to hazards such as mistreatment, the infant may develop *mistrust*, later reflected in hostility, suspiciousness, and a general feeling of dissatisfaction.
2. *Early Childhood* (18 months to 3 years)
   a. In this stage, *autonomy* results from reassuring, constructively guided experiences in which the child is allowed to exercise self-control of his behavior without being subjected to experiences beyond his capabilities.
   b. Socially acceptable behaviors of holding and letting go, on which toilet training focuses during this stage, become generalized to other aspects of living.
   c. The development of autonomy leads to self-control without loss of self-esteem, a sense of pride and good will, the ability to initiate activities yet be cooperative, and to be appropriately generous and withholding.
   d. Difficulties, such as from external overcontrol, can lead to *shame and doubt;* i.e., feelings of being exposed, lack of a belief in being able to control one's life, and a lack of self-worth.
3. *Late Childhood* (3 to 5 years)
   a. The child develops *initiative,* the ability to undertake and plan tasks, the pleasure of being active, and the experience of a sense of purpose.
   b. Pleasure in attack and conquest aid in developing sexual identity and roles.
   c. Initiative is controlled by a developing conscience. The person grows to develop and strives to utilize his potentials in a socially appropriate manner.
   d. *Guilt,* accompanied by self-restriction and denial, can result from an unsuccessful negotiation of this stage. The person fails to develop his potential.
4. *School Age* (6 to 12 years)
   a. The major task is *industry* characterized by involvement in the world, constructing and planning things, developing relationships with peers, developing specific skills, and identifying with admired others.
   b. A sense of competence and the pleasure of diligence develops.
   c. *Inferiority,* the feeling that one is unworthy and inadequate, can result from hindrances.
5. *Adolescence* (12 to 20 years)
   a. The developmental task is *identity,* a confident sense of self, commitment to a career, and finding one's place in society.
   b. Successful resolution leads to the ability to work toward long-term goals, self-esteem, and emotional stability.
   c. The danger is *role confusion,* characterized by feelings of confusion, lack of confidence, indecision, alienation, and possibly acting-out behavior.
   d. Unsuccessful resolution may require the adult to spend life-long energies attempting to resolve remaining conflicts.
6. *Young Adulthood* (18 to 25 years)
   a. *Intimacy* is the major developmental task. The person develops the ability to love, to develop commitments to other persons, and to enter true mutual relationships.
   b. *Isolation* is the danger. The person remains distant from others, withdraws, enters into superficial relationships, or develops prejudices.
7. *Adulthood* (28 to 65 years)
   a. *Generativity* is the task. The adult becomes responsible for guiding children or in the development and creativity of productive and constructive tasks.
   b. Failure leads to *stagnation,* personal impoverishment and self-indulgence.
8. *Old Age* (65 years to death)
   a. The last stage is characterized by feelings of acceptance, importance, and self-worth about the value of one's life, *integrity.*
   b. *Despair,* the negative outcome of this stage, is the sense of loss, a feeling of life's meaninglessness, and the feeling that life's goals have not been achieved and that it is too late to start over.

C. *Therapy*

Focus is on establishing trust not obtained early in life and assisting patient to gain insight into unconscious motivations, thus reducing anxiety.

Family System Approach (Bowen Theory)

Emphasizes variables of anxiety and level of integration and their influence on the family system. Illness is viewed as an aspect of human adaptation in which person experiences a level of undifferentiation.

A. *Theoretical Basis*

1. *Sibling position*—Personality characteristics are related to sibling position (10 have been identified) and provide predictive data.
2. *Triangles*—The basic unit of the emotional system, i.e., a twosome and an outsider. When tension is experienced, each person will attempt to obtain the outside position. If the tension increases, one of the persons will triangle another; a larger and larger interlocking system is thus formed.
3. *Family projection process*—Anxiety is experienced by the mother who may respond by becoming sensitive to the child and overconcerned. Mother's overattachment to the child is supported by the father. Child becomes anxious, demanding, and unable to function alone. Schizophrenia develops following several generations of lower levels of differentiation as a result of the family projection process.
4. *Multigenerational transmission process*—The family projection process involves multiple generations with one child in each generation becoming less differentiated and less able to function.

5. *Emotional cut-off*—Concept describes the process of separation from parents as people resolve the emotional attachments. The more intense the cut-off from parents, the more likely a person and his children will have similar problems in life.
6. *Differentiation*—Concept is related to a state of being and to the process of becoming more responsible for self at emotional and intellectual levels. Profiles are developed for different levels of differentiation.
7. *Nuclear family emotional system*—Patterns of functioning of mother, father, and children are identified. Major patterns include marital conflict, dysfunction in one spouse, projection of problems to a child, and/or a combination of the above patterns.
8. *Societal regression*—When a society is exposed to chronic anxiety, it responds with emotionality to relieve the anxiety; thus, functioning regresses. An example of regression response is overuse of drugs in society.

B. *Therapy*

1. Focused on reducing reactivity and increasing one's differentiation.
2. Expression of feelings is not encouraged or interpreted, but person is assisted in thinking about processes.
3. Exploration of family's past history is encouraged.
4. Re-establishment of contact with family is supported.
5. Therapist uses his skill to remain out of the interlocking triangles, thereby increasing flexibility and ability to decrease anxiety.

BIBLIOGRAPHY

Books

American Psychiatric Association. Diagnostic and Statistical Manual of Mental Disorders, 3rd ed. Washington, D.C., American Psychiatric Association, 1980

Bandura A. Principles of Behavior Modification. New York, Holt, Reinhart & Winston, 1969

Bowen M. Family Therapy in Clinical Practice. New York, Jason Aronson, 1978

Brenner C. An Elementary Textbook of Psychoanalysis, Rev. ed. New York, Anchor Press, 1974

Erikson E. Childhood and Society. New York, WW Norton & Co., 1964

Erikson E. Identity and the Life Cycle. New York, WW Norton & Co., 1979

Erikson E. Insight and Responsibility. New York, WW Norton & Co., 1968

Erikson E. Identity: Youth and Crisis. New York, WW Norton & Co., 1968

Erikson E. Toys and Reasons: Stages in the Ritualization of Experience. New York, WW Norton & Co., 1977

Ford DH and Urban HB. Systems of Psychotherapy. New York, John Wiley & Sons, 1963

Hansen J and Himes B. Normality. In Woody RH (ed). Encyclopedia of Clinical Assessment, Vol I. San Francisco, Jossey–Bass, 1980

Harmatz MG. Abnormal Psychology. New Jersey, Prentice–Hall, 1978

Jahoda M. Current Concepts of Positive Mental Health. New York, Basic Books, 1958

Kovel J. A Complete Guide to Therapy. New York, Pantheon Books, 1976

Nicholi A (ed). The Harvard Guide to Modern Psychiatry. Cambridge, Mass., Belknap Press, 1978

Offer D and Sabskin M. Normality. New York, Basic Books, 1966

Rogers C. A Theory of therapy, personality, and interpersonal relationships as developed in the client-centered framework. In Koch S (ed). Psychology, A Study of Science. New York, McGraw-Hill, 1963

Sullivan HS. The Interpersonal Theory of Psychiatry. New York, WW Norton & Co., 1953

United States, National Center for Health Statistics. Health, United States. DHEW Publication, No. (PHS) 78-1232, 1978

Williams A and Johnson J. Mental Health in the 21st Century. Lexington, Lexington Books, 1979

Wolpe J. The Practice of Behavior Therapy. Oxford, Pergamon Press, 1969

Articles

Weissman MM and Myers JK. Psychiatric disorders in a US community. Acta Psychiatr Scand 1980; 62:99–111

Pamphlets

Witkin MJ. Trends in patient care episodes in mental health facilities, 1955–1977. Mental Health Statistical Note No. 154. U.S. Department of Health and Human Services, September 1980

Survey and Reports Branch. Additions and resident patients at end of year state and county mental hospitals by age and diagnosis, by state, United States 1977. Unpublished material, Division of Biometry and Epidemiology, NIMH, April 1980

Survey and Reports Branch. Provisional data on federally funded community mental health centers 1977–1978. Unpublished material, Division of Biometry and Epidemiology, NIMH, May 1980

Conceptual Framework for Psychiatric Nursing Practice

See Figure 24-1.
1. The human being is in continuous interplay with his/her environment.
2. The human being possesses the potential ability to cope with stressors, meet his/her needs, and attain goals through adaptive strategies, skills, and processes.
3. Adaptive strategies, skills, and processes include:
   a. Factor I: Interaction—exchanging, interchanging, or linking matter, energy, persons, or objects between the person and the environment.
      (1) *Exchanging*—matter and energy interchange.
      (2) *Communicating*—information interchange.
      (3) *Relating*—person or object linkage(s).
   b. Factor II: Action—assigning value, selecting alternatives, and taking action.
      (1) *Valuing*—assigning value, worth, or meaning.
      (2) *Choosing*—setting priorities and selecting alternatives.
      (3) *Moving*—taking action within one's environment.
   c. Factor III: Awareness—alertness, feeling, knowing/perception.
      (1) *Waking*—level of alertness.
      (2) *Feeling*—sensation and mood.
      (3) *Knowing*—ability to accurately perceive, store, and use information.

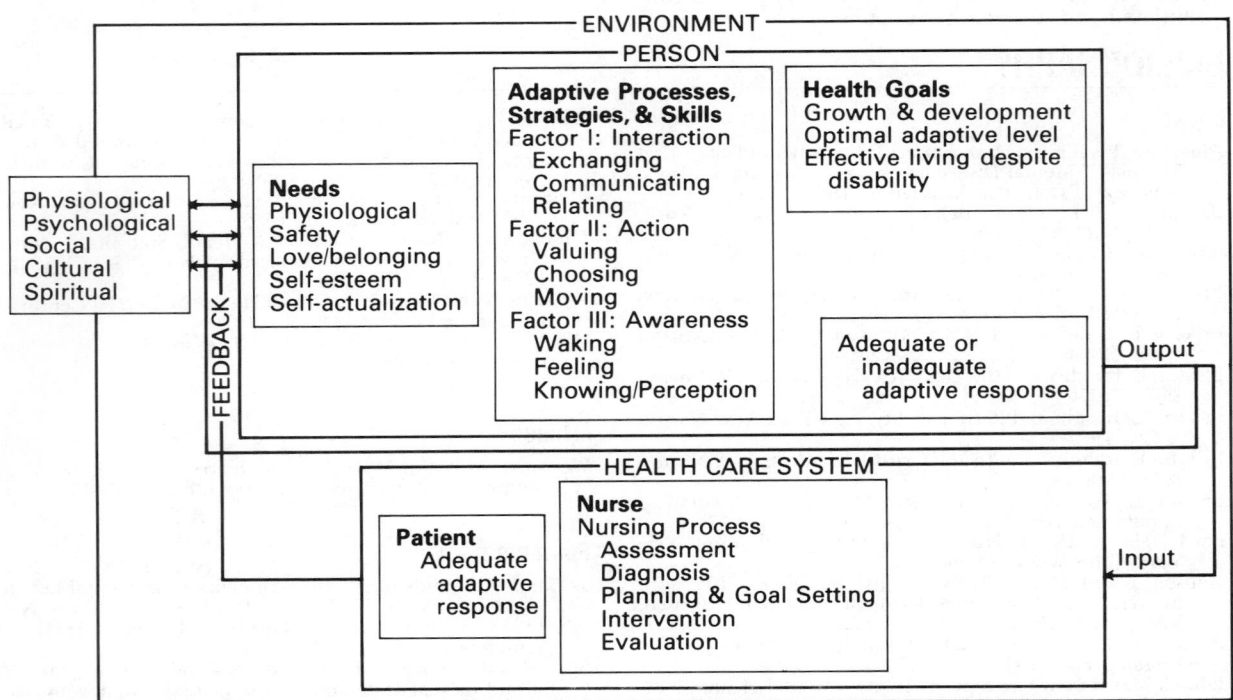

FIGURE 24-1. *A Conceptual Framework for Psychiatric Nursing Practice. (Adapted from Nursing Education Section: Conceptual Framework. Washington, D.C., St. Elizabeths Hospital, 1979 [unpublished]; Maslow A: Toward a Psychology of Being. New York, Van Nostrand Rheinhold, 1968; Riehl J and Roy C: Conceptual Models for Nursing Practice. New York, Appleton–Century–Crofts, 1974; Kim M, Moritz D: Classification of Nursing Diagnoses: Proceedings of Third and Fourth National Conference. New York, McGraw–Hill, 1981.)*

Psychiatric Nursing Assessment of the Adult Patient

I. Factor I: Interaction

	Self-care abilities	Limitations/problems
Eating/drinking	_____	_____
Eliminating	_____	_____
Breathing	_____	_____
Circulation	_____	_____
Grooming/hygiene	_____	_____
Other (specify)	_____	_____

Current physical problems _____

Current treatments & medications _____

Current ways help sought with health problems _____

Current drug or alcohol abuse _____

Previous mental or physical illness _____

General level of growth & development _____

Verbal/nonverbal interchange	Strengths	Limitations
With staff	_____	_____
With spouse	_____	_____
With children	_____	_____
With others (specify)	_____	_____

Relating	Strengths	Limitations
Ability to trust	_____	_____
Expression of sexuality	_____	_____
Self-control	_____	_____
Manner of expression of needs/goals	_____	_____
Degree of social interaction	_____	_____
Style of social interaction	_____	_____

Attitude toward perceived current role status _____

_____

Significant others' response to patient's illness _____

_____

Recreational activities & hobbies _____

Arrests, court dates, probation _____

II. Factor II: Action

Patient's perception/meaning of current mental illness & cause(s) _____

_____

Beliefs about illness & health & personal health goals _____

(continued on next page)

Psychiatric Nursing Assessment of the Adult Patient (cont.)

Patient's attitudes/beliefs toward hospitalization & health care personnel _____

Patient's expectations & goals for current hospitalization _____

Previous use of health care resources/type of help sought _____

Past & current compliance with prescribed treatment & health instructions _____

Coping skills used to resolve emotional problems _____

Religion/spiritual beliefs _____

Decision-making abilities/limitations _____

Attitudes toward future worth/value of own life _____

Suicidal thoughts/behaviors _____

Activity pattern _____

III. Factor III: Awareness

Arousal level _____

Sleep/rest pattern _____

Anxiety: Mild _____ Moderate _____ Severe _____

Degree & nature of ambivalence _____

Guilt & source _____

Type & change of mood _____

Frequency & types of physical complaints _____

Patient's adjustment to types, number, & recency of stressors _____

Type & use of defense mechanisms _____

Patient's opinion of himself (who he is, self-worth, etc.)_____

Patient's concerns about his physical appearance _____

Knowledge about present illness (prevention, treatment, self-care responsibilities) _____

Unusual beliefs _____

Unusual sensations & perceptions _____

The Mental Status Review

The mental status review is usually performed by the psychiatrist or the psychiatric nurse.

OBJECTIVE: To assess the mental functioning and present emotional state of the patient.

A. *General Appearance*—Observe the patient's:

1. Grooming and dress (slovenly, neat, unkempt, overly meticulous, disheveled, inappropriate, unusual).
2. Facial expression (calm, perplexed, stressed, tense, alert, dazed).
3. Physical appearance (noticeable physical deformities, thin, obese, average weight).
4. Posture (normal, rigid, slouching).
5. Eye contact (eyes closed, eyes open, good contact, avoids contact, stares).

B. *Motor Behavior*—Observe for unusual bodily movements as:

1. *Choreiform movements*—irregular, involuntary actions of muscles of face and extremities.
2. *Waxy flexibility*—holding body posture, which is imposed by another person, for a long time.
3. *Hyperkinesia*—excessive movement, destructive, or assaultive activity.
4. *Compulsion*—unwanted urge to perform repetitive actions.
5. *Automatism*—not consciously controlled, automatic, undirected motor activity.
6. *Cataplexy*—temporary loss of muscle tone precipitated by strong emotions.
7. *Catalepsy*—a trancelike state with loss of voluntary motion.
8. *Stereotypy*—repetitive, persistent motor activity or speech.
9. *Echopraxia*—repetitive imitation of another person's movements.
10. *Psychomotor retardation*—decreased, slowed activity.
11. *Catatonic stupor*—extreme underactivity.
12. *Catatonic excitement*—extreme overactivity.
13. *Impulsiveness*—outbursts of activity that are unpredictable and sudden.
14. *Tics and spasms*—twitching and jerking of muscles, usually above the shoulders, which is involuntary.

C. *Speech*—Observe for speech activity, unusual patterns, or unusual use of words, such as:

1. *Verbigeration*—repetitive, meaningless expression of sentences, phrases, or words.
2. *Rhyming*—interjecting into the conversation regular, recurring, corresponding sounds at the end of phrases or sentences, as in poetry.
3. *Punning*—interjecting into the conversation the clever and humorous use of a word or words.
4. *Mutism*—no expression of words or uncommunicative over a period of time.
5. *Aphasia*—partial or total loss of the ability to express self through language or the ability to understand the verbal communication of another person.
6. Unusual rate of speech, volume of voice, or intonation and modulation.

D. *Intellectual Functioning*—Assess patient for the following:

1. Orientation
   a. Orientation to time
      Ask the patient what year it is, what month, what day of the week, what time, and how long he/she has been in the hospital.
   b. Orientation to place
      Ask the patient: Where are you now located? What is the name of this place? What is the address of this place?
   c. Orientation to person
      Does patient know his name? Does patient know who the person conducting the interview is?
2. Memory
   a. Memory for remote events—Ask the patient:
      (1) Date(s) of marriage(s) and divorce(s), if any;
      (2) Birthdate(s) of child(ren), if any;
      (3) Birthdates of parents;
      (4) Name of grade, high school, and college attended;
      (5) Type of position and month and year of employment of first job after high school or college graduation.
   b. Memory for recent past events—
      (1) Ask where patient lived during past three months. Whom living with? Where working?
      (2) Ask patient which types of recreational activities he/she is involved in.
   c. Memory for recent events—
      (1) Ask what patient ate for breakfast, lunch, dinner today.
      (2) Ask how patient spent today, yesterday.
   d. Immediate memory and recall
      (1) Administer digit span test. Ask patient to repeat three digits in order presented, then backwards. Repeat procedure for 4, 5, and 6 digits.
      (2) Other assessment techniques include asking patient same question several times during the interview to determine whether same or different answer is given.
      (3) In another technique, instruct patient to count to 28, stop for 45 seconds, instruct to count from where left off to 39, stop again for 3 minutes and engage in neutral conversation, then instruct to count from where left off to 50.
   e. Abnormal memory or symptoms related to impaired memory, such as amnesia, anterograde amnesia, hysterical amnesia, confabulation, déjà vu, hypermnesia, clang association, and retrospective falsification.
3. Level and Fund of Knowledge
   a. To determine fund of knowledge, ask such questions as: What are the names of 3 countries in Europe? The colors in the American flag? The distance between any 2 major U.S. cities?
   b. Request listing of as many items in different categories, such as U.S. state capitols, fruits, etc.
   c. Overall responses to total interview questions are used to assess level of knowledge appropriate to patient's age and socioeconomic, cultural, occupational, and educational background
4. Ability for Calculation
   Have patient subtract 7 from 100 and keep subtracting 7s, allowing up to 30 seconds between calculations.
5. Ability to Think Abstractly or to Make Generalizations
   a. Ask patient to interpret a proverb particular to his/her subculture.
   b. Or, use object sorting test by having patient group toy objects according to use.

E. *Perception*—Observe for altered or abnormal awareness of self or environment as:

1. *Hallucinations*—sensory perceptions for which there are no external stimuli. These can be visual, olfactory, auditory, tactile, gustatory, or kinesthetic.
2. *Hypnagogic hallucinations*—misperceptions occurring as patient is falling asleep for which there is no basis in reality.
3. *Hypnopompic hallucinations*—misperceptions occurring as patient is waking up for which there is no basis in reality.
4. *Illusion*—misinterpretation of an actual, existing external stimuli by any of the senses.

F. *Attitude*—Observe for changes in patient's general manner of feeling, thinking, or behavior during the interview as evidenced by being any one or more of the following: cooperative, outgoing, withdrawn, evasive, sarcastic, aggressive, perplexed, hostile, arrogant, dramatic, ingratiating, submissive, fearful, seductive, uncooperative, impatient, remote, resistant, unfeeling, apprehensive, or apathetic.

G. *Affective State*—Observe for unusual mood or expression of emotions, such as:

1. *Euphoria*—excessive feeling of emotional and physical well-being inappropriate for actual environmental stimuli.
2. *Flat affect*—less than normal expression of feelings.
3. *Blunting*—loss of affective capacity.
4. *Elation*—a high degree of confidence, boastfulness, uncritical optimism and joy accompanied by increased motor activity.
5. *Exultation*—an affective reaction extending beyond elation and accompanied by feelings of grandeur.
6. *Ecstasy*—an overpowering feeling of joy and rapture.
7. *Anxiety*—an apprehensive, uneasy, and worried feeling, usually of unconscious, intrapsychic origin.
8. *Fear*—an apprehensive, uneasy, and worried feeling related to a known source of danger, usually externally based.
9. *Ambivalence*—expressing the existence of two opposing feelings or emotions at the same time.
10. *Depersonalization*—feeling unreal about oneself or the environment.
11. *Irritability*—feeling characterized by impatience, annoyance, and easy provocation to anger.
12. *Rage*—furious, uncontrolled anger.
13. *Lability*—quickly changing expression of mood or feelings.
14. *Depressed*—a feeling characterized by being sad, dejected, and gloomy.

H. *Thought Processes and Content*—Observe patient for:

1. *Blocking*—sudden ceasing of flow of thinking and speech related to strong emotions.
2. *Flight of ideas*—rapid conversation with logically unconnected shifting of topics.
3. *Word salad*—a combination of phrases, words, and sentences that are disconnected and incoherent.
4. *Perseveration*—pathologial repetition of a sentence, phrase, or word.
5. *Neologisms*—the use of new expressions, phrases, or words or making up a new meaning for accepted expressions, phrases, or words.
6. *Circumstantiality*—interjecting into the conversation great detail and incidental material which is of no primary significance to the central idea.
7. *Echolalia*—repetitive imitation of another person's speech.
8. *Condensation*—the process of reducing several ideas into one symbol.
9. *Delusion*—a false belief kept despite nonsupportive evidence.
10. *Phobia*—a strong, persistent, abnormal fear of an object or situation.
11. *Obsession*—persistent, unwanted, recurring thought.
12. *Hypochondriasis*—morbid concern for one's health and feeling ill without any actual medical basis.

I. *Judgment*—Observe patient's ability to problem solve and choose among alternatives based on reality.

J. *Alertness*—Observe patient for levels of alertness (drowsy, hyperalert, somnolent, intermittent alertness and drowsiness, stupor).

Psychological Testing

A. *Intelligence Testing*—To assess cognitive and intellectual abilities, usually administered by a psychologist.
Wechsler Adult Intelligence Scale (WAIS)
Most widely used standardized test of general intelligence.

B. *Personality Testing*—To assess personality functioning and psychodynamics, usually administered by a psychologist.

1. *Thematic Apperception Test (TAT)*
A projective test consisting of a series of 30 pictures. A number of these are presented to the patient with instructions that a story be constructed or created about the picture.
2. *Rorschach Test*
A projective test consisting of a set of 10 inkblots. The patient is asked what he sees in the inkblot, what it looks like, and what it suggests.
3. *Draw a Person Test (DAP)*
The patient is asked to draw a person(s) and possibly also a house, tree, the family, or an animal. The clinician may also question the patient about the drawing. It is a projective test used for personality analysis and in screening for organic brain damage.
4. *Bender-Gestalt Test*
The patient is presented with 9 cards, 1 at a time, and is asked to copy the geometric designs on them. The test is used to detect organic pathology and, also, as a projective technique to assess personality functioning.
5. *Sentence Completion Test (SCT)*
The patient is presented with 75 to 100 sentence stems which he is asked to complete with the first response that comes into mind. The test taps much conscious data and can identify the patient's preocupatons, concerns, fears, and goals.
6. *Minnesota Multiphasic Personality Inventory (MMPI)*
A 500-item questionnaire designed to measure major aspects of personality related to hypomania, paranoia, hypochondriasis, hysteria, psychopathic deviation, psychasthenia, schizophrenia, masculinity-femininity, and depression.

BIBLIOGRAPHY

Books

Arieti S (ed). American Handbook of Psychiatry. New York, Basic Books, 1974

Butler R and Lewis M. Aging and Mental Health: Positive Psychosocial Approaches. St. Louis, CV Mosby, 1977

Diagnostic and Statistical Manual of Mental Disorders, 3rd ed. Washington, D. C., The American Psychiatric Association, 1980

Freedman A, Kaplan H, Sadock B. Modern Synopsis of Comprehensive Textbook of Psychiatry II. Baltimore, Williams & Wilkins, 1978

Goble F. The Third Force. New York, Grossman Publishers, 1975

Kim M and Moritz D. Classification of Nursing Diagnoses. Proceedings of Third and Fourth National Conference. New York, McGraw-Hill, 1981

Kolb L. Modern Clinical Psychiatry. Philadelphia, WB Saunders, 1977

Manfreda M and Krampitz S. Psychiatric Nursing. Philadelphia, FA Davis, 1977

Maslow A. Toward a Psychology of Being. New York, Van Nostrand Rheinhold, 1968

Nicholi A (ed). The Harvard Guide to Modern Psychiatry. Cambridge, Harvard University Press, 1978

Orem D. Nursing: Concepts of Practice. New York, McGraw-Hill, 1971

Riehl J and Roy C. Conceptual Models for Nursing Practice. New York, Appleton–Century–Crofts, 1974

Articles

Clarke R. Assessment in psychiatric hospitals. Nurs Times 1979 April; 75(14):590–592

Coryell W, Cloninger C, Reich T. Clinical assessment: Use of nonphysician interviewers. J Nerv Ment Dis 1978 Aug; 166(8):599–605

Dodd M. Assessing mental status. Am J Nurs 1978 Sept; 78(9):1501–1503

Green N. A psychiatric assessment tool for staff and students. J Psychiatr Nurs 1979 Apr; 17(4):28–31.

Kleh J, Lange P, Karu E et al. Differential diagnosis of the disturbed elderly patient. Hosp Community Psychiatry 1978 Nov; 29(11):735–738

Marano H. The new psychiatry, getting in step with scientific medicine. Med World News 1980 Jan 21; 21(2):45–46, 51–54, 59

Morgan S and Macey M. Three assessment tools for family therapy. J Psychiatr Nurs 1978 Mar; 16(3):39–42

Reynolds J and Logsdon J. Assessing your patient's mental status. Nursing '79 1979 Aug; 9(8)26–33

Whitley M and Willingham D. Adding a sexual assessment to the health interview. J Psychiatr Nurs 1978 Apr; 16(4):17–22, 27

Unpublished Material

Nursing Education Section. Conceptual framework. Washington, D. C., St. Elizabeths Hospital, 1979

COMMUNICATION AND THERAPEUTIC RELATIONSHIP

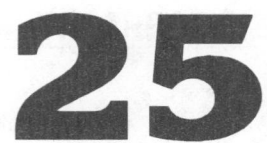

Developing Effective Communication and a Therapeutic Relationship

A. *Develop and improve self-awareness*

1. Develop awareness of own verbal and nonverbal communication patterns.
2. Recognize, explore origin, and attempt to work through stereotyping, prejudices, and negative attitudes.
3. Develop awareness of own cultural and subcultural values and customs and their influence on personal behavior, as well as on one's own perception and interpretation of another's behavior.
4. Identify common personal stressors and typical behavioral responses.
5. Identify and increase own adaptive coping patterns in response to stress.
6. Identify and develop constructive personal ethical values in relation to care of the adult psychiatric patient and health care in general.
7. Validate perceptions and interpretations of patient's behavior with patient or with professional colleague as indicated.
8. Examine own motives, feelings, and behavior.
   a. Develop self-acceptance, self-esteem, and self-respect.
   b. Develop ability to clearly differentiate between own feelings and those belonging to the patient.
   c. Recognize, accept, analyze origin of negative feelings.
9. Seek qualified supervision, as needed, especially when providing one-to-one nurse therapy.
10. Operate on facts rather than on assumptions or misperceptions.
11. Identify awareness of anxiety developed in self during a nurse-patient interaction and seek to gain information about the patient's anxiety level using self as guide.

B. *Demonstrate acceptance of patient*

1. Convey acceptance of patient as a person, while at the same time not approving inappropriate behavior.
2. Remain objective in observing and identifying reasons for patient's behavior.
3. Make self available.
   a. Do not reject patient.
   b. Offer presence and spend time with patient.
   c. Demonstrate concern, understanding, and interest.
4. Develop and use open-minded, accurate, and flexible interpersonal perceptions.

a. Be aware that the accuracy of one's perceptions of a patient could be influenced by:
   (1) *Assimilation effect*—viewing a person's opinions more similar to one's own than they are.
   (2) *Contrast effect*—viewing a person's opinions more unlike one's own than they are.
   (3) *Primacy effect*—making judgments on first impressions.
   (4) *Halo effect*—tendency to assume a person possesses positively valued traits if generally impressed with person, or the converse.
   (5) *Concern with central traits*—perceiving others on the basis of whether or not they possess traits one positively values.
   (6) *Stereotyping*—assigning selected traits to a person because he belongs to a certain group.
   (7) *Self-defense mechanisms*—especially if overused.
   (8) *Assumed liking*—assuming that people we like will like us and our preferences, or the converse.
5. Permit expression of negative feelings.
   Avoid retaliation and punishment for behavior expressed.
6. Focus on strengths and potential of patient.
7. Avoid increasing anxiety unnecessarily.

C. *Provide consistency of experience.*
1. Enforce consistent restrictions.
2. Provide consistency in attitude.
3. Provide patient with information about the availability of time to spend with him.
   Meet with patient at agreed-upon time(s).
4. Give patient information about changes in his schedule or surroundings.

D. *Demonstrate respect for patient.*

1. Show honesty and moral integrity.
2. Allow for privacy as needed.
3. Listen actively to what patient is saying.
4. Permit decision-making within limits of safety to self and others.
5. Encourage self-care and use of capabilities.
6. Communicate value of the patient's being and potential.
   a. Preserve patient's individuality, opinions, uniqueness, and feelings.
   b. Be nonevaluative and nonjudgmental.
   c. Avoid reducing self-esteem of patient.
7. Demonstrate sincere and nonpossessive caring and concern.
8. Communicate openness and willingness to engage in a therapeutic nurse-patient relationship.

9. Create an atmosphere enabling patient to freely express himself.
10. Convey hope, optimism, and expectation for patient's ability to change, grow, and develop a more adaptive behavioral response.
    Support healthy parts of patient's personality.
11. Explain and provide information to the patient about his condition and the health care setting in which he is being treated in words that he can understand.
    Use informational booklets and other teaching materials as appropriate.

E. Show sensitivity to patient.

1. Don't attempt to negate patient's perception of an experience by comments such as, "Oh, it can't be that bad!"
2. Demonstrate availability to patient by taking time to assist him therapeutically.
3. Attempt to understand patient's perspective and feelings.
4. Demonstrate awareness and understanding of differences in cultural and subcultural values and customs.
5. Demonstrate flexibility; i.e., a responsiveness to change in conditions.

F. Express empathy.

1. Perceive and recognize patient's private, inner experiences and feelings.
   a. Use open-ended questions focusing on feelings.
   b. Reflect patient's feelings.
   c. Focus on "being with" patient.
2. Develop awareness of own response to patient.
   a. Recognize interaction of own experiences and those described by patient.
   b. Develop awareness of own response, to assist in grasping dynamic meaning, significance, and purpose of patient's experiences and feelings.
   c. Develop sense of meaning for that which patient is not fully aware.
   d. Achieve an on-going awareness of perceptual, cognitive, and affective aspects of patient.
3. Communicate accurate, sensitive understanding.
   a. Selectively use self-disclosure.
      Share experiences that model expression of feelings and exploration, as well as help patient recognize that he is not alone.
   b. Communicate understanding of feelings expressed by patient.
   c. Communicate understanding of underlying feelings and assumptions implied by patient.
4. Express highest level of empathy possible (i.e., at least Level 3. At Levels 4 and 5 even more empathy is expressed. Levels 1 and 2 are not therapeutic and are therefore not described. For Levels 3, 4, and 5 see below.)
   a. Characteristics of Level 3 expression of empathy:
      (1) Communicate understanding of patient's feelings at the same level as he expresses them.
      (2) Respond by accurately reflecting patient's state of being.
      (3) Seek to explore meaning of feelings that are expressed in a vague manner.
   b. Characteristics of Level 4 expression of empathy:
      (1) Communicate understanding of underlying feelings of patient, somewhat deeper than actual level expressed.
      (2) Communicate verbally in a manner adding somewhat deeper meaning than that which is verbally expressed by patient.
   c. Characteristics of Level 5 expression of empathy:
      (1) Respond by adding significantly to the meaning and affect which patient expresses explicitly.
      (2) Communicate accurately the meaning and affect of the patient's deeper feelings.

G. Develop trust—confidence and security in the reliability of oneself and others.

1. Be consistently truthful.
2. Offer patient clear understanding of purpose of nurse-patient relationship, or one-to-one nurse therapy.
3. Be consistent, reliable, and open.
4. Demonstrate interest in and commitment to patient over a period of time.
5. Consistently communicate trustworthiness and credibility.
6. Be sensitive to patient's needs and his being.
7. Give information as needed by patient. Do not try to control patient.
8. Create interpersonal relationship in which patient can freely communicate his feelings, needs, and problems.
9. Communicate a warm, positive regard for patient.
10. Don't make promises unless they can be kept.
11. Try to respond to reasonable requests.

H. Be genuine, congruent, and authentic.

1. Demonstrate consistency between actual feelings, thoughts, verbalizations, and behavior.
2. Be natural, spontaneous, real, open, sincere, and nondefensive.
3. Admit own errors to patient, when appropriate.
4. Communicate negative feelings to patient if:
   a. They are truly generated by patient, not from one's own past.
   b. The patient is capable of distinguishing the feedback to an aspect of his behavior and not to his total being.
   c. It can be done within the context of a therapeutic objective.
5. Share own personal reactions and feelings with patient if this serves a therapeutic purpose.
   a. Avoid constant and total disclosure of feelings.
   b. Express negative feelings to patient in a nondestructive way that encourages further discussion.
6. Be as natural and spontaneous as possible in the use of therapeutic interventions.
   Avoid artificial, mechanical use of interpersonal techniques.

I. Use confrontation appropriately.

1. Communicate to patient growth-defeating discrepancies in his behavior, feelings, perceptions, and thinking.
2. Encourage examination of these discrepancies.
3. Assist patient in becoming more fully aware of an aspect of his behavior or problem.
4. While using confrontation, convey a constructive interest, caring, and a high level of respect for patient's ability to grow.
5. Use appropriate timing when using confrontation.
6. Utilize empathy, authenticity, respect, etc. to facilitate self-confrontation.
   Avoid overuse of nurse-initiated confrontation.

J. *Use personal self-disclosure appropriately.*
Characteristics include:
1. Patient's levels of self-disclosure have been positively correlated with the ability to deal with his illness.
2. If the nurse or patient discloses self at a certain level in the relationship, the other person tends to respond with a similar or greater degree of self-disclosure.
3. The higher the level of trust, the higher the level of self-disclosure.

Facilitating Nurse-Patient Communication

A. *Definition of Communication*
1. *Communication* is a dynamic, complex, constantly changing process which occurs over time, in which human beings send and receive verbal and nonverbal messages, in order to understand and to be understood by others, adapt to the environment, and transfer ideas to another.
2. It is impossible not to communicate, because all behavior communicates something.

B. *Characteristics and Elements of Communication*
1. Communication includes:
   a. Sender—transmits message.
   b. Message—meaning which is communicated, intentionally or unintentionally.
   c. Code, channel, or media—the way in which a message is sent.
   d. Receiver—recipient of message.
   e. Response or feedback—behavior of receiver (verbal and nonverbal) in relation to message received.
2. Communication can be:
   a. Verbal—use of written or spoken words, or
   b. Nonverbal—use of facial expression; eye contact; posture; bodily movements; touch; appearance and dress; pitch, rate, and volume of voice; gestures.
   c. Digital—the verbal mode of communication, or
   d. Analogic—the nonverbal mode of communication including the context.
   e. Symmetrical—communication characterized by equality in the right to initiate communication, to criticize, and to offer advice; or
   f. Complementary—communication characterized by one person giving and the other receiving in the interaction.
3. The communication process can be affected by:
   a. Culture, customs, education, social background, physical and mental status, intellectual ability, and past experiences of the participants.
   b. Channel, language, and words used to transmit message.
   c. Context in which communication occurs.
   d. Perceptions, feelings, thoughts, and motivations of receiver and sender prior to communication.
   e. Nature of the relationship between sender and receiver.
   f. Intentions or goals of sender.
   g. Self-concept or self-perception of sender and receiver.
   h. Anxiety or stress level of sender or receiver.
   i. Sensory organ impairment or physical disorder interfering with mechanical ability to produce sound.
   j. Discrepancies between the sender's and receiver's punctuation of the communication sequence of events—i.e., the particular aspect of the communication on which each focuses—can affect the relationship.

4. Communication includes a:
   a. Content aspect of message—verbal message, and
   b. Relationship aspect of message—verbal and/or nonverbal aspect of message about the relationship between the sender and the receiver.
   Nonverbal communication can qualify or disqualify verbal message.

C. *Communication techniques include:*
1. Understanding response—a response which conveys sincere effort to understand how the patient views his world, his experiences, and the meaning he attaches to his experiences.
2. Open-ended questions—questions which present the patient with options for response other than just answering "yes" or "no."
   a. Avoid closed questions—questions in which nurse implies what answer is expected.
   b. Questioning can be useful in obtaining information, clarification, and offering assistance.
3. Reflection—letting patient know through feedback what he has overtly or covertly said or the feelings that he has conveyed.
   Use same key words used by patient.
4. Active listening—listening characterized by attending to patient's communications (not on own personal responses to be made), interpreting what is communicated, and responding selectively.
   a. Communicate concern, caring, and understanding.
   b. "Pick up on" feelings and needs expressed verbally and nonverbally.
   c. In responding selectively, use communication techniques as reflection, summarizing, etc.
   d. After communicating understanding, use problem-solving approach to help patient explore alternatives.
   e. Use silence constructively and appropriately.
5. Seeking validation—requesting feedback from patient to check understanding and interpretation of his communication or of his perceptions.
6. Sharing observation—verbalizing what is observed about a patient's behavior; e.g., "You appear rather sad."
7. Clarifying—requesting feedback to make certain that patient's communications are accurately understood; e.g., "By telling me . . . do you mean . . .?" or "To whom are you referring when you say 'they'?"
8. Picking up on themes expressed—providing feedback on ideas or feelings repetitively expressed; e.g., "You seem to be feeling that your family can't be trusted."
   Avoid switching conversation to superficial topics.
9. Restating—repeating a main thought, using words much like those used by the patient in order to encourage expansion.
10. Encouraging verbalization—verbal and nonverbal means to assist patient to keep talking; e.g., "Go on," or "You were saying?" or nodding head.
11. Focusing—asking questions or using other communication techniques to help patient stick to important subject matter or theme.
12. Feedback—describing some aspect of patient's communication and its impact on the receiver.
13. Summarizing—giving patient feedback on general content and theme of conversation in a condensed version.

14. Confrontation—describing discrepancies in behavior of patient and encouraging exploration.

D. *Causes of communication breakdown or distortion include:*
1. Unintelligible messages—using terms the patient does not understand, especially psychiatric or medical terminology or jargon.
2. Incomplete messages—assuming that the patient already has the knowledge and therefore leaving the patient's questions unanswered.
3. Inadvertent messages—unintentionally transmitting a message, as by giving too much detail, which the patient then misinterprets.
4. Omitted messages—failing to explain something the patient should know.
5. Contradictory messages—transmitting a message in which the verbal and nonverbal aspects are contradictory, or several different staff members give different messages to the patient.
6. Unfulfilled messages—making promises which are not kept.
7. Failure to listen actively.
8. Failure to interpret message accurately.
9. Failure to focus on patient's concerns.
10. Ineffective or inappropriate reassurance.
11. Lecturing, moralizing, pep talks.
12. Switching topic of conversation to superficial aspects.
13. Judgmental attitude, prejudice, stereotyping.
14. Stress perceived or faced by nurse in work situation.
15. High level of fear and anxiety patient may have about his illness and its treatment. (Items 1 through 13 can increase patient's anxiety.)

The One-to-One Nurse-Patient Relationship

Definition and characteristics include:
1. Focusing attention on the patient and his emotional and behavioral concerns through a mutually defined professional relationship.
2. Using goal-directed therapeutic communication, including active listening, in order to foster exploration of problem areas, learning, change, and personal growth.
   Includes a series of nurse-patient interactions occurring over time.
3. Can range from brief counseling to more lengthy forms of treatment as individual nurse psychotherapy.

The Nursing Process

The nursing process should be utilized throughout the one-to-one nurse-patient relationship.

A. *Interviewing and assessment*
1. A nursing history guide is useful in collecting data in an interview.
2. Provide for privacy, physical comfort, and freedom from interruption during the interview.
3. Conduct interview with sensitivity so as to facilitate the beginning of a positive nurse-patient relationship.
4. Explain the purpose, nature, and length of the interview.
   Inform patient that information gained will be utilized to assist in his treatment and shared with appropriate staff.
5. Ask about the nature of the patient's problem and current life situation. (See Chapter 24, chart on Psychiatric Nursing Assessment of the Adult Patient.)
6. Observe for both verbal and nonverbal expressions, changes in mood, and difficulties in answering any questions.
7. Ask questions in a concrete and simple way.
   Do not delve into complex issues in depth during the first interview.
8. Utilize a conceptual framework for nursing practice to guide observations, interviewing, and assessment.
9. Follow health care agency guidelines for charting observations and assessment.
10. *Process recordings*—a written record of the communication of both the nurse and the patient, especially during individual nurse psychotherapy. In addition, can include:
    a. An analysis of the nurse's feelings and interventions (including the treatment goal)
    b. An analysis of the patient's response
    c. An evaluation of the total interaction
       Often used by a nurse expert to review and supervise the one-to-one nurse-patient relationship developed by the nurse or nursing student being supervised.

B. *Nursing Diagnosis*
Formulated from an analysis of patient assessment and the data collected. (See Chapter 26.)

C. *Planning*
1. Behavioral goals are developed after adequate assessment and formulation of the nursing diagnosis. (See Chapter 26.)
2. Plan with input from patient, as much as possible.

D. *Intervention*
1. Should be designed to help patient achieve formulated behavioral goals. (See Chapter 26.)
2. A conceptual framework for nursing practice serves to guide planning and design intervention strategies.

E. *Evaluation*
1. Determine extent to which goals have been met.
2. Data resulting from evaluation is used to plan and redesign intervention strategies to meet goals, to revise goals, or to formulate new goals, as necessary.

Phases of the Nurse-Patient Relationship

A. *Phase I (Beginning or Orientation Phase)*
1. Patient uses primarily cognitive words and phrases; e.g., when describing personal history, patient recounts primarily factual material.
2. Patient will often reach a point at which he will state that he has nothing more to say.
   a. For therapeutic progress, patient must move beyond this plateau into the affective domain and into Phase II of the relationship.
   b. To assist him in moving into the affective domain, focus on an identified cognitive theme which is linked with affective material.
3. Nurse therapist becomes acquainted with patient.
   The patient is assessed and nursing diagnoses are formulated.
4. A mutually agreed upon contract for the one-to-one nurse-patient relationship is established.
   a. The nurse therapist's role and responsibilities in the one-to-one nurse-patient relationship are explained.
   b. The overall purpose of the one-to-one nurse-patient relationship is described.

c. Initial, mutually defined, behavioral goals are identified.
d. The place, time, and length of the meeting are agreed upon.
e. The actual or tentative length of the entire therapy is stated.
f. Arrangements are made to deal with missed appointments.
g. The responsibilities of the patient in the one-to-one nurse-patient relationship are discussed.

5. Of great importance is the formation of a working relationship with the patient.
   a. Patient begins to demonstrate a sense of confidence in and liking for the nurse therapist.
   b. The nurse therapist senses an ability "of making contact" with patient and an ability of being able to facilitate change and growth.

6. Discuss confidentiality of information discussed by patient.
   a. Inform patient that progress in therapy will be reported to health care team members in general terms, maintaining confidentiality of specific information, except that
   b. Information about harmfulness to self or others will be shared with appropriate professional staff.

7. Build trusting relationship by maintaining the stipulations of the contract and informing patient of any changes; e.g., unavoidable absences.

B. *Phase II (Middle or Working Phase)*

1. Phase in which patient discusses his problems and feelings and in which behavioral change and growth occur.

2. Affective material will dominate. Patient will use cognitive words and phrases to describe or emphasize material from affective domain.

3. Attend to frequency of affective word(s) used and to behavioral trends and patterns described.

4. Encourage expression and analysis of emotional concerns and self-defeating behavioral patterns and trends.
   a. Mutually determine the behavioral dynamics of the patient; i.e., explore origin, operation, and consequences of behavioral patterns.
   b. Facilitate patient's own assessment of self-defeating behavioral patterns.

5. Be aware of the possibility of resistance occurring.
   a. Behavioral manifestations of patient can include rejection, avoidance, denial, hostility, and reaching a plateau in therapy.

6. Facilitate resolution of emotional conflicts, reduction in self-defeating behavioral patterns, and the attainment of the mutually defined behavioral goals of the patient.

a. Identify forces with patient that hinder behavioral change.
b. Facilitate problem-solving strategies to formulate behavioral alternatives and to select a behavioral alternative for testing.
c. Create atmosphere in which the testing of new behaviors can readily occur and any associated anxiety can be worked through.

C. *Phase III (Termination or Resolution Phase)*

1. The patient makes increasing use of cognitive words and themes in relation to future planning.

2. Patient responses to the actual termination with the nurse therapist are variable and are related to prior termination experiences, type of treatment, present problems, and personality.
   Reactions to impending loss can include grief, sadness, displacement, reaction formation, dependency, or frank hostility.

3. Interventions or tasks to be achieved in termination include:
   a. Assist patient to identify his responses to impending loss of therapist.
   b. Encourage expression of feelings.
   c. Assist patient to work through and resolve his feelings about the impending separation from the therapist.
   d. Encourage patient to explore and evaluate his total experience in the one-to-one nurse-patient relationship.
   e. Give feedback to patient on his accomplishments and areas for further growth.
   f. Help patient tolerate the discomfort involved in termination.
   g. Mutually determine exact termination date.
   h. Encourage patient's emotional investment in others significant to him.
   i. Assist patient in planning for the future.

4. To facilitate termination and closure of relationship in a mutually planned, satisfying manner, instruct patient to:
   a. Spend some time (at least a half hour) alone and without interruptions.
   b. Think about the relationship with the nurse therapist during the entire course of therapy.
   c. Stay with the feelings that are generated as long as needed.
   d. Imagine and practice how he wants the last session to be, until the last session is satisfying for him.
   e. Actually share thoughts, feelings, and fantasies with nurse in the therapy session. (The nurse therapist will also have gone through the above process and will share her thoughts and feelings.)

BIBLIOGRAPHY

Books

Carkhuff R. Helping and Human Relations: Practice and Research. New York, Holt, Rinehart, & Winston, 1969
Collins M. Communication in Health Care: Understanding and Implementing Effective Human Relationships. St. Louis, CV Mosby, 1977
Danziger K. Interpersonal Communication. New York, Pergamon Press, 1976

Fromm–Reichmann F. Principles of Intensive Psychotherapy. Chicago, University of Chicago Press, 1971
Hammond D, Hepworth D, Smith V. Improving Therapeutic Communication. San Francisco, Jossey–Bass Publishers, 1977
Lewis G. Nurse-Patient Communication. Dubuque, Wm C Brown Co., 1978
O'Brien M. Communications and Relationships in Nursing. St. Louis, CV Mosby, 1978

Peplau H. Basic Principles of Patient Counseling. Philadelphia, Smith, Kline, & French Laboratories, 1964

Pluckhan M. Human Communication; The Matrix of Nursing. New York, McGraw-Hill, 1978

Purtilo R. Health Professional–Patient Interaction. Philadelphia, WB Saunders, 1978

Robinson L. Psychiatric Nursing as a Human Experience. Philadelphia, WB Saunders, 1977

Rogers C, Gendlin E, Kiesler D et al. The Therapeutic Relationship and Its Impact: A Study of Psychotherapy with Schizophrenics. Madison, University of Wisconsin Press, 1967

Ruesch J. Therapeutic Communication. New York, WW Norton, 1973

Sierra–Franco M. Therapeutic Communications in Nursing. New York, McGraw-Hill, 1978

Simmons J. The Nurse-Client Relationship in Mental Health Nursing. Philadelphia, WB Saunders, 1976

Topalis M and Aguilera D. Psychiatric Nursing. St. Louis, CV Mosby, 1978

Truax C and Carkhuff R. Toward Effective Counseling and Psychotherapy: Training and Practice. Chicago, Aldine–Atherton, 1967

Watzlawick P, Beavin J, Jackson D. Pragmatics of Human Communication. New York, WW Norton, 1967

Wiedenbach E and Falls C. Communication, Key to Effective Nursing. New York, Tiresias Press, 1978

Wilson H and Kneisl C. Psychiatric Nursing. Menlo Park, Addison–Wesley Publishing Co., 1979

Articles

Almore M. Dyadic communication. Am J Nurs 1979 June; 79(6):1076–1078

Asken M. Communicating in a medical setting. J Pract Nurs 1978 Apr; 28(4):22–23, 35

Authier J, Authier K, Lutey M. Clinical management of the tearfully depressed patient: communication skills for the nurse practitioner. J Psychiatr Nurs 1979 Feb; 17(2):34–41

Blount M, Green S, Hamory A et al. Documenting with the problem-oriented record system. Am J Nurs 1978 Sept; 78(9):1539–1542

Boettcher E. Nurse-client collaboration: Dynamic equilibrium in the nursing care system. J Psychiatr Nurs 1978 Dec; 16(12):7–15

Brink T. Is TLC contraindicated for geriatric patients? Perspect Psychiatr Care 1977 July–Aug–Sept; 15(3):129–131

Carser D and Doona M. Alienation: A nursing concept. J Psychiatr Nurs 1978 Sept; 16(9):33–40

Cosper B. How well do patients understand hospital jargon? Am J Nurs 1977 Dec; 77(12):1932–1934

Daubenmire M, Searles S, Ashton C. A methodologic framework to study nurse–patient communication. Nurs Res 1978 Sept–Oct; 27(5):303–310

Doona M, Annino S, Kelleher M. Professional affirmation in nursing care. J Psychiatr Nurs 1977 Aug; 15(8):16–23

Fahrner B, Ellis N, Stark S et al. Record-keeping in a state hospital: A modification of the Weed system. Hosp Community Psychiatry 1977 Dec; 28(12):907–908

Frenkel S, Greden J, Robinson J et al. Does patient contact change racial perceptions? Am J Nurs 1980 July; 80(7):1340–1342

Friedrich R, Scandrett S, Turock A. Innovation in continuing education: A statewide program for systematic training in interpersonal skills. J Cont Ed Nurs 1979 Mar–Apr; 10(2):29–35

Gifford S and Maberry D. An integrated system for computerized patient records. Hosp Community Psychiatry 1979 Aug; 30(8):532–535

Gluck J. The computerized medical record system; meeting the challenge for nursing. J Nurs Admin 1979 Dec; 9(12):17–24

Grazette H. An anatomy of communication. Nurs Times 1978 Oct 12; 74(41):1672–1679

Hall B. The effect of interpersonal attraction on the therapeutic relationship: a review and suggestions for further study. J Psychiatr Nurs 1977 Sept; 15(9):18–23

Johnson M. Self-disclosure: A variable in the nurse-client relationship. J Psychiatr Nurs 1980 Jan; 18(1):17–20

Jungman L. When your feelings get in the way. Am J Nurs 1979 June; 79(6):1074–1075

Kalisch B. What is empathy? Am J Nurs 1973 Sept; 73(9):1548–1552

Kaplan N and Levy K. An approach for facilitating the passage through termination. J Psychiatr Nurs 1978 June; 16(6):11–14

Karshmer J, Kornfeld–Jacobs G, Carr A. Causal attributions: bias in the nurse–patient relationship. J Psychiatr Nurs 1980 May; 18(5):25–30

Kauffman M. On developing empathy; sharing the patient's experience. Am J Nurs 1978 May; 78(5):860–861

Lego S. The one-to-one nurse–patient relationship. Perspect Psychiatr Care 1980 Mar–Apr; 18(2):67–89

McCann J. Termination of the psychotherapeutic relationship. J Psychiatr Nurs 1979 Oct; 17(10):37–46

McFarland G and Apostoles F. The nursing history in a psychiatric setting: Adaptations to a variety of nursing care patterns and patient populations. J Psychiatr Nurs 1975 July–Aug; 13(4):12–17

McNeill D. Developing the complete computer-based information system. J Nurs Adm 1979 Nov; 9(11):34–46

Norton C. Can you hear between the lines? RN 1978 Sept; 41(9):117–118, 120, 122

Ramaekers M. Communication blocks revisited. Am J Nurs 1979 June; 79(6):1079–1081

Rawnsley M. Toward a conceptual base for affective nursing. Nurs Outlook 1980 Apr; 28(4):244–247

Rieder K and Wood M. Problem-orientation: An experimental study to test its heuristic value. Nurs Res 1978 Jan–Feb; 27(1):25–29

Roseman E. Correcting communication faults. MLO 1978 Nov; 10(11):37–41

Ruditis S. Developing trust in nursing interpersonal relationships. J Psychiatr Nurs 1979 Apr; 17(4):20–23

Scheideman J. Problem patients do not exist. Am J Nurs 1979 June; 79(6):1082–1084

Seeger P. Self-awareness and nursing. J Psychiatr Nurs 1977 Aug; 15(8):24–26

Smith L. Communication skills. Nurs Times 1979 May 31; 75(22):926–929

Sparks S, Vitalo P, Cohen B, Kahn G. Teaching of interpersonal skills to nurse practitioner students. J Cont Ed Nurs 1980 May–June; 11(3):5–16

Sparling S and Jones S. Setting: A contextual variable associated with empathy. J Psychiatr Nurs 1977 Apr; 15(4):9–12

Swearingen D, Messick J, May P et al. Improving patient care through measurement: Goal importance and achievement scaling. J Psychiatr Nurs 1977 Sept; 15(9):30–36

Wallston K, Cohen B, Wallston B et al. Increasing nurses' person-centeredness. Nurs Res 1978 May–June; 27(3):156–159

Wyatt M and Withersty D. Teaching interpersonal management for effective professional nursing practice. J Psychiatr Nurs 1979 June; 17(6):23–27

NURSING DIAGNOSES IN CARING FOR THE ADULT PSYCHIATRIC PATIENT

Definition and Characteristics of Nursing Diagnoses

1. *Nursing diagnosis* is a word or phrase summarizing a set of empirical indicators linked to contributing factors or etiology, when possible, and representing actual or potential altered patterns of human functioning, which nurses are licensed to treat.*
2. Nursing diagnoses accepted at National Conferences on the Classification of Nursing Diagnoses especially useful in the care of the psychiatric patient include:†
   a. Impaired verbal communication
   b. Ineffective individual coping
   c. Ineffective family coping—compromised
   d. Ineffective family coping—disabling
   e. Family coping—potential for growth
   f. Fear
   g. Anticipatory grieving
   h. Dysfunctional grieving
   i. Disturbance in self-concept
   j. Sensory perceptual alterations
   k. Spiritual distress
   l. Alterations in thought processes
   m. Potential for violence
3. The nursing diagnoses identified in this Chapter relate primarily to the individual adult psychiatric patient. They are not family, group, or community diagnoses. Under each diagnosis is discussed:

   * Task Force of the National Group for the Classification of Nursing Diagnoses. Subcommittee report on definition of nursing diagnosis. The Fourth National Conference on Classification of Nursing Diagnoses, St. Louis, April 9–13, 1980.

   † Kim M and Moritz D.: Classification of Nursing Diagnoses: Proceedings of Third and Fourth National Conference. New York, McGraw-Hill, 1981.
   Gebbie K and Levin M (eds). Classification of Nursing Diagnoses. St. Louis, C.V. Mosby, 1975.
   Gebbie K. Summary of the Second National Conference—Classification of Nursing Diagnoses. St. Louis, The Clearinghouse, St. Louis University, 1976.

   a. *Characteristics*—includes the empirical indicators or behavioral manifestations. Key concepts or etiological factors will be discussed for some diagnoses.
   b. *Nursing Assessment*—initial or ongoing diagnosis-specific assessment factors supplemental to the overall assessment parameters outlined in Chapter 24. The questions and statements listed serve as guidelines for assessment and should be adapted as necessary.
   c. *Nursing Management Goals and Treatment Interventions*—includes goals followed by nursing interventions designed to achieve each specific goal.
      (1) In designing an individual patient care plan, goals can be restated in patient behavioral outcome terms, if desired.
      (2) Select interventions from among those listed to individualize the nursing care plan for a specific patient.
   d. *Health Education and Prevention*—diagnostic-specific content useful in patient teaching or as preventive measures.
4. There are differences in the conceptual level of abstraction of the listed diagnoses. The best diagnosis(es) for a patient should be determined on the basis of an analysis of the available assessment data collected.
5. Nursing diagnosis can be changed as more data, warranting the change, become available.
6. The established nursing diagnosis(es) for a patient gives direction to the next phases of the nursing process—planning, intervention, and evaluation.
   a. The etiological or contributing factor(s) should be identified, if possible, and added to the main phase of the nursing diagnosis.
   b. The two parts are linked with the words "related to."

      This is done to clarify documentation of the relationships of the components of the nursing conceptual framework which, in turn, affects nursing care planning and intervention.

c. For example, on admission, the initial nursing diagnosis may be "suicide, attempted." After ad-

ditional data is collected, the diagnosis may be changed to "suicide, attempted, related to dealing with symbiotic relationship with mother."

INAPPROPRIATE EXPRESSION OF AGGRESSION

Characteristics

1. *Aggression*—a forceful goal-directed verbal or physical action which may result from such feelings/emotional states as anger, anxiety, tension, guilt, and hostility, in turn resulting from a variety of precipitating factors.
2. Inappropriate assaultive behavior may be:
   a. learned and perpetuated by motives, attitudes, and rationalizations supported by subculture;
   b. produced or perpetuated by hospital social structure (e.g., coercion, regimentation, personal space invasion).
3. *Violence*—pursuit of own interests by force; at extreme end of aggression continuum.
4. See Table 26-1, Model of Aggression.

Nursing Assessment

1. What is the nature of the patient's aggressive behavior? Preceding events? Precipitants? Place of occurrence? Actual behavior including intensity, target, degree of inner controls?
2. What is the patient's perception of self, environment?
3. What is the meaning behind the aggressive behavior?
4. Determine patient's prior methods of coping with stress-producing situations and ways used to gain self-control.
5. How does the patient cope with anger?
   a. Internalizes, becomes depressed?
   b. Unable to identify source, displacement?
   c. Able to identify source but unable to express directly, so is passive aggressive?
   d. Identifies source along with direct and appropriate or inappropriate expression?
6. Assess potential for violent behavior by considering factors such as:
   a. Past history of arrests and violent behavior
   b. History of life stressors resulting in bitterness
   c. Unstable family situation characterized by quarreling
   d. Violence displayed by significant others, especially parental brutality
   e. High interest in and availability of weapons
   f. Low self-esteem without involvement in constructive activities
   g. Toxic state from alcohol or drug abuse
   h. Presence of persecutional delusions
   i. History of physical impairment, such as minimal brain dysfunction
   j. Organization and rehearsal of plans for violent act
   k. Absence of reliable significant other(s)
   l. Degree of reversibility of predisposing conditions
   m. Methods of dealing with similar past situations
7. Continue observations for:
   a. Behavioral changes indicating increasing anxiety, guilt, anger
   b. Homicidal or suicidal ideation

TABLE 26-1. MODEL OF AGGRESSION

Possible Causes	Possible Resulting Feelings	Possible Resulting Responses
Frustration Loss of dignity Fear Need to test reality	Anxiety	*Adaptive Response* Use of coping skills and strategies resulting in resolution, including constructive expression of aggression as in problem-solving or realistic defense. OR
Physical impairment (e.g., minimal brain dysfunction)	Guilt	*Inadequate Adaptive Response—Inappropriate Expression of Aggression*
Inferiority and low self-esteem		Defensive actions—designed to meet needs, achieve goals and protect self and includes both inappropriate verbal or physical expression of aggression.
Repressed resentment, hate, or hostility	Tension	Offensive actions—designed to punish or destroy and includes verbal hostility, physical assault, or violence.
Grief (anger phase)	Anger	Direct action against cause—includes other or self-directed physical or verbal aggression.
Perceived threat		
Threat of intimacy	Hostility	Indirect action against cause—includes scape-goating; acting-out; overuse of displacement, projection, introjection, reaction-formation, or somatization; or passive-aggressive behavior, such as gossiping, round-about jokes, derogatory jokes, slamming doors, temper tantrums, negativism, resentment, irritability, or postponements.
Perceptual or cognitive distortion		
Social milieu (e.g., rejection from significant others or subculture expression of aggression)		
Helplessness		
Thwarting of goals as career progression		
Thwarting of needs for power, control, authority, attention		
Ward milieu (e.g., staff conflict, over-crowding, etc.)		

c. Inappropriate aggression
(1) What were the preceding events including ward milieu?
(2) What were the precipitating factors?
(3) What actually happened?
(4) How does the patient perceive the event?
d. Ward milieu, including staff ability to deal effectively with own emotions
e. Possession of any weapons
f. Change in ability to resolve anxiety, anger, tension, or guilt in an acceptable way

Nursing Goals and Interventions

A. *To reduce/eliminate inappropriate aggression and to help patient identify feelings and to express them appropriately.*

1. Assist patient to deal with anger.
   a. Provide feedback on nonverbal behavior to help patient identify anger.
   b. Develop relationship in which patient can be angry and can learn to distinguish between feelings and actions.
   c. Have patient practice verbalizing angry feelings in a minimally threatening situation.
   d. Assist in identifying sources of anger.
   e. Explore and aid in developing alternate methods of expressing anger, including using direct approach.
2. Reduce passive–aggressive behavior.
   a. Observe and document behavior.
   b. After having developed positive relationship with patient, confront, pointing out behaviors and their consequences.
   c. Set limits and give positive reinforcement for appropriate behavior.
3. Develop therapeutic ward milieu.
   a. Provide opportunity through group meetings for staff and patients to discuss reactions and feelings about inappropriate aggression.
   b. Settle conflict.
   c. Work through phases of planned change.
4. Mutually develop goals with patient for more appropriate expression of anger, hostility, anxiety, tension, or guilt.
   Seek alternatives that can be used after discharge.
5. Analyze own perceptions of patient.
   Avoid stereotyping or "expecting" physical aggression.
6. Assist patient in reducing cognitive distortion and developing alternative perspective about himself and the causes of his aggression.
7. Help reduce anxiety. (See pp. 926–927).
8. Point out consequences of inappropriate aggression.
9. Prevent suicide (see pp. 949–950) or homicide.
10. Evaluate need for group or family therapy.
11. Provide outlets for feelings engendered (e.g., activity groups, punching bags, clay, sports, art, music).
12. Help patient recognize cause and effect among cause, emotions, and aggressive behavior displayed.
13. Develop behavior-modification approaches for selected aggressive behaviors.
14. Explore patient's past experiences with aggressive behavior as demonstrated by significant others and what rewards his current aggressive behavior achieves for him.

15. Provide peer role models who demonstrate more adaptive behavioral responses.

B. *To provide protection from injury to self and others, to recognize potential for inappropriate aggression, and to intervene prior to expression.*

1. If patient possesses a weapon:
   a. Don't attempt to grab it, unless there are enough staff members present.
   b. Request that weapon be deposited in a neutral place.
   c. If threatened with weapon, place protective barrier between self and weapon, such as mattress or chair.
2. Support ego.
   a. Use honest, empathic, firm approach.
   b. Avoid accusatory approach and increasing guilt.
3. Recognize potential for inappropriate aggression and intervene prior to expression.
4. Be cautious and avoid facade of bravado. Do convey security and don't exhibit fear or panic.
5. Provide opportunity for verbalization of feelings, especially anger: Attempt to "talk down."
6. Do not be hasty in attempts to uncover precipitants, but acknowledge patient's tension and state desire to help him regain control.
7. Set consistent limits on type and degree of inappropriate aggression that is tolerated.
8. Pose well-timed questions about what the patient may be experiencing.
9. Be aware of potentially stressful situations for patient and document and communicate any change in behavior.
10. If physical aggression is imminent or occurring, approach quietly with staff and, if indicated, use a well-planned method of physical restraint.
11. Do not ignore threats of physical aggression.
12. Be available to patient during periods of increasing tension, etc.
13. Respect patient's need for personal space.
14. Provide consistent set of expectations for patient to develop self-control.
15. Explore options for more constructive outlets for inappropriate aggression.
16. Be as truthful as possible.
17. Remove external object that patient fears, if possible.
18. Recognize need for clear-cut staff-patient boundaries.
19. When therapist is verbally threatened:
    a. Continue patient contact.
    b. Explore precipitants of threat.
    c. Permit verbalizations of feelings associated with threat.
    d. Assist patient in realizing link between cause, subsequent feelings, and verbal threat.
20. When verbal and nonverbal cues indicate physical aggression:
    a. Do not avoid patient but interact early with him.
    b. Convey acceptance of person but not of physical aggression.
    c. Avoid retaliatory behaviors.
    d. Permit verbalization of feelings.
    e. Suggest constructive physical outlets, such as punching bag, etc.
    f. Suggest use of a quiet area until self-control is fully regained.

C. *To provide protection from injury to self and others and to use appropriate protective measures.*

1. Maintain stable, therapeutic ward milieu for brain-damaged patients.
2. Develop and implement well-planned, orderly method of restraint for violent patient.
3. Be aware of potential target for patient's physical aggressions.
4. Determine and anticipate need for medications, physical restraints, seclusion, or mechanical restraints and utilize, following physician's protocol or requests. (See Chapter 28.)
5. Ask patient whether medications are desired.
6. If medications are refused, reoffer them a short time later.
7. If agitated, administer medications after patient has been physically restrained in flat position.
8. Discuss violence and physical aggression with patient after the episode.
9. Communicate that staff is attempting to solve the immediate problem.
10. Avoid sudden movements with a violent patient.
11. To control violence:
    a. Observe, plan, and act.
    b. One staff member is given final authority on method of restraint to be used.
    c. Staff is given specific instructions.
    d. Use institutional policy as guideline.
    e. Have more staff present than needed to communicate strength.
    f. Do not use force.
    g. Use pillows, mattress, or chair to ward off blows.
12. Use self-protective devices to deal with actual physical aggression: Do not inflict pain or injury.

a. Controlled breathing—inhale and exhale deeply and sharply before physical action to protect self.
b. Movement—move while speaking to agitated patient so he can't predict exact location.
c. Stance—place feet shoulder-width apart, forward foot in front, and back foot at 90° angle from forward foot.
d. Utilize protective fall.
e. Observation—observe patient's eyes for he will observe body part that will be attacked.
f. Protective actions:
    (1) Deflect patient action by self-defense techniques.
    (2) Use counter-pressure.
    (3) Use body pressure points.
    (4) Seek assistance as soon as possible.

Health Education and Prevention

1. To prevent inappropriate aggression, teach patient to:
    a. Recognize warning signs, symptoms, and feelings preceding occurrence.
    b. Avoid toxic substances, such as alcohol, which can impair judgment.
    c. Practice self-control and appropriate expression of feelings and aggression beginning with precipitants evoking minor tension, anger, guilt, or anxiety.
    d. Seek psychiatric assistance when he feels need for help in establishing self-control.
2. List phone numbers of Hot Line and professionals who can be contacted when need arises.
3. Use relaxation techniques.

MILD ANXIETY, MODERATE ANXIETY, SEVERE ANXIETY, EXTREME ANXIETY (PANIC)

Characteristics

1. *Anxiety*—an uncomfortable warning of varying intensity of an impending subjective danger for which the source of danger is unknown.
    a. Can be experienced at conscious, preconscious, or unconscious level.
    b. Causes include threats to one's biological integrity (e.g., diminished food supply) or threats to one's self-security (e.g., unmet needs for belonging, unmet goals, or guilt).
    c. Response to anxiety can be constructive (task-oriented behavior) or destructive (defensive-oriented reactions).
    d. When anxiety level exceeds person's adaptive coping strategies, maladaptive patterns of behavior may result.
    e. The same stressor will not lead to anxiety or to the same level of anxiety in all persons.
2. *Normal anxiety*—does not involve repressive or other defensive mechanisms.
3. *Neurotic anxiety*—involves repression and other defensive mechanisms.

Can manifest itself in phobic disorders, anxiety states, or other maladaptive behaviors.
4. *Mild anxiety*—characterized by:
    a. Slight discomfort
    b. Enhanced ability to deal with stressor
    c. Increased awareness, problem-solving abilities, perceptual field, and alertness as well as the ability to see more connections between events.
    d. Sleeplessness
    e. Curiosity, repetitive questioning
    f. Constant attention seeking, belittling
    g. Misunderstandings, idle hostility, restlessness, irritability
    h. Increased attention on problem situation
5. *Moderate anxiety*—characterized by:
    a. Moderate discomfort
    b. Increased ability to concentrate, focus attention on problem situation; concentrate on sensory data relevant to problem, and verbalize; more alert
    c. Narrowing of perceptual field, selective inattention, some ability to perceive and understand connections between events

d. Voice tremors, change in voice pitch
e. Increased respiratory rate, heart rate, and muscle tension
f. Shakiness
6. *Severe anxiety*—characterized by:
   a. Tendency to dissociate anxious feelings from self; denial of existence of uncomfortable feelings to protect self
   b. Range of perception greatly reduced; focus on small or scattered detail; inability to see connections between events or details
   c. Selective inattention, interference with effective functioning
   d. Difficult and inappropriate verbalizations; inability to concentrate, purposeless activity; inability to learn
   e. Sense of impending doom
   f. Hyperventilation; tachycardia; frequency and urgency
   g. Nausea, headache, dizziness
7. *Extreme (panic) anxiety*—characterized by:
   a. Extreme discomfort
   b. Unrealistic perception of situation
   c. Distortion and enlargement of detail, disruption of perceptual field
   d. Inability to speak, unintelligible communication
   e. Vomiting, feeling of personality disintegration, immobility

Nursing Assessment

1. What level of anxiety does the patient manifest?
2. Observe adaptive or maladaptive behavioral responses to anxiety.
3. Observe for stressors or threats generating anxiety.
4. What behavioral changes indicating anxiety are present?
5. What has patient done in past to reduce anxiety?

Nursing Goals and Interventions

A. *To prevent or reduce anxiety to a level at which problem-solving can be effective.*

1. Be a good listener.
2. Engage in recreational and diversional activities aimed at reducing anxiety: group singing, volley ball, ping-pong, walking, swimming, simple concrete tasks, simple games, routine tasks, housekeeping chores, grooming, puzzles, cards, etc.
   a. Seek out staff members' advice in developing ways to lower patient's anxiety.
   b. Identify constructive ways patient has reduced anxiety in the past.
3. Develop a positive interpersonal relationship with the patient.
4. Administer tranquilizers or sedative drugs as prescribed.
5. Encourage ventilation of feelings, considering readiness of patient.
6. Do not probe.
7. Be calm.
   a. Avoid becoming anxious reciprocally.
   b. Recognize anxiety in own self and develop control over one's own responses.
8. Use short, simple sentences and a calm, firm tone in speaking with a highly anxious patient.
9. Provide simple, brief, and clear information about experiences to be encountered while hospitalized. Provide, clarify, or validate information as necessary.

10. Avoid requests for decision-making, asking for cause of behavior, or making interpretations when patient is highly anxious.
11. Convey empathy, unconditional positive regard, and congruence.
12. Offer reassurance, including use of nonverbal behavior such as quiet physical presence, use of touch, etc.
13. Intervene early to prevent escalation of anxiety to severe or extreme levels.
14. Keep highly anxious patient in a calm milieu: remove patient from stress until he/she is less sensitive to situation if anxiety level is high.
15. Limit contact with other anxious patients.
16. Convey matter-of-fact attitude that problem is not catastrophic and that a constructive resolution can be found.
17. Avoid anxiety-provoking situations, e.g., threats, insincerity, focus on weakness, indiscriminate use of psychiatric or medical terminology, unreasonable demands, indiscriminate use of confrontation of behavior, indifference or unconcerned attitude, blocking patient's rights or goals, judgmental attitude, impatience, etc.
18. Mutually develop daily schedule of activities incorporating patient's preferences and strengths.
19. During short-term hospitalization offer additional support and assistance in dealing with anxiety on admission, on about the fifth day, and upon notification of discharge.
20. Permit crying.
21. Reduce guilt by resolving psychodynamics involved.

B. *To help patient recognize presence of anxiety, develop insight into cause, and develop adaptive coping strategies and behavioral responses.*

1. If anxiety is at low or moderate level:
   a. Help patient to identify his anxiety by asking questions such as, "Are you uncomfortable right now?" Point out your awareness of his discomfort by providing feedback on nonverbal behaviors that indicate anxiety.
   b. Assist in discovering similarity of the immediate situation and past experiences in which similar discomfort was experienced. Ask questions such as, "Have you, in the past, ever felt like you feel right now? What was happening then to you? What did you do to feel less anxious?"
   c. Ask patient to describe what was desired, thought, or expected before becoming anxious and to discover the relationship of his state of anxiety to consequent adaptive or maladaptive behavior.
   d. Explore possible reasons for anxiety with patient: help patient to realistically clarify nature of problem.
   e. Assist in developing alternative solutions and methods to reduce anxiety; choose solutions for use and encourage trying out solutions.
   f. Evaluate results with patient. Encourage task-oriented versus self-oriented evaluation. Seek additional information and alternative action if plan was unsuccessful.
2. Encourage new interests and hobbies.
3. After anxiety is lowered and relationship with staff member is established:
   a. Encourage social activities despite reluctance and fears.
   b. Accompany patient first few times to activity and permit him to leave if he becomes too anxious.

c. Gradually encourage attendance independent of staff support.
4. Utilize and assist patient in choosing objective environmental interventions to deal with anxiety if he is basically optimistic, open to experience, and flexible.
5. Assist patient in developing a more optimistic and constructive world view if his subjective world is deadened, closed, or distorted.
   Assist in reducing life-style of negative expectations.
6. Allow patient freedom to work at his own level and pace in solving his problems.
7. Reduce secondary gains patient achieves from maladaptive behavioral responses.

Health Education and Prevention

1. Explore upcoming events.
   Use role play to help cope with anxiety-provoking encounters.

2. Teach patient:
   a. That some anxiety is part of living and that enduring mild and moderate anxiety can enhance learning, problem solving, and movement towards self-actualization
   b. To observe what is happening, describe it, analyze what he expected and how it differs from the actual situation, develop alternatives to solve problem or change expectations, and validate situation with others.
   c. Assertive communication skills
   d. Progressive muscular relaxation
3. Instruct patient to reduce severe or extreme anxiety through talking to someone; walking; simple games; simple, concrete tasks; sports; or, if anxiety is extreme, by seeking professional help.

DYSFUNCTIONAL COMMUNICATION

Characteristics

1. Poor communication practices such as:
   a. Monopolizing conversation
   b. Not discussing problems
   c. Poor listening skills
   d. Unclear messages
   e. Difficulty in dealing with anger or other feelings
   f. Nagging
   g. Sulking and pouting
   h. Lack of selective communication
   i. Not expressing feelings
   j. Lack of understanding
   k. Irritating tone of voice
   l. Interrupting
   m. Lack of empathy
   n. Lack of deliberate and frequent efforts to communicate
   o. Minimal use of clarification and feedback
   p. Overuse of generalizations
   q. Not fitting the metacommunications (the message *about* the message) with the communication
   r. Not fitting the message sent with the context within which it is sent
2. Using dysfunctional communication responses such as:
   a. *Impervious response*—outright failure to acknowledge another's attempt to communicate, suggesting that the speaker is unimportant and does not merit attention; e.g., irrelevant response, no response, interrupting.
   b. *Tangential response*—response that is only to an incidental part of speaker's communication; e.g., shifting focus, responding with "yes" or "no," and then talking about something else.
   c. *Ambiguous response*—response that is meaningless because more than one, often conflicting, message is contained; e.g., straddling the fence by saying both yes and no, use of nonverbal communication which is incongruous with verbal communication.
   d. *Inadequate response*—response that is meaningless because the message is lost in trivia, is incomplete, or is overqualified.

   e. *Projective response*—a mystifying response in which the speaker implies that he knows what is going on inside the other person or is qualified to judge the correctness of the other's feelings.
   f. *Crossed transaction*—the response received is not appropriate, is unexpected, and does not follow the natural order of healthy human interactions, as opposed to complimentary transactions.
   g. *Ulterior transaction*—the transaction occurs at two levels simultaneously, the social and the psychological.
3. Using dysfunctional communication patterns such as:
   a. *Games*—a well-structured series of ulterior transactions leading to a well-defined, predictable but often painful outcome.
   b. *Symmetrical escalation*—one person seeks to make the other conform to expectations that are met with defiance.
   c. *Rigid complementarity*—one person is strong and overprotective of the other.

Nursing Assessment

1. Carefully note patient's communication abilities and limitations during the interview.
2. What are the patient's perceptions about his ability to communicate with others?
3. Does patient have a network of significant others?
4. What are the perceptions of significant others regarding patient's ability to communicate?
5. Observe for dysfunctional communication responses such as impervious, tangential, ambiguous, inadequate, and projective responses in patient's interactions.
6. Observe for frequency of crossed transactions, of ulterior transactions, and of type of games in which patient involves himself.
7. Observe for symmetrical escalation and rigid complementarity.
8. Observe for other factors characteristic of poor communication.

Nursing Goals and Interventions

To reduce dysfunctional communication.

1. Involve patient in transactional analysis group or program in which he can increase his understanding of his transactions and games and analyze these.
2. Describe to patient and encourage him to use active listening skills.
3. Ask patient to examine the effect his communication skills and patterns have.
   Suggest patient request honest feedback on his effect on others.
4. Help patient develop insight into dynamics of relationships.
5. Support use of assertive communication skills.
6. Increase patient's acceptance of positive and negative feedback.
7. Request patient to ask for feedback as he is communicating with others.
8. Increase patient's awareness of areas in which he can be hurt and of what he is willing to share with others.
9. Teach and support patient's use of communication techniques.
10. Increase patient's awareness of the feelings of others.
11. Reduce patient's need to be overprotective in a relationship.
12. Reduce patient's need to attempt to make others conform to his expectations.
    Teach patient to accept the right of others to have their own attitudes.
13. Help patient develop honest, open way of getting needs met.
14. Increase self-esteem.
15. Increase awareness of strengths and limitations in communicating with others.
16. Increase participation in groups.
17. Develop the ability to give and receive in a relationship.
18. Practice reducing use of dysfunctional communication responses.
    Increase use of assertive communication skills. (See pp. 916–919.)
19. Help patient tolerate disagreement and resolve conflict.
20. Reduce nagging.
21. Encourage initiation of interactions and communication.
22. Decrease use of generalizations.
23. Point out discrepancies in message and the metacommunication sent.
24. Point out discrepancies in the message sent and the context within which it is sent.
25. Use role playing to practice improved communication skills and techniques.

Health Education

Teach patient communication techniques. These can include teaching patient to:

1. Request feedback from the other person to make certain that communications are accurately understood; e.g.,
   "By telling me . . . do you mean . . . ?"
2. Let other person know through feedback what he has overtly or covertly said or the feelings that he has conveyed; e.g.,
   "You're telling me that the whole experience makes you 'livid'."
3. Respond to other person in a manner that conveys a sincere effort to understand how the other person perceives his world; e.g.,
   "As you see it, I just shouldn't have purchased that fur coat without discussing it with you. You feel left out and in a way, 'put-upon'."
4. Listen actively to what the other person is saying. Do not focus on own personal response to be made.
5. Request feedback from the other person to check patient's own perception and interpretation of the other person's communication; e.g.,
   "You're giving me the impression that you're totally bored with the movie."
6. Encourage verbalization by verbal and nonverbal means to assist other person to keep talking; e.g.,
   "Go on."
   "You were saying?"
   Nodding head.
7. Provide feedback by describing some aspect of the other person's communication and its impact on the patient.
8. Confront other person by describing discrepancies between what he says and does.

MATURATIONAL CRISIS, SITUATIONAL CRISIS

Characteristics

1. *Crisis*—a state of disequilibrium resulting from an imbalance between a person's perceived difficulty of a hazardous event and the person's current coping mechanisms and situational supports to deal with this stressor.
2. *Maturational crisis*—occurs as a result of transitional periods during the psychosocial developmental periods, which require the person to make many character changes.
3. *Situational crisis*—occurs as a result of environmental stressors.
4. Additional characteristics of maturational and situational crises include the following crisis phases:
   a. Denial—may last for several hours.
   b. Increased free-flowing anxiety—activities of normal living continued but with much difficulty. Some hyperactivity or psychomotor retardation.
   c. Disorganization—activities of normal living limited or ceased. May include severe anxiety, fear, guilt, shame, helplessness, depression, or anger. Preoccupation with current hazardous event and earlier symbolically linked events.
   d. Attempted reorganization—use of familiar coping mechanisms and situational supports lasting several weeks, if successful. If unsuccessful, may lead to escape mechanisms such as blaming others for difficulty, resulting in unsuccessful crisis resolution.

e. Local and general reorganization—lower, same, or improved functioning, as compared to precrisis level, usually attained in 6 weeks from onset of crisis.
5. Hazardous events or stressors may represent:
   a. Threat to integrity of self or instinctual needs
   b. A real or perceived loss
   c. A challenge
6. Self-limiting with average duration of 6 weeks. Precipitating event often occurs 10–14 days before client comes for assistance.
7. Maladaptive resolution of crisis may lead to violence, suicide, or prolonged mental illness.
8. Offers opportunity for personal growth if successfully resolved.
9. Can occur as individual crisis or family crisis.

Nursing Assessment

1. What are the current behavioral manifestations? Are any suicidal or homicidal impulses present? What is the current level of role functioning?
2. What is the nature of the crisis? Onset? Intensity and duration of precipitating factor(s) or event(s)?
3. How does patient perceive difficulties?
4. What coping mechanisms and problem-solving skills does he possess?
5. Are there situational supports available such as family or friends?
6. Does the patient's crisis affect other family members? How?

Nursing Goals and Interventions

A. *To reduce level of anxiety and resolve other emotions.*

1. Establish rapport through warm, empathic, supportive, caring, trustworthy, nonjudgmental approach.
2. Assist patient in recognizing and expressing feelings such as anxiety, anger, and sadness.
3. Reduce anxiety (see pp. 926–927).
4. Support active grieving process (see p. 935).
5. Offer careful, simple explanations during early crisis phases.
6. Reinforce coping mechanisms used effectively by patient in past to reduce tension.
7. Help patient to decrease blaming others.

B. *To foster realistic perception of precipitating event and subsequent experiences in order to restore level of functioning to precrisis state or better.*

1. Ask patient to describe sequence of events in process of adjusting to stressor.
2. Help patient gain intellectual understanding of crisis by discussing effect of stressor(s) and link to subsequent behaviors.
3. Offer ego support.
4. Convey to patient that his difficulties can be understood, that others have undergone similar problems, and that ways for solving the difficulty can be explored.
5. Focus on present, not past, difficulties.

6. Outline target behaviors and goals for therapy, using feasible patient input.
7. Clearly define problem with patient.
8. Clarify experiences by restating previously unconnected facts.

C. *To support use of and to increase repertoire of coping skills in order to restore level of functioning to precrisis state or better.*

1. Encourage use of existing problem-solving skills.
2. Encourage patient to describe own accomplishments in dealing with crisis.
3. Summarize positive changes during therapy.
4. Promote individual responsibility for problem solving.
5. Explore and examine alternate ways of coping with stress.
6. Suggest and give direct advice and guidance as needed.
7. Formulate action plan:
   a. Use situational supports.
   b. Identify and mobilize use of inner strengths and problem-solving skills.
   c. Develop a number of options for action.

D. *To encourage use and development of situational supports in order to restore level of functioning to precrisis state or better.*

1. Make home visits as needed.
2. Offer information about community resources, such as residential housing, make referrals, or assist patient in contacting agencies.
3. Provide easy access to therapist, within limits.
4. Encourage and use phone as communication link.
5. Encourage use of and reliance on community supports, social service agencies, or significant others.
6. Reduce patient's dependency on therapist after establishing initial rapport.
7. Share treatment plan with patient.
8. Assist patient in increasing his social sphere.
9. Explore resources known by patient.

Health Education and Prevention

1. Teach patient problem-solving skills:
   a. Clearly defining problem
   b. Generating potential solutions
   c. Describing projected consequences of proposed solutions
   d. Selecting best alternative
   e. Testing behavior or action
   f. Evaluating results
   g. Redefining problem, if necessary
2. Use preventive technique of anticipatory planning, tailored to the patient's unique circumstances; describe potential future crises and possible coping strategies.
3. Provide immediate therapy in crises to reduce disorganization, enhance optimal resolution, and prevent psychopathology.

DEMANDING BEHAVIOR

Characteristics

1. Intrusiveness
2. Constantly seeking and insisting on input from others
3. Requesting help when able to do for self
4. Interfering with activities of others
5. Critical of others

Nursing Assessment and On-going Observations

1. Determine patient's ability to perform activities he insists others do for him.
2. Identify anger at being helpless.
3. Note hostility generated in environment.

Nursing Goals and Interventions

A. *To assist in perceiving self as able to satisfy needs.*

1. Help in identifying fears and frustrations in environment.
2. Convey trust in patient's ability to act.
3. Provide direction and assistance in areas where he needs help.
4. Give feedback about reality and, especially, identify distortions of reality.
5. Identify carefully the areas in which he cannot act or over which he has little control or less control than he desires.

B. *To provide alternative ways of dealing with helplessness.*

1. Set limits on irrational demands.
2. Refrain from judging too quickly that patient cannot do a task; explore requests made by patient.
3. Validate the feelings being experienced by patient.
4. Support staff since they frequently see the patient as the "difficult one."
5. Discuss consequence of continued demanding behavior.
6. Use structured, vigorous activities to assist in dealing with anger.
7. Help identify one thing patient can do by and for himself.

Health Education

Teach patient:

1. To identify stress areas of daily living, such as inability to be self-sufficient, fear of failure, or inability to attain one's goals.
2. How to make requests of others; have patient practice making requests.
3. Difference between a demand and a request, especially in relation to the effect on relationships.
4. How to deal with feelings of helplessness by identifying what can be done by self.

DENIAL

Characteristics

1. Response of "I don't know; nothing matters; don't care; no problems; not me"
2. Frequent expressions of anger
3. Ignoring statements made, walking away, changing the subject
4. Laughing or crying inappropriately

Nursing Assessment and On-going Observations

1. Determine if someone or something of emotional significance has been lost.
2. Ascertain effectiveness of patient's use of denial in dealing with his problems.
3. Identify self-defeating aspects of the use of denial behaviors.
4. Note which basic needs are threatened.
5. Establish meaning of situation or illness for the patient.

Nursing Goals and Interventions

A. *To establish a safe environment for expression of thought and feelings about reality.*

1. Convey respect and concern for patient's feeling of loss.
2. Assist in lowering level of anxiety (see pp. 926–927).
3. Focus on what is occurring in the immediate present.
4. Be prepared to change topic of interaction, if patient becomes more resistive or anxious.
5. Have consistent, brief, honest exchanges.
6. Verbalize own feelings in relationship as model for patient.
7. Avoid interaction with focus on "You do have a problem—I don't."
8. Respond to verbal tirade about wanting no treatment or having no problem by making calm, brief statement about present reality.
9. Begin with a small piece of reality, i.e., "You can go home to mother on the weekend," rather than "mother does not want you to live at home any more."
10. Empathize with patient, especially in area of greatest threat.
11. Explore reality by helping patient to describe present situation, i.e., who, what, why, when, where, how.

B. *To assist in setting a goal.*

1. Help patient with struggle to discover what he wants to do for himself.
2. Assist in identifying needs and ways to cope with them.
3. Promote discoveries of self rather than constantly confronting reality.

C. *To protect self from being overwhelmed by situation.*

1. Identify what patient has done to help himself.
2. Give feedback when reality is dealt with appropriately.
3. Listen to expressions of fear and helplessness.
4. Assist him in mobilizing others for emotional support.

Health Education

Teach patient:

1. The problem-solving process:
   a. Defining the problem
   b. Constructing several solutions and expected results
   c. Selecting best solution for oneself
   d. Trying the solution in one situation
   e. Evaluating the results
2. The common reactions to threats to self or loss: depression, withdrawal, anger
3. Ways to check reality, such as asking others, reading, listening carefully
4. To begin to deal with emotional issues by examining relationships

DEPRESSIVE BEHAVIOR

Characteristics

1. Lack of activity for long periods of time
2. Not caring for personal hygiene
3. Little conversation with others
4. Physical complaints
5. Sleep disturbance
6. Verbalization of feelings of worthlessness, hopelessness, helplessness
7. Frequent crying spells
8. Change in appetite or weight

Nursing Assessment and On-going Observations

1. Ascertain whether there has been:
   a. A recent loss of significant other
   b. An insult to self-esteem
   c. A change in sexual or socioeconomic status
2. Determine extent of withdrawal from family and friends.
3. Identify person with whom the patient feels he can talk.
4. List physical complaints and identify actions taken by patient to cope with them.
5. Note changes in physical complaints and determine relationship to level of anxiety.
6. Establish current sleep pattern and inquire what might help to extend the period of sleep, if short.
7. Observe current eating pattern and potential for weight loss.
8. Note verbal indications of appetite.
9. Identify which activities patient does for himself.
10. Note recurring thought content and verbalizations (e.g., thoughts about self-worth, fear, worries; expressions of worthlessness, hopelessness, helplessness).
11. Determine suicide potential. It is increased as patient becomes agitated or experiences loss of significant person.
12. Determine homicidal potential. It is increased as patient becomes agitated.
13. Observe for suicidal and homicidal ideation.
14. Observe changes in coping strategies or ability to plan activities for the day.

Nursing Goals and Interventions

A. *To meet basic needs while reducing pervasive feelings of worthlessness, hopelessness, and helplessness.*

1. Respond to expressions of feelings; i.e., if patient states, "I'm no good," or "There is nothing to live for," a response would be, "I understand you feel worthless."
2. Begin to question the statement "I am no good" by responding, "In what area?"
3. Spend time with patient, even though he says nothing.
4. Avoid arguments or making moral judgments regarding what patient should or should not do.
5. Prevent isolation from others.
6. Confront irrational demands.

B. *To redefine situation or expand coping strategies.*

1. Set limits on physical abuse of self or others.
2. Listen to angry expressions and assist in constructive expression of anger.
3. When patient begins ruminating, redirect him to other activities or ask for further information about a part of the story.
4. Assist patient to focus on activity that he has to do now rather than on a physical complaint.
5. Support and give positive feedback for the small decisions made by the patient.
6. Set realistic limits on behavior.

C. *To structure activities of daily living.*

1. Use firmness when patient hesitates to do things for himself.
2. Encourage physical activity.
3. Set realistic limits on behavior.
4. Assist patient in setting small goals and experiencing success.
5. Assist him as needed in areas of self-care deficits, such as personal hygiene.

Health Education

1. Teach patient:
   a. To recognize tension within oneself
   b. To identify the thoughts that occur just before feelings of helplessness and hopelessness, which are associated with depression
   c. The importance of doing activities associated with basic needs regardless of how he feels
   d. To begin thinking about future plans
   e. Common effects and precautions related to antidepressant medications
   f. Ways of developing and maintaining a positive self-attitude
   g. Need to recognize highly stressful situations
2. Suggest reading material: e.g., Burns DD: Feeling Good. The New Mood Therapy. New York, William Morrow Co., 1980.

DRUG MISUSE

Characteristics

1. Pathological use of a drug(s):
   a. Frequent need and use of drug for personal functioning
   b. Difficulty in reducing or stopping amount of drug used
   c. Periodic, unsuccessful efforts to stop use of drug
   d. Episodes of complications from drug misuse
2. Impaired physical, emotional, occupational, or social functioning resulting from pathological use of drug(s)—can include:
   a. Interpersonal difficulties with family, friends, co-workers
   b. Maladaptive behavior patterns such as impulsiveness, irrational behavior, manipulative behavior, grandiosity, withdrawal, inappropriate aggression, etc.
   c. Arrests for inappropriate behavior, criminal behavior, or traffic accidents

d. Absenteeism, difficulty in performing work effectively, job loss
e. Depending on length and severity of drug misuse, as well as nature of drug, can develop:
   (1) Tolerance—the need for more of the drug to produce the same desired effect
   (2) Physical dependence or addiction—characterized by withdrawal, a syndrome that follows cessation or reduction in drug use and that can include joint and muscle aches, restlessness, inability to sleep, dilated and sluggish pupils, runny nose, chills, fever, perspiration
   (3) Marked physical or psychological deterioration (malnutrition, vasculitis, toxic or allergic reactions, nasal septum erosion, septicemia, tetanus, hepatitis, infective endocarditis, embolic phenomena, organic brain syndrome, mood lability, suspiciousness, violent behavior, depressive behavior, suicidal attempts or threats, suicide)
3. Frequent use of drug(s) causing impairment in functioning for at least 1 month.
4. Other characteristics can include low self-concept, mistrust, low tolerance for stress, lack of ability to communicate well, values conflicting with social standards, and high level of dependency.
5. Biological, sociological, cultural, and psychological factors interrelate to cause and perpetuate drug misuse; e.g.,
   a. Problem drug users often have low tolerance for frustration, tension, or anxiety and turn to drugs to escape.
   b. The "reinforcer" received from the "high" that is experienced from the use of many drugs often perpetuates drug misuse.
   c. The need to belong to a group, with its own unique life-style, may both contribute to and perpetuate drug misuse.
6. Drugs frequently misused include:
   a. Barbiturates and other similarly acting hypnotics or sedatives:
      (1) Barbiturates—butabarbital sodium, hexobarbital, pentobarbital sodium, phenobarbital, secobarbital sodium
      (2) Hypnotics—paraldehyde, chloral hydrate, methaqualone, ethchlorvynol, flurazepam, glutethimide, methyprylon
      (3) Minor tranquilizers—oxazepam, diazepam, chlordiazepoxide
   b. Opioids
      (1) Natural opioids—heroin, morphine
      (2) Synthetics with morphine-like action—meperidine, methadone
   c. Amphetamine and other sympathomimetics—amphetamine, methamphetamine, dextroamphetamine, methylphenidate
   d. Cocaine
   e. Cannabis
      (1) Substances derived from cannabis plant or synthetic substances that are chemically similar
      (2) Marijuana, hashish, delta-9-tetrahydrocannabinol (THC).
   f. Hallucinogens—e.g., dimethyltryptamine (DMT), lysergic acid diethylamide (LSD), mescaline
   g. Phencyclidine hydrochloride (PCP) or a similarly acting arylcyclohexylamine
      Phencyclidine (PCP), ketamine (Ketalar), thiophene analogue of phencyclidine (TCP)

Nursing Assessment

1. What drug(s) was(were) misused most recently? When? How much?
   a. Describe behavior on admission.
      Assess for depression, suicidal threats and attempts.
   b. Assess physical condition, including nutritional state and habits. Any evidence of withdrawal?
2. What was the pattern of drug misuse during the last month? Kinds of drug(s) used? Amounts? Frequency? Source? Effects on personal functioning?
   a. Current role performance in school or on job?
   b. Interpersonal relationships with family and with friends?
   c. Any financial difficulties?
   d. Legal difficulties? Arrests?
   e. Describe general life-style.
3. In what way does patient perceive drug misuse as problematic?
4. At what age did patient start misusing drugs? What kinds of drugs were used? Frequency? Amounts? Effects on personal functioning?
5. What triggers misuse of drugs?
6. Do family members or friends misuse drugs?
      What are family members' attitudes towards patient's misuse of drugs?
7. Has patient received prior treatment for drug misuse? When? Where? Kind of treatment?
8. Assess strengths useful in developing alternative coping patterns.
9. Observe for signs of continued drug misuse.

Nursing Goals and Interventions

A. *To meet physiological and safety needs.*

1. Assist with activities of daily living as needed.
2. Observe for signs of withdrawal.
3. Eliminate environmental hazards.
4. Utilize protective measures during controlled withdrawal.
5. Observe for depressive behavior, suicidal threats and attempts.
6. Set limits on behavior harmful to self or others.
   a. Monitor attempts to secure a continuing supply of drugs.
   b. Offer continuous one-to-one observation when patient is unaware of dangers of his own behavior.
   c. Direct patient in reality-oriented activities when needed.
7. Provide planned and structured environment.
8. Use verbal reassurance to "talk down" patient experiencing "bad trips" from LSD.
9. Place patient experiencing "bad trip" from PCP in a quiet environment, protect from danger, and monitor unobtrusively. Do not attempt to "talk down."
10. Provide opportunity to assist, when possible, with self-care.
11. Prevent uncontrolled access to drugs.
    a. On admission, search patient and belongings for drugs.
    b. Monitor visitors, as necessary, to prevent access to drugs.
    c. Observe for attempts to secure additional drugs on unit.

B. *To develop alternative coping skills and life-style and to reduce or eliminate drug misuse.*

1. Assist in reducing manipulative behavior and impulsiveness.
   a. Increase patient's awareness of behavior.
   b. Explore with patient antecedents of behavior.
   c. Explore alternative ways of relating.
   d. Assist in testing alternative ways of relating.
   e. Use precaution with patient's manipulative attempts to obtain supply of drugs.
   f. Set limits on manipulative or impulsive behavior harmful to self or others. (See manipulative behavior, pp. 938–939 and impulsiveness, p. 937.)
   g. Orient patient to rules and regulations of unit as means to communicate expectations.
2. Assist in reducing grandiosity.
   a. Do not respond to grandiosity with verbal attack.
      (1) Point out reality, using appropriate timing.
      (2) Do not argue or laugh at grandiose notions.
   b. Reflect back feeling tone accompanying expressions of grandiosity.
   c. Increase patient's awareness of consequences to himself of his grandiosity.
   d. Work with patient to set realistic goals.
   e. Work with patient to develop schedule and method for achieving goals.
   f. Set limits for behavior harmful to self or others.
3. Assist in reducing emotional withdrawal from people and improving interpersonal relationships.
   a. Assist in finding satisfaction in relating to others.
   b. Involve in one-to-one and group conversations.
   c. Intervene with social withdrawal. (See pp. 951–952.)
   d. Assist in development of drug-free social network.
   e. Establish positive nurse-patient relationship.
      (1) Demonstrate acceptance.
      (2) Be consistent. Use rules consistently.
      (3) Show a nonjudgmental attitude toward drug misuse.
      (4) Offer positive reinforcement for appropriate interpersonal behavior.
      (5) Offer support as changes in self-identity occur.
      (6) Provide feedback on the consequences of acting-out behavior.
      (7) Set clear, consistent limits on passive-aggressive behavior.
      (8) Guide superficial talk into personal and meaningful conversation.
      (9) Avoid dependency; foster self-reliance.
4. Help patient develop appropriate ways to express and channel feelings.
   a. Encourage and support physical outlet through team sports, etc.
   b. Help patient recognize feelings such as anger, depression, guilt, suspiciousness.
   c. Help patient verbalize about feelings of anger, depression, guilt, suspiciousness.
   d. Help patient recognize antecedents to feelings such as anger, depression, guilt, suspiciousness.
   e. Increase patient's insights for the connection between feelings and behavior.
   f. Explore with patient adaptive ways to channel feelings of anger, depression, guilt, suspiciousness.
   g. Suggest biofeedback, relaxation training, group therapy, or meditation.
   h. Avoid critical and punitive approach or retaliation.
      i. Discuss with patient how he may be covering up and avoiding feelings through drug misuse.
5. Explore more adaptive coping strategies to deal with life stressors other than the misuse of drugs.
   a. Discuss with patient his reasons for misusing drugs.
      (1) Discover rewards gained from drugs.
      (2) Explore more adaptive ways to gain these rewards.
   b. Explore patient's perceptions of present problems caused by misuse of drugs.
   c. Encourage former drug abusers (or drug abusers in treatment) to join therapy groups or group counseling.
      Orient patient to what is expected from him and how to participate in groups.
   d. Counsel about problems that may be faced in living a drug-free role in the community.
   e. Provide opportunities or make appropriate referrals for patient to develop work habits and job skills.
   f. Provide opportunities or make appropriate referrals to develop interests in new hobbies and activities.
   g. Explore social, psychological, and physical consequences of drug misuse.
   h. Help motivate patient to develop a commitment to a drug-free life-style.
   i. Differentiate between expressions of real versus exaggerated physical symptoms.
   j. Rebuild self-esteem and self-concept.
   k. Offer opportunities to assume increased responsibility and earn positive rewards.
   l. Use behavior-modification techniques. (See Chapter 28.)
   m. Intervene in family addictive cycle.
      (1) Suggest referral to multiple family therapy, individual family therapy, or marital or couple therapy, as indicated.
      (2) Teach development of mutual attitude concerned with prevention methods rather than one of scapegoating and placing blame.
      (3) Observe family member's, especially mother's, expression of death wish for drug misuser.
      (4) Assist families to deal with anxiety related to separation, to sexual conflicts, and to behavior related to drug misuse, such as acting out.
   n. In methadone maintenance program:
      (1) Develop positive interpersonal relationship with patient. Work through resistance to interpersonal involvement.
      (2) Observe for continued misuse of drugs.
      (3) Assist patient in developing new social networks and new life-style.
   o. In therapeutic community, foster peer support and pressure to attain behavior that is free of drug misuse.

Health Education and Prevention

1. Encourage family treatment as a preventive modality, especially for families with any one of the following characteristics:
   a. Families experiencing crises
   b. Immigrant families
   c. Families in which one or more of the siblings misuse drugs
   d. Families in which the parents misuse drugs
2. Increase public awareness in all segments of the

community of the harmful consequences of drug misuse; e.g.,
  a. Offer preventive drug programs to 10- to 13-year-old youths, including teaching decision-making

and assertive communication skills, to deal with peer pressure.
  b. Teach parents signs and symptoms of substance abuse.

POTENTIAL DYSFUNCTIONAL GRIEVING, DYSFUNCTIONAL GRIEVING

Characteristics

1. *Grieving*—a normal process, which can last up to one year, by which a person adaptively adjusts to a significant loss which includes:
   a. Emotional emancipation from significant loss of object, person, or other established pattern of life
   b. Readjustment to environment
   c. Development of new relationships, emotional investment in new objects, etc. to restructure new life and achieve personal reorganization
2. Physical symptoms that do not last long frequently appear immediately after loss:
   a. Sighing respirations
   b. Choking sensation
   c. Empty feeling in stomach, digestive upsets
   d. Physical distress
   e. Shortness of breath
3. Any other combination of symptoms which may develop soon after the loss include:
   a. Apathy
   b. Depersonalization
   c. Numbness; pain; disorganization
   d. High degree of organization followed by collapse; shock; disbelief; hyperactivity; hypersomnolence; bewilderment; confusion; restlessness; lack of strength; aimless activity; meaninglessness of daily routine; withdrawal; immobile behavior
4. Stages of grieving:
   a. The exact nature of the grief reaction may vary from person to person.
   b. *Denial*—avoids acceptance of loss thereby developing a buffer against reality.
      (1) Acts as if deceased is still present or loss has not occurred. Searching behavior.
      (2) Other characteristics can include disinterest in environment, withdrawal, immobility, decreased responsiveness, occurrence of fantasies about loss.
      (3) Begins to mobilize other coping strategies.
   c. *Anger*—channeled toward lost object or person, toward self, or displaced toward other object or person.
      (1) Questions reasons for happening: "Why did this happen to me?"
      (2) Experiences guilt along with self-criticism and self-punishing behavior.
      (3) May place blame on health professionals or may misinterpret what is said by them.
      (4) Other characteristics can include irritability, fear, lack of sleep.
   d. *Bargaining*—last attempt to postpone realization of loss, which may include bargaining with a deity.
      (1) Seeks magical cures.
      (2) Attempts to negotiate for change in reality.
      (3) Preoccupied with image of deceased.
   e. *Realization of loss*—full awareness of loss, including meaning and value of person or object to self, awareness of lost or changed roles, realization of new responsibilities and roles.
      (1) Preoccupation with loss.
      (2) Can include symptoms of depressive behavior, such as despair, crying, inertia, withdrawal, emptiness, helplessness, hopelessness, loneliness.
   f. *Acceptance and reintegration*—problem-solving behavior initiated relative to loss and concomitant problems and change.
      (1) Renewal of energy in living
      (2) Development of new emotional investments
      (3) Ability to realistically remember both positive and negative aspects of the person, object, or life pattern lost
      (4) Restructuring and reordering of life
5. Normal grieving unaccompanied by mental problems does not usually require psychiatric referral but is facilitated by skilled interpersonal intervention to prevent the occurrence of dysfunctional grieving and such phenomena as post-bereavement morbidity.
6. *Dysfunctional grieving*—person becomes stuck in one phase of grieving, demonstrating excessive emotional reactions or excessive length of time in a phase.
   a. Is unable to attain acceptance phase and successful adaptation to loss.
   b. Can include prolonged, excessive denial; prolonged depression.
   c. Can lead to mental illness, especially clinical depression.
7. *Anticipatory grief*—grieving process taking place prior to an actual loss and occurring in preparation for actual loss.

Nursing Assessment

1. What is the nature of the loss? When did it occur?
2. How did the patient perceive the loss? Special meaning/value? Significance of loss in relation to patient's perceived and real abilities to meet his own needs?
3. What stage of grieving and behavioral manifestations does patient currently present?
4. Describe patient's behavior between actual occurrence of loss and present.
5. How has patient coped with loss in the past? What strengths were demonstrated in coping with loss?
6. Determine whether patient is at high risk for dysfunctional grieving, such as those with:
   a. Poor relationship with person prior to death
   b. Social isolation or poor social network
   c. History of multiple past losses and use of maladaptive coping strategies
   d. Presentation of a brave, stoic front
7. What is the nature of the social network present?
8. Assess degree of depression. Observe for suicidal tendencies.

9. What are significant others' reactions to patient's response to loss?

Nursing Goals and Interventions

A. *To facilitate normal grieving.*

1. Assist patient through denial phase.
   a. Help patient understand that others respond similarly when grieving a loss.
   b. Be genuine, honest, and realistic about loss.
   c. Permit visual and tactile contact with body of dead when possible.
   d. Use caring tone of voice.
   e. See Denial, pages 930–931.
2. Assist patient through anger phase.
   a. Demonstrate tolerance, patience, and empathy.
   b. Permit open expression of feelings. Do not become defensive.
   c. Assist patient in understanding reasons for feelings.
   d. If patient has difficulty in expressing anger, place him/her with patients who can express feelings openly. See also Aggression, Inappropriate Expression, pages 923–925.
   e. Reassure patient that feelings of guilt are part of the normal grieving process.
      Assist in working through feelings of guilt.
   f. Encourage patient to work out conflicting aspect of relationship with deceased.
      Work through any ambivalence.
3. Assist patient through bargaining phase.
   a. Permit patient's need to talk and reminisce about loss through active listening.
   b. Permit expression of feelings and thoughts. Gently point out reality.
4. Assist through realization of loss phase.
   a. Be physically present; offer support and enhance self-esteem.
   b. Offer acceptance and unconditional positive regard.
   c. Correct misinformation about cause of loss.
   d. Reinforce past and present strengths in dealing with difficulty.
   e. Through sympathetic understanding show that crying is acceptable.
   f. Encourage support for patient from family members and friends.
   g. Observe for and monitor depression.
   h. Facilitate review of positive and negative aspects of lost person, object, or life pattern.
   i. Clarify and offer missing factual information.
   j. Use touch to offer support.
5. Assist through acceptance phase.
   a. Explore nature of problems encountered that are linked to loss with patient.
   b. Raise questions regarding next steps in coping.
   c. Assist in thinking through adaptive coping strategies.
   d. Assist or coordinate resources to develop new skills, to make readjustments in life-style, and to make new emotional investments.
   e. Support patient when he is trying out new coping strategies.
6. Do not suppress symptoms of grieving with drugs, suggested use of willpower, or other verbal interventions.
7. Answer questions directly and tactfully.
8. Orient patient to new aspects of environment in a simple and clear way.
9. Foster environment in which loss can be placed in spiritual context by engaging patient in religious and spiritual rituals and practices as desired.
10. Be cognizant of the possibility of different stages of grieving occurring among family members.
    Help patient and family members communicate with each other.
11. Offer extensive support and guidance in performing activities of living during bewilderment experienced immediately after loss.
12. Demonstrate caring and concern, especially immediately after the loss.
13. Encourage patient to seek help and not be "too proud."
14. Use role play as a way to help work through feelings.
15. Do not abandon patient while he is experiencing loss.

B. *To resolve dysfunctional grieving.*

1. Apply interventions outlined for normal grieving.
2. Assist patient in getting through phase in which he is stuck.
   a. Assess present stage of grieving and the current objects or facts that patient still links to the loss.
   b. Use graded flooding approach.
      (1) Present patient with increasing significant facts about, or objects linked to, loss.
      (2) Rework feelings generated.
      (3) Use role play to work through feelings and preoccupations.
      (4) Apply principles of behavior modification, such as rewards for more adaptive behavior.

Health Education and Prevention

1. Provide anticipatory guidance and support anticipatory grieving.
   a. Assist in coping with expected and impending loss.
   b. Encourage open discussion of impending loss and expression of feelings.
   c. Teach use of problem-solving skills:
      (1) Define potential life changes and problems predicted from the loss.
      (2) Develop alternative potential strategies to deal with problems.
      (3) Map out possible consequences of each strategy.
      (4) Prioritize strategies in terms of usefulness for potential problem resolution.
2. Offer extra assistance in process of grieving to those at high risk for dysfunctional grieving:
   a. Those who had a traumatic, difficult relationship with person who is now deceased
   b. Those who present cheerful, brave, and stoic behavior
   c. Those who are socially isolated or who have a poorly developed social network
   d. Those who have a history of multiple past losses and have used maladaptive coping strategies
   e. Those who perceive their social network as nonsupportive
   f. Those with very traumatic circumstances surrounding death of spouse—anger- or guilt-provoking death, unexpected or untimely death
   g. Those with concurrent life crises.
3. Provide psychological intervention to person with loss, especially in bereavement, to reduce potential for dysfunctional grieving.

GUILT

Characteristics

1. Seeks punishment for self
2. Rejects self as a person of worth; feelings of worthlessness and failure, tearful
3. Constant recalling of events in which self was wrong; repetitive stories

Nursing Assessment and On-going Observations

1. Ascertain the presence of the shame-guilt cycle. Inhibition and inaction→passivity→sense of failure→shame and fear of rejection and disapproval→aggressive fantasies and impulses→guilt and fear of responsibility, punishment for wrong→inhibition, etc.
2. Recognize use of defenses:
   a. Denial frequently used to deal with shame.
   b. Projection or blaming others frequently used to deal with guilt.
   c. Guilt can be used to deal with shame. Guilt can explain degree of suffering being experienced and therefore give meaning to suffering.
3. Determine the appropriateness of the guilty feelings.

Nursing Goals and Interventions

A. *To maintain or enhance sensitiveness to deal with perceived failure.*

1. Support expression of feelings.
2. Discuss consequences of not dealing with guilt and shame.
3. Share experiences of self or others in dealing with shame and guilt.
4. Give feedback about the appropriateness of feelings.

B. *To offer opportunity to explore feelings of guilt.*

1. Avoid reinforcing patient's belief that he is guilty.
2. Do not argue over moral issues.
3. Refrain from giving or agreeing with "shoulds" or "should nots."
4. Raise questions about conclusions at which patient has arrived.
5. Listen to the expressions of anger and hostility.
6. Encourage patient to accept consequences of actions without a complete devaluation of himself.
7. Be sensitive to other's need to tell the patient to forget it or to be quiet.
8. Accept revelations in matter-of-fact manner.
9. Avoid giving false reassurance, for patient may feel more guilty.

Health Education

Teach patient:
1. How to think through the feelings of guilt and shame and to determine appropriateness
2. Consequences of constantly seeking perfection or the approval of others
3. The shame-guilt cycle
4. Constructive ways to deal with failure, such as identifying what needs to be changed to avoid a repeated failure

HYPERACTIVE BEHAVIOR

Characteristics

1. Excessive motor activity; short attention span
2. Difficulty in completing a task; distractable
3. Destructive tendencies

Nursing Assessment and On-going Observation

1. Determine if pattern of hyperactivity during the day is related to environmental stresses, presence of certain people, or possible biorhythm.
2. Identify sleep pattern and determine when it could be extended.
3. Note ability to carry out grooming skills.
4. Collect data related to eating pattern to determine potential for weight loss.
5. Determine presence of learning disability.
6. Ascertain responsiveness to nondemanding situations in contrast to conflict-laden situations.
7. Observe for signs of increasing hyperactivity and loss of self-control.
8. Collect data on the response to varying stimuli.
9. Check relatedness of fatigue and attention-seeking behaviors to hyperactivity.

Nursing Goals and Interventions

A. *To reduce responsiveness to environment.*

1. Set limits with hyperactivity when it interferes with others or the patient himself.
2. Decrease number of stimuli, including number of people, in the environment.
3. Offer warm baths and showers.
4. Monitor and reduce the noise level.

B. *To provide safe environment.*

1. Allow for movement of large muscles in safe, non-crowded area.
2. Provide a quiet area as needed.
3. Actively participate in games with patient.
4. Structure activities during the day.
5. Provide for physical safety; patient may be accident prone.

C. *To maintain consistency in relationships.*

1. Provide activities and warm relationships to assist in the reduction of anxiety.
2. Refrain from commenting about activity intensity, but intervene directly as needed.
3. Have short, frequent contacts; let patient know you are available.

Health Education

Teach patient:
1. Some structured, active games, such as volley ball, run-sheep-run, swimming
2. To focus on one thing for a set period of time
3. To complete one task before beginning another
4. The effects of hyperactivity on self and others
5. To reduce number of stressors in the environment as a way to maintain control.

IMPULSIVENESS

Characteristics

1. Unpredictable behavior
2. Frequently threatening or hurtful to others
3. Disregard for social customs
4. Irresponsible acts
5. Easily frustrated

Nursing Assessment and On-going Observations

1. Collect data on scope of impulsive behaviors.
2. Identify controls used by patient.
3. Determine what actions of staff assist patient in using his own controls.
4. Observe for precipitating factors.
5. Watch for changes in impulsive acts, especially any tendency toward suicide or homicide.
6. Note any expressions of responsible behavior.
7. Identify requests for assistance in maintaining control.

Nursing Goals and Interventions

A. *To increase patient's awareness of one's own limits.*

1. Discuss areas of life or specific people with whom he feels threatened or afraid.
2. Assist patient in protecting himself and others, if he loses control.
3. Recognize need for distance and provide it.
4. Avoid behaviors which contribute to feelings of being controlled.
5. Interrupt any impulsive act; patient may feel guilty or ashamed as a result of the act.
6. Give frequent feedback about observed behavior as a way to increase patient's awareness of it.

B. *To encourage patient to talk through problems rather than act on feelings.*

1. Discuss angry interactions with others.
2. Point out consequences of impulsive acts.
3. Assist in applying problem-solving process to problems such as where to live or where to find a job.
4. Assist in regaining control of activity level.
5. Help to increase tolerance for feelings.
6. Set limits on impulsive actions.

C. *To guide patient in being responsible for his own actions.*

1. Identify with patient the circumstances contributing to impulsive acts.
2. Explore alternative behaviors after each impulsive act.
3. Give positive feedback when responsible behaviors are noted, such as patient identifying how he is feeling and what he plans to do about it.
4. Discuss the consequences of impulsiveness on self.

Health Education

Teach patient:

1. To describe what is happening in interpersonal situations and then to identify problems needing a response
2. Ways to solve problems by defining, determining solutions, testing, and evaluating
3. To ask for help in identifying thoughts and feelings before acting on feelings
4. Ways to decrease anxiety by exercise, shower or bath, or by other means, as decreasing environmental stimuli.

INSTITUTIONALIZED BEHAVIOR

Characteristics

1. Passivity
2. Dependent compliance on rules and regulations
3. Little interest in environment
4. Hopelessness
5. Distorted sense of reality
6. Alienated feeling
7. Patterned behavior
8. Dependence
9. Pending plans of discharge result in increase of anxiety and recurrence of symptoms
10. Lack of change in patient's level of functioning
11. Lack of creativity

Nursing Assessment and On-going Observations

1. Note increase in complaints, demands, and refusal to go along with treatment programs as possible indication of an increase in patient's tension level.
2. Observe indications of increase in patient's compliance and passivity.
3. Check areas which patient feels cannot be changed.
4. Evaluate resistance to change in order to determine if he is afraid of change or trying to maintain some control over his life.
5. Watch for increasing isolation, resistance, and rejection.
6. Determine orientation to time, place, person.

Nursing Goals and Interventions

A. *To maintain or increase patient's ability to control his/her activities.*

1. Individualize ward routine as much as possible; e.g., times for bathing, bedmaking.
2. Refrain from labeling patient.
3. Protect patient's privacy.
4. Convey the expectation that patient will seek help with problems he is experiencing.
5. Be attentive to the communications given by the patient.
6. Provide for basic needs with acceptance of dependence and with encouragement of individual freedom and choice.
7. Encourage patient to help create a pleasant environment.
8. Maintain patient's interest in his treatment program.
9. Show willingness to change rules to increase independence of patient in hospital.
10. Assist in redefining relationships.
11. Help identify areas which patient can control.
12. Increase number of activities in the community.
13. Provide time for being alone.
14. Call patient by full name or name which he chooses.

B. *To promote development of therapeutic community among staff and patients.*

1. Provide opportunities for personal and professional growth.
2. Support peers and other staff members, especially in crisis situations.
3. Ensure that each person is aware of and is given frequent feedback concerning the importance of his role in the treatment process.
4. Avoid becoming absorbed in paperwork or just physical nursing care.

5. Have regular, scheduled community meetings.

Health Education

Teach patient:
1. Basic skills, such as bathing, care of clothing, table manners
2. Facts about present reality of own environment
3. Role of patient as an active participant and not as a passive, dependent receiver
4. The behaviors expected in one-to-one and group situations

MANIC BEHAVIOR

Characteristics

1. Euphoria
2. Hyperactivity
3. Diminished sleep
4. Disruptive
5. Distractible
6. Grandiose
7. Speech pressure
8. Sarcastic
9. Not eating
10. Demands response from others

Nursing Assessment and On-going Observations

1. Review life events in order to seek recent rejection by a mother figure.
2. Evaluate responsiveness to the environment, for the person may be hypersensitive to it.
3. Be alert to possible presence of such organic conditions as epilepsy, neoplasm, infections, or metabolic disturbance and reaction to such drugs as steroids, isoniazid, levodopa, or bromides.
4. Ascertain patient's ability to tolerate group interactions.
5. Collect data on sleeping pattern.
6. Note relationship between eating pattern and weight maintenance.
7. Determine range of hyperactive behavior.
8. Observe for signs of increasing agitation: increased loudness of voice, increased motor activity, increased irritability.

Nursing Goals and Interventions

A. *To assist patient in coping with rejection he may be experiencing in the environment.*

1. Provide protection from group response to disruptive behavior in group meetings by limiting these experiences or having staff sit with patient to provide support and control.

2. Set limits, particularly if patient is demanding, threatening, or seductive toward another.
3. Support involvement in limited number of activities to prevent rejection because of poor performance.
4. Respond to verbal abuse in matter-of-fact manner.

B. *To develop ways to decrease or control hyperactivity.*

1. Define limits and controls with patient.
2. Provide rest periods.
3. Formulate schedule of activities for the day.
4. Protect from overstimulation.
5. Attempt to distract as one way to deal with escalating situation.
6. Assist in substituting an activity for the purposeless hyperactivity.
7. Avoid any implication of personal rejection.

C. *To gain satisfaction from a less adventuresome life-style.*

1. Assist patient in dealing with fact of his illness.
2. Provide supervision or assistance with basic grooming activities.
3. Patiently support patient's efforts to be a group member and not the center of attention.
4. Encourage patient to verbalize the things he is not going to participate in with a change in behavior.

Health Education

Teach patient:
1. The importance of taking antimanic medication, as well as its side effects; toxic effects; precautions, routine blood levels; and long-term maintenance
2. The importance of learning to live with a state of mind that is less than constant euphoria
3. Ways to channel hyperactivity so as not to be disruptive
4. The importance of caring for health needs during periods of manic behavior, i.e., diet, rest, exercise, fluids, medication
5. That feelings of grandiosity may interfere with safety of self, or may cause one to overspend or overcharge money

MANIPULATION

Characteristics

1. Demanding behavior
2. Impersonal use of others to achieve own ends
3. Frequent use of flattery, of actions drawing attention to oneself, of seductive behavior, of forgetting
4. Involvement in other people's problems instead of one's own

5. Role reversal
6. Lack of frustration tolerance

Nursing Assessment and On-going Observations

1. Identify the range of manipulative behaviors being used by the patient.
2. Determine what problems the patient is avoiding.

3. Note what or who becomes the major focus of manipulative behaviors.
4. Observe what situational factors tend to increase the manipulation.
5. Watch for an increase in patient's ability to identify his own feelings and wants.

Nursing Goals and Interventions

A. *To reduce exploitation of others by decreasing feelings of insecurity and unworthiness.*

1. Allow testing of interpersonal limits.
2. Assist in changing patient's view of himself as a victim by defining one's rights.
3. Help in clarifying what he wants to do as opposed to doing something because another demands it.
4. Be nonjudgmental as patient examines his manipulative behaviors.
5. Give feedback regarding any type of manipulation attempted.
6. Discuss alternative ways of dealing with people, particularly those in authority.
7. Seek times to interact with patient when he is not demanding to be noticed.
8. Avoid rejective and retaliatory behaviors.
9. Help to delay the immediate satisfaction of every wish or need.

B. *To provide consistency in the milieu and to decrease the patient's use of manipulation.*

1. Ensure documentation of nursing care plan in order to foster a coordinated and consistent effort among health team members.
2. Be consistent in following the specified limits.
3. Demonstrate a willingness to admit to mistakes.
4. Clarify reasons for limit setting and consequences of breaking the limit.
5. Continuously direct patient's attention to his behavior.
6. Assist in exploring the meaning of the patient's behavior and avoid attempts to focus on the nurse's activities.

Health Education

1. Teach patient responsibilities of a person in a patient role, i.e., make requests clearly and to one member of team; attend therapies.
2. Teach patient to outline activities of the day and to concentrate on accomplishing these.
3. Demonstrate how to approach others in order to meet needs.
4. Assist patient in identifying when his needs or requests are met and the interactions in which he was given consideration and respect.

NONCOMPLIANCE

Characteristics

1. Missing clinic appointments; not taking medications; not following prescribed treatment; not carrying out instructions
2. Questioning the need for further treatment
3. Procrastination

Nursing Assessment and On-going Observations

1. Examine attitudes of significant others regarding the severity of patient's illness and the acceptance of it as a lifetime condition.
2. Collect data on the meaning of the patient's medication, on the act of taking the medicine, and on the act of refusing to take the medication. There may be social, cultural, and religious implications.
3. Determine personal discomfort experienced as result of noncompliance.
4. Identify health needs.
5. Observe consequences of noncompliance with health care system.
6. Note secondary gains sought.
7. Check accuracy of patient's knowledge about medications and psychotherapy.
8. Identify irrational fears and fantasies related to treatment process.
9. Note patient's record in keeping appointments.
10. Watch for expressions of patient's willingness and intent to follow treatment plan.
11. Ascertain behaviors that indicate patient is following health care advice.
12. Determine positive reinforcers of compliance for the patient.

Nursing Goals and Interventions

A. *To clarify health needs and behaviors required to meet these needs.*

1. Reinforce constructive patient decisions concerning his/her health needs.
2. Support use of educational materials.
3. Assist in simplifying treatment instructions.
4. Formulate with patient a list of things to be done.
5. Develop a method for patient to monitor his own progress and report to care-giver.
6. Be specific when identifying a behavior which needs changing.

B. *To assist in re-establishing a productive relationship with care-giver and health agency.*

1. Clarify misunderstanding of any aspect of treatment process.
2. Give feedback about behavior change resulting from not following directions.
3. Demonstrate respect for patient's views of his illness.
4. Provide weekly visits or more frequent contacts to give support when patient is discouraged.
5. Provide consistent interaction with patient.
6. Make a written contract with patient, clearly stating expectations.

C. *To explore relationship between emotional needs and noncompliance.*

1. Identify noncompliant behaviors and possible reasons for them.
2. Assist in exploration of mistrust and of threats to autonomy as possible emotional issues.
3. Promote decision-making and self-expression in as many areas as possible, such as the time to take medicine and ways to remember appointments.

Health Education

1. Explain expectations of health-care system.
2. Give information sheets about drugs and discuss patient's questions.
3. Provide educational material and instruction about patient's illness, including current treatment.

DYSFUNCTIONAL BEHAVIOR RELATED TO CHRONIC ORGANIC BRAIN DISEASE

Characteristics

Diffuse or localized cerebral damage resulting in the following changes:
1. Changes in cognitive functioning, which can include:
   a. Loss of memory, especially for recent events
   b. Various degrees of disorientation and confusion—patient may get lost
   c. Decreased ability to concentrate
   d. Impairment of language skills
   e. Reduced attention span
   f. Altered ability to think, learn, reason, abstract, conceptualize
   g. Poor judgment
2. Maladaptive coping patterns:
   a. Personality traits prevalent before illness often become exaggerated and maladaptive following chronic organic brain disease.
   b. Depressive behavior, withdrawal, ritualism, projection, aggression, or preoccupation with somatic complaints may be evident.

Nursing Assessment

1. Thoroughly assess mental status of patient:
   a. Observe patient's general appearance.
   b. Note any unusual bodily movements.
   c. Observe for unusual speech activity, speech patterns, or use of words.
   d. Assess patient's orientation to time, place, and person.
   e. Assess memory for remote events and especially for recent past events and immediate recall.
   f. Note level and fund of knowledge, ability to calculate, and ability to think abstractly.
   g. Observe presence of altered or abnormal perceptions.
   h. Observe for changes in attitude.
   i. Assess unusual mood or expression of emotions.
   j. Note thought processes and content.
   k. Observe patient's judgment.
   l. Note level of alertness.
2. From patient and significant other(s) find out nature of behavioral changes and when changes were first noted.
3. What supportive interpersonal network is available to the patient?
4. What is patient's personal reaction to his illness?

Nursing Goals and Interventions

A. *To prevent injury.*

1. Remove environmental hazards, such as loose rugs and small, movable furniture.
2. Keep furniture in same place.
3. Assist with ambulation as necessary.
4. Observe and assist with nutrition and elimination. May use behavior-modification techniques. (See Chapter 28.)
5. Assist with personal hygiene.
6. Use close observation and tact if prone to assaultive behavior.
   Avoid situations which precipitate assaultiveness. (See pp. 924–925.)

B. *To foster security, to maximize patient's strengths, and to attain the optimal adaptive behavior of which patient is capable.*

1. Communicate to patient that he is still a worthwhile human being.
   a. Be supportive.
   b. Show respect and interest in patient.
   c. Be sincere.
   d. Use active listening.
2. Be aware of special needs and attempt to find ways of meeting them.
3. Provide consistent, nonconfusing, quiet atmosphere.
4. Assist patient in being as comfortable and happy as possible.
5. Involve patient in simple, repetitive activities when he/she can tolerate this; e.g., simple activities in occupational therapy.
6. Provide a home-like atmosphere within limits of safety.
   a. Allow personal belongings.
   b. Encourage use of own clothing.
   c. Use appropriate music.
7. Develop a therapeutic milieu that provides for structure and routine.
   a. Provide appropriate level of environmental stimulation, maintaining basic daily routine for patient, as he is able to tolerate.
   b. Carefully assess new experiences introduced into patient's life: some patients will require more structure in routine.
   c. Provide consistency in attitude and approach.
8. Use touch when appropriate.
9. Reduce competition: emphasize individual achievement.
10. Increase confidence and self-esteem.
11. Encourage activities in which success is reasonable and failure minimal.
12. Involve patient in the planning of his own care as much as possible.
13. Involve friends and relatives in care as much as possible.
14. Provide liberal praise and positive reinforcers for accomplishments.
    Avoid punishment or negative reinforcers.
15. Approach issue of physical and mental limitations with calm, matter-of-fact acceptance.
16. Use quiet firmness.
17. Do not retaliate in response to poor social graces: recognize this as symptomatic.
18. Use remotivation group therapy as appropriate.
    a. Goals are:
       (1) To remotivate patient and focus on reality
       (2) To develop pleasant interpersonal relationships
       (3) To recognize things and people and become more aware and interested in surroundings
       (4) To utilize strengths and potential of patient.
    b. The steps of remotivation therapy include:
       (1) "The climate of acceptance"—patients are introduced and warmly welcomed to group.
       (2) "The bridge to reality"—reading of poetry or article in group.
       (3) "Sharing the world we live in"—the topic for

discussion is introduced using real objects, pictures, etc.

    (4) "An appreciation of the work of the world"—the patient is encouraged to relate his work and life experiences to topic.

    (5) "The climate of appreciation"—pleasure is expressed for the member's attendance.

19. Use reality orientation group therapy as appropriate.
    a. Goals are to reorient person to time, place, person, and things.
    b. Classroom group sessions are first held at third-grade level; in daily, 30-minute periods, for 2 weeks.
    c. Use clocks, calendars, and other educational materials to orient patient.
    d. When progress is evident, raise level of instructional materials to sixth grade level (optional). Use memory games.
20. Use reminiscing group therapy as appropriate.
    a. Goals are:
      (1) To identify and share accomplishments, tribulations, and viewpoints with others
      (2) To increase opportunities for socialization
      (3) To stimulate memories
      (4) To gain respect and support from group members
      (5) To provide for recreation
      (6) To facilitate putting life experiences into an acceptable meaningful whole
    b. Use mild physical exercise prior to group discussion.
    c. Use developmental framework to organize reminiscing.
      (1) Select initial content area for reminiscing.
      (2) Use real objects to facilitate reminiscing; e.g., use of maps to talk about birthplace.
      (3) Plan outings with group as part of therapy.

Health Education

1. Teach patient to care for his own activities of daily living, keeping within his capabilities.
2. Use behavior-modification techniques where appropriate. (See Chapter 28.)

ALTERATIONS IN PERCEPTIONS

Characteristics

1. Unpredictableness
2. Mumbling to self
3. Talking about unseen objects
4. Looking about in a frightened, guarded manner
5. Being unusually interested in T.V. or radio
6. Complaints of headache
7. Withdrawal

Nursing Assessment and On-going Observations

1. Collect data on patient's sleep pattern and prebedtime routines.
2. Determine if hallucinatory experience involves direction to do some harm to people or things.
3. Observe nonverbal behaviors to detect when patient is hallucinating.
4. Note high risk of suicide.
5. Relate hallucinatory experience to possible increase in anxiety, use of alcohol or psychedelic drugs, organic disease, injury, or high fever.
    a. More animal themes are in the hallucinations of patients experiencing alcoholism.
    b. More human content is in the hallucinations of patients experiencing functional psychosis.
6. Determine if voices are perceived as helpful, threatening, accusing, or terrorizing.
7. Ascertain which basic needs the hallucinatory experience helps the patient satisfy, such as dependence, acceptance, self-esteem.

Nursing Goals and Interventions

A. *To promote acceptance of patient as a valued human being and to assist his understanding that alterations in perceptions are part of his illness.*

1. Assist in describing hallucinatory experience.
2. Provide reassurance of safe, secure environment, especially at night when hallucinatory experiences are more frequent.
3. Leave light on at night if this promotes increased feeling of security.
4. Avoid arguments, proving you are right, or making jokes about voices.
5. Refrain from threats or hostile comments, for patient is already extremely fearful.

B. *To assist in orientation to present reality.*

1. Provide orientation to time, place, and person as needed.
2. Give clear, simple directions.
3. Validate reality of experience for the patient, rather than unreal aspects.
4. Assist patient in associating increased anxiety levels with increased alterations in perceptions.
5. Give feedback, especially about reality aspects of conversation.

C. *To provide external controls if patient feels he cannot stop responding to voices.*

1. Provide restraints or quiet area if patient is unable to control response to voices.
2. Ask patient to seek assistance from staff in controlling voices.
3. Stay with patient to assure him of being safe.
4. Explain carefully what is happening and what you are doing.
5. Verbalize any actions; do not rely on nonverbal communication, for it may be misinterpreted.
6. Help patient to use techniques to lower anxiety level.

D. *To decrease reliance on voices in order to deal with loneliness, anxiety, and fears.*

1. Assist patient in becoming involved in activities on clinical unit or in community.
2. Provide opportunities for him to listen to problems and concerns of others.
3. Help patient have labels for feelings he is experiencing.
4. Support patient when he begins to tell the voices "to

go away" or "be quiet" or begins to be consciously involved in other activities as a way of coping with them.
5. Provide opportunity for a consistent, supportive relationship.

Health Education
Teach patient:
1. That hallucinatory experiences can be a part of mental illness

2. To approach others and not to withdraw when experiencing hallucinations
3. Ways of dealing with anxiety, such as relaxation techniques, distraction (See Anxiety, pp. 925–927.)
4. To expect hallucinatory experience when in stressful environment or when there is a change in routine activities
5. To refrain from speaking out loud to voices in presence of others in recovery phase of illness

INAPPROPRIATE USE OF PHYSICAL SYMPTOMS

Characteristics
1. Numerous physical complaints with no organic bases
2. Overconcern with health
3. Nagging and demanding quality of complaints

Nursing Assessment and On-going Observations
1. Note carefully the character, duration, and frequency of symptoms.
2. Collect data on recent stressful life events.
3. Watch for potential health danger in presenting symptoms, because patients with psychiatric diagnoses may be at high risk for medical illness.
4. Determine which activities of daily living or life goals the symptoms are disrupting.
5. Identify patient's method of dealing with dependency needs: a denial of; a defending against; with extreme independency; an acceptance, with a clinging to others.
6. Examine environment to determine situational context symptoms.
7. Note expressions of anxiety.
8. Differentiate between involvement in activities of living versus preoccupation with physical illness.

Nursing Goals and Interventions
A. *To develop ability to express emotional needs more directly.*
1. Encourage expression of feelings.
2. Ask patient to describe feelings and thoughts when describing a body symptom.

3. Give feedback in terms of feelings when patient is noted to be free of symptoms and looks relaxed.
4. Assist in describing feelings, such as "feeling better, more relaxed," and help identify what is helpful in achieving that state.
5. Refrain from "doing something" in response to increased complaints as patient's anxiety mounts.

B. *To prevent further alienation from others by constant complaints.*
1. Redirect interest in body functions to an interest in the environment.
2. Listen to complaints to convey concern and to become knowledgeable in scope of complaints before setting limits on further expression.
3. Discuss consequences of constant focus on various aches and pains.
4. Verbalize how burdensome things must be for the patient.
5. Support patient's efforts to do something for someone else.

Health Education
Teach patient:
1. Relaxation techniques, such as visualizing vacation scenes, focusing on each body part in a progressive manner and relaxing it, exercise.
2. How to become aware of one's own feelings
3. The basic emotional needs of people and ways they are met
4. Consequences of overusing physical symptoms as a way of dealing with emotional needs

PROBLEM DRINKING

Characteristics
1. Excessive drinking of alcohol:
   a. At regular daily intervals
   b. On regular weekend intervals
   c. During *binges* (intoxicated for at least 2 successive days) interspersed with periods of nonexcessive drinking
2. Difficulty in stopping or reducing amount of alcohol used
3. Impaired physical, emotional, occupational, or social functioning resulting from excessive drinking of alcohol; e.g., can include:
   a. Absenteeism, difficulties at work, or job loss
   b. Arrests for inappropriate behavior or traffic accidents

   c. Interpersonal difficulties with spouse, children, or friends
   d. Depression, suicidal threats and attempts
   e. Divorce
   f. Alcoholic psychosis, hallucinosis, or delirium tremens
   g. *Blackouts*—amnesia for experiences occurring during intoxicated state
   h. Social isolation
   i. Loss of economic security
4. Depending on severity of problem drinking, patient can develop:
   a. *Tolerance*—the need for more alcohol to produce the same desired effect
   b. *Alcohol withdrawal*—symptoms can include "morn-

ing shakes," tremors, fever, perspiration, halluci-nations; relieved by resumption of alcohol intake
5. Use of inadequate coping skills to deal with stressors and problems; reliance on alcohol to "escape" anxiety, tension, depression, personal problems
6. Inappropriate aggression; withdrawn and depressed behavior; or silliness, loudness, and boisterousness—frequently expressed while drinking heavily
7. Etiological factors—may include genetic, psychological, sociological, cultural, and biological factors.

Nursing Assessment

1. Obtain data base by asking the following questions:
   a. At what age did you start drinking alcoholic beverages?
   b. When did you first experience problems with alcohol?
   c. When did you have your last drink? Drinking episode? What kind and how much alcohol did you drink daily during this time?
   d. Describe your drinking pattern during the past year.
   e. Has drinking alcohol created any problems for you? On your job? With your spouse, children, or other relatives? Any arrests? Auto accidents? Financial difficulties? Fights? Accidental falls?
   f. How do you view yourself presently?
2. Assess effect of alcohol on physical health status by asking patient:
   a. What is your general physical health like?
   b. Do you have any pain in your stomach? Changes in appetite? Changes in bowel habits? Weight changes? Nausea or vomiting? Throat or mouth irritation? Vomited blood?
   c. Are you having any trouble with your heart? Chest pain? Any swelling? Shortness of breath? Chronic cough? Coughed up any blood?
   d. Any difficulty maintaining your balance? Vision difficulties? Tremors? Seizures? D.T.s? Blackouts? Hearing or seeing things? Tingling, pain, or numbness in extremities?
   e. Are you taking any medications now?
   f. Have you been treated before for alcohol problems? Describe.
3. Determine if patient has been experiencing any stress or having any problems that may lead to drinking.

Nursing Goals and Interventions

A. *To help patient recognize and accept drinking problem and to reduce or eliminate problem drinking.*

1. Permit patient to describe his perception of the problem.
2. Encourage patient to mention those aspects he dislikes about his drinking behavior.
3. Upon offering such a statement, ask patient to elaborate and describe his feelings about this aspect.
4. Do not induce guilt but attempt to have patient tune in to any feelings of remorse stemming from those aspects he dislikes about his drinking.
5. Point out to patient those negative behavioral consequences caused by his problem drinking.
   a. Do not directly attack alibi system used by patient to explain negative consequences.
   b. Do not make patient feel blameworthy.
   c. Ask patient to state again what he dislikes about his drinking behavior.

d. Point out differences between what he is saying and reality.
6. Deal with drinking stories calmly and matter-of-factly.
7. Observe for suicidal tendencies if there is evidence of depression.
8. Meet protective needs.
9. Accept matter-of-factly, without retaliation, patient criticism, and hostility toward staff and institution.

B. *To decrease hopelessness, to improve self-concept, and to reduce or eliminate problem drinking.*

1. Avoid punitive attitude. Be nonjudgmental and understanding.
2. Help patient express feelings of helplessness and inadequacy.
3. Demonstrate concern for and interest in patient.
4. Set realistic goals with patient; e.g., encourage sobriety "one day at a time."
5. Avoid communicating expectations of failing: do communicate verbally and nonverbally so that patient *can* overcome difficulties.
6. Give patient tasks he can perform successfully. Increase responsibilities given to patient gradually.
7. Identify, verbalize recognition, and support use of assets and potential.
8. Establish therapeutic interpersonal relationship.
9. Support participation or leadership in groups and activities.

C. *To develop adaptive coping strategies, to reduce use of alcohol in order to "escape" unpleasant stimuli, and to reduce or eliminate problem drinking.*

1. Reduce social isolation.
   a. Serve as a link between patient and his attempts to establish relationships with other people.
   b. Support and strengthen family interest.
   c. Teach socialization skills.
   d. Encourage removal from groups that support excessive drinking and encourage the development of new relationships.
   e. Help set up social support system in community with patient.
   f. Facilitate patient interaction with other patients through social activities and conversation.
   g. Assist patient in recognizing how his behavior influences that of others.
   h. Support use of assertive communication skills.
2. Involve spouse in aspects of treatment program, along with patient, where possible.
3. Confront patient when responsibilities are avoided.
4. Suggest referral of spouse or relatives to Al-Anon and children to Alateen groups.
5. Assist in developing and participating in old or new enjoyable activities and interests.
6. Refer to Alcoholics Anonymous.
7. Suggest referral to treatment components, such as family therapy, couples counseling, occupational therapy, recreational therapy, vocational rehabilitation, religious counseling, group therapy, outpatient follow-up treatment program.
8. Assist in reducing anxiety. (See pp. 926–927.)
9. Involve patient in patient groups in which gripes can be aired and policies for ward living can be drawn up.
10. Ask patient to develop constructive plans for use of time that he usually spent drinking.
11. Use role play to teach patient how to refuse a drink when offered one in a social setting.

a. Decide whether or not and how much to drink before entering drinking social environment.
b. Establish eye contact.
c. Assertively make statement; e.g., "No, I do not want a drink."
d. Request a nonalcoholic beverage, if desired.
12. Confront and deal with manipulative behavior.
13. Use firm kindness to deal with unreasonable demands.
14. Encourage self-care.

Health Education and Prevention

Teach patient:
1. Principles for prevention of problem drinking, such as:
    a. Become aware and learn to distinguish between acceptable and unacceptable drinking; e.g., teach effects of alcohol intake on driving, etc.
    b. Develop "take it or leave it" attitude and decrease emotionalism associated with drinking alcohol.
    c. De-emphasize drinking for its own sake or as a means to escape problems.
    d. Encourage an emphasis on other activities and integrate drinking only as a secondary activity.
    e. Offer young people opportunities to drink in controlled settings.

2. Principles of behavioral self-control, to reduce problem drinking:
    a. Instruct patient to keep record of all drinking—type and amount of drink, location and time of drink, what was happening before taking the drink.
    b. Review records at regular intervals with patient. Show patient how to calculate blood alcohol concentrations for each drinking incident.
    c. Teach patient to examine record for antecedents to his drinking incidents.
        (1) Discuss strategies for any possible alteration of these antecedents.
        (2) Discuss strategies for alternative reactions to antecedents, other than turning to alcohol.
    d. Use role play to aid patient in learning new behavioral responses.
    e. Have patient practice new behaviors and reach eventual independence in self-monitoring.
3. Problem-solving skills:
    a. Recognize existence of a problem.
    b. Define nature of problem clearly.
    c. Develop alternatives for solution along with their anticipated consequences.
    d. Select best alternative, use it, and evaluate its results.

REGRESSIVE BEHAVIOR

Characteristics

1. Focus on self
2. Kicking; crying; biting; screaming
3. Vomiting; smearing feces; urinating on self
4. Masturbating; exposing self
5. Playing with food
6. Rocking; sleeping in fetal position
7. Distractible
8. Lack of sense of time and work
9. Stealing; destructive behavior; hoarding

Nursing Assessment and On-going Observations

1. Collect data on scope of regressive behaviors being used.
2. Determine what behavior means to patient and family members.
3. Observe behavior carefully to ascertain area in which patient is assuming more appropriate behaviors.
4. Note dependency behaviors.
5. Ascertain if fear of abandonment is present.

Nursing Goals and Interventions

A. *To prevent further development of more regressive behaviors.*

1. Respond to basic needs expressed, especially the need for survival, which may be threatened.
2. Give feedback on positive accomplishments even though they may seem small and irrelevant; i.e., "You ate without spilling on your dress." or "You looked upset when Betty threw the ashtray."
3. Explain any changes in daily activities.
4. Convey concern about present behavior.
5. Encourage discussion about happenings in the environment.
6. Assist in grooming activities if necessary.
7. Set limits on regressive behaviors that interfere with

living space of others or endanger patient's own well-being.
8. Establish daily routines.
9. Accept dependency expressed without insisting on confronting dependency needs.

B. *To promote the development of more mature ways to meet basic needs.*

1. Assist patient in verbally identifying what he wants.
    a. May have to make guesses at needs and ask patient for feedback.
    b. Patient may express very narcissistic needs or needs to please others.
2. Ask patient to observe what happens when others do not get what they want before opening a discussion of what happens when he does not get what he wants.
3. Help to schedule activities for the day or week.
4. Identify patient's responsibilities in areas of grooming and care of personal space, on patient unit and in community.
5. Suggest to patient that he ask questions so that he will know and understand for himself.
6. Expect testing of the relationship by the patient; reappearance of former regressive behaviors may occur.

Health Education

Teach Patient:
1. Skills associated with grooming, eating, cleaning living area, and talking with others
2. Daily and weekly routines for caring for self and health needs
3. What he can reasonably expect from others and what things cannot be expected from others
4. An interesting fact about his environment, then ask him to share with others
5. To become interested in one person or object at least once daily

RITUALISTIC BEHAVIOR

Characteristics

1. Manifestations of anxiety
2. Repetitive act or thought; inability to control act or thought; inflexibility
3. Overabundance of detail with little notation of feeling

Nursing Assessment and On-going Observations

1. Identify level of anxiety.
2. Evaluate for manipulation and suicidal behavior and any relationship between the two.
3. Note situations that tend to increase anxiety and lead to ritualistic acts.
4. Identify changes in the patient's view of himself and in his view of the repetitive thought or act as being alien to him.
5. Collect data on relief from urgency of repetitive act or thought provided by various activities.
6. Identify specific interpersonal relationships and health routines being adversely affected by repetitive thoughts or acts.
7. Observe for the expression of feelings.

Nursing Goals and Interventions

A. *To reduce anxiety level and conscious uncomfortableness with ritualistic behavior.*
1. Reward acceptable behavior.
2. Provide opportunities to express feelings.
3. Allow performance of ritual without making demeaning remarks or attempting to stop behavior.
4. Be consistent and time-conscious when making contacts and appointments or giving specific care.

5. Offer information about rituals and obsessions in everyday life.
6. Assist in increasing range of behaviors to decrease anxiety.
7. Support patient in talking about repetitive thoughts or acts.
8. Be aware of and take action to decrease anxiety level aroused in staff.
9. Assist patient in identifying his way of dealing with anxiety and resulting obsessive thoughts, such as being overly nice; washing hands; repeating a phrase; distracting self by singing, counting, praying; leaving immediate area; or avoiding a known trigger.
10. Give feedback about expressions of obsession and assist him in saying directly what he means.

B. *To provide range of normal activities during the day.*
1. Plan for additional time to complete rituals.
2. Assist in making schedule of daily activities.
3. Provide patient support in completing his activities, particularly any new ones.
4. Reassure and assist in enduring small periods of relaxation and pleasure.

Health Education

Teach patient:
1. Ways of dealing with anxiety, such as identifying the feeling, controlling thoughts, exercise (See Anxiety.)
2. Ways of dealing with consequences of ritualistic behavior
3. Simple games and recreational activities
4. To engage in normal activities and to allow for extra time for rituals

ALTERATIONS IN SELF-CARE ACTIVITIES

Characteristics

1. Irregular bathing; unshaven face; body odor; unkempt hair; dirty fingernails; clothes uncared for
2. Poor dental hygiene; bad breath
3. Unmade bed; spilling food on clothes and table; playing with food
4. Sleep disturbances; sleeping in clothes
5. Ignoring smoking rules; needing direction for simplest activity; forgetful
6. No energy to carry out activities; minimal talking

Nursing Assessment and On-going Observation

1. Make inventory of areas in which help is needed.
2. Determine other psychological needs the patient is meeting by not caring for himself.
3. Observe effects of praise, simple rewards, success, recognition, and group pressure on behavior.
4. Collect data on daily activities before illness.

Nursing Goals and Interventions

A. *To re-establish a pattern of living without total dependence on others.*
1. Give feedback about improvement in care of personal appearance or other activities.

2. Use consistent repetition of health routines as a means of establishing them.
3. Avoid showing rejection or belittlement as patient struggles with changing behavior.
4. Provide remotivation groups.
5. Assist patient in verbalizing what he is doing, as he does it.

B. *To assist in caring for self.*

1. Supervise daily activities, such as bathing, cleaning of teeth, bedmaking.
2. Make various creams and toilet articles easily available.
3. Give praise when activity is completed.
4. Allow adequate time for carrying out activities.
5. Do not make demands on patient that he cannot fulfill.
6. Offer support and give as needed; take care not to make patient totally dependent on you.

Health Education

Teach patient:
1. Basic grooming skills, i.e., how to care for own clothing, how to make bed
2. Table manners, i.e., how to hold silverware, how to ask for more

3. Simple conversational methods, i.e., to say "Good morning," to maintain eye contact, to speak slowly
4. How to ask for only a few things from others and to rely on self
5. Consequences of assuming responsibility for self

6. To question whether or not he can do something before asking another to do it for him
7. To look for written directions, try to follow them, and write down things for him to remember

ALTERATIONS IN SELF-ESTEEM

Characteristics

1. Devalues self through criticism and self-derision; judges own behavior harshly; low personal self-worth
2. Experiences numerous fears; fears failure; worries
3. Has feelings of disappointment, helplessness, hopelessness, guilt, inferiority, defeatism, frustration; feelings of being fragile and inadequate
4. Minimizes own real strengths and abilities; sense of self-defeat
5. Judges gap between self-ideal (patient's perception of what he would like to be or should be) and self as actually perceived
6. Fails to live up to self-expectations; self-contempt; inability to accept self; denies self pleasure
7. Discounts own opinion; hesitant to offer own opinions and viewpoints
8. Sets unreasonable, inflexible standards for self; preoccupied with real or imagined past failures
9. Ambivalent; procrastinates; self-destructive
10. May use poor self-esteem for secondary gains; failure to achieve goals
11. Failure to receive approval from others; lacks sources of love and respect from others; poor interpersonal relationships

Nursing Assessment

1. What is patient's present perception of himself?
2. What does the patient think he should be like? Or what would he be like?
3. What are patient's goals and how realistic are they?
4. What standards does patient set for himself? Are they realistic?
5. Assess patient's real strengths and potentials. In what ways has patient been successful in the past?
6. Describe patient's interpersonal relationships. Does he have a network of meaningful others with whom he relates well?
7. Observe for manifestations of depression

Nursing Goals and Interventions

To increase self-esteem.
1. Avoid judgmental attitude.
   Do not reject patient for expressing negative feelings.
2. Make patient aware of times he discounts his own opinions.
3. Show empathy.
4. Demonstrate unconditional positive regard.
5. Be congruent and genuine.
6. Communicate acceptance of patient as a worthwhile human being.
7. Show interest in and concern for patient.
   Spend time with patient in groups and in a one-to-one nurse-patient relationship.
8. Assist patient in developing the attitude of not always having to be perfect to feel adequate and good about himself.
   Point out that he is as worthwhile as anyone else.
9. Focus on patient's strengths and potential.
   a. Encourage patient to identify and list his strengths and potential.
   b. Discourage emphasis on failure.
   c. Offer experiences of success.
   d. Encourage participation in rewarding and satisfying experiences.
   e. Encourage patient in developing new skills and in initiating activities in which he can be reasonably successful.
   f. Find ways to utilize strengths.
10. Encourage patient to participate in group therapy in which the emphasis is to provide support.
    Through principle of universality, help patient recognize that he is not alone in experiencing fears and failures.
11. Work through feelings of disappointment.
    Problem-solve to seek constructive resolution to problems faced.
12. Encourage patient to begin taking responsibility for his own opinions.
13. Have patient list negative qualities and develop plans to change them.
14. Give compliments on neat appearance, activities well done, and other strengths.
    a. Offer positive reinforcers for actual achievements.
    b. Avoid false praise.
15. Teach patient to give himself positive reinforcement; e.g., treating himself to dinner after completing something successfully.
16. Accept patient as person regardless of his thoughts or his past failures.
17. Discourage use of poor self-esteem for secondary gains.
18. Encourage good grooming habits and personal appearance.
19. Encourage use of assertive communication skills.
20. Assist patient in developing defenses against attack on self.
21. Expand patient's self-awareness.
22. Encourage patient to explore feelings, thoughts, and behavior and to examine critically his own behavior.
23. Encourage patient to accept responsibility for his own behavior and to evaluate its outcome in relation to the options open to him.
24. Assist patient in developing solutions to problems and in setting realistic goals and plans.
25. Help patient begin to take action to meet goals.

Health Education

Teach patient assertive behavior and communication skills.
1. Characteristics:

a. Sensitive to others' feelings.
b. Use of "I" messages.
c. Behaviors, opinions, and rights of others respected.
d. Posture, facial expression, tone of voice consistent with verbal communication.
e. Expectations conveyed to others.
f. Negotiation viewed as viable tactic.
g. Firm but gentle; unyielding where appropriate.
h. Force used only when and where necessary.
 i. Threats not needed.
 j. Based on own human rights.
 k. Learning and competence are emphasized.
2. Components include:
a. Set goals and express to others your honest thoughts and feelings.
b. Act on set goals in clear, consistent way.
c. Accept personal responsibility for consequences of actions.
d. Remain sensitive to rights and feelings of others.

INAPPROPRIATE SEXUAL BEHAVIOR

Characteristics

1. Making sexually provocative remarks; flirting; trying to touch and pinch others; hugging and kissing
2. Masturbating in public places; disrobing; exposing genitals
3. Reciting sexual activities or fantasies
4. Magical expectations of others

Nursing Assessment and On-going Observations

1. Ascertain meaning of sexual behavior as release of sexual needs or anxiety, aggressive act, fear of loss of identity, powerlessness, means of obtaining punishment, or need for closeness.
2. Note increase of anxiety during period of sexual acting-out.
3. Identify situations in which sexual acting-out occurs.
4. Check medications patient is taking; sedatives, narcotics, psychotropics, antidepressants, antihypertensives, antispasmodics, and alcohol affect sexual function.
5. Evaluate knowledge and beliefs regarding sexual function.

Nursing Goals and Interventions

A. *To regain control over sexual impulses.*

1. Identify when level of anxiety increases.
2. Openly discuss sexual behaviors to arrive at understanding of meaning and ways to assist in coping.
3. Provide structured, active games.
4. Give feedback about uncomfortableness created in self or others.

5. Discuss appropriate ways in which sexual needs can be met; i.e., drawing, listening to music, dancing, reading, participating in sports.
6. Point out what behaviors are sexually provocative.
7. Reassure patient that sexual behavior is not needed to maintain nurse's interest and concern in him as a person.
8. Suggest shower to assist in controlling impulse.

B. *To maintain identity of self as person, man or woman.*

1. Provide opportunities to express feelings of impotence or loss of control.
2. Recognize the fear of homosexuality which may be expressed; support patient in his choice of sex role.
3. Assist patient in identifying his/her areas of strength.
4. Explore meanings of being a man or woman.
5. Discuss and negotiate ways to provide privacy in long-term hospitalization.

Health Education

Teach patient:
1. Appropriate ways of dealing with sexual impulses, i.e., intercourse with appropriate person, time, and place; cold showers; vigorous physical activity; masturbation
2. Major structure and function of the reproductive system
3. The different meanings associated with the sexual act
4. The effect of certain tranquilizers on sexual drive
5. Consequences of sexually provocative behavior

SPIRITUAL DISTRESS

Characteristics

1. *Spiritual*—encompasses those all-pervasive needs and forces that, if met, can lead to and include:
a. The formulation of a positive personal meaning and purpose of existence
b. The development of meaning in suffering
c. A positive, dynamic relationship to a deity characterized by faith, trust, and love
d. Personal integrity and self-worth
e. A sense of direction in life characterized by hope
f. The development of positive human relationships
2. *Spiritual distress*—behavioral manifestations that can
 include behaviors listed in stages of spiritual distress and any other of the following:
a. Demonstrates stages of spiritual distress:
(1) Disillusioned
(a) Questions, "Why did God permit this to happen?"
(b) Jokes about heaven and hell.
(c) Questions worth or credibility of religious beliefs.
(d) Questions relationship with God.
(e) Questions reasons for or meaning of existence.

(f) Unable to develop meaning or begins to lose the meaning which has been developed about the suffering.

(2) Investigation
  (a) Wonders, "Can I blame God?"
  (b) Begins to blame God for illness or other difficulties experienced.
  (c) Feels anger towards God.
  (d) Desire to depend on and trust God decreases.
  (e) Faith in God or spiritual beliefs decreases.

(3) Idolatry
  (a) Asks, "Where can I find a God?"
  (b) Usual religious practices and rituals change.
  (c) Searches for alternative beliefs.
  (d) Expresses conflict or concern about own religious beliefs/values.

(4) Resolution
  (a) Inadequate—spiritual distress continues.
  (b) Adequate—spiritual distress resolved.

b. Lack of will to live
c. Restlessness
d. Loneliness
e. Mild, moderate, or severe anxiety
f. Decreased hope
g. Unhappiness
h. Views people as less helpful, fair, trustworthy, or expresses less concern for others
i. Fear
j. Withdrawal or silence
k. Expression of guilt or shame
l. Decrease in zest for life
m. Depression or expressions of worthlessness
n. Discontent or disillusioned

3. Etiology of spiritual distress can include:
a. Separation from own religious community and culture
b. Challenged religious beliefs
c. Encountered difficulties or stress in life, such as illness
d. Inability to carry out usual religious rituals and practices
e. Unresolved feelings about death
f. Moral/ethical nature of therapy
g. Lost belief in God and religion
h. Inescapable predicament which appears to have no solution

4. Patients may respond to illness with spiritual distress followed by inadequate resolution or adequate resolution and growth.

5. Spiritual beliefs and meeting spiritual needs can be helpful in overcoming physical and mental illness and in restoring health.

Nursing Assessment

1. Obtain data based on following questions:
a. What do you worship?
b. How do you perceive your relationship with God now?.
c. How does religion or spiritual beliefs influence your life?
d. In what ways are religion or spiritual beliefs helpful or not helpful to you in your present illness?
   Determine whether religion is viewed as a supportive or unrealistic resource.

e. What/who offers you strength and hope right now?
f. What religious practices, symbols, rituals, or literature are important or helpful to you? Has being ill affected any of these?
g. What effect does your present illness have on your spiritual beliefs and needs? What effect do your spiritual beliefs have on your views about your present illness?
h. Do you need any spiritual assistance now? Tell me what would be helpful to you? Does your pastor know you are in the hospital? Would you like to have him contacted?

2. Observe for evidence of religious commitment; e.g., religious articles in room; behaviors as prayer, reading Bible; verbalizations about religious topics; visits from minister.

3. Observe for behaviors indicating stages of spiritual distress.

Nursing Goals and Interventions

A. *To establish or maintain a dynamic involvement with religion and to adequately resolve spiritual distress.*

1. Permit patient to keep religious articles, unless harmful to self or other.
2. Permit patient to continue beneficial religious practices and rituals as much as feasible.
3. Listen carefully to patient's communication and develop a sense of timing for prayer.
4. Be honest and offer informed understanding.
5. Encourage talk with other patients who have similar religious beliefs.
6. Don't attempt to change patient's religious affiliation.
7. Contact religious advisor for assistance as needed. Share with clergy information that is necessary and useful in helping the patient.

B. *To develop, support the use of, or strengthen spiritual values or beliefs in order to adequately resolve spiritual distress.*

1. Communicate willingness to talk about spiritual beliefs.
   Avoid idle curiosity.
2. Develop or support meaning in life or suffering.
   a. Listen nonjudgmentally and with understanding.
   b. Show tolerance, respect, concern, care, and empathy.
   c. Assist patient in recognizing that spiritual longing, or a desire to search for meaning in life or suffering, is acceptable.
   d. Convey belief that life is worth living.
   e. Support patient's will to live.
   f. Develop nurse-patient relationship in which patient can be comfortable in exploring meaning in life or suffering.
   g. Encourage patient to develop realistic hope and a constructive philosophy that helps deal with suffering.
   h. Assist in facing pain or suffering.
3. Share personal strengths and beliefs as one means of offering support and assistance.
4. Determine and discuss aspects of hospitalization or treatment which may run counter to patient's spiritual beliefs.
5. Offer support and understanding.
6. Reaffirm and mobilize patient's own internal resources and strengths.

7. Provide environment in which patient is free to choose and make his own decision about spiritual beliefs and values.
8. Respond naturally to expressed spiritual needs.
   Don't avoid conversation about spiritual matters.
9. Assist in exploring spiritual concerns and needs and feasible alternatives.
   Ask questions to assist in verbalizing beliefs.
10. Avoid statements that increase conflict or stress regarding beliefs or values.
11. Maintain conversation about spiritual matters at patient's level.
12. Avoid social stereotyping.

Health Education

Teach patient to:

1. Recognize own personal stages of spiritual distress—disillusioned, investigation, idolatry, and resolution
2. Discuss spiritual concerns with concerned significant other(s) and seek support
3. Seek religious counseling
4. Discuss concern with clergy
5. Seek psychiatric therapy
6. Continue to seek and use ways to develop or build on a constructive spiritual belief system by:
   a. Participating in discussion groups focusing on spiritual concerns
   b. Attending and participating in religious or spiritual rituals and practices
   c. Reading religious literature

THREATENED SUICIDE, ATTEMPTED SUICIDE

Characteristics

1. *Threatened suicide*—verbalization of wish to die.
2. *Attempted suicide*—recent injury to body (cutting, burning, hitting, drug overdose, jumping off bridge) with intent to kill self.

Nursing Assessment

1. What is the nature of the patient's suicidal behavior leading to admission? Method? Clarity of plan? Place? Proximity of other people? Physical results? Actions to reverse physical results or obtain help?
2. Does patient verbalize desire to die (e.g., "I'm tired. It's no use. No one would care if I died." or "Death would solve everything.")?
3. Observe patient's nonverbal behaviors: isolating self, collecting harmful objects, making out wills
4. Does patient have a history of past suicidal behavior?
5. Observe for signs of depression: lack of interest in activities of daily living, insomnia, lack of appetite, sadness, physical complaints, hopelessness
6. Does patient exhibit impaired judgment that may result from drug abuse?
7. Has patient experienced delusions or auditory hallucinations?
8. Has patient experienced disorientation, memory impairment, confusion?
9. Has patient made any attempts at suicide? Method used? Place? Proximity of other people? Physical results?
10. Does patient show changes in level of depression?
11. Are any physical illnesses present that may be masked by other behaviors?

Nursing Goals and Interventions

A. *To provide protection from self-destruction or injury.*

1. Provide safe environment, which includes freedom from sharp objects and other harmful items.
   Discuss with team members and decide what personal items to remove from patient and what specific environmental hazards to eliminate.
2. Evaluate with team members the necessity for close observation, area restriction procedures, or one-to-one observations for suicide prevention.
3. Observe patient closely; emphasize protective, not punitive, attitude.
4. Set limits in relation to destructive behavior towards self or others.
5. Permit expression of anger and hostility within these limits.
6. Offer support against self-destructive impulses and suggest alternative behaviors.
7. Prevent isolation. Seek out patient.
8. Do not dare patient to carry out a suicidal threat.
9. Assess impact of patient on staff or other patients.

B. *To meet activities of daily living.*

1. Assist in meeting activities of daily living, permitting as much independence as possible and keeping within the boundaries of patient's capabilities.
2. Allow simple decision making and progress within limitations of patient.

C. *To develop adaptive methods to cope with stress.*

1. Ask patient to postpone suicidal attempt.
2. Communicate opportunity to re-evaluate the situation when not overwhelmed by desire to die and that other ways are available to cope with what is happening.
3. Identify what patient believes will be helpful to him.
4. Help patient look at positive aspects of living that can be anticipated in the future.
5. Assist patient in identifying when he is anxious.
6. Seek ways to lower anxiety in patient.
7. Avoid interpreting remarks such as "I'll kill myself before I do that" as attention-seeking behaviors.
8. Listen with sensitivity to expressions of unworthiness, without insisting that words are false.
9. Avoid imposing own feelings, values, and moral judgments.
10. Convey message that having bad thoughts and

making mistakes does not mean one is a "bad person."
11. Assist patient in developing realistic personal goals.
12. Do not use jubilant, gay approach.
13. Help patient identify times when angry, sources of anger, and ways to channel anger.
14. Reflect a caring, concerned attitude.
15. Accept patient as a worthwhile person even though self-destructive behavior is not acceptable.

Health Education and Prevention

Teach patient life strategy skills, to prevent future suicidal threats, attempts, or actual suicide, as follows:
1. Establish realistic goals. Master daily activities and rely on self as much as possible.
2. Minimize distraction from immediate desires and self-indulgence by recognizing each day as an opportunity to increase self-confidence and movement toward realistic goals.
3. Reduce self-doubts about abilities by focusing on the involvement and satisfaction in the task and by maximizing the use of special skills and abilities.
4. Set a daily schedule, allowing for flexibility, but making the most out of each part of the day.

5. Be reasonably selfish so that other people's opinions do not prevent accomplishing new or original activities or meeting personal goals.
6. Learn to recognize fear and anxiety and their effects. Gather information and engage in focused activity to deal with fear. Evaluate the results of the focused activity. Find the best personal formula to reduce anxiety.
7. Demonstrate courage, persistence, and self-possession to prevent negative feedback from others.
8. Use personal goals as an overall frame of focus in order to put complex situations into perspective.
9. Develop relationships through shared objectives and activities. Don't compromise self-identity or try to remold others in case of differences.
10. Focus on positive, not negative, thoughts.
11. Do not feel obligated to continually reveal self to others.
12. Find solitude to gain strength and focus on personal direction.
13. Recognize that in future stressful situations, feelings of suicide may occur and that talking to someone is an important aspect of prevention. List Hot Line phone number and other numbers which may be useful in an emergency.

SUSPICIOUSNESS

Characteristics

1. Extreme distrust; belief in a conspiracy; feelings of being persecuted and misjudged
2. Frequently alone; may convey a superior attitude; concern about status and prestige
3. Inflexible in thinking
4. Misinterpretation of acts of others followed by an aggressive response

Nursing Assessment and On-going Observations

1. Determine extent of contact with significant others.
2. Identify areas in which patient accepts help.
3. Examine patient's fear of losing control.
4. Ascertain areas of daily activities and personal hygiene being avoided.
5. Note behaviors that indicate a seeking of relationships with others or continued isolation from others.
6. Observe for clues that patient is hallucinating; i.e., the way he looks and listens to something beside you.
7. Determine if there is a relationship between aggressiveness and the increased expression of suspicion.
8. Collect data on eating pattern.
9. Collect data on sleeping pattern.
10. Observe patient carefully for taking of medication, for he may pretend to take it.

Nursing Goals and Interventions

A. *To orient patient towards reality with a decreased need to control, have power, but to increase self-esteem.*

1. Give concrete tasks to increase relatedness to reality.

2. Give clear, concise information when answering questions or offering explanations of what is occuring. Avoid whispering.
3. Question gently the beliefs of the patient.
4. Convey understanding of patient's dilemma without arguing about his ideas.
5. Respond to a delusion by stating the theme or feeling symbolically expressed: "It must be very distressing to believe that." Further state, "I have not experienced him as threatening."
6. Give positive feedback when reality is presented in the conversation.
7. Avoid putting patient on the defensive so that he has to protect himself.
8. Refrain from correcting misinterpretations through reasoning. Instead, as a step in assisting patient to analyze the belief, raise a doubt by asking a question.
9. Inform patient of schedule changes as soon as possible.

B. *To decrease the aggressiveness in social contact, which further threatens patient's self-esteem.*

1. Make frequent, short interpersonal contacts by minimal number of staff.
2. Assist in identifying people with whom it is appropriate to share thoughts.
3. Discuss consequences of continued suspicion of others on self.
4. Give assurance that the environment is safe.
5. Listen, demonstrating an accepting attitude.
6. Set limits on aggressive acts towards others.
7. Give feedback when patient is noted to be insulting and threatening towards others.

Health Education

1. Teach patient:
   a. To become consciously aware of his feelings of suspiciousness and to make an effort to objectively check them out or to act appropriately despite the fear
   b. The importance of dealing with his feelings and his personal space and not the whole environment

c. Problem solving as one way of dealing with misinterpretations of reality
d. Steps in the formation of a trusting relationship, such as introducing self, spending time with another, being aware of the other's needs, sharing something in common
e. To validate perceptions with others
2. Demonstrate the consequences of suspiciousness.

DISTURBED THOUGHT PROCESS

Characteristics

1. Delusions; flight of ideas; disorganization
2. Word salad; neologisms; echolalia; condensation; perseveration
3. Circumstantiality
4. Difficulty in interacting with others; withdrawn; predictable

Nursing Assessment and On-going Observations

1. Carefully validate what is thought to be a delusion. Delusion may be of grandeur or persecution, or somatic delusions.
2. Ascertain if need for power or self-esteem is being met by a delusion or use of neologism or other type of disturbed thought process.

Nursing Goals and Interventions

A. *To provide opportunity for patient to correct delusional system.*
1. Give feedback concerning a delusion in terms of feeling tone expressed; i.e., the fear it may generate for the patient.
2. Do not expect rational explanations to change the patient's mind and correct the delusion. They may make the patient cling to his thoughts.
3. Refocus conversation to another topic after you have listened carefully to the delusion.
4. Provide experiences in the here and now that patient can talk to others about and have his experiences validated by others.
5. Have daily schedule that stimulates interest in what is occurring in the real world.

6. Protect patient from receiving too many new and stressful experiences too fast.

B. *To assist patient in communicating his thoughts more clearly.*
1. Seek clarification from patient when something is not understood.
2. Avoid nodding in agreement when being bombarded with word salad or rapid stream of disconnected phrases.
3. Ask patient to speak slowly.
4. Give frequent feedback as to what you understand patient to be saying.
5. State that you are trying to understand and want to understand what is being said.
6. Create a pleasant, friendly atmosphere for conversation to take place in.
7. Give feedback about "crazy talk" and assist patient in saying directly what he means.

Health Education

Teach patient:
1. Ways to control thoughts; i.e., to distract self from thinking same thought over and over, to become involved in concrete activities
2. To recognize when thoughts are becoming disorganized; i.e., people are not answering but staring, finding self jumping from subject to subject
3. To anticipate increased anxiety in a new situation and to think of a way to decrease the anxiety
4. To check out ideas and thoughts with others

WITHDRAWAL

Characteristics

1. Isolation from others; seclusiveness; seemingly unaware of environment
2. Disregard for social customs relating to interactions
3. Speaks in short phrases or does not respond verbally to comments or questions
4. Reduced motor activity; sleeping during the daytime

Nursing Assessment and On-going Observations

1. Note ways patient is testing interest of staff in him as a person.

2. Determine how he views himself.
3. Identify persons with whom he has established a relationship.
4. Identify what overprotective attitudes and actions of family or staff are affecting his behavior.
5. Note problems in his thinking and perceiving.
6. Observe interactions with others: how, what, when, where, why.
7. Determine which needs are verbally expressed.
8. Identify situations which tend to increase withdrawal.

9. Observe expressions of feelings of safety and security.
10. Watch for increase in willingness to share own thoughts and feelings.

Nursing Goals and Interventions

A. *To increase interaction with others and the environment.*

1. Be aware of where patient is in the environment.
2. Give verbal acknowledgment of any absence from meetings.
3. Provide ward activities so there is less time for daydreaming.
4. Change environment by going outside for walks, to movies.
5. Encourage group activity, but if there is a need to withdraw, support this decision.
6. Have a matter-of-fact approach to unrealistic expressions.
7. Expect testing of reality and negative responses.
8. Verbalize needs met through interpersonal contacts.
9. Give feedback about behavior which is not appropriately related to current happenings in environment.
10. Request and expect verbal communication.

B. *To provide security in interpersonal contacts.*

1. Maintain eye contact.
2. Explain self and reason for interaction.
3. Tolerate silences.

4. Assist with physical needs, if appropriate, as way to establish contact.
5. Convey concern about "his silence" or "not knowing his needs," and willingness to talk with him.
6. Offer own reactions to happenings in the environment.
7. Focus on what is occurring now.
8. Support positive opinions of self.
9. Avoid probing questions, for it increases anxiety and withdrawal.
10. Carry on a one-sided conversation, if necessary.
11. Reduce tendency of staff to withdraw from patient.

C. *To explore meaning of and to reduce withdrawal.*

1. Discuss what is conveyed to others by silence.
2. Use nonverbal techniques to encourage communication.
3. Point out the responsibility of each in a relationship.
4. Provide safe atmosphere to discuss fears of rejection and retaliation.
5. Give patient opportunities to discuss perception of himself.

Health Education

Teach patient:
1. The difference in being assertive, aggressive, and rejecting in communicating with others (also demonstrate)
2. The consequences of withdrawing from others
3. To begin association with others by contact through structured activities

BIBLIOGRAPHY

Books*

American Psychiatric Association. Diagnostic and Statistical Manual of Mental Disorders, 3rd ed. Washington, D.C., American Psychiatric Association, 1980
Doona M. Travelbee's Intervention in Psychiatric Nursing, 2nd ed. Philadelphia, FA Davis, 1979
Gebbie K. Summary of the Second National Conference—Classification of Nursing Diagnoses. St. Louis, The Clearinghouse, St. Louis University, 1976
Haber J, Leach AM, Schudy SM, Sideleau BF. Comprehensive Psychiatric Nursing. New York, McGraw-Hill, 1978
Joel L and Collins D. Psychiatric Nursing Theory and Application. New York, McGraw-Hill, 1978
Kalkman M and Davis A. New Dimensions in Mental Health—Psychiatric Nursing, 5th ed. New York, McGraw-Hill, 1980
Kreigh H and Perko J. Psychiatric–Mental Health Nursing: A Commitment to Care and Concern. Reston, Reston Pub. Co., 1979
Kyes J and Hofling CK. Basic Psychiatric Concepts in Nursing, 4th ed. Philadelphia, JB Lippincott, 1980
Madden J. A Guide to Alcohol and Drug Dependence. Bristol, John Wright & Sons Limited, 1979
Meldman M, McFarland G, Johnson E. The Problem-Oriented Psychiatric Index and Treatment Plans. St. Louis, CV Mosby, 1976
Mereness D and Taylor C. Essentials of Psychiatric Nursing, 10th ed. St. Louis, CV Mosby, 1978

  * These references were used for multiple diagnoses in this chapter.

Stuart GW and Sundeen SJ. Principles and Practice of Psychiatric Nursing. St. Louis, CV Mosby, 1979
Topalis M and Aguilera D. Psychiatric Nursing, 7th ed, St. Louis, CV Mosby, 1978
Wilson HS and Kneisl CR. Psychiatric Nursing. Menlo Park, Addison–Wesley Pub. Co., 1979

NURSING DIAGNOSES

Books

Gebbie K and Lavin M. (eds). Classification of Nursing Diagnoses. St. Louis, CV Mosby, 1975
Kim M, and Moritz D. Classification of Nursing Diagnoses: Proceedings of Third and Fourth National Conference. New York, McGraw-Hill, 1981
Soares C. Nursing and medical diagnoses: A comparison of variant and essential features. In Chaska N (ed). The Nursing Profession: Views through the Mist. New York, McGraw-Hill, 1978

Articles

Bircher A. On the development and classification of diagnoses. Nurs Forum 1975; 14(1):10–29
Bruce J. Implementation of nursing diagnosis: A nursing administrator's perspective. Nurs Clin North Am 1979 Sept; 14(3):509–515
Fortin J and Rabinow J. Legal implications of nursing diagnosis. Nurs Clin North Am 1979 Sept; 14(3):553–561
Fredette S and O'Connor K. Nursing diagnosis in teaching and curriculum planning. Nurs Clin North Am 1979 Sept; 14(3):541–552

Gebbie K and Lavin M. Classifying nursing diagnoses. Am J Nurs 1974 Feb; 74(2):250–253

Gordon M. Nursing diagnoses and the diagnostic process. Am J Nurs 1976 Aug; 76(8):1298–1300

Gordon M. Predictive strategies in diagnostic tasks. Nurs Res 1980 Jan–Feb; 29(1):39–45

Gordon M. The concept of nursing diagnosis. Nurs Clin North Am 1979 Sept; 14(3):487–495

Gordon M and Sweeney M. Methodological problems and issues in identifying and standardizing nursing diagnoses. Adv Nurs Sc 1979 Oct; 2(1):1–15

Guzzetta C and Forsyth G. Nursing diagnostic pilot study: Psychophysiologic stress. Adv Nurs Sc 1979 Oct; 2(1): 27–44

Mundinger M and Jauron G. Developing a nursing diagnosis. Nurs Outlook 1975 Feb; 23(2):94–98

Roy C. A diagnostic classification system for nursing. Nurs Outlook 1975 Feb; 23(2):90–94

Shoemaker J. How nursing diagnosis helps focus your care. RN 1979 Aug; 42(8):56–61

Weber S. Nursing diagnosis in private practice. Nurs Clin North Am 1979 Sept; 14(3):533–539

Unpublished Material

Task Force of the National Group for the Classification of Nursing Diagnoses. Subcommittee report on definition of nursing diagnosis. The Fourth National Conference on Classification of Nursing Diagnoses, St. Louis, April 9–13, 1980

INAPPROPRIATE EXPRESSION OF AGGRESSION

Books

Bandura A. Aggression: A Social Learning Analysis. Englewood Cliffs, Prentice-Hall, 1973

Blake K and Taylor C. The Prevention and Management of Aggressive Behavior. Columbia, South Carolina, Department of Mental Health, 1977

Fawcett J (ed). Dynamics of Violence. Chicago, American Medical Association, 1971

Lion J. Evaluation and Management of the Violent Patient. Springfield, Charles C Thomas, 1972

Stegne L. The Prevention and Management of Disturbed Behavior. Toronto, Ontario Government Book Store, 1977

Articles

Armstrong B. Conference report. Handling the violent patient in the hospital. Hosp Community Psychiatry 1978 July; 29(7):463–467

Bursten B. Using mechanical restraints on acutely disturbed psychiatric patients. Hosp Community Psychiatry 1975 Nov; 26(11):757–758

Buss A and Durkee A. An inventory for assessing different kinds of hostility. J Consult Psychol 1957; 21(4):343–349

Carney M and Nolan P. Management of the disturbed patient. Nurs Times 1979 Nov 1; 75:1896–1899

Cocozza J and Steadman H. Some refinements in the measurement and prediction of dangerous behavior. Am J Psychiatry 1974 Sept; 131(9):1012–1014

Edelman S. Managing the violent patient in a community mental health center. Hosp Community Psychiatry 1978 July; 29(7):460–462

Gutheil T. Observations on the theoretical basis for seclusion of the psychiatric inpatient. Am J Psychiatry 1978 Mar; 135(3):325–328

Harrington J. Violence: A clinical viewpoint. Br Med J 1972 Jan 22; 1(5794):228–231

Karhmer J. The application of social learning theory to aggression. Perspect Psychiatr Care 1978 Sept–Dec; 16(5–6):223–227

Lenefsky B, dePalma T, Locicero D. Management of violent behaviors. Perspect Psychiatr Care 1978 Sept–Dec; 16(5–6):212–217

Lathrop V. Aggression as a response. Perspect Psychiatr Care 1978 Sept–Dec; 16(5–6):202–205

Maynard C and Chitty K. Dealing with anger: Guidelines for nursing intervention. J Psychiatr Nurs 1979 June; 17(6):36–41

Moos R. Size, staffing, and psychiatric ward treatment environments. Arch Gen Psychiatry 1972 May; 26(5):414–418

Moritz D. Understanding anger. Am J Nurs 1978 Jan; 78(1):81–83

Murphy P and Schultz E. Passive–aggressive behavior in patients and staff. J Psychiatr Nurs 1978 Mar; 16(3):43–45

Penningroth P. Control of violence in a mental health setting. Am J Nurs 1975 Apr; 75(4):606–609

Rumpler C and Seigerman C. A behavior modification approach to dealing with violent behavior in an Intensive Care Unit. Perspect Psychiatr Care 1978 Sept–Dec; 16(5–6):206–211, 245

Stewart A. Handling the aggressive patient. Perspect Psychiatr Care 1978 Sept–Dec; 16(5–6):228–232

MILD ANXIETY, MODERATE ANXIETY, SEVERE ANXIETY, EXTREME ANXIETY (PANIC)

Books

Grosicki J (ed). Nursing Action Guide. Washington, D.C., Veterans Administration, 1972

Articles

Holderby R and McNulty E. Feelings feelings. Nursing '79 1979 Oct; 9(10):39–43

Kerr N. Anxiety: Theoretical considerations. Perspect Psychiatr Care 1978 Jan–Feb; 16(1):36–40, 46

Knowles R. Dealing with feelings: Managing anxiety. Am J Nurs 1981 Jan; 81(1):110–111

Kristic J. Anxiety levels of hospitalized psychiatric patients throughout total hospitalization. J Psychiatr Nurs 1979 July; 17(7):33–34, 37–42

Liebowitz M and Klein D. Case 1, Assessment and treatment of phobic anxiety. J Clin Psychol 1979 Nov; 40(11):486–492

Pfeiffer E. Handling the distressed older patient. Geriatrics 1979 Feb; 34(2):24–25, 28–29

DYSFUNCTIONAL COMMUNICATION

Books

Berne E. Games People Play. The Psychology of Human Relationships. New York, Grove Press, 1966

Berne E. What Do You Say After You Say Hello? New York, Bantam Books, 1973

Ruesch J. Disturbed Communication; The Clinical Assessment of Normal and Pathological Communication Behavior. New York, WW Norton, 1972

Satir V. Conjoint Family Therapy. Palo Alto, Science and Behavior Books, 1967

Watzlawick P, Beavin J, Jackson D. Pragmatics of Human Communication. New York, WW Norton, 1967

Articles

Bienvenu M. Measurement of marital communication. The Family Coordinator 1970; 19:26–31

Unpublished Material

Sieburg E. Dysfunctional Communication and Interpersonal Responsiveness in Small Groups. Unpublished Doctoral Dissertation, University of Denver, 1969

Wasli E. Dysfunctional Communication Response Patterns of Depressed Wives and Their Husbands in Relation to Activities of Daily Living. Unpublished Doctoral Dissertation, The Catholic University of America, 1977

MATURATIONAL CRISIS, SITUATIONAL CRISIS

Books

Aguilera D and Messick J. Crisis Intervention, Theory and Methodology. St. Louis, CV Mosby, 1978

Butler R and Lewis M. Aging and Mental Health. St. Louis, CV Mosby, 1977

Caplan G. Principles of Preventive Psychiatry. New York, Basic Books, 1964

Jacobson E. Modern Treatment of Tense Patients. Springfield, Charles C Thomas, 1970

Morrice J. Crisis Intervention Studies in Community Care. New York, Pergamon Press, 1976

Parad H. Crisis Intervention; Selected Readings. New York, Family Service Association of America, 1969

Articles

Baldwin B. Crisis intervention: An overview of theory and practice. Counseling Psychol 1979; 8(2):43–52

Chen M. Applying Yalom's principles to crisis work . . . some intriguing results. J Psychiatr Nurs 1978 June; 16(6): 15–22, 27

Cronin–Stubbs D. Family crisis intervention: A study. J Psychiatr Nurs 1978 Jan; 16(1):36–44

Finkelman A. The nurse therapist: Outpatient crisis intervention with the chronic psychiatric patient. J Psychiatr Nurs 1977 Aug; 15(8):27–32

Gaston S. Death and midlife crisis. J Psychiatr Nurs 1980 Jan; 18(1):31–35

Goldstein D. Crisis intervention: A brief therapy model. Nurs Clin North Am 1978 Dec; 13(4):657–663

Hatch C and Schut L. Description of a crisis-oriented psychiatric home visiting service. J Psychiatr Nurs 1980 Apr; 18(4):31–35

Jacobson G. Crisis-oriented therapy. Psychiatr Clin North Am 1979 Apr; 2(1):39–54

Johnston D. Crisis intervention skills. Part I: What is a crisis? J Pract Nurs 1978 Jan; 28(1):16–19

Johnston D. Crisis intervention skills. Part II: Putting the skills to work. J Pract Nurs 1978 Feb; 28(2):20–23

Lancaster B and Berkovsky D. An ecological framework for crisis intervention. J Psychiatr Nurs 1978 Mar; 16(3): 17–23

Phelan L. Crisis intervention: Partnership in problem solving. J Psychiatr Nurs 1979 Sept; 17(9):22–27

DENIAL

Articles

Elliott SM. Denial as an effective mechanism to allay anxiety following a stressful event. J Psychiatr Nurs 1980 Oct; 18(10):11–15

DEPRESSIVE BEHAVIOR

Books

Beck AT. Depression, Causes and Treatment. Philadelphia, University of Pennsylvania Press, 1972

Articles

Authier J, Authier K, Lutey B. Clinical management of the tearfully depressed patient: Communication skills for the nurse practitioner. J Psychiatr Nurs 1979 Feb; 17(2): 34–41

Beck A and Kovacs M. A new, fast therapy for depression. Psychology Today 1977 Jan; 10(8):94–102

Craig TJ and VanNatta PA. Recognition of depressed affect in hospitalized psychiatric patients: Staff and patient perceptions. Dis Nerv Syst 1976 Oct; 37(10):561–566

Rosenbaum M. Depression: What to do, what to say. Nursing '80 1980 Aug; 10(8):64–66

White CL. Nurse counseling with depressed patient. Am J Nurs 1978 Mar; 78(3):436–439

DRUG MISUSE

Books

Bennett J and Demos G. Drug Abuse and What We Can Do About It. Springfield, Charles C Thomas, 1972

Davis C and Schmidt M. Differential Treatment of Drug and Alcohol Abusers. Palm Springs, ETC Publications, 1977

Articles

Abruzzi W. The failure of therapeutic communities, drug treatment, and rehabilitation programs. Int J Addict 1979 Oct; 14(7):1023–1030

Coleman S and Davis D. Family therapy and drug abuse: A national survey. Fam Process 1978 Mar; 17(1):21–29

Family therapy helps addict. JAMA 1979 Feb 9; 241(6):546, 551

Gossop M. Drug dependence—1. The pattern of drug abuse. Nurs Times 1978 June 15; 74(23):996–998

Gossop M. Drug dependence—2. Treatment and nursing care. Nurs Times 1978 June 22; 74(25):1060–1061

Huberty D and Malmquist J. Adolescent chemical dependency. Perspect Psychiatr Care 1978 Jan–Feb; 16(1):21–27

Johnson E and Klotkowski D. Turning an addicted patient on to turning drugs off. RN 1978 May; 41(5):91–97

Klagsbrun M and Davis D. Substance abuse and family interaction. Fam Process 1977 June; 16(2):149–173

Lewin D. Care of the drug-dependent patient. Nurs Times 1978 Apr 13; 74(15):621–624

Panyard C and Wolf K. Attitudinal differences affecting participation in group counseling in outpatient drug treatment centers. Int J Addict 1979 Oct; 14(7):987–992

Personett J. Couples therapy: Treatment of choice with the drug addict. J Psychiatr Nurs 1978 Jan; 16(1):18–21

Quinones M, Doyle K, Sheffet A et al. Evaluation of drug abuse rehabilitation efforts: A review. Am J Public Health 1979 Nov; 69(11):1164–1169

Smith T. The dynamics in time-limited relationship therapy with methadone-maintained patients. Perspect Psychiatr Care 1978 Jan–Feb; 16(1):28–33

Stanton M. Family treatment approaches to drug abuse problems: A review. Fam Process 1979 Sept; 18(3):251–275

Stanton M. The addict as savior: Heroin, death, and the family. Fam Process 1977 June; 16(2):191–197

Vourakis C and Bennett G. Angel dust: Not heaven sent. Am J Nurs 1979 Apr; 79(4):649–653

Weller R and Halikas J. Objective criteria for the diagnosis of marijuana abuse. J Nerv Ment Dis 1980 Feb; 168(2): 98–103

POTENTIAL DYSFUNCTIONAL GRIEVING, DYSFUNCTIONAL GRIEVING

Books

Brown M and Hess P. Nursing and the Concept of Loss. New York, John Wiley & Sons, 1980

Caplan G. Principles of Preventive Psychiatry. New York, Basic Books, 1964

Doyle P. Grief Counseling and Sudden Death. Springfield, Charles C Thomas, 1980

Feifel H. New Meanings of Death. New York, McGraw–Hill, 1977

Glaser B and Strauss A. Awareness of Dying. Chicago, Aldine Publishing Co., 1965

Glaser B and Strauss A. Time for Dying. Chicago, Aldine Publishing Co., 1968

Glick I, Weiss R, Parkes C. The First Year of Bereavement. New York, John Wiley & Sons, 1974

Kubler–Ross E. On Death and Dying. New York, Macmillan, 1969

Lindemann E. Beyond Grief: Studies in Crisis Intervention. New York, Aronson, 1979

Simos B. A Time to Grieve. New York, Family Service Association of America, 1979

Simpson M. Dying, Death, and Grief. New York, Plenum Press, 1979
Werner–Beland J and Agee J. Grief Responses to Long-Term Illness and Disability. Reston, Reston Pub. Co., 1980

Articles

Asbury B, Barton D, Barton L et al. What can you give for grief? Care. Patient Care 1979 Mar; 13(6):100–102, 104, 108–110, 115–116, 121–122, 127–128, 131–132
Blanchard C, Blanchard E, Becker J. The young widow: Depressive symptomatology throughout the grief process. Psychiatry 1976 Nov; 39(4):394–399
Breu C and Dracup K. Helping the spouses of critical patients. Am J Nurs 1978 Jan; 78(1):50–53
Clayton P, Halikas J, Maurice W et al. Anticipatory grief and widowhood. Br J Psychiatry 1973 Jan; 122(566):47–51
Coles P. Breaking the grief barrier. Nurs Mirror 1979 May 31; 148(22):34–35
Courtemanche J. Death in emergency. Can Nurse 1978 Nov; 74(10):24–26
Dracup K and Breu C. Using nursing research findings to meet the needs of grieving spouses. Nurs Res 1978 July–Aug; 27(4):212–216
Engel G. Grief and grieving. Am J Nurs 1964 Sept; 64(9):93–98
Freihofer P and Felton G. Nursing behaviors in bereavement: An exploratory study. Nurs Res 1976 Sept–Oct; 25(5):332–337
Greenblatt M. The grieving spouse. Am J Psychiatry 1978 Jan; 135(1):43–47
Hodgkinson P. Treating abnormal grief in the bereaved. Nurs Times 1980 Jan 17; 76(3):126–128
Horowitz M, Wilner N, Marmar C et al. Pathological grief and the activation of latent self-images. Am J Psychiatry 1980 Oct; 137(10):1157–1162
Jackson E. Wisely managing our grief: A pastoral viewpoint. Death Education 1979 Summer; 3(2):143–155
Lamperelli P and Smith J. The grieving process of adoption; an application of principles and techniques. J Psychiatr Nurs 1979 Oct; 17(10):24–29
Lindemann E. Symptomatology and management of acute grief. Am J Psychiatry 1944 Sept; 101:141–148
McCawley A. Help patients cope with grief. Consultant 1977 Nov; 17(11):64–67
Pett D. Grief in hospital. Nurs Times 1979 Apr 26; 75(17):709–712
Raphael B. Preventive intervention with the recently bereaved. Arch Gen Psychiatry 1977 Dec; 34(12):1450–1454
Schlosser S. The emergency C-section patient. Why she needs help . . . what you can do. RN 1978 Sept; 41(9):52–57
Schmale A. Reactions to illness; convalescence and grieving. Psychiatr Clin North Am 1979 Aug; 2(2):321–330
Schultz C. The dynamics of grief. J Emerg Nurs 1979 Sept–Oct; 5(5):26–30
Stoller E. Effect of experience on nurses' responses to dying and death in the hospital setting. Nurs Res 1980 Jan–Feb; 29(1):35–38
Thompson D. Thoughts on bereavement. Nurs Times 1977 Aug 25; 73(34):1334–1335
Vachon M. Grief and bereavement following the death of a spouse. Can Psychiatr Assoc J 1976 Feb; 21(1):35–43
Weingourt R. Battered women: The grieving process. J Psychiatr Nurs 1979 Apr; 17(4):40–47

GUILT

Articles

Friesen VI. On shame and the family. Fam Therapy 1979 Jan; 6(1):39–58

HYPERACTIVE BEHAVIOR

Articles

Loney J. Hyperkinesis comes of age: What do we know and where should we go? Am J Orthopsychiatry 1980 Jan; 50(1):28–42

INSTITUTIONALIZED BEHAVIOR

Articles

Adelson PY. The back ward dilemma. Am J Nurs 1980 Mar; 80(3):423–425
Bachrach LL. A conceptual approach to deinstitutionalization. Hosp Community Psychiatry 1978 Sept; 29(9):573–578
Craig AE and Hyatt BA. Chronicity in mental illness: A theory on the role of change. Perspect Psychiatr Care 1978 May–June; 16(3):139–154
Haynes B. Institutionalization: What happens to patients in a long-term treatment center. Can Nurs 1980 Mar; 76(3):43–45
Slavinsky AT and Krauss JB. Mutual withdrawal . . . or Gwen Tudor Revisited. Perspect Psychiatr Care 1980 Sept–Oct; 18(5):194–203
Weinberg J. The chronic patient: The stranger in our midst. Hosp Community Psychiatry 1978 Jan; 29(1):25–28

MANIC BEHAVIOR

Articles

Bjork D, Steinberg M, Lindenmayer J, Pardes H. Mania and milieu; treatment of manics in a therapeutic community. Hosp Community Psychiatry 1977 June; 28(6):431–436
Hussey T. Manic–depressive psychosis with rapid and profound changes of mood. Nurs Times 1979 Feb; 75(5):193–195
Krauthammer C and Klerman GL. Secondary mania. Arch Gen Psychiatry 1978 Nov; 35(11):1333–1339
Young RC, Biggs JT, Ziegler VE, Meyer DA. A rating scale for mania: Reliability, validity and sensitivity. Br J Psychiatry 1978 Nov; 133(11):429–435

MANIPULATION

Articles

Schlemmer JK and Barnett PA. Management of manipulative behavior of anorexia nervosa patients. J Psychiatr Nurs 1977 Nov; 15(11):35–41
Carser D. The defense mechanism of splitting: Developmental origins, effects on staff, recommendations for nursing care. J Psychiatr Nurs 1979 Mar; 17(3):21–28
Neill JR. The difficult patient: Identification and response. J Clin Psychiatry 1979 May; 40(5):209–212

NONCOMPLIANCE

Articles

Amarasingham LR. Social and cultural perspectives on medication refusal. Am J Psychiatry 1980 Mar; 137(3):353–358
Baile WF and Engel BT. Behavioral strategy for promoting treatment compliance following myocardial infarction. Psychosom Med 1978 Aug; 40(5):413–419
Connelly CE. Patient compliance: A review of the research with implications for psychiatric–mental health nursing. J Psychiatr Nurs 1978 Oct; 16(10):15–18
McMorrow MJ, Cullinan D, Epstein MH. The use of the premack principle to motivate patient activity attendance. Perspect Psychiatr Care 1978 Jan–Feb; 16(1):14–18
Radius SM, Becker MH, Rosenstock IM et al. Factors influencing mother's compliance with a medical regimen for asthmatic children. J Asthma Res 1978 Apr; 15(3):133–149
Steckel SB and Swain MA. Contracting with patients to improve compliance. Hospitals 1977 Dec; 51:81–84
Tessler R and Mason JH. Continuity of care in the delivery of mental health services. Am J Psychiatr 1979 Oct; 136(10):1297–1301
Wiley L (ed). How can you improve patient compliance? Nursing '78 1978 May; 8(5):40–47

DYSFUNCTIONAL BEHAVIOR RELATED TO CHRONIC ORGANIC BRAIN DISEASE

Books

Dennis H. Remotivation therapy groups. In Burnside I (ed). Working with the Elderly: Group Process and Techniques, Chapt. 14. North Scituate, Duxbury Press, 1978

Ebersole P. Establishing reminiscing groups. In Burnside I (ed). Working with the Elderly: Group Process and Techniques, Chapt. 15. North Scituate, Duxbury Press, 1978

Freedman A, Kaplan H, Sadock B. Modern Synopsis of Comprehensive Textbook of Psychiatry. Baltimore, Williams & Wilkins, 1978

Taulbee L. Reality orientation: A therapeutic group activity for elderly persons. In Burnside I (ed). Working with the Elderly: Group Process and Techniques, Chapt. 13. North Scituate, Duxbury Press, 1978

Articles

Chivers T and Westwater J. Hospital care of confused elderly people. Nursing (Oxford) 1980 Jan; 9:393–396

Hansen L. Treatment of reduced intellectual functioning in alcoholics. J Stud Alcohol 1980 Jan; 41(1):156–158

Kiernat J. The use of life review activity with confused nursing home residents. Am J Occup Ther 1979 May; 33(5):306–310

Sidell M. Confused elderly people and community care. Nursing (Oxford) 1980 Jan; 9:399–402

Trockman G. Caring for the confused or delirious patient. Am J Nurs 1978 Sept; 78(9):1495–1499

ALTERATIONS IN PERCEPTIONS

Articles

Deiker T and Chambers HE. Structure and content of hallucinations in alcohol withdrawal and functional psychosis. J Stud Alcohol 1978 Nov; 39(11):1831–1840

Field WE and Ruelke W. Hallucinations and how to deal with them. Am J Nurs 1973 Apr; 73(4):638–640

Schwartzman ST. The hallucinating patient and nursing intervention. J Psychiatr Nurs 1975 Nov–Dec; 13(6): 23–36

Siegel RK. Hallucinations. Sci Am 1977 Oct; 237(4):132–140

INAPPROPRIATE USE OF PHYSICAL SYMPTOMS

Books

Altman N. Hypochondriasis. In Strain J and Grossman S (ed). Psychological Care of the Medically Ill. New York, Appleton–Century–Crofts, 1975

Articles

Hall RC, Gardner ER, Stickney SK et al. Physical illness manifesting as psychiatric disease. Arch Gen Psychiatry 1980 Sept; 37(9):989–995

Steinhart MJ and Dutton CB. Symptoms—physical or function, Part 1. Physical symptoms of psychological conditions. Consultant 1977 Mar; 17(3):38–44

PROBLEM DRINKING

Books

Estes N and Heinemann M. Alcoholism: Development, Consequences, and Interventions. St. Louis, CV Mosby, 1977

Ewing J and Rouse B. Drinking, Alcohol in American Society—Issues and Current Research. Chicago, Nelson–Hall, 1978

Glaser F, Greenberg S, Barrett M. A Systems Approach to Alcohol Treatment. Toronto, Addiction Research Foundation, 1978

Articles

Brown L and Ostrow F. The development of an assertiveness program on an alcoholism unit. Int J Addict 1980 Apr; 15(3):323–327

Caddy G, Addington H, Perkins D. Individualized behavior therapy for alcoholics: A third year independent double-blind follow-up. Behav Res Ther 1978 May; 16(5): 345–362

Crumbaugh J and Carr G. Treatment of alcoholics with logotherapy. Int J Addict 1979 Aug; 14(6):847–853

Finlay D. Alcoholism and systems theory: Building a better mousetrap. Psychiatry 1978 Aug; 41(3):272–278

Fischer J. The relationship between alcoholic patients' milieu perception and measures of their drinking during a brief follow-up period. Int J Addict 1979 Nov; 14(8): 1151–1156

Gareri E. Assertiveness training for alcoholics. J Psychiatr Nurs 1979 Jan; 17(1):31–36

Gilbert G, Parker J, Claiborn C. Differential mood changes in alcoholics as a function of anxiety management strategies. J Clin Psychol 1978 Jan; 34(1):229–232

Hirsch S, Rosenberg R, Phelan C et al. Effectiveness of assertiveness training with alcoholics. J Stud Alcohol 1978 Jan; 39(1):89–97

Intagliata J. Increasing the interpersonal problem-solving skills of an alcoholic population. J Consult Clin Psychol 1978 June; 46(3):489–498

Kennedy R, Gilbert G, Thoreson R. A self-control program for drinking antecedents: The role of self-monitoring and control orientation. J Clin Psychol 1978 Jan; 34(1):238–243

Kurtines W, Ball L, Wood C. Personality characteristics of long-term recovered alcoholics: A comparative analysis. J Consult Clin Psychol 1978 Oct; 46(5):971–977

MacDonough T. Evaluation of the effectiveness of intensive confrontation in changing the behavior of alcohol and drug abusers. Int J Addict 1978 May; 13(4):529–589

McCourt W and Glantz M. Cognitive behavior therapy in groups for alcoholics. J Stud Alcohol 1980 Mar; 41(3): 338–346

McFarland G and Apostoles F. The nursing history in a psychiatric setting: Adaptation to a variety of nursing care patterns and patient populations. J Psychiatr Nurs 1975 July–Aug; 13(4):12–17

Miller W. Behavior treatment of problem drinkers: A comparative outcome study of three controlled drinking therapies. J Consult Clin Psychol 1978 Feb; 46(1): 74–86

Moos R and Bromet E. Relation of patient attributes to perceptions of the treatment environment. J Consult Clin Psychol 1978 Apr; 46(2):350–351

Owen P. A multimodal treatment approach for incarcerated alcoholics. J Clin Psychol 1978 Oct; 34(4):1005–1009

Page R and Schaub L. EMG biofeedback applicability for differing personality types. J Clin Psychol 1978 Oct; 34(4):1014–1020

Parker J and Gilbert G. Reduction of autonomic arousal in alcoholics: A comparison of relaxation and meditation techniques. J Consult Clin Psychol 1978 Oct; 46(5): 879–886

Van Gee S. Alcoholism and the family: A psychodrama approach. J Psychiatr Nurs 1979 Aug; 17(8):9–12

Vannicelli M. Treatment contracts in an inpatient alcoholism treatment setting. J Stud Alcohol 1979 May; 40(5): 457–471

RITUALISTIC BEHAVIOR

Articles

Misik IM. Dr. Evans, obsessed with food, was starving himself. Nursing '80 1980 Mar; 10(3):54–56

Rachman S and de Silva P. Abnormal and normal obsessions. Behav Res Ther 1978 Apr; 16(4):233–248

ALTERATIONS IN SELF-ESTEEM

Books

Clark C. Assertive Skills for Nurses. Wakefield, Contemporary Publishing, 1978

Fitts W. The Self Concept and Performance. Nashville, Dede Wallace Center, 1972

Fitts W. The Self Concept and Psychopathology. Nashville, Dede Wallace Center, 1972

Hamachek D. Encounters with the Self. New York, Holt, Rinehart, & Winston, 1971

Lewis G. Nurse–Patient Communication. Dubuque, Wm C Brown Co., 1978

Moskowitz R. Assertiveness for Career and Personal Success. New York, American Management Association, 1977

Rosenberg M. Conceiving the Self. New York, Basic Books, 1979

Articles

Goldberg C and Stanitis M. The enhancement of self-esteem through the communication process in group therapy. J Psychiatr Nurs 1977 Dec; 15(12):5–8

Knowles R. Dealing with feelings: Control your thoughts. Am J Nurs 1981 Feb; 81(2):353

INAPPROPRIATE SEXUAL BEHAVIOR

Articles

Akhtar S, Crocker E, Dickey N et al. Overt sexual behavior among psychiatric inpatients. Dis Nerv Syst 1977 May; 38(5):359–361

Hampton PJ. Coping with the male patient's sexuality. Nurs Forum 1979 18(3):304–310

Paradowski W. Socialization patterns and sexual problems of the institutionalized chronically ill and physically disabled. Arch Phys Med Rehabil 1977 Feb; 58(2):53–59

Shaul S and Morrey L. Sexuality education in a state mental hospital. Hosp Community Psychiatry 1980 Mar; 31(3):175–179

SPIRITUAL DISTRESS

Books

Fish S and Shelly J. Spiritual Care: The Nurse's Role. Downers Grove, Inter-Varsity Press, 1978

Henderson V and Nite G. Principles and Practice of Nursing. New York, Macmillan, 1978

Spiritual Perspectives, Vols. I & II (Reprints from The Nurses Lamp). Madison, Nurses Christian Fellowship, 1969–1978

Stallwood J and Stoll R. Spiritual dimensions of nursing practice. In Beland I and Passos J (eds). Clinical Nursing, Pathophysiological and Psychosocial Approaches. New York, Macmillan Pub. Co., 1975

Articles

Carson V. Meeting the spiritual needs of hospitalized psychiatric patients. Perspect Psychiatr Care 1980 Jan–Feb; 18(1):17–20

Carson V and Huss K. Prayer—an effective therapeutic and teaching tool. J Psychiatr Nurs 1979 Mar; 17(3):34–37

Delgado M. Puerto Rican spiritualism and the social work profession. Soc Case 1977 Oct; 58(8):451–458

Dickinson C. The search for spiritual meaning. Am J Nurs 1975 Oct; 75(10):1789–1793

Ellison C. Psychology, christianity, and urban need. J Psychol Theol 1978 Fall; 6(4):283–290

Galanter M and Buckley P. Evangelical religion and meditation: Psychotherapeutic effects. J Nerv Ment Dis 1978 Oct; 166(10):685–691

Gibbs H and Achterberg–Lawlis J. Spiritual values and death anxiety; implications for counseling with terminal cancer patients. J Couns Psychol 1978 Nov; 25(6):563–569

Gilloway F and Donnelly L. Religion and patient care: The functionalist approach. J Adv Nurs 1977 Jan; 2(1):3–13

Hadaway C. Life satisfaction and religion: A reanalysis. Soc Forces 1978 Dec; 57(2):636–643

Heukelem J. Weep with those who weep: Understanding and helping the crying person. J Psychol Theology 1979 Summer; 7(2):83–91

Hynson L. Belief in life after death and societal integration. Omega: J Death and Dying 1978–79; 9(1):13–18

Paloutzian R, Jackson S, Crandall J. Conversion experience, belief system, and personal and ethical attitudes. J Psychol Theol 1978 Fall; 6(4):266–275

Piepgras R. The other dimension: Spiritual help. Am J Nurs 1968 Dec; 68(12):2610–2613

Pumphrey J. Recognizing your patients' spiritual needs. Nursing '77 1977 Dec; 7(12):64–70

Stoll R. Guidelines for spiritual assessment. Am J Nurs 1979 Sept; 79(9):1574–1577

Vaillot M. The spiritual factors in nursing. J Pract Nurs 1970 Sept; 20(9):30–31

THREATENED SUICIDE, ATTEMPTED SUICIDE

Books

Kiev A. The Suicidal Patient: Recognition and Management. Chicago, Nelson–Hall, 1977

Kiev A. The prevention of suicide. In Masserman J (ed). Current Psychiatric Therapies Vol. 18–1978, pp 91–95. New York, Grune & Stratton, 1979

Articles

Beck A and Kovacs M. Assessment of suicidal intention: The scale for suicide ideation. J Consult Clin Psychol 1979 Apr; 47(2):343–352

Bressler B. Depression and suicide. Consultant 1978 Mar; 18(3):123–126, 129

DiVasto P, West D, Christy J. A framework for the emergency evaluation of the suicidal patient. J Psychiatr Nurs 1979 June; 17(6):15–20

Eggland E. Dealing with tragedy: The aftermath of suicide. J Nurs Care 1978 Dec; 11(12):14–15

Gurrister L and Kane R. How therapists perceive and treat suicidal patients. Community Ment Health J 1978 Spring; 14(1):3–13

Hopper K and Guttmacher S. Re-thinking suicide notes toward a critical epidemiology. Int J Health Serv 1979; 9(3):417–438

Reubin R. Spotting and stopping the suicide patient. Nursing '79 1979 Apr; 9(4):82–85

Zung W. Suicide prevention by suicide detection. Psychosomatics 1979 Mar; 20(3):149, 153–159

SUSPICIOUSNESS

Articles

Modly MM. Paranoid states. J Psychiatr Nurs 1978 May; 16(5):35–37

DISTURBED THOUGHT PROCESS

Articles

Schroder RJ. Nursing intervention with patient with thought disorders. Perspect Psychiatr Care 1979 Jan–Feb; 17(1):32–39

WITHDRAWAL

Articles

Yoder SA. Alienation as a way of life. Perspect Psychiatr Care 1977 Mar–Apr; 15(2):66–71

Tudor G. A sociopsychiatric nursing approach to intervention in a problem of mutual withdrawal on a mental hospital ward. Perspect Psychiatr Care 1970 Jan–Feb; 8(1):11–35

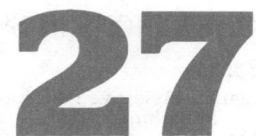
SELECTED MENTAL DISORDERS

The American Psychiatric Association's *Diagnostic and Statistical Manual of Mental Disorders** divides mental disorders into 17 major diagnostic categories. Disorders from 9 of the categories are presented below.

ORGANIC MENTAL DISORDERS

Organic mental disorders represent a group of mental disorders that present a variety of symptoms, especially a disturbance of cognition.

Incidence

1. Delirium is common in general hospitals, with an estimated 5% to 15% of patients exhibiting symptoms.
2. Dementia impairs about 1,000,000 people; Alzheimer's disease is the most common type.

Etiology

A number of factors are important:
1. Vascular disorders
2. Metabolic changes
3. Growth impairments
4. Nutritional deficiencies
5. Trauma
6. Drugs
7. Poison
8. Infections
9. Tumors
10. Epilepsy
11. Degenerative diseases
12. Stress

Clinical Features of Selected Types

A. *Delirium*—sudden onset of impairment of all cognitive functions.

* American Psychiatric Association. Diagnostic & Statistical Manual of Mental Disorders, 3rd ed. Washington, D.C., American Psychiatric Association, 1980.

1. *State of consciousness impairment*
   a. Mild—indecisiveness, weakness, problems in judging time, difficulty paying attention and thinking logically, episodes of untidiness.
   b. Severe—drowsy, sleeping most of day, unable to comprehend requests, frequently sleeping by day and experiencing a state of excitement at night.
2. *Psychomotor impairment*—varies from mild slowing (little spontaneous movement, apathy) to inactivity, to overactivity and noisiness.
3. *Thinking impairment*
   a. Early signs—problems in presenting complex ideas, increase in importance of own internal world, loss of insight.
   b. More severe signs—concreteness and disorganization, not knowing if one is inside or outside, sitting or standing; persecutory delusions, mixing of past and present experiences.
3. *Memory impairment*
   a. May at first be to time (e.g., a missing of sequences of time or not realizing that so much time has passed).
   b. Later impairment related to place and person with confabulations and false memories.
4. *Perception impairment*
   a. Occurs in visual field especially.
   b. Ranges from a blurring to changing shapes to hallucinations.
5. *Emotional impairment*—ranges from early depression to later apathy.

B. *Dementia*—a slow deterioration in cognitive functioning causing multiple changes.

1. Early signs include:
   a. Losing objects
   b. Mixing up appointments
   c. Not being aware of recent occurrences
   d. Making mistakes with money
   e. Being inefficient at work
   f. Not grasping important things
   g. Displaying poor social manners, social blunders

(stealing, exposing self), bizarre behavior (putting food in washing machine)
    h. Tiring easily
    i. Having poverty of ideas (cliches and set phrases said repeatedly)
    j. Showing forgetfulness, irritability, anxiety
2. Later signs include:
    a. Neglect of personal hygiene and disordered appearance
    b. Indifference, sloppy eating manners
    c. Incontinence
    d. Aimlessness
    e. No new thoughts, inflexible
    f. Paranoid ideation
    g. Speech broken and used to obtain food or other physical needs
    h. Disorientation, apathy
    i. Euphoria at times
    j. Increasingly flat in affect to complete inactivity
C. *Organic Delusional Syndrome*—a disorder with delusions related to an organic factor such as amphetamines, alcohol, and cocaine.
D. *Organic Affective Syndrome*—a disorder with mood disturbance related to organic factor, such as amphetamines and hallucinogens.
E. *Organic Disorders Associated with Circulatory Disturbances*
1. Lack of cellular oxygenation results in ischemia or infarction with localized (lacunae) or diffuse changes.
2. Transient Cerebral Ischemic Attacks (TIA) are episodes of dysfunction lasting 5 to 15 minutes and are risk factors for cerebral infarction.
F. *Senile Dementia*—a disorder of unknown cause characterized by severe impairment of intellectual functioning; if it occurs when person is under 65 years of age, it is called Alzheimer's Disease.
G. *Focal Cerebral Disorders*
1. *Frontal lobe*—Person has changes of personality with overfamiliarity, talkativeness, excitement, joking, punning tactlessness.
2. *Parietal lobe*—Person has variety of cognitive disturbances.
3. *Temporal lobe*—Person has disturbance of intellectual functioning associated with emotional instability and aggressive misconduct; epileptic phenomena.
4. *Occipital lobe*—Person has visual field effects.
5. *Corpus callosum*—Person has rapid intellectual deterioration.
6. *Diencephalon and brain stem*—Person has recent short-term memory loss and hypersomnia.
H. *Organic Mental Disorders Induced by Drugs or Poisons*
1. *Intoxication*
    a. Generally includes changes in perception, attention, thinking, wakefulness, judgment, emotional control, and psychomotor behavior.
    b. The changes are directly related to the ingestion of specific substances.
    c. Most symptoms are related to decrease in level of consciousness, interfering with sensory input.
2. *Withdrawal*
    a. Generally includes anxiety, restlessness, insomnia, irritability, impaired attention, GI symptoms, weakness, desire for drug, sleep-pattern disturbances, convulsions.
    b. The symptoms are related to the ingestion of the specific substance.

3. *Sedatives and hypnotics* are associated with half of the patients with disorders induced by drugs or poisons.

Treatment

A. *Delirium*

Treatment of delirium is focused on elimination of physical cause; symptom relief; prevention of complications, especially injuries from falling; nutritional supplements; psychotropics to assist in agitation; and environmental management.

B. *Dementia*

1. Treatment of dementia is also directed towards elimination of any physical cause; however, in the majority of cases there is no specific treatment.
2. Treatment includes symptom relief; medications to relieve anxiety, depression, or agitation; psychotherapy with focus on management of anxiety, loss, and changes in life-style; and rehabilitation techniques.

C. *Disorder Induced by Drugs or Poisons*

Treatment of disorders induced by drugs or poisons is directed at the removal of the toxic substance from the body, management of agitation with minimal medication, adequate nutrition, monitoring of vital signs, uncovering of the reasons for the ingestion of substance, and supportive psychotherapy.

Health Education

A. *Delirium*

Teach patient and family that outcome is generally a full return to previous functioning level.

B. *Dementia*

Show family ways to offer emotional support to each other and ways to cope with stress of seeing older family member change.

C. *Disorders Induced by Specific Causes*

Instruct persons involved in ways to avoid cause or deal with consequence.

Commonly Associated Nursing Diagnoses

Inappropriate expression of aggression
Anxiety
Depressive behavior
Drug misuse
Dysfunctional behavior related to chronic organic brain disease
Regressive behavior
Problem drinking
Alterations in self-care activities
Suspiciousness
Withdrawal
Disturbed thought processes

SUBSTANCE USE DISORDERS

Substance use disorders are a group of mental disorders manifested by impairments in social and occupational functions that are related to a regular use of specific substances that are intended to alter mood or behavior.

Definitions

A. *Intoxication*—a term used to indicate specific symptoms including disturbed behavior associated with ingestion of substance.

B. *Abuse*—a term used to indicate a daily use of substance in order to function, intoxication, inability to stop use, and disturbed social and work behaviors (arrests, car accidents, absences from work, fights) for at least a 1-month period.

C. *Dependence*—a term used to indicate the presence of physiological dependence.

1. *Tolerance*—a term used to indicate that more of the substance is needed to obtain the same effect or that the same amount of the substance is not producing the same effect.
2. *Withdrawal*—a term used to indicate a syndrome following the absence of the usual intake of the substance. Symptoms of anxiety, insomnia, irritability, restlessness, and impaired attention along with symptoms related to the lack of the specific substance are present.

Incidence

1. Alcoholism affects 9–10 million people and is considered by some to be the number one health problem.
2. Onset of alcoholism occurs in the teens to the 40s; other types of substance abuse begins in adolescence.
3. Heroin addicts number 1–3 million.
4. Substance abuse is more common in men.
5. Barbiturate overdose is related to 6% of deaths by suicide.
6. Diazepam (Valium), alcohol, and heroin are the top three drugs used by patients seen in emergency department.

Etiology

No known specific cause, but suggested hypotheses are:
1. Psychodynamic theory—emphasizes a fixation at oral stage of development, such as failure to develop internal controls and continued insistence on immediate gratification
2. Presence of a personality disorder
3. Family-relationship problems
4. Children having problems in school, having health problems, and being narcissistic
5. Overdependence on mother and hostility towards father
6. Peer pressure
7. Familial association noted in alcoholism
8. Physiological theories to explain dependence as the substance affecting the neurotransmittors or affecting cellular adaptation
9. Overprescribed medication

Clinical Manifestations of Selected Types Associated with Abuse and Dependence

A. *Opiates, Morphine, Heroin*
1. Taken orally, I.V. (needle tracts) and subcutaneously (skin pops and nodules).
2. Nonmedical use:
   To achieve pain relief and euphoria.
3. Intoxication:
   Pinpoint pupils, slow respirations, slow pulse, low blood pressure, hypothermia, drowsiness, euphoria, apathy, dysphoria, impairment in memory and attention.
4. Overdose:
   a. Coma, shock, pinpoint pupils, respiratory depression.

b. Treatment is with use of Naloxone.
5. Withdrawal:
   a. Symptoms occur within a week after last dose.
   b. Early signs: restlessness, dilatation of pupils, sweating, tearing, runny nose, yawning, fever.
   c. Later signs: muscle aches and spasms, G.I. symptoms, increased blood pressure, insomnia, anorexia, agitation.
6. Dependence:
   a. Persons use drug for an average of 9 years.
   b. There is a high death rate related to violent lifestyles and physical complications.

B. *Amphetamines*
1. Taken orally, I.V., or by inhalation.
2. Nonmedical use:
   To provide relief from fatigue, to assist with studying, to produce euphoria and sense of well-being, and to recover from hangover.
3. Intoxication:
   a. Elation, talkativeness, pacing, hypervigilance, dilatation of pupils, tachycardia, increased blood pressure, G.I. symptoms, chills, perspiration, and sometimes persistent delusions or hallucinations.
   b. Is similar to cocaine.
4. Overdose:
   Convulsions, cardiovascular shock, hyperpyrexia.
5. Amphetamine delirium:
   Includes symptoms of delirium, changing affect, and frequent aggressive, violent behavior.
6. Withdrawal:
   Depression, anxiety, lethargy, disorientation, irritability, muscle spasms, G.I. symptoms, sweating, headache.
7. Dependence:
   a. Pattern of use is characteristically heavy use for several days or weeks (a "run"), then abstinence, producing a "crash."
   b. This may continue for a year.

C. *Barbiturates* or similarly acting hypnotics (Valium, methaqualone)
1. Taken orally most frequently, but may be given I.V.
2. Nonmedical use:
   a. For nervousness, insomnia.
   b. To obtain a high or sense of well-being.
3. Intoxication:
   a. Slurred speech, unsteadiness, poor memory and attention, impaired judgment, talkativeness, irritability, hostility, sexual aggressiveness.
   b. Is similar to alcohol intoxication.
4. Overdose:
   Death is frequently by an accidental overdose.
5. Withdrawal:
   G.I. symptoms, weakness, increased blood pressure, sweating, anxiety, depressed mood, coarse tremors, convulsions.
6. Dependence:
   Person may eventually cease taking the drug.

D. *Cannabis (marihuana)*
1. Taken by smoking and ingested.
2. Nonmedical use:
   For a high and to enhance creativity.
3. Intoxication:
   a. May be initial anxiety for 10–30 minutes then euphoria, intensified perceptions, slowed time, apathy, tachycardia, dry mouth, increased appetite, passivity, drowsiness.

b. Always conjunctival injection (bloodshot eyes due to dilation of arterioles).
c. Lasts about three hours.
d. Experience is affected by expectations of users.
4. Death is rare.
5. Dependence:
a. Is a controversial issue.
b. Some people stop when impairment of functioning begins.

E. *Alcohol*

1. Taken orally in varying strengths in types of drinks.
2. Nonmedical use:
To relax, to be life of the party and to have sense of being "sharp."
3. Intoxication:
Slurred speech, unsteadiness, memory and attention problems, incoordination, talkativeness, irritability, depression, withdrawal, aggressive and sexual acts, nystagmus, flushed face, blackouts, blood level of alcohol 100–200 mg.%
4. Overdose:
a. Unconsciousness with blood level of 400 mg./dl. to 500 mg./dl.
b. Death with blood level of 600 mg./dl. to 800 mg./dl. with complications of respiratory depression.
5. Withdrawal:
a. Coarse tremors of hands, tongue, and eyelids; increased blood pressure and pulse; diaphoresis; hyperirritability; G.I. symptoms.
b. Occurs within several hours or days after alcohol use and continues about one week unless delirium develops.
6. Alcohol withdrawal delirium (delirium tremens):
a. Is a disorder including delirium delusions and visual hallucinations, tremors, and unpredictable or violent acts.
b. Occurs 2 to 3 days after last drinking episode and lasts about one week.
7. Dependence:
May continue throughout life span.

Clinical Manifestations of Selected Types Associated with Abuse

A. *Cocaine*

1. Taken by sniffing through nose, through injection, and through genitals.
2. Nonmedical use:
To achieve "rush" of well-being and confidence, to be more talkative and energetic, and to assist in performance of sports and music.
3. Intoxication:
Elation, talkativeness, pacing, hypervigilance, dilation of pupils, tachycardia, increased blood pressure and pulse, chills, perspiration, transient delusions and hallucinations.
4. Death is rare.
5. Abuse:
a. Pattern may continue 2 to 8 months.
b. Moral deterioration is frequently associated with its use.

B. *Phencyclidine (PCP)*

1. Taken orally, I.V., or by sniffing or smoking.
2. Nonmedical use:
To achieve some self-learning or social experience.
3. Intoxication:
Nystagmus, increased blood pressure and pulse,

ataxia, dysarthria, diminished responsiveness to pain, euphoria, agitation, anxiety, grandiosity, emotional lability, synesthesias, slowing of time, unpleasantness.
4. Death is possible but rare.

C. *Hallucinogens (LSD, DMT, mescaline)*

1. Taken orally or smoked.
2. Nonmedical use:
To elevate mood.
3. Hallucinogen hallucinosis:
Synesthesias, visual hallucinations, illusions, depersonalization, derealization, intensified perceptions, dilation of pupils, tachycardia, sweating, blurring of vision, tremors, incoordination.
4. Bad trips:
a. Is a panic state lasting 8 to 12 hours.
b. For guidelines of "talking down," see p. 894.
5. Flashbacks:
a. Are a repetition of an aspect of the drug-induced experience, such as a flash of light or seeing a figure lasting seconds or minutes occurring days to weeks after ingestion.
b. Marihuana smoking is frequently associated with flashbacks.
6. Abuse:
Generally occurs for brief periods only.

Treatment

A. *Varied Problems*

There is no one treatment to deal with varied problems.

B. *Complications*

Treatment of associated complications, such as malnutrition, infections from use of contaminated needles and syringes, allergic reactions, erosion of nasal septum from cocaine "snorting" (placement of cocaine in nose), hepatitis, gastritis, neuropathy, venereal disease, cirrhosis, pancreatitis, family disruption, and social problems.

C. *Detoxification Programs*

1. Alcohol user
Antianxiety drugs are given to assist patient in dealing with withdrawal symptoms, along with frequent evaluation and support by psychiatrists.
2. Opiate user
a. Methadone is given in progressively decreasing doses for help with the withdrawal symptoms.
b. Other therapies may be offered.

D. *Therapeutic Communities*

1. Alcoholics Anonymous
a. Group is organized to provide group support of abstinence based on a 12-step program.
b. There is also an organization for spouses of alcoholics, Al-Anon.
2. Synanon, Phoenix House
Are groups organized to assist the addict through a highly structured program and some degree of isolation from others.

E. *Maintenance Program for Addicts*

a. Is to assist patient in achieving a comfortable state, but without feelings of euphoria experienced with opiate use.
b. Controversy exists over the 2-year limit on the maintenance program for the individual addict.

F. *Use of Deterrents*

1. Disulfiram (Antabuse)
   a. Drug is taken daily and causes toxic reaction if alcohol is taken also.
   b. Symptoms include flushed feeling, weakness, nausea, low blood pressure.
2. Narcotic antagonists (Naloxone, Cyclazocine) A group of drugs used to block the effects of opiates.

G. *Anxiety and Depression*

Antianxiety and antidepressant medications to assist with the symptoms of anxiety and depression.

H. *Psychotherapy*

Psychotherapy for alcoholics in various forms to deal with problems of denial, reasons for drinking behaviors, and avoidance of sobriety.

I. *Delirium Tremens*

   a. Librium or Valium is used to prevent delirium tremens during alcoholic withdrawal.
   b. High-caloric and high-carbohydrate diet, multivitamins, antianxiety medications, fluids, and assistance to control agitated, aggressive behaviors are needed.

J. *Other Approaches*

1. Relaxation techniques.
2. Behavior modification to teach alternatives to drinking or to modify or stop drinking.
3. Crisis intervention.
4. Alcoholism is difficult to treat because of the patient's intense denial and associated behaviors, and the negative attitudes generated in the staff treating him.
5. Treatment of drug dependence is more frequently associated with achieving a drug-free state rather than with emotional problems preceding drug use.

Health Education

1. Drug and alcohol education programs in school system to prevent abuse.
2. Teach patient the numerous alcohol–drug interactions:
   a. Depressant effects of alcohol and barbiturates, minor and major tranquilizers, narcotics.
   b. Sedative effects enhanced by alcohol and antihistamines.
   c. Many other drugs have antagonistic, additive, or cross-tolerance interaction with alcohol; therefore, have patient carefully tell doctor all medications he is on, and encourage him to stop drinking.
3. Discuss with patient the increased risk for heart disease, tuberculosis, pneumonia, cirrhosis, neurological disorders, car accidents, committing murder, committing suicide, injury while falling, or being exposed to extremes of temperature.

Commonly Associated Nursing Diagnoses

Anxiety
Depressed behavior
Impaired self-care activities
Threatened or attempted suicide
Inappropriate expression of aggression
Problem drinking
Drug misuse
Noncompliance
Denial
Alterations in perceptions

SCHIZOPHRENIC DISORDERS

Schizophrenia represents a group of mental disorders that present varied symptoms of disordered thinking and bizarre social behaviors.

Incidence

1. About 1% of the total population is affected; is most prevalent of the major psychoses.
2. Affects adolescents and young adults.
3. There is an increased incidence in lower social class.

Risk Factors

1. Family member with schizophrenia
2. Difficult delivery with trauma to brain of child
3. Children who are:
   a. Highly individualistic in their thought processes
   b. Overly dependent and obedient
   c. Unable to enjoy life
   d. Shy, withdrawn, and loners
   e. Sensitive to separation
   f. Unmanageable; displaying destructive, aggressive behavior
   g. Truant from school
4. Parents who are:
   a. Hostile, very possessive, insensitive to needs of children
   b. Suspicious, and inclined toward disturbances in thinking
5. Illness
   a. Medical condition (e.g., temporal lobe epilepsy)
   b. Drug abuse (e.g., marihuana, PCP) and chemical factors (e.g., MAO-B in blood platelets).
6. Abnormal eye pursuit movements.

Etiology

No single cause, but hypotheses and research studies indicate several possible factors:
1. Environmental stress, such as crisis, migration
2. Genetic factors, especially in twins
3. Effects of early trauma on response to intrapsychic conflict
4. Learned behavior responses that are nonadaptive
5. Deviations of ego and superego development resulting in impairment of functioning; deviations may be related to:
   a. Increased sensitivity to stimuli
   b. Disturbances in mother–child relationship
   c. Problems in separation–individualization phases of development as child begins to walk
6. Close bond between mother and child
7. Disturbed family interaction patterns (double bind, pseudomutuality in relationships among family members, family projection process)
8. Dopamine hypothesis
   a. There is an increased sensitivity to dopamine by the postsynaptic receptor.
   b. There is an increased amount available at synapse.
   c. There is an imbalance in the neurotransmitters between inhibitory action (dopamine and GABA) and excitatory action (acetylcholine).

Clinical Manifestations

A. *Early signs:*

1. Blocking or cutting off conversation; not responding as usual to friends, appearing aloof
2. Experiencing blackouts or other spells
3. Expressing various body symptom concerns
4. Forgetting and abandoning plans or life goals
5. Disregarding social customs and talking about abstract ideas such as love, creation, equality

B. *Onset:*

An experience involving loss, separation, rejection; or use of LSD, marihuana, alcohol, amphetamine.

C. *Symptoms:*

1. Hallucinations, especially auditory.
   The voices are heard commenting in general about patient or making obscene, threatening remarks.
2. Sensory disturbances, especially optical (e.g., changing shapes and figures are seen).
3. Delusions of persecution, grandeur, or impending destruction.
4. Austistic thinking characterized by being highly personal and not logical with perseveration, blocking, concretization, and loosening of associations.
5. Speech characterized by incoherence, use of symbols, and concrete responses. Patient may exhibit echolalia, flight of ideas, or neologisms or may be mute.
6. Inappropriate behavior, such as grimacing, negativism, anergia (state of inaction), suggestibility, poor personal hygiene, few social manners.
7. Blunting, ambivalence, and inappropriateness of affect.

Selected Types

A. *Catatonic Schizophrenia*—a disorder characterized by:

1. Stuporous state in which person is mute, is negative or complains in response to a request; is immobile; displays waxy flexibility; may retain urine and feces
2. Excited state in which person is assaultive, aggressive, hyperactive, or agitated

B. *Disorganized Schizophrenia*—a disorder characterized by incoherence, foolishness, and regressive behavior.

C. *Paranoid Schizophrenia*—a disorder characterized by delusions of persecution or grandeur.

D. *Undifferentiated Schizophrenia*—a disorder characterized by a variety of symptoms found in several types.

Treatment

A variety of therapies are available and are used to meet treatment goals designed for the individual patient.

1. *Short hospitalization*—to assist with problems of dangerousness to self or others, of deviant behaviors that are increasingly abrasive to family and community, and of monitoring effects of drugs or other therapies.
2. *Day treatment and outpatient treatment*—to provide help with problems arising from familial, work, and social situations while remaining in the situations.
3. *Outpatient treatment*—to provide aftercare and maintenance therapy.
4. *Rehabilitation services*—to provide range of opportunities to increase skills in living, such as vocational rehabilitation, foster home care, half-way houses.
5. *Milieu therapy*—to assist in counteracting the chronic schizophrenic's withdrawal from society and dependence on an institutional life-style.
6. *Drug therapy with antipsychotics*—to assist in ameliorating symptoms and in increasing patient's availability for psychotherapy.
7. *Psychotherapy*—to assist patient in daily problems by exploration of relationships, sources of anxiety, and coping techniques.
8. *Group therapy*—to offer support with problems encountered in everyday life.
9. *Behavior therapy*—to assist with bizarre and disruptive behaviors in a variety of forms, such as token economy.
10. *Electroconvulsive therapy*—for patients with severe psychoses.
11. *Psychoanalysis*—is considered generally inappropriate because of intense relationship problems encountered and because of the relatively poor recovery rate.

Health Education

1. Teach patient and family the various ways to obtain help in improving work, educational, and social skills.
2. Explain that the potential for rehospitalization is around 20%; therefore, information and support is needed to continue aftercare plans and to be less discouraged, if rehospitalization becomes a reality.

Commonly Associated Nursing Diagnoses

Institutionalized behavior
Manipulation
Noncompliance
Alterations in perceptions
Inappropriate expression of aggression
Alterations in self-esteem
Dysfunctional communication
Anxiety
Regressive behavior
Alterations in self-care activities
Threatened suicide
Suspiciousness
Disturbed thought processes
Withdrawal
Impulsiveness

PARANOID DISORDERS

Paranoid disorders represent a group of mental disorders manifested by delusions of jealousy and of persecution that are not explained by other psychiatric disorders.

Etiology

No known specific cause, but hypotheses and research suggest several factors:

1. Psychodynamic theory—postulates the use of denial and projection as defenses against homosexual wishes as basis for delusions
2. Childhood developmental deficits of failure to develop basic trust—related to physical abuse, broken homes, and unpredictable parents or other forms of rejection
3. Parental expectations of perfection and high achievement
4. Stress situations involving lowering of self-esteem,

increasing distrust, envy, and isolation, and other factors leading to a delusional system that is frightening and partially comforting

Clinical Manifestations of Selected Type

Paranoia:
a. A disorder that has a clear, logical, lasting delusional system.
b. Interpersonal relationships are poor, for there is a basic mistrust of all.

Treatment

1. *Hospitalization*—is generally not indicated since person seldom seeks treatment and community develops a tolerance for the odd behaviors. If delusions are causing person to behave in ways dangerous to self or others, then hospitalization is indicated.
2. *Drug therapy* with antipsychotics.
3. *Psychotherapy*—initially deals with the problem of establishing a trusting relationship and with immediate, concrete problems; later discussion involves delusions and the mistrust of others.

Commonly Associated Nursing Diagnoses

Suspiciousness
Inappropriate expression of aggression
Disturbed thought processes

AFFECTIVE DISORDERS

Affective disorders are a group of mental disorders that present mainly symptoms of mood disturbance with associated changes in thinking and behavior.

Incidence

1. Most common disorder grouping in adults; bipolar disorder in about 600,000 cases per year and unipolar depressive disorder in 1.5 million cases per year.
2. There are only 20% to 25% of people with depression seeking treatment.
3. Bipolar disorder occurs before age 30; depression occurs at any age.

Etiology

No known specific cause, but hypotheses and research indicate several factors:
1. Genetic factor
2. Early experiences of separation and loss of parents
3. Psychodynamic view of depression and mania with hostility, turned against self or projected to others, being the primary factor
4. Ego adaptive view of depression as ego state response to separation and loss
   a. Avoidance of overt anger occurs because of the potential to endanger relationships in which dependency needs are met
   b. The idealization of another with consequence that there is no need for anger
   c. The implication of anger involving autonomy, which the depressed person does not understand
5. Cognitive view of depression with individual viewing himself, the future, and the current experience in a negative way
6. Family interaction patterns in which child experiences high expectations of achievement by parents and little approval for being self
7. Disturbance in the transmission of nerve impulses

related to norepinephrine deficiency or serotonin deficiency

Clinical Manifestation of Selected Types

A. *Major Depression*

Symptoms include sadness, apathy, feelings of worthlessness, self-blame, thoughts of suicide, desire to escape, avoiding simple problems, anorexia, weight loss, lessened interest in sex, sleeplessness, reduction in activity, or ceaseless activity.

B. *Bipolar Disorder*

A disorder in which there are alternating periods of depression and mania.
1. Bipolar Disorder Manic Episode
   Symptoms include hyperactivity, speech pressure, grandiosity, manipulativeness, irritability, euphoria, mood lability, hypersexuality, delusions, assaultiveness, and sleeplessness.
2. Bipolar Disorder Depressive Episode
   Symptoms are the same as major depression.

C. *Dysthymic Disorder*

A new diagnostic category for disorders in which person experiences for at least 2 years a depressed mood, no pleasure in activities of daily living, an impairment in social skills, and numerous bodily complaints.

Treatment

1. *Hospitalization*—in acute mania and in depression when there is evidence of poor judgment, weight loss, insomnia, and lack of emotional support
2. *Electroconvulsive therapy*—in severe depression or mania
3. *Drug therapy* with antidepressants or antimanic drugs; neuroleptics may be used to assist in controlling the violent behavior seen in manic state
4. *Psychotherapy*—in various forms, dealing with issues of dependency and manipulation, of need to detoxify loss experience, and of self-destructiveness
5. *Cognitive psychotherapy*—focusing on the correction of errors in thinking

Health Education

1. Teach patient that:
   a. Psychotherapy is an important aspect of the treatment program; support person's efforts to become involved in process.
   b. Antidepressants are continued for a 4- to 6-week period after symptoms of depression are absent.
   c. Generally the prognosis is good with only 1 out of 10 persons becoming chronically ill.
2. Assist patient in seeking information from self and others to identify the prodromal stage to manic state.

Commonly Associated Nursing Diagnoses

Threatened or attempted suicide
Inappropriate expression of aggression
Crisis
Manipulation
Disturbed thought processes
Inappropriate sexual behavior
Demanding behavior
Dysfunctional communication
Manic behavior

Depressive behavior

Impaired self-care activities

Noncompliance

Problem drinking

ANXIETY DISORDERS

Anxiety disorders are a group of mental disorders in which anxiety is the main concern.

Incidence

1. Panic disorder and generalized anxiety disorder may affect 5% of the population.
2. Obsessive–compulsive disorder may affect 0.05% of the population.
3. Phobic disorder may affect 1% of the population; agoraphobia is most common.

Etiology

1. Psychodynamic theory views anxiety as arising from conflicts which are usually sexual and aggressive.
   a. Types
      (1) Superego anxiety, e.g., fear of being found guilty
      (2) Castration anxiety, e.g., fear of bodily mutilation or decrease of abilities and skills
      (3) Separation anxiety, e.g., fear of loss of significant relationship
      (4) Impulse anxiety, e.g., fear of loss of contol of impulses
   b. Obsessive–compulsive disorder arises during anal developmental stage; mental mechanisms used are undoing, isolation, and reaction formation.
   c. Phobic disorder is characterized by use of mechanisms of displacement and avoidance to deal with castration anxiety and oedipal drives.
2. Behavioral theory views anxiety as the motivation for the person to relieve the pain after which avoidance behaviors are established.
3. Other theories stress the importance of separation anxiety and aggressive impulses.

Clinical Manifestations of Selected Types

A. *Panic Disorder*

Is characterized by acute anxiety episode of intense terror and dread, by awareness of palpitation and tachycardia, chest pain, and air hunger.

B. *Generalized Anxiety Disorder*

Is characterized by chronic anxiety (6 months) with restlessness, irritability, dry mouth, sweating of palms, G.I. symptoms, insomnia, and problems in concentration.

C. *Obsessive–Compulsive Disorder*

   a. Is characterized by a persistent idea or impulse that is neither acceptable nor controllable, anxious feelings, and attempts to resist the impulse.
   b. Compulsive acts may be one act or complex rituals.

D. *Phobic Disorder*

Is characterized by an intense fear of an object (simple phobia), situation (agoraphobia), or functioning in situations (social phobia).

Treatment

1. *Psychotherapy*—in various forms with focus on analyzing unconscious conflicts, or on interpersonal conflicts, or on only a supportive measure

2. *Behavioral therapy*—with use of desensitization techniques to deal with anxiety-provoking stimuli
3. *Drug therapy*—with antianxiety drugs
4. *Relaxation techniques*
5. *Hospitalization*—for short periods if symptoms become intense and family's ability to offer support at that time is limited

Health Education

1. Instruct patient with phobic disorder or obsessive–compulsive disorder that the condition may tend to be chronic.
2. Teach patient and family ways to deal with incapacities and inconveniences created by the disorders.

Commonly Associated Nursing Diagnoses

Anxiety

Ritualistic behavior

Depressive behavior

Guilt

Crisis

Threatened or attempted suicide

Inappropriate use of physical symptoms

Demanding behavior

SOMATOFORM DISORDERS

Somatoform disorders are a group of mental disorders characterized by multiple somatic complaints with no physical illness.

Etiology

1. Etiology in somatization disorders is unknown.
2. Etiology in conversion disorders involves:
   a. Fixation of development at Oedipus complex with resulting sexual conflicts and symptoms
   b. Self-preservation drives to be protected and to escape
   c. Pathological reactions and responses to environmental stress

Clinical Manifestations of Selected Types

A. *Somatization Disorder*

Is characterized by symptoms of fatigue, nausea and vomiting, bowel problems, headaches, fainting, and by the dramatics and emotionality involved in describing problems.

B. *Conversion Disorder*

Is characterized by abnormal movements or paralysis of parts with no relation to specific nerve involvement, anesthesias, and symptoms of physical illness.

Treatment

1. *Psychoanalysis*—with focus on dynamics of repression
2. *Psychotherapy*—with focus on symptom alleviation and supportive techniques
3. *Drug therapy*—with antianxiety drugs

Health Education

1. Teach patient that symptoms may recur in stressful situations.
2. Assist patient to focus on returning to independence and support family in allowing freedom of activities.
3. Instruct patient and families that having numerous

types of treatments focused on the physical illness are not useful.

Commonly Associated Nursing Diagnoses

Anxiety
Inappropriate use of physical symptoms
Crisis
Denial
Drug misuse
Noncompliance

DISSOCIATIVE DISORDERS

Dissociative disorders are a group of mental disorders presenting a temporary alteration in conscious awareness, identity, personality, and behavior.

Etiology

Psychodynamic theory states that dissociation is the mental mechanism used to deal with severe anxiety; also, conflicts arising from Oedipal and pre-Oedipal stages affect ego development.

Clinical Manifestations of Selected Type

Psychogenic amnesia
  a. Is the most common and is characterized by abrupt inability to recall pertinent information.
  b. It frequently is associated with physical injury.

Treatment

Brief, immediate psychotherapy with emphasis on assisting recall to prevent material from becoming inaccessible to recall.

Health Education

Assist patient in seeking the brief psychiatric help needed.

Commonly Associated Nursing Dignoses

Anxiety
Alterations in self-care activities

PERSONALITY DISORDERS

Personality disorders are a group of mental disorders characterized by life-long patterns of maladaptive responses to stress, by problems in developing work behaviors and intimate relationship behaviors, and by the capacity to perpetuate interpersonal problems and to annoy others.

Incidence

There is about 5% to 15% of the adult population with higher percentages in areas where socially impaired live, e.g., urban areas are affected by this disorder.

Etiology

1. Not much is known about the causes.
2. Possible genetic factor.
3. Disturbance in early childhood involving presence of inconsistent, neglectful parents.

Clinical Manifestations

1. Commonly used defense mechanisms are fantasy, isolation, dissociation, projection, somatization, splitting, and passive–aggression.
2. Person perceives self as extremely important and powerful. Others are unreal.

3. Formation of dependent and demanding relationships.
4. Creation of entangled interpersonal relationships.

Selected Types

A. *Paranoid Personality Disorder*
  Is characterized by a history of mistrust of others.

B. *Schizoid Personality Disorder*
  Is characterized by history of withdrawal from society.

C. *Histrionic Personality Disorder*
  Is characterized by history of dramatic displays of emotions that includes temper tantrums and suicide threats, of attention-seeking behaviors, of a desire for activity, and of brief relationships with others.

D. *Antisocial Personality Disorder*
  Is characterized by history of antisocial behavior involving courts, prisons, and health and welfare agencies.

E. *Boarderline Personality Disorder*
  Is characterized by history of instability of affect; of impulsivity; of periods of intense anger; of intense, clinging relationships; and of unpredictable self-destructive acts.

F. *Compulsive Personality Disorder*
  Is characterized by history of orderliness, obstinateness, parsimony, emotional constriction, rigidity, indecisiveness, devotion to a task, and overconcern with rules and morals.

G. *Passive–Aggressive Personality Disorder*
  Is characterized by history of resistance to most expectations involved in social and work settings by procrastinating, forgetting, delaying, and inefficiency.

Treatment

1. Treatment is very difficult, because of the anxiety generated with responses of anger, defensiveness, and authoritarianism in therapist and staff. In addition, patient does not perceive self as sick.
2. Psychotherapy deals with problems in living, especially the consequences of person's behaviors and learning to experience discomfort.
3. Self-help groups are useful, for person requires more support than any one person can provide.

Health Education

Instruct patient to become aware of the consequences of his behavior and support his attempts to be involved in psychotherapy.

Commonly Associated Nursing Diagnoses

Manipulation
Impulsive behavior
Withdrawal
Inappropriate expression of aggression
Problem drinking
Drug misuse
Denial
Demanding behavior
Noncompliance
Suspiciousness

SELECTED TREATMENT MODALITIES

Psychotherapy

A. *Psychoanalysis (Freud)*
1. Use of unconscious material, dream analysis, free association, interpretation, and transference to assist patient in achieving reorganization of his personality.
2. May extend over a period of 1 to 7 years.

B. *Psychotherapy (Sullivan)*
1. Use of relationship with analyst to focus on interpersonal relationship and communication process.
2. Dream analysis, free association, interpretation, and transference are also used to assist the individual.

C. *Psychotherapy (Rogers)*
   Use of empathetic understanding, concreteness, self-exploration and positive regard to encourage individual towards self-actualization.

D. *Cognitive Therapy (Beck)*
1. Use of guided discovery to assist patient in focusing on dysfunctional thoughts or behaviors and analyzing them, and in the assignment of tasks.
2. Strategy for behavior change is based on interrupting the sequence of cognition, imagery, and affect.
3. Method has been studied and proven useful in depression.

E. *Rational–Emotive Psychotherapy, RET (Ellis)*
1. Therapist teaches person to use an ABC method.
2. A is for activating experience by actively fantasizing experience to determine emotional consequence.
3. B is for belief system that a person notes as he allows self to feel uncomfortable.
4. C is for confronting irrational beliefs by using positive imagery.

F. *Interpersonal Therapy, IPT (Klerman)*
   Focus is on interpersonal transactions that have not gone well and on the development of specific strategies for coping with internal and external stress.

G. *Transactional Analysis (Berne)*
1. Use of concepts of parent, child, and adult to describe ego states; and transaction and games to view interactions with others.
2. Goal is to obtain the adult ego state of "I'm OK—You're OK" or a game-free relationship.

H. *Reality Therapy (Glaser)*
   Focus is on acceptance of reality and responsibility for self with the therapist who is involved in loving and teaching.

I. *Supportive Psychotherapy*
   Use of techniques to achieve other ways for control of impulses, to strengthen defenses, or to maintain adaptation.

J. *Crisis Therapy*
1. Focus is on offering emotional support, providing for catharsis, communicating hope, setting model for action, listening selectively for material for assessment, providing factual information, setting limits on acting-out behavior, writing out contract, and formulating problem in terms of precipitating factors, background problems, and available coping mechanism.
2. Duration of 1 to 6 sessions.

K. *Brief Psychotherapy*
1. Use of 1 to 20 sessions using techniques to help patient relate present situation to past experiences in order to assist him in removal of specific symptoms.
2. Outcome is related to experience of trust in the therapist relationship.

Group Psychotherapy

Selected persons are placed in a group (4–10) guided by a trained therapist to effect personality change or to assist with problems affecting mental health.
1. *Analytic Group*—Leader uses psychoanalytic concepts to produce change.
2. *Sullivanian Group*—Leader uses interpersonal theory to explore problems and eliminate maladaptations.
3. *Bion Group*—Leader uses concepts concerning group life, including basic assumptions, to interpret group phenomena.
4. *Transactional Group*—Leader focuses on games and not on causes of problems nor uncovering unconscious material to achieve "cure."
5. *Gestalt Group (Perls)*—Leader uses rules and games to assist person in acknowledging immediate feelings and to prevent their avoidance in order to restore the person to a sense of wholeness.
6. *Psychodrama (Moreno)*
   a. Is a treatment method offering opportunity for problem-solving through enactment of conflict situation.
   b. It involves a protagonist who acts out the situation, a director who assists in the exploration of the situation, an auxilliary who acts as a person in the protagonist's life, and an audience.
   c. Many techniques are used to promote involvement and analysis; some are soliloquy, self-presentation, mirror, role reversal, and double.

Family Therapy

1. *Structural model (Minuchin)*
   a. Therapist seeks to alter the family structure because changes in the family structure will alter behavior and the psychic processes.
   b. Therapist uses joining operations as he recreates communication patterns.
2. *Bowen therapy*
   Therapist assists family members in achieving differentiation and in reducing reactivity. (See Chapter 23, p. 909.)

Electroconvulsive Therapy (ECT)

ECT is a series of treatments given under anesthesia and muscle relaxants involving application of electrical current to the brain in order to produce convulsions. It is indicated in severe cases of depression, psychoses, catatonia, or mania.
1. Behavioral changes are probably the result of biochemical changes in brain function.
2. Treatment preparation involves physical examination; lab tests; x-ray of spine, if indicated; full, informed consent of patient; nothing by mouth after midnight; voiding prior to treatment; and removal of dentures.
3. Fractures or dislocations and pulmonary aspiration are the most frequent complications.

4. Patient will have amnesia for the treatment procedure.
   a. Memory impairment is related to number of treatments and will last for a couple of weeks after the series of treatments.
   b. Immediately afterwards the patient may be confused, drowsy, and euphoric or flat in affect.

Activity Therapy

1. *Occupational Therapy*
   Use of selected activities (painting, pottery, leather work, crocheting, hammering, shopping, washing clothes, budgeting, etc.) to improve general performance, to learn essential skills of living, and to assist in symptom reduction.
2. *Recreation Therapy*
   a. Use of recreational activities (social, sports, games, hobbies, arts, crafts, service activities, outdoor sports, etc.) in treatment of behavior.
   b. Special emphasis is given to resocialization, reality orientation, and involvement when working with psychiatric patients.
3. *Bibliotherapy*
   Use of literature, films, and person's own creative writing with group discussion to promote self-knowledge, and integration of thoughts and feelings.
4. *Dance Therapy*
   Use of rhythmic movements and interaction to express emotions, thereby increasing awareness of body and ego strength.

Other Modalities

A. *Sex Therapy (Masters & Johnson)*
Use of desensitizing techniques to increase sexual pleasure and arousal, and to demystify sex.

B. *Assertive Training*
Teaching of skills to assist people in getting what they want in a firm, effective, and useful manner as opposed to an aggressive manner in which emotions are expressed in destructive, aggressive ways.

C. *Biofeedback*
Feedback of functioning of autonomic system through instruments that pick up electrical potentials; assists patient in gaining control of heart rate, blood pressure, skin temperature, and muscle tension.

D. *Milieu Therapy*
Use of open door, home-like furnishings, high staff–patient ratio, patient government, democratic decision making, ward–staff initiative, high interaction level with patients, and shared responsibility among patients to improve patient behavior.

E. *Token Economy*
Use of positive reinforcement in form of tokens and extinction of undesirable behaviors by ignoring or being fined tokens to achieve behavior change.

F. *Hypnosis*
Therapist uses techniques such as repetitive suggestion to induce state of altered consciousness or intense concentration to provide additional data for diagnosis and treatment; it of itself is not treatment.

BIBLIOGRAPHY

Books

Aguilera AC and Mesnick JM. Crisis Intervention Theory and Methodology, 2nd ed. St. Louis, CV Mosby, 1974
Arieti S. The Intrapsychic Self. New York, Basic Books, 1967
Arieti S and Bemporad J. Severe and Mild Depression. New York, Basic Books, 1978
American Psychiatric Association. Diagnostic and Statistical Manual of Mental Disorders, 3rd ed. Washington, D.C., American Psychiatric Association, 1980
American Psychiatric Association. Electroconvulsive Therapy. Task Force Report No. 14. Washington, D.C., American Psychiatric Association, 1978
Beck AT. Cognitive Therapy and Emotional Disorders. New York, International Universities Press, 1976
Beck AT. Depression, Causes and Treatment. Philadelphia, University of PA Press, 1972
Berger MM (ed). Beyond the Double Bind. New York, Brunner/Mazel, 1978
Blatner HA. Acting-In. Practical Applications of Psychodramatic Methods. New York, Springer Pub. Co., 1973
Burns DD. Feeling Good, The New Mood Therapy. New York, William Morrow, 1980
Cole JO, Schatzberg AF, Frazier SH (eds). Depression: Biology, Psychodynamics, and Treatment. New York, Plenum Press, 1978
Ellis A and Harper RA. A New Guide to Rational Living. New Jersey, Prentice–Hall, 1975
Ford DH and Urban HB. Systems of Psychotherapy. New York, John Wiley & Sons, 1963
Greenberg IA (ed). Psychodrama, Theory and Therapy. New York, Behavior Publications, 1974
Guerin PJ (ed). Family Therapy, Theory and Practice. New York, Gardner Press, 1976
Hopkins HL and Smith HD (eds). Willard and Spackman's Occupational Therapy, 5th ed. Philadelphia, JB Lippincott, 1978
Kaplan HI and Sadock BJ (ed). Comprehensive Group Psychotherapy. Baltimore, Williams & Wilkins, 1971

Kaplan HI, Freedman AM, Sadock BJ (eds). Comprehensive Textbook of Psychiatry, Vol. II, 3rd ed. Baltimore, Williams & Wilkins, 1980
Kolb L. Modern Clinical Psychiatry, 9th ed. Philadelphia, WB Saunders, 1977
Lishinan W. Organic Psychiatry. London, Blackwell Scientific Publications, 1978
Minuchin S. Families and Family Therapy. Cambridge, Harvard University Press, 1974
Moreno JL. Psychodrama. New York, Beacon House, 1945
Nicholi A (ed). The Harvard Guide to Modern Psychiatry. Cambridge, Mass., Belknap Press, 1978
Paul GL and Lentz RJ. Psychosocial Treatment of Chronic Mental Patients. Cambridge, Harvard University Press, 1977.
Pradhan SN and Dutta SN (ed). Drug Abuse, Clinical and Basic Aspects. St. Louis, CV Mosby, 1977
Schecter A and Mule SJ (ed). Treatment Aspects of Drug Dependence. Boca Raton, Florida, CRC Press, 1978
Strider F. Psychoses/schizophrenia: Cues. In Woody RH: Encyclopedia of Clinical Assessment. San Francisco, Jossey–Bass, 1980
West LJ and Flinn DE. Treatment of Schizophrenia, Progress and Prospects. New York, Grune & Stratton, 1976
Wilshine H. The Impulsive Personality. New York, Plenum Press, 1977
Wolberg LR. The Techniques of Psychotherapy, Part 1. New York, Grune & Stratton, 1977
Yalom ID. The Theory and Practice of Group Psychotherapy, 2nd ed. New York, Basic Books, 1975

Articles

Covi L, Lipman RS, Derogatis LR et al. Drugs and group psychotherapy in neurotic depression. Am J Psychiatry 1974 Feb; 131(2):191–198
Friedman AS. Interaction of drug therapy with marital therapy in depressive patients. Arch Gen Psychiatry 1975 May; 32(5):619–637

SELECTED NURSING RESPONSIBILITIES **28**

BEHAVIOR MODIFICATION

Definitions

1. *Behavior modification* refers to the theory and treatment techniques based on the behavioral model. (See Chapter 23.)
2. *Operant behavior* refers to behavior that is increased by the events which follow the behavior.
3. *Reinforcers*—any event which strengthens or weakens a behavior; i.e., increases or decreases the probability that the behavior will occur again.

General Principles

1. In behavior modification, the patient is taught more adaptive ways to behave.
2. A treatment plan is developed specifically for each patient based on behavioral assessment and functional analysis.
3. Importance is placed on patient practice, when possible, of the desired behavior in his own community environment.
4. The desired behavioral goals are often jointly defined by the patient and the therapist.
5. The desired behavioral goals, as well as the treatment plan to reach them, are outlined to the patient.

Assessment and Goals

A. *Strategies for Assessing Patient Behavior*

1. Directly observe and record behavior of patient.
2. Observe patient's behavior while role playing or during staged interactions.
3. Patient provides self-report of behavior.
   a. Retrospective self-report.
   b. Self-monitoring by documenting on-going self-observations.
   c. Note patient reports of behavioral excesses—behaviors that occur too often, too long, and too intensely, or that occur at socially inappropriate times.
   d. Note patient reports of behavioral deficits—behaviors that occur too infrequently, not long enough, and with insufficient frequency, or that do not occur at expected appropriate times.

B. *Goal of Behavioral Assessment*—is functional analysis

1. Identify patient's primary problem behavior, also referred to as the *target behavior*.
2. Analyze the form or topography of the identified primary problem behavior (target behavior).
   a. How frequently and how long does the behavior occur?
   b. Does the behavior occur more frequently during one part of the entire day?
   c. What is the exact nature of the behavior? Does it vary in intensity, in duration, etc.?
3. Analyze the stimulus situation, that is, the environment in which the behavior occurs.
   a. What are the antecedents that maintain the identified primary problem behavior?
   b. Can a pattern be identified in the environmental stimuli that takes place prior to the occurrence of the target behavior?
   c. What are the consequences of the target behavior that maintain the behavior?
   d. Can a pattern be identified in the environmental stimuli that takes place following the occurrence of the target behavior?
4. Assess collateral factors.
   a. Behavioral strengths: What strengths or potential does the patient have that could be incorporated into the treatment plan?
   b. What limitations does the patient have that need to be considered in developing the treatment plan?
   c. What environmental strengths and limitations can be identified? For example, what kind of support can the patient potentially receive from significant others to help him change his behavior?
5. Identify potential positive reinforcers for the patient that could be incorporated into the treatment plan.
   a. Find out from the patient what he likes to do. A specific reinforcer does not have the same value for everyone.
   b. Observe for any change in preferences. Reinforcers have different value to the patient as situations in his life change, including changes in his mental health.

c. Strive to identify possible secondary reinforcers for incorporation into the treatment plan. Primary reinforcers, except for extra food, should not be used.

d. Identify for possible incorporation into the treatment plan secondary reinforcers that can be utilized upon discharge.

6. Identify potential negative reinforcers in the patient's environment that would impede achieving the desired behavior. Does the spouse, for example, have a stake in maintaining the target behavior?

Treatment

1. As much as feasible, jointly determine with patient the desired behavioral goal—that is, what behavior is desired, instead of the identified problem behavior or target behavior.
2. Clearly identify and describe what is expected in the desired behavior.
   a. When necessary, break desired behavior down into steps and teach patient to master each step in sequence.
      (1) Shaping can be used to positively reinforce a response that has not yet reached the level of the desired behavioral response.
      (2) In shaping, closer and closer approximations of the desired behavior are reinforced until the desired behavioral response is reached.
      (3) In shaping, the positive reinforcer must be given immediately after the response sought.
   b. Gradually increase the patient's time spent on the desired behavior.
   c. The desired behavioral goal should first be achieved in a nonstressful environment before it is expected in a stressful environment.
3. Use imitation or modeling to demonstrate to the patient the exact steps involved in performing the behavior.

4. Modify or change any environmental conditions which may prevent the desired behavioral goal; e.g., identify any sources of punishment for the desired behavioral goal and eliminate or reduce them.
5. Select positive reinforcers to be used with patient from assessment data.
   a. Activity reinforcers—going on trips, ground privileges, going for a walk, staying up late, watching TV, listening to radio, sleeping late.
   b. Social reinforcers—warm tone of voice, laughing with patient, nodding in agreement, smiling, turning face and body towards patient, touch, sitting next to patient, walking together.
   c. Verbal praise of behavior—"Good for you!" "It pleases me when you . . ."
6. At first reinforce each desired response immediately after its occurrence.
   Can tell patient exactly what response is being rewarded.
7. The desired behavioral response can later be reinforced intermittently.
   a. Fixed interval schedule—the same amount of time elapses before the next reinforcer is given for the desired behavioral response.
   b. Variable interval schedule—the amount of time elapsed varies around a mean before the next reinforcer is given for the desired behavioral response.
   c. Fixed ratio schedule—reinforcers follow a specified number of occurrences of the desired behavior.
8. Avoid using negative reinforcers or punishment to change behavior because:
   a. It teaches patient to avoid person giving punishment as well as to avoid the punished behavior.
   b. It can teach patient to hate person giving punishment.
   c. It can teach patient to lie, hide, and run away in order to avoid punishment.

GROUP THERAPY

Group therapy groups—overall emphasis, or goal, is re-education, remotivation, reorientation, or support.
Group psychotherapy groups—overall emphasis, or goal, is problem-solving, insight without personality reconstruction, or personality reconstruction.

Influencing Factors

Factors in group therapy and psychotherapy that facilitate patient's development of more adaptive behavioral patterns include:*

1. *Universality*—the patient discovers that he is not alone and that others in the group may experience problems similar to his own.
2. *Instillation of hope*—the patient develops hope for his own improvement as he sees others in the group coping more adaptively.
3. *Corrective reexperiencing of the primary family group*—group experiences provide the patient with the opportunity to work through conflicts stemming from his primary family group.
4. *Information gained*—the group provides the patient

---

* Yalom I. The Theory and Practice of Group Psychotherapy. New York, Basic Books, 1975.

with the opportunity to learn about mental health and mental illness.
5. *Altruism*—the patient benefits from being helpful to other group members; e.g., his self-esteem may be improved.
6. *Group cohesiveness*—group members are attracted to the group with a sense of "we-ness".
   Patients in the group develop a sense of belonging, acceptance, individual validation, and ability to express, but tolerate, intermember hostility.
7. *Catharsis*—patient is able to ventilate his emotions.
8. *Imitative behavior*—the patient observes the behavior of others in the group and experiments with the behavior's usefulness for himself.
9. *Gaining socializing techniques*—the group experience provides the patient with the opportunity to acquire social skills.
10. *Interpersonal learning*—the patient displays his behavior and through feedback and self-observation gains understanding of his impact on others and about the opinions others have of him.
    The patient gains awareness for his own responsibility in developing his interpersonal world.
11. *Existential factors*—the patient experiences being able to "be" with others and to belong to the group.

Phases of Group Development

A. *Beginning Phase*

1. Tasks confronting the group members are:
   a. Developing a method for achieving the purpose for which they joined the group
   b. Managing the social relationships so that each member gains a comfortable role for himself
2. Patient behavioral characteristics include:
   a. Seeking to clarify meaning of group therapy and what group membership entails
   b. Evaluating and testing other group members and seeking viable personal role
   c. Seeking acceptance, approval, domination, or respect
   d. Demonstrating dependency on leader, and seeking guidance, approval, and direction
   e. Restricted and stereotyped communication
   f. Searching for member similarities
   g. Providing description of symptoms, medications, former treatment
   h. Anxiety among members

B. *Second phase*

Patient behavioral characteristics include:
   a. Searching for power, control, dominance
   b. Engaging in conflicts between members and between members and leader
   c. Searching for appropriate amount of personal power: struggling for control
   d. Expressing criticism and negative comments
   e. Giving advice, judgments, and criticism, as means of jockeying for position
   f. Expressing hostility and rebellion towards therapist
   g. Engaging in fantasies of getting rid of leader

C. *Third phase*

Patient behavioral characteristics include:
   a. Development of group cohesiveness
   b. Increase in self-disclosure and mutual trust
   c. Increased concern about each other and missing members
   d. Appearance of issues of intimacy and closeness among group members
   e. Increased awareness of interpersonal interactions as they evolve in the group
   f. Final movement of the third phase: teamwork and focus on the purpose and work of the group
   g. Feelings about termination (emerge as group comes to the end)

Characteristics of Effective Groups

1. Problem-solving is frequently evidenced.
2. Creativity and innovation are supported.
3. Conflict is tolerated, examined, and resolved.
4. High levels of trust, open and two-way communication, support, and inclusion facilitate cohesion.
5. The group atmosphere is relaxed and comfortable.
6. Group members participate in the evaluation of the group's functioning.
7. Decisions are made by consensus.
8. Objectives and tasks are clarified and modified to foster group member commitment.
9. Emphasized are the three group functions—internal maintenance, developmental change, and goal achievement.
10. The leadership role changes among group members over time.

Initiating Group Therapy or Psychotherapy

1. Decide on type of group to be conducted: delineate the major emphasis and group goals.
   The specificity of the group goals depends on the type of group.
2. In selecting group members for the type of group, consider:
   a. The diagnosis and the degree of mental illness of the patient, before placing the patient in group therapy as opposed to group psychotherapy.
   b. Potential therapeutic value to patient; i.e., Will the group help the patient develop more adaptive behavioral patterns?
   c. Patient motivation and willingness.
   d. Factors such as age, sex, intelligence.
   e. The size of the group—depends to some extent on the type of group and the type of patients. A good range is from 6 to 10 members.
3. Select adequate meeting area.
   Should be adequate size for group and free from interruptions, have good ventilation, and be attractively furnished.
4. Select time and frequency of meeting.
   a. The actual frequency depends on type of group. A common frequency is once per week.
   b. In selecting the time, work around other patient therapies with less flexibility in scheduling, such as industrial therapy.
   c. Changes in meeting place, time, and frequency can adversely affect the group process.

Therapist's Role in Preparing Patient for Group Therapy

1. The therapist's role and interventions will be influenced by the type of group, the type of patients, and the therapist's own theoretical orientation.
2. Preparation of patient for group can vary as follows:
   a. Information about time, place, and frequency.
   b. Individual therapy followed by group therapy/psychotherapy.
   c. Brief individual orientation.
      (1) Time, place, frequency
      (2) Purpose of group
      (3) Brief description of group members
      (4) What is expected of patient in group; e.g., attendance
      (5) Behavior that will not be tolerated.
   d. In an open group (one in which new members can be added at any time), assist the new members in feeling comfortable.
      (1) Introduce the new member to the group and have group members introduce themselves.
      (2) Summarize what the group has been currently discussing.
      (3) Facilitate group support of new member, e.g., "Mrs. Jones may need our support in becoming a member of this group. We remember how we felt on our first day."

Interventions

A. *Beginning Phase*

1. Serve as a role model to demonstrate behavior expected in group.
2. Discuss with group members what is expected of them in group.
   Offer structure and direction.
3. Have members introduce themselves.

4. Foster and facilitate interaction.
   a. Do not permit monopolizing.
   b. Intervene to reduce *social* roles and interaction.
   c. Demonstrate congruence, empathy, and unconditional positive regard.
5. Answer questions in relation to time, place, frequency, and purpose of the group.
6. Do not reinforce group need for dependency on leader.
7. Reduce high anxiety.

B. *Second Phase*

1. Permit expression of criticism and hostility toward therapist.
2. Support fragile group member when needed during intermember conflict.
3. Foster and facilitate interaction.
4. Demonstrate congruence, empathy, and unconditional positive regard.

5. Focus on the here-and-now group experiences.
6. Begin to explore themes.

C. *Third Phase*

1. Foster and facilitate communication.
2. Encourage exploration of behavior, interactions among members, and topic areas discussed.
3. Provide feedback on group process.
4. Support development of group cohesiveness. Support self-disclosure.
5. Support and encourage problem-solving and working towards group goals.
6. Offer opportunity to work through feelings for loss or addition of group member (especially true for open groups).
7. Encourage members to respond to here-and-now experiences in the group.
8. Work through feelings related to termination of the group.

ADMINISTRATION OF DRUG THERAPY

Antipsychotic Drugs

Antipsychotic drugs are effective in treatment of psychoses and schizophrenias.

A. *Major Classes and Trade Names*

1. Phenothiazines
   a. Aliphatics:

Generic Name	Trade Name
Chlorpromazine	Thorazine
Triflupromazine	Vesprin
Promazine	Sparine

   b. Piperazines:

Generic Name	Trade Name
Acetophenazine	Tindal
Butaperazine	Repoise
Carphenazine	Proketazine
Fluphenazine	Prolixin
decanoate	decanoate
enanthate	enanthate
Perphenazine	Trilafon
Prochlorperazine	Compazine
Trifluoperazine	Stelazine

   c. Piperidines:

Generic Name	Trade Name
Mesoridazine	Serentil
Piperactazine	Quide
Thioridazine	Mellaril

2. Butyrophenones:

Generic Name	Trade Name
Haloperidol	Haldol

3. Thioxanthenes:

Generic Name	Trade Name
Thiothixene	Navane

4. Dibenzoxazepines

Generic Name	Trade Name
Loxapine	Loxitane, Daxolin

5. Indolics:

Generic Name	Trade Name
Molindone	Lidone
	Moban

B. *Mechanism of Action*—is probably the blocking of dopamine receptor.

C. *Drug Effectiveness*

1. Dosage may be divided throughout the day or be given at bedtime.
   a. Preferably it should be given at bedtime, because its sedative effect assists in establishing normal sleep pattern.
   b. Better compliance is achieved with bedtime dose.
   c. There are fewer extrapyramidal effects.
2. Rapid neuroleptization for acutely ill psychotic patients may be instituted.
   a. Patient is given intramuscular medication every 30 to 60 minutes over a 2- to 6-hour period.
   b. Monitor blood pressure for hypotension before each dose; withhold dose if B.P. is 90 or below systolic.
   c. Monitor sleep state to achieve a 6- to 7-hour period.
   d. Monitor for dystonia occurring 1 hour to 48 hours after beginning of treatment and treat with antiparkinson drug.
   e. Monitor for decrease in dangerousness to self and others.
3. Drug holidays of 1 to 3 days may be given when patient is on long-term use.
4. Trial withdrawals are recommended every 6 months or year.
5. Excretion of drugs from body occurs slowly. May be present in body for weeks after last dose.
   Recurring symptoms of mental illness may not be experienced for weeks or months, reinforcing patient's belief that no medication is needed.

D. *Responses to Treatment*

1. Initially the patient is drowsy and cooperative within hours to a week.
2. The patient becomes more sociable and less withdrawn during next 2 months.
3. The thought disorder generally disappears in 6 weeks or more.
4. Improvement is generally noted in hallucinations, acute delusions, sleeping habits, appetite, tension, combativeness, hostility, negativism, and dress.
5. Lack of response to treatment is frequently related to failure to take the drug.
6. Polypharmacy or use of more than 1 phenothiazine is not necessary nor recommended.
7. Geriatric patients respond to lower dosages and may have hypotension.

E. *Side Effects with Nursing Implications*

1. *Drowsiness*
   a. Is present especially when drug is started.
   b. Tolerance will develop in about 2 weeks.
   c. Avoid activities such as driving a car or repairing delicate equipment, because alertness and muscular coordination is needed.
   d. Medication may be given before bedtime thereby decreasing the awareness of this side effect.
2. *Orthostatic Hypotension*
   a. Occurs more often after I.M. injections.
   b. Symptoms are dizziness and weakness.
   c. B.P. is below normal; systolic B.P. 90 or below is dangerous.
   d. Have patient change positions slowly.
   e. Monitor B.P. while patient is standing and sitting if symptoms of hypotension exist.
   f. Dosage may be adjusted or medication changed or discontinued if symptoms persist.
   g. Head-down, feet-raised position may be used to raise B.P.

NURSING ALERT: Neo-synephrine may be administered to raise the B.P. when it is dangerously low. Epinephrine is *not* used as this will cause further lowering of blood pressure.

3. *Extrapyramidal Symptoms* (EPS)
   a. *Dystonia*—spasms of muscles of face, neck, back, eye, arms and legs.
      (1) *Oculogyric crisis*—fixed upward gaze from spasm of the oculomotor muscles.
      (2) *Torticollis*—pulling of head to the side from spasms of cervical muscles.
      (3) *Opisthotonus*—hyperextension of back from spasms of back muscles.
   b. *Akathesia*—continuous motor restlessness.
   c. *Pseudoparkinsonism*—shuffling gait; masklike facial expression; drooling; tremor; rigidity; and akinesia, which is experienced as weakness and fatigue.
   d. EPS may occur 2 hours following an antipsychotic drug.
   e. Dosage may be adjusted or medication changed or an antiparkinson drug may be given.

f. Relief from severe reactions should occur 15 minutes after I.M. dose of antiparkinson drug.

4. *Tardive Dyskinesia*
   a. Symptoms include involuntary movements of tongue, lips, and jaw; chorea; tics; athetosis; and dystonia.
   b. There is a relationship between the use of neuroleptic drugs and tardive dyskinesia.
      (1) Advantages and disadvantages of neuroleptics need to be discussed with patient.
      (2) It is suggested that documentation of agreement to take neuroleptics with full knowledge of the possible effects of tardive dyskinesia be done.
   c. Treatment:
      (1) Consists of lowering the dose of neuroleptics, or change of medication, or withdrawal of medication.
      (2) No treatment is uniformly effective.
      (3) Lithium or diazepam may be used.
   d. Evaluation of neuroleptic medication every 6 months, which includes a trial reduction of the medication, is recommended.
5. *Convulsive Seizures*—may occur, for the threshold is lowered.
6. *Autonomic Nervous System Effects*
   a. Tachycardia, dry mouth, constipation, blurred vision, paralytic ileus, bladder paralysis.
   b. Use of frequent fluids, sugarless gum, candy, or lozenges help the dry mouth.
   c. Diet, fluids, and laxatives may relieve constipation.
7. *Allergic or Toxic Effects*
   a. Agranulocytosis
      (1) Symptoms: Rapid onset of sore throat and fever.
      (2) Occurs in first 3 to 8 weeks of treatment.
      (3) Treatment: Stop the drug, use reverse isolation technique, and administer antibiotics.
   b. Oral monoliasis
   c. Dermatitis
   d. Jaundice
      (1) Note color of stool (pale) and urine (dark).
      (2) Treatment consists of discontinuing medication
8. *Endocrine or Metabolic Effects*
   a. Weight gain
   b. Menstrual irregularities and excessive secretion of mammary gland in females
   c. Decreased libido, impotence, impaired ejaculation in males
   d. Decreased thermoregulatory ability
      (1) Complaints of being too hot or too cold are heard.
      (2) Care should be taken in use of ice bag or hot water bottle.
9. *Miscellaneous*
   a. Toxic Retinopathy
      (1) Symptoms: Disturbed color vision, especially brown tones; decreased visual acuity.
      (2) Is believed to be related to Mellaril dosage of over 1200 mg daily.
   b. Phenothiazine Lens Disease
      (1) Does not affect visual acuity. Is partially reversible.

(2) Recommend eye exam every 3–12 months and minimal dosage of medication.
c. Photoxicity
(1) Excessive sun exposure may result in burn or rash.
(2) Sunscreens and adequate clothing are recommended.

F. *Contraindications*

Comatose states, glaucoma, prostatic hyperplasia, acute myocardial infarction.

G. *Drug Interactions*

1. Sedation and hypotension are potentiated when antipsychotics and alcohol, barbiturates, and other CNS are combined.
2. Dry mouth, postural hypotension, urinary retention, and constipation are increased when antipsychotics and antiparkinson or tricyclics are combined.

H. *Withdrawal Syndrome*

1. Sweating, diarrhea, nausea, vomiting, insomnia, restlessness, tremor.
2. May be associated to cholinergic rebound, CNS stimulation, emerging tardive dyskinesia, and great sensitiveness to stress.

Antidepressant Drugs

Antidepressant drugs are used to treat affective disorders.

A. *Major Classes and Trade Names*

1. Tricyclic antidepressants

Generic Name	Trade Name
Amitriptyline	Elavil
Desipramine	Norpramin
Imipramine	Tofranil
Nortriptyline	Aventyl
Protriptyline	Vivactil
Doxepin	Sinequan

2. Tetracyclic antidepressants

Generic Name	Trade Name
Maprotilene	Ludiomil

3. Monoamine oxidase inhibitors

Generic Name	Trade Name
Isocarboxazid	Marplan
Phenelzine	Nardil
Tranylcypromine	Parnate

B. *Mechanism of Action*—is probably the increasing of norepinephrine.

C. *Drug Effectiveness*

1. Dosage may be divided throughout the day or be given at bedtime because of the sedative effects.
2. A minimum dose is initially given and then gradually increased.
3. There may be no immediate changes in mood as there is a lag of 5 to 21 days.
4. Therapeutic effect may take 4 to 6 weeks to achieve.
5. Psychomotor activity increases before patient states he actually feels better.
6. Medication may be continued for 6 months after patient is free from depression.

D. *Side Effects*

1. Tricyclics
   a. Postural hypotension, fainting and dizziness, low blood pressure.
   b. Drowsiness
   c. Hallucinations and delusions
   d. Dry mouth, constipation
   e. Weight gain
   f. Impotence
2. Monamine oxidase inhibitors
   a. Postural hypotension
   b. Liver damage
   c. Hypertensive crises
      (1) Occurs 30 minutes to 24 hours after eating foods containing tyramine (cheese, wine, beer, sour cream, chocolate, liver, pickled herring, raisins, bananas, avocados, soy sauce, fava beans).
      (2) Symptoms: Severe headache, palpitation, neck stiffness, nausea, vomiting, increased B.P., chest pain, collapse.
      (3) Treatment: Medication is discontinued and medicine (Regitine) given to lower the blood pressure.

E. *Contraindications*

Glaucoma, agitated states, urinary retention, cardiac disorders, seizure disorders.

F. *Drug Interactions*

1. Sedative and hypotensive effects are potentiated when antidepressants are given with alcohol.
2. Monamine oxidase inhibitors have many drug interactions; therefore, check carefully before giving.

Antimanic Drugs

Antimanic drugs are used to treat bipolar disorder, manic phase, and periodic impulsive aggressiveness.

A. *Major Class and Trade Names*

Generic Name	Trade Name
Lithium salts	Lithane
	Lithonate
	Eskalith

B. *Mechanism of Action*—is not known, but may be related to changes in catecholamine metabolism.

C. *Drug Effectiveness*

1. Dosage is given 2 to 3 times a day because of its rapid excretion from body; given at mealtime to those sensitive to nausea.
2. Blood levels are monitored carefully.
   a. Acute manic states—blood level ranges 1.0 to 1.5 mEq.; measured 2 times weekly.
   b. Long-term control—blood level ranges 0.6 to 1.2 mEq.; measured monthly.
   c. Toxic state—blood level ranges above 1.5 mEq.; measured daily.
3. Therapeutic effect is seen in 4 to 10 days.
4. Adequate sodium intake is needed as lithium is excreted more slowly when diet is low in sodium.

D. *Side Effects*

1. Early effects, which subside after 1 to 2 weeks, are:

a. G.I. symptoms: nausea, vomiting, diarrhea, thirst, weight loss
b. Hand tremors, muscle weakness
c. Polyuria (may wet the bed at night), skin rashes
2. Other side effects
    a. Neurological: organic brain syndrome, extrapyramidal effects, seizures, ataxia, dysarthria, EEG changes
    b. Cardiovascular: pulse irregularities, low blood pressure
    c. Possible irreversible thyroid and renal damage
3. Toxicity
    a. Symptoms: muscle weakness, diarrhea, vomiting, lack of coordination, giddiness, tremor, slurring speech.
    b. Treatment: discontinuance of drug, giving fluids, correcting fluid and electrolyte imbalance, protecting kidney function.
    c. Response to treatment is monitored by daily electrolytes, hematocrit, lithium level, and body weight.

E. *Contraindications*

Cardiovascular disease, renal disorders, epilepsy, dehydration.

F. *Drug Interactions*

1. Nausea, which is a sign of lithium toxicity, may be decreased or blocked when antipsychotic drugs are given with lithium.
2. Electrolyte imbalance may be possible when lithium and diuretics or steroid prepartions are given together.

Antianxiety Drugs

Antianxiety drugs (minor tranquilizers, anxiolytics, relaxants) are used to treat psychoneurotic disorders.

A. *Major Classes and Trade Names*

1. Propanediols

Generic Name	Trade Name
Meprobamate	Equanil
	Miltown
Tybamate	Solacen
	Tybatran

2. Benzodiazepines

Generic Name	Trade Name
Clorazepate	Tranxene
Chlordiazepoxide	Librium
Diazepam	Valium
Oxazepam	Serax
Flurazepam	Dalmane

3. Diphenylmethanes

Generic Name	Trade Name
Diphenhydramine	Benadryl
Hydroxyzine	Atarax
	Vistaril

B. *Mechanism of Action*—is unknown.

C. *Drug Effectiveness*

1. Drug therapy is generally for a short period of time to relieve anxiety in neuroses and personality disorders.

2. Tolerance to drugs may develop in 3 to 4 weeks, or even in less time.
3. Physical dependence may occur.
4. Withdrawal syndrome includes nervousness, weakness, restlessness, convulsions.

D. *Side Effects*

1. There is low incidence of autonomic and extrapyramidal effects.
2. Sedation and hypotension may occur.

E. *Contraindications*

Severe depression, glaucoma, psychoses.

F. *Drug Interactions*

1. Sedative effects potentiated when antianxiety drugs are given with alcohol, barbiturates, and other CNS depressants.
2. Sedation, dry mouth, blurred vision, rapid pulse, flushed face, and urinary retention effects are potentiated when antianxiety drugs are given with antidepressants.
3. Antihypertensive effects are potentiated when Valium is given with diuretics and antihypertensive drugs.

Antiparkinson Drugs

Antiparkinson drugs are used to alleviate the side effects of antipsychotics.

A. *Major Class and Trade Names*

Anticholinergics

Generic Name	Trade Name
Trihexyphenidyl	Artane
Benztropine	Cogentin
Biperiden	Akineton
Procyclidine	Kemadrin

B. *Mechanism of Action*—is reduction of cholinergic activity.

C. *Drug Effectiveness*

1. Drug therapy is given in divided doses to treat drug-induced extrapyramidal symptoms.
2. Controversy over prophylactic use.
3. Drug may be discontinued after 1 to 3 months with only few patients requiring resumption of medication, even though they are still taking an antipsychotic.
4. Discontinuation of phenothiazines should occur before discontinuation of antiparkinson drug because of the slow excretion of phenothiazines.

D. *Side Effects*

Dry mouth, blurred vision, constipation, drowsiness, nausea, nervousness, urinary retention.

E. *Contraindications*

Glaucoma, prostatic hyperplasia.

F. *Drug Interactions*

1. Blurred vision, dry mouth, constipation, and other anticholinergic actions are additive when tricyclic antidepressants or antipsychotics are given with antiparkinson drugs.
2. Neurological symptoms are potentiated when monamine oxidase inhibitors are given with antiparkinson drugs.

GUIDELINES FOR PROTECTIVE INTERVENTIONS

GUIDELINES: 1:1 Observation for Suicide Prevention*

1:1 observation for suicide prevention is a procedure in which the nurse–patient relationship is continuously used to prevent suicide.

Purpose
1. To protect patient from self-injury or death.
2. To increase patient's control of self-destructive impulses.
3. To provide opportunity to talk about problems.

Procedure

NURSING ACTION	*RATIONALE/AMPLIFICATION*
1. Explain purpose of procedure to patient as way of offering support during time of crisis for him.	1. If procedure is perceived as "guard duty," patient may resort to being more subtle and less willing to talk about his ideas of suicide. If procedure is perceived as having someone to judge every act and to intervene, the patient may feel distrustful of staff and himself. He may conclude that no one has ability to prevent or to stop the act.
2. Stay with patient at arms length at all times during waking hours.	2. Patient may have difficulty in controlling sudden impulses to act, and nurse needs to remain close enough to the patient so that she can act quickly.
3. Have patient sleep in area that facilitates constant observation. Distance of nurse from the patient may increase.	3. Continuous observation is necessary even when patient is asleep; however, distance of nurse at 10 to 20 feet may be appropriate.
4. Discuss with patient the activities of the day, and plan for patient to attend as many activities as possible.	4. Maintenance of daily activity supports the continuance of life and involvement in it.
5. Encourage verbalization of thoughts and feelings.	5. Opportunity to assist patient to think through and validate ideas about self, stress situation, and the future will emerge.
6. Discuss with team members daily the continuance of the procedure. This assumes the presentation of data gathered during period of observation and a nursing assessment.	6. Nurse needs to actively participate in the team decision about the need for continuance. All staff members need to be consulted as to need for continuance of the procedure. The nurse providing the close observation needs opportunity to voice her concerns, and needs support from the staff to continue the relationship.

* Refer to Chapter 26, Threatened or Attempted Suicide.

GUIDELINES: Activity Area Restriction

Room restriction is a mechanism to limit movement of the patient to a specific room.
Area restriction is a mechanism to limit movement of the patient to a large room or rooms, such as a lounge or dayroom.

Purpose
1. To protect patient from self-injury or injury to others.
2. To assist patient in controlling impulses.
3. To provide time to think through current situation.

Procedure

NURSING ACTIONS	*RATIONALE/AMPLIFICATION*
1. Explain procedure, including purpose and time period of the restriction.	1. Understanding the purpose for restriction will decrease tendency to view restrictions as punishment.
2. Provide support to stay within area.	2. Restriction of movement can be anxiety producing as well as anxiety reducing. Interpersonal support will promote feelings of security.
3. Give feedback about inappropriate behavior immediately and assist to modify the behavior.	3. Increasing knowledge about behavior and reactions to others can be helpful in thinking about it more objectively. On-the-spot direction and support is frequently helpful in producing change, when anxiety level is high.

GUIDELINES: Seclusion*

Seclusion is placement of the patient in a protected room with a locked door.

> **NURSING ALERT:** Basic to the use of this controversial method of treatment is the assumption that other interventions were tried and did not succeed in reducing the behavior. Doctor's order is needed.

Purpose
1. To provide protection from self-injury and injury to others only when the danger is clearly recognized.
2. To prevent gross damage or disruption to the environment.

Procedure

NURSING ACTION	RATIONALE/AMPLIFICATION
1. Provide protected room that generally includes lack of furnishings, soundly constructed walls and floor, door that cannot be opened from the inside, mattress and blankets that cannot be destroyed easily, protected window, light fixture, and ventilation equipment.	1. A protective room limits area of motor activity and opportunities for loss of impulse control or other expressions of extremely impaired judgment. Limits opportunities for self-injury. Decreases stimuli, for there is sensory overload in psychotic states. Provides relief from interpersonal intensity and distortions.
2. Obtain additional staff to escort patient into seclusion, then to escort patient to bathroom, to provide opportunity to smoke, to give food at meal times, to take vital signs, etc. Give clear, brief explanations.	2. Increased number of staff is calming to some patients and it demonstrates that the patient will not be allowed to remain in an uncontrollable state. Explanations elicit greater cooperation.
3. Remove clothing and jewelry and provide gown or shorts and tee shirt. Clothing may have to be completely absent if patient is actively attempting to kill himself. Otherwise patient should have one layer of clothing to maintain some sense of privacy and respect.	3. Removal of clothing provides opportunity to check patient for other items that might be dangerous, such as ring with sharp edge, matches hidden under breasts, or pins in socks.
4. Tell patient what is happening to his personal belongings. List items removed from patient and place in locked area.	4. Patient is concerned about his things and has right to know that they will be protected.
5. Provide urinal or explain to patient how to let staff know that he needs to go to the bathroom.	5. Elimination needs are provided for in a manner showing respect for the person.
6. Offer fluids frequently or leave container in room.	6. Additional psychotropic medication given to assist in dealing with behavior increases thirst and need for fluids.
7. Make frequent and regular checks of patient (every 15 minutes is suggested; more frequent checks may be necessary if patient is very agitated).	7. Effects of seclusion need to be monitored closely.
8. Verbally acknowledge your presence to the patient at each check. For example, call his name, give time of day.	8. Patient needs to experience the continued concern of the nurse, and data about the effects of seclusion can be gathered through his response.
9. Serve food in paper containers and remove uneaten portions promptly.	
10. Check vital signs or at least blood pressure before administering antipsychotic medication.	10. Procedure not only gives physiological data, but information on ability to relate to reality.
11. Continue to give p.r.n. medications prescribed for agitation.	11. Patient's acute distress is relieved to a degree with seclusion, but continued medication increases ability to control behavior.
12. Investigate by entering room and talking or inspecting patient, if patient remains in one position for prolonged period or if unusual noise or activity is noted.	12. Maintain constant vigilance to ensure safety of patient.
13. Arrange for cleaning of room area daily.	13. Patient may spit, throw food, urinate or defecate on floor and area needs to be clean.
14. Evaluate continuance of patient's seclusion with treatment team.	14. A nursing assessment of the need to continue seclusion is shared with treatment team. It may include data about therapeutic alliance established between patient and staff, and ability of patient to control his behavior.
15. Provide opportunity to discuss staff's beliefs and feelings about seclusion of patient and also what can be done to prevent its use in future.	15. Use of seclusion is affected by staff's reaction and perceptions, such as a way to avoid interpersonal exchanges with disturbed, hostile, insulting and difficult patients; as a way to deal with anxiety in staff; or as a way to punish or teach a lesson to patient.

* Refer to Chapter 26, Inappropriate Expression of Aggression.

GUIDELINES: Restraints*

Handcuffs are two metal, ringlike devices connected by short chain and locked around the wrists.
Wristlets are wide, leather, padded cuffs which are secured with a leather strap and locking device.
They can be attached to wrists or ankles of the patient and then secured to the waist or to a bed.
Limb and body holders are special devices to hold a body part in a bed or chair.
Sheet restraint is a folded sheet placed over body part and fastened to bed or chair that is out of the
reach of the patient.

Purpose   To provide protection from self-injury and injury to others.

Procedure

NURSING ACTION	RATIONALE/AMPLIFICATION
1. Explain reasons for application of restraint.	1. Explanations elicit greater cooperation.
2. Provide continuous monitoring of patient's response to procedure.	2. Limits opportunities for self-injury.
3. Check skin areas for signs of irritation.	3. Maintains skin integrity.
4. Assure some movement of body part.	4. Maintains adequate circulation.
5. Release restraints prn (at least every 2 hours is suggested) or to allow patient to eat and to go to the bathroom.	5. Assists in evaluating patient's response to procedure and allows exercise of muscles.
6. Provide for limited activity.	6. A decrease in stimuli can assist patient to regain more control over impulses.
7. Encourage recognition by patient that a time-out period or activity restriction is needed and can be requested at another time.	7. Participation in the decision to restrict activities or stimuli is important in obtaining full cooperation from patient.

* Refer to Chapter 26, Inappropriate Expression of Aggression.

GUIDELINES: Protective Interventions in Violent Situations

A. *Sequence I: Interventions Using Interpersonal Techniques*

Procedure

NURSING ACTION	SUGGESTED COMMENT
1. Move other patients out of area.	1. "I believe some privacy is needed so Mr. X and I can work something out."
2. Allow increased distance between self and patient.	2. "I'll stay here." (Said in calm, respectful manner.)
3. Obtain additional help.	3. "Miss X is calling for some assistance."
4. Identify your concern.	4. "Something serious has happened to upset you so . . ."
5. Offer assistance.	5. "I would like to help . . ."
6. Give positive reassurance to patient that he will be assisted in maintaining control and prevented from hurting self or others.	6. "I do not want you to hurt anyone. I cannot allow that . . ."
7. Suggest alternatives to present behavior.	7. "Can you put down the chair so I can talk with you a bit more easily?" or "Can we walk down to my office?" or "How about a shower?"
8. Actively request verbalization of problem.	8. "What went on . . ."

B. *Sequence II: Interventions Using Physical Restraint*

Interventions using interpersonal techniques may not be successful in helping the patient achieve
more rational control of his behavior and physical restraint may be indicated.

1. Obtain additional help. At least four persons is suggested.
2. Explain to patient what type of restraint will be used to help him achieve control of his behavior.
3. Use necessary method to remove patient from the area, to place patient in seclusion or restraints, or to immobilize him.*
   a. One staff member with head lock and a half nelson.
   b. Two staff members using lever restraint. Each person rotates patient's wrist outward keeping patient's elbow straight and, with other hand under patient's arm, grasps his partner's hand.
   c. Two staff members using shoulder restraint. Each person grasps patient's wrist and shoulder and swings patient's straight arm backward and up keeping elbow joint up.
   d. Two staff members using straight-arm restraint. Each person rotates patient's wrist outward and places other arm over the patient's arm and under his elbow.
   e. Four staff members using one man on each extremity.
4. Use blanket or mattress to distract patient while others are achieving physical restraint.
5. See Guidelines: Restraints or Guidelines: Seclusion and, also, Chapter 26, Inappropriate Expression of Aggression.

* To ensure full understanding of these holds, arrange to see videotapes and demonstrations, and to practice.

C. *Interventions Using Measures to Protect Self*

1. Have confidence in own ability to manage based on skills in assessing, planning, and acting in violent situations.
2. Move slowly from side to side allowing distance from patient as you talk with him.
3. Use the left/right back stance to achieve greater stability and flexibility.
4. Observe eye movements of patient, for he will look at what he plans to attack, and you will have a chance to take preventive action.
5. Use objects in environment, such as a chair, to protect self from a blow with an object.
6. Avoid blows from patient who is sitting or lying on floor by kneeling on floor with knee close to patient in a bent position, but not touching floor.
7. Keep arms bent and in front of body to protect chest and face from blows.

BIBLIOGRAPHY

BEHAVIOR MODIFICATION

Books

Agras W (ed). Behavior Modification: Principles and Clinical Applications. Boston, Little, Brown, & Co., 1978

Bellack A and Hersen M. Behavior Modification: An Introductory Textbook. Baltimore, Williams & Wilkins, 1977

Carr J and Yule W (eds). Behavior Modification for the Mentally Handicapped. Baltimore, University Park Press, 1980

Hersen M and Bellack A (eds). Behavior Therapy in the Psychiatric Setting. Baltimore, Williams & Wilkins, 1978

Kazdin A. Behavior Modification in Applied Settings. Homewood, Dorsey Press, 1975

Leitenberg H (ed). Handbook of Behavior Modification and Behavior Therapy. Englewood Cliffs, Prentice–Hall, 1976

Marks I. Care and Cure of Neuroses: Theory and Practice of Behavioral Psychotherapy. New York, John Wiley & Sons, 1981

Marmor J and Woods S (eds). The Interface Between the Psychodynamic and Behavioral Therapies. New York, Plenum Medical Book Co., 1980

Quick E. Teaching Responsibility to Psychiatric Patients: A Behavioral-Humanistic Approach. Pittsburgh, Gateway Book Pub. Co., 1978

Rathus S and Nevid J. Behavior Therapy; Strategies for Solving Problems in Living. Garden City, Doubleday & Co., 1977

Reese E. The Analysis of Human Operant Behavior. Dubuque, Wm C. Brown, 1973

Reese E. Experiments in Operant Behavior. New York, Irvington, 1980

Rehm L. Behavior Therapy for Depression: Present Status and Future Directions. New York, Academic Press, 1980

Stolz S. Ethical Issues in Behavior Modification. San Francisco, Jossey–Bass Publishers, 1978

Wilson G and O'Leary K. Principles of Behavior Therapy. Englewood Cliffs, Prentice–Hall, 1980

Yates A. Biofeedback and the Modification of Behavior. New York, Plenum Press, 1980

Articles

Barker P. Behavior therapy in psychiatric and mental handicap nursing. J Adv Nurs 1980 Jan; 5(1):55–69

Butler R. The evolution of a token economy programme for female chronic schizophrenic patients. J Adv Nurs 1979 May; 4(3):307–318

Clark C. Combining therapeutic approaches. J Psychiatr Nurs 1977 Oct; 15(10):18–22

Forsland C and Errickson E. A behavioral approach to physical rehabilitation: A case study. J Psychiatr Nurs 1978 May; 16(5):48–51

Hauser M. Nurses and behavior modification: Resistance, ignorance or both. J Psychiatr Nurs 1978 Aug: 16(8):17–19

Mansdorf I, Bucich D, Judd L. Behavioral treatment strategies of institution ward staff. Ment Retard 1977 Oct; 15(5):22–24

Peterson K and Errickson E. Use of reinforcement principles to reinstate self-care activities in a deaf and blind psychiatric patient. J Psychiatr Nurs 1977 June: 15(6):15–18

Rumpler C and Seigerman C. A behavior modification approach to dealing with violent behavior in an Intensive Care Unit. Perspect Psychiatr Care 1978 Sept–Dec; 16(5–6):206–211, 245

Schlemmer J and Barnett P. Management of manipulative behavior of anorexia nervosa patients. J Psychiatr Nurs 1977 Nov; 15(11):35–41

Seidel H and Hodgkinson P. Behavior modification and long-term learning in Korsakoff's psychosis. Nurs Times 1979 Oct 25; 75(43):1855–1857

Weaver S, Armstrong N, Broome A, et al. Behavioral principles applied in a security ward. Nurs Times 1978 Jan 5; 74(1):22–24

GROUP THERAPY

Books

Benjamin A. Behavior in Small Groups. Boston, Houghton Mifflin, 1978

Bion W. Experiences in Groups, and Other Papers. New York, Basic Books, 1961

Burnside I. Group work with the mentally impaired elderly. In Burnside I (ed). Working with the Elderly: Group process and Techniques, Chapt. 12. North Scituate, Duxbury Press, 1978

Cartwright D and Zander A. Group Dynamics: Research and Theory. New York, Harper & Row, 1968

Dennis H. Remotivation therapy groups. In Burnside I (ed). Working with the Elderly: Group Process and Techniques, Chapt 14. North Scituate, Duxbury Press, 1978

Ebersol P. Establishing reminiscing groups. In Burnside I (ed). Working with the Elderly: Group Process and Techniques, Chapt. 15. North Scituate, Duxbury Press, 1978

Kaplan H, Freedman A, Sadock B. Comprehensive Textbook of Psychiatry III. Baltimore, Williams & Wilkins, 1980

Leveton E. Psychodrama for the Timid Clinician. New York, Springer Publishing, 1977

Marram G. The Group Approach in Nursing Practice. St. Louis, CV Mosby, 1978

Mullan H and Rosenbaum M. Group Psychotherapy: Theory and Practice. New York, Free Press, 1978

Paul G and Lentz R. Psychosocial Treatment of Chronic Mental Patients: Milieu Versus Social Learning Programs. Cambridge, Harvard University Press, 1979

Shapiro J. Methods of Group Psychotherapy and Encounter: A Tradition of Innovation. Itasca, FE Peacock Publishers, 1978

Slater P. Microcosm, Structural, Psychological, and Religious Evolution in Groups. New York, John Wiley & Sons, 1966

Starr A. Rehearsal for Living: Psychodrama. Chicago, Nelson Hall, 1977

Taulbee L. Reality orientation: A therapeutic group activity for elderly persons. In Burnside I (ed). Working with the Elderly: Group Process and Techniques, Chapt. 13. North Scituate, Duxbury Press, 1978

Topalis M and Aguilera D. Psychiatric Nursing. St. Louis, CV Mosby, 1978

Wilson H and Kneisl C. Psychiatric Nursing. Menlo Park, Addison–Wesley Pub. Co., 1979

Yablonsky L. Psychodrama. Resolving Emotional Problems Through Role-Playing. New York, Basic Books, 1976

Yalom I. The Theory and Practice of Group Psychotherapy. New York, Basic Books, 1975

Articles

Asimos C and Rosen D. Group treatment of suicidal and depressed persons. Bull Menninger Clin 1978 Nov; 42(6):515–519

Balgopal P and Vassil T. The group psychotherapist: A new breed. Perspect Psychiatr Care 1979 May–June; 17(3): 132–135

Bennis W and Shepard H. A theory of group development. Hum Rel 1956; 9(4):415–437

Benton D. The significance of the absent member in milieu therapy. Perspect Psychiatr Care 1980 Jan–Feb; 18(1): 21–25

Calicchia C and Governali J. Attitudes toward homosexuality: Does role-playing have an impact? Health Values 1980 July–Aug; 4(4):176–182

Frances A, Clarkin J, Marachi J. Selection criteria for outpatient group psychotherapy. Hosp Community Psychiatry 1980 Apr; 31(4):245–250

Hager R. Evaluation of group psychotherapy—a question of values. J Psychiatr Nurs 1978 Dec; 16(12):26, 31–33

Hankins–McNary L. The use of humor in group therapy. Perspect Psychiatr Care 1979 Sept–Oct; 17(5):228–231

Hellwig K and Memmott R. Partners in therapy: Using the co-therapists' relationship in a group. J Psychiatr Nurs 1978 Apr; 16(4):42–44

Horowitz J. Sexual difficulties as indicators of broader personal and interpersonal problems. Perspect Psychiatr Care 1978 Mar–Apr; 16(2):66–69

Janosik E. Reachable and teachable: Report on a prison alcoholism group. J Psychiatr Nurs 1977 Apr; 15(4):24–28

Kiernat J. The use of life review activity with confused nursing home residents. Am J Occup Ther 1979 May; 33(5): 306–310

Lyon G. Stimulation through remotivation. Am J Nurs 1971 May; 71(5):982–985

MacMillan M. Madness—or just a case of sadness? Nurs Times 1980 July 24; 76(30):1310–1313

McIvor D, and Rosario A. Group therapy for women going through divorce. Can J Psychiatr Nurs 1979 May–June: 20(3):11–13

McMordie W and Blom S. Life review therapy: Psychotherapy for the elderly. Perspect Psychiatr Care 1979 July–Aug; 17(4):162–166

Mitchell R. Establishing a therapy group. Nurs Times 1978 Mar 2; 74(9):352–354

Pullinger W. Remotivation. Am J Nurs 1960 May; 60(5): 682–685

Rioch M. The work of Wilfred Bion on groups. Psychiatry 1970 Feb; 33(1):56–66

Sanderson M and Blackley J. Problems displayed "in vivo"—a particular advantage of group therapy. Perspect Psychiatr Care 1979 July–Aug; 17(4):176–186

Slimmer L. Use of the nursing process to facilitate group therapy. J Psychiatr Nurs 1978 Feb; 16(2):42–44

Smith L. Finding your leadership style in groups. Am J Nurs 1980 July; 80(7):1301–1303

Stryker R. How to develop a therapeutic community. J Nurs Adm 1980 Apr; 10(4):14–17

Wise P. Methods of teaching—revisited character play and role play. J Cont Ed Nurs 1980 Jan–Feb; 11(1):37–38

Wynne A. Movable group therapy for institutionalized patients. Hosp Community Psychiatry 1978 Aug; 29(8): 516–519

DRUGS & PROTECTIVE INTERVENTIONS

Books

Blake K and Taylor CE. The Prevention and Management of Aggressive Behavior. Columbia, South Carolina Department of Mental Health, 1977

Klein DF, Gittelman R, Quitkin F, Rifkin A: Diagnosis and Drug Treatment of Psychiatric Disorders: Adults and Children, 2nd ed. Baltimore, Williams & Wilkins, 1980

Lipton MA, DeMascio A, Killam R, (eds). Psychopharmacology, A Generation of Progress. New York, Raven Press, 1978

Physicians' Desk Reference, 34th edition. New Jersey, Medical Economics, 1980

Schon M. Lithium Treatment of Manic–Depressive Illness. A Practical Guide. Basel, S Karger International, 1980

Tognon G, Latink R, Jusko W (eds). Frontiers in Therapeutic Drug Monitoring. New York, Raven Press, 1980

Wardell S. Acute Intervention: Nursing Process Through the Life Span. Reston, Reston Pub. Co., 1979

Articles

Anders BL. When a patient becomes violent. Am J Nurs 1977 July; 77(7):1144–1148

Appleton WS. Third psychoactive drug usage guide. Dis Nerv Syst 1976 Jan; 37(1):39–51

Burgess HA. When a patient on lithium is pregnant. Am J Nurs 1979 Nov; 79(11):1989–1990

Cohen M, Gordon R, Marlowe H et al. A single-bedtime-dose self-medication system. Hosp Community Psychiatry 1979 Jan; 30(1):30–33

DeGennaro MD, Hymen R, Crannell AM, Mansky PA. Antidepressant drug therapy. Am J Nurs 1981 July; 81(7):1304–1310

DiBella GA. Educating staff to manage threatening paranoid patients. Am J Psychiatry 1979 March; 136(3):333–335

Ghadirian AM and Lehnann HE: Neurological side effects of lithium: Organic brain syndrome, seizures; extrapyramidal side effects, and EEG changes. Compr Psychiatry 1980 Oct; 21(5):327–334

Gertz B. Training for prevention of assaultive behavior in a psychiatric setting. Hosp Community Psychiatry 1980 Sept; 31(9):628–630

Gutheil TG. Observations on the theoretical bases for seclusion of the psychiatric inpatient. Am J Psychiatry 1978 Mar; 135(3):325–328

Gutheil TG and Daly M. Clinical considerations in seclusion room design. Hosp Community Psychiatry 1980 Apr; 31(4):268–270

Harris E. Antipsychotic medications. Am J Nurs 1981 July; 81(7):1316–1323

Harris E. Extrapyramidal side effects of antipsychotic medications. Am J Nurs 1981 July; 81(7):1324–1328

Harris E. Lithium. Am J Nurs 1981 July; 81(7):1310–1315

Harris E. Sedative–hypnotic drugs. Am J Nurs 1981 July; 81(7):1329–1334

Hunn S, Miranda C, Moyneaux V, Warshaw C. Nursing care of patients on lithium. Perspect Psychiatr Care 1980 Sept–Oct; 18(5):214–220

Kuruca J and Fallon J. Dose reduction and discontinuation of antipsychotic medication. Hosp Community Psychiatry 1980 Feb; 31(2):117–119

Mason AS and Granacher RP. Basic principles of rapid neuroleptization. Dis Nerv Syst 1976 Oct; 37(10):547–551

Penningroth PE. Control of violence in a mental health setting. Am J Nurs 1975 Apr; 75(4):606–609

Redmond FC. Study on the use of the seclusion room. Quality Review Bulletin 1980 Aug; 6(8):20–23

Rosen H and Dibiacomo J. The role of physical restraint in the treatment of psychiatric illness. J Clin Psychiatry 1978 Mar; 39(3):228–232

Schwab PJ and Lahmeyer CB. The use of seclusion on a general hospital psychiatric unit. J Clin Psychiatry 1979 May; 40(5):228–231

Soloff PH and Turner SM. Patterns of seclusion, a prospective study. J Nerv Ment Dis 1981 Jan; 169(1):37–44

Task Force on Late Neurological Effects of Antipsychotic Drugs. Am J Psychiatry 1980 Oct; 137(10);1163–1172

MATERNITY NURSING

PART 3

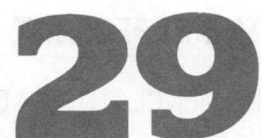

MATERNAL AND FETAL HEALTH

INTRODUCTION TO MATERNITY NURSING

Maternity nursing includes the care of and other activities relevant to maternity patients and their infants during all phases of the childbearing experience.

Such care is being increasingly provided by nurses with special education and experience. Among these is the *nurse midwife,* a registered nurse who has completed a recognized program of study and clinical experience and who works interdependently with others in the health care system under the ultimate direction of an obstetrician. She provides care for women throughout the reproductive years, focusing on, but not totally restricted to, the low-risk aspects of patient care.

Current Problems Affecting Maternal and Infant Morbidity and Mortality

1. Poor distribution or lack of care among disadvantaged low-income families living in urban industrial, rural, and ghetto areas.
2. Increased incidence of prematurity, congenital defects, and birth injuries in the newborn.
3. Nutritional problems among disadvantaged and adolescent mothers.
4. Shortage of professional personnel—physicians, nurses, midwives, and social workers.

Assessment of High-Risk Pregnancy

Factors associated with such pregnancy outcomes as infant and maternal mortality, low birth weight, premature or brain-damaged infants, and maternal complications (see also Chapter 32) include the following:
1. Maternal age factor
  a. Age 35 or older—tendency to have heavier babies with high rate of perinatal mortality; high incidence of infants with Down's syndrome.
  b. Adolescent pregnancy
    (1) Obstetrical and medical problems
      (a) Lack of prenatal care due to low socioeconomic background and to psychological factors such as lack of motivation, denial, ignorance, pride, or rebellion against authority.
      (b) Malnutrition with anemia and vitamin deficiency, excessive weight gain, toxemias, prolonged labor due to fetopelvic disproportion, drug abuse, repeated and recurrent infections.
2. Social problems
  a. Failure to complete education or vocational training.
  b. Dependence on others for support.
  c. Failure to establish a stable family life.
  d. High rate of marital failure.
  e. High incidence of repeated out-of-wedlock pregnancies.
3. Socioeconomic factors
  a. Low income mothers are more predisposed to lowered health status and consequently to obstetrical and neonatal complications.
    (1) Mothers unable or unwilling to maintain a balanced dietary intake display a higher incidence of toxemias.
    (2) Dietary deficiencies directly related to low birth weight of infants.
    (3) Low levels of maternal essential amino acids correlate with infant intelligence; there appears to be a direct correlation between malnutrition of the mother and mental retardation of the infant.
  b. Women who are using illicit or certain licit drugs on a chronic basis usually do not seek prenatal care, are poorly nourished, and produce drug-addicted infants.
  c. Women who smoke cigarettes or drink alcohol have infants with low birth weights and have a higher rate of abortions and stillbirths.
4. Obstetrical factors
  a. High-risk patients also include women who:
    (1) Have had difficulties with previous pregnancies, a previous fetal loss, or a history of premature births.
    (2) Are diabetic, hypertensive, anemic, or suffer from cardiac, renal, or respiratory disease.
    (3) Have had evidence of vaginal bleeding.
    (4) Are Rh negative.
    (5) Have psychiatric disorders.
    (6) Have been exposed to teratogens, chemical or environmental toxins, or radiation.

THE EXPECTANT MOTHER

NOMENCLATURE—GRAVIDA AND PARITY

Gravidity

1. *Gravida*—a pregnant woman
2. *Primigravida*—a woman pregnant for the first time
3. *Multigravida*—a woman who has been pregnant several times

Parity

1. *Para*—alludes to past pregnancies that have reached viability.
2. *Parity*—refers to number of past pregnancies that have gone to viability and have been delivered regardless of the number of children involved (NOTE: The birth of triplets increases the parity by 1).
3. *Primipara*—a woman who has had 1 pregnancy resulting in the delivery of a child that has reached viability, without regard to the child's being alive or dead at the time of birth.
4. *Multipara*—a woman who has had 2 or more pregnancies that terminated at the stage when the children were viable.

Gravida and Para

1. A woman pregnant for the first time is a primigravida and is described as Gravida 1, Para 0.
2. If she aborts before viability, she remains Gravida 1, Para 0.
3. If she delivers a fetus which has reached viability she becomes a Primipara regardless of whether the child is alive or dead—Gravida 1, Para 1.
4. During a second pregnancy she is Gravida 2, Para 1.
5. A patient with 2 abortions and no viable children is Gravida 2, Para 0.

MANIFESTATIONS OF PREGNANCY

Presumptive Signs and Symptoms

1. Cessation of menses—pregnancy is indicated if more than 10 days have elapsed since the missed period.
2. Breast changes
   a. Breasts enlarge and become tender. Veins in breast become increasingly visible.
   b. Nipples increase in size and pigmentation.
   c. *Colostrum*, a thin milky fluid, may be expressed after the first few months.
   d. Montgomery glands, small elevations on the areolae, may appear.
3. Vaginal and vulval color changes (Chadwick's sign)—a bluish discoloration and congestion.
4. Abdominal striae (striae gravidarum)—sometimes appear on the breasts, abdomen, and thighs due to the stretching, rupture, and atrophy of the deep connective tissue of the skin.
5. Nausea and vomiting (morning sickness)—may occur at any time of day, usually last a few hours.
6. Quickening (sensations of movement in the abdomen)—occurs between 16th and 19th week after the last menses.
7. Frequency of urination
   a. Caused by pressure of the expanding uterus on the bladder.
   b. Disappears when the uterus rises out of the pelvis.
   c. Reappears when the fetal head engages in the pelvis at the end of pregnancy.
8. Fatigue

Probable Signs and Symptoms

1. Enlargement of abdomen—near the end of the 3rd month, the uterus can be felt through the abdominal wall.
2. Changes in shape, size, and consistency of the uterus
   a. A soft, cushion-like consistency in early pregnancy contributes to the nourishment and protection of the implanted ovum.
   b. Uterine thickness gradually decreases as the stretching of later pregnancy occurs.
3. Changes in cervix
   a. Softening may not occur until much later in pregnancy.
      (1) Goodell's sign—softening of the cervix
      (2) Hegar's sign—softening of the lower uterine segment
   b. In certain pathologic conditions the cervix may remain firm.
4. Intermittent contractions of the uterus (Braxton Hicks sign)—painless, palpable contractions occurring at irregular intervals.
5. Ballottement—a sinking and rebounding of the fetus in its surrounding amniotic fluid as a response to a sudden tap on the uterus (occurs in 4th or 5th month of pregnancy).
6. Outlining of the fetus through the abdomen—abdominal palpation in the 2nd half of pregnancy.
7. Positive hormonal tests for pregnancy (test reactions produced by gonadotropin in maternal plasma and urine).

Positive Signs and Symptoms

1. Fetal heartbeat (separate and distinct from that of the mother)—usually heard between 16th and 20th week of gestation
2. Perception of fetal movements by the examiner
3. X-ray visualization of the fetus (after the 4th month)
4. Sonographic evidence

MATERNAL PHYSIOLOGY DURING PREGNANCY

Duration of Pregnancy

280 days, or 40 weeks, 9 calendar months, 10 lunar months, counting from the 1st day of the last menstrual period.

General Alterations in Function

1. Changes become recognizable shortly after first missed period.
2. Pregnancy imposes a stress on the maternal organism, particularly on the vascular circulation.
3. Many changes represent the response of the body to additional metabolic demands.
4. Physical and functional alterations involve all body systems.

Changes in Reproductive Tract

1. Uterus
   a. Uterus increases in size: 7–35 cm. in length;

60–1200 gm. weight at term—owing to hypertrophy, muscle cells attain 5–10 times normal size.

b. By 2nd month, uterus triples in size and weight—may cause shift in position and exaggerated antiflexion, retrocession, or retroversion.

c. By 3rd month, uterus occupies pelvic cavity; may be felt suprapubically—myometrium 2–3 cm. in thickness.

d. By 4th month, uterus becomes an abdominal organ—fundus has reached the level of the umbilicus.

e. By 36–38 weeks, fundal portion has reached the ensiform process.

f. Last 3–4 weeks, uterus recedes slightly—due to descent into pelvis. Walls of uterus become thinner (1–2 cm.).

g. Changes in contractility occur—during 1st trimester regular painless contractions occur (Braxton Hicks contractions)—result of combination of muscle stretch, increased actinomycin in the muscle cells, and changes in estrogen, progesterone, and electrolyte levels.

h. Blood flow remains fairly constant.
   (1) 10–15 ml./100 gm./minute
   (2) Total flow, 500–700 ml./minute at term

2. Cervix
   a. Pronounced softening and cyanosis—due to increased vascularity, edema, hypertrophy, and hyperplasia of the cervical glands.
   b. Common erosions of cervix—represent an extension of proliferating endocervical glands and columnar endocervical epithelium due to increased estrogen production.

3. Ovaries
   a. Ovulation ceases during pregnancy; maturation of new follicles is suspended. One large corpus luteum remains on 1 ovary.
   b. Ovarian veins increase in caliber from 0.9–2.6 cm. at term.

4. Vagina
   a. Chadwick's sign noted—characteristic violet color due to increased vascularity and hyperemia.
   b. Vaginal walls prepare for labor: mucosa increases in thickness, connective tissue loosens, and small muscle cells hypertrophy.
   c. Vaginal secretions increase; pH is 3.5–6—owing to increased production of lactic acid from glycogen in the vaginal epithelium by *Lactobacillus acidophilus*. (Acid pH probably aids in keeping vagina relatively free of pathogenic bacteria.)

Changes in the Abdominal Wall

Striae gravidarum often develop—reddish, slightly depressed streaks in the skin of abdomen, breast, and thighs. (Become glistening silvery lines after pregnancy.)

Breast Changes

1. Are tender and tingly in early weeks of pregnancy.
2. Increase in size by 2nd month—hypertrophy of mammary alveoli.
3. Nipples become larger, more deeply pigmented, and more erectile early in pregnancy.
4. Colostrum may be expressed by 2nd trimester.
5. Areolae become broader and more deeply pigmented. The depth of pigmentation varies with the individual's complexion.
6. Scattered through the areola are a number of small elevations (glands of Montgomery) which are hypertrophic sebaceous glands.

Metabolic Changes

1. Are numerous and intensive—response to rapidly growing fetus and placenta.
2. Weight gain averages 9.1 kg. (20 lbs.).
   a. Fetus, 3.4 kg. (7½ lbs.)
   b. Placenta, 0.454 kg. (1 lb.)
   c. Amniotic fluid, 0.91 kg. (2 lbs.)
   d. Hypertrophy of uterus, 0.91 kg. (2 lbs.)
   e. Breasts, 0.91 kg. (2 lbs.)
   f. Increase in blood volume, 1.60 kg. (3½ lbs.)
   g. Water retention; fat and protein deposition, 1.8 kg. (4 lbs.)
3. Water metabolism
   a. Increased water retention (fetus, placenta, amniotic fluid) comprises 3.5 liters; uterus, maternal blood volume, and breast tissue comprise 3.5 liters, producing intracapillary hydrostatic pressure which favors filtration from the vascular bed and increased capillary permeability.
   b. Increased sodium retention.
4. Protein metabolism
   a. Fetus, uterus, and maternal blood are rich in protein rather than in fat or carbohydrates.
   b. At term fetus and placenta weigh about 4 kg. and contain 500 gm. of protein.
   c. Approximately 500 gm. more of protein are added to maternal blood in form of hemoglobin and plasma proteins.
5. Carbohydrate and insulin metabolism
   a. Diabetes mellitus is aggravated by pregnancy.
   b. Clinical diabetes appears in some women only during pregnancy. Normal pregnancy level of plasma insulin is higher and destruction of insulin more rapid; thus secretion of insulin during pregnancy is increased.
6. Fat metabolism
   Plasma lipids increase during latter half of pregnancy. (Reasons are not known.)
7. Iron metabolism
   a. Iron requirements increase—often exceed amounts available.
   b. Total volume of circulating red blood cells increases by about 450 ml. during pregnancy; iron requirement increases to nearly 500 mg. (6–7 mg.)/day.
   c. Supplemental iron is valuable during latter half of pregnancy and for several weeks after pregnancy.

Changes in Cardiovascular System

1. Heart
   a. Diaphragm is progressively elevated during pregnancy; heart is displaced to the left and upward, with apex moved laterally.
   b. Pulmonic systolic and apical systolic murmurs are common—since lowered blood viscosity and displacement cause torsion in the great vessels.
2. Circulation
   a. Cardiac volume increases by 10%, causing slight hypertrophy of the heart and increased cardiac output—begins in first trimester, reaches maximum of 30–50% above normal about 7th to 8th lunar month, then falls toward normal near term.
   b. Blood pressure decreases slightly because of reduction in peripheral resistance.

c. Femoral venous pressure increases—owing to retardation of blood flow from lower extremities as a result of pressure of enlarged uterus on pelvic veins and inferior vena cava.
d. In the supine position, the large uterus of pregnancy compresses the venous system, thereby slowing cardiac filling and decreasing cardiac output.
e. Pulse rate usually increases; amount varies from almost no increase to 20%, or 15 beats per minute at term.
3. Hematologic changes
   a. Leukocyte count is elevated to values ranging between 6000–12,000/cu. mm. during pregnancy and rising to 25,000 or more during labor—cause unknown; probably represents the reappearance in the circulation of leukocytes previously shunted out of active circulation. Differential count should remain the same as for nonpregnant women.
   b. Fibrinogen levels increase 50%—influence of estrogen and progesterone.

Changes in Urinary Tract

1. Dilation of ureters and renal pelvis begins early in pregnancy—due to effect of progesterone.
2. Dilation later in pregnancy—mechanical pressure is greater on right side above the pelvic brim.
3. Glomerular filtration increases early in pregnancy and persists almost to term—due to pressure on the inferior vena cava and iliac veins.
4. Renal plasma flow increases early in pregnancy—may be due to effect of antidiuretic hormone, upright position, or vena cava congestion.
5. Glucosuria is evident—due to increase in glomerular filtration without increase in tubular reabsorptive capacity for filtered glucose.

Changes in Gastrointestinal Tract

1. Generalized softening of gingiva occurs—associated with bleeding or irritation.
2. Stomach and intestines are displaced upward and laterally by enlarging uterus.
3. Liver is displaced backward, upward, and to the right—hepatic blood flow remains unaltered and various liver function tests are within normal limits.
4. Alkaline phosphatase activity doubles during normal pregnancy—due to placental enzymes and maternal estrogen level.
5. Tone and motility of gastrointestinal tract decreases, leading to prolongation of gastric emptiness and relaxation of pyloric sphincter—these effects due to large amount of progesterone produced by placenta.

Changes in Respiratory Tract

1. Hyperventilation occurs—increase in respiratory rate, tidal volume (45%), and minute volume (40%); reasons remain obscure but probably result from increased consumption of oxygen, production of carbon dioxide by products of conception, and increased production of progesterone influencing the respiratory center.
2. Diaphragm is elevated during pregnancy—chiefly by the enlarging uterus.
3. Thoracic cage expands by means of flaring of the ribs—result of increased mobility of rib attachments.

Changes in Endocrine System

1. Pituitary enlarges slightly.

2. Thyroid is moderately enlarged due to hyperplasia of glandular tissue and increased vascularity.
   a. Basal metabolic rate increases progressively during normal pregnancy (as much as 25%)—due to metabolic activity of fetus.
   b. Level of protein-bound iodine and thyroxin rises sharply and is maintained until after delivery—owing to increased circulatory estrogen.
3. Adrenal secretions considerably increased—amounts of aldosterone increase as early as 15th week—due to augmented renin, renin-substrate, and angiotensin.

Changes in Integumentary System

1. Pigmentary changes occur due to melanocyte-stimulating hormone, level of which is elevated from the 2nd month of pregnancy until term.
2. *Chloasma gravidarum* (pigmentation of circumscribed areas of the skin during pregnancy) occurs.

Changes in Musculoskeletal System

1. The increasing mobility of sacroiliac, sacrococcygeal, and pelvic joints during pregnancy is result of hormonal (progesterone) changes.
2. This mobility contributes to alteration of maternal posture and to back pain.

PRENATAL ASSESSMENT AND NURSING SUPPORT DURING THE ANTEPARTAL PERIOD

Purposes

1. To ensure optimum health for both mother and infant.
2. To identify mothers and infants at risk.
3. To prevent complications or accidents during childbirth.
4. To educate the mother-to-be in self-care and infant care.
5. To provide medical, sociological, and psychological support as necessary.

History Taking

1. Interview to obtain relevant data—age; marital status; family setting; sources of income; cultural values and practices relative to childbearing and rearing; education; employment background.
2. Initial prenatal history
   a. Family history of health problems—mental, emotional, or psychiatric problems; congenital abnormalities or hereditary diseases; multiple pregnancies; diabetes; cardiovascular disorders; tuberculosis; epilepsy; allergies.
   b. Patient's medical history—immunization status; childhood diseases; major illnesses; surgery; blood transfusions; drug sensitivities and habits.
   c. Obstetrical history
      (1) Problems of infertility.
      (2) Relevant data of previous pregnancies and deliveries—dates; infant weights; length of labors; types of deliveries; multiple births; abortions; maternal, fetal, and neonatal complications.
   d. History of present pregnancy
      (1) Date of last menstrual period (LMP).

(2) Estimated date of birth. Expected date of confinement (EDC) is calculated by counting back 3 calendar months from the first day of the last menstrual period and adding 7 days. For specific delivery prediction data see Table 29-1.

3. Preliminary Physical Examination
   a. Observation for impression of physical and mental well-being
   b. Weight
      (1) The average woman may gain up to 11.3 kg. (25 lbs.) during normal gestation period.
      (2) A woman whose prepregnant weight was subnormal may safely gain more, and conversely, the overweight woman will be encouraged to gain less.
      (3) Marked weight gain or loss is a significant symptom and requires further follow-up.
   c. Blood pressure—any rise in systolic or diastolic blood pressure is cause for concern.
   d. Urinalysis
      (1) Urine is tested for sugar and albumin.
      (2) Glucose threshold is normally lower during pregnancy (the urine specimen should be taken before breakfast to avoid false positive reports of glucose).
      (3) Any sign of albumin in the urine should be reported immediately, since it is considered a serious sign of toxemia.
      (4) Specific gravity (1.015–1.025 is normal).
      (5) If bacteria or leukocytes are found, a urine culture is taken.
   e. Blood evaluation
      (1) Determination of hematocrit and hemoglobin levels, and description of the morphology of the red blood cells in an effort to find any evidence for certain states of anemia.
      (2) Sedimentation rate—at approximately the 10th or 12th week an acceleration of the rate begins; does not return to normal levels until 3rd or 4th week postpartum.
      (3) Biochemical determination—usually only glucose and urea nitrogen done; however, patients with renal disorders may require estimation of total protein with albumin and globulin ratios.
      (4) Serologic tests
         (a) Nonspecific antibody tests for syphilis (STS or VDRL) are usually done twice during pregnancy.
         (b) Rubella titre—immunity can be measured by a positive hemagglutination inhibition test.
         (c) Blood type and Rh factor—if the woman is found to be Rh negative the father's blood is typed; if he has Rh-positive blood, a Coombs test and antibody titre of the mother's blood is indicated.

Physical Examination

1. Patient should be asked to empty her bladder.
2. Examination of the eyes, ears, nose, teeth, and throat, with palpation of the thyroid gland (a slight degree of hyperplasia is considered normal).
3. Inspection of the breasts and nipples.
4. Auscultation and percussion of the heart and lungs.
5. Abdominal examination
   a. Examination for scars or striations, diastasis (or separation) of the rectus muscle, or umbilical hernia.
   b. Palpation of the abdomen for height of the fundus (palpable after 13 weeks of pregnancy); measurement recorded and used as guideline for subsequent calculations.
   c. Palpation of the abdomen for fetal outline (ascertained by 30 weeks of gestation).
   d. Fetal heart tone checked (heard by fetoscope at 20-24 weeks of gestation, earlier if a Doptone is used). Fetal position, presentation, and heart rate are recorded.
6. Pelvic examination
   a. Patient is placed in lithotomy position.
   b. External genitalia inspected.
   c. Vaginal examination done to rule out abnormalities of the birth canal and to obtain cytological smear (Papanicolaou and, if indicated, smears for gonorrhea, vaginal trichomoniasis, or moniliasis).
   d. Examination of the cervix for position, size, mobility, and consistency.
   e. Identification of the ovaries (size, shape, and position).
   f. Rectovaginal exploration to identify hemorrhoids, fissures, herniation or masses.
   g. Pelvimetry—may be done in early pregnancy but should be repeated prior to term for a more accurate evaluation of fetopelvic accommodation.

Pelvic Bones and Joints

A. *Bones*

The pelvis is composed of 4 bones.
1. 2 innominate bones
2. Sacrum
3. Coccyx

B. *Joints*

The bones articulate through 4 joints.
1. 2 sacroiliac joints—link the sacrum to the iliac part of the innominate bones.
2. Symphysis pubis—joins the 2 pubic bones.
3. Sacrococcygeal joint—attaches the sacrum to the coccyx.

C. *True and False Pelvis*

1. *False pelvis*—lies above the linea terminalis. Its obstetrical function is to support the enlarged uterus during pregnancy.
2. *True pelvis* lies below the pelvic brim or linea terminalis; it is the bony canal through which the infant must pass. It is divided into 3 parts (Fig. 29-1).
   a. Inlet
   b. Pelvic cavity
   c. Pelvic outlet

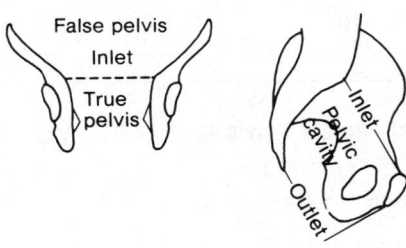

FIGURE 29-1. *The true pelvis.*

TABLE 29-1. DELIVERY PREDICTION DATES

Date of delivery (2) (3) (4) can be predicted when one of three dates (1) are known:

Example:

(1) Date of first day of last menstruation → (4)
(1) Date of first day life is felt for a primipara → (2)
(1) Date of first day life is felt for a multipara → (3)

(1) Jan. 1—Date of first day of last menstruation → (4) Oct. 8
(1) Jan. 1—Date of first day life is felt for a primipara → (2) June 4
(1) Jan. 1—Date of first day life is felt for a multipara → (3) June 18

Month		1	2	3	4	5	6	7	8	9	10	11	12	13	14	15
Jan.	(1)	1	2	3	4	5	6	7	8	9	10	11	12	13	14	15
June	(2)	4	5	6	7	8	9	10	11	12	13	14	15	16	17	18
June	(3)	18	19	20	21	22	23	24	25	26	27	28	29	30	1	2
Oct.	(4)	8	9	10	11	12	13	14	15	16	17	18	19	20	21	22
Feb.	(1)	1	2	3	4	5	6	7	8	9	10	11	12	13	14	15
July	(2)	5	6	7	8	9	10	11	12	13	14	15	16	17	18	19
July	(3)	19	20	21	22	23	24	25	26	27	28	29	30	31	1	2
Nov.	(4)	8	9	10	11	12	13	14	15	16	17	18	19	20	21	22
March	(1)	1	2	3	4	5	6	7	8	9	10	11	12	13	14	15
Aug.	(2)	2	3	4	5	6	7	8	9	10	11	12	13	14	15	16
Aug.	(3)	16	17	18	19	20	21	22	23	24	25	26	27	28	29	30
Dec.	(4)	6	7	8	9	10	11	12	13	14	15	16	17	18	19	20
April	(1)	1	2	3	4	5	6	7	8	9	10	11	12	13	14	15
Sept.	(2)	2	3	4	5	6	7	8	9	10	11	12	13	14	15	16
Sept.	(3)	16	17	18	19	20	21	22	23	24	25	26	27	28	29	30
Jan.	(4)	6	7	8	9	10	11	12	13	14	15	16	17	18	19	20
May	(1)	1	2	3	4	5	6	7	8	9	10	11	12	13	14	15
Oct.	(2)	2	3	4	5	6	7	8	9	10	11	12	13	14	15	16
Oct.	(3)	16	17	18	19	20	21	22	23	24	25	26	27	28	29	30
Feb.	(4)	5	6	7	8	9	10	11	12	13	14	15	16	17	18	19
June	(1)	1	2	3	4	5	6	7	8	9	10	11	12	13	14	15
Nov.	(2)	2	3	4	5	6	7	8	9	10	11	12	13	14	15	16
Nov.	(3)	16	17	18	19	20	21	22	23	24	25	26	27	28	29	30
March	(4)	8	9	10	11	12	13	14	15	16	17	18	19	20	21	22
July	(1)	1	2	3	4	5	6	7	8	9	10	11	12	13	14	15
Dec.	(2)	2	3	4	5	6	7	8	9	10	11	12	13	14	15	16
Dec.	(3)	16	17	18	19	20	21	22	23	24	25	26	27	28	29	30
April	(4)	7	8	9	10	11	12	13	14	15	16	17	18	19	20	21
Aug.	(1)	1	2	3	4	5	6	7	8	9	10	11	12	13	14	15
Jan.	(2)	2	3	4	5	6	7	8	9	10	11	12	13	14	15	16
Jan.	(3)	16	17	18	19	20	21	22	23	24	25	26	27	28	29	30
May	(4)	8	9	10	11	12	13	14	15	16	17	18	19	20	21	22
Sept.	(1)	1	2	3	4	5	6	7	8	9	10	11	12	13	14	15
Feb.	(2)	2	3	4	5	6	7	8	9	10	11	12	13	14	15	16
Feb.	(3)	16	17	18	19	20	21	22	23	24	25	26	27	28	1	2
June	(4)	8	9	10	11	12	13	14	15	16	17	18	19	20	21	22
Oct.	(1)	1	2	3	4	5	6	7	8	9	10	11	12	13	14	15
March	(2)	4	5	6	7	8	9	10	11	12	13	14	15	16	17	18
March	(3)	18	19	20	21	22	23	24	25	26	27	28	29	30	31	1
July	(4)	8	9	10	11	12	13	14	15	16	17	18	19	20	21	22
Nov.	(1)	1	2	3	4	5	6	7	8	9	10	11	12	13	14	15
April	(2)	4	5	6	7	8	9	10	11	12	13	14	15	16	17	18
April	(3)	18	19	20	21	22	23	24	25	26	27	28	29	30	1	2
Aug.	(4)	8	9	10	11	12	13	14	15	16	17	18	19	20	21	22
Dec.	(1)	1	2	3	4	5	6	7	8	9	10	11	12	13	14	15
May	(2)	4	5	6	7	8	9	10	11	12	13	14	15	16	17	18
May	(3)	18	19	20	21	22	23	24	25	26	27	28	29	30	31	1
Sept.	(4)	7	8	9	10	11	12	13	14	15	16	17	18	19	20	21

The Normal Female Pelvic Inlet and Planes

A. *Diameters of Female Pelvis*

Four diameters traverse the female pelvis (Fig. 29-2):

1. The anteroposterior diameter
   a. Extends from the middle of the promontory of the sacrum to the upper margin of the symphysis pubis.
   b. Is the most important diameter because it is the point of departure in estimating the size of the pelvis. *It is the true conjugate and measures 11 cm. or more.*

2. The transverse diameter

16	17	18	19	20	21	22	23	24	25	26	27	28	29	30	31	
19	20	21	22	23	24	25	26	27	28	29	30	1	2	3	4	July
3	4	5	6	7	8	9	10	11	12	13	14	15	16	17	18	July
23	24	25	26	27	28	29	30	31	1	2	3	4	5	6	7	Nov.
16	17	18	19	20	21	22	23	24	25	26	27	28				
20	21	22	23	24	25	26	27	28	29	30	31	1				Aug.
3	4	5	6	7	8	9	10	11	12	13	14	15				Aug.
23	24	25	26	27	28	29	30	1	2	3	4	5				Dec.
16	17	18	19	20	21	22	23	24	25	26	27	28	29	30	31	
17	18	19	20	21	22	23	24	25	26	27	28	29	30	31	1	Sept.
31	1	2	3	4	5	6	7	8	9	10	11	12	13	14	15	Sept.
21	22	23	24	25	26	27	28	29	30	31	1	2	3	4	5	Jan.
16	17	18	19	20	21	22	23	24	25	26	27	28	29	30	1	
17	18	19	20	21	22	23	24	25	26	27	28	29	30	1	2	Oct.
1	2	3	4	5	6	7	8	9	10	11	12	13	14	15	16	Oct.
21	22	23	24	25	26	27	28	29	30	31	1	2	3	4	5	Feb.
16	17	18	19	20	21	22	23	24	25	26	27	28	29	30	31	
17	18	19	20	21	22	23	24	25	26	27	28	29	30	31	1	Nov.
31	1	2	3	4	5	6	7	8	9	10	11	12	13	14	15	Nov.
20	21	22	23	24	25	26	27	28	1	2	3	4	5	6	7	March
16	17	18	19	20	21	22	23	24	25	26	27	28	29	30		
17	18	19	20	21	22	23	24	25	26	27	28	29	30	1		Dec.
1	2	3	4	5	6	7	8	9	10	11	12	13	14	15		Dec.
23	24	25	26	27	28	29	30	31	1	2	3	4	5	6		April
16	17	18	19	20	21	22	23	24	25	26	27	28	29	30	31	
17	18	19	20	21	22	23	24	25	26	27	28	29	30	31	1	Jan.
31	1	2	3	4	5	6	7	8	9	10	11	12	13	14	15	Jan.
22	23	24	25	26	27	28	29	30	1	2	3	4	5	6	7	May
16	17	18	19	20	21	22	23	24	25	26	27	28	29	30	31	
17	18	19	20	21	22	23	24	25	26	27	28	29	30	31	1	Feb.
31	1	2	3	4	5	6	7	8	9	10	11	12	13	14	15	Feb.
23	24	25	26	27	28	29	30	31	1	2	3	4	5	6	7	June
16	17	18	19	20	21	22	23	24	25	26	27	28	29	30		
17	18	19	20	21	22	23	24	25	26	27	28	1	2	3		March
3	4	5	6	7	8	9	10	11	12	13	14	15	16	17		March
23	24	25	26	27	28	29	30	1	2	3	4	5	6	7		July
16	17	18	19	20	21	22	23	24	25	26	27	28	29	30	31	
19	20	21	22	23	24	25	26	27	28	29	30	31	1	2	3	April
2	3	4	5	6	7	8	9	10	11	12	13	14	15	16	17	April
23	24	25	26	27	28	29	30	31	1	2	3	4	5	6	7	Aug.
16	17	18	19	20	21	22	23	24	25	26	27	28	29	30		
19	20	21	22	23	24	25	26	27	28	29	30	1	2	3		May
3	4	5	6	7	8	9	10	11	12	13	14	15	16	17		May
22	23	24	25	26	27	28	29	30	31	1	2	3	4	5	6	Sept.
16	17	18	19	20	21	22	23	24	25	26	27	28	29	30	31	
19	20	21	22	23	24	25	26	27	28	29	30	31	1	2	3	June
2	3	4	5	6	7	8	9	10	11	12	13	14	15	16	17	June
22	23	24	25	26	27	28	29	30	1	2	3	4	5	6	7	Oct.

a. Constructed at right angles to the true conjugate.
b. Joins the 2 most widely separated points of the pelvic inlet; measures approximately 13.5 cm.
3. Two oblique diameters
   a. Each extends from one of the sacroiliac synchondroses to the iliopectineal eminence on the opposite side of the pelvis.
   b. The oblique diameters measure approximately 12.75 cm.

Classification of the Pelvis

Name based on structure of the inlet (Fig. 29-3).
1. Gynecoid
2. Android
3. Anthropoid
4. Platypelloid

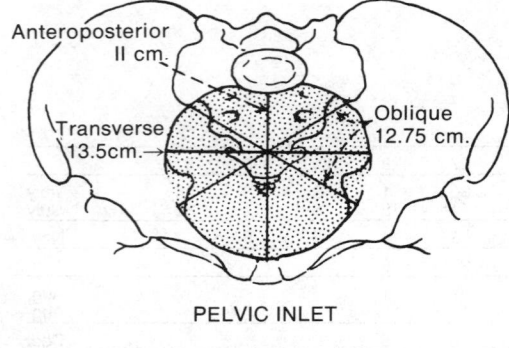

FIGURE 29-2. *The pelvic inlet.*

Pelvic Examination

A. *Manual determination of the pelvic architecture* (Fig. 29-4)

1. Determining the contour of the sacrum.
2. Estimating the size of the sacrosciatic notch and the prominence of the ischial spines.
3. Assessing the length of the bispinous diameter.
4. Assessing the splay of the pelvic side walls.

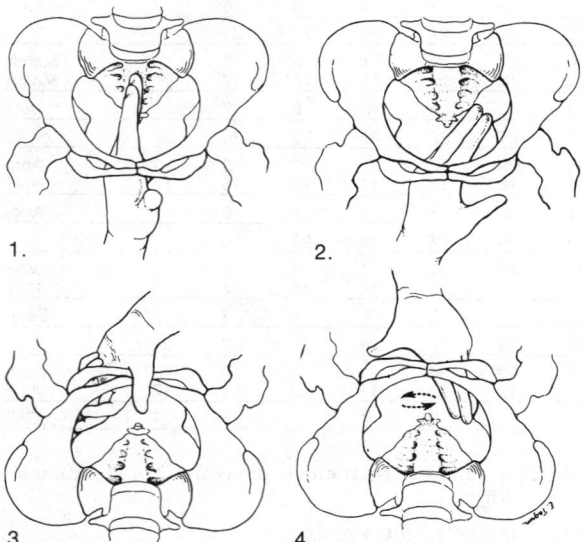

FIGURE 29-4. *Pelvic examination. (From Reid DE et al. Principles and Management of Human Reproduction. Philadelphia, WB Saunders.)*

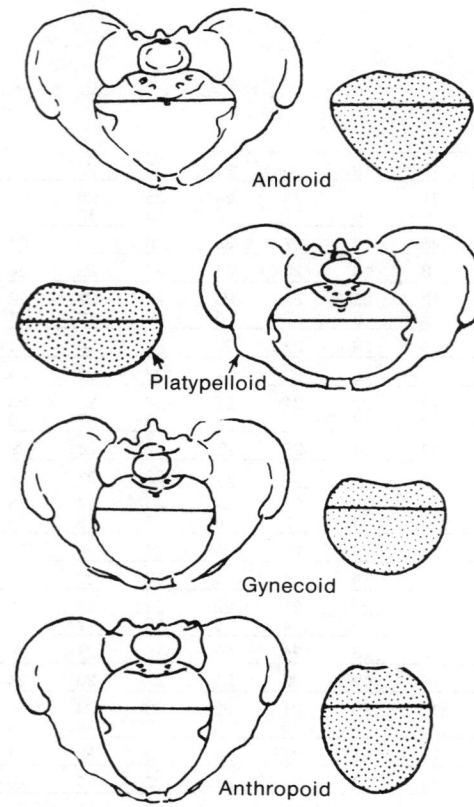

FIGURE 29-3. *The four types of female pelvis.*

B. *Pelvimetry*—methods of measuring pelvic dimensions (Fig. 29-5)*

1. The external conjugate or Baudelocque's diameter—the distance from the anterior-superior surface of the symphysis pubis to the depression below the spine of the last lumbar vertebra.
2. The intercristal diameter—the distance between the outermost portions of the iliac crests.
3. The interspinous diameter—the distance between the outer surface of the anterior-superior spines of the ilia.
4. The intertrochanteric diameter—the distance between the two great trochanters.
5. The bi-ischial diameter—or the transverse diameter of the outlet of the pelvis.
6. Manually determining the diagonal conjugate of the pelvis by vaginal examination.
7. Measuring with a pelvimeter the length of the diagonal conjugate as determined by manual examination

Subsequent Prenatal Assessments

Monthly visits are made for the first 7 months, then every 2 weeks, and weekly during the last month.

* Figures from Bookmiller and Bowen. Textbook of Obstetrics and Obstetrical Nursing. Philadelphia, WB Saunders, 1968.

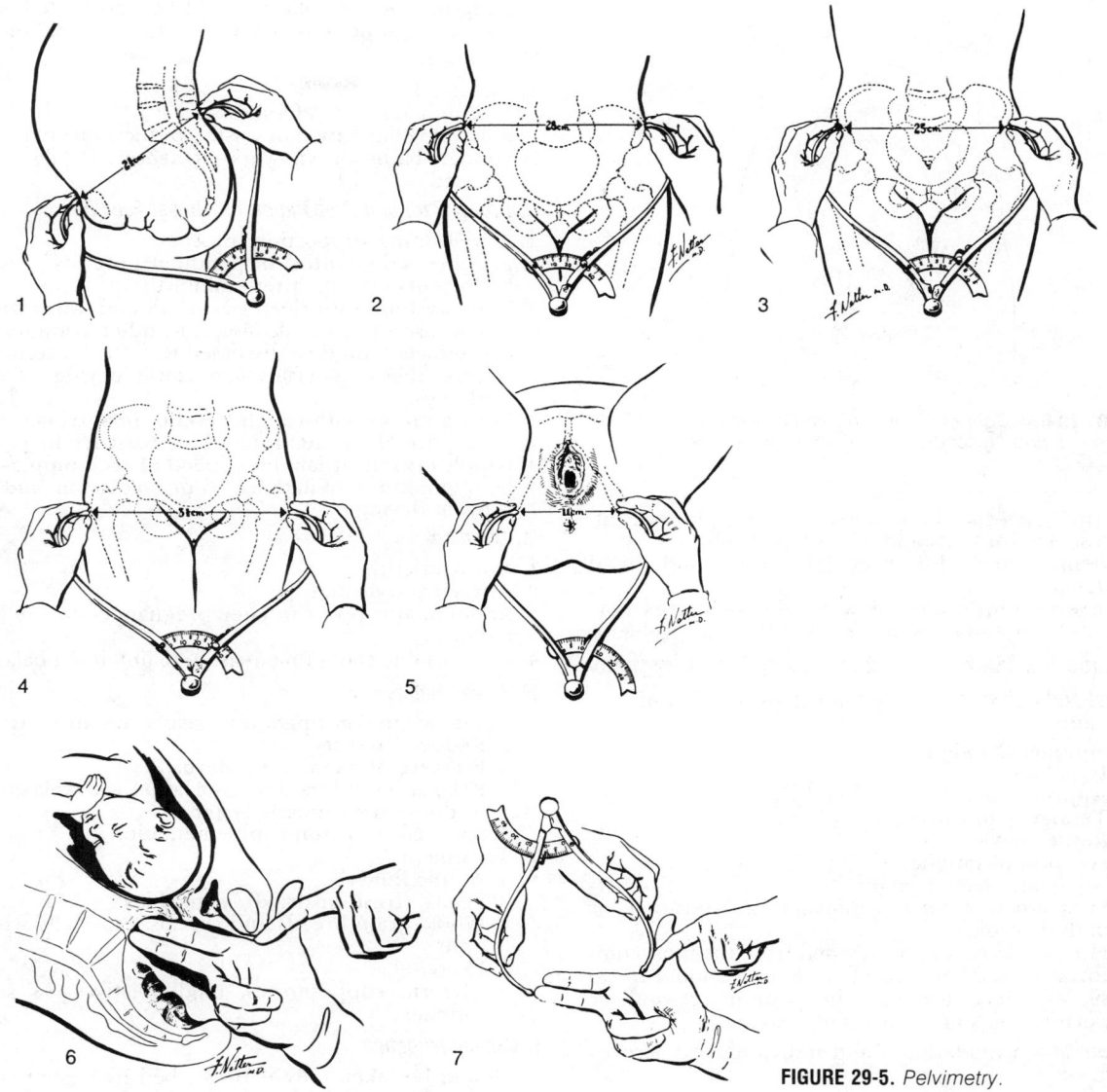

FIGURE 29-5. *Pelvimetry.*

1. Growth of the uterus and estimated fetal growth (Fig. 29-6):

   Fundus at symphysis pubis = 12 weeks gestation
   Fundus at umbilicus = 20 weeks gestation
   Fundus 28 cm. from top of symphysis pubis = 28 weeks gestation
   Fundus at lower border of rib cage = 36 weeks gestation
   Uterus becomes globular and drops = 40 weeks gestation

   a. A greater fundal height suggests:
      (1) Multiple pregnancy
      (2) Miscalculated due date
      (3) Ovarian or uterine tumor
      (4) Polyhydramnios
      (5) Hydatidiform mole
   b. A lesser fundal height suggests:
      (1) Intrauterine fetal growth retardation
      (2) Fetal or amniotic fluid abnormalities
      (3) Intrauterine fetal death
      (4) Error in estimating gestation

2. Fetal heart tones—palpate abdomen for fetal position; listen over anterior shoulder.
   a. Normal—120–160 beats per minute
   b. Very slow or accelerated rates are usually indicative of fetal distress (see Chapter 30).

3. Weight—Major increase in weight occurs during second half of pregnancy; not less than 0.22 kg. (½ lb.) per week and not more than 0.9 kg. (2 lbs.).

4. Tuberculosis test—tine test for initial screening; chest X-ray if needed, *with abdomen shielded.*

5. Blood pressure—should remain at normal baseline.

6. Hemoglobin—checked at 30 weeks.

7. Serology and smear or culture for gonorrhea at 36 weeks.

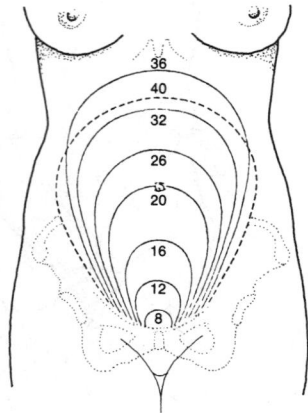

FIGURE 29-6. *Height of fundus. (From Danforth. Textbook of Obstetrics and Gynecology, 2nd ed. New York, Harper and Row, 1971.)*

8. Urinalysis—specific gravity, albumin, glucose, microscopic for casts and white blood cells.
9. Edema—check for pretibial, facial, and hand edema.
10. General appearance of well-being—changes may be indicative of physiologic or psychologic problems

Teaching the Maternity Patient Principles of Hygiene

A. *Rest and Relaxation*—aimed at the prevention of fatigue

1. Symptoms of fatigue
   a. Irritability
   b. Apprehension
   c. Tendency to worry
   d. Restlessness
2. Prevention of fatigue
   a. Adequate sleep at night
   b. Supplemental naps in morning or afternoon, or both if possible
   c. Household chores performed from the most comfortable position, expectant mother should try to sit, with feet elevated, when ironing, sewing, or performing some aspects of cooking.

B. *Exercise*—in moderation and individualized according to:

1. Age and physical condition
2. Customary amount of exercise (Exercise is never continued to the point of fatigue).
3. Stage of pregnancy

C. *Employment*—in moderation and individualized so as to:

1. Avoid fatigue
2. Prevent accidents to which the pregnant woman is especially vulnerable because of changes in center of gravity
3. Reduce environmental hazards, both physical and chemical
4. Exclude any job requiring manual labor, delicate balance, or inverted living hours.

D. *Traveling*—usually not contraindicated during pregnancy

1. The obstetrician's advice should be sought before any traveling is undertaken.

2. Long-distance traveling should be punctuated with frequent rest periods (10–15 minutes every 2 hours).

E. *Skin Care*

1. Daily bath
   a. Stimulates and refreshes
   b. Favors elimination of waste products through skin
2. Sponge baths or showers—if sense of balance is affected

F. *Breast Care and Preparation for Breast Feeding*

1. A well-fitting supporting brassiere
   a. Relieves discomfort of pendulous breasts
   b. Prevents sagging after childbirth
2. Daily washing with clean washcloth and warm water The use of soap, alcohol, and other commercial products should be discussed with the obstetrician since these materials can cause drying of the nipples.
3. Drying nipple with rough towel in final trimester—to help toughen the nipples for breast feeding
4. Nipple creams or lanolin applied to each nipple—to help minimize irritations from colostrum and to prevent drying

G. *Clothing*

1. Nonrestrictive
2. Attractive style and fit
3. Abdominal support in later pregnancy—to prevent fatigue
4. Comfortable shoes that assist in maintaining balance

H. *Bowel Habits*

1. Tendency to constipation increased because of:
   a. Reduced activity
   b. Pressure of expanding uterus
   c. Relaxation of bowel in association with relaxation of the smooth muscle system
   d. Side effect of iron supplementation
2. Treatment
   a. Ample fluids
   b. Fruits, (fresh or dried), vegetables
   c. Whole grain breads and cereals, especially whole bran
   d. Exercise
   e. Glycerin suppositories, mild laxatives, or stool softeners

I. *Vaginal Irrigation*

Should be taken only if prescribed by obstetrician. (See p. 541 for irrigation procedure.)

J. *Sexual Intercourse*

Individualized, but the following points may be noted:
1. Sexual desire may be unpredictable in the woman during early pregnancy.
2. If there is danger of abortion or premature labor, coitus is avoided.
3. During last few weeks before term, some obstetricians advise abstaining from sexual intercourse.
4. The male-superior position is avoided as the pregnancy progresses.

K. *Smoking*

1. Causes peripheral vasoconstriction affecting heart rate, blood pressure, and cardiac output.
2. Small birth weights, higher rates of prematurity, and higher neonatal mortality have been associated with smoking in pregnant women.

Teaching the Maternity Patient About Nutrition
A. *Diet*
1. Significant relationship found between maternal nutrition (especially protein intake) and well-being of infant.
2. Energy requirements—change during course of pregnancy; calorie intake regulated accordingly.
3. Meals—should be individually balanced and consumed on a regular schedule.
4. Best indices of nutritional needs are the condition of the patient, her body weight, and pregravid status of nutrition; particular attention should be directed to the following:
   a. Biologically immature mothers under age 17—stress of pregnancy added to the nutritional needs for baby's growth and maturation.
   b. Women who have low incomes—unable to purchase needed foods; history of poor diet and suboptimum health.
   c. Women with depleted nutritional stores due to rapidly successive pregnancies.
   d. Overweight women. Food selections tend to emphasize empty-calorie foods high in fat and carbohydrates, low in essential proteins, minerals, and vitamins.
   e. Women with low prepregnancy weight for their height and those with a limited weight gain during pregnancy show an increased incidence of toxemia, prematurity, and infants with low birth weights.
   f. Women with religious or philosophical reasons for limiting their food intake to certain groups of foods.
      (1) Vegetarian diets—adequate only if they are supplemented with dairy and poultry products. Symptoms of Vitamin B_{12} deficiency may be masked by folic acid until irreversible degeneration of the spinal cord has occurred. Iron-deficiency anemia and zinc deficiencies are also found.
      (2) Macrobiotic diets—may produce scurvy, hypoproteinemia, anemia, and hypocalcemia.
5. Total weight gain: 9–11.25 kg. (20–25 lbs.) with gain of 0.675–1.35 kg. (1.5–3 lbs.) in the first trimester and 0.36 kg. (0.8 lbs.) per week during the remainder of the pregnancy.
6. Calorie intake—sufficient to maintain calculated ideal body weight plus additional 200 calories per day during last 5 months of gestation.
7. Protein intake—needs should be met easily with additional 10 gm. to maintain level of 0.9 gm/kg. of ideal body weight, provided that at least ⅔ of total nitrogen component is of animal origin.
8. Fat intake—should constitute approximately 25% of total calories.
9. Carbohydrate intake—consists predominantly of complex polysaccharides.
10. Sodium intake—2.5–5 gm. daily intake allowed unless contraindicated by water retention.
11. Vitamins
    a. During pregnancy and lactation, vitamin needs increase.
    b. Best sources found in natural foods.
    c. Supplements usually recommended by most physicians.
       (1) Vitamin A
          (a) Essential for maintenance of body resistance to infection.
          (b) Sources—whole milk, dairy products containing butterfat, eggs, green leafy or yellow vegetables, and liver.
       (2) Vitamin B complex
          (a) Fetus depletes mother's reserves.
          (b) Sources—milk, eggs, lean meat, whole grains or enriched bread and cereals; riboflavin and nicotinic acid found in meat, milk, eggs, and green vegetables.
       (3) Vitamin C
          (a) Water-soluble vitamin, not stored—daily intake required.
          (b) Sources—fresh citrus fruits, berries, and green leafy vegetables are excellent sources—preferably taken raw since cooking destroys one-half vitamin content.
       (4) Vitamin D
          (a) Relationship of calcium and phosphorus metabolism important.
          (b) Sources—liver, eggs, fortified milk, and fish.
       (5) Vitamin E
          (a) Necessary for the normal development of the fetus.
          (b) Sources—leafy vegetables, whole grain products, and fats, especially vegetable oils.
       (6) Vitamin K
          (a) Needed to prevent hemorrhagic fever in the infant, given soon after birth if status in mother is unsatisfactory or unknown.
          (b) Sources—green leafy vegetables.
12. Iron—indicated for all pregnant women, especially those with history of anemia, multiple births, or frequent pregnancies.
    a. Hemoglobin below 11 gm. indicates iron deficiency.
    b. Iron is needed to maintain satisfactory hemoglobin concentration during pregnancy and to compensate for blood loss during delivery.
    c. Possibility of complicated deliveries and postpartal hemorrhage requires a reserve supply of iron.
    d. Adequate reserves of iron together with protein and other essential nutrients are conducive to rapid recovery and ability to breast feed.
    e. Oral preparation of 100 mg. of iron daily is usually effective.
       (1) During 3rd trimester, absorption increases 3-fold.
       (2) Ferrous gluconate may be recommended.
    f. Long-lasting, sustained-release preparations are useful for patients with impaired absorption.

NURSING ALERT: Parenteral administration of large doses of iron is frequently accompanied by adverse reactions and should be reserved for patients who have extremely low levels and are close to term. A large intake of milk may interfere with iron absorption.

13. Folic acid—requirements markedly increased during pregnancy due to rapid cell multiplication and DNA synthesis. RDA of 800 mg. may not be met by diet alone (cooking may reduce folic acid content of food).

14. Calcium and phosphorus intake of 1.2 gm. each per day needed for calcification and formation of fetal bone structure.
15. Magnesium, copper, potassium, and iodine—balanced diet provides adequate intake.

B. *Foods to be eaten daily* (see Table 29-2)

1. Milk—1 quart of whole milk (or 1 quart of skim milk if weight control desired).
   a. Powdered skim milk may be used as a substitute for or supplement to liquid milk (1-2 tablespoons to 1 glass of liquid).
   b. 1 oz. of cheddar cheese may substitute for 1 glass of milk.
2. Eggs—1 daily (if animal fats are restricted).
3. Meat—6 to 8 oz. lean meat (beef, veal, lamb, chicken, turkey, or fish—2 servings). Organ meats substituted 2 times weekly.
4. Fat—2 tablespoons butter, margarine, or vegetable oil.
5. Bread and cereal—2 slices of whole grain or enriched bread plus ½ cup enriched cereal or cooked whole grain cereal.
6. Vegetables
   a. Potato—1 medium; or ¾ cups cooked rice, noodles, spaghetti, or macaroni substituted 2 times weekly.
   b. 1 cup dark green or deep yellow vegetables.
   c. 1 cup of another vegetable, raw or cooked; or ½ cup of peas, beans, corn, or lentils.
7. Fruit
   a. Citrus fruit—2 oranges or 1 grapefruit, or 8 oz. of orange juice or tomato juice.
   b. 1 fresh fruit or ½ cup cooked, unsweetened fruit; 4–5 prunes or 5–6 dried apricots may be substituted.
8. Desserts—1 serving simple pudding made with milk, eggs, or fruit, if desired.
9. Water—4 glasses minimum requirement unless specifically restricted.

DISCOMFORTS OF PREGNANCY

Frequency of Urination

1. Cause—pressure of enlarging uterus on bladder.
2. Course—usually subsides spontaneously by the 2nd or 3rd month when the uterus rises into the abdominal cavity; returns in the last weeks of pregnancy when the vertex drops into the pelvic cavity (engagement).

Morning Sickness

Nausea, sometimes accompanied by mild vomiting—usually occurs in morning, but may occur at any time of day.
1. Possible causes
   a. Changes in hormonal balance
   b. Emotional upset
   c. Sluggish peristalsis
2. Duration (4–12 weeks)
3. Aim of treatment—to prevent exaggeration of symptoms (see hyperemesis gravidarum, p. 1040).
4. Treatment
   Instruct patient as follows:
   a. Before breakfast:
      (1) Eat dry toast or a cracker one-half hour before rising.
      (2) Drink hot tea, clear coffee, or hot milk.
      (3) Remain in bed and rest one-half hour before rising.
   b. Eat simple light foods 5–6 times a day, rather than 3 full meals.
   c. Avoid foods that are difficult to digest.

Heartburn

1. Causes
   a. May occur anytime during pregnancy—because of diminished gastric motility there is a reflux of stomach contents into the esophagus, with resulting irritation.

TABLE 29-2. SUMMARY OF MAJOR FUNCTIONS AND SOURCES OF NUTRIENTS

	Function	Source	
Protein	Growth of fetus and accessory tissues Production of breast milk	Animal Protein meat fish poultry eggs milk cheese	Vegetable Protein dried beans dried peas lentils nuts peanut butter
Iron	Maintains hemoglobin level of mother Maintains mother's stores of iron Provides iron for fetal development Furnishes infant with iron stores needed for blood formation during neonatal period before food sources of iron are added to diet	Good Sources pork liver kidney beef liver oysters clams canned dried beans prune juice liverwurst heart lean pork lean beef raisins cooked dried beans cooked dried peaches cooked dried apricots cooked dried prunes canned green peas	Fair Sources enriched pastas spinach canned mackerel enriched white bread kale mustard greens whole wheat bread canned string beans eggs brussels sprouts broccoli

	Function	Source	

Calcium	Skeletal structures of the fetus
	Production of breast milk
	Blood coagulation, neuromuscular irritability, and muscle contractility
		Good Sources
		skim milk
		buttermilk
		whole milk
		nonfat dry milk
		cheese
		ice milk
		ice cream
			Fair Sources
			dark green
			  leafy vegetables
			dried beans
			broccoli
			cottage cheese
			canned fish—
			  including bones
			oranges

Vitamin A	Tooth formation
	Normal bone growth
	Healthy skin
	Vision—light/dark adaptation
		Vitamin A
		butter
		egg yolk
		fortified margarine
		kidney
		liver
		whole milk
		cream
			Carotenes
			dark green and deep
			  yellow vegetables
			  and a few fruits
			apricots
			broccoli
			cantaloupe
			carrots
			chard
			collards
			kale
			mustard greens
			persimmons
			spinach
			pumpkin
			sweet potatoes
			turnip greens
			winter squash

Riboflavin	Functions in number of enzyme systems in tissue respiration Metabolism of amino acids and carbohydrates	Good Sources heart kidney liver milk ice milk	Fair Sources broccoli cheese dark green leafy vegetables eggs ice cream lean meat poultry

Thiamine	Maintains normal appetite and digestion
	Maintains health of nervous system
	Completion of carbohydrates
		Good Sources
		whole grain and enriched
		  bread
		whole grain and enriched
		  cereals
		dried peas
		dried beans
		oranges
		liver
		heart
		kidney
		lean pork
		nuts
		potatoes
		peas
		wheat germ
			Fair Sources
			eggs
			fish
			meat
			poultry
			milk
			many vegetables

Niacin	Helps translate sources of energy into usable form	Good Sources
		fish
		heart
		lean meat
		liver
		peanuts
		peanut butter
		poultry
			Fair Sources
			milk
			potatoes
			whole grain and
			  enriched bread
			whole grain and
			  enriched cereal

Ascorbic Acid	Production of intercellular substances necessary for the development and maintenance of normal connective tissue in bones, cartilage, and muscles
	Improves health of bones and teeth
	Increases absorption of iron
		Good Sources
		citrus fruits or juice
		broccoli
		brussels sprouts
		cantaloupe
		greens—collards,
		  mustard, turnip
		peppers
			Fair Sources
			asparagus
			cabbage, raw
			cauliflower
			chile, fresh or canned
			kale
			liver
			other melons
			potatoes or sweet
			  potatoes in jackets
			spinach
			tomatoes or prunes

Vitamin D	Promotes absorption and retention of calcium and phosphorus necessary for growth and formation of bones and teeth	butter egg yolk fish oils liver milk fortified with Vitamin D other foods may contain added vitamin D—check labels	

Source: Cross AT and Walsh HE. Prenatal diet counseling, J Reproductive Med, Dec 1971, 7:271–272.

b. Nervous tension and emotional disturbances contribute to heartburn.
2. Treatment
Instruct patient as follows:
a. Avoid fatty and fried foods.
b. Take antacid medications

> **NURSING ALERT:** Soda bicarbonate should not be used since it promotes retention of fluid.

Flatulence

1. Cause—gas-forming bacterial action in the intestines.
2. Treatment
Instruct patient as follows:
a. Chew food thoroughly.
b. Avoid gas-forming foods (fried foods, beans, corn).

Constipation

1. Cause—impaired intestinal peristalsis due to pressure of gravid uterus.
2. Treatment
Instruct patient as follows:
a. Take adequate fluids.
b. Establish regular patterns of elimination.
c. Eat an appropriate diet (fruits, vegetables, coarse bread).
d. Take laxatives only when prescribed by obstetrician.

Backache

1. Cause
a. Postural adjustments of pregnancy.
b. Relaxation of sacroiliac joints in late pregnancy.
2. Treatment
Instruct patient as follows:
a. Maintain good posture, avoid fatigue, use good body mechanics.
b. Wear appropriate clothing.
(1) Flat, wide-based shoes.
(2) Supporting maternity girdle.

Respiratory Discomfort

1. Cause—pressure of enlarged uterus on diaphragm.
2. Treatment
a. Spontaneous relief occurs with "lightening" (sensation of decreased abdominal distention caused by descent of uterus into pelvis) or with the birth of the baby.
b. Provide relief by semi-Fowler's position arranged with pillow.

NOTE: The possibility of heart disease may have to be ruled out.

Varicose Veins

1. May affect the lower extremities, vulva, and pelvis (Fig. 29-7).
2. Causes
a. Heredity
b. Pressure of gravid uterus on the great veins of the pelvis
c. Prolonged standing
d. Constrictive clothing

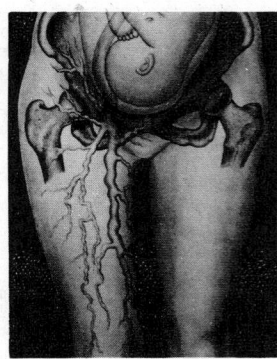

FIGURE 29-7. *Varicose veins due to gravid uterus. (Courtesy of Jobst Co.)*

3. Treatment
Instruct patient as follows:
a. Avoid restrictive clothing
b. Elevate legs and hips on pillows above the level of the heart.
c. Wear elastic stockings or bandages (support hose).
d. Take frequent rest periods.

Hemorrhoids

1. Causes
a. Pressure of gravid uterus interferes with venous circulation.
b. Aggravated by constipation.
2. Treatment
Instruct patient as follows:
a. Prevent and treat constipation.
b. Replace protruding internal hemorrhoids using lubricated finger.
c. Apply cold compresses with or without witch hazel or Epsom salts.
d. Use suppositories, if prescribed.

Leg Cramps

1. Causes
a. Increased pressure from gravid uterus
b. Fatigue
c. Chilling
d. Muscle tenseness
e. Excessive amounts of phosphorus
f. Inadequate dietary calcium
2. Treatment
Instruct patient as follows:
a. Provide for frequent rest periods with feet elevated.
b. Assure adequate intake of calcium (diet, medication, or both).
c. Wear comfortable, warm clothing.
d. *Push the toes upward while applying pressure to the knee to flatten the affected extremity; provides immediate relief.*

Edema of the Lower Extremities

1. Most common in hot weather.

> **NURSING ALERT:** Edema is one of the early signs of hypertensive disorders (see p. 1038).

2. Treatment
Instruct the patient as follows:
a. Take frequent rest periods.
b. Elevate legs.
c. Provide abdominal support.

Vaginal Discharge

1. Increased vaginal discharge is normal in pregnancy. Generally a perineal pad is all that is needed.
2. Excessive, or green, yellow, foul-smelling, or irritating vaginal discharge may be caused by any of the following:
a. Venereal disease
b. Trichomonas vaginalis
c. Moniliasis
3. Treatment—according to the cause (see pp. 538–539).

Danger Signals

1. Vaginal bleeding, no matter how slight
2. Swelling of the face or fingers
3. Severe continuous headaches
4. Dimness or blurring of vision, flashes of light or dots before the eyes
5. Abdominal pain
6. Persistent vomiting
7. Chills and fever
8. Sudden escape of fluid from vagina

Patient Instructions

As the patient, particularly a primigravida, approaches full term, instruction should be given on signs and symptoms of approaching labor, and when to notify the physician.

THE FETUS

FETAL DEVELOPMENT

1st Lunar Month

1. *Length* 0.75–1 cm. (0.3–0.4 inch)
2. Trophoblasts imbed in decidua.
3. Chorionic villi form.
4. Foundations formed for nervous system, genitourinary system, skin, bones, and lungs.
5. Buds of arms and legs begin to form.
6. Rudiments of eyes, ears, and nose appear.

4 weeks

2nd Lunar Month

1. *Length* 2.5 cm. (1 inch)
   Weight 4 gm.
2. Fetus is markedly bent.
3. Head is disproportionately large, owing to brain development.
4. Sex differentiation begins.
5. Centers of bone begin to ossify.

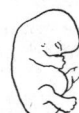

8 weeks

3rd Lunar Month

1. *Length* 7–9 cm. (2.8–3.6 inches)
   Weight 5.20 gm.
2. Fingers and toes are distinct.
3. Placenta is complete.
4. Fetal circulation is complete.

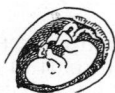

3 months

4th Lunar Month

1. *Length* 10–17 cm. (4–6.7 inches)
   Weight 55–120 gm. (1.9–4.2 oz.)
2. Sex is differentiated.
3. Rudimentary kidneys secrete urine.
4. Heart beat is present.
5. Nasal septum and palate close.

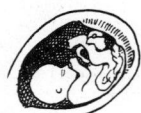

4th month

5th Lunar Month

1. *Length* 30 cm. (12 inches)
   Weight 280–300 gm. (9.9–10.6 oz.)
2. Lanugo covers entire body.
3. Fetal movements are felt by mother.
4. Heart sounds are perceptible with fetoscope.

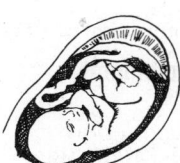

5th month

6th Lunar Month

1. *Length* 28–34 cm. (11.2–13.4 inches)
   Weight 650 gm. (1.4 lb.)
2. Skin appears wrinkled.
3. Vernix caseosa appears.
4. Eyebrows and fingernails develop.

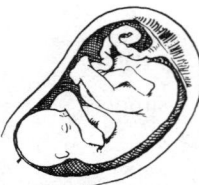

6th month

7th Lunar Month

1. *Length* 35–38 cm. (13.8–15 inches)
   Weight 1200 gm. (2.6 lb.)
2. Skin is red.
3. Pupillary membrane disappears from eyes.
4. If born, infant cries, breathes, but usually expires.

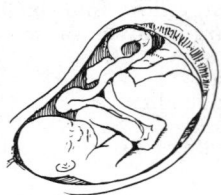

7th month

8th Lunar Month

1. *Length* 38–43 cm. (15–17 inches)
   Weight 2000 gm. (3.5–4.2 lb.)
2. Fetus is viable.
3. Eyelids open.
4. Fingerprints are set.
5. Vigorous fetal movement occurs.

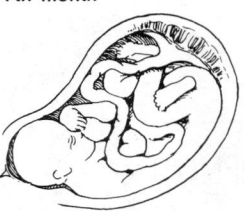

8th month

9th Lunar Month

1. *Length* 42–49 cm. (16.5–19.3 inches)
   Weight 1700–2600 gm. (3.7–5.7 lb.)
2. Face and body have loose wrinkled appearance due to subcutaneous fat deposit.
3. Lanugo disappears.
4. Amniotic fluid decreases somewhat.

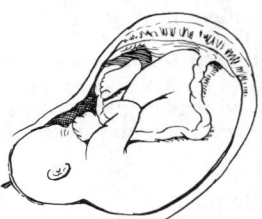

9th month

10th Lunar Month

1. *Length* 48–52 cm. (18.9–20.5 inches)
   Weight 3000–3600 gm. (6.6–7.9 lb.)
2. Skin is smooth.
3. Eyes are uniformly slate-colored.
4. Bones of skull are ossified and nearly together at sutures.

THE FETAL HEAD

From the obstetrical standpoint, the *fetal head* (Fig. 29-8), is the most important part of the fetus because (1) it is the largest part of the baby, (2) it is the least compressible, and (3) it is the most frequently presenting part.

Base of the Skull

1. Characteristics of Bones
   a. Large
   b. Ossified
   c. Firmly united
   d. Not compressible
2. Function is to protect vital centers on the brain stem.

Vault of the Skull (cranium)

1. Composed of:
   a. Occipital bone posteriorly
   b. 2 parietal bones on the sides
   c. 2 temporal bones anteriorly
   d. 2 frontal bones anteriorly
2. The cranium is thin, poorly ossified, and easily compressible; permits overlapping known as *molding*.

Sutures of the Skull

1. Aid in molding process and in identifying the position of fetal head during labor.
2. Sagittal suture—lies between the parietal bones.
3. Lambdoidal suture—lies between the occipital and 2 parietal bones.
4. Coronal suture—extends transversely from the anterior fontanelle; lies between the parietal and frontal bones.
5. Frontal suture—is between the 2 frontal bones and is an anterior continuation of the sagittal suture.

Fontanelles

1. Membrane space where the sutures intersect.
2. Anterior fontanelle—junction of the sagittal, frontal, and coronal sutures (3 × 2 cm.)—*closes by 18 months of age.*
3. Posterior fontanelle—located where the sagittal suture meets the lambdoidal (smaller than anterior)—*closes at 6–8 weeks of age.*

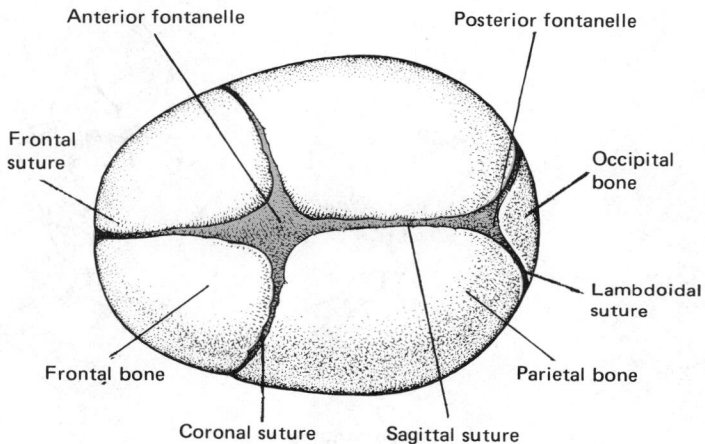

FIGURE 29-8. *Fetal skull.*

CHANGES IN FETAL CIRCULATION

See chart below.

PRESENTATIONS AND POSITION OF THE FETUS

General Terms

1. *Lie*—the relationship of the long axis of the fetus to the long axis of the mother. The 2 lies are longitudinal or transverse.
2. *Presentation*—the part of the fetus which lies over the inlet; may be vertex (Fig. 29-9); face (Fig. 29-9); breech (Fig. 29-9); or shoulder.
3. *Presenting part*—the part of the fetus that lies over the internal os of the cervix.
4. *Attitude*—the relation of the fetal parts to each other; basic attitudes are flexion and extension.
5. *Position*—the relation of the denominator to the front, back, or sides of the maternal pelvis.

Terms Describing Position

1. *Denominator*—an arbitrarily chosen spot on the presenting part of the fetus.
2. *Right or left*—depending on which side of the maternal pelvis the denominator is located.
3. *Anterior, posterior, or transverse*—according to whether the denominator is in the front, in the back, or at the side of the pelvis.

FETAL ASSESSMENT

Assessment of Fetal Well-being and Maturity

A. *Maternal History*

1. History of current pregnancy
2. Woman's general health
3. Outcome of previous pregnancies
4. Health during previous pregnancies

B. *Estimation of Fundal Height* (See Fig. 29-6).

Changes in Fetal Circulation*

Structure	Before Birth	After Birth
Umbilical vein	Brings arterial blood to liver and heart	Obliterated, becomes the round ligament of liver
Umbilical arteries	Bring arteriovenous blood to the placenta	Obliterated, become vesical ligament on anterior abdominal wall
Ductus venosus	Shunts arterial blood into inferior vena cava	Obliterated, becomes ligamentum venosum
Ductus arteriosus	Shunts arterial and some venous blood from the pulmonary artery to the aorta	Obliterated, becomes ligamentum arteriosum
Foramen ovale	Connects right and left atria	Usually obliterated
Lungs	Contain no air and very little blood	Filled with air and well supplied with blood
Pulmonary arteries	Bring little blood to lungs	Bring much blood to lungs
Aorta	Receives blood from both ventricles	Receives blood from left ventricle only
Inferior vena cava	Brings venous blood from body and arterial blood from placenta	Brings venous blood only to right atrium

* Adapted from Williams JF. Anatomy and Physiology, ed 7. Philadelphia, WB Saunders, 1976.

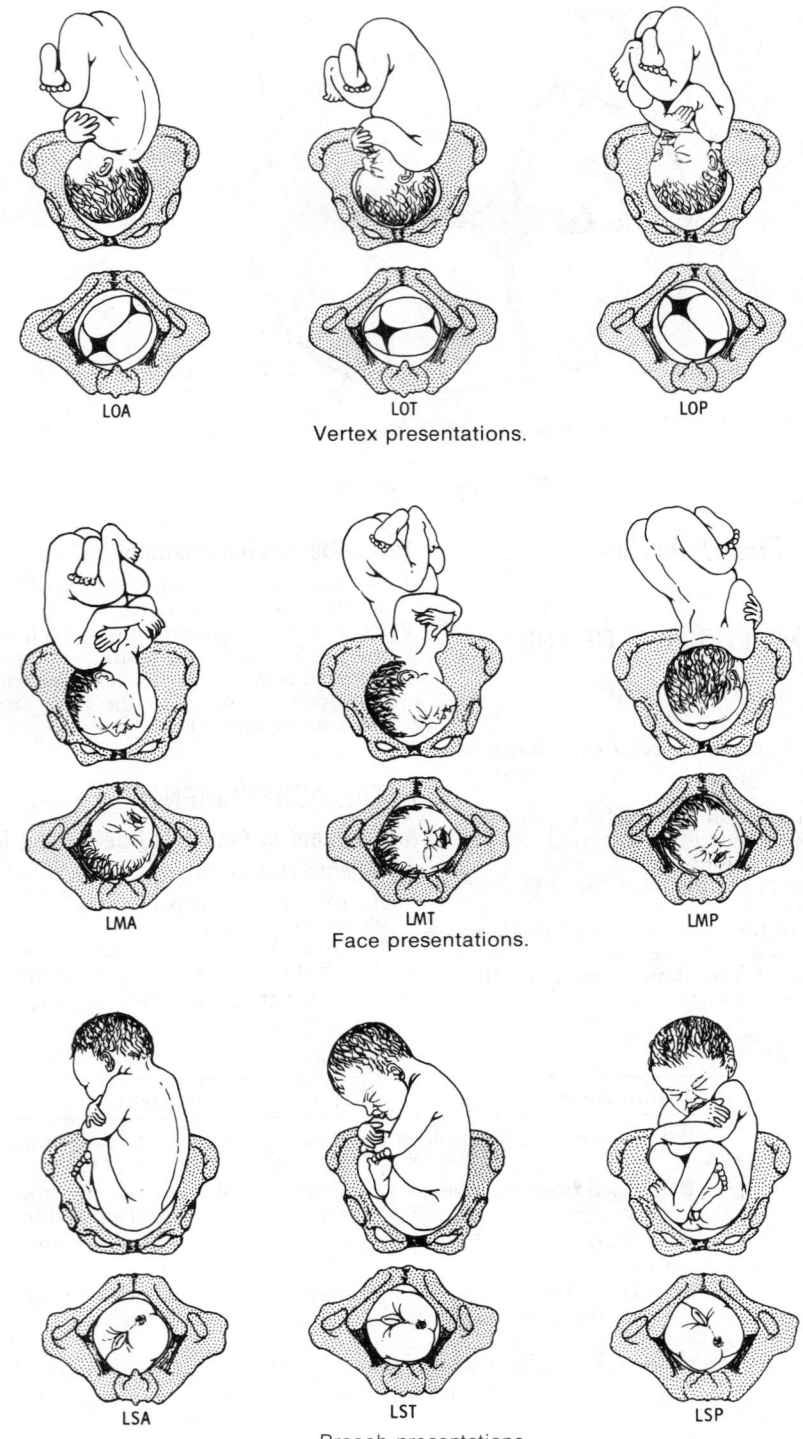

LOA   LOT   LOP

Vertex presentations.

LMA   LMT   LMP

Face presentations.

LSA   LST   LSP

Breech presentations.

FIGURE 29-9. *Fetal presentations. (From Benson RC. Handbook of Obstetrics and Gynecology. Los Altos, California, Lange Medical Publications, 1971.)*

C. X-Ray

Contraindicated during pregnancy; unreliable for estimating fetal age or assessing fetal health. X-ray at term may be helpful in determining maturity (if distal femoral and proximal tibial epiphyses are both present, fetus is considered mature). Fetal death established by x-ray of overriding skull bones and curved spine.

D. Ultrasound

1. Determines fetal size, position, and location of the placenta.
2. Useful in estimating head growth in a small-for-date fetus.

E. Fetal Heart Tones

1. Electrocardiography—may be recorded by 11th week, inaccurate before 5th month. Fetal cardiac electrical signal very weak and masked by mother's signal.
2. Doppler FHR (Fetal Heart Rate) detector.

F. Oxytocin Challenge Test (OCT) or Contraction Stress Test (CST)

Used to assess the placental reserve for transmitting oxygen to the fetus and to detect uteroplacental insufficiency by observation of the FHR response to spontaneous or oxytocin-induced contractions; tests usually begin at approximately 32–34 weeks and are repeated weekly until the patient delivers.

1. *Indications*—patients with hypertensive disorders, diabetes mellitus, prolonged pregnancy, Rh isoimmunization, cardiac or renal disease, intrauterine growth retardation, history of previous stillbirth, abnormal estriol values, or other evidence of potential fetal distress.
2. *Contraindications*—patients with previous cesarean section, 3rd trimester bleeding, multiple gestations, incompetent cervix, or premature rupture of membrane.
3. *Procedure*
   a. Patient placed in semi-Fowler's position (to avoid supine hypotension).
   b. External monitor (tokodynamometer) for measurement of uterine activity and ultrasonic transducer, or fetal electrocardiogram to record FHR is placed on patient's abdomen.
   c. Accelerations of the FHR associated with fetal movements are noted as well as base-line heart rate variability and base-line uterine activity.
   d. Intravenous dilute oxytocin infusion by constant fusion pump is begun and increased at 15–20 minute intervals until 3 uterine contractions of good quality are observed within a 10 minute period.
4. *Interpretation*
   a. Negative test—three contractions of good quality in 10 minutes lasting 40 seconds or more without late deceleration.
   b. Positive test—occurrence of repetitive late deceleration with more than 50% of contractions.

G. Nonstress Test

1. Observation of the FHR associated with fetal movements.
2. Used to screen for OCT or may be used on patient for whom the OCT is contraindicated.
3. Recordings of the FHR are obtained for approximately 30–40 minutes.
4. Notations are made of fetal activity, acceleration of the FHR with fetal and uterine activity, and interpreted as reactive or nonreactive.

H. Amniotic Fluid Studies

1. Determination of hereditary disease and congenital defects (early pregnancy).
   a. Determination of ABO blood groups and amounts of Rh-factor sensitization; identification of homozygous biochemical defect (inborn errors of metabolism in fetuses of known heterozygous parents).
   b. Determination, by biochemical analysis of cells, of whether fatal fetal disorders exist (Tay-Sachs disease or galactosemia).
   c. Cytogenetic evaluation—to detect trisomy 21 (mongolism) and to establish the fetal sex (important when sex-linked disorders such as hemophilia are anticipated).
   d. Purpose of these studies is to consider an elective abortion if abnormal fetus (generally not done unless patient willing to consider abortion).
2. Determination of fetal maturation (late pregnancy).
   a. Creatinine—measures amount of fetal skeletal muscle and kidney function, useful after 36 weeks gestation (fluid sample must be clear; blood and meconium interfere with creatinine determination).
   b. L/S ratio (lecithin/sphingomyelin ratio)—measures the maturity of the fetal lung.
   c. Purpose of these studies is to determine maturity of fetus for planned elective cesarean section delivery. Needed because EDC and sonography are approximate estimates of maturity.
3. Determination of fetal distress (late pregnancy)
   a. Nonspecific problems identified by gross examination of amniotic fluid
      (1) Fluid yellow—fetus may be suffering effects of erythroblastosis.
      (2) Fluid dark red–brown—indicates fetal death.
      (3) Presence of meconium—frequently indicates previous or present fetal distress from anoxia caused by placental failure, umbilical cord compression, or postmaturity (fetus delivered carefully with least possible risk of further anoxia).
   b. PCO_2—acid base measurement; fetal disease from hypoxia results in fetal acidosis with increase in amniotic fluid pH.
   c. Combine with FHR assessment of high-risk infants to determine need for immediate delivery.

I. Fetoscopy

The insertion of a fiberoptic instrument into the uterine cavity to visually examine the fetus or to obtain blood, placental or tissue samples for identification and diagnosis of:

1. Congenital anomalies or teratologically induced malformations.
2. Hemoglobinopathies
3. Sex-linked autosomal abnormalities or neural tube disorders
4. Metabolic disorders

J. Assay of Maternal Urine

1. Urinary pregnanediol—determines the efficiency of the placental production of progesterone.
2. Estriol levels (in 24 hour urine specimens)—measure the combined effort of the fetal adrenal glands and liver, the placenta, and the mother's liver and kid-

neys. During the third trimester it should show a steady increase; a downward trend indicates placental insufficiency.

NOTE: Fetal jeopardy cannot be detected by estriol excretion when the mother is sensitized to Rh or other blood factors or when she is eclamptic.

K. *Assay of Maternal Serum*
1. Electrophoretic protein band present in over 80%

of pregnant women during the third trimester; absence observed in some patients who deliver congenitally deformed infants.
2. Diamine oxidase—enzyme typically found at high levels in maternal blood and in placenta. When levels are lower, there appears to be a significant increase in fetal mortality.

GUIDELINES: Assisting with an Amniocentesis

Amniocentesis is the transabdominal aspiration of amniotic fluid (Fig. 29-10).

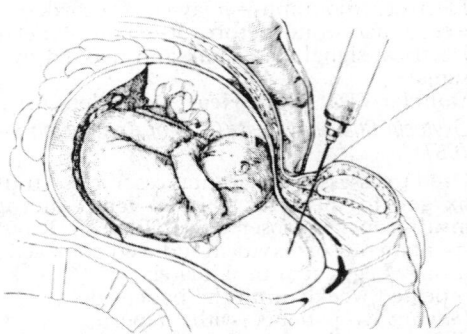

FIGURE 29-10. *Amniocentesis, as usually carried out at suprapubic site after localization and manual elevation of the fetus.** *

Purposes
1. Cytogenic evaluation
   a. To detect trisomy 21 (mongolism).
   b. To establish the fetal sex (important when sex-linked disorders such as hemophilia are anticipated).
2. Amniotic fluid studies
   a. To determine ABO blood groups and amounts of Rh factor sensitization.
   b. To assess fetal maturity.
   c. To identify homozygous biochemical defects (inborn errors of metabolism) in fetuses of known heterozygous parents.
   d. To determine through biochemical analysis of cells the presence of any fatal fetal disorders such as Tay-Sachs disease or galactosemia.
   e. To determine the possible need for intrauterine fetal transfusion.

Equipment
Sterile amniocentesis tray
   Draping towels
   Skin antiseptic
   No. 25 gauge needle on 3-ml. syringe for local skin injection
   Vial of local anesthetic (Xylocaine)
   No. 22-gauge spinal needle 12.5 cm. (5 inches) in length, with stylet in place
   10-ml. syringe
   Test tube
Sterile surgical gloves

Procedure

NURSING ACTION	RATIONALE/AMPLIFICATION
Preparatory Phase	
1. Identify patient's concerns and if necessary provide additional explanation of procedure.	1. Patient may consider procedure hazardous to self or fetus.
2. Assist patient to undress and put on patient gown.	2. Procedure will be done in delivery or operating room.
3. Have patient void.	3. To prevent injury to bladder.
4. Transfer the patient to delivery or operating room.	4. Procedure is performed under sterile conditions.
Performance Phase	
1. The physician determines fetal position by palpation.	1. Fetal position must be determined to prevent inadvertent fetal injury.

* (Figure reproduced with permission from VJ Freda. The control of Rh disease. Hospital Practice, Jan 1967, and from RA Good and DW Fisher (eds). Immunology. Sunderland, Simauer Associates, Inc., 1971)

Procedure	NURSING ACTION	RATIONALE/AMPLIFICATION
	2. The placenta is localized through ultra-sound.	2. This is a feasible technique after 13 weeks gestation. Puncture of fetal placental vessels could cause exsanguination and contamination of the fluid by blood, making specimen useless for chemical or cytogenic analysis.
	3. Carry out surgical skin preparation.	3. Since the needle will be inserted through the skin into the amniotic cavity, asepsis is carried out to prevent infection.
	4. Drape patient's abdomen using sterile technique.	4. Same as above.
	5. Local anesthesia is infiltrated in the site.	5. The site is determined by the position of the fetus and placenta.
	6. The 12.5-cm. (5-inch), 22-gauge spinal needle with stylet in place is introduced into the amniotic cavity.	
	7. The stylet is removed and the 10 ml. syringe attached; 2–10 ml. of fluid is slowly withdrawn and placed in test tube.	7. Shield fluid from light, which may cause a breakdown of the pigments to be measured. The fluid obtained is sent to the lab or shipped to a center equipped for the analysis: 2–4 weeks are required for cellular growth.
	8. The needle is withdrawn and a small dressing applied.	

Follow-up Phase

1. Be aware of complications (fetal or maternal hemorrhage, premature labor, infection).
2. Assess patient for fainting, pain, nausea, or onset of contractions.
3. Return patient to dressing room and outpatient clinic.

BIBLIOGRAPHY

Books

Barber HR, Fields DH, Kaufman SA. Quick Reference to Ob-Gyn Procedures, 2nd ed. Philadelphia, JB Lippincott, 1979

Benson RC. Current Obstetric and Gynecologic Diagnosis and Treatment. Los Altos, Lange Medical Publications, 1978

Bleier IJ. Bedside Maternity Nursing, 4th ed. Philadelphia, WB Saunders, 1979

Butnarescu G. Perinatal Nursing: Reproductive Health, Vol I. New York, John Wiley & Sons, 1978

Clark AL, Affonso DD, Harris TR. Childbearing: A Nursing Perspective, 2nd ed. Philadelphia, FA Davis, 1979.

Clausen JP, Flook MH, Ford B. Maternity Nursing Today. New York, McGraw–Hill, 1977

Danforth DN. Textbook of Obstetrics and Gynecology. New York, Harper & Row, 1977

Goodhart RS and Shils ME. Modern Nutrition in Health and Disease, 6th ed. Philadelphia, Lea & Febiger, 1980

Goodlin RC. Care of the Fetus. New York, Masson, 1979

Hafez ESE. Human Reproduction, 2nd ed. Hagerstown, Harper & Row, 1980

Hale NC. The New Role of the Father in Childbirth. New York, Anchor Press/Doubleday, 1979

Hassid P. Textbook for Childbirth Educators. Hagerstown, Harper & Row, 1979

Hunonen OP, Slone D, Shapiro S. Birth Defects and Drugs in Pregnancy. Littleton, Publishing Sciences Group, 1977

Insalls AJ and Salerno MC. Maternal and Child Health Nursing, 4th ed. St. Louis, CV Mosby, 1979

Insalls AJ and Salerno MC. Maternal and Child Health Nursing Study Guide, 2nd ed. St. Louis, CV Mosby, 1980.

Jensen MD, Benson RC, Bobak IM. Maternity Care: The Nurse and the Family. St. Louis, CV Mosby, 1977

Kaminetzky HA and Iffy L (eds.) New Techniques and Concepts in Maternal and Fetal Medicine. New York, Van Nostrand Reinhold, 1979

Kitzinger S. Education and Counselling for Childbirth. New York, Macmillan, 1977

Krause M and Mahan K. Food Nutrition and Diet Therapy. 6th ed. Philadelphia, WB Saunders, 1978

Krentner KK et al. Adolescent Obstetrics and Gynecology. Chicago, Year Book Medical Publishers, 1978

Lerch C and Bliss VJ. Maternity Nursing, 3rd ed. St. Louis, CV Mosby, 1978

MacDonald RP (ed). Scientific Basis of Obstetrics and Gynaecology, 2nd ed. New York, Churchill Livingstone, 1978

Malo-Juvera D et al. Obstetrical Nursing, 2nd ed. Garden City, Medical Examination Pub. Co., 1979

McNall LK (ed). Contemporary Obstetric and Gynecologic Nursing. St. Louis, CV Mosby, 1980

Milunsky A. Genetic Diseases and the Fetus: Diagnosis, Prevention and Treatment. New York, Plenum Press, 1979

Mitsunao K. Illustrated Manual in Obstetrics and Gynecology, 2nd ed. New York, Igaku–Shoin, 1980

Moore ML and Davis MS. Realities in Childbearing. Philadelphia, WB Saunders, 1978

Olds S et al. Obstetric Nursing. Menlo Park, Addison–Wesley Pub. Co, 1980

Percival R. Holland and Brews Manual of Obstetrics. New York, Churchill Livingstone, 1980

Philipp EE, Barnes J, Newton M. Scientific Foundations of Obstetrics and Gynecology. Chicago, Year Book Medical Publishers, 1977

Pritchard JA and Macdonald PC. Williams' Obstetrics, 16th ed. New York, Appleton–Century–Crofts, 1980

Reeder SR, Mastroianni L, Martin LL. Maternity Nursing, 14th ed. Philadelphia, JB Lippincott, 1980

Sandberg EC. Synopsis of Obstetrics, 10th ed. St. Louis, CV Mosby, 1978

Sciarra J. Gynecology and Obstetrics, Vol 2. Hagerstown, Harper & Row, 1978

Stevenson RE. The Fetus and Newly Born Infant, 2nd ed. St. Louis, CV Mosby, 1977

Taylor SE. Obstetrics and Fetal Medicine. Baltimore, Williams & Wilkins, 1977

Willson JR and Carrington ER. Obstetrics and Gynecology, 6th ed. St. Louis, CV Mosby, 1979

Wolman BB (ed). Psychological Aspects of Gynecology and Obstetrics. Oradell, Medical Economics, 1978

Wynn RM (ed). Obstetrics and Gynecology Annual, Vol 8. New York, Appleton–Century–Crofts, 1979

Ziegel EE and Cranley MS. Obstetric Nursing, 7th ed. New York, Macmillan, 1978

Articles

Ascher BH. Maternal anxiety in pregnancy and fetal homeostasis. JOGN Nurs 1978 May/June; 7(3):19–21

Bartsch F, Lundberg J, Wahldstrom JL. One thousand consecutive midtrimester amniocenteses. Obstet Gynecol 1980 Mar; 55(3):305–08

Bishop B. A guide to assessing parenting capabilities. Am J Nurs 1976 Nov; 76(11):1784–1787

Cranley MS. Fetal and maternal monitoring. Am J Nurs 1978 Dec; 78(12):2097–2102

Evertson LR et al. Antepartum fetal heart rate testing. I. Evolution of the nonstress test. Am J Obstet Gynecol 1979 Jan; 133(1):29–33

Flowers I et al. Ob-Gyn nurse practitioner program. JOGN Nurs 1976 Mar/Apr; 5(2):49–52

Goodlin RC. History of fetal monitoring. Am J Obstet Gynecol 1979 Feb; 133(3):323–347

Gottsfeld KR. Ultrasound in obstetrics. Clin Obstet Gynecol 1978 June; 21(1):311–327

Jimenez S and Jungman R. Supplemental information for the family with multiple pregnancy. Am J Mat Child Nurs 1980 Sept/Oct; 5(5):320–325

Klein L. Antecedents of teenage pregnancy. Clin Obstet Gynecol 1978 Dec; 21(4):1151–1159

Kretzschmar R. Smoking and health: The role of the obstetrician and gynecologist. Obstet Gynecol 1980 Apr; 55(4):403–406

Meyer MB. How does maternal smoking affect the birth weight and maternal weight gain? Am J Obstet Gynecol 1978 Aug; 131(8):888–893

Nadelson C, Notman M, Gillon J. Sexual knowledge and attitudes of adolescents: relationship to contraceptive use. Obstet Gynecol 1980 Mar; 55(3):340–345

Neutra RR et al. Effects of fetal monitoring on neonatal death rates. N Engl J Med 1978 Aug 17; 299(7):324–326

Petrella JM. The unwed pregnant adolescent. JOGN Nurs 1978 July/Aug; 7(4):22–26

Osofsky J and Osofsky HJ. Teenage pregnancy: Psychosocial considerations. Clin Obstet Gynecol 1978 Dec; 21(4):1161–1173

Smith D and Smith H. Toward improvements in parenting: A description of prenatal and postpartum classes with teaching goals. JOGN Nurs 1978 Nov/Dec; 7(6):22–27

Tyrer LB, Mazlen RG, Bradshaw L. Meeting the special needs of pregnant teenagers. Clin Obstet Gynecol 1978 Dec; 21(4):1199–1213

OBSTETRICAL AND NURSING MANAGEMENT DURING LABOR AND DELIVERY

30

THE LABOR PROCESS

Phenomena Preliminary to the Onset of Labor

1. Lightening (the settling of the fetus in the lower uterine segment) occurs 2–3 weeks before term in the primigravida and later or during labor in the multigravida.
   a. Respiration becomes easier as the fetus falls away from the diaphragm.
   b. Lordosis is increased as the fetus enters the pelvis and falls farther foreward.
   c. Frequency of urination due to pressure on the bladder occurs.
2. Vaginal secretions increase.
3. Some weight is lost—from excretion of body fluid and loss of appetite.
4. Mucus plug (protective mechanism which forms by the 7th month) is discharged from cervix.
5. Bloody show appears—effacement or thinning of the cervix causes capillary bleeding.
6. Cervix becomes soft and effaced (thinned).
7. Backache becomes persistent.
8. False labor pains occur with variable frequency; myometrium becomes irritable.

Stages of Labor

1. First stage of labor, or stage of cervical dilatation, begins with first true labor contractions and ends with complete dilatation of the cervix.
2. Second stage of labor, or stage of expulsion, begins with complete dilatation and ends with birth of the baby.
3. Third stage of labor, or placental stage, begins with delivery of the baby and ends with delivery of the placenta.
4. Fourth stage lasts from delivery of the placenta until the postpartum condition of the patient has become stabilized.

Signs of True Labor

1. Uterine contractions occur at regular intervals. They occur every 20–30 minutes at the beginning; later they appear closer together and increase in duration and intensity.
2. Uterine contractions are painful and hard.
3. Pain is felt in both back and front of abdomen.
4. Dilatation and effacement of the cervix are accomplished.
5. Presenting part descends.
6. Fetal head is fixed between contractions.
7. Bulging or rupture of the membranes at the cervix may occur.
8. Moderate sedation will not stop contractions.

False Labor

1. Caused by inefficient contractions of the uterus or painful spasms of the intestines, bladder, and abdominal wall muscles.
2. May appear a few days to a week before term.
3. May be brought on by digestive upset.
4. Contractions are irregular and short and are felt more in front.
5. May consist of slight uterine contractions which are not hard and which do not bring about dilatation and effacement.
6. Can be stopped by sedation.

Mechanisms of Labor

1. *Descent*—includes engagement of head; continues through labor.
2. *Flexion*—resistance to descent causes head to flex so that the chin approaches the chest, reducing the presenting diameter by 1.5 cm. (⅝ inch).
3. *Internal rotation*—takes place in 2nd stage of labor. Head enters pelvis in transverse diameter of the

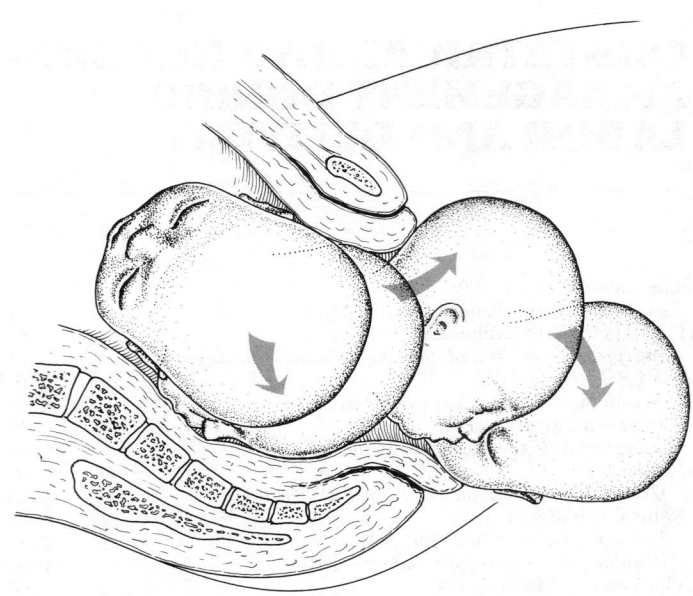

FIGURE 30-1. *L.A.O. positional changes of head in passing through birth canal. (From Fitzpatrick E et al. Maternity Nursing, 13th ed. Philadelphia, JB Lippincott, 1976.)*

inlet—occiput is at 3 o'clock and rotates 90 degrees to arrive under the pubic symphysis. The sequence is L.O.T. (left occipital transverse) to L.O.A. (left occipital anterior) to O.A. (occipital anterior). The shoulders are flexed 45 degrees in the left oblique.

4. *Extension*—birth is by extension. Back of neck pivots under the pubis; the vertex, bregma, forehead, face, and chin are born over the perineum.
5. *Restitution*—when the head has been delivered, the neck twists and the head turns back 45 degrees to the left, resuming the normal relationship with the shoulders—O.A. (occipital anterior) to L.O.A. (left occipital anterior).
6. *External rotation*—the shoulders now rotate 45 degrees to the left, which brings their bisacromial diameter into the anteroposterior diameter of the pelvis. The head follows the shoulder and rotates another 45 degrees to the left—L.O.A. to L.O.T. (See Fig. 30-1.)

ASSESSMENT OF THE PATIENT DURING LABOR

Abdominal Palpation

A. *Purpose*

Abdominal palpation is done to determine the following:
1. The presentation and position of the fetus
2. Whether engagement has occurred
3. If the vortex is in a normal state of flexion
4. The presence of multiple pregnancy or abnormalities of the fetus or uterus

B. *Leopold Maneuvers*

1. *First maneuver* (Fig. 30-2A)—to determine which fetal pole is in the uterine fundus.
   Hands are moved up the side of the uterus, and the fundus is palpated. In most cases, the breech is felt and is softer, more irregular, less globular, and less mobile than the head.
2. *Second maneuver* (Fig. 30-2B)—to determine the position of the fetal extremities, the fetal back, and the anterior shoulder.
   Hands are placed on the sides of the abdomen to identify the location of the back and small parts.
3. *Third maneuver* (Fig. 30-2C)—to determine the portion of the fetus that is presenting.
   The lower uterine segment is grasped between the thumb and fingers of 1 hand to feel the presenting part. The head is at the inlet or in the pelvis in 90% of cases.
4. *Fourth maneuver* (Fig. 30-2D)—to confirm the findings of the third maneuver and to determine the flexion of the vertex.
   Examiner turns and faces the patient's feet. Gently the fingers are moved down the sides of the uterus. The cephalic prominence is felt on the side where there is greater resistance to the descent of the fingers into the pelvis. In addition, it is noted whether the head is free and floating or fixed and engaged.

Vaginal Examination (Fig. 30-3)

1. Vaginal examination is preferable to rectal examination in several ways:
   a. Allows greater accuracy in determining the following:
      (1) Condition and dilatation of the cervix
      (2) Station and position of the presenting part
      (3) Relationship of the fetus to the pelvis
   b. Takes less time since it requires less manipulation.
   c. Causes less pain.
   d. Abnormal presentation can be diagnosed earlier.
   e. Accidents or complications can be identified.
      (1) Prolapse of the umbilical cord
      (2) Placenta previa
2. Examination is carried out as follows:

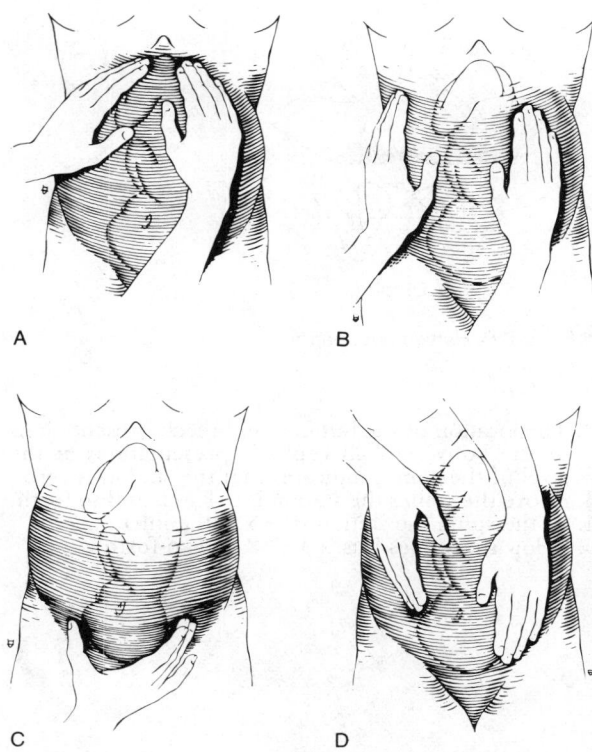

A   B

C   D

FIGURE 30-2. *Leopold maneuvers.*

   a. Gently and carefully
   b. Under aseptic conditions
   c. With patient in the lithotomy position
3. After palpation, condition of cervix is characterized as follows:
   a. Soft or hard

   b. Effaced and thin or thick and long
   c. Easily dilatable or resistant
   d. Closed or open (dilated) (and degree of dilatation)
4. Presentation
   a. Breech, cephalic (head), or shoulder
   b. Caput succedaneum (edema occurring in and under fetal scalp) present (small or large)
   c. Station identified
5. Position
   a. Cephalic presentation (identification of the sagittal suture and of its direction)
   b. Location of posterior fontanelle
6. Membranes
   a. Intact
   b. Ruptured
     (1) Drainage of fluid
     (2) Passage of meconium

Assessment of Fetal Position and Descent

Engagement—has taken place when the widest diameter of the presenting part has passed through the inlet (Fig. 30-4*A*). In cephalic presentations this diameter is the biparietal diameter of the head.

Floating—the presenting part is entirely out of the pelvis and is freely movable above the pelvic inlet (Fig. 30-4*B*).

Dipping—the presenting part has passed through the plane of the inlet but engagement has not occurred (Fig. 30-4*C*).

A. *Engagement*

1. The presence or absence of engagement is determined by abdominal and vaginal or rectal examination.
2. In primigravidas, engagement usually takes place 2–3 weeks before term.
   (Lack of engagement in primiparas calls for investigation to rule out disproportion, abnormal position, or some condition blocking the birth canal.)

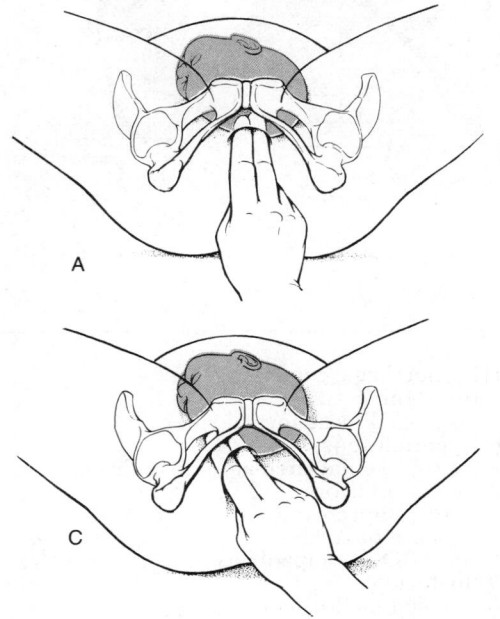

A

C

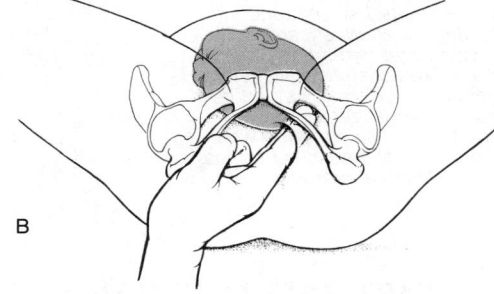

B

FIGURE 30-3. *Vaginal Examination. A. Determining the station and palpating the sagittal suture. B. Identifying the posterior fontanelle. C. Identifying the anterior fontanelle.*

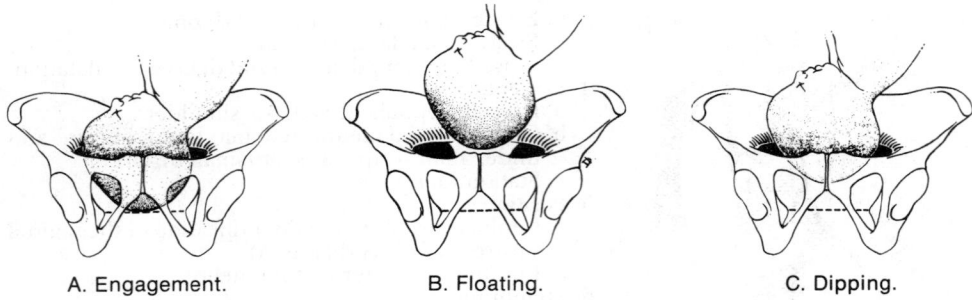

A. Engagement.   B. Floating.   C. Dipping.

FIGURE 30-4. *Engagement, floating and dipping. (From Oxorn H and Foote WR. Human Labor and Birth. New York, Appleton-Century-Crofts)*

3. In multigravidas, engagement occurs any time before or after onset of labor.

B. *Station* (Fig. 30-5)

1. The relationship of the presenting part to an imaginary line drawn between the ischial spines.

2. The location of the buttocks in breech presentations or the bony skull in cephalic presentations at the level of the spines indicates that the station is zero.
3. Above the spines the station is −1, −2 and so forth.
4. At the spine the station is −5 at the inlet.
5. Below the spines it is +1, +2 and so forth.

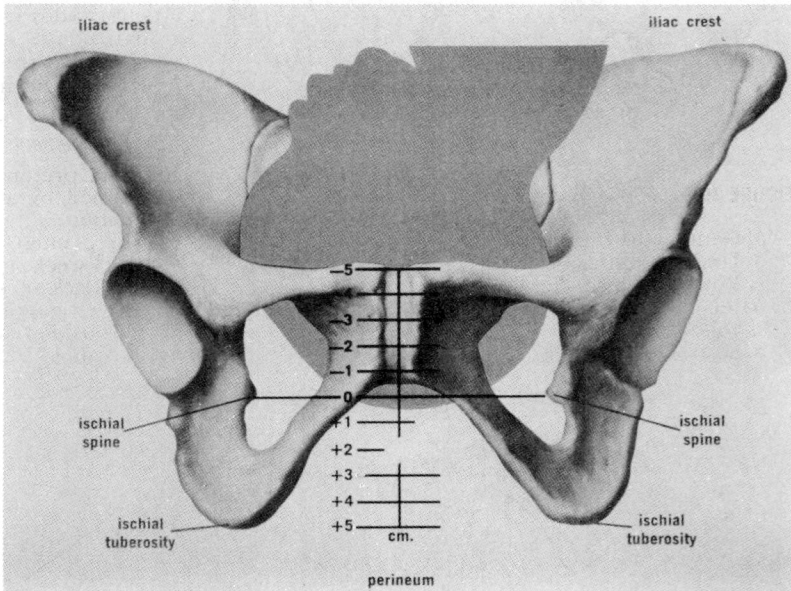

FIGURE 30-5. *Stations of presenting part. The location of the presenting part in relation to the level of the ischial spines is designated* station, *and indicates the degree of advancement of the presenting part through the pelvis. Stations are expressed in centimeters above (minus) or below (plus) the level of the ischial spines (zero). The presenting part is usually engaged when it reaches the level of the ischial spines. (Courtesy of Ross Laboratories.)*

FETAL HEART RATE EVALUATION

Purpose

1. To monitor the status of the fetus.
2. To detect fetal distress and provide appropriate nursing intervention.

Causes of Fetal Distress

1. Maternal complications
   a. Diabetes mellitus
   b. Heart disease
   c. Toxemias of pregnancy
   d. Hemorrhagic conditions
   e. Infection
   f. Prolonged or abnormal labor
   g. Hypertension
   h. Uteroplacental circulatory insufficiency
2. Mechanical factors
   a. Cord compression
   b. Prolapse of cord
3. Rh or ABO incompatibility
4. Prematurity
5. Congenital malformations

Methods of Evaluation

A. *Intermittent auscultation*

1. De Lees-Hollis fetoscope (see Fig. 30-6)
2. Leffscope (stethoscope with a large weighted bell)

B. *Continuous auscultation*

1. *Phonocardiography*—small amplifying microphones
2. *Ultrasonic sensor*—a small battery-operated unit which is held or taped to the patient's abdomen and which amplifies the fetal heart tones (Doptone or Doppler sensors)
3. *Indirect continuous monitor*—separate transducers are secured to the patient's abdomen; the transducers translate abdominal tension and fetal heart sounds into electrical signals that are recorded on a strip chart (Fig. 30-7)
4. *Direct continuous monitor*—a method of recording intrauterine pressure and the fetal heart rate (FHR) through internal measurements
   a. Fetal electrocardiograph—obtained by a small electrode clipped to the presenting part (membranes must be ruptured, the cervix must be dilated 3–4 cm. (1⅝ inches), and the station must be at −2 or lower).
   b. Uterine contractions are recorded by means of a catheter placed in the uterine cavity behind the presenting part.

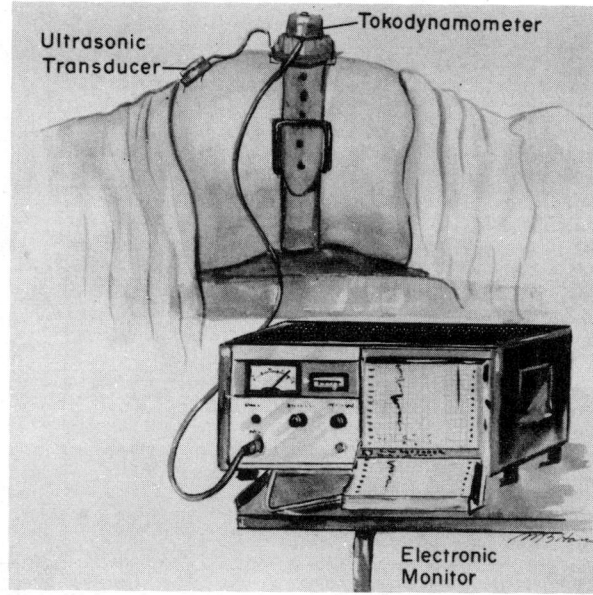

FIGURE 30-7. *Indirect continuous monitor. (From Roux, Jacques F. Monitoring of labor in high-risk centers. In Aladjem S and Brown AK (eds): Clinical Perinatology. St. Louis, CV Mosby, 1974.)*

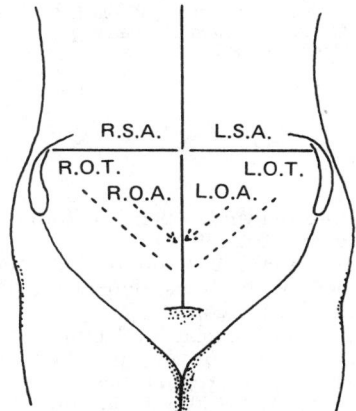

FIGURE 30-8. *Fetal heart tone locations on the abdominal wall indicating possible corresponding fetal positions and the effects of the internal rotation of the fetus.*

(1) The catheter is filled with distilled water and is connected to an external transducer which converts pressure values into an electric signal.
(2) Monitor strips record the quality of the uterine contractions and fetal heart patterns simultaneously (see Fig. 30-9).

C. *Nursing Activities*—intermittent auscultation

1. Explain the procedure to the patient.
2. Determine the position, presentation, and lie of the fetus by palpation. As internal rotation and descent occur, the location of the fetal heart tone (FHT) changes, swinging gradually from the right or left quadrant to the midline and dropping until imme-

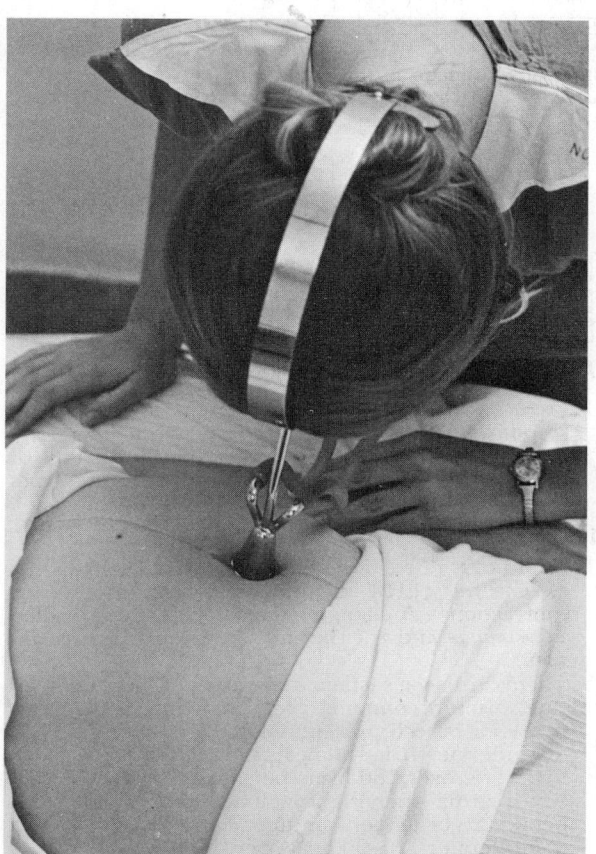

FIGURE 30-6. *Auscultation of the fetal heartbeat using the fetoscope.*

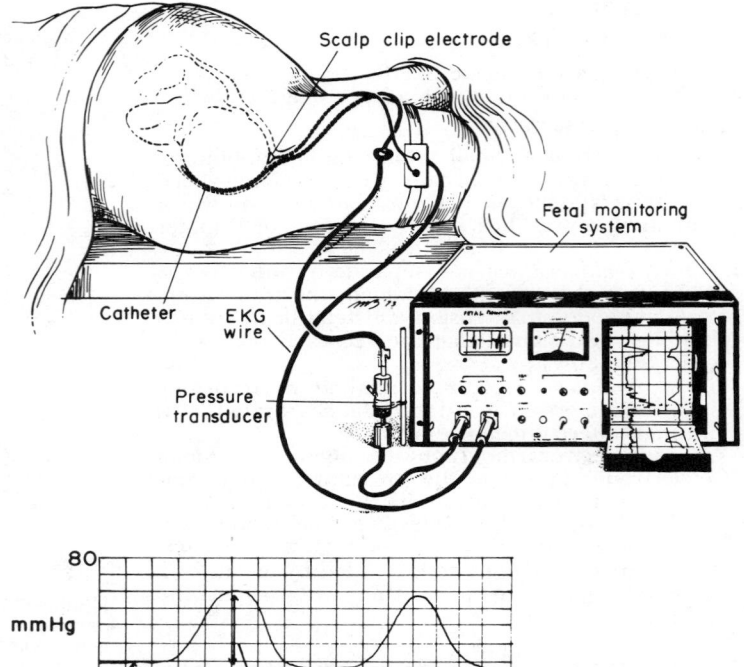

FIGURE 30-9. *Fetal monitoring system for intra-uterine determination of uterine pressure and fetal heart rate. (From Roux, Jacques F. Monitoring of labor in high-risk centers. In Aladjem S and Brown AK (eds): Clinical Perinatology. St. Louis, CV Mosby, 1974.)*

diately before delivery, when it is found above the pubic bone. (See Fig. 30-8.)

3. Place the fetal stethoscope on the abdomen over the back or chest of the fetus, depending on which is closer to the uterine exit.
4. Listen and count the beat for 1 minute.
5. Check the rate before, during, and after a contraction to detect slowing or irregularities.
    Normal rate: 120–160 beats/minute.
6. Avoid friction noises caused by fingers on abdominal surface area.
7. Differentiate between fetal heart tone (FHT) and other abdominal sounds.
    a. *Fetal heart tone*—a very rapid, somewhat muffled ticking sound.
    b. *Uterine bruit*—a soft murmur caused by the passage of blood through dilated uterine vessels; it is synchronous with the maternal pulse.
    c. *Funic souffle*—a hissing sound produced by passage of blood through the umbilical arteries; it is synchronous with the fetal heart rate (FHR).
8. Check fetal heart tones (FHT) immediately following the rupture of the membranes; sudden release of fluid may cause prolapse of the umbilical cord.
9. The ultrasonic transducer device should be applied over the area of the abdomen where the sharpest sound is heard. Lubricate the face of the transducer with a thin layer of ultrasonic jelly to aid in the transmission of sounds.

INTERPRETATION OF FETAL MONITORING DATA AND MANAGEMENT OF FETAL DISTRESS

Advantages of Electronic Monitoring

1. Provides an accurate measurement of the fetal heart's response to stress during uterine contractions.
2. Monitor strips provide a record of the quality of uterine contractions and of fetal heart rate from which evaluations and comparisons can be made.

Interpretation

1. Fetal heart rate (FHR) must be checked initially for *baseline rate* (FHR in the absence of or between contractions). A change from the baseline is termed a *fluctuation* and is either an *acceleration* or a *deceleration*.
2. Tachycardia—a sustained elevation of the fetal heart rate (often accompanies fetal hypoxia, fetal immaturity, or breech presentation).
    a. Moderate: 161–180 beats per minute.
    b. Severe: over 180 beats per minute.
3. Bradycardia—persistent fetal heart rate (FHR) levels below 120 beats per minute.
    a. Moderate: 120–90 beats per minute.
        (1) Not associated with significant fetal acidosis.
        (2) Congenital heart disease may be related to persistently slow fetal heart rate (FHR).

b. Marked: 89–70 beats per minute.
Associated with progressive fetal acidosis.
c. Severe: less than 70 beats per minute.
4. Short term fetal heart rate (FHR) fluctuations—reflect the state of the nervous mechanisms controlling the fetal heart and are indicative of a healthy fetus. A *lack* of this type of irregularity may indicate the following:
   a. A serious fetal compromise reflecting an acidotic fetal nervous system unable to make parasympathetic or sympathetic responses.
   b. Maternal use of central nervous system depressant drugs (narcotics, tranquilizers, anesthetic agents).
   c. Immature fetal nervous control mechanisms.
5. Periodic fetal heart rate (FHR) changes
   a. Accelerations or decelerations of the FHR are due to:
     (1) Mechanical effects or a uterine contraction applied directly to the fetus and/or umbilical cord.
     (2) Uterine pressure applied indirectly to the intervillous space, decreasing blood flow.
   b. Acceleration of more than 60 beats per minute above baseline is considered severe and indicates fetal compromise.
   c. Deceleration
    Early Deceleration (Fig. 30-10*A*)
     (1) Waveform approximates a mirror image of the pattern of intrauterine pressure.
     (2) Pattern is uniform in appearance from one contraction to another.
     (3) Early deceleration begins near the onset of the contraction.
     (4) Lowest level of the FHR deceleration occurs at the peak of the uterine contraction.

(5) FHR does not fall below 100 beats per minute and duration is less than 90 seconds.
(6) Early deceleration does not usually cause a change in fetal acid-base status.
(7) This type of deceleration is considered benign, caused by fetal head compression. No intervention is required.
Late Deceleration (Fig. 30-10*B*)
(1) Also manifests a smooth uniform heart rate pattern and reflects the pattern of uterine pressure.
(2) Begins later in contracting phase of uterus (as the contraction reaches its peak).
(3) Usually less than 90 seconds duration.
(4) Markedly altered by maternal hypoxia.
(5) Frequently associated with fetal tachycardia.
(6) Partially modified by administration of atropine.
(7) FHR irregularity and passage of meconium may occur.
(8) Associated with progressive fetal hypoxia and acidosis; if prolonged, hypoxia may have a direct effect on the fetal myocardium and possibly on the conduction system of the heart.
(9) Late deceleration pattern due to acute uteroplacental insufficiency as a result of a decreased intervillous space blood flow.
   d. Deceleration of the FHR may be avoided by the following measures:
     (1) Careful maintenance of the maternal blood pressure within normal limits.
     (2) Careful infusion of oxytocics.
     (3) Extremely careful administration of agents such as conduction anesthesia, which may produce maternal hypotension.

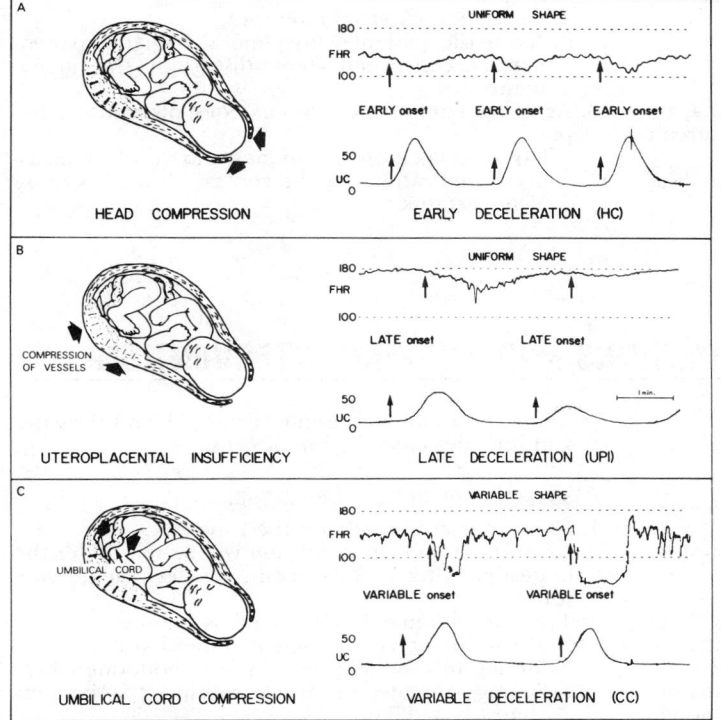

FIGURE 30-10. *Three FHR deceleration patterns. (From Hon E H. An Atlas of Fetal Heart Rate Patterns, New Haven, Harty Press.)*

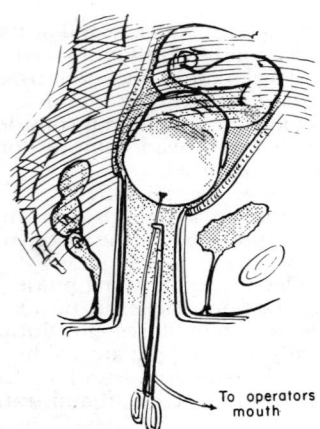

FIGURE 30-11. *Technique of obtaining samples from the fetal scalp during labor.*

e. Deceleration may be modified or corrected by measures which improve uteroplacental blood flow and oxygen transfer across the placenta.
   (1) Discontinue oxytocin if it is being given.
   (2) Change patient's position to the left side to facilitate emptying of the vena cava into the heart and to correct hypotension caused by supine position. Elevation of the patient's legs at a 90-degree angle to the bed may also be effective.
   (3) Administer oxygen by face mask.
   (4) Anesthetist may start IV fluids and administer ephedrine.
   (5) Obtain fetal blood sample to measure degree of fetal hypoxia (Fig. 30-11); fetal compromise causes the following changes:
   pH decrease (normal 7.30 to 7.40)
   PCO_2 increase
   PO_2 decrease
   (6) If ominous FHR pattern persists, labor may be terminated by forceps delivery or cesarean section.
   f. *Variable deceleration* (Fig. 30-10C)—due to umbilical cord compression.

(1) Nonuniform periodic changes in FHR bear no consistent relationship to the uterine contractions.
(2) Often preceded and followed by acceleration.
(3) FHR usually falls below 100 beats per minute and may fall as low as 50 to 60 beats per minute.
(4) Duration of deceleration varies from a few seconds to minutes.
(5) Usually associated with baseline FHR in normal or near-normal range.
(6) Condition corrected by changing patient's position so as to relieve pressure on the cord.
(7) When severe variable deceleration is present, prolapse of the cord should be suspected.
g. *Combined FHR deceleration patterns*—combination of 2 or 3 patterns may exist since a single uterine contraction may evoke all 3 types simultaneously; visual identification of the patterns thus becomes very difficult or impossible.

Nursing Activities During Fetal Monitoring

1. Provide explanations to the patient and her family; ideally these should be given during the prenatal period during tours or by means of films.
   Information should include the following:
   (1) Why the monitor is being used and the benefits derived from its use.
   (2) What the monitor does and what causes the "bleeps."
   (3) How the monitor is applied.
   (4) What limitations of movement will be necessary.
2. Provide comfort measures.
   a. Give back rubs.
   b. Assist patient to change position; changes should be noted on graph since slight variations may occur.
   c. Reposition external monitors.
   d. Assist the patient with general hygiene; patient may be concerned about disturbing the attachments.
3. Assist patient to cope with anxieties, discomfort, and pain.
   Utilize relaxation techniques and comfort measures; medication may be contraindicated because of fetal status.

ASSESSMENT OF UTERINE CONTRACTIONS AND NURSING INTERVENTION

Purposes

1. To determine progress of labor.
2. To detect deviations from normal pattern.
3. To intervene in pain anticipation and decrease anxiety levels.
4. To instruct patient in relaxation techniques and in timing of her contractions.

Physiology of Uterine Contractions

1. Maternal arterial pressure rises during contractions because of an increase in peripheral resistance.
2. Increase in peripheral arterial resistance means increase in the force opposing the moving of blood, which causes an elevation of arterial blood pressure and impedes oxygenation of cells.

Assessment of Uterine Contractions

1. Place fingertips gently on the fundus.
2. As contraction begins, tension will be felt under the fingertips. Uterus will become harder, then slowly soften.
3. The intensity may be described as follows:
   a. Mild—the uterine muscle is somewhat tense
   b. Moderate—the uterine muscle is moderately firm
   c. Strong—the uterine muscle is so firm that it seems almost boardlike

4. The frequency is measured in minutes—represents the time from the beginning of one contraction until the beginning of the next.
5. Duration of a contraction is timed from the moment the uterus first begins to tighten until it relaxes again.
6. As labor progresses, the character of the contractions changes and they last longer.
7. When the cervix becomes completely dilated (the transition stage) the contractions become very strong, last for 60 seconds, and occur at 2–3 minute intervals.

NURSING ALERT: If any contraction lasts longer than 70 seconds and is not followed by a period of uterine muscle relaxation, notify the attending physician immediately. Uterine rupture and fetal hypoxia may occur.

MANAGEMENT OF THE PATIENT DURING LABOR AND DELIVERY

Admitting the Patient to the Unit

1. Establish positive relationships by greeting and reassuring the patient and by providing supportive nursing care.
2. Assist the patient to undress and get into bed.
3. Provide for safekeeping of personal belongings.
4. Listen to fetal heart tones to identify location, rate and character. *Detection of fetal distress may require that the clinical management of the patient be adjusted*
5. Assess and evaluate the following by means of vaginal examination (p. 1006).
   a. Cervical dilatation
   b. Status of membranes
   c. Presentation, position, and station of the fetus
6. Accept father's presence or absence.
7. Ascertain patient's desires concerning the management of her labor and delivery (e.g., natural childbirth, type of analgesia and anesthesia).
8. Obtain pertinent information from the patient or from records previously submitted by the obstetrician.
   a. Expected date of delivery (may indicate complications of pre- or postmaturity of the fetus).
   b. Parity and character of previous labors.
   c. Time when contractions begin; their frequency, duration, and intensity
   d. If membranes are ruptured, time of rupture and general characteristics
   e. Food and fluid intake during the 6 hours prior to admission. (Digestion is inhibited during labor, which leads to danger of aspiration during delivery when inhalation anesthesia is used.)
   f. Rh-factor, blood type, hemoglobin, and hematocrit (obtained from patient's prenatal record)
   g. Contact lenses, dentures, or removable bridges—removed if the patient has general inhalation anesthesia
9. Record blood pressure and report any elevations of systolic pressure over 140 mm. Hg or diastolic pressure over 80 mm. Hg or any unusual reading in relation to the stage of labor.
10. Measure pulse, respiration rates, and temperature.
    a. Anxiety and exertion may cause increase in pulse and respiration rates, but temperature will remain normal.
    b. Elevated temperature suggests maternal infection—isolation techniques may be indicated and the infant may be placed in the observation nursery.
11. Carry out perineal preparations.
    a. Shaving the vulva and perineal areas promotes cleanliness and reduces possibilities of postpartum infection.
    b. Vaginal opening will be more easily visible.
12. Obtain urine specimen only if specifically requested. It is difficult to obtain an uncontaminated voided specimen if membranes have ruptured or if show is present.
13. Administer enema (soapsuds or Fleet).
    Emptying the lower large intestine has the following effects:
    (1) Increases space available for passage of the fetus.
    (2) Decreases fecal contamination of the field during delivery.
    (3) Usually increases frequency and intensity of uterine contractions.

NURSING ALERT: An enema is contraindicated when vaginal bleeding, premature labor, or abnormal fetal presentation or position is present.

First Stage of Labor

A. *Characteristics of Labor During First or Dilating Stage*

1. Cervix dilates to 3–4 cm. (1⅝ inches).
2. Uterine contractions occur regularly 5–10 minutes apart and are of short duration (20 seconds).
3. Patient usually experiences low back pain and abdominal discomfort with contractions.
4. Patient may feel anticipation, excitement, relief, or apprehension.
5. Patient usually appears alert and talkative; however, if she is unprepared and improperly informed, she may be fearful and withdrawn.

B. *Nursing Management During Latent Phase of First Stage*

1. Provide techniques of support and relaxation.
   a. Encourage patient to time her contractions.
   b. Provide reading materials.
   c. Teach breathing techniques to be used in active phase.
   d. If her partner is present, involve him in activities.
   e. Encourage patient to listen to fetal heart tones.
2. Provide explanations of nursing activities.
3. Share information about patient's progress following examinations.
4. Continue constant nursing surveillance.
   a. Major concern of most patients is being left alone and unattended.

b. Identify any deviations from the normal status of both mother and fetus.

5. Continue to monitor fetal heart tones every 30 minutes.
6. Evaluate vital signs every 2 hours, blood pressure every hour—more often if indicated.
7. Encourage patient to void every 3 hours—a full bladder will inhibit contractions and interfere with descent of fetus.

C. *Characteristics of Labor During the Active Phase of the First Stage of Labor*

1. Cervical dilation from 4–8 cm. (1⅝–3⅛ inches).
2. Labor becomes active—contractions occur at 2- to 5-minute intervals with greater intensity and duration of 30–40 seconds.
3. When cervical dilation reaches 6 cm. (2⅜ inches) there is noticeable change in character of labor and of patient reaction.
4. If membranes are intact, rupture usually occurs spontaneously.

NURSING ALERT: Monitor fetal heart tones following amniotomy or spontaneous rupture of membranes; flow of fluid may cause prolapse of cord.

---

5. Patient becomes serious, pays little attention to external stimuli, and is concerned with progress of labor.
6. Patient may feel unable to cope with contractions and may begin to lose control.

D. *Nursing Management During Active Phase*

1. Ascertain patient progress by vaginal examination.
2. Monitor fetal heart tones every 5 minutes if not attached to continuous monitoring equipment.
3. Observe contractions for frequency, intensity, and duration.
4. Assist patient with controlled abdominal breathing to reduce tension and prevent hyperventilation.
5. Encourage patient to assume Sims' position whenever possible.
   a. Favors anterior rotation of the fetal head.
   b. Prevents continual pressure of the gravid uterus on the inferior vena cava.
   c. Promotes relaxation between contractions.
6. Provide comfort measures.
   a. Provide sacral hand pressure and backrest.
   b. Change damp or soiled linen.
   c. Assist with mouth care.
   d. Give partial sponge bath.
   e. Continue to provide encouragement and information in accordance with the patient's needs.
7. Administer IV fluids as prescribed.
   a. Dehydration leads to acidosis—fetus may be born with respiratory acidosis.
   b. Electrolyte imbalance may occur.
   c. Drugs can be given more effectively if complications occur.
8. Administer analgesia as prescribed. Check dosage according to: (a) weight of patient, (b) status of labor, (c) size and stage of gestation of fetus.
9. Assist anesthesiologist in administering regional anesthesia (caudal or lumbar epidural block).
   a. For even distribution of agent, supine position is necessary following placement of catheter.

b. Since Carbocaine or Xylocaine are vasodilators, the blood pressure may drop rapidly.
   Turn on side immediately if blood pressure drops significantly.
c. Pressure of the gravid uterus in the supine position affects blood flow of the large vessels—also predisposes to hypotension.
d. Monitor blood pressure constantly until stabilized.
   (1) Adjust patient's position as indicated.
   (2) Elevate lower extremities to increase blood flow to vital centers.
   (3) Oxygen (5 liters by mask) may be used.

Transitional Stage of Labor

A. *Characteristics of the Transitional Stage*

1. Dilation progresses from 8 cm. (3⅛ inches) to full dilatation.
2. Average time is 40 minutes (with 20 contractions) in primigravidas; 20 minutes (with 10 contractions) in multigravidas.
3. Bloody show increases as more capillary vessels in the cervix rupture.
4. Nausea and vomiting may occur because of reflex action as the cervix stretches and retracts over the fetal head.
5. Patient experiences feelings of rectal pressure.
6. Patient may have partial amnesia between contractions; if narcotics have been given, she may be restless and may cry during contractions.

B. *Nursing Management During the Transitional Stage*

1. Assist with controlled chest (costal) breathing as contractions occur.
2. Discourage patient from bearing down until cervical dilatation is complete.
3. Encourage her to rest between contractions to conserve energy.
4. If epidural analgesia is being used, continue to monitor blood pressure and renew agent if hospital policy permits; if not, notify anesthesiologist when more medication is needed.
5. Continue to monitor fetal heart tones.
6. Observe for onset of second stage.

Second Stage of Labor

A. *Characteristics of the Second Stage of Labor*

1. Usually lasts 2–20 minutes; the primigravida has an average of 20 contractions and the multigravida an average of 10 contractions.
2. Pressure of the presenting part against the pelvic floor during contractions causes an involuntary bearing down of the abdominal wall.
3. The amount of mucoid vaginal discharge of blood and fluid increases because of the rupture of superficial capillaries.
4. Perineal muscles stretch and the central portion of the perineum thins; there is marked distention of the anus.
5. The perineal bulge increases in size with each contraction and recedes slightly between contractions.
6. The fetal head descends with each contraction and recedes slightly between contractions.
7. The vaginal entrance becomes an anteroposterior slit, then an oval, and finally a circular opening that exposes the fetal head.
8. The head continues to advance and recede with

contractions, passing through the pelvis in a diagonal position, then turning to an anteroposterior position under the symphysis pubis.

9. The presenting part of the head appears through the vulvar opening.
10. With the head in an extended position, the forehead, nose, mouth, and chin appear.
11. After the entire head has emerged, it turns to one side or the other of its own accord (restitution) as the shoulders rotate internally to the anteroposterior position.
12. The anterior shoulder emerges followed by the posterior shoulder.
13. Once the head and shoulders are delivered, the rest of the body slips out easily, usually with a gush of amniotic fluid.
14. Uterine contractions continue until placental separation is accomplished, usually within 15 minutes.

B. *Nursing Management During the Second Stage*

1. Transfer multigravida to the delivery room; primigravidas usually remain in the labor room until caput is observed.
2. Provide direction to the patient to accomplish effective pushing.
3. Provide encouragement with each effort.
4. Monitor fetal heart tones following each contraction and pushing effort; transient fetal bradycardia is not unusual at this stage because of pressure exerted upon the fetal head or compression of the cord.
5. Transfer primigravida to delivery room.
6. Assist the patient onto the delivery table and place in lithotomy position.

> **NURSING ALERT:** Fetal bradycardia is pathologic if (1) the recovery period is delayed beyond 20 seconds (2) it is preceded by a period of acceleration, 160 beats or more per minute, or (3) meconium is observed in the amniotic fluid.

7. Provide hand grips and wrist restraints; explain purpose if patient is awake.
8. Wait for instructions before adjusting position if inhalation anesthesia is to be given.
9. Elevate both of the patient's legs simultaneously (to avoid backache, injury, or ligament strain) and position in stirrups. Adjust stirrups to leg length and provide padding to prevent pressure on the popliteal veins.
10. Cleanse vulva and perineal area.
11. Uncover sterile table and check infant resuscitator. Attach sterile suction catheter and oxygen mask.
12. Check infant weight scale for correct balance.
13. Prepare silver nitrate ampule and sterile water for newborn eye care.
14. Assist practitioner to drape patient, using aseptic technique.
15. Adjust instrument table and provide additional materials as needed.
16. Observe delivery of the infant and complete written records of birth.
17. Administer oxytocics as requested.

GUIDELINES: CONDUCT OF NORMAL DELIVERY

Purpose   To provide a safe outcome for the mother and to deliver a healthy infant.

Equipment   Standard delivery room equipment
    Delivery table with stirrups
    Instrument table
    Anesthesia machine
    Resuscitator with heating unit for infant
Sterile packs containing drapes, leggings, towels, gowns, sponges, catheter
Sterile instruments
    2 scissors (1 for episiotomy, 1 for cutting the umbilical cord)
    1 cord clamp
    4 Allis clamps (for episiotomy repair)
    2 needle holders; curved, round, and cutting needles with sutures
    2 ring forceps (to aid in delivery of placenta and membranes)
    1 vaginal retractor (to aid in inspection of birth canal)
    4 hemostats

Procedure

NURSING ACTION	RATIONALE/AMPLIFICATION
1. Practitioner carries out aseptic technique of surgical scrub, gowning, and gloving while an assistant carries out the activities discussed above, under B.	1. To prevent introduction of organisms into the intrauterine cavity (small lacerations and trauma to the birth canal favor bacterial invasion).
2. Drape and cleanse perineal area.	2. To maintain asepsis.
3. Catheterize patient (only if necessary).	3. To prevent bladder trauma (may be difficult to pass the catheter because the infant's head may compress the urethra).
4. Instruct patient to "push."	4. This is a technique of using the abdominal muscles to assist in uterine expulsive effort during contractions.

GUIDELINES: CONDUCT OF NORMAL DELIVERY (cont.)

Procedure (cont.)

NURSING ACTION	RATIONALE/AMPLIFICATION
5. Wipe the perineum and anus with 4 × 4 sponges and antiseptic solution using a downward and backward motion.	5. To prevent fecal contamination.
6. Avoid the use of fundal pressure to hasten delivery.	6. Fundal pressure may cause uterine damage.
7. Avoid too rapid a delivery. Until the head crowns, the major function of the practitioner is to avoid hurrying the delivery.	7. To preserve the flexion of the fetal head.
8. Assess for severe leg cramps, which may occur when the head crowns. They are relieved by changing the position of the leg.	8. Caused by pressure of the fetal head on the pelvic nerves.
9. Assess the necessity for an episiotomy (perineal incision) when the head crowns slightly. If a tear seems inevitable, a midline or a right or left mediolateral episiotomy may be performed.	9. To prevent perineal laceration and disruption of endopelvic fascia caused by pressure of the fetal head.
10. Control the delivery by the following method, known as "Ritgen's maneuver" (Fig. 30-12). Consists of covering the anus with a sterile towel and exerting upward and forward pressure on the area beneath the fetal chin while maintaining pressure against the occiput with the other hand to control the emerging head and to effect delivery between contractions.	10. To prevent injury to mother and infant. This method delivers the fetal head by extension with the large occipitofrontal diameter presenting at the outlet.

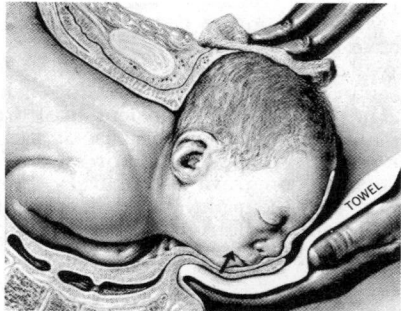

FIGURE 30-12. *Ritgen's maneuver, as it appears in median section. (From Reeder, et al. Maternity Nursing, 13th ed. Philadelphia, JB Lippincott, 1976.)*

NURSING ACTION	RATIONALE/AMPLIFICATION

11. Feel and look for loops of the cord around the neck of the infant as soon as the head is delivered.
  a. Loosen the cord and slip over the head.
  b. If unable to loosen coils, occlude the cord with 2 clamps and cut between them.
	11. To prevent interference with the infant's oxygen supply.

12. Remove mucus and fluid from the infant's face and suction oropharynx.	12. To prevent aspiration of mucus when infant gasps during initial respirations.
13. Do not hasten completion of the delivery. Wait until the head rotates externally.	13. As soon as the head is delivered there is usually a lull in contractions. Rotation of the head is an indication that the shoulders have rotated internally.

14. Observe for continued uterine contractions and for the shoulder to lie directly anteroposteriorly.
  a. Pull the head gently downward and backward until the anterior shoulder is behind and against the symphysis pubis.
  b. Lift the head for delivery of the posterior shoulder.	

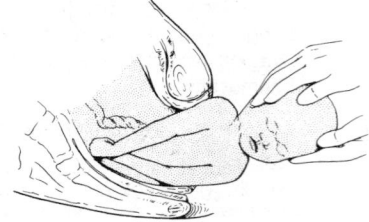

CAUTION: When depressing the head downward and backward, avoid traction, which may cause injury to the brachial plexus.

Procedure (cont.)

NURSING ACTION	RATIONALE/AMPLIFICATION
15. Clamp the cord about 2.5 cm. (1 inch) from umbilicus. (Clamp further down, if infant has an Rh incapability and if umbilical cord catheterization may be necessary for exchange transfusion.)	15. Whether sustained benefit is obtained by the infant by waiting for cessation of pulsation before clamping the cord has not been established.
16. Place infant in a heated crib.	16. To prevent heat loss and hypothermia.
17. Assistant administers oxytocin or ergonovine IM to the mother.	17. To initiate effective uterine contractions for the purpose of expelling the placenta and preventing uterine atony.

CAUTION: Oxytocin is contraindicated for use in combination with drugs that have a sympathomimetic action.

18. Observe for resumption of contractions and for indications that the placenta has separated from the uterine wall.	18. The uterus rises upward in the abdomen, the umbilical cord protrudes further out of the vagina, and the uterus changes from a discoid to a globular shape.
19. Express the placenta by pushing downward on the fundus with moderate pressure and with slight tension on the cord (Fig. 30-13*A, B*). If membranes begin to tear, grasp with clamp and tease out slowly (Fig. 30-13*C*).	19. Excessive pressure on a relaxed uterus may cause inversion.
20. Examine the placenta carefully.	20. a. To make certain that none of the placental and fetal membranes have been retained in the uterus. b. To identify any gross change that may have pathological significance.
21. Inspect the vaginal canal and cervix for lacerations or injury.	21. The examination is carried out before the episiotomy repair; otherwise, if bleeding should occur following repair, inspection at that time would cause tension on the recently placed sutures and could damage the episiotomy wound.
22. Repair the episiotomy (Fig. 30-14.)	
23. Estimate blood loss.	23. Observe the saturation of sponges and towels as well as the amount of bleeding.
24. Remove soiled linen, replace end of the delivery table, and lower the patient's legs from the stirrups simultaneously.	24. To prevent injury or muscle spasm.
25. Apply a sterile perineal pad, warm gown, and blanket.	25. Chilling accompanied by shaking often occurs immediately following delivery. The exact etiology is undetermined.
26. Help the mother to hold the infant and inspect it if she wishes.	26. Early contact with the infant assists in the mother-infant bonding process. One of the mother's first needs is to be reassured that her infant is normal.
27. Assist other personnel in transferring the patient to the recovery room and the infant to the newborn nursery.	

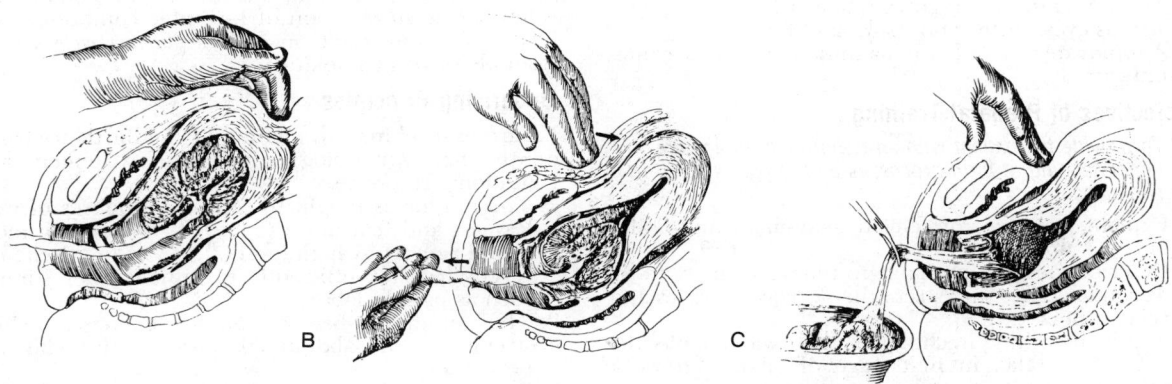

A   B   C

FIGURE 30-13. *Delivery of the placenta. (From Willson JR. Atlas of Obstetric Technic, 2nd ed. St. Louis, CV Mosby, 1969.)*

GUIDELINES: CONDUCT OF NORMAL DELIVERY (cont.)

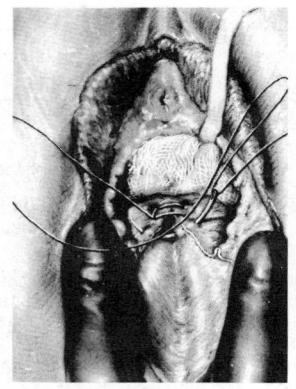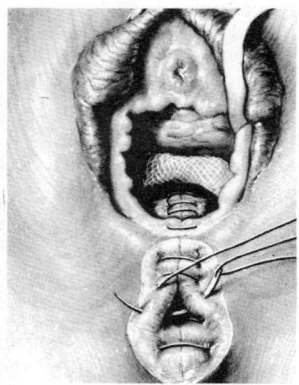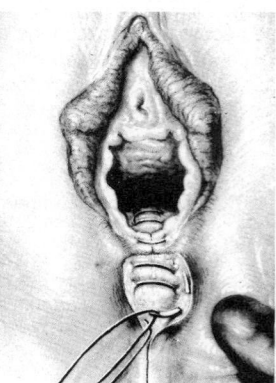

FIGURE 30-14. *Suturing the episiotomy. (From Reeder et al. Maternity Nursing, 13th ed. Philadelphia, JB Lippincott, 1976.)*

NATURAL CHILDBIRTH

Natural childbirth is a normal or natural process in which an infant is delivered without medical analgesia or anesthesia. The mother is prepared for this type of delivery through prenatal training.

Underlying Principles

(As advocated by Grantly Dick-Read and Herbert Thoms)
1. Fear stimulates the sympathetic nervous system and causes the circular muscles of the cervix to contract.
2. The longitudinal muscles of the uterus then have to act against increased cervical resistance, causing tension and pain.
3. Tension and pain aggravate fear, which produces a vicious cycle of tension, pain, and fear.
4. A minor degree of pain, magnified by fear, becomes unbearable.

Objectives of Prenatal Training

A. *To provide the patient with an opportunity to acquire understanding of birth processes and to gain self-confidence.*
1. Explain processes of fetal development and childbirth.
2. Describe methods available to relieve pain.
3. Teach exercises that strengthen certain muscles and relax others.
4. Teach breathing techniques that will enable the patient to relax in first stage of labor and work effectively with muscles used in the delivery.
5. Stress improvement of physical health and emotional stability.

B. *To eliminate fear.*
1. Never tell the patient that labor and delivery will be painless; indicate that analgesia and anesthesia are available if needed or desired.
2. Assure the patient that she will be given empathetic understanding and support during labor by her partner, the nurse, and the physician.

PSYCHOPROPHYLACTIC CHILDBIRTH

Psychoprophylactic childbirth is a version of natural childbirth which has a rationale based on Pavlov's concept of pain perception and his theory of conditioned reflexes (the substitution of favorable conditioned reflexes for unfavorable ones). The *Lamaze method* is an example of this technique.

Underlying Principles

Programs teaching this method of childbirth are based on the neurophysiology of cortical excitement and conditional response.
1. The mother is taught to replace responses of restlessness and fear and the loss of control with more useful activity. A high level of activity can excite the cerebral cortex efficiently to inhibit other stimuli, such as pain in labor.
2. The mother-to-be is taught exercises which strengthen the abdominal muscles and relax the perineum.
3. Breathing techniques to help the process of labor are practiced.
4. The mother is conditioned to respond with respi-

ratory activity and disassociation or relaxation of the uninvolved muscles, while controlling her perception of the stimuli associated with labor.

5. One method of control consists of breathing normally while silently mouthing the words to a song and simultaneously tapping the rhythm with the fingers.

Similarity Between Psychoprophylactic and Natural Childbirth Theories

1. Fear, which enhances the perception of pain, may diminish or disappear when the patient understands the physiology of labor.
2. Since psychic tension enhances perception of pain, relaxation is achieved more easily in a calm, agreeable atmosphere with supportive persons nearby.
3. Muscular relaxation and a specific type of breathing diminish or abolish the pains of labor.

BREATHING TECHNIQUES FOR CHILDBIRTH

During First Stage of Labor

1. A complete breath is taken—once at the beginning of a contraction and once again when the contraction is completed.

2. At the peak of each contraction breathing should be quiet and shallow.
3. The technique for complete breathing involves the following 3 steps:
   a. Breathing in as deeply as possible.
   b. Hissing or blowing the air out slowly.
   c. Allowing the whole body to go limp (relaxation phase).

During Second Stage of Labor

Pushing breath should augment uterine contractions and aid in the delivery of the baby.

1. The mother breathes in as deeply and quickly as possible.
2. She holds her breath. (This fixes the diaphragm and allows more effective downward pressure on the uterus.)
3. She takes catch-breaths as needed. Catch-breaths are taken whenever breath can no longer be held comfortably.
4. She pushes as if straining at defecation. (Pushing is not necessary during practice sessions.)
5. *Panting* may be necessary in the middle of a contraction during the 2nd stage of labor. Panting physically prevents pushing although it does not decrease the desire to push.

THE LEBOYER METHOD

The Leboyer method is based on the premise that the infant suffers psychological shock at the time of delivery. An effort is made to reduce the contrast between the intrauterine environment and the outside world.

Underlying Principles

1. Gentle, controlled delivery. Prenatal education, support from family and personnel to decrease anxiety, fear, and tension.
2. Emphasis on providing protection to the craniosacral axis by gently supporting the newborn infant's head,

neck, and sacrum. The craniosacral axis is completely relaxed, and lost body heat restored in a warm water bath.
3. Avoiding overstimulation of the newborn sensorium. The infant is allowed to breathe spontaneously; cutting the cord is delayed to permit placental blood transfusion for improved respiration.
4. Importance of maternal–infant bond. Skin-to-skin contact with mother provided, and infant is fondled and stroked.

HOME DELIVERY

Delivery of the infant in the home, though controversial, has won increasing support in recent years. It is essential that couples considering home delivery be informed of potential risks and be willing to accept responsibility for well-being of infant and mother.

Underlying Principles

1. Belief that home birth has significant advantages for the family and the newborn infant.
2. Objection to the impersonal and authoritarian atmosphere of the hospital environment with enforced separation of patient and family.
3. Desire to avoid such practices as routine cesarean delivery for breech presentation, episiotomy, forceps delivery, oxytocin stimulation, routine monitoring of the FHT, and other practices associated with hospitals.
4. Risk of in-hospital infections; belief that infant is immune to own-home bacteria.
5. Rising costs of hospitalization.

Contraindications

1. High-risk indications for infant or mother.
2. Patient with history of premature or post-date delivery in previous pregnancy.
3. Women with medical or emotional complications.
4. Patients who cannot be quickly transported to a hospital.

Hazards

1. Maternal—unpredictable intrapartum or postpartum hemorrhage.
2. Infant—premature separation of the placenta or cord prolapse in second stage of labor requiring immediate cesarean delivery, undiagnosed twins, prematurity with respiratory difficulty.

Possible Solutions

1. Alteration of hospital setting to a family-centered approach.
2. Birthing centers for low-risk patients with adequate facilities for emergency care.
3. Properly educated and motivated support personnel.

OPERATIVE OBSTETRICS

Operative obstetrics refers to a number of special procedures (episiotomy, forceps delivery, cesarean section, induction of labor) which the physician may use to assist the mother in labor and delivery.

EPISIOTOMY

An *episiotomy* is an incision of the perineum during delivery to facilitate the birth of the baby.

Types of Episiotomies

1. Median—incision is made in the middle and directed toward the rectum (Fig. 30-15).
2. Mediolateral—incision is begun in the middle and directed laterally and downward away from the rectum. A mediolateral episiotomy reduces incidence of third-degree laceration (extends through skin, mucous membrane, perineal body, and the rectal sphincter).

Purposes

1. To substitute a straight surgical incision for the laceration that otherwise frequently occurs.
2. To facilitate repair of laceration and to promote healing.
3. To spare the infant's head from prolonged pressure and pushing against the rigid perineum which may result in brain damage, especially in the premature infant.
4. To shorten the 2nd stage of labor.

Nursing Management

1. Assess the healing processes; inspect for signs of infection or pain.
2. Provide analgesics for pain relief or apply ice bag *early* to reduce edema and allay discomfort.
3. Evaluate degree of pain; *excessive pain may be a signal of vulval, paravaginal, or ischiorectal hematoma or abscess.*
4. Return patient to the operating room for ligation of bleeding vessels if hematoma is identified.
5. Provide antibiotic therapy for infection and incision and drainage of abscess.

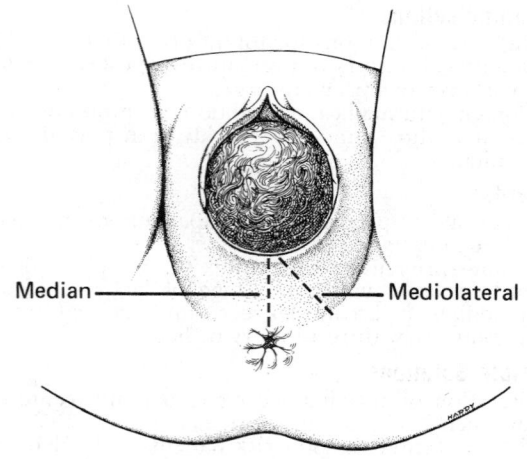

Median ———— Mediolateral

FIGURE 30-15. *Types of episiotomies.*

FORCEPS DELIVERY

The *obstetric forceps* is an instrument, consisting of 2 crossing blades, designed to extract the fetus by means of traction and rotation.

Types of Forceps Deliveries

1. *Low forceps operation*—forceps are applied after the head has reached the perineal floor with the sagittal suture in the anteroposterior diameter of the outlet.
2. *Midforceps operation*—forceps are applied before the criteria for low forceps are met but after engagement has taken place.
3. *High forceps operation*—forceps are applied before engagement has taken place (only used in modern obstetrics in very rare circumstances).

Prerequisites for Application of Forceps

1. Pelvis should be adequate, with no disproportion.
2. Fetal head must be engaged—preferably deeply engaged.
3. Cervix must be completely dilated.
4. Accurate diagnosis of position and station must be made (see p. 1008).
5. Membranes must be ruptured.
6. Some form of anesthesia should be used.
7. Rectum and bladder should be empty.

Indications

1. Fetal distress as identified by any of the following:
   a. Irregular fetal heart rate
   b. Bradycardia under 100 beats per minute
   c. Rapid fetal heart rate—more than 160 beats per minute
   d. Passage of meconium in cephalic presentation
   e. Prolapse of the cord
2. Maternal conditions
   a. Maternal exhaustion
   b. Maternal disease (cardiac or pulmonary disease, hemorrhage, intrapartal infection)
   c. Failure of progress in the 2nd stage due to poor uterine contractions, rigid perineum
   d. Failure of fetal head to rotate

Complications

1. Maternal complications
   a. Lacerations of the vagina and cervix, predisposing to hemorrhage and infection
   b. Rupture of the uterus
   c. Injury to bladder or rectum
2. Fetal complications
   a. Cephalohematoma
   b. Brain damage and intracranial hemorrhage
   c. Skull fracture
   d. Facial paralysis
   e. Cord compression

Nursing Management

1. Carry out surveillance during the postpartum period for signs and symptoms of complications.
2. Assess the newborn for indications of injury.
3. Provide explanation to parents if bruising is apparent.

CESAREAN SECTION

Cesarean section is removal of the infant from the uterus through an incision made in the abdominal wall and the uterus.

Indications

1. Cephalopelvic disproportion
2. Uterine dysfunction, inertia, inability of cervix to dilate, lack of progress
3. Neoplasm obstructing birth canal or pelvis
4. Malposition and malpresentation
5. Previous uterine surgery (cesarean section, myomectomy, hysterotomy) or cervical surgery
6. Complete or partial placenta previa
7. Certain cases of premature separation of the placenta
8. Certain cases of toxemia of pregnancy
9. Maternal diabetes (large infants)
10. Certain cases of older primigravida (35–40 years old)
11. Prolapse of the umbilical cord
12. Fetal distress
13. Post-term pregnancy
14. Failed forceps

Types of Cesarean Section

A. *Low Segment Cesarean Section* (operation of choice)

Incision made transversely in lower segment of uterus.
1. Incision is made in thinnest portion so that blood loss is minimal and uterus is easier to open.
2. Lower segment is area of least uterine activity.
3. Postoperative convalescence is more comfortable.
4. Possibility of later rupture is lessened.
5. Peritoneal flap is brought over uterine incision, preventing lochia from entering peritoneal cavity.
6. Incidence of postoperative adhesions and danger of intestinal obstruction are reduced.

B. *Classical Cesarean Section*

Vertical incision is made directly into the wall of the body of the uterus.
1. Useful when bladder and lower segment are involved in extensive adhesions.
2. Selected when anterior placenta previa exists.
3. Useful when fetus is in a transverse lie.

C. *Extraperitoneal Cesarean Section*

The tissue around the bladder is dissected, providing access to lower uterine segment without entering into the peritoneal cavity.
1. Devised to prevent peritonitis.
2. Availability of blood and antibiotics has reduced use of this method.

D. *Cesarean Section and Hysterectomy (Porro's operation)*

Cesarean section followed by removal of the uterus. Indications:
1. Hemorrhage due to uterine atony, after conservative therapy fails
2. Uncontrollable hemorrhage from placenta previa and abruptio placentae
3. Placenta accreta (abnormal attachment of placenta to uterine endometrium)
4. Rupture of the uterus, not repairable
5. Gross multiple fibromyomata

Nursing Management

A. *Preoperative Care*

1. Carry out physical examination.
2. Request routine laboratory studies, including type and cross-matching of blood.
3. Monitor fetal heart tones.
4. Shave abdomen and perineal area as directed.
5. Insert a retention urinary catheter.
6. Administer prescribed preoperative atropine. (Narcotic drugs are avoided.)
7. Start IV infusion with 19-gauge needle and double hook-up so that blood may be administered quickly if necessary.
8. Prepare oxytocic drugs to be added to the infusion following delivery of the infant.
9. Notify pediatrician or pediatric resident of surgery to provide initial care and resuscitation of infant.

B. *Postoperative Care*

1. Provide postoperative care similar to that following abdominal surgery.
2. Observe for hemorrhage
   a. Inspect perineal pads and abdominal dressings.
   b. Assess vital signs frequently.
3. Administer oxytocics as prescribed.
4. Check fundus frequently for firmness.
5. Continue IV fluids for 24 hours.
6. Check urinary output from indwelling catheter.
7. Provide medication for relief of pain.
8. Encourage patient to turn from side to side, to breathe deeply, and to cough.
9. Assist with ambulation during first postoperative day.

INDUCTION OF LABOR

Induction of labor is the bringing about of labor by amniotomy (surgical rupture of fetal membranes) or administration of oxytocin.

Indications

1. Maternal Condition
   a. Toxemia of pregnancy when medical therapy has been unsuccessful
   b. Uncontrollable antepartal bleeding in late pregnancy (premature separation of the marginal placenta previa)
   c. Premature spontaneous rupture of membranes (infant should be delivered within 24 hours)
   d. History of rapid labors
   e. Patients who live far from hospital
   f. Maternal diabetes (pregnancy terminated at approximately 37 weeks)
2. Fetal Condition
   a. Rh incompatibility with rising titer
   b. Excessive size of fetus or postmaturity

Prerequisites for Successful Induction

1. Normal cephalopelvic relationship
2. Single fetus with vertex engaged
3. Stage of pregnancy—the closer to term the easier the induction
4. Fetal maturity—chance of survival before 32 weeks is reduced
5. Cervix amenable to induction—effaced or partially effaced and dilated 1–2 cm. (⅜–¾ inch)

Nursing Management

A. *For Induction by Oxytocin*

1. Prepare infusion of 1000 ml. 5% glucose with pre-scribed units of Pitocin added.
2. Regulate number of drops per minute prescribed by physician—two-bottle system and constant infusion pump used to maintain accuracy and control.
3. Check rate of flow frequently; patient's movement may change rate of flow.
4. Observe uterine contractions—*keep hand on fundus to time beginning and termination of contractions.*
5. Turn off infusion if there are any abnormalities in contractions or fetal heart tones or if attending physician leaves labor suite.

B. *For Artificial Rupture of Membranes*

1. Explain procedures to patient.
2. Carry out antiseptic preparation of vulva.

> **NURSING ALERT:** Artificial rupture of membranes is usually done to assist a labor already begun by oxytocin rather than to initiate labor. The membranes serve as a barrier against bacterial invasion, so delivery should be accomplished as soon as possible after membranes have been artificially ruptured.

3. Carry out vaginal examination.
4. Insert amniohook or Allis clamp or orangewood stick to rupture membranes.
5. Allow as much fluid as possible to escape.
6. Note quality of fluid (normal, amber, clear).
7. *Check fetal heart tones immediately because there is a greater possibility of cord prolapse.*

OBSTETRICAL ANALGESIA AND ANESTHESIA

OBSTETRICAL ANALGESIA

Method	Comment	Precautions
Natural childbirth (Read, Lamaze methods)	Requires patient preparation and psychologic support, controlled breathing, voluntary muscle relaxation	Requires commitment of patient and partner and support of obstetric staff
Hypnosis		Requires specially trained obstetrician, a willing patient, considerable prenatal training
Narcotics (Demerol most frequently used)	Given IM or IV in 50–100 mg. doses (smaller doses given IV)	Must be withheld until active labor starts Not to be administered when delivery imminent lest depression of infant occur
Tranquilizers (ataractics)	May be used in combination with narcotics Reduced dose of narcotic required Allay anxiety Have antinauseant effect	
Barbiturates	Given in combination with analgesic Produce sedation and hypnosis	Produce excitement when given alone Depress infant for many hours after birth Caution must be exercised when there is maternal liver or renal impairment
Scopolamine	Depresses parasympathetic nervous system Produces amnesia	Must be given with narcotics or will produce excitation, delirium, hallucinations; used infrequently
Trichlorethylene (Trilene)	Usually is self-administered by cannister and face mask	Should not be given with another form of inhalation anesthesia for delivery Cardiac arrhythmias may occur For best results, the patient must be carefully instructed on how to use the equipment Prolonged use may cause confusion or drowsiness, indicating that the concentration should be reduced

GENERAL ANESTHESIA

Method	Comment/Precautions
Nitrous oxide with oxygen	Administered in low concentrations during period of expulsion
Halothane	Produces good uterine relaxation quickly Useful for intrauterine manipulations such as version and extraction Postpartum hemorrhage is a problem
Methoxyflurane (Penthrane)	Contraindicated in patients with a history of liver disease Slow-acting Rarely used in obstetrics
Thiopental (Pentothal sodium)	For rapid induction of anesthesia for vaginal deliveries and cesarean sections Fetal depression is a problem Maternal laryngospasm may lead to fetal and maternal hypoxia

REGIONAL ANALGESIA AND ANESTHESIA

See Table 30-1.

TABLE 30-1. REGIONAL ANALGESIA AND ANESTHESIA

Type	Method	Advantages	Disadvantages
Paracervical block	Transvaginal injection of a local anesthetic into the tissue on either side of the cervix Lasts 45 to 60 minutes	1. Started in the 1st stage of labor 2. Useful in a rapidly progressing labor 3. Causes cervix to dilate more rapidly	1. May cause transient fetal bradycardia 2. Danger of direct injection into maternal circulation or fetal tissue 3. Constant fetal heart monitoring required
Caudal	Blocking of nerves in the peridural space at the sacral hiatus Can be given as single or continuous injection	1. Provides analgesia in the 1st and 2nd stages of labor and anesthesia for delivery 2. Patient is awake 3. Has little effect on fetus 4. Better than narcotics for patients with metabolic diseases or lung or heart disease, and for some patients with toxemia	1. Specially trained anesthesiologist is needed 2. Produces hypotension (agents are vasodilators) 3. May prolong labor in primigravida 4. Higher incidence of forceps deliveries if unassisted with pushing 5. May prolong labor if administered too early 6. Sacral hiatus may be difficult to locate 7. Inadvertent puncture of dura mater into subarachnoid space with large needle—causes severe postanesthesia headache 8. Difficult to keep site clear
Local infiltration	Regional anesthesia produced by local infiltration of the nerves of the perineum	1. Simple to administer 2. Does not affect fetus 3. Toxic effects minimal	1. No value for analgesia during labor 2. Takes time for infiltration and for agent to take effect 3. Useful for perineal repair with natural childbirth
Lumbar epidural (see Fig. 30-17)	Extradural analgesia produced by injection of a local anesthetic into the epidural space in the lumbar region Can be given in single or continuous injection	1. Provides analgesia in the 1st and 2nd stages and anesthesia for delivery 2. Patient is awake and cooperative 3. No effect on fetus unless hypotension occurs 4. Useful when general anesthesia is contraindicated and when patient has diabetes, cardiovascular disease, or pulmonary, renal, or hepatic disease, or is in premature labor	1. Risk of dural puncture greater than in caudal 2. May cause hypotension 3. Requires expert administration by anesthesiologist 4. Patient requires assistance in pushing 5. Greater incidence of uterine atony following delivery 6. May prolong labor 7. Higher incidence of forceps delivery if patient unable to push effectively
Subarachnoid block (spinal anesthesia, saddle block) 1. Low spinal (saddle block) limited to the sacral segment 2. Midspinal analgesia extends to 10th thoracic dermatoma 3. High spinal analgesia to T5 or T6 used for cesarean section	Form of regional anesthesia produced by injection of a local anesthetic solution into the cerebrospinal fluid in the spinal canal	1. Relative simplicity of procedure 2. Is rapid and certain and has lasting action 3. Low failure rate 4. Low incidence of side effects when properly performed	1. Frequency and degree of hypotension higher than with either caudal or epidural block 2. Postspinal headache 3. Anesthesia from a single injection is of short duration (used primarily for delivery)
Pudendal block (Fig. 30-16)	Form of regional anesthesia produced by blocking the pudendal nerve with a local anesthetic agent	1. Simple and safe method of securing perineal analgesia for normal deliveries 2. Does not depress infant	1. Short duration, may be done in patient's room 30 minutes before delivery (may need to be repeated) 2. May fail to produce adequate pain relief 3. Patient must be cooperative

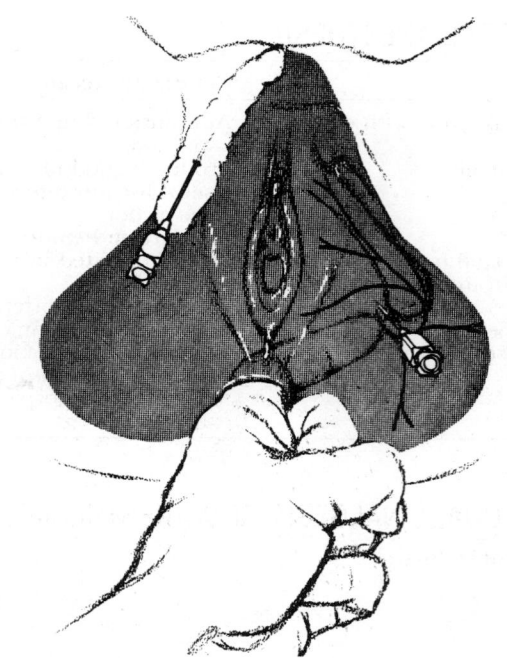

FIGURE 30-16. *The pudendal block is used for perineal anesthesia in uncomplicated obstetrical procedures. The pudendal nerve lies medial to the ischial tuberosity, and the physician inserts his index finger into the rectum to guide the needle point to the tuberosity.*
The other part of the block is done to anesthetize the iliohypogastric, ilioinguinal and genitocrural nerves which innervate the skin over the mons pubis and the labia. (From Nealon TF. Fundamental Skills in Surgery. Philadelphia, WB Saunders, 1971.)

GUIDELINES: Assisting with a Continuous Lumbar Epidural Block

Continuous lumbar epidural block is a form of analgesia achieved by blocking the nerves in the epidural space (Fig. 30-17).

Purpose　　To provide pain relief during labor and delivery.

Equipment　Sterile surgical gloves
Vials of Xylocaine 1% and 2% and Carbocaine 1.5%
Adhesive tape 4 cm. (1½ inches) wide.
Vinyl plastic epidural catheter in sterile package
Antiseptic solution for skin preparation
Sterile epidural tray containing
　　2 medicine glasses (1 for antiseptic solution and 1 for anesthetic agent)
　　10-ml. glass syringe
　　3-ml. glass syringe with 4 cm. (1½-inch) 25-gauge needle
　　No. 17 Touhy spinal needle with stylet in place
　　Draping towels
　　Sponge forceps with sponges for applying antiseptic solution for the skin preparation

Procedure

NURSING ACTION	RATIONALE/AMPLIFICATION
Preparatory Phase	
1. Provide explanation of procedure to the patient.	1. Cooperation by the patient is essential. She must not move while the needle and catheter are being positioned.
2. Have the patient void.	2. It is difficult, if not impossible, to void after the anesthesia has taken effect.
3. Take blood pressure.	3. Anesthetic agent usually causes some degree of hypotension. (Anesthesiologist should be aware of blood pressure levels before proceeding.)
4. Assist the patient to lie on the left side with shoulders parallel, head flexed toward chest, and knees drawn upward.	4. The spinal column should not be too convex or the epidural space will be reduced and the dura stretched, making it more susceptible to puncture.
5. Open the outer covering of the surgical gloves and the epidural tray.	

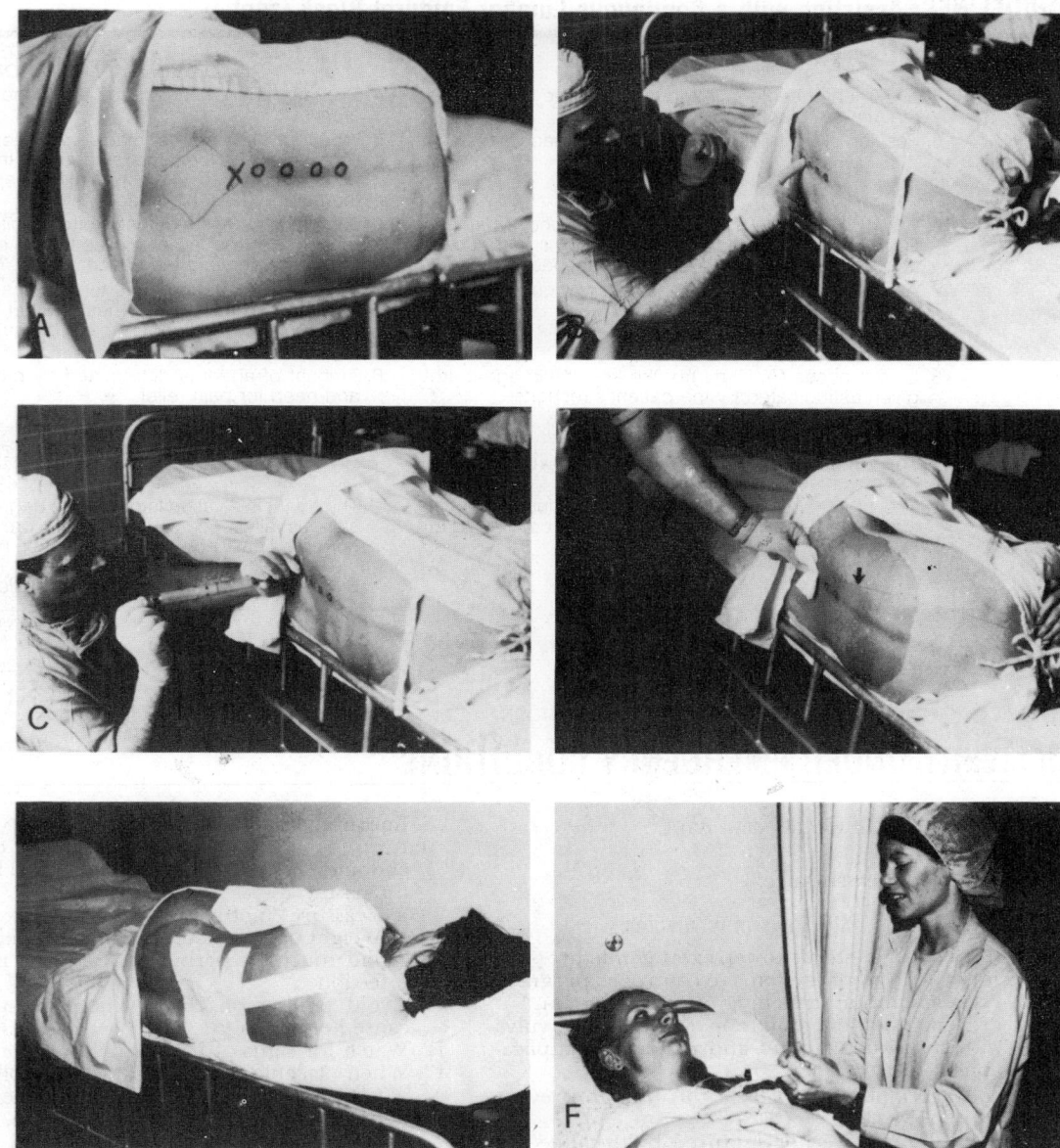

FIGURE 30-17. *Epidural block. A. The X marks the L_{4-5} interspace where epidural needle is to be inserted. B. The anesthesiologist is pointing to the needle puncture site. C. He uses the loss of resistance test to identify the epidural space. D. The epidural catheter has been threaded into the needle and is in position (arrow). The needle is removed and the catheter is folded over a sponge to prevent kinking. E. The catheter is taped in place so it will not become dislodged. F. The delivery room nurse is giving a maintenance dose. (Photographs, courtesy of John O'Connor, M.D.)*

Procedure (cont.)

NURSING ACTION	RATIONALE/AMPLIFICATION
***Performance Phase** (by the anesthesiologist)*	
1. Put on surgical gloves and open inner sterile covering. (Assistant fills the medicine glasses with anesthetic agent and antiseptic solution for skin preparation.)	1. Aseptic technique is required since needle is injected through the skin into the epidural space.
2. Skin is cleansed with solution and area draped as for a spinal puncture (see p. 704).	
3. Skin, interspinous ligament, and the ligamentum flavum are infiltrated with the same anesthetic solution used for the continuous block.	

GUIDELINES: Assisting with a Continuous Lumbar Epidural Block (cont.)

Procedure (cont.)

NURSING ACTION	RATIONALE/AMPLIFICATION
4. The Touhy needle is introduced into the 3rd, 4th, or 5th lumbar interspace.	4. The largest epidural spaces are found in the lumbar area.
5. Position of the needle in the epidural space is tested.	5. When an attempt is made to inject air into the ligamentum flavum, the plunger of the syringe rebounds; when air is injected into the epidural space, the plunger falls into space.
6. When the needle is properly placed and no spinal fluid is aspirated, the plastic catheter is introduced through the needle into the epidural space.	6. The passage of the catheter often elicits a neurologic response in the leg or hip as the tip of the catheter touches a nerve in the space.
7. A test dose of 5–8 ml. of anesthetic agent is given.	7. If catheter has been inadvertently placed in subarachnoid space, spinal anesthesia rather than epidural will result. The patient will have difficulty moving her legs.
8. Larger doses (8–12 ml.) of the anesthetic agent are given as indicated by the patient's response.	8. Amount of agent is determined by process of labor and need for pain relief.

Follow-up Phase

NURSING ACTION	RATIONALE/AMPLIFICATION
1. The catheter is held in place by adhesive tape, and the patient is turned on her back.	
2. The blood pressure is monitored continuously until stabilized. Systolic pressure should not be allowed to fall below 100 mm.Hg.	2. The agent is a vasodilator—some degree of hypotension usually occurs. The fall of pressure can be corrected easily by turning patient on her side so that the gravid uterus falls away from large vessels. Elevation of legs will also aid circulation.

DELIVERY UNDER EMERGENCY CONDITIONS

Immediate Needs of Mother and Baby

1. Baby must breathe.
2. Mother needs reassurance.

Essentials of Care until Physician Arrives

1. Using a clean or sterile towel, exert gentle pressure against the head of the fetus to control its progress.
   a. Prevents undue stretching of the perineum.
   b. Prevents sudden expulsion through the vulva with subsequent infant and maternal complications.
2. Encourage mother to pant at this time to prevent bearing down.
3. If membranes have not ruptured by the time the head is delivered, they must be removed immediately by tearing them at the nape of the infant's neck.
4. Holding the baby's head in both hands, gently exert downward pressure toward the floor, thereby slipping the anterior shoulder under the symphysis pubis (Fig. 30-18B).
5. If the cord is looped around the baby's neck, gently slip it over the head. If the cord is too tight to permit this, it must be clamped in 2 places and cut between the clamps before the rest of the body is delivered.
6. Support the infant's body and head as it is born.
7. Pick baby up gently by feet, with head down to prevent aspiration of fluid. Drainage of mucus is stimulated when the infant cries; gentle rubbing of the back may stimulate breathing.
8. Encourage mother.
9. After baby cries, place him gently on mother's abdomen where she can see him. This serves 2 purposes:
   a. Reassures mother.
   b. Weight over the uterus will help uterus contract.
10. Avoid touching perineal area so as not to cause infection.
11. Avoid pulling on cord, which might break and cause hemorrhage.
12. Watch for signs of placental separation.
13. When placenta is delivered, do the following:
   a. Clamp cord with surgical clamp when cord stops pulsating. If clamp is not available, tie off cord with any suitable material several centimeters from the infant's abdomen.
   b. Do not cut cord; the physician will cut it later under more stable conditions.
   c. Wrap the baby and placenta in a blanket.
14. Check fundal contractions; massage if indicated. *Putting the baby to breast may help the uterus to contract.*
15. Give mother fluids.
16. Encourage mother to move; if she is not in bed or in a place where she can lie down, she may move to a more suitable environment.
17. Do not leave mother alone until help arrives. Mother should never be alone during the first hour and a half after delivery.
18. Instruct mother so that she may care for herself and her newborn.
19. Explain why cord has not been cut.
20. Keep accurate record of delivery.

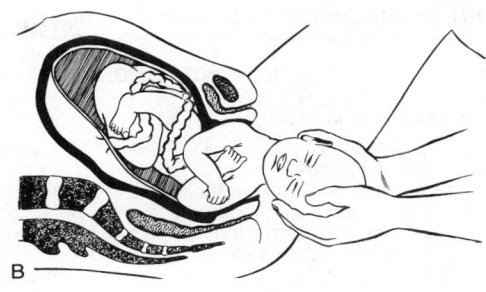

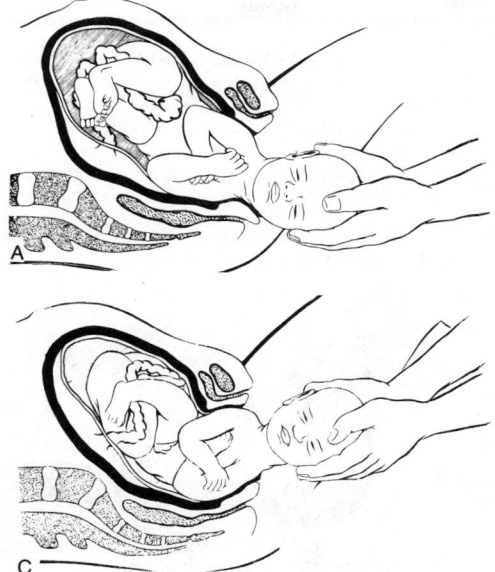

FIGURE 30-18. *Emergency delivery by the nurse. A. Controlling the head during delivery. B. Delivering the upper shoulder. C. Delivering lower shoulder while maintaining support of the head. (From Emergency Birth in Disaster. US Army Film and Equipment Exchange.)*

IMMEDIATE CARE OF THE NEWBORN INFANT

GUIDELINES: Immediate Care of the Newborn Infant

Purpose   To support the infant in adjusting to extrauterine life.

Equipment
Radiant warmer, oxygen, and vacuum suction with sterile catheter
Oxygen analyzer
Oxygen masks of 3 different sizes
Warm receiving blankets
Laryngoscope with premature blade
Oropharyngeal airways

Endotracheal tubes of 3 different sizes with stylets
ECG electrodes and heart rate monitor
Sterile pack containing equipment for umbilical vessel catheterization

Procedure

NURSING ACTION	RATIONALE/AMPLIFICATION
1. Immediately after delivery, blot infant dry while placing in radiant warmer.	1. Minimizes heat loss by evaporation; acidosis and hypoxia, if present, are increased by cold stress.
2. Place infant in modified Trendelenberg position.	2. Gravity aids in drainage of mucus and fluid from the naso-oral cavity.
3. Aspirate mucus from mouth and pharynx with suction catheter; low vacuum and gentle manipulation required.	3. Insure patent airway. Stimuli may produce laryngeal spasm or cause pharyngeal edema.
4. Evaluate infant's condition by the Apgar scoring system; observe at 1 and 5 minutes after birth.	4. Reflects infant's condition and, if present, degree of asphyxia.

APGAR SCORING CHART

Sign	0	1	2
Heart rate	absent	slow (less than 100)	over 100
Respiratory effort	absent	slow, irregular	good, crying
Muscle tone	flaccid	some flexion of extremities	active motion
Reflex irritability	no response	cry	vigorous cry
Color	blue, pale	body pink, extremities blue	completely pink

GUIDELINES: Immediate Care of the Newborn Infant (cont.)

Procedure (cont.)

NURSING ACTION	RATIONALE/AMPLIFICATION

Interpretation of Apgar Scoring:

1. Apgar score of 7–10 indicates infant's condition is good.
2. Score of 4–6 means the infant is in fair condition—baby may have moderate central nervous system depression, some muscle flaccidity, cyanosis, and poor respiratory effort.
3. Score of 0–3 indicates infant is in extremely poor condition.
   a. Insert endotracheal tube and begin ventilation with 60% oxygen.*

1. No special procedures necessary.
2. Air passages must be cleared and oxygen given.
3. Resuscitation required immediately.

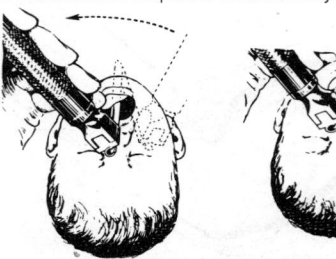

   b. Apply electrocardiographic electrodes and monitor heart rate. If there is no electrical activity or no audible heart beat, begin cardiac massage.
   c. Catheterize the umbilical artery and draw a sample of blood for determination of pH, oxygen and carbon dioxide tensions.
   d. Begin a slow infusion of sodium bicarbonate (given only when acidosis is very severe and ventilation is being assisted).
   e. Epinephrine may also be given by slow infusion through the umbilical catheter and is followed by glucose solution.
   f. After initial resuscitation, maintenance electrolytes are added to parenteral fluids.
   g. Transfer infant to intensive care nursery.

   b. Irreversible brain damage and cell death will occur unless circulation is restored.
   c. Other blood tests may be prescribed.
   d. To correct the metabolic acidosis.
   e. To increase the force and rate of heartbeat.
   f. Hypocalcemia and hypokalemia are common after successful resuscitation of infant with neonatal asphyxia.
   g. For continued observation and monitoring.

Basic Data
Collect data for initial assessment.

1. Weigh and measure infant.
2. Inspect oral cavity.
3. Pass a catheter through esophagus down to stomach.
4. Aspirate gastric contents.

5. If no meconium has been passed, a soft catheter may be inserted into the rectum.
6. Count the number of vessels in the umbilical cord.

Procedures are done only after infant has established respiration.
1. To establish gestational age.
2. To rule out cleft palate.
3. To rule out esophageal atresia.
4. To reduce the amount of fluid that may later be regurgitated and possibly aspirated (15–20 ml. of fluid aspirated may indicate intestinal obstruction).
5. To rule out anal atresia.
6. Any abnormal finding may indicate congenital anomalies.

Prophylactic Measures
1. Instill silver nitrate 1% in the conjunctival sac according to drug manufacturer's package insert directions. Subsequent irrigation is not necessary.

2. Administer Vitamin K.

1. Prophylactic treatment against ophthalmia neonatorum (gonorrheal conjunctivitis); mandatory in all states. The infant of a mother with known gonococcal disease should receive intramuscular penicillin.
2. To prevent hemorrhagic tendencies since liver's ability to produce clotting factors is dependent on Vitamin K.

Identification
Provide identification of the infant.
1. Apply I.D. band or bracelet to infant's arm; include mother's name, hospital number, infant's sex, and time and date of birth.

1. Affords assurance to mother.

* (Figures from Silverman WA. Dunham's Premature Infants, p. 97. New York, Harper & Row)

Procedure (cont.)	NURSING ACTION	RATIONALE/AMPLIFICATION
	2. Apply bracelet with same information to mother's wrist.	2. Legal requirement. Bracelets of mother and infant are compared each time infant is brought from nursery to mother.
	3. If hospital policy indicates, take prints of infant's foot, palms, and fingers and mother's palms and fingers.	
	Mother-Infant Bonding	
	If condition of mother and infant is satisfactory, assist mother to hold infant.	Helps promote a positive mother-child relationship and allays mother's anxiety.
	Transfer to Nursery	
	1. Transfer infant to nursery in warm blankets or in a heated covered bassinet.	1. Reduces heat loss.
	2. Provide nursery personnel with written record of birth information and check infant's identification.	2. Insures continuity of care.

BIBLIOGRAPHY

Books

Abouleish E. Pain Control in Obstetrics. Philadelphia, JB Lippincott, 1977

Dick–Read G. Childbirth Without Fear. New York, Harper & Row, 1972

Friedman EA. Labor: Clinical Evaluation and Management, 2nd ed. New York, Appleton–Century–Crofts, 1978

Kitzinger S and Davis JA. The Place of Birth. New York, Oxford University Press, 1978

Leboyer F. Birth Without Violence. New York, Alfred A Knopf, 1975

Lipkin GB. Parent–Child Nursing: Psychological Aspects, 2nd ed. St. Louis, CV Mosby, 1978

Malenowski JS et al. Nursing Care of the Labor Patient. Philadelphia, FA Davis, 1978

Moir DD. Anaesthesia and Analgesia. Baltimore, Williams & Wilkins, 1976

Oxorn H and Foote WR. Human Labor and Birth, 3rd ed. New York, Appleton–Century–Crofts, 1980

Phillips CR and Anzalone SJ. Fathering: Participation in Labor and Birth. St. Louis, CV Mosby, 1978

Serafetinides EA. Methods of Behavioral Research. New York, Grune & Stratton, 1979

Shnider SM and Levinson G. Anesthesia for Obstetrics. Baltimore, Williams & Wilkins, 1979

Articles

Adamson GD and Gare DJ. Home or hospital births? JAMA 1980 May 2; 243(17)1732–1736

Anderson J. A clarification of the Lamaze method. JOGN Nurs 1977 Mar/Apr; 6(2):53–58

Angelini DJ. Nonverbal communication in labor. Am J Nurs 1978 July; 78(7):1220–1222

Barton JJ et al. Alternative birthing center: Experience in a leading obstetric service. Am J Obstet Gynecol 1980 June; 137(3):377–384

Boyd ST and Mahan P. Family centered cesarean delivery. Am J Mat Child Nurs 1980 May/June; 5(3):176–180

D'Affonso D and Stichler J. Cesarean birth: Women's reaction. Am J Nurs 1980 Mar; 80(3):468–470

Foxel AM. The birthing room concept at Phoenix Memorial Hospital. Part I. JOGN Nurs 1980 May/June; 9(3)151–154

Gimbel J and Nocon J. The physiological basis for the Leboyer approach to childbirth. JOGN Nurs 1977 Jan/Feb; 6(1):11–15

Hedahl K. Cesarean birth: A real family affair. Am J Nurs 1980 Mar; 80(3):471–472

Johnson JM. Teaching self-hypnosis in pregnancy, labor and delivery. Am J Mat Child Nurs 1980 Mar/Apr; 5(2):98–101

Kassar N, Aldridge J, Quirk B. Rollover test. Obstet Gynecol 1980 Apr; 55(4):411–413

Kieffer M. The birthing room concept at Phoenix Memorial Hospital. Part II: Consumer satisfaction during one year. JOGN Nurs 1980 May/June; 9(3):154–159

L'Esperance CM. Home birth: A manifestation of aggression. JOGN Nurs 1979 July/Aug; 8(4):227–230

Lieber MT. "Nonstress" antepartal monitoring. Am J Mat Child Nurs 1980 Sept/Oct; 5(5):335–339

Lubeck RW and Ernst EKM. The child bearing center: An alternative to conventional care. Nurs Outlook 1978 Dec; 26(12):754–760

Maloni J. The birthing room: Some insights into parents' experience. Am J Mat Child Nurs 1980 Sept/Oct; 5(5):314–319

Mozingo JN. Pain in labor: A conceptual model for intervention. JOGN Nurs 1978 July/Aug; 7(4):47–49

Oliver C and Oliver G. Gentle birth: Its safety and its effect on neonatal behavior. JOGN Nurs 1978 Sept/Oct; 7(5):35–40

Stichler J and D'Affonso D. Cesarean birth. Am J Nurs 1980 Mar; 80(3):466–468

OBSTETRICAL AND NURSING SUPPORT OF THE MOTHER AND NEWBORN DURING THE POSTPARTAL PERIOD

31

PHYSIOLOGY OF THE PUERPERIUM

Physiologic Changes

A. *Involution of the Uterus*

Rapid shrinking or contraction of the uterus to its nonpregnant shape.
1. Process requires 5–6 weeks. Rate of decrease in size of fundus is about 1.2 cm. (½ inch) a day.
2. Affected by muscle contraction and autolytic processes.
3. Outer layer of the decidua is cast off along with blood, mucus, and cellular debris from placental site (lochia rubra, lochia serosa, and lochia alba).
4. Process includes regeneration of endometrial lining.

B. *The Pelvis*—vaginal walls and vulval ligaments undergo process of involution.

C. *Abdominal Wall*—involution requires at least 6 weeks; muscle tone restored by rest, diet, exercises, good body mechanics, and good posture.

D. *The Breasts*

1. Colostrum secreted by 2nd postpartal day; nutritive value low in comparison to breast milk. Both contain defense factors that promote normal bacterial colonization of the gastrointestinal tract and suppress certain pathogenic microorganisms.
2. Breast milk secreted by 3rd or 4th postpartal day.
3. Primary engorgement may occur because of increased amounts of milk and because circulation of blood and lymph increases, producing tension in surrounding tissues.

Psychologic Changes

A. *Phases of the Restorative Period*

1. *"Taking-in" Phase*
   a. Mother is passive and dependent.
   b. Sleep and food are primary needs.
2. *"Taking-hold" Phase*
   In this phase the mother acts as follows:
   a. Begins to initiate action
   b. Moves toward independence
   c. Requires explanations and reassurance that she is performing well
   d. Requires assistance in setting realistic goals; anxiety may lead to fatigue and exhaustion

B. *Postpartal "Blues"*

1. A temporary depression due to any or all of the following:
   a. Hormonal change
   b. Ego regression caused by increased dependency needs and responsibilities
   c. Discomfort and fatigue
2. If condition persists, postpartum psychosis may develop and may require psychiatric treatment.

POSTPARTUM CARE

Immediate Postpartum Care

The first hour after delivery of placenta ("fourth stage of labor") is a critical period; postpartum hemorrhage is most likely to occur at this time.
1. Check fundus frequently and massage gently if not firm.
2. Inspect perineum frequently for visible signs of bleeding.
3. Evaluate vital signs at frequent intervals as determined by mother's condition.
4. Avoid leaving mother alone at this time since changes in condition can occur precipitously.

Subsequent Postpartum Care

A. *For Postpartum Bleeding*
1. Check firmness of the fundus at regular intervals.
2. Inspect the perineum regularly for frank bleeding.
   a. Note color, amount, and odor of the lochia (perineal discharge).
   b. Count the number of perineal pads that are saturated in each 8-hour period.
3. Assess vital signs at least once daily and more frequently if indicated.

B. *For Comfort and Healing*
1. Provide perineal care.

a. Pour warm water gently over the perineum while cleansing the labia, always from front to back.
b. Avoid separating the labia for this procedure (to prevent infection).
c. Wash the anal region separately.

2. Sitz baths are frequently used to promote perineal hygiene.
3. Teach the mother to handle the perineal pad from the outside so that the fingers do not come in contact with the side that will touch the perineum.
4. Provide perineal heat lamp (20 minutes, 2–3 times a day) to promote healing.
5. Use anesthetic sprays or ointment to alleviate perineal discomfort.
6. Some patients feel that foam rubber rings offer some relief.

C. Ambulation

1. Normally patients are out of bed within the first 24 hours after childbirth.
2. The mother should be assisted in her first effort out of bed to prevent accidents caused by weakness.

D. Diet

1. After the first postpartum hour, the mother may eat or drink as desired provided she is not nauseated.
2. The diet of a lactating mother should contain somewhat increased amounts of protein, calories and fluids.

E. Voiding

1. The patient should be encouraged to void within 8 hours after delivery.
2. Catheterize the patient if she is unable to void and the bladder is distended.
3. Evaluate urinary output.

F. Breast Care

1. Observe nipples for fissures daily.
2. Wash nipples at least once a day to remove dried and seeping colostrum.
3. Give the following care to nursing mothers.

a. Cleanse nipples with warm water before each feeding; soap may be drying to the nipples.
b. Lotion or ointment may help to prevent cracks or drying and may be applied after the baby's feedings.

4. Treat breast engorgement as follows:
a. A well-fitting supportive brassiere or breast binder should be worn night and day.
b. Hot packs 15–20 minutes before nursing may be helpful
c. For removal of milk
(1) Oxytocin encourages the "let down" reflex.
(2) Express milk manually or with breast pump.

G. Suppression of Lactation

1. Administer hormones as prescribed; estrogen, progesterone, or testosterone may be administered alone or in combination. (A single IM injection may be given.)
2. Apply ice bags to breasts.
3. Offer mild analgesic agent as needed.
4. Advise the patient to wear a supporting brassiere.
5. Avoid pumping the breasts.

H. Menstruation

1. For non-nursing mothers, menstrual flow usually returns within 6–8 weeks.
2. For nursing mothers, menstruation does not usually recur until after the child is weaned from the breast.

I. Follow-up Examination

A routine examination is usual within 3–6 weeks postpartum.

1. General physical condition is evaluated.
2. Vital signs are checked.
3. Urine is examined for sugar and protein.
4. Muscle tone is checked, particularly that of the abdominal wall.
5. Pelvic examination is conducted.
6. Counseling and information regarding birth control methods are provided as indicated or requested.

GUIDELINES: Teaching the Mother Breast Feeding Procedure

Procedure TEACHING POINTS	RATIONALE/AMPLIFICATION
1. Wash hands before breast feeding.	1. Protects infant and breast from infection.
2. Prepare to nurse shortly after birth and at least every 4 hours.	2. Regular feeding (every 4 hours) establishes nursing pattern.
3. Nurse infant at night feeding.	3. Prevents engorgement and helps bring in milk supply quickly.
Position of the Mother	
1. Lie on left side with pillow under head. Position left arm above head—or	1. The mother should be relaxed and comfortable.
2. Use a chair with a back support. Place pillow on lap to hold infant.	2. The infant's head should be higher than his abdomen to prevent regurgitation.
Nursing Technique	
1. With the right hand, press darkened area around nipple into infant's mouth.	1. This maneuver is necessary for adequate suction.
2. If breast is full and firm, use 1 finger to press breast away from infant's nose.	2. Prevents obstruction of airway; infant breathes mainly through his nose.
3. Use both breasts at each feeding; 5 minutes on each breast, then increase nursing time to 10 minutes.	
4. At each feeding, alternate the breast that is used first. Pin a safety pin to the bra as a reminder of which breast to start with at the next feeding.	4. The infant will empty the first breast; nursing at the second breast will increase milk production.

GUIDELINES: Teaching the Mother Breast Feeding Procedure (cont.)

Procedure (cont.)	NURSING ACTION	RATIONALE/AMPLIFICATION
	5. Break the suction by putting a finger into the corner of infant's mouth.	5. Pulling the nipple abruptly away from the infant will result in sore nipples.
	6. "Burp" infant midway through the feeding. Pat gently on the back or hold in upright position.	6. Helps infant to release air bubbles in stomach.
	7. Uterine cramps may occur.	7. Nursing stimulates release of oxytocin hormone, causing uterine contractions.
	Other Considerations for Mother	
	1. Drink water for two. Continue to eat a balanced, nutritious diet. (Nursing mother may require 1000 more calories and an additional 8–10 gm. of protein daily.)	1. Necessary for adequate milk production.
	2. Get adequate rest.	
	3. Avoid emotional stress and do not become discouraged.	3. It takes time to establish a good nursing routine.
	4. Avoid taking medications and drugs unless approved by the physician.	4. Cold or allergy medication will limit fluid output. Birth control medication may suppress milk production.

PHYSIOLOGY OF THE NEWBORN

Transitional Stages

The first 24 hours of life constitute a highly vulnerable time during which the infant must make several adjustments to extrauterine life. During this period of transition, 6 overlapping stages have been identified:

Stage 1. Receives stimulation (during labor) from the pressure of the uterine contractions and from changes in pressure when the membranes rupture.

Stage 2. Encounters a variety of foreign stimuli—light, cold, gravity, and sound.

Stage 3. Initiates breathing.

Stage 4. Changes from fetal to neonatal circulation.

Stage 5. Undergoes alteration in metabolic processes with activation of liver, renal and gastrointestinal tracts for passage of meconium.

Stage 6. Achieves a steady level or equilibrium in metabolic processes (production of enzymes, increased blood oxygen saturation, decrease in acidosis associated with birth, and recovery of the neurologic tissues from the trauma of labor and delivery).

Respiratory Changes

A. *Initiation of Respiration*

A combination of physical, sensory, and chemical factors.

1. *Physical*—sudden change from intrauterine life produces stimulation needed to initiate respiration.
2. *Chemical*—changes in the blood as a result of transitory asphyxia include the following:
   a. Lowered oxygen level
   b. Increased carbon dioxide level
   c. Lowered pH—if asphyxia is prolonged, depression of the respiratory center (rather than stimulation) occurs, and resuscitation is necessary
3. *Sensory*—maximum effort is required to expand the lung and fill the collapsed alveoli.
   a. Surface tension in the respiratory tract, resistance in the lung tissue, the thorax, the diaphragm, and the respiratory muscles must be overcome.
   b. First active inspiration comes from a strong contraction of the diaphragm, which creates a high negative intrathoracic pressure causing a marked retraction of the ribs and distention of the alveolar space. (Any remaining fluid is reabsorbed rapidly if the pulmonary capillary blood flow is adequate, since the fluid is hypotonic and passes easily into the capillaries.)

B. *Character of Normal Respirations*

1. The infant begins life with intense activity; diffuse, purposeless movements alternate with periods of relative immobility.
2. Respirations are rapid, as high as 80 breaths per minute, accompanied by tachycardia, 140–180 beats per minute.
3. Relaxation occurs and the infant usually sleeps; he then awakes to a second period of activity. Oral mucus may be a major problem during this period.
4. Respirations are reduced to 35–50 breaths per minute and become quiet and shallow; respiration is carried out by the diaphragm and abdominal muscles.
5. Period of dyspnea and cyanosis may occur suddenly in an infant who is breathing normally and may indicate an anomaly or a pathologic condition.

Circulatory Changes

A. *Anatomic Changes* (see Chapter 29)

B. *Blood Volume*

85–100 ml./kg. at birth

Factors that influence blood volume:

1. Maternal blood volume (affected by maternal diseases and iron intake)
2. Placental function
3. Uterine contractions during labor
4. Amount of blood loss associated with delivery
5. Placental transfusion at birth—increase in blood volume of 60% if cord is clamped and cut after pulsation ceases.

C. *Peripheral Circulation*

Residual cyanosis in hands and feet for 1–2 hours after birth due to sluggish circulation.

D. *Pulse Rate*

1. Generally follows pattern similar to that of respiration.
2. Apical pulse rate is more accurate.
3. Normal rate 120–150 beats per minute.
4. May rise to 180 when baby is crying or drop to 70 during sleep.

E. *Blood Pressure*

70/45 at birth; 100/50 by 10th day

F. *Blood Coagulation*

Coagulability is temporarily diminished owing to absence of bacteria in the intestinal tract that contribute to the synthesis of Vitamin K.

1. Coagulation time 3–4 minutes.
2. Bleeding time 2–4 minutes.
3. Prothrombin 50% decreasing to 20–30%.

G. *Blood Elements*

Values for blood components in the neonate
1. Hemoglobin 16–22 gm.
2. Reticulocytes 2.5–6.5%.
3. Leukocytes 15,000–20,000 cu. mm.
(See Appendix III, p. 1493, for detailed pediatric hematology table.)

Temperature Regulation

1. Mechanism not fully developed; heat production low.
2. Infant responds readily to environmental heat and cold stimuli.
3. Heat loss of 2 to 3 degrees C. at birth by evaporation, convection, conduction, and radiation.
4. The infant develops mechanisms to counterbalance heat loss.
   a. Vasoconstriction—blood directed away from skin surfaces.
   b. Insulation—from subcutaneous adipose tissue.
   c. Heat production—by nonshivering thermogenesis elicited by the sympathetic nervous system's response to decreased temperatures; activated by adrenalin.

Basal Metabolism

1. Surface area of infant is large in comparison with weight.
2. Basal metabolism per kg. of body weight is higher than that of adult.
3. Calorie requirements are high—117 calories per kilogram of body weight per day.

Renal Function

Low arterial blood pressure and increased renal vascular resistance lead to the following effects:
1. Decreased ability to concentrate urine because of low tubular reabsorption rate and low levels of antidiuretic hormone.
2. Limited ability to maintain water balance by excretion of excess water or retention of needed water.
3. Decreased ability to maintain acid-base mechanism; slower excretion of electrolytes, especially sodium and the hydrogen ions, results in accumulation of these substances, which predisposes the infant to dehydration, acidosis, and hyperkalemia.
4. Excretion of large amount of uric acid during newborn period—appears as "brick dust" stain on diaper.

Hepatic Function

Function limited because of lack of gastrointestinal tract activity and limited blood supply; consequences include the following:
1. Decreased ability to conjugate bilirubin (rationale for physiologic jaundice).
2. Decreased ability to regulate blood sugar concentration (rationale for neonatal hypoglycemia).
3. Deficient production of prothrombin and other coagulation factors that depend on Vitamin K for synthesis (rationale for neonate's predisposition to hemorrhage).

Endocrine Function

Endocrine glands are better organized than other systems; disturbances are most often related to maternally provided hormones, which can cause the following:
1. Vaginal discharge (and/or bleeding) in female infants.
2. Enlargement of mammary glands in both sexes—related to increased estrogen, luteal, and prolactin activity.
3. Disturbances related to maternal endocrine pathology—e.g., diabetic mother or mother with inadequate iodine intake.

Gastrointestinal Changes

The newborn's intestinal tract is proportionately longer than the adult's; however, elastic tissue and musculature are not fully developed, and nervous control is variable and inadequate.
   a. Most digestive enzymes are present with the exception of pancreatic amylase and lipase. Protein and carbohydrates are easily absorbed, but fat absorption is poor.
   b. Limitations relate primarily to anatomic structures and neutrality of the gastric contents.
   c. Imperfect control of the cardiac and pyloric sphincters and immaturity of nervous control cause mild regurgitation or slight vomiting.
   d. Irregularities in peristaltic motility slow stomach emptying.
   e. Peristalsis increases in the lower ileum, resulting in stool frequency—1–6 stools per day. Absence of stool within 48 hours after birth is indicative of intestinal obstruction.

Neurologic Changes

Neurologic mechanisms are immature; they are not fully developed anatomically or physiologically, and as a result, uncoordinated movements, labile temperature regulation, and poor control over musculature are characteristic of the infant. Reflexes are important indices of infant neural development. (See Chapter 34, pages 1086–1088, for a detailed discussion of the pediatric neurological examination. See also Chapter 35, Pediatric Concepts, Growth and Development [pp. 1093–1098], which describes reflexes of the newborn and traces appearance and disappearance of the various reflexes.)

GUIDELINES: Physical Appraisal of the Newborn

Purpose To collect data for the assessment of the newborn by observation and routine screening techniques so that any abnormalities or injuries may be identified early.

Procedure

NURSING ACTION	RATIONALE/AMPLIFICATION
1. Carry out 3-minute washing of hands and arms with an antiseptic detergent or soap before handling infant or equipment.	1. Major route of bacterial contamination of the newborn is by direct contact rather than by airborne route.
2. Take apical heart rate and rhythm with stethoscope.	2. Provides baseline norms. Rate at birth ranges from 100–180; within 30 minutes it is usually 120–140. May be rapid but should be regular in rhythm.
3. Take blood pressure by arteriosound transducer or Doppler ultrasonic flow detector.	3. Hypotension is most frequent blood pressure abnormality found in newborn; may not be present until 20% of the blood volume is lost.
4. Count respiration rate and observe characteristics of respiration bilaterally with stethoscope. Observe rise and fall of abdomen.	4. Fluctuations in rate and pattern are normal, 35–60 per minute. Infants breathe predominantly with the diaphragm.
5. Observe frequency and type of cry.	5. Crying, necessary for lung aeration in normal infant, is lusty and easily provoked. A feeble cry is most often due to general depression of the central nervous system. A shrill, high-pitched cry is a major sign of meningeal or brain stem irritation or kernicterus. A hoarse cry may be due to injury to the recurrent laryngeal nerve during delivery.
6. Observe position and movements.	6. The newborn usually lies with arms and legs flexed. When awake—yawns, sneezes, blinks, makes sucking motions with mouth, moves extremities purposelessly.
7. Observe skin color and character. Note signs of rash, jaundice, cyanosis, or pallor. Loss of turgor indicates dehydration.	7. Should be pink except for hands and feet, which may appear bluish because of slower peripheral circulation.
8. Obtain measurements. Weight: 2500 to 4300 g. (5½ to 9½ lbs). Length: 48–53 cm. (19–21 inches). Head circumference: 33–35 cm (13–14 inches). Chest circumference: 30–33 cm. (12–13 inches).	8. To identify any disproportionate growth.
9. Observe symmetry of body parts.	9. Lack of symmetry may indicate congenital defects or birth trauma.
10. Take initial body temperature rectally; take temperature by axilla thereafter.	10. To assure anal patency; not recommended routinely, since it may cause rectal mucosa irritation.
11. Examine extremities. a. Feel for tenderness in clavicular area. b. Check arms for Erb's palsy. c. Check for congenital hip.	11. a. To rule out fracture of clavicle. b. In this condition, the arm is held in adduction and external rotation, with forearm pronated. c. Hips should be in frog-position (flexed to 90° and abducted to 60° without resistance or a click), and skin folds on posterior upper leg should be symmetrical.
12. Inspect head. a. *Moulding*—overlapping of skull bones caused by compression (disappears in a few days). b. *Caput succedaneum*—swelling of the soft tissues of the scalp due to pressure (lasts a few days). c. *Cephalohematoma*—subperiosteal hemorrhage with collection of blood beneath the periosteum and the bone. d. Resolution of swelling confined to an individual bone may take up to 6 weeks. Anterior fontanelles usually closes in 18 weeks.	12. Variations in shape due to pressure during vaginal delivery.
13. Examine eyes. a. Check for scleral color. b. Observe for edema of the lids or purulent discharge.	13. Infant can see and discriminate patterns. Limited by imperfect oculomotor coordination and inability to accommodate for varying distances. a. Icterus seen first in the sclera. Small areas of subconjunctival hemorrhage will disappear spontaneously. b. Caused by silver nitrate. Subsides within 2-7 days.
14. Examine ears for position.	14. Top of ear should be at the same level as the eyes. Low-set ears may indicate chromosomal abnormalities or congenital renal disorder.

Procedure (cont.)

NURSING ACTION	RATIONALE/AMPLIFICATION
15. Inspect neck for position and movement.	15. Excessive folds and hyperextension may be associated with abnormalities.
16. Observe abdomen.	
a. Note contour.	a. Distention may indicate bowel obstruction, enlarged kidneys, weak abdominal muscles, and/or umbilical hernia.
b. Inspect umbilical stump.	b. Normally bluish-white. By 24 hours yellowish-brown, dull, and dry; then blackish-brown.
c. Listen for bowel sounds with stethoscope.	c. To identify peristalsis.
d. Palpate abdomen. Feel for edge of liver, tip of spleen, position of kidney.	d. To identify any structural defect or abnormal masses or lumps.
e. Peripheral circulation.	e. Feel for pulsation of femoral arteries.
f. Observe bladder area.	f. Rule out abnormal distention.
17. Examine genitalia and rectum.	17. Observe males for phimosis, undescended testicles or hypospadias. Female structures may be edematous due to maternal hormones.
18. Observe basic automatic reflexes. See Chapter 34, pp. 1086–1088, for oral, grasping, traction, Moro-tonic neck and extremity responses.	

GUIDELINES: Nursing Care of the Newborn

Purposes

1. To continue appraisal of the newborn by observing and recording vital signs, daily weight loss or gain, bowel and bladder function, activity or sleep.
2. To provide safeguards against infection.
3. To initiate feeding.
4. To provide health counseling to the parents

Procedure

NURSING ACTION	RATIONALE/AMPLIFICATION
General Considerations	
1. Carry out hospital policy for gowning and 3-minute scrub.	1. Utilize basic principles of nursing care.
2. Never leave infant alone.	2. Ensure safety factors.
3. Prevent undue exposure; provide warm environment (24°–27°C. or 75°–80°F.) and bath water (37°–38°C. or 98°–100°F.).	3. Prevent cold stress. Neonates have little adipose tissue to protect them.
Weight, Temperature, and Blood Pressure	
1. Weigh infant and record weight.	1. Infant may lose 5–10% of birth weight because of minimal intake of nutrients and fluid and loss of excess fluid.
2. Take axillary temperature by placing thermometer in axilla and pressing infant's arm gently but firmly against it for 3 minutes.	2. Use of rectal thermometer predisposes to irritation of rectal mucosa.
3. Take blood pressure.	3. Hypotension may be present and require remedial action.
Bathing Technique	
1. Use cotton balls or soft disposable wash cloths to wipe eyes, face, and outer ear. Eyes are wiped from inside corner outward.	1. Start from cleanest areas to most soiled.
2. Use a neutral soap—check pH. Clear water may be used if infant's skin is dry.	2. Prevents irritation of skin. The use of hexachlorophene to prevent staphylococcal infection is controversial. Hexachlorophene may cause brain damage if a sufficient quantity is absorbed through the skin.
3. Wash infant's head, using gentle circular motions.	3. Prevents cradle cap from forming, especially over the frontal areas.
4. Hyperextend neck to cleanse.	4. Exposes neck folds for more thorough cleansing.
5. Bathe torso and extremities quickly.	5. Prevents unnecessary exposure and chilling.
6. Inspect umbilical cord. Check area for bleeding or foul odor. A drying agent such as 70% alcohol or merthiolate is applied several times daily. Dressings are not used.	6. Minimizes colonization by bacteria.
7. Cleanse genital area of male infants.	
a. Retract foreskin gently for cleaning, and replace quickly.	a. Replacing foreskin quickly prevents edema.
b. Circumcision care—keep area clean. Place sterile petrolatum gauze over area for first 24 hours; change after voiding. Observe hourly for bleeding. Position infant and diaper to avoid friction.	b. Prevents infection and promotes healing. Bleeding can be controlled by pressure or by application of adrenalin solution. Prevents discomfort.

GUIDELINES: Nursing Care of the Newborn (cont.)

Procedure (cont.)

NURSING ACTION	RATIONALE/AMPLIFICATION
8. Cleanse genital area of female infants.	a. Vaginal discharge and smegma must be removed.
a. Gently separate folds of the labia and remove secretions.	b. Front-to-back cleansing prevents contamination of vagina.
b. Wipe vaginal area with cotton ball, using 1 stroke in a front-to-back direction.	
9. Bathe buttocks, using a gentle patting motion. Keep area clean and dry.	9. Area is susceptible to skin breakdown due to acid reaction of urine and feces.
10. Prevent diaper rash. If rash does occur, protective ointment (zinc oxide or A & D) may be used. Exposure of buttocks to air or heat lamp is helpful.	

Stool Observation

NURSING ACTION	RATIONALE/AMPLIFICATION
1. Observe stool pattern. Meconium—first 2–3 days.	1. Material composed of epithelial and epidermal cells, lanugo and bile pigments.
2. Transitional stools—change from tarry-black to greenish-black, to greenish-brown to brownish-yellow to greenish-yellow.	2. Changes reflect intake of milk—stools are composed of both meconium and milk stools.
3. Number, color, and consistency are recorded daily.	3. For early identification of abnormalities.
	a. No stool within 48 hours indicates an intestinal obstruction.
	b. Passage of meconium only (without other stool) suggests obstruction in the ileum.
	c. Thick, putty-like meconium may indicate cystic fibrosis.
	d. Diarrhea may be caused by overfeeding or by gastroenteritis.
	e. Blood in the stool is an indication of intestinal bleeding.

Nutritional Considerations

NURSING ACTION	RATIONALE/AMPLIFICATION
1. Provide for nutritional intake.	1. Infants vary in their readiness to feed.
2. Promote feeding method of choice. (See page 1031 for Guidelines for breast feeding.)	
3. Test urine glucose utilizing reagent strip test and blood glucose using enzymatic strip test.	3. Infant may be hypoglycemic and require feeding sooner than usual 4–6 hour wait.
4. First feeding is sterile water. If retained, formula is given at next feeding.	4. Glucose water, if aspirated, is dangerous to lung tissue. Most hospitals use prepared milk mixture in disposable containers. Various formulas are available.
5. Instruct parent in technique of bottle feeding.	5.
a. Hold baby in semi-upright position.	a. Gravity assists flow of milk into stomach.
b. Position bottle so that neck of bottle is filled.	b. Prevents the baby from swallowing air.
c. Insert nipple into baby's mouth so that baby's tongue is under nipple.	c. Sucking and swallowing reflexes are used in feeding.
d. Burp during feeding by holding infant upright.	d. Allows air to escape from stomach, preventing distention or milk regurgitation.
6. PKU testing. Usually done on 3rd day before discharge from hospital.	6. Most states require by law routine testing of newborn infants for phenylketonuria (abnormal amino acid metabolism). For test to be accurate, infant must be receiving formula or breast milk in order to provide a supply of phenylalanine-containing protein.

Discharge Planning

NURSING ACTION	RATIONALE/AMPLIFICATION
1. Preparation for home care. Instruction is given concerning infant bathing and care, preparation of formula, and infant feeding. Written formula with instructions for preparation is provided to parents.	1. Instruction for infant care is a combined responsibility of the medical and nursing staffs.
2. Provide ample opportunity for parent contact.	2. Early attachment results in improved parent-child relationships.

BIBLIOGRAPHY

Books

Roberts FB. Perinatal Nursing. New York, McGraw–Hill, 1977

Smith AN. Physical examination of the newborn. In Clausen JP et al (eds): Maternity Today, 2nd ed. New York, McGraw–Hill, 1977

Smith C and Nelson N. The Physiology of the Newborn Infant, 4th ed. Springfield, Charles C Thomas, 1979

Stave U (ed). Perinatal Physiology. New York, Plenum Medical Books, 1978

Articles

Binzley V. Overlooked factor in newborn nursing. Am J Nurs 1977 Jan; 77(1):102–103

Brown MS and Hurlock JT. Mothering the mother. Am J Nurs 1977 Mar:77(3):439–441

Dingle R et al. Continuous transcutaneous O_2 monitoring in the neonate. Am J Nurs 1980 May: 80(5):890–893

Erikson MP. Trends in assessing the newborn and his parents. Am J Mat Child Nurs 1978 Mar/Apr; 3(2):99–103

Grams KE. Breast feeding: A means of imparting immunity. Am J Mat Child Nurs 1978 Nov/Dec; 3(6):340–344

Gruis M. Beyond maternity: Postpartum concerns of mothers. Am J Mat Child Nurs 1977 May/June; 2(3):182–188

Hall JM. Influencing breast feeding success. JOGN Nurs 1978 Nov/Dec; 7(6):28–32

Jones D. Home early after delivery. Am J Nurs 1978 Aug; 78(8):1378–1380

Kyndely K. The sexuality of women in pregnancy and postpartum: A review. JOGN Nurs 1978 Jan/Feb; 7(1):28–31

Lum B, Batzel RL, Barnett E. Reappraising newborn eye care. Am J Nurs 1980 Sept; 80(9):1602–1603

Nicholas MG. Effective help for the nursing mother. JOGN Nurs 1978 Mar/Apr; 7(2):22–30

Rosen E and Dupuis H. Comparison of temperatures of neonates born vaginally and by cesarean section. Am J Nurs 1978 Oct; 78(10):1693

Schroeder MA. Is the immediate postpartum period crucial to the mother–child relationship? JOGN Nurs 1977 May/June; 6(3):37–40

Smith D and Smith HL. Toward improvement in parenting. JOGN Nurs 1978 Nov/Dec; 7(6):22–27

Stokan RE. The right formula for the right infant. Am J Mat Child Nurs 1977 Mar/Apr; 2(2):101–103

Stranik MK et al. Transition into parenthood. Am J Nurs 1979 Jan; 79(1):90–93

Swanson J. Nursing intervention to facilitate maternal–infant attachment. JOGN Nurs 1978 Mar/Apr; 7(2):35–38

Whitley N. Preparation for breast feeding. JOGN Nurs 1978 May/June; 7(3):44–48

THE MATERNITY PATIENT WITH COMPLICATIONS

32

HYPERTENSIVE DISORDERS OF PREGNANCY

Hypertensive disorders are major complications of pregnancy responsible for significant mortality and morbidity of the fetus, newborn infant, and mother, but largely preventable by early detection and appropriate management.

Types of Hypertensive Disorders

The American College of Obstetricians and Gynecologists has classified the hypertensive states of pregnancy as:

A. *Gestational edema*

The occurrence of a general and excessive accumulation of fluid in the tissues of greater than 1+ pitting edema after 12 hours' rest in bed, or of a weight gain of 5 lbs. (2½ kg.) or more in one week caused by pregnancy.

B. *Gestational proteinuria*

The presence of proteinuria during pregnancy, in the absence of hypertension, edema, renal infection, or known intrinsic renovascular cause.

C. *Gestational hypertension*

The development of hypertension during pregnancy or within the first 24 hours postpartum in a previously normotensive woman.

D. *Preeclampsia*

1. The development of hypertension with proteinuria, edema, or both caused by pregnancy or a recent pregnancy.
2. It occurs after the 20th week of gestation but may develop before this time in the presence of trophoblastic disease.
3. Preeclampsia is predominantly a disease of primigravidas.

E. *Eclampsia*

The occurrence of one or more convulsions, not attributable to other cerebral disorders such as epilepsy or cerebral hemorrhage, in a patient with preeclampsia.

F. *Superimposed preeclampsia or eclampsia*

1. The development of preeclampsia or eclampsia in a patient with chronic hypertensive, vascular, or renal disease.
2. When the hypertension antedates the pregnancy, as established by previous blood pressure recordings, the following criteria are used to establish the diagnosis.
   a. A rise in the systolic pressure of 30 mm. Hg
   b. A rise in the diastolic pressure of 15 mm. Hg
   c. The development of proteinuria, edema, or both

G. *Chronic hypertensive disease*

The presence of persistent hypertension, of whatever cause, before pregnancy or prior to the 20th week of gestation, or persistent hypertension beyond the 42nd day of the postpartum period.

Incidence

1. Hypertension occurs in 6 to 7% of all pregnancies in the United States.
2. Third among major complications responsible for maternal and fetal deaths.

Predisposing Factors

1. Age and gravida—higher incidence among younger primigravida and those with multiple gestation.
2. Diet—high carbohydrate, high salt, and low protein—influenced by socioeconomic status, racial and

1038

cultural patterns, geographic location, and psychologic state of patient.
3. Coexisting conditions—hypertensive vascular disease, chronic renal disease, diabetes mellitus, polyhydramnios, and hydatidiform mole.

Etiology

1. Unknown.
2. Current research suggests:
   a. Decreased uterine and placental blood flow—result of vascular spasm caused by hormonal influence.
   b. Overstimulated adrenal cortex due to hypertrophic anterior pituitary and placental function. This activity decreases upon reduction of the oxygen tension caused by uterine ischemia—observed when there is overdistention of the uterus (twins, hydramnios), increased tension on abdominal walls (primigravida) or constricted blood vessels (preexisting hypertension).

Clinical Manifestations

1. Weight gain—first indication, over 0.45 kg. (1 lb.) per week, as early as the 20th week.
2. Ankle edema, digital swelling, periorbital edema, then pretibial fluid collection.
3. Optic fundi—reveal segmental or generalized arteriolar spasms.
4. Hypertension—140/90 or increase of 30 mm. systolic or 15 mm. diastolic.
5. Proteinuria—may develop into oliguria.
6. Cerebral and neurological involvement—frontal headache, vertigo, tinnitus, visual disturbance, drowsiness, hyperreflexia, apprehension, excitability, nausea and vomiting.
7. Positive rollover test—a simple procedure carried out between the 28th and 32nd weeks in which the blood pressure is checked with the patient first on her side and then on her back. A test is positive when there is an increase of 20 mm. Hg in diastolic pressure. Ninety percent of patients with a positive rollover test develop pregnancy-induced hypertension.

NURSING ALERT: Feelings of thoracic pressure or epigastric pain due to liver pathology may herald onset of convulsions or coma.

8. Poor prognostic signs
   a. Increasing number of convulsions
   b. Prolonged interval between first convulsion and delivery
   c. Persistence of coma, high fever, pulse rate of 120 or over, cyanosis, and hemoglobinuria
9. Complications associated with severe forms of preeclampsia and eclampsia:
   a. Abruptio placentae
   b. Hypofibrinogenemia
   c. Hemolysis
   d. Necrosis of the liver
   e. Cerebral hemorrhage (most common cause of death)
   f. Pulmonary edema
   g. Ophthalmologic abnormalities
   h. Glomeruloendotheliosis (toxic lesions in the kidney)

Objectives of Management

A. *To provide frequent periods of observation and assessment during the antepartal period, and to attempt to prevent the development of severe preeclampsia or eclampsia.*

1. Emphasize the importance of bed rest, encouraging the side position which decreases blood pressure, increases uterine and renal blood flow, and may cause diuresis resulting in a decrease in proteinuria.
2. Evaluate blood pressure readings and report any sudden or persistent elevations; diastolic measurement is a significant indication of severity of condition.
3. Encourage adequate dietary and fluid intake:
   a. Sodium is not restricted except when pitting edema occurs or cardiac conditions coexist.
   b. Ample protein required for production of plasma protein that influences intra and extravascular fluids.
4. Weigh patient weekly:
   a. The most constant sign of preeclampsia is a sudden excessive weight gain due to accumulation of water in the tissues (usually appears before face and finger edema).
   b. Sudden gains of 2 lbs. (1 kg.) or more a week are viewed with suspicion.
5. Test urine weekly for proteinuria; urinary estriol determinations may be done to evaluate condition of the fetus.

B. *To provide medical management for further control of signs and symptoms.*

1. Barbiturates and analgesics—provide sedation by depressing the central nervous system; sodium phenobarbital is frequently prescribed; sodium amobarbital (Amytal) is fast-acting.
2. Antihypertensive agents—Hydralazine (Apresoline) provides both adrenalytic and sympatholytic action.

C. *To provide care and therapy for the patient with severe preeclampsia or eclampsia so as to prevent maternal and fetal pathology.*

1. Provide hospitalization and therapy to prevent seizures by decreasing blood pressure, establishing adequate renal function, and continuing the pregnancy until the fetus is viable.
2. Provide strict bed rest.
3. Promote rest with sedatives; narcotics must be used with caution since they may cause marked depression of fetus.
4. Hypotensive drugs
   a. Magnesium sulfate (administered intramuscularly in 50% solution with 1% procaine; injection painful and may cause abscess formation. Continuous IV infusion may be preferred; depresses myoneural junction, increases hyperreflexia, and increases vasodilatation.

NURSING ALERT: Repeat doses of magnesium sulfate only if (1) deep tendon reflexes are present, (2) respirations are above 12 per minute and (3) urine output is at least 100 ml. per 6 hours. Calcium gluconate 10% IV must be available to counteract magnesium toxicity.

b. Hydralazine (Apresoline)
c. Cryptenamine tannates (Unitensen), a slower acting agent. (Ephedrine or atropine should be on hand for IV administration to counteract severe hypotension.)
d. Diazoxide (Hyperstat).
5. Anticonvulsants—phenytoin (Dilantin) or diazepam (Valium).
6. Digitalis—indicated by signs and symptoms of cardiac failure.
7. Broad spectrum antibiotics—prophylactic measure to prevent pneumonitis.
8. IV fluids—type of solution and flow rate based on urinary output, oral intake, and laboratory findings.
9. Indwelling catheter—ascertain exact renal output for comparison with fluid intake.
10. Oxygen—administered by nasal catheter or mask (6 liters per minute) to increase oxygen supply to compromised fetus.
11. Regional anesthesia (epidural) may be utilized if medical management fails to control hypertension.

Nursing Management

1. Provide quiet, restful environment; prevent any stimuli that could provoke seizures.
2. Monitor patient's physical condition; evaluate and record vital signs and FHR.
3. Evaluate patient's response to medications.
   a. Observe for early signs of magnesium intoxication; patient may become flushed, feel hot, perspire, become thirsty, show hypotension and depression of reflexes; later signs are CNS depression accompanied by anxiety, nausea, headache, drowsiness, lethargy, respiratory depression, and circulatory collapse.
   b. Check deep tendon reflexes hourly.

4. Provide safety measures; be prepared for sudden seizures.
   a. Have padded side rails in place.
   b. Have rolled washcloth to place between teeth (better than padded tongue blade).
   c. Have emergency equipment (oxygen, suction, airway, tracheostomy tray) ready for immediate use.
   d. Have emergency medications immediately available; IV sedation and inhalation anesthesia may be needed to control convulsions.
   e. Observe for indications of uterine contractions; convulsions may initiate labor.
   f. Provide continuous observation and care during period of coma following convulsions.
   g. Position patient to promote drainage of respiratory passage; maintain clear airway, observe for pulmonary edema.

Treatment During Labor and Delivery

1. Management is based on assessment of the disease and viability of the fetus.
2. If fetus is thought to be viable and disease is not controlled, induction or cesarean section is usually recommended.
3. Delay may result in fetal death.

Management During Postpartum

1. Signs and symptoms usually decrease rapidly after delivery, however, danger of seizures does not pass until 48 hours following delivery.
2. Sedation is continued.
3. Hypertension may exist indefinitely or recur with next pregnancy.
4. Follow-up care is essential.

HYPEREMESIS GRAVIDARUM

Hyperemesis gravidarum is exaggerated nausea and vomiting during pregnancy.

Incidence

Fewer than 1 in 300 pregnancies (becoming more rare due to lessened fear of pregnancy and early correction of ordinary nausea and vomiting).

Predisposing Factors

1. Hormonal changes of pregnancy—chorionic gonadotropin levels are high during the first trimester.
2. Emotional factors—uncontrollable vomiting more common in neurotic women.
3. Psychopathology—vomiting may symbolize subconscious rejection of the pregnancy.

Clinical Manifestations

1. Weight loss—due to anorexia
2. Alkalosis—due to loss of hydrochloric acid
3. Acidosis—from starvation
4. Hypokalemia—due to electrolyte imbalance
5. Increased pulse rate—due to anemia
6. Increased blood concentration—due to dehydration
7. Oliguria—due to dehydration

Treatment and Nursing Management

A. *Initial Step*

Rule out other diseases—gastroenteritis, hepatitis, cholecystitis, peptic ulcer, or brain tumor present similar signs and symptoms.

B. *Management of Mild Disease*

1. Provide understanding support; often the only therapy required is discussion of the patient's concerns.
2. Prevent morning nausea by instructing the patient to:
   a. Eat 2 or 3 crackers and remain in bed 15 minutes after awakening. (Dry carbohydrates have an effective antiemetic action.)
   b. One-half hour after rising, eat a small, dry breakfast.
3. Give prochlorperazine (Compazine) on awakening and every 6–8 hours (acts as an antiemetic).

C. *Management of Moderately Severe Disease*

(When nausea and vomiting extend throughout the 24 hours without remission, or if the patient has a weight loss of more than 4.5 kg. or 10 lbs.)

1. Restrict solid food and give orange or lemon juice

over cracked ice—supplies fluid and vitamin C and is acceptable to the patient.
2. Provide for bed rest—at home if facilities are adequate (or patient may need to be hospitalized).
3. Administer Compazine suppositories—for antiemetic and sedative action.
4. Provide 6 small dry meals per day—give only if nausea and vomiting have subsided.
5. Provide fluids—offer hot fluids or very cold fluids.
6. Decrease sedation and allow patient activity.

D. *Management of Severe Disease*—vomiting very severe
1. Provide hospitalization in quiet private room and permit no visitors (including husband)—prevents stimuli.
2. Restrict the patient's activity by complete bed rest—conserves energy.
3. Repeat laboratory evaluation of patient's electrolyte and chemical balance. Tests of carbon dioxide, chlorides, and total proteins, as well as diacetic acid and acetone in the urine, are done. (They aid in replacement therapy and indicate the patient's condition.)
4. Allow nothing by mouth for 24 hours—provide parenteral fluids (1500 ml. of 5% glucose followed by 1000 ml. of 5% glucose in saline).

5. Give B complex factor with vitamin C in IV fluids—prevents avitaminosis.
6. Give promazine hydrochloride (Sparine) in IV fluid, and Compazine IM, t.i.d.—provides sedative and antiemetic action.

NURSING ALERT: Antiemetic and antihistaminic agents may have teratogenic effects during early pregnancy (proven with laboratory animals).

7. Allow oral feedings when patient no longer experiences nausea.
8. Arrange for psychiatric interview—indicated if patient does not improve with therapeutic regimen.
9. Consider therapeutic abortion—recommended if following conditions occur:
   a. Jaundice.
   b. Delirium
   c. Rising pulse rate—to 130
   d. Fever of 38.3°C. (101°F.) despite adequate hydration
   e. Retinal hemorrhage

HEMORRHAGIC DISORDERS

ECTOPIC PREGNANCY

In an *ectopic pregnancy*, gestation is located outside the uterine cavity. Although the majority of ectopic pregnancies are tubal implantations, other types include cervical, abdominal, or ovarian implantations.

Contributing Causes

1. Salpingitis
2. Pelvic inflammatory disease
3. Endometriosis
4. Infantile tubes or imperfect development
5. Spasm of the tubes with muscular insufficiency

Clinical Manifestations

1. Vary with the site of implantation and usually occur after tubal rupture
2. Early signs and symptoms
   a. Abnormal menstrual period
   b. Symptoms of early pregnancy
   c. Dull pain on affected side
3. Signs and symptoms of tubal rupture (Fig. 32-1)
   a. Pain: sudden, severe, and unilateral—later generalized and radiating to shoulder and neck due to diaphragmatic irritation
   b. Nausea, vomiting, faintness
   c. Shock manifested by pallor with slight cyanosis around the lips, yawning, rapid weak pulse
   d. Normal or low temperature—fever important in distinguishing ruptured tubal pregnancy from acute salpingitis
   e. Leukocyte count—normal if rupture is old or if only leakage is occurring, but after sudden hemorrhage usually exceeds 15,000
   f. Tenderness over abdomen upon palpation
   g. Pelvic mass—posterior or lateral to uterus

   h. Cervical pain during vaginal examination and motion of the cervix
   i. Distention of the posterior fornix with blood in the cul-de-sac

Treatment and Nursing Management

OBJECTIVE: to establish the diagnosis without delay and to initiate immediate surgical intervention.
1. Provide constant nursing surveillance—note any changes in patient's condition.
2. Monitor vital signs—assess for indications of impending shock.
3. Start IV fluids with 19-gauge needle—in preparation for administration of blood.
4. Observe for vaginal bleeding—may indicate a uterine abortion rather than ectopic pregnancy.
5. Give narcotics or analgesic agents as prescribed—shock may be due to pain rather than blood loss.
6. Request hematology reports—CBC, type, and cross-matching (blood replacement often necessary).
7. Offer intelligent support and provide explanation of nursing activities—reduces fear and anxiety.
8. Prepare patient for vaginal examination or surgery—to establish or confirm diagnosis and to institute surgical correction.
   a. *Culdocentesis*—aspiration of fluid from the cul-de-sac of Douglas. Presence of bloody fluid indicates intraperitoneal bleeding.
   b. *Culdoscopy*—visualization of the pelvic organs through the punctured posterior fornix.
   c. *Colpotomy*—incision through the posterior fornix to remove the tube. (If the tube is observed to be ruptured, the incision is closed and a laparotomy and salpingectomy are performed.)
9. Provide postoperative care—this is the same as for the patient who has an abdominal laparotomy.

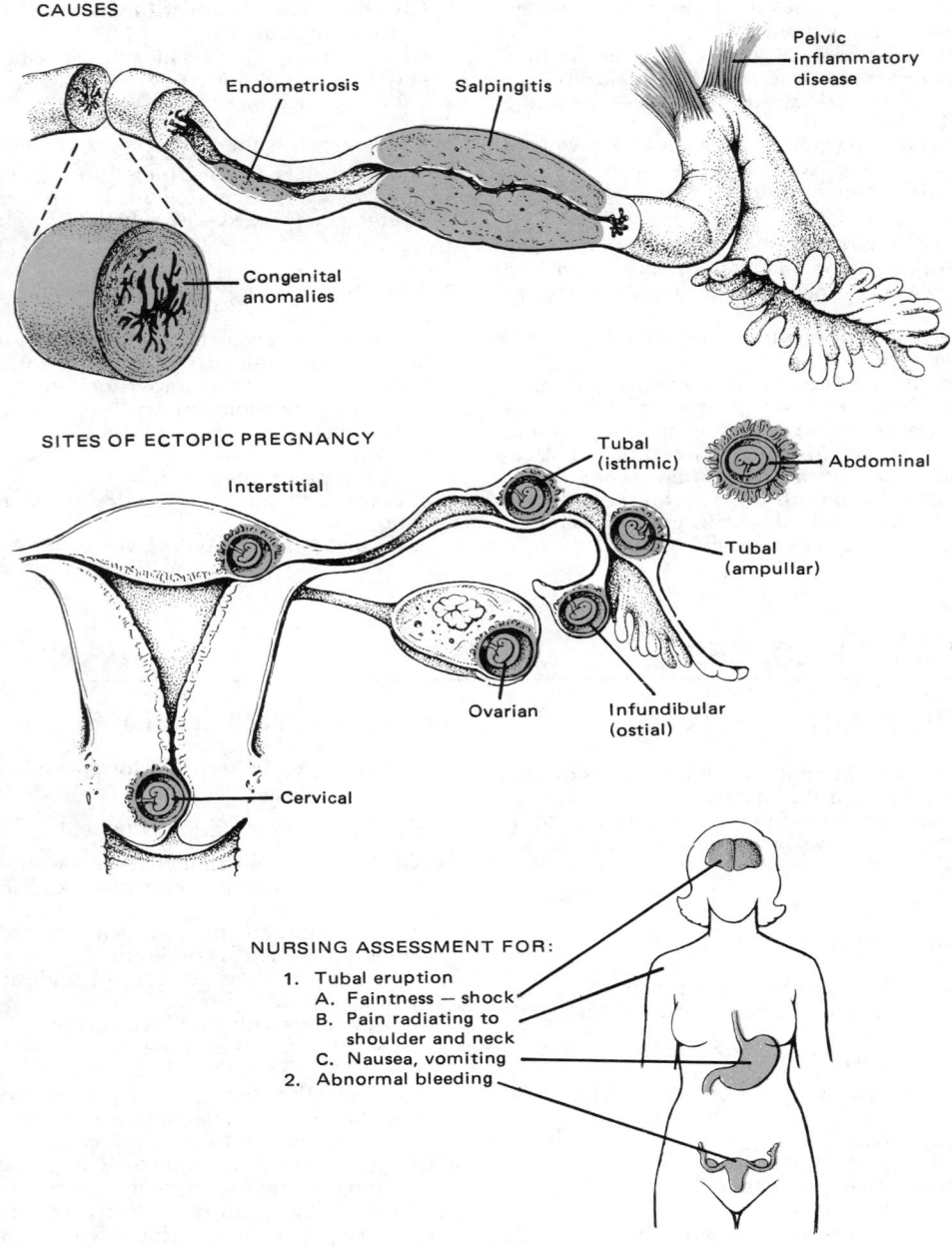

CAUSES

Endometriosis

Salpingitis

Pelvic inflammatory disease

Congenital anomalies

SITES OF ECTOPIC PREGNANCY

Interstitial

Tubal (isthmic)

Abdominal

Tubal (ampullar)

Ovarian

Infundibular (ostial)

Cervical

NURSING ASSESSMENT FOR:

1. Tubal eruption
   A. Faintness — shock
   B. Pain radiating to shoulder and neck
   C. Nausea, vomiting
2. Abnormal bleeding

FIGURE 32-1. *Ectopic pregnancy.*

PLACENTA PREVIA

Placenta previa is the development of the placenta in the lower uterine segment, partially or completely covering the internal cervical os (Fig. 32-2).

Incidence

1. Common cause of bleeding during the last trimester.
2. Occurs once in every 200 deliveries.
3. 3 out of 4 women with placenta previa are multigravidas.

Contributing Causes

1. Largely unknown, although multiparity and advancing age favor occurrence.
2. Unfavorable decidua in upper uterine segment (fibroid tumors, old cesarean section scars).

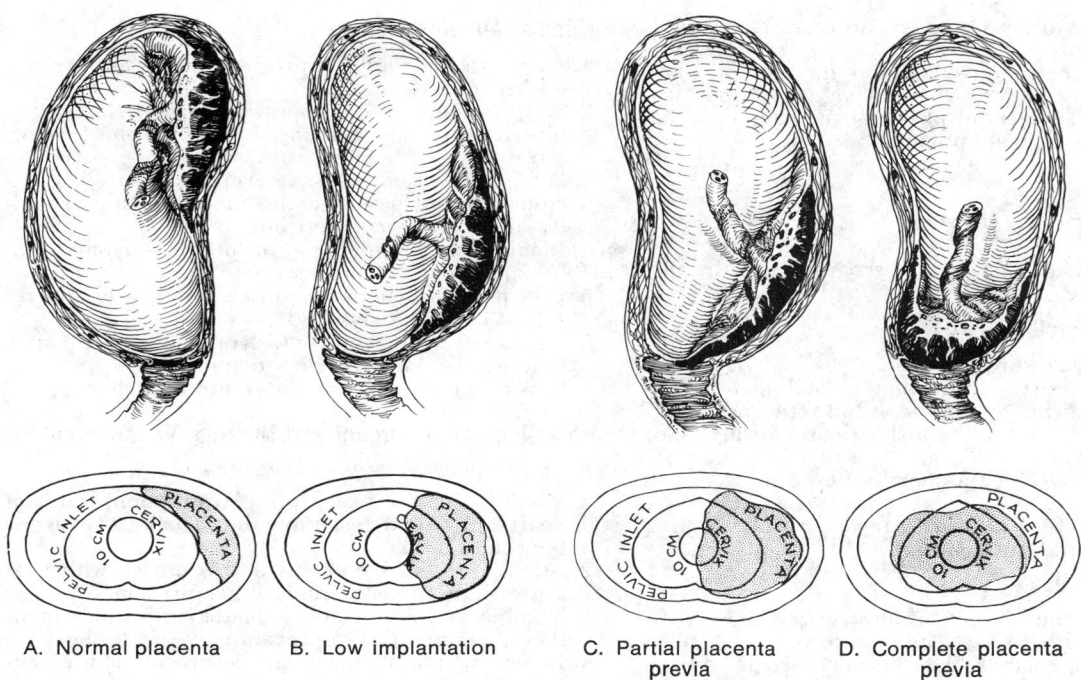

A. Normal placenta   B. Low implantation   C. Partial placenta previa   D. Complete placenta previa

FIGURE 32-2. *Placenta previa. (From Benson RC. Handbook of Obstetrics and Gynecology. Los Altos, California, Lange Medical Publications, 1971.)*

Clinical Manifestations

Hemorrhage—first and most constant symptom
  a. *Painless, causeless bleeding*—not accompanied by uterine contraction.
  b. Occurs most frequently in 8th month—dilation of the internal os causes tearing of placental attachments.
  c. Each succeeding hemorrhage is greater—further dilation is taking place.
  d. Constant seepage of blood-stained serum—indicates a large clot is forming in lower uterine segment.
  e. Partial placenta previa may not cause bleeding until labor begins or until complete dilation has occurred.
  f. Bleeding occurs earlier and is more profuse with total placenta previa.

Treatment and Nursing Management

1. Provide constant nursing surveillance during critical phase.
  a. Provide hospitalization—delivery is recommended except when bleeding is slight and the fetus is not viable.
  b. Prepare for blood replacement—obtain hemoglobin and hematocrit, type and cross-matching of blood.
  c. Prepare patient for pelvic examination. (For 8th month pregnancy, examination must be done in operating room prepared for emergency cesarean section since this maneuver may induce profuse hemorrhage.)
  d. Differentiate between total and partial placenta

previa if fetus is immature and delay in delivery is advisable.
  (1) Ultrasonography—simplest, most precise, and least hazardous procedure.
  (2) Radiology—soft tissue x-ray—least accurate.
  (3) Radioactive isotope scan—localization of placenta by noting area of maximal count.
  (4) Amniography—contrast material injected into amniotic sac.
  (5) Angiography—injection of contrast material into maternal femoral artery.
  e. Reduce patient's fear and anxieties—explain nursing activities and x-ray procedure.
2. Provide for rest and diversional activities—if fetus is immature and hemorrhage moderate, the patient is managed with supportive therapy and bed rest.
3. Prepare patient for vaginal delivery—if pregnancy is near term, the cervix favorable, and partial placenta identified, labor is induced by amniotomy.
4. Provide constant nursing surveillance during labor.
  a. Correct anemia—be prepared for further blood loss.
  b. Start IV fluids—avoid dehydration and hypoglycemia during labor.
  c. Assess vaginal bleeding—cesarean section may be indicated.
  d. Assess progress of labor—malposition of fetus and slow descent are common with placenta previa.
  e. Monitor fetal heart tones—use of cardiotocograph monitor or corometric fetal monitor is indicated for more accurate fetal assessment.
  f. Provide continuing observation during 3rd and 4th stages of labor and delivery—lower uterine segment may be atonic, leaving venous sinuses

open. Oxytocins are given and uterine packing is placed.

g. Provide meticulous attention to antiseptic and aseptic precautions—hemorrhage predisposes to postpartal infection; placental site slower to heal than with normal implantation.

ABRUPTIO PLACENTAE

Abruptio placentae is premature separation of the placenta (Fig. 32-3).

Predisposing Factors

1. Hypertensive disorders
2. Trauma (severe coughing, blow on abdomen, coitus)
3. Delivery of twins—placenta of 2nd fetus disturbed
4. Traction on placenta by a short cord during labor contractions
5. Sudden rupture of the membranes, especially with hydramnios
6. Injudicious use of pitocin during labor with resulting hard and long contractions

Altered Physiology

Separation of the placenta is always accompanied by hemorrhage, either concealed or external.

a. Concealed hemorrhage usually occurs during pregnancy—placental separation occurs centrally; large amount of accumulated blood is stored under the placenta.
b. External hemorrhage usually occurs during labor—blood flows outward from the edge of the placenta, under the membranes, and through the cervix.

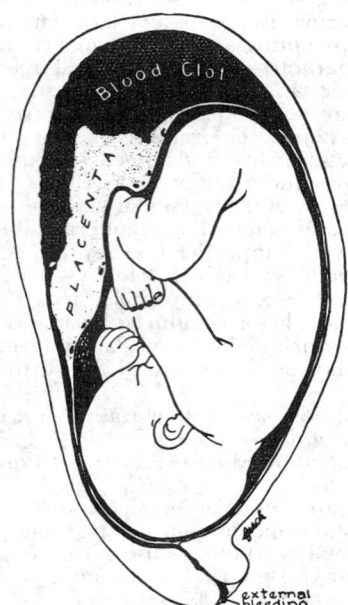

FIGURE 32-3. *Abruptio placentae with large blood clot between placenta and uterine wall.*

Clinical Manifestations

1. Hemorrhage, slight or profuse—blood escapes under the decidua basalis.
2. Shock—often out of proportion to blood loss; manifested by hypotension, rapid pulse, dyspnea, pallor, syncope.
3. Pain, usually sudden and severe—produced by accumulation of blood behind the placenta and infiltration into the myometrium.
4. Rigidity and tenderness of uterus—myometrium becomes board-like (Couvelaire uterus).
5. Uterine contractions—begin spontaneously as a result of uterine irritability.
6. Excessive fetal movement with onset of severe pain—indicates fetal distress due to anoxia.
7. Loss of fetal heart tone—indicates fetal death.

Objectives of Treatment and Nursing Management

A. *To control hemorrhage and overcome shock.*

1. Monitor blood pressure, pulse, respiration, and fetal heart tones—to detect impending shock and to assess fetal condition.
2. Assess external blood loss and compare with vital signs—indications of internal hemorrhage.
3. Administer IV fluids or whole blood—replacement therapy imperative to prevent irreversible shock.
4. Determine plasma fibrinogen levels frequently—entry of thromboplastin into the circulation from the uterus and placenta causes small fibrin clots in the capillaries and consumes fibrinogen, leaving the patient with nonclotting blood.

> **NURSING ALERT:** Human fibrinogen (Cohn Fraction I) has been responsible for transmitting hepatitis more frequently than other blood components.

B. *To relieve the patient's pain and anxiety.*

1. Give analgesic medications with caution—central nervous system depressant may intensify shock symptoms.
2. Provide intelligent explanation of activities.

C. *To accomplish delivery of infant as promptly as possible.*

1. Prepare patient for amniotomy and vaginal delivery (treatment of choice) if cervix is dilated, bleeding moderate, and shock minimal.
2. Prepare patient for cesarean section—immediate delivery desirable for best chance of fetal survival and for control of hemorrhage.

D. *To prevent postpartal complications.*

1. Provide nursing surveillance during the puerperium—early detection of complications.
2. Monitor vital signs and uterine muscle tone—traumatized myometrium may cause uterine atony, necessitating hysterectomy.
3. Be alert for indications of postpartum infections—blood loss and shock greatly reduce resistance to infections.
4. Observe urinary output for oliguria or hematuria—renal failure may result from acute tubular necrosis or bilateral cortical necrosis.

HYDATIDIFORM MOLE

Hydatidiform mole is a developmental anomaly of the placenta resulting in the conversion of the chorionic villi into a mass of clear vesicles. It is the most common lesion anteceding choriocarcinoma, a malignant tumor of the trophoblast with a tendency toward rapid and widespread metastasis.

Incidence

1. Occurs in 1 of every 2000 pregnancies.
2. Relatively high frequency in women over 45.

Clinical Manifestations

1. Enlargement of the uterus out of proportion to the duration of pregnancy.
2. Continuous or intermittent brownish bloody discharge about the 12th week of pregnancy.
3. Signs and symptoms of preeclampsia, proteinuria, hypertension, or edema occurring earlier than usual in pregnancy.

Diagnostic Evaluation

1. Absence of fetal parts on palpation or by x-ray.
2. High chorionic gonadotropin level in serum 100 days or more after last menstrual period.
3. Care must be taken in differential diagnosis to rule out multiple pregnancy.

Objectives of Treatment and Nursing Management

A. *To prepare patient for immediate abortion or evacuation of the mole.*

1. Administer oxytocic agents—stimulates uterine contractions.
2. Evaluate blood loss—have ample blood for transfusion; hemorrhage may be severe.
3. Prepare patient for surgery—abortion of mole is either completed or followed by D & C or suction curettage (deferred for several days until uterus is firmer, to prevent perforation).
4. Prepare patient for hysterotomy or hysterectomy— if the mole is not passed spontaneously, surgical intervention is indicated.
5. Request microscopic examinatin of curetted tissue— for identification of residual or proliferative trophoblastic tissue.

B. *To provide follow-up for detection of malignant change.*

1. Measure chorionic gonadotropin levels—levels become negative within a week after normal pregnancy; within 50-60 days following a hydatidiform mole.
2. Assess chorionic gonadotropin titer—if titer is rising, D & C is performed and tissue is examined.
3. Give chemotherapy if malignant cells are found— methotrexate is usually drug of choice.
4. Assess for indication of impending perforation of the uterus by the tumor—hysterectomy is recommended.

MEDICAL COMPLICATIONS OF PREGNANCY

CARDIAC INVOLVEMENT

The most common form of heart disease in pregnancy is *rheumatic heart disease* (90% of patients). Arteriosclerotic, hypertensive, and congenital types of heart disease account for the other 10%.

Normal Cardiopulmonary Symptoms During Pregnancy

1. Shortness of breath on effort—due to increased ventilation rate and elevated diaphragm.
2. Tachycardia and palpitations at rest or on mild exertion—heart rate increases, gradually reaching a peak 1-2 months before term; average increase—15 beats per minute.
3. Cardiac enlargement—increased plasma volume 30-50% greater during 25th and 35th week, causing increased pulmonary blood flow.
4. Edema of lower extremities—disproportionate increase in venous pressure in the lower extremities as compared with upper extremities, predisposing to dependent edema, varicosities, and hemorrhoids.
5. Functional heart murmurs—due to overactive heart, increased blood velocity, and anemia.

Pathological Cardiopulmonary Signs and Symptoms

1. Dyspnea, increasing at rest or with mild exertion.
2. Diastolic murmur at the heart apex—indicative of mitral stenosis.
3. Tachycardia, increasing with activity.
4. Cough, hemoptysis, and rales at the lung bases— indicates development of pulmonary edema and congestive heart failure.

Treatment and Nursing Management

A. *General Considerations*

1. Obtain history and physical examination—to establish functional classification and determine prognosis and diagnosis of specific heart lesions.
2. Provide frequent observation throughout pregnancy—note evidence of increasing pulmonary, arterial, and venous pressures and venous congestion, particularly from 20th to 30th week.
3. Prevent venous congestion and fluid retention or provide therapy if they occur.
4. Prevent precipitating causes of heart failure such as infection, nutritional deficiencies, physical stress, and anemia; if any of these occur, treat immediately.

NURSING ALERT: A serious anemia (hemoglobin, 8 gm./100 ml. or less) may produce all of the signs simulating congestive heart failure, especially if a functional heart murmur is present.

B. *Specific Aspects of Management*

1. Limit patient's activities.
   Instruct the patient as follows:
   a. Obtain adequate rest—10 hours sleep at night, frequent rest periods during the day, and ½ hour of rest after each meal.
   b. Secure housekeeping help—arrange with social worker if necessary.
   c. Avoid crowds—at social functions or in shopping areas—to avoid infection.
   d. Avoid stress.
   e. Should any signs of decompensation appear, notify physician and remain in bed.
2. Set down diet guidelines for patient.
   a. Prevent excessive weight gain with lower calorie intake—excessive weight increases load on heart and predisposes to hypertension, toxemia, venous stasis, edema, and dyspnea.
   b. Prevent excessive fluid retention by restricting salt intake—retention of water and electrolytes, which occurs in normal pregnancy due to adrenocortical hormone changes, is exaggerated in cardiac patients.

C. *Medical Management*

1. Diuretic therapy—to increase the excretion of sodium, chlorides, and water to counteract the predisposition for congestive failure; however, recent studies indicate that diuretics decrease both placental and renal clearance.
2. Anticoagulant—heparin may be used if coagulation problems develop (does not cross the placenta).
3. Antibiotics—to control infection, which is often a precipating cause of pulmonary edema; antibiotics are often used as a prophylactic measure.
4. Digitalis—to exert a depressant effect. See page 299. Use with discretion since digitalis can be teratogenic to fetus.
5. Oxygen therapy—to facilitate breathing.

Physiologic Changes in the Heart and Circulation During Labor and Delivery

1. Oxygen consumption is greatly increased during periods of uterine contractions, and there is a parallel acceleration of pulse and respiratory rate.
2. Cardiac output increases 20% during each contraction.
3. Blood pressure rises; there are increases in both systolic and diastolic pressures, usually at the peak of uterine contraction.
4. Venous pressure is usually elevated during labor and 24 hours postpartum—increased venous return is associated with muscular exercise of labor and the physiological changes involved.
5. Heart rate increases during early seconds of a uterine contraction, then slows as the contraction continues, because of reduction of placental blood flow; during delivery there is a persistent tachycardia.

Management During Labor and Delivery

1. Provide hospitalization for most cardiac patients for several days (or even weeks, if necessary) before "due date"—to evaluate signs and symptoms of cardiac decompensation.
2. Perform cesarean section only when absolutely necessary—to avoid hazards:
   a. Risk of infection
   b. Prolonged need of anesthesia

c. Greater blood loss
d. Higher incidence of postoperative thromboembolic complications
3. Insure constant nursing surveillance to:
   a. Provide support and encouragement, allay anxiety, and evaluate progress of labor.
   b. Take and record vital signs and fetal heart rate.
   c. Observe for evidence of obstetric or cardiac complications.
   d. Assist the respiratory effort of the patient by placing her in semi-Fowler's position.
   e. Apply elastic stockings to help prevent venous congestion in the lower extremities.
4. *Analgesia*—to relieve pain and apprehension, avoid hypotension, and maintain good oxygenation (essentially the same as for the noncardiac patient).
   a. Early labor
      Barbiturate therapy—to control restlessness.

NURSING ALERT: These agents are slowly metabolized by the fetus and may cause central nervous system depression in the newborn.

   b. Advanced labor
      (1) Meperidine or morphine IM—use with caution since they depress respiratory and vasomotor centers and may cause hypoxia.
      (2) Meperidine given IV may cause vomiting and create unwanted stress.
5. *Anesthesia*
   a. Inhalation anesthesia with high level of oxygen is considered safe for a short period.
   b. Regional anesthesia, especially epidural or caudal, is a superior alternative which provides excellent anesthesia while eliminating the need for barbiturates and narcotics during labor.
   c. Note that hypotension may occasionally occur. This can be corrected by:
      (1) Positioning patient on her side.
      (2) Elevating her legs.
      (3) Administering oxygen and vasopressor drugs, if necessary.

Management During the Postpartum Period

Continue observation and assessment.
1. Evaluate blood loss—excessive blood loss or hypotension may cause shock.
   a. Massage uterine fundus.
   b. Record vital signs.
   c. Administer oxytocic drugs.
2. Administer fluids slowly by mouth or intravenously—to replace fluid loss.
3. Provide narcotics and sedatives as prescribed—to relieve pain and provide comfort following episiotomy and trauma to tissues.
4. Prepare for discharge; plan activity schedule.

NURSING ALERT: Patient may show no signs of difficulty during 1st and 2nd stages of labor, BUT may collapse following delivery because of the sudden decrease in intraabdominal pressure, with consequent engorgement of vessels.

THE DIABETIC AND PREDIABETIC PREGNANT PATIENT

Diabetes mellitus is a chronic hereditary disease characterized by hyperglycemia (abnormally high level of blood sugar) due to a relative insufficiency or lack of insulin which leads to abnormalities in the metabolism of carbohydrates, protein, and fat.

Predisposing Factors

1. Heredity factor—recessive trait
2. Obesity—increases demand on the secretory activity of the beta cells of the islands of Langerhans in the pancreas
3. Stress—emotional and physical (e.g., infections, trauma, surgery, pregnancy)

Mortality

1. Maternal mortality rate
   a. More than 50% before insulin therapy
   b. Currently comparable to nondiabetic rate
2. Infant mortality rate
   a. 40–50% before insulin therapy
   b. Currently 15–20% in mothers with preexisting diabetes
   c. High rates of spontaneous abortion, extrauterine and neonatal deaths, and congenital abnormalities
   d. Figures lower but still substantial for mothers with diabetes diagnosed for the first time during pregnancy

Metabolic Changes During Normal Pregnancy

1. Lowered glucose tolerance—alteration in metabolic rate and increased secretion of adrenocortical and pituitary hormones.
2. Decreased glucose utilization—insulin antagonists are produced by the fetus.
3. Loss of reactivity to insulin—insulin tolerance tests performed throughout pregnancy show a significant reduction in effectiveness because of insulin degradation influenced by the placenta as it increases in size.
4. Hypoglycemic patients return to normal levels during pregnancy—islands of Langerhans increase in size and number during pregnancy.

Altered Physiology

1. Insulin requirements usually increase during the 1st trimester, remain stable during the 2nd and increase considerably during the 3rd—due to increased basal metabolic rate.
2. Increased tendency to ketosis and acidosis—nausea and vomiting during 1st trimester and diminished CO_2-combining power of the blood.
3. Spontaneous abortion—vascular complications affect placental circulation.
4. Diabetic nephropathy and retinopathy may develop or be aggravated during pregnancy—arteriosclerotic changes.
5. Hydramnios—excessive accumulation of amniotic fluid—mechanism unknown.
6. Rapid fetal growth with acceleration of skeletal development, excessive deposition of fat and water retention because of the following:
   a. Excessive supply of glucose from maternal hyperglycemia
   b. Increased production of growth hormone from maternal pituitary
   c. Increased secretion of insulin from fetal pancreas
   d. Increased action of adrenocortical hormones which favor passage of glucose from mother to fetus
7. High fetal and neonatal death rate because of the following:
   a. Ketoacidosis—a single episode can cause fetal death—because of electrolytic imbalance with severe circulatory alteration
   b. Hyaline membrane disease—combination of prematurity and water retention
   c. Birth injuries—cephalopelvic disproportion
   d. Hypoglycemia
   e. Respiratory distress syndrome
   f. Congenital anomalies
   g. Hyperbilirubinemia
   h. Hypocalcemia

Objectives of Treatment and Nursing Management

A. *To identify and diagnose the prediabetic or diabetic patient as early as possible.*

1. Obtain complete history.
   a. Signs and symptoms of diabetes
   b. Diabetes within family
   c. Previous unexplained stillbirths
   d. Large babies weighing over 9 pounds (4000 gm.)
   e. Habitual spontaneous abortions
   f. Delivery of infants with multiple congenital anomalies
   g. Presence of hydramnios
   h. Excessive obesity
2. Carry out thorough physical examination.
   a. Determine patient's medical and obstetrical status.
   b. Assess patient's individual needs and plan management with her.

B. *To provide best possible outcome for mother and newborn by rigid control of the diabetes.*

1. Observe and examine patient frequently—patient should be seen every week (alternately) by the internist and obstetrician; pediatrician must also be aware of patient's progress.
   a. Provide continuing education of the patient regarding diet, medications, signs and symptoms of diabetes and its complications.
   b. Keep record of weight and blood pressure.
   c. Examine ocular fundus.
   d. Observe for signs of edema or hydramnios.
   e. Assess whether diet or medication is controlling disease; adjust as necessary.
2. Laboratory tests
   a. Urinalysis for sugar and protein at each visit—indicates effectiveness of medication or diet and renal function.
   b. Frequent glucose tolerance tests—test results may change from normal to abnormal as pregnancy progresses.
   c. Monthly hemoglobin determination—increased need for iron is same as that of nondiabetic patient.

NURSING ALERT: Tes-Tape and Diastix are specific for glucose and should be used for urine testing in preference to Benedict's solution or clinitest tablets, which give a positive reaction for sugar in such benign melliturias as pentosuria, fructosuria, and lactosuria late in pregnancy and during lactation.

Management of Delivery

1. Pregnancy may be terminated 2–4 weeks before term
   a. Major concern is fetal size and viability (determined by sonogram, nonstress test, amniocentesis, level of plasma, or urine estriol).
   b. Earlier delivery is recommended if there is evidence of:
      (1) Excessive fetal size
      (2) Difficulty in controlling diabetes
2. Pediatrician should be notified of patient's status—to plan management of newborn.
3. Patient hospitalized several days before delivery—to prepare for delivery; long-lasting insulin is changed to regular, and fractional urinalysis is begun for early detection and prevention of hypoglycemic reactions while patient is in labor or undergoing cesarean section.
4. Labor is induced by stripping of membranes, amniotomy, and IV pitocin drip.
5. Patient is given nothing by mouth; continuous IV 10% glucose, covered by regular insulin, is usually administered.
6. Cesarean section is indicated if induction of labor fails.
7. Patient is maintained on regular insulin until able to eat, then returned to long-lasting insulin; dosage usually decreases in the postpartum period.

THYROID DYSFUNCTION

Hyperthyroidism

A. *Incidence*

This is an uncommon complication of pregnancy; the condition may be aggravated by pregnancy and if uncontrolled can cause spontaneous abortion or premature labor.

B. *Etiology*

1. Unknown
2. May appear after emotional shock or infection

C. *Clinical manifestations*

1. In mild cases, diagnosis is difficult since some thyroid enlargement and confusing symptoms occur in normal pregnancy; suggestive symptoms are resting pulse rate greater than 100 beats per minute and muscle wasting, particularly of the quadriceps.
2. Laboratory studies may be confusing because of increased protein binding of thyroid hormone in pregnancy.
3. Major risk is thyroid storm.
4. Patients with exophthalmic goiter produce a substance called LATS (long-acting thyroid stimulator) a gamma-g globulin which crosses the placenta and can cause hyperthyroidism in the newborn.

D. *Treatment*

1. Drug Therapy
   a. Medical management with antithyroid drugs is used with caution since antithyroid drugs also cross the placenta and if doses are excessive, the fetal thyroid can be suppressed, leading to fetal goiter or cretinism.
   b. It has been suggested that therapy with methimazole or propylthiouracil be combined with thyroid extract to prevent adverse effects to the fetus.
2. Surgical Intervention
   a. Indicated if patients do not respond to medical management.
   b. All or part of the thyroid gland is resected.
   c. This is best carried out in the second trimester to decrease untoward fetal effects.

Hypothyroidism

A. *Incidence*

1. Patients with severe hypothyroidism rarely become pregnant.
2. With milder form, although menstrual disturbances are common, conception may occur.

B. *Clinical manifestations*

1. Iodine deficiency may cause mother and fetus to develop colloid enlargement.
2. Thyrotoxicosis may develop from nodular goiter.

C. *Treatment*

Administration of thyroid hormone, thyroglobulin, liotrix, or levothyroxine.

INFECTIONS DURING PREGNANCY

There are numerous types of infections which the mother can contract during pregnancy. The implications of many of these infections in terms of maternal effects, fetal effects, and nursing management are presented in Table 32-1.

URINARY TRACT INFECTION

Incidence and Effect

1. Urinary tract infection is the most common renal problem encountered in pregnancy.
2. Chronic renal disease, especially if accompanied by hypertension, may cause fetal growth retardation and increases risk of perinatal mortality.

Predisposing Factors

1. Hormonal changes, mainly the effect of progesterone, cause dilatation of the upper ureters and renal pelvis and narrowing of the lower ureters, which leads to delayed emptying.
2. Mechanical pressure caused by the uterus pressing the ureters against the pelvic brim results in urinary stasis and increased risk of infection.

Clinical Manifestations

1. Chills and fever
2. Frequency
3. Dysuria
4. Nausea and vomiting

TABLE 32-1. EFFECTS OF INFECTIONS DURING PREGNANCY

Disease	Maternal Effects	Fetal Effects	Prevention or Treatment
Scarlet fever	High fever Puerperal infection	Abortion	Isolation Penicillin
Erysipelas	Puerperal infection Septicemia	Fetal infection Fetal death	Isolation Penicillin or erythromycin
Typhoid fever	High fever	Abortion Premature labor	Antityphoid vaccine Isolation Chloramphenicol
Urinary tract infections	Fever with chills Hematuria Pyuria Dysuria Pain	No effects from maternal infection Large doses of antibiotics in late pregnancy may cause kernicterus in newborn	Sulfonamides Furadantin Ampicillin Tetracycline
Syphilis	Increased resistance with pregnancy Primary and secondary lesions May be asymptomatic	Infection of fetus occurs from 3 months to day of delivery Untreated—premature stillbirth 20% surviving newborns have congenital syphilis	Prevention—treat prior to pregnancy Procaine penicillin G, 2.4 million units In late syphilis, 6 million–9 million units IM in divided doses
Gonorrhea	Infection of genitourinary tract Closure of fallopian tubes May be asymptomatic during pregnancy	Ophthalmia neonatorum acquired during birth	Preventive—silver nitrate 1% eye drops at birth

Rubella	Fever and rash	If infected during first 8 weeks:
		  Congenital cataracts
		  Heart anomalies
		  Deafness
		  Central nervous system damage
			12 ml. of rubella convalescent gamma globulin IM for exposure
			Prevention—immunization of mother more than 3 months before start of pregnancy

Cytomegalovirus disease	Asymptomatic	Hydrocephaly Microphthalmia Seizures Encephalitis Hepatosplenomegaly Hematologic changes Microcephaly Blindness	Various antiviral agents now under study (very toxic) include cytosine arabinoside and idoxuridine
Herpes simplex	Gingivostomatitis Vulvovaginitis	May be lethal to fetus Skin eruptions on newborn Septicemia with respiratory and circulatory failure	Cesarean section if maternal vaginal canal infected
Varicella (chickenpox)	Skin lesions Fever; may be severe	Fetus may have varicella in utero Infant may develop herpes zoster	If mother has disease shortly before delivery, zoster immune globulin is given to infant at birth
Coxsackie virus	Minor illness	Fatal to fetus—myocarditis Encephalomyelitis	No effective treatment
Mumps	Parotitis	Abortion Premature labor Congenital defects Fetal death	Intradermal mumps skin test used to determine immunity If susceptible, convalescent gamma globulin given
Measles (rubeola)	Rash and fever	Abortion Premature labor If late in pregnancy, infant born with infection in same stage as mother's	Gamma globulin if exposed
Smallpox	Skin lesions Fever	Abortion Premature labor Born with disease	If vaccination indicated (exposure to smallpox), Vaccinia Immune Globulin is given with the vaccine (particularly in primary vaccine cases)
Poliomyelitis	More susceptible during pregnancy Labor proceeds normally even in presence of paralysis	Abortion Infant may develop poliomyelitis or be completely normal	Both inactivated vaccine (Salk) and attenuated live vaccine (Sabin) are safe for immunization during pregnancy Antibodies may be transmitted from mother to fetus
Influenza	Prognosis excellent in uncomplicated influenza, serious if pneumonia develops	Abortion Premature labor Congenital defects	Vaccination with specific immune serum
Toxoplasmosis	Asymptomatic	Abortion Death Chorioretinitis Mental retardation Cerebral calcification Anomalies of head size Convulsions	Diagnosis verified by rising antibody titer Pyrimethamine (an antiprotozoal agent)

(Continued on next page)

TABLE 32-1. EFFECTS OF INFECTIONS DURING PREGNANCY (cont.)

Disease	Maternal Effects	Fetal Effects	Prevention or Treatment
Malaria	Fever and chills	Abortion May involve placenta extensively	Commonly used antimalarial drugs
Common cold	More susceptible during pregnancy Becomes serious if hemolytic streptococci infect upper respiratory system	Not known	Symptomatic
Hepatitis B	If progressive may lead to hepatic failure	Fetal death Jaundice and hepatosplenomegaly may develop Liver damage or portal fibrosis	Immune globulin Experimental vaccine has been developed but is not yet available

5. Pain in the area of kidney
6. Abdominal distention
7. Uterine irritability (may result in premature labor)

Treatment

1. Urine culture and antimicrobial sensitivity studies are carried out.
2. Appropriate antimicrobial is given for 2 weeks, then urine is recultured since recurrences are common.
3. Long-term suppressive antimicrobial therapy may be recommended.
4. Adequate fluid intake must be maintained, parenterally if necessary.

NURSING ALERT: The usual antibiotics and sulfonamides may be contraindicated since they may produce hemolysis, hyperbilirubinemia, or kernicterus in the fetus.

DRUG EFFECTS ON THE FETUS

During pregnancy and labor, the mother may be exposed to a variety of drugs for a variety of reasons. The effects of these drugs on the fetus are indicated in Table 32-2.

TABLE 32-2. DRUGS REPORTED TO AFFECT THE FETUS*

Drug	Effect		
	Morphological	*Functional*	*Delayed*
Analgesics			
Narcotics		Withdrawal syndrome ↓ Hyperbilirubinemia	?
Salicylates	↑ Minor anomalies	Platelet dysfunction ↓ Factor XII	
Anesthetics			
General		Depression	
Local		Depression Bradycardia Acidosis Methemoglobinemia	
Antidiabetic Agents			
Tolbutamide	Anomalies	Thrombocytopenia	?
Chlorpropanide	Anomalies	Severe hypoglycemia	?
Cyclamates		?	?
Saccharin		?	?
Hormones			
Cortisone	Cleft palate ?	? Hemorrhages ? Hypoglycemia Normal adrenal activity	
Prednisolone	Anencephaly ? Low birth weight ?	? Hemorrhages ? Hypoglycemia Normal adrenal activity	
Androgens	Masculinization female	Tomboyish behavior	Higher I.Q.
Progestins	Masculinization female	Tomboyish behavior	Higher I.Q.
Diethylstilbestrol	Clitoris hypertrophy		Adenocarcinoma vagina (adolescence)
Smoking	Low birth weight ↑ Stillborn		Smaller at 1 year of age
Alcohol			
Chronic intake	Intrauterine growth failure		
Acute administration		Withdrawal symptoms	?
Pollutants and Pesticides			
Mercury		Severe neurologic defects	Severe handicaps Mental retardation
Lead	Low birth weight	↑ Abortions Anemia Enzyme induction	

* From GB Avery. Neonatology, Pathophysiology and Management of the Newborn. Philadelphia, JB Lippincott, 1975

Drug	Effect		
	Morphological	*Functional*	*Delayed*
DDT and metabolites			
Parathion	? Teratogen		
Fungicides	?	?	
Herbicides	?	?	
Miscellaneous			
Atropine		Tachycardia	
Hexamethonium		Ileus	
Tubocurarine	? Arthrogryposis Multiplex Congenita	Muscular paralysis	
LSD	? Minor limb deformities		
Cloroquine		Deafness	
Antimicrobials			
Sulfonamides		Kernicterus	
Nitrofurantoin		Hemolysis	
Tetracyclines	Teeth staining Enamel hypoplasia		
Streptomycin		8th nerve damage	Deafness
Isoniazid		Encephalopathy	
Anticonvulsants			
Phenytoin	Cleft-lip and palate	Coagulation defects	?
Phenobarbital		Coagulation defects Enzymes induction	?
Barbiturates		Addiction Enzymes induction ↓ Sucking	
Anticoagulants			
Coumarin		↓ Prothrombin time Hemorrhages	
Diuretics			
Thiazides		Thrombocytopenia Hyponatremia ? Electrolyte imbalance	? ?
Antihypertensive Drugs			
Reserpine		Nasal stuffiness	
Cancer Chemotherapeutic Drugs			
Aminopertin	Bone defects Intrauterine growth retardation		Retarded growth
Methotrexate	Malformation of head		
Chlorambucil	Unilateral absence of kidney and ureter		
Immunosuppressants			
Azathioprine	?	?	?
Psychopharmacologic Drugs			
Phenothiazine		?	? Behavioral changes
Chlorpromazine	? (Eyes)	Extrapyramidal dysfunction	
Imipramine	? Limb defects		
Lithium	?	Toxicity	
Diazepam		? Temperature	
Antithyroid			
Potassium iodide	Goiter		
Thiouracil	Goiter	↓ Thyroxine synthesis	?
I131		Hypothyroidism	? Malignant changes

TERMINATION OF PREGNANCY

ABORTION

Abortion is the termination of pregnancy at any time before the fetus has attained viability (20 weeks gestation or fetal weight of 400 gm., or 14 oz.).

Incidence

1. Frequent complication of pregnancy.
2. One pregnancy in every 10 terminates in spontaneous abortion.

Predisposing Factors

1. Faulty germ plasm—imperfect ova or sperm cells.
2. Decrease in production of progesterone—insufficient progesterone leads to increased uterine sensitivity and contractions which cause expulsion of the ovum or embryo.
3. Incompetent cervix—mechanical defect in the cervix causes dilatation and effacement in early pregnancy (women with history of induced abortion have increased incidence of incompetent cervix).

4. Acute infections—cause fetal death by:
   a. Transmission of bacterial toxins from mother to fetus
   b. Passage of microorganisms from mother to fetus
   c. High temperature, which stimulates uterine contractions
   d. Excessive carbon dioxide in blood (as associated with respiratory infections)

Types of Abortion
See chart, below.
1. Threatened abortion
2. Inevitable abortion
3. Habitual abortion
4. Incomplete abortion
5. Missed abortion
6. Induced abortion
7. Therapeutic abortion

Induced Abortion
Termination of a pregnancy by the patient or others. The nurse should encourage a woman contemplating such an abortion to seek medical advice and counseling; many agencies are set up to assist in such situations.

Therapeutic Abortion
According to U.S. Supreme Court ruling of January 22, 1973, pregnancy may be terminated as follows:
1. In the first trimester of pregnancy, the abortion decision is to be left to the woman and her physician.
2. During the next trimester, the state may not prohibit abortion, but may regulate its practice in the interest of protecting the woman's health.
3. During the final weeks of pregnancy, the state may choose to protect the potential life of the fetus by prohibiting abortion except where necessary to preserve the life or health of the woman.
4. The religious beliefs of the patient are always respected.

NURSING ALERT: Serious hemorrhage from alteration in the blood clotting mechanism may occur with prolonged retention of a dead fetus. Fibrinogen concentrations should be measured weekly. If concentrations are reduced to 150 mg./100 ml. of blood, the uterus should be emptied; fibrinogen and whole blood may have to be administered.

Nursing Management
1. Provide constant nursing surveillance.
   a. Measure and record vital signs—to determine presence of shock.
   b. Assess amount of blood loss—perineal pad count.
   c. Save all tissue and clots—for examination by pathologist for presence of decidua or embryo.
2. Relieve the patient's pain and anxiety—uterine contractions may be as severe as those experienced during childbirth.
   a. Give analgesic medication within prescribed limit.
   b. Monitor the blood pressure, pulse, and respiratory rate before administering or repeating narcotics—

Types of Abortion

Classification	Clinical Manifestations	Management
1. Threatened	Vaginal bleeding or spotting Mild cramps Cervix closed or slightly dilated Symptoms subside or develop into an inevitable abortion	Vaginal examination Pregnanediol test if progesterone low Bed rest Pad count
2. Inevitable	Bleeding more profuse Cervix dilated Painful uterine contractions	Embryo delivered, followed by D & C
3. Habitual abortion	Spontaneous abortion occurs in successive pregnancies (3 or more)	Hysterogram to rule out uterine abnormalities, infections Complete bed rest Medical management Hormones to prevent sloughing of endometrium (controversial) Thyroid extract therapy Surgical constriction of the cervix if incompetent cervix is causative factor D & C
4. Incomplete abortion	Fetus usually expelled Placenta and membranes retained	D & C
5. Missed abortion	Fetus dies in utero and is retained Maceration occurs No symptoms of abortion, but malaise, anorexia, and headache are common	D & C and oxytocin contraindicated Intra-amniotic injection of saline usually successful in expulsion of retained material

narcotics are central nervous system depressants and may contribute to development of shock.

c. Offer intelligent reassurance—avoid statement that would imply a favorable outcome for the fetus even with threatened abortion—prognosis very uncertain.

3. Be alert for complications that could develop.
   a. Assess for signs of shock from excessive blood loss.
      (1) Reduced blood pressure
      (2) Rapid weak pulse
      (3) Cool moist skin
      (4) Restlessness
      (5) Apathy
   b. Provide emergency measures to combat shock

(1) Elevate patient's legs.
(2) Notify physician.
(3) Start IV fluids with 19 gauge needle.

c. Prepare patient for surgical completion of the abortion—patient will continue to bleed or hemorrhage until uterus is emptied and able to contract.

d. Observe patient postoperatively for signs of infection—hemorrhage lowers resistance to infection, and retained tissue or blood clots provide excellent bacterial media.

e. Prepare patient for artificial termination of the pregnancy by intra-amniotic instillation of hypertonic solution.

GUIDELINES: Saline Infusion into the Amniotic Cavity

Saline infusion is replacement of the amniotic fluid with a hypertonic saline solution which chemically stops fetal and placental function and thus initiates labor.

Purpose Interruption of pregnancy after 12 weeks gestation

Equipment A receptacle for the amniotic fluid
200 ml. of a 20% solution of sodium chloride
Skin antiseptic
Sterile infusion tray
   Draping towel
   Container for saline solution
50-ml. syringe for removal of amniotic fluid and injection of the saline solution
20-ml. syringe, a 25 gauge 3.8-cm. (1½-inch) needle and a 20 gauge 3.8 cm. (1½-inch) needle for anesthetizing the anterior abdominal wall
10-cm. (4-inch), 14-gauge spinal needle with stylet
A No. 5 teflon catheter, 1 meter (approximately 36 inches) long with 3 holes at the tip
Vial of local anesthetic agent
Surgical gown and gloves

Procedure

NURSING ACTION	RATIONALE/AMPLIFICATION
Preparatory Phase	
1. Obtain history and assist with general physical examination.	1. Problems elicited may indicate referral to an appropriate specialist or decision to perform procedure in hospital rather than office or clinic.
2. Discuss present pregnancy.	2. Identifying patient's feelings toward abortion is important. Further counseling may be indicated.
3. Have patient void.	3. To avoid injury to the bladder.
4. Assist patient to disrobe, put on examining gown, and assume supine position.	
5. Expose the abdomen and wash with antiseptic solution.	5. Since the needle will be inserted through the skin into the amniotic cavity, asepsis is carried out to prevent infection.
Performance Phase	
The physician does the following:	
1. A skin wheal is made with local anesthesia using the 25-gauge needle.	1. The site chosen for injection is usually the mid-uterus.
2. A 20-gauge 3.8-cm. (1½-inch) needle is used to anesthetize the other layers of the anterior abdominal wall.	
3. For actual amniocentesis, a 10-cm. (4-inch) No. 14 gauge spinal needle with stylet is placed at the site of anesthesia and firmly inserted through the abdominal wall into the uterus.	3. A loss of resistance may be felt when the needle enters the amniotic cavity. The needle will be inserted to a depth of 7.6 cm. (3 inches) before fluid is reached.
4. Stylet is removed and amniotic fluid returns through the needle.	

GUIDELINES: Saline Infusion into the Amniotic Cavity (cont.)

Procedure (cont.)	NURSING ACTION	RATIONALE/AMPLIFICATION
	5. The No. 5 teflon catheter is threaded slightly beyond the needle top, and the needle is withdrawn.	
	6. Approximately 150 ml. of amniotic fluid is withdrawn through the catheter.	
	7. 200 ml. of 20% solution of sodium chloride is injected through the catheter.	7. The first 20–30 ml. of solution is injected slowly and patient is observed for any unusual symptoms such as pain at the site of injection, feeling of warmth, thirst, headache, or numbness, which indicate that the catheter is no longer in the amniotic space and that adjustments must be made.
	8. One million units of aqueous penicillin are instilled through the catheter.	8. This is a prophylactic measure to prevent intrauterine infection.
	9. The catheter is withdrawn and a small dressing applied.	

Follow-up Phase

1. The patient may be discharged with the following instructions:
   a. Drink at least 2 liters (quarts) of water sometime during the afternoon following the procedure.
   b. When contractions become uncomfortable, return for completion of abortion.
   c. If fever develops or bleeding commences, call physician and plan to return to hospital.

   a. To combat hypernatremia and to promote diuresis.
   b. Labor contractions should begin within 12–24 hours.
   c. Fever may be caused by chorioamnionitis, or by chemical necrosis of tissue. Tetracycline or ampicillin may be prescribed. Bleeding is usually due to partial placenta separation.

2. After the abortion the patient should be instructed:
   a. To abstain from intercourse and avoid tampons for 2 weeks.
   b. Resume normal activity in 1–2 days.

   a. To prevent trauma and infection.

3. Evaluate psychological status and refer for psychological follow-up if indicated.

   3. Depression related to hormonal changes is common.

Complications

1. Complications of saline infusions include hemorrhage, infection, and retained placental tissue.
2. Among occasional serious complications are hypernatremia, amniotic fluid embolism, disseminated intravascular coagulation, and necrosis of the myometrium.

COMPLICATIONS OF LABOR

DYSTOCIA

Dystocia, or difficult labor, may be due to either mechanical or functional factors or to a combination of both.

Mechanical Dystocia

1. *Maternal Causes*
   a. Contracted pelvis
   b. Obstructive tumors (ovarian or uterine fibromyoma
2. *Fetal Causes*
   a. Failure of the vertex to rotate, as in occiput posterior or occiput transverse
   b. Malpresentations (shoulder, brow, face, or breech)
   c. Malformation of the fetus (as in hydrocephalus) or excessive size of the infant

Functional Dystocia (Uterine Dysfunction or Inertia)

Conditions in which uterine contractions deviate from the normal.

1. *Types of Uterine Inertia*
   a. Primary inertia—occurring at onset of labor
   b. Secondary inertia—occurs later; prolongation of the active phase of labor
2. *Contributing Conditions*
   a. Uterine abnormalities (such as double uterus)
   b. Minor degrees of pelvic contraction and fetal malposition
   c. Overdistention of the uterus, associated with multiple pregnancy, polyhydramnios
   d. Postmaturity or delayed labor
   e. Grand multiparity
   f. Excessive cervical rigidity, as with the older primigravida
   g. Excessive or too early administration of analgesic drugs
   h. Unknown causes
3. *Complications of Uterine Dysfunction*
   a. Fetal injury and death
   b. Maternal exhaustion and dehydration if labor is greatly prolonged

c. Intrauterine infection

d. Deleterious effect on future childbearing

Treatment and Nursing Management

A. *For Mechanical Dystocia*

1. Re-evaluate pelvis with X-ray pelvimetry.
2. Prepare for cesarean section if vaginal delivery appears to be hazardous to either mother or infant.
3. Plan nursing intervention if occiput posterior presentation is identified.
   a. Relieve back pain as much as possible by sacral pressure, back rubs, frequent change of position from side to side (may also assist fetal head to rotate).
   b. Observe the character and frequency of contractions and monitor fetal heart rate constantly and critically.
   c. Assess the amount of discomfort the mother is experiencing and her general condition.
   d. Prevent dehydration during the lengthened labor by starting IV fluids.
   e. Rotate fetal head manually or by forceps when cervical dilation is complete.
4. Plan obstetrical and nursing intervention if breech presentation is identified.
   a. Provide explanation and appropriate reassurance.
   b. Identify type of breech presentation.
      (1) Complete breech—when feet and legs are flexed on the thighs and the thighs are flexed on the abdomen so that the buttocks and feet present.
      (2) Footling—when one or both feet present through the cervix.
      (3) Frank breech—when legs are extended and lie against the abdomen and the chest, with the feet meeting the shoulders; the buttocks present.
   c. Provide comfort measures.
      (1) Labor is generally longer since in a breech delivery the soft buttocks do not aid in cervical dilation as well as the head does in a vertex presentation.
      (2) Analgesia may be limited so as not to interfere with the mother's ability to push effectively.
      (3) Amniotomy is not done until breech is well engaged as there is greater danger of prolapse of the cord with footling presentation.
   d. Assist with delivery
      (1) Breech cases may be delivered spontaneously with strong contractions, particularly in multiparae.
      (2) More aid is indicated (manual extraction of the head or application of Piper forceps to the aftercoming head) for the majority of patients, especially primigravidae.
      (3) Cesarean section is a better approach than difficult extraction.
   e. Assess newborn's condition.
      One in every 15 breech deliveries results in the death of the infant because of tentorial tears and subsequent intracranial hemorrhage, lesions of the spinal cord, and extrusion of the medulla into the foramen magnum.
   f. Assess condition of the mother and observe for postpartum bleeding; lacerations of birth canal are more frequent.

B. *For Functional Dystocia*

1. *Hypertonic uterine dysfunction*—muscle of the uterus is in a state of greater than normal tension, so that contractions are ineffective for accomplishing dilatation.
   a. Provide rest with aid of sedatives. (Morphine, 16 mg., usually stops contractions.)
   b. Provide fluids to maintain hydration and electrolyte balance.
   c. Observe for normal contractions when patient awakens.
2. *Hypotonic uterine dysfunction*—tone or tension of the uterine muscle is defective or inadequate—usually occurs during the active phase of labor.
   a. Confirm diagnosis with x-ray pelvimetry and sterile vaginal examination to ascertain the following:
      (1) Accurate pelvic measurements
      (2) Abnormalities of presentation and position
      (3) State of cervical dilation
      (4) Level of presenting part
   b. Prepare for cesarean section if indicated.
   c. Provide comfort measures to promote relaxation if cesarean section not indicated.
   d. Provide explanations and continue supportive care.
   e. Administer enema to stimulate contractions.
   f. Perform amniotomy—rupture of membranes often stimulates contractions.
   g. Start IV fluids to prevent dehydration.
   h. Administer intravenous infusion of oxytocin.
   i. Provide continuous surveillance.
      (1) Observe contractions for character and frequency. If contractions last more than 60-70 seconds, adjust infusion. (Tetanic contractions may cause premature separation of the placenta or rupture of the uterus.)
      (2) Observe IV drip; be certain infusion is running at prescribed rate (drops per minute).
      (3) Report any maternal or fetal aberrations immediately.
      (4) Record observations and nursing activities.

PRECIPITATE LABOR

Precipitate labor is a labor which lasts 2 hours or less and which may possibly include precipitate delivery (sudden and unexpected delivery without professional attendance).

Predisposing Factors

1. Multiparity
2. Large pelvis
3. Lax and unresistant soft tissue
4. Tumultuous contractions
5. Small baby in good position
6. Induction of labor by rupture of membranes and oxytocin infusion

Complications

1. Impaired blood flow may have hypoxic effect on fetus. (May be an etiologic factor in cerebral palsy.)
2. Rapid transit of fetus through bony pelvis may produce cerebral trauma.
3. Delivery may be unattended and baby may not receive the benefit of immediate resuscitation.
4. Maternal birth canal may be lacerated.
5. Uterus may rupture.

Treatment and Nursing Management

1. Obtain obstetrical history. Patients with previous

rapid labors may be candidates for elective induction of labor and control of labor.
2. Provide constant surveillance.
3. If contractions become excessively strong, anesthesia is given to decrease strength of contractions.
4. Administer oxygen by mask to aid fetus.

UTERINE RUPTURE

Uterine rupture is a spontaneous or traumatic rupture of the uterus.

Causes

1. Excessive strain on the myometrium
2. Rupture of the scar from a previous cesarean section or hysterotomy
3. Prolonged or obstructed labor
4. Faulty presentation
5. Forced delivery of fetus with abnormalities, e.g., hydrocephalus
6. Ill-advised podalic version
7. Application of forceps and extraction before cervical os has completely dilated
8. Injudicious use of oxytocin
9. Excessive manual pressure applied to the fundus during delivery

Clinical Manifestations

1. Complete rupture
   a. Sudden sharp abdominal pain during contractions
   b. Abdominal tenderness
   c. Cessation of contractions
   d. Bleeding into the abdominal cavity and sometimes into the vagina
   e. Fetus easily palpated; fetal heart tones cease
   f. Signs of shock—rapid, weak pulse; cold, clammy skin; pale color; flaring of nostrils due to air hunger
2. Incomplete rupture—develops over a period of a few hours
   a. Abdominal pain during contractions
   b. Contractions continue but cervix fails to dilate
   c. Slight vaginal bleeding
   d. Rising pulse rate and skin pallor
   e. Loss of fetal heart tones

Treatment and Nursing Management

1. Fetal prognosis is grave, fetus often dies of asphyxia prior to delivery or suffers permanent damage from effects of hypoxia.
2. Maternal prognosis is guarded, especially in uterine rupture of traumatic origin (5-10% mortality rate).
3. Treatment begins with prevention of spontaneous rupture:
   a. Accurate evaluation of maternal pelvis
   b. Identification of fetal position
   c. Avoidance of prolonged labor
   d. Judicious use of oxytocin
   e. Cesarean section for subsequent deliveries
4. Prepare for immediate hysterectomy after rupture.
   a. Obtain complete hemostasis at earliest possible moment.
   b. Ensure adequate amount of blood by 1 or 2 venous cutdowns.
   c. Ligation of the hypogastric arteries may be considered preliminary to hysterectomy.
   d. Administer antibiotics to combat peritonitis.

AMNIOTIC FLUID EMBOLISM

Amniotic fluid embolism is the escape of amniotic fluid containing debris such as meconium, lanugo, and vernex caseosa into the maternal circulation, usually resulting in deposition of fluid or debris in the pulmonary arterioles (rare; usually fatal).

Clinical Manifestations

1. Sudden dyspnea
2. Cyanosis
3. Pulmonary edema
4. Profound shock due to:
   a. Anaphylaxis, which causes vascular collapse
   b. Uterine bleeding with development of hypofibrinogenemia

Treatment and Nursing Management

1. Treatment initially directed to relief of respiratory difficulties.
2. Administer oxygen therapy and provide assisted ventilation (see pp. 171–199).
3. Start fresh whole blood transfusion immediately.
4. Give IV administration of fibrinogen.
5. Administer heparin to control intravascular coagulation, especially in the pulmonary circulation.
6. Prepare for immediate sterile vaginal examination. If cervix is dilated, forceps delivery may salvage fetus and reduce maternal respiratory difficulty.

PROLAPSED UMBILICAL CORD

Prolapsed umbilical cord—descent of the cord following rupture of the membranes.

Causes

1. Rupture of membranes when the presenting part is not engaged in the pelvis.
2. More common in shoulder and foot presentations.
3. Prematurity—small fetus allows more space around presenting part.
4. Hydramnios—causes greater amount of fluid to be released with greater force when membranes rupture.

Clinical Manifestations

1. Cord may be seen protruding from vagina.
2. Fetal distress occurs following rupture of membranes.
3. Cord can be palpated in the vaginal canal or cervix.

Treatment and Nursing Management

1. Place mother in deep Trendelenburg position.
2. Administer oxygen (5 liters) by mask.
3. Place sterile gloved hand in vagina and push baby's head upward to relieve compression of the cord.
4. Prepare for immediate vaginal delivery if cervix is dilated.
5. Prepare for immediate cesarean section if cervix is incompletely dilated.
   General anesthesia is administered to prevent uterine contractions while preparation for cesarean section is being made.

INVERTED UTERUS

Inverted uterus—uterus inverted, or turned inside out, usually during the delivery of the placenta.

Causes

1. Excessive traction on the cord when the placenta is firmly attached to the uterine wall
2. Markedly lax or thin uterine walls
3. Fundal pressure when the uterus is relaxed
4. May occur spontaneously

Clinical Manifestations

1. Shock with faintness, severe uterine pain, and hemorrhage

POSTPARTUM COMPLICATIONS

PUERPERAL INFECTION

Puerperal infection is a postpartum infection of the genital tract, usually of the endometrium, that may remain localized or may extend to various parts of the body.

Causes

Bacterial organisms either are introduced from external sources or are normally present in the generative tract.

Predisposing Factors

1. Prolonged labor
2. Postpartum hemorrhage
3. Premature rupture of membranes
4. Urinary tract infections
5. Intrauterine manipulation
6. Anemia
7. Retention of placental fragments

Clinical Manifestations

Symptoms depend on site and degree of extension.
1. Sustained fever of 38°C. (100.4°F.) or higher
2. Pain
3. Profuse, foul-smelling vaginal discharge, sometimes frothy
4. Burning on urination
5. Secondary abscesses elsewhere in the body
6. Thrombophlebitis, caused by extension of infection along veins
7. Pyemia

Complications

1. Pulmonary embolism
2. Peritonitis
3. Pelvic cellulitis

Preventive Measures

1. Prompt treatment of anemia
2. Well-balanced diet
3. Avoidance of coitus in late pregnancy
4. Strict asepsis during labor and delivery
5. Sterile perineal pads changed every 4 hours
6. Separation of infected from noninfected patients

Treatment and Nursing Management

1. Antibiotic therapy
2. Warm sitz baths, warm compresses or heat lamp
3. Drainage—established when possible (Fowler's position is helpful.)
4. Maintenance of fluid and electrolyte balance

2. Mild symptoms observed with incomplete version in the later postpartum period

Treatment and Nursing Management

1. Uterus is replaced manually while the patient is under anesthesia.
2. Treatment for shock is given.
3. Uterus may have to be replaced surgically.

MASTITIS

Mastitis is inflammation of the breasts.

Etiology

Usually due to *Staphylococcus aureus* derived from the nursing infant's nose and throat.

Clinical Manifestations

Usually appears in 3rd or 4th week of puerperium.
1. Marked breast engorgement
2. Chills
3. Elevated temperature
4. Increased pulse rate
5. Hardness and reddening of breasts
6. Pain in breasts

Preventive Measures

1. Nursery routine
   a. Careful handscrubbing between handling of infants
   b. Prompt isolation of any infant who appears to be developing an infection
   c. Exclusion from the nursery of all personnel with infections
2. Proper care of maternal breasts
   a. Limit nursing times for initial feedings
   b. Prompt attention to fissures and cracks in nipples

Treatment

Antibiotic therapy

POSTPARTUM HEMORRHAGE

Postpartum hemorrhage involves a loss of 500 ml. or more of blood; it occurs most frequently in the first hour following delivery.

Causes (in order of frequency)

1. Uterine atony—relaxation of the uterus secondary to:
   a. Multiple pregnancy—causes overdistention of uterus and a larger placental site
   b. Polyhydramnios
   c. High parity
   d. Prolonged labor with maternal exhaustion
   e. Deep anesthesia
   f. Fibromyomata—prevents uterus from contracting
2. Laceration of the vagina, cervix or perineum secondary to:
   a. Forceps delivery, especially rotation forceps
   b. Large infant

c. Multiple pregnancy
d. Unsutured vessel in the episiotomy site
e. Breech extraction
3. Retained placental fragments secondary to:
a. Manual removal of the placenta
b. Abruptio placentae
c. Placenta previa
4. Tumors of the uterus

Clinical Manifestations

1. Effects of hemorrhage depend on maternal blood volume and degree of anemia previous to delivery.
2. Bleeding from lacerations is bright red and usually occurs with a firm fundus.
3. Moderate blood loss is often not reflected by depression of blood pressure or pulse.
4. Blood loss usually occurs by constant seepage rather than in a sudden massive hemorrhage episode.
5. Excessive blood loss is indicated by pallor, restlessness, dyspnea, thready pulse, lowered blood pressure, chills, and air hunger.
6. Soft uterus that is difficult to palpate indicates uterine atony.

Treatment and Nursing Management

A. *For Uterine Atony*

1. Massage the uterus firmly.

NURSING ALERT: Overmassage of the uterus will contribute to muscle fatigue and cause further relaxation and increased bleeding.

2. Administer oxytocins as prescribed.
3. Start IV fluids to increase blood volume.
4. Replace blood loss by transfusion.
5. Examine uterine cavity for blood clots or placental fragments which would keep the uterus from contracting.

B. *For Lacerations*

1. Return patient to delivery room for inspection and repair.
2. Administer IV fluids and blood transfusion if necessary.

C. *For Retained Placental Fragments*

1. Symptoms usually occur late after the patient has been discharged from the hospital.
2. Patient is returned to the hospital for dilatation of the cervix and curettage of the uterus.

BIBLIOGRAPHY

Books

Aladjem S and Brown AK. Perinatal Intensive Care. St. Louis, CV Mosby, 1977

Bennington JL (ed). Pathology of the Placenta, Vol 2. In Major Problems of Pathology. Philadelphia, WB Saunders, 1978

Benson RC. Current Obstetric and Gynecologic Diagnosis and Treatment. Los Altos, Lange Medical Publishers, 1978

Bolognese RJ and Schwarz RH. Perinatal Medicine: Management of the High Risk Fetus and Neonate. Baltimore, Williams & Wilkins, 1977

Buchsbaum HJ. Trauma in Pregnancy. Philadelphia, WB Saunders, 1979

Butnarescu GF et al. Perinatal Nursing, Vol 2, Reproductive Risk. New York, John Wiley & Son, 1980

Campbell JA. Obstetrical Diagnosis by Radiographic, Ultrasonic and Nuclear Methods. Baltimore, Williams & Wilkins, 1977

Cavanagh D et al. Obstetric Emergencies, 2nd ed. Hagerstown, Harper & Row, 1978

Cavanagh D et al. Septic Shock in Obstetrics and Gynecology. Philadelphia, WB Saunders, 1977

Chesley LC. Hypertensive Disorders in Pregnancy. New York, Appleton–Century–Crofts, 1978

Coid CR. Infections and Pregnancy. New York, Academic Press, 1977

Dickason EJ et al. Maternal and Infant Drugs and Nursing Intervention. New York, McGraw–Hill, 1978

Donaldson JO. Neurology of Pregnancy. Philadelphia, WB Saunders, 1978

Friedman EA and Neff RK. Pregnancy Hypertension: A Systematic Evaluation of Clinical Diagnostic Criteria. Littleton, Publishing Sciences Group, 1977

Gluck L (ed). Intrauterine Asphyxia and the Developing Fetal Brain. Chicago, Year Book Medical Publishers, 1977

Heinonen OP et al. Birth Defects and Drugs in Pregnancy. Littleton, Publishing Sciences Group, 1977

Johnson SH. High Risk Parenting: Nursing Assessment and Strategies for the Family at Risk. Philadelphia, JB Lippincott, 1979

Lindheimer MD et al. Hypertension in Pregnancy. New York, John Wiley & Sons, 1975

Lindheimer MD and Katz AI. Kidney Function and Disease in Pregnancy. Philadelphia, Lea & Febiger, 1977

Novak ER and Woodruff JD. Novak's Gynecologic and Obstetric Pathology. Philadelphia, WB Saunders, 1979

Paul RH et al. Fetal Intensive Care I: An Introduction. North Haven, William Mark, 1979

Paul RH et al. Fetal Intensive Care II: Case Management. North Haven, William Mark, 1979

Pederson J. The Pregnant Diabetic and Her Newborn: Problems and Management. Baltimore, Williams & Wilkins, 1977

Sabbagha R. Ultra Sound in High Risk Pregnancy. Philadelphia, Lea & Febiger, 1979

Sandler M (ed). Mental Illness in Pregnancy and the Puerperium. New York, Oxford University Press, 1978

Sciarra J (ed). Gynecology and Obstetrics, Vol 2, Clinical Obstetrics. Hagerstown, Harper & Row, 1980

Sciarra J (ed). Gynecology and Obstetrics, Vol 3, Maternal and Fetal Medicine. Hagerstown, Harper & Row, 1980

Stevenson RE. The Fetus and the Newly Born Infant: Influences of the Prenatal Environment, 2nd ed. St. Louis, CV Mosby, 1977

Taber B. Manual of Gynecologic and Obstetric Emergencies. Philadelphia, WB Saunders, 1979

Tucker SM. Fetal Monitoring and Fetal Assessment in High Risk Pregnancy. St. Louis, CV Mosby, 1978

Tulchinsky D and Ryan K. Maternal and Fetal Endocrinology. Philadelphia, WB Saunders, 1980

Tunnadine D and Green R. Unwanted Pregnancy: Accident or Illness. New York, Oxford University Press, 1978

Articles

Butts P. Magnesium sulfate in the treatment of toxemia. Am J Nurs 1977 Aug; 77(8):1294–1298

Bills B. Nursing considerations: Administering labor-suppressing medication. Am J Mat Child Nurs 1980 July/Aug; 5(4):252–256

Charache S et al. Management of sickle cell disease in pregnant patients. Obstet Gynecol 1980 Apr; 55(4):407–410

Cranley MS. Corinne: A mother at risk. Am J Nurs 1978 Dec; 78(12):2117–2121

Davison JM and Lindheimer MD. Renal disease in pregnant women. Clin Obstet Gynecol 1978 June; 21(2):411–427

De Alvarez RR. Preeclampsia–eclampsia and renal diseases in pregnancy. Clin Obstet Gynecol 1978 Sept; 21(3):881–905

Diamond F. High risk pregnancy screening techniques: A nursing review. JOGN Nurs 1978 Nov/Dec; 7(6):15–20

Evertson LR et al. Antepartum fetal heart rate testing. I. Evolution of the nonstress test. Am J Obstet Gynecol 1979 Jan; 133(1):29–33

Gable SG. Diabetes in pregnancy: Clinical controversies. Clin Obstet Gynecol 1978 June; 21(2):443–452

Gauthier RJ et al. Antepartum fetal heart rate testing. II. Intrapartum fetal heart rate observation and newborn outcome following a positive contraction stress test. Am J Obstet Gynecol 1979 Jan; 133(1):34–39

Gibbs R. Clinical risk factors for puerperal infection. Obstet Gynecol 1980 May; 55(5):178–184

Hanson MS. Abortion in teenagers. Clin Obstet Gynecol 1978 Dec; 21(4):1175–1190

Haukkamaa M et al. Screening, management and outcome of pregnancy in diabetic mothers. Obstet Gynecol 1980 June; 55(5):596–602

Jones MB. Hypertensive disorders of pregnancy. JOGN Nurs 1979 Mar/Apr; 8(2):92–96

Ledger WJ. Bacterial infections complicating pregnancy. Clin Obstet Gynecol 1978 June; 21(2):455–475

Longo LD. Environmental pollution and pregnancy: Risks and uncertainties for the fetus and infant. Am J Obstet Gynecol 1980 May; 137(2)162–173

Luke B. Understanding pica in pregnant women. Am J Mat Child Nurs 1977 Mar/Apr; 2(2):97–100

Marchant DJ. Urinary tract infections in pregnancy. Clin Obstet Gynecol 1978 Sept; 21(3)921–927

Mocarski V. Asymptomatic bacteriuria: A silent problem in pregnant women. Am J Mat Child Nurs 1980 July/Aug; 5(4):238–241

Neutra RP et al. Effects of fetal monitoring on neonatal death rates. N Engl J Med 1978 Aug 17; 299(7):324–326

Nyman JES. Thrombophlebitis in pregnancy. Am J Nurs 1980 Jan; 80(1):90–93

Pardue S. Hydatidiform mole: A pathological pregnancy. Am J Nurs 1977 May; 77(5):836–838

Rosen S. Pathology of renal disease during pregnancy. Clin Obstet Gynecol 1978 Sept; 21(3):875–880

Ryan GM and Schneider JM. Teenage obstetric complications. Clin Obstet Gynecol 1978 Dec; 21(4):1191–1199

Schular K. When a pregnant woman is diabetic: Antepartal care. Am J Nurs 1979 Mar; 79(3):448–450

Sever JL. Viral infections in pregnancy. Clin Obstet Gynecol 1978 June; 21(2):477–487

Ueland K. Cardiovascular disease complicating pregnancy. Clin Obstet Gynecol 1978 June; 21(2):429–442

Vogel M. When a pregnant woman is diabetic: Care of the newborn. Am J Nurs 1979 Mar; 79(3):458–460

Wimberly D. When a pregnant woman is diabetic: Intrapartal care. Am J Nurs 1979 Mar; 79(3):451–456

PEDIATRIC NURSING

PART 4

33

PEDIATRIC HISTORY TAKING

Identifying Information

A. *Type of Information Needed*

1. Date and time
2. Hospital number, if known
3. Patient's name, address, phone number, birth date
4. Referring health care source (e.g., physician, nurse practitioner, health care agency, etc.)
5. Insurance data

B. *Method of Collecting Data*

1. Identify the "care person" in charge of the patient by name and relationship to patient; obtain care person's address and phone number, if different from those of the patient.
2. To make the informant feel more at ease, the questions should begin in a friendly, nonthreatening manner. Questions addressed to the parent should be phrased appropriately.
3. Casual, friendly responses or remarks on the part of the interviewer may also help break the ice.
   a. "Whoever takes care of this baby certainly does a good job."
   b. "That's a lovely outfit the baby is wearing." (Remember that families will often put a new dress or suit on a baby for a visit to a health care agency.)
4. Sometimes repeat the information in order to verify data. This will give you a better judgment of the care person's cooperation and reliability.

Chief Complaint

A. *Method of Recording*

1. Write an exact description of the complaint.
2. Use quotation marks to clearly indicate that the informant's words are being used. It is helpful to explain:
   a. "I'll write it down so there will be no mistake."
   b. "Let me read this back to you to be sure it is correct."
3. Quotation of the care person's exact words may give an indication of how he/she feels about the symptoms; may reflect fear, guilt, defensiveness, etc.

B. *Method of Collecting Information*

1. Begin with a helpful question. That is the first overture made to this patient.

a. "How may I help you?"
b. "Please tell me the reason for your coming here today."
c. "What do you think is wrong with the baby?"
2. Avoid confusing questions that may elicit funny-sounding or "smart" answers.
   a. "What brings you here?" (Answer: "The bus.")
   b. "Why are you here?" ("That's what I came to find out.")

C. *Duration of Complaint*

1. The information obtained may indicate the natural history of the disease, if one is present, and its gradual evolution. Pursue the information with a series of probing questions.
   a. "How long has the baby (child) had this problem?"
   b. If the informant cannot remember, try another route.
      "When did he last act well?"
      "Do you remember last Christmas? Did the baby have the trouble then?"
2. Write down the responses; try to assess, as more questions are asked, how accurate the informant's answers may be.

History of Present Illness

A. *Type of Information Needed*

When patient is an infant or a preverbal child, information will consist mainly of what the informant has been able to observe. Having established what the chief complaint is, identify further problems, if any. Obtain the following information for each problem:
1. Body location—of pain, itching, weakness, etc.
2. Quality of complaint—both type (a burning pain) and severity (knife-like, comes and goes).
3. Degree of symptom—(e.g., pain, how severe; cough, day and night; eye drainage, how much).
4. Chronology—indicate time sequence and whether problem is episodic (lasts for a while and then clears up completely).
5. Environment or setting—where and when the symptoms occur.
6. Aggravating and alleviating factors—what makes the pain worse or better?
7. Associated manifestations or symptoms—accompanied by vomiting, blurred vision, etc.

B. *Importance of Detail*

1. A carefully written description of a symptom will frequently be the source of a future diagnosis and will serve all who are involved in helping the patient.
2. Do not worry about large volume of notes at first.
3. You will be able to recheck this information when you do the review of systems.

Past History

A. *Prenatal*

1. Pregnancy—planned or not; source of care; date (approximate) of seeking care; birth order of this pregnancy, including miscarriages. This area of the history may be one of great sensitivity. Try to make the questions gentle and supportive.
   a. "Did you plan a baby around this time?"
   b. "When did you manage to get your first check-up for the pregnancy?"
2. Maternal health—includes illnesses and dates, abnormal symptoms, e.g., fever, rash, vaginal bleeding, edema, hypertension, urine abnormalities, venereal disease. Avoid technical words, if possible.
   a. "Did you have trouble with swollen feet?"
   b. "Were your rings tight?"
   c. "Do you know if your blood pressure went up?"
   d. "Did you have trouble with your urine?"
3. Weight gain—Validate by trying to get a figure for nonpregnant weight and weight at delivery.
4. Medicines taken—e.g., vitamins, iron, calcium, aspirin, cold preparations, tranquilizers (nerve medicine), antibiotics; use of ointments, hormones, injections during pregnancy, special or unusual diet, radiation exposure, sonography, amniocentesis.
5. Quality of the fetal movements; when felt, how brisk.

B. *Natal*

1. Expected date of delivery and approximate duration of pregnancy.
2. Place of delivery and who conducted the delivery.
3. Labor—spontaneous or induced; duration and intensity.
4. Analgesia or anesthesia.
5. Presentation—vaginal, breech, or vertex; C-section; forceps.
6. Episiotomy.
7. Complications, e.g., blood transfusion, delay in delivery, etc.

C. *Neonatal*

1. Condition of infant
2. Color (if seen) at delivery
3. Activity of infant
4. Crying heard
5. Breathing abnormality
6. Birth weight and length
7. Problems occurring immediately at birth

D. *Postnatal*

1. Duration of hospitalization of mother and infant
2. Problems with baby's breathing or feeding
3. Need of supportive care; e.g., oxygen, incubator, special care nursery, isolation, medications
4. Weight changes, weight at discharge if known
5. Color—cyanosis or jaundiced
6. Bowel movements—when
7. Problems—seizures, deformities identified, consultation required
8. Mother's contact with the baby and her first impression
   a. "How did the baby look to you?"
   b. "What did the baby do when you were first together?"

E. *Nutrition*

1. Breast or bottle fed; what formula? how prepared?
2. Amounts offered and consumed
3. Frequency of feeding; weight gain
4. Addition of juice and/or solid foods
5. Food preferences or allergies
6. Feeding problems—variations in appetite
7. Age of weaning
8. Vitamins—type, amount, regularity
9. Pattern of weight gain
10. Current diet; frequency and content of meals

F. *Growth and Development*

1. Past weights and lengths if available
2. Milestones—sat alone unsupported; walked alone; used words, then sentences
3. Teeth—eruption, difficulty, cavities
4. Toilet training
5. Current motor, social, and language skills
6. Sexual development
   a. Infant—swollen breast tissue, vaginal discharge, hypertrophy of the labia
   b. Toddler or school child—early development of breasts or pubic hair
   c. Prepubertal or pubertal child—in females, time of development of breasts, pubic hair; onset of menstruation. In males, time of enlargement of testes, penis; development of pubic and facial hair; voice changes; acne

G. *Health Maintenance*

1. Immunizations—smallpox, rubella, rubeola, mumps, polio, diphtheria, pertussis, tetanus toxoid, BCG, influenza
   Indicate number and dates.
2. Screening Procedures—hematocrit, tuberculin testing, visual and auditory acuity, rubella antibodies, syphilis testing, gonorrhea screen, Pap smear
3. Dental Care—source and frequency of care, dental hygienist visits, fillings or extractions

H. *Acute Infectious Diseases*

   Rubella, rubeola, mumps, chicken pox, scarlet fever, rheumatic fever, hepatitis, infectious mononucleosis, venereal disease, tuberculosis. Recent exposure to communicable disease.

I. *Hospitalizations and Operations*

1. Dates, hospital, physician
2. Indications, diagnosis, procedures
3. Complications

J. *Injuries*

1. Emergency room visits—frequency and diagnosis
2. Fractures—location and treatment
3. Trauma, burns, bruises
4. Ingestions

K. *Medications*

1. For general use such as vitamins, antihistamines, laxatives
2. Special or fad diets
3. Recent antibiotics
4. Routine use of aspirin
5. Oral contraceptives—types and dose, duration
6. Drugs, narcotics, marijuana, hallucinogens, mood elevators, tranquilizers

L. *Radiation*

1. Diagnosis requiring, number and occasion of exposures
2. Accidental exposure
3. Routine x-rays (chest, dental)
4. For injury, follow-up of fracture, etc.

Personal History

A. *Type of Information Needed*
1. Hygiene, exercise
2. Activities and hobbies, special talents
3. Friends
4. Sibling and parent relationships
5. Expression of emotions
   a. Blows up easily
   b. Rather quiet
6. Idiosyncratic behavior and habits, e.g., thumb sucking, nail biting, temper tantrums, head banging, pica, breath holding, rituals, tics, etc.

B. *Method of Collecting Data*
1. Straightforward questions to a child, e.g., "What grade are you in?" "Who are your friends?"
2. Three wishes offered to the child:
   a. "If Christmas were here, what would you ask for?"
   b. "If you had your way, who would you like to be?"
   c. "What would be the best thing that could happen to you?"
3. "Who's your best friend?"

School History

A. *Type of Information Needed*
1. Present and past schooling, grade, and performance
2. Favored and least favored subjects
3. School-related behavior—anxious to go, anxious to stay home
4. General attitude towards school and any career plans

B. *Method of Collecting Data*

Emphasize the positive, e.g., "What's your best subject?" "Have you repeated a grade?" "Do you see your friends after school?"

Social History

A. *Type of Information Needed*
1. Environment—rural, urban
2. Housing—type, location, heating, sewage, water supply, family pets, other animal exposure
3. Parents' occupations (employment) and marital status
4. Number of individuals living in home, sleeping arrangements
5. Any religious affiliations
6. Utilization of social agencies previously
7. Health insurance and usual source of care

B. *Method of Collecting Data*

Parents are a proud race, so be careful with some of the questions. Ask permission.

1. "Can you tell me a little bit about your home?"
2. "I need to know more about how you live in order to help you with your child's problem."

Review of Systems

A. *Type of Information Needed*
1. General—activity, appetite, affect, sleep patterns, weight changes, edema, fever
2. Allergy—eczema, hay fever, asthma, hives, food or drug allergy, sinus disorders
3. Skin—rash or eruption, nodules, pigmentation or texture change, sweating or dryness, infection, hair growth, itching
4. Head—headache, head trauma, dizziness
5. Eyes—visual acuity, corrective lenses, strabismus, lacrimation, discharge, itching, redness, photophobia
6. Ears—auditory acuity, earaches (frequency), infection, drainage
7. Nose—cold and runny nose (frequency), infection, drainage
8. Teeth—hygiene practices, general condition
9. Throat—sore throat, tonsillitis, difficulty swallowing
10. Speech—peculiarity of or change in voice; hoarseness, clarity, enunciation, stammering
11. Respiratory—difficulty breathing, shortness of breath, chest pain, cough, wheezing, croup, pneumonia, TB or exposure
12. Cardiovascular—cyanosis, fainting, exercise intolerance, murmurs
13. Hematologic—pallor, anemia, tendency to bruise or bleed
14. Gastrointestinal—appetite (amount, frequency, cravings), nausea, vomiting, abdominal pain, abnormal size, bowel habits and nature of stools, parasites, encopresis (incontinence of feces), colic
15. Genitourinary—age of toilet training, frequency of urination, straining, dysuria, hematuria (or unusual color or odor of infant's soiled diaper), previous urinary tract infection, enuresis; urethral or vaginal discharge. Females: last menses, cramps, changes in interval and duration.
16. Musculoskeletal—deformities, fractures, sprains, joint pains or swelling, limitation of motion, abnormality of nails
17. Neurologic—weakness or clumsiness, coordination, balance, gait, dominance, fatigability, tone, tremor. Seizures or paroxysmal behavior. Personality changes.

BIBLIOGRAPHY

Books

Alexander M and Brown M. Pediatric History Taking and Physical Diagnosis for Nurses, New York, McGraw–Hill, 1979

Bernstein L, Bernstein RS, Dana RH. Interviewing: A Guide for Health Professionals, 3rd ed. New York, Appleton–Century–Crofts, 1980

Department of Medicine and Department of Pediatrics. Clinical History and Physical Examination. Baltimore, Johns Hopkins University School of Medicine, 1976

Elstein A et al. Medical Problem Solving: An Analysis of Clinical Reasoning. Cambridge, Mass, Harvard University Press, 1978

Enelow A and Swisler S. Interviewing and Patient Care. New York, Oxford University Press, 1979

Ferholt JD. Clinical Assessment of Children: A Comprehensive Approach to Primary Pediatric Care. Philadelphia, JB Lippincott, 1980

Weed LL. Medical Records, Medical Education and Patient Care: The Problem Oriented Record as a Basic Tool. Cleveland, Case Western Reserve University Press, 1969

Articles

Harris R. Facilitating change to the problem-oriented medical record system. J Nurs Admin 1978 Aug; 8(8):35–38

Margolis C. Effects of the problem-oriented record system on care in a pediatric clinic. Pediatr Res 1979 Sept; 13(9):1047–1051

Ruth D. An integrated family-oriented problem-oriented medical record. J Fam Pract 1979 June; 8(6):1179–1184

Schneggenberger C. History-taking skills: How do you rate? Nursing '79 1979 Mar; 9(3):97–101

General Principles

1. Establish the order of all data collection according to the needs of the patients. For example:
   a. An exhausted mother with a screaming baby will not give a careful comprehensive history.
   b. Alternative care may not be available for preschoolers when the newborn comes in for the first check.
2. If the mother has come in with more than 1 child, try to organize some supervision of the other children so that you can have a little time with the mother alone.
3. Remember that the safest place for any child is on the mother's knee. Privacy may not be possible because of the presence of other children.
4. Attempt to develop rapport with the young patient from the moment you first see or meet him or her.

Approach to the Patient

1. Begin the examination with the patient on the mother's knee.
2. To evaulate the chest properly, you need to listen through 10 heartbeats when the child is not screaming; therefore, the chest is a good place to begin the examination.
3. The part to be examined should be completely exposed, but if an apprehensive child objects to having his clothes removed, slip your stethoscope under the shirt.
4. Forget the orderly and systematic approach, but remember to examine everything. Fortunately, children are small and one can check several systems very quickly over a small area.
5. As you examine each region, be aware that everything is confined to a small space.
6. Gradually remove the child's clothes, if you can; look for asymmetry very carefully in the bodies of all children.
7. Develop a pattern appropriate to the patient's age.
   a. Whistling is a great distraction.
   b. Keep a small music box or toy readily available.
8. A cold stethoscope may result in a frightened and screaming child, so warm the stethoscope before bringing it into contact with the child.

Equipment

1. Have equipment ready and in working order before beginning.
2. Equipment is similar to that used in the adult physical examination:

Thermometer	Stethoscope
Oto-ophthalmoscope	Reflex hammer
Flashlight	Tuning fork
Tongue depressor	Disposable gloves
Cotton applicator stick	Lubricant

3. Additional equipment:
    Sphygmomanometer cuffs in different sizes
    Denver Developmental Test materials (see p. 1090)
    Items for distraction—music box, toys

Vital Signs

Vital signs will vary; they require careful evaluation in children. Excitement, crying, feeding, the need to burp, all make a difference in color, respiration, and pulse rate.

If an abnormality is found, recheck a few minutes later when the baby is quiet, if possible.

BODY TEMPERATURE (oral, rectal, infrequently axillary)

1. Delay until end of examination for younger child, who will be upset by technique.
2. Oral temperature
    a. Is inaccurate, especially in child who will not hold thermometer under tongue.
    b. Requires about 8 minutes to get an accurate temperature.

BLOOD PRESSURE

1. Use the correct cuff size:
    a. For the upper arm, cuff should be no more than ⅔ of the distance between the elbow and the shoulder and no less than ½ of this length.
    b. Standard cuff sizes are 6.25 cm. (2.5 inches), 12.5 cm. (5 inches), 20.0 cm. (8 inches) and 30.0 cm. (12 inches).
2. Record the point at which the sounds are first heard, the point at which these sounds become muffled, and the point at which they disappear.

PULSE

1. Palpate radial pulses in both arms, noting rate and equality at the wrist.
2. To obtain strip rate from the ECG, multiply by 20 the number of complexes between 2 vertical lines (3 seconds) at the top of the strip. If the rate is slow or irregular, a more accurate reflection of rate is obtained by multiplying by 10 the number of complexes between 3 vertical lines (6 seconds).
3. Record atrial and ventricular rates when AV block is present

RESPIRATORY RATE

1. Count and record while the child is quiet, if possible.
2. Remember that younger children and infants mainly use the diaphragm, not the intercostal muscles, so that the abdomen tends to rise and fall as they breathe in and out.

RECTAL TEMPERATURE—is the best and most accurate

Normal—around 37° C. (98.6° F.)
Fluctuations are due to:
a. Too much or too little clothing.
b. Excessive activity (child racing around clinic).
c. Ingestion of hot or cold drink within previous 30 minutes.

NORMAL BLOOD PRESSURE FOR VARIOUS AGES

Ages	Mean systolic ± 2 S.D.	Mean diastolic ± 2 S.D.
Newborn	80 ± 16	46 ± 16
6 months–1 year	89 ± 29	60 ± 10
1 year	96 ± 30	66 ± 25
2 years	99 ± 25	64 ± 25
3 years	100 ± 25	67 ± 23
4 years	99 ± 20	65 ± 20
5–6 years	94 ± 14	55 ± 9
6–7 years	100 ± 15	56 ± 8
8–9 years	105 ± 16	57 ± 9
9–10 years	107 ± 16	57 ± 9
10–11 years	111 ± 17	58 ± 10
11–12 years	113 ± 18	59 ± 10
12–13 years	115 ± 19	59 ± 10
13–14 years	118 ± 19	60 ± 10

(Adapted from Haggerty, R. J., et al: Essential hypertension in infancy and childhood. AMA Journal of Diseases of Children, 92:536, 1956. Copyright 1956, American Medical Association.)

HEART RATE AT VARIOUS AGES

Age	Heart Rate	
	Mean	*Range*
0–24 hours	145	80–200
1–7 days	138	100–188
8–30 days	162	125–188
1–3 months	161	115–215
3–6 months	149	100–215
6–12 months	147	100–188
1–3 years	130	80–188
3–5 years	105	68–150
5–8 years	105	68–150
8–12 years	88	51–125
12–16 years	83	38–125

(Adapted from Ziegler, RF: Electrocardiographic Studies in Normal Infants and Children. Springfield, Charles C Thomas; from a table appearing originally in Homans J: A Textbook of Surgery, 6th ed. Courtesy of Charles C Thomas, Publisher, Springfield, Ill.)

Age	Normal Respirations
Newborn	30–50
6 months	20–30
2 years	20–30
Adolescent	12–20

TECHNIQUE		*FINDINGS*

STANDING HEIGHT, HEAD CIRCUMFERENCE, AND CHEST CIRCUMFERENCE

1. Must be measured accurately (use tape measure).

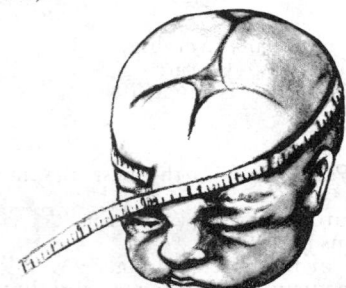

HEAD AND CHEST CIRCUMFERENCE

Age	Head Circumference		Chest Circumference	
Yr. Mo.	Inch	Cm.	Inch	Cm.
Birth	13.8	35.0	13.0	33.0
3	15.9	40.4	15.8	40.2
6	17.1	43.4	17.1	43.4
9	17.8	45.3	18.0	45.7
1–0	18.3	46.6	18.6	47.3
1–6	18.9	47.9	19.4	49.2
2–0	19.3	48.9	19.8	50.4
3–0	19.6	49.8	20.6	52.5
3–6	—	—	20.8	52.8
4–0	19.8	50.4	21.0	53.4
5–0	20.0	50.8	21.5	54.6

(From Studies at Harvard School of Public Health.)

2. Increments of growth are as important as the basic measurements.
3. Weight should be recorded at every visit.

General Appearance

1. Begin observations with the first contact with the patient, taking into account that there are at least 2 people to observe (child and parent).
2. The patient's interaction with the caretaker, whether it be the mother, a baby-sitter, an older sibling, or a friend of the family, is vital in the assessment of the child.

As you observe for race, sex, general physical development, nutritional state, mental alertness, evidence of pain, restlessness, body position, clothes, apparent age, hygiene, and grooming, remember that many of these things are part of the parent's caretaking.

1. If the child is easily distracted or sleepy, it may be naptime.
2. Careful observation of the general state of the child will provide many clues about the child's relationship to the family and their response to the child.

Skin

Examine as you move through each body region. (Include hair as well as skin.)

Inspection
Inspection of the skin is the same as for the adult (see p. 20).

1. Observe for: skin color, pigmentation, lesions, jaundice, cyanosis, scars, superficial vascularity, moisture, edema, color of mucous membranes, hair distribution.
2. Describe any variation in color, particularly in children with increased pigmentation. Absence of pigment, or vitiligo, in darker children can be noted.
3. Birthmarks of any type are recorded. (May change as child grows older.)
4. Bruises or unusual marks of any kind, wounds or insect bites, scratch marks, scars, etc., may have particular significance.
5. Draw a picture of anything unusual like a scar, and measure the dimensions of the lesion when recording the findings.
6. To ascertain suspected jaundice, take the child to the window to get a true picture of the color of the skin.
(A room with yellow walls and artificial lighting may create a wrong impression when jaundice is suspected.)

1. In young babies, the skin is soft, smooth, velvety in texture.

2. Pigmentations vary in children, depending on race, and will change as child gets older.

3. A suntan, freckles, small, light-brown patches or café-au-lait spots may occur.
4. Bruises are particularly important because of possibility of child abuse.

5. If you have difficulty in describing something, use ordinary words rather than inaccurate technical terms.
6. Carotenemia, which causes the nose and palms of the hands to have a yellowish tinge, may lead the parents to suspect jaundice; however, carotenemia is due to eating an excessive amount of yellow vegetables (carrots, sweet potatoes, squash, etc.). In carotenemia, the sclerae are clear; this is not so in jaundice.

TECHNIQUE	**FINDINGS**

TECHNIQUE

7. The skin of newborn infants will still be covered with vernix caseosa, the oily material that covers the fetus's body while in utero.

8. Postmature infants may have scaliness which persists for several weeks after birth, particularly around the feet. The color of the skin may change as the child gets a little older.

9. Note the presence of striae.

Palpation

1. Use the tips of the fingers to palpate. (Fingertips are more sensitive.)

2. Feel the tension of the skin by pinching up a fold of skin.
Normal skin quickly falls back, but dehydrated skin remains in the pinched position.

3. Feel the skin for texture, moisture, temperature, turgor, elasticity, masses, tenderness.

NAILS

1. Observe for color, shape, irregularities in surface and general nail care—cleanliness, evidence of biting, etc.

2. Check the angle between the nails and the finger, normally about 160 degrees.

3. Palpate the skin around the fingernails for firmness. Palpate any part that appears inflamed.

HAIR

1. Observe for color and distribution.
   a. Note according to the age of the child and race.
   b. Be aware that tufts of hair over the spine or sacral area may mark an underlying abnormality.

2. Note any change in pigmentation.

3. Palpate the hair for texture and thickness.

4. Examine to see if there are any patches where hair is missing on the head.

5. Separate thick hair on the head to get a good view of the scalp. Check for dandruff or scaliness in older children.

6. Check scalp for any signs of lice infestation.

7. Inspect in the axillae and over the pubis as well as the extremities for the presence and quantity of hair, to gauge the development and level of puberty.

FINDINGS

7. Swollen sebaceous glands over the nose and chin are frequently seen right after birth and are called *milia*.

8. The blotchy, pink patches over the eyelid, bridge of the nose and the back of the neck may persist until the child is nearly two.

9. May indicate rapid weight gain.

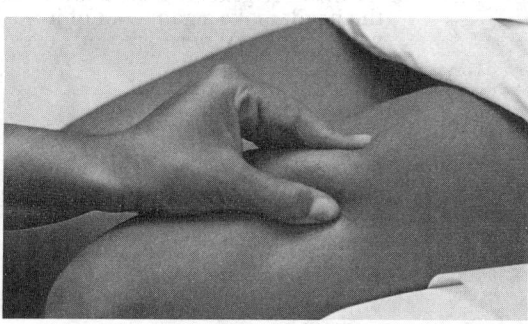

3. Skin that is rough and dry in texture may actually have a discrete rash that can be felt but not seen.

1. The nailbeds should be pink, the nails convex.

2. The nail should not be split, infected, or bitten

3. General care of the child is frequently reflected in good care of the nails.

1. *Newborn:* Normally varies from no hair to a thick bush.
   Infant: Consists of lanugo, a soft, downy covering frequently seen over the shoulders, back, arms, face, and sacral area, especially in dark-skinned children.
   Race: Variations in hairiness.

2. Remember, children frequently experiment with mother's hair dye or rinse.

3. Texture may be thick or thin, coarse or fine, straight or curly.

4. May denote underlying skin infection; however, some children pull their hair out; sometimes the hair is braided so tightly that it falls out.

5. Look carefully for broken hairs, for scaliness on the scalp or cradle cap in infants.

6. Nits (louse eggs) appear on the hair as little white dots. Lice may be seen on the scalp; they move quickly and may jump.

7. The child need not be totally undressed; a prepubertal child will usually be embarrassed if all of his or her clothes are removed.

<table>
<tr><td>**TECHNIQUE**</td><td>**FINDINGS**</td></tr>
</table>

Head and Neck

1. Unless specifically requested to do otherwise, examine the eyes and ears at the very last, especially in the younger child.
2. Also, examine the throat toward the last, unless the child exhibits concern about the "throat stick." It is then best to examine the throat right away in order to "get it over with."
3. To avoid frightening the child when palpating the head, make a game out of it—ask "Where's your nose?" "Where are your eyes?"

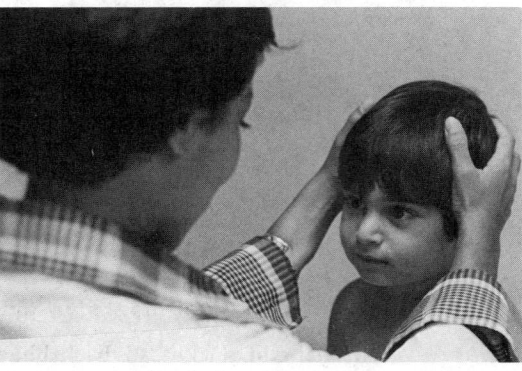

Head Shape in Newborns and Infants

Inspection

1. Observe the face and skull for asymmetry, deformity, and abnormal or limited movements.

1. A baby's head may be asymmetrical due to pressure during pregnancy and delivery.

   The rounded head of the baby born by breech delivery contrasts with the long, pointed head of a baby who is a firstborn and whose head was moulded during a prolonged labor.

2. Closely observe facial expressions, blinking, etc., if the child is not crying. This may be one of your few moments to see the child when he is not crying.
   If you are examining a crying baby, watch particularly for asymmetry of the face.

2. In a baby born by forceps delivery, there may be signs of weakness of the facial nerve caused by pressure of the forceps over the front of the ear where the facial nerve emerges. When the baby cries, the involved side will show weakness and downturning of the mouth.

3. Observe the movement of the head on the neck as the baby looks around. When turning an infant over, observe the head for control, position, and movement.

3. There should be very little head lag beyond the age of 3 months.

4. Since an infant's neck is often short and there are often several folds of skin under the chin, it is necessary to lift the chin a little to observe the skin completely—to see that it is clear and free of perspiration rash or irritation.

4. In the back, the neck should be free of webbing or extra folds of skin extending from just beneath the ear toward the shoulder.

Palpation

1. Palpate the skull for the fontanelles and suture lines. Feel the face for any masses, noting size, consistency, surface, temperature, and tenderness.

1. The suture lines of the skull may be felt to override as a result of the pressure applied when contractions occurred during labor. This is usually most marked between the frontal and the parietal bone where the coronal suture

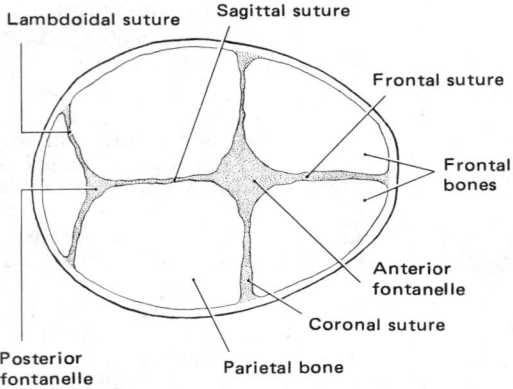

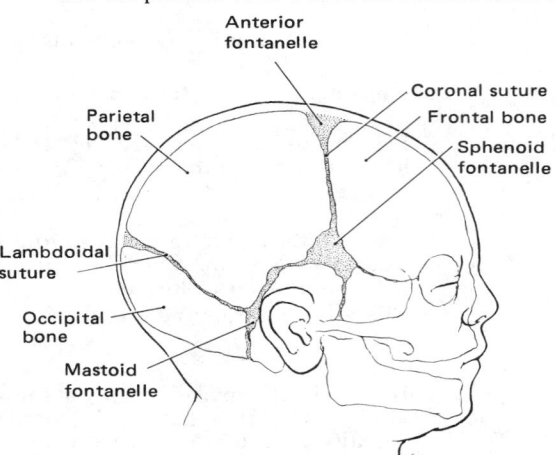

TECHNIQUE	**FINDINGS**

2. Measure the anterior fontanelle for size.
3. Palpate along the lambdoidal suture at the back of the head between the parietal bones and the occipital bone.
4. Palpate the neck for swollen lymph nodes, noting tenderness, mobility, location, and consistency.

4. Palpation of the lymph nodes may reveal slightly enlarged nodes in the anterior cervical chain secondary to sore throat.

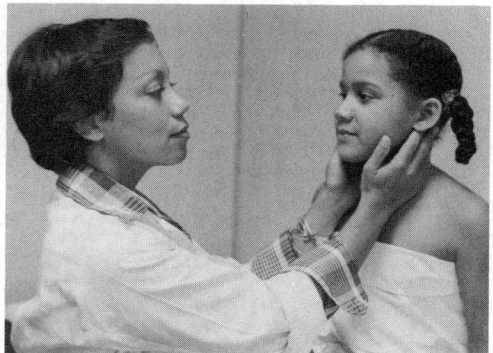

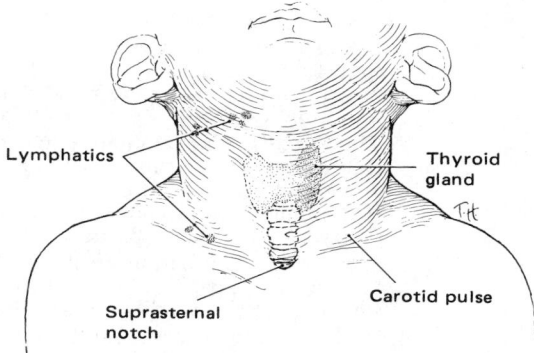

5. Note that there are other nodes, which are normally not palpable.

5. These include the pre- and postauricular, the posterior cervical (behind the sternomastoid), the submental and submandibular (under the jaw), and the occipital nodes (along the prominence of the occiput).

6. Feel the pulses in the neck for location, strength, and equality.
7. Check the thyroid for enlargement, position, texture, and tenderness.
8. Locate the trachea in the suprasternal notch for position in the center of the neck.

Percussion
1. Percussion of the face may elicit tenderness over the sinuses.
2. Percuss over the head and neck directly with the fingertips, usually the middle finger of the right hand.
3. Percuss over the forehead for tenderness in the sinuses and across the zygoma, or cheekbone.

1. Tenderness may be due to a tooth cavity.
2. Gentle tapping over the skull elicits a typical noise when the sutures are open and a different sound when the sutures are closed.
3. This is to determine underlying tenderness in the maxillary sinus.

Auscultation
Auscultate the skull and carotid arteries in the neck.

To determine presence of bruits.

Eye and Vision

Equipment

Ophthalmoscope and pen light. Be sure batteries are new and lights are bright.

Inspection
(Similar to adult examination; p. 21)
1. Pay particular attention to the lacrimal duct.

1. Discharge from the eyes along the lower lid or from the lacrimal duct can occur as a result of infection or reaction to silver nitrate administered to the neonate.

2. Note the distance between the eyes and the distribution of the eyebrows.

2. Hypertelorism denotes a wider area between the eyes than normal. Excessively long and full eyebrows that meet in the midline and extra long eyelashes may signify a developmental abnormality.

TECHNIQUE	FINDINGS

3. Test the eyes for light perception.

3. It is difficult to prevent children from blinking their eyes or closing them when testing light response.

Palpation

If the child is old enough, have him squeeze his eyes tightly. (Not possible in younger children.)

Weakness of the muscles around the eyes is difficult to demonstrate in the young child. Muscle strength or weakness can be evaluated when the child cries.

Fundoscopic Examination

1. Check to see that the child's eyes move in conjugate fashion.
Ask the mother if she has noticed any signs of squinting, especially when the child is tired.

2. This is a difficult examination to conduct since children tend to watch the light and stare directly at you, which constricts their pupils. If the child cannot cooperate, it may be necessary to dilate the pupil to see the fundus.

3. Start your examination at about ⅓ meter (1 foot) from the patient. Look for the red reflex, which should be readily observable.

4. Look for any opacities and then slowly approach the patient, turning the ophthalmoscopic dial to the smaller plus (+) numbers. Start originally at +8 to +10.
(Wearing glasses or contact lenses may make a difference in the type of lens you use in the ophthalmoscope.)

5. To help guide your gaze, put your hand on top of the child's head, with your thumb at the corner of the eye at the outer edge. If you lose the fundus, you can return to your thumb and get your bearings by directing your gaze medial to the tip of your thumbnail.

1. Loss of vision can occur if the eyes are not working together properly. Squinting can indicate vision problems.

2. A picture can be pinned to the wall opposite the child, who is then instructed to look at the picture during the examination. If the child is examined while lying down, a picture can be placed on the ceiling.

4. The red reflex is diminished if there is something obstructing your view. A cataract or an opacity in the retina can cause this, as would a tumor filling the posterior chamber. If there is any paleness in the red reflex or difficulty in identifying it, a consultation should be sought immediately.

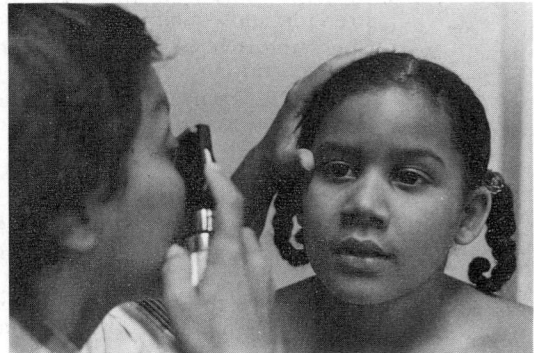

Ear and Hearing

Equipment

Tuning fork and otoscope
Small speculum for child's ear

Fresh batteries to assure a bright light

Inspection

1. When examining the external ear, the auricle, or the pinna, be sure to note the position of the ear.
The top of the ear should cross an imaginary line drawn between the edge of the eye and the back of the occiput. If the ear is positioned more obliquely or is low-set, some underlying abnormality, particularly of the genitourinary system, may be present.

2. If you cannot get the child to cooperate by offering an explanation or by playing a game, the child will have to be restrained.

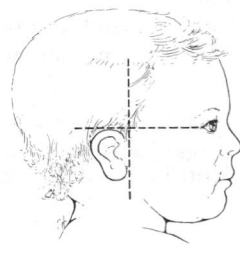

TECHNIQUE	**FINDINGS**

a. The child can be seated on the mother's knee with the child's legs wedged between her knees and the head held firmly with one hand while the baby's hands are controlled with the other hand.

b. An older child may be held in a supine position, with the mother holding the child's arms above the head and controlling the head.

c. If the child is very restless and apprehensive, examine the child from the top while the mother leans over the child's body, holds the arms down with her elbows, and at the same time grasps the child's head with her hands.

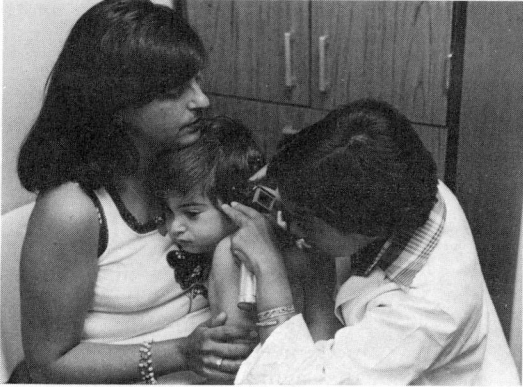

If the child is in a supine position, be sure to remove the shoes, because some children will kick when frightened.

Inspection with Otoscope

1. Hold the otoscope gently with the handle between the thumb and forefinger. This will enable you to control the head of the otoscope while keeping your hand steady on the child's head.

2. With your free hand, pull the pinna back and slightly upward to straighten the canal. Examine the canal.

3. Inspect the eardrum and test for mobility by means of the pneumatoscope (the tube attachment of the otoscope).

   a. Attach one end of the tube to the otoscope and place the other end in your mouth.

   b. Blow gently through the tube.
   By blowing through plastic tubing it is possible to see the normal eardrum move back and forth. If the eardrum does not move, this may be indicative of infection behind the drum (serous otitis media).

   c. This method is preferred to the squeeze bulb because it allows for greater control of the force with which the air is introduced into the ear.

   d. The normal ear drum moves slightly when a soft breath is blown into the ear canal.

1. Small children will jerk about, so be careful not to push the speculum into the drum.

2. Cerumen or wax may interfere with your view of the eardrum.

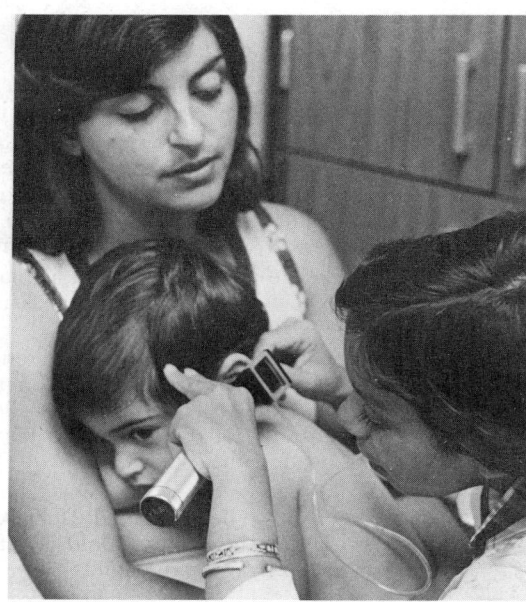

Palpation

Palpate behind the ear over the mastoid process.

Mechanical

1. Most children will be able to respond to a test of gross hearing.

2. More specific tests using an electric screening device are used prior to school age.

Tenderness behind the ear denotes infection. Sometimes a lymph node can be felt in this area.

A small bell, such as the kind found in the Denver kit, can be used to determine hearing ability by noting if the child stops moving when the bell is rung and turns his head toward the sound.

TECHNIQUE

Nose and Sinuses

Equipment

Nasoscope, small speculum

Inspection

1. Observe for general deformity.
2. With nasoscope, examine nasal septum, mucous membranes and turbinates, and for discharge and nasal obstruction (see Adult Physical Examination, p. 24).
3. Check for presence of any foreign body. Always remember that any child who has a "strange" odor may have a foreign body in the nose or ear. (In a female child, do not forget the vagina.)
4. Look for scratch marks about the nose and be alert to a child picking his nose.

Palpation

Palpate the sinuses, remembering the order of development.

Mouth and Throat

Equipment

Penlight, tongue depressor

1. Shining the light into the mouth or around the lips and teeth is not a threatening gesture.
2. However, the tongue blade, which is used to press against the inside of the cheek to allow for examination of the mucous membranes and which is also used to push the tongue out of the way, is a threatening instrument.
3. When the tongue depressor is placed on the tongue it can have the unpleasant effect of making the child gag.
4. To avoid this unpleasant occurrence, encourage the child to stick out his tongue, breathe deeply, and say "ah." This may allow for easy visualization of the palate and uvula, without the need of the "stick."
5. If these steps are not feasible, then the child may need to be restrained. If such is the case, examining the throat should be left to last, so as not to frighten the child.

Inspection

1. Observe the lips, noting the color. (Remember that cyanosis is difficult to detect in a black child.)

2. Count the teeth and note any extra or missing teeth, and any evidence of caries, staining, tartar, and malocclusion.

FINDINGS

2. Dry mucous membranes may bleed and cause clots of blood to form in the nares. Scratches may also occur if child picks at nose or scratches when itching occurs.
3. A foreign body in the nose will cause a foul odor, purulent discharge, and may possibly cause bleeding.

4. Children frequently have "itchy" noses.

Sinuses develop in a set order; the ethmoid and maxillary sinuses are present at birth; the frontal sinus develops at around 7, and the sphenoid after puberty.

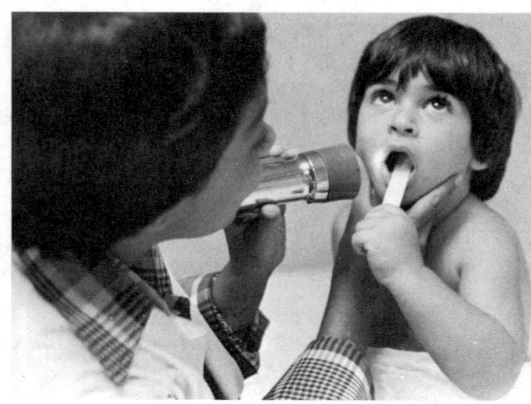

A child may also be allowed to place the tongue blade directly on his own tongue while you guide him with your hand.

1. *Infants:* There may be a protuberance on the upper lip, the so-called "sucking blister."

Children: May have dry lips and redness around the lips due to an allergy or to some such activity as blowing bubble gum.

TECHNIQUE

Time of eruption of deciduous teeth

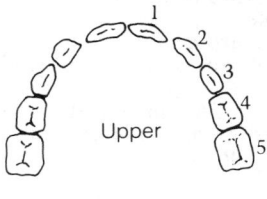

Upper

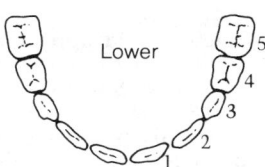

Lower

		(Upper)	(Lower)
1	Central incisor	8–12 mos.	5–9 mos.
2	Lateral incisor	8–12 mos.	12–18 mos.
3	Cuspid		18–24 mos.
4	First molar		12–18 mos.
5	Second molar		24–30 mos.

FINDINGS

Time of eruption of permanent teeth

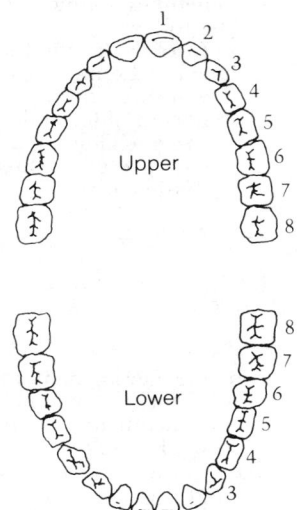

Upper

Lower

		(Upper)	(Lower)
1	Central incisor	6–7 yr.	7–8 yr.
2	Lateral incisor	7–8 yr.	8–9 yr.
3	Cuspid	9–10 yr.	11–12 yr.
4	First bicuspid	10–11 yr.	10–11 yr.
5	Second bicuspid	11–12 yr.	10–12 yr.
6	First molar	6–7 yr.	6–7 yr.
7	Second molar	11–13 yr.	12–13 yr.
8	Third molar	17 yr.	17–18 yr.

3. Check the gums for swelling and signs of easy bleeding. Also note mouth odor.
4. Check the tongue for movement, color, and the presence of taste buds on the surface. Check to see that the frenulum under the tongue is of the proper length.

5. As the gag reflex is elicited, note how the palate moves upward and the uvula springs into view.
6. Examine the roof of the mouth.

7. Inspect the height of the arch of the palate.

8. Note the tonsils on each side of the uvula and immediately posterior to it for position, surface, size, equality, and color.
9. As the baby cries, note the odor of the breath and any hoarseness of the voice; note difficulty on inspiration, as in croup, or wheezing on expiration.

Palpation

1. Palpate the lips and cheeks manually using a finger cot or glove.
2. Note any evidence of swelling.

4. If the frenulum is too short, the child may be tongue-tied (meaning that the baby cannot advance the tip of the tongue beyond the lips), although this is not thought to interfere with sucking or speech.
5. It should be midline and single, although occasionally it will be divided or bifid.

6. The roof of the mouth at the junction of the hard and soft palate will frequently reveal whitish lesions, or Epstein's pearls, which persist through infancy.
7. With experience, an unusually high arch is easily recognizable.
8. Any coating with pus or ulcers or a pocket or cryptic appearance should be recorded.

9. These signs may be indicative of throat and chest disturbances.

1. By comparing one side with the other, differences due to abnormality can be detected.

| *TECHNIQUE* | *FINDINGS* |

Breast and Thorax

1. Sometimes young children object to having their clothes removed.
2. The following approaches may overcome this problem:
   a. Distract the child by having him listen to a few heartbeats.
   b. Have the mother (while the child is on her knee) remove the underclothing while you stand by.
   c. For an older child entering puberty, provide an examining sheet, but stay in the room while the child puts on the gown, provided he or she is not embarrassed by your presence. During such preparation, you are able to make a superficial appraisal of the chest.

BREAST

1. Check to see if there are any small extra nipples present.	1. These would appear along a line extending from the anterior axillary line through the normal nipple down toward the symphysis pubis.
2. In the newborn infant the nipples appear a little darker than normal, and breast tissue underneath may form a small knot with occasional leakage of milk.	2. This leakage is a secondary effect of the hormone level in the mother; instruct the mother not to try to express the milk, because of the danger of infection.
3. In the older child a lump found under the nipple in either male or female may cause some concern for cancer.	3. Such lumps are usually secondary to hormone stimulation and occur toward puberty.
4. Occasionally, the breasts begin to develop earlier than normal, at around 5 or 6 years.	4. This should be a reason for referral to a physician.

THORAX

Inspection

1. Observe the entire thorax as the child breathes; note symmetry and equal expansion of both sides as the lungs inflate.	1. In babies and young children (especially an infant lying on mother's knee), diaphragm excursion is more marked than intercostal expansion. Thus the abdomen goes up and down more than the chest expands.
2. Confirm the respiratory rate as you observe the child with his shirt off.	

Percussion

Percussion of the child's chest is difficult. Because the underlying structures are crowded, not too much is elicited. The heart edge is difficult to outline, and percussing the chest is frightening.	Very light percussion is necessary; a hyperresonant note may be elicited over air, particularly of a stomach bubble which projects up into the left side of the chest.

Palpation

1. Use warmed hands as you palpate the shape and angle of the sternum. Note if there is any sinking in of the sternum.	1. The shape of the sternum may vary, although there may be a sinking in of the sternum (funnel sternum) which may cause subsequent trouble due to pressure on underlying structures. This should be referred to the pediatrician.
2. Palpate the costochondral junctions for tenderness and enlargement.	2. May suggest an underlying inflammatory response.
3. Warm the stethoscope before using by placing it in your pocket.	3. A cold stethoscope will startle the child and make him pull away.
4. As you palpate, hoarse sounds (as in bronchitis) may be felt through your hands.	4. Normal inspiration and expiration do not give a sensation under the fingers, except for the expansion of the chest.
5. Vocal fremitus is difficult to elicit in the smaller child since it is difficult to have him make repetitive sounds on command.	5. In the older child it is worth trying, in order to obtain transmission of sound through the lung tissue.

Auscultation

The difficulty with examining a child is that everything sounds muddled and mixed. The examiner has to sort out breathing which is rapid from a heart rate which is also rapid

TECHNIQUE	FINDINGS

and must also differentiate between inspiration and expiration and the 1st and 2nd heart sounds.

1. Try to examine a baby before he begins crying.

2. Be aware that breathing is louder in younger children with slightly increased length of inspiration, almost to the point of bronchovesicular breathing in the adult.

3. Rales with their fine crackling sound can also be heard much more easily in children.

1. Note, however, that crying increases lung expansion.

2. Bronchial breathing with equal inspiration and expiration is very loud and easy to hear if the patient has pneumonia.

3. Added coarse-quality sounds in the chest are commonly associated with mucus in the trachea or even in the back of the nose.

Heart

Inspection

In thin children, the apical beat or the point of maximal impulse (PMI) can easily be seen, particularly if you look obliquely across the chest wall.

Palpation

The apical beat may be felt in the 6th intercostal space about 5 cm. (2 inches) from the midline in the school-age child. It is more difficult to feel in the baby, particularly a plump child, and would not be so far out towards the anterior axillary line.

As in all areas of the pediatric examination, measurement and documentation of the distance from the midline and the exact rib space are worth noting.

The apical beat will be deviated to the left with cardiac enlargement or if there is a collapsed lung on that side.
The apical pulse could be pushed toward the right by a tumor or collapse of the lung on the right.
Pneumothorax under tension will push the heart away from the side of the increased pressure.

Auscultation

1. Identify the 1st heart sound (S_1). (Occurs during systole.)
   a. Locate the apical beat (closing of the mitral valve) by placing the stethoscope over the maximum impulse area, concentrating on the first heart sound. (As the ventricle on the left contracts, pushing the blood up into the aorta, the sound of the mitral valve closing is heard.)
   b. That sound can be identified by placing the thumb on the carotid pulse of the neck, which will coincide very closely with the heart sounds.
2. Identify the 2nd heart sound (S_2).
   a. Move the stethoscope up toward the sternum and to the left.
   b. At the base of the heart, both over the aortic and pulmonic areas, S_2 is louder than S_1.

1. Consists of the "lub" portion of the "lub-dub" heart sound.

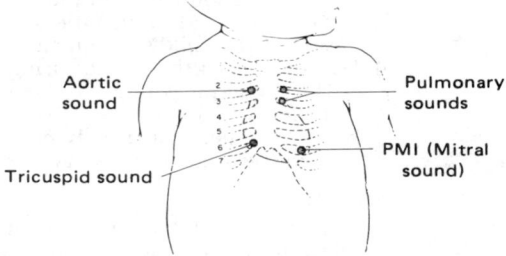

2. Represents the "dub" portion of the "lub-dub" heart sound.

   b. In a child, S_2 can be heard as 2 heart sounds, since the 2 valves in the aorta and pulmonary vessels do not close at quite the same time. The "dub-dub" will disappear if you can get the child to cooperate and breathe deeply.
3. This represents the area of maximum intensity of sound of the pulmonary vessels.

3. Move the stethoscope in small jumps from the apical area medially towards the sternum. Go up the left side of the sternum, listening at each interspace next to the sternum.

4. Move next to the patient's right second intercostal space—again next to the sternum.

5. Descend down the right side of the sternum to the lower end where you will hear best the tricuspid valve from the right of the heart.

6. Listen only to 1 sound; concentrate on that to the exclusion of all others. Can you identify this sound? Is it clear? Compare it with your own heart sound or that of the mother's.

4. It is at this area that you will hear the aortic sound best.

6. The child will enjoy this comparison if he is allowed to listen.

TECHNIQUE	*FINDINGS*
7. If there is any question of a heart murmur or added sounds, refer to the physician.	
8. As you listen to the heart sounds, you are also listening to the rhythm to confirm your findings on pulse. a. If he breathes in and out deeply, the sinus arrhythmia will be obvious. b. If a child holds his breath, the sinus arrhythmia will disappear.	8. The typical rhythm of a child is called *sinus arrhythmia*. As the heart speeds up, the child is breathing in; the heart slows down on expiration.
9. Be sure to count a rapid heart that is heard even when the child is quiet.	9. This may be indicative of a tachycardia that requires further investigation.
10. In the infant, heart sounds are just a series of taps; they occur so fast that it is impossible to make out which sound is the 1st heart sound.	10. In the infant, the 1st and 2nd heart sounds are equal in intensity.

Abdomen

1. For examination of the abdomen, the child should be lying down, relaxed, and not crying.
   Placing a small child, particularly around the age of 1 to 3 years, on a high table on cold paper, can be very frightening; as a result, the abdomen will not be relaxed.
2. Babies up to about 1 year do not seem to be perturbed and will often lie down and play very nicely as long as they can see the mother, who should be stationed at the head of the child while you examine the abdomen.
3. Having the child lie across the mother's knees with the legs dangling on one side and the head cradled in her arms, will enable you to feel the abdomen quite well.
   a. You may find that with the baby's head in the mother's left arm, you can use your left hand to examine the baby's abdomen on the right, feeling up under the right costal margin and into the right hypochondrium.
   b. You may need to turn the baby around and use your right hand to examine the left side of the child's abdomen.
4. Do not discard the idea of using the floor.
   a. If the child is young, ask the mother if she minds putting the child on the floor on a sheet.
   b. The toddler will usually enjoy crawling around the floor and has probably been doing so while the history was being taken

Inspection

1. Observe the abdomen for contour and any markings both while the child is standing and when he is lying down. As you inspect, you may see some abdominal movement with respiration. (Remember that the diaphragm, as it goes up and down, will move the contents of the abdomen.)	1. Sometimes superficial veins are seen on the abdomen, particularly in a very blond infant. Striae are often noticed on the flank following rapid loss or gain of weight.
2. Check for early signs of puberty as evidenced by pubic hair over the symphysis pubis.	2. Early pubic hair in younger children (8–10) may appear long and silky. This will ultimately become curly towards the onset of puberty.
3. Carefully inspect the umbilicus for cleanliness and the presence of any scar tissue.	3. A deep umbilicus may be difficult to keep clean. Immediately after the cord has dropped off, scar tissue or a granuloma may occur.

Auscultation

1. Since percussion and palpation will stimulate the small bowel and increase bowel sounds, auscultation should precede these 2 techniques.	1. Bowel sounds are heard as tinkling, irregular sounds that indicate that fluid is moving from one section of the bowel to the next.
2. To obtain the child's cooperation, you can conduct a running commentary as you listen, saying such things as "I can hear the Cheerios in there."	2. In a quiet baby who has just eaten, not many bowel sounds will be heard. In a hungry child, noisy bowel sounds can be heard, even without a stethoscope.

TECHNIQUE

Percussion

1. On the right side, percuss for the liver. Confirm on palpation.
2. Percuss over the left upper quadrant.

3. Percuss the lower abdomen, particularly above the symphysis pubis.

Palpation

1. Divide the abdomen into 4 imaginary quadrants, palpating each with the fingertips.
2. In the right upper quadrant, palpate for the liver edge.
   a. Although the liver is easily palpable in most children, you may have to press quite firmly.
   b. The liver is frequently felt about 1 cm. (⅜ inch) below the right costal margin and in some instances as low as 2 cm. (¾ inch). This is a common finding in the newborn and through the early school-age years.

3. In the left upper quadrant, palpate for the spleen. Less resistance is encountered as you feel up under the left costal margin.

4. In the upper quadrants also try to palpate for the kidneys. Deep palpation for both kidneys should routinely be a part of the examination to make sure there is no enlargement of the kidney. Normally, the kidney is not palpable.

5. In the iliac fossa or the left lower quadrant, palpate for the descending bowel.

6. Palpate on the right lower quadrant where the appendix is located.

7. If the child has pain in any area or has pointed to the umbilicus when asked to show where the pain is, avoid the area demonstrated and leave it until last.
8. Palpate around the umbilicus for any masses which may indicate a hernia, especially in black children.
   As you press over the protruding hernia you can feel the sensation of gurgling under your fingers as the bowel returns to the abdomen.

FINDINGS

1. Liver dullness can frequently be outlined.

2. Percussion over a gas-filled bowel or stomach gives a high pitched, hollow sound.
3. Above the symphysis pubis, a filled bladder can produce a confusing sound, as does a pregnant uterus. (A mass in the abdomen of a girl over 10 may be a fetus.)

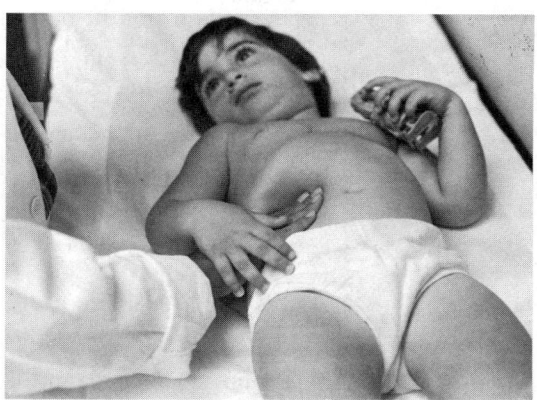

3. Only the tip of the spleen can be felt in the upper outer left quadrant, in the early months of life and in very thin children of preschool age.
4. Kidney palpation is difficult, but during the newborn period, the lower pole of the right kidney can frequently be felt and sometimes the left as well. (This applies to the period immediately following delivery, when the infant's abdomen is relaxed and the bowel is not distended.)
5. The descending colon can be felt, particularly if filled with firm stool. It may be slightly tender, but it should not cause severe pain on gentle palpation.
6. In the RLQ, usually the only sensation is that of gas-filled bowel. Tenderness in this area could be related to an inflamed appendix.
7. If the painful area is palpated first, the child may tense up when the other areas of the abdomen are examined.
8. Most of these hernias heal naturally by the age of 6 years.
   A hernia above the umbilicus can be revealed by asking the child to lift his head from the table. (Widening of the muscles above the umbilicus is called *diastasis recti*.)

Rectum and Anus

1. Rectal examination in the young is not indicated very often.
   a. Studies have shown that not much is achieved by carrying out a rectal examination in young children.
   b. However, the importance of detecting acute appendicitis in school-age children requires that the procedure be followed.

TECHNIQUE	**FINDINGS**

2. When the child is extremely anxious and will not cooperate by relaxing the rectal muscles, it is best to put off the rectal examination unless the expected findings are considered essential.
3. If the child is going to need a consultation with a physician who will have to do a rectal examination anyway, it is only fair to consider that one rectal examination is sufficient.
4. If a rectal examination must be performed, the child can be told that the procedure is much like taking a rectal temperature, although some children will not accept this explanation.
5. Frequently it is necessary to sedate the child if he is acutely distressed.
6. Positioning the child may also require special consideration.
   a. Infants and toddlers present little trouble; they can be placed on their abdomens on a flat surface, and the buttocks can be parted.
   b. An older child should be lying on the left side. If a child cannot be persuaded to cooperate, the mother should be asked to help by flexing the child's legs and holding them steady while the examiner parts the buttocks.
   c. Another technique to use with a reluctant child is to have the youngster lean over the mother's knee in a standing position, while you gently pull the underclothing down. (You may have to talk to the child to divert his attention.)
   d. For the teenager, the utmost care must be taken to avoid embarrassment. When the child is adequately draped in front with an opening in the back, you can examine with the least amount of embarrassment. In fact, the child may be unaware of the extent of your examination if the drape obstructs his view.

Inspection

1. When examining a baby or toddler, place the child on a flat surface so that the weight is evenly distributed on the front of the pelvis. As the baby moves about on his abdomen, observe the entire back, the lower back, the upper thigh, and the tightening of the buttocks.	1. If one buttock is larger than the other, you will see that side projected above the other. Weakness of one side will be obvious as the baby moves around, although a child in the early stages of crawling will normally tend to use one knee as a predominant leader, dragging the other behind.
2. Notice particularly the lower part of the back for hairiness.	2. This may indicate an underlying abnormality of the vertebrae.
3. As the child moves away, part the buttocks and look at the cleft between them.	3. A pilonidal dimple or sinus may be seen over the lip of the coccyx at the superior end of the internatal cleft. This is a common finding, but mothers should be told about it for cleaning purposes.
4. Pay careful attention to the outer appearance of the anus and the perineal body, the underside of the scrotum in the male, and the labia majora in in the female. (Male genitalia, below and to pp. 1081–1083) (Female genitalia, pp. 1083–1084)	4. The anus is inspected for blood, fissures, or splitting in the external tissue, redness, swelling, or pads of extra flesh. On occasion, small, white pinworms may be seen adhering to the anal skin.

Palpation

1. Take into consideration the child's age and feelings; ask the mother to assist if need be.	1. This is the time when the "gift of gab" is most useful because you are really talking the child into cooperating.
2. Start by parting the buttocks with the left hand and introducing a well-lubricated finger (with finger cot) into the anus.	2. When an infant is being examined, the small finger should be used.
3. Gently apply pressure on the anal sphincter to allow the muscles to relax and the finger-tip to slide into the rectum.	3. Apply pressure with the pulp of the finger rather than jab at the anus with the finger-tip.
4. Gently palpate the inner ring, feeling for areas of thickening and tenderness and simultaneously judging the sphincter tone.	4. As the perianal area is pressed upon from the inside, tenderness will be elicited if a deep fissure exists or if an infection has occurred around a fissure.
5. If the rectum is full of feces, it will be impossible to feel any other mass.	5. In the young child, particularly the infant, dilatation provided by the finger will result in a bowel movement. In the older child, a suppository or even an enema may be required.

TECHNIQUE	*FINDINGS*
6. Palpate the walls of the rectum.	6. Within the rectum, the mucosal walls should be smooth, and deep palpation should elicit mild tenderness and no acute pain.
7. As the finger reaches up from the rectum towards the right iliac fossa, place your other hand over the right iliac fossa, trying in effect to roll the appendix between your hands.	7. With an acutely inflamed appendix, this will elicit a great deal of pain and thus constitutes a significant finding.
8. In the male, gently turn your finger through 180 degrees and feel the posterior surface of the prostate. Note size, consistency, tenderness, and contour.	
9. In the female, perform a bimanual examination and palpate the cervix.	

Male Genitalia

1. This part of the examination, especially when carried out by a female, requires the greatest tact and care.
2. The infant and toddler can be distracted or persuaded to cooperate, but the older child will require a direct, matter-of-fact approach which stresses the fact that this area must be examined.

    "I will keep you covered up as much as possible, but it is important for me to examine you down here."
3. The adolescent male must be approached in the same way as an adult. If a young man refuses to undress, it may be necessary to request the help of a male colleague.

Inspection

1. Before touching the child, determine by observation of the testes whether they are in the scrotum.	1. Retraction of the testes into the abdomen occurs very frequently in young children; the development of the scrotum depends on the presence of the testes.
2. Observe the skin over the scrotum for color and surface appearance, noting the presence of wrinkles, or rugae.	2. The skin over the scrotum varies in color, being a darker brown to black in the more pigmented races and reddish in the fair-skinned. The wrinkles, or rugae, are more developed as the child grows older.
3. Next inspect the penis, noting the position of the meatus and the presence or absence of the foreskin. If you are in doubt about it, ask the mother of the child if he has been circumcised.	3. The meatus is usually located at the tip of the penis. The part of the penis that is observed is the anterior surface unless there is an erection. (Remember in a young pre-toilet-trained child, an erection indicates voiding. Be prepared!)

Palpation
SCROTUM AND TESTES

1. Check the scrotum wall for swelling or sensitivity. Gently feel the testes, palpating across the upper pole and feeling for the epididymis. (Remember the scrotum is extremely sensitive to pressure.)	1. The epididymis is a ridge of soft, bumpy tissue extending from the superior pole and running down and behind the testis.
2. Estimate the size of the testes and identify the spermatic cord, tracing it from the testis up toward the groin.	2. The spermatic cord, with the vas deferens, feels firm and is accompanied by softer nerves, arteries, veins, and a few muscle fibers.
3. Make a special effort to locate the testis in a young child whose testes may be retracted into the abdomen via a hyperactive cremasteric reflex. a. If the testes cannot be felt in the scrotum, gently run the skin of the upper scrotum between your fingers, moving superiorly and approaching the external inguinal ring. b. Try to milk the testis down towards the scrotum from above with your hand. c. If this fails, have the child sit cross-legged to abolish the reflex of the cremaster muscle.	3. The presence of the testes in the scrotum is vital in the preschool or early school-aged child. Nondescent of the testes requires that the child be referred to a physician. During this period the testis is about 1.5–2 cm. (½–¾ inch) in length. In the quiescent period prior to puberty the male genitalia remain fairly infantile.

TECHNIQUE	FINDINGS

TECHNIQUE

4. When examining a boy in the early stages of puberty, it is important to note the size of the testis as well as the greater number of rugae on the scrotum and the appearance of pubic hair around the penis.

PENIS

1. Evaluate the penis on all sides by lifting up the shaft in order to see the undersurface.
If the child is not circumcised, gently retract the foreskin and evaluate as to the possibility of infection. Take this opportunity to instruct the mother about cleanliness and care.

2. Observe the position of the meatus and gently pinch the lips of the meatus to reveal an adequate orifice.

The meatus may occur anywhere along the ventral surface of the glans or the shaft of the penis underneath.

3. Note and palpate the urethra.

4. In the older child, inspect the penis for ulcers or other signs of infection and discharge from the meatus.

INGUINAL AREA

1. Palpate for hernia over the external inguinal ring. Have the child cough to enhance your observation.

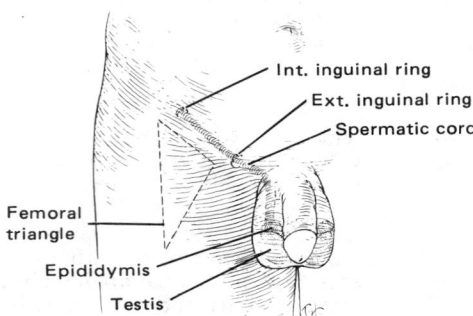

Int. inguinal ring
Ext. inguinal ring
Spermatic cord
Femoral triangle
Epididymis
Testis

2. An increased cough reflex or swelling in the area should be checked by carefully placing the finger on the scrotal skin and invaginating the skin over your fingers toward the external ring. You are trying to follow the course of a hernia which would descend into the scrotum while you feel the external ring from below.
A hernia in the inguinal region presents as a bulge which can be either seen or felt from below by placing the finger in the scrotum pointing up toward the external inguinal ring.

FINDINGS

4. In early puberty, the testes start to grow. Onset of puberty varies, occurring in some boys by age 10 and in others as late as 14. In most teenagers, the findings are similar to those in adults.

1. The shaft of the penis contains the urethra on the under, or ventral, surface; it should be easily palpable.
In an uncircumcised infant, circumcision may be necessary because of tightness of the foreskin. Regular stretching on a daily basis may stretch the foreskin enough so that it will come back over the entire glans.
In an older child, failure of the foreskin to retract may result in inflammation and difficulty in keeping the glans clean.

2. The meatus may be positioned off-center on the undersurface at the junction of the glans and the shaft. This degree of hypospadias is usually not operated upon, but must be noted and reported.
Very rarely the meatus occurs on the dorsal or anterior surface. Surgical correction is essential or the child will not be able to stand when urinating.

3. The urethra is located on the under, or ventral, surface of the penis and should be easily palpable.

4. Suspicion of sexual activity despite a young age is an important consideration.

1. Having the child stand either with the mother holding him or placing him against her knee will help you in locating a hernia in the inguinal area.

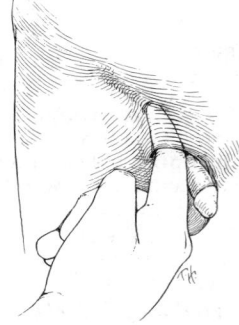

TECHNIQUE	FINDINGS
3. Also palpate for the inguinal lymph nodes.	3. The inguinal lymph nodes in an infant are palpable as small and "shotty." Anything more than this should alert you to possible infection, since the perianal area drains into the superficial inguinal lymph nodes. Thus, any signs of diaper rash will explain enlargement of the lymph nodes, which should be noted and reported.

FEMORAL AREA

Palpate the femoral triangle carefully for a hernia and for lymph nodes

In the femoral area, a swelling which can be reduced with a gurgling sound is an unusual finding.

Auscultation

If you are trying to reduce a mass, listen over the scrotum to see if there is a gurgling sound.

This will locate the bowel for you and confirm the presence of a hernia.

Transillumination

1. To locate the testis, darken the room and shine a bright light from behind the scrotum. In a normal child, the testis will stand out as the darker area.
2. Transilluminate any suspicious mass to help locate a hernia.

1. Testes which are swollen by fluid (hydrocele) will transilluminate. Fluid around the testes or cord must be differentiated from a hernia.
2. Any mass in this area must be reported to a physician immediately.

Female Genitalia

1. Place the infant or toddler on the table or on the mother's knee while she holds the knees in an abducted and flexed position.
2. A preschool child can be allowed to lean over her mother's knee. However, remember that the structures are being visualized upside down.
3. The older child or teenager should be draped as an adult would and should be placed in a lithotomy position with the aid of stirrups.

Equipment

Disposable gloves, speculum, light source

1. Carefully inspect the perineal area for cleanliness, inflammation, and abnormality.
2. Fold back the labia majora and note the labia minora.
3. Part the labia and note the clitoris and the meatus at the anterior end. (The clitoris is a hook-like structure that extends over the opening of the urethral meatus.) The meatus appears as a slit which is slightly darker in color against the pink of the mucosa about 2 cm. (¾ inch) posterior to the clitoris.
4. Having parted the labia, check for any signs of inflammation, discharge, tenderness, or infection. Include the urethral meatus, periurethral glands, the vagina, and the greater vestibular glands (Bartholin's). (Tenderness of these glands is unusual in young children, but may occur in adolescents.)

1. This includes the mons pubis, clitoris, labia, urethra, and perineal body.
2. The labia minora are seen as 2 slender folds of tissue inside the labia majora.
3. In some instances, adhesions of the labia minora occur because of the lack of natural hormones. The opening of the vagina is obscured by the two lateral flaps, which stick together, sometimes to the degree that urination is difficult because the urethral meatus is covered.
4. Inflammation and pus-like discharge from the urethra may be noted on palpation. The periurethral glands may be tender because of infection—possibly due to gonococci. If discharge is collected from the vagina, it should be cultured.

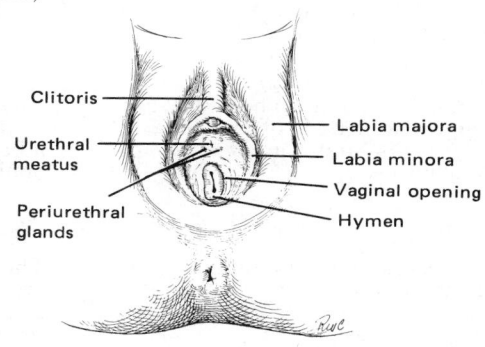

Clitoris — Labia majora
Urethral meatus — Labia minora
Periurethral glands — Vaginal opening
— Hymen

TECHNIQUE	***FINDINGS***
5. If the mother of a newborn infant has noted a bloody discharge from the infant's vagina during the first few days of life, reassure her that this is not an uncommon occurrence; the discharge will disappear, as will any swelling of the labia majora and clitoris and any enlargement of the infant's breasts.	5. Hormone stimulation from the mother's body accounts for this occurrence. The discharge usually stops once the hormones are excreted. The bloody appearance on the diaper may be confused with the presence of urates, which are also orange-red and which appear quite normally in the urine.
6. Note the vaginal opening, which may vary in size due to the presence of a thin membrane, the hymen. The hymen varies in appearance according to the age of the child.	6. The lack of an opening into the vagina may result in the retention of menstrual fluid when the child reaches puberty. In the sexually active adolescent, vestigial remains of the hymen may appear as small particles (caruncles) at the fringe of the vagina.
7. In the young child, it is usually unnecessary to examine inside the vagina. Should you suspect the presence of a foreign body, insert a finger into the rectum and milk anteriorly to allow you to feel the lower part of the cervix and any firm foreign body within the vagina.	7. A foreign body may be suspected if there is vaginal discharge (of any quantity) that is blood-tinged or has an odor. In the older child, vaginal discharge of this type may be due to gonorrhea.
8. In an older child, the little finger can be inserted gently into the vagina and anterior pressure applied.	8. Anterior pressure and milking downwards palpates the urethra towards the meatus. The periurethral glands are located on each side of the urethra.
9. Turn the finger gradually, sweeping down the right side of the vagina, back over the rectum, and up on the left side of the vagina. Turn your finger, arm, and wrist so that undue pressure is not made on the child's tissues.	
10. Once the genitalia are examined, lower the child's legs somewhat so that the femoral and inguinal areas can be palpated the same way as in the male.	10. Enlargement of the lymph nodes in the presence of a hernia in the femoral triangle may be found. Similarly, enlargement of the inguinal nodes may occur.

Musculoskeletal System

1. Evaluation of the musculoskeletal system can be done both in an informal manner while watching the child at rest and at play and in a formal manner as specific findings are methodically checked.
2. In the newborn, observe the position of the limbs during sleep and the quality of movement when the infant is awake.
3. Various aspects of size, shape, and movement are evaluated as the baby is observed pushing up on his arms and turning his head towards his mother.
4. The infant in the early stages of walking offers many opportunities for evaluation of muscle strength and movement.
   At the same time, rapport with the mother can be reinforced by your admiring the baby's ability and by inquiring if she is concerned about the manner in which the baby is walking.
5. A more mobile child can be evaluated as you watch him play and explore the room.
6. Having the older child reach for crayons, run after a ball, or walk around the room enables you to evaluate the musculoskeletal system and the child's sense of balance.

UPPER EXTREMITIES

1. In the infant, evaluate the status of the clavicles when examining the skull and neck.	1. During a difficult delivery, the clavicle that has been exposed to traction may snap. A lump can be felt on the bone at about 3 weeks of age.
2. Carefully examine the hands to note shape of the hand, shape and length of the fingers, changes in the nails, and the presence of creases on the palms.	2. Any variation in the hands or unusual length of the fingers should be noted. An incurved little finger or low-set thumb with the single Simian crease may reflect Down's syndrome, or mongolism.

LOWER EXTREMITIES

1. Examine the appearance of the infant's foot, noting arch formation.	1. The foot of an infant is usually flat and appears broad since the arch on the inside of the foot is covered by a fat pad. Parents may need reassurance in this regard.

TECHNIQUE	**FINDINGS**

2. Inspect the angle of the foot and lower leg and then manipulate the ankle to evaluate the range of motion.

2. Full flexibility of the foot (plantar flexion) rules out underlying abnormality. The foot should return to the neutral position after manipulation. Frequently, the foot will turn in, or adduct. Such a finding should be recorded.

3. Place the knees together and see how far the ankles are separated.

3. Normally there is only a small space between the ankles when the knees are held together. Marked bowing of the legs will be demonstrated by a wide distance between the ankles. This is particularly important following assumption of the upright position.

4. Evaluate the baby's ability to walk, noting the appearance of the legs and foot placement. Remember to look at the child's shoes and see which side of the sole is worn down.

4. When babies first start to walk, their legs appear bowlegged. The feet are kept wide apart and turn slightly in, so that the ankles seem curved when viewed from behind.

HIP

1. When examining children under 1 year of age, check to see if there are signs of hip dislocation.
2. Place the baby on his back and grasp the knees with your thumbs, spreading your fingers up the lateral sides of the femora, so that the tips of your middle and 3rd fingers rest over the hip joints.
3. As the legs are flexed to a right angle at the hips and knees, they should be slowly pressed outwards and abducted. The tips of the examining fingers are palpating the heads of the femora as they rotate in the acetabula.

1. Any difficulties with hip examination call for immediate medical consultation because of possible congenital dislocation of the hip.

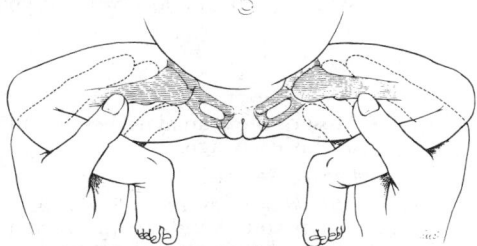

In the normal infant, the lateral aspect of each knee will touch the examining table without difficulty.

SPINE

1. Check the spine for any signs of abnormal curvature. If any doubt exists in your mind about the presence of a curve, mark each spinous process with a dot made by a felt pen.
2. Note any signs of forward curving of the shoulders.
   Have the child lean forward with the arms hanging down.

1. The normal child has a curve inward at the lumbar region (lordosis), but this should not be exaggerated.
   Abnormal curvatures include the following:
   Kyphosis: Forward curvature of the shoulders.
   Scoliosis: Side-to-side curvature of the spine.

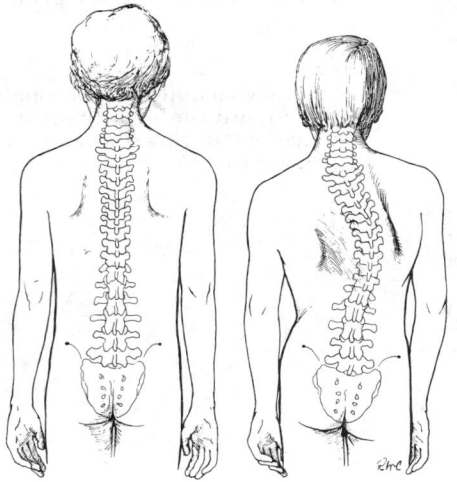

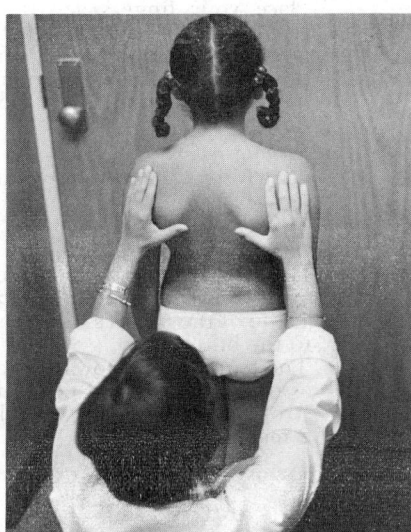

TECHNIQUE   *FINDINGS*

Neurological Examination

1. The neurological system in infancy is different from that of the baby of a few months. There is an even greater contrast between the baby on the one hand and children and adults on the other.
2. The central nervous system at birth is underdeveloped and the functions tested are below the level of the cortex.

Equipment

Flashlight, noisemaker, ophthalmoscope, tongue depressor, tuning fork

Procedure for the Newborn and Young Infant

(See Guidelines: Physical Appraisal of the Newborn, p. 1034.)

1. Observe the newborn for general appearance, positioning, activity, crying, and alertness. Take note of the posture—including head, neck, and extremities.

2. Note the pitch, volume, and character of the cry.

3. Observe the infant's facial expression and the symmetry of the face when crying or sucking.

1. Stiffness of the neck or marked attraction of the head will cause a position of opisthotonos.

2. The high-pitched cry of the infant who has intracranial irritation is very distinctive.

3. Poor sucking, with dribbling, is abnormal. Transient weakness of the mouth due to 7th cranial nerve paralysis is frequently seen as a result of a forceps delivery in which the forceps is pressed on the facial nerve where it emerges from the ear.

4. Most of the cranial nerves are difficult to check at this early age.

Automatic Reflexes

1. *Blinking reflex due to loud noise*
   Clap your hands or produce a loud clicking noise, being careful not to clap near the baby so that a wave of air passes over his eyes and causes him to blink them anyway.

2. *Blinking reflex due to bright light*
   Shine a bright light into the infant's eyes to elicit blinking reflex.
   a. Cranial nerve 10 can be checked by using a tongue depressor to gag the infant.
   b. Cranial nerve 12 (hypoglossal) can be tested by pinching the nose closed as the baby sucks.

3. *Palmar grasp reflex*
   Place your fingers across the baby's palm from the ulnar side. The baby needs to be in a relaxed position with his head in a central position. Reinforcement may be offered by having the baby suck on the bottle at the same time.

4. *Rooting reflex*
   Touch the edge of the baby's mouth.

5. *Incurving of the trunk*
   Hold the baby horizontally and prone in one arm while using the other hand to stimulate 1 side of the infant's back from the shoulders to the buttocks.
   The trunk curves toward the stimulated side as the shoulders and pelvis move toward the stroking hand (persists until infant is about 2 months old).

1. Lack of a blink in response to a loud noise may indicate deafness.

2. Failure to blink may indicate blindness.

   a. Palate moves.

   b. The infant opens the mouth and raises the tip of the tongue reflexly.

3. Both hands will flex and can be compared for strength.
   Weakness on 1 side may be indicated by a failure to grasp when the palm is stimulated.

4. The baby's mouth will open and the head will turn toward the side stimulated. This reflex is marked during the early weeks of life. (Persistence time varies.)

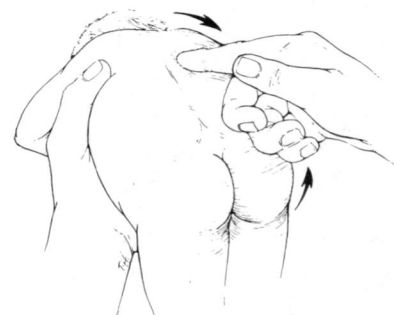

TECHNIQUE	FINDINGS

TECHNIQUE

6. *Vertical suspension position*
   Place your hands under the baby's axillae with thumbs supporting the back of the head and hold the baby upright.

7. *Stepping response*
   Hold the baby under its axillae with thumbs supporting the back of the head. Allow baby's foot to touch firm surface.

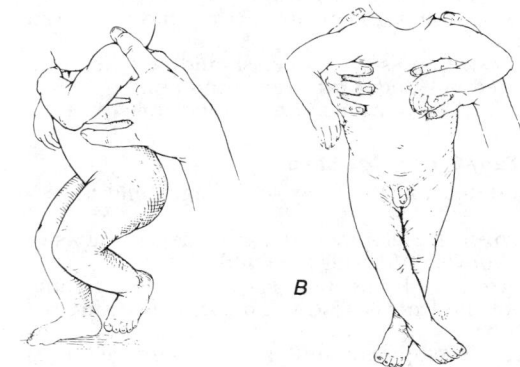

8. *Tonic neck reflex*
   Hold the baby in a supine position with the head turned to one side and the jaw held in place over the shoulder.

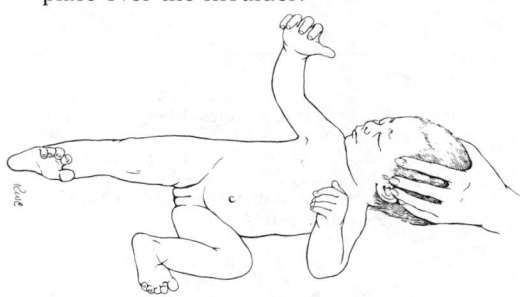

9. *Mass reflexes (Moro or startle reflex)*
   Hold the baby along your arm with the other hand below the lower legs. Lower the feet and body in a sudden motion.

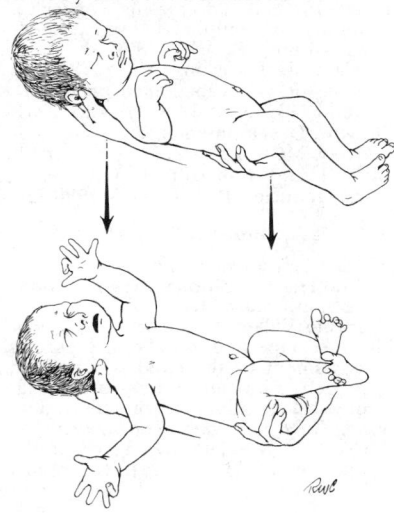

FINDINGS

6. The legs flex at the hips and knees. (Persists for about 4 months.)

7. Normally the baby responds by lifting 1 knee and hip into a flexed position and moving the opposite leg forward—making a series of stepping movements (A).
   a. Difficulty with the stepping reflex and stiffness or spasticity connected with crossing of the feet and scissoring (B) is indicative of spastic paraplegia or diplegia.
   b. It should be noted that the stepping response may be affected by breech delivery. (It may also be affected by weakness.)
   c. The stepping response is evident toward the end of the 1st week and persists for a variable time.

8. a. The arm and leg on the side to which the head is turned will extend, whereas those on the other side will flex (the so-called "bow and arrow position").
   b. This reflex persists for about 6 months; it may be present at birth or delayed until the baby is 6 or 8 weeks old.
   c. Persistence beyond 6 months suggests major cerebral damage.

9. The arms will spring up and out, abducting and extending; the fingers are also extended. The arms then return forward over the body with a clasping motion. At the same time, the legs flex slightly and the hips abduct.
   a. The Moro reflex is present at birth and disappears at about the end of the 3rd month. Persistence beyond 6 months is significant.
   b. Asymmetric response may be due to paralysis of the arm following a difficult delivery, tension and injury to the brachial plexus, or a fracture of the clavicle or humerus. A dislocated hip would produce an asymmetrical response in the lower limbs.

TECHNIQUE	*FINDINGS*
10. *Perez reflex* Hold the baby in a prone position along your arm; place the thumb of the other hand on the sacrum and move it firmly toward the head, along the entire length of the spine.	10. The head and spine will extend and the knees will flex upward. The baby will frequently cry and urinate. (Can be used as a method for collecting a clean voided specimen.)

Summary

1. Some of the jerking and shaking movements seen in infants are normal, but they should be rechecked frequently during the first few weeks of life.
2. Plantar stimulation will elicit a Babinski response (toes curl upward) in most children until the age of 2; this is a normal finding.
3. Variants in the findings due to the baby's sleepiness or hunger should be taken into account and reevaluations should be carried out under different conditions.
4. Severe neurological damage may be completely asymptomatic and impossible to detect during the first few weeks of life.

Neurological Examination of the Toddler and Early School-Age Child

1. The neurological examination for the toddler and the early school-age child is very similar to that for the adult.
2. The Draw-A-Person Test* and the Denver Developmental Assessment† are both excellent methods for testing areas in the development of the child.
3. Beyond the newborn period, specific gross and fine motor coordination testing, accompanied by appropriate evaluation of the Denver test, will assist in assessing the child's level of development.
4. These tests also assess social and language development and are important screening devices.
5. Interview technique‡ can also be useful in assessing development in the preschool child.

* See Appendix A, page 1089. † See Appendix B, page 1090. ‡ See Appendix C, page 1092.

BIBLIOGRAPHY

Books

Alexander MN and Brown MS. Pediatric Physical Diagnosis for Nurses, 2nd ed. New York, McGraw–Hill, 1979

Barness LA. Manual of Pediatric Physical Diagnosis, 4th ed. Chicago, Year Book Medical Pub., 1972

Bates B. A Guide to Physical Examination, 2nd ed. Philadelphia, JB Lippincott, 1979

Brown MS and Murphy MA. Ambulatory Pediatrics for Nurses. New York, McGraw–Hill, 1975

Chrispin AR et al. Current Diagnostic Pediatrics. New York, Springer–Verlag New York, Inc., 1980

Ewerbeck H. Differential Diagnosis in Pediatrics. New York, Springer–Verlag New York Inc., 1980

Ferholt JDL. Clinical Assessment of Children. Philadelphia, JB Lippincott, 1980

Fowkes VC and Hunn VK. Clinical Assessment for the Nurse Practitioner. St. Louis, CV Mosby, 1973

Goodenough FL. Measurement of Intelligence by Drawings. Chicago, World Book, 1926

Green M. Pediatric Diagnosis, 2nd ed. Philadelphia, WB Saunders, 1980

Green M and Haggerty RJ (eds). Ambulatory Pediatrics, 2nd ed. Philadelphia, WB Saunders, 1977

Harris DB. Children's Drawing as a Measure of Intellectual Maturity. New York, Harcourt, Brace and Jovanovich, 1963

Heagarty M et al. Child Health: Basics for Primary Health Care. New York, Appleton–Century–Crofts, 1980

The Johns Hopkins Hospital. The Harriet Lane Handbook, 8th ed. Chicago, Year Book Medical Pub., 1978

Judge RA and Zuidema GD. Methods of Clinical Examination: A Physiologic Approach, 3rd ed. Boston, Little, Brown and Co., 1974

Kempe CH et al. Current Pediatric Diagnosis and Treatment, 6th ed. Los Altos, California, Lange Medical Pub., 1980

Articles

Blosser C. Avoiding potential behavior problems in children. Pediatr Nurse 1979 May–June; 5(3):11–15

Brown JB. Child health maintenance. Nurse Pract 1980 Jan–Feb; 5(1):33–34, 36–38 passim

Critchley DL. Mental status examinations with children and adolescents. Nurs Clin North Am 1979 Sept; 14(3): 429–441

Freis PC. Sounds of a healthy heart. Issues Compr Pediatr Nurs 1979 Dec; 3(7):1–4

Holt SJ and Robinson TM. The school nurses's "family assessment tool." Am J Nurs 1979 May: 79(5):950–953

Levine MD et al. The pediatric examination of educational readiness: Validation of an extended observation procedure. Pediatrics 1980 Sept; 66(3):341–349

Mitchell JR. Male adolescents' concern about a physical examination conducted by a female. Nurs Res 1980 May–June; 29(3):165–169

Oberklaid F, Dworkin PH, Levine MD. Developmental–behavioral dysfunction in preschool children. Am J Dis Child 1979 Nov; 133(11):1126–1131

O'Pray M. Developmental screening tools: Using them effectively. MCN 1980 Mar–Apr; 5(2):126–130

Wolf WJ and Bancroft B. Early detection of childhood malignancies. Pediatr Nurs 1980 Jan–Feb; 6(1):43–46

Audio-Visual Materials

Pediatric Physical Assessment, 1976
Blue Hill Educational Systems, Inc
52 South Main Street
Spring Valley, New York 10977

This video tape and workbook presentation of the physical assessment of the child is a programmed learning approach to introduce the professional or student to doing physical examinations on children.

A Visual Guide to Physical Examination
(No. 12) Special Procedures of the Pediatric Physical Examination, Bates B., J. B. Lippincott, 1974

APPENDIX A: Goodenough—Harris Draw-a-Person Test

This test provides one of the methods of measuring the level of mental development of children between 3 and 10 years of age. It was originally described in 1926 and appears to be a sound one; there is a significant degree of correlation in the results of this test and IQ. Subsequently Harris brought the test up-to-date with specific scoring for drawings of a man or a woman.

1. *Procedure:* The child is supplied with a pencil (preferably a No. 2 with eraser) and a sheet of blank paper and instructed to "Draw a person," "Draw the best person you can." No additional directions are necessary. Encouragement may be supplied if necessary. Under no condition should the examiner suggest that the child's production needs to be supplemented or changed in any way—the only exception being the drawing of the stick figure. In this case the examiner is permitted to encourage the child to "draw a whole person."

2. *Scoring:* The child receives one point for each detail present according to the following scoring guides:

Drawing of a Woman

1. Head present
2. Neck present
3. Neck, 2 dimensions
4. Eyes present
5. Eye detail: brow or lashes
6. Eye detail: pupil
7. Nose present (not round ball)
8. Nose, 2 dimensions
9. Bridge of nose (straight to eyes, narrower than base)
10. Nostrils shown
11. Mouth present
12. Lips, 2 dimensions
13. Both nose and lips in 2 dimensions
14. Both chin and forehead shown
15. Hair I (any scribble)
16. Hair II (more detail)
17. Necklace or earrings
18. Arms present
19. Fingers present
20. Correct number of fingers shown
21. Opposition of thumb shown (must include fingers)
22. Hands present
23. Legs present
24. Feet (any indication)
25. Shoe "feminine" (any attempt such as high heels, open toe, strap)
26. Attachment of arms and legs I (to trunk anywhere)
27. Attachment of arms and legs II (to trunk at correct point)
28. Clothing indicated (any)
29. Sleeve
30. Neckline (any indication)
31. Trunk present
32. Trunk in proportion, 2 dimensions (length greater than breadth)

Drawing of a Man

1. Head present
2. Neck present
3. Neck, 2 dimensions
4. Eyes present
5. Eye detail: brow or lashes
6. Eye detail: pupil
7. Nose present
8. Nose, 2 dimensions (not round ball)
9. Mouth present
10. Lips, 2 dimensions
11. Both nose and lips in 2 dimensions
12. Both chin and forehead shown
13. Bridge of nose (straight to eyes; narrower than base)
14. Hair I (any scribble)
15. Hair II (more detail)
16. Ears present
17. Fingers present
18. Correct number of fingers shown
19. Opposition of thumb shown (must include fingers)
20. Hands present
21. Arms present
22. Arms at side or engaged in activity
23. Feet: any indication
24. Attachment of arms and legs I (to trunk anywhere)
25. Attachment of arms and legs II (at correct point of trunk)
26. Trunk present
27. Trunk in proportion, 2 dimensions (length greater than breadth)
28. Clothing I (anything)
29. Clothing II (2 articles of clothing)

3. *Norms:* Minimum score for child to be within one standard deviation of age–appropriate mean.

Age	Drawing of man		Drawing of Woman	
	by boys	by girls	by boys	by girls
3	4	5	4	6
4	7	7	7	8
5	11	12	11	14
6	13	14	13	16
7	16	17	16	19
8	18	20	20	23

APPENDIX B: Denver Developmental Screening Test

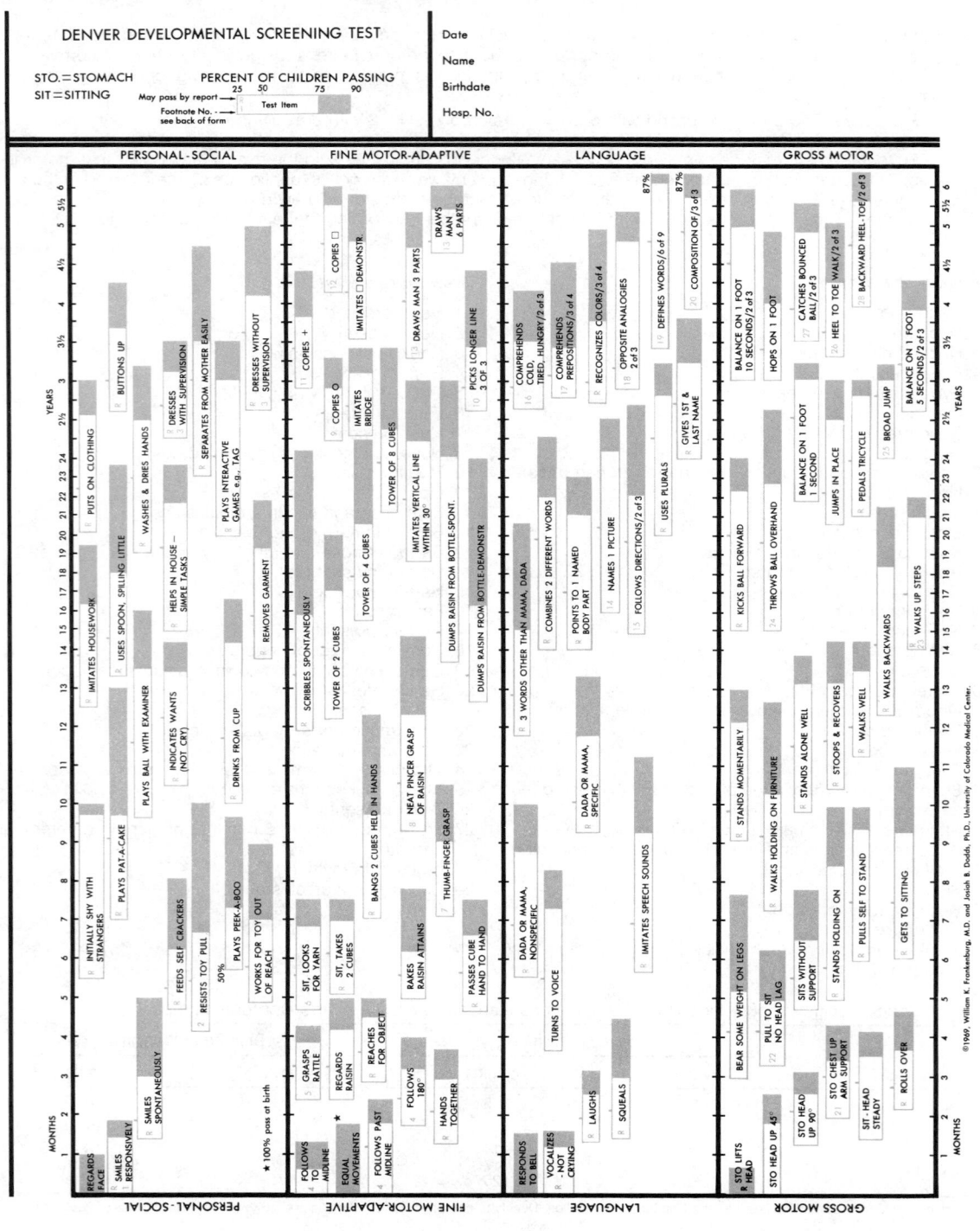

The Denver Developmental Assessment method developed by William K. Frankenburg, M.D., and his colleagues, is presented in a manual called Denver Developmental Screening Test. The test materials can be ordered from: Lodaco Project & Publishing Foundation, Inc., East 51st Avenue and Lincoln Street, Denver, Colorado 80216.

DIRECTIONS	DATE NAME BIRTHDATE HOSP. NO.

1. Try to get child to smile by smiling, talking or waving to him. Do not touch him.
2. When child is playing with toy, pull it away from him. Pass if he resists.
3. Child does not have to be able to tie shoes or button in the back.
4. Move yarn slowly in an arc from one side to the other, about 6″ above child's face. Pass if eyes follow 90° to midline. (Past midline; 180°)
5. Pass if child grasps rattle when it is touched to the backs or tips of fingers.
6. Pass if child continues to look where yarn disappeared or tries to see where it went. Yarn should be dropped quickly from sight from tester's hand without arm movement.
7. Pass if child picks up raisin with any part of thumb and a finger.
8. Pass if child picks up raisin with the ends of thumb and index finger using an over hand approach.

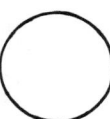   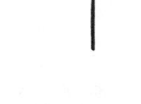   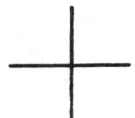   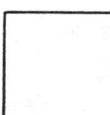

9. Pass any enclosed form. Fail continuous round motions.
10. Which line is longer? (Not bigger.) Turn paper upside down and repeat. (3/3 or 5/6)
11. Pass any crossing lines.
12. Have child copy first. If failed, demonstrate

When giving items 9, 11 and 12, do not name the forms. Do not demonstrate 9 and 11.

13. When scoring, each pair (2 arms, 2 legs, etc.) counts as one part.
14. Point to picture and have child name it. (No credit is given for sounds only.)

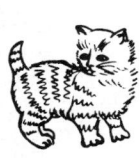   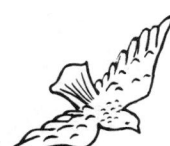   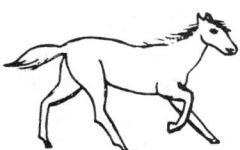   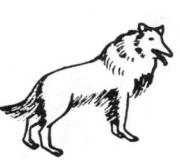   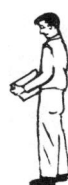

15. Tell child to: Give block to Mommie; put block on table; put block on floor. Pass 2 of 3. (Do not help child by pointing, moving head or eyes.)
16. Ask child: What do you do when you are cold? . .hungry? . .tired? Pass 2 of 3.
17. Tell child to: Put block <u>on</u> table; <u>under</u> table; in <u>front</u> of chair, <u>behind</u> chair. Pass 3 of 4. (Do not help child by pointing, moving head or eyes.)
18. As child: If fire is hot, ice is ?; Mother is a woman, Dad is a ?; a horse is big, a mouse is ?. Pass 2 of 3.
19. Ask child: What is a ball? . .lake? . .desk? . .house? . .banana? . .curtain? . .ceiling? . .hedge? . .pavement? Pass if defined in terms of use, shape, what it is made of or general category (such as banana is fruit, not just yellow). Pass 6 of 9.
20. Ask child: What is a spoon made of? . .a shoe made of? . .a door made of? (No other objects may be substituted.) Pass 3 of 3.
21. When placed on stomach, child lifts chest off table with support of forearms and/or hands.
22. When child is on back, grasp his hands and pull him to sitting. Pass if head does not hang back.
23. Child may use wall or rail only, not person. May not crawl.
24. Child must throw ball overhand 3 feet to within arm's reach of tester.
25. Child must perform standing broad jump over width of test sheet. (8½ inches)
26. Tell child to walk forward, ⌐○⌐○⌐○→ heel within 1 inch of toe. Tester may demonstrate. Child must walk 4 consecutive steps, 2 out of 3 trials.
27. Bounce ball to child who should stand 3 feet away from tester. Child must catch ball with hands, not arms, 2 out of 3 trials.
28. Tell child to walk backward, ←○⌐○⌐○ toe within 1 inch of heel. Tester may demonstrate. Child must walk 4 consecutive steps, 2 out of 3 trials.

<u>DATE AND BEHAVIORAL OBSERVATIONS</u> (how child feels at time of test, relation to tester, attention span, verbal behavior, self-confidence, etc,):

APPENDIX C: Developmental Assessment by Interview

A method has been developed of evaluation by utilizing an interview technique asking parents a list of questions regarding milestones in achievements which most will remember. Developed by Drs. Capute and Biehl, it has been very successful in its use at the John F. Kennedy Institute for the Habilitation of Handicapped Children at Johns Hopkins.

Age	Gross Motor	Fine Motor	Language	Social
3 mo.	A. Does he support himself on forearms when lying? B. Does he hold his head up steadily while on his stomach?	A. Are his hands usually open at rest? B. Does he pull at his clothing?	A. Does he laugh or make happy noises? B. Does he turn his head to sounds?	A. Does he smile at you? B. Does he reach for familiar people or objects?
6 mo.	A. Does he lift his head when lying on his back? B. Does he roll from back to front?	A. Does he transfer a toy from one hand to the other? B. Does he pick up small objects?	A. Does he "babble," repeat sounds together (i.e., mum-mum-mum)? B. Is he frightened by angry noise?	A. Does he stretch his arms out to be picked up? B. Does he show his likes and dislikes?
9 mo.	A. Does he sit for long periods without support? B. Does he pull up on furniture?	A. Does he pick up objects with his thumb and one finger? B. Does he finger-feed any foods?	A. Does he understand "no-no," "bye-bye"? B. Will he imitate any sounds or words if you make them first?	A. Does he hold his own bottle? B. Does he play any nursery games ("peek-a-boo," "bye-bye")?
12 mo.	A. Is he walking (alone or with hand held)? B. Does he pivot when sitting?	A. Does he throw toys (objects)? B. Does he give you toys (let go) easily?	A. Does he have at least one meaningful word other than "mama," "dada"? B. Does he shake his head for "no"?	A. Does he cooperate in dressing? B. Does he come when you call him?
18 mo.	A. Does he walk upstairs with help? B. Can he throw a toy while standing without falling?	A. Does he turn book pages (2 or 3 at a time)? B. Does he fill spoon and feed self?	A. Does he have at least 6 real words besides his "jargon"? B. Does he point at what he wants?	A. Does he copy you in routine tasks (sweeping, dusting, etc.)? B. Does he play in the company of other children?
2 yr.	A. Does he run well without falling? B. Does he walk up and down stairs alone?	A. Does he turn book pages one at a time? B. Does he remove his own shoes, pants?	A. Does he talk in short (2–3 word) sentences? B. Does he use pronouns ("me," "you," "mine")?	A. Does he ask to be taken to the toilet? B. Does he play in company of other children?
2½ yr.	A. Does he jump, getting both feet off the floor? B. Does he throw a ball overhand?	A. Does he unbutton any buttons? B. Does he hold a pencil or crayon adult fashion?	A. Does he use plurals or past tense? B. Does he use the word "I" correctly most of the time?	A. Does he tell his first and last name if asked? B. Does he get himself a drink without help?
3 yr.	A. Does he pedal a tricycle? B. Does he alternate feet (one stair per step) going upstairs?	A. Does he dry his hands (if reminded)? B. Does he dress and undress fully including front buttons?	A. Does he tell little stories about his experiences? B. Does he know his sex?	A. Does he share his toys? B. Does he play well with another child? Take turns?
4 yr.	A. Does he attempt to hop or skip? B. Does he alternate feet going downstairs?	A. Does he button clothes fully? B. Does he catch a ball?	A. Does he say a song or a poem from memory? B. Does he know all his colors?	A. Does he tell "tall tales" or "show off"? B. Does he play cooperatively with a small group of children?
5 yr.	A. Does he skip, alternating feet? B. Does he jump rope or jump over low obstacles?	A. Does he tie his own shoes? B. Does he spread with a knife?	A. Can he print his first name? B. Does he ever ask what a word means?	A. Is he a "mother's helper"—likes to do things for you? B. Does he play competitive games and abide by the rules?

(From Johns Hopkins Hospital: The Harriet Lane Handbook, 8th edition, Dennis L. Headings, Editor. Copyright © 1978 by Year Book Medical Publishers, Inc., Chicago. Used by permission.)

PEDIATRIC HEALTH MAINTENANCE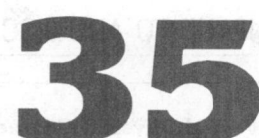

GROWTH AND DEVELOPMENT

Reflexes of the Newborn

1. *Pupillary reflexes*—ipsilateral (pertaining to the same side) constriction to light.
2. *Rooting*—when corner of mouth is touched and object is moved toward cheek, infant will turn head toward object and open mouth.
3. *Palmar grasp*—pressure on palm of hand will elicit grasp.
4. *Plantar grasp*—pressure on sole of foot behind toes will cause flexion of toes.
5. *Tonic neck reflex*—sudden jolt will cause head to turn to one side with leg and arm on that side extended, while the extremities on the other side flex.
6. *Neck righting*—when head is turned to one side, the shoulder and trunk, followed by the pelvis, will turn to that side.
7. *Moro reflex*—response to sudden loud noise, causing body to stiffen and arms to go up and out, then forward and toward each other. Thumb and index finger will assume C-shape.
8. *Positive-supporting reflex*—when held in an erect position, baby will stiffen lower extremities and support his weight.
9. *Babinski's sign*—scratching sole of foot causes great toe to flex and toes to fan.
10. *Crossed extensor reflex*—when one leg is extended and the knee is held straight, while the sole of foot is stimulated, the opposite leg will flex.
11. *Landau's sign*—when baby is suspended horizontally with head depressed against trunk and neck flexed, legs will flex and be drawn up to trunk.
12. *Optical blink reflex*—when light is suddenly shone into open eyes, the eyes will close quickly with a quick dorsal flexion of head.
13. *Auditory blink reflex*—eyes quickly close if examiner loudly claps her hands about 30 cm. (11.5 inches) from infant's head.
14. *Recoil of arm*—when both arms are extended simultaneously by pulling outward grasping wrists, both arms will flex at the elbows when released.
15. *Withdrawal reflex*—pricking sole of foot will result in the baby's leg being flexed at hip, knee, and ankle.
16. *Stepping reflex*—when infant is held upright with dorsum of foot gently touching edge of table, he will bend his hips and knees and put foot on table. This will elicit stepping response in the opposite foot. Series of alternating stepping actions will result when infant is moved forward so that 1 foot at a time touches the firm surface.
17. *Parachute reflex*—while the infant is held prone and lowered quickly toward a surface, he will extend arms and legs.
18. *Side-turning*—placing baby prone with head in midline will elicit the baby's turning his head to the side.
19. Other characteristics of the newborn:
    a. Cries
    b. Sucks
    c. Has extremely sensitive skin
    d. Makes discriminating sounds
    e. Sleeps for long intervals
    f. Has little head control (head lag)

Infant to Adolescent

See table on pages 1094–1105.

Childhood Diseases

See table on pages 1106–1111.

Nutrition of Pediatric Patients

See table on pages 1112–1117.

INFANT TO ADOLESCENT: GROWTH AND DEVELOPMENT

Age and Physical Characteristics	Behavior Patterns	Nursing Implications/Parental Guidance
Birth—4 weeks (1 month)	*Motor Development* Momentary visual fixation on objects and adult face. Eyes follow bright moving objects. Lies awake on back with head averted. Immediately drops objects placed in hands. Responds to sounds of bell and other similar noises. Keeps hands fisted. *Socialization and Vocalization* Mews and makes throaty noises. Shows interest in human face. *Cognitive and Emotional Development* Reflexive. External stimuli are meaningless. Responses are generally limited to tension states or discomfort. Gains satisfaction from feeding and being held, rocked, fondled, and cuddled. Has an intense need for sucking pleasure. Quiets when picked up.	*Play Stimulation* Use human face—smile and talk. Dangle bright and moving object in field of vision (mobile). Hold, touch, caress, fondle, kiss. Rock, pat, change position. Play soft music or have infant listen to ticking clock, sing. Talk to infant, call him by name. *Parental Guidance* Begin to expose infant to different household sounds. Change crib location in room. Use bright-colored clothing and linen. Keep infant nearby. Allow him to sleep. Play with him when he is awake. Hold him during feeding.
8 weeks (2 months) Crossed extensor reflex disappears.	*Motor Development* Reflexive behavior is slowly being replaced by voluntary movements. Turns from side to back. Begins to lift head momentarily from prone position. Shows eye coordination to light and objects. If bell is sounded near him, he will stop activity and listen. Eyes follow better, both vertically and horizontally. *Socialization and Vocalization* Begins vocalization—coos, especially to a voice. Crying becomes differentiated. Visually looks for sounds. May squeal with delight when stimulated by touching, talking, or singing. Begins social smile. Eyes follow person or object more intently. *Cognitive and Emotional Development* Recognizes familiar face. Becomes more aware and interested in environment. Anticipates being fed when in feeding position. Enjoys sucking—puts hand in mouth.	*Play Stimulation* Arrange mobile over crib so infant's movement will set it in motion. Hang wind chimes near infant. Hang bright-colored pictures on wall (yellow and red-colored stripes, for example). Use cradle gym and infant seat. Use rattles. Hold infant and walk around room. Allow freedom of kicking with clothes off. *Parental Guidance* Talk to him and smile, get excited when he coos. Place infant seat near mother's activities but where he cannot fall off or tip over. Put in prone position in bed or on floor. Expose infant to different textures. Exercise infant's arms and legs. Sing to infant. Provide tactile experience during bathing, diapering, feeding. First DTP and TOPV immunization should be given.
12 weeks (3 months) Landau reflex appears at 3–4 months; stepping reflex disappears.	*Motor Development* When prone, he will rest on forearms and keep head in midline—makes crawling movements with legs, arches back, and holds head high, he may get chest off surface.	*Play Stimulation* Encourage socialization, smiling, laughing. Place on mat on floor. Continue to introduce new sounds.

Age and Physical Characteristics	Behavior Patterns	Nursing Implications/Parental Guidance
Positive support reflex disappears. Posterior fontanelle closes.	Indicates preference for prone or supine position. Discovers hands—strikes at objects while watching hands. Holds objects in hands and brings to mouth. Has fairly good head control. *Socialization and Vocalization* Smiles more readily. Babbles and coos. Stops crying when mother enters room or when he is caressed. Enjoys playing during feeding. Stays awake longer without crying. Turns head to follow familiar person. *Cognitive and Emotional Development* Shows active interest in environment. Recognizes familiar faces and objects. Focuses and follows objects. Shows repetitiveness in play activity. Is aware of strange situations. Derives pleasure from sucking—purposefully gets hand to mouth. Begins to establish routine preceding sleep.	*Parental Guidance* Take on daily outing as weather permits. Bounce on bed. Play with infant during feeding. Rattles can be used effectively for visual following and for hand play.
16 weeks (4 months) Stepping reflex disappears. Rooting reflex disappears. By 4–5 months infant's weight approximately doubles birth weight.	*Motor Development* Eyes focus on small objects; he may pick a dangling ring. Holds head up (when being pulled to sitting position). Becomes more interested in environment. Hand comes to meet rattle. Listens—turns head to familiar sound. Sits with minimal support. Intentional rolling over, back to side. Reaches for offered objects. Grasps objects with both hands and everything goes into mouth. *Socialization and Vocalization* Laughs and chuckles socially. Demands social attention by fussing. Recognizes mother. Begins to respond to "No, no." Enjoys being propped in sitting position. *Cognitive and Emotional Development* Actively interested in environment. Enjoys attention; becomes bored when alone for long periods of time. Recognizes bottle. More interested in mother. Indicates increasing trust and security. Sleeps through night; has defined nap time.	*Play Stimulation* Encourage mirror play. Provide soft squeeze toys in vivid colors of varying texture. Allow infant to splash in bath. Infant still enjoys holding and playing with rattles. Enjoys old-fashioned clothespins and playing pat-a-cake, peek-a-boo. *Parental Guidance* Be certain button eyes on toys and other small objects cannot be pulled off. Hold rattle for him and let him reach and grasp it. When baby is in highchair, strap in. Let him play with food; give finger foods. Move mobile out of reach—he may grab it and cause injury. Repeat child's sounds to him. Talk in varying degrees of loudness. Begin looking at and naming pictures in book. Begin roughhousing play by both parents. Second DTP and TOPV immunization should be given.
26 weeks (7 months)	*Motor Development* Shows momentary sitting, with hand support.	*Play Stimulation* Enjoys social games, hide-and-seek with adult, toys, large blocks.

(continued on next page)

Age and Physical Characteristics	Behavior Patterns	Nursing Implications/Parental Guidance
By 5–6 months, tonic neck reflex disappears. By 6–7 months, palmar grasp disappears. By 7–9 months, develops eye-to-eye contact while talking; engages in social games. 2 central lower incisors erupt.	Bounces and bears some weight when held in standing position. Transfers and mouths objects in one hand. Discovers feet. Bangs objects together. Rolls over well. May begin some form of mobility. *Socialization and Vocalization* Discriminates between strangers and familiar figures. Crows and squeals. Starts to say "Ma," "Da." Self-play is self-contained. Laughs out loud. Makes "talking" sounds in response to others' talking. *Cognitive and Emotional Development* Secures objects by pulling on string. Searches for lost objects that are out of sight. Inspects objects; localizes sounds. Likes to sit in highchair. Drops and picks up objects. Displays exploratory behavior with food. Exhibits beginning fear of strangers. Becomes fretful when mother leaves. Shows much mouthing and biting.	Likes to bang objects. Plays in bounce chair, walker. Enjoys large nesting toys (round rather than square). Likes to drop and retrieve things. Likes metal cups, wooden spoons, and things to bang with. Loves crumpled paper. Enjoys squeeze toys in bath. Likes peek-a-boo, bye-bye, and pat-a-cake. *Parental Guidance* Will play as long as you can. Tie toys to chair with short string. Let play with extra spoon at feeding. Give soft finger foods. Since infant puts everything in mouth, *use safety precautions.* Keep small items away from him; he could choke on them. Show excitement at his achievements. Supply kitchen items for toys. Third DTP and TOPV immunization at 6 months.
40 weeks (10 months) 4 upper incisors erupt around 7–9 months. By 9–12 months, plantar reflex disappears. By 9–12 months, neck-righting reflex disappears.	*Motor Development* Sits without support. Recovers balance. Manipulates objects with hands. Unwraps objects. Creeps. Pulls self upright at crib rails. Uses index finger and thumb to hold objects. Rings a bell. Can feed himself a cracker and can hold bottle. Can control lips around cup. Does not like supine position. Can hold index finger and thumb in opposition. *Socialization and Verbalization* Claps hands on request. Responds to own name. Is very aware of social environment. Imitates gestures, facial expressions, and sounds. Smiles at image in mirror. Offers toy to adult, but does not release it. Begins to test parental reaction during feeding and at bedtime. Will entertain self for long periods of time. *Cognitive and Emotional Development* Begins to imitate. Shows more interest in picture books. Enjoys achievements. Has strong urge toward independ-	*Play Stimulation* Encourage use of motion toys— rocking horse, stroller. Water play. Imitate animal sounds. Allow exploration outdoors. Provide for learning by imitation. Offer new objects (blocks). Child likes freedom of creeping and walking, but closeness of family is important. Good toys: milk carton; bean bag for tossing; fabric books; things to move around, fill up, empty out; pile-up and knock-down toys. *Parental Guidance* Do things with him. Protect him from dangerous objects—cover electrical outlets, block stairs, remove breakable objects from tables. Use plastic bottle. Have child with family at mealtime. Offer cup.

Age and Physical Characteristics	Behavior Patterns	Nursing Implications/Parental Guidance
	ence—locomotion, feeding, dressing.	

12 months
(1 year)
 	
By 12–18 months, Babinski sign disappears.
By 12–24 months, Landau reflex disappears.
By 10–14 months, anterior fontanelle closes.
Weight should approximately triple birth weight.
2 lower lateral incisors appear.
4 first molars appear by 14 months.
 	
Child Development Theories
Freudian: Behavior
  Birth–1 year—Oral Stage
Eriksonian: Emotion/Personality
  Birth–1 year—Sense of Trust vs. Mistrust
Piagetian: Intellectual Activity (Thought Process)
  Birth–2 years—Sensorimotor period
	Motor Development
	Cruises around furniture.
	Beginning to stand alone and toddle.
	Turns pages in book.
	Tries tossing object.
	Shows hand dominance.
	Navigates stairs; climbs on chairs.
	Builds a tower of 2 blocks.
	Puts balls in box.
	May use spoon.
	Can release objects at will.
	Has regular bowel movements.
	
	Socialization and Verbalization
	Uses jargon.
	Points to indicate wants.
	Loves give-and-take game.
	Responds to music.
	Enjoys being center of attention and will repeat laughed-at activities.
	
	Cognitive and Emotional Development
	Shows fear, anger, affection, jealousy, anxiety, and sympathy.
	Experiments to reach new goals.
	Displays intense determination to remove barriers to action.
	Begins to develop concepts of space, time, and causality.
	Has increased attention span.
		Play Stimulation
		Ball play
		Cloth doll
		Motion objects and toys
		Transporting objects
		Name and point to body parts.
		"Put-in" and "take-out" toys
		Sand box with spoons and other similar objects.
		Blocks
		Music
		
		Parental Guidance
		Allow self-directed play rather than adult-directed play.
		Continue to expose to foods of different textures, taste, smell, substance.
		Offer cup.
		Show affection and encourage child to return affection.
		Tuberculin test as well as measles, mumps, and rubella immunization should be given at 15 months.

18 months NOTE: Between 1 and 3 years the child is called a "toddler." Anterior fontanelle closed. Abdomen protrudes Big muscles become well developed 4 cuspids appear by 18 months. Fine muscle coordination begins to develop.	*Motor Development* Walks up stairs with help, creeps downstairs. Walks without support and with balance. Falls less frequently. Throws ball. Stoops to pick up toys, look at bug. Turns pages of book. Holds and lifts cup. Builds 3-block tower. Picks up and places small beads in container. Begins to use spoon. *Cognitive and Emotional Development* Has vocabulary of 10 words which have meanings. Uses phrases, imitates words. Points to objects named by adult. Follows directions and requests. Imitates adult behavior. Retrieves toy from several hiding places. Is beginning to develop symbolic thought. *Psychosocial Development* Develops new awareness of strangers. Wants to explore everything in reach. Plays alone, but near others. Is dependent upon parents, but begins to reach out for autonomy. Finds security in a blanket, toy, or thumbsucking.	*Play Stimulation* Allow unrestricted motor activity (within safety limits). Offer push-pull toys. Child selects favorite toy. Child likes blocks, pyramid toys, teddy bears, dolls, pots and pans, cloth picture books with colorful large pictures, telephone, musical top, nested blocks. *Parental Guidance* Begin to teach tooth brushing to establish good dental habits. Safety teaching: Child gets into everything within his reach. Place medications in safe, locked place. Create a safe environment for child. DTP and TOPV booster immunization. Limits need to be set that give toddler sense of security, yet encourage exploration. Identify behavior changes common in toddler.

(continued on next page)

Age and Physical Characteristics	Behavior Patterns	Nursing Implications/Parental Guidance
2 years Protruding abdomen less noticeable. Landau reflex disappears. During first 2 years 35 cm. (14–15 inches) are added to height.	*Motor Development* Walks up and down stairs. Opens doors; turns knobs. Has steady gait. Holds drinking cup well with 1 hand. Uses spoon without spilling food (may prefer fingers). Kicks a ball in front of him without support. Builds a tower of 4–6 blocks. Scribbles. Rides tricycle or kiddie car (without pedals). *Cognitive Development* Has 200–300 words in vocabulary. Begins to use short sentences. Refers to self by pronoun. Obeys simple commands. Does not know right from wrong. Begins to learn about time sequences. *Psychosocial Development* Uses word "mine" constantly. Is possessive with toys. Displays negativism—uses "no" as assertion of self. Routine and rituals are important. Begins cooperation in toilet training. Resists restrictions on freedom. Has fear of parents' leaving. Shows parallel play. Dawdles. Resists bedtime—uses transitional objects (blanket, toy). Vacillates between dependence and independence.	*Play Stimulation* Shows parallel play, although he enjoys having other children around him. Has very short attention span. Enjoys same toys as child of 18 months. Likes doll play, ball. Imitates parents in domestic activities. Likes swing, hammering, paper, large crayons. *Parental Guidance* Has need for peer companionship, although he displays his immaturity by his inability to share and take turns. A decrease in appetite normally occurs at this stage. Toilet training should be started (each child follows his own pattern). Begin to have child eat his meals with family if he has not already done so. Begin to read to child; child likes storybooks with large pictures.
2–3 years Height approximates half his adult height. Legs are about 34% of body length. Begins 2+ kg (5 lb.) weight gain per year until 5 years old. At 2½ years has full set (20) of baby teeth. 4 second molars appear by 2½ years.	*Motor Development* Throws objects overhead. Pedals tricycle. Walks backward. Washes and dries hands. Begins to use scissors. Can string large beads. Can undress himself. Feeds himself well. Tries to dance. Jumps in place. Builds tower of 8 blocks. Balances on one foot. Swings and climbs. Can eat an ice cream cone. Drinks from a straw. Chews gum without swallowing it. *Cognitive Development* Shows increased attention span. Gives first and last name. Begins to ask "why." Is egocentric in thought and behavior Beginning ability to reflect on own behavior. Talks in short sentences. Uses plurals. May attempt to sing simple songs. Has vocabulary of 900 words.	*Play Stimulation* Plays simple games with other children. Enjoys story-telling and dress-up play. Plays "house." Colors. Uses scissors and paper. Rides tricycle. Read simple books to him. Will assist in developing memory skills, visual discrimination skills, and language. *Parental Guidance* From 2–3 years the child develops a seeming maturity; do not expect more of him than he is able to do. Arrange first visit to the dentist to have teeth checked. Be aware that negativistic and ritualistic behavior is normal. Be consistent in discipline. Control temper tantrums. Begin to teach traffic safety. Supervise outdoor play.

Age and Physical Characteristics	Behavior Patterns	Nursing Implications/Parental Guidance
	Begins to understand what it means to take turns. Can repeat 3 numbers. Shows interest in colors.	
Child Development Theories Freudian: 1–3 years—Anal Stage Eriksonian: 1–3 years—Sense of autonomy vs. shame and doubt Piagetian: 2–7 years—Preoperational Period; shows egocentrism and centering	*Psychosocial Development* Negativism grows out of child's sense of developing independence—says "no" to every command. Ritualism is important to toddler for his security (follows certain pattern, especially at bedtime). Temper tantrums may result from toddler's frustration in wanting to do everything himself. Shows parallel play as well as beginning interaction with others. Engages in associative play. Fears become pronounced. Continues to react to separation from parents but shows increasing ability to handle short periods of separation. Has daytime bladder control and is beginning to develop night-time bladder control. Becomes more independent. Begins to identify sex (gender) roles. Explores environment outside the home. Can create different ways of getting desired outcome.	
3–4 years NOTE: Between 3 and 5 years the child is called a "pre-schooler."	*Motor Development* Drawings have form and meaning, not detail. Buttons front and side of clothes. Laces shoes. Bathes self, but needs direction. Brushes teeth. Shows continuous movement going up and down stairs. Climbs and jumps well. Attempts to print letters. *Cognitive Development* Awareness of body is more stable; child becomes more aware of own vulnerability. Is less negativistic. Learns some number concepts. Begins naming colors. Can identify longer of 2 lines. Has vocabulary of 1500 words. Uses mild profanities and name-calling. Uses language aggressively. Asks many questions. Can be given simple explanation as to cause and effect. Thinks very concretely; demonstrates irreversibility of thought. Has beginning understanding of past and future. Is egocentric in thought. *Psychosocial Development* Is more active with peers and engages in cooperative play.	*Play Stimulation* Plays and interacts with other children. Shows creativity. "Helps" adults. Likes costumes and enjoys dramatic play. Toys and games: record player, nursery rhymes, housekeeping toys, transportation toys (tricycle, trucks, cars, wagon), blocks, hammer and peg bench, floor trains, blackboard and chalk, easel and brushes, clay, crayon and finger paints, outside toys (sandbox, swing, small slide), books (short stories, action stories), drum, scrapbook. *Parental Guidance* Base your expectations within child's limitations. Provide limited frustrations from environment to assist him in coping. Give small errands to do around the house (putting silverware on table, drying a dish). Expand child's world with trips to the zoo, to the supermarket, to restaurant, etc. Prevent accidents. Provide for brief, nonthreatening separation from parents and home.

(continued on next page)

Age and Physical Characteristics	Behavior Patterns	Nursing Implications/Parental Guidance
	Performs simple tasks. Frequently has imaginary companion. Dramatizes experiences. Is proud of accomplishments. Exaggerates, boasts, and tattles on others. Can tolerate separation from mother longer without feeling anxiety. Is keen observer. Has good sense of "mine" and "yours." Behavior still frequently ritualistic. Becomes curious about life and sex. Often indulges in masturbation.	Reinforce correct use of language. Utilize opportunities for simple sexual education as child's needs arise. Accept masturbation as a normal phenomenon to be discouraged in public. Provide consistent discipline, motivated by love not anger. Prepare child for nursery school.

4–5 years
 	
By 2–5 years adds 25 cm. (9–10 inches) to height.
At age 4, legs comprise about 44% of body length.
 	
Child Development Theories
Freudian:
  3–6 years—Phallic Stage
Eriksonian:
  3–6 years—Sense of Initiative vs. Guilt
Piagetian:
  2–7 years—Preoperational Period; shows egocentrism and centering
	Motor Development
	Hops 2 or more times.
	Dresses without supervision.
	Has good motor control—climbs and jumps well.
	Walks up stairs without grasping handrail.
	Walks backwards.
	Washes self without wetting clothes.
	Prints first name and other words.
	Adds 3 or more details in drawings.
	
	Cognitive Development
	Has 2100-word vocabulary.
	Talks constantly.
	Uses adult speech forms.
	Participates in conversations.
	Asks for definitions.
	Knows age and residence.
	Identifies heavier of two objects.
	Knows weeks as time units.
	Names days of week.
	Begins to understand kinship.
	Knows primary colors.
	Can count to 10.
	Can copy a triangle.
	Has high degree of imagination.
	Questioning is at a peak.
	Begins to develop power of reasoning.
	
	Psychosocial Development
	May have an imaginary companion.
	Has a sense of order (likes to finish what he has started).
	Is obedient and reliable.
	Is protective toward younger children.
	Begins to develop an elementary conscience with some influence in governing his behavior.
	Has increased self-confidence.
	Accepts responsibility for acts.
	Is less rebellious.
	Has dreams and nightmares.
	Is cooperative and sympathetic.
	Shows generosity with toys.
	Begins to question parents' thinking.
	Identifies strongly with parent of same sex.
		Play Stimulation
		Demonstrates gross motor activity—likes to jump rope, skip, climb on jungle gyms, etc.
		Prefers group play and cooperates in projects.
		Plays simple letter, number, form, and picture games.
		Plays with cars and trucks.
		Still likes being read to.
		Continues to enjoy fantasy play.
		
		Parental Guidance
		Child no longer takes an afternoon nap.
		Prepare child for kindergarten.
		Tell him stories.
		Provide opportunities and reassurance for group play; have his friends visit for lunch and an afternoon of playing.
		Prevent accidents.
		Between 4 and 6 years DTP and TOPV booster immunizations are needed.
		Encourage child's participation in household activities.

Age and Physical Characteristics	Behavior Patterns	Nursing Implications/Parental Guidance

Middle Childhood
(5–9 years)
 	
Growth rate is slow and steady. Child gains an average of 3.18 kg. (7 lb.) per year. Height increases approximately 6.25 cm (2½ inches) per year.
Among children there is considerable variation in height and weight.
Child appears taller and slimmer.
Early lordosis disappears.
Child begins to lose baby teeth; permanent teeth appear at a rate of about 4 teeth per year from 7–14 years.
Neuromuscular and skeletal development allows improved coordination.
Eyes become fully developed; vision approaches 20/20.
 	
Child Development Theories
Freudian:
  5–9 years—Beginning of latency period
Eriksonian:
  5–9 years—Industry vs. Inferiority
Piagetian:
  5–9 years—Enters stage of concrete operations
	Motor Development
	6 years
	  Is active and impulsive.
	  Balance improves.
	  Uses hands as manipulative tools in cutting, pasting, hammering.
	  Can draw large letters or figures.
	7 years
	  Has lower activity level.
	  Capable of fine hand movements; can print sentences.
	  Nervous habits such as nail biting are common.
	  Muscular skills such as ball throwing have improved.
	8 years
	  Moves with less restlessness.
	  Has developed grace and balance, even in active sports.
	  Has developed coordination of fine muscles, allowing him to write in script rather than to print.
	9 years
	  Uses both hands independently.
	  Has become skillful in manual activities because of improved eye-hand coordination.
	
	Cognitive Development
	6 years
	  Begins to learn to read. Defines objects in terms of use. Time sense is as much in past as present.
	  Is interested in relationship between home and neighborhood; knows some streets.
	  Uses sentences well; uses language to share other's experiences; may swear or use slang.
	  Distinguishes morning from afternoon.
	7 years
	  More reflective and has deeper understanding of meanings.
	  Interested in conclusions and logical endings. Begins to have scientific interests in cause and effect.
	  More responsible in relation to time; is more punctual. Sense of space is more realistic; child wants some space of own.
	  Knows value of coins.
	8 years
	  Thinking is less animistic. Is aware of impersonal forces of nature. Begins to understand logical reasoning, conclusions, implications.
	  Less self-centered in thinking.
	  Personal space is expanding,
		Family atmosphere continues to have impact on child's emotional development and his future response within the family.
		
		The child needs ongoing guidance in an open, inviting atmosphere. Limits should be set with conviction. Deal with only one incident at a time. When punishment is necessary, the child should not be humiliated. He should know that it was the *act* that the adult found undesirable, not the child.
		
		Needs assistance in adjusting to new experiences and demands of school. Should be able to share experiences with family. Parents need to have communication with the teacher in order to work together for the health of the child.
		Convey love and caring in communication. The child understands language directed at feelings better than at intellect. Get down to eye level with the child.
		Focus attention on child's abilities and accomplishments rather than his shortcomings and limitations.
		
		Child is sex-conscious. He should be able to discuss his questions at home rather than with his friends. Requires simple, honest answers to questions.
		Common problems include teasing, quarreling, nail-biting, enuresis, whining, poor manners, swearing. These are usually fleeting phases and should not be handled negatively. The causes for such behavior should be investigated and dealt with constructively.
		
		The child needs order and consistency in his life to help him cope with doubts, fears, unacceptable impulses, and unfamiliar experiences.
		Encourage peer activities as well as home responsibilities and give recognition to child's accomplishments and unique talents.
		Television may stimulate learning in several spheres, but should be monitored.
		Accidents are a major cause of disability and death. Safety practices should be continued. (Refer to section on safety, pp. 1119–1123.)
		Exercise is essential to promote mo-

(continued on next page)

Age and Physical Characteristics	Behavior Patterns	Nursing Implications/Parental Guidance
	goes places on own. Aware of time; plans events of day. Understands right from left.	tor and psychosocial development. The child should have a safe place to play and simple pieces of equipment.
	9 years Intellectually energetic and curious. Realistic; reasonable in thinking. Able to plan in advance. Breaks complex activities into steps. Focuses on detail. Sense of space includes the entire earth. Participates in family discussions. Likes to have secrets.	A school health program should be available and concerned with the child's physical, emotional, mental, and social health. This should be augmented by information and example at home. Medical supervision should continue with yearly examination to detect developmental delay, disease. Appropriate immunizations should be administered. Child frequently has "quiet days"—periods of shyness, which should be tolerated as part of growing up and deciding who he is. Child may be subject to nightmares, a situation which requires reassurance and understanding.
	Psychosocial Development (The following characteristics apply to the child in the 5–9 year group.) Still requires parental support, but pulls away from overt signs of affection. Peer groups provide companionship in widening circle of persons outside the home. Child learns more about self as he learns about others. "Chum" stage occurs at about 9–10 years of age. Child chooses a special friend of same sex and age in whom to confide. This is usually child's first love relationship outside of home, when someone becomes as important to him as himself. Play teaches the child new ideas and independence. He progressively utilizes tools of competition, compromise, cooperation, and beginning collaboration.	Parents, teachers, and health professionals should be available and able to provide information and answer questions about the physical changes which occur.
	Patterns of Play 6–7 years Child acts out ideas of family and occupational groups with which he has contact. Painting, pasting, reading, simple games, watching T.V., digging, running games, skating, riding bicycle, and swimming, are all enjoyed activities. 8 years Child enjoys collections; loosely formed, short-lived clubs; table games; card games; books; T.V.; records. Body image and self-concept are	

Age and Physical Characteristics	Behavior Patterns	Nursing Implications/Parental Guidance
	quite fluid because of rapid physical, emotional, social changes. Latency stage-sexual drive is controlled and repressed. Emphasis is on the development of skills and talent.	
Late Childhood (9–12 years) Vital signs approach adult values. Loses childish appearance of face and takes on features that will characterize him as an adult. Growth spurt occurs, and some secondary sex characteristics appear: in females, at age 10–12 years; in males, at age 12–14 years. Physical changes of puberty: Increased height and weight, increased perspiration, activity of sebaceous glands, vasomotor instability, increased fat deposition. Physical changes in female: Pelvis increases in transverse diameter; hips broaden; tenderness in developing breast tissue; enlargement of areola diameter; appearance of pubic hair. Physical changes in male: Size of testes increases; scrotum color changes; breasts enlarge, temporarily; height and shoulder breadth increase. Appearance of lightly pigmented hair at base of penis. Increase in length and width of penis. *Child Development Theories* Freudian: 9–12 years—Latency period continues Eriksonian: 9–12 years—Industry vs. Inferiority continues Piagetian: 9–12 years—Stage of concrete operations continues	*Motor Development* Energetic, restless, active movements such as finger-drumming or foot-tapping appear. Has skillful manipulative movements nearly equal to those of adults. Works hard to perfect physical skills. *Cognitive Development* 10 years Likes to reason, enjoys learning. Thinking is concrete, matter of fact. Wants to measure up to challenge. Likes to memorize, identify facts. Attention span may be short. Space is rather specific (i.e., where things are). Can write for relatively long time with speed. 11 years Likes action in learning. Concentrates well when working competitively. Can understand relational terms such as weight and size. Perceives space as nothingness that goes on forever. Able to discuss problems. Can describe some abstract terms. 12 years Enjoys learning. Considers all aspects of a situation. Motivated more by inner drive than by competition. Able to classify, arrange, generalize. Likes to discuss and debate. Begins conceptual thinking. Verbal, formal reasoning now possible. Can recognize moral of a story. Defines time as duration; likes to plan ahead. Understands that space is abstract. Can be critical of own work. *Psychosocial Development* Gang becomes important, and gang code takes precedence over nearly everything. Often gang codes are characterized by collective action against the mores of the adult world. Here, children begin to work out own social pat-	Continue appropriate nursing interventions related to early childhood. Continue sex education and preparation for adolescent body changes. Understanding is important. Encourage participation in organized clubs, youth groups. Democratic guidance is essential as child works through a conflict between dependence (on his parents) and independence. Child needs realistic limits set. Needs help channeling energy in proper direction—work and sports. Requires adequate explanation of body changes. Special understanding required for the child who lags in physical development. Continue consistent disciplinary style.

(continued on next page)

Age and Physical Characteristics	Behavior Patterns	Nursing Implications/Parental Guidance
	terns without adult interference. Early gangs may include both sexes; later gangs are separated by sex. May strive for unreasonable independence from adult control. Often interested in religion, morality. Has increased interest in sexuality. *Patterns of Play* Continues to enjoy reading, T.V., table games. More interested in active sports as a means to improve skills. Creative talents may appear; may enjoy drawing, modeling clay. By age 10, sex differences in play become profound. Occasional privacy is important. May reach puberty; resurgence of sexual drives causes recapitulation of oedipal struggle. Begins to have vocational aspirations.	
Early Adolescence (females: 12–14 years; males: 14–18 years) Phase of development begins when reproductive organs become functionally operative; phase ends when physical growth is completed. Skeletal system grows faster than supporting muscles. Hands and feet grow proportionally faster than rest of body. Large muscles develop more quickly than small muscles. Females: Physical changes include appearance of menarche; growth of axillary and perineal hair; deepened voice; ovulation; further development of breasts. Male: Physical changes include growth of axillary, perineal, facial, chest hair; deepening of voice; production of spermatozoa; nocturnal emissions. *Child Development Theories* Freudian: 12–14 years—Begins stage of sexuality Eriksonian: 12–14 years—Identity vs. role diffusion Piagetian: 12–14 years—Begins stage of formal operations	*Motor Development* Often uncoordinated; has poor posture. Tires easily. *Cognitive Development* Mind has great ability to acquire and utilize knowledge. Categorizes thoughts into usable forms. May project thinking into the future. Is capable of highly imaginative thinking. *Psychosocial Development* Interest in opposite sex increases. Often revolts from adult authority to conform to peer-group standards. Continues to rework feelings for parent of opposite sex and unravel the ambivalence toward parent of same sex. Affection may turn temporarily to an adult outside of the family (for example, crush on family friend, neighbor, or teacher). Utilizes peer group dialect—highly informal language or specially coined terminology. Peer groups are especially important and help adolescent to define own identity, to adapt to changing body image, to establish more mature relationships with others, and to deal with heightened sexual feelings. Cliques may develop. Dating generally progresses from groups of couples to double dates and finally single couples.	Stresses frequently result from conflicting value systems between generations. Parents may need help to see that the adolescent is a product of the times and that his actions reflect what is happening around him. Parents' limits and rules should be realistic and consistent. They should convey the love and concern of parents and should be a source of comfort and reassurance, protecting the child from activities for which he is not ready. The home should be an accepting, emotionally stable environment. Continue sex education, including discussion of ovulation, fertilization, menstruation, pregnancy, contraception, masturbation, nocturnal emissions, and hygiene. Adolescents have an increased need for rest and sleep, because they are expending large amounts of energy and are functioning with an inadequate oxygen supply. Recreational interests should be fostered. Favorite activities include sports, dating, dancing, reading, hobbies, and T.V. Talking on the telephone, listening to records are favorite pastimes. Adolescent health problems which require preventive education are accidents, obesity, acne, pregnancy, venereal disease, drug abuse. Allow adolescent to handle his own affairs as much as possible, but be aware of physical and psychoso-

Age and Physical Characteristics	Behavior Patterns	Nursing Implications/Parental Guidance
	Teenage "hangouts" become important centers of activity. Begins questioning existing moral values.	cial problems with which he will need help. Encourage independence but allow child to lean on parents for support when frightened or unable to attain his goals. Adolescents with special problems should have access to specialists such as adolescent clinics, and psychologists. Requires reassurance and help in accepting his changing body image. Parents should make the most of his positive qualities. Give gentle encouragement and guidance regarding dating. Avoid strong pressures in either direction. Understand his conflicts as he attempts to deal with social, moral, and intellectual issues. Provide opportunities for adolescents to earn their own money; allow some financial independence. Provide safety education—especially regarding driving. Provide assistance to develop good attitudes toward health—smoking, drinking, drugs, nutrition, etc.
Late Adolescence Begins when physical growth is completed and extends from age 15–18 years for females and from 18–20 for males. Wisdom teeth erupt. Males: Genitals and pubic hair are adult in appearance. Physique is that of mature male. Females: Breasts and pubic hair are adult in appearance. *Child Development Theories:* Freudian: 15–18 years—Stage of adult sexuality Eriksonian: 15–18 years—May begin intimacy vs. isolation Piagetian: 15–18 years—Stage of formal operations	*Motor Development* Energy is increased as growth spurt ends. Muscular ability and coordination increase. *Cognitive Development* Spends large amount of time in abstract and analytical thinking. Begins to develop workable philosophy of life. May accept or reject the family religion. *Psychosocial Development* Tasks include achievement of ego identity, establishment of heterosexual relationships, planning for the future and for occupational and marital choices. Dating emphasis shifts to sharing and to intimate relationship. Sexual experimentation is common in various forms—masturbation, necking, petting, intercourse. May seek alternatives to marriage—"living together," communes, etc. Ability to love becomes a major concern. Values include fidelity, friendship, cooperation. Ability to work is the culmination of the developmental life that began with play. Achieves emotional independence from parents and other adults.	Continue appropriate nursing interventions related to early adolescence. Provide guidance in selection of and preparation for a vocation. Encourage discussion regarding mate selection and alternatives to marriage. Parents themselves may require assistance facing the loss of a child once dependent on them.

CHILDHOOD DISEASES

Disease: a. Agent. b. Mode of transmission. c. Age when most common.	Incubation (I) and Communicability (C) Periods	Symptoms
Rubella (German/3-day-measles) a. Rubella virus b. Droplets or direct contact with infected persons or articles freshly contaminated with nasopharyngeal secretions, feces, urine c. School age, young adult *Diagnostic Tests:* Tissue culture of throat, blood or urine *Passive Immunity:* Birth to about 1 year of age if mother is immune prior to pregnancy	*I:* 14–21 days after exposure *C:* Virus can be passed from 7 days before to 5 days after rash appears.	a. Rash—enlarged lymph nodes in postauricular, suboccipital and cervical areas b. In adolescents—headache, anorexia, low-grade fever, sore throat, coryza, conjunctivitis, generalized malaise 1–5 days before rash appears *Duration:* 3–5 days *Rash Characteristics:* Pinpoint (or larger) red spots on soft palate (Forchheimer's spots) spread to face and downward toward the feet, covering entire body at end of first day; maculopapular eruption; Rash begins to subside on second day in same order
Roseola infantum (exanthema subitum) a. Presumably caused by virus b. Transmission not known c. 6 months–2 years	Not known—believed not to be highly contagious	a. Fever of 40–40.5°C (104–105°F), either intermittent or sustained 3–4 days; decrease in appetite; slightly irritable b. Fever suddenly drops and rash of red measles or maculopapules 2–3 mm. appears *Duration:* 1–2 days Rash fades on pressure. It appears first on trunk and spreads upward and downward.
Rubeola (hard, red, 7-day measles) a. Measles virus, RNA-containing paramyxovirus b. Direct contact with droplets from infected persons *Diagnostic Tests:* Serologic procedures *Passive Immunity:* Birth to about 1 year of age if mother is immune prior to pregnancy	*I:* 10–12 days *C:* 5th day of incubation to first 5–7 days of rash	a. Fever, lethargy b. 48 hours—Koplik's spots on buccal mucosa (spots are reddened areas with grayish-blue center) c. 2 days later, rash appears at hairline and spreads to feet in one day, maculopapular eruption d. Lymphadenopathy e. Anorexia f. Pruritus
Mumps a. Mumps virus, paramyxovirus b. Urine, blood, and saliva by direct contact or droplets *Diagnostic Tests:* Complement fixation *Passive Immunity:* Birth to 3–4 months of age if mother had antibodies against mumps prior to pregnancy	*I:* 14–21 days *C:* 7 days before to 9 days after swelling appears; virus in saliva greatest just before and after parotitis onset	a. Headache, anorexia, generalized malaise; fever 1 day before glandular swelling; fever lasts 1–6 days. b. Glandular swelling, usually of parotid c. Enlargement and reddening of Wharton's duct and Stensen's duct

Treatment	Complications	Special Considerations
Symptomatic	In adolescent and adult: Arthritis Encephalitis Purpura	Exposure of nonimmune pregnant women in first trimester results in high percentage of affected fetuses and infants born with various birth defects: cataracts, heart murmur, deafness
Symptomatic—antipyretic	Convulsions due to high fever	
Bed rest; isolation from onset of catarrh through 3rd day of rash *Treatment of Itching:* Cornstarch bath, mitt hands, application of calamine lotion to lesions, keeping fingernails trimmed	Otitis media, pneumonia, laryngitis, mastoiditis, encephalitis	
Isolation until swelling has subsided	Meningoencephalitis Auditory nerve involvement, resulting in deafness Orchitis (if disease occurs after puberty)	

(continued on next page)

Disease: a. Agent. b. Mode of transmission. c. Age when most common.	Incubation (I) and Communicability (C) Periods	Symptoms
Chickenpox a. Varicella-zoster b. Highly communicable; acquired via direct contact, indirect contact, droplet spread, airborne transmission c. 2–8 years *Diagnostic Tests:* Scrapings from vesicle; staining reveals multinucleated giant cells. *Passive Immunity:* Best accomplished by Varicella-Zoster Immune Globulin	*I:* 14–21 days after exposure *C:* Onset of fever (one day prior to first lesion) until last vesicle is dried (5–7 days)	a. General malaise and fever for 24 hours b. Rash—macules to papules and vesicles to crusts within several hours c. Itching of lesions may be severe and scratching may cause scarring *Rash Characteristics:* Rash appears first on head and mucous membranes, then becomes concentrated on body and sparse on extremities, papulovesicular eruption
Diphtheria a. *Corynebacterium diphtheriae* b. Acquired through secretions of carrier or infected individual by direct contact with contaminated articles and environment c. Incidence increased in autumn and spring *Diagnostic Tests:* Cultures of nose and throat	*I:* 2–6 days *C:* 2–4 weeks untreated; 1–2 days with antibiotic treatment	a. Pharyngeal and tonsillar diphtheria: (1) General malaise, low-grade fever, anorexia (2) 1–2 days later, whitish-gray membranous patch on tonsils, soft palate, and uvula (3) Lymph node swelling, fever, rapid pulse b. Nasal diphtheria: (1) Coryza with increasing viscosity, possibly epistaxis, low-grade fever (2) Whitish-gray membrane may appear over nasal septum c. Laryngeal diphtheria: (1) Usually spread from pharynx to larynx (2) Fever, harsh voice, barking cough; respiratory difficulty with inspiratory retraction d. Nonrespiratory diphtheria: affects eye, ear, genitals or, rarely, skin
Pertussis (whooping cough) a. *Bordetella pertussis* b. Direct contact, droplet spread; indirect contact with contaminated articles c. Infants and young children; incidence higher in spring and summer	*I:* 5–21 days *C:* 7 days after exposure (greatest just before catarrhal stage) to 3 weeks after onset of paroxysms	a. Stage I (catarrhal stage) (1) Lasts 1–2 weeks (2) Coryza, sneezing, tearing, tickling/dry cough, fever, loss of appetite b. State II (paroxysmal stage) (1) Lasts 4–6 weeks (2) Severe, violent coughing attacks occurring in clusters leading to vomiting, cyanosis, and exhaustion c. Stage III (convalescent stage) (1) Lasts 4 months–2 years (2) Coughing attacks decrease, but return with each respiratory infection *Duration:* 9 months–2 years

Treatment	Complications	Special Considerations
Symptomatic: Short fingernails to prevent scratching Oral antihistamines to decrease pruritus Isolation until all lesions have crusted—about 5–6 days Treatment of itching: Mix baking soda (sodium bicarbonate) with warm water and pat on lesions	Complications are rare in normal children Hemorrhagic varicella, encephalitis, pneumonia, and bacterial skin infection are not common, but they can occur Reye's Syndrome	Severe in neonate and pregnant women Varicella-Zoster Immune Globulin (VZIG) is available from Center for Disease Control (Atlanta, Ga.) for high-risk susceptible children who have been exposed to varicella zoster. This should be given within 72 hours of exposure to Varicella-Zoster. If VZIG is unavailable, Immune Serum Globulin (ISG) at a dose of 0.6–1.2 ml./kg. body weight; Promptly given may modify Varicella
Diphtheria antitoxin Antibiotic therapy (penicillin, erythromycin) Supportive treatment Respiratory support Isolation until 2–3 cultures are negative after antibiotic therapy is completed	Myocarditis Neuritis	

Supportive:
  Bed rest
  Suctioning
  Antipyretics
  Antibiotics: erythromycin, ampicillin
Increase fluids; nutrition and electrolyte balance
Place in an environment with reduced stimuli to reduce coughing
Sedation
Isolation 4 weeks after coughing begins
	Respiratory: pneumonia, atelectasis, emphysema
	Neurologic: brain damage	

(continued on next page)

Disease: a. Agent. b. Mode of transmission. c. Age when most common.	Incubation (I) and Communicability (C) Periods	Symptoms
Tetanus (lockjaw) a. *Clostridium tetani*—prevalence in soil and animal feces; can be introduced into body through any break in skin or intestinal tract b. Direct or indirect contact with wound c. All ages *Diagnostic Tests:* Wound culture anaerobically for *Clostridium tetani*	*I:* 3 days to 3 weeks *C:* None	a. Stiffening of striated muscles, usually the jaw b. 1–2 days later, stiffening leads to spastic rigidity and spreads down body to the extremities
Poliomyelitis (polio) a. Virus serotypes 1−3+2; incidence is higher in summer and fall b. Virus is harbored in GI tract and is transmitted through saliva, vomitus and feces c. Predisposing factors that increase risk of disease: recent tonsillectomy, tooth extraction or DTP injections, pregnancy, physical exhaustion *Diagnostic Tests:* Isolation of polio virus from feces and throat	*I:* 7–14 days, paralytic or nonparalytic; 3–5 days for prodromal or minor illness *C:* Increases around onset when virus is in throat and is excreted in feces; virus is present in throat 1 week after onset, in stool 4–6 weeks after	a. Nonparalytic polio: (1) Headache, lethargy, anorexia, vomiting, fever (2) Muscle pain and stiffness b. Paralytic polio: (1) Same as nonparalytic type, lasting about a week (2) Then 1–2 days of CNS symptoms: loss of deep tendon reflexes, positive Kernig's and Brudzinski's signs, lethargy (3) 1–2 days later, weakening of muscles and paralysis
Streptococcal pharyngitis ("Strep Throat") a. Beta hemolytic streptococcus—group A strain b. Direct or indirect contact with nasopharyngeal secretion of infected person or recently established carrier c. Not under 3 years of age, 5–16 years, incidence higher in winter and spring *Diagnostic Tests:* nasopharyngeal (throat) culture	*I:* 2–5 days *C:* Greatest during acute phase of illness	a. Onset is generally acute: high fever, headache, vomiting, scarlatina rash b. After 12–24 hours—sore throat of varying degrees of severity, dryness of throat, cervical lymphadenopathy, white tongue coating that gives way to strawberry-red tongue
Impetigo a. Group A Streptococcus (more common in older children)—Bullous Staphylococcus aureus (more common in younger children) b. Usually direct contact often initiated by abrasions/insect bites; Streptococcal skin lesions often precede URI colonization *Diagnostic Tests:* Lesions cleansed; culture on blood agar fluid from intact bleb or base of crusted lesion, no active or passive immunity	*I:* 2–5 days *C:* Until lesions healed	Lesions: Vesicular, become confluent and rapidly progress to pustular and crusting stage; do not appear in crops. Commonly involves nasolabial area and others easily scratched; typical lesion is a thick, adherent amber-colored crust Bullous impetigo usually caused by staphylococci Purulent crusting lesions caused by hemolytic streptococci or staphylococci

Treatment	Complications	Special Considerations
Reduce muscular spasm with medication, quiet, dark room Antibiotics: penicillin or tetracycline Tetanus immune globulin or antitoxin Debridement of wound Fluid and nutrition	Convulsion with laryngospasms leading to death Asphyxia from dysphagia and secretions	
Supportive, i.e., relief of pain Analgesics, heat Enteric isolation	Respiratory paralysis Hypertension	
Isolation for 1 day while starting prescription Antibiotic therapy: penicillin G Symptomatic	Acute glomerulonephritis, 1–2 weeks after acute stage Rheumatic fever, 2–3 weeks after acute stage Peritonsillar abscess, cervical adenitis Pneumonia, otitis media, meningitis	Throat cultures of entire household (i.e., parents, siblings) 2–3 days after patient started therapy and treated if culture was positive Repeat throat culture done 2–3 days after completion of 10-day course of oral antibiotic
Specific: Systemic antimicrobial therapy for extensive impetigo—oral Pen V or Penicillin G for injection; others as indicated *Symptomatic:* Careful cleansing of lesions with soap and water; short fingernails to prevent scratching	Glomerulonephritis	Isolation necessary for hospitalized child; observe for skin lesions and treat promptly

NUTRITION IN CHILDREN*

Age and Developmental Influence on Nutritional Requirements and Feeding Patterns	Feeding Pattern/Diet	Nursing Implications/Parental Guidance

Neonate (birth-4 weeks)
 	
 Newborn's rapid growth makes him especially vulnerable to dietary inadequacies, dehydration, and iron deficiency anemia.
 Feeding process is basis for infant's first human relationship, his formation of trust. Feeding reinforces mother's sense of "motherliness."
 Because of limited nutritional stores, neonates require vitamin and mineral supplements.
 Neonates require more fluid relative to their size than do adults.
 Sucking ability is influenced by individual neuromuscular maturity.
	Breast milk or formula is generally given in 6–8 feedings per day, spaced 3–4 hours apart.
	 Feeding schedules should be individualized according to infant's needs.
		Provide information to help parents make decision concerning breast or bottle feeding.
		 Support parents in their decision.
		 Breast-fed infant (See p. 1031):
		 1. Help mother assume comfortable and satisfying position for self and baby.
		 2. Help mother to determine schedule, timing, and when infant is satisfied.
		 3. Provide specific information about the following:
		   a. Feeding technique: position, "bubbling"
		   b. Care of breasts
		   c. Manual expression of milk from breast
		   d. Maternal diet
		 Bottle-fed infant:
		 1. Provide specific information concerning
		   a. Type of formula
		   b. Preparation of formula: measuring and sterilization
		   c. Equipment—types of bottles, nipples, etc.
		   d. Sterilization of equipment
		   e. Technique of feeding: position, "bubbling"
		 2. Help mother to determine when infant is satisfied; develop schedule for feeding.
		 Provide information concerning normal characteristics of stools, signs of dehydration, constipation, colic, milk allergy.
		 Discuss need for vitamin supplements and how to administer.
		 Discuss need for additional fluids during periods of hot weather, and with fever, diarrhea, and vomiting.
		 Observe for evidence of common problems and intervene accordingly:
		 1. Overfeeding
		 2. Underfeeding
		 3. Difficulty digesting formula because of its particular composition.
		 4. Improper feeding technique; holes in nipples too large or too small; formula too hot or too cold; uncomfortable feeding position; failure to "bubble"; improper sterilization.
		 5. Emotional problems in family may cause irritability, colic and other similar disturbances.

* For recommended daily dietary allowances, refer to Appendix II, page 1489.

Age and Developmental Influence on Nutritional Requirements and Feeding Patterns	Feeding Pattern/Diet	Nursing Implications/Parental Guidance
Infant (3 months–1 year) Increased neuromuscular development allows infant to make transition from a totally liquid diet to a diet of milk and solid foods as well as to more active participation in the feeding process. 3–6 months Sucking reflex becomes voluntary and chewing action begins; infant can approximate lips to rim of cup and may begin drinking from cup at 6 months. 6–12 months Eyes and hands can work together; infant is able to sit without support and has developed grasp; able to feed self a biscuit; bangs objects on table; able to hold own bottle at 9–12 months; has "pincher" approach to food; able to be weaned as child becomes developmentally able to take sufficient fluids from the cup. Food provides the infant with a variety of learning experiences; motor control and coordination in self-feeding; recognition of shape, texture, color; stimulation of speech movement through use of mouth muscles. Mealtime allows the infant to continue his development of trust in a consistent, loving atmosphere. The infant is forming his lifetime eating habits; it is therefore important to make mealtime a positive experience.	Number of feedings per day decreases through the first year. By a year of age, most infants are satisfied with 3 meals and additional fluids throughout the day. By 4–6 months of age, the infant is generally ready to begin eating strained foods. The usual sequence of foods is cereal followed by fruits, vegetables, and meats. This sequence may vary according to individual preferences of pediatrician and family. Mashed table foods or junior foods generally are started at 6–8 months, when infant begins chewing action. Infant begins to enjoy finger foods at 10–12 months. The transition from iron fortified formula or breast milk to cow's milk is usually advised at about 12 months of age.	New foods should be offered one at a time and early in the feeding while the infant is still hungry. The person feeding should be calm, gentle, relaxed and patient in approach. When the child is first offered puréed foods with a spoon, he expects and wants to suck. The protrusion of his tongue, which is needed in sucking, makes it appear that he is pushing the food out of his mouth. This response should not be interpreted as dislike for the food; it is a result of immature muscle coordination and surprise at the taste and feel of the new food. The baby foods selected should be those which are high in nutrients without providing excessive calories. Personal and cultural preferences should be considered. Infants should be observed for allergic reactions when new foods are added. Common allergies are to citrus juices and egg white. Finger foods should be selected for their nutritional value. Good choices include teething biscuits, cooked vegetables, meat, cheese sticks, and enriched cereals. Avoid nuts, raisins and raw vegetables, which can cause choking. Parents can be taught to prepare their own strained or junior foods using a commercial baby food grinder or blender. Weaning is a gradual process. 1. Assist parents to recognize indications of readiness. 2. Do not expect the infant to completely drop his old pattern of behavior while learning a new one; allow overlap of old and new techniques. 3. Evening feedings are usually the most difficult to eliminate, because the infant is tired and in need of sucking comfort. 4. During illness or household disorganization, the infant may regress and return to sucking to relieve his discomfort and frustration. SPECIAL CONSIDERATIONS: Hospitalized infant Obtain a thorough nursing history that includes the following: Feeding pattern and schedule; types of foods that have been introduced; likes and dislikes; breast or bottle-fed, type of bottle; temperature at which infant prefers foods and fluids. (continued on next page)

Age and Developmental Influence on Nutritional Requirements and Feeding Patterns	Feeding Pattern/Diet	Nursing Implications/Parental Guidance
Toddler (1–3 years) Growth slows at the end of the first year, and weight gain is small. The slower growth rate is reflected in a decreased appetite. The toddler has a total of 14–16 teeth, making him more able to chew foods. Increased self-awareness causes the toddler to want to do more for himself. Refusals of food or of assistance in feeding are common ways in which the toddler asserts himself. Since body tissues, especially muscles, continue to grow quite rapidly, protein needs are high.	Appetite is sporadic; specific foods may be favored exclusively or refused from time to time. Child may be ritualistic concerning food preferences, schedule, manner of eating, etc. Diet should include a full range of foods: milk, meat, fruits, vegetables, breads, and cereals. Older toddler can be expected to consume about one-half the amount of food that an adult consumes.	Provide foods with a variety of color, texture, and flavor. Toddlers need to experience the feel of foods. Offer small portions. It is fun for the child to ask for more. It is more effective to give small helpings than to insist that he eat a specified amount. Maintain a regular mealtime schedule. Provide appropriate mealtime equipment: 1. Silverware scaled to size. 2. Dishes—colorful, unbreakable; shallow, round bowls are preferable to flat plates. 3. Plastic bibs, placemats, and floor coverings permit a relaxed attitude toward child's self-feeding attempts. 4. Comfortable seating at good height and distance from table. Adults who help toddlers at mealtime should be calm and relaxed. Avoid bribes or force feeding because this reinforces negative behavior and may lead to a dislike for mealtime. Encourage independence, but provide assistance when necessary. Do not be concerned about table manners. Avoid the use of soda or "sweets" as rewards or between-meal snacks. Instead, substitute fruit, juice, or cereal. Toddlers who show little interest in eggs, meat, or vegetables should not be permitted to appease their appetite with carbohydrates or milk because this may lead to iron-deficiency anemia (see page 1275). SPECIAL CONSIDERATIONS: Hospitalized toddler Nursing history should include the following: Feeding pattern and schedule; food likes and dislikes; food allergies; special eating equipment and utensils; whether or not child is weaned and whether he takes bottle to bed; what child is fed when ill.
Preschooler (3–5 years of age) Increased manual dexterity enables child to have complete independence at mealtime. Psychosocially, this is a period of increased imitation and sex identification. The preschooler identifies with parents at the table and will enjoy what parents enjoy. Additional nutritional habits are	Appetite tends to be sporadic. Child requires the same basic 4 food groups as the adult, but in smaller quantities. Generally likes to eat one food from plate at a time. Like vegetables that are crisp, raw, and cut into finger-sized pieces. Often dislikes strong-tasting foods.	Emphasis should be placed on the quality rather than the amount of food ingested. Foods should be attractively served, mildly flavored, plain, as well as being separated and distinctly identifiable in flavor and appearance. Nutritional foods (e.g., crackers and cheese, yogurt, fruit) should be offered as snacks. Desserts should be nutritious and

Age and Developmental Influence on Nutritional Requirements and Feeding Patterns	Feeding Pattern/Diet	Nursing Implications/Parental Guidance
developed which become part of the child's lifetime practices. Slower growth rate and increased interest in exploring his environment may decrease the preschooler's interest in eating. Eating assumes increasing social significance. Mealtime promotes socialization and provides the preschooler with opportunities to learn appropriate mealtime behavior, language skills, and understanding of family rituals.		a natural part of the meal, not used as a reward for finishing the meal or omitted as punishment. Unless they persist, periods of overeating or not wanting to eat certain foods should not cause concern. The overall eating pattern from month to month is more pertinent to assess. Frequent causes of insufficient eating: 1. Unhappy atmosphere at mealtime 2. Overeating between meals 3. Parental example 4. Attention-seeking 5. Excessive parental expectations 6. Inadequate variety or quantity of foods 7. Tooth decay 8. Physical illness 9. Fatigue 10. Emotional disturbance Measures to increase food intake: 1. Allow child to help with preparations, planning menu, setting table, and other simple chores. 2. Maintain calm environment with no distractions. 3. Avoid between-meal snacks. 4. Provide rest period before meal. 5. Avoid coaxing, bribing, threatening. SPECIAL CONSIDERATIONS: Hospitalized preschooler Consider cultural differences. Allow parents to bring in favorite foods or eating utensils from home. Encourage family members to be present at mealtime. Place children in small groups, preferably at tables during mealtime. Provide simple foods in small portions. Peanut butter and jelly sandwiches are often favorites. Allow and encourage children to feed themselves. Utilize nursing histories as described for toddlers (See p. 1114). Do not punish children who refuse to eat. Offer alternative foods.
School-Age Child Slowed rate of growth during middle childhood results in gradual decline in food requirements per unit of body weight. The preadolescent growth spurt occurs about age 10 in girls and	By this time, food practices are generally well established, a product of the eating experiences of the toddler and preschool period. Many children are too busy with other affairs to take time out to eat. Play readily takes priority unless a firm understanding is	Nutrition education should help the child to select foods wisely and to begin to plan and prepare meals. Parental attitudes continue to be important as the child copies parental behavior (e.g., skipping breakfast, not eating certain foods).

(continued on next page)

Age and Developmental Influence on Nutritional Requirements and Feeding Patterns	Feeding Pattern/Diet	Nursing Implications/Parental Guidance
about age 12 in boys. At this time energy needs increase and approach those of the adult. Intake is particularly important, since reserves are laid down for the demands of adolescence. The child becomes dependent on peers for approval and makes food choices accordingly. The child experiences increased socialization and independence through opportunities to eat away from home—for example, at school and homes of peers.	reached and mealtime is relaxed and enjoyable.	Most children require a nutritious breakfast to avoid lassitude in late morning. Mealtime should continue to be relaxed and enjoyable. Diversions such as T.V. and other children should be avoided. Calcium and vitamin D intake warrant special consideration. They must be adequate to support the rapid enlargement of bones. Parents and health professionals should be alert to signs of developing obesity. Intake should be altered accordingly. Table manners should not be overemphasized. The young child often stuffs his mouth, spills foods, and chatters incessantly while eating. Time and experience will improve his habits. Provide some companionship and conversation at the child's level during meals. Peers should be invited occasionally for meals. SPECIAL CONSIDERATIONS: Hospitalized child Nursing history should include the following: Food preferences; mealtime patterns and snacks; food allergies; food preferences when ill. Provide opportunities for children to eat in small groups at tables. Consider cultural differences. Allow parents to bring in favorite foods from home. Allow child to order his own meal.

Adolescent
(approximately 11–17 years of age)
 	
Dietary requirements vary according to stage of sexual maturation, rate of physical growth, and extent of athletic and social activity.
When rapid growth of puberty appears, there is a corresponding increase in energy requirements and appetite.
	Previously learned dietary patterns are difficult to change.
	Food choices and eating habits may be quite unusual and are related to the adolescent's psychological and social milieu.
	Generally, a significant percentage of the daily caloric intake of the adolescent comes from snacking.
		Continue nutrition education, with special emphasis on the following:
		1. Selecting nutritious foods.
		2. Nutritional needs related to growth.
		3. Preparing favorite "adolescent foods."
		4. Kinds of foods that may aggravate acne.
		5. Foods and physical fitness.
		Informal sessions are generally more effective than lectures on nutrition.
		Special problems requiring intervention:
		  Obesity
		  Excessive dieting
		  Extreme fads—eccentric and grossly restricted diets
		  Anorexia
		  Adolescent pregnancy
		Provide nutritious foods relevant to the adolescent's life style.

Age and Developmental Influence on Nutritional Requirements and Feeding Patterns	Feeding Pattern/Diet	Nursing Implications/Parental Guidance
		Discourage cigarette smoking, which may contribute to poor nutritional status by decreasing appetite and increasing the body's metabolic rate.
		SPECIAL CONSIDERATIONS: Hospitalized adolescent
		Allow patient to choose own foods, especially if on a special diet.
		Provide a refrigerator in the recreation room for snacks, or utilize a snack cart.
		Serve foods that appeal to adolescents.
		Utilize a nursing history similar to that for the school-age child.

PREVENTIVE PEDIATRICS

IMMUNIZATION

Active Immunization Schedule for Infants and Children[1]

Age	Immunization
2 months	DTP[2], TOPV[3]
4 months	DTP, TOPV
6 months	DTP, TOPV[6]
15 months	Tuberculin test, measles, mumps, rubella[5]
18 months	DTP, TOPV
4–6 years	DTP, TOPV
14–16 years	Td[4] and every 10 years thereafter

[1] From 1977 Report of the Committee of Infectious Diseases of the American Academy of Pediatrics.
[2] DTP—Diphtheria and tetanus toxoids, and pertussis vaccine combined.
[3] TOPV—Trivalent oral polio vaccine. Recommended for breast- and bottle-fed infants.
[4] Td—Adult type combined tetanus and diphtheria toxoids, containing less diphtheria component than DT (Diphtheria and Tetanus toxoid) for those more than 6 years old.
[5] May be given as measles and rubella or measles–mumps–rubella (M–M–R).
[6] 3rd dose of TOPV is optional but recommended for infants in areas where there is a high incidence of poliomyelitis.

Recommended Schedule for Active Immunization of Children Who did not Receive Vaccines During First Year of Life[1]

Time Interval	Under 6 years old	6 years and older
1st visit	DTP, TOPV, Tuberculin test	Td, TOPV, Tuberculin test
1 month later	Measles*, rubella, (mumps)	Measles, (mumps), rubella
2 months later	DTP, TOPV	Td, TOPV
4 months later	DTP	—
10–16 months later	DTP, TOPV	8–14 months later Td, TOPV
ages 14–16	Td—continue every 10 years	Td—continue every 10 years

* Not recommended to be given before 15 months of age.
[1] From 1977 Report of the Committee of Infectious Diseases of the American Academy of Pediatrics.

General Considerations

1. Immunizations may be started at any age. If an immunization program is not begun in infancy, a slightly different schedule may be followed, depending upon the child's age and the prevalence of specific infections at the time.

2. An interrupted primary series of immunizations need not be restarted; it need only be continued, regardless of the length of time that has elapsed.

3. The immunoresponse is limited in a significant proportion of young infants, and the recommended booster doses are designed to ensure and maintain immunity.

4. A time lapse of 8 weeks is recommended between the first 3 DTP injections for desirable maximum effects.
   a. The combination of depot antigens is preferred, because it is more immunogenic.
   b. Because of the increased risk of possible reactions to either diphtheria or pertussis antigen, Td (adult-type tetanus and diphtheria toxins) is recommended for children over 6 years of age.
   c. For contaminated wounds, a booster dose of tetanus should be given if more than 5 years have elapsed since the last dose. No booster is needed for clean, minor wounds if immunizations are up to date and no more than 10 years has elapsed since last dose.
5. *Pertussis*
   a. Protection of infants against pertussis should begin early.
   b. In newborn infants, the best protection against pertussis is avoidance of household contacts by adequate immunization of older siblings.
6. *Tuberculin Test*
   a. It is recommended that the tuberculin test be given before or simultaneously with the measles vaccine.
      (1) The measles vaccine may invalidate the tuberculin test, giving a false negative, if given within 6 weeks after measles immunization.
      (2) Theoretically, measles vaccine could activate latent tuberculosis.
   b. Frequency of repeated tuberculin testing depends upon the following:
      (1) Risk of exposure of the child.
      (2) Prevalence of tuberculosis in the population group.
      (3) High-risk situations; intervals between routine testing should not exceed 6 months.
7. *Measles vaccine* is most effective when given at about 12–15 months of age. At this age all maternal transplacental antibody has been catabolized.
   Measles vaccine may be administered at 6 months of age when child is at a high risk of contact with natural measles. A second dose should be given at 12–16 months of age if the original vaccine was given prior to 1 year of age, since rate of seroconversion before 1 year of age is variable.
8. Live trivalent oral polio virus vaccine is preferred to the inactivated form, because administration is easier and the immunologic effects are broader and longer.
9. *Mumps vaccine*—all preadolescent or older males who have not had mumps should be immunized.
10. *Rubella vaccine*
    a. Live vaccine is recommended for boys and girls between 1 year of age and puberty.
    b. Children in kindergarten should be given priority, because they are the major source of viral dissemination.
    c. A history of rubella illness is not reliable enough to exclude children from immunization.
11. Immunizations should be deferred if child has an acute febrile infection or illness. The common cold, without fever, is not a contraindication to immunization.
12. Contraindications to receiving measles-mumps and rubella vaccines include the following: pregnancy; generalized malignancy; cell-mediated immunodeficiency disorders; current immunodepressive therapy; sensitivity to animal species used in vaccine preparation; transfusion of immune serum globulin, plasma, or blood.
    If any of these contraindications exist, immunizations may be temporarily deferred or an alternative vaccine preparation may be used.
13. *Smallpox vaccination*
    a. No longer recommended in U.S.
    b. Where indicated (i.e., while traveling), initial smallpox vaccine may be given at any time between 12–24 months of age (after age 12, it may be given every 3–10 years).
14. A good nursing history will include determining whether or not the child has been exposed to any communicable disease or has experienced such. Surveillance in this area will prevent unnecessary disease and allow for proper immunization for the child and his family.
15. Strict adherence to the manufacturer's storage recommendations is vital. Failure to observe these precautions and recommendations may reduce the potency and effectiveness of the specific vaccine. Read manufacturer's package insert for volume of individual dose.

DENTAL CARE
Primary Teeth

1. Eruption
   a. Two lower central incisors—appear by 6–7 months
   b. Four upper incisors—appear by 9 months
   c. Two lower lateral incisors—appear by 1 year
   d. Four first molars—appear by 14 months
   e. Four cuspids—appear by 18 months
   f. Four second molars—appear by 2–2½ years
2. Importance of primary teeth and dental care for primary teeth
   a. At about 2 years of age, toothbrushing should be started. At this age, most of the primary teeth have erupted, and the child's muscle coordination has developed enough to allow some form of brushing.
   b. By age 3, the child should be examined by a dentist when all primary teeth have erupted.
   c. When decayed primary teeth are neglected, they endanger the child's health and may cause abscesses, fever, and excessive pain. The infected teeth may damage the permanent tooth that is forming within the jaw. A child with advanced tooth decay finds it difficult to chew some foods that are essential to a well-balanced diet.
   d. Primary teeth act as a guide for the proper positioning of permanent teeth. Each primary tooth is holding the space for a permanent tooth that will replace it. If a primary tooth is lost prematurely there will be a loss of space. This can result in crowding of permanent teeth, ultimately requiring orthodontic work when a child is older.
   e. Primary teeth serve as a stimulus for growth of the jaws, aid in the development of speech, and serve a cosmetic function.
      (1) A young person can become very self-conscious when he loses a tooth in the front of his mouth and realizes that he looks different.
      (2) Indirectly, a child's speech may be affected if self-consciousness about his loss of teeth prevents him from opening his mouth for proper talking.

(3) Ability to use the teeth for pronunciation is acquired entirely with the aid of the primary teeth. Early loss of front teeth may lead to difficulty in pronouncing "s," "f," "l," "z," and "th."

(4) Even after the permanent teeth erupt, difficulty in pronouncing "s," "z," and "th" may persist to the point that the child requires speech correction.

Permanent Teeth

1. Eruption
   a. Four "6-year molars" appear between the age of 6 and 7 years.
   b. From this point onward, until 12–13 years of age the primary teeth loosen, one by one, and each is replaced by a permanent tooth.
   c. Four additional molars appear at 12–13 years of age.
   d. Four molars ("wisdom teeth") appear at 17–21 years.
2. Importance of early dental care
   Care of teeth during infancy and childhood is necessary in order to:
   a. Promote proper development of the teeth.
   b. Prevent dental caries and periodontal disease.
   c. Establish good dental habits for optimal dental health.

Nursing Management

1. Take advantage of incidental opportunities to teach children and their parents information that will promote dental health.
   a. Emphasize that inflammatory periodontal disease and dental caries are the results of dental plaque. *Dental plaque* is a mass composed primarily of microorganisms that adhere to the tooth surface. As these microorganisms grow, they form products that are destructive to the underlying tissue. Removal of this plaque and prevention of its collection is a major part of dental care.
   b. Provide a well-balanced diet that is necessary for tooth development. Stress the importance of diet control in dental care. The microorganisms that form dental plaque need a sucrose substrate which comes from refined sugars for rapid growth. Therefore, decreasing the intake of such refined sugars is important.
   c. Start child on the correct procedure by having a good attitude toward brushing. Parents serve as role models as well as assist the young child to care for his teeth.
2. Provide supplemental fluoride if the local drinking water supply does not contain fluoride. Fluoride makes the tooth surface more resistant to disease.
   a. Topical application of fluoride should be done twice a year.
   b. Daily fluoride rinse after brushing is effective in decreasing dental caries in children.
   c. Daily use of a dentifrice containing fluoride is another source of protection.
3. Maintain the child's general health.
4. Encourage parents to arrange a dental visit when child is 2½–3 years old.
5. Teach child and parents good brushing technique and dental habits.
   a. Use soft-bristle nylon brush with polished ends. Brushes for small children should be ¼–⅓ smaller than adult brushes with a flat brushing surface, firm, resilient bristles, and head sufficiently small to allow access to all surfaces of the teeth.
   b. Place bristles at the gingival margin at a 45-degree angle to the tooth. The brush rotates from gingival toward occlusal surface. Occlusal surfaces are brushed with scrubbing motion with small strokes in every direction.
   c. Stress that the length of time and thoroughness of brushing are important.
   d. Disclosing tablets can be used during teaching program to show the location of dental plaque before and after brushing.
6. The adolescent needs special encouragement and attention to maintain good dental habits.
   a. Stress importance of diet control of refined sugars.
   b. Encourage proper brushing technique. The circular motion method: the brush is carried up, back, and forward, then up again without twisting hand.
   c. Encourage daily flossing in which floss is used correctly. (Improper use can cause traumatic injury to the gingiva.) Flossing is accomplished by passing the floss between the teeth with a back and forth motion. Place floss against tooth and move it up and down 6–7 times against the tooth as far as the gingiva permits. Repeat process on side of adjacent tooth. Repeat until all sides of all teeth are cleansed.
7. Practice measures that will aid in avoiding cavities.
   a. Bottle-mouth syndrome—high incidence of dental caries in child 18 months–3 years is the result of taking bottle of milk or juice to bed. This syndrome can be prevented. Do not let child take a bottle to bed with him; if child does take a bottle, put plain water in it.
   b. Have the child brush teeth after every meal and at bedtime. If brushing is not possible after meals, rinse mouth with water.
   c. Reduce the amounts of sugar and sweets eaten by the child.
   d. Beware of foods that contain large amounts of sugar:
      Bubble and chewing gum
      Cola drinks
      Peanut butter and jelly on white bread
      Candies, cookies, cakes
      Jelly, jam, honey
      Malted and sweet chocolate drinks
      Synthetic orange juice (artificially sweetened)
      White bread and raisin bread
      Sugar-coated cereals

SAFETY

Incidence of Childhood Accidents

1. Accidents are the leading cause of death for children in the United States.
2. Approximately 1 of every 3 children in the United States is injured seriously enough each year to require medical treatment.

Role of the Nurse

1. Identify environmental hazards and take action to reduce or eliminate them.
2. Identify behavioral characteristics in individual children which may be related to accident liability and

caution parents accordingly. Pay particular attention to children who show the following:

  a. Characteristics which increase exposure to hazards, such as: excessive curiosity, inability to delay gratification, hyperactivity, and daring.
  b. Characteristics which reduce the child's ability to cope with hazards, i.e., aggressiveness, stubbornness, poor concentration, low frustration threshold, lack of self-control.

3. Provide anticipatory guidance about child development as it relates to accidents. Direct preventive teaching toward individuals or groups, toward children or adults.
4. Participate in policy-setting for accident prevention in institutions and communities

Principles of Safety

1. The child's developmental stage influences the types of accidents that are likely to occur.

   Potential accident situations may be foreseen by parents who have knowledge of their own child's typical patterns of growth and development.

2. Children are naturally curious, impulsive, and impatient. The young child needs to touch, feel, and investigate.

   a. Patient, adult supervision will enable the child to learn what he wants to know within the limits of safety for his stage of growth and development.
   b. Young children should never be left alone at home.

3. Children copy the behavior of their parents and absorb parental attitudes.

   Parents and other adults should be certain that their ways of doing things are safe.

4. Children become less careful and less willing to listen to warnings and to observe routine safety precautions when they are tired or hungry.

5. An estimated 90% of all accidents are preventable.

General Areas of Adult Safety Responsibility

A. *Motor Vehicle*

1. All automobiles should be maintained in good mechanical condition.
2. Seat belts should be worn at all times.
3. Driver should look carefully in front of and in back of the car before accelerating.
4. All car doors should be locked when a child travels in the vehicle.
5. Young children should never be left alone in a car.
6. Heavy or sharp objects should not be placed on the same seat with a child.

B. *Sports and Recreation*

1. Keep equipment in good condition and proper working order.
2. Wear appropriate clothing for the activity.
3. Do not attempt activities beyond one's physical endurance.
4. Keep firearms and ammunition locked up.

C. *Electrical and Mechanical Equipment*

1. Only underwriter-approved devices should be installed; they should be inspected periodically.
2. Dry hands before touching appliances.

   Keep radios, fans, portable heaters, and hair dryers out of the bathroom.

3. Disconnect appliances after use or before attempting minor repairs.

4. Keep garden equipment and machinery in a restricted area.

   Teach proper use of the equipment as soon as the child is old enough.

5. Avoid overloading electrical circuits.
6. Discourage children from playing with or being in area where appliances or power tools (e.g., washing machine, clothes dryer, saw, lawn mower) are in operation.

D. *Prevention of Falls*

1. Keep stairs well lighted and free from clutter.
2. Provide sturdy railings.
3. Anchor small rugs securely.
4. Use rubber mats in the bathtub and shower.
5. Use only sturdy ladders for climbing.

E. *Poisonings and Ingestions*

1. Do not mix bleaches with ammonia, vinegar, and other household cleaners.
2. See section on ingested poisons, page 889; poisoning (pediatric), page 1449.

F. *Fire*

1. Maintain an adequate fire escape plan and routinely conduct home fire drills.

   Teach the child escape routes as soon as he is old enough.

2. Keep a pressure-type hand fire extinguisher on each floor.

   Instruct all family members who are old enough in its use.

3. Fit fireplaces with snug fireplace screens.
4. Store gasoline and other flammable fluids in tightly covered containers that are clearly labeled and away from heat and sparks.
5. Dispose of paint- and oil-soaked cloth quickly.
6. Utilize flame-retardant sleepwear.
7. Mark children's rooms so that they are obvious to firemen.
8. Teach children about the danger of smoke inhalation.

G. *Swimming Pools*

1. Completely enclose pool with a fence that complies with local regulations. The gate should be self-closing and have a lock.
2. Indicate water depth with numbers on the edge of the pool. Place a safety float line where the bottom slope begins to deepen.
3. Install at least 1 ladder at each end of the pool. Ladders should have handrails on both sides, and the diameter of the rails should be small enough for a child to grasp.
4. Use nonslip materials on ladders, deck, and diving boards.
5. Install underwater lighting as well as outdoor lights if the pool is used at night. A ground fault circuit interrupter should be installed on the pool circuit to cut off electrical power and thus prevent electrocutions should electrical fault occur.
6. Instruct children about safety rules such as not swimming alone, and not running around the pool or pushing others. Avoid using radios or other electrical appliances near the pool.
7. Keep essential rescue devices and first-aid equipment close to the pool.

H. *Emergency Precautions*

1. Record emergency phone numbers in an obvious and easily accessible place.

2. Keep a well-stocked first-aid kit immediately available for emergencies.
3. Give instruction in principles of first aid to all family members who are old enough.
   a. Responsible adults should enroll in first-aid courses offered by the Red Cross, adult education programs, etc.
   b. Be aware of first-aid procedures for:
      Burns
      Electric shock
      Poisoning
      Bites and stings
      Cuts, scrapes and punctures
      Drowning
      Fractures
4. Know the location of gas, water, and electrical switches and how to turn them off in an emergency.

I. Miscellaneous

1. Take advantage of preventive health care.
   a. Obtain recommended immunizations.
   b. Have regular physical examinations.
2. Seek immediate treatment of all diseases and health problems.
3. Balance periods of work, rest, and exercise in daily living.

Specific Safety Concerns Related to Child's Stage of Growth and Development

A. Infants

Newborn babies are helpless and need absolute protection. When they begin to move about they need close supervision.
1. Infants may wiggle, roll, and shift position.
   a. The crib should conform to the requirements of the Consumer Product Safety Commission.
   b. The sides of the crib should be kept up at all times.
   c. The crib should not be placed near a radiator or heating unit.
   d. The crib should be away from windows with venetian blinds, because the infant may become fatally entangled in a dangling cord.
   e. Babies should not be left unattended on anything from which they might fall.
      Infant seats should not be left on tables, beds, or other furniture.
   f. Infants should be strapped carefully in feeding chairs, infant seats, etc.
      A means should be provided to prevent the child from slipping down and being strangled by his waist strap.
   g. No strings should be placed around the infant's neck.
   h. Well-constructed infant carriers should be used for traveling.
      (1) *For all children under 4 years of age or weighing less than 40 pounds, the standard seat belt is not safe.* Special restraint devices should be used, beginning with the ride home from the nursery.
      (2) Infant car seats and car beds should meet the vehicle safety standards of the Department of Transportation for child-seating systems.
         (a) There should be a means of anchoring the device to the seat of the vehicle with the standard lap belt.

(b) A harness should keep the child contained within the device.
(c) The device should include a head support to minimize the danger of whiplash injury.
      (3) For older infants and toddlers, special devices are available which dispense with the harness and instead surround the child with a protective shield that distributes collision forces evenly.
   i. Diaper pins should always be kept closed, even when not in use.
2. Infants may start to suck on toys, crib slats, and other objects.
   a. Paints containing lead should not be used on toys, furniture, or any other objects that the child is likely to put into his mouth.
   b. Stuffed toys should be checked carefully to be certain that button eyes and other small, attached parts cannot be pulled off and eaten by the child.
   c. Small objects should not be left within the reach of the infant.
   d. All plastic bags should be tied in knots and discarded to avoid danger of suffocation. Under no circumstances should mattresses be covered with thin plastic.
3. Children are helpless in water for the next several years.
   a. The temperature of the bath water should be checked carefully to avoid scalding.
   b. The child should never be left unattended in the bathtub for any reason.
4. They are frequently victims of rats in highly populated metropolitan areas.
   a. The rats should be exterminated before the baby is discharged from the hospital.
   b. Infant beds should be high above the floor.
5. They should be carried from one place to another.
   a. The adult who carries the infant should avoid walking on slippery floors or where toys or other small objects have been scattered.
   b. *Hospitalized infants* should always be transported in cribs or strollers and never carried from place to place in the arms of the nurse.

B. Toddlers

Toddlers are adventurous and are eager to explore everything around them. Although they sometimes seem very mature and independent, they still require close adult supervision.
1. They want to roam all over the house.
   a. Gates should be used at the head and foot of stairways to prevent falls.
   b. Fireplaces should be screened.
   c. Radiators should be enclosed or covered.
   d. Cords on blinds or draperies should be tied or cut so that children cannot get their heads through the loops.
2. They poke and probe with their index fingers.
   a. Sharp objects such as scissors, and nail files should be kept out of reach.
   b. Bureau drawers and cabinets with anything potentially dangerous in them should be locked.
   c. Unused light sockets should be taped or capped.
   d. Electric fans or heaters should be out of reach.
   e. Electrical cords should be kept in good repair.
3. They are curious about many things, especially those things higher than their eye level.
   a. They should be lifted occasionally to satisfy their curiosity.

b. Furniture should be balanced to prevent the child from pulling it over on himself.

c. Hot, scalding foods should be kept out of the reach of the children.

d. All handles of pots and pans should be turned to the back of the stove.

e. Tablecloths should not hang over the edge of the table.

f. A small child should never be left alone in the kitchen. Appliances such as hot ovens, toasters, coffee pots, and irons pose a special threat to small children.

4. A child puts almost anything into his mouth.

a. Medicines, lye, and household cleaning products should be locked up out of the reach of children.

b. Pins, buttons, and needles should be put away.

c. Unbreakable toys that have no small removable parts should be used.

d. The child should be closely supervised if he plays with a balloon. Aspiration of rubber from broken balloons can be fatal.

e. Foods such as popcorn, peanuts, and carrot sticks should not be offered to toddlers because of the danger of aspiration.

5. They climb onto things.

a. Toddlers should be protected from falls.

(1) Windows should have guards on them.

(2) Screens should be firm and securely fastened.

b. Car doors should be locked.

c. Special equipment for climbing (e.g., small wooden grates) should be provided, and climbing should be done under adult supervision.

6. They like to play outside and in water.

a. The toddler must have close supervision while playing outside.

b. His play yard should be fenced.

c. Ponds, pools, wells, and other similar outdoor structures should be fenced or covered. Wading pools should be emptied immediately after use.

d. The child should never be left alone in a wading pool.

e. Caution should be used in allowing the toddler to play with older children. He may easily be injured by bats, hard balls, bicycles, and rough play.

C. Preschool Children

Preschool children are very active and inquisitive. They begin to develop increased self-control, but still have an immature understanding of danger. They are at an ideal age to learn simple safety routines.

1. They can reach doorknobs and are eager to explore the world beyond.

a. Doors that open to potential danger should be locked.

b. Bathroom doors should have locks which can be opened from the outside to prevent the child from locking himself in the room.

c. Unused refrigerators, freezers, and trunks should have doors, handles and/or hinges removed to prevent small children from climbing into them and becoming trapped inside.

2. They enjoy taking things apart, putting them together again and experimenting with their use.

a. Dangerous items such as knives and electrical equipment should be put away.

b. Matches and lighters should be kept well out of the child's reach.

3. They are nimble on their feet and usually in a hurry.

a. The child should not be allowed to walk or run while eating a lollipop.

b. Stairs should have strong railings. They should be clear of objects or defective coverings on which a child can trip.

c. Stairs and floors should not be highly waxed.

d. Area rugs should be fixed.

4. They often enjoy cooperative play with others.

a. Toy trucks or wagons should be strong enough to bear their weight as well as that of their playmates.

b. They should be taught to ride tricycles on the sidewalk and to watch for cars in driveways.

c. They should be cautioned not to run after the ball if it rolls into the street or driveway.

d. Clothes should allow the child freedom of action and shoes should be suitable for running and climbing.

e. The play area should be checked for such hazards as old refrigerators, deep holes, construction, broken glass, and trash heaps.

f. Swings and other equipment should be properly installed and maintained.

5. They are proud to run simple errands.

They should not be asked to do anything hazardous such as crossing the street or carrying a knife or glass container.

6. They can take verbal directions and their attention span is lengthening. They can be instructed in the following areas:

a. Personal safety

(1) To supply information such as their name, address, and telephone number.

(2) To identify firemen, policemen, and other safety officials.

(3) Not to accept gifts or rides from strangers.

b. Home safety

(1) The reasons for various safety measures such as keeping the floor clear of their toys.

(2) The safe way to use tools.

(3) Kitchen safety.

(4) The danger of matches, open flames, hot objects, and gas and electric equipment.

c. Recreational safety

Swimming instructions

d. Motor vehicle and pedestrian safety.

(1) Safety rules and the dangers of traffic.

(2) Obedience to the rules.

(3) Appropriate use of automobile restraint systems.

D. School-age Children

School-age children are usually fairly independent. They still need discipline and rules but they also need to know *why* precautions are necessary and what the consequences are for failing to follow the rules.

1. They are eager to make things and participate in household activities.

a. They should be taught the proper use and storage of equipment such as those listed below:

(1) Saws

(2) Nails and hammer

(3) Kitchen implements

(4) Sewing machines

(5) Gas and electric appliances

b. They should be taught to wear protective devices over their eyes when doing anything potentially dangerous to their vision.

2. They enjoy holding and attending parties, carnivals, and other similar gatherings.
    Party costumes and equipment should be checked to be certain that they are flameproof.
3. They enjoy sports and outdoor play.
    a. Their whereabouts should be known at all times.
    b. The play areas should be inspected for broken glass, rusty nails, etc.
    c. They should be instructed regarding the dangers of playing in sand pits, old refrigerators, excavations, rickety shacks, and deserted buildings.
    d. They must learn the rules of the sports that they play. They should have the proper equipment and keep it in good working condition.
    e. Ice skating and other water sports should always be closely supervised.
    f. They should be taught how to climb a tree safely. Tree houses that are sturdily constructed under adult supervision may help prevent falls from trees.
4. Areas for teaching:
    a. The rules of cycling safety should be emphasized. A child with a bicycle must learn the rules of the road as well as respect for the traffic officers and their directions.
    b. Pedestrian safety rules should also be stressed because motor accidents are the most common cause of accidental injury in this age group.
    c. Swimming instruction should be continued.
    d. The older child should be taught respect for fire, its uses, and its dangers.
    e. Safety with firearms should be discussed.
    f. Children should be taught to read labels and recognize symbols indicating poisons.

E. *Adolescents*

   Adolescents are increasingly independent. They should be able to build on their past experiences and accept responsibility for their own safety. Limits must still be set and direction given by adults because adolescents may lack emotional maturity.
1. They may obtain driving licenses.
    a. They should learn to maintain their automobiles in good mechanical condition.
    b. Seat belts should be worn at all times.
    c. They must be aware of traffic regulations and the penalty for not obeying them.
    d. They should be encouraged to participate in driver education and safety programs at school.
    e. Proper clothes should be worn while riding on motorcycles, motor scooters, or motorbikes. A safety helmet is essential.
2. They enjoy competing in competitive sports.
    Safeguards should be taken to prevent physical trauma when they want to do something beyond their physical endurance.
3. Their values and habits are greatly influenced by their peer groups and cliques.
    a. Parents should be aware of their child's activities.
    b. Constructive group activities should be encouraged.
    c. Formal instructions should be continued in the areas of sex education, drug and alcohol abuse, and smoking.
        Open discussions with responsible adults should be encouraged.
4. Older adolescents are capable of assuming some responsibility for family safety measures.
    a. They should be included in safety planning.
    b. Their opinions and suggestions should be considered.
    c. Specific areas of responsibility may be delegated to them.

BIBLIOGRAPHY

GENERAL
Books

Chinn P. Child Health Maintenance: Concepts in Family Centered Care, 2nd ed. St. Louis, CV Mosby, 1979
Clark AL and Affonso DD. Childbearing: A Nursing Perspective, 2nd ed. Philadelphia, FA Davis, 1979
Furholt JDL. Clinical Assessment of Children: A Comprehensive Approach to Primary Care. Philadelphia, JB Lippincott, 1980
Headings D (ed). The Harriet Lane Handbook: A Manual for Pediatric House Officers, 8th ed. Chicago, Year Book Medical Pub., 1978
Johnson SH. High-Risk Parenting: Nursing Assessment and Strategies for the Family at Risk. Philadelphia, JB Lippincott, 1979
Scipien G et al. Comprehensive Pediatric Nursing, 2nd ed. New York, McGraw-Hill, 1979
Silver HK et al. Handbook of Pediatrics. Los Altos, Lange Medical Publications, 1977
Waechter E and Blake F. Nursing Care of Children. Philadelphia JB Lippincott, 1976
Whaley L and Wong D (eds). Nursing Care of Infants and Children. St. Louis, CV Mosby, 1979

GROWTH AND DEVELOPMENT
Books

Bigner J. Parent–Child Relations: An Introduction to Parenting. New York, Macmillan, 1979
Chinn P and Leitch C. Child Health Maintenance: A Guide to Clinical Assessment. St. Louis, CV Mosby, 1979
Elkind D. A Sympathetic Understanding of the Child: Birth to Sixteen. Boston, Allyn & Bacon, 1974
Erickson M. Assessment and Management of Developmental Changes in Children. St. Louis, CV Mosby, 1976
Ginsburg H and Opper S. Piaget's Theory of Intellectual Development, 2nd ed. Englewood Cliffs, Prentice-Hall, 1979
Howe J. Nursing Care of Adolescents. New York, McGraw-Hill, 1979
Hymovich D and Barnard M. Family Health Care, vol 2. New York, McGraw-Hill, 1979
Kaluger G and Kaluger M. Human Development: The Span of Life, 2nd ed. St. Louis, CV Mosby, 1979
Manaster GJ. Adolescent Development and the Life Tasks. Boston, Allyn & Bacon, 1977
Matthews UF (ed). Manual of Pediatric Nursing Care Plans. Boston, Little, Brown & Co., 1979

Mercer R. Perspectives in Adolescent Health Care. Philadelphia, JB Lippincott, 1979

Murray R and Zentner J. Nursing Assessment and Health Promotion Through the Life Span, 2nd ed. Englewood Cliffs, Prentice-Hall, 1979

Mussan P, Conger J, Kagen J. Child Development and Personality, 5th ed. New York, Harper & Row, 1979

Articles

American Academy of Pediatrics, Committee on Adolescence. On the terminology of adolescent/adolescence. Pediatrics 1978 Nov; 62(5):838

Bell RS. The Gesell developmental schedules: Arnold Gesell (1880–1961). J Abnorm Child Psychol 1977, Sept; 5(3):233–239

Brown RT. Assessing adolescent development. Pediatr Ann 1978 Sept; 7(9):587–595

Connolly C. Counseling parents of school age children with special needs. J Sch Health 1978 Feb; 48(2):115–117

Coyner AB. Meeting developmental needs of neonates. Family and Community Health 1978 Nov; 1(3):79–90

Erickson CJ et al. Understanding and evaluating adolescent behavior problems. J Sch Health 1978 May; 48(5):293–297

Fleming R. Developing a child's self-esteem. Pediatric Nursing 1979 July/Aug; 5(4):58–60

Gardner H. The developmental psychology after Piaget: An approach in terms of symbolization. Hum Dev 1979; 22:73–88

Gibbons M. When parents ask about play. Pediatric Nursing 1977 Nov/Dec; 3(6):19–22

Hart H et al. The value of a developmental history. Dev Med Child Neurol 1978 Aug; 20(4):442–452

Kover MG. Some indicators of health related behavior among adolescents in the United States. Public Health Rep 1979 Mar/Apr; 94(2):109–118

Largo RH and Howard JA. Developmental progression in play behavior of children between nine and thirty months. Dev Med Child Neurol 1979 June; 21(3):299–310

Leppirk MA. Adolescent sexuality. Matern Child Nurs J 1979 Fall; 8(3):153–161

Manaster G. The ideal self and cognitive development in adolescence. Adolescence 1977 Winter; 12(48):547–558

Miller SR. Children's fears: A review of the literature with implications for nursing research and practice. Nurs Res 1979 July/Aug; 28(4):217–223

Natapoff JN. Children's view of health: A developmental study. Am J Public Health 1978 Oct; 68(10):995–1000

Parcel GS. Health education for kindergarten children. J Sch Health 1979 Mar; 49(3):129–131

Peach E. Counseling sexually active very young adolescent girls. MCN 1980 May/June; 5(3):191–195

Peautti L. An exploration of adolescent feminine and occupational behavior development. AJOT 1979 Feb; 33(2):84–91

Rapheal D. Identity status in high school females. Adolescence 1978 Winter; 13(52):729–734

Riesch S. Enhancement of mother–infant social interaction. JOGN Nurs 1979 July/Aug; 8(4):242–246

Segal SJ. Contraceptives and the young: Present status and future prospects. Pediatrics 1978 Dec; 62(6):1211–1215

Shirreffs JH et al. Adolescent perceptions of sex education needs: 1972–1978. J Sch Health 1979 June; 49(6):343–346

Siemon M. Promoting mental health in school-aged children. MCN 1978 July/Aug; 3(4):211–218

Taft LT. Child development: Prenatal to early childhood. J Sch Health 1978 May; 48(5):281–287

Vipperman J and Rager P. Childhood coping: How nurses can help. Pediatric Nursing 1980 Mar/Apr; 6(2):11–21

Wood D. Children and health: Can they be taught, should they and will it have any effect? Can Med Assoc J 1979 Feb 3; 120(3):341 +

NUTRITION

Books

Lansky V. Feed Me, I'm Yours. New York, Bantam Books, 1979

Pipes P. Nutrition in Infancy and Childhood. St. Louis, CV Mosby, 1977

Articles

Braham RL et al. Nutrition and its importance in dental health. J Fam Pract 1978 Jan; 6(1):49–50

Getchell E and Howard R. Nutrition in development. In Scipien G et al (eds). Comprehensive Pediatric Nursing, 2nd ed. New York, McGraw–Hill, 1979

Mowery B. Family oriented approach to childhood obesity. Pediatric Nursing 1980 Mar/Apr; 6(2):40–46

Nutt HH. Infant nutrition and obesity. Nurs Forum 1979 Spring; 18(2):130–157

Pearson G. Nutrition in the middle years of childhood. MCN 1977 Nov/Dec; 2(6):378–384

Rowe N. Childhood obesity: Growth charts vs. calipers. Pediatric Nursing 1980 Mar/Apr; 6(2):24–29

Weidman WH et al. Nutrient intake and serum cholesterol level in normal children 6–16 years of age. Pediatrics 1978 Mar; 6(3):354–359

PREVENTIVE PEDIATRICS

Books

Arena J and Bachar M. Child Safety Is No Accident. Chapel Hill, Duke University Press, 1978

Dunning JM. Principles of Dental Public Health, 3rd ed. Cambridge, Harvard University Press, 1979

Krugman S et al. Infectious Diseases of Children. St. Louis, CV Mosby, 1977

McCormick R and Gilson–Parkevich T. Patient and Family Education: Tools, Techniques and Theory. New York, John Wiley & Sons, 1979

Steigman A (ed). Report of the Committee on Infectious Disease, 18th ed. Evanston, The American Academy of Pediatrics, 1977

Articles

Godwin RH. Child resistant locks in poison control. Pediatrics 1978 May; 6(5):750–752

Gratz RR. Accidental injury in childhood: A literature review on pediatric trauma. J Trauma 1979 Aug; 19(8):551–555

Helfner RE et al. Injuries resulting when small children fall out of bed. Pediatrics 1977 Oct; 60(4):533–535

Herbertt RM and Innes JM. Familiarization and preparatory information in reduction of anxiety in child dental patients. ASDC J Dent Child 1979 May/June; 46(3):219–225

Hobson P. Dietary control and prevention of dental disease in chronically sick children. J Hum Nutr 1979; 33(2):140–145

Johnson N. Teaching dental health to children. Pediatric Nursing 1978 Mar/Apr; 4(2):20–23

Pern JH et al. Bathtub drownings: Report of seven cases. Pediatrics 1979 July; 64(1):68–70

Pless IB. Accident prevention and health education: Back to the drawing board. Pediatrics 1978 Sept; 62(3):431–435

Randolph MF. Streptococcal pharyngitis in children: Diagnosing with throat cultures. Consultant 1979 Feb; 19(2):153–154 +

Reinhard S. Nursing responsibility in infant car safety. MCN 1980 Jan/Feb; 5(1):26–27, 64

Reisinger KS et al. Evaluation of programs designed to increase the protection of infants in cars. Pediatrics 1978 Sept; 62(3):280–287

SUGGESTED ADDITIONAL READING FOR STAFF AND PARENTS

Becker, W. Parents Are Teachers. Champaign, Research Press, 1971

Brazelton TB. Infants and Mothers. New York, Dell Publishing Co, 1969

Brazelton TB. Neonatal Behavioral Assessment Scale. Philadelphia, JB Lippincott, 1973

Brazelton TB. Toddlers and Parents. New York, Dell Publishing Co, 1974

Caplan F. The First Twelve Months of Life. New York, Grossett & Dunlap, 1973

Christophersen, ER. Little People. Lawrence, H&H Enterprises, 1977

Dodson F. How to Parent. New York, New American Library, 1971

Fraiberg S. The Magic Years. New York, Charles Scribner's Sons, 1959

Gordon I. Baby Learning Through Baby Play. New York, St. Martin's Press, 1970

Holt J. How Children Learn. New York, Dell Pub. Co, 1967

Infant Developmental Program. Johnson and Johnson Baby Products, 175 Community Dr, Great Neck, New York 11025

Painter G. Teach Your Baby. New York, Simon & Schuster, 1971

THE HOSPITALIZED CHILD

GENERAL PRINCIPLES OF CARE

Emotional and Social Needs

1. The child has the same basic emotional and social needs during hospitalization as he does at home.
   a. He needs a chance to develop the following:
      (1) Motor skills
      (2) Social skills
      (3) Language skills
      (4) Psychological strengths
         (a) A sense of autonomy
         (b) Ego strength
         (c) A sense of identity
      (5) Patterns of behavior
   b. To help him accomplish these skills and strengths, he needs:
      (1) The continuing and reliable presence of someone who is important to him.
      (2) An appropriately stimulating environment.
      (3) Opportunities to explore and play.
      (4) Information and explanations concerning the hospital, treatments, procedures, routines, people, and expectations of him both before and during hospitalization. The child needs to know and to be able to predict how he will interact with his environment. Thus when he knows what to expect in an unfamiliar situation, he will be better able to cope and not feel so helpless.
2. The hospitalized child has special needs—to deal with the many new problems that confront him.
   a. Separation from home—implying loss of:
      (1) Consistent person who nurtures
      (2) Family associations
      (3) Familiar environment
      (4) Daily activities and routines
      (5) Peer associations
      (6) Independence
   b. Problems concerning the illness itself
   c. Hospital rules and regulations
   d. Surgery
   e. Death

Essential Elements

1. Parents must be closely involved with the child's hospitalization and the plan for his care. Parent participation is to be encouraged.
2. Nursing care should allow the child dependence, thereby helping him to develop confidence and trust in the situation and at the same time assisting him to develop independence. (Refer to Chapter 35.)
3. Nursing histories should be taken when the child is admitted to the hospital. Specific questions should be asked to obtain information related to the following:
   a. Family home situation
   b. Toilet habits and means of communicating
   c. Dietary habits
   d. Home routines and rituals
   e. Schooling
   f. Friends, peers
   g. Experience with illness
   h. Preparation for hospitalization
   i. Favorite toy, object, etc.
   j. How child handles frustration or stressful situations
   k. Disciplinary practices at home
   l. Comforting practices at home
   m. Parental plans for visiting
4. Attempt to maintain home ties. Continuation of the ties within the existing family unit is a critical aspect of meeting the psychological needs of the child. (Refer to Family-Centered Care, pp. 1131.)
   a. Continue established rituals—rocking and story before bedtime.
   b. Have family photograph at child's bedside.
   c. Use tape recorder to listen to tapes made of family conversations.
   d. Encourage use of the telephone, sending letters and pictures home, incoming cards.
   e. Talk about the people at home with the child.
   f. For the adolescent: assign roommate of same age, encourage use of telephone, encourage socializa-

tion with communal meal-times and recreation periods.

5. Thorough explanations of the treatment plan and preparation for special tests, procedures, and surgery are essential. Unless the child is prepared for these experiences, he has minimal chance to mobilize his coping mechanisms to help him through his hospital experience.
   a. Listen to him repeat descriptions of his experience and continue to correct any misconceptions with factual information. Negative preparation of the child results in chaos, panic, doubt or fear.
   b. Make sure preparation is appropriate to:
      (1) Child's age
      (2) Level of comprehension
   c. Be creative; avoid using terminology that may have unintended alternate meanings to the child, and that may cause him undue stress because of an inability to understand what is being said.
   d. Use metaphors appropriate for cognitive age.
   e. Include parents in the preparation process. Children through age 6 are dependent upon their parents for identity and a sense of well-being, and will need their support. The parents know their child better than anyone and can serve as interpreters for child and health-care personnel.
6. Play is a natural part of nursing care. It is a means to help the child cope with an unpleasant experience; it allows him to project his fears to the outside world, and it helps him to attain a feeling of independence and control of the situation. It is important for the child's physical, emotional, and social development.
7. Nursing care should relate illness to the child's personality, individual reaction, and previous experiences. Recognition must be given to:
   a. What the child comes from
   b. What he is returning to
   c. What he is experiencing during his hospitalization
8. The ultimate goal in pediatric nursing is directed toward:
   a. Reduction of stress
   b. Increasing the child's feeling of well-being
9. Nursing care is successful when its outcome is therapeutic and encompasses growth.

Parental Support

1. Parental presence and involvement with the hospitalized child will decrease anxieties of the child.

Parents, however, need encouragement, support, and education to be of the greatest help possible to their hospitalized child.
   a. Identify anxieties the parents may have regarding hospitalization of the child:
      (1) Relinquishing their child's care to others
      (2) Preparation for surgery or surgical outcome
      (3) Opinions they feel others have of their child
      (4) Guilt feelings regarding disciplining the sick and hospitalized child
      (5) Dealing with the child upon return to the home
   b. Establish at an early stage the degree to which parents are able and want to participate in the care of their child. Reassess this periodically, and provide opportunities for parents to give continuity of care thus promoting continued close parent–child relationships. (Refer to Family-Centered Care, p. 1131.)
      (1) Keep the family informed regarding the condition of the child.
      (2) Reassure parents that someone is available to help them.
      (3) Answer questions regarding hospital policy, procedures, or other concerns.
2. Begin early preparation and education of parents for possible post-hospital behavior of their child.
   a. Frequently there are behavior changes following hospitalization, especially in the child 18 months through 6 years of age. Behavioral changes seen may include: increased demands for attention, withdrawal, violent reactions to temporary separation, changes in sleep patterns, shyness, increased clinging, bedwetting, temper tantrums, new fears, and change in eating habits.
   b. Assist parents in anticipating these changes in their child's behavior. Help them to feel more adequate in coping with and responding to these temporary changes. Parents' reactions to post-hospital behavior can either help to reinforce, prolong, and perpetuate these behaviors or gradually diminish these behaviors. Aid parents in identifying their reactions and feelings towards any post-hospital alterations in their child's behavior.
      (1) Establish a parent–teacher, anticipatory–guidance program for parents.
      (2) Provide staff support to parents during and following hospitalization.

IMPACT OF HOSPITALIZATION ON THE CHILD'S STAGE OF DEVELOPMENT

Neonate

Birth–1 Month

A. *Primary Concern*

1. Bonding: Hospitalization interrupts the early stages of the development of a healthy mother-child relationship, thus early stages of the development of trust are missing.
2. Sensory-motor deprivation: Tactile, visual, auditory, kinesthetic.
3. Sensory bombardment.

B. *Reactions*

1. Impairment of maternal-child attachment.
2. Impairment of mother's ability to love and care for her baby.
3. Risking of infant's emotional and physical well-being.

C. *Nursing Intervention*

1. Provide for continual contact between baby and his parents (eye-to-eye contact and touch).
2. Minimize isolation and strangeness by explaining and re-explaining equipment, procedures, etc., to parents.

3. Actively involve parents in caring for their baby.
4. Foster good neonate-sibling relationships if appropriate.
5. Identify areas of infant deprivation and/or overstimulation.
6. Provide sensory-motor stimulation as appropriate.
7. Allow individuality to begin to emerge.

Infant

1–4 Months

A. *Primary Concern*

1. Separation: Mother is learning to identify and meet the needs of her infant. Infant is learning to make his needs known and to trust his mother to meet them.
2. Sensory-motor deprivation.

B. *Reactions*

Separation anxiety is different from that of older child, because for the infant, his mother seems to be a part of him. Development of trust is disturbed when infant is separated from mother.

C. *Nursing Intervention*

1. Encourage mother to stay and care for her baby, thus minimizing separation. When mother is absent, give infant attention and frequent handling from a limited number of personnel.
2. Provide opportunity for sensory stimulation, motor development, and social responsiveness.
3. Help parents to work through their anxieties. Remember, a mother's touch communicates her comfort or discomfort to her infant.

4–8 Months

A. *Primary Concern*

Separation from mother: Infant now recognizes his mother as a separate person from himself. He rejects strangers.

B. *Reactions*

Separation anxiety: crying, terror, somatic upset, blank facial expression, extreme preoccupation.

C. *Nursing Intervention*

1. Encourage mother to stay and care for her baby.
2. Attempt to adjust schedule to home routines.
3. Become friends with the infant through the mother.
4. The infant is beginning to develop purposeful activities and to strive toward independence. Provide opportunities and encouragement for this development to continue and provide ways for him to use newly acquired skills.

8–12 Months

A. *Primary Concern*

Separation: Infant becomes more possessive of mother and clings to her at the time of separation.

B. *Reactions*

Separation anxiety: tolerance is very limited. Fear of strangers, excessive crying, clinging, and overdependence on mother.

C. *Nursing Intervention*

1. Have mother stay and care for her child.
2. Relieve some of his tensions and loneliness with "transference" object (i.e., blanket, toy).

3. Prepare child for procedures; allow him to become familiar with simple equipment. Have mother comfort child during procedures.
4. Provide for sensory stimulation and motor development appropriate for age. Provide opportunities for child to continue using skills he has acquired, such as feeding himself and drinking from cup.

Toddler (1–3 years)

A. *Primary Concerns*

1. Separation anxiety: Relationship with mother is intense. Separation represents the loss of family and familiar surroundings, resulting in feelings of insecurity, grief, anxiety, and abandonment. The toddler's emotional needs are intensified by his mother's absence.
2. Changes in rituals and routines, all of which are important to his sense of security, become a source of concern.
3. Inability to communicate: Beginning use and understanding of language affords him limited communication between himself and the world. Limited capacity to understand reality, passage of time.
4. Loss of autonomy and independence: His egocentric view of life helps him develop a sense of autonomy. He expresses himself as a separate being with some potential control of his body and environment.
5. Body integrity: Incomplete and inaccurate understanding of the body results in fear, anxiety, frustration, and anger.
6. Decrease in mobility: Restricting his mobility causes frustration. He wants to keep moving for the pleasure it gives him as well as for the feeling of independence, the opportunity to learn about his world, and the route it provides for coping with frustrations that cannot be verbally expressed. Physical interference with this freedom results in a sense of helplessness.

B. *Reactions*

1. Protest:
   a. Has urgent desire to find mother.
   b. Expects that she will answer his cries, "I want mommy."
   c. Frequently cries and shakes crib.
   d. Rejects attention of nurses.
   e. When with mother, child shows signs of distrust and anger, tears.
2. Despair:
   a. Feels increasingly hopeless about finding his mother.
   b. Becomes apathetic, anorectic, listless; looks sad.
   c. May cry continuously or intermittently.
   d. Uses comfort measures—thumbsucking, fingering lip, tightly clutching a toy.
3. Denial:
   a. Represses all feelings and images of his mother.
   b. Does not cry when she leaves.
   c. May seem more attached to nurses—will go to anyone.
   d. Finds little satisfaction in relationships with people.
   e. Accepts care without protest.
   f. Regresses to an earlier state of development.
4. Regression:
   Temporarily ceases use of newly acquired skills in an attempt to retain or regain control of a stressful situation.

C. *Nursing Intervention*

1. Rooming-in, unlimited visiting.
   Parental visits provide:
   a. Opportunity for child to express some of his feelings about his situation.
   b. Assurance that his parents are not abandoning him or punishing him.
   c. Periods of comfort and reassurance that allow for the reestablishment of family bonds.
2. Attempt to continue routines used at home, especially with regard to sleeping, eating, and bathing. Reestablish trust through body contact and comfort.
3. Set limits.
4. Obtain from parents key words in communicating with child. Find out about his non-verbal behavior as well.
5. Allow child to make choices when possible. Arrange physical setting to encourage independence. Allow child to explore the environment.
6. A Band-Aid may give the child security of wholeness after an injection.
7. Replace lost mobility with another form of motion: moving about in a wheelchair, cart, or bed. Exercise restrained extremity. Provide opportunity for the child to release energy suppressed by decreased mobility, i.e., by pounding, throwing. Provide opportunity to continue learning about world through sensory modalities such as water play and diversional play.
8. Discharge:
   If rooming-in has not occurred during hospitalization, parents must be prepared for the possible post-hospital behavior of their toddler. They will need support in understanding and handling these behaviors. The child may do any of the following:
   a. Show lack of affection or resist close physical contact. Parents may interpret this as rejection.
   b. Regress to an earlier stage of development.
   c. Cling to mother, unable to tolerate any separation from her. Show excessive need for love and affection.
9. Parents' response to child's behavior is vital if relationships are to be reestablished.
   a. Extra love and understanding will help restore child's trust.
   b. Hostility and withdrawal of love will cause child further loss of trust, self-esteem, and independence.

Preschool Child (3–5 years)

A. *Primary Concerns*

1. Separation: Although cognitive and coping capabilities have increased and the child responds less violently to separation from parents, separation and hospitalization represent stress beyond the coping mechanisms and adaptive capabilities of the preschool child. Loneliness and insecurities are experienced. Language is important; although the child may not verbally express what he is feeling, there is an attempt at this in the 4- and 5-year-old.
2. Unfamiliar environment: This requires coping with a change in daily routine and represents a loss of control and security.
3. Abandonment and punishment: Fantasies and thought may contain vengeful wishes for other persons, for which the child expects retribution. Illness may be interpreted as punishment for thoughts.

Enforced parental separation may be interpreted as loss of parental love and represents abandonment by them.
4. Body image and integrity: Hospitalization and intrusive procedures provide a multitude of threats of both bodily mutilation and loss of identity, which are just beginning to develop along with the acquisition of autonomy.
5. Immobility: Mobility is the child's dominant form of self-expression and adaptation to the environment. He has a great urge for locomotion and exercise of large muscles. It represents his main expression of emotion and release of tension.
6. Loss of control: This influences the preschooler's perception of and reaction to separation, pain, and illness.

B. *Reactions*

1. *Regression:* Child temporarily stops using newly acquired skills in an attempt to retain or regain control of a stressful situation. Preschooler may return to behavior of the infant or toddler.
2. *Repression:* Child may attempt to exclude the undesirable and unpleasant stresses from consciousness.
3. *Projection:* Preschooler may transfer his own emotional state, motives, and desires to others in his environment.
4. *Displacement/sublimation:* Emotions are permitted to be redirected and expressed in other situations such as art or play.
5. *Identification:* The child assumes characteristics of the aggressor in an attempt to reduce fear and anxiety and to feel that he is in control of the situation.
6. *Aggression:* Hostility is direct and intentional; physical expression takes precedence over verbal expression.
7. *Denial and withdrawal:* The child is able to ignore interruptions and disavow any thought or feeling that would result in a painful experience.
8. *Fantasy:* A mental activity to help the child to bridge the gap between reality and fantasy through imagination. The child has difficulty separating reality from fantasy because of lack of experience.
9. The preschooler may simply show similar behaviors (protest, despair, denial) to those of the toddler, although the stage of protest is usually less aggressive and direct.

C. *Nursing Intervention*

1. Minimize stress of separation by providing for parental presence and participation in care. Strive to shorten the hospital stay. Help parents understand what hospitalization means to the child.
2. Identify defense mechanisms apparent in the child and help him through the stressful situation by accepting him, showing him love and concern, and being alert to his readiness to relinquish them.
3. Set limits for child. Let him know that someone is there. Help child become master of something in the situation.
4. Provide opportunity and encouragement for child to verbalize.
5. Careful preparation for all procedures should be done on the child's level of development and comprehension.
6. Be sure child has opportunities for play. Play is one important medium through which the child can overcome his fear and anxiety. A body outline, doll, and simple visual aides are appropriate teaching tools.

7. Provide consistency in nursing personnel and approach to care.
8. Encourage child to participate in his care and self-hygiene as appropriate.
9. Deal specifically with castration and mutilation fears. If the child is having surgery, describe exactly which body part will be repaired, and provide reassurance that nothing else will be removed or repaired.
10. Whenever appropriate, reassure the child that no one is to blame for his illness or hospitalization.

School-Age Child (5–12 years)

A. *Concerns*
1. Many fear loss of recently mastered skills.
2. Many worry about separation from school and peers. They may fear loss of former roles.
3. Mutilation fantasies are common.
4. Some may believe that they or their parents magically caused the illness merely by thinking that the event would occur.
5. Often they have increased concerns related to modesty, privacy.
6. The imposed passivity may be interpreted as punishment.
7. Children may feel their body no longer is their own, but rather is controlled by doctors and nurses.

B. *Reactions*

(See "Reactions" regarding the preschool child for a more complete description of these responses.)
1. Regression.
2. Conscious attempts at mature behavior.
3. Suppression or denial of symptoms.
4. Repression.
5. Depression.
6. Obsessive-compulsive behavior (common).
7. Sublimation.
8. Tendency to be phobic (normal).
   a. Fears include that of the dark, doctors, hospitals, medication, and death.
   b. Unrealistic fears are commonly attached to needles, x-ray procedures, and blood.

C. *Nursing Intervention*
1. Obtain a thorough nursing history, including information regarding health and physical development, hospitalizations, social-cultural background, and normal daily activities. Utilize this information to plan care.
2. Provide for continuity of nursing personnel.
3. Provide order and consistency in the environment whenever possible.
4. Establish and enforce reasonable policies to protect the child and to increase his sense of security in his environment.
5. Arrange the environment to allow for as much mobility as possible (i.e., make sure articles are appropriately placed; move the bed if the child is immobilized).
6. Respect the child's need for privacy and respect modesty during examinations, bathing, etc.
7. Utilize treatment rooms whenever possible when performing painful or intrusive procedures.
8. Help young children identify problems and questions (often through play). Then help them to find the answers.
9. Provide information about the illness and hospitalization based on assessment of what facts the child needs and wants and how this information can be made readily understandable to him.
10. View all nursing care activities as teaching situations. Explain the function of equipment and allow the child to handle it. Teach scientific terminology for body parts, procedures, etc.
11. When explaining a procedure, make sure that the child knows its purpose, what will be done, and what will be expected of him. Reassure the child during the procedure by continuing the explanations and support.
12. Reassure the child having surgery; explain where the organ to be removed or repaired is located, and that no other body part will be removed.
13. Utilize play whenever appropriate to provide information about the hospital experience and to identify and decrease the child's fantasies and fears.
14. Reassure the child that he or his parents are not to blame for his illness.
15. Facilitate discharge of energy and aggression through appropriate play activities or through sharing aspects of ward management.
16. Encourage the child's participation in his care and self-hygiene.
17. Support intellectual potential through the use of games, books, puzzles, school work, and drawings.
18. Assist the child's family to understand his reactions to illness and hospitalization so that family members can facilitate positive coping patterns.
19. Let the child know that his normal status as a family member remains intact during his hospitalization. Encourage a consistent visiting pattern and allow sibling visits.
20. Help parents to deal with their own anxieties about hospitalization and assist them to help their child cope with the situation.
21. Encourage parental participation in the child's care when appropriate. Discourage rooming-in with the child except in cases of acute illness and initial regression.
22. Encourage written communication with peers, and allow peer visiting when appropriate.
23. Begin discharge planning early, including plans for physical and emotional needs. Alert families to possible behavioral changes, including phobias, nightmares, regression, negativism, and disturbances in eating and learning.

Adolescent

A. *Concerns*

1. Physical illness, exposure, and lack of privacy may cause increased concern about body image and sexuality.
2. Separation from security of peers, family, and school may cause anxiety.
3. Interference with his struggle for independence and emancipation from his parents is a concern.
4. The adolescent may be very threatened by helplessness. He may see illness as a punishment for feelings not mastered or for breaking rules imposed by his parents or physician.

B. *Reactions*
1. May be anxious about or embarrassed by loss of control.
2. May be insecure.

3. May intellectualize about details of the disease to avoid addressing actual concerns.
4. May reject treatment measures, even if they had been previously accepted.
5. May be angry because goals are being thwarted. This anger may be directed toward staff.
6. Depression may occur.
7. Increased dependence on staff and parents may occur.
8. May show denial or withdrawal.
9. May assert control by being demanding and uncooperative.
10. May capitalize on gains from illness or pain.

C. Nursing Intervention

1. Assess the impact of illness on the adolescent by considering factors such as timing, nature of illness, new experiences imposed, changes in body image, and expectations for the future.
2. Introduce the adolescent to the hospital staff and to regular routines soon after admission.
3. Obtain a thorough nursing history that includes information about hobbies, school, family, illness, hospitalization, food habits, and recreation.
4. Encourage adolescents to wear their own clothes, and allow them to decorate their beds or rooms to express themselves.
5. Have drawers and closets available to store personal items.
6. Allow the adolescent access to a telephone.
7. Allow adolescents control over appropriate matters, i.e., timing of bath, selection of food, etc.
8. Respect their need for periodic isolation and privacy.
9. Have a well-supervised recreational and activities program available that is planned by a professional child care worker.
10. Accept adolescent's level of performance. Allow regression with expectation of growth.
11. Involve adolescent in planning his care so that he will be more accepting of restrictions and receptive to health teaching. He should be accepted as a vital member of the health-care team. His consent should be obtained for procedures and surgery.

12. Explain clearly all procedures, routines, expectations, and restrictions imposed by illness. If necessary, clarify the adolescent's interpretation of illness and hospitalization. Plan separate teaching sessions for parents.
13. Facilitate verbal rejection of treatment measures to protect adolescent from harming himself physically by stopping treatment.
14. Assess the adolescent's intellectual skills and provide him with the necessary information to allow him to use problem-solving to deal with his illness and hospitalization.
15. Recognize positive and negative coping behaviors as attempts to adjust to a threatening situation. Attempt to deal with the feeling that caused the behavior as well as with the behavior itself.
16. Be a good listener. Maintain a sense of humor.
17. Provide opportunities such as writing, art work, and recreational activities to allow nonverbal adolescents to express themselves.
18. Foster interaction with other hospitalized adolescents and continuation of peer relationships with outside friends.
19. Establish regular group meetings to allow patients to meet with staff members and with each other to comment and to ask questions about their hospital experiences.
20. Set necessary limits to encourage self-control and ensure the rights of others.
21. Help adolescents work through sexual feelings. Avoid behavior which could be interpreted as provocative or flirtatious. Masturbation, unless excessive, may be considered a psychologically healthy way to discharge sexual tension.
22. Interpret the needs and reactions of hospitalized adolescents to parents. Emphasize the adolescent's need to be respected as a unique individual, separate from his parents.
23. Assist parents to cope with the illness and hospitalization as well as to deal effectively with the adolescent's response to related stress.
24. Encourage continuation of education.
25. Stress the confidential nature of conversations between nurse and patient and doctor and patient.

FAMILY-CENTERED CARE

Family-centered care provides an opportunity for the family to care for the hospitalized child with nursing support.

The *goal* of family-centered care is to maintain or strengthen the roles and ties of the family with the hospitalized child in order to promote normality of the family unit.

Benefits for Parents and Child

1. Continued close family interactions during stress.
2. Absence of separation anxiety.
3. Reactions of protest, denial, and despair are decreased or nonexistent.
   a. There is little inconsolable crying.
   b. Sleep is more relaxed.
4. Greater sense of security for the child.
5. Opportunity for family to fulfill their needs to care for their child physically and emotionally.
6. Allows parents to feel useful and important rather than making them dependent and destroying their confidence.
7. Lessening of parental guilt feelings.
8. Opportunities for parents to increase their competence and confidence in caring for the sick child.
9. Comfort for the family provided by other families.
10. Greater absorption of staff teaching by the family.
11. Posthospitalization reactions are diminished.

Implementation Strategies

Implementation of family-centered care will depend on regulations of the particular health-care setting as well as the capabilities of the individual family unit. Examples of activities that can facilitate and strengthen family ties include:
1. Rooming-in for parents of young children
2. Parent participation in the child's physical care
3. Flexible visiting regulations for family members, including siblings

4. Having pictures of family members available at the hospital
5. Encouraging telephone contact
6. Use of family tape recordings

General Principles of Family-Centered Care

1. The nurse must be equipped with a broad knowledge base from the physical and behavioral sciences. Special emphasis is required in such areas as growth and development, family dynamics, socialization, and communication. Continuing education programs must be designed to support and improve family-centered care.
2. Staff must realize that parents are not time savers for nurses when they are participating in their child's care. The parents are not there to relieve the nurse of her routines and care.
   Additional nursing time is necessary to answer questions, to orient parents to the unit, to teach child care, and to comfort parents.
3. Family-centered care places a great deal of responsibility on the nurse and offers an opportunity to administer total patient care to the child and his family.
4. Family-centered care units should present a relaxed, comfortable atmosphere.
   a. Do not require parents to stay, but allow them to stay if they desire.
      (1) Some mothers may feel too anxious or guilty to participate.
      (2) Outside responsibilities may prohibit parents' staying.
   b. Provide physical comfort for participating parents.
      (1) Folding chair or bed in child's room.
      (2) Comfortable lounge or waiting room.
      (3) Eating facilities.
      (4) Bathroom facilities, including showers.
   c. Encourage parent(s) to take appropriate breaks from attending to the child.
      (1) Provides rest for the parent.
      (2) Helps child learn parent(s) will return and not abandon him.
5. When parents are active participants in their child's care, they too have certain needs, because they are concerned about their ill child.
   a. They want to care for their child as they would do at home.
   b. They are interested in working with the staff and learning from the staff how they can help their child.
   c. They like to have something to do for the child while visiting. This lessens their feeling of helplessness.
   d. Supports should be available (e.g., parent advocates, child care for well siblings, parent surrogates for times when parents cannot stay).
6. If parents know what is expected of them and what they can expect of the staff, many problems can be avoided. It helps parents feel more comfortable.
   a. Nursing and medical observations and care will be continued with or without the parents (or mother) present.
   b. Parents should be encouraged to assume a nurturing, comforting role. They should also be allowed to participate in the child's physical care to the extent that they desire or that will be necessary after the child's discharge. This requires encouragement, support, and education from the nurse.
   c. Parents should allow child to become involved with peers on the unit.
   d. Parents should not ask for personal services.
7. Families of hospitalized children can offer a great deal of support to one another. Many times they have similar problems.
   a. Allow families to gather in groups—informal or formally planned group meetings.
   b. Formal group meetings usually provide a professional mental health team composed of social worker, psychiatrist, physician and nurse, as needed.

Role of Parents

1. To serve as the child's primary resource of security and support so that he will be better able to tolerate unfamiliarity and discomfort and will be able to emerge from the experience with less likelihood of posthospitalization reactions.
2. To serve as the child's advocate in order to ensure that his basic human rights will be respected.
3. To teach nurses specific ways in which they can support the child.
4. To serve as role models and to support other families who may be dealing with similar problems.

Role of Nurse

1. To create an environment conducive to maintaining family integrity and unity. The nurse should do each of the following:
   a. Help to maintain healthy mother-child relationship. (Mother should not be threatened by the nurse.)
   b. Help father establish or maintain his role of supporting mother and child, of keeping things going at home, and of relieving mother in the hospital.
   c. Include siblings in planning and intervention as appropriate.
   d. Supplement the family in the common goal of the child's welfare.
2. To assist parents to make decisions about when to stay with their child.
   a. Parents' presence is especially important if the child is 5 years or younger, is especially anxious or upset, or is in medical crisis.
   b. The parents' decision is influenced by needs of other family members, as well as by job and home responsibilities.
   c. The nurse should try to alleviate guilty feelings of parents who are unable to stay with their child.
3. To develop trusting, goal-directed relationship with families.
   a. Obtain a thorough nursing history that provides information to assess strengths, relationships, and concerns.
   b. Plan with the family toward mutual, realistic goals.
   c. Recognize good care that the child receives from parents.
4. To observe the parent-child relationship in order to do the following:
   a. Evaluate the degree of participation of the parents in physical and emotional care.
   b. Observe parents' attitudes, skills, and techniques and the child's behavior and response to them.

c. Assess what teaching needs to be done.

d. Detect problems in parent-child relationships.

5. To teach parents knowledge, understanding, and skills necessary to function effectively with the hospitalized child. The nurse should do the following:

   a. Perform nursing techniques safely and efficiently.

   b. Interpret the behavior of the hospitalized child to parents so that they can understand it and intervene appropriately (refer to the section, "Impact of Hospitalization on the Child's Stage of Development").

   c. Interpret and reinforce what physician has told parents. Answer questions thoroughly and honestly as knowledge permits.

   d. Interpret medical procedures and diagnostic tests.

   e. Provide health teaching.

   f. Offer anticipatory guidance.

6. To help parents adapt to the situation and to develop their own feeling of value by coping with the child's illness.

   a. Be aware of common parental reactions to the stress experienced by families of children who have severe or chronic illness.

   b. Be aware that defense mechanisms, if employed in moderation, are constructive and may facilitate optimal coping.

   c. Help parents recognize their own feelings.

   d. Identify parental support systems as well as adaptive and maladaptive coping.

   e. Be perceptive of parents' physical and emotional needs and limitations.

      (1) Do not allow parents to become fatigued.

      (2) Allow parents to leave, take a break.

7. To assist families as appropriate in dealing with normal family developmental tasks.

   a. Be aware that the child's hospitalization is often only one of many stresses a family experiences at a given time. Others frequently include:

      (1) Interpersonal problems.

      (2) Debt, unemployment, job change.

      (3) Recent changes in dwelling place and consequent disruption.

      (4) Problems associated with child care and discipline.

      (5) Concurrent illness of other family members.

8. To ensure continuity of family-centered care between the hospital and home.

CHILD LIFE PROGRAMS

Many hospitals have established programs with a specially trained staff whose job it is to concern themselves solely with the social and emotional welfare of every pediatric patient. Such programs are called by a variety of names, including "Child Life," "Children's Activities," "Recreational Therapy," "Play Therapy," and others.

Rationale for Child Life Programs

1. Hospitalization separates a child from his home, family, and all that is familiar, and places him in an institution where he may experience intrusive, embarrassing, painful, and mutilating invasion of his body.

2. The short-term and long-term effects of illness and hospitalization on the intellectual, social, and emotional development of children has been documented by observations and research.

3. A separate child life department to meet the social and emotional needs of patients is justified, because such work requires the following:

   a. Special expertise and training.

   b. Adequate time that is free of other responsibilities.

   c. A special role definition of staff member so that the child knows that this is a person who will not become involved in his medical care.

Staffing of Child Life Programs

1. Staffing of child life departments differs among institutions according to their needs and resources. In most settings, they are staffed entirely by professionals who work with aides and volunteers.

2. Most child life workers have bachelor's or master's degrees in child-related professions such as preschool, kindergarten, and elementary education; nursing; social work; child development; and speech pathology.

   a. Various educational institutions offer courses and areas of concentration in "The Hospitalized Child."

   b. Most child life departments offer their own in-service training programs so that the staff may learn to work with the hospitalized child.

Goals of Child Life Programs

1. To prevent some of the emotional pain and fear associated with illness and hospitalization.

   a. Child life workers may assume primary responsibility or a supportive role in the preparation of patients for hospitalization, surgery, and/or particular procedures.

   b. In many hospitals, child life workers arrange preadmission tours, puppet shows, and similar activities to which all children who are planned pediatric admissions are invited.

2. To provide a comfortable, accepting, and nonthreatening environment where the child may play and interact with other children and with an adult who is not involved with his medical needs.

   a. Ideally, there is a separate child life playroom in every unit. However, there may be only an open area at the end of a corridor or in the middle of the ward.

   b. Generally, there is a specific regulation that no medical procedures (even relatively benign ones such as taking a child's temperature) are to be carried out in the play area.

   c. In many settings, children are encouraged to have their meals in the playroom. Generally, they not only enjoy the opportunity to eat with others but also seem to eat better.

3. To provide the child with an opportunity for choice.

   a. The child may choose whether or not he wishes to come to the playroom. Once there, he may choose what to do.

b. A variety of craft and play materials, including real and miniature medical equipment is available.

c. Should the child choose to sit and watch or be held and rocked, these activities are seen as acceptable choices.

4. To provide a continuing educational program.
   a. In some settings teachers are paid by the hospital and are an integral part of the child life program. In others, teachers are provided by the local public schools, and they work in close cooperation with the child life department.
   b. In most hospitals, the educational program includes special activities for preschoolers and toddlers as well as a program of infant stimulation.

Role and Responsibilities of the Child Life Worker

1. To serve as advocate for the child.
   a. The worker serves as spokesperson for the child in his interaction with the health care delivery system.
   b. Serves as an instrument of change when the delivery system does not seem to be in the best interests of a large group of children.
2. To alleviate distress.
   a. Supports and tries to help children who have already been traumatized by their illness, surgery, and hospitalization.
   b. Is available for immediate crisis intervention such as comforting children during painful or frightening procedures, consoling children when expected visits from parents do not occur, and in other similar situations.
3. To provide therapeutic and recreational activity programs.
   a. The worker provides programs on the unit—both for individuals (at bedside) and for groups of children able to come to the play area.
   b. Utilizes play to allow the child to do the following:
      (1) Master his fears about an anticipated procedure or one that he has already experienced.

(2) Express his feelings.
(3) Give life to his fantasies and clarify misconceptions.
(4) Try other roles (particularly those of doctor and nurse).
(5) Distract himself.
(6) Relieve boredom and simply have fun.

c. The nature of such programs, the facilities for them, and the time allowed will necessarily vary from one hospital to the next.

4. To serve as a diagnostic observer.
   a. As a trained observer of the development and behavior of children, the child life worker acts as a member of the diagnostic team.
   b. Records observations and shares them with other members of the health team.
5. To participate in patient planning.
   Acts as a member of the health team to ensure that consideration is given to the child's social and emotional needs during and after hospitalization.
6. To serve as a source of support for parents.
   a. Is available to parents as needed to help them deal with their own anxieties as well as those of their children.
   b. In most settings, parents are encouraged to join their children in the play area.
7. To serve as teacher to physicians, nurses, and other hospital personnel.
   Teaches others in the areas of child development and behavior and the reactions of children to illness and hospitalization.

Shared Goals and Responsibilities

1. A child life department can exist only as one part of a hospital's total commitment to the social and emotional welfare of all children who enter the hospital.
2. Child life staff and nursing staff must work closely together and must complement each other's efforts.

INTENSIVE CARE NURSERY

Nurse's Role and Responsibilities in an Intensive Care Nursery

1. The nurse is an active, integral part of the essential nurse-physician team in caring for the sick newborn.
   a. The nurse has a major responsibility in caring for the sick newborn. Much credibility is given to her observations because of continual contact with and care of the infant and past experience in making similar observations.
   b. It is not enough to follow the written prescription of the physician. The nurse must use initiative (i.e., must employ independent nursing judgment) in evaluating the infant's condition and must make changes in therapy when there are signs of deterioration or be able to handle a medical emergency. Subtle changes in behavior or condition of the infant detected early by the nurse and related to the physician often result in treating the infant before he is critically ill or beyond the point where permanent damage may have occurred.

2. The nurse must have an understanding of pathogenesis of diseases of the newborn in order to program nursing activities in caring for the infant. The nurse must be informed about the following:
   a. Specific diseases of the newborn
   b. The treatment of their problems
   c. The uses of the equipment employed in caring for these infants
3. In addition, the nurse must possess the following qualities:
   a. Improved clinical awareness
   b. Increased diagnostic skills
   c. Ability to make nursing assessments
   d. Skills in performing special procedures
4. Working with the critically ill infant requires technical skills in several areas. Some of these include:
   a. Respiratory care
      (1) Endotracheal suctioning
      (2) Oxygen administration and monitoring
      (3) Ventilatory management
   b. Cardiac and vascular monitoring

(1) Blood pressure assessment
(2) Exchange transfusion and blood administration
(3) Umbilical catheterization
(4) Blood-gas monitoring
c. Other treatment and assessment modalities
(1) Laboratory and roentgen studies
(2) Phototherapy
(3) Temperature control
d. Equipment control
Equipment working properly, etc.
5. The knowledge acquired in caring for the critically ill newborn will equip the nurse to compare signs such as respiration, fluctuating blood pressure, heart rate, subtle movement or lack of movement, and provide:
a. Cardiopulmonary support
b. Respiratory management
c. Fluid and nutritional assessment and management
d. Observation for complications and other illnesses
6. Infection control is within the realm of nursing responsibilities. Constant surveillance and strict adherence to procedures directed toward preventing infection must be practiced.
a. Good handwashing technique:
(1) 2–3 minute scrub with a brush and hexachlorophene or iodophor at the start of each shift
(2) 10 second scrub before and between infants
b. Consider contact with Isolette or bassinet the same as contact with the infant himself.
c. Nonhuman areas of contact and sources of possible contamination might be scales, examining table, and washing areas.
d. Need for adequate and appropriate nurse-baby ratio.
e. Surveillance of infant to recognize evidence of illness and source of infection to others.
f. Removal from the area of staff experiencing viral or bacterial illness.
g. Effective cord care of the newborn—application of antiseptic dye (triple dye) or neomycin-polymyxin-bacitracin ointment.
h. If staphylococcal or streptococcal infection develops in the area, the following procedures should be followed:
(1) Periodic bathing of infants with a 0.1N dilution (0.3%) of hexachlorophene solution is effective in controlling infection by these organisms. Blood levels of hexachlorophene are lower if this solution is used rather than the 3% solution.

NURSING ALERT: Hexachlorophene should be used cautiously and under strict and specific medical supervision in order to prevent neurotoxicity in the infant.

(2) The Isolette and incubator serve as effective isolation when good handwashing is practiced.
7. The nurse must begin to help form a bond between infant and his mother as well as to build cohesiveness of the family immediately upon the infant's admission to the intensive care unit (see "Caring for Parents of Infant in Intensive Care Nursery").
8. Research indicates that to enhance the quality of the life saved and to provide the best chance for the child to achieve his potential, early environmental, emotional and psychosocial stimulation is essential. By virtue of involvement, the nurse has a tremendous responsibility and opportunity in this area (see p. 1136).
9. It is vitally important that the nurse practice meticulous recording and documentation for the protection of the infant as well as the nurse:
a. Always record routine procedures, i.e., hourly ventilator care.
b. Record physician visits to infant and any contact by nurse with physician.
c. Never erase. Errors should be crossed out with a single line, marked "error," and initialed.
d. Record events accurately, e.g., emergency treatment.

Classification of High-Risk Neonate Requiring Intensive Care

1. Premature
Problems are related to general immaturity: feeding, respiratory distress and/or apneic spells, hyperbilirubinemia
2. Small for Gestational Age
Problems include: hypoglycemia, poor temperature control, and high susceptibility to infection
3. Medical Problems
These include: respiratory distress, hypoglycemia, hyperbilirubinemia, erythroblastosis, sepsis neonatorum, hypocalcemia, infant of diabetic mother (IDM), drug withdrawal, and neurologic conditions
4. Surgical Problems
These include: tracheoesophageal fistula, myelomeningocele, cleft palate, imperforate anus, and distended abdomen
5. Congenital Malformations
These include: cardiac problems, genetic defects

Caring for Parents of Infant in Intensive Care Nursery

Research has documented that infant-mother bonding is significantly influenced by events before and immediately after delivery and may greatly influence later maternal behavior and the infant-mother relationship. Mother's attachment to her infant is critical for his optimal growth and development, since he depends entirely upon his mother to satisfy his needs.

A. *Barriers to healthy mother-infant bonding*

1. Grief, guilt, anger, fear, and anxiety felt by the mother at the birth of a child she expected to be perfect. Mother may mourn over loss of this child.
2. Maternal background factors—socioeconomic status, educational training, own childhood experiences, emotional stability.
3. Expectations and attitudes of the mother toward her infant.
4. Separation of mother and her infant at a time when her sensitivity may be at a maximum for attachment to her infant.
5. Anticipatory grieving for possible loss of this infant and emotional withdrawal from infant.
6. Maternal attitude about herself—her lack of self-confidence in her ability to care for her infant; her negative feelings about her inability to carry her infant to term or to produce a normal child.

7. Disruption of care-eliciting behaviors by the infant; the infant serves as a stimulus for mother in helping her identify her offspring and promote her caretaking behaviors.
8. Stress elicited by physical presence of infant in intensive care nursery, i.e., realization of severity of illness of infant, emergency atmosphere, sensory deprivation—all tend to diminish her self-confidence—since she cannot give her own infant the special care he needs.

B. *Nursing intervention to help foster mother-infant bonding as well as eventual appropriate parenting behaviors*

1. Allow mother to see and touch her infant immediately after delivery and again as soon and as often as possible.
2. Describe in detail all the equipment surrounding the infant in the intensive care nursery, prior to the mother's seeing the infant and again when she is near him.
3. Talk with mother on a personal basis; call her by name; make personal comments. Encourage parents to name their baby and refer to him by that name.
4. Encourage mother to enter the intensive care nursery as soon as possible and allow unlimited visiting except during specialized procedures. If daily visits are not always possible, encourage phone contact with nursery staff. The nurse should also call the mother.
5. Carefully consider the mother's concerns and feelings. Being the parent of a critically ill infant is emotionally devastating. Communicate to her your caring concern.
6. Encourage mother to touch her infant.
   a. This will help her to see him as real and will decrease some of her fears.
   b. Touching is the first step in the mother's developing her own self-confidence.
   c. Show mother how she can gradually assume more of baby's care and is better at mothering than the nurse.
7. Open communication channels with parents early.
   a. Meet parents in hospital of origin.
   b. Reinforce information given.
   c. Share good news—first feeding, physical activity, less oxygen needed, etc.
   d. Support them when discouraging news (e.g., discontinued feedings, increased apneic spells) is given.
   e. Often there develops a closeness between the mother and nurse that allows her to participate knowledgeably and confidently with the nurse in evaluating the infant's progress.
8. Observe the intensive care nursery physical setting in terms of parental needs, i.e., need for rocking chairs, bright pictures on the walls, parents' visiting area inside the nursery, pictures of past ICN babies that are growing and thriving.
9. Encourage active participation by the mother in the care of her infant (as the infant's condition permits). For example, instruct the mother on how to enter the Isolette; allow her to visit during feeding and to do something in connection with feeding.
   a. Explain how her visits and contact will benefit the baby.
   b. Assist her in touching and talking to her infant as necessary.

c. Show her that increasing her physical contact with infant will increase her involvement and confidence in caring for the child.
   d. Continually assess the parents' (the mother's, in particular) ability to be involved; be sensitive to their tolerance for handling the infant and their degree of emotional tolerance.
10. There should be continuous focus on the family. Parents and infant must be treated as a unit.
   a. Priorities for this are:
      (1) Crisis intervention.
      (2) Continual parent contact.
      (3) Encouragement of parenting behaviors.
   b. Goals are:
      (1) To develop mother's self-confidence and ability to rely on her own instincts and common sense in caring for her infant.
      (2) To assist the father in becoming involved emotionally and in developing competence in taking care of his family after discharge as well as in taking pleasure in his infant.
11. There is a necessity to decrease the social isolation that is often inherent in the birth of a critically ill baby.
   a. Initiate social service and community health nurse support early.
   b. Provide mother (parents) with an opportunity to talk with other mothers (or parents) of infants with similar conditions, thus affording them the opportunity to express their feelings and concerns and to realize that they are not alone in feelings of guilt, failure, and fear.
   c. Permit visits to infant and parents by others who will be a support to them.
12. Provide some mechanism by which information concerning parents can be evaluated and trouble areas can be recognized early. Document information such as the following:
   a. Parental involvement (phone calls, visits, handling and caring for infant).
   b. Specific or special procedures observed by, taught to, and performed by parents.
   c. Specific information discussed with parents—by whom and when.
   d. Discharge teaching and plans.

Stimulation: The Infant in Intensive Care Nursery

Every infant has the emotional need and right to recognize his mother's face, touch, and voice. The sick infant or premature infant is forced to accept less. Research documents that problems can arise from early sensory deprivation. The intensive care nursery is devoid of much sensory and perceptual stimuli—a situation that is harmful to the infant, the mother, and the mother-infant interactions. To maximize the potential to which the infant can develop, an early stimulation program should be planned.
1. Each stimulation program should be individualized for the specific infant-parent unit, based upon:
   a. Familiarization with the baby's physical condition and limitations.
   b. Assessment of the baby's behavioral skills, developmental status, areas of deprivation, or overstimulation.
   c. Assessment of the parents' abilities to be involved in stimulating their child.
   d. A program of infant stimulation adds specific sensory–motor activities and techniques to daily

care activities for a specific area of development. It is not random activity meant to excite the infant.

2. Some general guidelines for establishing a psychosocial stimulation environment to be adapted for each infant include the following:
   a. Provide for the continuity of the same caretaker each day, each shift. This will benefit both infant and parents.
   b. Make the baby as attractive as possible—clean, colorful linen, lotion on skin, ribbon in hair. The general appearance of a "preemie" or sick infant makes it difficult for mother to relate to her infant.
   c. Help infant establish a day/night cycle. Dim lights or cover infant's eyes.
   d. Place an active mobile or colorful object in baby's line of vision, and adjust as his vision accommodation changes with age—about 23 cm. (9 inches) for newborn. This will increase visually directed reaching.
   e. Encourage personnel to talk to and touch infant when caring for him. Hold him at feedings as well as between feedings when infant's condition allows this. Have personnel attempt to have infant focus upon their face and follow their head movement with his eyes.
   f. Encourage personnel to follow specific procedure when feeding if infant is able to tolerate it.
      (1) Hold infant in nursing position to aid in establishing enface.
      (2) Rock, talk to, fondle, and pat infant before, during, and after feeding. Hold infant in upright position when burping to aid in this visual orientation.
   g. Encourage parent participation in this program.
      (1) Assist the parents so they become emotionally involved with the baby.
      (2) Point out specific responses and behavior of the infant they can look for and what these responses mean. This will help them learn to pay attention to the baby's behavior and to respond to his needs. Talk about this behavior and the parents' feelings about it.
      (3) Encourage parents to visit during feeding time and to participate in the procedure. Even if gavage feedings are done, parents can hold infant, give him a pacifier, fondle him, and relate to him in many ways.
   h. Be aware of specific sensory stimulation for the infant.
      (1) Olfactory—mother's article of clothing near infant.
      (2) Visual—change position of infant; change location of Isolette; use of mobiles or bright objects.
      (3) Auditory—music box, tape of mother's voice.

Discharge Planning Begins Early

1. Maternal behaviors are learned. In order to provide the mother with an opportunity to build self-confidence and to develop to her potential, active participation with her infant during the infant's hospitalization is essential. Mother-infant bonding must be started and allowed to grow during this time for the well-being of both infant and mother.
2. Detailed preparation for home care is essential and must be given in advance.
   a. Specific or special procedures and medications.
   b. Information concerning routine baby care.
   c. Crying pattern of the newborn.
3. Initiate social service and/or community nurse referrals long before discharge.
   a. This provides parents with continual support by someone they know.
   b. Initiating these referrals also gives the nurse feedback about the home situation and possible areas where problems can be averted.
   c. Continual support by the community health nurse is important. Follow-up care can be directed also at assessing family interaction and parenting behaviors as well as development of the baby.
4. Evaluate the parents' willingness and ability to accept the child into their total care.
   Permit the mother a special nesting period when she can have close physical contact with her infant in privacy and can provide complete care for her infant. Nursing support and help are readily available for the mother to call on if needed.
   a. Instructions, demonstrations, and practice of procedures should have occurred prior to this time.
   b. It is possible that this period may enhance normal maternal attachment behaviors days or weeks after birth.
5. Encourage parents to continue psychosocial and intellectual stimulation of their infant at home
   Provide a resource for parents so that they can assess child's readiness for the next step and promote it.

Realities of Nursing in the Intensive Care Nursery

Nursing in an intensive care nursery can be an emotionally draining experience; it can be difficult and depressing as well as hopeful and rewarding. Nurses frequently become surrogate mothers, grieving and rejoicing as the infant's condition changes. To minimize the personal agony frequently encountered, certain areas should be explored and opened to discussion.

1. Each nurse working in the intensive care nursery setting must be completely and totally educated to work in the area.
2. Discussions on grief and grieving should be open and frequent to allow each nurse to explore her own feelings.
3. Patient-centered discussions should be part of the routine to allow the nurse to express feelings about a particular patient.
4. Parent-centered discussions should focus on the parent's coping behaviors and stages of grief.
5. Each nurse must explore and acknowledge her feelings about the work in which she is involved.

PEDIATRIC INTENSIVE CARE UNIT

Nursing Role and Responsibilities in a Pediatric Intensive Care Unit

1. To provide continuing, comprehensive physical care and supportive treatment required to maintain life and to aid recovery of acutely ill children.
2. To provide emotionally supportive care to acutely ill children.
3. To provide empathetic support to parents and families of children in the intensive care unit.
4. To act as an integral and essential member of the

health care team by assessing patient needs as well as by planning care and evaluating its effectiveness.

5. To act as child advocate by ensuring that basic human rights are respected.

6. To serve as nursing care consultants when children who require some intensive care nursing skills are admitted to regular pediatric units.

7. To serve as members of appropriate hospital committees (e.g., committees that decide policy on emergency care, protocol for admission to the pediatric ICU, etc.).

8. To teach intensive care nursing principles and skills to appropriate groups (e.g., nursing students, resident physicians, persons in continuing education programs).

9. To function effectively and safely, the ICU nurse should demonstrate the following capabilities:
   a. Good physical and emotional health required to withstand the strain of continually nursing critically ill patients
   b. Understanding of pathophysiology underlying disease
   c. Knowledge and understanding of sophisticated monitoring equipment and special apparatus
   d. Ability to reason objectively and to judge and be aware of rapidly changing situations
   e. Ability to interpret data and to take rapid, decisive action
   f. Ability to perform complex technical skills correctly and in an organized manner
   g. Understanding of the impact of illness and hospitalization on the life of the child
   h. Understanding of parental responses and ways of coping with the stress of a critically ill child
   i. Ability to record data concisely, accurately, and thoroughly

Physical Care of the Child

1. Apply understanding of the pathogenesis of the disease in assessing patient needs and in planning care.

2. Perform complex technical skills to monitor and support the child (see text for specific procedures). These may include:
   a. Cardiac, respiratory, and blood pressure monitoring
   b. Basic interpretation of ECG tracing
   c. Endotracheal suctioning
   d. Oxygen administration and monitoring
   e. Tracheostomy care
   f. Ventilator management
   g. Monitoring central venous pressure
   h. Monitoring intracranial pressure
   i. Measuring arterial pressure
   j. Hyperalimentation
   k. Collection of specimens
   l. Chest drainage

3. Perform nursing activities related to life support of the child (see text for specific procedures). These activities include the following:
   a. Cardiopulmonary support
   b. Respiratory management
   c. Observation of neurologic signs
   d. Fluid and nutritional assessment and management
   e. Observations for complications and changing status

4. Apply general nursing measures for patient comfort and prevention of complications:
   a. Positioning—to prevent contractures, to drain secretions from the lungs, and to minimize pressure effects on skin
   b. Monitoring and regulation of body temperature
   c. Skin care—to prevent breakdown
   d. Eye care—to prevent conjunctivitis and injury to the cornea in unconscious children
   e. Fluid balance—record daily fluid intake by all routes and losses of urine, stool, vomit, blood, and other drainage; be sensitive to weight loss and gain
   f. Mouth care—to cleanse mouth of secretions, vomitus, especially in unconscious patient or patient with endotracheal tube
   g. Control of infection

5. Provide careful, continuous clinical observations of the child.

Emotional Support of Child

1. Refer to the section on the impact of hospitalization on the developmental stage of the child, page 1127.

2. If possible, familiarize the child with the unit before admission.

3. Provide immediate physical care that communicates strength and facilitates trust.

4. Be alert to behavioral changes that may indicate physical distress.

5. Facilitate parent–child interaction.

6. Question parents concerning the child's own way of responding to emotional stress. Utilize particular comforts that are most soothing to the child.

7. Support parents so that they will be best able to support their child.

8. Time activities; dim lights to allow for adequate sleep whenever possible.

9. Do everything possible to reduce the amount of pain that the child must endure.

10. Provide age-appropriate stimulation when indicated by the child's condition (TV, games, books, toys, etc.).

11. Provide opportunities for the child to express his fears and concerns.

12. If possible, avoid exposing an alert child to the death or resuscitation of another child. If the child is exposed, provide adequate explanation. The child must also be helped to express and work through the experience.

13. Prepare the child for transfer from the intensive care unit by implementing a nursing care plan similar to that which the child will experience on a regular unit (e.g., decrease frequency of monitoring of vital signs, encourage independence). Give a thorough report to the receiving nurse during transfer.

Emotional Support to Family

1. Orient parents to the unit and its waiting areas. Clarify visiting policies and hospital expectations.

2. Encourage liberal visiting hours and unlimited phone calls from parents to the intensive care unit.

3. Assure parents that everything possible is being done for their child. Whenever possible, allow them to see child receiving treatment.

4. Make certain that parents are informed of important changes in the child's clinical status. Reinforce medical interpretations.

5. Explain special equipment and changes in nursing management.
6. Provide opportunities for parents to ask questions and have them answered.
7. Encourage parents to interact verbally and physically with their child. Support them in this endeavor.
8. Facilitate expressions of parental grief.
9. Provide opportunities for parents to talk with a person with whom they can share their concerns and fears. Be sure this person can see them as often as they require.
10. Provide opportunities for parents to meet together to share experiences and offer mutual support.
11. Be sensitive to parents' additional commitments to family and home as well as to their need to remain with their child. Whenever possible, allow visiting at a mutually convenient time.
12. Help parents provide anticipatory guidance for siblings and extended family members.
13. Refer parents to appropriate community resources for help with financial, environmental, or psychologic problems.
14. Offer follow-up contact to parents if appropriate.
15. Refer to section on Family-Centered Care.

THE CHILD UNDERGOING SURGERY

Preoperative Care

1. Provide emotional support, psychological preparation, and preoperative teaching appropriate for the age of the child. Such preparation and support will minimize stress and will help the child cope with his fears.
   a. Potential threats for the hospitalized child anticipating surgery are:
      (1) Physical harm—body injury, pain, mutilation, death
      (2) Separation from parents
      (3) The strange and unknown—possibility of surprise
      (4) Confusion and uncertainty about his limits and expected behavior
      (5) Relative loss of control of his world, his autonomy
      (6) Fear of anesthesia
      (7) Fear of the surgical procedure itself
   b. All preparation and support must be based upon the child's age, developmental stage, and level; personality; past history and experience with health professionals and hospitals; background—including religion, socioeconomic group, culture, and family attitudes.
      (1) Know what information the child has already received.
      (2) Determine from the child what he knows or expects.
   c. Orient patient and family to the unit, room, location of playroom, operating room, and recovery room and introduce them to other children, parents, and some of the personnel.
      Make arrangements for child to meet anesthesiologist as well as the operating room nurse and recovery room nurse.
   d. Allow and encourage questions. Give honest answers.
      (1) Such questions will give the nurse a better understanding of the child's fears and perceptions of what is happening to him.
      (2) Infants and young children need to form a trusting relationship with those who care for them.
      (3) The older child tends to be reassured by the information he receives.
   e. Provide opportunity for child and parent to work out concerns and feelings (play, talk).

Such supportive care should result in less upset behavior and more cooperation.
   f. Prepare child for what to expect postoperatively (i.e., equipment to be used or attached to child, different location, how he will feel, what he will be expected to do, diet).
2. Assist in physical preparation of patient for surgery.
   a. Assist with necessary laboratory studies. Explain to child what is going to happen prior to procedure and how he can respond. Give continual support during procedure.
   b. See that patient has nothing by mouth (NPO) (from Latin *nil per os*).
      Explain to child and parents what NPO means.
   c. Assist with fever reduction.
      (1) Fever will result from some surgical diseases, i.e., intestinal obstruction.
      (2) Fever increases risk of anesthesia and need for fluid and calories.
   d. Administer appropriate medications as prescribed.
      Sedatives and drugs to dry the secretions are often given on the unit.
   e. Establish good hydration.
      Parenteral therapy may be necessary to hydrate the child, especially if he is NPO, vomiting or febrile.
3. Support parents during this time of crisis. The attitudes of the parents towards hospitalization and surgery largely determine the attitudes of their child.
   a. The experience may be emotionally distressing.
   b. Parents may have feelings of fear or guilt.
   c. The preparation and support should be integrated for parent and child.
   d. Give individual attention to parents; explore and clarify their feelings and thoughts; provide accurate information and appropriate reassurance.
   e. Stress parents' importance to the child. Help mother understand how she can care for her child.
4. Special considerations should be made for the mentally retarded child requiring surgery. (See section on the mentally retarded child.)
   a. Remember that the parents know their child and his behaviors best and should be encouraged to share this knowledge with staff. Continue to work closely with parents throughout the hospitalization.

b. Encourage parent(s) to remain with child to help him maintain a sense of security and to decrease his fears.

c. Do not isolate the child. When placing him with others, explain his behavior to his peers in preparation for this social contact.

d. Design play activities for his behavioral age.

e. Communicate your knowledge of his behaviors, handicaps, etc. to others who will care for him.

Postoperative Care

A. Immediate

1. Maintain a patent airway and prevent aspiration.
   a. Position child on his side or abdomen to allow secretions to drain and prevent tongue from obstructing pharynx.
   b. Suction any secretions present.
2. Make frequent observations of general condition and vital signs.
   a. Take vital signs every 15 minutes until child is awake and his condition stable.
   b. Note respiratory rate and quality, pulse rate and quality, blood pressure, skin color.
   c. Watch for signs of shock.
      (1) All children in shock have signs of pallor, coldness, increased pulse and irregular respirations.
      (2) Older children have decreased blood pressure and perspiration.
   d. Change in vital signs may indicate airway obstruction, hemorrhage or atelectasis.
   e. Restlessness may indicate pain or hypoxia.
      Medication for pain is not usually given until anesthesia has worn off.
   f. Check dressings for drainage or constriction and pressure.
3. See that all drainage tubes are connected and functioning properly.
   Gastric decompression relieves abdominal distention and decreases the possibility of respiratory embarrassment.
4. Monitor parenteral fluids as prescribed. (See p. 1171.)
5. Be physically near the child as he awakens to offer soothing words and a gentle touch. Rejoin parents and child as soon as possible after child recovers from anesthesia.

B. After Recovery from Anesthesia

After undergoing simple surgery and receiving a small amount of anesthesia, the child may be ready to play and eat in a few hours. More complicated and extensive surgery debilitates the child for a longer period of time.

1. Continue to make frequent and astute observations in regard to behavior, vital signs, dressings or operative site and special apparatus (IV, chest tubes, oxygen).
   a. Note signs of dehydration.
      (1) Dry skin and membranes
      (2) Sunken eyes
      (3) Poor skin turgor
      (4) Sunken fontanelle in infant
   b. Record any passage of flatus or stool, bowel sounds.

c. Record voiding time, amount, characteristics.
2. Record intake and output accurately.
   a. Parenteral fluids and oral intake.
   b. Drainage from gastric tubes or chest tubes, colostomy, wound, and urinary output.
      Dressing may need to be weighed for more accurate estimate of output.
   c. Parenteral fluid is evaluated and prescribed by considering output and intake.
      Parenteral fluid is usually maintained until child is taking adequate oral fluids.
3. Advance diet as tolerated, according to child's age and the physician's directions.
   a. First feedings are usually clear fluids; if tolerated, advance slowly to full diet for age.
      Note any vomiting or abdominal distention.
   b. Since anorexia may occur, offer child what he likes in small amounts and in an attractive manner.
4. Prevent infection.
   a. Keep child away from other children or personnel with respiratory or other infections.
   b. Change the child's position every 2–3 hours—prop infants with a blanket roll.
   c. Encourage patient to cough and breathe deeply—let infant cry for short periods of time, unless contraindicated.
   d. Keep operative site clean.
      (1) Change dressing as needed.
      (2) Keep diaper away from wound.
5. Provide good general hygiene.
   a. Good skin care will increase circulation and prevent pressure sores.
   b. Provide proper rest and sleep periods.
   c. Allow child exercise and movement out of bed when he feels better.
      Advance gradually.
   d. Allow diversional activity at intervals appropriate for age.
6. Offer the child measures of comfort.
   a. See that child is warm and changes position as needed.
   b. Provide mouth care.
   c. Allow child to have and hold favorite toy or object.
   d. Anticipate his needs.
   e. Holding and rocking the infant or young child may be comforting.
7. Provide emotional support and psychological security.
   a. Encourage child to talk about his operation.
   b. Allow child to play out his feelings.
   c. Return often to see and talk to the child.
   d. Reassure him that things are going well. Talk about going home, if appropriate.
8. Continue to offer support to the parents.
   a. Help to maintain healthy family relationships. (Encourage parents to care for their child.)
   b. Encourage parents to talk about their concerns.
   c. Begin early to prepare for discharge.
      (1) Teach any special procedures to be continued at home.
      (2) Arrange for community nurse referral.
      (3) Determine limits of activity for the child.
      (4) Make follow-up appointments.
      (5) Anticipate reactions of the child as a result of the hospitalization.

TRANSCULTURAL NURSING IN PEDIATRICS (CROSS-CULTURAL KNOWLEDGE OF HEALTH–ILLNESS BEHAVIOR)

General Principles

1. Comprehensive nursing should include being alert and responsive to the many cultural cues present in daily nursing situations. A conscious effort should be made to become knowledgeable about cultural diversity, and distinctiveness and similarities of the culture most likely to be served in nursing practice so that cues will be more meaningful and will be incorporated into patient assessment and care.
2. The nurse should be aware that cultural beliefs affect how a family perceives, experiences, and copes with illness. Culture influences how a family communicates about its health problems, the manner in which symptoms are presented, when and to whom members go for care, how long they remain in care, and how the care is evaluated.
3. It is possible that some health behaviors generated from cultural beliefs may be anxiety-producing and threatening to the nurse. Knowledge of and sensitivity to cultural diversity will decrease these anxieties thus facilitating effective interactions and relationships with the child and his family.
4. The nurse should be aware of the beliefs of the popular (family, community) and folk (nonprofessional healers) domains of health care available to her client as well as the accepted views of the medical profession so that discrepancies can be discussed and resolved.
5. Knowledge of the cultural beliefs of the patient will assist the nurse in understanding behaviors that may seem negative, confusing, illogical, or primitive, and help in producing a response that is more appropriate for the client's condition.

Assessment

Cultural background determines issues nurses should be aware of when caring for a child and his family.

1. Areas to consider when involved in cultural assessment:*
   a. Patterns or life-style of an individual or cultural group
   b. Specific cultural values, norms, and experiences of the client regarding health and illness
   c. Cultural taboos and myths
   d. The world view or ethnocentric tendencies

   e. The extent of assimilation into the mainstream cultural group
   f. Health and life-care rituals or rights of passage to maintain health and avoid illness
   g. Folk and professional approaches to healing
   h. Objectives and methods of caring for self and others
   i. Indicators of cultural change or adaptive behavior
2. In an attempt to become knowledgeable about cultural beliefs relating to pediatric nursing, the nurse must determine the following:
   a. What is the meaning of children in the culture?
   b. Do cultural patterns determine infant or child care? What are these patterns?
   c. Do cultural patterns determine parental responses to behaviors and appearances of the infant or child?
   d. What meaning does language or nonverbal communication have in the culture?
3. The acceptance of health care by a family or subculture may depend upon the nurse's knowledge of the cultural beliefs and behaviors and her attempt to understand their values while working within given guidelines. It is essential to know how the family unit is culturally defined, the family's functions, and the functions of the child in order to work effectively with that unit.
4. The following questions may be helpful in eliciting the family's perception of the illness and related cultural beliefs:†
   a. What do you think caused the problem?
   b. Why do you think it started when it did?
   c. What do you think your child's illness does to him?
   d. How severe is your child's illness? Will it have a short or long course?
   e. What kind of treatment do you think your child should receive?
   f. What results do you hope to receive from this treatment?
   g. What are the major problems your child's illness has caused you?
   h. What do you fear most about your child's illness?
5. In addition to health care, cultural patterns and bereavement behaviors must also be understood in order to provide effective psychological services and support for family.

* Leininger M. Transcultural Nursing: Concepts, Theories and Practices, p 88+. New York, John Wiley & Sons, 1978

† Kleinman A, Eisenberg L, Good B. Culture, illness and care. Ann Intern Med 1978 Feb; 88(1):251–258

BIBLIOGRAPHY

Books

Avery G. Neonatology. Philadelphia, JB Lippincott, 1980

Duvall E. Marriage and Family Development, 5th ed. Philadelphia, JB Lippincott, 1977

Fochtman D and Raffensperger J. Principles of Nursing Care for the Pediatric Surgery Patient. Boston, Little, Brown & Co, 1976

Gellert E. Psychosocial Aspects of Pediatric Care. New York, Grune & Stratton, 1978

Hardgrove C and Dawson RB. Parents and Children in the Hospital. Boston, Little, Brown & Co, 1972

Hymovich D and Barnard M. Family Health Care, vol 2. Developmental and Situational Crises. New York, McGraw–Hill, 1979

Hofman AD, Becker RD, Gabriel HP. The Hospitalized Adolescent. New York, Free Press, 1976

Khan AV. Psychiatric Emergencies in Pediatrics. Chicago, Year Book Medical Pub, 1979

Klaus M and Fanaroff A. Care of the High-Risk Neonate. Philadelphia, WB Saunders, 1973

Klaus MH and Kennell JH. Maternal–Infant Bonding. St. Louis, CV Mosby, 1976

Klinzing D and Klinzing D. The Hospitalized Child: Communication Techniques for Health Personnel. Englewood Cliffs, Prentice–Hall, 1977

Lindheim R et al. Changing Hospital Environments for Children. Cambridge, Harvard University Press, 1972

Mercer R. Nursing Care for Patients At Risk. Thorofare, New Jersey, Charles B. Slack, 1978

Mortenson I et al. Psychosocial Caring Throughout the Life Span. New York, McGraw–Hill, 1979

Oremland E and Oremland J (eds). The Effects of Hospitalization on Children. Springfield, Charles C Thomas, 1974

Petrillo M and Sanger S. Emotional Care of Hospitalized Children. Philadelphia, JB Lippincott, 1980

Schulmann J. Coping With Tragedy: Successfully Facing the Problems of A Seriously Ill Child. Chicago, Follett Pub. Co., 1978

Scipien G et al. Comprehensive Pediatric Nursing. New York, McGraw–Hill, 1979

Woods NF. Human Sexuality in Health and Illness, 2nd ed. St. Louis, CV Mosby, 1979

Pediatric and Neonatal Intensive Care

Klaus M and Fanaroff A. Care of the High-Risk Neonate. Philadelphia, WB Saunders, 1979

Levin D, Morriss F, Moore G. A Practical Guide to Pediatric Intensive Care. St. Louis, CV Mosby, 1979

Child Going to Surgery

Fochtman D and Raffensperger J. Principles of Nursing Care for the Pediatric Surgery Patient. Boston, Little, Brown & Co., 1976

Transcultural Nursing in Pediatrics

Leininger M. Transcultural Nursing: Concepts, Theories and Practices. New York, John Wiley & Sons, 1978

Schmidt VE and McNeil E. Cultural Awareness. Washington, D.C., The National Association for the Education of Young Children, 1978

Articles

Al Agel MSC. Reactions of a hospitalized school-age child to separation and restricted mobility. Matern Child Nurs J 1978 Fall; 7(3):163–173

Allen J. Influencing school-age children's concept of hospitalization. Pediatric Nursing 1978 Nov/Dec; 4(6):26–28

Altsshuler A and Seidl A. Teen meetings: A way to help adolescents cope with hospitalization. MCN 1977 Nov/Dec; 2(6):348–353

Arneson S and Triplett J. How children cope with disfiguring changes in their appearance. MCN 1978 Nov/Dec; 3(6):366–370

Blumberg ML. Depression in children on a general pediatric service. Am J Psychother 1978 Jan; 32(1):20–32

Calkin JD. Are hospitalized toddlers adapting to the experience as well as we think? 1979 MCN Jan/Feb; 4(1):18–23

Chadwick BJ, Pflederer D, Ray MA. Maintaining the hospitalized child's home ties. Am J Nurs 1978 Aug; 78(8):1360–1366

Clark D. Parents' meetings in a pediatric unit: helping parents cope with their child's hospitalization. JACCH 1979 Fall; 8(2):32–35

Demaio DJ. Body image concerns of a six year old boy. Matern Child Nurs J 1978 Fall; 7(3):175–184

Droske SC. Children's behavior changes following hospitalization—have we prepared the parents? JACCH 1978 Fall; 7(2):3–7

Elmasisian BJ. A practical approach to communicating with children through play. MCN 1979 July/Aug; 4(4):238–240

Ferguson F and Robertson J. Making hospital preparation child-centered—with a little help from Emily. JACCH Fall; 8(2):27–31

Frauman A and Sypert N. Sexuality in adolescents with chronic illness. MCN 1979 Nov/Dec; 4(6):371–375

Galligan AC. Using Roy's concept of adaptation to care for young children. MCN 1979 Jan/Feb; 4(1):24–28

Gelhard H. Drawing and development. Pediatric Nursing 1978 Nov/Dec; 4(6):23–26

Gerhart SM. A preschool child's use of language in coping with hospitalization. Matern Child Nurs J 1979 Spring; 8(1):39–47

Gohsman B and Yunck M. Dealing with the threats of hospitalization. Pediatric Nursing 1979 Sept/Oct; 5(5):32–35

Hardgrove CB and Kermoian R. Parent-inclusive pediatric units: A survey of policies and practice. AJPH 1978 Sept; 68(9):847–850

Harper DC et al. Personality profiles of physically impaired adolescents. J Clin Psychol 1978 July; 34(3):636–642

Hill CJS. The mother on the pediatric ward: Insider or outlawed? Pediatric Nursing 1978 Sept/Oct; 4(5):26–29

Jackson PB, Bradham RF, Burwell HK. Child care in the hospital—a parent/staff partnership. MCN 1978 Mar/Apr; 3(2):104–107

Johnson M. Toward a culture of caring: Children, their environment and change. MCN 1979 July/Aug; 4(4):210–215

Johnson M and Salazar M. Preadmission program for rehospitalized children. Am J Nurs 1979 Aug; 79(8):1420–1422

Kerr NJ. The effect of hospitalization on the developmental tasks of childhood. Nurs Forum 1979 Summer; 18(2):108–130

Klein CB and Satterthwaite M. Preparation and the hospitalized child. JACCH 1980 Winter; 8(3):60–63

Korsch BM. Editorial. Issues in humanizing care for children. AJPH 1978 Sept; 68(9):831–832

Lincoln L. Effects of illness and hospital procedures on body image in adolescents. Matern Child Nurs J 1978 Summer; 7(2):55–60

McGuire M, Shepherd R, Greco A. Hospitalized children in confinement. Pediatric Nursing 1978 Nov/Dec; 4(6):31–35

McLeavey K. Children's art as an assessment tool. Pediatric Nursing 1979 Mar/Apr; 5(2):9–14

Neill K. Behavioral aspects of chronic physical disease. Nurs Clin North Am 1979 Sept; 14(3):443–456

Neuhauser C, Amsterdam B. Hines P, Steward M. Children's concept of healing: Cognitive development and locus of control factors. Am J Orthopsychiatry 1978 April; 48(2):335–341

Parker G. Development of the hospitalized adolescent anxiety tool. J Psychiatr Nurs 1977 Dec; 15(12):21–24

Peters BM. School-aged children's beliefs about causality of illness: A review of the literature. Matern Child Nurs J 1978 Fall; 7(3):143–154

Pomarico C, Marsh K, Doubrave P. Hospital orientation for children. AORN J 1979 April; 29(5):864–875

Rappazzo JA. Psychoesthetic environmental design for pediatric care facilities. JACCH 1980 Spring; 8(4):85–93

Ritchie JA. Preparation of toddlers and preschool children for hospital procedures. Can Nurs 1979 Dec; 75(11):30–32

Roskies E, Mongeon M, Gagnon–Lefebvre B. Increasing maternal participation in the hospitalization of young children. Med Care 1978 Sept; 16(9):756–777

Seegal VF. The divorced parent and the hospitalized child: Implications for the hospital staff. JACCH 1978 Fall; 7(2):16–18

Schrader ES. Preparation play helps children in hospitals. AORN J 1979 Aug; 30(2):36–41

Suran BG et al. Rights of children in pediatric settings. Pediatrics 1977 Nov; 60(5):715–720

Terry G. A five-year-old boy's aggressive and compensatory behavior in response to immobilization. Matern Child Nurs J 1979 Spring; 8(1):29–38

Vardaro JA. Preadmission anxiety and maternal–child relationships. JACCH 1978 Fall; 7(2):8–16

Vipperman JF and Rager PM. Childhood coping; how nurses can help. Pediatric Nursing 1980 Mar/Apr; 6(2):11–18

Whitt JK et al. Children's conceptions of illness and cognitive development: Implications for pediatric practitioners. Clin Pediatr 1979 June; 18(6):327–339

Wolfer JA et al. Prehospital psychological preparation for tonsillectomy patients: Effects on children's and parent's adjustment. Pediatrics 1979 Nov; 64(5):646–655

Wolfgang CH and Bolig R. Play techniques for helping preschool children under stress. JACCH 1979 Winter; 7(3):3–10

Family-Centered Care

Association for the Care of Children in Hospitals. Position statement on involvement of parents and families in health care settings. Washington, DC, ACCH, 1977

Ayer A. Is partnership with parents really possible? MCN 1978 March/April; 3(2):107–110

Chadwick B, Pflederer D, Ray MA. Maintaining the hospitalized child's home ties. Am J Nurs 1978 August; 78(8):1361–1362

Hardgrove C and Kermoian R. Parent-inclusive pediatric units: A survey of policies and practices. Am J Public Health 1978 Sept; 68(9):847–850

Hill C. The mother on the pediatric ward: Insider or outlawed? Pediatric Nursing 1978 Sept/Oct; 4(5):26–29

Jackson P, Bradham R, Burwell H. Child care in the hospital—a parent/staff partnership. MCN 1978 Mar/Apr; 3(2):104–107

Korsch B. Editorial. Issues in humanizing care for children. Am J Public Health 1978 Sept; 68(9):831–832

Lavigne JV et al. Psychologic adjustment of siblings of children with chronic illness. Pediatrics 1979 Apr; 63(4):616–627

Marino B. When nurses compare with parents. JACCH 1980; 8(4):94–98

Smitherman C. Parents of hospitalized children have needs too. Am J Nurs 1979 Aug; 79(8):1423–1424

Vermillion BD et al. The effective use of the parent care unit for infants on the surgical service. J Pediatr Surg 1979 June; 14(3):321–324

Pediatric and Neonatal Intensive Care

Arney WR, Nagy JN, Little GA. Caring for parents of sick newborns. Clin Pediatr 1978 Jan; 17(1):35–39

Carry R. Observed behaviors of preschoolers to intensive care. Pediatric Nursing 1980 July/Aug; 6(6):21–26

Cataldo MF et al. Behavioral assessment for pediatric intensive care units. J Appl Behav Anal 1979 Spring; 12(1):83–97

Cooperman EM. Hexachlorophene in the nursery. Can Med Assoc J 6 Aug 1977; 117(3):205–206

Czarniecki L. Developmental nursing care: Infant stimulation for high-risk children. Pediatric Nursing 1978 Sept; 4(5):32–38

Gardner D and Stewart N. Staff involvement with families of patients in critical care units. Heart Lung 1978 Jan/Feb; 7(1):105

Grant P. Psychosocial needs of the family of high-risk infants. Family and Community Health 1978 Nov; 1(3):91–102

Green M. Parent care in the intensive care unit. Am J Dis Child 1979 Nov; 133(11):1119–1120

Huckaboy LM et al. Nurses' stress factors in the intensive care unit. J Nurs Adm 1979 Feb; 9(2):21–26

Jay SS. Pediatric intensive care—involving parents in the care of their child. Can Nurs 1978 May; 74(5):28–31

Jones CL. Criteria for evaluating infant environments in hospitals. JACCH 1979 Spring; 7(4):3–11

Kopelman AE et al. Does a photograph of a newborn about to be transferred to an intensive care center promote mother–infant bonding? Clin Pediatr 1978 Jan; 17(1):15–16

Mangurtan HH, Slade C, Fitzsimon D. Parent–parent support in the care of high-risk newborns. JOGN Nurs 1979 Sept/Oct; 8(5):275–277

Miller C. Working with parents of high-risk infants. Am J Nurs 1978 July; 78(7):1228–1230

Potter P. Stress and the intensive care unit: The family's perception. Missouri Nurse 1979 July; 48:5

Rasie S. Meeting families' needs help you meet ICU patients' needs. Nursing '80 1980 July; 10(7):32–35

Smith DH. Epidemics of infectious diseases in newborn nurseries. Clin Obstet Gynecol 1979 June; 22(2):409–423

Spikes J and Bowen T. Nursing care plans for the special care nursery. Super Nurs 1979 Jan; 10(1):23–26

Vanek C. How school-age children perceive the intensive care unit environment. J NY State Nurses' Assoc 1979 Dec; 10(4):30–33

Waggoner SK. Nursing care of the infant in surgery. AORN J 1978 Nov; 28(5):827–839

Waller DA, Todres D, Cassen NH, Arderten A. Coping with poor prognosis in the pediatric intensive care unit. Am J Dis Child 1979 Nov; 133(11):1121–1125

Child Going to Surgery

Kaisling PM and Kalafatich AJ. Caring for the mentally handicapped child undergoing surgery: A parent's point of view. JACCH 1978 Winter; 6(3):15–16

Nahigian EG. Minor procedure becomes major for child, mother. AORN J 1979 Oct; 30(4):230–234

Robinson SJ. A nurse's role in preparing children for surgery. AORN J 1979 Oct; 30(4):619–623

Schrader ES. Megan copes with surgery. AORN J 1979 Oct; 30(4):624–629

Trelour DM. Ready, set–No: Something is missing from pediatric preop preparation. MCN 1978 Jan/Feb; 3(1):50–51

Vermilion BD, Ballantine TV, Grosfeld JL. The effective use of the parent care unit for infants on the surgical service. J Pediatr Service 1979 June; 14(3):321–324

Transcultural Nursing in Pediatrics

Beliefs that can affect therapy. Pediatric Nursing 1979 May/June; 5(3):40–43

Brownlee A. The family and health care: Explorations in cross-cultural settings. Social Workers in Health Care 1978 Winter; 4(2):179–198

Hautman MA. Folk health and illness beliefs. Nurse Practitioner 1979 July/Aug 4(4):23–34

Kleinman A et al. Culture, illness and care—clinical lessons from anthropologic and cross-culture research. Ann Intern Med 1978 Feb; 88(2):251–258

Leininger M. Changing foci in American nursing education: Primary and transcultural nursing care. J Adv Nurs 1978 Mar; 3(2):155–166

Pumphrey J. Recognizing your patients' spiritual needs. Nursing '77 1977 Dec; 7(12):64–70

Walker R. Developing cultural awareness. AORN J 1978 June; 27(7):1302–1304

Books For Children

Clark B. Pop-up Going to the Hospital. Westminster, Md., Random House, 1971

Froman R and Veno J: Let's Find Out About the Clinic. New York, Franklin Watts, 1968

Greene C and Kessler L. Doctors and Nurses—What Do They Do? New York, Harper & Row, 1963

Howe J. The Hospital Book. New York, Crown Publishers, Inc., 1981

Morel E, Izawa T, Hijikata S. Teddy Goes to the Doctor. New York, Grosset & Dunlap, 1973

Rey H. Curious George Goes to the Hospital. New York, Scholastic Book Services, 1968

Shay A. What Happens When You Go to the Hospital? Chicago, Henry Regnery, 1969

Sobol HL, and Agre P. Jeff's Hospital Book. New York, Henry Z. Walck, 1975

Stein SB. A Hospital Story. New York, Walker & Co. 1974

Weber A and Blass J. Elizabeth Gets Well. New York, Thomas Y. Crowell, 1969

Films

Care Through Parents
   University of California Extension Media Center, Berkeley, Calif. 94720. Color, 14 minutes.
Emphasizes the role of parents in caring for the young, hospitalized child. Depicts a program where parents are actively involved in the care of their children.

Play in the Hospital
   Campus Films Distribution Corporation, 14 Madison Ave., Valhalla, N.Y. 10595. Color, 55 minutes.
Portrays many ways in which hospitalized children are helped by a special play program. Filmed in a variety of settings. Gives a good picture of children's special concerns and needs and offers particular ways of dealing with these.

To Prepare a Child
   Media Center, Children's Hospital National Medical Center, Washington, D.C. 20010. Color, 32 minutes (available in 16 mm. sound and video casette).
This is an account of one hospital's approach to the preparation of children for hospitalization and surgery. Three children (one is an out-patient emergency case and the other two are surgical in-patients) are followed through their preparation for surgery and diagnostic procedures.

A Hospital Visit with Clipper
   Media Center, Children's Hospital National Medical Center, Washington, D.C. 20010. Color, 15 minutes (available in 16 mm. sound and video cassette).
A professionally produced puppet show about a little girl coming into the hospital for a tonsillectomy. The script pays special attention to the most common concerns children have about hospitalization and surgery.

Hospital Adventure
   Media Resources Librarian, Naval Health Sciences Education and Training Command, National Naval Medical Center, Bethesda, Md. 20014. Color, 15 minutes.
This cartoon takes the child through a typical hospital and presents some of the most common experiences and procedures. It focuses on the misconceptions and concerns that children may have.

Let's Talk About
. . . .*Going to the Hospital;* . . . .*Having an Operation;* . . . .*Wearing a Cast*
Mr. Rogers—Family Communications, Arthur Greenwald, Project Director, 4802 Fifth Ave, Pittsburgh, PA 15213. Videocassettes, 20 minutes each.
. . . . .*Going to the Hospital:* A general introduction to the hospital and to the sights, sounds, and feelings children may experience there.
. . . . .*Having an Operation:* A more specific program for children scheduled for simple surgery. Helping them know what to expect and encouraging them to express their feelings in words and play.
. . . . .*Wearing a Cast:* A program about how casts are applied and removed, and how children can do many things for themselves while wearing a cast.

Preparing A Child for O.R., Anesthesia, Recovery Room and I.C.U.
   Campus Film Distributors Corporation, 14 Madison Ave., Valhalla, NY, 10595. Filmstrips, 8 minutes.
Filmstrips for staff development when preparing children for procedures. Developed and written by Madeline Petrillo.

Additional Information

Association for the Care of Children's Health, 3615 Wisconsin Ave, Washington, DC 20016.
For information and listings regarding films and books related to children's health issues.

MEASURING VITAL SIGNS IN CHILDREN

Normal Vital Sign Ranges in Children

Temperature
  Oral 36.4–37.4°C. (97.6–99.3°F.)
  Rectal 36.2–37.8°C. (97–100°F.)
  Axillary 35.9–36.7°C. (96.6–98°F.)

Pulse and Respiratory Rates

Age	Pulse	Respirations
Newborn	70–170	30–50
11 months	80–160	26–40
2 years	80–130	20–30
4 years	80–120	20–30
6 years	75–115	20–26
8 years	70–110	18–24
10 years	70–110	18–24
Adolescence	60–110	12–20

Blood Pressure* (Figs. 37-1, 37-2)

  *Blood pressure measurement percentiles prepared by the National Heart, Lung and Blood Institute's Task Force on Blood Pressure Control in Children. Pediatrics 1977 (Suppl.) Vol. 59, No. 5, Part 2, May 1977, p. 803.

General Considerations for Measuring Vital Signs

1. Vital sign values provide the nurse with only rough estimates of physiological activity. It is important to identify trends, sudden discrepancies and wide deviations from normal.
2. Vital signs should be taken as often as the nurse thinks necessary. They should not be delayed until the next scheduled time if it is suspected that a trend is developing.

Temperature

1. Normal body temperature represents a balance between the body heat produced and body heat lost.
2. The mode for taking the temperature should be kept as constant as possible. (Refer to Table 37-1 for methods of measuring body temperature in infants and children.)
3. Never leave the child alone when taking his temperature.
4. For security, safety, and accuracy keep 1 hand on the thermometer when it is in place.

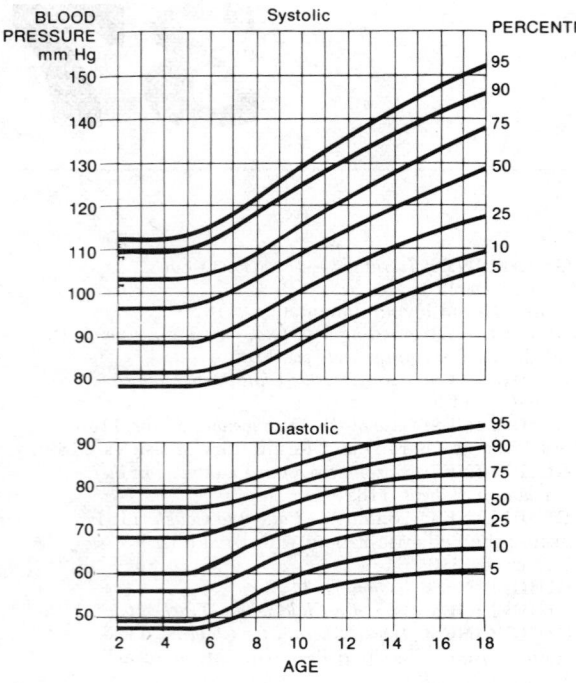

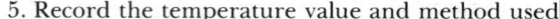

FIGURE 37-1. *Percentiles of blood pressure measurements in boys (right arm, seated).*

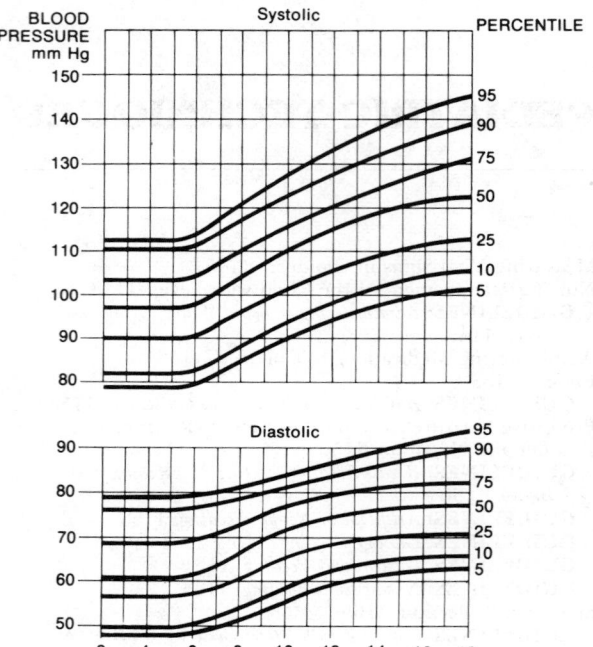

FIGURE 37-2. *Percentiles of blood pressure measurement in girls (right arm, seated).*

5. Record the temperature value and method used.
6. Report an elevated or subnormal temperature and initiate whatever nursing measures are indicated by the child's condition.
7. If using an electronic thermometer, follow manufacturer's directions explicitly.
8. Question the accuracy of any temperature reading that does not correlate with the child's signs and symptoms.

Pulse

1. Take apical rate on an infant.
   a. Place stethoscope between left nipple and sternum.
   b. Take heart rate for 1 full minute.
2. With an older child, the pulse rate may be obtained easily at the radial, temporal, or carotid locations. (The pulse may be taken for 30 seconds and multiplied by 2.)
3. Take pulse rate prior to taking temperature because child may cry when temperature is taken; this increases the pulse rate and makes it more difficult to hear the apical rate.
4. Record accurately the following:
   a. Rate
   b. Rhythm (regular or irregular)
   c. Strength of beat (full, bounding, weak, faint)
   d. Activity of child at time pulse is taken (sleeping, crying, etc.)
5. Report immediately any changes in pulse characteristics, and initiate whatever nursing measures are indicated by the child's condition.

Respirations

1. Count respirations on an infant for 1 full minute.

Observe chest movement as well as abdominal movements.
2. Respirations may be counted for 30 seconds and multiplied by 2 in the older child.
3. Obtain respiratory rate prior to taking temperature and pulse since child may cry during these procedures.
4. Note and record accurately the following:
   a. Respiratory rate.
   b. Depth of respirations.
      (1) Feel exhaled air to estimate adequacy of tidal volume.
      (2) Observe excursions of the chest and diaphragm.
   c. Quality of respirations.
      (1) Determine if respirations are predominantly costal or abdominal. Dyspnea should be suspected in a school-age child who is breathing primarily with the abdomen.
      (2) Listen for unusual noises such as expiratory grunts, crowing noises, wheezing, or inspiratory stridor.
      (3) Observe for signs of dyspnea:
         (a) Restlessness
         (b) Retractions—sternal or intercostal
         (c) Nasal flaring
         (d) Cyanosis
   d. Activity of the child during the procedure.
5. Report immediately any change in respiratory status. Initiate whatever nursing measures are indicated by the child's condition.

Blood Pressure

Generally, the technique for taking the blood pressure

TABLE 37-1. METHODS OF MEASURING BODY TEMPERATURE IN INFANTS AND CHILDREN

Method	Advantages	Disadvantages	Length of time required for accurate measurement with mercury-in-glass thermometer
Rectal	1. Safe for children who are unable to cooperate and who may bite the thermometer. 2. Not directly influenced by the ingestion of hot or cold fluids, smoking. 3. Method of choice if: child has seizures or breathing difficulties; is receiving oxygen therapy; has had oral surgery.	1. Values may be altered by the presence of stool. 2. Emotional response may be negative. 3. Damage to rectal mucosa may occur. 4. Replication of thermometer placement is difficult. 5. Contraindicated when child has diarrhea and following rectal surgery.	3–5 min.
Oral	1. Easily accessible. 2. Replication of thermometer placement is easy. 3. Responds more quickly and regularly to changes in arterial temperature than does rectal method. 4. More aesthetically pleasing.	1. Value is readily influenced by ingestion of hot or cold fluids, oxygen therapy. 2. Requires child's cooperation to keep mouth closed and not to bite the thermometer. 3. Contraindicated if child has had oral injuries or surgery.	6–9 min.
Axillary	1. Safe and easily accessible. 2. Avoids the danger of rectal or colon perforation. 3. Avoids initiating the defecation stimulus. 4. Often recommended for infants under one year.	1. Value is more readily influenced by environmental temperature and airflow. 2. Requires a relatively long period of time to obtain accurate reading.	9–11 min.

of a child is the same as for the adult. The following principles are important to observe when dealing with the pediatric patient.

A. *General Considerations*

1. The cuff should cover no less than ½ and no more than ⅔ the length of the upper arm or leg. Even small variations in cuff size may produce significant differences in blood pressure reading.
   a. A cuff that is too narrow will produce an apparent increase in blood pressure.
   b. A cuff that is too wide will produce an apparent decrease in blood pressure.
   c. Using a flexible blood pressure cuff that can be folded to the correct size is frequently easier and more effective for the nurse than choosing among several assorted premeasured cuffs.
   d. The cuff should be of consistent width each time that a child's blood pressure is measured during hospitalization.
2. If the child is excited or uncomfortable or if he distrusts the person taking the blood pressure, the systolic pressure may rise significantly.
   a. The blood pressure should be taken when the child is at rest and in a consistent position.
   b. The procedure should be explained to the child before it is done.
      (1) He should know that it will not hurt.
      (2) He should be allowed to handle the equipment, pump the cuff, etc.
      (3) It may be helpful for the child to use the equipment on his parents, the nurse, or a doll in order for him to overcome his fears and understand its use.

B. *Methods Used in Obtaining Blood Pressure Measurements in Pediatrics.*

1. *Auscultatory Method* (Method of choice whenever possible)
   a. Center the bladder of the cuff over the artery.
   b. Apply the cuff evenly and snugly over the bare arm with the lower edge about 1.25 cm. (½ inch) above the antecubital space.
   c. Support the arm in a slightly flexed and abducted position at the level of the child's heart.
   d. Palpate the brachial artery and inflate the cuff until the palpated pulse is lost. Then pump for an additional 20–30 mm. Hg beyond that.
   e. Deflate the cuff slowly at a rate of about 5 mm. Hg/second.
   f. Deflate the cuff rapidly and completely when all sounds disappear.
   g. Record the reading and compare it with previous values.
      There continues to be a controversy as to what best indicates diastolic pressure. Therefore, it is good practice to record all 3 readings: (1) systolic—point at which pulse becomes audible; (2) diastolic—point of muffling of sound; and (3) point of disappearance of sounds.
   h. The blood pressure may be obtained by the same method in the leg, using the popliteal artery.
2. *Palpatory Method* (This method provides only an approximate mean pressure which lies between the systolic and diastolic pressures obtained by the auscultatory method.)
   a. Follow Steps 1-3 of the auscultatory method.
   b. Inflate the cuff to about 200 mm. Hg.
   c. Take the reading when the pulse distal to the cuff becomes palpable in the course of deflation.
3. Flush Method (This method is especially useful with infants, but also has the disadvantage of providing only an approximate mean pressure.)
   a. The infant should be quiet and in the supine position.
   b. Apply a blood pressure cuff to the upper or lower extremity, just above the wrist or ankle.
   c. Squeeze the extremity distal to the cuff with a hand or firm wrapping to force blood into the upper extremity. This will blanch the child's arm or leg below the cuff.
   d. Pump the manometer to 120–140 mm. Hg.
   e. Release the hand or the wrapping.
   f. Slowly deflate the cuff.
   g. Take the reading at the point at which blood

reenters the hand or foot, causing a sudden flushing.

4. *Electronic Methods*
   a. Electronic equipment utilizes a tiny microphone within the cuff to amplify the Korotkoff sounds or to convert them to another type of signal such as a flashing light.
   b. More sophisticated equipment is available which can inflate and deflate the cuff and either hold or automatically record the measurement.
   c. Advantages of electronic methods:
      (1) Observer bias is minimized as electronic circuitry rather than the human ear analyzes the Korotkoff sounds. Therefore, blood pressure readings are more consistent.
      (2) The child is subjected to minimal handling despite frequent monitoring of the blood pressure.
   d. Nursing considerations
      (1) Read specific instructions carefully before operating an electronic device since each unit has a slightly different operating procedure.
      (2) Note whether the equipment measures muffling or silence, or both, as the diastolic pressure.

5. Ultrasonic Equipment
   a. Utilizes an ultrasonic transducer in the cuff to detect and amplify blood pressure sounds.
   b. Some equipment is capable of measuring only systolic pressure, while other instruments can sense both systolic and diastolic sounds.
   c. Advantages of ultrasonic methods
      (1) Measurements correlate closely with intra-arterial pressures.
      (2) Especially useful in infants when the Korotkoff sounds may be inaudible by ordinary methods.
   d. Nursing considerations
      (1) Read specific instructions carefully before operating an ultrasonic device
      (2) Note specifically what sounds are being measured and whether the equipment measures muffling or silence, or both as the diastolic pressure.

C. *Principles Related to Pediatric Blood Pressure Values*

1. The blood pressure varies with the age of the child and is closely related to his height and weight.
2. Variability of blood pressure among children of approximately the same age and body build is normal.
3. The pressure in the legs with the cuff technique is ordinarily 20 mm. Hg higher than in the arms in children over 1 year of age.

NURSING MANAGEMENT OF THE CHILD WITH FEVER

Fever is any abnormal elevation of body temperature. Prolonged elevation of temperature above 40°C.(104°F.) may produce dehydration and harmful effects on the central nervous system.

Causes

1. Infection
2. Inflammatory disease
3. Dehydration
4. Tumors
5. Disturbance of temperature regulating center
6. Extravasation of blood in the tissues
7. Drugs or toxins

Assessment

1. Consider basic principles related to temperature regulation in pediatric patients.
   a. Usually an infant's temperature does not stabilize before the first week of life. A newborn's temperature varies with the temperature of his environment.
   b. The degree of fever does not always reflect the severity of the disease. A child may have a very serious illness with a normal or subnormal temperature.
   c. Fever, itself, may cause convulsions in some children when the temperature goes very high, very fast.
   d. The range for normal temperature varies widely in children. A common explanation for "fever" is misinterpretation of a normal temperature reading. (Refer to Measuring Vital Signs in Children, p. 1145)
   e. The child's temperature is influenced by activity and by time of day; temperatures are highest in late afternoon.
2. Be certain that accurate technique is used for temperature measurement. The mode should be appropriate for the child's age and condition, and the thermometer should be left in place for the required period of time. (Refer to Measuring Vital Signs in Children, p. 1145).
3. Assist the physician in determining the cause of the illness.
   a. History
      Information should be elicited regarding:
      Age of the child
      Pattern of the fever
      Length of the illness
      Change in normal patterns of eating, elimination, recreation, etc.
      Other symptoms
      Exposure to any illnesses
      Recent immunizations or drugs
      Treatment of the fever and effectiveness of treatment
      Previous experiences with fever and its control
   b. Physical examination
      Of special significance are:
      General appearance of the child
      Inspection of the skin for rashes, sores, flushed appearance
      Inspection of eyes, ears, nose and throat for redness and/or drainage
      Auscultation of lungs for abnormal sounds
      Neurological observation for changes in state of consciousness, pupillary reaction, strength of grip, abnormal muscle movement or lack of movement

Inspection of the external genitals for redness and/or drainage

Presence of abdominal or flank pain

(Refer to Pediatric Physical Assessment, p. 1066)

c. Laboratory Tests

Initial tests frequently include: complete blood count, urinalysis, cultures of the throat, nasopharynx, urine, blood, and spinal fluid, and x-ray of the chest.

4. Attempt to identify the pattern of the fever. Take the child's temperature by the same method every hour until stable, then every 2 hours until normal, then every 4 hours for 24 hours.

Nursing Measures to Reduce Fever

Fever itself does not necessarily require treatment. The presence of fever should not be obscured by the indiscriminate use of antipyretic measures. However, if the child is uncomfortable or appears toxic because of fever, an attempt should be made to reduce it by any of the following nursing measures or by a combination of these measures (see below).

Nursing Action	Rationale/Amplification
1. Increase the child's fluid intake to prevent dehydration.	1. Fever increases the child's fluid requirements by increasing the metabolic rate.
2. Expose the skin to the air by leaving the child lightly dressed in an absorbent material. Avoid warm, binding clothing and blankets.	2. Loss of heat from the skin by radiation is the main temperature regulating mechanism available to the infant or small child.
3. Administer a tepid sponge bath. (See Guidelines: Administering a Tepid Water Sponge, below.)	3. The temperature is lowered by evaporation of water from the surface of the skin.
4. Administer antipyretic drugs.	4. Although effective in reducing fever, antipyretic drugs may obscure the clinical picture and cause numerous side effects including: diaphoresis, skin eruptions, nausea, vomiting, hematologic changes, and fever.
5. Utilize a hypothermia blanket.	5. This is often the method of choice for older children.
6. Utilize ice bags for local comfort.	6. These should not be used for infants since they may produce chilling.

GUIDELINES: Administering a Tepid Water Sponge for Fever

A tepid water sponge is bathing of the body for a period of time to reduce fever.

Equipment Basin of tepid water (21.1–27° C. or 70–80° F.)
Plastic sheet
2 bath blankets
Hot water bottle with cover
Towels
6 washcloths

NURSING ALERT: Cold water or alcohol sponges should not be administered to pediatric patients. Cold water may produce vasoconstriction and shivering, which raise central body temperature. Alcohol sponges may reduce the temperature too rapidly, leading to convulsions in small children. In addition, the fumes may be toxic.

Procedure

NURSING ACTION	RATIONALE/AMPLIFICATION
Preparatory Phase	
1. Secure the child's cooperation.	1. This helps to increase the effectiveness of the procedure. A tub bath in tepid water is less frightening and is the preferred method for reducing a fever if the child is able to cooperate.
a. Explain the procedure to the child in language he can understand.	
b. A small infant may be held during sponging.	
c. Allow the child or his parent to participate in the procedure.	
d. Discontinue sponging if the child is extremely upset and uncooperative.	
2. Take temperature, pulse, and respiration before starting the sponge.	2. This serves as a baseline for comparison to determine the effectiveness of treatment.
3. Give antipyretic medication as prescribed 15-20 minutes before starting the sponge.	3. There is a more rapid reduction of fever when sponging is combined with administration of antipyretic medication.

GUIDELINES: Administering a Tepid Water Sponge for Fever (cont.)

Procedure (cont.)	NURSING ACTION	RATIONALE/AMPLIFICATION
	Performance Phase	
	1. Place a plastic sheet covered with a bath blanket under the child.	
	2. Place a bath blanket over the child, and remove top bedding.	
	3. Place a warm water bottle at the child's feet.	3. Aids in combating chills and shivering.
	4. Place cold, moist cloths over the superficial blood vessels in the axillae and the groins.	4. This aids in lowering body temperature.
	5. Expose the body area to be sponged. Place a towel under the area.	
	6. Slowly stroke the extremities with long, soothing strokes of the washcloth. a. Stroke each arm from the neck to the axilla and down to the palm of the hand. b. Stroke each leg from the groin to the foot. c. Bathe the back and buttocks.	
	7. Use gentle friction to bring the blood to the surface.	7. This increases the effectiveness of the treatment and prevents chilling.
	8. Change the water as often as necessary to maintain a water temperature of 21.1–27° C. (70–80° F.)	
	9. Continue this procedure until temperature is adequately reduced, more drastic measures are prescribed, or the child's condition indicates that it should be discontinued.	9. Generally, the sponge should not last more than 30 minutes. Observe for shivering. If this occurs, cover the child and wait a few minutes before proceeding. Stop the sponge if cyanosis, mottling, or chilling do not stop when friction is applied to the skin. These symptoms indicate a change in vasomotor tone.
	10. Pat dry with towel.	
	Follow-up Phase	
	1. Remove bath blankets and plastic sheet. Place a dry gown on the child.	
	2. Record vital signs 30 minutes after the sponge is finished.	2. Postsponge values indicate whether or not treatment has been effective.

ADMINISTERING MEDICATIONS TO CHILDREN

Purpose

To safely administer medications to the child as prescribed by the physician.

Important Considerations

1. The nurse's manner of approach should indicate that she firmly expects the child to take the medication. This manner often convinces the child of the necessity of the procedure. Establishing a positive relationship with the child will allow him to express feelings, concerns, and fantasies regarding medications.
2. Explanation about the medication should appeal to the child's level of understanding (i.e, color, comparison to something familiar).
3. The nurse must mask her own feelings regarding the medication.
4. Always be truthful when the child asks, "Does it taste bad?" or "Will it hurt?" Respond by saying, "The medicine does not taste good, but I will give you some juice as soon as you swallow it," or "It will hurt for just a minute, like a mosquito bite."
5. It is often necessary to mix distasteful medications or crushed pills with a small amount of coke or cherry syrup, honey, or applesauce.
6. Never threaten a child with an injection if he refuses an oral medication.
7. Medications should not be mixed with large quantities of food or with any food that is taken regularly (e.g., milk).
8. Medications should not be given at mealtime unless specifically prescribed.
9. The nurse must know the following about each medication she is administering: common usages and dosages, contraindications, side effects, and toxic effects.
10. When preparing intramuscular injections, draw in 0.2 ml. of air after the correct amount of solution is in the syringe. This serves to clear all medication from the needle upon injection and prevents backflow and the depositing of medication in subcutaneous fat upon withdrawal of the needle.

Calculating the Pediatric Dosage

It is not the nurse's responsibility to determine the dosage of a drug.

1. Know what factors determine the amount of drug prescribed.
   a. Action of the drug, absorption, detoxification, excretion are related to the maturity and metabolic rate of the child.
   b. Neonate and premature infants require a reduced dosage because of:
      (1) Deficient or absent detoxifying enzymes
      (2) Decreased effective renal function
      (3) Altered blood-brain and protein-binding capacity
   c. Dosages recommended according to age groups are not satisfactory since a child may be much smaller or larger than the average child in his age group.
   d. Dosage calculations based on weight have limitations.
2. Be alert to a prescription that would be inappropriate for a child.
3. Consult drug literature for recommended dosage and other information.

Body Surface Area

The following formulas are used to estimate the pediatric dosage based on the child's body surface area. Body surface area (BSA) calculations are generally preferred because many physiologic processes in the child (i.e., blood volume, glomerular filtration) are related to BSA.

1. Surface area in sq. meters × dose per sq. meter = approximate child dose
2. $\dfrac{\text{Surface area of child}}{\text{Surface area of adult}} \times$ dose of adult = approximate child dose
3. $\dfrac{\text{Surface area of child in sq. meters}}{1.75} \times$ adult dose = child dose

Clark's Rule

The following rule may be used as an estimate of the pediatric dosage based on the child's weight in respect to the adult dose of the drug.

$$\dfrac{\text{Child's Weight in Pounds}}{150} \times \text{Adult Dose} = \text{Approximate Dose for Child}$$

Identifying the Patient

Always check a child's identification bracelet before administering a medication. Ask the older child his name.

Oral Medications

A. *Infants*

1. Draw up medication in a plastic dropper or disposable syringe.
2. Elevate infant's head and shoulders; depress chin with thumb to open mouth.
3. Place dropper or syringe on the middle of the tongue and slowly drop the medication on the tongue.
4. Release thumb and allow child to swallow.
5. Once the correct amount of medication has been measured, it can be placed in a nipple and the infant can suck the medication through the nipple.
6. If the nurse feels comfortable managing the infant in her lap it is acceptable to hold him for medication administration.

B. *Toddlers*

1. Draw up liquid medication in syringe or measure into medicine cup. Medications may be placed in medicine cup or spoon after being measured accurately in a syringe.
2. Elevate the child's head and shoulders.
3. Squeeze cup and put it to the child's lips; or place the syringe (without the needle) in the child's mouth and slowly expel the medicine. Child may prefer using the familiar teaspoon.
4. Allow the child time to swallow.
5. Allow the child to hold the medicine cup by himself, if he is able, and to drink it at his own pace. (This may be a more agreeable method.) Offer his favorite drink as a "chaser," if not contraindicated.
6. The small, safe, disposable medicine cups can be given to the child for play.

C. *School-age children*

1. When a child is old enough to take medicine in pill or capsule form, he should be taught to place the pill near the back of his tongue and immediately swallow fluid such as water or fruit juice. If the swallowing of the fluid is emphasized, the child will no longer think about the pill.
2. Always praise a child after he has taken his medication.
3. If the child finds it particularly difficult to take oral medications, the nurse must let him know that she understands some of his fear and displeasure and that she wants to help him.

Intramuscular Injections (Fig. 37-3)

A. *Infants*

1. Site selection
   Vastus lateralis, rectus femoris (see below), ventrogluteal—there are no major nerves and blood vessels in this area.
2. Administration
   a. Place the child in a secure position to prevent movement of the extremity.
   b. Do not use a needle longer than 2.5 cm. (1 inch).
   c. Use upper outer quadrant of the thigh.
   d. Insert needle at a 45-degree angle in a downward direction, toward the knee.
   e. Hold and cuddle the infant following the injection.
   f. This site is also used on the older child who may be difficult to restrain.

B. *Toddlers and School-age Children*

1. Site selection
   a. Posterogluteal-upper outer quadrant
      (1) Gluteal muscles do not develop until the child begins to walk; they should be used only when the child has been walking for 1 year or more.
      (2) Upper outer quadrant of the young child's buttock is smaller in diameter than an adult's; thus accuracy in determining the area comprising the upper outer quadrant is essential.
      (3) Administration
         (a) Do not use a needle longer than 2.5 cm. (1 inch).
         (b) Position the child in a prone position.
         (c) Place thumb on the trochanter.
         (d) Place middle finger on the iliac crest.

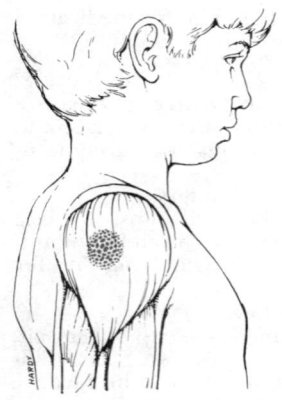
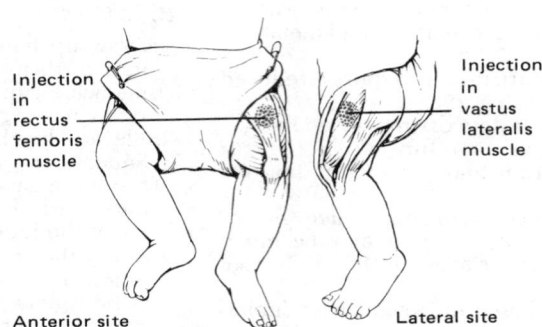

FIGURE 37-3. *Sites for IM injections in children.*

(e) Let index finger drop at a point midway between the thumb and middle finger to the upper outer quadrant of the buttock.

(f) Insert needle perpendicular to the surface on which the child is lying, not perpendicular to the skin.

b. *Ventrogluteal*

(1) This site provides a dense muscle mass which is relatively free of the danger of injuring the nervous and vascular systems.

(2) The disadvantage is that the injection site is visible to the child.

(3) Administration

(a) Place child on his back.

(b) Place index finger on the anterosuperior spine.

(c) With the middle finger moving dorsally, locate the iliac crest; drop finger below the crest. The triangle formed by the iliac crest, index finger, and middle finger is the injection site.

(d) Inject needle perpendicular to the surface on which child is lying.

c. *Deltoid*

(1) May be used for older, larger children.

(2) Determine injection site as with an adult.

d. *Lateral and anterior aspect of the thigh*

(1) Do not use a needle longer than 2.5 cm. (1 inch).

(2) Use the upper outer quadrant of the thigh.

(3) Insert needle at a 45-degree angle in a downward direction, toward the knee.

2. Nursing support

a. Explain to the child where you are going to give him the injection (site) and why he must receive the injection.

b. Allow the child to express his fears.

c. Carry out procedure quickly and gently. Have needle and syringe completely prepared and ready prior to contact with child.

d. Numb site of injection by rubbing skin with cleansing swab or with ice, and change needle after drawing up medication through rubber stopper on medicine vial. Minimize pain of intramuscular injection by injecting needle into muscle with a quick, darting motion.

e. Always secure the assistance of a 2nd nurse to help immobilize the child and divert his attention as well as to offer him support and comfort.

f. Praise the child for his behavior after the injection. Often, allowing him to assist with applying a Band-Aid will give him some feeling of comfort.

g. Also encourage activity that will use the muscle site of injection—promotes dispersal of medication and decreases soreness. This can also be done by firmly massaging muscle following injection, unless contraindicated.

h. Record accurately the injection site to ensure proper site rotation.

Intravenous Medications

(See intravenous infusions, p. 1171.)

A. *Intravenous Drip*

1. Selecting the proper site for injecting medication into an intravenous line depends upon the correct dilution for the drug, the rate of fluid administration, and the amount of intravenous fluid tolerated by the child.

a. *Piggyback*—a second container holding the drug and a relatively small volume of fluid and administration set are attached at the injection site of the primary administration set tubing, and allowed to flow over a period of time from 20 minutes to 2 hours. This method maintains fluid schedule without fluid overload.

b. *Bolus*—a rapid injection of a small volume of drug directly into the intravenous tubing or cannula by means of a syringe and needle.

2. Prepare mixtures aseptically (laminar-flow hood) and use sterile technique when violating the line. (Sepsis is a constant threat when a child is receiving intravenous medications.)

3. Be aware the exaggerated pharmacologic effect may exist with intravenous medications. As with any medication, know the use, side effects, and toxic effects of the drug, as well as the pharmacologic effect upon the body.

4. Dilute intravenous medications and inject slowly—never less than 1 minute (this allows peripheral blood flow through the entire circulating system to dilute the medication and prevent high concentrations of the drug from reaching the brain and heart).
5. Be knowledgeable regarding compatibilities of drugs, electrolytes in IV solutions, and the fluid itself.
6. Observe IV site frequently. Restrain child, as needed, to prevent infiltration. Infiltration of fluids containing medications can cause rapid and severe tissue necrosis.

B. *Heparin Lock* (see adult, p. 106).

Venipuncture setup with 3½-inch tubing ending in a resealing rubber diaphragm creating a closed system.

1. The use of a heparin lock allows children who need repeated doses of chemotherapeutic agents to be fully mobile while reducing the trauma of repeated injections.
2. Heparin solution (0.25 heparin, 1000 USP/ml. to 10 ml. sterile water) is administered prior to and following instillation of medication, and regular heparin flushing is done every 8 hours to maintain patency.
3. The heparin lock can be connected to standard pediatric administration sets so that larger volumes of vehicle solutions can be used for dilution of medications.
4. The heparin lock should be securely taped in place to prevent dislodgement. Patency of vein must be determined prior to administration of fluids or medications.

ENEMA

An *enema* is the insertion of fluid into the rectum for the purpose of cleansing the lower bowel. An enema for an infant or a young child is based on the same principles as for an adult and is essentially the same, except that *less fluid and pressure are used than in an adult.*

GUIDELINES: Administering an Enema to a Child

Equipment Solution measurements:
Soap suds enema—add 8 ml. (2 drams) soap jelly to 500 ml. (1 pint) of water
Saline enema—add 4 ml. (1 dram) salt to 500 ml. (1 pint) of water

Procedure

NURSING ACTION	RATIONALE/AMPLIFICATION
Preparatory Phase	
1. Explain procedure to the child according to his level of understanding.	1. Even though the child may not fully understand, an explanation will soothe him and build his trust in you.
2. Position	
a. *Older child:* Have him lie on his left side with his upper leg flexed.	a. This position places the descending colon at the lowest point.
b. *Infant:* Place infant in supine position, with a pillow under his head and back and a small bedpan under his buttocks. Gentle restraint may be needed—diaper placed under the bedpan, brought over thighs, and then pinned.	b. Infants and small children cannot retain enema fluid. Pillows provide for body alignment.
Performance Phase	
1. Insert rectal tube 3.7–10 cm. (1½–4 inches) into the rectum just within the anal sphincter.	
2. Hang solution reservoir no higher than 30–45 cm. (12–18 inches) above the infant's hips.	2. This allows the solution to run slowly with minimum pressure.
3. Do not administer more than 300 ml. (10 oz.) of solution to infant unless otherwise prescribed.	3. Fluid volume may range from 30–300 ml. (1–10 oz.) depending on the size of the child.
4. Once the rectal tube is removed, the abdomen can be gently massaged, if there are no contraindications.	4. This gentle massage will help relax the infant and assist in expelling the solution.
5. If young child is "potty trained," have a small potty chair available for his use.	5. The familiarity of a potty chair will provide great comfort for the child and eliminate the possible embarrassment of soiled bed or pants.
6. When a retention enema is administered, the buttocks may be held or taped together to assist retention of fluid. Keep child as quiet as possible.	

PROTECTIVE MEASURES TO LIMIT MOVEMENT (Restraints)

Protective measures to limit movement are mechanisms for restraining children (Fig. 37-4).

Purpose

1. To maintain the child's safety and protect him from injury.
2. To facilitate examination and minimize the child's discomfort during special tests, procedures, and specimen collections.

Underlying Principles

1. Protective devices should be used only when necessary and never as a substitute for careful observation of the child.
2. The reason for using the protective device should be explained to the child and his parents to prevent misinterpretation and to ensure their cooperation with the procedure. Restraints are often interpreted as punishment by children.
3. Any protective device should be checked frequently to make sure that it is effective. It should be removed periodically to prevent skin irritation or circulation impairment.
4. Protective devices should always be applied in a manner that maintains proper body alignment and ensures the child's comfort.
5. Any protective device that requires attachment to the child's bed should be secured to the bed springs or frame, *never* the mattress or side rails. This allows the side rails to be adjusted without removing the restraint or injuring the child's extremity.
6. Any knots that are required should be tied in a manner that permits their quick release. This is a safety precaution.
7. When a child must be immobilized, an attempt should be made to replace the lost activity with another form of motion. For example, even though restrained, a child can be moved in a stroller, wheelchair, or in his bed. When arms are restrained, the child may be allowed to play kicking games. Water play, mirrors, body games, and blowing bubbles are helpful replacements.

Mummy Device

The mummy device involves securing a sheet or blanket around the child's body in such a way that his arms are held to his sides and his leg movements are restricted (see Fig. 37-4).

A. *Purpose*

To restrain infants and small children during treatments and examinations involving the head and neck.

B. *Equipment*

Small sheet or blanket
Several large safety pins

C. *Nursing Action*

1. Place the blanket or sheet flat on the bed.
2. Fold over 1 corner of the blanket.
3. Place the child on the blanket with his neck at the edge of the fold.
4. Pull the right side of the blanket firmly over the child's right shoulder.
5. Tuck the remainder of the right side of the blanket under the left side of the child's body.
6. Repeat the procedure with the left side of the blanket.
7. Separate the corners of the bottom portion of the sheet, and fold it up toward the child's neck.
8. Tuck both sides of the sheet under the infant's body.
9. Secure by crossing 1 side over the other in the back and tucking in the excess, or by pinning the blanket in place.

D. *Special Precautions*

Make certain that the child's extremities are in a comfortable position during this procedure.

Jacket Device

The *jacket device* is a piece of material that fits the child like a jacket or halter. Long tapes are attached to the sides of the jacket (see Fig. 37-4).

A. *Purpose*

To keep the child in his wheelchair, highchair, or crib.

B. *Nursing Action*

1. Put the jacket on the child so that the opening is in the back.
2. Tie the strings securely.
3. Position the child in his highchair, wheelchair, or crib.
4. Secure the long tapes appropriately:
   a. Under the arm supports of a chair.
   b. Around the back of the wheelchair or highchair.
   c. To the springs or frame of the crib.

C. *Special Precautions*

The child in a crib must be observed frequently to make certain that he does not entangle himself in the long tapes of the jacket device.

Belt Device

The belt device is exactly like the jacket method of restraining, except that the material fits the child like a wide belt and buckles in the back (see Fig. 37-4).

Elbow Device

The elbow device consists of a piece of material into which tongue depressors have been inserted at regular intervals. It is especially useful for infants receiving a scalp-vein infusion, those with eczema or cleft lip repair, and children having eye surgery.

A. *Purpose*

To prevent flexion of the elbow.

B. *Equipment*

Elbow cuff
Tongue depressors
Safety pins, tapes, or string

C. *Nursing Action*

1. Insert tongue depressors into the appropriate places in the elbow cuff.

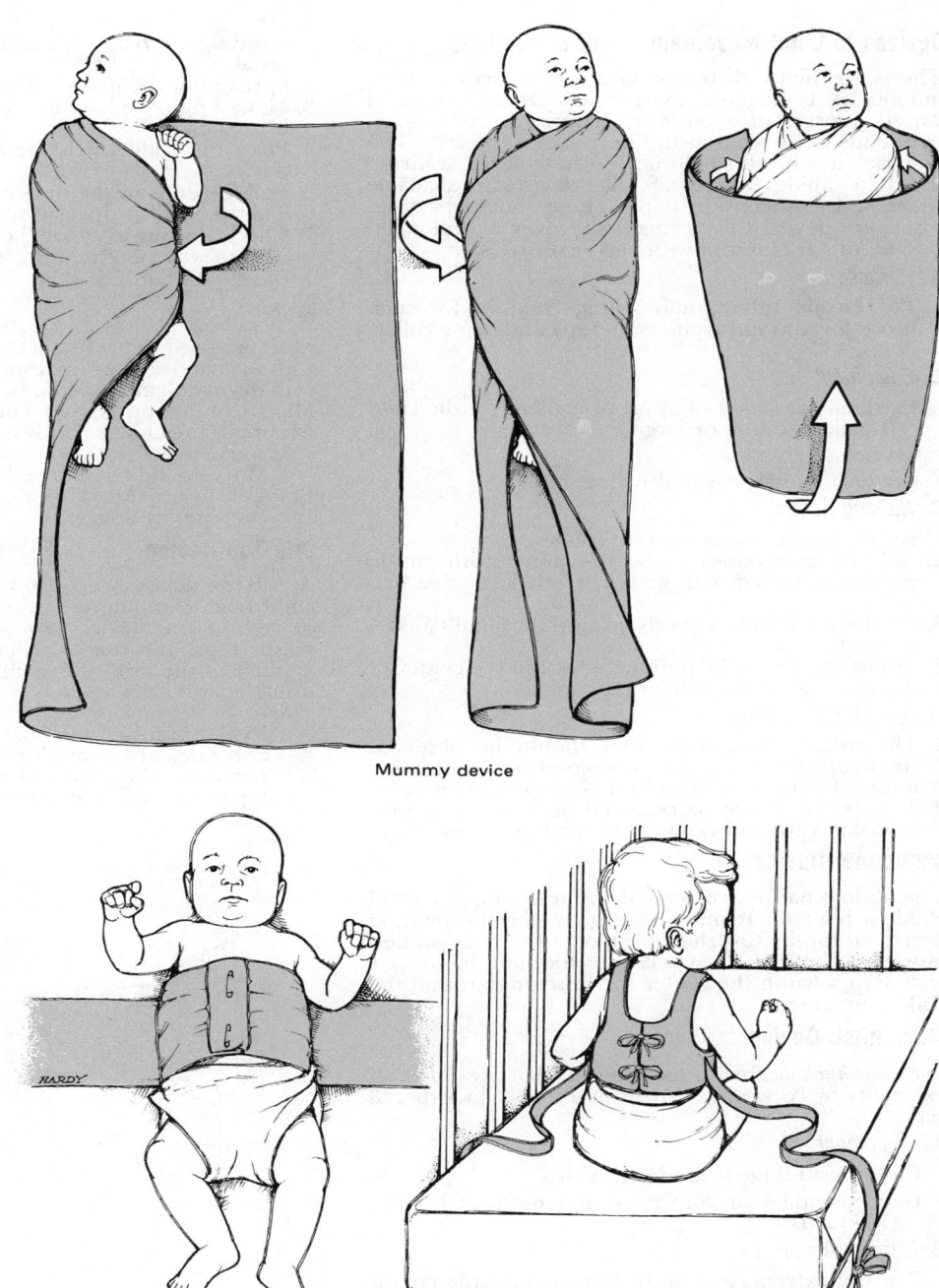

FIGURE 37-4. *Types of restraints*

2. Place the child's arm in the center of the elbow cuff.
3. Wrap the cuff around the child's arm.
4. Secure the cuff with pins, tapes, or string.

D. *Special Precautions*

1. The tongue depressors should be cut to about 10 cm. (4 inches) in length if the elbow cuff is to be used for an infant—for greatest comfort.

2. Additional security may be provided by dressing the child in a long-sleeved shirt prior to the application of the elbow cuff. The ends of the shirt can then be turned back over the cuff and pinned securely.

Devices to Limit Movement of the Extremities

There are many different kinds of devices to limit motion of 1 or more extremities. One commercial variety consists of a piece of material with tapes on both ends to be secured to the frame of the crib. The material also has 2 small flaps sewn to it for securing the child's ankles or wrists. Similar devices are available which utilize sheepskin flaps. These should be used when the device will be necessary over a prolonged period, or for children with very sensitive skin.

A. *Purpose*

To restrain infants and young children for such procedures as intravenous therapy and urine collection.

B. *Equipment*

Extremity restraint of appropriate size for the child (small, medium, or large)

Several safety pins

Cotton wadding covered with gauze

C. *Nursing Action*

1. Secure the device to the crib frame.
2. Pad the extremities to be restrained with cotton wadding covered with gauze or other suitable material.
3. Pin the small flaps securely around the child's ankles or wrists.
4. Adjust the device by pinning a tuck in the center of the material, if it is too large.

D. *Special Precautions*

1. The infant's fingers or toes should be observed frequently for coldness or discoloration and the skin under the device checked for signs of irritation.
2. The device should be removed periodically to provide skin care and range of motion exercises.

Abdominal Device

The abdominal device is used for restraining a small child in his crib. It operates exactly like the method described for limiting the movement of the extremities. However, the strip of material is wider and has only 1 wide flap sewn in the center for fastening around the child's abdomen.

Clove-hitch Device

The clove-hitch device is a mechanism for restraining an extremity by tying gauze strips or a diaper in a special way.

A. *Equipment*

Cotton wadding covered with gauze

Gauze bandage or diapers cut in lengths of 1.37 m. (1½ yards)

B. *Nursing Action*

1. Pad the extremity to be restrained with the cotton wadding covered with gauze or other suitable material.
2. Spread out the gauze strip or diaper on the bed.
3. Make a figure-8 loop in the center of the gauze strip or diaper.
4. Place the child's wrist or ankle in the loop of the device
5. Pull the ends of the device to the desired tightness.
6. Tie the ends to the crib springs or frame.
7. Check the device to make certain that it does not tighten when both ends are pulled taut or slip over the child's hand or foot.

Mitts

Mitts are used to prevent a child from injuring himself with his hands. They are especially useful for children with dermatologic conditions, such as eczema or burns. Mitts can be purchased commercially or made by wrapping the child's hands in Kling gauze.

Special Precaution

Mitts should be removed at least twice during each shift to provide skin care and to allow the child to exercise his fingers.

Crib Top Device

A crib top device is used to prevent an infant or small child from climbing over the crib sides. Several types of commercial devices are available, including nets, plastic tops, and domes. A crib top device should be applied to the crib of any infant capable of climbing over the crib sides.

Special Precaution

In all instances, it is essential to be certain that the crib sides are kept all of the way up and latched securely. There should be no space between the top of the crib sides and the bottom of the crib top device.

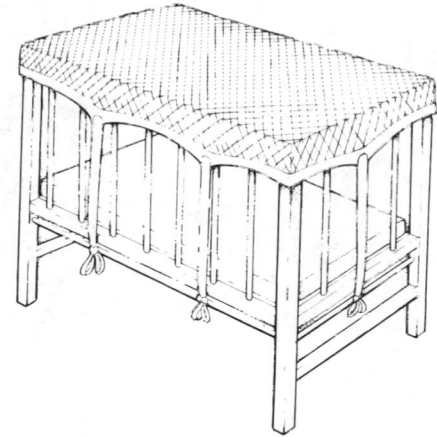

FEEDING AND NUTRITION

GUIDELINES: Breast Feeding the Ill or Hospitalized Infant*

Breast feeding is suckling of an infant at the mother's breast to provide him with nourishment.

Purposes
1. To provide psychological and emotional satisfaction for the infant and the mother.
2. To feed the infant a natural and ideal food that will supply him with adequate nutrition.

* See page 1031 for breast feeding the newborn.

Purposes (cont.)

3. To have milk always available, at the right temperature.
4. To prevent chance of gastrointestinal disturbances and development of allergies.
5. To provide physical closeness of baby to mother during feeding.
6. To provide comfort after a frightening or painful procedure.

Points to Consider

1. The breast-fed infant up to 6 months of age may not have been started on solid foods.
2. The mother (at home) may only give other liquids by spoon or cup, not bottle and nipple.
3. The infant may nurse frequently if mother is available.
4. Because breast milk is more easily and quickly digested, shorter periods of NPO both pre- and post-operatively may be used with the breast-fed infant.
5. Stress of hospitalization and illness experienced by the mother may decrease her milk supply and inhibit her "let down" reflex, as well as increase or decrease the infant's desire to suckle.

Equipment

Clear water
Cotton balls

Procedure

NURSING ACTION	RATIONALE/AMPLIFICATION
Preparatory Phase	
1. When an infant who is nursing is hospitalized, it is the nurse's responsibility to encourage the mother to continue breast feeding if the infant's condition does not contraindicate it. Explain to the mother that: a. Supplemental artificial formula can be given to the infant if she is not available; or b. She can pump her breasts and bring in her milk to be given to the infant via bottle when she is not available.	1. Some mothers have very strong feelings about wanting to nurse their baby. It gives them an emotional satisfaction that is vitally important to the mother-child relationship since it is an integral part of the total mothering process. The nurse must help to foster this relationship as much as she can.
2. When nursing is to be done in the hospital pediatric setting, the physical surroundings may need to be altered somewhat. Provide the mother and infant with a relatively quiet area that is as private as possible and free from interruption.	2. This will provide the mother and infant with an opportunity to continue to develop their relationship during the crisis of illness and hospitalization.
3. Provide the mother with a comfortable armchair or pillow so that she can assume a comfortable position during the feeding. A footstool should also be available so that she can support her feet and the infant.	3. Proper and comfortable position of the mother will enable her to hold the baby correctly and support him while he is at the breast.
4. The infant should be awake and dry before the feeding is started.	4. If the infant is awake and comfortable he will settle down and feed better.
5. Dress the infant appropriately so that he is not too warm or too cool during the feeding. The infant should also be hungry.	5. If he is too warm, he may fall asleep after the first few sucks of milk. A sleepy baby will not nurse well. If he is too cool, he may be fussy and restless.
6. Have mother wash her hands. Then she should wash her nipples with clear water and cotton balls.	6. Washing the nipples will remove any old milk that may have leaked and dried on them, providing a good medium for the growth of bacteria that can cause gastrointestinal disturbance in the infant.
7. Position the baby at breast. Put him in a semi-sitting position with his face close to the breast and supported by 1 arm and hand. A pillow may be used under the baby to support him. The breast may need to be supported by mother's other hand.	7. Proper positioning will provide the infant with comfort and security and make it easier for him to suck and swallow. This makes the nipple more easily accessible to the infant's mouth and prevents obstruction of nasal breathing.
Performance Phase	
1. When the feeding is to start, let the breast touch the infant's cheek. Do not hold his cheek and try to help him find the nipple.	1. The rooting reflex will take over and the infant will turn his head toward the breast with his mouth open. If his cheek is touched with a hand, he will become confused, perhaps turning toward the hand.
2. The infant's lips should be out over the areola and not just around the nipple before he begins to suck.	2. Since the nipple is so small, suction cannot be achieved merely by grasping it. The areola must be in the infant's mouth in order to establish suction and make the suck effective.
3. Note the presence or absence of the "let-down" reflex during the nursing period.	3. Milk flowing from the other breast during nursing is quite normal. It is not usually present when the mother is worried.
4. The length of feeding time may vary from 5–20 minutes. Let the infant nurse until he is satisfied.	4. When the infant is satisfied and has nursed well, he is relaxed and usually falls asleep. He will stop sucking.

GUIDELINES: Breast Feeding the Ill or Hospitalized Infant* (cont.)

Procedure (cont.)	NURSING ACTION	RATIONALE/AMPLIFICATION
	5. Instruct the mother to bubble the baby during and at the end of the feeding.	5. When the infant is sucking he swallows some air. Bubbling will help prevent abdominal distention and discomfort as well as regurgitation.
	6. One or both breasts may be used at each feeding. It makes no difference as long as (a) baby is satisfied at the end of the feeding and (b) one breast is completely emptied at the feeding.	6. Regular and complete emptying of the breast is the only stimulation for the production of milk.
	7. Once the infant has stopped sucking, he likes to cling to the breast. To break this suction, instruct mother to put her finger to the corner of the baby's mouth and gently pull.	7. Gentle pulling will not hurt mother or infant.

Follow-up Phase

	1. When the infant has finished feeding, change his diaper if it is wet or soiled.	1. To provide comfort for a restful sleep and to prevent diaper rash.
	2. Position infant on his right side or on his abdomen in his bed.	2. This facilitates emptying of the stomach and decreases the possibility of regurgitation.
	3. Note if baby appears satisfied or still seems to be hungry.	3. Mother may not have enough milk to satisfy the baby. Supplemental formula may be necessary.
	4. Record descriptively and accurately: a. How baby fed b. How baby went to breast c. Satiety or hunger after feeding d. Breast or breasts used; which breast was emptied and which breast was nursed from thereafter.	d. If both breasts were used, the second breast is not usually emptied and should be used first at the next feeding.
	5. For the new mother-infant nursing team: a. Provide the mother with anticipatory guidance for possible problems (i.e., breast engorgement). b. Promote maternal confidence in handling and nursing her infant. c. Increase mother's knowledge about the mechanics of breast feeding. d. Provide mother with literature and resources: (1) Resources for Nursing Mothers: Eigor M and Olds SW. The Complete Book of Breast Feeding. Des Plaines, Illinois, Bantam Books, 1973 Pryor K. Nursing Your Baby. New York, Harper & Row, 1973 The Womanly Art of Breast Feeding, 2nd ed. LaLeche League International, 9616 Minneapolis Ave., Franklin Park, Illinois, 60131 (2) Agency: LaLeche League International, 9616 Minneapolis Ave., Franklin Park, Ill. 60131	5. To help establish and maintain successful breast feeding that will be continued following discharge.

GUIDELINES: Artificial or Nipple Feeding

Artificial or nipple feeding is a method of supplying nutrition to the infant by oral feedings, using a bottle and nipple set-up.

Purposes
1. To provide the baby adequate fluid and calorie intake for appropriate growth.
2. To supplement breast feeding with formula or water.
3. To provide additional fluid intake between feedings.

Equipment
Sterile nipple and bottle
Sterile formula or feeding fluid

Procedure	NURSING ACTION	RATIONALE/AMPLIFICATION
	Preparatory Phase	
	1. Baby should be awake and hungry. Change wet or soiled diaper.	1. A sleepy baby will not feed well. A dry diaper will provide comfort so that the baby will settle down and eat more easily.
	2. Check formula for correct type and amount.	2. To prevent error.

Procedure (cont.)

NURSING ACTION	RATIONALE/AMPLIFICATION
3. Sit in a comfortable chair. Cradle baby with one hand and arm, while supporting baby against your body or lap.	3. Proper position will provide the baby with comfort and security and will make it easier for him to suck and swallow. Holding infant will enhance trust-building and provide sensory stimulation.

Performance Phase

NURSING ACTION	RATIONALE/AMPLIFICATION
1. Let the baby root for the nipple by touching the corner of his mouth with the nipple. When he opens his mouth, insert the nipple.	1. Place the nipple on top of the tongue and far enough in his mouth so suction can be created when he sucks.
2. Hold the bottle at an angle to completely fill the nipple with fluid.	2. This prevents the baby from sucking and swallowing excessive amounts of air.
3. NEVER prop the bottle or leave the baby unattended during feeding.	3. This is unsafe. Should vomiting occur, aspiration is more likely.
4. The bottle should be handled so as not to contaminate the nipple or fluid.	4. Contamination will increase the chances of gastrointestinal disturbances.
5. Baby's feeding time will vary from 10–25 minutes.	5. The length of time will depend on the age of the baby and how vigorously he sucks.
6. Bubble the baby at least once during the feeding and at the end of the feeding. 　a. Place the baby in sitting position in nurse's lap, tilt him slightly forward, and gently rub or pat his back or abdomen. 　b. Place baby in prone position on nurse's shoulder and gently pat or rub his back. 　c. Place baby in prone position on nurse's lap and gently rub or pat his back.	6. Most babies swallow some air during feeding. These positions aid in expelling air and thus prevent abdominal distention, discomfort, and regurgitation. Vigorous handling or patting may result in the infant spitting up or regurgitating feeding.
7. Take nipple out of mouth periodically.	7. To allow baby to rest and to let air into the bottle so that the nipple does not collapse.

Follow-up Phase

NURSING ACTION	RATIONALE/AMPLIFICATION
1. After final bubbling, change wet or soiled diaper and place baby in crib on his abdomen or right side.	1. This position aids in emptying the stomach and prevents regurgitation.
2. Check baby in a few minutes. If he is restless, pick him up and bubble him. Note if any spitting-up has occurred.	2. Some babies relieve themselves of air when in the crib and also bring up small amounts of formula at the same time.
3. Accurate and descriptive recording: 　a. What was fed and amount 　b. How feeding was tolerated 　c. Any regurgitation or emesis—amount and material 　d. Length of time of feeding 　e. How baby sucked and took the feeding	

NOTE: When feeding a premature infant, the same principles apply. The premature infant, however, will tire more easily and fall asleep. Allow him frequent rest periods and use a soft nipple so that less energy is needed to suck. To stimulate this infant to suck, the nurse can brush the infant's cheek with her finger, place thumb or finger under the infant's chin or move the nipple slowly back and forth in his mouth. Feeding time should not exceed 30 minutes.

GUIDELINES: Gavage Feeding

Gavage feeding is a means of providing food via a catheter passed through the nares or mouth, past the pharynx, down the esophagus, and into the stomach, slightly beyond the cardiac sphincter.

Purposes

1. To provide a method of feeding or administering medications that requires minimal patient effort, when the infant is unable to suck or swallow (i.e., infant under 32 weeks gestation or under 1650 gm).
2. To provide a route that allows adequate calorie or fluid intake.
3. To prevent fatigue or cyanosis which is apt to occur from nipple feeding.
4. To provide a safe method of feeding a limp and listless patient.

Equipment

Sterile rubber or plastic catheter, rounded-tip, size 5–10 (French Argyle feeding tube)
Clear, calibrated reservoir for feeding fluid
Syringe
Stethoscope
Water for lubrication
Tape—hypoallergenic
Feeding fluid
Pacifier

GUIDELINES: Gavage Feeding (cont.)

Procedure

| NURSING ACTION | RATIONALE/AMPLIFICATION |

Preparatory Phase

1. Position infant on his side or back with his neck hyperflexed with a diaper roll placed under neck. A mummy restraint may be necessary to help maintain this position.

2. Measure feeding catheter and mark with tape.

    a. *Premature infant and neonate:* measure from bridge of nose to umbilicus.
    b. *Older child:* measure from tip of nose past the ear, to tip of sternum.

1. This position allows for easy passage of the catheter, facilitates observation, and helps avoid obstruction of the airway.

2. Premeasuring the catheter provides a guideline as to how far to insert catheter.

Performance Phase

1. Lubricate catheter with water.

2. Stabilize patient's head with one hand; use the other hand to insert catheter.
    a. *Insertion through nares:* slip the catheter into nostril and direct toward the occiput in a horizontal plane.
    b. *Insertion through the mouth:* pass the catheter through the mouth toward the back of the throat.

3. If patient swallows, passage of the catheter may be synchronized with the swallowing.

4. If there is no swallowing, insert the catheter smoothly and quickly.

5. In the infant, especially, observe for vagal stimulation, i.e., bradycardia (slow heart rate) and apnea.

6. Once the catheter has been inserted to the premeasured length, tape the catheter to the patient's face (Fig. 37-5).

1. Do not use oil because of danger of aspiration.

2. a. This direction will follow the nares passageway into the pharynx. Do not direct the catheter upward.

3. Swallowing motions will cause esophageal peristalsis, which opens the cardiac sphincter and facilitates passage of the catheter.

4. Because of cardiac sphincter spasm, resistance may be met at this point. Pause a few seconds, then proceed.

5. The vagus nerve pathway lies from the medulla through the neck and thorax to the abdomen. Above the stomach, the left and right branches unite to form the esophageal plexus. Stimulation of these nerve branches with the catheter will directly affect the cardiac and pulmonary plexus.

6. This prevents movement of catheter from the premeasured, preestablished correct position. Alternative method: loop narrow cloth tape around tube just below nostril, then secure it above lip or nose with tape. Some movement of tube may be seen with swallowing.

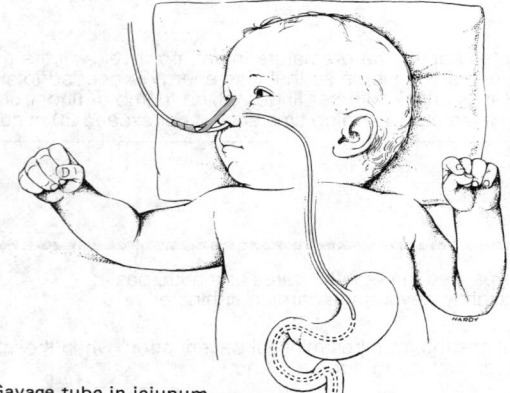

Gavage tube in jejunum

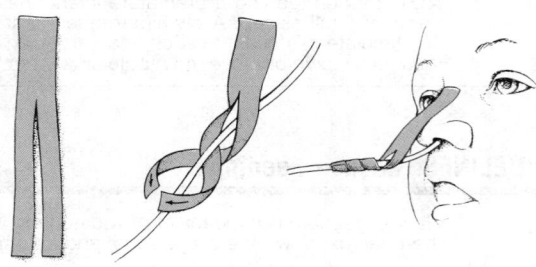

Steps in preparing adhesive tape to retain gavage tube

FIGURE 37-5. *Gavage feeding.*

7. Test for correct position of the catheter in the stomach:
    a. Inject 0.5–1 ml. air into the catheter and stomach. At the same time listen to the typical growling stomach sound with a stethoscope placed over the epigastric region.
    b. Aspirate injected air from the stomach.
    c. Aspirate small amount of stomach content.

a. Aids in insuring proper location of catheter.

b. This prevents abdominal distention.

c. Failure to obtain aspirate does not indicate improper placement; there may not be any stomach content or the catheter may not be in contact with the fluid.

Procedure (cont.)

NURSING ACTION	RATIONALE/AMPLIFICATION
d. Avoid inserting catheter into infant's trachea. (An infant's anatomy makes it relatively difficult to enter the trachea since esophagus is behind the trachea.)	d. If improper placement occurs and the catheter enters the trachea, the patient may cough, fight, and become cyanotic. Remove the catheter immediately and allow the patient to rest before attempting intubation again.
8. The feeding position should be supine or right side-lying, with head and chest slightly elevated. Attach reservoir to catheter and fill with feeding fluid. Allow infant to suck on pacifier during feeding.	8. This position allows the flow of fluid to be aided by gravity. The use of the pacifier will relax the infant, allowing for easier flow of fluid as well as provide for normal sucking needs. Sucking will help develop muscles, and provide a positive association between sucking and relief of hunger.
9. Aspirate tube before feeding begins. a. If over ½ the previous feeding is obtained, withhold the feeding. b. If small residual of formula is obtained, return it to stomach and subtract that amount from the total amount of formula to be given.	9. This is done to monitor for appropriate fluid intake, digestion time, and overfeeding that can cause distention.
10. The flow of the feeding should be slow. Do not apply pressure. Elevate reservoir 15–20 cm. (6–8 inches) above the patient's head.	10. The rate of flow is controlled by the size of the feeding catheter: the smaller the size, the slower the flow. If the reservoir is too high, the pressure of the fluid itself increases the rate of flow.
11. Food taken too rapidly will interfere with peristalsis, causing abdominal distention and regurgitation.	11. The presence of food in the stomach stimulates peristalsis and causes the digestive process to begin.
12. Feeding time should last approximately as long as when a corresponding amount is given by nipple, 5 ml/5–10 minutes or 15–20 minutes total time.	
13. When the feeding is completed, the catheter may be irrigated with clear water. Before the fluid reaches the end of the catheter, clamp it off and withdraw it quickly.	13. Clamp the catheter before air enters the stomach and causes abdominal distention. Clamping also prevents fluid from dripping from the catheter into the pharynx, causing patient to gag and aspirate.
14. Discard feeding tube and any leftover solution.	

NOTE: Intermittent gavage feeding is often preferred to indwelling gavage feeding. An indwelling catheter may coil and knot, perforate the stomach, and cause nasal airway obstruction, ulceration, irritation of the mucous membranes, incompetence of esophageal-cardiac sphincter, and epistaxis. However, if intermittent intubation is not well tolerated and the indwelling method is used, the catheter should be changed every 48–72 hours. (Use alternate sides of the nares.) Constant alertness to the above problems should be stressed. Indwelling method may be preferred with older infant or child.

Follow-up Phase

1. Burp or bubble patient.	1. Adequate expulsion of air swallowed or ingested during feeding will decrease abdominal distention and allow for better tolerance of the feeding.
2. Place patient on right side or on abdomen.	2. To facilitate gastric emptying and minimize regurgitation and aspiration.
3. Observe condition after feeding; bradycardia and apnea may still occur.	3. Because of vagal stimulation as mentioned above.
4. Note any vomiting or abdominal distention.	4. Due to overfeeding or too rapid feeding. Regurgitation of 1–2 ml may occur in the premature infant as the musculature of the sphincter of the gastrointestinal tract is relaxed and allows for easy reflux.
5. Note infant's activity.	5. Fatigue or peaceful sleep.
6. Accurately describe and record procedure, including time of feeding, type of gavage feeding, type and amount of feeding fluid given, amount retained or vomited, how patient tolerated feeding, and activity following feeding.	6. Observe for readiness of the infant to feed by nipple—note sucking activity and sleep–wake cycle in relation to feeding.

GUIDELINES: Gastrostomy Feeding

Gastrostomy feeding is a means of providing nourishment and fluids via a tube that has been surgically inserted via a stab wound through the abdominal wall into the stomach.

Purposes

1. To provide a method of nutrition and fluids that requires minimal effort when the patient is unable to suck or swallow for long periods of time.
2. To allow for better decompression of stomach (because of large tube size) following a surgical procedure.

GUIDELINES: Gastrostomy Feeding (cont.)

Purposes (cont.)

3. To provide a safe method of feeding a hypotonic patient or one who cannot tolerate alternative methods. Specific indications may include duodenal atresia, tracheal esophageal fistula, and omphalocele.
4. To provide a route that allows adequate calorie and/or fluid intake in a child with chronic lung disease or in one who does not have continuity of the gastrointestinal tract, i.e., esophageal atresia.

Equipment

Warm feeding fluid
Pacifier
Reservoir syringe or funnel
Syringe for aspirating

Procedure

NURSING ACTION	RATIONALE/AMPLIFICATION
Preparatory Phase	
1. Gastrostomy tube may be in one of 3 positions between feedings: a. Lowered and open to start drainage. b. Open, connected to reservoir (funnel, syringe) that is elevated 10–12 cm. (4–4¾ inches). c. Clamped.	a. Constant decompression. b. To serve as safety valve outlet to prevent esophageal reflux and increased stomach pressure. c. Most "normal" physiologic setup; preparation for home care or tube removal.
2. The nurse may be directed to check residual stomach contents prior to any feeding. a. Attach syringe and aspirate stomach contents. b. Measure. c. Residual fluid may be returned to stomach or discarded depending on amount.	2. This is done to monitor for appropriate fluid intake, digestion time, and overfeeding that can cause distention.
3. A Y-tube which is connected at the point where reservoir and gastrostomy tube join may be used during feeding.	3. To provide simultaneous decompression during feeding.
4. When feeding is about to begin, infant/child should be placed in comfortable position in bed—either flat or with head slightly elevated. If condition permits, the nurse should hold infant. A pacifier can be given to him.	4. When infant/child is comfortable and relaxed, feeding fluid will flow more easily into stomach. Pacifier will satisfy normal sucking activity, provide exercise for jaw muscles, and relax musculature as well as provide pleasure normally associated with feeding.
Performance Phase	
1. Attach reservoir syringe to tube (if not already open to continuous elevation) and fill reservoir with feeding fluid prior to unclamping tube.	1. Prevents air from entering tube (and then stomach), which may cause distention.
2. Elevate tube and reservoir to 10–12 cm. (4–4¾ inches) above abdominal wall. Do not apply any pressure to start flow.	2. This elevation level will allow for slow, gravity-induced flow. Pressure may cause a backflow of fluid into the esophagus.
3. Feed slowly, taking 20–45 minutes. Fill reservoir with remaining fluid before it is empty to avoid installation of air.	3. Too rapid a feeding will interfere with normal peristalsis and will cause abdominal distention and backflow into reservoir or esophagus.
4. Continue to provide infant with pleasant feelings associated with feeding.	
5. When feeding is completed: a. Instill clear water (10–30 ml., or 0.3–1 oz.) if tube is to be clamped. Apply clamp before water level reaches end of reservoir. b. Leave tube unclamped and open to continuous elevation.	a. This rinses tubing and will prevent clogging. b. Feeding fluid is allowed to return to reservoir if infant cries or changes position, and thus decreases pressure on the stomach.
6. Often when oral feedings are started, they are given simultaneously with gastrostomy feedings.	6. This allows the infant to learn or reestablish the sucking–swallowing process as well as to build up tolerance to eating without compromising nutritional intake.
Follow-up Phase	
1. Check dressing and skin around point of tube entry for wetness. Clean skin and apply skin barrier (petrolatum, Maalox, aluminum paste, etc.). See that there is no pull on tube.	1. Skin breakdown is caused by continued exposure to stomach contents that may be leaking out around tube causing excoriation and infection. Constant pulling on tube can cause widening of skin opening and subsequent leakage.
2. Leave infant dry and comfortable. If unable to hold him during feeding, this may be a good time to hold, fondle, and provide him with warmth and love. Place him on right side or in Fowler's position.	2. To promote relaxation and improved digestion of feeding.

Procedure (cont.)

NURSING ACTION	RATIONALE/AMPLIFICATION
3. Accurately describe and record procedure, including time of feeding, type and amount of feeding fluid given, amount and characteristics of residual (if any) and what was done with it, how patient tolerated feeding, any abdominal distention, and activity following feeding.	

NOTE: Should infant pull gastrostomy tube out, cover ostomy site with sterile dressing and tape, notify physician, and accurately record events.

GUIDELINES: Nasojejunal Feeding

Nasojejunal feeding is a means of providing full enteral feeding via a catheter passed through the nares, past the pharynx, down the esophagus, bypassing the stomach through the pylorus into the jejunum.

Purposes

1. To provide a method of feeding that requires minimal patient effort when the infant is unable to tolerate alternative feeding methods (i.e., low birth weight, persistent respiratory distress).
2. To provide a route that allows for adequate calorie or fluid intake (a full enteral feeding) via intermittent or continuous drip.
3. To provide a method of feeding a critically ill infant that minimizes regurgitation, aspiration, and gastric distention.
4. To provide a route for administration of oral medications (controversial).

Equipment

*Sterile radiopaque silicone or polyvinyl nasojejunal tube, 1 meter (39 inches), No. 19, No. 21, or No. 23—may or may not have weighted tip.
Tape
pH paper
Reservoir for feeding
Possibly an infusion pump
3-way stopcock
Syringe—0.5 ml. normal saline or sterile water
Equipment for N-G tube insertion

Procedure

NURSING ACTION	RATIONALE/AMPLIFICATION
Preparatory Phase	
1. Attach cardiac monitor to infant.	1. To allow for continuous monitoring of heart rate and rhythm. The vagus nerve pathway lies from the medulla through the neck and thorax to the abdomen. Above the stomach, the left and right branches unite to form the esophageal plexus. Stimulation of these nerve branches with the catheter will directly affect the cardiac and pulmonary plexus.

2. Tube is generally inserted by a physician
  a. Measure from glabella (prominent point between eyebrows) to the heel for estimated length.
  b. Measure and mark the remaining length of tubing and record.
	b. This serves as a double check to ensure that tube has not advanced farther than intended.

3. Place infant on his right side with hips slightly elevated. Gentle restraint or soft mittens may have to be applied.	3. Facilitates passage of tube. Restraints prevent infant from pulling out tube before the tip passes the pylorus.
4. Tube is inserted through a nostril into the stomach—allowing adequate length so that it can pass the pylorus into the jejunum. Securely tape tube in place so as not to block nasal canal or cause pressure necrosis or irritation.	
5. Check intestinal aspirate for pH every 1-2 hours. Infant may be positioned on right side, back, or abdomen. Once the tube is past the pylorus, abdominal posteroanterior and lateral x-rays are taken to confirm that tip of catheter is at the ligament of Treitz.	5. When aspiration fluid reaches a pH of 5-7 or bile colored fluid is obtained, the tip of the tube has passed the pylorus into the jejunum.
6. A No. 5 French nasogastric feeding tube may be passed through the other nostril at this time and left indwelling. This is used to check stomach for residual fluid and regurgitation through the pylorus.	6. If gastric residual is significant, it will interfere with prescribed feeding. Notify physician. 4 ml./kg. (0.12 oz./2.2 lbs.) reflux in stomach is tolerated. Do not remove N-G tube since it will adhere to N-J tube during withdrawal and pull out N-J tube also.

* See Gavage Feeding, page 1159.

GUIDELINES: Nasojejunal Feeding (cont.)

Procedure (cont.)

NURSING ACTION	RATIONALE/AMPLIFICATION
7. N-J feedings can generally be started following this progression: a. D₅W for 6–12 hours. b. ½ strength formula with low osmolality for 6–12 hours. c. Full strength low osmolality formula. d. The volume of feeding is increased 2 ml. (0.06 oz.) at a time until infant's daily calorie and fluid requirements are being administered. e. Medications may be given via the N-J tube if prescribed. A 3-way stopcock will have to be placed at the connection of the N-J tube and the line from the feeding fluid. Alternative method for administering oral medications is by passing an oral–gastric or nasogastric feeding tube; in this way the stomach and process of digestion and absorption are not by-passed.	b. Low solute formulas include SMA, Similac, Enfamil; (20 calories/30 ml., or 20 calories/1 oz.). c. Low osmolality formula is used to prevent loss of fluid into intestine and possible necrotizing enterocolitis. d. 150 ml./kg. (4.5 oz./2.2 lbs.) fluid requirement is generally used (130–150 cal./kg.). e. Flush tubing with 0.5 ml. (.015 oz.) normal saline or sterile water after medication is administered to ensure that infant receives entire dosage prescribed and to prevent any sediment from remaining in tubing.

Performance Phase

NURSING ACTION	RATIONALE/AMPLIFICATION
1. N-J feedings can be given as follows: a. Intermittently (i.e., every 1-3 hours) b. In a continuous slow drip 2. If intermittent feeding is the method used, the feeding techniques are the same as for nasogastric (gavage) feeding. 3. If slow continuous drip method is used, the setup used is similar to the pediatric IV infusion using an infusion pump and small (100–250 ml., or 3.0–7.5 oz.) closed chamber for reservoir. a. Reservoir chamber and tubing should be changed every 8–24 hours. b. Record input every hour. Fill reservoir as needed, with no more than 3 hours worth of feeding fluid.	b. Generally the preferred method to minimize the satiety-hunger cycle and large-volume instillation. 2. Feeding is given at room temperature. Avoid cold fluid, which may cause infant discomfort. If breast milk is used, gently rotate reservoir periodically to mix settled-out fat content. a. To prevent growth of bacteria. b. To ensure a constant flow and minimize overinfusion directly into the jejunum.

Follow-up Phase

NURSING ACTION	RATIONALE/AMPLIFICATION
1. Be constantly alert for mechanical problems: a. Check for abdominal distention due to infant's inability to handle ingested amount of fluid: • palpate abdomen; • observe for ripple of intestines; • measure abdominal girth every 3–8 hours; • check residual formula in jejunum every 3–8 hours; • discard or refeed as prescribed. b. Check stools for occult blood, pH, and sugar every void or 4–8 hours to determine tolerance of feeding fluid. c. Check emesis for blood and report to physician immediately—may be a sign of necrotizing enterocolitis. 2. Observe infant closely to avoid potential dangers as tube passes the pylorus. a. Close attention to amount, type, concentration and osmolality of feeding fluid is stressed. b. Check heart rate and BP. 3. Hold, fondle, and give positive stimulation to the infant if conditions permit. (See Premature Infant, p. 1224) 4. Accurately describe and record condition of infant and procedure, including type and amount of feeding given, amount of residual and characteristics, any signs of impending infant distress or problems.	1. Tube clogging due to inadequate rinsing. Tube advancing too far into jejunum. Check protruding tube measurement. Fluid overload, causing aspiration. 2. Diarrhea; as the tube passes through the pylorus it (the tube) becomes stiff due to the change in pH. A stiff tube has been reported to cause intestinal perforation. If tube becomes clogged or dislodged, it must be removed. 3. This procedure limits the normal pleasures associated with feeding. Infant needs some attention to his psychological needs in order to thrive.

SPECIMEN COLLECTION

GUIDELINES: Assisting with Blood Collection

Blood collection from a venous puncture in the extremity of an infant or young child is the same as for an adult, with the following exceptions or additions.

Equipment   No. 23–19 gauge short needle or scalp-vein needle
Smaller volume or micro blood-collecting tubes
Smaller tourniquet (rubber band may be used with infant)

Procedure

NURSING ACTION	RATIONALE/AMPLIFICATION
Preparatory Phase	
1. Immobilize the child by placing him in a mummy restraint if necessary (see p. 1154).	1. Infants and young children squirm. Immobilizing them allows easier access to the venipuncture site. It also helps keep infant warm.
2. Position the patient. a. *Femoral venipuncture:* place child on his back with legs in frog-like position. Nurse places her hands on child's knees. (See position for bladder puncture, p. 1167.) b. *External jugular venipuncture:* place child in mummy restraint and lower his head over the side of the bed or table. Turn head to side and stabilize. Crying will make external jugular vein visible and causes blood to flow more readily. c. *Antecubital fossa venipuncture:* place the child in a supine position. The nurse stands on the side opposite the site to be used (across from the person drawing the specimen). The nurse positions her right arm across the upper part of the child's chest and grasps the shoulder at the axilla position. Her left arm is placed across the lower part of the child's chest and is used to extend the child's arm at the wrist.	2. These positions allow for optimum visualization and stabilization of the patient. Cover perineum to protect site and operator, should infant void. 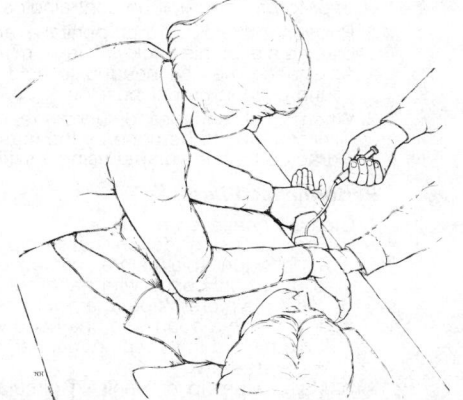
d. *Infant—heel, toe, or digital stick:* warm area with warm compress for 5–10 minutes.	d. This dilates vessels allowing blood to flow more freely.
Performance Phase	
1. After the specimen is collected and the needle is removed, apply pressure to the site with dry gauze for 3–5 minutes. a. *Jugular venipuncture:* while applying pressure to the site, place the patient in an upright sitting position. Do not apply excessive pressure that may compromise circulation or respiration. b. *Capillary:* clean area with antiseptic and dry with dry sterile 2 × 2 gauze. Hold heel firmly and with free hand quickly puncture with microlancet or sterile 21-gauge needle on most medial or lateral part of plantar surface. Puncture deeply enough to get free-flowing blood—never deeper than 2.4 mm. Discard first drop of blood; rapidly collect specimen in proper capillary tube.	1. Both the femoral and jugular veins are large vessels. Since respiratory pressure is great, bleeding, oozing, and hematoma formation may result. External pressure prevents this from happening.
2. When the bleeding has been stopped, soothe and comfort the child before leaving him.	2. Crying and thrashing about may initiate bleeding.
Follow-up Phase	
1. Check patient frequently for an hour after the procedure for oozing, bleeding, or evidence of a hematoma.	1. Reapply pressure and report if oozing continues.
2. Record carefully and accurately: a. Site of venipuncture b. How patient tolerated procedure c. Bleeding stopped or continued and for how long d. What test the specimen was collected for	

GUIDELINES: Collecting a Urine Specimen from the Infant and Young Child

Urine collection is a safe method of obtaining urine for a specified purpose.

Purposes
1. To check urine for presence of sugar, acetone, bacteria, and other urinary products.
2. To aid in diagnosis.
3. To determine the condition of the patient.
4. To determine effectiveness of therapy.

Equipment
Collecting device—plastic, disposable urine bag or collector (Hollister, Inc. U-Bag, double chamber)
Cleansing agent
Wiping material—4 × 4's or cotton balls
Clean or sterile water
Containers for solutions
Specimen container

Procedure

NURSING ACTION	RATIONALE/AMPLIFICATION
Preparatory Phase	
1. Offer young child fluids he likes to drink 30–60 minutes prior to procedure, if no contraindications.	
2. Position patient so that genitalia are exposed by placing him on his back with legs in frog-like position. Assistance may be needed to hold the legs of the young child in proper position.	2. Proper positioning will facilitate cleansing and allow for proper placement of collection device.
3. When small samples of urine are needed for pH, Clinitest, etc., to be done by the nurse, urine can be extracted from the diaper using a syringe or dropper.	
Performance Phase	
1. Cleanse genital area.	1. This method of cleansing the female will prevent contamination of the genitalia from the anus, and will prevent contamination of the urine specimen obtained.
a. *Female:* using cotton balls, dip into cleansing agent, wipe labia majora from top to bottom (clitoris to anus) only once with each cotton ball. Repeat this once more. Wipe again with clear water. Then spread labia apart with one hand while wiping the labia minora in the same manner with other hand. Wipe area dry.	
b. *Male:* wipe tip of penis in circular motion down towards the scrotum. Be certain to retract foreskin, if present. Wipe first with cleansing agent 2–3 times, then clear water. Dry the area.	During the cleansing, be gentle to avoid any injury or possible stimulation of urination.
2. Apply collecting bag firmly so that the opening is exposed to receive urine.	2. If collecting bag is properly and securely placed, the procedure will not have to be repeated.
a. Female—stretch perineum taut during application. Attach bag to perineum first, then proceed up to symphysis.	a. This should ensure leak-proof contact.
b. Male (small boys)—place penis and scrotum inside bag.	
3. Diaper patient and comfort him; possibly give him additional clear fluids.	
4. Check the patient frequently (30–45 minutes) to see if he has voided. When patient has voided, remove bag gently. Clean area and rediaper the child. If child has not voided within 45 minutes, procedure must be repeated.	4. The adhesive on the collecting bag may tend to be sticky. Careful removal of the bag will prevent skin injury on and around genitalia. Also avoid spilling urine out of the bag during removal.
	Reapplication of bag will decrease the possibility of unreliable test results.
Follow-up Phase	
1. Pour specimen into proper collecting container. Send specimen to the laboratory within 30 minutes or refrigerate.	1. Prompt delivery of specimen to the laboratory will prevent growth of organisms in an uncontrolled environment and distortion of the test results.
2. Accurately chart and describe the following in the nurse's notes:	
a. Time specimen collection was started and ended	
b. Amount of urine voided	
c. Color of urine (cloudy, clear, any sediment)	
d. Type of test to be done	
e. Condition of skin of perineal area	

GUIDELINES: Assisting with a Percutaneous Suprapubic Bladder Aspiration

Percutaneous bladder aspiration is an aseptic method of entering the bladder in the suprapubic location with a needle to obtain a urine specimen.

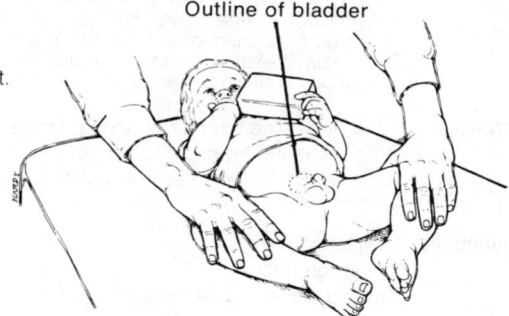

Outline of bladder

Purposes
1. To obtain urine in an aseptic manner for culture.
2. To aid in diagnostic workup.
3. To determine condition of the patient and aid in treatment.

Equipment
Skin cleansing solution
Sterile 4 × 4's
Sterile gloves
Sterile needle, No. 21 gauge, 3.7 cm. (1½ inches) long
Sterile syringe, 20-ml.
Sterile specimen container
Band-Aid
Antiseptic skin cleansing solution

Procedure

NURSING ACTION	RATIONALE/AMPLIFICATION
Preparatory Phase	
1. Check diaper for wetness. If child has just voided, report this to the physician or report last voiding time.	1. In order to perform a successful bladder aspiration, enough urine must be present to distend the bladder up above the pubic symphysis—so that bladder is accessible.
2. Position child on his back on the examining table. His head should be toward nurse, his feet toward the physician. Spread his legs apart in a frog-like position. Place hands on his knees and thumbs along his side at the hip level.	2. This position allows the nurse to stabilize the child. It also gives a full view of the child, making it easier to observe him, talk to him, and soothe him.
3. Ensure that the skin over the puncture site is cleansed in an antiseptic manner.	3. To prevent infection from being introduced into the bladder by inserting the needle through unclean skin which would contaminate the specimen.
Performance Phase	
1. While the procedure is being performed, note the condition of the patient and any signs of distress. Comfort him by talking to him and smiling at him.	1. Report any changes in color or respiration rate or other signs. Soothing the child will help him to relax so that he will not move about so much. Crying increases the muscle tone of the lower abdomen, making it more difficult to insert the needle.
2. When urine has been obtained or the procedure is discontinued and the needle is removed, apply pressure over the puncture site with a 4 × 4 and fingers.	2. This prevents any bleeding from occurring either internally or externally. Pressure should be maintained about 3 minutes or until oozing ceases and coagulation has taken place.
3. Apply a Band-Aid if necessary. Rediaper child. Hold and comfort him for a few minutes.	3. Holding the child will help to restore and maintain a good nurse-patient relationship and will help the child to relax after a frightening and painful procedure.
Follow-up Phase	
1. Check child periodically for 1 hour after procedure to see that bleeding or oozing has not occurred.	1. This is not likely if pressure was applied properly after procedure and patient was left quiet.
2. Note time of first voiding after procedure. Note color of urine (it may be pink). Bloody urine should be reported to the physician.	2. It is important to note any changes in voiding pattern following the procedure, since change might indicate injury. The first voided urine may be bloody due to a small amount of local capillary bleeding at the time of the procedure.
3. Accurately describe and chart the procedure, including: a. Time of procedure b. Whether or not a specimen was obtained c. How the patient tolerated the procedure d. Description and amount of urine obtained e. Patient's condition and activity following the procedure	

GUIDELINES: Continuous Urine Collection Using a Metabolic Bed

A *metabolic bed* is a bed modified to allow urine to pass through a hole in the mattress into a collection bottle placed below the bed. It may also be a specially constructed crib with a mesh hammock in place of a mattress, which allows urine to pass into a collection bottle.

Continuous urine collection is a method of accurate collection of urine excreted within a specific time frame. (Continuous urine collection in the older child is based on the same principles and is essentially the same as for an adult. The importance of saving all the urine and keeping it separate from stool must be stressed.)

Purposes
1. To determine the rate of urine production.
2. To measure the excretion of specific chemicals produced by the body.
3. To eliminate the need for restraints and give child freedom to move around and partake in play or pleasant activities.

Equipment
Metabolic bed
Collection bottle
Any special equipment specific to test being done

Procedure

NURSING ACTION	RATIONALE/AMPLIFICATION
Preparatory Phase	
1. If child is old enough, explain at his level of understanding what is going to happen and why.	1. Being placed in this strange-looking bed can cause increased anxiety and frustration. Tell the child if he will be allowed to get out of bed for short periods, i.e., for meals. Tell him how long he will be in the bed.
2. Remove diaper and note time when child is placed in the metabolic bed.	2. Collection timing begins after the first voiding, which is discarded.
Performance Phase	
1. Be certain that collection bottle remains in proper position to receive specimen from funnel of bed.	1. Lost specimen will necessitate restarting test; will increase time the child will have to remain in the metabolic bed.
2. Immediately remove any stool from the area.	2. Stool-contaminated urine may result in altered, unreliable test results.
3. Meticulous skin care must be given to prevent any breakdown or irritation.	3. Frequently the material composition of the metabolic bed is irritating to tender skin, especially when it may be wet from voiding.
4. Offer the child diversional activities. The child continues to need physical contact and reassurance. If there are no contraindications, a disposable urine collecting bag may be applied to the child for short periods of time.	4. Mobiles, colorful pictures, squeak toys for infant; games, books, etc., for young child—consider playthings that can be washed. An ideal time to be out of bed might be mealtime—especially important for infant to be held and fondled.
5. At the end of specified collection time, collect last voiding, if possible, and add to the total collection.	5. This will insure an accurate output of the timed collection specimen.
Follow-up Phase	
1. Send specimen to laboratory immediately or follow specific instructions.	1. Inappropriate handling may distort test results.
2. Bathe child and dress him as usual. Return him to his own crib or bed. Give him extra psychological comfort. Leave him happy and comfortable.	2. Bathing will usually relax child as well as give you a chance to examine his skin for any irritation while giving him some extra attention.
3. Record accurately and describe the following in nurse's notes: a. Time specimen collection was started and ended b. Amount of urine collected c. Type of test to be done d. Condition and activity of child during and following collection of specimen	

GUIDELINES: Collecting a Stool Specimen

Stool collection is a method of obtaining a stool specimen from the patient.

Purposes
1. To check stool for presence of specific material, i.e., blood, ova, and parasites or bacteria.
2. To aid in diagnosis.

Purposes (cont.)	3. To determine condition or status of the patient. 4. To determine effectiveness of therapy.
Equipment	Diaper Cellophane or plastic liner (used when stool is loose or watery) Tongue blade Specimen container

NOTE: Collecting a stool specimen from an older child who is toilet-trained is the same as collecting such a specimen from an adult.

Procedure

NURSING ACTION	RATIONALE/AMPLIFICATION
Preparatory Phase	
1. If a specimen is needed from a patient whose stools are loose or watery enough to be absorbed in the diaper, line the diaper with a piece of cellophane or plastic. Place this liner between the diaper and the skin. Then diaper the child and position him so that his head is slightly elevated. If stools are soft or formed, simply diaper the child.	1. The liner and position will allow the loose stool specimen to collect in the liner and not be absorbed by the diaper.
Performance Phase	
1. Check child frequently to see if stooling has occurred.	1. A fresh specimen should be obtained so that test results will not be distorted by time-lapse. This will also decrease the chance of contamination of the stool with urine and will prevent skin irritation from the stool.
2. Remove soiled diaper from child. Clean perineal area, apply clean diaper, and leave child comfortable.	
3. Remove small amount of stool from diaper with the tongue blade and place it in the specimen container.	
4. Send labeled specimen to the laboratory promptly.	4. Prompt delivery to the lab will prevent changes from taking place in the specimen that could alter the test results.
Follow-up Phase	

1. Accurately describe and record the following:
  a. Time specimen was collected
  b. Color, amount, and consistency of stool (Note any foul smell.)
  c. Type of specimen collected
  d. Nature of test for which the specimen was collected
  e. Condition of the skin	

GUIDELINES: Assisting with a Spinal Tap—Lumbar Puncture

A *spinal tap* in an infant or young child is based on the same principles and is essentially the same as for an adult, with the following exceptions.

Equipment No. 21–20 gauge, 3.5 cm. (1½-inch) long spinal needle

Procedure

NURSING ACTION	RATIONALE/AMPLIFICATION
Preparatory Phase	

1. Position the patient.
  a. *Side position* (similar to the adult): wrap the lower extremities in a sheet, if an older child; place the patient on his side facing the nurse; flex knees and neck by placing one hand on his shoulders and head and the other hand on buttocks and upper thigh.
  b. *Sitting position:* this position is primarily used with small infants. Place infant in sitting position; extend legs and arms in front of the infant; flex his neck so chin is almost resting on chest; back is rounded by placing thumbs on his shoulders and hands along side of his hips.
	1. In either position the patient may squirm. Hold him securely to prevent him from moving and causing injury to himself or causing the spinal needle to be inserted too far, resulting in a traumatic tap.

GUIDELINES: Assisting with a Spinal Tap—Lumbar Puncture (cont.)

Procedure (cont.)	NURSING ACTION	RATIONALE/AMPLIFICATION

NURSING ALERT: Observe for signs of respiratory distress. Because the trachea in the infant is so soft, it can kink very easily when the neck is flexed. If this happens and the airway is obstructed, the infant will stop breathing. This is an emergency situation.

Follow-up Phase

1. It is not usually necessary to keep the infant or young child flat in bed following the procedure unless there are contraindications to his being up and physician has prescribed that he be kept in bed. It may be helpful to institute play activity and offer fluids to the child.

FLUID AND ELECTROLYTE BALANCE IN CHILDREN

Basic Principles

1. Infants and small children have different proportions of body water and body fat than do adults (Table 37-2).
   a. The body water of a newborn infant approaches 80% of his body weight, compared to that of an average adult male, which approaches 60%.
   b. The normal infant demonstrates a rapid physiological decline in the ratio of body weight to body water during the immediate postpartum period.
   c. Proportion of body water declines more slowly throughout infancy and reaches the characteristic value for adults by approximately 2 years of age.
2. Compared to adults, a greater percentage of the body water of infants and small children is contained in the extracellular compartment.
   a. Infants—approximately ½ of the body water is contained in the cell.
   b. Adults—approximately ⅔ of the body water is contained in the cell.
3. Compared to adults, the water turnover rate per unit of body weight is 3 or more times greater in infants and small children.
   a. The child's metabolic rate is about 3 times that of an adult.
   b. The child has more body surface in relation to weight.
   c. The immaturity of kidney function in infants may impair their ability to conserve water.
4. Electrolyte balance is dependent on fluid balance and cardiovascular, renal, adrenal, pituitary, parathyroid, and pulmonary regulatory mechanisms.

5. Infants and children are more vulnerable to disorders of hydration than are adults.
   a. The basic principles relating to fluid balance in children make the magnitude of fluid losses considerably greater in children than in adults.
   b. Children are prone to severe disturbances of the gastrointestinal tract that result in diarrhea and vomiting.
   c. Young children cannot independently respond to increased losses by increased intake. They depend on others to provide them with adequate fluid.

Common Fluid and Electrolyte Abnormalities

See Table 37-3, page 1171.

General Goals of Fluid and Electrolyte Therapy

1. Repair of preexisting deficits which may occur with prolonged or severe diarrhea or vomiting.
   a. Deficits are estimated and corrected as soon and as safely as possible.
      (1) Initial therapy is aimed at restoring blood and extracellular fluid volume in order to relieve or prevent shock and restore renal function.
      (2) Intracellular deficits are replaced slowly over 8–12 hour period after the circulatory status is improved.
2. Provision of Maintenance Requirements
   a. Maintenance requirements occur as a result of normal expenditures of water and electrolytes due to metabolism.
   b. Maintenance requirements bear a close relationship to metabolic rate and are ideally formulated in terms of caloric expenditure.
3. Correction of concurrent losses which may occur via the gastrointestinal tract by vomiting, diarrhea, or drainage of secretions
      Replacement should be similar in type and amount to the fluid being lost.
      Replacement is usually formulated as ml. of fluid and mEq. of electrolyte replaced per ml. of fluid and mEq. of electrolyte lost.

TABLE 37-2. BODY FLUIDS EXPRESSED AS PERCENT OF BODY WEIGHT

Fluid	Adult		Infant
	Male	*Female*	
Total Body Fluids	60%	54%	75%
(1) Intracellular	40%	36%	48%
(2) Extracellular	20%	18%	27%

TABLE 37-3. COMMON ABNORMALITIES OF FLUID AND ELECTROLYTE METABOLISM

Substance	Major Function	Abnormality	Cause	Clinical Manifestation	Lab Data
Water	Medium of body fluids, chemical changes, body temperature, lubricant	Volume deficit	1. Primary—inadequate water intake 2. Secondary—loss following vomiting, diarrhea, excessive gastrointestinal obstruction, etc.	Oliguria, weight loss, signs of dehydration including: dry skin and mucous membranes, lassitude, sunken fontanelles, lack of tear formation, increased pulse, decreased blood pressure	Concentrated urine azotemia, elevated hematocrit, hemoglobin and erythrocyte count
		Volume excess	1. Failure to excrete water in presence of normal intake such as in congestive heart failure, renal disease 2. Water intake in excess of output	Weight gain, peripheral edema, signs of pulmonary congestion	Oliguria, concentrated urine with reduced sodium chloride concentration
Potassium	Intracellular fluid balance, regular heart rhythm, muscle and nerve irritability	Potassium deficit	1. Excessive loss of potassium due to vomiting, diarrhea; prolonged cortisone, ACTH or diuretic therapy; diabetic acidosis 2. Shift of potassium into the cells such as occurs with the healing phase of burns, recovery from diabetic acidosis	Signs and symptoms variable, including weakness, lethargy, irritability, abdominal distention and eventually cardiac arrhythmias	Low plasma K^+ level (may be normal in some situations); polyuria with very dilute urine; hypochloremic alkalosis
		Potassium excess	Excessive administration of potassium-containing solutions, excessive release of potassium due to burns, severe kidney disease, adrenal insufficiency	Variable, including: listlessness, confusion, heaviness of the legs, nausea, diarrhea, ECG changes, ultimately paralysis and cardiac arrest	Elevated potassium plasma level
Sodium	Osmotic pressure, muscle and nerve irritability	Sodium deficit	Water intake in excess of excretory capacity; replacement of fluid loss without sufficient sodium; adrenal insufficiency; malnutrition	Headache, nausea, abdominal cramps, confusion alternating with stupor, diarrhea, lacrimation, salivation, later hypotension; early polyuria, later oliguria	Low sodium plasma level, oliguria with concentrated urine except in severe K^+ depletion or simple overhydration
		Sodium excess	Inadequate water intake especially in the presence of fever or sweating; severe, watery diarrhea; hyperventilation in warm, dry air; diabetes insipidus	Thirst, oliguria, weakness, muscular pain, excitement, dry mucous membranes, hypotension, tachycardia, fever	Elevated Na^+ plasma level, high specific gravity of urine
Bicarbonate	Acid-base balance	Primary bicarbonate deficit	Diarrhea (especially in infants); diabetes mellitus; starvation; infectious disease; shock or congestive heart failure producing tissue anoxia	Progressively increasing rate and depth of respiration—ultimately becoming Kussmaul respiration: flushed, warm skin, weakness, disorientation progressing to coma	Urine pH usually less than 6 Plasma bicarbonate less than 20 mEq./L. Plasma pH less than 7.35
		Primary bicarbonate excess	Loss of chloride through vomiting, gastric suction, or the use of excessive diuretics; excessive ingestion of alkali	Depressed respiration, muscle hypertonicity, hyperactive reflexes, tetany and sometimes convulsions	Urine pH usually above 7.0; plasma bicarbonate above 25 mEq./L. (30 mEq./L. in adults); plasma pH above 7.45

GUIDELINES: Intravenous Fluid Therapy

Intravenous therapy refers to the infusion of fluids directly into the venous system. This may be accomplished through the use of a needle or by venous cutdown and insertion of a small catheter directly into the vein (Fig. 37-6).

Purpose   To restore and maintain the child's fluid and electrolyte balance and body homeostasis when his oral intake is inadequate to serve this purpose.

GUIDELINES: Intravenous Fluid Therapy (cont.)

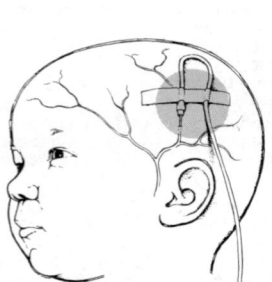
Venipuncture of scalp vein

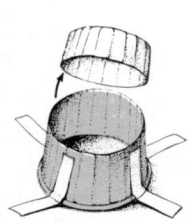
Paper cup taped over venipuncture site for protection

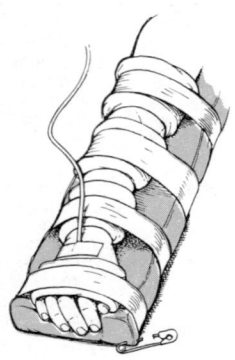
Restraint of arm when hand is site of infusion

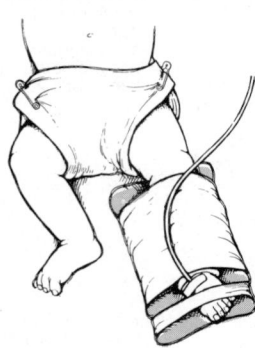
Infant's leg taped to sandbag for immobilization

FIGURE 37-6. *IV fluid therapy.*

Equipment

A. *Needle Method*

IV solution

> The kind of solution is specified by the physician.
> For small children, 250-ml. bottles should be used for purposes of safety.

IV pole

IV administration set

> The set should include a closed reservoir with a minidropper to ensure that the child will not receive an excessive amount of fluid in a brief period of time.

Micropore filter

Syringe, 5 or 10 ml.—approximately ½–⅔ filled with normal saline

Butterfly needle or catheter of appropriate gauge

> The size of the needle depends on the age and size of the child and the type of fluid to be administered.

Alcohol sponges, dry sponges

Betadine or other antibacterial cleansing solution

Normal saline

Small tourniquet or rubber band

Adhesive tape, 1.2 cm. (½ inch), 2.5 cm. (1 inch), 5 cm. (2 inches)

Padded armboard

Gauze bandage for securing the extremity to the armboard

Restraining devices—bath blanket, extremity restraint, covered sandbags

> The type of restraint depends on the child's age, his level of cooperation, and the kind of IV to be started.

Safety razor (if scalp vein is to be used)

B. *Cutdown Method*

IV solution, IV pole, IV administration set

Alcohol sponges

Adhesive tape, 1.2 cm. (½ inch), 2.5 cm. (1 inch), 5 cm. (2 inches)

Padded armboard

Dry sponges

Gauze bandage

Sterile cutdown tray

> The tray should include the following equipment: medicine cups, treatment towels, wound towel, syringe, No. 1–25 gauge 1.5-cm. (⅝-inch) needle. No. 1–20 gauge 2.5-cm. (1-inch) needle, knife handle and No. 15 blade, forceps, scissors, gauze sponges, 4–0 black silk suture, needle holder.

Assorted sizes of sterile polyethylene tubing and Luer adapters.

5–0 black silk suture with a straight eye needle

1–2% procaine

Normal saline

Tourniquet

Sterile gloves

Restraining devices

Procedure

NURSING ACTION	RATIONALE/AMPLIFICATION

Preparatory Phase

1. Obtain the IV solution.

1. Although the type of solution and the rate of flow are prescribed by the physician, the nurse should be aware of the composition of common parenteral solutions and should know how to calculate maintenance therapy. (Table 37-4).

2. Check the IV fluid for sediment or contaminant by holding the bottle up to the light.

2. Contaminant is most easily identified with the bottle in this position. If sediment is observed, the solution should be discarded.

3. Check the bottle for cracks.

3. If a flash of light can be seen through the bottle, it has a razor-thin crack and should be discarded.

4. Attach a micropore filter to the end of the infusion tubing which attaches to the needle. Use aseptic technique.

4. A 0.45 micron filter prevents entry into the vein of larger particles, air emboli, and most bacterial and fungal organisms except some pseudomonas organisms. A 0.22 micron filter prevents entry of any organisms but requires the use of an IV pump.

5. Remove the metal seal from the IV bottle without touching the rubber top.

5. Do not use the solution if the seal has been broken. It is not necessary to cleanse the sterile, rubber top with alcohol unless it has been accidentally contaminated.

6. With the IV bottle upright, insert the end of the administration set into the bottle's opening. Use aseptic technique.

7. Hang the bottle from the IV pole and allow the fluid to fill the tubing. Make sure that there are no air bubbles present.

7. Filling the drip chamber halfway by compressing the chamber will prevent air from entering the tubing.

8. Shut off the fluid flow and keep the end of the tubing sterile until ready to connect it to the needle.

9. Promote the cooperation of the child.
   a. *Infant.* Provide with a pacifier.
   b. *Older child:* Explain the procedure and its purpose.

9. The procedure will be least traumatic for the child if he is able to cooperate and is not frightened or resistant.

10. Transport the child to the treatment room.

10. Since this is often a traumatic procedure for the child, it should not be done in his room or in front of other children on the unit.

11. Position the child so that he is comfortable.

12. Restrain the child as necessary.
   a. *Infant or young child:* Restraints may include mummy wrappings, jacket or elbow restraints, or small sandbags.
   b. *Older child:* The extremity to be used should be comfortably restrained on the armboard. Free extremities may also require light restraints to remind the child not to move.

12. Protective devices may be necessary to prevent the child from dislodging the IV needle. The type and size of such devices should be appropriate for the child's age and the position of the IV.
   b. Toes and fingers should be visible to avoid compromising blood flow. The restraint board must be padded and the main pressure points (heel, palm), padded with gauze. Before strapping an extremity to the armboard, back the adhesive with tape or gauze wherever it touches the skin. (See Fig. 37-6.)

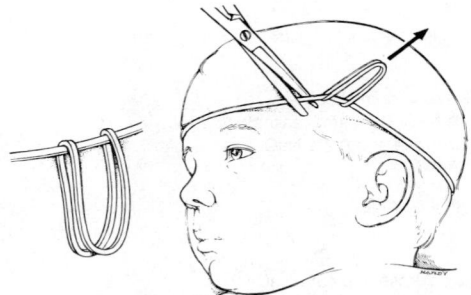

Performance Phase

1. Assist the physician as necessary. This may involve holding the child, cutting tape, regulating fluid flow, applying the tourniquet, etc.

2. A simple method of applying a rubber band tourniquet is illustrated here.
   a. When applying the tourniquet, a second rubber band is placed crosswise under it.
   b. To remove the tourniquet, grasp the unstretched rubber band, pull up, and cut the tourniquet.

3. Check the restraints at intervals and adjust them as necessary.

3. The restraints may become loose after a period of time and must be secured to ensure the child's safety. They may also become too tight and require loosening to maintain adequate circulation.

4. Comfort and reassure the child.

4. The procedure is usually disturbing for the child. This should be acknowledged. If crying and upset, the child should be reassured that his behavior is acceptable.

5. Regulate the IV flow at the designated rate.

GUIDELINES: Intravenous Fluid Therapy (cont.)

Procedure (cont.)

NURSING ACTION	RATIONALE/AMPLIFICATION

6. Record:
    Type of solution being used
    Reading on the bottle or reservoir
    Rate of flow
    Time that the infusion began
    Name of the physician who started the IV
    Site of administration
    Reaction of the child to the procedure
7. Return the child to his room	

Follow-up Phase

NURSING ACTION	RATIONALE/AMPLIFICATION

1. Check the child at least hourly.
    a. Note the location of the IV
    b. Note the color of the skin at the needle point.
    c. Check for swelling of the skin at the needle point.
       (1) If in a hand or foot, compare with the opposite extremity.
       (2) If in the head, look at the face to determine asymmetry.
    d. Feel the area around the IV site for sponginess or leakage.
    e. Check for blood return into the tube when the flow of fluid is stopped.
    f. Make certain that the child is adequately restrained.
	1. The child must be observed frequently to make certain that the IV is not infiltrating and is functioning properly. Report any swelling, discoloration or leakage.

2. Observe closely for complications.
    a. *Local reactions:*
       (1) Compromised circulation
       (2) Pressure sores
       (3) Thrombophlebitis
    b. *Fluid and/or electrolyte disturbances.*
       (1) Maintain an accurate record of intake and output.
          (a) Total the intake and output every 8 hours.
	2. Complications associated with the administration of intravenous fluids to infants and children are very serious and may have fatal consequences. Any signs of complications must be reported immediately.
	
	    b. Refer to Table 37-3, page 1171.

TABLE 37-4. COMPOSITION AND USES OF FREQUENTLY USED PARENTERAL FLUIDS*

Fluid	Calories per liter	Electrolytes, mEq./liter			Use
		Na	K	Cl	
Water with 5% dextrose	200	0	0	0	1. Correction of water deficits in excess of salt, due to inadequate water intake and/or excessive water losses in urine or perspiration
Water with 10% dextrose	400	0	0	0	2. Promotion of sodium diuresis following the excessive use of electrolyte solutions 3. Prophylaxis and treatment of ketosis in starvation, diarrhea, vomiting, or high fever
0.9% NaCl (normal saline)	0	154	0	154	Correction of dehydration
0.45% NaCl (½ normal saline)	0	77	0	77	
5% dextrose and 0.2% NaCl in water	200	34	0	34	Standard solution for initial therapy, e.g., after surgery or before lab results are available, etc.
Ringer's solution	0–400	147	4	155.5	1. Hypotonic dehydration (also contains Ca 4 mEq./L.) 2. Mild alkalosis 3. Hypochloremia
2.5% dextrose in 0.45% NaCl	85	77	0	77	Repair of dehydration while still providing calories and water
5% dextrose in 0.45% NaCl	170	77	0	77	
Ringer's lactate	0–44	130	4	109	1. Dehydration of any type 2. Restoration of normal fluid balance following distributional shifts of extracellular fluid due to burns, fractures, infection, etc. 3. Moderate metabolic acidosis as occurs with infant diarrhea, mild renal insufficiency

* (From Johns Hopkins Hospital: The Harriet Lane Handbook, 8th ed. Copyright © 1978, Year Book Medical Publishers, Chicago. Used by permission.)

Procedure (cont.)

NURSING ACTION	RATIONALE/AMPLIFICATION
(b) Describe carefully the amount and consistency of all stools and vomiting.	
(c) Collect all urine and weigh diapers if more accurate measurement of the child's output is necessary	
(2) Weigh the child at regular intervals, using the same scales each time.	(2) An increase or decrease of 5% within a relatively brief period of time is usually significant and should be reported.
(a) Record the amount of clothes the child is wearing, etc.	
(3) Report:	
(a) Decreased skin turgor	
(b) Marked increase or decrease in urination	
(c) Fever	
(d) Sunken or bulging fontanelles in an infant	
(e) Sudden change in weight or vital signs	
(f) Diarrhea	
(g) Weakness, apathy, or lethargy	
c. Pyrogenic Reactions	c. If severe, the IV should be discontinued. The solution should be saved for possible analysis.
3. Record essential information.	
a. Reading on the bottle or reservoir	
b. Amount of fluid absorbed in the hour	
c. Total amount of fluid absorbed (compare with the total amount of fluid intended to have been absorbed)	
d. Rate of flow	
e. Apparent condition of the child	
4. Regulate the rate of flow as necessary by any of the following methods:	
a. Raising the height of the bottle	
b. Adjusting the flow regulator	
c. Adjusting the position of the extremity	
d. Removing excess tubing or coiling it on the bed	d. If excess tubing falls below the level of the bed, the flow is slowed because the fluid must run uphill.
e. Adjusting the restraint.	e. If an extremity is restrained too snugly, the restraint acts as a tourniquet and the flow of solution will be slowed or stopped.
5. Irrigate the IV as necessary.	5. Irrigation may be required to dislodge small clots in the needle or to maintain the infusion rate of a sluggish IV.
a. Gather equipment:	
(1) Syringe with 1–3 ml. of normal saline	
(2) Several alcohol wipes	
b. Clamp off the IV solution.	
c. Disconnect the IV tubing at the needle insertion site. Keep it sterile.	
d. Remove the needle from the syringe.	
e. Connect the syringe to the tubing at the needle insertion site.	
f. Slowly inject the normal saline.	f. Great force of injector should be avoided as this may cause the vein to rupture or the needle to become dislodged from the vein.
g. Disconnect the syringe and reconnect the IV tubing to the needle insertion site.	
h. Unclamp the IV and regulate the flow of the solution.	
i. Check frequently to make certain that the IV is functioning properly.	
6. Change the IV bottle and tubing every 24 hours.	6. The IV set-up should be changed daily to maintain sterility and prevent contamination of the IV fluid during IV therapy.
7. If a catheter is used, change the dressing and apply an antibiotic ointment to the insertion site at least once every 24 hours.	7. This reduces the incidence of infection and other local complications.
8. Disconnect the IV when ordered or if it is obviously infiltrated.	
a. Gather equipment.	
(1) Scissors	
(2) 4 × 4 gauze square	
(3) Band-Aid	
b. Explain the procedure to the child, depending on his age.	
c. Clamp off the flow of the IV fluid.	
d. Determine the location of the needle.	

GUIDELINES: Intravenous Fluid Therapy (cont.)

Procedure (cont.)	NURSING ACTION	RATIONALE/AMPLIFICATION
	e. Loosen the tape around the needle, holding the needle firmly in position so that it does not slip out.	
	f. Hold the 4 × 4 lightly over the insertion site and remove the needle quickly and carefully.	f. Inspect an intracath or plastic needle to insure that no portion has been left in the vein. If this is suspected, notify the physician. Alcohol sponges should not be used for removing IV needles because the stinging of alcohol on the puncture site causes unnecessary discomfort.
	g. Apply pressure to the site immediately and hold until bleeding stops.	
	h. Apply Band-Aid.	h. The Band-Aid should not be applied until all bleeding has stopped to minimize the possibility of prolonged or unnoticed bleeding.
	i. Remove the tape and armboard from the extremity.	
	j. Comfort the child as required.	
	k. Note the fluid level on the bottle or reservoir and complete recordings.	
	l. Record that the IV was discontinued.	

For additional information relating to intravenous therapy, including criteria for selecting a suitable vein for venipuncture, guidelines for administering an infusion using the cubital fossa, and complications of intravenous therapy, refer to: The Patient Receiving Intravenous Therapy, pages 93–112.

INFUSION PUMPS

Infusion pumps are often used in pediatrics to provide a constant, slow rate of infusion. Several units are available and can be used with standard, commercial IV administration sets.

Types of Pumps

1. Peristaltic pumps—Move fluid by compressing IV tubing.
2. Piston and cylinder pumps—Move fluid by pushing it through a cylinder.

Indications for Use

1. When a constant rate of infusion is necessary, such as for administration of medication with a short half-life, (e.g., insulin, lidocaine, catecholamines)
2. When a constant volume must be assured per unit of time (e.g., prevention of volume overload in small infants, administration of parenteral hyperalimentation)
3. When patency of a vessel, usually an artery, must be preserved

Nursing Responsibilities

1. All nurses who operate a pump should be educated to do so correctly. Manufacturer's operating manuals and instruction sheets should be available.
2. Follow manufacturer's recommendations:
   a. In assembling equipment, initiating and maintaining infusion
   b. Before using an IV filter; some filters will blow out at infusion pump pressures, others can cause rate inaccuracies
   c. Before using a pump to infuse blood; some models can cause hemolysis
   d. In checking all parts of the pump frequently
3. Every hour, check:
   a. Delivery rate
   b. For infiltration, as many pumps will continue to infuse solution even if infiltration has occurred
4. Restart the pump promptly after it has been turned off to prevent the catheter from becoming clogged.
5. Turn off pump as soon as the infusion is completed. Failure to do so may damage some machines.
6. Be certain that the pump is tested for current leakage at least every 6 months to reduce electrical hazard.

GUIDELINES: Total Parenteral Nutrition (Hyperalimentation)

Hyperalimentation is a method of providing complete nutrition entirely by the intravenous route. It involves the infusion of hypertonic solutions of glucose, a nitrogen source, water, vitamins, minerals, and electrolytes at a constant rate.

Types of Hyperalimentation

1. *Central line TPN*: Infusion occurs through an indwelling catheter placed in the central vein, usually the superior vena cava. It is the method of choice for long-term therapy or if a high concentration of infused glucose (20–25 gm./100 ml.) is necessary.
2. *Peripheral line TPN*: Infusion occurs through a single needle set, catheter, or cutdown into a peripheral vein, usually in the scalp or extremities. It is the method of choice for intralipid infusion, but generally restricts infused glucose concentrations to 10–12 gm./100 ml.

Purpose To sustain life and promote growth in patients when oral or gastrointestinal tube intake is either impossible, potentially hazardous, or insufficient for an extended period of time.

1. The procedure has been used successfully in children with gastrointestinal diseases such as chronic diarrhea, malabsorption syndrome, bowel fistulas, esophageal atresia or obstruction, and omphalocele.
2. It is also useful when a child's condition produces excessive nutritional needs, as in the case of burns, neurosurgical procedures, major trauma, large wound infections, and cancer.
3. Hyperalimentation has been successful in the treatment of premature infants of very low weights and infants with malnutrition or failure to thrive.

Equipment   Hyperalimentation solution

The type, amount, and composition of the solution is prescribed by the physician.

The initial solution provides adequate daily fluid and minerals but less than optimal calories and nitrogen. The concentrations of caloric substances are increased daily over 3 to 5 days as the child tolerates higher glucose loads.

Micropore filter

IV extension tubing

Silastic catheter of appropriate size

Constant infusion pump

Acetone

Betadine

Benzoin

Antibacterial ointment

All of the equipment listed in the procedure for intravenous fluid therapy by cutdown method; see IV Fluid Therapy, cutdown method, page 1172.

Procedure—Central Line TPN

Nursing activities for all phases of the administration of hyperalimentation solution are the same as those specified in the procedure for intravenous fluid therapy, with the following additions:

NURSING ACTION	RATIONALE/AMPLIFICATION
Preparatory Phase	
1. Mix the components of the hyperalimentation solution under strict aseptic conditions. Culture each bottle to assure the adequacy of the technique.	1. It is essential to prevent microbial contamination of the infusate in order to protect the child from septicemia.
a. Mixing should be done in the pharmacy, using a closed system such as a laminar flow filtered air hood. Solutions should be prepared every 24 hours and refrigerated until used.	
b. In hospitals without a laminar flow system, a closed system for mixing the glucose and protein should be used.	b. This can be done safely by carefully following package directions and using the cleanest area possible for mixing.
Performance Phase	
1. Assist the physician with the insertion of the hyperalimentation catheter. This may involve obtaining equipment, positioning and restraining the child, etc.	
a. The hyperalimentation catheter should be inserted under sterile surgical conditions.	a. Violation of aseptic techniques at the time of insertion can result in overwhelming septicemia and death.
b. In infants and small children the vena cava is usually approached through one of the common facial, internal jugular, or (usually) external jugular veins. The free end of the catheter is passed through a subcutaneous tunnel and is anchored in place at the parietal scalp, (Fig. 37-7).	b. This prevents catheter displacement by the child's movements, and allows asepsis to be maintained away from the child's oral and nasal secretions.
Follow-up Phase	
1. Until x-ray confirmation of the location of the catheter tip, infuse only isotonic solutions at a slow, "keep open" rate.	1. A chest x-ray confirms proper placement of the line and rules out complications such as pneumothorax or hemothorax which may be associated with catheter insertion. Infusing an isotonic solution minimizes the possibility of complications arising from the infusion of solution through a misplaced catheter.
2. Do not use the catheter for the administration of medications or for blood sampling.	2. This increases the risk of infections and the possibility of dislodging the catheter.
3. Check the infusion rate every ½–1 hour to make certain that the solution is infused continuously and at a constant rate.	3. Continuous infusion is necessary to prevent such metabolic complications as osmotic diuresis, hypoglycemia, and pulmonary edema.
a. Use a constant-infusion pump	
b. Reset the rate to that prescribed by the physician as necessary, but do not slow or increase the drip to make up for an excess or deficit without consulting the physician.	b. Increasing the rate may cause hyperglycemia with osmotic diuresis. Slowing the rate may cause hypoglycemia.

GUIDELINES: Total Parenteral Nutrition (Hyperalimentation) (cont.)

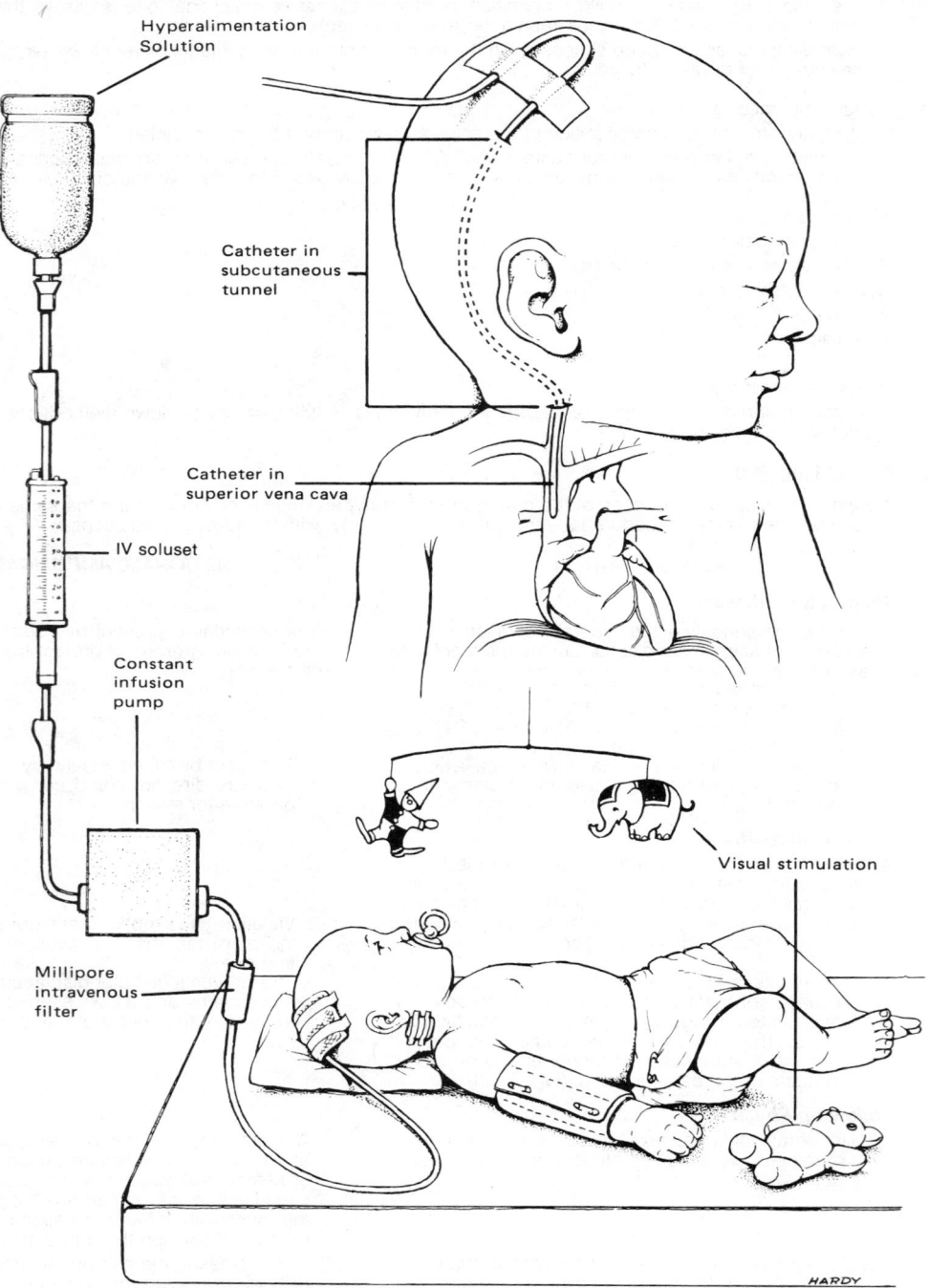

Hyperalimentation
Solution

Catheter in
subcutaneous
tunnel

Catheter in
superior vena cava

IV soluset

Constant
infusion
pump

Visual stimulation

Millipore
intravenous
filter

HARDY

FIGURE 37-7. *Hyperalimentation.*

Procedure (cont.)

NURSING ACTION	RATIONALE/AMPLIFICATION

4. Change the bottle, tubing, and filter at least once each day.

   a. Remove the tape which secures the filter to the dressing.
   b. Attach a new infusion set to the new bottle.
   c. Prime tubing and tap the end gently.
   d. Connect the infusion set to the new filter housing carefully.
   e. Hang the new bottle on the pole.
   f. Remove the protective covering from the distal end of the filter and discard.
   g. Hold the filter parallel to the floor and run solution through the entire line.
   h. Gently tap the filter housing to dispel air and tap the end to free glucose droplets. Be careful not to contaminate the end of the filter.
   i. Change the IV line at the catheter union rapidly with the patient flat in bed or in low Fowler's position. Use a sterile Kelly clamp to grasp the catheter hub for leverage during the tubing change.
   j. Anchor the filter to the dressing.
   k. Cleanse all connection sites with Betadine, allow to dry, and wrap with sterile 2 × 2 gauze pads.
   l. Secure all IV tubing joints with adhesive tape.

   m. Readjust flow rate.
   n. Write time and date on new tubing.
   o. Culture the filter each time it is changed.

4. This is another attempt to prevent contamination and reduce the possibility that the child will develop infection.

   b. Prep each connecting point with Betadine.
   c. This dislodges any glucose droplets.
   d. Avoid contamination of the filter.

   g. This position allows for complete filling of the filter housing.
   h. Air bubbles will cause difficulty in maintaining constant flow.

   i. This technique minimizes the danger of air embolism. Using a Kelly clamp helps reduce traction on the catheter and the chance of dislocation.

   j. This prevents tension on the catheter.

   l. This prevents accidental separation of the tubing from the catheter and prevents air embolus.

   o. It is possible, by culturing the filter, to detect microbial contamination prior to the development of clinical signs. Cultures should include fungal studies since a special danger of hyperalimentation is fungal septicemia.

5. Change the dressing around the catheter at least 3 times each week, using strict aseptic technique. Face masks should be worn by all persons at the head of the bed to prevent airborne contamination of the insertion site by nasopharyngeal organisms. If possible, the child should also wear a mask and turn his head away from the dressing.
   a. Remove the dressing carefully.

   b. Using acetone or ether on a sterile 4 by 4 inch gauze square, scrub a large area surrounding the insertion site. Move in a circular motion from the center to the periphery.
   c. Paint the skin with Betadine solution.
   d. Apply a prescribed antibacterial ointment directly to the catheter insertion site and 2–3 cm. down the catheter.
   e. Apply a small dressing around the catheter. Using sterile scissors, cut a slit in the lower piece of a small nonadhering dressing, enabling it to fit around the catheter at the insertion site.
   f. Apply benzoin to the area where tape will be applied.
   g. Apply sterile dressings.

   h. Cover the entire sterile dressing and the union of the catheter and tubing with 5 cm. (2 inch) adhesive tape.
   i. If the dressing is exposed to moisture such as tracheal secretions or humidified oxygen, protect it with a plastic adhesive.
   j. Record the dressing change, how the child tolerated the procedure, and any relevant condition.

5. This reduces the possibility of infection at the catheter site.

   a. Extreme care is necessary to avoid dislodging the catheter.
   b. This removes surface skin fats that might harbor organisms and removes remaining traces of adhesive tape that have adhered to the skin.

   f. Even nonirritating tape may produce damage to the underlying skin with prolonged use.
   g. In infants and small children, the catheter is coiled to reduce tension on the site, and a small, sterile gauze sponge is applied. A generous length of the catheter is left to facilitate head and body movements without undue tension on the catheter. In older children, the entire catheter is included in the dressing.
   h. This provides a totally occlusive dressing. Neither the sterile dressing nor the tubing union is exposed to air.
   i. In this situation, use paper tape to secure all tubing connections and anchor the filter, because adhesive will tear holes in plastic.
   j. Consider condition of the skin, drainage, catheter placement, placement of needle guard, and presence of suture.

GUIDELINES: Total Parenteral Nutrition (Hyperalimentation) (cont.)

Procedure (cont.)

NURSING ACTION	RATIONALE/AMPLIFICATION
6. In infants with a cutdown site on the neck, change the dressing as needed, using aseptic technique. Discontinue the dressing when the wound is healed.	6. Since this site is closest to the vascular bed, it should be observed closely for signs of infection. Wound sepsis can easily lead to bacteremia.
7. Monitor fractional urines for glucose and acetone every 6 hours. Report any glucosuria to the physician.	7. Some children require supplemental parenteral insulin to utilize the required amount of infused glucose. Children receiving certain drugs may show false positive results. Positive urine sugars are confirmed by blood glucose levels.
8. Keep an accurate record of the child's total intake and output, including bowel movements, emesis, and gastric drainage. If the child is allowed oral intake, a calorie count should be kept.	8. This helps to provide a clear picture of the child's fluid and electrolyte balance.
9. Monitor the child's weight daily. Weigh at the same time each day, with the same amount of clothing, and on the same scales.	9. Weight gain is one of the most reliable indications of a positive response to therapy.
10. In infants, measure length and head circumference weekly.	10. Hyperalimentation promotes growth in these dimensions.
11. Observe for signs of complications resulting from therapy. a. Complications related to the catheter: (1) Septicemia (2) Thrombosis of a major blood vessel (3) Plugging or dislodging of the catheter (4) Local skin infection (5) Cardiac arrhythmia (6) Leak around catheter or hole in catheter (7) Air embolism b. Metabolic Complications (1) Hyperglycemia (2) Hypoglycemia (3) Dehydration (4) Metabolic acidosis (5) Electrolyte imbalances (6) Amino acid imbalance (7) Postinfusion hypoglycemia	a. Three-fourths of the major complications of therapy are of this variety. Sepsis accounts for more than half of these problems. b. Careful clinical and chemical monitoring, especially during the initial period of hyperalimentation, can greatly reduce the incidence of these types of complications.
12. Provide mouth care. a. If allowed, use a variety of mouthwashes to provide some change in taste. b. Apply lip balm flavored with fruit or mint. c. Offer crushed ice flavored with juice or syrup.	12. In patients who are NPO, the tongue, throat, and mouth tend to become dry, inflamed and uncomfortable. The total absence of taste is unpleasant for older children.
13. Provide the infant with a pacifier.	13. It is especially important to meet the sucking needs of the infant since hyperalimentation therapy may be necessary for several weeks or months.
14. Discontinue the infusion when directed to do so by the physician. (In many hospitals this is the responsibility of the physician.) a. Turn the flow rate off. b. Remove the dressings. c. Cut and remove the stay suture. d. Pull the catheter out. e. Apply pressure with a sterile 4 by 4 inch gauze for a minute or two. f. Cover the site with a Band-Aid. g. Record time and date procedure was discontinued, by whom, cultures sent, and child's condition. h. Send the tip of the catheter, the filter, and the fluid in the tubing for culture.	14. The child is gradually tapered off from hyperalimentation to allow for adjustment to decreased levels of glucose. Final cessation is often followed by isotonic glucose infusion for at least 12 hours to protect against rebound hypoglycemia from still high insulin levels. During the weaning process, the child's oral intake is gradually increased as the hyperalimentation solution is proportionally decreased.

Procedure—Peripheral Line TPN

Nursing activities are essentially the same as for central line TPN although dressing changes are not indicated. However, peripheral sites should be checked and cared for at regular intervals to avoid infiltration and vascular inflammation. For additional information, refer to the following procedure for the administration of intralipids.

GUIDELINES: Intralipids—Intravenous Fat Emulsion

(See adult, pp. 409.)

Purpose   Used in conjunction with partial parenteral (peripheral) nutrition (PPN) as an additional source of calories and fatty acids.

Equipment   *Intralipid 10% fat emulsion—Isotonic emulsion composed of 10% soybean oil (a triglyceride), 1.2% egg yolk phospholipids, 2.2% glycerin and water for injection. Total caloric value is 1.1 calorie/ml. Intralipid 10%.

Antiseptic wipe	Constant infusion pump
IV tubing and sterile needle	Tape
Complete infusion IV line	

Procedure   Nursing activities for the administration of Intralipid 10% are the same as those specified in the procedure for intravenous fluid therapy and total parenteral nutrition, with the following exceptions.

NURSING ACTION	RATIONALE/AMPLIFICATION
Preparatory Phase	
1. Prior to therapeutic administration of Intralipid 10%, a test dose of 0.1 ml./min. (10 mg.) is given in 10–15 minutes; afterwards, the rate is increased to permit 1gm./kg. to run over 4 hours.	1. To identify any sensitivity the child may have to the emulsion
a. Observe for immediate reactions of dyspnea, flushing, rash, sweating, sleepiness, headache, tachycardia, bradycardia, acidosis in infants.	**NURSING ALERT:** Treatment of premature and low-birth-weight infants with IV fat emulsions must be based upon careful evaluation of the potential benefits weighed against the potential risks of fat accumulation in the lungs.†
b. Should any of these signs appear, stop infusion and notify physician.	
2. Ensure that prescribed lab studies are done prior to commencement of test dose, i.e., cholesterol, triglycerides, platelets baseline. Once testing has been accomplished, Intralipid 10% is administered as part of PPN.	2. To serve as baseline before test dose.
3. Ensure that nothing is added to emulsion, (i.e., drugs, electrolytes, vitamins, or other nutrients).	3. May cause lipid to separate or cause a fat embolus.
4. Be aware of conditions that may contraindicate the use of Intralipid 10%—sepsis, hyperbilirubinemia, severe respiratory distress.	4. Prevent further compromise of the child: Fat is taken up by the reticuloendothelial system; it displaces bilirubin from albumin and can plug small vessels in the lungs.
Performance Phase	
1. Once the IV lines have been purged with the emulsion, connect the line to the existing peripheral or central line via piggyback or Y-connector just proximal to the infusion site. Tape connection. Do not pass solution through a bacterial filter, as this can clog filter and break down emulsion.	1. Infuse emulsion as a separate line that is added into the existing IV. The emulsion is administered in the self-contained solution bottle from manufacturer, syringe, and tubing or pediatric infusion set. The emulsion is not added to the TPN solution bottle so as to avoid disturbing the stability of the emulsion. It is administered with another fluid to decrease the high concentration of fat.
2. Administer emulsion using separate continuous flow pump from that of PPN. (Pumps with electric eye may not be effective due to the opaque solution).	2. Allows flow rate of each solution to be controlled independently.
3. Monitor hourly the amount of emulsion infused.	3. To control fluid intake. Emulsion can be infused continuously or in 4–5 separate doses over 2- to 4-hour time periods.

4. Change bottle and tubing:
  a. Intermittent administration—each administration
  b. Continuous administration—every 8 hours.
	4. To assist in preventing infection

Follow-up Phase	
1. Once prescribed emulsion has been infused, discontinue. Check to be sure there is no leaking at point where connection was made.	1. To prevent infection and inaccurate account of fluid intake as a result of the line being violated.
2. Record time procedure was discontinued, by whom, amount given, and child's condition.	

* Cutter laboratories
† Levene MI, Wigglesworth JS, Desai R. Pulmonary fat accumulation after intralipid infusion in preterm infant. Lancet 8199:815–818, 1980

GUIDELINES: Intralipids—Intravenous Fat Emulsion (cont.)

Procedure (cont.)	NURSING ACTION	RATIONALE/AMPLIFICATION
	3. Ensure that prescribed laboratory studies are done at designated times—usually 2–6 hours after emulsion is discontinued or weekly, (i.e., lipid and triglyceride levels.)	3. To see if fat has been metabolized and utilized and to detect any early signs of complications.
	4. Continue to observe child for any delayed adverse reactions: hepatomegaly, splenomegaly, thrombocytopenia, transient increase in liver function tests, system overload.	4. To detect any early signs of complications in addition to physical assessment of the child, serum studies may include: liver function, bilirubin, alkaline phosphatase, CBC or platelet count.

PEDIATRIC HOME HYPERALIMENTATION

Home hyperalimentation programs have been developed to provide an alternative to hospitalization for children who require long-term TPN.

Benefits of Home Hyperalimentation

1. The child is able to maintain a more normal lifestyle in his home environment.
2. Stress is reduced for the child and his family.
3. Cost is greatly reduced.

Resources Necessary for an Effective Program

1. A pharmacy to prepare the solution
2. A physician available to deal with problems
3. A reliable microchemistry laboratory
4. Someone to deal with equipment procurement, maintenance, and problems
5. An insurance agency willing to cooperate with such a program
6. Effective community health nursing support

Criteria for Determining Family Readiness and Ability to Cope with Home TPN

1. Does the family comfortably participate in the technical procedures in the hospital?
2. Do the parents state a desire to perform the TPN procedure in the home?
3. Do the parents respond to cues from the child and deal with them appropriately?
4. Do the parents interact effectively with the child by providing nurturing care and comfort measures, which they will have to continue at home?
5. Do parents have support from the nuclear and extended family in conducting home TPN?
6. Are community support systems available?

Health Education

1. Explain the principles and concepts of TPN.
2. Instruct parents concerning the methods, procedures, and prevention of complications of TPN administration.
3. Demonstrate TPN procedures to the parents.
4. Have parents demonstrate their ability to perform TPN procedures.
5. Encourage parents to carry out complete care of TPN until the child is discharged.
6. Provide means for continued education and problem solving during home TPN.
7. Evaluate treatment and follow-up.

GUIDELINES: Assisting with Exchange Transfusion

Exchange transfusion is replacement of circulating blood by withdrawing blood and injecting donor's blood in equal amounts.

Purposes

1. To prevent accumulation of bilirubin in the blood above a dangerous level.
2. To prevent kernicterus (brain damage—occurs when there is yellow staining of brain tissue from deposits of indirect bilirubin).
3. To prevent accumulation of other by-products of hemolysis from hemolytic disease, i.e., ABO incompatibility.
4. To raise a very low hemoglobin.
5. To replace red blood cells which have poor oxygen releasing capacity and poor carbonic anhydrase activity, i.e., as in a premature infant.
6. To remove toxic metabolites.

Equipment

Fresh donor blood
Monitoring equipment
Sterile disposable exchange transfusion set containing:
  Stopcock with extension tubing
  Extra extension tubing
  Umbilical catheters sizes 5 and 8, French
  2 20-ml. syringes
  1 5-ml. syringe and No. 23-gauge needle
  Waste-blood container
  Blood administration set

Gauze sponges
Transfusion record
Cleansing solution
Means of warming infant
Means of warming blood
Calcium gluconate in 5-ml. syringe
50% glucose solution in 10-ml. syringe
Sodium bicarbonate in 10-ml. syringe
Sterile gown and gloves for physician
Resuscitative equipment

Procedure

NURSING ACTION	RATIONALE/AMPLIFICATION

Preparatory Phase

1. Place infant under heat lamps or radiant heating unit to keep his temperature within the thermoneutral zone. Environment temperature of 32° C. (86° F.) will usually maintain correct infant body temperature, depending on size of infant.

1. Chilling of the infant during the procedure can result in apnea and in increased caloric need and oxygen consumption, which can be exhausting to a baby with already limited amount of energy. Abnormal decrease in blood pH leading to acidosis can result from the stress of prolonged chilling. Hypothermia may also hinder albumin and bilirubin binding capacity.

2. If the infant has not been NPO for 3–4 hours it may be necessary to empty stomach content via stomach tube.

2. To prevent aspiration, should vomiting occur during the procedure.

3. Albumin (1gm./kg.) may be given 1–2 hours prior to exchange transfusion.

3. The albumin may increase the effectiveness of the transfusion by yielding more bilirubin binding sites.

4. Attach electronic cardiac monitoring device to infant if available. Otherwise place stethoscope over apex of heart. Also attach temperature monitoring device. Monitor continuously.

4. Apnea, bradycardia, and cardiac arrest are complications of an exchange transfusion. Close monitoring will allow for immediate observation of signs of trouble.

5. Place infant on his back. Restrain all 4 extremities.

5. This will prevent the infant from moving and inadvertently pulling out the exchange catheter.

6. Have resuscitative equipment ready for immediate use: oxygen supply, mask, intubation equipment, laryngoscope, breathing bag, suction, sodium bicarbonate, and 50% glucose solution.

6. Should the infant develop bradycardia, hypoglycemia, or cyanosis during procedure, these items will be necessary for immediate and supportive treatment.

7. Check donor blood for type, age, and other identifying data. Check blood pH. It should be corrected to pH 7.1 or as specified by physician.

7. Heparinized blood must be used within 24 hours of collection. Optimal age of ACD (heparin, acid-citrate-dextrose) or CPD (citrate-phosphate-dextrose) blood is less than 3 days old. CPD lasts longer—has better carbonic anhydrase level. Acidemia may result when fresh blood is not used due to the acid metabolites. Cardiac arrest may also occur from elevated potassium in donor blood.

8. Assist the physician in setting up blood and exchange equipment. Blood should be run through a coil of tubing through a water bath at 38° C., (100° F.). Ensure that lines and connections are securely closed.

8. Although hypothermia, i.e., rapid chilling of the infant, is a primary concern, increased blood viscosity and ventricular fibrillation can also result from administering cold blood.

Performance Phase

1. The infant's skin is cleansed with soap and water followed by an antiseptic solution. Sterile drapes are applied by the physician who is gowned and gloved. Strict attention should be paid to maintaining aseptic technique.

1. To prevent infection or sepsis. A foreign body introduced into the blood vessel is always a potential for infection due to an infected cord stump or contaminated equipment.
   The unbilicus can be grossly contaminated and is impossible to sterilize.

2. Once the umbilical catheter is in place in the umbilical vein, the initial venous pressure is measured (although it is not usually accurate) and the exchange is begun. (Preferred site is the umbilical vein; jugular or femoral vessels may be used.)

2. Record the venous pressure. This will be maintained at about 10–12 cm. by equal volume exchanges. An increase in pressure during the procedure is an indication to stop and assess the infant.

3. Note and record the time the exchange started. Record each successive withdrawal and infusion of blood stating exact amount and time. Report to the physician when each 100 ml. of blood is exchanged. (See Record Chart, p. 1184.)
   This will prevent system overload from excessive infusion—resulting in cardiac failure and shock from too-rapid removal of infant's blood.

3. Blood is exchanged slowly in amounts of 5–20 ml., depending on the infant's size and condition. The total amount exchanged is about 170 ml. of blood/kilogram of body weight (80 ml./pound). About 75–93% of the infant's total blood volume is exchanged.
   The exchange should take about an hour. Rapid exchange can aggravate cardiovascular changes and prevent normal metabolism of infused acid and citrate.

4. After each 100 ml. of blood is exchanged, 0.5–1.0 ml. 10% calcium gluconate is injected to prevent hypocalcemia. Blood-bank donor blood is calcium-deficient. Monitor cardiac rate very carefully during the injection.

4. Calcium decreases the irritability and irregularity of the heart. Too rapid an injection will cause bradycardia.

5. Constant monitoring of the cardiac rate is imperative. Also note respirations, skin color, and color of withdrawn blood.
   Keep transfusion lines tightly secured to prevent air embolus or exsanguination.

5. Observation and monitoring will allow immediate treatment if untoward signs appear. Bradycardia may occur at any time during the procedure due to a low pH of donor blood or old blood.

6. Protamine sulfate may be given after the transfusion is completed.

6. Because heparinized blood will affect the coagulation potential of the infant from 4–6 hours postexchange.

GUIDELINES: Assisting with Exchange Transfusion (cont.)

EXCHANGE TRANSFUSION RECORD

HOSPITAL NO. _____

DATE OF DELIVERY: *8-29-81*

NAME OF BABY: *Johnson, Clarence David*

TIME: *4:10 am*

NAME OF MOTHER: *Marsha Johnson*

APGAR SCORE AT DELIVERY: *8 at 1 min / 9 at 5 min*

BIRTH WEIGHT: *3580 grams*

INITIAL HEMOGLOBIN: *42*

BLOOD GROUP: *O pos*

BILIRUBIN: *16.3*

TIME COMMENCING EXCHANGE: *3:45 pm*

POST-EXCHANGE BILIRUBIN: *11.8*

TIME FINISHING EXCHANGE: *4:17 pm*

AGE OF BABY IN HOURS: *30*

TIME	OUT		IN		PULSE	RESPI-RATION	VENOUS PRESSURE	MEDI-CATION	COMMENTS
	Amount	Total	Amount	Total					
3:45	20	20	20	20					
3:48	20	40	20	40					
3:51	20	60	20	60					
3:55	20	80	20	80					
3:58	20	100	20	100	150	48		Ca 1ml	
4:02	20	120	20	120					
4:06	20	140	20	140					
4:10	20	160	20	160					
4:13	20	180	20	180					
4:17	20	200	20	200	160	56			

Procedure (cont.)	NURSING ACTION	RATIONALE/AMPLIFICATION

Follow-up Phase

1. When transfusion is completed, umbilical catheter may be:
   a. Left in place with an IV plug or intravenous infusion or
   b. Removed.

1. If catheter is left in place, it is usually done for future exchange transfusions, easy withdrawal of blood for blood studies, administration of intravenous fluids and medications. Keep infant restrained. If catheter is removed, apply small pressure dressing and observe for any bleeding. Check the area every hour for 3 hours, then every 3 hours for 24 hours.

2. Finish charting by recording accurately:
   a. Time transfusion was completed
   b. Total amount blood withdrawn and infused
   c. Any changes in vital signs
   d. Medications administered during exchange
   e. Infant's color and current vital signs
   f. Catheter removed or left indwelling
   g. How infant tolerated the procedure
   h. Any blood samples taken before or after exchange

3. Monitor infant for any signs of post-exchange transfusion complications:
   a. Hypoglycemia—Dextrostix test every hour × 4.

   a. Hypoglycemia frequently occurs with erythroblastosis fetalis. Incidence is also increased because of fasting prior to and during procedure.
   b. Hemolytic reaction.
   b. Reaction from donor blood.
   c. Thrombocytopenia and hemorrhage. Check for bleeding at catheter site and petechiae.
   c. This results from overheparinized blood or when citrated blood is given without calcium replacement.
   d. Intestinal perforation. Observe for bloody stools, bile-stained vomitus, abdominal distention, respiratory distress, pallor.
   d. Ischemia of bowel.
   e. Metabolic acidosis. Observe for deep, increased respirations; decreased consciousness; acid' urine.
   e. Resulting from old donor blood.

THE CHILD UNDERGOING DIALYSIS

Dialysis refers to the process of separating substances in solution by the differences in their rates of diffusion through a semipermeable membrane. Dialysis is used in the treatment of renal failure to remove uremic toxins from the body fluids by allowing blood to equilibrate across a semi-permeable membrane with fluids lacking these toxins.

Purpose

To preserve life by acting as a substitute for kidney function during renal failure.
1. Aids in the removal of toxic substances and metabolic wastes.
2. Removes excessive body fluid.
3. Assists in regulating the body's fluid and electrolyte balance.

Types of Dialysis

A. *Peritoneal Dialysis*
1. Mechanism
   a. The peritoneal lining is used as the semipermeable membrane.
   b. A catheter is inserted through the anterior abdominal wall and the dialysate is instilled into the abdominal cavity.
   c. After an equilibration time (about 30 minutes), the fluid is drained by gravity and fresh dialysate is instilled.
2. Major uses
   a. Acute, reversible uremic episodes such as those due to sudden illness, trauma, poisoning, or drug intoxication.
   b. In terminal illness, to keep the child comfortable for as long as possible.
   c. Prior to acceptance in a long-term hemodialysis and transplantation program.
   d. In selected cases of chronic renal failure.
      The child is dialyzed at night through a semipermanently implanted abdominal cannula by an automatic, continually recycling machine.
3. Advantage
   Relatively safe and readily available.
4. Disadvantages
   a. Long periods of time required to effectively remove waste products.
   b. May cause abdominal pain and discomfort.
   c. Sterile dialysate is required.
   d. Complications
      (1) Peritonitis
      (2) Bowel perforation during insertion of the catheter
      (3) Respiratory distress caused by upward displacement of the diaphragm by fluid in the peritoneal cavity
      (4) Shock due to excessive fluid loss
      (5) Protein loss because serum proteins pass through the peritoneal membrane during dialysis
      (6) Bleeding and leakage at the catheter insertion site

(7) Inadequate fluid return
(8) Nausea, vomiting, diarrhea

B. *Hemodialysis*

1. Mechanism
   a. The semipermeable membrane is located in a machine through which the child's blood is directed.
   b. Access to the circulation is provided via a Teflon-Silastic arteriovenous shunt or a subcutaneously implanted arteriovenous fistula.
   c. The child's blood is diverted through the machine adjacent to the semipermeable membrane to equilibrate with dialysate on the other side of the membrane.
   d. Selection of the dialyzer depends on the size of the child. Considerations include:
      (1) Amount of blood the machine holds relative to the amount that the child can safely spare from the body at one time.
      (2) Efficiency of the machine relative to the child's weight.
      (3) Speed with which fluid can be removed by the machine.

   NOTE: Dialysis can be dangerous if it is too rapid.

2. Major Uses
   a. Long-term therapy for chronic renal failure.
   b. Holding procedure prior to kidney transplant.
3. Advantages
   a. Shorter period of time required to effectively remove waste products (about 4 times more efficient).
   b. Does not require sterile dialysate.
   c. Is less traumatic to initiate once access to the circulation is made.
   d. Home dialysis is available in selected situations.
4. Disadvantages
   a. Is costly.
   b. There are inherent moral, legal, logistical, and technical problems.
   c. Complications
      (1) Clotting, infection, accidental separation of shunt
      (2) Anemia—because a small amount of blood remains behind in the machine with each run
      (3) Malaise, headache, nausea, and vomiting during dialysis
      (4) Hepatitis due to transfusions necessitated by uremic anemia
      (5) Rickets, growth failure, and delayed or absent sexual maturation

GUIDELINES: Caring for the Child Undergoing Dialysis

Nursing Care

NURSING ACTION	RATIONALE/AMPLIFICATION

1. Prepare the child for the procedure.
  a. Explain the procedure to the child in terms that he can understand.
    (1) Allow the child to handle equipment similar to that which will be used during dialysis.
    (2) Encourage the child to express his fears so that misinterpretations can be corrected.
    (3) Provide simple pictures and diagrams, if appropriate.
    (4) Allow the child to talk with peers who have undergone dialysis.
  b. Explain the procedure to the family and answer questions so that they will be in the best position to support their child.
	1. Dialysis is threatening to most children and may evoke fears of pain, mutilation, immobilization, helplessness, and dependency. Many children have fears of losing all of their blood in this process. A child who is well prepared will be less frightened and better able to cooperate during the procedure.

2. Protect the child from infection.
  a. Keep the dressings and area around the catheter or shunt clean and dry.
  b. Use aseptic technique throughout the dialysis procedure.
  c. Avoid exposure to children or adults with infection.
  d. Provide supplemental vitamins since a protein-restricted diet is poor in vitamins.
  e. Provide meticulous daily hygiene.
	2. These children are prone to infection because of their general debilitated state and because of protein loss and anemia.

3. Provide a high calorie diet which is low in sodium and protein. Since the child often experiences anorexia, it may be helpful to allow him to choose foods from his allowances and offer small, frequent meals.	3. Calorie intake is increased since growth failure is observed in children while on dialysis. Sodium and protein are limited to prevent the blood pressure and BUN from going too high between dialyses. The child may see dietary restrictions as punishment and must be helped to realize the purpose of the restrictions.
4. Maintain careful records of intake and output, vital signs, blood pressure, and daily weights.	4. These provide valuable information about the effectiveness of the therapy.

Procedure

NURSING ACTION	RATIONALE/AMPLIFICATION

5. Support the child during the dialysis procedure.
  a. Provide symptomatic relief of nausea, vomiting, malaise, or headache.
    Notify the physician if these symptoms are severe.
  b. Be alert to clues from the child for helpful methods of offering support.
    (1) Young children often cling to stuffed toys or blankets or depend on parent's presence at the bedside.
    (2) Older children may benefit from radio, television, magazines, or contact with peers.	

6. Provide an environment that is as normal as possible.
  a. Encourage the family to bring in articles that will make the child's room appear more homelike, i.e., pictures, posters, etc.
  b. Encourage the child to be as independent as possible in his daily care.
  c. Provide for age-appropriate recreation and/or diversion.
  d. Help the child to keep up with his school work by initiating a referral to a tutor, providing study times, etc.
	6. Although life is preserved, it is by no means normal during the time on dialysis or between dialyses. These measures may increase the child's feeling of self-esteem and diminish regression and social isolation. By serving as role models, health professionals may encourage parents to recognize and foster the normal, healthy aspects of the child's daily life.

7. Offer appropriate support to the family.
  a. Provide opportunity for family members to discuss their feelings, fears, and frustrations and to ask questions.
  b. Allow family members to become involved in the child's care to the extent that they wish and that is helpful for the child and family.
  c. Provide for continuity of personnel.
  d. Initiate appropriate referrals. These may include referrals to a social worker, psychiatrist, dietitian, community health agency, other families who are coping with dialysis.
	7. Families often need extensive support from many health professionals to cope with the physical, psychological, financial, and logistical aspects of renal failure and dialysis. Attention must be focused on siblings as well as parents since sibling relationships are often strained and difficult.

8. Teach the child and family about all of the important aspects of renal failure and dialysis, including:
  a. Signs and symptoms of uremia
  b. Shunt care and protection
  c. Protection from infection
  d. Dietary restrictions and recommendations; ways of incorporating the special diet into the family meal plan
  e. Dialysis schedule
  f. Medications
  g. Emergency procedures
	8. The family should be prepared to care for the child at home well before the day of discharge. Learning about the child's care also helps restore some sense of control in a frightening situation.

Peritoneal Dialysis: Specific Nursing Responsibilities

Refer to Guidelines: Assisting the Patient Undergoing Peritoneal Dialysis, pages 494–497. In addition, the following principles should be considered by the nurse working with pediatric patients.

1. Because of the child's smaller size, the volume of dialysate required is less. Generally, 1000 ml. of dialysate is instilled at one time.
2. Because the child may be unable to hold still, it may be necessary to apply protective measures to limit motion in order to avoid contamination of the sterile field or injury to the child. (See p. 1154.)
3. Because of the possibility of nausea and vomiting, oral intake should be limited to ice chips and small amounts of fluids during the first 12–24 hours of dialysis. Frequent mouth care should be provided.
4. Because the child may develop fears and fantasies about the equipment, it should be stored out of sight when not in use.

Hemodialysis: Specific Nursing Responsibilities

1. Care for the arteriovenous shunt. (Refer to Guidelines, p. 1188.)
2. Assist in teaching the child and/or family proper care and protection of the shunt.
3. When possible, avoid giving subcutaneous or intramuscular injections because the child is anticoagulated with heparin at least twice weekly during dialysis and extensive bleeding could occur as a result of such injections.
4. Care for the child during dialysis. (This aspect of nursing care is not presented since it is generally provided by specially trained personnel in a dialysis unit.)

GUIDELINES: Care of the Arteriovenous Shunt

Purpose To preserve shunt function and prevent separation of the cannulas.

Equipment 2 shunt clips
Dressing tray with:
  2 sterile plastic basins
  Sterile 2 × 2-inch sponges
  Sterile 4 × 3-inch sponges
  Kling bandage
  Hydrogen peroxide
  Alcohol
  Antibiotic ointment
  Sterile applicators
  Sterile scissors
  Mask
  Sterile gloves

Procedure

NURSING ACTION	RATIONALE/AMPLIFICATION
1. Place shunt clips on the dressing and keep with the child at all times.	1. The clamps are used to close the shunt in case it separates at its connection.
2. Use another extremity for:	2. Disturbing the shunt in any way can encourage clotting and infection.
a. Taking blood pressure	a. Inflation of blood pressure cuff may precipitate clotting by slowing the flow of blood through the tubing.

b. Giving medications
  c. Giving infusions
  d. Taking blood samples.
	b, c. Injections in the extremity increase the possibility of thrombosis of the vein.
	  d. A rubber puncture site may be added to the shunt. This can be punctured with a needle to obtain blood specimens.

NOTE: The silastic tubing should never be punctured since it will not seal.

NURSING ACTION	RATIONALE/AMPLIFICATION
3. Cleanse the area around the shunt and change the dressing daily or p.r.n. a. Remove old dressing.	a. Never use scissors to remove the dressing so as to avoid accidentally cutting the cannulas.
b. Observe the shunt for malalignment or kinks.	b. These factors increase the possibility of clot formation and must be corrected.
c. Observe the area around the cannula insertion sites for signs of inflammation (redness, swelling, drainage).	c. If noted, report signs of inflammation, and take culture before cleansing the area.
d. Using aseptic technique, clean the venous insertion site first with hydrogen peroxide and then with alcohol. Take new swabs and clean the arterial site in the same manner.	d. Do not use the same swabs to clean both sites as this may cause cross-infection.
e. Apply an antibiotic ointment to the insertion sites, using a new sterile applicator for each application. f. Apply dry sterile dressing to the areas of cannula insertion.	f. A 2 × 2 gauze pad under the cannula at each insertion site will lessen tension at the site and increase comfort.
g. Wrap arm with compression bandage firmly, but not tightly, leaving a small section of the shunt in view. h. Retape shunt clips to outer dressing in full view.	g. Leave a section small enough that it cannot be pulled out by the child. If protective devices to limit movement are indicated, apply below the shunt.

4. Check frequently for shunt obstruction.
  a. Use stethoscope or place fingertips on area between cannula insertion points to detect bruit.
  b. Observe child for signs of pain in the extremity.
  c. Observe color of blood in tubing.
	a. Presence of bruit indicates free flow of blood through shunt.
	
	  c. Blood should appear smooth and should be of uniform color. Fibrin may appear as white specks along the cannula wall.

d. Report clotting immediately to the physician.	d. Clotting is indicated by separation of blood, i.e., presence of a darkened clot and clear serum. The shunt feels cool rather than warm to the touch. Delay in declotting may necessitate replacement of the entire shunt.
5. Be prepared for emergency action if the shunt should separate or the cannula should become dislodged. a. Identify source of bleeding by unwrapping bandage.	5. These are emergency situations which may result in severe hemorrhage and possible exsanguination.

Procedure (cont.)	NURSING ACTION	RATIONALE/AMPLIFICATION

NURSING ACTION

b. Separation of shunt:
  (1) Clamp tubes with shunt clips and rejoin shunt—or
  (2) Pinch off tubes with fingers and rejoin shunt.
c. Dislodgment of arterial or venous cannula:
  (1) Apply firm pressure over bleeding cannula site and clamp remaining cannula.
  (2) Notify physician.
6. Teach the child and parents how to care for the shunt.
  a. Dressing changes and cleansing of area around shunt.
  b. Observation for signs of inflammation, infection, obstruction.
  c. Bathing
    (1) Some children are permitted to bathe the shunted extremity, soaping the area at the beginning and at the end of the shower or bath.
    (2) Swimming may be permitted if the extremity is completely protected with a waterproof covering.
  d. Prevention of clotting.
    (1) Avoid constricting clothing which may impair blood flow through the shunt.
    (2) Avoid keeping the extremity acutely flexed for long periods of time.
    (3) Avoid sleeping on the shunted arm.
  e. Emergency measures in case of accidental separation or dislodging of the cannula.

RATIONALE/AMPLIFICATION

c. These activities are allowed at the discretion of the individual physician.

CHEST PHYSICAL THERAPY AND RESPIRATORY MEASURES

GUIDELINES: Promoting Postural Drainage in the Pediatric Patient

Postural drainage is the positioning of the patient so that gravity will assist in the movement of secretions from the smaller bronchial airways to the main bronchus and trachea, from which the secretions can be removed by coughing or suctioning.

Procedure

NURSING ACTION

Preparatory Phase

1. Assess the child's respiratory status.
  a. Obtain a baseline respiratory rate.
  b. Observe for respiratory distress, retractions, nasal flaring, etc.
2. Identify the involved portion(s) of the lung by auscultation, percussion, and/or examination of the x-ray report.
3. Explain the procedure to the child and/or the parent.
4. Make the child comfortable.
  a. Remove constricting clothes.
  b. Flex the child's knees and hips.

  c. Have tissues and an emesis basin available.
  d. Have several pillows available.
5. Provide bronchodilator and/or nebulization therapy if indicated.

Performance Phase

1. Place the child in a series of appropriate positions.
  a. The area to be drained should be elevated and its respective bronchus placed in a vertical position. (Specific drainage positions are described in Table 37-5, p. 1190.)
  b. The spine should be as straight as possible to permit optimal expansion of the rib cage.

RATIONALE/AMPLIFICATION

1. This is necessary in order to evaluate the effectiveness of the therapy.

2. The positions selected for drainage will depend on what portion of the lung is involved.

3. This allays anxiety and helps to secure the child's cooperation.

  b. To assist in relaxing and decreasing strain on the abdominal muscles during coughing.
  c. To collect mucus.
  d. To facilitate positioning.
5. It is easier to raise mucus mechanically after the bronchi are dilated and the secretions are thinned.

1. The positions are selected and modified according to the lung area involved, the child's age and general condition, and equipment such as IV, tracheostomies, monitors, ventilators, etc.

  b. Infants are positioned on the nurse's lap, in the isolette or in the crib; older children may be treated on a tilt board or in bed.

GUIDELINES: Promoting Postural Drainage in the Pediatric Patient (cont.)

TABLE 37-5. POSTURAL DRAINAGE POSITIONS

Area of Lung to be Drained	Position	Area of Percussion
Upper lobes, left and right anterior apical segments	Child sitting, leaning slightly backward	Percuss over the top of shoulder and anterior thorax. Hand, in cupped position, should be over the clavicle
Upper lobes, left and right posterior apical segments	Child sitting, leaning slightly forward	Percuss over the upper posterior thorax. Fingers should be contoured over the top of the child's shoulders
Upper lobes, left posterior segment	Child sitting, slightly reclined and rotated to the right. (Infant may be positioned on stomach with left shoulder elevated on therapist's arm)	Percuss over the left scapula
Upper lobes, right posterior segment	Child lying flat and rotated onto the left side. (Infant may be positioned on stomach with right shoulder elevated on therapist's arm)	Percuss over the right scapula
Upper lobes, left and right anterior segments	Child lying flat on back	Percuss the anterior chest directly under the clavicles. Avoid direct pressure on the sternum
Upper lobe, lingular segment	Child lying on right side, rotated back one-quarter turn and tilted 30 degrees	Percuss over the left breast
Right middle lobe	Child rotated one-quarter turn from supine position onto the left side and tilted 30 degrees	Percuss over the right breast
Lower lobes, left and right apical segments	Child lying flat in prone position	Percuss below the inferior angle of the scapula
Lower lobes, left and right anterior basal segments	Child lying on back, tilted about 45 degrees	Percuss slightly above the lower ribs
Lower lobe, left lateral basal segment	Child lying on right side, tilted about 45 degrees	Percuss the left lateral thorax at the level of the 8th rib
Lower lobe, right lateral basal segment	Child lying on left side, tilted about 45 degrees	Percuss the right lateral thorax at the level of the 8th rib
Lower lobes, left and right posterior basal segment	Child lying on stomach, tilted about 45 degrees	Percuss just above the 11th and 12th ribs

Procedure (cont.)

NURSING ACTION	RATIONALE/AMPLIFICATION
2. Unless contraindicated, cup the chest wall for 1–2 minutes. (Description of cupping and vibration can be found below.)	2. More secretions can be raised in a shorter period of time when cupping and vibration are added to posturing.
3. Have the child inhale deeply; then, as he exhales, vibrate the chest wall during 3–5 exhalations.	
4. Encourage the child to cough.	4. Infants and young children may require suctioning.
5. Allow the child to rest for a minute, then repeat cupping, vibration, and coughing until no more mucus is produced or the child's condition indicates that the procedure should be stopped.	5. Total treatment time should generally not exceed 20–30 minutes.
	a. In acute conditions such as atelectasis, postural drainage may be done for 5 minutes out of every hour.
	b. In chronic conditions such as cystic fibrosis, postural drainage may be done 2–5 times per day for 15–30 minutes.

> **NURSING ALERT:** Postural drainage should not be done immediately after meals since it may induce vomiting.

6. Provide for patient safety.	6. Stay with the child during the procedure, especially when he is in a head-down position.

Follow-up Phase

1. Assist the child to slowly resume a normal position.	1. It may take a few minutes for the child to regain his equilibrium.
2. Provide oral hygiene.	2. This removes residual mucus from the child's mouth and promotes comfort.
3. Assess and record the effectiveness of the procedure and how well it was tolerated by the child.	

Cupping and Vibrating the Pediatric Patient

1. Cupping, or percussion, should be performed with a cupped hand, contoured to the thorax. For infants, it may be more effective to use cupped fingers or a small face mask from a self-inflating bag. (If this method is used, the rim should be filled with air so that it is firm.)
2. Light clothing or a single thickness diaper may be used between the therapist's hand and the child's chest to minimize discomfort during the procedure.

Procedure (cont.)

3. A hollow sound should be produced by the trapped air between the cupped hand and the patient. A slapping sound indicates that the hand is not cupped enough.
4. Cupping should not be performed directly over recent incisions, open wounds, or drainage tubes.
5. Cupping should be discontinued immediately if the percussion site is noted to be reddened.
6. To do vibration, the nurse must first observe the child for exhalation. With the upper arm stiffened, gently shake child's chest; keep upper arm stiff and extend wrist. The older the child, the more force should be applied.
7. For infants who are breathing rapidly it is usually easier to vibrate with every second or third exhalation rather than with each exhalation. Hand electric vibrators may be easier to use with small infants.
8. For additional information, including the purpose, indications, contraindications, and procedure for administering cupping and vibration, refer to Guidelines: Percussion and Vibration, page 165.

GUIDELINES: Assisting the Patient to Cough

Coughing is the process of expelling air suddenly and noisily from the lungs through the glottis.
Purpose: **To clear secretions from the airways.**

Procedure

NURSING ACTION	RATIONALE/AMPLIFICATION
Preparatory Phase	
1. Position the child to help loosen and drain secretions.	1. a. Turn side to side b. Position for postural drainage as indicated. (See p. 1190).
2. Administer appropriate medications and allow time for them to take effect.	2. Medications may be utilized to loosen secretions or decrease pain awareness.
3. Explain the procedure to the child and/or parents.	3. This helps to secure the child's cooperation.
4. Position the child for optimal chest expansion.	4. The head should be elevated as high as possible.
Performance Phase	
1. If the child has had surgery, splint the operative area with a pillow or by placing your hands on either side of the operative site.	1. This decreases the pain associated with the procedure by decreasing movement in the area.
2. Have the child take 3–4 deep breaths with emphasis on complete exhalation. Have him attempt to cough at the end of a series of deep breaths.	2. This helps to stimulate the cough reflex. Full exhalation causes secretions to be moved into the larger airways where mechanical cough receptors are present.
3. Repeat the procedure according to the child's tolerance until the airways are cleared.	3. Suctioning may be indicated if the child is unable to produce an effective cough.
4. Additional techniques for stimulating a cough in pediatric patients: a. Offer cold fluids or ice chips. b. Have the child swallow several times in sequence. c. Apply manual pressure by using an up-and-down movement of the finger with firm, steady pressure over the trachea above the manubrial arch. d. Pass a sterile suction catheter to produce endotracheal stimulation.	4. These techniques cause an irritating sensation in the trachea, triggering the cough reflex. d. The catheter is introduced through the child's nose and advances until coughing occurs. (Refer to the procedure for suctioning, p. 1192.)
Follow-up Phase	
1. Provide oral hygiene.	1. This removes residual mucus from the child's mouth and promotes comfort.
2. Assess and record the effectiveness of the cough, the amount and nature of the secretions, and successful techniques for stimulating the child to cough.	2. Auscultate the lungs to determine the extent of airway clearing.

ASSISTING THE PEDIATRIC PATIENT WITH BREATHING EXERCISES

Nursing Considerations*

1. Breathing exercises must be performed routinely and diligently to be effective. Whenever possible, the same nurse should instruct and work with the child.
2. The respiratory tract should be free of secretions. If indicated, aerosol treatments, postural drainage, coughing, or suctioning should be done prior to deep breathing exercises.
3. The child should be relatively free of pain. If necessary, pain medication should be administered and time allowed for it to take effect before breathing exercises are initiated.
   Operative incisions should be splinted.
4. The nurse should be relaxed and unhurried. Her tone of voice, approach, and mannerisms affect the child's ability to relax.
5. The child should be positioned to eliminate excessive muscular activity.

* For additional information, including the purpose of and instructions for diaphragmatic and pursed-lip breathing, refer to pages 166–167.

a. Flexion of the hips and knees reduces tension of the abdominal muscles, aiding inspiration.

b. Supporting the upper extremities on pillows relieves the thorax of this additional weight during inspiration.

c. The position for breathing exercises depends on the specific pulmonary problem and its severity as well as on the child's age and general condition.

6. Techniques to facilitate diaphragmatic breathing
Have the child place a book on his abdomen. Instruct him to make the book fall off as he takes air in and makes his abdomen round. Have him watch his abdomen get flat as he blows all the air out. The chest should move as little as possible.

7. Techniques to facilitate pursed-lip breathing

a. Blow cotton balls or Ping-Pong balls across a bedside table.

b. Blow bubbles.

c. Blow a harmonica or party favor.

d. Blow a pinwheel.

e. Suspend a Ping-Pong ball on a string from a doorframe. Have the patient see how long he can keep it propelled away before he needs to inhale. He should attempt to increase his time.

8. Techniques to facilitate deep breathing

a. Rebreathing tube

b. Incentive spirometry (see p. 183)

c. Blowing up balloons or examining gloves

d. Blowing bubbles

GUIDELINES: Suctioning

Suctioning is a method for removing excessive secretions from the airway. Suction may be applied to the oral, nasopharyngeal, or tracheal passages.

Procedure   To provide a patent airway by keeping it clear of excessive secretions.

Equipment
1. Suction source
2. Suction catheter with vent
3. Connecting tube
4. Sterile basin (for tracheal and tracheostomy suctioning)
5. Sterile distilled water
6. Tissues
7. Sterile towel
8. Sterile gloves (for tracheal and tracheostomy suctioning)
9. Collection bottle
10. Manometer to measure amount of vacuum applied
11. Padded tongue blades, p.r.n.

Procedure

NURSING ACTION	RATIONALE/AMPLIFICATION
ORAL SUCTIONING	
Preparatory Phase	
1. Gather equipment, including extra catheters of the appropriate size. Connect collection bottle and tubing to vacuum source.	1. Since suctioning is often done on an emergency basis, it is mandatory that the nurse keep the necessary equipment at the bedside.
2. Establish the need for suctioning by observing respirations and auscultating lungs.	2. The frequency of suctioning will vary with each patient. The need will be evidenced by noisy, moist respirations in a child who is unable to cough adequately.
3. Wash hands thoroughly.	
4. Turn on suction to check system and regulate pressure if indicated and if equipment makes it possible.	4. Recommendations for *negative pressure*

Wall suction

Infants	60–100 mm. Hg
Children	100–120 mm. Hg

With excessive suction, catheter may adhere to the mucosa and cause trauma as it is withdrawn.

NURSING ACTION	RATIONALE/AMPLIFICATION
5. Fill basin with sterile distilled water.	
6. Position child on his side, with his head slightly lowered. If necessary, seek an assistant to help maintain the child in this position.	6. This position aids in pooling and draining, secretions.
7. Attach catheter to suction tubing; use a glove when handling catheter.	7. Wear a glove to keep the catheter clean and to keep the nurse's hand clean.
8. Place catheter tip in the basin and draw sterile distilled water through it.	8. This checks the patency of the system, lubricates catheter, and allows some water in the collection bottle which will prevent aspirated secretions from sticking to it.

**Procedure
(cont.)**

NURSING ACTION	RATIONALE/AMPLIFICATION

Performance Phase

1. Use padded tongue blades to separate the teeth, if necessary

2. Leave vent open to air and introduce catheter into the area to be suctioned.

3. Occlude vent with thumb and slowly withdraw catheter while rotating it between the thumb and finger. If catheter "grabs," remove thumb to stop suction.

4. Dip catheter in and out of the basin, drawing sterile distilled water through it to clean it.

5. Repeat steps 1–4 as necessary, suctioning no longer than 10 seconds at a time and allowing 1–3 minutes between suctioning periods (unless abundance of secretions makes this impossible).

1. This prevents the child from biting the catheter.

2. Area may include cheeks, beneath the tongue, and back of mouth. Avoid overstimulation of the gag reflex to prevent vomiting.

3. If catheter is allowed to remain in one place, the mucous membrane will be drawn against it. This will occlude the catheter and injure the tissues.

4. Use 50–100 ml. of water to adequately clean catheter. The bubbles created by the interrupted flow of water through the catheter increase the mechanical cleansing action.

5. Prolonged suctioning can produce laryngospasm, profound bradycardia and/or cardiac arrhythmias from vagal stimulation and loss of oxygen.

Follow-up Phase

1. Turn off suction source, detach catheter from tubing, and wrap tubing in sterile towel. Discard disposable catheter.

2. Make child comfortable and give mouth care.

3. Assess effectiveness by observing respirations and auscultating lungs.

4. Record the following:
   a. Amount, color, and consistency of secretions
   b. Coughing
   c. Dyspnea
   d. Cyanosis
   e. Frequency of suctioning
   f. Any bleeding
   g. Response of child to suctioning

5. Empty and rinse collection bottle before it fills completely and at the end of each tour of duty.

1. Preferably, a new catheter is used each time suctioning is required. The connecting tube should be changed at the end of each tour of duty, or more often if necessary.

3. Respirations should be quiet and occur with less effort.

NASOPHARYNGEAL SUCTIONING

Preparatory Phase

This is the same as for oral suctioning.
In addition, the nurse should:
   Measure the distance between the tip of the child's nose and the tragus of the ear to determine how far to insert catheter.

The catheter tip will reach the nasopharynx.

Performance Phase

1. Leaving the vent in the catheter open, elevate the tip of the nose and introduce the catheter along the floor of the nose (with the patient facing straight ahead).

2. If obstruction is encountered, do not force, but remove and insert at another angle or try the other nostril.

3. Follow steps 3–5 of the procedure for oral suctioning. Alternate nostrils when introducing the catheter.

1. This position will facilitate introduction of the catheter.

2. Some resistance should be expected when the catheter reaches the nasopharynx.

3. Alternating nostrils will ensure cleaning of both nasal passages and will minimize trauma to either side.

Follow-up Phase

This is the same as for oral suctioning.

TRACHEOSTOMY SUCTIONING

1. Refer to Guidelines: Aspirating the Tracheostomy Tube, pp. 189–191.
2. Additional considerations for the pediatric patient include:
   a. Wall suction should be set at 50–95 mm. Hg for infants or at 90–115 mm. Hg for children.
   b. If sodium chloride solution is used to dilute secretions, the amount should be less (generally 1 ml. for infants and 1–5 ml. for children).
   c. The infant or young child should not be suctioned for more than 5 seconds at a time.
   d. The child's heart rate and color should be monitored throughout the procedure. In the event of irregularity, suctioning should be discontinued and oxygen or assisted ventilation administered.

GUIDELINES: Suctioning (cont.)

Procedure (cont.)

NURSING ACTION	RATIONALE/AMPLIFICATION
NASOTRACHEAL SUCTIONING	

Preparatory Phase

1. Follow steps 1–4 of the Guidelines for oral suctioning.
2. Set wall suction at 50–95 mm. Hg for infants and 95–115 mm. Hg for children.
3. Make certain that an oxygen source is available.

   3. This procedure may produce hypoxia and necessitate oxygen therapy.

4. Using aseptic technique, fill a sterile basin with sterile distilled water.

   4. Tracheal suctioning should be done with sterile equipment to minimize the danger of infection.

5. Position child facing straight ahead with his neck slightly hyperextended. The infant should be placed in the "sniffing" position with chin up, head tipped slightly backward.

   5. This position facilitates introduction of the catheter.

6. Open the package containing the sterile catheter. Wear a sterile glove on the hand that will handle the catheter. Attach the catheter to the suction tubing.

   6. From now until termination of the procedure, this hand should touch only the catheter.

7. Place catheter tip in the basin and draw sterile distilled water through it.

   7. This checks the patency of the system, lubricates catheter, and allows some water in the collection bottle which will prevent aspirated secretions from sticking to it.

Performance Phase

1. Leaving the vent in the catheter open, elevate the tip of the nose and introduce the catheter along the floor of the nose (with the patient facing straight ahead).

   1. This position will facilitate introduction of the catheter.

2. If obstruction is encountered, do not force, but remove and insert at another angle or try the other nostril.

   2. Some resistance should be expected when the catheter reaches the nasopharynx.

3. Move catheter forward slowly until it enters the trachea—when the following may happen:
   a. Child may cough
   b. Air will be felt from vent in catheter on expiration.
   c. Voice or cry may change.
   d. Child may show marked anxiety.

   3. Attempt to enter the trachea carefully and on inspiration only. Tracheal tickle may be applied to stimulate coughing and ease the passage of the catheter into the trachea. Gentle pressure at the level of the vocal cords may also be helpful.

4. When catheter is in the trachea, occlude vent with the thumb of the ungloved hand and slowly withdraw catheter while rotating it between the thumb and finger.

   4. If catheter grabs, remove thumb from vent to stop suction.

5. Remove thumb from vent for several seconds between inspirations.

   5. Suctioning must be stopped at intervals to prevent hypoxia. During normal suctioning, 4 liters of air will be pulled out of the lungs in 15 seconds. Never suction for longer than 5 seconds.

6. Dip catheter in and out of the basin, drawing sterile distilled water through it to clean it.

   6. Use 50–100 ml. of water to adequately clean catheter. The bubbles created by the interrupted flow of water through the catheter increase the mechanical cleansing action.

7. Repeat steps 1–6 as required, suctioning no longer than 5 seconds at one time and allowing 1–3 minutes between suctioning periods (unless the secretions are too abundant).

   7. If child is receiving oxygen, provide oxygen during these rest periods.

8. Monitor the child's heart rate and color throughout the procedure.

   8. Discontinue suctioning and administer oxygen or assisted ventilation in the event of any irregularity.

NURSING ALERT: Tracheal suction can result in laryngospasm. This may be recognized as obstructed respiration (rapid and labored with inspiratory stridor) and may rapidly progress to complete apnea. The nurse should call for assistance; she should straighten the airway by hyperextending the patient's neck and pulling his jaw forward and should administer oxygen.

Follow-up Phase

1. Follow the same procedure as for oral suctioning.
2. Administer oxygen if it is required by the patient's condition.

GUIDELINES: Care of a Child with a Tracheostomy

For information concerning purposes for tracheostomy, kinds of tracheostomy tubes, techniques for performing a tracheostomy, and nursing management, refer to the section on tracheostomy in adults, pages 188–194.

Kinds of Tracheostomy Tubes for Pediatric Patients

1. Plastic (polyvinyl chloride or silastic) tubes, usually without an inner cannula.
2. Silver tubes consisting of 3 parts: obturator, inner cannula, and outer cannula.
3. Cuffs are not generally used for infants and small children since the tracheostomy tube itself is big enough relative to the size of the trachea to act as its own sealer.

Common Reasons for Performing Tracheostomies in Pediatric Patients

1. Laryngotracheal bronchitis
2. Congenital abnormalities such as laryngeal stenosis, choanal atresia, and various anomalies of the heart and lung
3. Foreign bodies lodged in the hypopharynx or larynx
4. Severe chest trauma
5. Burns of the head and neck
6. Laryngeal edema from prolonged intubation
7. Management of secretions and provision of assisted ventilation postoperatively
8. Problems requiring ventilatory support

Nursing Management

NURSING ACTION	RATIONALE/AMPLIFICATION
Physical Care of the Patient	
1. Provide adequate humidity, usually via a ventilator, humidifier, or tent.	1. The natural humidifying pathway of the oropharynx is no longer used. Mist will loosen mucus and secretions and reduce the chances of a mucus plug.
2. Aspirate secretions (using sterile technique) whenever indicated by noisy respiration, retractions, poor color, or change in vital signs. (Refer to procedure for aspirating a tracheostomy, pp. 189–191.)	2. It takes a very small amount of secretions to obstruct a small tube.
3. Suction the child after he has had nebulization therapy, chest therapy, and postural drainage.	3. The secretions will be more liquid, more copious, and more easily removed following these procedures.
4. Observe closely for rising pulse rate and restlessness.	4. These are the first clinical signs of respiratory insufficiency and should be followed by careful tracheobronchial toilet.
5. Monitor respirations frequently and observe for unequal chest expansion.	5. This might indicate the development of a pneumothorax.

6. Keep the area around the tube clean and dry:
  a. Cleanse area with an applicator dipped in hydrogen peroxide.
  b. Observe the site for bleeding and irritation.
  c. Coat area with antibiotic cream.
  d. Place an unfrayed sterile dressing around the tube and under the tapes that hold the tube in position.
	6. To minimize irritation and the risk of infection.

7. Observe the child closely to prevent accidental removal of the tube. Arm restraints may be necessary.
  a. Have necessary equipment available at the bedside:
    Duplicate tracheostomy tubes with tapes attached
    Tracheostomy set for emergency tracheostomy
    Materials for suctioning and cleansing tubes
    Materials for cleansing stomal site
  b. Never immerse the child in a full bath.
	7. These are safety precautions.
	
	b. To prevent fluids from entering the airway.

8. Make certain that the tapes which hold the tube in place are tied securely with the proper amount of tension.	8. This prevents the tube from slipping out of place as the child becomes distressed or frightened or moves about.
9. Change ties as needed.	9. The knot should be at the back of the neck to minimize the chance of it becoming untied. Two nurses should be involved in changing the ties to prevent the tube from slipping out.

GUIDELINES: Care of a Child with a Tracheostomy (cont.)

Procedure		
	NURSING ACTION	**RATIONALE/AMPLIFICATION**

10. If an inner cannula is used it should be removed and cleaned of debris as needed, about every 4 hours.

SPECIAL CONSIDERATIONS FOR THE INFANT

1. Position the infant with his neck extended by placing a small roll under his shoulders.
2. Support the infant's head when moving him.

3. When feeding, cover the tracheostomy with a moist piece of gauze. A bib may be used for older infants and young children.

1. An infant has a tendency to occlude the tube with his chin when his neck is flexed.
2. Sudden movements of the head and neck can cause the tube to slip out.
3. This prevents food particles from dropping into the tube.

Psychosocial Care of Patients

1. Explain, at the level of the child's understanding, the reasons for the tracheostomy and for all procedures and treatments.
2. Allay fears and anxieties of parents by explanations and support.
3. Provide some means of communication such as gestures, lip reading, magic slate, pad and pencil. An older child may enjoy alphabet letters or a word board.
4. Make sure that a call bell is within easy reach of the child, and answer it promptly.

5. Whenever possible, provide continuity of direct nursing care.

6. Provide an environment that will support the child's developmental potentials.

1. The child's fantasies about what is happening and why may be more frightening than the truth.

2. Parental attitudes are conveyed to the child.

3. The child is unable to communicate verbally.

4. The child is dependent on others to meet even his most basic needs. Prompt attention to his needs will help the child build trust in the nursing personnel.
5. It takes time for a child to develop trust in strangers. He will be frightened by constantly changing personnel.
6. The child's developing sense of identity is threatened. He may be deprived of performing tasks that he has recently mastered.

Nursing Considerations if the Child is Discharged with a Tracheostomy Tube in Place

1. Involve the parents with the child's care as soon as possible. First, explain procedures and their rationale, and have them observe. Gradually turn more of the procedure over to them under nursing supervision.
2. Teach at the parent's level and pace of understanding.
3. Help parents to obtain necessary equipment. Make sure that they have a very specific list of the equipment (and the amounts needed).
4. Be alert to financial difficulties associated with securing equipment or nursing services. Refer to social worker if appropriate.
5. Make certain that parents know what to do and where to go in an emergency.
6. If possible, put parents in contact with other families who have managed children at home with tracheostomies.
7. If appropriate, initiate a community health nursing referral for nursing intervention after discharge.
8. Provide the parents with a written procedure to study and take home.
9. Assist parents to appreciate the normality of their child and to recognize his needs for an environment that will support developmental potentials.
10. References for parents include:
    Kaler J and Kaler H. Michael had a tracheostomy. Am J Nurs, 74:852–855, May 1974
    Tracheotomy Handbook for Parents. Chevalier Jackson Pediatric Tracheotomy Unit, St. Christopher's Hospital for Children, Philadelphia, Pa. 19133.

GUIDELINES: Oxygen Therapy for Children

For additional information concerning the purpose, general considerations, and procedures for administering oxygen therapy, refer to Oxygen Therapy, pages 171–181.

General Nursing Responsibilities

NURSING ACTION	**RATIONALE/AMPLIFICATION**

1. Explain the procedure to the child and allow him to feel the equipment and the oxygen flowing through the tube, mask, etc.
2. Maintain a clear airway by suctioning, if necessary.

1. The child will be reassured if he understands the procedure and knows what to expect.
2. The delivery of oxygen requires a clear airway.

NURSING ACTION	RATIONALE/AMPLIFICATION
3. Provide a source of humidification.	3. Oxygen is a dry gas and requires the addition of moisture to prevent drying of the tracheobronchial tree and thickening and consolidation of secretions.
4. Measure oxygen concentrations every 1–2 hours when a child is receiving oxygen via incubator hood, tent, or Croupette. a. Measure when the oxygen environment is closed. b. Measure the concentration close to the child's airway. c. Record oxygen concentrations and simultaneous measurements of the pulse and respirations.	4. It is desirable to keep the oxygen concentration as low as possible while still providing for physiologic requirements. This minimizes the danger of the child's developing retrolental fibroplasia or pulmonary oxygen toxicity. (Desired oxygen concentrations are determined by the arterial oxygen tension measurement.) The oxygen analyzer itself should be calibrated daily on both room air and 100% oxygen. The concentration of oxygen within the space is determined by the liter flow, the efficiency of the equipment, and the frequency with which it is opened to the external environment.
5. Observe the child's response to oxygen.	5. Desired response includes: a. Decreased restlessness b. Decreased respiratory distress c. Improved color d. Improved vital sign values
6. Organize nursing care so that interruption of therapy is minimal.	6. Interruption of therapy may result in the return of anoxia and defeat the goals of therapy.
7. Periodically check all equipment during each tour of duty.	7. For optimum functioning, the equipment should be clean, undamaged, and in good working order.
8. Clean equipment daily and change it at least once each week. (Tubing and nebulizer jars should be changed daily.) Take cultures of oxygen tubing, water, nebulizers, and the interior of incubators at least every 3 days.	8. Unclean equipment may be a source of contamination.
9. Keep combustible materials and potential sources of fire away from oxygen equipment. a. Avoid using oil or grease around oxygen connections. b. Do not use alcohol or oils on a child in an oxygen tent. c. Do not permit any electrical devices in or near an oxygen tent. d. Avoid the use of wool blankets and those made from some synthetic fibers because of the hazards resulting from static electricity. e. Prohibit smoking in areas where oxygen is being used. f. Have a fire extinguisher available.	9. Oxygen supports combustion.
10. Terminate oxygen therapy gradually. a. Slowly reduce liter flow. b. Open air vents in incubators. c. Open zippers or flip a section of the canopy over the top of the tent.	10. This allows the child to adjust to normal atmospheric oxygen concentrations.
11. Continually monitor the child's response during weaning. Observe for: restlessness, increased pulse rate, respiratory distress, cyanosis.	11. These are indications that the child is unable to tolerate reduced oxygen concentration.

Specific Methods for Administering Oxygen to Pediatric Patients

NURSING ACTION	RATIONALE/AMPLIFICATION
Oxygen by Nasal Cannula or Catheter 1. Refer to Guidelines: Administering oxygen by nasal cannula or catheter, pages 172–174.	1. Infants and small children rarely tolerate administration of oxygen by these methods.
Oxygen by Mask 1. Choose an appropriate size mask that covers the mouth and nose but not the eyes.	1. Extra space under the mask and around the face is added dead space and decreases the effectiveness of the therapy.
2. Use a mask that is capable of delivering the desired oxygen concentration. (Refer to Table 37-6, p. 1198.)	2. Venturi masks, available for use in pediatrics, deliver low to moderate concentrations of oxygen: 24%, 28%, 35%, or 40%.
3. Place the mask over the child's mouth and nose so that it fits securely. Secure the mask with an elastic head grip.	3. Make sure that the mask is adjusted properly over the mouth and nose. Do not allow the oxygen to blow in child's eyes. Small pieces of cotton may be placed above the ears to help relieve pressure and discomfort caused by the head strap.

GUIDELINES: Oxygen Therapy for Children (cont.)

TABLE 37-6. OXYGEN FLOW REQUIRED TO ACHIEVE DESIRED OXYGEN CONCENTRATION IN MASK THERAPY*

Oxygen Flow Required L./minute	Oxygen Concentration Desired†	
	Non-rebreathing Oxygen Mask	*Pediatric Medium Concentration Oxygen Mask*
6–8	40–50%	35–45%
8–10	50–60%	45–55%
10–12	60–95%	55–60%

* Tables from Lough, M. D., and Doershuk, C. F.: Respiratory therapy, in Lough, M. D., Doershuk, C. F., and Stern, R. C.: Pediatric Respiratory Therapy. Copyright © 1979 by Year Book Medical Publishers, Inc., Chicago. Used by permission.
† Indicates approximate figures.

NURSING ACTION	RATIONALE/AMPLIFICATION
4. Remove the oxygen mask at hourly intervals; wash the face and apply a cream to area where mask contacts the face.	4. Makes the patient feel more comfortable.
5. Do not use masks for comatose infants or children.	5. Such children are more apt to vomit. The risk of aspiration may be increased with mask therapy because of obstruction of the flow of vomitus.
6. For additional information, refer to Guidelines: Administering Oxygen by Face Mask and by Venturi Mask, pp. 174–178.	
Face Tent	
1. Face tents are available in the adult size only. They can be used effectively in pediatric patients if inverted to create a smaller reservoir and better fit.	1. Face tents combine the positive qualities of aerosol masks and mist tents. The child is accessible and may continue to play without feeling confined.
2. A flow of 8–10 L. should be used to flush the system and provide a stable oxygen concentration.	2. Larger children will require higher flows.
T-Bars and Tracheostomy Masks	
1. These devices are used to deliver oxygen to intubated patients.	
2. The flow rate must be set to meet the minute volume requirements of the child and to provide a 100% source gas.	2. T-bars require a short, flexible tube on the distal end to act as a reservoir and prevent room-air entrapment.
Oxygen Tent	
1. Tents are being used less frequently because of their limitations.	1. Tents are cumbersome, patient access is limited, canopies must be kept tightly sealed, and they are frequently frightening to the child.
2. Select the smallest tent and canopy which will achieve the desired concentration of oxygen and maintain patient comfort.	2. This increases the efficiency of the unit.
3. Pad the metal frame which supports the canopy.	3. This protects the child from injury.
4. Maintain the tent temperature at 17.8–21.1° C. (64–70° F).	4. This is done by placing ice in a trough on the back of the tent. It should be checked periodically and replaced as needed. Open-top tents do not require ventilation.
5. Analyze and record the tent atmosphere every 1–2 hours. Concentrations of 30–50% can be achieved in well maintained tents.	5. The concentration varies with the efficiency of the tent, the rate of flow of oxygen, and the frequency with which the tent is opened to the outside environment.
6. Maintain a tight-fitting canopy. Whenever possible, provide nursing care through the sleeves or pockets of the tent.	6. This prevents oxygen leakage and disruption of the tent atmosphere. a. Fastening the canopy to the bedsprings with wooden clothespins may be helpful. b. If the child is extremely restless or uncooperative it may be useful to permit a parent to hold the child's hand through a small opening in the zipper of the canopy.
7. Make certain that the cribsides are up.	7. The canopy, when tucked into the mattress, often gives the illusion of a safe, confined environment.
8. Select toys that retard absorption, are washable, and will not produce static electricity.	8. The child needs toys for stimulation and diversion. They should be safe and practical.

TABLE 37-7. INCUBATOR OXYGEN THERAPY*

Red Flag in Horizontal Position		Red Flag in Vertical Position	
Flow of Oxygen L./minute	*Concentration of Oxygen*	*Flow of Oxygen L./minute*	*Concentration of Oxygen*
4	28–31%	4	Flow not sufficient for high concentration
6	32–36%	8	70–75%
8	37–40%	10	75–80%
		12	80–85%

* Tables from Lough, M. D., and Doershuk, C. F.: Respiratory therapy, in Lough, M. D., Doershuk, C. F., and Stern, R. C.: Pediatric Therapy. Copyright © 1979 by Year Book Medical Publishers, Inc., Chicago. Used by permission.

NURSING ACTION	RATIONALE/AMPLIFICATION
Croupette	
1. This is an oxygen tent equipped with a high humidification system. (Refer to procedure under oxygen tent.)	1. If the child's condition requires high humidity but not oxygen, the unit can be operated with compressed air.
2. Change the child's clothing and bed linen when damp. Cover the child with a cotton blanket.	2. This prevents chilling in an environment of cooled, supersaturated, aerated mist.
3. Check the child frequently.	3. Condensation on the canopy may make it difficult to visualize the child.
4. If possible, remove the child from the mist periodically.	4. This prevents maceration of the skin. Mist may be delivered via nebulizer tubing or mask during these periods.
5. Promote postural drainage and suction the child as necessary.	5. Rapid mobilization of secretions may follow initiation of mist tent therapy.
6. Observe the small infant for signs of overhydration.	6. This occasionally results from intensive use of an ultrasonic nebulizer especially if a saline solution is nebulized.
Closed Incubators/Isolettes	
1. The incubator is used to provide a controlled environment for the neonate.	1. The unit is able to provide precise environmental control of temperature, oxygen, humidity, and isolation.
2. Adjust the oxygen flow to achieve the desired oxygen concentration.	2. Refer to Table 37-7, above.
a. An oxygen limiter prevents the oxygen concentration inside the incubator from exceeding 40%.	a. This is desirable since it reduces the hazard of the child's developing retrolental fibroplasia.
b. Higher concentrations (up to 85%) may be obtained by placing the red reminder flag in the vertical position.	b. This operates by reducing the air intake.
3. Secure a nebulizer to the inside wall of the incubator if mist therapy is desired.	3. This should be cleaned and autoclaved daily. Sterile solutions are used to keep the bacteria count at a minimum.
4. Keep sleeves of incubator closed to prevent loss of oxygen.	4. When incubator or sleeves are opened, supply supplemental oxygen with oxygen mask to face and nose.
5. Periodically analyze the incubator atmosphere.	5. To be certain that the child is receiving the desired concentration of oxygen.
Oxygen Hood	
1. Warmed, humidified oxygen is supplied via a plastic container that fits over the child's head (Fig. 37-8).	1. This is especially useful when high concentrations of oxygen are desired. The hood may be used in an incubator or with a warming unit.
2. Continuously monitor the oxygen concentration, temperature, and humidity inside the hood.	2. Oxygen should be warmed to 31–34° C. (87.8–93.2° F.) to prevent a neonatal response to cold stress—including oxygen deprivation, metabolic acidosis, rapid depletion of glycogen stores, and reduction of blood glucose levels.
3. Open the hood or remove the baby from it as infrequently as possible.	3. This prevents fluctuations of heat and oxygen which may further debilitate the young infant.
4. Several different designs are available for use. The manufacturer's directions should be carefully followed.	4. This is a safety consideration.

GUIDELINES: Oxygen Therapy for Children (cont.)

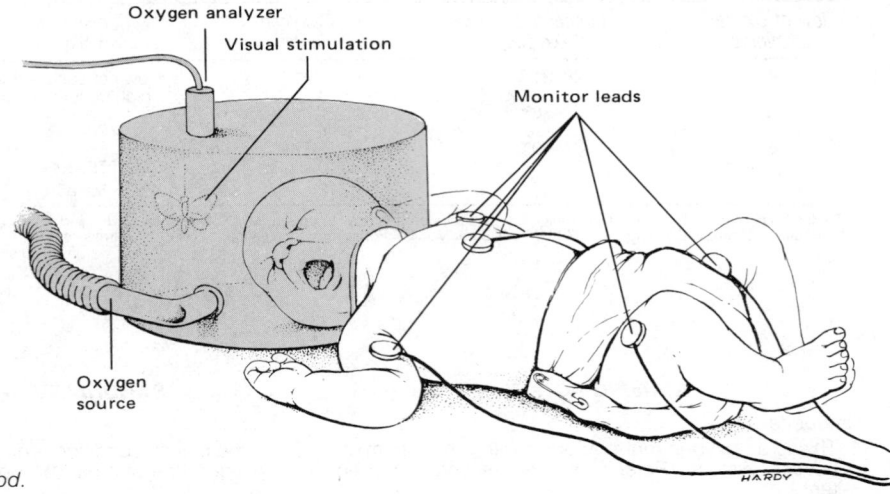

Oxygen analyzer

Visual stimulation

Monitor leads

Oxygen source

FIGURE 37-8. *Oxygen hood.*

NURSING CARE OF THE CHILD REQUIRING MECHANICAL VENTILATION

Characteristics of the Ventilator

Available ventilators have a wide range of capabilities, versatility, and clinical application. Some are more suitable for use with infants, others with children. It is wise for the nurse to be well acquainted with the characteristics of the machine that is being used and to be able to answer the following questions.

A. *Rate Control*

1. How is the rate controlled?
2. Can the patient initiate the cycle? (assisted ventilation)
3. What is the response time? (time elapsed between the initiation of respiration and response of the ventilator) This must be rapid in infants.
4. Is there a sensitivity control which allows the machine to be more or less sensitive to the patient's efforts to initiate respiration?
5. Is an IMV (intermittent mandatory ventilation) feature present? This allows the patient to breathe on his own and, at certain intervals, a mandatory inspiration is provided by the ventilator.

B. *Volume Control*

1. How is the volume controlled?
   a. Automatically preset (i.e., the Bennett MA–1, Ohio 560 and Bourn LS 104–150)
   b. Variable, with a preset pressure
2. What is the range of inspiratory flow rate capability? A very low flow rate is required by neonates; the rate will increase with the size of the child.

C. *Cycling*

1. What controls the cycle of the machine?
   a. Time cycle
   Inspiration is terminated at the end of a preset period that is controlled by a timing device. The volume delivered is usually a function of flow per unit of time.
   b. Volume cycle
   The inspiratory phase is terminated after the predetermined volume of gas has been delivered. The pressure generated is dependent on the characteristics of the lung.
   c. Pressure cycle
   The inspiratory phase ceases when a preset pressure is achieved. The volume of gas delivered and the time required to achieve the preset pressure are dependent on the characteristics of the lungs.
   d. Mixed cycle
   Many ventilators have 2 or more cycling modes.

D. *Humidification*

1. How is moisture added to the inspired air?
   a. Humidification
   b. Nebulization
2. Is there a means of controlling the temperature of the inspired air?
   Many models provide an adjustable thermostat on the humidifier controls.

E. *Oxygen Control*

1. What is the oxygen source?
2. How is the oxygen concentration controlled?

F. *Pressure Control*

1. How is the pressure controlled?
   a. Automatically preset (i.e., the Bennett Pr–2, Bird Mark 7, 8, and 14, Baby-bird, and Bourns P200 infant ventilator)
   b. Variable, with a preset volume
2. What do the pressure guages indicate and how are they read?
   a. Airway pressure indicator
   b. Machine pressure indicator
3. What is the peak effective pressure capability?

G. *Ratio of Inspiration to Expiration* (I/E ratio)

1. Is this variable?
2. How is it controlled?

H. *PEEP* (positive end expiratory pressure)

Does the ventilator have this feature? How is it controlled?

1. Involves exhalation against a threshold resistance.
2. Inspiratory pressure is increased by PEEP; in addition, back pressure remains throughout the expiratory phase.
3. This keeps the lungs in an expanded state and elevates the lung's resting volume, which prevents excessive alveolar collapse.

I. *CPAP* (continuous positive airway pressure)

Does the ventilator have this feature? How is it controlled? Refer to pages 1202–1205.

J. *Sigh*

Does the ventilator have this feature? How is it regulated?

1. Works by adding additional volume to the established tidal volume.
2. Has the effect of taking a deep breath and may expand alveoli, which tend to be collapsed at low volume ventilation.

K. *Alarm Systems*

What are the alarm systems to warn of possible problems?

1. Low pressure or disconnect alarm system.
2. High pressure alarm system to indicate rising pressures within the lung.
3. Electrical failure alarm system.
4. Volume and rate monitor
   a. Acceptable low and high rates and tidal volumes are set for the alarm.
   b. If either rate or tidal volume are outside acceptable parameters, an alarm sounds.

Nursing Management

Refer to Guidelines for managing the patient requiring mechanical ventilation, pages 194–196. In addition, the following considerations should be kept in mind by the nurse who is caring for a pediatric patient.

A. *Setting Controls*

In setting controls, inspiratory flow rate will be less, and the respiratory rate will be greater than in the adult patient. These depend on the patient's size and condition and are determined by the physician and/or respiratory therapist.

B. *Humidification*

1. Because of their small diameters, pediatric endotracheal tubes easily become obstructed by thickened secretions. Therefore, adequate humidification must be maintained to keep secretions loose.
2. During ventilation of an infant in an incubator, the amount of ventilator tubing outside the incubator should be kept to a minimum. The warm temperature inside the incubator helps decrease the amount of condensation in the tubing and thus provides higher water content in the inspired gas.

C. *Oxygen Concentration*

1. Inspired concentrations of oxygen should always be kept as low as possible (while still providing for physiologic requirements), to prevent the develop-

ment of retrolental fibroplasia or pulmonary O_2 toxicity.
2. The oxygen concentration should be checked periodically with an analyzer.

D. *Blood Gases*

1. The arterialized capillary sample method is inaccurate for infants in respiratory distress because the constricted peripheral circulation may not reflect the arterial blood gases accurately.
2. An umbilical artery catheter is most frequently used to obtain arterial blood samples.

E. *Sterile Precautions*

The newborn has only those antibodies transferred across the placenta from the mother. Therefore sterile precautions are essential.

1. Ventilator tubing should be changed every 24 hours.
2. Routine cultures should be taken after intubation; there should be daily Gram staining of secretions.
3. Suctioning requires aseptic technique.

F. *Tubing Support*

1. Special frames are available to support ventilator tubing; this helps to prevent accidental decannulation in infants and small children.
2. Infants may require folded diapers or padding on either side and at the top of their heads to decrease mobility and take up space between the head and the frame.

G. *Monitoring the Ventilator*

1. Pressure gauges should be checked at frequent intervals since this gives an indication of changing compliance or increased airway resistance.
2. Volume measurements are difficult to obtain in infants since most spirometers incorporated into ventilators and meters (such as the Wright respirometer) do not read accurately at low volumes and flows. However, they are helpful with older children.
3. Measure respiratory rates of the machine and the patient at least every hour.

Weaning the Pediatric Patient From the Ventilator

A. *Method I*—Permits the patient to breathe spontaneously for short periods of time:

1. Often used when ventilation has been solely for apnea.
2. The length of time without ventilator assistance is gradually increased, while insuring that the infant does not become fatigued.
3. This method is often facilitated by applying continuous positive pressure to the airway when the infant is off the ventilator.
4. The CPAP (continuous positive airway pressure) can then be gradually decreased until the infant can breathe without assistance. (See pp. 1202–1205.)
5. Humidified gas is provided during the weaning process.

B. *Method II*—Switches from the "control" to the "assist" mode to permit the child to trigger respiration by his own effort.

1. This method is preferred for children with lung disease.
2. The ventilator is switched to the "assist" mode.
3. The trigger sensitivity is gradually decreased as the patient is encouraged to provide greater effort until he is able to ventilate adequately without the assistance of the machine.

4. The patient is then taken off the ventilator for progressively longer periods until use of the ventilator can be discontinued completely.
5. CPAP can be used with this method during the periods that the patient is off the ventilator.

C. *Nursing Management*

1. Weaning children from a ventilator is frequently a long and tedious process. The child and/or his parents may need a lot of support and encouragement.
2. Frequent blood gas determinations are necessary to determine if the child is maintaining adequate oxygenation.
3. The child should be observed closely for signs of respiratory difficulty including fatigue, nasal flaring, increased pulse, sweating, facial pallor and cyanosis, and rising blood pressure.
4. A calm atmosphere should be maintained.
5. Whenever possible, the ventilator should remain at the bedside until the child is satisfied that he can breathe without it.

GUIDELINES: CPAP (Continuous Positive Airway Pressure)

CPAP is a system of applying a constant distending or gas pressure which is greater than atmospheric pressure to the airway during spontaneous breathing. The real mechanisms of action are unknown. This system is also referred to as CPPB (continuous positive pressure breathing).

Purposes

1. To prevent alveolar collapse during expiration by keeping the alveoli open with pressure while avoiding over-distending already-expanded alveoli.
2. To prevent intrapulmonary right-to-left shunting.
3. To increase the oxygenation of the lungs, which in turn decreases potential for hypoxia, bradycardia, or apnea.
4. To decrease the work of breathing on the part of the infant.
5. To increase FRC (functional residual capacity).

Equipment (Fig. 37-9)

1. A source of gas—mixture of air and oxygen; warmth and humidity device for varying the pressure in the system
2. Means of connecting the system to the infant's airway
   Endotracheal tube
   Nasal prongs (cannula)
   Face mask
   Head hood
   Negative pressure in NP respirator around chest
3. Extra equipment for administering mechanical ventilation
4. Equipment for immediate treatment of pneumothorax

Procedure

NURSING ACTION	RATIONALE/AMPLIFICATION
Preparatory Phase 1. The CPAP system is generally set up by the physician and/or respiratory therapist. The accepted early criteria for initiating CPAP are: a. Infant breathing spontaneously b. P_aO_2 (arterial O_2 tension) < 60 mm. Hg (breathing) in 60–65% oxygen less than 24 hrs. of age c. F_1O_2 (inspired oxygen) > 80% at any time 2. The connecting systems used may be nasal cannula or endotracheal tube.	1. The nurse must be in attendance to monitor the infant during application and must know and understand the workings of the CPAP system.

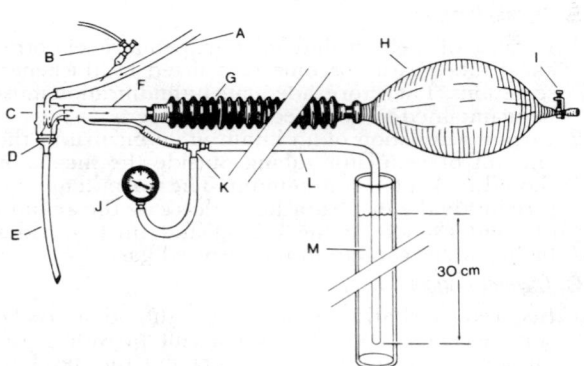

FIGURE 37-9. *System for Applying Continuous Positive Airway Pressure through an Endotracheal Tube. (A) represents gas inflow, (B) oxygen sampling port, (C) Norman elbow (modified T piece), (D) endotracheal tube connector, (E) endotracheal tube, (F) Sommers T piece, (G) corrugated anesthesia hose, (H) reservoir bag (500 ml.) with open tail piece, (I) screw clamp, (J) aneroid pressure manometer, (K) plastic T connector, (L) plastic tubing (1-cm. internal diameter), and (M) underwater "pop-off." Arrows indicate direction of gas flow. (From Gregory, et al.: New Engl. J. Med. 284: 1333, 1971.) (Note: Although newer ventilator equipment can provide CPAP, the principles are the same.)*

Procedure
(cont.)

NURSING ACTION	RATIONALE/AMPLIFICATION

NASAL CANNULA

Orogastric tube is inserted and opened to straight drainage to allow for gastric decompression.

1. Lubricate cannula with a hydrocortisone cream before insertion. This helps to decrease the inflammatory reaction.
2. Prepare headband and place around infant.

ENDOTRACHEAL TUBE

1. Lubricate endotracheal tube with hydrocortisone cream prior to insertion.
2. Set up sterile suction equipment.

Performance Phase

1. Infant's status can change quickly. Carefully observe the condition of infant:
   a. Skin color—cyanotic, dusky, or too pink.

       a. Changes may be signs of pneumothorax, reduced cardiac output, low P_aO_2, too much O_2 administration, infant too hot or cold.

   b. Respiratory pattern—rate, retractions, grunting, apnea, decreased breath sounds.

       b. Change in respirations may indicate that patient is not tolerating CPAP or that pneumothorax has occurred.

   c. Cardiac pattern—rate, especially bradycardia, blood pressure, femoral pulses.

       c. Hypocalcemia, hypoglycemia, or opening of ductus arteriosus should be suspected when changes occur.

   d. Activity—sudden increase or decrease in movement.

       d. Check for hypocalcemia, hypoglycemia, respiratory obstruction.

2. Observe closely for problems or malfunctions connected with CPAP system.
   a. Check inspired O_2 levels being delivered to the infant.

       a. O_2 needs are determined by the P_aO_2 values and the infant's condition. Allowing elevated levels is detrimental to the infant.

   b. Blood gases are checked frequently and always 20 minutes after any change is made in the system. O_2 changes are usually made in 5% increments unless the P_aO_2 is > 100 mg./dl.

   c. Pressure levels should be maintained as prescribed. Check all lines and connections.

       c. Any change in the pressure should be observed immediately and the cause determined. Increase in pressure indicates an obstruction in the baby or in the system tubing. Decrease in pressure indicates a leak in the system. Keep patient's mouth closed when administering nasal CPAP. CPAP levels are usually increased or decreased by 1–2 cm. H_2O increments.

   d. Maintain O_2 humidification and temperature.

       d. The air/O_2 mixture must be properly humidified for the following reasons:
       (1) To prevent drying of mucous membranes and thick secretions caused by too little moisture.
       (2) Possible aspiration or water intoxication can occur from a collection of droplets accumulating on walls of tubing and flowing to infant.
       Proper humidification is present when the tubing is evenly fogged with a fine mist.

NURSING ALERT: Improper temperature of the air-oxygen mixture can lead to hypo- or hyperthermia and can increase oxygen consumption, resulting in acidosis and apnea. Proper temperature is just below body temperature and is not warm or cold when passing over one's skin.

---

3. Observe for signs of complications inherent with a premature infant (see p. 1225), respiratory distress syndrome (see p. 1268), and ventilation.
   a. Spontaneous tension pneumothorax

       a. Presenting signs include decreased chest movements and breath sounds on affected side; tachypnea; cyanosis; bradycardia, inspiratory pressure elevated on manometer; decrease in systolic blood pressure.

GUIDELINES: CPAP (Continuous Positive Airway Pressure) (cont.)

Procedure (cont.)	NURSING ACTION	RATIONALE/AMPLIFICATION

Procedure (cont.)

NURSING ACTION	RATIONALE/AMPLIFICATION
b. Metabolic acidosis	b. The blood pH is less than 7.3. This occurs because of tissue hypoxia and anaerobic metabolism.
c. Hyperbilirubinemia	c. See page 1242.
d. Infection, systemic	d. Temperature instability may be first indication of infection. Apnea, irritability, vomiting, diarrhea, change in status should be reported immediately.
e. Cardiac output reduction	e. Results from CPAP set at too high levels for improving compliance of lungs. CPAP is transmitted through the lungs to the large vessels of mediastinum. The increasing pressure may cause the vessels to partially collapse, affecting the return of blood to the heart; this causes a decrease in cardiac output.
f. Hypocalcemia (blood calcium less than 8 mg./100 ml.) Hypoglycemia (blood sugar less than 20 mg./100 ml.)	f. Symptoms are nonspecific: jitteriness, sweating, tachypnea or apnea, lethargy, convulsions, cyanosis.
g. Hypovolemia (1) Accurate records should be kept of blood removed. (2) Watch blood pressure.	g. This occurs from placenta previa or abruptio, loss of blood into the placenta due to rapid clamping, or iatrogenically from too much sampling without replacement.
h. Abdominal distention—caused by inflation of air. (1) To decompress stomach use an NG (nasogastric) tube or aspirate air prior to NG (gavage) feedings. (2) Elevate infant's head if possible during feeding and attempt to burp him. (3) NG (nasogastric) tube may be kept in place and connected to elevated open reservoir between feedings to serve as overflow safety valve.	h. Most common when using nasal, mask, or hood CPAP. Abdominal distention and increasing gastric residuals may be first sign of necrotizing enterocolitis.
4. Additional nursing care responsibilities to consider when caring for infant being treated with CPAP. a. Provide and maintain thermal stability of infant (p. 1231). b. Provide adequate fluid and caloric intake to meet infant's needs via intravenous fluids and/or nasojejunal (N-J), gavage, or other methods. c. Administer proper and adequate physical therapy to infant to help reduce the potential for pneumonia.	c. Physical therapy includes percussion or vibrating, postural drainage, suctioning, and position change. This prevents airway obstruction as a result of the presence of mucus anywhere along the respiratory tract.
d. Mechanical ventilation with anesthesia bag may be administered at specific times.	d. To help decrease PCO_2, assist a tiring infant, increase O_2 levels prior to any CPAP change or suctioning.
e. Assist in obtaining blood gases at appropriate times. (1) Observe infant for signs that would indicate need for special blood gas studies. Also done after CPAP settings are changed and to monitor infant's progress and condition. (2) When drawing blood use a needle and syringe that have been rinsed with heparin. Avoid too much heparin since it will alter pH value. Store blood sample in ice while transporting to laboratory. Know normal blood gas values as well as patient's "normal" values.	e. Blood gases are always taken 20–30 minutes after CPAP settings are changed—this allows infant to stabilize with new settings. Arterial capillary blood is obtained from warmed heel blood. Arterial blood is drawn from umbilical artery indwelling catheter, radial or temporal artery puncture.
f. Avoid irritation and drying of mouth and nares. The mouth should be cleansed frequently with lemon-glycerin or normal saline swabs.	f. Prevent crust formation, which can lead to breakdown, by using an antibiotic ointment.
g. Keep skin clean and dry. Massage reddened areas gently. Change position every 1–2 hours. Avoid using large quantities of tape.	g. Give good skin care to prevent breakdown and eventual ulceration and infection.
h. Provide infant with pleasant stimulation and love.	h. Colorful objects or pictures can be placed around infant. Small musical toys and a pleasant, soothing voice combined with gentle touching can provide the necessary stimulation.

Follow-up Phase

1. When the infant can maintain adequate arterial oxygenation with CPAP at 1–2 for 2–4 hours he is ready to come off CPAP.

Procedure (cont.)

NURSING ACTION	RATIONALE/AMPLIFICATION
2. Once CPAP is discontinued, the infant is placed in an environment which provides 10–20% more oxygen than he was breathing while on CPAP. Blood gases are checked as O_2 concentration is decreased as tolerated. See Respiratory Distress Syndrome (RDS), page 1268, for further in-depth discussion.	

CARDIAC AND RESPIRATORY MONITORING

Cardiac and respiratory monitoring refers to electrical surveillance of heart and respiratory rates and patterns. It is indicated in all patients whose conditions are unstable or potentially unstable.

Nursing Management

1. Select a monitor that is appropriate for the child's needs. This will depend on the child's age, ability to cooperate, purpose for monitoring, information desired, and equipment available.
2. Stabilize the device to reduce the amount of mechanical noise and for safety considerations.
3. Reduce the child's anxiety:
   a. Provide age-appropriate explanations of the equipment.
   b. When possible, involve the child in his own care, including change of electrodes.
4. Select lead placement sites according to equipment specifications:
   a. Cardiac monitors frequently employ 3 leads located at:
      (1) right upper lateral chest wall below clavical
      (2) left lower chest wall in the anterior axillary line
      (3) upper left chest wall
   b. Respiratory monitors frequently employ 3 electrodes located:
      (1) on either side of the chest (anterior axillary line in fourth or fifth intercostal space)
      (2) at a reference electrode placed on the manubrium or other suitable distal point
5. Apply electrodes by:
   a. Cleaning the appropriate areas on the chest with alcohol
   b. Placing a small amount of conductive gel at each area of contact unless pre-gelled, disposable electrodes are used
   c. Applying the electrode firmly to completely dry skin
6. Plug the leads into the lead cable at appropriate insertion points.
7. Be certain that the monitor alarms are in the "on" position. High and low alarm limits should be set according to the child's age and condition so that apnea, tachypnea, bradycardia, and tachycardia can be readily detected.
8. Avoid skin breakdown by changing lead placement sites as needed. Clean and dry old sites and expose them to the air.
9. Check integrity of the entire system at least once each tour of duty.
   a. Carefully inspect lead wires and cable for breaks and proper attachment.
   b. If malfunction is suspected, change equipment and notify the engineering department immediately.
10. Continue to count respiratory and apical rates at frequent intervals.
   a. Compare with monitor rates to verify accuracy of equipment.
   b. It must be remembered that monitors cannot substitute for close observation of the child.
11. Apnea mattresses or pads that employ sensing devices may be used for infants, eliminating the need for electrodes.
   a. Although less susceptible to cardiovascular artifact, these devices may record physical impact, vibrations, or body movements as breaths.
   b. In addition, older infants can easily roll or crawl off the pad.

CARDIOPULMONARY RESUSCITATION

Cardiopulmonary resuscitation involves measures instituted to provide effective ventilation and circulation when the patient's respiration and heart have ceased to function.

Underlying Considerations

A. *Cardiac Arrest*
1. Signs—absence of heartbeat and absence of carotid and femoral pulses.
2. Causes—asystole, ventricular fibrillation, or cardiovascular collapse related to arterial hypotension.

B. *Respiratory Arrest*
1. Signs—apnea and cyanosis.
2. Causes—obstructed airway, depression of the central nervous system, neuromuscular paralysis.

C. *Emergency Preparation*
1. Every hospital should have a well-defined and organized plan to be carried out in the event of cardiac or respiratory arrest.
2. Emergency carts should be placed in strategic locations in the hospital and checked daily to ensure that all equipment is available.

Equipment

Emergency Cart—assembled and ready for use
   Positive pressure breathing bag with nonrebreathing valve and universal 15 mm. adaptor

Masks (premature infant, infant, child, adult sizes)

Oropharyngeal airways, sizes No. 0 to No. 4

Laryngoscope with blades of various sizes

Extra batteries and light bulbs for laryngoscope

Endotracheal tubes with connectors (complete sterile set, 2.5–8.0 mm. I.D.)

Portable suction equipment and sterile catheters of various sizes

Bulb syringe, DeLee trap

Oxygen source—portable supply gauge and tubing, masks of various sizes

Cardiac board (30 by 50 cm.)

Emergency drugs
  Sodium bicarbonate
  Epinephrine
  Isoproterenol
  Dextrose
  Saline (for dilution)
  Calcium chloride 10%
  Dextrose 50%
  Lidocaine (xylocaine)
  Atropine
  Diphenhydramine hydrochloride (Benadryl)
  Diazepam (Valium)
  Hydrocortisone Sodium Succinate
  Digoxin
  Naloxone (Narcan)
  Calcium gluconate

Intracardiac needles, 20 and 22 gauge, 6–8 cm. (2⅜–3⅛ inches) long

IV equipment
  Fluids
  Infusion set
  Tourniquet
  Armboards
  Tape
  Scalp vein needles of various sizes
  Longdwell catheters of various sizes
  3 way stopcock
  Cutdown set
  Pole
  Labels

Nasogastric tubes of various sizes

Equipment
  Syringes of various sizes
  Needles of various sizes
  Alcohol wipes
  Tongue blades
  Sterile 4 by 4 gauze sponges
  Sterile hemostat
  Sterile scissors
  Blood specimen tubes

Electrocardiograph and monitor

Lubricating jelly

Defibrillator and paddles (pediatric and adult)

ARTIFICIAL VENTILATION

Technique for Artificial Ventilation

A. *Mouth to mouth*

1. Infants
   a. Clear mouth of mucus or vomitus with finger or suction.
   b. Extend neck by placing a rolled towel or diaper under the infant's shoulders, or use one hand to support the neck in an extended position. Do not hyperextend the neck since this narrows the airway.
   c. Take a breath.
   d. Make a tight seal with your mouth over the infant's mouth and nose.
   e. Gently blow air from the cheeks and observe for chest expansion.
   f. Remove your mouth from infant's mouth and nose and allow the infant to exhale.
   g. Repeat approximately 20 times per minute (one breath every 3 seconds).

2. *Older Children and Adolescents*
   a. Clear mouth of mucus or vomitus with finger or suction.
   b. Hyperextend neck with one hand or a rolled towel.
   c. Clamp the nostrils with the fingers of one hand which also continues to exert pressure on the forehead to maintain the neck extension.
   d. Take a deep breath.
   e. Make a tight seal with your mouth over the child's mouth.
   f. Force air into the lungs until chest expansion is observed.
   g. Release your mouth from the child's mouth and release nostrils to allow the child to exhale passively.
   h. Repeat approximately 12 times per minute (one breath every 5 seconds).

B. *Hand-operated ventilation devices*

1. Remove secretions from mouth and throat and move mandible forward.
2. Appropriately extend the neck with one hand or a diaper roll.
3. Select an appropriate size mask to obtain an adequate seal, and connect mask to the bag.
4. Hold the mask snugly over the mouth and nose, holding the chin forward and the neck in extension.
5. Squeeze the bag, noting inflation of the lungs by chest expansion.
6. Release the bag, which will expand spontaneously. The child will exhale and the chest will fall.
7. Repeat 12–20 times per minute (depending on size of the child).
8. Since this technique is often difficult to master, it should be practiced in advance, under supervision.

Indications of Effective Technique

1. Victim's chest rises and falls.
2. Rescuer can feel in his own airway the resistance and compliance of the victim's lungs as they expand.
3. Rescuer can hear and feel the air escape during exhalation.
4. Victim's color improves.

Management of Complications

1. Gastric distention (occurs frequently if excessive pressures are used for inflation)
   a. Turn victim's head and shoulders to one side.
   b. Exert moderate pressure over the epigastrium between the umbilicus and the rib cage.
   c. A nasogastric tube may be used to decompress the stomach.
2. Vomiting
   a. Turn patient on side for drainage.

b. Clear the airway with fingers or suction.

c. Resume ventilations.

ARTIFICIAL CIRCULATION

General Principles Related to Artificial Circulation

(Technique of Artificial Circulation [Table 37-8, Figure 37-10])

1. A backward tilt of the head lifts the back in infants and small children. A firm support beneath the back is therefore essential if external cardiac compression is to be effective.

2. A supine position on a firm surface is mandatory. Only in this position can chest compression squeeze the heart against the immobile spine enough to force blood into the systemic circulation.

3. External cardiac compression must always be accompanied by artificial ventilation for adequate oxygenation of the blood.

4. Compressions must be regular, smooth, and uninterrupted. Avoid sudden or jerking movements.

5. Relaxation must immediately follow compression; relaxation and compression must be of equal duration.

TABLE 37-8. TECHNIQUE OF ARTIFICIAL CIRCULATION

Size of Child	Preparatory Phase	Action Phase	Distance of Compression	Rate
Neonate, Premature or Small Infant	1. Place in supine position 2. Encircle the chest with the hands, with thumbs over the midsternum or Use method for a larger infant, at a rate of 100–120/min.	1. Compress midsternum with both thumbs, gently but firmly	2/3 distance to the spine or 1.3–1.8 cm. (½–¾ inch)	100–120/minute
Larger Infant	1. Place on a firm, flat surface 2. Support the back with one hand or use a small blanket under the shoulders 3. Place the tips of the index and middle fingers of one hand over the midsternum	Compress the midsternum with the tips of the index and middle fingers.	1.3–1.8 cm. (½–¾ inch)	100 per minute
Small Child	1. Place on a firm, flat surface 2. Support the back by slipping one hand beneath it, or use a small blanket under the shoulders 3. Place the heel of one hand over the midsternum, parallel with the long axis of the body	1. Apply a rapid downward thrust to the midsternum, keeping the elbow straight 2. Hold for approximately 0.4 second 3. Instantly and completely release the pressure so the chest wall can recoil 4. Do not remove the heel of the hand from the chest	1.8–3.8 cm. (¾–1½ inches)	80–100/minute
Larger Child Adolescent	1. Place on a flat, firm surface or place a board under the thorax 2. Place the heel of one hand on the lower half of the sternum, about 2.5–3.8 cm. (1–1½ inches) from the tip of the xiphoid process and parallel with the long axis of the body 3. Place the other hand on top of the first one (may interlock fingers) 4. Place shoulders directly over child's sternum, in order to use own weight in application of pressure	1. Exert pressure vertically downward to depress lower sternum, keeping elbows straight 2. Hold for approximately 0.4 second 3. Instantly and completely release the pressure so the chest wall can recoil 4. Do not remove the hands from the chest	2.5–5.0 cm. (1–2 inches)	80 per minute

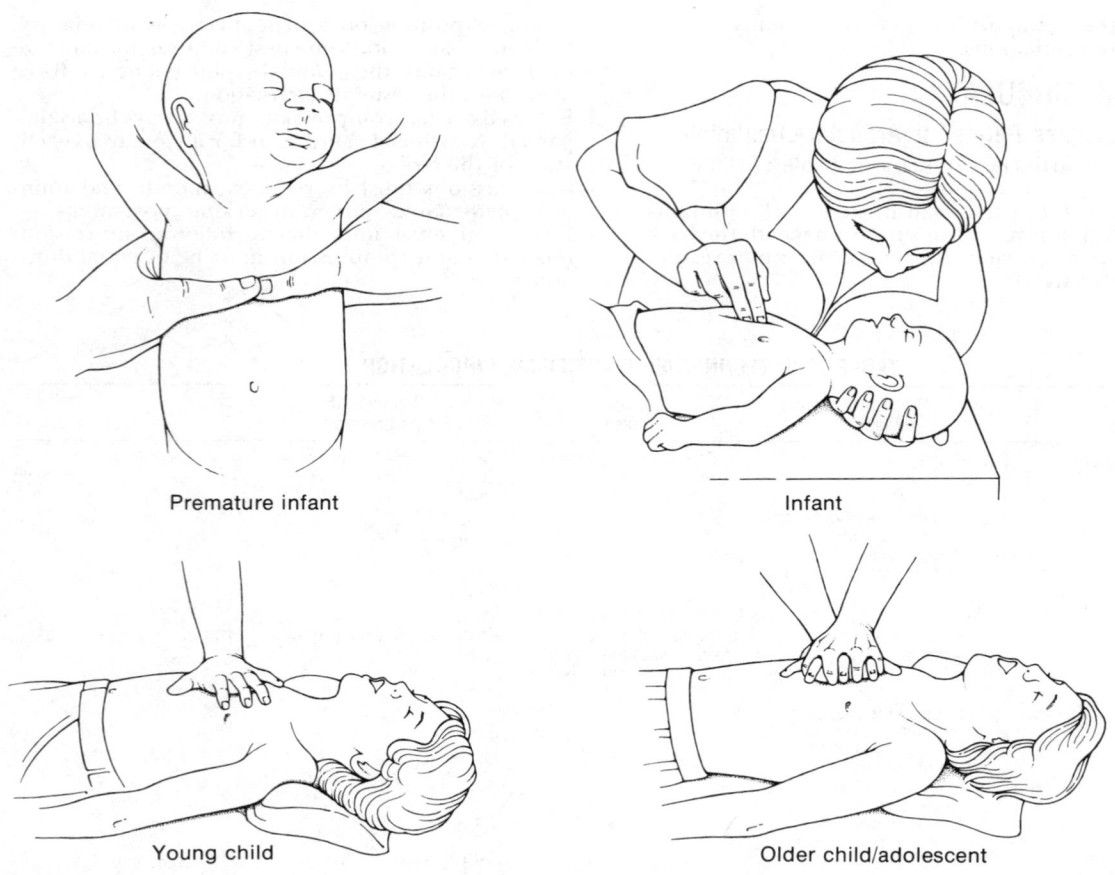

Premature infant   Infant

Young child   Older child/adolescent

FIGURE 37-10. *Cardiopulmonary resuscitation in children. In the young child, the heel of the hand is placed over the lower sternum. In older children and adolescents, both hands are used.*

6. Between compressions, the fingers or heel of the hand must completely release their pressure but should remain in constant contact with the chest.
7. Fingers should not rest on the patient's ribs during compression. Pressure with fingers on the ribs or lateral pressure increases the possibility of fractured ribs and costochondral separation.
8. Never compress the xiphoid process at the tip of the sternum. Pressure on it may cause laceration of the liver.
9. Indications of effective technique include: (1) a palpable femoral or carotid pulse; (2) decrease in size of pupils; (3) improvement in patient's color.

Nursing Management in Cardiopulmonary Resuscitation

1. Recognize cardiac and/or respiratory arrest.
2. Send for assistance and note time.
3. If alone:
    a. First ventilate the child's lungs rapidly 4 times, using appropriate technique (p. 1206), then palpate the carotid or precordial pulse. If a pulse is palpated, continue ventilatory support.
    b. If no pulse is felt, institute artificial circulation using appropriate technique (p. 1207).

series of 5 compressions. For a child or adolescent, interpose 2 breaths after each series of 15 compressions.
    d. Continue repeating this cycle until help arrives.
4. When help arrives:
    a. One rescuer performs mouth-to-mouth resuscitation or institutes bag breathing.
    b. Another rescuer performs cardiac compressions.
    c. A ratio of 5 compressions to 1 breath is maintained for both infants and children.
    d. Cardiac compression should not be stopped for respiration. Breaths should be interposed on the upstroke of each fifth cardiac compression.
5. Anticipate and assist with emergency procedures and medications.
    a. Assist with intubation, monitoring, placement of cutdown, administration of intravenous fluids, defibrillation, and other definitive measures.
    b. Prepare and administer emergency medications as prescribed. Record dose and time.
6. After resuscitation:
    a. Care for the child as required.
    b. Determine if family members have been notified and are being cared for.
    c. Record all events.
    d. Restock emergency cart.

TRACTION

Traction refers to the extension of an injured extremity in the direction and position which will promote healing and optimal functioning. It is accomplished by the use of weights which pull a part in the desired direction in the presence of countertraction.

Purpose

1. To maintain the approximation of fractured segments of a bone until union occurs.
2. To prevent deformities from resulting in the presence of injury or inflammation.
   a. Fractures
   b. Arthritis
   c. Trauma
3. To correct existing deformities.
   a. Congenital dislocation of the hip
   b. Flexion contractures of the knees
4. To lessen muscle spasm.
5. To immobilize a part.
6. To reduce dislocation.

Types of Traction

1. Skin Traction
   a. Used for younger children when the condition of the skin is good and mild forces of traction are sufficient.
   b. Traction is applied to the skin of the affected body part:
      (1) Moleskin, adhesive, or foam rubber extensions are fastened firmly to the skin.
      (2) Elastic bandages are applied to hold them in place.
      (3) Weights are attached to the extensions by cords which pass over one or more pulleys.
2. Skeletal Traction
   a. Used in children when greater traction force is required or if the skin is damaged.
   b. Force is exerted against the bone by means of a metallic device such as a pin, wire, or Crutchfield tongs.
3. Traction may be continuous or intermittent, depending on its purpose.
   a. Continuous traction cannot be interrupted for dressing or other activities.
   b. Intermittent traction may be temporarily disconnected as specified by the physician.

GUIDELINES: Care of a Child in Traction

Equipment   Strips of moleskin
Adhesive tape
Ace bandages
Square wooden blocks
Ropes, weights, pulleys
Traction bars
Slings

Procedure

NURSING ACTION	RATIONALE/AMPLIFICATION
1. Explain the procedure to the child and his parents.	1. If the traction is to be effective, it is essential that the parents understand the procedure and cooperate while the child is in traction.
2. Maintain even, constant traction: a. Do not add or remove weights. b. Allow the weights to hang free at all times. Do not allow them to touch the floor or bed. c. Be certain that the ropes are in the wheel grooves of the pulleys. d. Keep the weights out of the child's reach. e. Wrap knotted areas of the ropes with adhesive tape to prevent slipping. f. Do not elevate the head or foot of the bed without consulting the physician. g. Supervise the child's position so that the purpose of the traction is accomplished.	2. Traction must be kept constant in order to achieve the desired results. Any change in the amount of weights or countertraction affects the entire traction system.
3. Check for disturbance of circulation by observing: a. Skin color—for redness, pallor, cyanosis b. Joint motion c. Skin temperature d. Tingling, numbness e. Swelling	3. Compare the affected limb with the unaffected one.
4. Provide skin care. a. Pad bony prominences (ankles) with cotton padding before wrapping with ace bandages. b. Wash and dry all exposed areas thoroughly. c. Massage the child's back and sacral area at least 2–3 times daily. If indicated, apply cornstarch.	4. Immobilized children readily develop areas of pressure unless meticulous skin care is provided. a. Protects skin from injury. c. Cornstarch absorbs moisture and prevents maceration of the skin.

GUIDELINES: Care of a Child in Traction (cont.)

Procedure (cont.)

NURSING ACTION	RATIONALE/AMPLIFICATION
d. Inspect the heels, ankles, popliteal space, and top of the foot for signs of pressure from ace bandages.	d. These are the areas most prone to breakdown.
e. Keep the linen clean, dry, and free from wrinkles and crumbs.	e. When a large bed is used, two folded sheets are often more easily managed than one large sheet. One is used to cover the upper half of the bed, and one to cover the lower half. This facilitates changing the bed and makes the procedure less uncomfortable for the child.
f. Do not allow any traction cords to dig into the child's skin.	
g. Utilize a fracture bedpan.	g. This is less awkward and more comfortable for the child.
5. Plan for short periods of muscle exercise every day.	5. Disuse of muscles can result in atrophy and deformities.
a. Encourage the child to move and exercise his unaffected extremities. Provide diversional therapy which requires the use of these muscles.	
b. Assist the child to exercise his toes.	
6. Have the child breathe deeply at intervals. Provide him with soap bubbles, whistles, or party favors to make this more fun. An older child may use blow bottles.	6. Prolonged periods of immobilization may cause the child to develop hypostatic pneumonia.
7. Keep a record of the child's intake and output and do periodic urinalyses.	7. Immobilization renders the child prone to developing urinary retention and renal calculi.
8. Provide a diet high in roughage and fluids (especially fruit juices) and low in calcium.	8. This helps to prevent constipation and the development of renal calculi.
9. Provide daily diversion and encourage the child's family to visit frequently.	9. Enforced bed rest makes time pass very slowly and can be very traumatic for a small child.
a. Attempt to replace the lost activity with another form of motion.	a. Water play, mirrors, body games are helpful replacements. Often the child can be moved in his bed into the playroom or hall.
b. Suspend toys over the child's head so he can reach them. (Punching bag can help child relieve hostility.)	
c. Provide continuing education for the school-age child.	
d. Encourage projects that will allow child a feeling of accomplishment: painting, puzzles, knitting, ceramics.	
e. Patients who are immobilized in traction or casts should be grouped together.	
10. If not contraindicated, supply the child with an overhead trapeze.	10. This will facilitate movement and self-help.
11. Record:	
a. Color, temperature, and appearance of the affected extremity	
b. Skin condition	
c. Evidence of local edema	
d. Body alignment	
e. Functioning of traction ropes, weights, and pulley	
f. Response of the child to therapy	
12. Make certain that countertraction is provided.	12. Usually, the patient's body acts as the counterweight which keeps the limb aligned and immobilized.
a. The foot of the child's bed may have to be raised or placed on shock blocks to counteract the traction weight and prevent the child from being pulled to the end of the bed.	a. The child's weight is often insufficient to provide countertraction.
13. Never disturb the traction device.	13. If it appears to need adjustment, notify the physician.
14. Avoid jarring the bed or swinging the weights.	14. This may cause pain and is upsetting to the child.
15. Do not allow the weights to hang directly over the child's body.	15. This is a safety precaution.

SKIN TRACTION

1. Shave the area if hair is present and paint the skin with tincture of benzoin.	1. This allows the adhesive to grasp the skin more firmly. Benzoin also disinfects the skin, allays itching, and prevents skin breakdown under the tape.

Procedure (cont.)

NURSING ACTION	RATIONALE/AMPLIFICATION

SKELETAL TRACTION

1. Treat all entry sites, pins, wires, or tongs as surgical wounds.
   a. Wipe the insertion site with betadine and apply an antibiotic ointment at least daily. Cover with a sterile 4 × 4 gauze—or
   b. Dress the insertion site with a 4 × 4 sterile gauze treated with an antiseptic prescribed by the physician.
   c. Check the entry site regularly for any signs of infection and to be certain that the pin has not slipped through the bone.
2. Place corks or plastic guards over the exposed ends of the pins.

a. This is an attempt to reduce the hazard of infection along the track of the pin. Some physicians prefer to let these areas crust over or cover them with plaster.

c. Notify the physician of either of these conditions.

2. This is a safety precaution to prevent injury to the nurse or patient.

BRYANT'S TRACTION (Fig. 37-11)

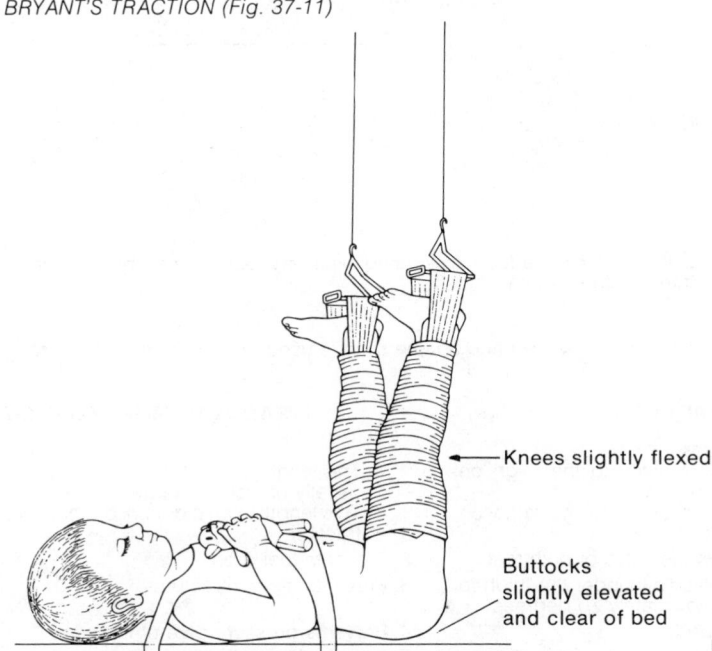

Knees slightly flexed

Buttocks slightly elevated and clear of bed

FIGURE 37-11. *Bryant's traction.*

Purpose

Used to reduce fractured femurs in small children.

Mechanism of Action

Involves bilateral, vertical extension of the child's legs. The child's weight serves as countertraction to the vertical pull of the weights. Skin traction is applied to both legs in order to minimize potential trauma to the affected leg and maintain the stability of the position.

NURSING ACTION	RATIONALE/AMPLIFICATION

1. Maintain the child in the appropriate position.

   a. The legs are extended at right angles to the body.
   b. The hips are elevated slightly from the bed.
   c. The buttocks are elevated and clear of the bed.
   d. The heels and ankles are free from pressure.
   e. The child is flat in bed and unable to turn from side to side.
2. Check the position of the ace bandages and rewrap as necessary.

1. This position is essential in order to achieve the desired results.

e. A jacket or abdominal restraint is usually necessary.

2. The bandages should be wrapped snugly around the legs without compromising circulation. They should not slip and cause pressure on the dorsa of the feet.

GUIDELINES: Care of a Child in Traction (cont.)

RUSSELL'S TRACTION (Fig. 37-12)

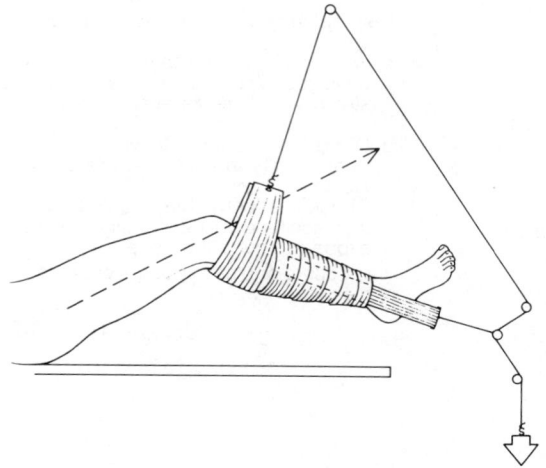

FIGURE 37-12. *In Russell's double traction.*

Purpose

To reduce contractures of the knee or hip, reduce dislocated hips, immobilize the knee or hip postoperatively, or reduce fractures of the femoral shaft.

Mechanism of Action

Force is exerted on the long axis of the lower leg and a knee sling is used under the distal thigh to provide flexion of the knee and hip.

NURSING ACTION	RATIONALE/AMPLIFICATION

1. Application of ace bandages.
  a. Wrap bandages from the ankle to the thigh on patients under 18 months of age.
  b. Wrap bandages from the ankle to the knee on patients over 18 months of age.
	a. The length of the leg from the knee to the foot is usually not long enough to maintain traction.
	b. This length in an older child is sufficient to maintain traction.

2. Place foot supports against the soles of both feet.	2. Prevents foot drop.
3. If necessary, place a small pillow under the thigh to maintain hip flexion at approximately 20 degrees.	3. Prevents hip contractures.
4. Keep the heel free of the bed.	4. Prevents pressure sore of the heel.
5. Carefully check the popliteal space for pressure sores. Make certain that the knee sling is positioned so that it does not exert pressure on the space.	5. Line the knee sling with a piece of felt or sheepskin for additional protection against sores.
6. Make certain that the bandages do not exert pressure over the dorsalis pedis artery (inside of top of foot) or the Achilles tendon (back of heel).	6. Prevents discomfort, pressure sores, and circulatory complications.
7. Make certain that the footplate or spreader is wide enough to prevent irritation of the skin but not so wide that the tapes tend to pull from the skin.	

90-DEGREE–90-DEGREE TRACTION (90–90 TRACTION) (Fig. 37-13)

Purpose

Used to reduce a fractured femur when skin traction is not adequate.

Mechanism of Action

Both the affected knee and hip are flexed at a 90-degree angle. Traction is applied by a skeletal pin drilled through the distal femur. A short leg cast or polyfoam boot is used to suspend the lower leg.

BUCK'S EXTENSION

Purpose

Used to correct knee and hip contractures, to rest the leg, and for other short-term immobilization. For additional information, refer to Guidelines: Application of Buck's Extension Traction, page 764.

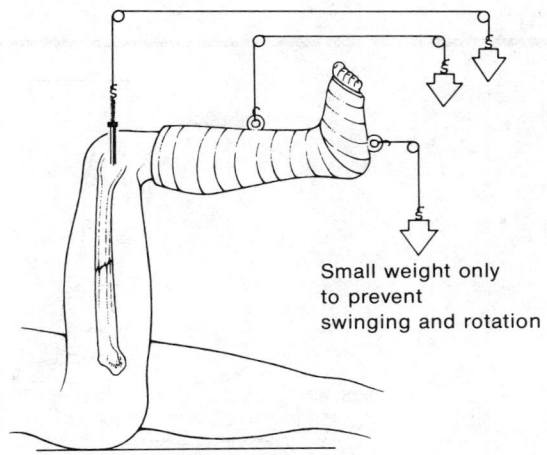

Small weight only
to prevent
swinging and rotation

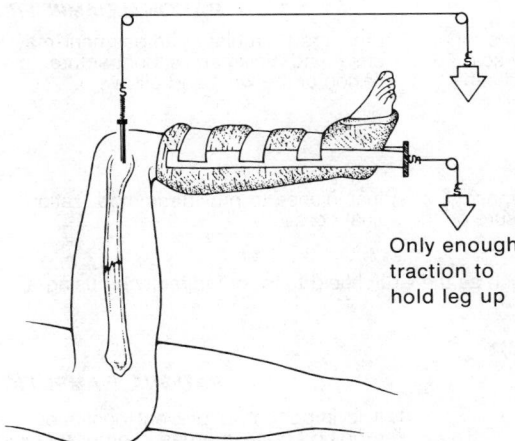

Only enough
traction to
hold leg up

FIGURE 37-13. *90–90 traction.*

BALANCED TRACTION WITH THOMAS SPLINT AND PEARSON ATTACHMENT

Purpose

Used in older children and adolescents for fractured femurs, to rest the hip and knee, or to immobilize the hip and knee postoperatively.
Refer to Fracture of the Femur, page 1413.

DUNLOP TRACTION (Fig. 37-14)

Purpose

Used to treat fractures or injuries of the humerus, shoulder, or shoulder girdle.

Mechanism of Action

Longitudinal traction on the humerus is applied using a soft sling to pull against the forearm or using a pin drilled through the olecranon. A suspension apparatus is applied to the forearm with traction straps and an elastic bandage, using only enough weight to hold the forearm upright and the elbow just touching the bed. The elbow is kept flexed at slightly more than 90 degrees.

NURSING ACTION	RATIONALE/AMPLIFICATION
1. Be certain that the sling at the proximal forearm is well padded and that the margin does not create a ridge at the bend of the elbow.	1. This is a precaution to avoid pressure on the ulnar nerve.

GUIDELINES: Care of a Child in Traction (cont.)

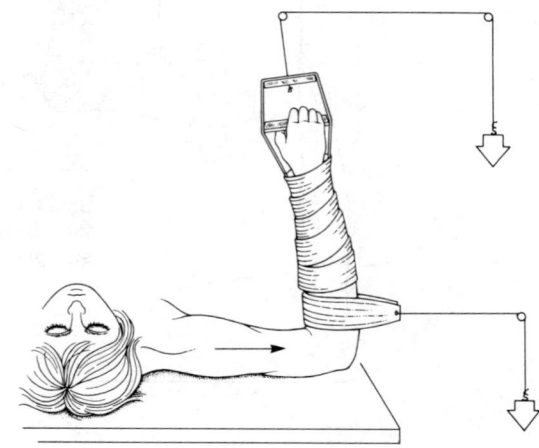

FIGURE 37-14. *Dunlop's traction.*

NURSING ACTION	RATIONALE/AMPLIFICATION
2. Check the child's fingers frequently for signs of circulatory impairment. Immediately report any coldness, pallor, cyanosis, swelling, pain, or limited sensation.	2. Prolonged circulatory impairment may lead to ischemia and Volkmann's contracture (clawhand) and flexion at the wrist and elbow.

CERVICAL TRACTION

Purpose

Used for children with spinal fractures, muscle spasms, or spinal injuries to provide immobilization in a neutral position which causes the least pressure on the spinal cord.

Mechanism of Action

Applied directly to the skull bone by a device such as the Crutchfield tong, or indirectly by using a head halter.

Cervical Skin (Head Halter) Traction (Fig. 37-15)

NURSING ACTION	RATIONALE/AMPLIFICATION
1. Check the position of the head halter frequently: a. The halter should not press on the ears. b. The rope should not rest against the skin. c. The chin piece should not press on the throat. d. Protect the chin halter when feeding the child.	1. It is important to prevent continuous pressure and rubbing on these areas in order to avoid skin breakdown.
2. Keep the position of the bed flat unless otherwise prescribed by the physician. Avoid lifting the child's head or flexing the neck.	2. Raising the head increases countertraction, which may be undesirable.
3. Keep the child flat on his back	
4. Diversion a. Position an adjustable mirror at the head of the bed so that the child can see around the room. b. Encourage companionship: (1) Place the child in a room with other children his age. (2) Allow liberal visiting by parents, older siblings and friends. c. Place colorful objects, cards, pictures, etc. within sight of the child. d. Utilize audiovisual stimulation—records, radio, television, etc. e. Provide for continuing education for the child of school age.	

Cervical Skeletal Traction

NURSING ACTION	RATIONALE/AMPLIFICATION
1. If possible, place the child on a Stryker frame or CircOlectric bed.	1. Allows the child to be turned in one motion.

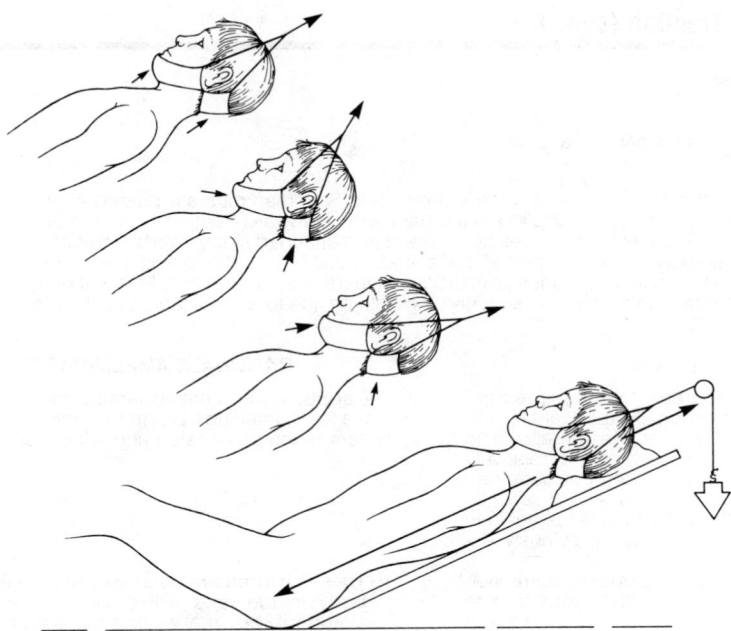

FIGURE 37-15. *Cervical traction.*

NURSING ACTION	RATIONALE/AMPLIFICATION
2. Make certain that the neck is held in steady longitudinal traction. 　　When the child is lying on his abdomen, support his arms on pillows at his sides and at the level of the bed.	2. The neck should never be flexed since this may cause permanent spinal cord injury. 　　The head should be in a neutral position in relation to the spine. The arms should not droop and the shoulders should not be hunched.
3. Do not allow the patient to reach for objects.	3. Reaching can disrupt spinal alignment.
4. Provide the child with adjustable mirrors at the head of the bed, and with prism glasses.	4. These aids enable the child to look around the room, watch television, or read while on his back.
5. Brush the child's teeth and frequently rinse his mouth with an antiseptic mouthwash. 　a. Instruct the child to try not to breathe through his mouth since this may cause dryness of the mucosa. 　b. Apply lemon and glycerin or a lip balm to his lips to prevent dryness and cracking.	5. This prevents mouth sores and is refreshing.

COTREL'S TRACTION

Purpose

To provide distraction of the spine prior to surgery or to the application of a scoliotic brace.

Mechanism of Action

Traction is applied primarily to the occipital bone by means of a head harness which fits onto the chin and reaches around to the occiput. Pelvic straps maintain the pelvis in a fixed position.

NURSING ACTION	RATIONALE/AMPLIFICATION
1. Check the head halter for proper placement. 　a. The chin pad should not compress the child's throat. 　b. The hair should be free from entanglement. 　c. The halter should not pinch the ears.	1. This helps to ensure effectiveness of the treatment and prevents skin breakdown.
2. Check the facial skin, chin, occiput, and iliac crests for possible irritation and breakdown.	
3. Check the child frequently for maintenance of alignment.	3. It is relatively easy for the child to become malaligned in this type of traction.

GUIDELINES: Care of a Child in Traction (cont.)

HALO-FEMORAL TRACTION

Purpose

Utilized to correct severe and resistant spinal curvatures.

Mechanism of Action

An aluminum halo is fixed to the cranium with 4 threaded pins and Steinman pins are placed in the distal ends of the femur. Upward traction is applied to the halo and downward traction to the femurs to pull the spine into alignment. Frequently, a suspension assembly is attached to the halo by threaded traction rods, the entire assembly being supported by a hoop attached to the pelvic pins. This apparatus allows control of position in all 3 planes plus progressive traction application. Femoral pins may be removed and countertraction applied by securing the halo device to a body jacket cast. This allows the child to be ambulatory.

NURSING ACTION	RATIONALE/AMPLIFICATION

1. Prepare the child and the parents for the procedure.
  a. Explain the purpose, method of application, and approximate time required for the therapy. The child should know that the treatment is relatively pain-free and that the device does not penetrate the brain.
  b. If possible, introduce the child to other patients in the apparatus or those who have previously experienced it.
  c. Emphasize that this will provide optimal correction of the deformity and allow the child to appear more normal.
	1. The appearance of the apparatus may be overwhelming and frightening. Diagrams and visual aids will enhance comprehension and allay fear.
	
	  c. These children are often very sensitive about their body image, and will develop a more positive attitude if they realize that the deformity is being improved.

2. Observe the child carefully while traction is being increased for:
  a. Neck pain
  b. Respiratory distress
  c. Nerve injury
	2. Alteration of neurological or respiratory status is regarded as a warning sign and a release of several turns on the extension bars may be carried out by the physician as an emergency measure. Neck pain is a less serious sign. The amount of traction is usually not increased until the pain disappears.

3. *Symptoms of injury*
  a. Spinal cord
    (1) Weakness, numbness in legs
    (2) Loss of bladder function
    (3) Up- or downturning of toes
    (4) Clonus of ankles or knees
  b. Cranial nerves
    (1) Double vision
    (2) Difficulty in swallowing
    (3) Difficulty in coughing
    (4) Voice changes
    (5) Tongue weakness
  c. Upper extremities
    (1) Difficulty in moving hand, shoulder, or arm
    (2) Numbness or weakness in hand (check grip)	

4. Make certain that all of the fixtures on the apparatus are tightened.	4. Looseness and excessive movement of the apparatus may cause pain and infection. The physician should be notified.
5. Report complaints of pain or drainage at the pin sites.	5. Most children have mild pain and headache for the first few days. Thereafter, pain at the pin site usually means that the pin is loose or infected, and it may be necessary to change the pin.

GUIDELINES: Assisting the Child on a Bradford Frame

A *Bradford frame* is a piece of equipment which facilitates the nursing of young children who must be immobilized for extensive periods of time. It is frequently used for young infants with meningoceles, children in hip–spica casts, and children with extensive burns.

Purposes
1. To ensure correct positioning.
2. To facilitate the collection of urine and stools.
3. To protect the child from injury.

Equipment   Frame of appropriate size for the child
2 pieces of canvas of appropriate size to cover the head and foot of the frame

Equipment (cont.)

Plastic sheeting
2 crib sheets or draw sheets
Bedboard
Linen for the bed
Plastic draw sheet
Heavy blocks for supporting the frame
Material such as canvas strips for attaching the frame to the bed
Protective device to limit the child's movement

Procedure

NURSING ACTION	RATIONALE/AMPLIFICATION
Preparatory Phase	
1. Select frame according to the size of the child.	1. Frame should be approximately 15 cm. (6 inches) longer and 5 cm. (2 inches) wider than the patient.
2. Cover the head and foot areas with canvas. 　a. Leave an open area between the head and foot sections for the drainage of urine and feces. 　b. Stretch the canvas tightly over the frame.	a. Make sure that the size of the opening is adequate for the size of the child. 　b. If the canvas is not tight, it will stretch.
3. Cover the top and bottom sections of the canvas with heavy plastic sheeting.	3. This protects the canvas from becoming soiled.
4. Place a small sheet tightly over each section of the frame.	
Performance Phase	
1. Place a bedboard on the mattress.	1. A firm base is required for proper use of the frame.
2. Place 2 draw sheets on the bed, one at each end.	2. The entire bed will not require changing when only one part is soiled.
3. Place a plastic draw sheet under the center opening of the frame.	3. This is the area most likely to become soiled by urine or feces.
4. Place blocks on the bed. Place the frame on the blocks.	4. The position of the blocks and frame will be prescribed by the physician. The blocks should always be placed under the child's shoulders, never directly under his head if the head of the frame is to be elevated.
5. Secure the frame to the bed at the head and foot.	5. This is a safety precaution to prevent slipping.
6. Place the bedpan below the center opening. 　a. Plastic sheeting may be draped over the top and bottom edges of the opening of the frame. 　b. Place diapers over the plastic.	a. This permits urine and feces to drain into the bedpan if the child is incontinent. 　b. This prevents irritation of the skin.
7. Place the child on the frame. 　a. Maintain his position by use of a jacket restraint. (See procedure for protective measures to limit movement.)	
8. Place pillows at the sides of the frame to support the child's arms.	8. It is important to maintain proper body alignment.
Follow-up Phase	
1. Check the following frequently: 　a. Position of the frame on the blocks. 　b. Security of all knots and materials which are used to fasten the frame to the bed. 　c. Position of the child on the frame.	1. These are principles of safety. (See procedure for protective devices to limit movement.)
2. Provide meticulous general hygiene: 　a. Empty the bedpan frequently. 　b. Check the linen for soiling by urine or feces and change it if necessary. 　c. Cleanse the buttocks after each bowel movement and apply lotion or cornstarch. 　d. Bathe daily and provide skin care frequently.	2. See procedure for traction and for care of a child in a spica cast.
3. Provide for the prevention of contractures, muscle wasting, and the development of hypostatic pneumonia.	3. See procedure for traction.
4. Provide diversion 　a. Move the child's bed from room to room for a change of scenery or out into the hall so that he can watch unit activities.	4. See procedures for traction and care of a child in a spica cast.
5. Reconstruct the child's frame as necessary 　a. The child can usually be placed on a firm bed or stretcher while his frame is being changed. 　b. If a second frame is available, this can be prepared and placed on another bed. The child can then be easily transferred from one frame to another.	a. Special care must be taken to ensure correct body alignment during this procedure.

CASTS

Nursing Considerations

Nursing activities related to the application and care of casts are essentially the same for pediatric and adult patients. The following points of consideration are important.

1. The child is usually more troubled by immobilization than the adult. A special attempt should be made to ensure that his activities are as normal as possible and that full use is made of his unaffected joints and muscles.
2. The younger child may not be able to understand why the cast is necessary. He may attempt to remove it, put pieces of toys or food under it, etc.

   a. An attempt should be made to allow the child to work through his questions and feelings via play (e.g., give him a doll with a cast).

   b. Close supervision is necessary to prevent the child from destroying the cast or injuring himself.

3. There is danger of soiling a long-leg or hip-spica cast with feces or urine. (The area of the cast near the buttocks and genitalia should be protected with waterproof material.)
4. For additional information, including types of casts, methods of application, complications, etc., refer to pages 757–763.

GUIDELINES: Care of a Child in a Spica Cast

Procedure NURSING ACTION	RATIONALE/AMPLIFICATION
1. If possible, prepare the child for the application of the cast.	1. This can best be acccomplished by allowing the child to put a cast on a doll. Older children should see a picture of the cast that is going to be applied and receive an explanation of the method of application.
2. Facilitate drying and accurate molding of the cast.	2. About 24-48 hours are required for a cast to dry completely. A cast dries from the outside to the inside. It may feel dry to the touch but still be wet on the inside.
a. Place a bedboard under the mattress.	a. Prevents sagging of the bed from pressure of the cast.
b. Support the curves of the cast with small, plastic-covered pillows.	b. Prevents cracking while the cast is drying.
c. Avoid placing a pillow under the head and shoulders.	c. Causes pressure on the chest by thrusting it forward in the cast.
d. Keep the cast uncovered and turn the child every 1-2 hours.	d. Allows moisture to evaporate from the surface.
e. Handle moist cast with the palms of hands.	e. Fingers may cause indentation in the moist plaster.
3. Observe for complications resulting from pressure of the cast.	3. Vascular insufficiency due to unrelieved swelling can cause necrosis and pressure sores. It may be necessary to bivalve the cast.

a. Impaired circulation to the toes.
   (1) Discoloration or cyanosis
   (2) Impaired movement
   (3) Loss of sensation
   (4) Edema
   (5) Temperature change
   (6) Absent pedal pulses	

b. Complaints of pain or pressure in any area where the cast fits closely over the body.	
4. Provide good skin care.	4. Prevents the development of pressure sores.
a. Bathe accessible skin and massage with emollient lotion. Pay special attention to the buttocks and genital area.	
b. Massage the skin underneath the cast with alcohol.	

c. Inspect the skin for signs of irritation:
   (1) Around cast edge.
   (2) Under the cast—pull skin taut and inspect under the cast, using a flashlight for illumination.	

d. Investigate complaints of pain or burning or an offensive odor from the inside of the cast.	d. These may indicate that a pressure sore is forming or has become infected. It may be necessary to create a "window" in the cast.
e. Relieve itching by blowing cool air through the cast with an asepto syringe or hair dryer.	e. Some physicians insert a strip of gauze through the cast which can be used to gently massage the skin. Do not use sharp objects such as coat hangers or knitting needles.

Procedure (cont.)

NURSING ACTION	RATIONALE/AMPLIFICATION

f. Do not allow a small child to put objects inside his cast.
   (1) Keep small toys away from the child
   (2) Pad the edges of the cast with cotton padding or cover it with a towel to prevent food particles and foreign objects from being inserted by the child.

f. A small hand vacuum cleaner may be used to remove crumbs from inside the cast.

5. Prevent the skin around the edge of the cast from becoming excoriated.
  a. Smooth the edges of the cast and petal it with waterproof adhesive tape.

a. This prevents flakes of plaster from breaking off and slipping under the cast. It also facilitates cleansing of the cast.

  b. Do not lift infants by their legs to change diapers.

6. Prevent urine and feces from soiling the cast.
  a. Offer the bedpan frequently.
   (1) Elevate the child's head slightly higher than his feet to prevent urine from running under the cast.
   (2) Place a sheet of plastic under the front and back edges of the cast opening for the buttocks and genitalia.
   (3) Slip the fracture pan beneath the buttocks.
   (4) Allow the ends of the plastic strips to hang into the pan.
  b. Place the child who is not toilet-trained on a Bradford frame.
   (1) See procedure for care of the child on a Bradford frame, page 1216.
   (2) Line the edges of the cast with waterproof material such as plastic or cellophane.
   (3) Tuck a folded diaper or perineal pad under the cast edges and change it frequently.
  c. Keep the perineum clean.
   (1) Wash the skin under the edge of the cast whenever necessary and dry it thoroughly.
   (2) Change diapers immediately after they become soiled.
  d. Clean the cast by rubbing it with a small amount of scouring agent on a damp cloth, then dry it promptly.

6. A soiled cast will cause skin irritation, become odorous, and may mildew or partially disintegrate.

d. A solution of zephiran chloride 1:750 may be used sparingly to eliminate odor-causing bacteria from cast.

7. Plan for short periods of muscle exercise every day.

  a. Encourage the child to move and exercise his unaffected extremities. Provide diversional therapy which requires the use of these muscles.
  b. Exercise the child's toes.

7. Disuse of muscles can result in atrophy and deformities.

8. Have the child breathe deeply at intervals. Provide him with soap bubbles, whistles, or party favors to make this more fun. An older child may use blow bottles.

8. Prolonged periods of immobilization may cause the child to develop hypostatic pneumonia.

9. Turn the child at least every 4 hours.
  a. Move the child to the side of the bed, using a steady, pulling motion.
  b. Place 1 hand under the head and back and 1 hand under the leg portion of the cast, and turn the child on his side.
  c. Second nurse accepts support of the child and cast as he is turned completely.

9. Do not use the supporting bar between the legs as a lever when turning the child.

10. Assess the child's bowel and bladder function.
  a. Provide an adequate fluid intake, especially fruit juices.
  b. Check the urine for signs of infection.

10. Immobilization may cause constipation and poor urinary drainage. Suppositories or mild laxatives may be necessary for the constipated child.

11. Maintain correct position of the cast.
  a. Support the contour of the cast with pillows. Allow the heel to extend beyond the pillow to avoid pressure sores.

11. This prevents cracking or flattening of the cast.

12. Provide as normal an environment as possible.

12. Enforced immobility is often traumatic for the child and may cause regression.

GUIDELINES: Care of a Child in a Spica Cast (cont.)

Procedure (cont.)

NURSING ACTION	RATIONALE/AMPLIFICATION

NURSING ACTION

a. Place the child on a cart or a stretcher so that he may leave his room. The child may be taken outdoors if the weather is suitable.

b. Allow the child to be dressed. (Wide, flared pants are especially suitable.)

c. Encourage contact with peers.

d. Provide for play activities.
 (1) Provide the young child with large toys which he cannot put into his cast.
 (2) Television is a good method of diversion if used with discretion.
 (3) Older children often enjoy checkers, sewing, art work, building models, etc.

e. Provide for education.
 (1) Refer the child to a visiting teacher service.
 (2) Provide for study time during each day.

13. Evaluate the home situation for feasibility of home care.
 a. The child's place in the family and the number of siblings
 b. Additional needs of the parents, such as pursuing their vocations
 c. Physical setup of the home
  (1) Number of stairs
  (2) Sleeping arrangement (type of bed, etc.)
 d. Financial situation
 e. Ability of the family to keep follow-up appointments

14. Assist the family in caring for the child after discharge.
 a. Initiate the appropriate referrals.
  (1) Community health nurse
  (2) Social service agency
  (3) Home tutoring service
  (4) Physical therapy
 b. Begin teaching early.
  (1) Instruct the parent on all aspects of the child's care.

RATIONALE/AMPLIFICATION

(1) Teach only a few aspects of care each day. Have the parent(s) participate in the child's care until capable of providing total nursing care under supervision.

  (2) Emphasize safety measures such as elevating the child's head during meals to prevent choking; preventing the small child from dropping objects into his cast; using good body mechanics when lifting and transporting the child, etc.
  (3) Provide with detailed, written instructions.

15. Assist with cast removal.
 a. Prepare the child for the procedure.
  (1) Describe the sensations that the child will feel (warmth, vibration, etc.) as well as the procedure itself.
  (2) Allow the child to observe as the saw is lightly touched to the operator's palm.
 b. Immobilize the child as necessary so that the procedure can be carried out quickly and safely.

15. Children often believe that the saw will cut off a limb, and are frightened by the loud noise.

16. Care for the child after cast removal.
 a. Support the part with pillows.

 b. Move the extremity gently.
 c. Wash the skin gently with mild soap and apply oil or lanolin.

 d. Encourage the child to do prescribed exercises.

 e. Elevate the extremity when sitting.

a. Maintain the same position that existed in the cast.
b. It will be very weak and stiff.
c. An accumulation of sebaceous material and dead skin causes the skin to appear brown and flaky. Vigorous rubbing will cause skin trauma.
d. These will strengthen muscles and relieve joint stiffness.
e. Minimizes the development of edema.

BIBLIOGRAPHY

GENERAL

Books

Avery GB. Neonatology. Philadelphia, JB Lippincott, 1981

Leiter G. Principles and Techniques in Pediatric Nursing, 3rd ed. Philadelphia, WB Saunders, 1977

Levin DL et al. A Practical Guide to Pediatric Intensive Care. St. Louis, CV Mosby, 1979

Marlow DR. Textbook of Pediatric Nursing, 4th ed. Philadelphia, WB Saunders, 1977

Matthews UF (ed). Manual of Pediatric Nursing Careplans. Dept. of Nursing, Hospital for Sick Children, Toronto, Canada, Boston, Little, Brown & Co, 1979

Montague A. Touching. New York, Harper & Row, Perennial Library, 1971

Schuberth K and Zitelli B (eds). The Harriet Lane Handbook, A Manual for Pediatric House Officers, 8th ed. Chicago, Year Book Medical Publishers, 1978

Scipien G et al. Comprehensive Pediatric Nursing, 2nd ed. New York, McGraw–Hill, 1979

Shirkey HC. Pediatric Therapy, 5th ed. St. Louis, CV Mosby, 1975

Steele S (ed). Nursing Care of the Child with Long-Term Illness. New York, Appleton–Century–Crofts, 1977

Waechter EH and Blake FG. Nursing Care of Children, 9th ed. Philadelphia, JB Lippincott, 1976

Whaley LF and Wong DL. Nursing Care of Infants and Children. St. Louis, CV Mosby, 1979

Whitson BJ and McFarlane J. The Pediatric Nursing Skills Manual. New York, John Wiley & Sons, 1980

VITAL SIGNS

Books

Assessing Vital Signs Accurately (Nursing Skillbook Series). Horsham, Intermed Communications, 1978

Articles

Abbey J et al. How long is that thermometer accurate? Am J Nurs 1978 Aug; 78(8):1375–1376

Haddock N. Blood pressure monitoring in neonates. MCN 1980 Mar/Apr; 5(2):131–135

Hill M. What can go wrong when you measure blood pressure. Am J Nurs 1980 May; 80(5):942–946

Patient assessment: Pulses, programmed instruction. Am J Nurs 1979 Jan; 79(1):115–132.

Reynolds J. How to take a temperature. Pediatric Nursing 1978 Nov/Dec; 4(6):67

Spitz P and Sweetwood H. Kids in crisis, Part 1: Bedside assessment—special considerations. Nursing '78 1978 Mar; 8(3):70–79

FEVER

Articles

Castle M and Watkins J. Fever: Understanding a sinister sign. Nursing '79 1979; 9(2):26–33

MEDICATIONS

Books

Sager DP and Bomar SK. Intravenous Medications. Philadelphia, JB Lippincott, 1980

Articles

Campbell J. The BSA Method of calculating pediatric drug dosages. MCN 1978 Nov/Dec; 3(6):357–360

Foster SD. Administering medications to children. Issues Compr Pediatr Nurs 1978 Nov; 3(5):1–14

Kimmell R. Keys to using the heparin lock. Nursing '74 1974 Nov; 4(11):52–53

Newton DW and Newton M. Route, site and technique: Three key decisions in giving parenteral medications. Nursing '79 1979 July; 9(7):18–25

PROTECTIVE DEVICES TO LIMIT MOVEMENT

Articles

Dowd E, Novak J, Ray E. Releasing the hospitalized child from restraints. MCN 1977 Nov/Dec; 2(6):370–373

McGuire M, Shepherd R, Greco A. Hospitalized children in confinement. Pediatric Nursing 1978 Nov/Dec; 4(6):31–35

FEEDING AND NUTRITION

Articles

Bishop WS and Bishop PA. Father-assisted breastfeeding. Pediatric Nursing 1978 Jan/Feb; 4(1):39–40

Choi MW. Breast milk for infants who can't breast-feed. Am J Nurs 1978 May; 78(5):852–855

Cruse P, Yudkin P, Baun JD. Establishing demand feeding in hospital. Arch Dis Child 1979 Jan; 53(1):76–78

Dutton MA. A breastfeeding protocol. JOGN Nurs 1979 May/June; 8(3):151–155

Grassley J and Davis K. Common concerns of mothers who breast-feed. MCN 1978 Nov/Dec; 3(6):347–351

Gunn S. The bottlefeeding mother needs your help too. RN 1979 Feb; 42(2):53

Henderson KJ and Newton LD. Helping nursing mothers maintain lactation while separated from their infants. MCN 1978 Nov/Dec; 3(6):352–356.

Measel CP and Anderson GC. Nonnutritive sucking during tube feedings: Effect on clinical course in premature infants. JOGN Nurs 1979 Sept; 8(5):265–272

Olson J. Breastfeeding: Common problems and practical answers. Pediatric Nursing 1978 Jan/Feb; 4(1):32–35

Price E and Gyotoku S. Using the nasojejunal feeding technique in a neonatal intensive care unit. MCN 1978 Nov/Dec; 3(6):361–365

Stewart D and Gaiser C. Supporting lactation when mothers and infants are separated. Nurs Clin North Am 1978 Mar; 13(1):47–61

McConnell EA. 10 problems with nasogastric tubes and how to solve them. Nursing '79 1979 Apr; 9(4):78–81

Simkins T. Feeding the premature infant: More questions than answers. Perinatology/Neonatology 1978 Jan/Feb; 2(1):30–36

SPECIMEN COLLECTION

Articles

Karna P and Poland RL. Digital capillary blood monitoring: An alternative. J Pediatr 1978 Feb; 92(2):270–273

FLUID AND ELECTROLYTE BALANCE

Books

Burgess A. The Nurse's Guide to Fluid and Electrolyte Balance. New York, McGraw–Hill, 1979

Fischer JE (ed). Total Parenteral Nutrition. Boston, Little, Brown & Co., 1976

Gans SL. Surgical Pediatrics—Nonoperative Care. New York, Grune & Stratton, 1980

Monitoring Fluid and Electrolytes Precisely (Nursing Skillbook Series). Horsham, Intermed Communications, 1978

Plumber A. Principles and Practice of I.V. Therapy, 2nd ed. Boston, Little, Brown & Co., 1975

Winters RW (ed). Body Fluids in Pediatrics. Boston, Little, Brown & Co., 1973

Articles

Principles

Aspinall M. A simplified guide to managing patients with hyponatremia. Nursing '78 1978 Dec; 8(12):32–35

McGrath B. Fluids, electrolytes and replacement therapy in pediatric nursing. MCN 1980 Jan/Feb; 5(1):58–62

Methany N and Snively W. Perioperative fluids and electrolytes, Am J Nurs 1978 Mar; 78(3):840–845

Shrake K. The ABC's of ABG's or how to interpret a blood gas value. Nursing '79 1979 Sept; 9(9):26–33

Twombly M. The shift into the third space. Nursing '78 1978 June; 8(6):38–41

Intravenous Infusion

Beaumont E. The new IV infusion pumps. Nursing '77 1977 July; 7(7):31–35

Fundamentals of I.V. maintenance, programmed instruction. Am J Nurs 1979 July; 79(7):1274–1287

Guhlow LJ et al. Pediatric IVs: Special measures you must take. RN 1979 Mar; 42:40–51

Manzi C and Masoorli S. Troubles with I.V.'s? Try these tips and techniques. Nursing '78 1978 Oct; 8(10):78–84

Milliam D. How to insert an I.V. Am J Nurs 1979 July; 79(7):1268–1271

Morris M. Intravenous drug incompatibilities. Am J Nurs 1979 July; 79(7):1288–1291

Total Parenteral Nutrition

Bjeletick J and Hickman R. The Hickman indwelling catheter. Am J Nurs 1980 Jan; 80(1):62–65

Colley R and Wilson J. Meeting patients' nutritional needs with hyperalimentation. How to begin hyperalimentation therapy. Nursing '79 1979 May; 9(5):76–83

Colley R and Wilson J. Managing the patient on hyperalimentation. Nursing '79 1979 June; 9(6):57–61

Colley R and Wilson J. Providing hyperalimentation for infants and children. Nursing '79 1979 July; 9(7):50–53

Colley R and Wilson J. Administering peripheral and enteral feedings. Nursing '79 1979 Sept; 9(9):62–69

Colley R and Wilson J. Teaching patients to administer hyperalimentation infusions at home. Nursing '79 1979 Aug; 9(8):56–63

Guild RT and Cerda, JJ. Total parenteral nutrition. J Fla Med Assoc 1979 Apr; 66(4):401–408

Ivey MF. The status of parenteral nutrition. Nurs Clin North Am 1979 June; 14(2):285–304

Lawson M, Bottino J, McCredie K. Long-term I.V. therapy: A new appraoch. Am J Nurs 1979 June; 79(6):1100–1103

Parfitt D and Thompson V. Pediatric home hyperalimentation: Educating the family. MCN 1980 May/June; 5(3):196–202

Product Information—Intralipid 10%. Berkley, Cutter Laboratories, 1975 Sept

Schloesser L, Hryciuk L, Hoffman DM. Parenteral nutrition: A team concept from the pharmacist's viewpoint. Am J Intravenous Therapy 1978 Jan; 5(1):42–53

CHEST PHYSICAL THERAPY AND RESPIRATORY MEASURES

Books

Lough M, Doershuk C, Stern RC (eds). Pediatric Respiratory Therapy, 2nd ed. Chicago, Year Book Medical Publishers, 1979

Providing Respiratory Care (Nursing Photobook Series). Horsham, Intermed Communications, 1979

Using Monitors (Nursing Photobook Series). Horsham, Intermed Communications, 1979

Articles

Chest Physical Therapy

Curran C and Kachoyeanos M. The effects on neonates of two methods of chest physical therapy. MCN 1979 Sept/Oct; 4(5):309–313

Lagerson J. The cough—its effectiveness depends on you. Respiratory Care 1979 Feb; 24:142–149

Segmental Bronchial Drainage, Professional Education Committee of the Cystic Fibrosis Foundation, Atlanta, Georgia, 1978

Tecklin J. Positioning, percussing and vibrating patients for effective bronchial drainage. Nursing '79 1979 Mar; 9(3):64–71

Suctioning

O'Malley P and Zankofski M. Disposable suction catheters. A Nursing '79 product survey. Nursing '79 1979 May; 9(5):70–75

Sandham G and Reid B. Some Q's and A's about suctioning. Nursing '77 1977 Oct; 7(10):60–65

Tracheostomy Care

Aradine C. Home care for young children with long-term tracheostomies. MCN 1980 Mar/Apr; 5(2):121–125

O'Donnell B and Gilmore B. How to change tracheostomy ties easily and safely. Nursing '78 1978 Mar; 66–69

Oxygen Therapy

Donahue LM et al. A comparison of arterial oxygenation in infants receiving CPAP by nasal prongs or by hood chamber. Respir Ther 1978 Sept/Oct; 8(6):61–62

Fuchs P. Getting the best out of oxygen delivery systems. Nursing '80 1980 Dec; 10(12):34–43

Glassanos MR. Infants who are oxygen dependent—sending them home. MCN 1980 Jan/Feb; 5(1):42–45

Glover DW. Infant oxygen hoods. Respir Ther 1978 Sept/Oct 8(6):49+

Hildebrand W et al. Use and abuse of oxygen in the newborn. Am Fam Physician 1978 Sept; 18(3):125–132

Ventilatory Support and Monitoring

Adams N. The nurse's role in systematic weaning from a ventilator. Nursing '79 1979 Aug; 9(8):35–41

Dingle R et al. Continuous transcutaneous O_2 monitoring in the neonate. Am J Nurs 1980 May; 80(5):890–893

Durand O. Equipment survey: Infant respirators and respirator–incubators. Respir Ther 1979 Jan/Feb; 9:46

Fuchs P. Understanding continuous mechanical ventilation. Nursing '79 1979 Dec; 9(12):26–33

Nielsen L. Mechanical ventilation: Patient assessment and nursing care. Am J Nurs 1980 Dec; 80(12):2191–2217

Schroeder BD. A creative approach to caring for the ventilator-dependent child. MCN 1979 May/June; 4(3):165–170

Shrake K. The ABC's of ABG's or how to interpret a blood gas value. Nursing '79 1979 Sept; 9(9)26–33

CARDIOPULMONARY RESUSCITATION

Articles

Boychuck RB and Boychuck TC. Resuscitation of the newborn, Part I. Respir Technology 1979 Aug; 15:9–13

Boychuck RB and Boychuck TC. Resuscitation of the newborn, Part 2. Respir Technology 1979 Oct;15:5–6

Hart R. CPR review. Nursing '78 1978 June; 8(6):48–53

LeFort S. Cardiopulmonary resuscitation: Step-by-step. Can Nurs 1978 Feb; 74(2):38–47

Melker R. CPR in neonates, infants and children. CCQ 1978 May; 1(5):49–65

Proctor A. Pediatric arrest: Scaling down CPR. RN 1979 Sept; 42(9):58–64

Wilson SE. Neonatal resuscitation. AANA J 1979 Oct; 47(10):548–555

DIALYSIS

Books

Jungers P et al. The Essentials in Hemodialysis. Boston, Martinus Nijhoff Publishers, 1978

Articles

Denniston D and Burns K. Home peritoneal dialysis. Am J Nurs 1980 Nov; 80(11):2022–2026

Gorrell JF. Hemolytic–uremic syndrome: An overview and pediatric case report. MCN 1978 July/Aug; 3(4):235–241

Irwin B. Hemodialysis means vascular access and the right kind of nursing care. Nursing '79 1979 Oct; 9(10):49–53

McDaid TK. Chronic hemodialysis in children. Compr Pediatr Nurs 1978 Mar/Apr; 2(2):53–70

Neff E. Orienting, resistive and adaptive responses of children undergoing hemodialysis for kidney failure. Matern Child Nurs J 1978 Winter; 7(4):195–254

Sampson N. Peritoneal dialysis as a treatment modality. Nephrol Nurse 1980 Jan/Feb; 2(1):15–17

Spinozzi NS. Teaching nutritional management to children on chronic hemodialysis. J Am Diet Assoc 1979 Aug; 75(2):157–159

TRACTION AND CASTS

Books

Hilt N and Schmitt W. Pediatric Orthopedic Nursing. St. Louis, CV Mosby, 1975

Lewis R. Handbook of Traction, Casting and Splinting Techniques. Philadelphia, JB Lippincott, 1977

Articles

Farrell J. Casts, your patients and you. Part I: A review of basic procedures. Nursing '78 1978 Oct; 8(10):65–69

Farrell J. Casts, your patients and you. Part II: A review of arm and leg cast procedures. Nursing '78 1978 Nov; 8(11)57–61

Farrell J. Casts, your patients and you. Part III: A review of hip–spica procedures. Nursing '78 1978 Dec; 8(12):53–57

McGuire M, Shepherd R, Greco A. Hospitalized children in confinement. Pediatric Nursing 1978 Nov/Dec; 4(6):31–35

Moratz VA. Adapting shirts to fit over a halo vest. Am J Occup Ther 1979 Aug; 33(8):524–525

Nursing care of the patient in traction, a programmed instruction. Am J Nurs 1978 Oct; 78(10):1771–1798

Prilook ME (ed). Keeping up with the best in casting, photolecture with Carl E. Anderson. M.D. Patient Care 1979 July; 13(7):24–27

Rutecki B and Seligson D. Caring for the patient in a halo apparatus. Nursing '80 1980 Oct; 10(10):73–77

38

PROBLEMS OF INFANTS

MANAGEMENT OF THE PREMATURE INFANT

The *premature infant* is a viable infant born before the completion of 37 weeks' gestation.

Low Birth Weight (LBW) infant is one whose birth weight is 1501–2500 gm. (3 lbs. 5 oz.–5 lbs. 8 oz.) without regard to gestational age.

Very Low Birth Weight (VLBW) infant is one whose birth weight is below 1500 gm. without regard to gestational age.

Etiology

1. Unknown
2. Maternal factors associated with prematurity:
   a. Chronic poor nutrition
   b. Diabetes
   c. Multiple births
   d. Drug abuse
   e. IUD in gravid uterus
   f. Chronic disease
      (1) Heart disease
      (2) Kidney disease
      (3) Infection
   g. Complications of pregnancy
      (1) Toxemia
      (2) Bleeding
      (3) Placenta previa or abruptio placentae
      (4) Incompetent cervix
      (5) Premature rupture of membranes
      (6) Polyhydramnios
   h. Multigravida under 18 years of age; primigravida over 35 years of age
3. Fetal factors associated with prematurity:
   a. Chromosomal abnormalities
   b. Anatomic abnormalities
      (1) Tracheoesophageal atresia or fistula
      (2) Intestinal obstruction
   c. Fetoplacental unit dysfunction

Clinical Manifestations

1. Physical appearance
   Hair—lanugo, fluffy
   Poor ear cartilage
   Skin—very thin; capillaries are visible (may be red and wrinkled)
   Lack of subcutaneous fat
   Sole of foot is smooth
      (36 weeks' gestation—anterior ⅓ of foot is creased)
      (38 weeks' gestation—⅔ of foot is creased)
   Breast buds 5 mm
      (36 weeks' gestation—none)
      (38 weeks' gestation—3 mm.)
   Testes—undescended
   Labia minora—undeveloped
   Rugae of scrotum—very fine
   Fingernails—softer
   Abdomen—relatively large
   Thorax—relatively small
   Head—appears disproportionately large
   Facies resembles "an old man"
   Muscle tone poor—reflexes weak
2. Generally, maturation and growth rate increase after birth

Pathophysiology

The premature infant has altered physiology due to immature and often poorly developed systems. The severity of any problem that occurs depends upon the gestational age of the infant.

A. *Respiratory system* *

1. Alveoli begin to form at 26–28 weeks' gestation; therefore, lungs are poorly developed.
2. Respiratory muscles are poorly developed.
3. Chest wall lacks stability.
4. Production of surfactant is reduced.
5. There is reduced compliance and low functional residual capacity of the lung.
6. Breathing may be labored and irregular with periods of apnea and cyanosis.

---

* Systems and situations that are most likely to cause problems in the premature.

7. Infant is prone to atelectasis.
8. Gag and cough reflexes are poor; thus, aspiration is a problem.

B. *Digestive system**

1. Stomach is small and vomiting is likely to occur because of poor muscle tone at cardiac sphincter. It is difficult to provide caloric requirement in early days.
2. Tolerance is decreased and there is impaired ability to absorb fat, vitamin D, and all fat-soluble vitamins.

C. *Poor thermal stability**

1. Has very little subcutaneous fat; thus, there is no heat storage or insulation.
2. Limited ability to shiver; has poor vasomotor control of blood flow to skin capillaries.
3. There is a relatively large surface area in comparison to body weight.
4. Sweat glands are decreased; infant cannot perspire, under 32 weeks' gestation.
5. Has reduced muscle and fat deposits that restrict metabolic rate and heat production.
6. Usually is less active.

D. *Renal function*

1. Sodium excretion is probably increased, which may lead to hyponatremia; there is difficulty in excreting potassium.
2. Ability to concentrate urine decreases; thus, when vomiting or diarrhea occur, dehydration is likely to follow.
3. Ability to acidify urine decreases.
4. Glomerular tubular imbalance accounts for sugar, protein, amino acids, and sodium present in urine.

E. *Nervous system*

1. Response to stimulation is slow.
2. Suck, swallow, and gag reflexes are poor; feeding and aspiration therefore are problems.
3. Cough reflex is weak or absent.
4. Centers that control respirations, temperature, and other vital functions are poorly developed.

F. *Infection** (see p. 1247, Sepsis Neonatorum)

1. Actively formed antibodies are absent at birth (active immunity).
2. No IgM is present at birth (passive immunity).
3. Limited chemotaxis (reaction of cell to chemical stimuli).
4. Decreased opsonization (preparation of cells for phagocytosis).
5. Limited phagocytosis (digestion of bacteria by cells).
6. Hypofunctioning adrenal gland contributes to a decreased anti-inflammatory response.

G. *Liver function*

1. Does not have ability to handle and conjugate bilirubin.
2. Does not store or release sugar well; thus, there is a tendency toward hypoglycemia.
3. There is a steady decrease in hemoglobin after birth and in the production of blood; therefore, anemia may occur.
4. Does not make or store vitamin K; thus, infant is susceptible to hemorrhagic disease.

* Systems and situations that are most likely to cause problems in the premature.

H. *Eyes*

1. Oxygen given beyond the point of infant need will cause retinal arteries to constrict, resulting in anoxic damage.
2. The retinae detach from the surface of posterior chambers and a fibrous mass forms, resulting in an inability to receive visual stimulation. This is retrolental fibroplasia (RLF).
3. There are many stages of RLF.
4. The exact amount and level of oxygen needed to produce RLF is unknown.

Complications in Premature Infants

1. The severity of any problem that occurs in the premature infant depends upon the gestational age of that infant.
   a. Hyaline membrane disease (respiratory distress syndrome)
   b. Aspiration
   c. Infection
   d. Hypoglycemia
   e. Hypocalcemia
   f. Patent ductus arteriosus
   g. Persistent fetal circulation
2. Major complications related to low birth weight infants include:
   a. Hypoxia, hyperoxia
   b. Hypoglycemia, hyperglycemia
   c. Difficulty feeding
   d. Dehydration

Assessment

A. *Accurate body measurements (Fig. 38-1)—including:*

1. Head circumference—Frontal–Occipital (FOC) one finger above eyebrows, using parallel lines of tape around head.
2. Chest circumference—at nipple line.
3. Abdominal girth—one finger above umbilicus, mark location.
4. Heel–Crown—used to calculate nasotracheal tube length.
5. Shoulder to umbilicus—used to calculate proper length of catheter for umbilical arterial catheter placement.

B. *Assessment to determine gestational age (Table 38-1)*

1. Physical Assessment of Maturity (i.e., sole creasing, presence of lanugo, skin transparency)
2. Neurologic Assessment
   a. Maturation of the nervous system progresses at its own pace and is not increased by birth.
   b. The value of a neurologic evaluation increases after 48 hours of life.
   c. This examination is used primarily to estimate the infant's gestational age.
   d. The examination should be done when the infant is awake and quiet.
   e. Examination includes evaluation of muscle tone and evaluation of reflexes and reactions.
3. Assessment for appropriateness of size for gestational age
   a. Once weight, length, head circumference, and gestational age have been determined, these criteria are plotted on the intrauterine growth curve to determine if the infant is small, appropriate, or large for his gestational age (Figure 38-2).
   b. This knowledge will aid in anticipating potential problems that may occur in the infant.

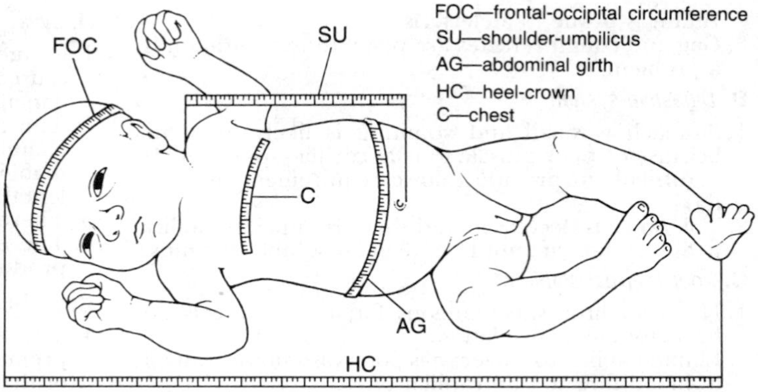

FIGURE 38-1. *Infant measurements: FOC,* frontal-occipital circumference; *SU,* shoulder-umbilicus; *AG,* abdominal girth; *HC,* heel-crown; *C,* chest. (Adapted from: Levin D.C., Morriss F.C., and Moore G.C. A Practical Guide to Pediatric Intensive Care. St. Louis, C.V. Mosby, 1979, p. 8.)

FOC—frontal-occipital circumference
SU—shoulder-umbilicus
AG—abdominal girth
HC—heel-crown
C—chest

c. Laboratory data as appropriate:
  (1) Blood gases
  (2) Blood sugar or Dextrostix
  (3) CBC or Hb and Hct
  (4) Lecithin/sphingomyelin ratio (L/S ratio) assessment of lung maturity
  (5) Electrolytes
d. Brazelton Neonatal Assessment Scale—can assist in identifying interactive capabilities of the infant and in assessing the impact of these capabilities upon the parents. Use of this information can enhance parent–infant interactions and relationships.

Nursing Objectives and Management

Admission to the Nursery

A. *To observe for any gross abnormalities as in the case of a full-term infant on admission, and to pay special attention to respirations, heart rate, blood pressure, muscle tone, and activity.*

1. Respirations above 40/minute over a period of time may be indicative of respiratory difficulty.
  a. Expiratory grunting, retractions, chest lag, or nasal flaring should be reported immediately (Silverman chart, Fig. 38-3).
  b. Cyanosis (other than acrocyanosis-coldness and cyanosis of hands and feet) should be watched for along with other signs of respiratory distress.
2. Increased (above 120/minute) or irregular heart rate may indicate cardiac or circulatory difficulties.
3. Muscle tone and activity should be evaluated.
4. Hypotension, indicated by blood-pressure measurement, may be due to hypovolemia.

B. *To maintain a patent airway.*

1. Have oxygen, suction, and resuscitation equipment readily available.
2. Suction mouth and pharynx if mucus is present—to prevent aspiration. Premature infants often have an excess amount of mucus as well as poor cough, swallow, and gag reflexes.
3. Position infant in Isolette or radiant heater to allow for easy drainage of mucus from his mouth.
  a. Very small premature infants—place on side.
  b. Larger premature infants—place on abdomen.
  c. Head may be tilted down—this may be contraindicated because of increased intracranial pressure or increased respiratory distress due to liver pushing against diaphragm decreasing lung expansion.

4. Administer emergency oxygen to just barely relieve cyanosis.

C. *To provide and maintain thermal neutrality of the premature infant.*

1. Obtain weight and temperature; then attach cardiac monitor leads quickly and place infant in warm environment (Isolette, radiant heater). Omit bath until infant's temperature has stabilized.
2. The premature infant's ability to control his own body temperature is inhibited by many factors related to his immaturity (see p. 1224).

D. *To ensure that prophylactic measures have been administered against ophthalmia neonatorum and that vitamin K_1 has been administered.*

Since the premature infant is frequently taken from the delivery room as soon as possible after birth, prophylactic measures may have been omitted.

E. *To be aware of early complications that may arise as a result of complications of the pregnancy, labor or delivery.*

1. Maternal medication.
  a. Drugs pass quickly from mother's blood, across the placenta into the infant's blood.
  b. Infant may be drowsy and have slowed respirations.
  c. Because of poor development, respiratory difficulty may occur.
2. Blood incompatibility of mother and infant.
  a. Premature infant is more susceptible to jaundice, even without incompatibilities.
  b. Observe closely for early signs of jaundice (see p. 1242, hyperbilirubinemia).
3. Maternal conditions that may predispose to infant problems.
  a. Infection or illness
  b. Diabetes
  c. Drugs
4. Neonatal asphyxia
  a. Apgar score of less than 5 at 1 minute and less than 7 at 5 minutes
  b. Asphyxia may be defined as any of the following:
    (1) Hypoxia (reduced oxygen available)
    (2) Anoxia (total lack of oxygen)
    (3) Hypercapnia (inability of eliminate CO_2)
    (4) Acidosis
  c. Causes of asphyxia or hypoxia can originate in the mother, the placenta, the infant, or may be a result of the delivery.

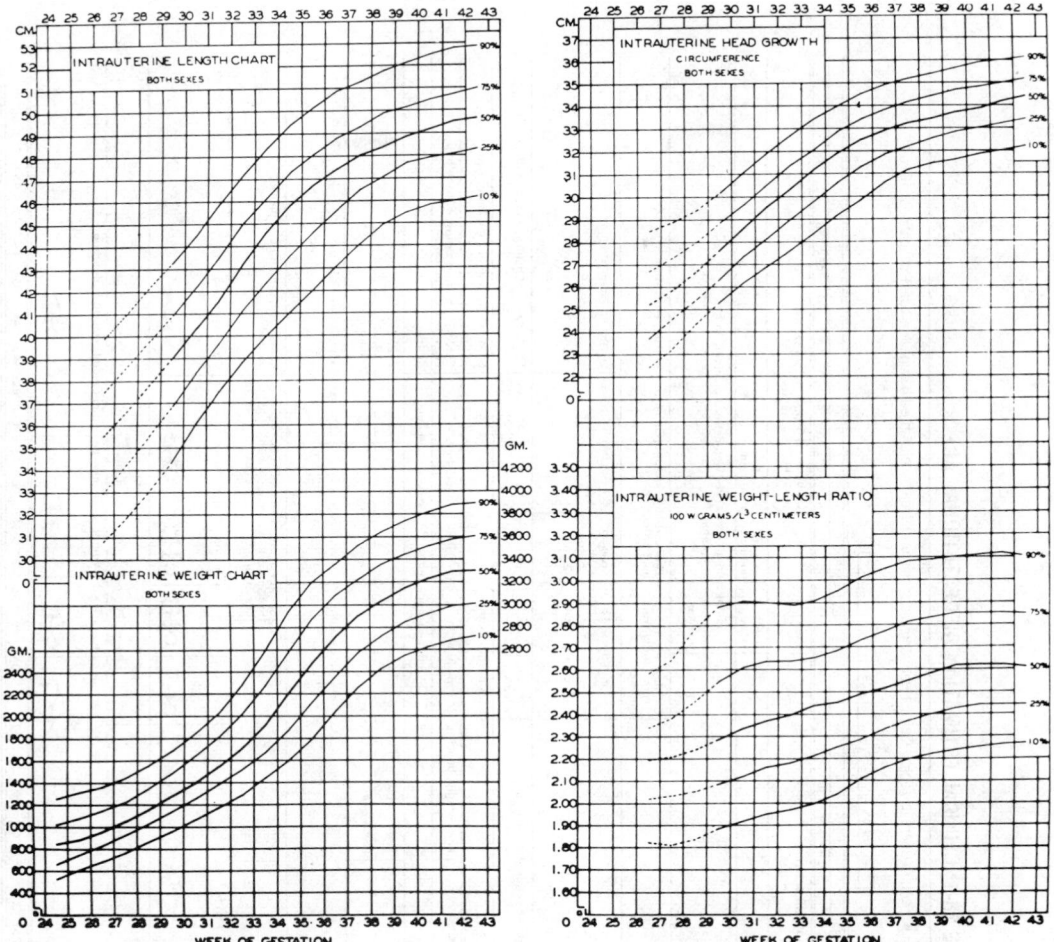

FIGURE 38-2. *Percentiles of intrauterine growth in weight, length, head circumference and weight-length ratio. (Lubchenco, L.O., Hansman, C., and Boyd, E.: Pediatrics 37:403, 1966.)*

The First 24–48 Hours of Life

This period after birth is the most critical time for the premature infant.

A. *To be constantly aware of the infant's condition and to make frequent observations.*

1. This poorly developed, immature infant is prone to sudden and rapid changes in condition.
2. Early recognition of symptoms and reporting observations to physician are the most valuable contributions the nurse can make in caring for and saving the premature infant's life.
3. Note bleeding from the umbilical cord.
   a. Should bleeding occur, apply pressure.
   b. Estimate amount of bleeding and record.
   c. Notify the physician immediately—replacement transfusion may be necessary.
4. Note first voiding.
   a. This may occur up to 36 hours after birth, but it usually occurs within the first 24 hours. Report any 4- to 6-hour period when voiding does not occur.
   b. Note amount, color, and frequency of voidings.

   c. Lack of voiding may indicate renal system anomalies, shock, or poor circulation
5. Note stools.
   a. Note when first stool occurred and its characteristics.
   b. Abdominal distention and lack of stool may indicate intestinal obstruction or other intestinal tract anomalies. Measure abdominal girth at regular intervals.
6. Note activity and behavior.
   a. Note amount of lethargy or activity or need for stimulation.
   b. Look for sucking movement, hand-to-mouth maneuver. This can help to determine oral feeding initiation.
   c. Note quality of cry.
7. Observe for a tense and bulging fontanelle; feel suture lines noting separation or overriding.
   a. Full fontanelle may indicate hydrocephalus or intracranial hemorrhage.
   b. Be alert to twitching and seizures.
8. Note color of skin.
   a. Cyanosis

TABLE 38-1. CLINICAL ESTIMATION OF GESTATIONAL AGE

(Reproduced with permission from Kempe, C.H., Silver, H.K., and O'Brien, D. (eds): Current Pediatric Diagnosis and Treatment, 4th ed. Lange Medical Publications, 1976.)

WEEKS GESTATION — columns: 20 21 22 23 24 25 26 27 28 29 30 31 32 33 34 35 36 37 | **Examination First Hours** — 38 39 40 41 42 43 44 45 46 47 48

PHYSICAL FINDINGS	Progression across weeks of gestation
Vernix	Appears (~20); Covers body, thick layer (24–37); On back, scalp, in creases (38); Scant, in creases (40–41); No vernix (43)
Breast tissue and areola	Areola and nipple barely visible, no palpable breast tissue (~22); Areola raised (35); 1–2 mm nodule (36–37); 3–5 mm (38–39); 5–6 mm (39–40); 7–10 mm (41); ?12 mm (44)
Ear — Form	Flat, shapeless (~22); Beginning incurving superior (34–35); Incurving upper 2/3 pinnae (36–37); Well-defined incurving to lobe (40)
Ear — Cartilage	Pinna soft, stays folded (~22); Cartilage scant, returns slowly from folding (33); Thin cartilage, springs back from folding (38); Pinna firm, remains erect from head (42)
Sole creases	Smooth soles without creases (~22); 1–2 anterior creases (32); 2–3 anterior creases (34–35); Creases anterior 2/3 sole (36–37); Creases involving heel (40); Deeper creases over entire sole (43)
Skin — Thickness & appearance	Thin, translucent skin, plethoric, venules over abdomen, edema (~22–30); Smooth, thicker, no edema (34); Pink (36); Few vessels (38–39); Some desquamation, pale pink (40–41); Thick, pale, desquamation over entire body (43–45)
Skin — Nail plates	Appear (~22); Nails to finger tips (34); Nails extend well beyond finger tips (45)
Hair	Appears on head (~26); Eye brows and lashes (~27); Fine, woolly, bunches out from head (29); Silky, single strands, lays flat (35); ?Receding hairline or loss of baby hair, short, fine underneath (44)
Lanugo	Appears (~22); Covers entire body (24); Vanishes from face (35); Present on shoulders (38); No lanugo (42)
Genitalia — Testes	Testes palpable in inguinal canal (~28); In upper scrotum (37–38); In lower scrotum (41)
Genitalia — Scrotum	Few rugae (28); Rugae, anterior portion (37); Rugae cover (40–41); Pendulous (42)
Genitalia — Labia & clitoris	Prominent clitoris, labia majora small, widely separated (30); Labia majora larger, nearly cover clitoris (37); Labia minora and clitoris covered (43)
Skull firmness	Bones are soft (~22); Soft to 1" from anterior fontanelle (30); Spongy at edges of fontanelle, center firm (36); Bones hard, sutures easily displaced (39–40); Bones hard, cannot be displaced (44)
Posture — Resting	Hypotonic, lateral decubitus (~22); Hypotonic (25–26); Beginning flexion, thigh (31); Stronger hip flexion (32); Frog-like (34–35); Flexion, all limbs (36); Hypertonic (38–39); Very hypertonic (43)
Recoil – leg	No recoil (~20); Partial recoil (33); Prompt recoil (39)
Recoil – Arm	No recoil (~20); Begin flexion, no recoil (34–35); Prompt recoil, may be inhibited (37–39); Prompt recoil after 30" inhibition (43)

Bottom scale (weeks): 20 21 22 23 24 25 26 27 28 29 30 31 32 33 34 35 36 37 38 39 40 41 42 43 44 45 46 47 48

Confirmatory Neurologic Examination To Be Done After 24 Hours

Weeks Gestation

Physical Findings	20	22	24	26	28	30	32	34	36	38	40	42	44	46	48
Tone															
Heel to ear					No resistance		Some resistance		Impossible						
Scarf sign	No resistance							Elbow passes midline		Elbow at midline		Elbow does not reach midline			
Neck flexors (head lag)	Absent										Head in plane of body		Holds head		
Neck extensors								Head begins to right itself from flexed position	Good righting cannot hold it	Holds head few seconds	Keeps head in line with trunk >40″		Turns head from side to side		
Body extensors								Straightening of legs	Straightening of trunk		Straightening of head and trunk together				
Vertical positions				When held under arms, body slips through hands				Arms hold baby, legs extended?	Legs flexed, good support with arms						
Horizontal positions				Hypotonic, arms and legs straight					Arms and legs flexed	Head and back even, flexed extremities			Head above back		
Flexion angles															
Popliteal	No resistance				150°		110°		100°	90°					
Ankle							60°	45°	20°	30°		A pre-term who has reached 40 weeks still has a 40° angle			
Wrist (square window)						90°	60°	45°		30°	0				
Reflexes															
Sucking				Weak, not synchronized with swallowing			Stronger, synchronized	Perfect			Perfect				
Rooting				Long latency period slow, imperfect	Hand to mouth		Extension, no adduction	Brisk, complete, durable			Perfect, hand to mouth		Complete		
Grasp				Finger grasp is good, strength is poor			Stronger			Can lift baby off bed, involves arms				Hands open	
Moro			Barely apparent	Weak, not elicited every time			Complete with arm extension, open fingers, cry		Arm adduction added					?Begins to lose Moro	
Crossed extension				Flexion and extension in a random, purposeless pattern			Extension, good support on sole	Still incomplete	Extension, adduction, fanning of toes		Complete				
Automatic walk					Minimal	Begins tiptoeing	Begins tiptoeing, good support on sole	Fast tiptoeing			Heel-toe progression, whole sole of foot	A pre-term who has reached 40 weeks walks on toes		?Begins to lose automatic walk	
Pupillary reflex	Absent				Appears										
Glabellar tap	Absent					Appears	Appears								
Tonic neck reflex	Absent					Appears	Present								
Neck-righting	Absent							Appears		Present after 37 weeks					

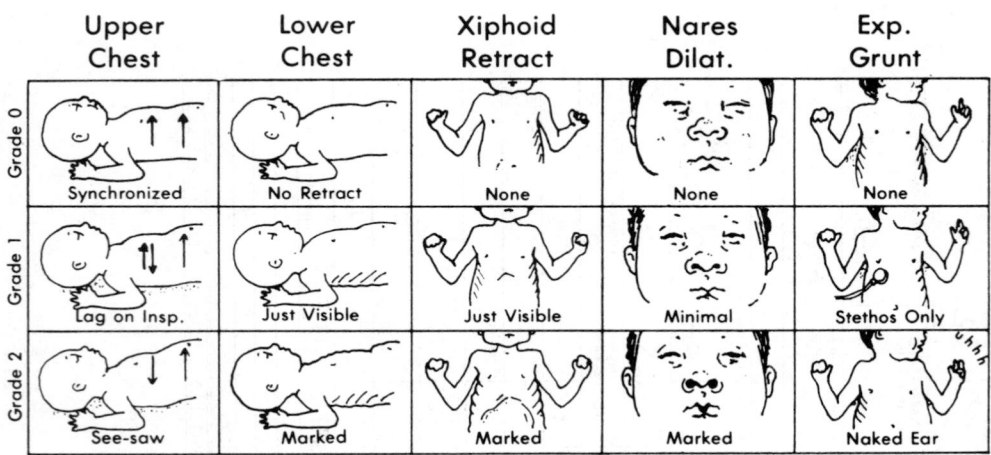

	Upper Chest	Lower Chest	Xiphoid Retract	Nares Dilat.	Exp. Grunt
Grade 0	Synchronized	No Retract	None	None	None
Grade 1	Lag on Insp.	Just Visible	Just Visible	Minimal	Stethos Only
Grade 2	See-saw	Marked	Marked	Marked	Naked Ear

FIGURE 38-3. *Observation of retractions. An index of respiratory distress is determined by grading each of five arbitrary criteria; grade 0 indicates no difficulty, grade 1 moderate difficulty, and grade 2 maximum respiratory difficulty. The "retraction score" is the sum of these values; a total score of 0 indicates no dyspnea, whereas a total score of ten denotes maximal respiratory distress. (Adapted from W.A. Silverman and B.H. Andersen. Pediatrics 17:4, 1956. Courtesy of Mead Johnson.)*

  (1) Circulatory or cardiac difficulties may be present.
  (2) Respiratory effort may be ineffective.
 b. Jaundice
  (1) May indicate infection.
  (2) Erythroblastosis fetalis is another possible difficulty.
9. Carefully monitor, record, and report vital signs.

B. *To maintain respirations.*

1. Immediate emergency support may be necessary, since respiratory system is poorly developed and ability to control respirations is often barely sufficient.
2. Have available resuscitative equipment, oxygen, and suction apparatus.
 a. Mucus may not be handled well, because of poor gag, cough, and swallowing reflexes.
  (1) Clearing the airway is of major importance.
  (2) A rubber ear bulb syringe is often all that is necessary for clearing the mouth.
  (3) Frequent suctioning of the pharynx may not be necessary.
3. Position infant to allow for easy ventilation.
 a. Supine position permits free expansion of the thoracic cage (infant's body weight is on the chest and abdomen when he is prone).
 b. Elevate head and trunk to decrease pressure on diaphragm from abdominal organs.
 c. Slight neck extension affords opening of trachea; place small roll under shoulders.
 d. Do not constrict abdominal area, since abdominal muscles are used to aid respiratory effort.
 e. Flex and abduct arms to enhance chest expansion.
 f. Change position from side to side. Perform postural drainage every 2 hours to aid in draining fluid accumulation in thoracic cavity.
4. Use only the percentage of oxygen necessary to relieve cyanosis or maintain color.
 a. Oxygen is used with moisture to prevent mucous membranes from drying and becoming irritated.
 b. Monitor oxygen with analyzer every hour to ensure consistency in percentage used.

5. Note any changes in respiratory effort and report these to physician.
 a. Note quality and rate particularly.
 b. Use Silverman score for continual, consistent assessment of the respiratory status (see Fig. 38-3).
 c. Hyaline membrane disease or respiratory distress syndrome occurs during the first 24–48 hours of life. Observe for and report immediately any signs and symptoms of respiratory difficulty:
  (1) Increased respiratory rate (usually above 60/minute)
  (2) Thoracic retractions
  (3) Nasal flaring
  (4) Cyanosis
  (5) Expiratory grunting
  (6) Developing exhaustion
  (7) Periods of apnea
6. Hypoxemia is associated with birth asphyxia and recurrent apneic episodes. Serum P_aO_2 less than 40 mm. Hg.
7. Hypoventilation—tendency to retain CO_2 due to irregular breathing, poor respiratory muscle activity, and flexible thoracic cage. PCO_2 greater than 50 mm. Hg.
8. Identify periodic breathing versus apneic episodes.
 a. *Periodic breathing*—cessation of breathing for short periods (5–10 seconds) followed by ventilation for 10–15 seconds at an increased rate.
 b. *Apneic episodes*—nonbreathing periods of more than 20 seconds' duration may be accompanied by bradycardia and cyanosis, and is related to immature respiratory center. Infant is hypotonic and unresponsive.
  (1) Stimulation or resuscitation is required to restart breathing and increase heart rate.
  (2) Provocative conditions that increase apneic spells include:
   (a) Hyperthermia
   (b) Hypoglycemia
   (c) Hypocalcemia
   (d) Acidosis

(e) Hypobilirubinemia
(f) CNS disease—intraventricular hemorrhage
(g) Pulmonary insufficiency
(h) Infection
(i) PDA (patent ductus arteriosus)
(j) Sodium disturbances
(k) Hypoxemia
(3) Theophylline or aminophylline may be given to reduce the frequency of apneic episodes. It is believed that the drug acts centrally by increasing the respiratory center activity and lowering the infant's sensitivity to CO_2.
   (a) Observe for tachycardia (heart rate of 180–190/min), toxicity.
   (b) Ensure that serum theophylline levels are checked frequently, since excretion of the drug is limited and toxic levels may be quickly reached.
(4) Waterbed or tactile stimulation schedule every hour may help decrease frequency of apnea.
(5) Keep infant's temperature close to the low range of the thermal neutral zone.

C. *To conserve the infant's energy while providing necessary care.*

1. Be organized in caring for the infant. Collect all equipment before starting care, do what needs to be done, and then let the infant rest. Infant's position will affect his ability to rest.
2. Premature infants tire very easily.
   a. Any activity increases oxygen need, thus increasing respiratory rate, taxing already limited energy. Holding the infant often causes lowering of the P_aO_2.
   b. Adjust infant's environment so that rest and sleep are not hindered. Decrease the risk of causing hypoxia.
   c. Interventions must be evaluated for their relative value versus the trauma they entail.

D. *To provide and maintain thermal neutrality of the premature infant.*

1. Maintain infant's temperature at the thermo-neutral zone, i.e., at the environmental temperature in which the resting infant maintains normal body temperature and still utilizes minimum energy-oxygen consumption and calories.
   a. Infant's core temperature (rectal temperature) should be maintained at 36.8–37.2° C. (98.6° F.). Abdominal skin temperature should be 36.0–36.8° C. (96.8–97.2° F.).
   b. Keep environmental (ambient) temperature ranges from 32–35° C. (89.6–95.0° F.). Smaller premature infants may need higher temperature, 35° C. (95° F.); larger premature infants, around 32° C. (89.6° F.). Generally ambient temperature is 1.5° C. warmer than abdominal skin temperature, thus oxygen consumption is minimal.
2. Be aware that the infant loses heat by radiation, conduction, convection, and evaporation; thus, the nurse must be alert to conditions that influence heat loss or gain by the infant.
   a. Note location of warming unit in relation to air conditioners, direct sunlight, and drafts. Move the unit, if necessary.
   b. Minimize porthole entrance activities into Isolette; keep portholes tightly closed when they are not in use or tightly fitting around arm when entering Isolette.
   c. Infant should be undressed to allow direct body contact with warm air.
   d. To minimize heat loss by radiation, consider the possibility of partially lining the Isolette with foil, being careful not to obstruct view of infant. Covering infant from shoulders to feet with a plastic (kitchen plastic material) bubble may also aid in maintaining a stable temperature.
   e. A goose-neck lamp will provide additional heat. Care must be used to prevent overheating or burning the infant.
3. Avoid constant or drastic changing of temperature-control dial.
   a. If ambient temperature rises, skin and core temperature of the infant will rise resulting in increased metabolic rate and insensible water loss. The infant may exhibit weight loss, abdominal distention, regurgitation of feeding, and irritability.
   b. Decrease in ambient temperature will result in a decrease of infant's skin temperature and an increase in metabolic rate in an attempt to increase heat production.
      (1) If the infant cannot compensate for the increased heat loss, his body temperature will drop.
      (2) Hypothermia results in tachycardia, hypoglycemia, metabolic acidosis, apnea, and inactivity.
4. Skin temperature probe should be placed on trunk of infant rather than extremities which are more susceptible to changes in peripheral circulation.
   a. Prevent infant from lying on thermistor.
   b. Cover skin probe with a heat-reflecting material (foil) to decrease influence of ambient temperature on sensor.
5. Monitor both infant's temperature and Isolette or radiant warmer temperature. Temperature control centers are poorly developed in the premature infant, and his temperature is easily influenced by his environment. Hypermetabolic state and inadequate peripheral circulation predispose premature infant to hyperthermia. When caring for the premature infant under the radiant warmer:
   a. Use white linen to increase efficiency of the unit.
   b. Monitor temperature every 30–60 minutes to determine specific temperature needed to keep infant at correct temperature. Start unit setting at 37–37.5° C. and adjust slowly (1.5° C. warmer than skin temperature) until infant temperature is stable. Then monitor every 1–4 hours.
   c. Keep alarm for overheating on.
   d. Be aware of the complications associated with the use of radiant warmer:
      (1) Overheating—increase in infant's oxygen consumption
      (2) Flash burns—avoid oil on infant's skin
      (3) Cataracts—observe closure of eye lids
      (4) Excess drying of skin and tissue breakdown
6. When assessing temperature regulation of the premature infant, consider the following:
   a. Note if infant's body or extremities are cool to touch—possibly due to underheated incubator or heat loss due to radiation.
   b. Note activity—restlessness or hyperactivity may indicate inappropriate temperature for comfort.
   c. Be aware of reasons for increased temperature of

infant—overheated incubator, early sign of illness, incorrect placement of sensor.

    d. Be aware of causes for drop in temperature of infant—underheated incubator, infection, faulty sensor–skin contact from feces or bony prominence, vasoconstriction, iatrogenic (cold O_2).

7. When humidity is increased in the incubator, it will reduce infant heat loss and insensible water loss.

E. *To prevent infection of this very susceptible premature infant.*

1. The premature infant is particularly susceptible to viral, fungal, and gram-negative bacterial infections. Septicemia, meningitis and urinary tract infections are a constant hazard postnatally.
2. Specific techniques should be employed to ensure the control of infection (see p. 1135).
    a. Scrupulous handwashing by all personnel handling the infant and entering the nursery must be practiced.
    b. Use gown and mask technique as prescribed by health agency. Short-sleeved gowns allow for proper handwashing up to the elbows.
    c. Minimize infant's contact with unsterile equipment; equipment should be individualized.
    d. Minimize number of persons who come in contact with infant.
    e. Exclude from nursery any person who is febrile, has draining lesions, or has acute respiratory or gastrointestinal infections.
    f. For infant care such as bathing or cord care, antiseptic solutions or soaps that are effective against gram-negative and gram-positive organisms might be considered.

> **NURSING ALERT:** Routine use of hexachlorophene for infant bathing is to be avoided. Data indicate a marked association between its use and neuropathologic lesions.

3. Early symptoms of infection may include (see p. 1248):
    a. Hypothermia or hyperthermia
    b. Jaundice
    c. Lethargy
    d. Poor eating
    e. Apneic spells
4. Predisposing factors of infection
    a. Maternal infection
    b. Difficult and prolonged labor
    c. Prolonged rupture of membranes
    d. Manipulative measures—resuscitation, umbilical catheterization, surgery

F. *To be aware of complications that occur in the premature infant and to be alert for early signs indicating a change in condition.*

1. *Hypoglycemia*
    a. Hypoglycemia—serum sugar levels are less than 25 mg./100 ml.
    b. Hypoglycemia is most likely to occur in first 12 hours after birth and as late as 48 hours after birth.
    c. Hypoglycemia is likely to occur in the premature infant because of the reduced glycogen storage he has at birth and his limited carbohydrate tolerance.

    d. Symptoms are nonspecific.
      (1) Jitteriness
      (2) Tachypnea or apnea
      (3) Lethargy
      (4) Cyanosis
      (5) Convulsions
      (6) High-pitched or weak cry
      (7) Pallor
      (8) Temperature instability
      (9) Sweating
    e. Predisposing factors include:
      (1) Infant of diabetic mother—2–72 hours
      (2) Erythroblastosis fetalis—4–72 hours
      (3) Sepsis
      (4) Intrauterine malnutrition—2 hours–1 week
      (5) Development defects
      (6) Asphyxia
      (7) Respiratory distress
      (8) Hypothermia
    f. Blood sugar levels should be accurately monitored. Dextrostix screening can be done by the nurse.
      (1) When a blood specimen is collected, ideally a capillary tube should be used to prevent the reactive tip from coming in contact with the skin, which may give a false reading.
      (2) Specimen should remain on reactive tip for 60 seconds, then forcefully rinsed with clear running water.
      (3) Check urine for excess levels of sugar.
    g. Treatment is to increase blood sugar intake by oral feeding or intravenously. If IV glucose is given too rapidly, it will stimulate insulin production, resulting in rebound hypoglycemia. Maintain blood sugar at greater than 45 mg./100 ml.
2. *Hypocalcemia*
    a. Hypocalcemia—serum calcium levels are less than 7 mg./100 ml. (3.5mEq./L.)
    b. Low blood calcium is reached the first day of life.
    c. Symptoms are nonspecific:
      (1) Twitching
      (2) Convulsions (late sign)
      (3) Hypotonia
      (4) Lethargy
      (5) High-pitched cry
      (6) Increased apneic spells
      (7) Abdominal distention with ileus
    d. Hypocalcemia occurs in the premature infant because of reduced calcium storage at birth
    e. Predisposing factors:
      (1) Hypoglycemia
      (2) Previous maternal abortion
      (3) Low infant Apgar rating—asphyxia
      (4) Hyaline membrane disease
      (5) Lack of intake
      (6) Treatment of acidosis with bicarbonate
      (7) Decreased renal capacity for phosphorus excretion
    f. Try to maintain serum calcium above 8 mg./100 ml.
    g. Treatment is to give calcium intravenously or orally.
      Intravenous calcium given too rapidly will cause bradycardia.
3. *Hypoxia* or anoxia at birth
    a. The degree of asphyxia is judged immediately after delivery by Apgar scores and blood gas changes.
    b. Specific problems to be anticipated include:

(1) Hyaline membrane disease
(2) Profound acidosis
(3) Hypoglycemia
(4) Abnormal clotting function
(5) Hyperbilirubinemia
(6) Apneic episodes
(7) Poor temperature control
(8) Intracranial hemorrhage
(9) Cardiac failure
4. Patent ductus arteriosus (PDA)
  a. PDA occurs occasionally in premature infants with respiratory distress syndrome and in less mature infants (24–30 weeks' gestation) with associated congestive pulmonary failure.
    Majority of very-low-birth-weight infants recovering from respiratory distress syndrome develop serious signs of this disease.
  b. Clinical signs include:
    (1) Bounding peripheral pulses
    (2) Chest retractions with mild cyanosis
    (3) Diminished breath sounds on auscultation
    (4) Moist rales
    (5) Elevated PCO_2
    (6) Apneic periods
    (7) Systolic murmur—clicking sound
    (8) Tachypnea
    (9) Deterioration of general condition
  c. Treatment:
    (1) Medical—fluid restriction, maintenance of normal blood pH, oxygen as needed, maintenance of adequate hemoglobin levels, digitalization, diuretics, indomethacin for closure.
      When indomethacin is used, the nurse should observe for diminished urine output, azotemia, and creatinemia. It may not be used if infant has bilirubin levels greater than 10 mg. (drug binds to albumin), bleeding tendencies (may alter platelet formation), or renal problems.
    (2) Surgical—ligation of ductus arteriosus
  d. Spontaneous closure of the PDA in the premature infant is likely to occur 2–6 weeks after birth.
5. *Sodium disturbances*
  a. Hypernatremia—serum sodium level above 150 mEq./L.; generally occurs because of inadequate hydration or overuse of $NaHCO_3$ for acidosis.
  b. Hyponatremia—serum sodium level below 125–130 mEq./L. is generally secondary to administration of hypotonic intravenous solutions.
6. *Intracranial hemorrhage* (most likely to occur in sick premature infants)
  a. Intracranial hemorrhage is a common cause of death in extremely premature infants.
  b. Factors predisposing infant to CNS bleeding
    (1) Immaturity
    (2) Respiratory distress syndrome
    (3) Hypoxia in fetus or neonate
  c. Clinical signs
    (1) Labored respirations
    (2) Hypoventilation
    (3) Cyanosis
    (4) Apnea
    (5) High-pitched cry
    (6) Convulsions
    (7) Bulging fontanelle
    (8) Clinical deterioration; shocklike appearance
  d. Prevention of intraventricular hemorrhage is the best treatment, because once bleeding begins, it is difficult to control.
    (1) Keep infant adequately oxygenated. Prevent asphyxia and hypercapnia.
    (2) Maintain thermoneutral environment.
    (3) Maintain normal acid-base balance.
7. *Hypertension*
  a. Hypertension may occur in infants with a history of indwelling artery catheter, patent ductus arteriosus, or perinatal hypoxia. These conditions put infant at risk for renal artery thrombosis and hypertension.
  b. Signs include:
    (1) Increasing blood pressure and considerable fluctuation in blood pressure
    (2) Tachypnea and cyanosis
    (3) Lethargy
    (4) Tremors
    (5) Apnea
  c. Treatment:
    (1) Diuretics and/or antihypertensive medications
    (2) Nephrectomy for unilateral involvement
8. *Hypotension*—indicative of hypovolemia

G. *To offer support to the parents of the premature infant during this crucial period.*

1. Most parents, particularly mothers, are physically and emotionally unprepared for the early arrival of their baby.
2. Allow parents to see their infant and touch him if this is feasible, and they are able to cope with doing so.
3. Listen to parents talk and express their concerns. Encourage them, but do not give them false hope.
  a. Assess where they are in their grief, in coping, and in accepting their infant.
  b. Be alert to the father who may be overwhelmed with concern for the infant and mother (who also is hospitalized) and who may not know how to help or meet the needs of the mother at this time. Provide appropriate support.
4. If this pregnancy occurred outside of marriage, the premature birth may precipitate other feelings of guilt or punishment in the parents. The parents may need help in identifying and working through these feelings in order to progress towards a more healthy attitude.

The Growing or Older Premature Infant
After the first few days have passed without any complications, the premature infant is very busy growing. During this time, however, it must be remembered that other complications can occur. The areas of concern mentioned above are still important, along with the following:

A. *To be constantly alert to signs and symptoms of complications.*

1. Aspiration
  a. The growing premature infant may still have poor gag and cough reflexes.
  b. The premature infant will show signs of respiratory distress.
    Suction mouth and pharynx immediately and get medical assistance.
2. Neonatal tetany (see hypocalcemia, p. 1232)
  a. Onset is between 5 and 10 days.
  b. Formula with a low phosphorus content is used in treatment.

(1) Regular infant formula has a high phosphorus content.

(2) Immature kidneys cannot handle the high phosphorus load that results when calcium level is low in the infant.

3. Latent acidosis of prematurity (developing after 3 days of life)

a. Metabolic acidosis occurring during first few weeks (pH and bicarbonate or base excess drops) is associated with immaturity of the kidneys and is unrelated to major cardiovascular or respiratory problems.

(1) Infant may hyperventilate to blow off excess CO_2.

(2) Urine pH varies from 6.0–7.5; blood pH ranges from 7.25–7.30 with base deficit.

b. Symptoms are subtle:

(1) Infant begins to feed poorly and takes longer to eat. He is sleepy and needs stimulation to keep awake; he displays lethargy.

(2) Infant shows increased frequency and severity of apneic spells.

(3) Infant may remain vigorous and take adequate fluid and calories, yet fail to gain weight.

(4) Inadequate weight gain or loss when there is large caloric intake.

(5) Stools become watery.

(6) Skin may take on a gray pallor.

c. Treatment consists of replacing bicarbonate lost through excretion and adjusting amino acid intake via formula as well as via a decrease in amount of protein load and total calories.

4. Fluid retention

a. Abnormal fluid retention results from infant's inability to excrete solutes or to excrete water.

b. Symptoms include:

(1) Excessive weight gain

(2) Pitting edema of feet, then body

(3) Chest retractions

(4) Inspired air diminished on auscultation with possible rales

(5) Increase in oxygen need; increase in PCO_2

c. Treatment consists of giving diuretic agent and possibly decreasing fluid intake.

d. Predisposing factors that lead to fluid retention include:

(1) Patent ductus arteriosus with borderline heart failure

(2) Bronchopulmonary dysplasia

(3) Postventilator therapy

(4) Low total serum proteins

5. Wilson-Mikity syndrome

a. Chronic form of respiratory distress. Infant may or may not have had respiratory distress syndrome.

b. Insidious symptoms include:

(1) Gradual increase in chest retractions

(2) Decrease in inspired air on auscultation

(3) Slowly increasing need for oxygen to about 30–40%

(4) Characteristic streaky pattern of lungs, progressing to soap-bubble appearance on x-ray

6. Hyperbilirubinemia (see p. 1242)

a. Bilirubin concentrations are generally higher in the premature infant because of the impaired ability to conjugate bile in the liver.

b. If infant is bruised from delivery or is plethoric, the risk of hyperbilirubinemia is increased.

c. Hypoproteinemia and acidemia increase risk of low bilirubin kernicterus.

7. Necrotizing enterocolitis (NEC)

a. Iatrogenic disease of the intestine of uncertain etiology; the bowel has patches of necrotic mucosa, with intramural gas (pneumatosis intestinalis).

(1) It is thought to result from hypoxia leading to bowel ischemia, ileus, and stasis.

(2) This, in turn, allows for bacterial invasion, proliferation, and damage to intestinal wall.

b. Predisposing factors

(1) Prematurity

(2) Shock of any type

(3) Perinatal or neonatal asphyxia, low Apgar score

(4) Exchange transfusion

(5) Association with postnatal infection

(6) Mother having had prolonged ruptured membranes or fever at delivery

(7) Nasojejunal tube feeding

(8) Respiratory distress

(9) Polycythemia

(10) Patent ductus arteriosus

(11) Umbilical artery catheterization

(12) Early milk feeding

c. Signs and symptoms—the onset of symptoms occurs suddenly between 1 and 14 days of life, most often between 4 and 7 days of life; infant has generally been tolerating feedings.

(1) Abdominal distention, delayed gastric emptying, vomiting, increased gastric residuals

(2) Jaundice

(3) Apnea

(4) GI bleeding; bloody diarrhea

(5) Toxic-looking, lethargic

(6) Temperature instability

(7) X-ray findings show distended, thickened bowel loops; they may show streaks of intramural gas in bowel wall and sometimes peritoneal air from perforation.

d. Supportive treatment

(1) Gastric decompression with nasogastric tube

(2) Antibiotic therapy—intravenously and orally to treat sepsis

(3) IV hyperalimentation

(4) Cultures to determine causative agent

(5) Blood work-up:

(a) hyponatremia

(b) decreased platelet count

(c) increased bleeding times

(d) metabolic acidosis

(6) Surgery—resection of gangrenous bowel

e. Nursing responsibilities

(1) Acute, constant observations—place child in Isolette or radiant warmer.

(2) Close monitoring of vital signs and general condition; report even minute changes in infant.

(a) Abdominal girth measurement; note distention or rigidity, redness or shininess, erythema, observable bowel loops.

(b) Check bowel sounds with stethoscope with minimal abdominal palpation.

(c) Check stools for occult blood; save specimen as appropriate for examination by physician.

(3) Prevent additional stress to infant by maintain-

ing stability in environment, IV intake, and gastric decompression.

(4) Minimize handling and trauma to abdomen—x-rays may be taken frequently to evaluate status.

(5) Do not take rectal temperatures.

(6) Provide meticulous skin care when diarrhea and vomiting are present.

8. Bronchopulmonary dysplasia (BPD)

a. Chronic lung disorder characterized by coarse cystic-appearing lungs with hyperinfiltration, obstructive brochiolitis, and pulmonary fibrosis resulting from respiratory distress syndrome with high concentrations of oxygen and positive-pressure ventilation.

b. Other factors associated with BPD include:

(1) Endotracheal tube

(2) Patent ductus arteriosus

(3) Pulmonary edema from increased fluid loads in first days of life

(4) Smaller premature infant with severe respiratory distress syndrome

c. Signs and symptoms include:

(1) Tachycardia

(2) Difficulty weaning from oxygen or ventilator

(3) Respiratory distress

(4) Cyanosis

d. Nursing responsibilities include:

(1) Support respiratory effort with gentle airway suctioning, chest physical therapy, and positioning.

(2) Observe and record frequency of persistent apnea, cyanotic episodes, tachypnea, retractions, and rales.

(3) Allow infant to rest during feeding regardless of method used (nipple or gavage). He will tire easily and respond with apnea.

(4) Exercise constant vigilance to avoid respiratory infection in the infant, which could lead to death.

(5) Help to maintain a meaningful parent–infant relationship through the long duration of treatment.

B. *To provide and maintain adequate nutrition to allow for growth and development.*

1. The growth rate of the premature infant should parallel the expected in utero growth rate: about 20 gm./24 hours after 30 weeks' gestation and 30 gm./24 hours as the infant approaches term.

From birth to 5–10 days of age there will be a 5–10% weight loss; then the infant should begin to gain weight.

2. The premature infant has a small gastric capacity but a great need for calories.

110–140 Kcal./kg./24 hours (40–45% of total calorie intake should be provided by carbohydrates)

120–150 ml./kg./24 hours of fluid

2–4 gm. protein/kg/24 hours

a. Generally the premature infant has adequate gastric capacity, intestinal motility, and absorption to tolerate small, frequent feedings.

b. The gastric capacity expands during the first few weeks of life; this enables the infant to tolerate larger feedings.

c. Overfeeding increases the risk of vomiting.

Vomiting can lead to dehydration, loss of hydrochloric acid, and alkalosis.

d. The premature infant regurgitates feedings easily because of poor muscle tone at the cardiac sphincter. Expect small amount after feeding, especially with burping.

e. Bubble infant frequently during feeding.

f. Formula should be adequate in calories, fluid, electrolytes, iron, and vitamins to meet the needs of the infant.

3. Inappropriate weight gain in relation to caloric intake can indicate problems.

a. Unusually large weight gain for caloric intake may indicate excessive fluid retention.

b. No weight gain or a loss with adequate caloric intake may indicate acidosis, sepsis or malabsorption

4. Allow the infant to rest prior to feeding. The premature infant tires easily from procedures and will eat better if rested.

5. Feed appropriately for individual patient.

a. Gavage is indicated for very small premature infant who does not demonstrate good sucking or synchronized sucking and swallowing. Diarrhea may result from malabsorption if feeding is advanced too rapidly.

b. Dropper or nipple feeding is indicated for a vigorous premature infant with good suck, gag, and swallowing reflexes.

6. Anemia, although not a significant problem, does occur.

a. Premature infants develop anemia (hemoglobin less than 8–10 gm./100 ml.). Reasons for the development of anemia include the following:

(1) Total body iron content is less.

(2) There is a proportionately larger blood loss from sampling.

(3) Relative body growth is more rapid and there is an expanding blood volume.

b. Supplemental iron is needed to supply new iron stores. Eventually hemoglobin is needed for the increasing blood volume during growth. The iron is generally started when the infant is 1.5–2 times birth weight.

c. Blood transfusions are indicated to replace sampling blood. Keep accurate records of blood output.

C. *To meet the psychological needs of the premature infant, who is an individual in his own right.*

1. At first, even though handling is minimal, the nurse should talk to and caress the infant while performing procedures.

a. Stroking and gentle handling will provide necessary sensory stimulation.

b. A soft musical sound may also be comforting.

2. Once the premature infant is able to leave the Isolette even for short periods of time, he should be held for feedings.

a. While holding him, stroke him and talk to him.

b. Keep him warmly wrapped; this will also give him a feeling of security.

3. If the infant is restless in his incubator, he may be calmed by propping him against a blanket or diaper roll.

The freedom of movement, restrained only by the mattress, cannot offer much security to the infant.

4. Remember that the infant's ability to hear, see, smell, and touch are intact. Give him the opportunities to develop these capabilities and encourage the devel-

opment of his interaction potential by providing sensory input.

    a. Physical contact is important for a sense of security.

    b. Arrange environment so eye-to-eye contact can be established between caretaker or mother and infant.

    c. Allow infant freedom of movement for self-stimulation.

    d. Change infant's position and location of Isolette to encourage him to see his environment.

5. Include parents in this activity to help them get to know their infant and incorporate these activities into their behavior so they will continue this at home.

D. *To provide the premature infant with an environment that will help him to emerge successfully into a state of well-being and into a healthy growing baby.*

1. Conserve his energy.
   a. Promote rest and sleep by the following:
      (1) Appropriate handling.
      (2) Organizing and controlling interruptions.
      (3) Proper positioning of infant.
   b. Support physiologic functions and provide assistance as necessary-i.e., monitor respiration, temperature, and nutrition.
2. Change position every 2 hours. This does the following:
   a. Stimulates circulation.
   b. Facilitates respirations.
   c. Prevents stasis of accumulated secretions.
   d. Minimizes skin irritation.
   e. Provides infant with opportunity for different stimulation input.
3. Provide for physical safety and comfort.
   a. Bathing—gives nurse opportunity to observe infant thoroughly.
   b. Protect infant from injury self-inflicted by own random movements.
   c. Protect from injury by equipment.
   d. Use protective devices as necessary but allow infant some unrestricted self-stimulation.
   e. Keep portholes of Isolette closed.
   f. Keep infant warm when out of the Isolette—wrap with blanket and cover head with bonnet.

E. *To foster healthy family relationships with the premature baby.*

1. Encourage parents to make frequent visits to the nursery so they can become familiar with all aspects of care of their infant.
   a. When they visit, explain the equipment and procedures that may be foreign to them.
   b. Help them to feel comfortable and confident in handling their infant.
   c. Parents may lose interest in the infant if the hospitalization is long. If parents cannot visit daily, encourage them to call, or call them at predetermined times.
2. Help mother to see infant as an individual and to develop mothering behaviors based on the infant's behavior.
   a. The infant's size and physical characteristics are generally unexpected and are different from those of the expected full-term baby.
   b. The premature infant's reflexes and responses to his environment are immature. Mother's expectations of his responses are based on those of a full-term baby.

    c. Explain these discrepancies between expectations and reality. Mother may associate infant's responses with her inadequacies rather than the baby's.

    d. Be aware of what reflexes and responses may elicit reactions in the mother. For example:
   (1) Uncoordinated sucking and swallowing—mother experiences disappointment in not being able to feed, especially if she wanted to breast-feed her infant.
   (2) Gag reflex—mother fears choking of infant.
   (3) Respiratory immaturity—periodic breathing frightens her.
   (4) Grasp reflex—mother is disappointed if infant does not grasp her finger.
   (5) Moro reflex—exaggerated Moro reflex may make mother feel she has frightened her infant.

    e. Reassure mother that as the infant matures, he will change his response and reflex behavior.

3. The support and help given to parents during hospitalization will make home care easier.
   a. Observe and assess behaviors as an aid to assessing attachment or bonding relationships and ability to relate to infant.
   b. Teach mother how to care for her infant. Thorough and careful preparation of the mother in feeding and caring for her infant often means earlier discharge.
   c. The small size of the infant often is the single factor that frightens parents the most.
4. Initiate community-nurse referral if parents seem anxious about caring for their baby at home.
   a. If this premature infant is the first baby, the referral may be particularly helpful to the mother.
   b. Home follow-up will enable the nurse to assess family interactions, parenting behaviors, and infant developmental screening.
5. Encourage parents to talk about their feelings or fears concerning their infant and how they will care for him.
   a. By listening, the nurse can gain some insight as to what to talk about or to teach the parents.
   b. Parents' feelings can frequently interfere with appropriate home care.
   c. Parents often treat the "preemie" as if he were fragile and more prone to illness. Overconcern is potentially harmful.
   d. Parents worry about how to feed and protect the infant.
6. Help the family prepare for the time when their new baby will arrive home.
   a. Because of the early, unexpected arrival of the infant, things such as clothing, bed, and bottles may not be ready.
   b. If there are other children at home they need to be prepared for the homecoming of the premature infant. This preparation should begin early—using, for example, pictures of infant and conversations about him.
   c. The readiness for the premature infant to go home is evaluated and assessed in terms of the following:
      (1) The infant's weight and progress
      (2) Maternal attachment to the infant
      (3) Maternal competence in caring for the infant

Parental (Family) Education

1. Help the family to understand that caring for the premature infant at home should not be any different from caring for a full-term infant.
   a. Special treatment may lead to behavior problems later.
   b. At first a little extra caution should be practiced. Cyanotic spells and severe infection are major concerns for premature infant during first few weeks at home.
      (1) Keep room temperature fairly constant—about 25–26° C. (77–79° F.).
      (2) Sponge-bathe infant instead of bathing in tub and keep him warm during procedure.
      (3) Feed him the recommended amount of formula to be certain he receives the necessary calories for continual growth. Maintain iron therapy.
      (4) Keep him away from crowds and people who have colds.

2. Spend enough time with the mother teaching her how to feed and care for her infant.
   Show her how, then watch her and help her improve and gain confidence.
      (1) Infant needs gentle, firm handling.
      (2) He needs to be mothered and kept comfortable with minimal tension.
      (3) A soothing voice can be comforting.
      (4) Sucking provides a pleasant experience.
3. Stress the importance of medical follow-up for the baby after discharge from the hospital.
   Anemia and failure to thrive are common long-term side effects of prematurity.
4. Help mother understand the importance of good, early prenatal care for subsequent pregnancies.
   Once a woman has had one premature infant, this classifies her as high-risk for another premature delivery with future pregnancies.

SMALL FOR GESTATIONAL AGE INFANT

The "small for gestational age infant" (SGA) is a newborn who shows a discrepancy between growth and gestational age or whose weight is 2 standard deviations below expected weight for duration of gestation, or plot below the 10th percentile on intrauterine growth chart.

Intrauterine growth retarded (IUGR) is used interchangeably with SGA.

Etiology

IUGR may be due to reduction of total number of cells in the body (hypoplastic), to a reduction in cell size (hypotrophic), or to both.

While the etiological factors are unknown in many cases, other cases may result from the following causes.

A. *Maternal factors*

1. Undernutrition
2. Diminished uterine blood flow
   a. Preeclampsia
   b. Toxemia
   c. Chronic hypertensive vascular disease
   d. Diabetes mellitus
3. Small stature
4. Smoking
5. Inadequate prenatal care
6. Low socioeconomic class
7. Heart disease
8. Low maternal age
9. Primiparity
10. Grand multiparity
11. Low prepregnant weight
12. Narcotic usage
13. Hemoglobinopathy
14. Phenylketonuria

B. *Environmental factors*

1. High altitude
2. Teratogens
3. Irradiation

C. *Placental lesions*

1. Infarcts
2. Premature placental separation

3. Hemangiomas
4. Thrombosis of fetal vessels
5. Single umbilical artery
6. Avascular terminal villi

D. *Fetal causes*

1. Genetic dwarfs
2. Anencephaly
3. Infections (rubella, cytomegalovirus, toxoplasmosis, herpes simplex)
4. Chromosomal aberrations
   a. Turner's syndrome
   b. Down's syndrome
   c. Trisomy syndromes
   d. Cri-du-chat syndrome
5. Congenital anomalies
   a. Osteogenesis imperfecta
   b. De Lange's syndrome
   c. Cystic fibrosis
   d. Galactosemia

Clinical Manifestations

Clinical manifestations of the SGA infant are related to the duration, intensity, and time of onset of the influence (factors) causing intrauterine growth retardation.

1. Chronic IUGR—growth of fetus has been curtailed by insult for weeks or months prior to birth. Note the following characteristics (hypoplastic stage):
   a. Body proportions remain unaltered—weight, length, and possibly head circumference are below normal for gestational age.
   b. Creases on soles of feet
   c. Coarse, straight, silky hair
   d. Well-developed ear cartilage
   e. Firm skull bones
2. Subacute IUGR—growth of fetus has been curtailed by insult only a few days or weeks prior to birth (hypotrophic stage).
   a. Weight is diminished; length of body and head circumference may be normal.
   b. Wasted look with loose, thin skin
   c. Long, thin appearance
   d. Face has look of "worried little old man"

e. Scaphoid abdomen
f. Skin dry, cracked, and peeling
g. Thin umbilical cord that dries and hardens rapidly
h. Widened skull sutures

Pathophysiology

Although, in general, the physiologic maturity of fetal organs develops according to gestational age, there are exceptions to organ maturation being consistent with gestational age that result in problems (conditions) associated with IUGR.
  1. Poor glucose control
     a. Hyperglycemia related to severe IUGR—"transient neonatal diabetes." Symptoms include weight loss, dehydration, fever, and glucosuria.
     b. Hypoglycemia is probably due to rapid depletion of hepatic glycogen stores and to ineffective functioning of hepatic enzyme system responsible for glyconeogenesis.
  2. Limited temperature control
     a. Infant has relatively large surface area per unit of body weight.
     b. He lacks energy stores and subcutaneous fat insulation.
     c. Infant can assume position of flexion of extremities—reduces surface area exposed to environment and decreases heat loss by radiation and convection.
     d. Has vasomotor control over peripheral circulation to dilate or constrict capillaries as needed.
     e. Sweating mechanism is intact.
  3. High hemoglobin, increased plasma volume, and enlarged extracellular fluid volume per kilogram of body weight, putting the infant at risk for respiratory distress, cardiac, and circulatory problems.
  4. Minimal weight loss with rapid initial weight gain.
     a. Weight gain is not maintained throughout first year.
     b. Rapid initial weight gain may suggest rehydration as well as tissue growth.
  5. Late anemia
     Secondary to rapid weight gain and poor iron stores present at birth, especially in the premature infant.
  6. Elevated immunoglobulin (IgM) in infants with intrauterine infection.
  7. High nonprotein nitrogen levels, possibly due to:
     a. Increase in fetal catabolism—or
     b. Impaired placental excretion of fetal waste products
  8. Prone to postasphyxial problems
     a. The asphyxial process of normal labor is associated with metabolic acidosis.
     b. Fetal malnutrition, in addition to birth process, predisposes infant to asphyxia neonatorum.
  9. Limited oxygen, fat, and glycogen reserves due to intrauterine growth retardation.
 10. X-ray findings:
     a. Atrophy of thymus
     b. Thin ribs

Diagnostic Evaluation

  1. Evaluate general appearance of infant.
  2. Determine gestational age using physical characteristics and neurologic examination (see Table 38-1, pp. 1228–1229).
  3. Infant can be SGA and preterm or SGA and term.
  4. Measure weight, length, and head circumference; plot on Colorado intrauterine growth chart and compare relative percentiles.
  5. Determine blood sugar.
  6. Obtain hematocrit (HCT) and hemoglobin to determine polycythemia and hyperviscosity (venous HCT over 65%).

Complications

  1. Problems associated with asphyxia neonatorum and meconium aspiration syndrome
  2. Hypoglycemia and hypocalcemia
  3. Polycythemia
  4. Pulmonary hemorrhage
  5. Prematurity with intrauterine growth retardation
  6. Infection associated with maternal conditions
  7. Hypothermia
  8. Congenital infection
  9. Congenital anomalies
 10. Late anemia
 11. Future growth retardation

Nursing Objectives and Management

The nursing management of the SGA infant in many aspects is similar to that for the premature infant (see p. 1226). The following are major objectives of the nurse caring for the SGA neonate:

A. *To observe for any gross and less obvious congenital anomalies as in the case of the full-term infant upon admission to the nursery.*

  1. Congenital anomalies are often associated with intrauterine growth retardation.
     Genitourinary and cardiovascular complications are the most common problems.
  2. Certain types of intrauterine infection account for intrauterine growth retardation and may present signs of skin rash, petechiae and ecchymoses, hepatomegaly, splenomegaly, early-onset of obstructive jaundice, chorioretinitis, lethargy, and irritability.
  3. Report any suspicious findings and observations to physician immediately.

B. *To observe for problems associated with asphyxia neonatorum.*

The SGA neonate has an increased incidence of asphyxia neonatorum. His lessened metabolic stores of carbohydrates lower his ability to handle the stresses of delivery. Acidosis may develop quickly.
  1. Be aware of the Apgar scores which will help in determining degree of asphyxia (Apgar less than 5 at 1 minute or less than 7 at 5 minutes).
  2. See that blood gas studies are done to confirm adequate oxygenation and acidosis. Frequent monitoring should be continued.
  3. Observe for signs of respiratory distress.
     a. Adequate oxygenation is imperative for improving prognosis.
     b. Suction and oxygen equipment should be available and ready for immediate use.
     c. Aspiration pneumonia and pulmonary hemorrhage are postasphyxiation problems.
  4. Check vital signs frequently and note behavior, i.e., reflex responses, irritability; cardiac function can be affected and CNS damage can occur with severe asphyxia.
  5. Check and record intake and output. Renal damage is a common sequel of severe asphyxia.
  6. Observe for abnormal clotting function and hyper-

bilirubinemia—liver damage from severe asphyxia may be manifested by postasphyxial hypoglycemia.
7. Postasphyxial hypocalcemia may occur.
8. Record and report all observations appropriately.

C. *To screen for hypoglycemia, beginning soon after birth.*

1. The SGA infant has reduced carbohydrate stores at birth. Glycogen reserves are depleted almost immediately after birth. Gluconeogenesis is inadequate because of reduced stores of muscle protein and fat tissue, as well as reduced hyperglycemic response to norepinephrine and glucagon, which activate the gluconeogenesis process.
2. Hypoglycemia is most likely to occur from 12 to 48 hours after birth.
   Severely hypoxic, hypothermic SGA infants can become hypoglycemic as early as 6 hours after birth.
3. Blood sugars should be monitored frequently (every 30–60 minutes) by Dextrostix during the critical time after birth and during IV glucose therapy.
   a. If Dextrostix evaluation is below 40 mg./100 ml., report this to physician immediately as measurement of serum glucose should be done.
   b. Keep Dextrostix bottle tightly covered and out of direct sunlight to avoid false reading on Dextrostix.
4. When IV infusion of glucose is used to prevent or treat hypoglycemia, particular care must be given to prevent infiltration and subsequent slough and necrosis of tissue.
5. With the infant at risk for hypoglycemia, oral feeding should be started as early as 2 hours after birth (if there are no contraindications).
6. Signs of hypoglycemia include:
   a. Jitteriness
   b. Sweating
   c. Tachypnea or apnea
   d. Cyanosis
   e. Convulsions
   f. Respiratory distress
7. Report all observations to the physician and record accurately.

D. *To prevent hypothermia and maintain thermal stability of the SGA neonate* (see p. 1226–1231).

1. Insure that adequate environmental heat is provided

to maintain infant's abdominal skin temperature at 36.0–36.5° C. (96.8° F.).
2. Prevent infant from lying on thermistor.

E. *To take measures to combat polycythemia.*

Polycythemia, which is increased red blood cell volume, is frequently seen in SGA infants when growth retardation is due to placental insufficiency.
1. Polycythemia is identified by a high hematocrit or hemoglobin level, i.e., venous blood HCT over 65%; Hgb of 20–22 gm./100 ml. Hyperviscosity can result from this condition.
2. Signs and symptoms of viscosity include:
   a. Plethora
   b. Jaundice
   c. Tachypnea
   d. Tachycardia
   e. Peripheral cyanosis
   f. Grunting
   g. Nasal flaring, intercostal retractions
   h. Scrotal edema
   i. Priapism (persistent, abnormal erection of penis)
   j. Tremors, irritability, possibly seizures
3. Ensure that the HCT or Hgb is monitored during the first 6–12 hours after birth in the high-risk infant.
4. Treatment for HCT above 70% usually consists of partial exchange transfusion. The nurse must be prepared to assist with this by using fresh frozen plasma or whole blood.

F. *To accurately measure and record daily weights and to monitor length and head circumference.*

Rapid weight gain is expected the first few days and weeks.

G. *To support the parents of the infant* (see Premature Infant, p. 1233).

1. The long-term outcome of the SGA infant often represents an increase in long-range sequelae frequently manifested in lowered intellectual achievement resulting from malnutrition during peak intrauterine brain growth.
2. Long-term prognosis depends upon adequate treatment of problems encountered immediately after birth, etiology of problems, and subsequent home environment.

POSTMATURE INFANT

The *postmature infant* is one whose gestation is 42 weeks or longer and who may show signs of weight loss with placental insufficiency.

Etiology

1. Not known in many cases.
2. Maternal factors associated with postmaturity:
   a. Primigravida and high-parity mother at any given age.
   b. Prolonged gestation in preceding pregnancies.

Clinical Manifestations

Physical appearance—the following characteristics are most often seen in infant of 44 weeks' gestation or more:

1. Reduced subcutaneous tissue—loose skin, especially buttocks and thighs
2. Long, curved fingernails and toenails
3. Reduced amount of vernix caseosa
4. Abundant scalp hair
5. Wrinkled, macerated skin; possibly pale, cracked, parchment-like skin.
6. Having the alert appearance of a 2- to 3-week old infant following delivery
7. Greenish-yellow staining of skin, indicating fetal distress

Pathophysiology

1. The postmature infant appears to have suffered from intrauterine malnutrition and hypoxia.

Before the termination of the pregnancy, but at the point when birth should have occurred, the placental function begins to diminish, resulting in impaired oxygen exchange and inadequate nutrient transfer to the fetus.
2. There are stages of postmaturity—severity of associated problems is determined by length of gestation, i.e., the longer the gestation, the more severe the problems.

Diagnostic Evaluation

1. Evaluate general appearance.
2. Determine gestational age—give neurological examination.
3. Measure weight, length, and head circumference, and plot on Colorado intrauterine growth chart. Compare percentiles (see chart, p. 1227).
4. Determine blood sugar. In hypoglycemia the serum sugar level is below 30 mg./100 ml.
5. Assessment of asphyxia neonatorum.
   a. Apgar score
   b. Blood gas analysis

Complications

1. Meconium aspiration
2. Hypoglycemia and hypocalcemia
3. Polycythemia
4. Pulmonary hemorrhage
5. Problems associated with asphyxia neonatorum
6. Pneumonia
7. Pneumothorax

Nursing Objectives and Management

Problems and nursing care encountered in the postmature infant may include the metabolic disturbances of the SGA and complications of asphyxia neonatorum as well as polycythemia (see p. 1239, SGA). Massive meconium aspiration causes specific problems for the postmature infant. (Refer to nursing objectives for the premature infant, p. 1226 and SGA, p. 1238).

A. *To be alert for respiratory distress that may indicate meconium aspiration.*

1. The stage is set for meconium aspiration when placental function diminishes and oxygen transport to the fetus decreases, leading to cerebral hypoxia.
   a. The anal sphincter relaxes and meconium passes into the surrounding amniotic fluid.
   b. The asphyxiated fetus gasps and aspiration occurs.
2. Signs and symptoms of meconium aspiration—severity depends upon amount and thickness of meconium aspirated, as well as the location of the aspirate in the respiratory tract.
   a. Tachypnea, increasing signs of cyanosis; difficulty breathing, with need for ventilation
   b. Tachycardia
   c. Inspiratory nasal flaring and retraction of chest
   d. Expiratory grunting
   e. Increased anteroposterior diameter of the chest
   f. Palpable liver
   g. Rales and rhonchi on chest auscultation
   h. Concomitant cerebral irritation—jittery, hypotonia, seizures
   i. X-ray—classical coarse, patchy, irregular pulmonary infiltrates ranging in severity
   j. Other additional signs: metabolic acidosis, hypotension, hypoglycemia, hypocalcemia
3. Mainly supportive treatment

a. Warmth—maintain thermally neutral environment so infant uses fewer calories and less oxygen
b. Adequate oxygenation and humidification to maintain P_aO_2 at 50–70 mm. Hg.
   (1) Be aware that metabolic disturbances often accompany respiratory problems.
   (2) Ensure that monitoring of blood gases and pH is done.
   (3) Carefully record blood sampling.
c. Adequate administration of calories and fluid Accurately record intake and output.
d. Antibiotics
   (1) Prophylactically—meconium can lead to a chemical pneumonia and the growth of gram-negative bacteria. Therefore antibiotics specifically for gram-negative bacteria may be used.
   (2) Treatment—antibiotics used only when clinical evidence indicates infection.
e. Corticosteroids may be given to minimize irritating effects of meconium on respiratory epithelium, although clinical evidence for this is nonconclusive.
f. Pulmonary physical therapy—every 30–60 minutes first few hours
   (1) Postural drainage (p. 1189).
   (2) Pulmonary lavage—using nonirritating solution and immediate suctioning of mouth, pharynx, and trachea; bag ventilate using high concentrations of oxygen between lavage procedures.
   (3) Change position from side to side frequently and elevate or lower head by adjusting the mattress to a 20-degree angle.
   (4) Complications of meconium aspiration
      (a) Pneumothorax and/or pneumomediastinum
      (b) Secondary pneumonia
      (c) Pulmonary hypertension with persistent fetal circulation
      (d) Respiratory failure
      (e) Death
   (5) Prevention
      Most cases of meconium aspiration can be prevented if meconium is removed from the mouth and trachea by proper suctioning, prior to infant's taking his first breath.

NOTE: If ventilator management is indicated, treatment is similar to that of infant with hyaline membrane disease (p. 1269).

B. *To be aware that the postmature infant is particularly prone to hypoglycemia within hours after birth (see SGA, p. 1239).*

1. Oral feeding or IV glucose is generally initiated soon after birth. If oral feedings are not contraindicated they can begin 1–2 hours after birth.
2. Close and careful monitoring of blood sugar should be done with Dextrostix every hour until condition stabilizes.
3. Persistent hypoglycemia may contribute to CNS problems.
4. Be alert to signs and symptoms of hypoglycemia and report to physician.

C. *To support the parents of the infant* (see Premature Infant, p. 1135 and ICN, p. 1233).

The long-term sequelae common in the postmature infant are associated with central nervous system (neurologic) problems.

INFANT OF DIABETIC MOTHER

The *infant of a diabetic mother (IDM)* is the infant born to a mother with diabetes. The mother may be a diabetic or gestational diabetic. The severity of infant problems depends on classification of the maternal diabetes (Table 38-2).

Clinical Manifestations

1. Macrosomia (gigantism)
2. Cardiomegaly
3. Hepatomegaly
4. Large umbilical cord and placenta
5. Plethora
6. Full-face
7. Tendency to be large for gestational age; some may be normal weight or SGA
8. Abundant fat, hair, and vernix caseosa

Pathophysiology

1. Increased amount of body fat, not edema.
   a. Total body water is somewhat reduced at birth.
   b. High urinary output during first 2 days of life, probably due to freeing of intracellular water.
2. Hypoglycemia
   a. Occurs within first 2–12 hours of life; may occur within minutes after birth.
   b. Infant's response to glucose is excessive, i.e., insulin blood level will have a slight elevation, will drop and then peak within 1 hour. This is probably due to maternal hyperglycemia.
   c. Infant's cord insulin levels may not be higher than in a normal infant unless a large amount of glucose is given.
   d. IDM may be symptomatic or asymptomatic with blood sugars below 20 mg./100 ml.
3. Hypocalcemia
   a. Associated with prematurity, difficult labor and delivery, and/or asphyxia at birth.
   b. Generally occurs during first 24–48 hours of life.
4. Hyperbilirubinemia
   a. Most likely to occur within 48–72 hours after birth.
   b. Immature liver results in inability to conjugate bilirubin.
   c. HCT is higher on the third day after birth and extracellular volume is decreased.
   d. Because of large size, birth trauma may increase risk of enclosed hemorrhage.
5. Prematurity
   a. May be premature or small for gestational age when associated with placental insufficiency.
   b. Respiratory function is similar to that of other premature infants—thus infant is prone to hyaline membrane disease.
6. Polycythemia
   a. Venous hematocrit greater than 65% or venous Hgb 22 gm./100 ml.
   b. Polycythemia increases the risks of occurrence of renal vein thrombosis, respiratory distress, hypoglycemia, and hypocalcemia.
7. Congenital anomalies
   a. Increased incidence of congenital anomalies may be due to:
      (1) Divergent gene pattern
      (2) Abnormal intrauterine environment
   b. Most common anomalies are skeletal and cardiac
8. Infection
   a. Prematurity and lowered passive immunity
   b. Possible maternal urinary tract infection and bacteria crossing the placenta

Diagnostic Evaluation

1. Maternal history of diabetes
2. Physical assessment of infant and determination of gestational age
3. Blood studies
   a. Glucose
   b. Calcium
   c. HCT and Hb
   d. Blood gas analysis
   e. Magnesium (if indicated)
   f. C-peptide immunoreactivity (indicates beta cell activity)

Complications

1. Hypoglycemia
2. Hypocalcemia
3. Hyaline membrane disease
4. Polycythemia and renal vein thrombosis
5. Infection
6. Hyperbilirubinemia
7. Hypermagnesium or hypomagnesium
8. Congenital anomalies
9. Birth injuries—cephalohematomas, facial nerve paralysis, fractured clavicles, brachial nerve plexus
10. Prematurity
11. Congestive heart failure

Nursing Objectives and Management

Except for specific considerations discussed below, the nursing care of the infant of a diabetic mother (IDM) is the same as for the premature infant (p. 1226).

A. *To observe closely for hypoglycemia.*
   Report any irregularities immediately to physician.
1. Monitor by Dextrostix every 30–60 minutes begin-

TABLE 38-2. WHITE'S CLASSIFICATION OF DIABETES*

Class A—Glucose tolerance test diabetes	Class D—Onset under age 10 Duration 20-plus years Vascular disease Calcification in legs Retinitis
Class B—Onset over age 20 Duration 0–9 years No vascular disease	
Class C—Onset age 10–19 Duration 10–19 years No vascular disease	Class E—Calcified pelvic vessels
	Class F—Patients with diabetic renal impairment

* From Nelson, B. Gillespie, L., and White, P.: Pregnancy complicated by diabetes mellitus. Obstet. Gynecol., 1:219, 1953, with permission.

ning immediately after birth for 24 hours or every 4–8 hours until stabilized. Glucose levels are lowest 1–2 hours after birth; at 2–6 hours, glucose levels even off and gradually increase. Warm the extremity prior to capillary sampling to prevent false low values resulting from stasis.

2. The infant with hypoglycemia (premature infant: below 20 mg./100 ml.; term infant: below 30 mg./100 ml.) may be symptomatic or asymptomatic. Signs include:
   a. Jitteriness
   b. Tremors
   c. Convulsions
   d. Sweating
   e. Cyanosis
   f. Weak or high-pitched cry
   g. Refusal to eat
   h. Hypotonia (reduced muscle tone)
   i. Apnea
   j. Temperature instability
   k. Rotating eye movements
3. Hypoglycemia may be prevented or treated by early feedings of 10–20% glucose or formula by nipple or gavage.
   a. IV glucose may be given for very low serum glucose levels or when infant's condition prevents oral feeding.
   b. Glucose levels should be maintained in the low–normal range.
   c. Overfeeding or excessive IV infusion of glucose may result in a rebound effect causing insulin levels to increase and hypoglycemia to reappear.
   d. IV glucose must not be discontinued abruptly in order to prevent rebound hypoglycemia.

B. *To monitor infant closely for changes in acid-base status, respiratory distress, temperature, hypocalcemia, and sepsis.*

C. *To observe for hyperbilirubinemia.*

1. Infants of diabetic mothers have a higher incidence of hyperbilirubinemia.
   Other predisposing factors include prematurity and polycythemia, which increases the load of bilirubin from the natural process of RBC breakdown to be cleared, and decreased extracellular fluid.
2. The infant may need an exchange transfusion at relatively lower bilirubin levels (as in the premature infant) to prevent kernicterus.
3. The blood sugar must be monitored during and following exchange transfusion. ACD (acid citrate

dextrose) and CPD (citrate phosphate dextrose) contain large amounts of dextrose which may subsequently cause rebound hypoglycemia.

D. *To assist in the prevention of dehydration and maintenance of fluid and electrolyte balance.*

1. Because of the increase in fatty tissue and decrease in total amount of body water, protein and carbohydrate breakdown after birth will increase urinary output. This, along with inability to concentrate urine, increases the risk of dehydration. Dehydration increases risk of polycythemia.
2. Accurately record intake and output; administer prescribed fluids and evaluate lab studies to determine current status.

E. *To be aware of the infant who is predisposed to hypomagnesemia or hypermagnesemia and observe for signs and symptoms of each.*

1. Hypermagnesemia may occur when the preeclamptic mother was treated with magnesium sulfate.
   a. Signs and symptoms may include:
      (1) Hypotonia
      (2) Weak or absent cry
      (3) Severe respiratory distress with apnea or cyanosis
   b. Treatment is an exchange transfusion.
2. Hypomagnesemia may accompany hypocalcemia or follow an exchange transfusion.
   a. Severe neuromuscular excitability may be the presenting symptom.
   b. IM magnesium sulfate is the treatment.

F. *To be alert for development of renal vein thrombosis in the infant during the first few days of life.*

1. Polycythemia, transient dehydration, and decreased extracellular fluid may be causes.
2. Observe for hematuria and proteinuria.
3. Flank masses may be palpable.

G. *To observe the infant for possible cardiac anomalies* (see p. 1285).

Monitor cardiac and respiratory rates.

H. *To support the mother who may have feelings of severe guilt or inadequacy, since she is directly related to the problems her infant may be having.*

1. Encourage and allow mother to talk about these feelings.
2. Encourage her, when appropriate, to have close obstetrical care for subsequent pregnancies.
3. Stress importance of a periodic evaluation for diabetes in her child.

JAUNDICE IN THE NEWBORN (HYPERBILIRUBINEMIA)

Hyperbilirubinemia (jaundice) in the newborn is an accumulation of serum bilirubin above normal levels.

Etiology

1. Increased bilirubin load
   a. Hemolytic disease—Rh and ABO incompatibility
   b. Morphologic abnormalities of red blood cells
   c. Red blood cell enzyme defects
   d. Physiologic jaundice (see later discussion of "physiologic jaundice")
2. Extravascular blood
   a. Cephalohematoma

   b. Pulmonary or cerebral hemorrhage
   c. Any enclosed occult blood
3. Decrease or inhibition of bilirubin conjugation
   a. Inherited bilirubin conjugation defect: Crigler–Najjar syndrome (deficiency of glucuronyl transferase).
   b. Acquired bilirubin conjugation defect: breast-milk jaundice, Lucey–Driscoll syndrome, infant of diabetic mother, asphyxiated infant with respiratory distress
4. Increased extrahepatic circulation
   Intestinal obstruction

5. Polycythemia
   a. Twin-twin transfusion
   b. Maternofetal transfusion
   c. Infant of diabetic mother
   d. Small for gestational age infant.
6. Mixed jaundice—increased bilirubin load and decreased clearance resulting in elevated indirect and direct bilirubin levels
   a. Sepsis
   b. Severe hemolytic disease
   c. Intrauterine transfusion
   d. Galactosemia
   e. Biliary atresia—absence of extrahepatic ducts or presence of cordlike structures without a lumen
7. Hypothyroidism
8. Familial, transient—associated with inhibiting factor in plasma
9. Unknown

Clinical Manifestations

1. Onset of clinical jaundice seen when serum bilirubin levels are less than 5–7 mg./100 ml.
   a. Physiologic jaundice—occurs 3–5 days after birth
      (1) Increase in unconjugated bilirubin levels; levels must not exceed 5 mg./100 ml. per day.
      (2) Peak bilirubin levels not to exceed 12 mg./100 ml. in full-term infant and 15 mg./100 ml. in premature infant.
      (3) Full term peak levels (6 mg./100 ml.) are reached by 48–72 hours after birth; clinical jaundice declines in 1 week and normal bilirubin levels are reached in 2 weeks.
      (4) Premature peak levels (10–15 gm./100 ml.) are reached by 4–6 days of age; clinical jaundice declines in 2 weeks and normal bilirubin levels are reached in 3–4 weeks.
   b. Erythroblastosis—may occur within 24 hours after birth
2. Signs and symptoms may include:
   a. Sclerae appearing yellow before skin appears yellow
   b. Skin appearing light to bright yellow
   c. Lethargy
   d. Dark amber, concentrated urine
   e. Poor feeding
   f. Dark stools

Pathophysiology

A. *Bilirubin Production*

1. 75% of the bilirubin present in the newborn is from RBC breakdown.
   a. The red blood cell is broken down into protein and globin combined with heme, which is an iron-porphyrin complex.
   b. In the presence of the enzyme called heme oxygenase:
      (1) Globin is reduced to amino acids.
      (2) Iron is broken off and stored.
      (3) Porphyrin moiety is broken into biliverdin, which is reduced to bilirubin.
   c. This bilirubin is unconjugated or indirect and is fat soluble.
   d. Indirect bilirubin, bound to albumin, is present in circulating blood and tissues.
   e. The liver selectively removes this albumin-bound bilirubin from the blood.
   f. Once the unconjugated bilirubin is in the liver, it is converted to direct or conjugated water-soluble bilirubin with the aid of enzymes, one of which is glucuronyl transferase.
   g. From the liver, conjugated bilirubin is excreted via the bile into the intestine and is excreted in the stool or is hydrolyzed to unconjugated bilirubin in the intestine and reabsorbed across the intestinal mucosa into the circulation (enterohepatic circulation).
2. 25% of the bilirubin present in the newborn is from non-erythrocyte-containing heme proteins.

B. *Physiologic Jaundice*

1. Increased load of bilirubin on liver cells.
   a. Increased bilirubin production—more rapid hemolysis because of higher level of circulating RBCs per kg. (2.2 pounds) of body weight and a shorter RBC life span.
   b. Enterohepatic circulation—reabsorption of unconjugated bilirubin.
2. Decreased clearance of bilirubin from plasma.
   a. Predominant bilirubin-binding protein in liver cells may be deficient the first days of life.
   b. Glucuronyl transferase enzyme activity may be decreased, resulting in impaired conjugation of bilirubin.
   c. Liver may show decreased ability to excrete large amounts of conjugated bilirubin.
   d. Poor portal blood supply may decrease the liver's capacity to act effectively.
   e. Open ductus venosus may allow blood to bypass liver.

C. *Hemolytic Disease*

1. Erythroblastosis fetalis (isoimmunization due to Rh factor or ABO incompatibility).
   a. Immune hemolysis or Rh/ABO blood group incompatibility; mother's and infant's blood are different.
      Rh factor; different ABO blood groups (see Coombs' test, p. 1244).
   b. Mother produces antibodies against the antigen of baby's blood. Fetal cells frequently cross placenta.
   c. Antibodies of mother's blood are present in baby's blood at birth, causing the following conditions:
      (1) There is hemolysis of infant's red blood cells.
      (2) Hemolysis leads to rising level of indirect bilirubin.
2. Glucose–6–phosphate dehydrogenase deficiency (G–6–PD)—nonimmune hemolytic disease.
   a. Deficiency results in reduced stability to oxidative destruction from substances that act as oxidizing agents (i.e., vitamin K, naphthalene, salicylates).
   b. X-linked recessive disease that affects primarily Negro and Mediterranean–Oriental groups.
   c. Screen maternal blood for carrier state and screen neonate blood in high-risk groups.

D. *Other Considerations*

1. Each gram of hemoglobin breakdown forms 35 mg. of bilirubin.
2. An unmeasurable amount of bilirubin does not bind to albumin. Free indirect bilirubin is very toxic to the cells of the CNS.
3. The enzyme system responsible for conjugation of bilirubin is oxygen-dependent and altered by infant's pH, temperature, etc. Thus infants who are acidotic, hypoxic, or hypothermic tend to present with higher levels of bilirubin.

Diagnostic Evaluation

1. All infants who have clinical signs of hyperbilirubinemia should be given the following work-up:
   a. Serum bilirubin levels—total and direct
   b. Peripheral smear—for evidence of red blood cell morphology and reticulocyte count
   c. Reticulocyte count—to determine rate of hemolysis
   d. Coombs' test—to check for Rh and ABO group incompatibility between mother and baby—direct Coombs' test on infant serum
   e. Blood typing of mother and infant
   f. Total serum protein—to measure binding capacity
   g. Hematocrit or hemoglobin
   h. Acid-base status
   i. Albumin-binding test—to measure reserve binding sites (if available)
2. There are 3 current approaches to measuring risk of bilirubin toxicity:
   a. Sephadex G–25 level
   b. HBABA dye-binding
   c. Salicylate saturation index
3. Measuring the bilirubin-albumin binding capacity of the plasma can also be valuable in determining the risk of kernicterus (see below) and the need for an exchange transfusion. This test defines the upper limits to which serum bilirubin is allowed to rise when an exchange transfusion is done.
   a. $\dfrac{\text{Total bilirubin}}{\text{Total serum protein}} =$
      1. if less than 3.7—no danger of kernicterus
      2. if greater than 3.7—treatment by exchange transfusion is indicated.
   b. Total serum protein × 3.7 = level of bilirubin at which to do exchange transfusion.
4. The level of bilirubin at which the infant is at risk for brain damage depends upon the degree of prematurity, presence of acidosis, hypoxia, or drugs which bind albumin. (20 mg. of bilirubin/100 ml. of blood in term infant is not necessarily the upper limit of bilirubin as formerly thought).
5. Appropriate cultures when infection is suspected.

Complications—Kernicterus

Kernicterus is a yellow discoloration of specific areas of brain tissue by unconjugated bilirubin; can be confirmed only by death and autopsy.

Bilirubin encephalopathy best describes the occurrence of the syndrome and the accompanying neurologic sequelae in neonates.

1. Early signs of kernicterus
   a. Poor feeding
   b. Vomiting
   c. Lethargy
   d. High-pitched cry
   e. Hypotonia
   f. Decrease of normal reflexes, Moro reflex
2. Later signs
   a. Opisthotonus
   b. Apnea
   c. Irritability
   d. Seizures
   e. Deafness to high-pitched sounds
3. Occurrence of kernicterus at low levels of bilirubin may be seen in infants with
   a. Previous asphyxia (acidosis)
   b. Respiratory distress
   c. Sepsis
   d. Hypothermia
   e. Prematurity
   f. Hypoglycemia
4. Bilirubin is nephrotoxic and especially compromises renal concentrating capacity.
5. Bilirubin increases affinity of RBC for oxygen.

Treatment

1. Exchange transfusion—to mechanically remove bilirubin.
2. Phototherapy—to allow for utilization of alternate pathways for bilirubin excretion.
3. Enzyme induction agent—to reduce bilirubin levels by inducing hepatic enzyme system involved in bilirubin clearance (i.e., phenobarbital, Ethanol).

Nursing Objectives and Management

A. *To observe infant's skin for appearance of or increase in jaundice.*

1. Make observations in daylight, sunlight, or white fluorescent light.
2. Blanch the skin during the observation to clear away capillary coloration: forehead, cheeks and clavical sites allow for clear view. Record findings at least twice daily.
3. Be aware of any blood incompatibility between infant's and mother's blood.
4. Be alert to the infant's age in connection with the appearance of jaundice.

B. *To note any changes in urine pigmentation and frequency of urination.*

Careful notation of frequency, amount, and color of urine should be made so changes will be noticed immediately. Test for presence of bilirubin (urobilinogen).

C. *To maintain adequate fluid intake.*

1. Be aware of feeding history and amount of fluid taken.
2. If infant is a slow eater, feed small amounts frequently.
3. The amount of fluid intake determines the amount of hydration and in turn determines the excretion of bilirubin. Early feeding is a good preventive prescription for hyperbilirubinemia.
4. If infant is receiving intravenous fluid, keep an accurate hourly record of fluid intake. Do not allow intake to fall behind prescribed rate. Observe IV site for infiltration so IV can be discontinued and restarted immediately.

D. *To be alert to any behavior changes and to report them to physician.*

Note particularly increasing lethargy, change in sucking activity or quality; or vomiting.

E. *To be alert to signs of kernicterus (bilirubin encephalopathy) and to report them to physician.*

Observe for signs of decreased muscle tone, no sucking, no hand grasp, or regurgitation of feedings not previously observed. In time, the infant becomes opisthotonic and irritable.

F. *To administer the treatment of phototherapy safely and properly, should it be prescribed.*

It is generally not used for nonhemolytic disease.

1. The shining of daylight fluorescent bulbs or blue light directly on the exposed skin of the infant

reduces tissue bilirubin, which in turn reduces serum bilirubin by:

a. Photo-oxidizing tissue bilirubin to biliverdin, to secondary yellow pigments, to colorless, nontoxic compounds excreted in bile and urine.

b. Causing tissue-serum bilirubin equilibrium, or as the bilirubin decreases in tissue, pulling bilirubin from the serum into the tissue to maintain this equilibrium. The *flux*, which is the unit of measurement of energy output of lamps, at 425–475 nm. is important in bilirubin degradation.

   (1) Distance of infant from light should be 60 cm.

   (2) Check light intensity for therapeutic range daily.

2. The physician will determine the length of time the infant is to be under the lights based on serum bilirubin levels and clinical condition of the infant.

3. Nursing care peculiar to phototherapy:

a. Have infant completely undressed so entire skin surface is exposed to light.

b. Keep infant's eyes covered to protect them from the constant exposure to high intensity light which may cause retinal injury. Do not apply pressure when the eyes are covered as this may cause corneal ulceration. Be certain both eyes are occluded with protective cover and that eyelids are closed. Change protective covers routinely and check for conjunctivitis. Make sure nose is not occluded. Cover scrotum.

c. Develop a systematic schedule of turning infant so all surfaces are exposed, (i.e., every 2 hours).

d. Maintain thermoneutrality—measure incubator or Isolette temperature as well as infant's. Light affects the ambient temperature.

   (1) Do not expose the thermistor probe to the lights without the probe's being covered with an opaque tape.

   (2) Avoid hyperthermia. Monitor temperature every 2–4 hours.

e. Adequate fluid intake should be provided either orally or intravenously. Vasodilatation increases the insensible water loss and there is excess stool loss from occasional diarrhea. Keep urine specific gravity below 1.015.

f. The infant should be shielded (by plexiglass) from direct exposure of the lights to filter out and protect him from the ultraviolet radiation of daylight and cool white fluorescent lights. This shield will also protect infant from injury should the lights break.

g. Ensure that serum bilirubin levels are obtained as prescribed. The diminishing icterus, i.e., the lowering of unconjugated bilirubin from cutaneous tissue, does not reflect the serum bilirubin concentration.

   (1) Lights should be turned off when blood is being collected to eliminate false bilirubin levels.

   (2) When phototherapy has been discontinued, check serum bilirubin levels within 4 hours to determine rebound.

h. Side effects of phototherapy:

   (1) Lethargy

   (2) Loose green stools

   (3) Dark urine

   (4) Temperature elevation

   (5) Skin changes—greenish color; rash due to capillary dilatation

   (6) Priapism—turn infant on abdomen for short periods of time and this will cease.

   (7) Dehydration from increased skin evaporation

i. If possible, remove infant from under the lights, remove eye covers, and hold infant for feedings. This will allow for some human contact and pleasure during feeding, a chance to open his eyes and look around and perhaps encourage parental involvement in the infant's care.

j. Note sleeping and eating patterns. The feeding schedule may need to be adjusted to the infant's pattern for better feeding. Obtain daily weight. Increased metabolic rate may increase caloric needs.

k. Develop a schedule for changing light bulbs. The effectiveness of light of this wavelength decreases after 800 hours of use; thus, the bulbs should be changed at that time. A record of hours of use will be helpful. Measure effective light life with light meter.

l. The nurse should wear sunglasses and hair cover when caring for an infant under blue lights for her own protection.

G. *To be aware of drugs that may compete with bilirubin for binding to albumin* (fat emulsion, sulfonamides, chloramphenicol, salicylates, caffeine, novobiocin).

Their administration will result in increasing serum level of "free" unconjugated bilirubin.

H. *To observe for hypoglycemia in infant with erythroblastosis resulting from islet cell hyperplasia, increased pancreatic and cord blood insulin.*

Hypoglycemia may occur shortly after birth or exchange transfusion.

I. *To assist in the treatment of exchange transfusion* (see p. 1182).

J. *To foster a healthy family–child relationship.*

1. Encourage parents to visit infant as much as possible during hospitalization.

2. Allow parents to fondle, care for, hold, and feed infant as much as possible or as his condition permits.

3. Initiate a community nursing referral if parents are particularly anxious about caring for infant at home after discharge.

4. If breast feeding is temporarily discontinued, encourage mother to pump breasts; be supportive.

Parental Education

1. Help family to understand what is wrong with their baby. Explain in simple terms what the doctor has already told them. Allow them to ask questions about the baby and treatment.

2. If the baby has erythroblastosis fetalis, help parents understand the importance of prenatal care and monitoring should another pregnancy occur.

3. Stress the importance of close follow-up of the baby after hospital discharge. Anemia is a common long-term side effect of red blood cell hemolysis and exchange transfusion. The baby's hemoglobin level should be monitored for some time after illness so appropriate treatment can be initiated if necessary.

4. Unsensitized Rh-negative mother, after delivery of Rh-positive infant, should receive Rho immune globulin (Rho GAM)* to prevent isoimmunization with subsequent pregnancies.

* Orthodiagnostics, Raritan, N.J.

FAILURE TO THRIVE

"Failure to thrive" syndrome is a term used to identify infants characterized by growth and developmental failure along with psychosocial disruption.

Etiology

1. Unknown
2. Organic
   a. Central nervous system
   b. Cardiovascular
   c. Renal
   d. Gastrointestinal
   e. Respiratory
   f. Endocrine
   g. Metabolic
3. Nonorganic
   a. Inadequate caloric intake; disturbed feeding patterns
   b. Maternal deprivation or faulty mother-child relationship
   c. Family problems (socioeconomic problems)
   d. Environmental deprivation

Clinical Manifestations

1. Weight measurement falls below 2 standard deviations from mean for age (weight and length fall below that expected for gestational and postnatal age).
2. Infant fails to gain weight or loses subcutaneous fat and muscle.
3. Possible presenting manifestations that are associated with maternal deprivation:
   a. Developmental retardation
   b. Disturbed psychosocial development
      (1) Inappropriate response for age to strangers
      (2) Avoidance of eye contact with another person
      (3) Exaggerated self-comfort measures
      (4) Withdrawn—no interest in environment
4. Somatic manifestations
   a. Gastrointestinal
      (1) Anorexia
      (2) Vomiting
      (3) Diarrhea
      (4) Rumination
      (5) Dehydration
   b. Respiratory—coughing

Diagnostic Evaluation

1. Detailed history—including dietary and family (social)
2. Physical examination—accurate measurements of length, weight, and circumference—general condition
3. Laboratory data—preliminary tests should be minimal, unless history or examination indicates a specific line of inquiry. Include the following tests:
   a. Complete blood count
   b. Urinalysis and culture
   c. Bone age
   d. Stool for fat, occult blood, O + P (ovum and parasites), and pH, trypsin
   e. Levels of serum sodium, potassium, CO_2, chlorides, creatinine, calcium
   f. Tine test
4. Cessation of somatic clinical manifestations
5. Weight gain

Treatment

(When no organic reasons have been found)
1. Adequate caloric intake for weight gain (130–150 cal./kg./day based on appropriate weight for gestational and postnatal age). Significant weight gain will usually occur within 10–14 days.
2. Appropriate "mothering"—nurturing activities and environmental stimulation. Investigation has suggested that weight gain will occur when adequate nutrition is taken independent of nurturing activities; however, one is also dealing with a hospitalized child who is subjected to parental separation or deprivation.
3. If, after a trial of adequate caloric ingestion, the infant does not gain weight, intensive investigation is done. Trial period may have to be 7–10 days in some instances.
4. Provide a nurturing environment that will enhance positive patterns of behavior toward interaction of the family unit.

Prognosis

1. Prognosis generally depends upon the etiology, severity, and duration of the condition, as well as on the home situation into which the child returns.
2. Long-term—continued impaired growth rate and failure to thrive, lowered intelligence, and emotional disorders.

Nursing Objectives and Management

A. *To make an assessment of the infant's general condition, level of development, coping mechanisms, and behavior.*
1. Carefully note what behaviors need attention and/or modifying.
2. Accurately record findings in nursing notes.
3. Obtain and record accurate height, weight, and head circumference.

B. *To develop a detailed nursing care plan that is workable based upon:*
1. Infant's physical condition and limitations
2. Medical management
3. Nursing history
4. Input from other multidiscipline team members

C. *To understand that the reason for this child's condition may not totally be the mother's fault.*
1. Lack of food availability may be a result of socioeconomic situation.
2. Disturbed feeding patterns may have continued despite attempts by mother to correct them.
3. Disturbed mother–infant relationship resulting from separation at neonatal period.

D. *To provide and maintain nutritional intake that will allow for weight gain.*
1. Determine if a feeding problem does exist. Document feeding behaviors (i.e., sleep/wake cycle related to eating, clues of hunger, response to offered food).
2. Infant may need to be taught to eat appropriately for his age, i.e., cup, solids, spoon, finger food.
3. If child vomits, then smaller, more frequent feedings may be necessary; prop him up in sitting position for feeding.
   a. Assess what effect environment, position, and

other factors have on vomiting and feeding behavior.

b. Prevent ruminating or self-induced vomiting.

c. Daily weights and accurate input and output are necessary to evaluate progress.

E. *To gently and warmly provide nurturing to this infant.*

1. Assess what the infant can tolerate and base activities on this, slowly increasing TLC and physical contact as infant can accept it.
2. Encourage the development of a trusting relationship between 1 or 2 persons and the infant.
3. Use each opportunity presented by daily care to develop the relationship, help infant become interested and enjoy his environment and eventually reach out to explore himself, people and things around him.
4. Part of nurturing activities include the therapeutic use of tactile, visual, and auditory stimulation through play. Do not force this upon child if he is unable to tolerate it. Have items within reach, occasionally showing infant how they operate.
5. Talk to infant, use his name; slowly help him to tolerate eye-to-eye contact.
6. Document infant's reactions and responses to handling, playing, etc.

F. *To establish a relationship with the mother (parents) that will allow for open communication and cooperative efforts.*

1. Accept the mother as a person, one who may have problems with which she cannot cope. She may be young and inexperienced or have doubts about her ability to be a mother, as well as other socioeconomic problems.
2. A trusting relationship between the nurse and mother will enhance identifying infant care problems the mother may be experiencing as well as make her more receptive to any teaching or information the nurse may pass on to her.
3. The mother (parents) must be allowed to express her (their) feelings.

G. *To work as a contributing integral part of the multidiscipline team caring for this infant and family.*

1. The physician—responsible for overall diagnosis and management of the family.
2. The social worker—helps parents handle the stress

that prevents them from assuming their parenting roles.

3. The nurse—coordinates infant care and participates in teaching infant care to the mother.
4. The parents—they must be included in the team as the plan of approach must be acceptable and understood in order to be used by them.
5. Other members of the team may include psychiatrist, child life worker, physical therapist, occupational therapist.

H. *To help mother and infant establish a healthy relationship that will continue to grow when the infant is discharged* (see also ICN, p. 1135).

1. Encourage the mother to be active in the plan of treatment. Identify areas of involvement in nursing care plan.
2. Praise her positive efforts; gradually redirect negative aspects.
3. Identify and interpret for the mother the infant's behavior pattern.
   a. Help her to understand the discrepancies between her expectations and reality.
   b. Teach her expected growth and development.
4. Help her to understand her importance to the infant and that the relationship is based on reciprocal needs and responses between mother and infant.
5. Observe and document mother-infant interactions.
   a. Mother—holding, interest in infant, comforting activities
   b. Infant—response to mother (i.e., looking at mother, squirming, cuddling, crying, cooing).
6. Mother may actually need to be taught "mother craft"—how to cuddle, feed, play, and react to her child.

I. *To initiate community nurse referral before discharge and/or communicate with community nurse already involved.*

1. Provides parents with continual support by someone they know.
2. Gives feedback as to the home situation and possible areas where problems can be avoided.

J. *To help the mother (parents) understand and accept the need for continual follow-up care of her (their) infant.*

1. Be certain mother knows where and when to obtain this care.
2. Encourage her to seek support from appropriate resources as necessary.

SEPTICEMIA NEONATORUM

Septicemia neonatorum (sepsis) is a generalized infection which may occur in the neonate and is characterized by the proliferation of bacteria in the bloodstream and frequently involves the meninges (as distinguished from simple bacteremia, congenital infection, septicemia following major diseases or surgery, or major congenital anomalies).

Etiology

1. The distribution of etiologic agents varies from year to year and from institution to institution.
2. Gram negative organisms:
   E. coli
   Klebsiella (enterobacteriaceae)
   Pseudomonas

   Proteus
   Salmonella
   H. influenzae
3. Gram positive organisms:
   Group B beta-hemolytic *streptococcus*
   Listeria monocytogenes
   Staphylococcus aureus—coagulase negative and coagulase positive
   Staphylococcus epidermidis
   Streptococcus pneumoniae
   Streptococcus faecalis
4. Predisposing factors
   a. Sex—male predominance
   b. Perinatal factors
      (1) Maternal complications

Prolonged rupture of membranes
Prolonged and difficult labor; precipitous delivery
Chorioamnionitis
Endometritis
Urinary tract infection
Toxemia
Abruptio placentae
Maternal illness
Cardiovascular disease
Colonization of organisms in genital tract
(2) Infant complications
Prematurity or low birth weight
Congenital heart disease
Intracranial bleeding
Respiratory distress syndrome
Skin infections
Difficult/traumatic labor or delivery
c. Iatrogenic or environmental factors
(1) Related to type of equipment used in caring for infant
Catheters
Oxygen and humidity
Resuscitative
(2) Defective or unclean equipment
(3) Obstetric and nursery practices
5. Mode of entry
a. Infection may gain access into the amniotic sac either prior to or after rupture of the membranes; the fetus may aspirate some of this infected fluid.
b. Bacteria may enter the fetal circulation following invasion of the decidua from the amniotic cavity.
c. After birth, bacteria may enter the infant's circulation by a variety of routes. Infection may originate in the skin, umbilical stump, or mucous membranes of the eyes, nose, pharynx, and ear as well as the respiratory, gastrointestinal, and renal tracts.
d. Iatrogenic—equipment, resuscitation.

Assessment and Clinical Manifestations

1. The early signs of sepsis are usually vague and subtle. The infant is often described as not doing well. The signs often include:
   a. Poor feeding
   b. Lethargy, limpness
   c. Temperature alteration—generally hypothermia, but infant may have hyperthermia
2. Later signs and symptoms may include any of the following:
   a. Pallor, cyanosis or apneic episodes, respiratory distress
   b. Jaundice
   c. Abdominal distention
   d. Vomiting and/or diarrhea
   e. Paronychia
   f. Petechiae or purpura
   g. Vesicles or pustules
   h. Hepatosplenomegaly
   i. Irritability, convulsion
   j. Bulging fontanelles

Pathophysiology

1. Temporary breakdown or depression of infant's defense mechanisms for unknown reason
   a. Possibly due to stress of labor and delivery
   b. Predisposing factors (see under Etiology)
2. The defense systems of the newborn, especially the

low birth weight infant, are ineffective with regard to:
a. Active immunity
(1) Significant formation of IgG (immunoglobulin G) begins at 1–3 months of age
(2) Significant formation of IgM (immunoglobulin M) begins at birth to 7 days
b. Passive immunity
Born without IgM antibodies and bactericidal protection against gram-negative organisms
c. Phagocytosis and minimal inflammatory response Neutrophils are less active in response to chemotactic stimuli and migrate more slowly to areas of inflammation
d. Unknown factors

Diagnostic Evaluation

1. History of predisposing factors
2. Physical findings
3. Laboratory: recovery of organism from blood cultures must be obtained for a diagnosis of sepsis neonatorum
   a. Cultures to detect specific organism
   (1) Blood
   (2) Urine
   (3) Spinal fluid
   (4) Umbilical stump
   (5) Skin lesions
   (6) Nose, throat, rectal
   (7) External auditory canal
   (8) Gastric fluid
   b. WBC and differential—nonspecific test; may be difficult to interpret
   c. Blood chemistries—sugar, calcium, pH, electrolytes
   d. C-reactive protein and erythrocyte sedimentation rate
   e. Acid-base studies
   f. Bilirubin
   g. Serum immunoglobulin estimation
   h. CIE (counterimmunoelectrophoresis)—to detect bacterial agents in body fluid
   i. TORCH (toxoplasmosis–rubella–cytomegalic inclusion virus—herpes—other)—detect antibodies against common intrauterine-infective agents.
4. Chest x-ray—may demonstrate pulmonary infection

Complications

1. Meningitis—very common complication
2. Shock
3. Adrenal hemorrhage
4. Disseminated intravascular coagulation
5. Metabolic derangements
6. Pneumonia
7. Urinary tract infection
8. High mortality rate

Treatment

A. *Antibacterial Therapy*—based on the identified organism

1. Before the specific organism is identified, and after cultures have been obtained, the antibacterial therapy is based on the more common causative agents and their anticipated susceptibilities
   a. Knowledge of particular nursery offenders and their antibiotic susceptibilities is needed for proper drug selection

b. Therapy duration is generally 5–10 days after clinical improvement, but may be as long as 3–4 weeks with complicated infections

B. *Supportive Therapy*

1. Observation
2. Isolation, if indicated
3. Fluid and caloric maintenance
4. Oxygen therapy
5. Regulation of thermal environment
6. Blood transfusion to correct anemia, shock
7. Others, as indicated

Nursing Objectives and Management

(See also ICN, p. 1135)

A. *To practice measures which will prevent the transmission of infection in the nursery.*

1. Practice careful handwashing technique and serve as a model of good technique.
2. Personnel with infection should avoid contact with infants.
   a. Seek medical care for infection. (Cultures should be done.)
   b. Remain out of the nursery.
   c. Wear a mask when it is necessary to enter the nursery.
3. Teach parents and other persons entering the nursery proper handwashing and gown technique.
4. Maintain sterile technique when procedures demanding this technique are performed.
5. Promote general cleanliness of the nursery environment.
   Infected equipment and stagnant water provide excellent conditions for bacterial growth.

B. *To observe infants for the vague symptoms which appear early in the course of sepsis.*

1. Observe for the following:
   a. Lethargy, decreased activity, and loss of muscle tone
   b. Poor feeding or refusal to feed
   c. Temperature alterations, especially hypothermia
2. Be consistent in planning for the care of infants to provide a means whereby these early symptoms may be detected.
   a. Accurate charting of the infant's previous behavior
   b. Assigning the same nurse to care for an infant on successive days
3. Report to the physician the symptoms observed.
4. When neonatal sepsis is caused by B group streptococci, the disease may take one of two courses:
   a. Early onset—within 12–24 hours after birth and within 3 days of age.
      (1) Acute septicemia with fulminant clinical course; high mortality and severe neurological sequelae in survivors.
      (2) There is generally a history of obstetric complications and the serotype of streptococci from mother's birth canal and infant are the same.
      (3) Signs and symptoms include respiratory symptoms—in particular, acute respiratory distress, hypoxia, leading to shock.
   b. Delayed onset—occurs 10 days after birth to 6–12 weeks
      (1) Illness is severe and associated with meningitis.
      (2) Normal obstetric history; probably acquired infection from environment.
      (3) Disease is characterized by meningeal symptoms, including bulging fontanelle and seizures.
5. Observe for signs of complications—meningitis, urinary tract infection, pneumonia.

C. *To observe for episodes of apnea and initiate measures to stimulate respiration.*

1. Observe the infant closely for apnea or place infant on a respiratory monitor.
2. Stimulate infant when apnea does occur.
   a. Slap feet and provide more vigorous stimulation if necessary.
   b. Apply hand pulmonator or mouth-to-mouth resuscitation when spontaneous respiration does not occur within 15 to 30 seconds.
3. Report frequent periods of apnea to physician.
4. Report length of apneic episode and response to stimulation.

D. *To observe the infant for convulsions which may occur with sepsis.*

1. Immediately report to the physician any twitching or convulsive activity.
   a. Remain with infant.
   b. Suction mouth and nose if infant has secretions or vomitus in his mouth.
   c. Turn head to side.
   d. Protect infant from banging against side of Isolette or incubator or falling from radiant warmer.
   e. Provide oxygen if cyanosis or respiratory distress occurs.
   f. Administer any medication prescribed to control the convulsions.
2. Record the length of and the type of convulsion, the parts of the body involved, the infant's general appearance before and following the convulsion, and response to any therapy given.

E. *To ensure that evaluation and diagnostic tests be initiated promptly and correctly to avoid altered results from contamination.*

1. Tests should be completed prior to starting antibiotics.
2. Since the infective organism must be recovered in blood cultures, strict aseptic technique in obtaining cultures is vital.
   a. Peripheral venipuncture is site of choice (umbilical vessels are already contaminated and femoral vein offers possible contamination from perineum).
   b. Cleanse skin with aseptic solution (e.g., iodine solution). For maximal aseptic effect, allow solution to dry.

F. *To provide for the nutritional needs of the infant in order to provide for his caloric needs.*

1. During the acute phase of the illness the infant may not be able to take or tolerate oral feedings.
   a. Monitor the administration of intravenous fluids. Nasogastric tube may be in place to aid in preventing abdominal distention.
   b. Provide for the sucking needs of the infant by providing him with a pacifier.
   c. Gavage feedings may be given to the infant.
2. Initiate oral feedings of formula as soon as the infant's condition improves.
   a. Begin by offering small feedings and observe following responses:
      Vomiting
      Abdominal distention

Infant's interest in feeding and ability to suck
Whether the infant tires with feeding
b. Nipple feedings may be supplemented with gavage feedings.
c. Gradually increase amount of feeding.
Do not force feedings—vomiting associated with diarrhea may result, leading to dehydration.
d. Resume regular feeding schedule based on infant's ability to tolerate feeding.
3. Hold the infant for feedings as soon as his condition warrants it.

G. *To provide measures to maintain the infant's temperature within normal range.*

1. Take infant's temperature at hourly intervals.
2. Adjust the Isolette temperature to maintain infant's temperature between 36–37° C. (96.8–98.6° F.).
3. When infant is placed in an open crib, maintain temperature and cover the infant appropriately.
4. Report hypothermia or hyperthermia to the physician.

H. *To administer the prescribed antibiotic therapy to control the infection.*

1. Administer the prescribed medications.
a. Be aware of the action and side effects of the specific medications.
b. Be aware of the route of excretion.
c. Be aware of drug incompatibilities.
2. Observe the infant's apparent response to therapy.
a. Note child's activity, feeding behavior and weight.
b. Observe for the development of new symptoms.

I. *To be prepared to assist with blood transfusions used to correct anemia and shock* (see Exchange Transfusions, p. 1182).

Adult whole blood also provides specific factors which enhance the phagocytic abilities of neonate leukocytes.

J. *To observe for the occurrence of septic shock and report immediately.*

1. Monitor blood pressure.
2. Check peripheral resistance in pulses in all extremities; note color and temperature.
3. Monitor hourly urine output for evaluation of renal function.

K. *To provide for the emotional needs of the infant.*

1. Place bright, colorful objects in the crib or Isolette.
2. Talk gently and quietly while caring for the infant.
3. Touch and gently stroke the infant.
4. Encourage the parents to visit and allow them to hold the infant as soon as possible.

L. *To involve the parents in the infant's care in the hospital and prepare them for the infant's discharge.*

1. Encourage parents to visit the infant.
a. Allow them to hold and feed the baby.
b. Answer questions they may have regarding the infant's progress and care.
c. Provide them with an opportunity to explain their concerns.
2. Discuss symptoms of complications which may occur and should be watched for following discharge.
3. Give specific instruction regarding medications to be given at home.

INFANT OF ADDICTED MOTHER

An *infant of an addicted mother* is one who is born to a mother who is narcotic- or methadone-dependent and who takes the drug or drugs in varying dosages for varying periods during her pregnancy.

Etiology

Maternal use of narcotics or methadone or both drugs during pregnancy.
1. The drugs cross the placental barrier and enter the fetal circulation.
2. The supply to the infant is abruptly terminated at delivery.
3. Other agents (i.e., phenobarbital, alcohol, propoxyphene) are capable of causing withdrawal symptoms.

Clinical Manifestations (of neonatal withdrawal)

1. The degree of withdrawal symptoms the infant manifests may be related to the duration of the mother's habit, the type and dosage requirements of her addiction, and her drug level immediately prior to delivery.
a. The closer to delivery the mother received her last dose, the longer her addiction and the higher her dose need, the longer the delay of withdrawal symptoms, and the more severe the symptoms in the infant.
b. Although heroin and methadone produce similar withdrawal symptoms in the infant, those same symptoms are generally more severe with methadone withdrawal—probably because of the high level of the mother's dose, the pharmacologic characteristics of the drug itself, and the use by the mother of other drugs simultaneously.
2. Onset of symptoms
a. Heroin—several hours after birth to 3–4 days of life
b. Methadone—7–10 days after birth to several weeks of life
3. Cardinal signs of neonatal narcotic withdrawal
a. Coarse, flapping tremors
b. Irritability; hyperactivity
c. Prolonged, persistent, high-pitched cry
d. Restlessness; sleepiness
4. Other signs and symptoms of acute withdrawal:
a. Vigorous, ineffective sucking; poor feeding
b. Excessive tearing; excessive sweating
c. Increased salivation
d. Sneezing, nasal stuffiness
e. Vomiting and/or diarrhea
f. Muscle rigidity
g. Yawning
h. Convulsions—with methadone withdrawal
i. Tachypnea with associated respiratory alkalosis
j. Exaggerated reflexes
k. Hyperpyrexia
5. Prematurity
High incidence of infants born to addicted mothers are premature and/or small for gestational age.

Diagnosis

1. Thorough maternal history, including drug habits.
2. Physical assessment; Kahn's* criteria of tremulousness and irritability:
   a. Grade I—signs recognizable but mild
   b. Grade II—signs marked but only when infant is disturbed
   c. Grade III—signs marked and occurring at frequent intervals, even when infant is undisturbed
3. Laboratory
   a. Urine for toxicologic studies
   b. Blood glucose
   c. Serum calcium, pH, and total protein
   d. Acid-base status studies, respiratory alkalosis
   e. Serologic studies for syphilis
   f. Appropriate cultures if systemic bacterial infection is suspected
4. Many of the clinical signs of neonatal narcotic withdrawal are nonspecific and may indicate other problems: hypoglycemia, hypocalcemia, CNS disorders or hemorrhage, infection, other, nonnarcotic drug withdrawal

Treatment

1. Narcotic antagonist for narcotic-induced respiratory depression at birth (morphine addiction)
2. Drug therapy for alleviation of signs of narcotic withdrawal. Duration of therapy using decreasing dosages may be from 4–40 days
   a. Paregoric (camphorated tincture of opium) orally
   b. Phenobarbital, orally
   c. Chlorpromazine (Thorazine) orally
   d. Diazepam (Valium) intramuscularly
3. Supportive therapy as appropriate

Complications

1. Prematurity
2. Intrauterine growth retarded infant (IUGR); small for gestational age infant (SGA)
3. Fetal anoxia with meconium aspiration
4. Infection-associated maternal venereal disease or hepatitis

Prognosis

1. The long-term biologic effects on the infant of a drug-dependent mother are not fully known. These children may have:
   a. Abnormal psychomotor development associated with intrauterine growth retardation
   b. Behavioral disturbances such as hyperactivity, brief attention spans, temper tantrums
2. The unstable environment which the drug-addicted mother (or parents) may provide is a major threat to the child's health and development.

Nursing Objectives and Management

A. *To be familiar with withdrawal symptoms in order to facilitate early diagnosis, which in turn will decrease incidence of morbidity and mortality of high-risk infants.*

1. Recognize cardinal as well as other symptoms.
2. Identify infants likely to have symptoms.
3. Report to physician any suspicious behavior.

* Kahn EJ et al. The course of heroin withdrawal syndrome in newborn infants treated with phenobarbital or chlorpromazine. J Ped 75:495, 1969

B. *To ensure that prophylactic measures have been administered against ophthalmia neonatorum.*

There is a high incidence of gonococcal infection in drug-addicted pregnant women.

C. *To ensure that diagnostic measures are carried out.*

Collect urine for toxicologic studies within 24 hours after birth, since narcotic metabolites disappear rapidly.

D. *To administer nursing care appropriate for the symptoms of withdrawal the infant is experiencing.*

1. Irritability and restlessness, high-pitched crying
   a. Swaddle (be aware that this may increase infant's temperature).
   b. Minimize handling—holding may aggravate irritability; some infants respond well to close contact and body movement.
   c. Decrease environmental stimuli (i.e., light, noise).
   d. Organize care to allow for periods of uninterrupted sleep.
2. Floppy tremors
   Protect skin from irritation and abrasions:
   (1) Use sheep skin.
   (2) Change position frequently.
   (3) Give good frequent skin care—keep infant clean and dry.
3. Frantic sucking
   a. Give pacifier between feedings.
   b. Protect infant's hands from excoriation.
4. Poor feeding—similar to premature infant's inability to take adequate amount at feedings
   a. Give small, frequent feedings.
   b. Maintain caloric and fluid intake requirement for infant's weight.
5. Vomiting/diarrhea
   a. Position infant to prevent aspiration.
   b. Provide good skin care to areas exposed to vomitus or stool.
6. Muscle rigidity—hypertonicity
   a. Change position frequently to minimize development of pressure areas.
   b. Use sheep skin.
   c. Skin care.
7. Increased salivation and/or nasal stuffiness
   a. Aspirate nasopharynx; suction tracheal mucus.
   b. Provide frequent nose and mouth care.
   c. Note respiration rate and characteristics and infant's color.
8. Tachypnea
   a. Note onset and severity of accompanying signs of respiratory distress; place infant on respiratory monitor.
   b. Position infant for easier ventilation—semi-Fowler's position; hyperextend head slightly.
   c. Minimize handling.
   d. Have resuscitative equipment available.

E. *To record accurately and in detail all symptoms, including the following:*

1. Time of onset
2. Duration and frequency
3. Severity
4. Treatment initiated and infant's response
   Example: extent of irritability, changes in feeding behavior, tolerance of handling, characteristics and frequency of stool
5. Vital signs

F. To maintain caloric and fluid requirement and balance.

1. Keep accurate intake and output records to prevent dehydration.
2. Maintain IV fluid as appropriate when infant experiences vomiting or diarrhea.
3. Infant may feed better on demand schedule.
4. Infant may need increased calories due to increased activity.

G. To support drug therapy when used to control symptoms of withdrawal.

1. When diazepam (Valium) is used, be alert for the appearance of jaundice.
   Sodium benzoate is used as a preservative in preparation and interferes with binding of albumin with unconjugated bilirubin.
2. Methadone withdrawal symptoms are frequently more difficult to control than those of heroin withdrawal.
3. Note appearance of side effects of depression from oversedation
   a. Respiratory distress
   b. Lethargy
   c. Decreased sucking activity
   d. Hypotonia

H. To protect the infant from pathophysiologic processes to which he is predisposed because of prematurity or being small for gestational age.

1. Hypoglycemia
2. Hypocalcemia
3. Hypothermia
4. Anoxia
5. Sepsis

I. To encourage multidisciplinary conferences in an attempt to treat the whole family.

1. Initiate early referrals as needed to social services, child welfare agency, and/or community nurse to provide for continuity of care after discharge.
   a. The unstable environment into which the infant may be discharged offers a threat to the child's future well-being and development.
   b. Discharge to foster home may be considered.
2. Evaluate mother's attitude toward her infant.
   a. She may be able to accept the responsibility of her child and to accept help offered her.
   b. She may become nonfunctioning as a result of the birth of her infant; she may feel inadequate, angry, guilty or see the infant as an added economic burden.

J. To encourage parental involvement in the care of this infant.

Frequently the infant may not be discharged with the mother. Promote early mother-infant attachment and foster their relationship.

1. Encourage frequent mother–infant contact.
2. Have mother feed infant.
3. Pace the growth of the relationship between infant and mother based on the infant's progress and the mother's positive reactions.
4. Keep in mind that methadone and heroin can be detected in breast milk and may lead to permanent addiction of the infant should the mother breast feed.

Parental Guidance

1. Carefully planned follow-up care for the infant is essential.
   a. Explain to the mother the need for consistent follow-up care of her infant.
   b. Infants of drug-dependent mothers are at risk; they may show failure to thrive, experience battering, or succumb to sudden infant death syndrome.
   c. Involve the community health nurse in the planning early in hospitalization. This early involvement may offer mother some security.
   d. It is often difficult to maintain contact for follow-up.
2. The mother may be accepting of rehabilitation during the postpartum period. Contact appropriate people or provide appropriate information for her.
3. Help the mother understand what she should expect in infant's behavior upon discharge.
   a. Many infants are irritable and restless for several months after birth.
   b. Discuss with the mother the feelings she may have as a result of a strained mother–child relationship.

NEONATAL OR PROLONGED SLEEP APNEA OF INFANCY (NEAR-MISS SIDS)

Nonfatal apnea of infancy is the cessation of breathing for more than 20 seconds, or a shorter episode associated with bradycardia, cyanosis, or pallor.

Near-miss SIDS is the term used to identify an infant, usually between 2 weeks and 6 months of age, who is brought to medical attention because of an unexplained frightening respiratory or cardiac event, usually occurring while the infant is asleep.

Etiology

1. Unknown—may result from many different pathological processes.
2. Apnea related to organic disorders:
   a. Seizure disorders
   b. Gastroesophageal reflux
   c. Significant anemia
   d. Sepsis, severe infection
   e. Hypoglycemia
   f. Impaired regulation of breathing
3. Current theories relating to the cause of SIDS:
   a. Prolonged sleep apnea
   b. Chronic oxygen deficiency
   c. Enzyme abnormalities
   Although many feel that some near-miss infants or those with prolonged sleep apnea are at risk for SIDS, a definitive causal relation between the two has not been scientifically established.
4. Characteristics that may identify infants at risk for SIDS include:
   a. Prematurity
   b. Neonatal conditions with apnea
   c. History of aborted SIDS
   d. History of SIDS in family
5. Characteristics of SIDS pattern include:
   a. Prematurity
   b. Preceding cold or URI
   c. Peak age 2–4 months
   d. Occurs in males in a ratio of 3:2

Clinical Manifestations

1. Infant is usually found by parents or caretaker to be:
   a. Limp
   b. Cyanotic
   c. Pale
   d. No respiration
   e. Cool to touch
   f. Normal muscle tone
2. Some form of resuscitation may be required—mouth-to-mouth respiration or cardiopulmonary assistance.
3. Infant usually exhibits symptoms when asleep, although the syndrome may occur during waking hours.
4. Types of sleep apnea include:
   a. Central or diaphragmatic—chest movement ceases.
   b. Upper airway—chest and diaphragm move but there is no air-exchange.
   c. Mixed—upper airway apnea follows one of central apnea. Bradycardia is associated with upper airway and mixed apnea.

Diagnostic Evaluation

It must be established that a primary life-threatening failure in physiologic homeostasis has occurred, ruling out other medical problems that could result in respiratory failure as a secondary cause. To accomplish this the following procedures are generally included:

1. Detailed history of the event including information concerning what happened, appearance of infant, type of intervention, how infant responded, conditions prior to the event, special past medical history, special family history
2. Medical evaluation of infant (physical examination)
3. Laboratory data—generally minimal unless history or examination indicates a specific line of inquiry
   a. Complete blood count with differential
   b. Serum glucose
   c. Electrolytes
   d. Calcium and phosphate
   e. Magnesium
   f. Blood gases, as indicated
4. Chest x-ray
5. Electrocardiogram
6. Electroencephalogram (may not be routine) and neurological exam
7. Respiratory studies—a pneumogram 12- to 24-hour tape recording of small changes in electrical resistance with each breath or respiratory pattern; multichannel sleep test with continuous print-out
8. Continuous cardiac and apnea monitoring for recurrence of event, prolonged apnea, or bradycardia
9. Barium swallow for gastroesophageal reflux

Management

1. Cardiopulmonary monitoring—is critical
2. Specific treatment of any underlying cause
3. Consultation with SIDS-near-miss team
4. Theophylline—may be used to decrease apneic spells
5. Long-term follow-up for physiologic and neurologic behavioral functions

Prognosis

1. Infants who have experienced near-miss SIDS may be at risk for recurrent apnea, hypoxia, and sudden death.

2. Because of hypoxemia that may have occurred, child should be assessed for learning difficulties (hearing, eyesight), discrete neurological impairments, personality disorders, etc.

Nursing Objectives and Management

A. *To be prepared for the infant's admission.*

Have all equipment, including apnea monitor, ready for use.

1. Select a room that is clearly visible from the nursing station; the room should be quiet in order to reduce sensory stimulation, which may reduce the likelihood of a recurring episode.
2. The family has just experienced the extreme stress of feeling that their infant has almost died. Professional efficiency and empathy at the time of admission is reassuring and builds parental confidence in nursing care.

B. *To obtain a nursing history with special attention to:*

1. Parents' description of the events that preceded hospitalization, and their understanding of prolonged apnea.
   a. This information may provide clues for factors to observe during hospitalization and provides data for the development of a teaching plan.
   b. It also allows for the correction of misinformation and misconceptions.
2. Have parents describe sleep patterns, feeding habits, prior health problems, immunizations, and medications; this information may provide data regarding possible influencing factors or causes of the condition.
3. Have parents describe a typical day in the life of the infant and the family unit. This provides important data on how home-monitoring may affect family life, and contributes to the effective development of home management and family teaching plans; it also provides a basis for continuity of care for the infant.

C. *To orient the parents to the unit and the equipment used in the infant's care.*

Explain the visiting policy and encourage parents to visit as much as possible.

1. Parents must be willing and available for comprehensive instruction in their infant's condition and necessary interventions so that they feel competent in the infant's care prior to discharge.
2. Assignment of consistent nursing (primary nurse) is helpful so that families can develop a trusting relationship that will help them deal with the emotional aspects of the diagnosis and the complexities of the treatment plan.
3. Preparing the parents for all diagnostic tests that will be performed helps reduce the fear surrounding these procedures.

D. *To monitor constantly, and document any apneic event the infant may experience.*

1. Condition of infant
   a. Awake/asleep
   b. Respirations—none, normal, shallow; color of infant
   c. Monitor reading—apnea, bradycardia and rate, read off
   d. Position of infant—limp, vomited, etc.
2. Intervention
   a. Nothing—infant ok or self-corrected
   b. Gentle stimulation

c. Vigorously shaken
d. Resuscitation

E. *To serve as a role model for the family in the following areas of infant care.*

1. Use of the infant monitor (i.e., electrode placement, operation of controls, care of lead wires to prevent damage, etc.). Discussion of home-monitoring should not take place until it has been determined that this procedure will be used.
2. Methods of responding to alarms. Respond to all alarms immediately according to established procedures (i.e., observation and assessment of infant, stimulation, resuscitation, etc.).
3. Recording procedure—complete documentation of any apneic episode; record each time alarm sounds.
4. Administration of theophylline, if prescribed.
   a. Observe for signs of toxicity: apical rate above 200, vomiting, and agitation.
   b. Although the mechanism by which theophylline reduces or prevents apnea in some infants is not understood, research indicates it may act by:
      (1) Inducing rapid shallow breathing
      (2) Increasing metabolic rate with an increase in alveolar ventilation in proportion to increased CO_2 production.
5. Continue the infant's normal activities whenever possible (i.e., holding him for feedings, playing with him, disconnecting him from monitor for bathing); allow for continuation of usual eating or sleeping patterns. Simulating the home environment as much as possible will encourage deep-sleep patterns, which may stimulate apnea in some infants (valuable diagnostic information).

F. *To effectively prepare parents for eventual discharge of infant.*

Since the parents have experienced at least one apneic episode prior to hospitalization, the fear of their infant's sudden death has been heightened. When discharged, the parents have direct and full responsibility for appropriate action should infant's breathing cease.

1. Assess what parents know and understand about apnea. Correct any misconceptions and provide accurate information.
2. Make sure parents know about feeding precautions—frequent burping, no bottle in bed, upright position after feeding, elevation of the head of the bed, position on abdomen for sleep.
3. Have parents contact local emergency service to discuss prolonged apnea of infancy and CPR, and to be certain they have infant resuscitation equipment. It may be possible to arrange for the power company to notify parents if power supply is to go off.
4. Instruct parents in the administration of any medications (i.e., theophylline).
5. Teach CPR to parents as well as to another responsible person, relative, or friend, to provide some relief for parents from infant care.

G. *To teach and prepare parents for home-monitoring, if necessary.*

1. Show parents how to operate and maintain the monitor. Reinforce teaching by equipment supplier. Be sure they know how to contact monitor technician.
2. Describe apnea recording procedure to be used (see D).

3. Teach methods of responding to alarms—what to observe (i.e., color, presence or absence of breathing) and how to respond (gentle and vigorous stimulation, CPR).
4. Discuss adjustments in daily living that will be necessary. Start by identifying a typical family day, then discuss anticipated changes.
   a. Emphasize that this responsibility must be shared by both parents.
   b. Discuss the possible impact on siblings.
   c. Caution parents to eliminate noises that would interfere with their ability to hear the alarm (i.e., showering, vacuum cleaning) when only one parent is present. Someone must always be available to hear and respond to the alarm.
   d. Avoid traveling long distances alone with infant.
   e. Encourage parents to maintain their relationship with one another by using another trained person in CPR to assume infant care occasionally.
5. Use anticipatory guidance in preparing parents for complication of home monitoring:
   a. Increased anxiety and tension
   b. Constant worry about the alarm—even when it does not go off
   c. Fatigue
   d. The financial and emotional burdens encountered by the entire family
   e. Loss of "normal, healthy child"—parents then grieve when given the diagnosis
6. Emphasize the healthy aspects of the infant. Encourage parents to continue as many usual routines as possible. Provide specific things parents can do to encourage normal development and a healthy parent–child relationship.
7. Encourage parents to provide total care for their infant for 24 hours prior to discharge.

H. *To continue to observe family dynamics.*

1. Assess for family conflicts or problems that can be alleviated.
2. Families who are overly stressed or demonstrate a maladaptive response may require social service or psychiatric consultation.
3. Modification of the management plan may be indicated.

I. *To document patient/family progress in order to facilitate comprehensive care and discharge planning.*

Daily notes should include:
1. Frequency and type of monitor alarms; intervention required
2. Teaching
3. Family dynamics
   a. Who visited and for how long
   b. Description of parent–child interaction
   c. Description of parent interaction
   d. Amount of care done by parents
   e. Assessment of parental competence in providing care.

J. *To ensure adequate follow-up support.*

Most families are frightened by the responsibility of home-monitoring and will require support after discharge.
1. Some may need a community health nurse—homemaker/home health aide.
2. Instruct parents regarding when and how to obtain assistance for medical, technical, and psychosocial problems.

3. Facilitate contact with other parents of infants with prolonged apnea.
4. Assist parents with arrangements for competent babysitting help.

K. *To be aware that successful outcome for every baby with prolonged apnea cannot be certain, despite continuous surveillance with or without monitors and appropriate intervention.*

L. *To participate in community education regarding prolonged apnea and SIDS.*

Available Resources

National Sudden Infant Death Syndrome Foundation (NSIDF), 310 South Michigan, Chicago, Ill. 60604, (312) 663-0650.

The International Guild for Infant Survival, Inc., 1515 Reisterstown Rd., Suite 300, Baltimore, Md. 21208, (301) 484-0111.

BIBLIOGRAPHY

Books

Avery GB. Neonatology. Philadelphia, JB Lippincott, 1981

Babson S et al. Diagnosis and Management of the Fetus and Neonate at Risk, 4th ed. St. Louis, CV Mosby, 1980

Butnarescu GF, Tillotson DM, Villarreal PP. Perinatal Nursing, Vol. 2: Reproductive Risk. New York, John Wiley & Sons, 1980

Clark AL and Affonso DD. Childbearing: A Nursing Perspective. Philadelphia, FA Davis, 1976

Evans HE and Glass L. Perinatal Medicine. Hagerstown, Harper & Row, 1978

Johnson SH. High-Risk Parenting: Nursing Assessment and Strategies for the Family at Risk. Philadelphia, JB Lippincott, 1979

Klaus MH and Fanaroff AA. Care of the High-Risk Neonate. Philadelphia, WB Saunders, 1979

Krones SB. High-Risk Newborn Infant: The Basis for Intensive Nursing Care. St. Louis, CV Mosby, 1976

Levin DL, Morriss CF, Moore GC. A Practical Guide to Pediatric Intensive Care. St. Louis, CV Mosby, 1979

Lubchenco LO. The High-Risk Infant, Vol. XIV: Major Problems in Clinical Pediatrics. Philadelphia, WB Saunders, 1976

Moore ML. Newborn, Family and Nurse, 2nd ed. Philadelphia, WB Saunders Co., 1981

Scipien GM et al. Comprehensive Pediatric Nursing, 2nd ed. New York, McGraw-Hill, 1979

Whaley LF and Wong DL. Nursing Care of Infants and Children. St. Louis, CV Mosby, 1979

Articles

Adelman RD. Neonatal hypertension. Pediatr Clin North Am 1978 Feb; 25(1):99–110

Bell EF. Combined effect of radiant warmer and phototherapy on insensible water loss in low-birth weight infants. J Pediatr 1979 May; 94(5):810–813

Boychuk RB. Meconium aspiration syndrome and pulmonary hypertension. Respir Technology 1978 Fall; 14(3):10–15+

Black L, Hersher L, Steinschneider A. Impact of the apnea monitor on family life. Pediatrics 1978 Nov; 62(5):681–685

Corcoran MM. Nursing role and management of failure-to-thrive clients. Issues Comp Pediatr Nurs 1978 Oct; 3(4):29–40

Darnall RA and Ariagno RL. Resting oxygen consumption of premature infants covered with a plastic thermal blanket. Pediatrics 1979 Apr; 63(4):547–551

Deal AW and Bordeaux BR. The phenomenon of SIDS. Pediatric Nurs 1980 Jan/Feb; 6(1):48–50

Eager M and Exoo R. Parents visiting parents for unequalled support. MCN 1980 Jan/Feb; 5(1):35–36

Eisner V, Brazie J, Pratt MW, Hexter AC. The risk of low birth weight. Am J Public Health 1979 Sept; 69(9):887–893

Favorito J, Pernice JM, Ruggiero P. Apnea monitoring to prevent SIDS. Am J Nurs 1979 Jan; 79(1):101–104

Fedrick J and Adelstein P. Factors associated with low birth weights of infants delivered at term. Br J Obstet Gynecol 1978 Jan; 85(1):1–7

Flores RN. Necrotizing enterocolitis. Nurs Clin North Am 1978 March; 13(1):39–45

Friedman WF et al. Prostaglandins: Physiological and clinical correlations. Adv Pediatr 1978; 25:151–204

Gerhardt T, McCarthy J, Bancalari E. Effects of aminophylline on respiratory center activity and metabolic rate in premature infants with idiopathic apnea. Pediatrics 1979 Apr; 63(4):537–542

Goldson E. Parents' reactions to the birth of a sick infant. Children Today 1979 July/Aug; 8(4):13–17

Gould JB and James O. Management of the near-miss infant: A personal perspective. Pediatr Clin North Am 1979 Nov; 26(4):857–865

Guilleminault C and Korobkin R. Sudden infant death: Near miss events and sleep research. Sleep 1979; 1(4):423–433

Haddock N. Blood pressure monitoring in neonates. MCN 1980 Mar/Apr; 5(2):131–135

Halliday HL, Hirata T, Brady JP. Indomethacin therapy for large patent ductus arteriosus in the very low birth weight infant: Results and complications. Pediatrics 1979 Aug; 64(2):154–159

Hawkins–Walsh E. Diminishing anxiety in parents of sick newborns. MCN 1980 Jan/Feb; 5(1):30–34

Kelly DH, Shannon DC, O'Connell K. Care of infants with near-miss sudden infant death syndrome. Pediatrics 1978 Apr; 61(4):511–514

Kennell JH and Klaus MH. Early mother–infant contact. Bull Menninger Clin 1979 Jan; 43(1):69–77

Klijanowicz A. Protocol for the nursing care of hospitalized infants with prolonged apnea. Infant Apnea Center Handbook. Rochester, University of Rochester School of Medicine and Dentistry and School of Nursing, 1980

Maisels MJ. Neonatal jaundice. Part II: An approach to the jaundiced infant. Perinatal Press 1979 Jan; 3(1):3–6

McAteer J. Diabetic pregnancy and neonatal outcome. CCQ 1979 Dec; 2(3):61–72

McBride BH. Babies with necrotizing enterocolitis—what to watch for. Can Nurse 1979 Dec; 75(11):41–44

McCracken GH. Neonatal septicemia and meningitis. Hosp Pract 1976 Jan; 11:89–97

McElroy E, Ruginis B, Shaefer SJM. Sudden infant death syndrome. Nurs Clin North Am 1979 Sept; 14(3):391–403

Meir P. "Wee" babies. QRB 1978 Sept; 4(9):22,26–27

Meir P and Wendorf B. Assessment of nursing care for extremely premature infants. QRB 1978 Sept; 4(9):24–25

Michie MM. The quality of neonatal care and intensive care units. Midwives Chronicle 1979 Jan; 92(1):13–15

Opirhory GJ. Counseling the parents of a critically ill newborn. JOGN Nurs 1979 May/June; 8(3):179–182

Porth CM and Kaylor LE. Temperature regulation in the newborn. Am J Nurs 1978 Oct; 78(10):1691–1693

Sills RH. Failure to thrive. Am J Dis Child 1978 Oct; 132(10):967–999

Silver S. A mother's guide to breastfeeding and mothering the premature or hospitalized sick infant. Clin Pediatr 1978 May; 17(5):425–427

Sosa R. Maternal–infant interaction during the immediate post-partum period. Adv Pediatr 1978; 25:451–465

Speidel BD. Adverse effects of routine procedures on preterm infants. Lancet 1978 Apr 22; 1(8069):864–865

Stern L. Physiology of the newborn infant: Bilirubin metabolism. Progr Pediatr Surg 1978; 12:1–21

Stevens D and Schreiner RL. Infants of diabetic mothers. J Indiana State Med Assoc 1978 Apr; 71(4):409–410

Sullivan R, Foster J, Schreiner RL. Determining a newborn's gestational age. MCN 1979 Jan/Feb; 4(1):38–45

Task Force on Prolonged Apnea. American Academy of Pediatrics. Pediatrics 1978 Apr; 61(4):651

Tufts F and Johnson F. Neonatal jaundice and phototherapy. Can Nurse 1979 Dec; 75(11):45–47

Turner BS and Merenstein GB. Hemodynamic monitoring of the critically ill neonate. CCQ 1979 Sept; 2:77–78

Vogel M. When a pregnant woman is diabetic: Care of the newborn. Am J Nurs 1979 Mar; 79(3):458–460

Weinstein SF. Sudden infant death syndrome: Impact on families and a direction for change. Am J Psychiatry 1978 July; 135(7):831–834

Whiteside D. Proper use of radiant warmers. Am J Nurs 1978 Oct; 78(10):1694–1696

Feeding infants of low birth weight. Br Med J 1979 Nov 3; 2(6198):1092–1093

Additional Pertinent References

Beckwith JB. The Sudden Infant Death Syndrome. Washington, D.C., U.S. Government Printing Office, 1975

Cagan J and Meier PA. A discharge planning tool for use with families of high-risk infants. JOGN Nurs 1979 May/June; 8(3):146–148

Garrand S et al. A parent-to-parent program. Family and Community Health 1978 Nov; 1(3):103–113

Goldberg S. Premature birth: Consequences for the parent–infant relationship. Am Scientist 1979 Mar/Apr; 67(2):214–220

Metcalf SC. Getting to know your premature baby. Louisville, The National Foundation March of Dimes

Schraeder BD. Attachment and parenting despite lengthy intensive care. MCN 1980 Jan/Feb; 5(1):37–41

Whaley PA, Gosling CG, Schreiner RL. Relieving parental anxiety—A booklet for parents of an infant in NICU. JOGN Nurs 1979 Jan/Feb; 8(1):49–55

Audio-Visual Materials

Brazelton Film No. 1: An Introduction

Education Development Center,
39 Chapel Street,
Newton, Mass 02160

In this 16 mm.–20-minute film, Dr. T. Berry Brazelton briefly describes the Neonatal Behavioral Assessment Scale while he examines a 2-day-old normal infant. In this film he assesses the infant's initial state of rest, and then tests its habituation to various stimuli and its responses to different experiences.

Inservice education modules:
Series I—First Six Hours of Life, Neonatal Thermoregulation, Hypoglycemia, Early Parent–Infant Relationships, Assessment of Risk in the Newborn

March of Dimes—Birth Defect Foundation,
1275 Mamaroneck Ave.,
White Plains, N.Y. 10605

CHILDREN WITH CONDITIONS OF THE RESPIRATORY TRACT

39

OVERVIEW OF CHILDHOOD RESPIRATORY DISORDERS

Common Types of Respiratory Disorders

Examples of common childhood respiratory disorders can be found in Table 39-1. The following disorders are included:
1. Bacterial Pneumonia
2. Viral Pneumonia
3. Pneumocystis Carinii Pneumonia
4. Mycoplasma Pneumonia
5. Bronchiolitis
6. Croup

Nursing Objectives and Management

A. *To determine the severity of the respiratory distress that the child is experiencing.*

Make an initial nursing assessment.
1. Observe the respiratory rate and pattern.
   a. Count the respirations for 1 full minute.
   b. Observe child for retractions, and note severity and location.
   c. Listen to the chest with a stethoscope to determine if rales are present and to evaluate the breath sounds.
2. Observe the child's color, and note any presence of cyanosis.
3. Observe for nasal flaring.
4. Evaluate the child's degree of restlessness, apprehension, and motor tone.
5. Note any wheezing, stridor, or hoarseness.

B. *To provide a humidified environment enriched with oxygen in order to combat anoxia and to liquefy secretions.*

1. Place child in a Croupette with cool mist or use ultrasonic mist in tent (see Oxygen Therapy, p. 1196).

> **NURSING ALERT:** At no time should the mist be allowed to become so dense that it obscures clear visualization of the patient's respiratory pattern.

2. Observe the child's response to this environment.

3. Place child in comfortable position to promote easier ventilation.
4. Frequent changing of clothing and bed linen will prevent chilling and will provide comfort.

C. *To provide the child with adequate hydration.*

1. Maintain the administration of intravenous fluids at the prescribed rate.
2. When the child is in severe respiratory distress, he is given nothing by mouth because of the danger of aspiration.
3. Offer the child small sips of a clear fluid when the respiratory status improves.
   a. Note any vomiting or abdominal distention after the oral fluid is given.
   b. As the child begins to take more fluid by mouth, notify physician so that intravenous fluid rate may be adjusted in order to prevent fluid overload.
   c. Do not force child to take fluids orally that he does not want, as this may cause increased distress and possible vomiting. Anorexia often accompanies acute febrile infection. Generally do not awaken a sleeping child just to give frequent fluids.
4. Record child's intake and output.
   a. Measure urinary output and record.
   b. Check specific gravity of urine.

D. *To provide the child with both physical and psychological rest.*

1. Disturb the child as little as possible by organizing nursing care, and protect him from unnecessary interruptions from other personnel.
2. Be aware of the age of the child and be familiar with his level of growth and development as it applies to hospitalization.
3. The presence of the child's parents will alleviate some of his apprehension.
4. Provide opportunities for quiet play as the child's condition improves.
5. Explain procedures and hospital routine to child as appropriate for his age.
6. Reduce anxiety and apprehension to aid in decreasing psychological distress, which will help the child relax and ease respiratory effort.

TABLE 39-1. RESPIRATORY DISORDERS

Condition and Causative Agent	Age and Incidence	Clinical Manifestations

I. Bacterial Pneumonia
A. Streptococcus pneumonia
Streptococcus pneumoniae
(gram-positive)
This type of bacterial pneumonia is most frequent in children.
	Birth–4 years
	Winter and spring
	(especially in patients with sickle cell disease and patients without spleens)
		Mild upper respiratory infection (URI) with sudden symptoms
		Infants:
		    Refusal to eat
		    Vomiting; diarrhea
		    Hypo- or hyperthermia
		May be:
		    Tachypnea
		    Grunting
		    Retractions
		    Nasal flaring
		Older child:
		    Prodromal upper respiratory infection
		    Headache
		    Anorexia
		    Malaise
		    Dry cough
		    Fever
		    Restlessness
		    Pleuritic pain
		    Grunting with shallow, rapid respirations
		    Possibly abdominal pain

B. Streptococcal pneumonia Beta-hemolytic streptococcus, Group A (gram-positive)	3–5 years	Commonly superimposed on febrile respiratory infection in a child already ill with a viral exanthem Shows sudden increased fever, worsening cough, chills, pleuritic pain, respiratory distress
C. Staphylococcal pneumonia Coagulase-positive *Staphylococcus aureus* (gram-positive)	Birth–2 years	History of predisposing factors: Gradual onset with respiratory symptoms or sudden onset with systemic involvement (very toxic child) Presence of coarse, bubbly crepitations
D. *Haemophilus influenzae*	6 months–3 years	Similar to other lobar pneumonias and bronchopneumonia with spasmodic cough; "toxic" appearance
II. Viral Pneumonia Respiratory syncytial virus (RSV) (most common) Parainfluenza virus Adenoviruses	Birth–2 years; higher incidence in females than in males Winter and early spring	Gradual onset following an upper respiratory infection RSV turns into extension of bronchiolitis Parainfluenza virus causes coryza, pharyngitis, cough; may succeed pneumonia Adenovirus causes pharyngitis and cervical adenitis; may succeed pneumonia
III. Pneumocystis Carinii Pneumonia *Pneumocystis carinii*—parasite of uncertain systemic status	Predisposing factors: Prematurity; immature debilitated infant; infectious disease, especially cytomegalic inclusion disease; serious compromising disease, e.g., cystic fibrosis Children receiving immunosuppressive medication for malignant diseases Immunodeficiency disease, especially in children under 1 year of age	Onset is generally slow, taking 3–6 weeks to peak, with increasing tachypnea, extreme grayish cyanosis, and dyspnea Presence of predisposing factors
IV. Mycoplasma Pneumonia *Mycoplasma pneumoniae* (pleuropneumonia-like organism) Microorganisms with properties between bacteria and viruses	5–15 years Late fall and winter	Onset is insidious: Malaise, headache, low-grade fever, sore throat, irritating cough, vomiting, possible crepitation

Diagnostic Evaluation	Medical Treatment and Nursing Management	Complications

X-ray—patchy area around bronchi
Positive cultures
  Sputum
  Nasopharyngeal secretions
  Blood
	Penicillin G
	Symptomatic:
	  Rest, with gradually increasing exercise
	  Fluids—I & O
	  Antipyretics
	  O$_2$ mist
	  Position change
		Rare with antibiotic prescription
		May see:
		  Otitis media
		  Sinusitis
		  Empyema
		  Bacteremia

X-ray—usually patchy, but may show disseminated infiltrate
WBC increased—polymorphic leukocytosis
Erythrocyte sedimentation rate (ESR) increased
Positive culture from:
  Respiratory secretions
  Empyema fluid
	Penicillin G
	Symptomatic
		Empyema
		Pneumatocele to pneumothorax
		Permanent pulmonary fibrosis and pleural thickening (fibrothorax)

X-ray—patchy consolidation of one or more lobes; pneumatocele abscesses
Culture: sputum or gastric aspirate, pulmonary fluid or lung aspirate
WBC—elevated in older child
	Methicillin or Penicillin G
	  Rapid treatment is important
	  Symptomatic: special attention to fluid balance, treatment of pleural complications, treatment of anemia
	Be alert to signs of tension pneumothorax: abrupt onset of pain; cyanosis, dyspnea, diminished chest movement on one side
		Empyema
		Pneumothorax
		Lung abscess
		Osteomyelitis
		Staphylococcal pericarditis
		Bronchiectasis

	Ampicillin—if organism is not resistant Other: Penicillin G, chloramphenicol	Empyema Bronchiectasis (rare)
Culture: Blood, nasal secretions; WBC shows an increase—lymphocytosis X-ray—lobar consolidation (may also have pleural effusion)	Symptomatic: cough suppression	
X-ray—infiltration of one or more lobes is more extensive than clinical picture would suggest Culture: nasopharyngeal Increase titer of specific antibody	Broad-spectrum antibiotic therapy (until confirmation of organism is established) Symptomatic and supportive	

X-ray shows bilateral diffuse alveolar densities, especially perihilar
Observe cysts in special stained smear in material obtained from lung biopsy (not reliable)
Lung aspiration by needle
Endotracheal brush catheter technique
	Pentamide isethionate
	Trimethroprim-sulfamethoxazole
	Supportive: Maintain oxygen and respirations; administer immunoglobins; possibly withhold immunosuppressive chemotherapy; maintain fluid, electrolyte, and acid-base balance; maintain nutrition
	Be alert to early signs and predisposing factors that will aid in early diagnosis
	Carefully observe for adverse effects of drug therapy: abscess formation and necrosis of injection site
	  Hypoglycemia
	  Nephrotoxicity
	  Hypotension
	  Tachycardia
	  Hypocalcemia
	  Nausea and vomiting
	  Skin rash
	  Anemia
	  Hyperkalemia
	  Thrombocytopenia
		Pneumothorax from diagnostic tests, concomitant bacterial pneumonia or sepsis
		Death

X-ray shows peribronchial infiltrate in lower lobes Increase in complement fixation test Positive sputum culture	Erythromycin Supportive: antipyretic cough suppression	

TABLE 39-1. RESPIRATORY DISORDERS (cont.)

Condition and Causative Agent	Age and Incidence	Clinical Manifestations

V. Bronchiolitis
  Respiratory syncytial virus (RSV)
  Adenovirus
  Parainfluenza virus
  Influenza virus
	Most common in infants and children under 6 months; may occur in child up to 2 years of age
	Greater incidence in males than in females
	Winter-spring
		Onset is often gradual and associated with exposure to respiratory infection
		Coryza of 1–3 days; tachypnea
		Intercostal and suprasternal retraction
		Expiratory rhonchi
		Dry cough
		Fever
		Cyanosis
		Possible dehydration
		Tachypnea

VI. A. Croup (see box, p. 1261)
    Acute laryngitis, laryngotracheobronchitis (LTB)
    Parainfluenza virus 1-2-3 (most common virus)
    Respiratory syncytial virus
    Influenza virus
    Enterovirus
    Adenovirus
	6 months–3 years
	Winter
		Generally onset is gradual and progresses slowly, following 1 to several days after an upper respiratory infection
		Coryza
		Croupy cough, barking cough
		Inspiratory stridor
		Hoarseness
		Low-grade fever
		Increasing respiration and pulse rate
		Apprehension, restlessness, anxiety

B. Epiglottitis—supraglottitis
    Bacterial:
    Haemophilus influenzae type B (most common)
    Pneumococci
    Staphylococcus aureus
    Beta-hemolytic streptococcus
	3–10 years
	Seasonal variations
		Onset and progression are rapid—may follow short duration of coryza
		Severe inspiratory stridor with marked supraclavicular and intercostal retractions
		Sore throat—refusal to eat, dysphagia
		High fever 39–40°C. (102–104°F.)
		Drooling; respirations may be shallow; hoarseness; paleness and exhausted appearance; may insist on sitting up—condition worsens when lying down; cherry-red epiglottis; apprehension; restlessness; anxiety

E. *To provide good skin care to prevent skin excoriation from secretions, accompanying diarrhea, and breakdown from confinement to bed.*

F. *To provide measures to improve ventilation of affected portion of the lung.*

1. Change position frequently.
2. Provide postural drainage if prescribed.
3. Relieve nasal obstruction that contributes to breathing difficulty.
     Instill saline solution or other nose drops and apply nasal suctioning.
4. Crying can be an effective method for ventilating the lungs.
5. Coughing is a normal tracheobronchial cleansing procedure. Constant coughing can be relieved temporarily by allowing the child to sip water; use extreme caution to prevent aspiration.
6. Abdominal distention frequently accompanies respiratory infection and can be painful and a hindrance to respiration.
     a. Place in semi-Fowler's position.
     b. Rectal tube, small enema, or suppository may give relief.
     c. Nasogastric tube may be prescribed to relieve distention.

G. *To assist in the control of fever.*

1. Antipyretics
2. Increase evaporation from skin with cool sponges.

H. *To provide for adequate nutrition to meet the growth and development needs of the child.*

1. Determine the child's food preferences.
2. Offer the child small meals.

I. *To administer appropriate antibiotic therapy.*

1. Observe for drug sensitivity.
2. Observe child's response to therapy.

J. *To be alert for the appearance of specific complications that may accompany respiratory infection and notify physician immediately* (see Table 39-1).

K. *To include parents in the planning of care and in caring for the child.*

Recognize parents' anxieties. The mother may be exhausted from caring for her sick child prior to his hospitalization.

Parental Education

Direct parents according to the pointers on page 1261.

Diagnostic Evaluation	Medical Treatment and Nursing Management	Complications
X-ray demonstrates overinfiltration of lungs Virological or serological studies to isolate virus on throat swab P_aO_2 decreases; P_aCO_2 increases (late finding)	Antibiotic therapy given to severely ill child until lab confirmation is established Humidified O_2 to relieve arterial hypoxemia Monitoring blood gases and correction of acidosis Possible ventilatory assistance Maintain fluid-electrolyte-acid/base and nutritional balance Keep nasal airway open and clear of mucus to decrease respiratory difficulty, because infant is an obligatory nose breather Position baby in infant seat inside Croupette; it may provide some respiratory assistance Be alert to signs of impending respiratory acidosis and dehydration	Exhaustion and anoxia Secondary bacterial infection Pneumothorax and pneumomediastinum (occasional) Apneic spells Circulatory collapse Increase—predisposed to asthma
History and clinical evaluation— Lab findings: PCO_2 increased (late finding), PO_2 decreased Normal—mild leukocytosis X-ray of neck—subglottic edema (below vocal cords) Normal supraglottic structures	Supportive: High humidification with oxygen, as necessary; hydration; nebulized racemic epinephrine with or without IPPB; antibiotic therapy; minimal handling; allow undisturbed sleep; monitor vital signs Teach parents home management of croup (see below) Syrup of ipecac may be beneficial in reducing coughing in spasmodic croup	Airway obstruction Anorexia
History and clinical evaluation— Lab findings: PCO_2 increased (late finding); PO_2 decreased Leukocytosis X-ray of neck—epiglottic edema (above vocal cords); normal trachea and larynx	Medical Emergency: Endotracheal/nasotracheal intubation or tracheostomy; "cool humidified oxygen" Antibiotic therapy: Chloramphenicol Observe carefully for signs and symptoms of increasing respiratory distress; have in readiness equipment for intubation or tracheostomy (see p. 1195) Teach parents home care of tracheostomy Community health nurse referral	Airway obstruction Death

---

WHEN YOUR CHILD HAS A CROUP ATTACK*

If your child develops hoarseness and a croupy cough with a cold, or if he wakes up in the middle of the night with a croup attack, here is the way to handle it:

1. Take your child into the bathroom and close the door. Turn on the hot water in the shower or tub, and let the room fill up with steam. Sit with your child in the steam-filled bathroom, with the water still running, for 10 minutes. If he is still making croupy noise as he breathes, call the doctor.
2. After breathing has improved, use a cold-air vaporizer. If your child sleeps in a crib, place a sheet or umbrella over the top of the crib and direct the stream of vapor under the sheet. If he sleeps in a bed, place a card table over his head, and drape a sheet over the card table. Keep one side of the crib or table open so he won't get too hot.
3. Give your child liquids that you know he likes every hour he's awake. Drinking plenty of fluids is very important in helping him get over croup.
4. Let him choose the position in which he is most comfortable. Don't make him lie down. An infant seat may be comfortable for a small baby.
5. If your child continues to make noise as he breathes, keep watch over him. Call the doctor immediately if any of the following things happen:
   - His symptoms get worse fairly fast—more noise, higher fever.
   - He becomes very restless—sitting up, lying down, jumping about trying to find a comfortable position.
   - You notice sharp movement of the soft area around his collar bones or just below the ribs.
   - His lips or fingernails become bluish in color.
   - He appears to be very sick regardless of the degree of breathing difficulty.

TONSILLECTOMY AND ADENOIDECTOMY

Tonsillectomy and *adenoidectomy* is the surgical removal of the adenoidal and tonsillar structures, part of the lymphoid tissue that encircles the pharynx. (The function of the tonsils and adenoids is to serve as a first line of defense against respiratory infection.)

Etiology

1. Because the growth of the tonsils and adenoids in the first 10 years of life exceed general somatic growth, these structures appear especially large in the child.
2. Acute or chronic infection of tonsils and adenoids
3. Hypertrophy produces obstruction to:
   a. Breathing
   b. Swallowing
   c. Eustachian tube

Clinical Manifestations

Tonsillectomy and adenoidectomy are separate procedures with separate indications. Controversy exists among experts as to indications, necessity, and benefits of surgery.

A. *Indications for Tonsillectomy*
1. Conservative:
   a. Recurrent or persistent tonsillitis with documented streptococcal infection
   b. Marked hypertrophy of tonsils, which distorts speech, causes swallowing difficulties, and causes subsequent weight loss
   c. Tonsillar malignancy
   d. Diphtheria carrier
   e. Cor pulmonale due to obstruction
2. Controversial:
   a. Peritonsillar abscess or retrotonsillar abscess
   b. Suppurative cervical adenitis with tonsillar focus
   c. Persistent hyperemia of anterior pillars
   d. Enlarged cervical nodes

B. *Indications for Adenoidectomy*
1. Conservative:
   a. Adenoid hypertrophy resulting in obstruction of airway leading to hypoxia, pulmonary hypertension, and cor pulmonale
   b. Hypertrophy with nasal obstruction accompanied by breathing difficulty and severe speech distortion
   c. Hypertrophy associated with chronic suppurative or serous otitis media and sensorineural or conductive hearing loss, chronic mastoiditis, or cholesteatoma
   d. Mouth-breathing due to hypertrophied adenoids
2. Controversial:
   Enlarged adenoids, chronic otitis media, and no evidence of complications

Contraindications to Surgery

1. Bleeding or coagulation disorders
2. Uncontrolled systemic disorders (i.e., diabetes, rheumatic fever, cardiac, renal disease)
3. Child under the age of 5–6 years—unless life-threatening situation
4. Presence of upper respiratory infection in child or immediate family

5. Specific for adenoidectomy—certain palate abnormalities (i.e., cleft palate or submucus cleft palate)

Diagnostic Evaluation

Since bleeding is a likely complication of surgery to this highly vascular area, preoperative blood studies must be completed.
   a. Clotting time
   b. Smear for platelets
   c. Prothrombin time
   d. Partial prothrombin time

Nursing Objectives and Management

Preoperative Care

A. *To assess upon admission the psychological preparation of the child for hospitalization and surgery.*
1. The child should know why he has been admitted to the hospital and what will happen to him.
2. When parents have not told the child about hospitalization, it may be because they cannot.
   a. They do not know what will happen.
   b. They do not know how to tell the child because of their own anxieties.
   c. They do not understand the importance of telling the child the truth in order to perpetuate the child's trust in the parents.
3. Help parents in preparing the child by talking at first in general terms about hospitalization.
4. Child may have preconceived ideas from parents and peers about what to expect. (These may pose a threat to the child.)
   a. Expose child to other children on the unit, especially those who have had and are recovering from surgery.
   b. Correct any misunderstandings the child may have.
5. The preschool child is very vulnerable to psychological trauma as a result of this experience.
   a. Tell the child the truth.
   b. Include parents when helping the child.

B. *To take nursing history from parents at the time of admission to obtain any pertinent information that would contraindicate surgery.*
1. Infection
   a. When was last recent infection?
   b. Has child been exposed to any contagious diseases?
2. Safety
   a. Does the child have any loose teeth?
   b. Are there any bleeding tendencies in child or family?

C. *To maintain adequate hydration prior to surgery, since blood loss may be extensive during surgery.*
1. Encourage the child to drink fluids the night before surgery.
2. Child usually is NPO a few hours prior to surgery.

D. *To prepare the child specifically (appropriate for age) for what to expect postoperatively.*
1. Where he will wake up.
2. Sore throat, emesis of blood, position
3. Ice collar, medications
4. Fluid regimen

E. *To encourage mother to stay with her young child the day and night of surgery or at least before surgery and when the child returns to his room and is waking up.*

Prepare the mother as to what to expect when she sees the child postoperatively.
a. Vomiting
b. Color
c. Crying, angry or frightened

F. *To know if the child has a history of chronic infection or rheumatic fever so antibiotics may be given pre- and postoperatively.*

Postoperative Care

A. *To administer good postoperative care based on general principles and to observe for usual postoperative complications* (see p. 1140).

B. *To assist the child in maintaining a patent airway, by draining secretions and preventing aspiration of vomitus.*
1. Place child prone or semiprone before he becomes alert with head turned to side.
2. Allow the child to assume position of comfort when he is alert. (Mother may hold child.)
3. Child may vomit old blood initially.

C. *To observe the child constantly until he is awake, and then frequently thereafter; monitor vital signs and be alert to signs of hemorrhage.*
1. Indications of hemorrhage (the most frequent complication)
a. Increasing rapid pulse
b. Frequent swallowing
c. Pallor
d. Restlessness
e. Clearing of throat and vomiting of blood
f. Continuous slight oozing of blood over a number of hours postoperatively
2. Have emergency equipment readily available.
a. Suction equipment
b. Packing material

D. *To offer measures of comfort to the child.*
1. Cool liquids offer some relief from sore throat, as well as prevent dehydration and temperature elevation.
a. Give ice chips 1–2 hours after awakening.
b. Advance to clear liquids cautiously until vomiting has ceased.
c. Offer cool, synthetic fruit juices and milk at first as they are best tolerated.

2. Ice collar to neck may provide some comfort. (Remove ice collar if child becomes restless.)
3. Give analgesic, especially to older child.
4. Rinse mouth with cool water or alkaline solution.

E. *To provide opportunity for child to have as much rest as possible.*
1. Encourage mother to be with the child when he awakens as he is usually frightened. (Mother's presence can be very comforting.)
2. When mother must leave, reassure child she will return.
3. Keep child in bed in a quiet room.

Parental Education

1. Explain and write instructions as to the care of the child at home after discharge (usually the day after surgery).
a. Diet should still consist of large amounts of fluids as well as soft, cool nonirritating foods. (Supply list of suggestions.)
b. Bed rest should be maintained for a couple of days, then daily rest periods for about a week. Resume normal activities about 2 weeks following surgery.
c. Discourage child from frequent coughing and clearing of throat.
d. Avoid gargling. Mouth odor may be present for a few days after surgery; only rinsing mouth is acceptable.
e. If signs and symptoms of impending trouble occur, the physician should be called immediately.
(1) Earache accompanied by fever
(2) Any bleeding, often indicated only by frequent swallowing
f. How to give any medications the physician may prescribe.
g. The telephone number of the physician or emergency room if trouble occurs.
2. Discuss with the mother (parents) what results they can expect from the surgery.
a. Decreased number of sore throats
b. Improvement in obstructive symptoms
c. Decreased incidence of cervical lymphadenitis
d. Improvement in nutritional status
3. Guide parents in helping child make the hospital experience a positive one once he has returned home.
a. Talk about what happened.
b. Let child play out his feelings.

ASTHMA

Asthma is a recurrent, reversible condition of the lungs in which there is airway obstruction due to spasm of the bronchial smooth muscle, edema of the mucosa, and increased mucus secretions in the bronchi and bronchioles that has been brought on by various stimuli.

Classification of Asthma

1. *Acute attack*—sporadic in nature, with varying intervals of freedom from difficulty and with precipitating factors often readily defined.
2. *Latent asthma*—no outward signs or symptoms of asthma, but there is some shortness of breath on

occasion, transitory wheezing on strenuous exercise, and wheezy rales heard during deep inspiration.
3. *Intractable asthma*—persistent wheezing requiring regular, daily medication, for either the control of symptoms or the ability to function.
4. *Status asthmaticus*—severe attack in which the patient deteriorates in spite of adequate treatment with sympathomimetic drugs.

Etiology

The stimuli responsible for triggering attacks of asthma are as follows:

1. Antigen-antibody reaction (allergy to pollen, animal dander, feather pillows, foods)
2. Infection: respiratory syncytial virus, para influenza virus (Types I and II), mycoplasmal pneumonia
3. Physical factors
   a. Cold
   b. Meteorological factors (i.e., humidity, sudden changes in temperature and barometric pressure)
4. Heritable tendencies
5. Irritants
   a. Dust
   b. Chemicals
   c. Air pollutants (e.g., sulfur dioxide, carbon monoxide, particulate matter)
6. Psychic or emotional factors (i.e., tension, fear, anxiety)
7. Physical stress—fatigue, excessive exercise

Clinical Manifestations

1. The onset of an asthmatic attack may be gradual with nasal congestion, sneezing and a watery nasal discharge present before the attack.
2. Attacks may occur suddenly, often at night, when the child awakens with the following symptoms.
   a. Wheezing which occurs primarily with expiration
   b. Anxiety and apprehension
   c. Diaphoresis
   d. Uncontrollable cough
   e. Dyspnea, with increased effort during expiration
3. With treatment the attack may be controlled. The asthmatic attack may progress, however, and the child will develop the following symptoms.
   a. Increasing dyspnea
   b. Thick, tenacious mucus
   c. Coarse and fine musical rales
   d. Flaring of the alae nasi
   e. Use of accessory muscles for respiration
   f. Cyanosis
   g. Hypercapnia
   h. Increased heart and respiratory rates
   i. Abdominal pain from severe coughing
   j. Vomiting
   k. Extreme anxiety and apprehension

Incidence

1. The incidence of asthma in infancy exists but increases in children 3 years and older.
   a. In younger children, the incidence is greater in males.
   b. Incidence is equal in males and females during adolescence.
2. Childhood asthma may cease at puberty.

Altered Physiology

1. The turbinates warm and moisten all air which passes into the lung.
2. Inspired air contains particulate matter which is removed by the blanket of mucus present in the tracheobronchial tree. This mucus is kept moistened by inspired moist air.
3. The blanket of mucus is moved constantly upward by the propelling action of the cilia, and if mucus becomes thickened or inspissated it cannot be moved.
4. An increased local deposition and concentration of allergens occurs.
5. This produces intrabronchial accumulation and stagnation of mucus which is the primary cause of the respiratory embarrassment.

6. Chemical mediators in asthma:
   a. Primarily involved are histamine and SRS-A (slow-reacting substance of anaphylaxis). SRS-A appears after histamine release, and persists for a longer period. It is not inhibited by the action of the antihistamines.
   b. These materials are primarily responsible for changes in the blood vessels and mucous membrane in the bronchi and bronchioles, as well as for the initiation of bronchospasm.
7. During an asthma attack, abnormal constriction of muscles surrounding the bronchioles (spasm) results in narrowed bronchiolar lumen and decreased oxygen supply in alveoli.
   a. In addition, edema, inflammation, and increased mucus production further compromise respirations.
   b. Hyperresonance and decreased breath sounds may be observed.

Diagnostic Evaluation

1. Eosinophilia in peripheral blood, nasal secretions, and sputum
2. Polymorphonuclear leukocytosis in the presence of infection
3. Pulmonary function studies—diminished maximal breathing capacity, tidal volume and timed vital capacity
4. Determination of blood gases and pH—respiratory acidosis and later metabolic acidosis
5. Gross and microscopic examination of sputum—bronchial casts and eosinophilia
6. Serum CBC
7. Chest x-ray—to exclude presence of other diseases; child may show hyperventilation during asthma attack
8. Routine skin testing may help determine allergic causes

Complications

1. Bronchiectasis
2. Emphysema
3. Cor pulmonale
4. Infants (up to 2 years)—serious respiratory failure due to the stage of development of their anatomic structures and physiologic mechanisms which are not able to cope with the insult and compensatory demands of the disease.

Treatment

1. Removal of suspected stimulus: allergen, irritant, exercise, emotional factors
2. Desensitization in order to build up child's resistance to his allergens
3. Drug therapy to control symptoms
4. Chest physical therapy—bronchial drainage, breathing exercises
5. Supportive:
   a. Adequate hydration
   b. Adequate oxygenation
   c. Appropriate treatment of any existing infection
   d. Correct acid-base balance
   e. Relieve fatigue

Nursing Objectives and Management

A. *To become informed regarding the child's symptomatology and the medical plan of care.*

1. Make a base-line nursing assessment of the child's

condition in order to determine the severity of the attack and the degree of respiratory distress.

a. Observe the child's breathing pattern:
  (1) Determine whether the expiratory phase of respiration is increased.
  (2) Determine whether the child is wheezing. (In severe attacks wheezing is audible at a distance from the child.)
  (3) Determine whether the child is using accessory muscles for breathing.
b. Listen to the child's chest with a stethoscope to determine whether rales and rhonchi are present, and to determine whether all areas of the lung fields are being aerated.
c. Assess the child's level of anxiety and apprehension.
d. Observe for flaring of the alae nasi.
e. Observe the child for the development of cyanosis, utilizing adequate light.

2. Determine the heart and respiratory rates; record and report to the physician any significant change.
3. Discuss with the physician the plan of medical care.

B. *To provide measures to relieve the respiratory distress the child is experiencing.*

1. Position the child in high Fowler's position to allow maximum lung expansion.
  a. Raise the head of the bed to achieve high Fowler's position.
  b. Place an overbed table padded with a pillow in front of the child and have him extend his arms over the table—this provides a comfortable position and allows maximum utilization of accessory muscles for breathing.
2. Administer oxygen when signs of air hunger are present.
  a. Do not wait for the appearance of cyanosis before administering oxygen.
  b. Oxygen must be administered with caution since the child with severe respiratory distress may be dependent upon his low PO_2 to stimulate spontaneous respiration. In the face of a rising PCO_2 and a potential CO_2 narcosis, the administration of oxygen may remove the last stimulus to spontaneous respirations.
3. Explain to the child the purpose of the oxygen equipment before oxygen is administered and allow the child to feel and touch the equipment.
4. Use aerosolized bronchodilators.

C. *To relieve the anxiety and apprehension which results from the respiratory embarrassment.*

1. Place the child in a quiet, clean room, where he can be closely observed.
2. Provide the child with maximum reassurance.
  a. Allow parents to remain with the child.
    (1) Keep the parents informed as to the child's progress—what is being done and why—in order to relieve their apprehension. Parental anxiety is readily transmitted to the child.
    (2) Talk calmly and quietly to the child.
    (3) Assure the child that you will not leave him alone.
    (4) Allow the child to have his favorite security object.
3. Organize care so as to avoid disturbing the child any more than necessary.
4. When the child falls asleep, allow him to continue to sleep and do not disturb him unless absolutely necessary.
5. Evaluate the need for sedation.

D. *To provide adequate hydration in order to liquefy and mobilize bronchial secretions and maintain electrolyte balance.*

Dehydration occurs secondary to decreased fluid intake, excessive perspiration, vomiting, increased respiration and infection.

1. Observe for signs of dehydration.
  a. Lack of skin turgor
  b. Lack of tears
  c. Dry parched lips
  d. Depressed fontanelle
  e. Decreased urinary output—high specific gravity; concentrated appearance.
2. Maintain parenteral fluid administration.
3. Encourage oral fluid intake.
  a. Determine child's fluid preferences.
  b. Offer small sips of fluid frequently.
  c. Avoid iced fluids which may provoke bronchospasm.
  d. Avoid carbonated beverages when wheezing.
4. Allow the child to return to a regular diet as soon as possible.
5. Observe for signs of overhydration and pulmonary edema.

E. *To be aware of the action and side effects of drugs used in the treatment of asthma.*

1. *Aminophylline*—bronchodilator
  a. Toxic reaction may occur, but it is more likely to happen with prolonged overdose or when given in conjunction with epinephrine or ephedrine without reducing aminophylline dosage.
    (1) Serum drug levels should be done.
    (2) Toxic reactions include:
      Fever, restlessness, nausea and vomiting, hypotension, abdominal distention.
  b. Side effects—irritability, excitability, continued dehydration, vomiting, hematemesis, proteinuria, stupor, convulsions, coma, death. Hypotension occurs with IV use. Avoid ingestion of stimulants.
  c. Occasionally cyanosis and syncope may appear after only a small amount of the prescribed dose. This is considered an idiosyncracy, and the drug should be discontinued.
2. *Epinephrine*—relaxes bronchial smooth muscle and constricts bronchial mucosal vessels, thereby reducing congestion and edema; acts as a bronchodilator.
  a. The smallest dose affording relief should be used.
  b. Side effects—insomnia, headache, nervousness, palpitations, precordial pain, hypertension, hypoxemia, tachycardia, nausea, sweating, urinary retention. (It may potentiate aminophylline toxicity.)
3. *Ephedrine*—relaxes bronchial smooth muscle and constricts bronchial mucosal vessels, thereby reducing congestion and edema. Acts as a bronchodilator.
  a. Has the advantage of prolonged action and oral administration.
  b. Side effects—same as for epinephrine.
  c. Do not allow child to drink coke, tea, or coffee, as they may increase nervousness.

4. *Pseudoephedrine*
   a. Has prolonged action and can be administered orally.
   b. Side effects—relatively free
5. *Isoproterenol (Isuprel)*—bronchodilator
   a. Toxic reaction—headache, flushing, dizziness, tremors, nausea and vomiting.
   b. Side effects—nervousness, palpitations, pink saliva or sputum if administered orally.
   c. Do not use concurrently with epinephrine.
6. *Expectorants*—given as an adjunct to hydration; thins secretions and helps the child to cough productively (i.e., saturated solution of potassium iodide, Robitussin).
7. *Aerosolized bronchodilator*—Bronkosol.
8. *Corticosteroids*—anti-inflammatory agents; diminish the inflammatory component of asthma, thus reducing airway obstruction.
   a. Produce beneficial effects only after several hours.
   b. Used when other drugs fail to bring beneficial relief from an asthmatic attack.
   c. Side effects—use for mild attacks may lead to suppression of adrenal activity. Prolonged use may lead to growth retardation and steroid dependency.
9. *Cromolyn sodium prophylaxis*—adjunct to existing treatment, especially for steroid-dependent child. It inhibits the release of histamine and the slow-reacting substance of anaphylaxis (SRS-A). It has prophylactic action; it should not be used in acute attack.
10. During the transition from intravenous to oral bronchodilators, respirations should be monitored carefully and frequently.

F. *To encourage the child and his parents to practice measures which will help to maintain optimal health, to prevent acute attacks, to ameliorate chronic symptoms, and to prevent onset of progression of respiratory disabilities.*

1. General health measures
   a. Provide a well-balanced diet and increased fluid intake.
   b. Assure sleep, rest, and reasonable exercise; avoid fatigue and chilling.
   c. Avoid known irritants.
2. Psychologic measures
   a. Attempt to keep child emotionally calm and at ease.
   b. Maintain optimistic attitude.
3. Regular medical follow-up
   a. Assure strict adherence to medication regimen.
   b. Give prompt attention when infection is present and new or progressive respiratory symptoms appear.

G. *To teach the child and involve the parents in the teaching of proper breathing habits.*

The exercises strengthen the diaphragm so that breathing will become much better and the total lung capacity will be increased. Breathing exercises used with postural drainage may lessen the need for continuous medication and contribute to increased expectoration of mucus that causes respiratory difficulty.

1. Instruct the child to clear his nasal passages before beginning exercises.
2. Each exercise should start with a short gentle inspiration through the nose, followed by a prolonged expiration through the mouth.
3. During inspiration, the upper portion of the thorax should be kept immobilized.
4. During expiration, abdominal muscles should be pulled in.
5. On no account should the child take a deep inspiration during the exercise, but instead he should see how long he can continue the expiration.

Exercise I—Abdominal Breathing
1. Lie on back with knees drawn up, body relaxed and hands resting on upper abdomen.
2. Exhale slowly, gently sink the chest and then upper abdomen until retracted at end of expiration (through mouth).
3. Relax upper abdomen (bulges forward) while taking brief inspiration through nose (chest is not raised).
Repeat 8–16 times; rest 1 minute; repeat.

Exercise II—Side Expansion Breathing
1. Sit relaxed in a chair and place palms of hands on each side of lower ribs.
2. Exhale slowly through mouth, contracting upper part of thorax, then lower ribs, then compress palms against ribs. (This expels air from base of lungs.)
3. Inhale, expanding lower ribs against slight pressure from hands.
Repeat 8–16 times; rest 1 minute; repeat.

Exercise III—Forward Bending
1. Sit with feet apart, arms relaxed at sides.
2. Exhale slowly, drop head forward and downward to knees, while retracting abdominal muscles.
3. Raise trunk slowly while inhaling and expand upper abdomen.
4. Exhale quickly, sinking chest and abdomen, but remain erect.
5. Inhale, expanding upper abdomen.

Exercise IV—Elbow Arching
(This exercise is performed between breathing exercises.)
1. Sit leaning slightly forward, back straight, fingers on shoulders.
2. Move elbows in circles forward, upward, backward, and downward.
Repeat 4–8 times; rest; repeat.

General Instructions
Perform exercises:
1. In the morning before breakfast when child is feeling fresh
2. At night, before getting into bed to clear the lungs before sleep, and
3. At the first sign of an impending attack to prevent asthma from developing.

NOTE: Many patients can abort their attacks entirely by doing simple exercises gently. Should child become short of breath or wheeze slightly, take single dose of whatever medication relieved him before beginning the exercises. Exercise may occasionally produce wheezing or coughing at the end of exercise. It may distress the child, but with perseverance the mucus in the bronchial tubes becomes loosened and the patient may be able to cough it up with consequent relief of attack.

H. *To assist the parents to develop a realistic attitude toward the child's illness.*

1. Try to treat the child as a completely normal child

who needs only a few additional restrictions imposed because of his illness.

   a. Accept him as a unique individual with unique contributions to make.

   b. Let him know he is capable, loved, and respected.

   c. Set consistent behavior limits. Do not accept child triggering attack to gain secondary rewards.

2. Allow child the same duties and rights as other children in the family.
3. Try to explain why he must watch for certain things and why he is restricted in some ways.
4. Teach child the symptoms of an asthma attack and how to relax.

   a. Give explanations instead of orders and show him confidence and respect.

   b. Be honest with him and express empathy.

   c. Help him to express his feelings rather than use his illness as an excuse for physically aggressive hostility or manipulative behavior.

5. Avoid overprotection and unnecessary surveillance.
6. Teach child to gradually manage for himself rather than to be dependent on parents.

   a. Allow him to actively explore his limitations and capabilities.

   b. Teach him all the symptoms of asthma—will aid in early treatment.

   c. Encourage him to keep a daily diary of symptoms, activity, environment, etc., noting any changes.

   d. Explain to him what medications he is taking and why and when they are taken.

   e. Show him the importance of a regular exercise program.

   f. Teach him to recognize signs of respiratory infection and to seek medical attention when appropriate.

   g. Encourage him to become involved in hyposensitization (if used). Perhaps he can even administer his own medications.

   h. Teach him the importance of increasing fluid intake, especially during an asthma attack when fluid is needed to compensate for fluid loss resulting from dyspnea and diaphoresis.

7. If child is too much engrossed with his illness, he can be diverted with kindly scolding, friendly minimizing of his ailments, or by encouraging other interests, so that he forgets his troubles as much as possible.

   a. Encourage him to build on his interests; help him to find activities that will not hurt him.

   b. Child's ability to control his breathing problems, in addition to learning that he can participate in some way with his peers, will increase his self-confidence and self-value, and result in beneficial physical and attitudinal changes.

   c. Involvement in physical activity should be encouraged, as should rest at signs of fatigue.

8. Do not talk about child's illness any more than necessary—do not allow secrecy or whispering. Recognize the child's feelings about his illness and allow him to talk about them with parents and family.
9. Inform friends and relatives of problems so that the necessary consideration is given him. Plan a team conference involving mother, school nurse, and teacher.
10. Create an atmosphere at home that is not full of nervousness or unrest—but is still not artificially calm.
11. Prepare child for approaching events (if bursts of emotions have an effect on his illness).
12. Teach child special skills.

   a. Let him develop special hobbies and interests that can be combined with his illness.

   b. Remember that accomplishments that develop respect and admiration in peers are particularly desirable and aid in building self-confidence and a feeling of security.

13. Both parents and child feel greater assurance if they are aware of how the child should be treated at certain stages of the disease.

   Have special instructions and medications on hand.

14. If child takes medications for his allergy or specific symptoms, administer them in a matter-of-fact manner without making any fuss. Encourage taking medication when stomach is empty, drinking adequate amount of fluid.
15. Child needs security, self-confidence, and love. (Do not force these on the child.) Exaggeration is never beneficial.
16. Provide information and literature for the family. Encourage contact with the local chapter of the American Lung Association for information on existing programs in which other children with asthma and their parents come together.

I. *To teach the child and his parents protective measures which will encourage environmental control and help to avoid the offending allergen, as well as practice measures that will help control asthma attacks.*

1. Keep child's bedroom as free from dust as possible.

   a. Keep in bedroom only the furniture which is absolutely necessary.

   b. Remove upholstered furniture, draperies, carpets, pictures, books, toys, and unnecessary dust-collecting objects.

   c. Use washable curtains and cotton or synthetic rugs.

   d. Use cotton or synthetic blankets and washable bedspreads (not chenille or tufted types).

   e. Do not use insect or other sprays in the bedroom.

   f. Do not store outer clothing or household articles in bedroom closets.

   g. Enclose mattresses, box-springs, and pillows in dustproof covers (unless they are synthetic).

   h. Blankets and clothing that have been stored should be thoroughly aired before use.

2. Avoid irritating odors such as paint, tobacco smoke, insect powders, pine oils and jellies, and irritating cooking odors.
3. If possible, use an exhaust fan in the kitchen to remove cooking odors.
4. Remove all overstuffed furniture and rugs.
5. Avoid sitting and playing on overstuffed furniture and down pillows.
6. Avoid carbonated drinks, such as ginger ale and colas (especially when wheezing).
7. Avoid any physical exertion that causes wheezing or excessive shortness of breath.
8. Avoid using irritating salves on chest or in nose.
9. Avoid dusty and musty places (basements, storerooms, etc.).
10. Avoid felt rug pads because of animal hair content.
11. Purchase foam furniture and foam rubber pads if possible when refurnishing the home.
12. If home is heated by a circulating hot-air system,

shut it off in the bedroom (use electric heater if necessary). A central air filter in the furnace is desirable; clean or replace it frequently.

13. Take only drugs prescribed by the physician.
14. Report for treatment as directed by physician.

J. *To help foster a healthy mother–child relationship by*

understanding the feelings of anxiety, guilt, or frustration the mother may have.

1. Remember that the mother's life-style may have changed with the diagnosis of asthma in her child, resulting in loss of sleep, constant care, etc.
2. Listen to her and provide appropriate support.
3. Initiate social service referral as indicated.

RESPIRATORY DISTRESS SYNDROME (HYALINE MEMBRANE DISEASE)

Respiratory distress syndrome is a syndrome of immature infants that is characterized by a progressive and frequently fatal respiratory disorder resulting from atelectasis and immaturity of the lungs.

Etiology

The exact etiology of respiratory distress syndrome is not clearly defined.
1. Adequate pulmonary function at birth depends upon the following:
   a. Adequate amount of surfactant (a lipoprotein mixture) lining the alveolar cells, which allows for alveolar stability and prevents alveolar collapse at the end of expiration.
   b. Adequate surface area in air spaces to allow for gas exchange, i.e., sufficient pulmonary capillary bed in contact with this alveolar surface area.
2. Respiratory distress syndrome is the result of decreased pulmonary surfactant.
3. Contributing factors—any factor that decreases surfactant, such as
   a. Prematurity and immature alveolar lining cells
   b. Acidosis
   c. Hypothermia
   d. Hypoxia
   e. Hypovolemia
   f. Unknown factor

Clinical Manifestations

Symptoms are usually observed soon after birth and may include

A. *Primary Signs and Symptoms*

1. Expiratory grunting or whining (when infant is not crying)
2. Sternal, suprasternal, substernal, and intercostal retractions progressing to paradoxical seesaw respirations (see Silverman Score, Problems of Infants, Fig. 38-3, p. 1230)
3. Inspiratory nasal flaring
4. Tachypnea
5. Hypothermia
6. Cyanosis when child is in room air (infants with severe disease may be cyanotic even when given oxygen), increasing need for oxygen
7. Decreased breath sounds and dry "sandpaper" breath sounds—on auscultation of chest
8. As the disease progresses:
   a. Seesaw retractions become marked with marked abdominal protrusion on expiration.
   b. Peripheral edema increases.
   c. Muscle tone decreases.
   d. Cyanosis increases.
      (1) Body temperature drops.
      (2) Short periods of apnea occur.
      (3) Bradycardia may occur.

   e. Asphyxia becomes more severe
      (1) Apneic episodes develop.
      (2) Changes in distribution of blood throughout body result in pale gray skin color.

B. *Secondary Signs and Symptoms*

1. Hypotension
2. Edema of hands and feet
3. Bowel sounds absent early in the illness
4. Urine output decreased

Pathophysiology

1. Immature lung—underdeveloped and uninflated alveoli, immature pulmonary capillary bed.
2. Surfactant lowers surface tension at alveolar surface, giving alveoli stability; at end of expiration, some of the air remains in the lung (called the functional residual capacity or FRC), thus requiring less negative pressure and exertion to take next breath. When surfactant is deficient, surface tension is higher and alveoli are unstable and collapse at end of expiration. There is decreased FRC; thus, the next breath requires almost as much effort as the first breath after birth.
3. Sequence of events resulting in hyaline membrane disease:
   a. Deficient surfactant.
      (1) Alveoli inflate unequally on inspiration and collapse on expiration.
      (2) More oxygen is required by the infant to expand the alveoli with each breath than he inhales, causing him to tire.
      (3) The number of alveoli that expand progressively decreases.
   b. Alveolar instability and atelectasis.
      (1) Pulmonary vascular resistance increases—hypoperfusion of lung.
      (2) Fetal circulation right-to-left shunt results leading to hypoxemia and hypercapnia, which lead to respiratory and metabolic acidosis.
   c. Hypoxemia and pulmonary vascular pressure causes ischemia in the alveoli.
      (1) Effusion of plasma through capillary walls (transudate) into alveoli.
      (2) Necrotic cells and fibrin form a membranous layer in alveoli.
      (3) Gas exchange becomes inhibited.
      (4) Lungs become stiff (decreased compliance), requiring more pressure to expand them.
   d. Airway obstruction leads to increased asphyxia and vasoconstriction, and the cycle continues.
4. RDS is usually a self-limited disease and symptoms peak in about 3–4 days, at which time surfactant synthesis begins to accelerate and pulmonary function and clinical appearance begin to improve.

a. Moderately ill infants or those who do not require assisted ventilation show the following:
   (1) Slow improvement by about 48 hours.
   (2) Rapid recovery over next 3–4 days; few complications.
b. Severely ill and very immature infants who require some ventilatory assistance:
   (1) Demonstrate rapid deterioration (see Clinical Manifestations).
   (2) Ventilatory assistance may be required for several days; chronic lung disease is a frequent complication.
   (3) Iatrogenic harm more likely (i.e., infection, necrotizing enterocolitis, etc.).

Incidence

Respiratory distress syndrome occurs most frequently in:
1. Premature infants (primarily weighing between 1000–1500 gm. [2.2–3.3 lbs.]) and between 28–37 weeks gestation
2. Infants of diabetic mothers
3. Infants delivered by cesarean section—probably related to underlying indication for surgery
4. Infants of mothers who have experienced intrauterine vaginal bleeding

Diagnostic Evaluation

1. Laboratory tests
   a. PCO_2—elevated
   b. PO_2—low
   c. Blood pH—low due to metabolic acidosis
   d. Potassium—elevated
   e. Calcium—low
   f. L/S ratio—for lung maturity
2. Chest x-ray—demonstrates a diffuse, fine granularity; air bronchograms show "ground glass" appearance representing atelectasis of some alveoli, surrounded by hyperdistended bronchioles.
3. Pulmonary function studies—demonstrate stiff lung with a reduced effective pulmonary blood flow.

Treatment

1. Early recognition is imperative so that treatment may be instituted immediately.
2. Transportation to a facility providing specialized care is desirable when possible.
3. The objectives of treatment include supportive measures:
   a. Maintenance of oxygenation—P_aO_2 at 60–80 mm. Hg—to prevent hypoxia
   b. Maintenance of respiration with ventilatory support if necessary
   c. Maintenance of thermoneutral state—to prevent hypothermia
   d. Maintenance of fluid, electrolyte, and acid-base balance
   e. Maintenance of nutrition
   f. Prophylactic or specific antibacterial therapy
   g. Constant observation for complications
   h. Care appropriate for small premature infant

Complications

1. Complications related to respiratory therapy:
   a. Air leak: pneumothorax—pneumomediastinum, pneumopericardium, and pneumoperitoneum
   b. Pneumonia—especially gram-negative organisms
   c. Pulmonary interstitial emphysema

2. Patent ductus arteriosus
3. Cerebral hemorrhage—especially in infant less than 1500 gm. (3.3 lbs.)
4. Disseminated intravascular coagulation
5. Chronic problems associated with long-term use of oxygen:
   a. Bronchopulmonary dysplasia—lungs cystic-appearing with hyperinfiltration, obstructive bronchiolitis, dysplastic changes, and pulmonary fibrosis
   b. Chronic respiratory infections
6. Tracheal stenosis
7. Other complications related to prematurity

Nursing Objectives and Management

The reader is referred to specific areas throughout this text for in-depth discussion of certain subjects.

A. *To check the birth history for pertinent information to assist in determining the intensity of observation and care that the infant may require.*

1. The Apgar score 1 minute after birth and 5 minutes after birth (see p. 1027).
2. The type of resuscitation required
3. Any treatment or medication administered
4. Any medication or anesthesia the mother received during labor
5. Estimated gestational age

B. *To make a generalized nursing assessment of the infant's condition immediately upon admission.*

Early diagnosis is critical to increasing survival rate.
1. Record and report any findings to physician immediately.
2. Determine the degree of respiratory distress.
   a. Observe the type of retraction.
      (1) Determine the type of retraction (see Silverman score p. 1230).
      (2) Determine the degree and severity of retractions.
   b. Count the respiratory rate for 1 full minute.
      (1) Observe and determine if respirations are regular or irregular.
      (2) Observe to determine if the infant experiences any periods of apnea.
         (a) Note the length of apnea.
         (b) Note what type of stimulation initiates breathing.
      (3) Note the infant's activity at the time respirations are recorded (e.g., crying, sleeping).
   c. Listen for expiratory grunting or whining sounds from the infant when he is not crying. This partial Valsalva maneuver is expiration against a partially closed glottis in an attempt to maintain a positive end-expiratory pressure and FRC (functional residual capacity) to prevent alveoli from collapsing.
   d. Observe for nasal flaring.
   e. Observe for cyanosis.
      (1) Note location of cyanosis.
      (2) Note if cyanosis improves with oxygen administration.
   f. Listen to the chest with a stethoscope.
      (1) Note diminished breath sounds and location.
      (2) Note the presence of rales.
3. Determine the infant's cardiac rate and rhythm.
   a. Count the apical pulse for 1 full minute.
   b. Note any irregularity in the heart rate.
4. Observe the infant's general activity.
   a. Determine if the infant is lethargic or listless.

b. Determine if the infant is active and responds to stimuli.

c. Determine if the infant cries.

5. Observe the infant's skin color.
   a. Note cyanosis as to degree and location.
   b. Note evidence of jaundice.
   c. Note skin mottling.
   d. Note paleness or grayness.

6. Observe the general appearance of the infant's body.
   a. Note edema and location (face, hands, feet, etc.).
   b. Note any other abnormal appearance of body.

7. Check infant's body temperature.

8. Listen to abdomen with a stethoscope to determine if bowel sounds are present. Note any stool passed and observe and record type of stool.

9. Note any urinary output.
   a. Apply urine collector to obtain sample of urine.
   b. Observe color of urine.
   c. Check specific gravity of urine and frequency.
   d. Record amount of urine and frequency

C. *To provide measures to relieve respiratory distress.*

1. Have emergency equipment readily available for use in the event of cardiac or respiratory arrest.

2. Provide measures for monitoring ECG and respiratory rate.

3. Place the infant in an oxygen-rich environment.
   a. Incubator with oxygen at prescribed concentration.
   b. Plastic hood with oxygen at prescribed concentration.
   c. Plastic hood with oxygen at prescribed concentration when using radiant warmer.
   d. Measure oxygen concentration every hour and record.

4. Observe the infant's response to oxygen.
   a. Observe for improvement in color, respiratory rate and pattern and nasal flaring (see Silverman score p. 1230).
   b. Note response by improvement in pH, PO_2, PCO_2 (arterial), or capillary blood gas.

5. Observe closely for apnea.
   a. Stimulate infant if apnea occurs.
   b. If unable to produce spontaneous respiration with stimulation within 15–30 seconds:
      (1) Call for help.
      (2) Clear airway.
      (3) Tilt head back.
      (4) Apply hand resuscitator attached to an oxygen supply, or apply mouth-to-mouth resuscitation (see pp. 1205–1206).
      (5) Intubation may be necessary:
         (a) Obtain heart rate during intubation by physician.
         (b) Initiate cardiac massage if severe bradycardia or asystole occurs.
         (c) Listen to breath sounds once intubated; make sure that they are equal bilaterally and that x-ray for position is taken and checked.
         (d) Attach infant to appropriate ventilator.
            Secure endotracheal tube.
            Suction tube to maintain patency.
         (e) Continue to monitor vital signs.
   c. Record events.

D. *To be familiar with the methods of providing assisted or controlled ventilation and the nursing implications for each.*

The objective of ventilation therapy is to ventilate the infant effectively, using the lowest possible F_1O_2 pressures and cycling frequency to eliminate oxygen toxicity and to minimize mechanical trauma thus reducing complications of treatment.

1. Positive end expiratory pressure (PEEP)
2. Continuous positive airway pressure (CPAP)
3. Positive or negative pressure respirator
4. Face mask and bag

E. *To maintain the method used for the administration of intravenous fluids necessary to meet the metabolic demands of the infant.*

Hypovolemia can affect pulmonary perfusion by associated metabolic acidosis resulting in pulmonary vasoconstriction.

1. Monitor flow.
2. Observe site for infiltration or infection.
3. If umbilical–artery catheter is in place, observe for bleeding.
4. Record the amount of blood drawn for laboratory analysis (small infants can become anemic from having large amounts of blood removed for samples).
5. Prepare and administer prescribed medications.

F. *To provide adequate caloric intake (80–120 kcal./kg./24 hours) as indicated.*

1. Nasojejunal
2. Nasogastric
3. Parenteral nutrition

G. *To maintain the infant's abdominal skin temperature between 36.0–36.5° C. (97–98° F.), thus minimizing oxygen consumption rate.*

Hypothermia may result in vasoconstriction and acidosis increasing complications in the already compromised infant.

1. Adjust Isolette or radiant warmer accordingly.
2. Prevent frequent opening of Isolette.

H. *To constantly and carefully observe for any complications that may occur from ventilatory assistance, prematurity, or the disease itself.*

Record and report observations to physician immediately.

I. *To assist the physician in other supportive measures used to treat the infant.*

1. Ventilatory assistance, oxygen therapy
2. Endotracheal tube, suctioning, physical therapy
3. Monitoring blood values
4. Monitoring vital signs, including blood pressure, and general condition
5. Monitoring machines

J. *To provide an environment that allows infant rest and minimal disturbance balanced with necessary procedures and treatment based upon the infant's condition.*

Infants undergoing multiple procedures lasting 45 minutes to 1 hour have shown a moderate decrease in PO_2 on continuous PO_2 measurement.

K. *To provide for the psychological needs of the infant with respiratory distress syndrome.*

Do not neglect his need for tactile, visual, and auditory stimulation.

L. *To support the parents of this critically ill infant.*

1. Help them work through their grief.
2. Assist them with psychological, emotional, and physical attachment to the infant as appropriate.

M. *To prepare the family for long-term follow-up as appropriate.*

Infants with BPD (Bronchopulmonary Dysplasia) may eventually go home on oxygen therapy.

NOTE: The premature infant with respiratory difficulty should continue to be observed very closely and his therapy should be adjusted as his condition changes. When his condition stabilizes, resume care as for a premature infant. (See p. 1224.)

CYSTIC FIBROSIS

Cystic fibrosis is a generalized disorder affecting the exocrine glands so that the substances they secrete are abnormally viscous, affecting primarily pulmonary and gastrointestinal function.

Etiology

1. Condition is inherited as a mendelian recessive trait.
2. Underlying cause of the abnormal secretions is unknown.

Clinical Manifestations

1. Diagnosis is frequently made prior to 6 months of age—can be made at any age.
2. Meconium ileus is found in newborn.
3. Other presenting signs:
   a. Salty taste when skin is kissed
   b. Cough, wheezing
   c. Failure to gain weight or grow in the presence of a good appetite
   d. Frequent, bulky, and foul-smelling stools
   e. Protuberant abdomen—pot belly
   f. Wasted buttocks
   g. Vomiting following coughing
   h. Recurrent pulmonary infection
   i. Clubbing of fingers—in older child
   j. Increased anteroposterior chest diameter

Pathophysiology

1. The secretions of the exocrine glands are thick and sticky rather than thin and slippery.
2. Pulmonary involvement
   a. Thick mucus clogs bronchi and bronchioles.
      (1) Lungs overinflate.
      (2) Atelectasis results.
   b. Associated infection occurs in lungs.
   c. Fibrotic changes occur in lungs.
3. Gastrointestinal involvement
   a. Thick mucus plugs pancreatic ducts.
      (1) Prevents pancreatic digestive enzymes from reaching the small intestine; thus, there is abnormality of stools, loss of foodstuff in feces (fat and nitrogen [protein])—malabsorption syndrome.
      (2) Digestion is impaired, especially of fats; nutritional failure results.
   b. Meconium ileus in infant—bowel obstructed by thick intestinal secretions.
   c. Biliary cirrhosis—intrahepatic biliary tract obstructed by thick secretions.
4. Involvement of sweat glands
   Secretions contain excessive amount of sodium and chloride, leading to excessive loss of these substances—especially in hot weather, when child experiences fever or becomes overheated with activity.

Diagnostic Evaluation

1. Check for family history of cystic fibrosis, failure to thrive, and unexplained infant death; check child's history and physical condition. Carefully listen for subtle information that may be suggestive of cystic fibrosis.
2. Measurement of sodium and chloride level in sweat—chloride level of more than 60 mEq./l. is virtually diagnostic.
   a. 40–60 mEq./l. is borderline and repeated.
   b. Sodium levels greater than 70 mEq./l. is diagnostic.
3. Measurement of trypsin concentration in duodenal secretions—absence of normal concentration is virtually diagnostic.
4. Analysis of digestive enzymes (trypsin) in stool
   Level is lower—used for initial screening for cystic fibrosis.
5. Chest x-ray
   a. May be normal initially.
   b. Later shows increased areas of infection, overinflation, atelectasis, and fibrosis.
6. Analysis of stool for steatorrhea.
7. BMC (Boehringer–Mannheim Corp.)—meconium strip test includes lactose and protein content, both present in babies with cystic fibrosis, used for screening.

Treatment

1. Establish and maintain good nutrition.
   a. Pancreatic enzyme supplement with each feeding.
   b. Increased caloric (carbohydrates) and protein intake.
   c. Decrease in fat intake.
   d. Daily intake of water-soluble vitamins.
   e. Supplementary fat soluble vitamins.
   f. Adequate fluid and salt intake.
2. Prevent and control pulmonary infection.
   a. Antimicrobial therapy as indicated for pulmonary infection.
   b. Bronchodilators and vasoconstrictors—for relief of bronchospasm.
   c. Aerosol mist tent, expectorants, and mucolytic agents—decrease viscosity of secretions.
   d. Antihistamines (controversial)—for hayfever-like symptoms.
3. Promote normal growth and development.
   a. Treat child as a normal person.
   b. Encourage normal relationships with peers and family.
   c. Promote positive self-image.

NURSING ALERT: Mist therapy may cause airway resistance to increase in some patients.

d. Physical therapy—bronchial drainage
   (1) Postural drainage
   (2) Breathing exercises
e. Bronchopulmonary lavage—treatment of atelectasis and mucoid impaction, using large volumes of saline (used in some institutions in country).
f. Lobectomy—resection of symptomatic lobar bronchiectasis to retard progression of lesion to total pulmonary involvement.

Complications

1. Pulmonary or respiratory infections—(emphysema, atelectasis, pneumothorax, bronchiectasis)
2. Pancreatic fibrosis
3. Cor pulmonale
4. Biliary cirrhosis—portal hypertension, esophageal varices, splenomegaly
5. Chronic sinusitis
6. Nasal polyps
7. Heat prostration
8. Fibrosis of epididymis and vas deferens in male; aspermia
9. Diabetes
10. Hemoptysis

Nursing Objectives and Management

A. *To assist in the diagnosis and assessment of the child being evaluated for cystic fibrosis by careful observation, recording, and reporting.*

1. Characteristics of stool
2. Respiratory status
3. General behavior and activity

B. *To establish and maintain adequate nutrition to allow for growth and development.*

1. Diet composed of food that is high in calories, high in protein, and low to moderate in fat is usually recommended. (Absorption of food is incomplete.) Infant may receive medium-chain triglyceride supplement in formula.
2. Fat-soluble vitamins in water-miscible solution are given in quantities that are 2–3 times the normal dose. (Child shows difficulty in absorption.)
3. Absent pancreatic enzymes are replaced with extracts of animal pancreas to obtain normal stools, nutrition, and growth.
   a. Give with each meal.
   b. Mix with small portion of food for infant or small child (e.g., mashed banana, applesauce). Never mix in formula.
   c. Offer the older child capsules or tablets.
   d. May not be given if child is only taking a clear liquid diet (e.g., post-op, vomiting).
4. Salt intake will need to be increased during hot weather or during excessive exercise when sweating increases, to prevent salt depletion and heat prostration and cardiovascular collapse. During periods of profuse sweating, infant may become hyponatremic and alkalotic.
5. Use patience when feeding child.
   a. Child may be irritable and fussy.
   b. Breathing may be difficult; coughing and vomiting may be common.
6. Supplemental diet that is readily absorbed and requires a minimum of digestive enzymes may be prescribed.

C. *To assist in preventing or treating lung infection and to support respirations by thinning secretions and clearing them from the respiratory tract.*

1. Intermittent aerosol therapy
   a. Usually done prior to postural drainage. (Treatment may also be done following drainage.)
   b. Provides small amount of medication in droplet form to penetrate respiratory tract.
   c. Treatment is 3–4 times daily.
2. Mist tent (controversial)
   a. Frequently used only with patients that have already used mist; not started on newly diagnosed patients.
   b. High humidity loosens secretions.
   c. Used primarily at night or nap time.
   d. Check temperature often and maintain below 26.6° C. (80° F.).
3. Postural drainage
   a. Usually follows aerosol therapy 3–4 times per day.
   b. Treatment ideally done 1 hour after eating to prevent vomiting or discomfort.
   c. Place child in position that gives greatest access to affected lobes of lung and facilitates gravity drainage of mucus from specific lung area. The following positions are useful:
      (1) Leaning over side of bed
      (2) Infant held in lap
   d. Clapping with cupped hands and vibrating for 1–2 minutes in each area loosens plugs of mucus.
   e. A relaxed patient will cough more easily; coughing should be encouraged after postural drainage.
      Suctioning of an infant or young child may be necessary when child will not cough.
4. Breathing exercises
   Have child exhale slowly to increase the duration of exhalation.

D. *To understand what medications are given in treatment and why they are given.*

1. Antibiotics
   a. Frequently given when a child is not doing well generally
   b. Broad-spectrum antibiotics to treat specific organism causing infection
   c. Specific antibiotics to treat specific organism causing infection
2. Expectorants are used to thin bronchial mucous secretions.
3. Bronchodilators are used to increase width of bronchial tubes, allowing free passage of air into lungs.

E. *To give meticulous attention and care in hygiene to the patient and prevent infection.*

1. Provide good skin care and position changes to prevent skin breakdown of malnourished child.
2. See that diaper area is clean to reduce offensive odor from stool and to prevent diaper rash.
3. Because child may perspire freely, change clothing as often as necessary to keep him dry.
4. Mouth care is important, since mucus is present so frequently.
5. Shampooing and bathing will provide comfort by removing sticky residue from mist and aerosol therapy.
6. Restrict contact with person with respiratory infection.

F. *To aim at supporting the child's emotional, psychological, and intellectual needs and development.*

1. Explain each procedure (new or routine), medica-

tions, etc. to child in a manner that is appropriate for his age.
2. Allow child to show his frustrations, fears, and feelings by talking, complaining, or crying.
   a. Support him during these times.
   b. Comfort him by talking to him and holding him.
3. Provide diversional activities appropriate for age, during or in between treatments.
4. Older child may begin to take responsibility for treatments with minimal supervision.
   a. Teach him about his disease (i.e., food, medications, treatments, equipment).
   b. Help him identify his strengths and limitations, and to feel good about himself as a person.
   c. Foster independence.
5. Frequently the child will manifest his anger, fear, and other emotions by resistance to chest-physical therapy. Allowing child to engage in normal activities (e.g., swimming) within his physical tolerance can help to redirect these feelings as well as to improve respiratory function.

G. *To make and record observations of the child and his condition and behavior which will give information concerning his condition.*

1. Characteristics of stools: color, size, consistency, frequency
2. Eating habits
   a. Foods taken or refused
   b. Appetite—good or poor
3. Coughing and description of secretions produced
4. Daily weight to determine weight gain or loss
5. General behavior
   a. Irritability
   b. Cooperativeness
6. Conservation of energy—periods of rest, nonstrenuous activity

H. *To encourage parental participation in learning to care for and handle the child and to foster acceptance of the child and his illness by his parents and family.*

1. Provide opportunities for the parents to learn all aspects of care of their child.
2. Note that all the support and help given the parents during hospitalization will make home care easier.
3. Initiate community nurse referral, which provides the following:
   a. Facilitates preparing the home for child's entry, both emotionally and physically.
   b. Can assist family in properly carrying out treatments.
4. Initiate social work referral. The social worker can help parents to better understand their family situation and their feelings about their child and cystic fibrosis; she can arrange for financial assistance if appropriate. The worker can be an emotional support to the mother who may be physically and emotionally exhausted from caring for the child with cystic fibrosis.
5. Inform friends and relatives of the child's illness so that necessary consideration is given him. Plan a team conference including mother, school nurse, teacher, and physical education teacher, as appropriate.
6. Assist with interpretation of the disease to family and patient. Help them to talk about their feelings and fears. Be honest with parents and child; help them understand there may be gradual lung involvement.

7. Initiate a teaching program for the child and his family early. Offer them available literature and help them to become familiar with the National Cystic Fibrosis Research Foundation and the nearest chapter.*
   a. Multidiscipline team approach and cooperation is vital.
   b. Incorporate teaching program into nursing care plan. Be consistent with information and methods.

Parental Education

Education of parents is important in preparing them to continue the child's care at home.
1. Parents must have a thorough understanding of the dietary regimen. Help them to know what types of foods the child is allowed to have and which foods are restricted. Talk about ways to make each meal or certain foods attractive. Discuss need for salt replacement.
2. Help parents to become thoroughly familiar with the pulmonary therapy regimen. Do not rush your explanation; take time to demonstrate and explain procedures. Then allow parents to demonstrate all the treatments to be done at home.
3. Help the family to plan the most normal family pattern of living in relation to treatment of their child.
   a. Consider the marriage needs of the parents and the needs of other members of the family.
   b. Encourage family activities, vacations, etc. during child's remission of symptoms.
4. Help parents to understand and to provide emotional support of their child. Explain that he will experience the usual problems of growing up as well as the problems of cystic fibrosis and hospitalizations. The child needs love, understanding, and security—not overprotection. He needs growing independence, peer relationships, and personal achievements.
5. Help parents understand the rebellious and uncooperative behavior of their adolescent. It is a normal part of this age; however, it may be directed toward the illness and treatment. Be firm with the child—optimistic, yet realistic, understanding, and loving.
6. Help the parents understand the value of genetic counseling and support the information given to them through counseling.
7. Impress upon the parents the importance of regular medical follow-up care:
   a. Routine immunizations—measles vaccine and influenza given early in infancy.
   b. Continuing evaluation and supervision in home management.
   c. New developments through research that may change therapy.
   d. Detection or prevention of complications.
8. Inform parents of the future of their child in society.

* National Cystic Fibrosis Research Foundation, 3379 Peachtree Road N.E., Atlanta, Ga. 30326.
Publications of the National Cystic Fibrosis Research Foundation:
   Your Child and Cystic Fibrosis.
   Living with Cystic Fibrosis—A Guide for the Young Adult.
   A C/F Child in Your Class.
   Cystic Fibrosis—Most Serious Lung Problem of Children.
   A Teacher's Guide to Cystic Fibrosis.
   Listing of Publications and Educational Materials for Physicians and Scientists.

a. With the medical advancements that have occurred, there is every reason to believe that, depending upon pulmonary involvement and complications, the child with cystic fibrosis may grow to adulthood. When child grows up, he may be smaller and shorter than expected.

b. Play and school participation depends upon severity of illness.

c. Have parents discuss the child's problem with the school nurse, teacher, and other responsible adults who have close contact with the child.

d. Encourage parents to allow the child to participate in as well as take additional responsibility for his own care and treatment as he gets older.

BIBLIOGRAPHY

Books

Avery GB. Neonatology. Philadelphia, JB Lippincott, 1980

Avery ME and Fletcher BD. The Lung and Its Disorders in the Newborn Infant. Philadelphia, WB Saunders, 1974

Butnarescu GF, Tillotson DM, Villarreal PP. Perinatal Nursing, Vol. 2. New York, John Wiley & Sons, 1980

Freeman BA. Textbook of Microbiology. Philadelphia, WB Saunders, 1979

Klaus MH and Fanaroff AA. Care of the High-Risk Neonate. Philadelphia, WB Saunders, 1979

Levin DL, Morriss CF, Moore GC. A Practical Guide to Pediatric Intensive Care. St. Louis, CV Mosby, 1979

Lough MD, Williams TJ, Rawson JE. Newborn Respiratory Care. Chicago, Year Book Medical Publishers, 1979

Moffet HL. Pediatric Infectious Diseases. Philadelphia, JB Lippincott, 1975

Roberts KB (ed). Manual of Clinical Problems in Pediatrics. Boston, Little, Brown & Co., 1979

Scipien GM et al. Comprehensive Pediatric Nursing, 2nd ed. New York, McGraw–Hill, 1979

Thibeault DW and Gregory GA. Neonatal Pulmonary Care. Reading, Addison–Wesley Pub. Co., 1979

Whaley LF and Wong DL. Nursing Care of Infants and Children. St. Louis, CV Mosby, 1979

Wistreich GA and Lechtman MD. Microbiology and Human Disease. Beverly Hills, Glencoe Press, 1976

Cystic Fibrosis

Anderson CM and Burke J. Pediatric Gastroenterology. Oxford, Blackwell Scientific Publications, 1975

Mangos JA and Talamo RC. Cystic Fibrosis: Projections into the Future. Miami, Symposia Specialists, 1976

Roberts KB. Manual of Clinical Problems in Pediatrics. Boston, Little, Brown & Co., 1979

Articles

Barker GA. Current management of croup and epiglottitis. Pediatr Clin North Am 1979 Aug; 26(3):565–579

Barr PA. Weaning very low birth weight infants from mechanical ventilation using intermittent mandatory ventilation and theophylline. Chron Dis Child 1978 July; 53(7):598–600

Bridgewater SC, Voignier RR, Smith CS. Allergies in children: Recognition. Am J Nurs 1978 Apr; 78(4):614–616

Bridgewater SC and Voignier RR. Allergies in children: Testing and treating. Am J Nurs 1978 Apr; 78(4):620–621

Buckley RH. Advances in asthma/allergy. Pediatr Nurs 1979 Mar/Apr; 5(2):39–42

Carden TS. Tonsillectomy—trials and tribulations (commentary). JAMA 1978 Oct 27; 204(8):1961–1962

Crummette B. The maternal care of asthmatic children. Matern Child Nurs J 1979 Spring; 8(1):23–27

Davison FW et al. Croup: When quick decisions count. Patient Care 1974 Nov; 8(19):104–139

Ennis S and Harris TR. Positioning infants with hyaline membrane disease. Am J Nurs 1978 Mar; 78(3):398–401

Fendrick GM, Hansel FK, Pararella MM, Richards W. When should tonsils and/or adenoids go? Patient Care 1979 Nov 30; 13(20):116–117 +

Ferguson RG and Webb A. Childhood asthma. Can Nurs 1979 Feb; 75(2):36–39

Freis PC. Nursing skills in the outpatient management of childhood inhalant allergy. Issues Compr Pediatr Nurs 1978 Aug; 3(2):24–34

Fried MP. Controversies in the management of supraglottitis and croup. Pediatr Clin North Am 1979 Nov; 26(4):931–942

Glassanose MR. Infants who are oxygen dependent—sending them home. MCN 1980 Jan/Feb; 5(1):42–45

Katten M. Long-term sequelae of respiratory illness in infancy and children. Pediatr Clin North Am 1979 Aug; 26(3):525–535

LaBelle G. The nurse practitioner and the allergic child. Pediatric Nurse 1979 Mar/Apr; 5(2):43–44

Landau LI. Outpatient evaluation and management of asthma. Pediatr Clin North Am 1979 Aug; 26(3):581–601

McBride MM and Sack WH. Emotional management of children with acute respiratory failure in the ICU. Heart Lung 1980 Jan/Feb; 9(1):98–106

Menachof LW. Croup or epiglottitis—a vital distinction. Consultant 1979 Mar; 19(3):27–30

Munoz AI. Hemophilus influenzae infections. Clin Pediatr 1980 Feb; 19(2):86–90

Organ AE. Lower respiratory tract infections in children. Issues Compr Pediatr Nurs 1978 Aug; 3(2):12–23

Paige P. Teaching the asthmatic child. Respir Ther 1979 Sept–Oct; 9(5):57–60

Sedlacek K. Helping the asthmatic child in school. MCN 1978 July/Aug; 3(4):207–210

Spector SL. Asthma: Current pathophysiologic and therapeutic aspects. Hosp Med 1979 Apr; 15(4):80–83 +

Voignier RR and Bridgewater SC. Allergies in children: Testing and treating. Am J Nurs 1978 Apr; 78(4):617–619

Voors BB. Pneumocystis carinii in the immunosuppressed child. Cancer Nurs 1979 Feb; 2(1):14–18

White LW. Handling the asthmatic child. Respir Ther 1979 July/Aug; 9(4):45–48

Wieczorek RR and Horner–Rosner B. The asthmatic child: Preventing and controlling attacks. Am J Nurs 1979 Feb; 79(2):258–262

Cystic Fibrosis

Anfenson M. The school-age child with cystic fibrosis. J School Health 1980 Jan; 50(1):26–28

Beckerman RC and Taussig LM. Hypoelectrolytemia and metabolic alkalosis in infants with cystic fibrosis. Pediatrics 1979 Apr; 63(4):580–583

Gurwitz D et al. Perspectives in cystic fibrosis. Pediatr Clin North Am 1979 Aug; 26(3):603–615

Jordan DA. Managing cystic fibrosis patients. Respir Ther 1979 Mar/Apr; 9(2):59–66

Kucia C et al. Home observation of family interaction and childhood adjustment to cystic fibrosis. J Pediatr Psychology 1979 June; 4(2):189–195

Pinney MA. Review of cystic fibrosis. Issues Compr Pediatr Nurs 1978 Aug; 3(2):54–65

ANEMIA

Anemia refers to a deficit of red blood cells or hemoglobin in the blood. It is the most frequent hematologic disorder encountered in children.

Etiology

1. Blood loss
2. Impairment of red blood cell production
   a. Nutritional deficiency
      (1) Iron deficiency
      (2) Folic acid deficiency
      (3) Vitamin B_{12} deficiency
      (4) Vitamin B_6 deficiency
   b. Decreased erythrocyte production
      (1) Pure red cell anemia
      (2) Secondary hemolytic anemias associated with infection, renal disease, chronic disorders
      (3) Aplastic anemias
      (4) Invasion of bone marrow
         (a) Leukemia
         (b) Tumors
3. Increased erythrocyte destruction
   a. Drugs and chemicals
   b. Infections
   c. Antibody reactions
   d. Burns
   e. Poisons, including lead poisoning
   f. Abnormalities of the red cell membrane
   g. Enzymatic defects
      G6PD (glucose-6-phosphate dehydrogenase) deficiency
   h. Hemolytic disease of the newborn
   i. Abnormal hemoglobin synthesis
      (1) Abnormal hemoglobins—sickle cell disease
      (2) Thalassemic syndromes

Clinical Manifestations

1. Condition may be acute or chronic
2. Early symptoms
   a. Listlessness
   b. Fatigability
   c. Anorexia
3. Late symptoms
   a. Pallor
   b. Weakness
   c. Tachycardia
   d. Palpitations
4. Eventual symptoms
   a. Mental and physical sluggishness
   b. Cardiac enlargement and symptoms of congestive heart failure
   c. Inability to carry out the usual childhood activities
5. Prognosis
   a. Varies with the type of anemia
   b. Death may result because of cardiac failure

Altered Physiology

A. *General Considerations*

1. Red cells and hemoglobin are normally formed at the same rate at which they are destroyed.
2. Whenever formation of red cells or hemoglobin is decreased or their destruction is increased, anemia results.
3. The ability of the red blood cell to carry hemoglobin is decreased.
4. The ability of hemoglobin to oxygenate the tissues and remove carbon dioxide for excretion by the lungs is also decreased.
5. Less hemoglobin is available to act as a buffer in regulating the pH of the blood.

B. *Specific Anemias*

1. Iron Deficiency Anemia (hypochromic anemia)
   a. Iron deficiency occurs most commonly between the age of 6 months and 2 years, but it also occurs frequently during adolescence.
   b. Initially the neonate's iron requirements are usually met by reserves acquired during fetal life, but after 3–4 months of age, additional iron must be derived from the diet.
   c. A positive iron balance is necessary for optimal formation of red blood cells.
   d. Results of iron deficiency:
      (1) Decreased hemoglobin formation
      (2) Red cells with less color and smaller in size
      (3) Low plasma iron
      (4) Low body stores
      (5) Low levels of transferrin, which binds and transports iron
   e. Causes of iron deficiency
      (1) Insufficient supply
         (a) Dietary insufficiency (most common)
         (b) Inadequate stores at birth (in premature infants, twins)
      (2) Excessive demands
         (a) Growth requirements
         (b) Chronic illness

(3) Blood loss
  (a) Hemorrhage
  (b) Parasitic infection
(4) Impaired absorption (rare)
  (a) Diarrhea
  (b) Malabsorption syndrome
2. Megaloblastic Anemias
  a. Folic acid and vitamin B_{12} are necessary for the synthesis of nucleoproteins which are essential for the maturation of red blood cells.
  b. Deficiencies of folic acid or vitamin B_{12} or disturbances in their normal metabolism interfere with the synthesis of nucleoproteins.
  c. Red blood cells are immature and larger than normal at every stage of their development.
  d. The number of circulating red blood cells is decreased.
  e. Each red blood cell may carry a normal amount of hemoglobin.
3. Hypoplastic Anemias
  The bone marrow is unable to manufacture new red blood cells and hemoglobin at a rate necessary to maintain a normal concentration of these substances in the circulating blood.
4. Aplastic Anemia
  a. Formation of red blood cells stops altogether.
  b. There is usually an associated defective synthesis of other elements in the blood such as platelets and white blood cells.
5. Anemia of Infection
  a. Life span of the red blood cell is moderately decreased.
  b. The ability of the bone marrow to produce red blood cells is significantly decreased. (This is the principal factor in determining the degree of anemia.)
6. Hemolytic Anemias
  a. The red blood cells are destroyed at abnormally high rates.
  b. The activity of the bone marrow increases to compensate for the shortened survival time of the red blood cells.
  c. Products of red cell breakdown increase with hemolysis.
  d. Jaundice results when the liver is unable to clear the blood of the pigment resulting from the breakdown of hemoglobin from destroyed red cells.
  e. Bone marrow hypertrophies and occupies a larger than normal share of the inner structure of bones.
7. Sickle Cell Anemia (see p. 1278).

Nursing Objectives and Management

A. *To make a baseline assessment of the child's condition.*

1. Examine skin and mucous membranes for evidence of pallor.
2. Estimate the child's current functional level, including exercise tolerance and level of frustration.
3. Question parents regarding the child's normal level of activity, any symptoms that they have observed (pallor, decreased appetite, excessive fatigue, etc.), ways that their child indicates frustration, fatigue.
4. Obtain a history related to possible causative factors:
  a. Dietary habits
  b. Persistent infection, chronic disease
  c. Access to drugs, poisons, etc.

B. *To prevent infection and assess for signs of infection.*

1. See that child maintains good general body hygiene.
2. Provide a diet high in vitamins, calories, and iron.
  a. Be aware of the child's food preferences and plan his diet accordingly.
  b. Offer small amounts of food at frequent intervals.
  c. Reward the child for positive attempts to eat.
  d. Allow the child to participate in selection of foods and in preparation of his meal tray.
  e. Avoid tiring activities and unpleasant procedures at mealtime.
  f. Make mealtime as pleasurable as possible. (Refer to section on Nutrition, p. 1112.)
  g. Provide food supplements and vitamins when necessary.
3. Ensure adequate rest.
  a. Plan nursing care to allow for lengthy periods when the child is not disturbed by hospital routines, procedures, treatments, etc.
  b. Observe for early signs of fatigue such as irritability, hyperactivity, etc.
  c. Encourage sedentary rather than active projects.
4. Avoid exposure to other children with colds, infections, etc.
5. Always be sure to wash hands thoroughly and advise visitors to do the same.
6. Report any temperature elevation to the physician.

C. *To administer blood and maintain the transfusion.*

1. The procedure is similar to the administration of IV fluids (see p. 1171).
  The blood administration set contains a filter in the drip chamber. The blood level should cover the filter.
2. Packed cells are frequently administered to enable the child to receive a high concentration of erythrocytes in a small quantity of fluid.
  The bag should be squeezed every 20–30 minutes during the transfusion to prevent settling of the red cells.
3. Take special precautions.
  a. The patient's name, physician's name, hospital number, and blood type must correspond with the information on the blood container from the blood bank.
  b. Identifying information such as donor type and number, patient's name on the blood label, kind of blood, and expiration date should always be checked by 2 people.
  c. The blood should be checked for abnormal cloudiness or color and for gas bubbles.
  d. The child's temperature should be taken as a baseline measurement before the transfusion is begun.
  e. Normal saline should be hung so that the tubing can be flushed before and after blood is administered and when medications must be given (a separate infusion line for IV medications is preferable).

NURSING ALERT: Medications should not be given in the infusing blood itself. Blood should never be given with a dextrose and water solution because hemolysis and clotting in the IV tubing can occur.

f. Blood should be run through new IV tubing, and after blood administration, the tubing should be changed before IV fluids are resumed.

g. The rate of flow should be carefully regulated to prevent circulatory overload, especially in those children receiving multiple transfusions. Blood is administered slowly at first as a precautionary measure in case of transfusion reaction, and to allow the blood to reach room temperature.

h. The same blood should not be left running over a long period of time (usually over 4 hours).

i. Recommendations of the blood bank for storage and administration of blood should be followed explicitly.

4. Observe the child for signs of transfusion reaction.
   a. Reaction usually occurs within 15–20 minutes from the start of the transfusion.
      Stay with the patient during this time.
   b. Signs and symptoms:
      (1) Restlessness
      (2) Irritability
      (3) Chills
      (4) Elevation of temperature
      (5) Sudden changes in pulse and respiration
      (6) Rash or change in the color of the skin
      (7) Changes in the appearance or quantity of urine output
      (8) Hemorrhagic phenomena
      (9) Pain, sensation of tightness in the chest
   c. Notify the physician immediately if a transfusion reaction is suspected. Discontinue the transfusion, but keep the intravenous line open with saline solution.

5. For additional information, refer to Transfusion Therapy and Guidelines: Administering Blood Transfusions (Adult), pp. 236 and 237.

D. *To minimize the child's anxieties and ensure his cooperation during hospitalization.*

1. Allow the child to handle equipment used for tests and procedures (tourniquets, syringes, etc.).
2. Explain all procedures and the treatment plan to the child in a way that he can understand.
3. Allow the older child to look through a microscope at a blood smear.
4. Permit the child to cleanse the area for a venipuncture or finger stick.

Nursing Management of Specific Anemias

A. *Iron Deficiency Anemia*

1. Administer iron as prescribed by the physician.
   a. Oral iron preparations
      (1) Administer shortly after meals to minimize gastric distress.
      (2) Administer with a dropper or straw, or dilute with water or fruit juice to prevent staining of teeth.
         Dental stains can be removed by brushing the teeth with sodium bicarbonate or hydrogen peroxide and then rinsing with water.
      (3) Observe for side effects.
         (a) Gastric distress
         (b) Colic pain
         (c) Diarrhea
      (4) Caution the mother that iron medication causes the child's stools to be dark green or black.

(5) Stress to parents the importance of continuing the iron therapy according to the physician's directions even though the child may not appear ill.

(6) Warn parents that medications containing iron are a leading cause of poisoning in children. The medication should always be stored well out of reach.

> **NURSING ALERT:** There is a great deal of variation in the elemental iron content of the commercially available liquid preparations containing iron. To avoid confusion, the dosage should be expressed in terms of elemental iron and then converted to the proper amount of the therapeutic agent selected.

   b. Intramuscular iron preparations
      (1) Dosage
         (a) Calculated by the physician
         (b) Depends on the child's weight and hemoglobin level
      (2) Special precautions
         (a) Should be injected into a large muscle, preferably the buttock.
         (b) Injection sites should be recorded and rotated.
         (c) The injection site should not be massaged. Any pressure on the site may force the medication out of the muscle into the subcutaneous tissue.
            Walking will help absorption.
         (d) Parenteral iron should be administered with discretion and only to those children whose anemia is not amenable to oral iron therapy.
         (e) Parenteral iron is contraindicated in children sensitive to the preparation or in anemias other than iron-deficiency anemia.
      (3) Technique of administration
         (a) Use a separate needle to withdraw the medication from the ampule and for injection.
         (b) Use a needle which is 5 cm. (2 inches) long. Medication must be injected deeply into the muscle to avoid staining the tissue.
         (c) Allow 0.5 ml. of air in the syringe before injecting.
         (d) Retract the skin over the muscle laterally before inserting the needle.
         (e) Insert the needle and withdraw the plunger to check against entry into a blood vessel.
         (f) Inject the medication and the 0.5 ml. of air following the injection—to clear the needle and prevent leakage of the medication along the injection track when the needle is withdrawn.
         (g) Wait 10 seconds after injection before removing the needle.
      (4) Observe for side effects
         (a) Local
            Pain at the injection site
            Skin discoloration
            Local inflammation with lymphadenopathy
         (b) Systemic toxicity (occurs within 10 minutes of injection)

Headache
Muscle and joint pain
Nausea and vomiting
Sweating
Tachycardia
Bronchospasm with dyspnea
Circulatory collapse, hypotension and dizziness

> **NURSING ALERT:** Because of the possibility of anaphylaxis, a test dose should be given before initiating parenteral iron therapy.

2. Initiate and reinforce good dietary habits.
   a. Determine from parents the type and amount of foods customarily eaten, the feeding methods, and the child's reaction to eating.
   b. Introduce foods rich in iron such as meat, fortified cereals, vegetables, and fruits.
   c. Do not allow the child to drink excessive quantities of milk at the exclusion of other foods that contain more iron. Limit milk intake to 1 liter (1 quart) per day.
   d. Provide vitamin supplements if necessary. Vitamin C appears to enhance the absorption of iron.
   e. Explain the reasons for diet change to parents in language they can understand. Visual aids and pictures may be helpful.
   f. Assist parents to select iron-rich foods that are acceptable to the child, within the family's food budget, and culturally acceptable.
   g. Make mealtime a pleasurable experience. (Refer to section on nutrition, p. 1112).
3. Investigate social and economic problems which may contribute to the child's disease.
   Complete a referral to a community health nurse if it appears that the mother will need support in dealing with the child's chronic disease.

B. *Anemia of Infection*

1. Provide supportive care relative to the underlying disease.
2. Administer antibiotics as directed by the physician.

C. *Megaloblastic Anemias*

Administer folic acid or vitamin B_{12} as directed by the physician.

1. Folic acid (pteroylmonoglutamic acid)
   a. Dosage—must be determined by trial for each patient.
   b. Route
      (1) Oral route is preferred.
      (2) May be administered intramuscularly if malabsorption is suspected.
   c. Toxic effects—none.
2. Vitamin B_{12} (cyanocobalamin)
   a. Dosage—regulated by individual trial for each patient
   b. Route
      (1) Intramuscular injection is preferred.
      (2) Oral administration is also possible. (This method is more expensive and less reliable).
   c. Side effects—none
   d. Points of emphasis
      Regular administration of the medication is essential. Patients may be tempted to miss injections because they are not in distress before the injection or do not feel significantly better after it.

Patient or Parental Education

1. Discuss general hygiene measures, including adequate rest, diet, sunshine, fresh air.
2. Encourage regular medical and dental evaluations.
3. Explain that infection may be prevented by dressing the child according to the weather and keeping him away from persons with colds, sore throats, and other infections.
4. Teach parents how to administer medication.
5. Alert parents to signs of disease progress.

SICKLE CELL DISEASE (SICKLE CELL ANEMIA)

Sickle cell disease is a severe, chronic hemolytic anemia occurring in persons homozygous for the sickle gene. The clinical course is characterized by episodes of pain due to the occlusion of small blood vessels by sickled red cells. Persons heterozygous for the sickling gene are said to possess sickle cell trait which is associated with a benign clinical course.

Etiology

1. Genetically determined, inherited disease
2. Each person inherits 1 gene from each parent which governs the synthesis of hemoglobin (Table 40-1.)

Incidence

1. Found almost entirely in American blacks and persons of Spanish-American ancestry.
2. Approximately 8% of black Americans have sickle cell trait.
3. Approximately 1 out of every 600 black infants born in the U.S. has sickle cell anemia.

Clinical Manifestations

A. *Symptoms*

1. Children are rarely symptomatic until late in the first year of life.
2. Clinical manifestations are sporadic.
   a. Child may be asymptomatic for several months.
   b. Periods of crisis occur at variable intervals.
   c. Precipitating factors of crisis include:
      (1) Dehydration
      (2) Infection
      (3) Trauma
      (4) Strenuous physical exertion
      (5) Extreme fatigue
      (6) Cold exposure
      (7) Hypoxia
3. Signs of crisis
   a. Loss of appetite
   b. Paleness
   c. Weakness

TABLE 40–1. TRANSMISSION OF SICKLE CELL DISEASE

Genotype of Parents	Probability of Abnormal Hemoglobin in Offspring		
	Normal	*Trait*	*Disease*
1 parent with trait	50%	50%	0%
Both parents with trait	25%	50%	25%
1 parent with trait, 1 parent with disease	0%	50%	50%
Both parents with disease	0%	0%	100%

d. Fever
e. Pain in abdomen, back, joints, and/or extremities
f. Swelling of joints, hands, or feet ("hand–foot syndrome")
g. Irritability
h. Jaundice

B. *Thrombocytic Crisis*

(most common form of crisis)
1. Small blood vessels are occluded by the sickle-shaped cells, causing distal ischemia and infarction.
2. Extremities
   a. Bony destruction
   b. Periosteal reaction
   c. Ulcers
3. Spleen
   Abdominal pain
4. Cerebral occlusion
   a. Strokes
   b. Hemiplegia
   c. Blindness
5. Pulmonary infarction
6. Pulmonary thromboses
7. Cardiac decompensation
8. Impaired liver function
9. Convulsions, cerebral infarction
10. Retinal damage, blindness
11. Growth failure

C. *Sequestrian Crisis*

1. Large amounts of blood become pooled in the liver and spleen.
2. Spleen becomes massively enlarged.
3. Signs of circulatory collapse develop rapidly.
4. Frequent cause of death in infant with sickle cell disease.

D. *Aplastic Crisis*

Bone marrow ceases production of red blood cells.

E. *Chronic Symptoms*

1. Jaundice
2. Gallstones
3. Progressive impairment of kidney function
4. Fibrotic spleen
5. High susceptibility to salmonella, osteomyelitis, and pneumococcal septicemia
6. Delayed puberty
7. Decreased life span

F. *Prognosis*

1. Depends on severity of the disease
2. No known cure
3. Decreased life span
   Death occurs frequently before age 20

Altered Physiology

1. Each hemoglobin molecule consists of 4 molecules of heme folded into 1 molecule of globin.

2. Each globin molecule consists of 2 alpha chains and 2 beta chains.
3. The amino acid sequence on the beta chain is altered in sickle cell hemoglobin.
   Valine is substituted for glutamic acid in the 6th position.
4. Sickle cell hemoglobin aggregates into elongated crystals under conditions of low oxygen concentration.
5. This distorts the membrane of the red blood cell causing it to assume a crescent or sickle shape. The cells easily become entangled and enmeshed leading to increased blood viscosity.
6. Sickled red cells are fragile and are rapidly destroyed in the circulation.
7. Anemia results when the rate of destruction of red cells is greater than the rate of production.

Diagnostic Evaluation

1. Stained blood smear
   a. Done by finger stick.
   b. Sickle cells are viewed under the microscope on a stained smear of blood.
   c. Cells are seen only in persons with sickle cell anemia (not sickle cell trait).
2. Sickle cell prep
   a. Done by finger stick.
   b. Oxygen is removed from a drop of blood.
   c. The blood is observed under the microscope for the presence of sickle-shaped cells.
   d. Does not distinguish between persons with sickle cell trait and disease.
3. Sickledex
   a. Done by finger stick.
   b. A small amount of blood is placed in a solution containing a chemical reducing agent.
   c. The presence of sickle hemoglobin is indicated if the solution turns cloudy.
   d. Also does not distinguish between persons with sickle cell trait and disease.
4. Hemoglobin electrophoresis
   a. Requires venipuncture.
   b. Hemoglobin is subjected to an electric current which separates the various types and determines the amounts present.
   c. A person is diagnosed as having sickle cell trait if 2 types of hemoglobin are demonstrated in approximately equal amounts.
      A person is diagnosed as having sickle cell anemia if the majority of his hemoglobin is sickle hemoglobin.
5. Antenatal diagnosis is available to the high-risk group through amniocentesis and gene mapping.

Preventive Measures

1. Every black child admitted to the hospital should be tested for sickle cell anemia.

2. Parents at risk should be counseled regarding the genetic aspects of sickle cell anemia.
3. All siblings of any child who is admitted to the hospital with sickle cell anemia should be tested for the disease.

Nursing Objectives and Management

A. *To dilute the blood and reverse the agglutination of sickled cells within the small blood vessels.*

1. Maintain intravenous therapy if indicated. (See procedure for the administration of intravenous fluids, p. 1171)
2. Increase the amount and frequency of liquid intake.
   a. Offer fruit juice, water, milk, etc.
   b. Offer child a choice in selection of fluids and method of drinking (straw, etc.).
3. Record the child's intake and output accurately. (Total his intake and output every 8 hours.)
4. Assist with a partial exchange transfusion if required. This technique is designed to remove some of the sickled cells and replace them with normal ones.

B. *To reduce the child's fever which may aggravate dehydration.*

1. Make frequent assessments of the child's temperature.
2. Administer antipyretic drugs as prescribed by the physician.
3. Refer to the section on fever, p. 1148

C. *To alleviate the child's pain during a crisis.*

1. Identify effective measures to alleviate pain by questioning parents and by personal trial and error. Consider any of the following measures:
   a. Carefully position and support painful areas.
   b. Hold or rock the infant.
   c. Distract child by singing to him, reading him stories, providing play activities.
   d. Provide familiar objects, persons.
   e. Bathe child in warm water, applying local heat or massage.
   f. Give suitable medications.
   g. Maintain bed rest.
2. Share effective methods of reducing pain with other nursing staff and family.

D. *To treat associated or precipitating infections.*

1. Treatment will depend on the specific nature of the infection.
2. Administer antibiotics as prescribed by the physician.

E. *To provide an optimal environment for the child during hospitalization.*

Be certain that the child is kept warm and protected from infection.

F. *To administer blood in cases of severe anemia.*

1. Refer to information on blood transfusion, p. 1276.
2. Be especially alert for signs of transfusion reaction, which is a very serious problem.

G. *To decrease surgical risk.*

1. Administer preoperative blood transfusion(s) as prescribed.
   Preoperative blood is usually prescribed to suppress the formation of new sickle cells and to reduce the threat of anoxia.
2. Prepare the child emotionally for surgery.

3. Maintain adequate hydration before and after surgery.
4. Avoid sedatives and analgesics which depress the respiratory center.
5. Observe the child closely for evidence of infection, especially of the respiratory tract.

H. *To provide emotional support to the child and his parents.*

1. Encourage parents to talk about their child, his disease, and how they feel about it.
   a. Expect such feelings as guilt, shock, frustration, depression, and resentment.
   b. Accept negative feelings.
   c. Counsel parents concerning ways to recognize and alleviate their child's apprehension.
   d. Provide factual information so that parents are prepared to answer their child's questions.
      (1) The recessive nature of the inheritance should be explained.
      (2) Make certain that parents understand the difference between sickle cell trait and sickle cell anemia.
2. Alleviate the child's anxieties concerning his illness.
   a. Role playing and play activities are useful in identifying his fears.
   b. Explain what is happening to him in a way that he can understand.
      Numerous teaching tools such as coloring books are available for this purpose.
   c. Adolescents should be assured that although sexual development is delayed, they will eventually catch up with their peers.
3. Stress the positive aspects of his disease.
   a. Sickle cell disease does not affect intelligence.
   b. Between periods of crisis the child can usually participate in peer group activities with the exception of some strenuous sports.
   c. Discuss the positive achievements of recent research and correct misconceptions.
4. Encourage quiet activities in which the child can excel—art, painting, leather work, metal and woodworking, chess, etc.
5. Plan for the child to continue his education.
   a. Encourage parents to bring school work to the child during a lengthy hospitalization.
   b. Refer the child to a home teacher if necessary.
   c. Be certain that the child receives vocational guidance if appropriate.
6. Inform parents of community resources, such as the school nurse or groups for parents and/or children, that may contribute to their child's well-being.

I. *To make certain that the child receives coordinated and continuous care.*

Send a nursing care summary to the community health nurse or school nurse who will work with the child after he is discharged from the hospital.

Patient or Parental Health Education

1. Provide factual information about the disease and its cause. Encourage questions.
2. Discuss the genetic implications of sickle cell disease and offer genetic counseling to the family.
3. Instruct parents in ways that they can help their child to avoid sickling episodes.
   a. Do not allow the child to become chilled or to wear tight clothing that might impede circulation.

b. Maintain adequate hydration. Give the parents written instructions regarding the minimum amount of fluid required by their child each day. Discuss implications of abnormal fluid loss (i.e., vomiting, excessive sweating). Instruct parents how to recognize signs of dehydration.

c. Instruct child to avoid strenuous physical activity.

d. Provide prompt treatment of cuts, sores, mosquito bites, etc. Notify the physician if the child is exposed to a contagious disease.

e. Maintain good dental hygiene and be certain that the child receives frequent dental checkups.

f. Be certain that the child receives regular medical supervision, including all the normal childhood immunizations and a PPD (purified protein derivative) every 2–3 years. In addition, children over 2 years of age should be immunized against pneumococcal infection.

g. Teach child to avoid undue emotional stress.

h. Instruct child to avoid areas of low oxygen concentration (i.e., high mountains and unpressurized airplanes).

4. Teach parents that the child has the same needs as a normal, healthy child for a balanced diet, good fluid intake, adequate rest, and daily exercise. The child will learn his own activity limitations and will rest when he becomes fatigued. He should not be pampered, but should receive the same love, discipline, privileges, and responsibilities of a normal child his age.

5. Sexually active adolescents should receive contraceptive information and should be helped to make informed choices.

6. Teach parents how to recognize the signs of mild crisis:
   a. Fever
   b. Decreased appetite
   c. Irritability
   d. Pain or swelling in abdomen, extremities, back

7. Instruct parents regarding home management of mild crisis.

a. Encourage adequate hydration. Teach techniques for increasing fluid intake.

b. Administer antipyretic medications.

c. Encourage rest.

d. Keep the child warm.

e. Hospitalize child if pain becomes severe or if IV hydration is required.

8. Teach parents the signs of severe crises:
   a. Pallor
   b. Lethargy and listlessness
   c. Difficulty in awakening
   d. Irritability
   e. Severe pain
   f. High fever or a moderate fever that persists for 2 days.

9. Instruct parents to have emergency information available to those involved in the child's care (school nurse, teacher, babysitter, family members, etc.).
   a. Name and phone number of physician and alternate
   b. Closest emergency facility and ambulance number
   c. Child's blood type, allergies, medications, and hospital chart number
   d. Name of informed neighbor or relative to be notified in an emergency
   e. Discuss the genetic implications of sickle cell disease with the child early, so that when he is old enough, he can avail himself of counseling concerning marriage and family planning.

10. Stress the benefit of wearing a medic-alert tag.

Teaching Aids

The following may be useful in providing information to the parents and child:

1. "Where's Herbie?" A Sickle Cell Anemia Story and Coloring Book. Publication No. 0–470–030. U.S. Dept. of HEW, U.S. Government Printing Office, Washington, D.C., 1972.

2. National Sickle Cell Disease Program. National Institutes of Health, Bethesda, Maryland 20014.

HEMOPHILIA

Hemophilia is an inherited, congenital blood dyscrasia which is characterized by a disturbance of blood clotting factors. It appears in males but is transmitted by females.

Etiology

1. Hereditary (about 80% of patients)
2. Sex-linked, recessive trait
   a. Caused by a gene carried on the X chromosome, one of the sex chromosomes.
   b. Transmitted by asymptomatic females who carry the hemophilic gene on 1 of their X chromosomes.
   c. Appears in males who have the hemophilic gene on their only X chromosome.
   d. Affected males may carry a latent form of the disease to female offspring.
   e. May appear in females if a female carrier mates with a male hemophiliac.
3. Spontaneous mutations may cause the condition when the family history is negative for the disease (about 20% of patients).

Transmission of Hemophilia

See Table 40-2.

Clinical Manifestations

A. *General Considerations*

1. Seldom diagnosed in infancy unless excessive bleeding is observed from the umbilical cord or after circumcision.
2. Usually diagnosed after the child becomes active.
3. Varies in severity depending on the plasma level of the coagulation factor involved.
   a. Children with factor levels of less than 1% of normal are considered severe hemophiliacs and often demonstrate severe clinical bleeding.
   b. Children with factor levels of above 5% but less than 25% of normal are considered moderately afflicted. These children may be free of spontaneous bleeding, and may not manifest the potentially severe bleeding disorder until after trauma.
   c. Children with factor levels of 25–50% of normal

TABLE 40–2. TRANSMISSION OF HEMOPHILIA

	Probability of Abnormality in Offspring				
	Female			Male	
Genotype of Parents	Normal	Carrier	Hemophiliac	Normal	Hemophiliac
Female carrier/Normal male	50%	50%	0%	50%	50%
Noncarrier female/Hemophiliac male	0%	100%	0%	100%	0%
Female carrier/Hemophiliac male	0%	50%	50%	50%	50%

are considered mildly afflicted. They usually lead normal lives and bleed only with severe injury or surgery.
   d. Degree of severity tends to be constant within a given family.

B. *Clinical Signs and Symptoms*

1. Easily bruised
2. Prolonged bleeding from the mucous membranes of the nose and mouth or from lacerations
3. Spontaneous soft-tissue hematomas
4. Hemorrhages into the joints—especially elbows, knees, and ankles (hemarthrosis)
   a. Causes pain, swelling, limitation of movement
   b. Repeated hemorrhages may produce degenerative changes with osteoporosis and muscle atrophy
5. Spontaneous hematuria
6. Gastrointestinal bleeding

C. *Complications*

1. Airway obstruction due to hemorrhage into the neck and pharynx.
2. Intestinal obstruction due to bleeding into intestinal walls or peritoneum.
3. Compression of nerves with paralysis due to hemorrhaging into deep tissues.
4. Intracranial bleeding.
5. Secondary complications associated with therapy— liver disease, immunologic problems, thrombotic complications.

D. *Prognosis*

1. Uncertain—a normal life span is possible for many hemophiliacs because of advances in therapy.
2. Cycles may occur with periods of little bleeding followed by periods of severe bleeding.
3. Death may result from intracranial hemorrhage or from exsanguination following any serious hemorrhage.

Diagnostic Evaluation

1. Routine bleeding and clotting tests—often normal
2. Partial thromboplastin time (PTT)—prolonged
3. Prothrombin consumption—decreased
4. Thromboplastin generation—increased
5. Specific assays for clotting factors—abnormal

Altered Physiology

1. Hemophilia results from the absence or malfunction of any one of the blood clotting factors from the plasma.

Most Common Types of Hemophilia

2. These blood clotting factors are necessary for the formation of prothrombin activator, which acts as a catalyst in the conversion of prothrombin to thrombin.
   a. The rate of formation of thrombin from prothrombin is almost directly proportional to the amount of prothrombin activator available.
   b. The rapidity of the clotting process is proportional to the amount of thrombin formed.
3. The most common types of hemophilia and the clotting factors involved are shown in the chart below.

Nursing Objectives and Management

A. *To provide emergency care for bleeding wounds.*

1. Cleanse wound thoroughly.
2. Immobilize the affected part and elevate above the level of the heart.
3. Apply local measures for control of bleeding.
   a. Apply pressure on the area for 10–15 minutes to allow clot formation.
   b. Place fibrin foam or absorbable gelatin foam in the wound.
4. Administer cryoprecipitate or plasma concentrate containing the necessary factor. (See procedure for the administration of intravenous fluid, p 1170, and for blood transfusion, p. 1276.)
   a. Avoid rapid administration to minimize the possibility of transfusion reaction.
   b. Stop the transfusion if hives, headaches, tingling, chills, flushing, or fever occur.
5. Keep the child quiet during treatment.
   a. Remain calm.
   b. Sedate the child if necessary.
6. Take special precautions.
   Suturing and cauterization should be avoided.

B. *To provide supportive care for the child with hemarthroses.*

1. Control bleeding.
   a. Immobilize the joint in a position of slight flexion.
   b. Elevate the affected part.
   c. Apply ice packs.
   d. Administer plasma or therapeutic concentrate as directed by the physician.
2. Alleviate pain.
   a. Administer sedatives or narcotics as prescribed by the physician.
   b. Avoid excessive manipulation of the child.

Type of Hemophilia	Clotting Factor
Hemophilia A (classic hemophilia)	Factor VIII (antihemophilic globulin)
Hemophilia B (Christmas disease)	Factor IX (plasma thromboplastin component)
Hemophilia C	Factor XI (plasma thromboplastin antecedent)

c. Use a bed cradle to keep the weight of the bedcovers off the affected part.

3. Prevent further bleeding.
   a. Continue immobilization of the joint. (A bivalve plaster cast may be necessary.)
   b. Maintain the child on bed rest. (Careful handling of the child is essential.)

4. Prevent permanent deformities and crippling.
   a. Begin gentle, passive exercise after the acute phase. Progress to active exercises.
   b. Refer the child for physical therapy on an outpatient basis if this is indicated by:
      (1) Presence of persistent deformity.
      (2) Need to use orthopedic devices such as crutches, braces, splints, etc.
      (3) Need for specialized programs such as whirlpool baths, electrical stimulation, increased physical exercises.
   c. Reconstructive orthopedic surgery may be required.

5. Assess the child for evidence of disease progress:
   a. Increased pain
   b. Further swelling of joints
   c. Limitation of movement
   d. Flexion contractures

C. *To prevent hemorrhage during nursing procedures.*

1. Temperature measurement
   Insert the thermometer very gently.
2. Injections
   a. Administer medications orally whenever possible.
   b. Choose intramuscular injection sites carefully and rotate them.
   c. Inject the medication slowly
   d. Apply pressure to the area for 5 minutes.

> **NURSING ALERT:** Children with hemophilia should not receive aspirin or compounds containing aspirin because this medication affects platelet function and prolongs bleeding time.

D. *To maintain a safe environment during hospitalization.*

1. Pad crib rails.
2. Inspect toys for sharp or rough edges.
3. Offer foods and fluids in plastic or paper containers.
4. Supervise small children when they are ambulatory.
5. Utilize protective devices which the child brings from home. (Many children wear helmets, knee pads).
6. Continually assess environment for potential hazards.

E. *To provide emotional support to the child and his family.*

1. Permit the child to participate in as many normal activities as possible within the realm of safety.
2. Allow the child to handle equipment used in his care.
   Use play to help the young child adjust to his illness by "transfusing" his teddy bear, etc.
3. Encourage the child's continuing education.
   a. Have parents bring assignments from the child's teacher.
   b. Refer to a home teacher if indicated.
   c. Investigate the possibility of a school-to-home telephone service.
4. Encourage parental participation in the child's care.
   a. Refer to section on family-centered care, page 1131.

b. Assess parents' attitudes and understanding about the disease. Clarify information if necessary.
c. Teach parents aspects of their child's care which must be continued after discharge. Have them practice appropriate techniques with nursing supervision until they achieve competence and are comfortable in the situation. (See Patient or Parent Health Teaching below.)

5. Counsel the parents concerning:
   a. Financial problems caused by repeated hospitalizations and transfusions.
   b. Feelings of guilt at having given birth to the child or resentment at having to care for him.
   c. Refer the parents to a social worker or psychiatrist if indicated.

6. Introduce the child and his family to other hemophiliac families.
   a. Information concerning the location of parent groups may be obtained from the National Hemophilia Foundation, 25 West 39th St., New York, N.Y. 10018.
   b. Numerous specialized hemophilia centers have been established in the United States.

7. Convey confidence to the patient and his family; they often are fearful of the diagnosis and need support.

8. Initiate a community health nursing referral if appropriate.

Patient or Parental Health Education

1. Protecting the child from trauma
   a. Select toys which are soft and without rough edges.
   b. Pad the sides of cribs, playpens, etc.
   c. Offer food and liquids in plastic containers to avoid laceration.
   d. Guard against child's falling when he is learning how to stand and walk.
      (1) Remove potential sources of injury from furniture.
      (2) Pad child's knees and buttocks.
      (3) Use a helmet for the child's head.
   e. Supervise play closely.
   f. Inform the child's teacher and playmates, the school nurse, and other adults of his condition so that they can be supportive of the child's needs and know what to do in an emergency.
   g. Have the child wear a medic-alert bracelet.
   h. Do not administer aspirin to the child.

2. Emergency treatment for hemorrhage
   a. Immobilize the part.
      This may be done with splints or an elastic compression bandage. (These materials should be immediately available in the home.)
   b. Apply ice packs.
      Parents should keep 2 or 3 plastic bags of ice immediately available in the freezer.
   c. Consult the child's physician and initiate additional recommended therapy.

3. Regular medical and dental supervision
   Preventive dental care is important; dental care may require prophylactic treatment to prevent bleeding. Hospitalization may be necessary for extensive dental work and extractions.

4. Diet
   Diet is important to avoid overweight which places additional strain on the child's weight-

bearing joints and predisposes him to hemarthrosis.
5. Information concerning the disease itself
The child should be helped to understand the exact nature of his illness as early as possible. Special attention should be given to the signs of hemorrhage, and the child should be told of the need to report even the slightest bleeding to an adult immediately.
6. Preventing emotional crippling by overprotection—this can be more disabling than the effects of the disease itself.
   a. Promote a sense of independence and self-care within the patient's limitations.
   b. Encourage healthful activity and reasonably aggressive pursuits. Reinforce self-judgment of child or teenager in selection of safe physical activities.
   c. Help parents understand the importance of vocational guidance for their child—emphasis given to occupations using intellect or skills rather than physical effort.
7. Genetic counseling and family planning services
These should be offered to the family and to the adolescent patient.
8. Home care program
   a. Home care programs teach parents and children to administer infusion therapy at home when a hemorrhage episode begins.
   b. Advantages of home treatment:
      (1) Can be initiated immediately
      (2) Earlier recovery of joint functions
      (3) Greater self-sufficiency for patient and family
      (4) Fewer absences from school or work
      (5) Less anxiety related to traveling

   (6) Decrease in the cost of treatment
   c. General criteria for acceptance into program:
      (1) Adequate knowledge of the disease
      (2) Willingness to learn venipuncture technique
      (3) Demonstrated ability to follow directions
      (4) Ability to manage infusions
      (5) Acceptance of the necessity for follow-up care
      (6) Emotional stability sufficient to accept the responsibility
   d. Teaching is usually done by the nurse in the specialty clinic and includes instruction and practice in the following:
      (1) Storage and preparation of replacement factors
      (2) Venipuncture technique
      (3) Transfusion management
      (4) Record keeping
      (5) Awareness of signs of transfusion reaction
      (6) Recognition of indications of need for subsequent transfusions
   e. Hospital nursing responsibilities:
      (1) Screen patients and families who may be eligible for home care programs.
      (2) Facilitate appropriate self-management by children and families enrolled in home care programs if hospitalization becomes necessary. Establish communication with the clinic nurse.
9. Reference:
Understanding Hemophilia—A Guide for Parents (1979), Hemophilia Foundation of Illinois, 327 South LaSalle St., Chicago, Ill. 60604
10. Agency:
National Hemophilia Foundation, 25 West 39th Street, New York, N.Y. 10018

BIBLIOGRAPHY

Books

Biggs R (ed). The Treatment of Haemophilia A and B and von Willebrand's Disease. London, Blackwell Scientific Publications, 1978

Boone DC (ed). Comprehensive Management of Hemophilia. Philadelphia, FA Davis, 1978

Johnson SH. High Risk Parenting. Philadelphia, JB Lippincott, 1979

Lichtman MA. Hematology for Practitioners. Boston, Little, Brown & Co., 1978

Tetrault S. A Child with Sickle Cell Disease—His Hobbies and Activities. Washington, D.C., Center for Sickle Cell Disease, Howard University, 1977

Whaley L and Wong D. Nursing Care of Infants and Children. St. Louis, CV Mosby, 1979

Williams WJ (ed). Hematology. New York, McGraw–Hill, 1977

Articles

Biggs R. Recent advances in the management of hemophilia and Christmas disease. Clin Haematol 1979 Feb 8(1):95–114

Buickus B. Administering blood components. Am J Nurs 1979 May; 79(5):937–941

Cullins L. Preventing and treating transfusion reactions. Am J Nurs 1979 May; 79(5):935–936

Flanagan C. Home management of sickle cell anemia. Pediatric Nursing 1980 Mar/Apr; 6(2):Update for Pediatric Nurses, B–D

Hilgarther MW. Managing the child with hemophilia. Pediatr Ann 1979 June; 8(6):68–84

Houghton GR et al. Orthopedic problems in hemophilia. Clin Orthop 1979 Jan/Feb; 138:197–216

Inwood MJ. Aids for hemophiliac children on a self-infusion program. J Pediatr 1978 Jan; 92(1):78–79

Kellaher TI and Fisher JM. A review of iron therapy. U.S. Pharm 1978 Jan; 3:36–44

Legarde MC et al. Surgery in patients with hemoglobin-S disease. J Pediatr Surg 1978 Dec; 13(60):605–607

McFarlane J. Sickle cell disorders. Am J Nurs 1977 Dec; 77(12):1948

McIntosh S et al. Fever in young children with sickle cell disease. J Pediatr 1980 Feb; 96(2):199–204

Oski FA et al. The effects of therapy on the developmental scores of iron-deficient infants. J Pediatr 1978 Jan; 92(1):21–25

Reindorf C. Sickle cell anemia: Current concepts. Pediatric Nursing 1980 Mar/Apr; 6(2):Update for Pediatric Nurses, E–G

Robinson L, Brown A, Underwood T. Iron therapy, helps and hazards. Pediatric Nursing, 1978 Nov/Dec; 4(6):9–13

Rowley PT. Newborn screening for sickle cell disease—benefits and burdens. NY State J Med 1978 Jan; 78(1):42–44

Saariner UM. Need for iron supplementation in infants on prolonged breast feeding. J Pediatr 1978 Aug; 93(2):177–180

Scarlato M. Blood transfusions today—what you should know and should do. Nursing '78 1978 Feb; 8(2):68–72

Tetrick A. Ambulatory care of the hemophiliac. JACCH 1978 Fall; 7(2):19–28

CONGENITAL HEART DISEASE

Congenital heart disease is a structural malformation of the heart or great vessels, present at birth.

Incidence

1. Congenital heart disease occurs in approximately 0.6–1.0% of all live births in the U.S.
2. Approximately 35,000 infants are born each year with congenital heart disease.
3. As a category, congenital heart disease is the most common congenital malformation.

Etiology

1. Exact cause is unknown
2. Results from abnormal embryonic development or the persistence of fetal structure beyond the time of normal involution
3. Possible causes
   a. Fetal and maternal infection occurring during first trimester (primarily rubella)
   b. Teratogenic effects of drugs
   c. Maternal dietary deficiencies
   d. Genetic factors
4. Frequently associated with other congenital defects

Common Congenital Heart Malformations (Table 41-1)

A. *Acyanotic*

1. Obstructive lesions
   a. Pulmonary stenosis
   b. Aortic stenosis
   c. Coarctation of the aorta
2. Left-to-right shunts
   a. Atrial septal defect
   b. Ventricular septal defect
   c. Patent ductus arteriosus

B. *Cyanotic*

   Right-to-left shunts
1. Tetralogy of Fallot
2. Tricuspid atresia
3. Transposition of great arteries

AORTIC VALVULAR STENOSIS

Aortic valvular stenosis occurs when there is obstruction to the left ventricular outflow at the level of the valve. This is the most common form of aortic stenosis, others being hypertrophic subaortic stenosis and supravalvular stenosis.

Pathophysiology

1. Blood flows from the left ventricle through the obstructed aortic valve into the aorta.
2. Left ventricular pressure increases to overcome the resistance of the obstructed valve.
3. Myocardial ischemia may occur as a result of an imbalance between the increased oxygen requirements of the hypertrophied left ventricle and the amount of oxygen that can be supplied to the myocardium.

Clinical Manifestations

1. Rarely symptomatic during infancy; in severe cases, infants may demonstrate evidence of decreased cardiac output, such as faint peripheral pulses or exercise intolerance.
2. Older children may experience chest pain, dyspnea, and fatigue with exertion.
3. Narrow pulse pressure.
4. Weak peripheral pulses.

Diagnostic Evaluation

1. Auscultation:
   a. Harsh, low-pitched systolic ejection murmur, maximal at the second right intercostal space, radiates to apex, back, neck.
   b. Ejection click at fourth interspace to the left of the sternum (mild or moderately severe cases).
2. Chest x-ray—dilated ascending aorta and varying degrees of left ventricular enlargement
3. Electrocardiogram—left ventricular hypertrophy: strain pattern (T-wave inversion) is evidence of severe stenosis

TABLE 41–1. CONGENITAL HEART ABNORMALITIES*

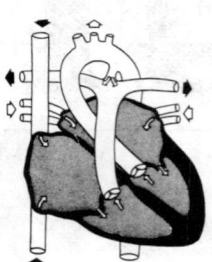

Patent Ductus Arteriosus

The patent ductus arteriosus is a vascular connection that, during fetal life, short circuits the pulmonary vascular bed and directs blood from the pulmonary artery to the aorta. Functional closure of the ductus normally occurs soon after birth. If the ductus remains patent after birth, the direction of blood flow in the ductus is reversed by the higher pressure in the aorta.

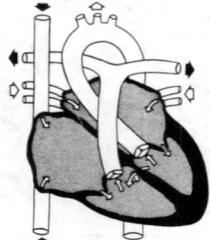

Ventricular Septal Defects

A ventricular septal defect is an abnormal opening between the right and left ventricle. Ventricular septal defects vary in size and may occur in either the membranous or muscular portion of the ventricular septum. Due to higher pressure in the left ventricle, a shunting of blood from the left to right ventricle occurs during systole. If pulmonary vascular resistance produces pulmonary hypertension, the shunt of blood is then reversed from the right to the left ventricle, with cyanosis resulting.

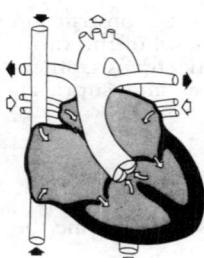

Truncus Arteriosus

Truncus arteriosus is a retention of the embryologic bulbar trunk. It results from the failure of normal septation and division of this trunk into an aorta and pulmonary artery. This single arterial trunk overrides the ventricles and receives blood from them through a ventricular septal defect. The entire pulmonary and systemic circulation is supplied from this common arterial trunk.

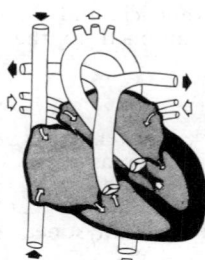

Subaortic Stenosis

In many instances, the stenosis is valvular with thickening and fusion of the cusps. Subaortic stenosis is caused by a fibrous ring below the aortic valve in the outflow tract of the left ventricle. At times, both valvular and subaortic stenosis exist in combination. The obstruction presents an increased work load for the normal output of the left ventricular blood and results in left ventricular enlargement.

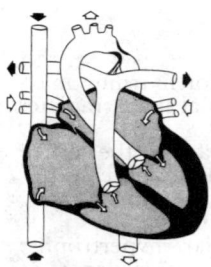

Coarctation of the Aorta

Coarctation of the aorta is characterized by a narrowed aortic lumen. It exists as a preductal or postductal obstruction, depending on the position of the obstruction in relation to the ductus arteriosus. Coarctations exist with great variation in anatomical features. The lesion produces an obstruction to the flow of blood through the aorta causing an increased left ventricular pressure and work load.

* Courtesy, Ross Laboratories.

Tetralogy of Fallot

Tetralogy of Fallot is characterized by the combination of 4 defects: (1) pulmonary stenosis, (2) ventricular septal defect, (3) overriding aorta, (4) hypertrophy of right ventricle. It is the most common defect causing cyanosis in patients surviving beyond 2 years of age. The severity of symptoms depends on the degree of pulmonary stenosis, the size of the ventricular septal defect and the degree to which the aorta overrides the septal defect.

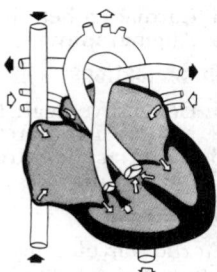

Complete Transposition of Great Vessels

This anomaly is an embryologic defect caused by a straight division of the bulbar trunk without normal spiraling. As a result, the aorta originates from the right ventricle, and the pulmonary artery from the left ventricle. An abnormal communication between the 2 circulations must be present to sustain life.

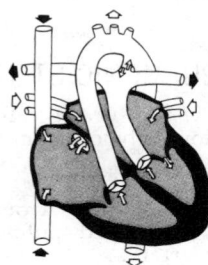

Atrial Septal Defects

An atrial septal defect is an abnormal opening between the right and left atria. Basically, 3 types of abnormalities result from incorrect development of the atrial septum. An incompetent foramen ovale is the most common defect. The high ostium secundum defect results from abnormal development of the septum secundum. Improper development of the septum primum produces a basal opening known as an ostium primum defect, frequently involving the atrioventricular valves. In general, left to right shunting of blood occurs in all atrial septal defects.

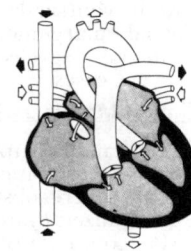

Tricuspid Atresia

Tricuspid valvular atresia is characterized by a small right ventricle, large left ventricle and usually a diminished pulmonary circulation. Blood from the right atrium passes through an atrial septal defect into the left atrium, mixes with oxygenated blood returning from the lungs, flows into the left ventricle and is propelled into the systemic circulation. The lungs may receive blood through 1 of 3 routes: (1) a small ventricular septal defect, (2) patent ductus arteriosus, (3) bronchial vessels.

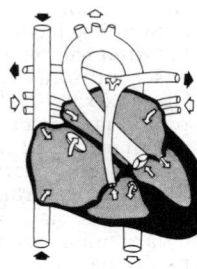

Anomalous Venous Return

Oxygenated blood returning from the lungs is carried abnormally to the right heart by one or more pulmonary veins emptying directly, or indirectly through venous channels, into the right atrium. Partial anomalous return of the pulmonary veins to the right atrium functions the same as an atrial septal defect. In complete anomalous return of the pulmonary veins, an interatrial communication is necessary for survival.

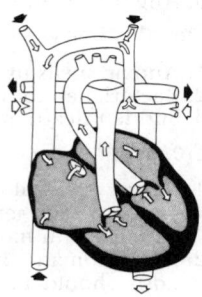

4. Cardiac catheterization
5. Angiography

Complications

1. Congestive heart failure
2. Myocardial infarction
3. Bacterial endocarditis
4. Sudden death

Treatment

Aortic valvulotomy or prosthetic valve replacement (indicated for children who are symptomatic or have evidence of left ventricular strain on electrocardiogram).

PULMONIC STENOSIS

Pulmonic stenosis refers to any lesion that obstructs the flow of blood from the right ventricle.

Pathophysiology

1. Blood flows from the right ventricle through the obstructed pulmonary valve into the pulmonary artery.
2. Right ventricular pressure increases to maintain normal cardiac output.
3. Right ventricular hypertrophy and occasionally left atrial enlargement occur.
4. Various degrees of tricuspid insufficiency occur in severe cases.

Clinical Manifestations

1. Generally asymptomatic; child may have decreased exercise tolerance.
2. With severe obstruction, child may have dyspnea, generalized cyanosis.
3. May complain of precordial pain.

Diagnostic Evaluation

1. Auscultation
   a. Systolic ejection murmur over pulmonic area
   b. Often will hear an ejection click and a widely split second sound
2. Chest x-ray—right ventricular enlargement, main pulmonary artery enlargement, normal pulmonary vascularity, and normal left side. In severe stenosis, right atrial hypertrophy is also observed.
3. Electrocardiogram—right ventricular hypertrophy
   a. Marked right axis deviation and right atrial enlargement are common in severe cases.
   b. T-wave inversion may be present.
4. Cardiac catheterization
5. Angiocardiography

Complications

1. Anoxic spells in infants with severe lesions
2. Bacterial endocarditis
3. Sudden death at any age

Treatment

1. Surgery (valvulotomy) is generally indicated for all patients with severe stenosis and for symptomatic patients with moderate stenosis.
2. Asymptomatic children with moderate pulmonic stenosis should be evaluated at regular intervals for progression of the lesion.

COARCTATION OF THE AORTA

Coarctation of the aorta is a narrowing or constriction of the vessel at any point. Most commonly, the constriction is located just distal to the origin of the left subclavian artery in the vicinity of the ductus arterious.

Altered Physiology

1. The narrowing of the aorta obstructs blood flow through the constricted segment of the aorta, thus increasing left ventricular pressure and work load.
2. Collateral vessels develop, arising chiefly from the branches of the subclavian and intercostal arteries, bypassing the coarcted segment of the aorta and supplying circulation to the lower extremities.

Clinical Manifestations

1. Usually asymptomatic in childhood—growth and development are normal.
2. May demonstrate:
   a. Occasional fatigue
   b. Headache
   c. Nose bleeds
   d. Leg cramps
3. Absent or greatly reduced femoral pulsations.
4. Hypertension in upper extremities and diminished blood pressure in lower extremities.
5. Symptoms secondary to hypertension (rare in children).
6. Severe anomalies cause symptoms in infants, including growth failure, tachypnea, dyspnea, peripheral edema, and severe congestive heart failure.

Diagnostic Evaluation

1. Auscultation—nonspecific systolic murmur heard along the left sternal border
2. Chest x-ray:
   a. Prominent aorta.
   b. Rib notching is a common finding in children over 10 years of age.
   c. Seriously ill infants demonstrate significant cardiomegaly with increased pulmonary vascularity.
3. Electrocardiogram—normal or varying degrees of left ventricular hypertrophy resulting from associated defects
4. Cardiac catheterization
5. Angiography

Complications

1. Cerebral hemorrhage
2. Rupture of the aorta
3. Infective endocarditis
4. Congestive heart failure

Treatment

1. Infants—vigorous management of congestive heart failure and surgical correction is indicated for infants who present in the first 6 months of life with heart failure.
2. Asymptomatic older child—surgical resection is recommended for children between the ages of 3 and 6 years with significant coarctation.
3. Surgery—resection of the coarcted segment and end-to-end anastomosis or graft.

PATENT DUCTUS ARTERIOSUS

Patent ductus arteriosus is the persistence of a fetal connection (ductus arteriosus) between the pulmonary artery and the aorta.

Altered Physiology

1. During fetal life, the ductus arteriosus allows most of the right ventricular blood to bypass the non-functioning lungs by directing blood from the pulmonary artery to the aorta.
2. After birth, with the initiation of respiration, the ductus arteriosus is no longer necessary. It should functionally close within several hours after birth and anatomically close within several weeks after birth.
   a. The smooth muscle in the wall of the ductus arteriosus contracts to obliterate the lumen.
   b. Within several weeks after birth, degenerative changes occur in the ductus arteriosus and it becomes a cord of fibrous connective tissue (ligamentum arteriosum).
3. When the ductus arteriosus remains patent, oxygenated blood from the higher pressure systemic circuit (aorta) flows to the lower pressure pulmonary circuit (pulmonary artery) through the patent ductus arteriosus.
4. The volume of blood that the heart must pump in order to meet the demands of the peripheral tissues is increased. A greater volume burden is placed on the lungs and eventually on the left heart.

Clinical Manifestations

1. Small patent ductus arteriosus—usually asymptomatic
2. Large patent ductus arteriosus—may develop symptoms in very early infancy
   a. Slow weight gain
   b. Feeding difficulties
   c. Frequent respiratory infections
   d. Congestive heart failure

Diagnostic Evaluation

1. Auscultation—continuous machinery-like murmur at the left intraclavicular area is heard in most older children. Neonates with patent ductus have a variety of murmurs.
2. May have a wide pulse pressure and/or bounding posterior tibial and dorsalis pedis pulses.
3. Chest x-ray:
   a. Symptomatic infants usually demonstrate gross cardiomegaly and increased pulmonary vasculature.
   b. Older children show normal or slightly increased pulmonary arterial markings and prominant main pulmonary artery.
4. Electrocardiogram—may be normal; may demonstrate left ventricular hypertrophy.
5. Cardiac catheterization
6. Angiocardiography

Complications

1. Congestive heart failure
2. Infective endocarditis

Treatment

Surgical division of the patent ductus arteriosus:
1. In early infancy if congestive heart failure develops and cannot be controlled
2. Electively by 2–3 years of age

NOTE: Indomethacin appears to trigger the natural closing of the ductus. It has been used successfully in some premature infants. If this success is sustained, this approach may replace surgery as the treatment of choice for a large proportion of infants.

ATRIAL SEPTAL DEFECT

Atrial septal defect is an abnormal opening in the septum between the left atrium and the right atrium.
1. *Ostium secundum type*—located in the center of the atrial septum (most common).
2. *Ostium primum type*—large gap at the base of the atrial septum frequently associated with deformities of the mitral and tricuspid valves and/or a small, high ventricular septal defect (endocardial cushion defects).

Altered Physiology

1. The pressure in the left atrium is greater than the pressure in the right atrium and promotes the flow of oxygenated blood from the left atrium to the right atrium.
2. The oxygenated blood that flows through the defect enters the right atrium and mixes with the systemic venous blood returning to the lung. The blood flow through the shunt recirculates through the lung, thus increasing the total blood flow through the lung.
3. The major hemodynamic abnormality is volume overload of the right ventricle.
4. If the pulmonary resistance is great, this may increase right atrial pressure, thus causing a reversal of the shunt, with unoxygenated blood flowing from the right atrium to the left atrium. (This situation will produce cyanosis.)

Clinical Manifestations

1. Ostium secundum type—generally asymptomatic even when this defect is large
2. Ostium primum type—generally asymptomatic, although the following may occur:
   a. Slow weight gain
   b. Fatigability
   c. Dyspnea with exertion
   d. Frequent respiratory infections
   e. Congestive heart failure

Diagnostic Evaluation

1. Auscultation
   a. Systolic, medium-pitched ejection murmur heard best at the second left interspace.
   b. Fixed widely split second sound.
   c. May have mid-diastolic filling sound at the lower left sternal border.
   d. A holosystolic murmur of mitral insufficiency is often heard at the apex in patients with primum defects.
2. Chest x-ray—prominent main pulmonary artery, right atrial and right ventricular enlargement, increase in vascular markings of the lungs. Radiologic findings are influenced by associated lesions in primum defects.
3. Electrocardiogram may demonstrate right ventricular hypertrophy and right axis deviation (ostium secundum defect); left axis deviation, P-wave changes indicating atrial enlargement, and prolonged P–R interval are common in ostium primum defects.
4. Cardiac catheterization
5. Angiocardiography

Complications

(Rare in children.)
1. Infective endocarditis
2. Cardiac failure
3. Pulmonary hypertension
4. Coronary artery disease
5. Atrial fibrillation

Treatment

Surgical closure with cardiopulmonary bypass by suture or patch

VENTRICULAR SEPTAL DEFECT

Ventricular septal defect is an abnormal opening in the septum between the right and left ventricles. It may vary in size from very small defects (Roger's defect) to very large defects, and may occur in either the membranous or muscular portion of the ventricular septum.

Altered Physiology

1. The pressure in the left ventricle is greater than the pressure in the right ventricle and promotes the flow of oxygenated blood from the left ventricle to the right ventricle.
2. The oxygenated blood that flows through the defect mixes with the blood returning from the right atrium. The blood flow through the shunt recirculates through the lungs, thus increasing the total blood flow through the lungs.
3. The major hemodynamic abnormalities are:
   a. Increased right ventricular and pulmonary arterial pressure.
   b. Increased blood flow to the right ventricle, pulmonary arteries, left atrium, and left ventricle.
4. If the pulmonary resistance is great, this may increase right ventricular pressure, thus causing a reversal of the shunt with unoxygenated blood flowing from the right ventricle to the left ventricle (this situation, termed Eisenmenger's complex, will produce cyanosis).

Clinical Manifestations

1. Small ventricular septal defects—usually asymptomatic (many close spontaneously)
2. Large ventricular septal defects—may develop symptoms as early as 1 to 2 months of age
   a. Slow weight gain
   b. Feeding difficulties
   c. Pale, delicate-looking, scrawny appearance
   d. Frequent respiratory infections
   e. Tachypnea
   f. Excessive sweating
   g. Congestive heart failure

Diagnostic Evaluation

1. Auscultation—harsh holosystolic murmur, heard best at the fourth interspace to the left of the sternum. Elevated pulmonary resistance is manifested by a loud, banging, pulmonic component of the second sound.
2. Chest x-ray—ranges from normal (small defect) to varying degrees of biventricular hypertrophy, left atrial enlargement, pulmonary artery enlargement, and increased pulmonary vascular markings.
3. Electrocardiogram—normal or biventricular hypertrophy, left atrial enlargement

4. Cardiac catheterization
5. Angiocardiography

Complications

1. Infective endocarditis
2. Congestive heart failure

Treatment

1. Medical management of congestive heart failure if this occurs in infancy.
2. If congestive heart failure is intractable to medical management, surgical closure is indicated.
3. Patients with pulmonary arterial hypertension require early surgery (before 2 years of age) to avoid irreversible pulmonary bed changes.
4. Surgery is contraindicated in patients with Eisenmenger's complex.

TETRALOGY OF FALLOT

Tetralogy of Fallot consists of 4 abnormalities: (1) right ventricular-outflow stenosis or atresia, (2) ventricular septal defect, (3) overriding of the aorta, and (4) right ventricular hypertrophy.

Altered Physiology

1. Obstruction of the blood flow from the right ventricle to the pulmonary circulation is caused by obstruction at the pulmonary valve level or the infundibular area of the right ventricle below the pulmonary valve.
2. Unoxygenated blood is shunted from the right ventricle through the ventricular septal defect directly into the aorta.
3. The right ventricle is hypertrophied because of high right ventricular pressure.

Clinical Manifestations

1. The clinical manifestations are variable and depend on the size of the ventricular septal defect and the degree of right ventricular outflow obstruction.
2. Cyanosis
   a. Initially, the shunt through the ventricular septal defect is mainly from left to right. Many infants with this defect are not cyanotic at birth, but they develop cyanosis as they grow and as the stenosis becomes relatively more severe.
   b. Cyanosis may at first be observed only with exertion and crying, but during the first few years of life, the child may become cyanotic even at rest.
   c. Infundibular stenosis may be minimal so that cyanosis never develops ("pink tetralogy").
3. Clubbing of the fingers and toes
4. Squatting (a posture characteristically assumed by children with this defect once they have reached the walking stage)
5. Slow weight gain
6. Dyspnea on exertion
7. Hypoxic spells, transient cerebral ischemia

Diagnostic Evaluation

1. Auscultation
   a. Single second sound (aortic component)
   b. Systolic ejection murmur at the second and third interspaces to the left of the sternum
   c. Prominent ejection click heard immediately after the first heart sound
2. Inspection—prominent left chest with right ventricular heave

3. Chest x-ray
   a. Heart size normal
   b. Pulmonary segment small and concave ("boot-shaped heart")
   c. Diminished pulmonary vascular markings
4. Electrocardiogram—right axis deviation; right ventricular hypertrophy
5. Cardiac catheterization
6. Angiocardiography
7. Laboratory data
   a. Polycythemia
   b. Increased hematocrit

Complications

1. Congestive heart failure—may occur in newborn but is uncommon beyond infancy
2. Infective endocarditis
3. Cerebral vascular accident (due to thrombosis or severe hypoxia)
4. Brain abscess
5. Iron deficiency anemia

Treatment

OBJECTIVE: to improve oxygenation of arterial blood.
1. Palliative
   a. *Waterston shunt*—anastomosis between the posterior lateral aspect of the ascending aorta and the right pulmonary artery
   b. *Blalock-Taussig shunt*—anastomosis between the right or left subclavian artery and the right pulmonary artery
2. Total correction
   a. Removal of shunt if previously performed.
   b. With cardiopulmonary bypass, ventricular septal defect is repaired and right ventricular-outflow obstruction is relieved.
   c. Total correction is increasingly being advocated for all infants in whom pulmonary arteries are of sufficient size.

TRANSPOSITION OF THE GREAT ARTERIES

Transposition of the great arteries occurs when the pulmonary artery originates posteriorly from the left ventricle and the aorta originates anteriorly from the right ventricle.

Altered Physiology

1. This defect results in 2 separate circulations; the right heart manages the systemic circulation and the left heart manages the pulmonary circulation.
2. In order for life to be sustained, there must be an accompanying defect which provides for the mixing of oxygenated and unoxygenated blood between the 2 circulations.
3. The mixing of oxygenated and unoxygenated blood occurs through one or more of the following shunts:
   a. Atrial septal defect
   b. Ventricular septal defect
   c. Patent ductus arteriosus
   d. Patent foramen ovale

Clinical Manifestations

Influenced predominantly by the extent of intercirculatory mixing:
1. Cyanosis, usually developing shortly after birth (degree dependent upon the type of associated malformations)

2. Congestive heart failure manifested by tachypnea, cardiomegaly, hepatomegaly
3. Fatigability
4. Slow weight gain
5. Clubbing of the fingers and toes

Diagnostic Evaluation

1. Auscultation—murmurs may be absent in infancy; may be murmur of an associated defect.
2. Chest x-ray—cardiomegaly, narrow mediastinum, egg-shaped cardiac silhouette, increased vascular markings (decreased vascular markings in children with associated pulmonary stenosis). Neonatal x-ray is often normal.
3. Electrocardiogram—right axis deviation, right atrial hypertrophy, right ventricular hypertrophy. Variable findings depending on age and anatomic factors.
4. Laboratory tests
   a. Polycythemia
   b. Thrombocytopenia
5. Cardiac catheterization
6. Angiocardiography

Complications

1. Congestive heart failure
2. Infective endocarditis
3. Brain abscess
4. Cerebral vascular accident (due to thrombosis or severe hypoxia)

Treatment

1. Vigorous medical management of congestive heart failure
2. Palliative procedures
   a. *Rashkind procedure*—the creation of an atrial septal defect with a balloon catheter during cardiac catheterization
   b. *Blalock-Hanlon procedure*—surgical creation of an atrial septal defect
   c. Pulmonary artery banding (indicated for infants with ventricular septal defects with large pulmonary blood flow)
3. Complete correction
   a. *Mustard procedure*—with cardiopulmonary bypass, the atrial septum is removed and a baffle of dacron velour and/or pericardium is sutured in place in such a way that the pulmonary venous blood is directed toward the right ventricle and the systemic venous blood is directed toward the left ventricle (usually done before 2 years of age, before pulmonary vascular disease develops).
   b. *Rastelli procedure*
      (1) Surgery of choice for transposition with ventricular septal defect and left ventricular outflow-tract obstruction.
      (2) With cardiopulmonary bypass, the ventricular septal defect is closed in such a way that the left ventricle communicates with the aorta. The pulmonary artery is ligated, and the right ventricle is connected to the distal portion of the pulmonary artery by means of a valve bearing tubular graft.
   c. Recent procedures have been developed for anatomic correction of transposition of the great arteries by direct contraposition of the transposed vessels. This may become the preferred treatment in the future.

d. As with other types of congenital cardiac surgery, the question of optimum timing for surgery is controversial. Increasingly, total correction is recommended when feasible.

TRICUSPID ATRESIA

Tricuspid atresia is a condition in which there is: (1) atresia of the tricuspid valve so that there is no communication between the right atrium and right ventricle, (2) interatrial septal defect, and (3) a hypoplastic right ventricle.

Pathophysiology

1. Blood from the systemic circulation is shunted from the right atrium through an interatrial communication to the left atrium and then to the left ventricle.
2. Pulmonary blood flow is established either through a patent ductus arteriosus, bronchial circulation, or a ventricular septal defect.

Clinical Manifestations

1. Severe cyanosis in the neonatal period
2. Respiratory distress
3. Clubbing
4. Hypoxic spells
5. Delayed weight gain
6. Right heart failure (may occur)

Diagnostic Evaluation

1. Auscultation
   a. First sound single and accentuated
   b. Commonly no murmur or murmur of associated defect
2. Chest x-ray—patients with diminished pulmonary blood flow have a normal to mildly increased cardiac silhouette, concavity in the region of the main pulmonary artery, and diminished pulmonary vascular markings; those with increased pulmonary flow have cardiac enlargement and plethoric pulmonary vasculature.
3. Electrocardiogram—right atrial, left atrial, left ventricular hypertrophy, left axis deviation
4. Echocardiogram—demonstrates diminutive right ventricular chamber and no tricuspid valve
5. Cardiac catheterization
6. Angiocardiography

Complications

1. Cerebrovascular accidents
2. Brain abscess
3. Bacterial endocarditis

Treatment

1. Palliative procedures to increase pulmonary blood flow:
   a. *Waterston shunt*—anastomosis between the ascending aorta and right pulmonary artery
   b. *Glenn procedure*—side-to-end anastomosis of the superior vena cava to the right pulmonary artery
   c. *Blalock–Taussig shunt*—subclavian to pulmonary artery anastomosis
2. Complete correction:
   a. Has been done successfully in a limited number of older, symptomatic patients with diminished blood flow.
   b. Involves placement of a tubular conduit with a valve between the right atrium and main pulmo-

nary artery. The atrial defect is closed and the main pulmonary artery is ligated just above the pulmonary valve.

TREATMENT AND NURSING MANAGEMENT OF THE CHILD WITH A CONGENITAL HEART DEFECT

Nursing Objectives and Management

A. *To become informed concerning the child's symptomatology and the plan of medical care.*

1. Obtain a thorough nursing history to become familiar with the child and his family in order to recognize normal and abnormal patterns (color, respirations, murmur, feeding, exercise tolerance, etc.).
2. Discuss with the physician his plan for medical care.
3. Make a baseline nursing assessment of the child's condition.
   a. Observe and record information relevant to the child's growth and development (motor coordination, muscular development, emotional maturity.)
      (1) Compare data with that for siblings, other family members.
      (2) Plot appropriate information on growth chart.
   b. Observe and record the child's level of exercise tolerance.
      (1) Observe the child at play:
         Is play interrupted to rest?
         How does he play as compared with his peers?
         Does he squat during play? (Squatting is a characteristic position a cyanotic child assumes when resting after exertion.)
      (2) Observe infants while feeding.
         Does the infant stop feeding to rest or does he fall asleep during feeding?
   c. Observe the child's skin and mucous membranes for color changes.
      (1) Skin
         Color changes vary from pink, dusky, mottled, to cyanotic.
         Earlobes are good indicators of the degree of oxygen saturation.
         Circumoral cyanosis occurs with oxygen deprivation.
         Nailbeds are good indicators of color change.
      (2) Mucous membranes
         Lips and tongue indicate color change because they are very vascular areas and contain superficial blood vessels; *mucous membranes are the best places to observe for cyanosis.*
      (3) Record where cyanosis was observed (localized or generalized), when it was observed and the duration (continuous or intermittent, whether variable with exercise).
   d. Observe for clubbing (rounding) of the fingers, especially the thumbnails, with thickening and shininess of the terminal phalanges—may occur in cyanotic children by 2–3 months of age.)
   e. Observe for chest deformities.
      (1) Visible pulsations
      (2) Left- or right-sided prominence
   f. Observe respiratory pattern.

(1) Remove any clothing or covers which obscure visualization of the chest.

(2) Count respirations for at least 30 seconds.

(3) Count respirations while a child is at rest; if unable to soothe the child, document that he is crying, irritable, etc.

(4) Observe for increased respiratory rate, grunting, retractions, nasal flaring, irregularity of respirations.

(5) Record all signs of respiratory distress including change from usual pattern, when it occurred, duration, etc.

g. Palpate the child's pulses.

(1) Radial or dorsalis pedis is difficult to feel in newborn.

(2) Femoral pulsations are easily felt in the inguinal region and can be compared with brachial pulsations.

(3) Record the strength of the pulse (full, bounding, weak, or faint).

(4) When a pulse is difficult to locate, mark its location with a pen to facilitate locating it the next time.

h. Auscultate the child's heart to:

(1) Count apical pulse rate.

(2) Determine cardiac rhythm or change in rhythm.

(3) Become familiar with a known murmur.

(4) Determine the presence of new murmurs.

i. Record vital signs (apical pulse, blood pressure, respirations)

(1) Have child quiet for base-line vital signs.

(2) Record which extremity is used for blood pressure measurement.

(3) Refer to vital sign procedure (see p. 1145).

B. *To provide adequate nutritional and fluid intake to maintain the growth and developmental needs of the child.*

1. Feed slowly in a semierect position; burp infants after each ounce.

2. Utilize soft nipples with large holes which make it easier for the infant to suck.

3. Provide small frequent feedings.

4. Feeding should generally be completed within 45 minutes or sooner if infant tires.

5. Provide foods which have high nutritional value.

6. Determine the child's likes and dislikes and plan meals with the dietitian, taking into consideration the child's preferences.

7. Observe the child at mealtime; does a poor appetite represent a lack of interest in food or does the child become fatigued while eating?

8. Report vomiting and specify the amount, type, relationship to feeding or to medications.

9. Report diarrhea and specify type and amount.

10. Maintain adequate hydration in the cyanotic child when he is vomiting, has diarrhea or fever, or is exposed to high environmental temperatures since polycythemia predisposes him to thrombosis.

C. *To prevent infection.*

1. Prevent exposure to communicable disease, including exposure to children with upper respiratory infections, diarrhea, wound infections, etc.

2. Check with parents to be certain the child's immunizations are up to date.

3. Practice careful handwashing technique and teach this to the child.

4. Report temperature elevation, diarrhea, vomiting, and upper respiratory symptoms promptly.

5. Be certain that the child receives prophylactic medication for infective endocarditis before genitourinary instrumentation or dental work. (Refer to American Heart Association recommendations.)

D. *To prepare the child for diagnostic and treatment procedures.*

1. Explain to the child what is going to be done in simple terms (refer to section on hospitalized child, p. 1126).

2. Encourage the child to express his fears and fantasies verbally or through play.

3. Diagnostic procedures may include:

a. Electrocardiogram

b. Vectorcardiogram

c. Phonocardiogram

d. Echocardiogram

e. Chest x-ray

f. Barium swallow

g. Cardiac catheterization and angiocardiography

h. Complete blood count

i. Platelet count

j. Blood gases

E. *To explain to the child about his heart condition as early as the child can understand.*

1. Discuss with the parents the importance of being truthful with the child about his heart condition.

2. The time to tell the child is generally when the child begins asking questions as to why he visits the doctor so frequently and why the doctor listens to his heart so closely.

3. The child's questions should be answered truthfully in a simple way.

F. *To relieve the respiratory distress associated with increased pulmonary blood flow or oxygen deprivation.*

1. Determine the degree of respiratory distress.

a. Infants—respirations greater than 60 per minute are indicative of respiratory difficulty.

b. Young children—respirations greater than 40 per minute are indicative of respiratory difficulty.

c. Observe the regularity of the respiratory pattern.

d. Observe for retractions (drawing in of soft tissue in the rib interspaces or below the costal margin with each inspiration; may be barely visible, mild or severe).

e. Observe for nasal flaring, listen for grunting.

2. Include specific information in nursing record.

a. Number of respirations per minute

b. Regularity of respirations

c. Type and severity of retractions

d. Presence of nasal flaring, grunting

e. Response to oxygen therapy

f. Response to positioning

g. Color changes

h. Irritability or anxiety observed

3. Position child at 45-degree angle to decrease pressure of the viscera on the diaphragm and increase lung volume.

a. Infant—place in an infant seat.

b. Children—elevate head of the bed and support the arms with pillows.

4. Pin diapers loosely; provide loose fitting pajamas for older children.

5. Feed slowly allowing frequent rest periods.

a. Rapid respirations and frequent coughing predispose the child to aspiration.
b. May require gavage feeding.
c. Observe for abdominal distention which may increase respiratory difficulty.
6. Hyperextend the infant's or child's head.
7. Suction the nose and throat if the child is unable to adequately cough up secretions.
8. Provide oxygen therapy as indicated.

G. *To relieve the hypoxic spells associated with cyanotic types of congenital heart disease (primarily tetralogy of Fallot).*

1. Observe for hypoxic spells (attacks of acute oxygen deprivation), characterized by:
    a. Increased rate and depth of respiration
    b. Increasing cyanosis
    c. Murmur that becomes less intense, may disappear
    d. Bradycardia
    e. Progressive limpness and syncope
    f. May result in convulsions
2. Be aware that these attacks frequently occur in the morning after awakening from sleep, during or after crying, during or after defecation, or during or immediately following feeding.
3. Once an attack is recognized, call for assistance and immediately:
    a. Place child in knee-chest position.
    b. Administer oxygen via mask.
    c. Be prepared to administer medications as prescribed.
        Morphine sulfate
        $NaHCO_3$ to correct acidosis
        Propranolol
    d. Assume a calm, reassuring attitude
4. Observe child closely following recovery from an attack. Encourage fluid intake.
5. Record observations in the following areas:
    a. Condition and activity before the attack
    b. Response to positioning and medication
    c. Vital signs during and after attack

H. *To improve oxygenation so that body functions may be maintained.*

1. Provide a safe, effective oxygen environment (refer to procedure on oxygen therapy, p. 1196).
2. Explain to the child how oxygen will help; orient him to equipment before it is used on him (e.g., tent, mask).
3. Observe the child's response to oxygen therapy.
    a. Improvement of color
    b. Change in rate and character of respiration
    c. Change in anxiety level
4. Observe the child's response while he is being weaned from oxygen.
    Reduce liter flow gradually and observe response after each reduction.
5. Measures which are directed to relieve respiratory distress will aid in improving oxygenation.

I. *To reduce the work load of the heart since decreased activity and expenditure of energy will decrease oxygen requirements.*

1. Organize nursing care to provide periods of uninterrupted rest.
2. Avoid unnecessary activities such as frequent, complete baths and clothing changes.
3. Prevent excessive crying.
    a. Use pacifier.

b. Hold baby.
c. Feed when hungry.
d. Keep baby comfortable.
4. Explain to the child the need for rest.
5. Provide diversional activities that require limited expenditure of energy.
6. Avoid discussing the child's condition or the condition of other children in the presence of the patient in order to prevent unnecessary anxiety.
7. Support the child during diagnostic and therapeutic procedures.

J. *To observe the child for symptoms of congestive heart failure which occur frequently as a complication of congenital heart disease.* (For nursing management, refer to section on congestive heart failure, p. 1295.)

1. Respiratory distress (tachypnea, retractions, nasal flaring, grunting, voice changes)
2. Tachycardia, gallop heart rhythm
3. Fatigue (as evidenced by poor feeding in infants)
4. Edema
    Periorbital edema is often observed in infants; older children develop swelling of the hands and feet.
5. Weight gain
6. Irritability
7. Sweating
8. Liver enlargement
9. Splenomegaly
10. Orthopnea
11. Neck vein distention (rarely seen in infants)
12. Murmurs (may appear, or the characteristics of previously heard murmur may change)
13. Cyanosis (may occur)
14. Pulmonary rales (may occur)

K. *To observe for the development of symptoms of infective endocarditis which may occur as a complication of congenital heart disease.*

1. Be aware of the symptoms of infective endocarditis.
    a. Spiking fever
    b. Petechiae
    c. Anorexia
    d. Pallor
    e. Fatigue
2. Be aware of the need for infective endocarditis prophylaxis for selected children undergoing surgery, dental work, and laceration repair.
3. For nursing management, refer to section on infective endocarditis, p. 1303.

L. *To observe for the development of thrombosis which may occur as a complication of cyanotic heart disease.*

1. Be aware of the signs and symptoms of thrombosis:
    a. Irritability and restlessness
    b. Convulsion, coma, neurologic signs
    c. Paralysis
    d. Rapid onset of edema
    e. Anuria, oliguria, hematuria
2. Be aware that thrombosis is more likely to occur during phases of acute dehydration, fever, and vomiting.

M. *To prepare the parents to care for the child following discharge.*

1. Instruct family in necessary measures to maintain child's health:
    a. Complete immunization

b. Adequate diet and rest
c. Prevention and control of infections
d. Regular medical and dental checkup
  Child should be protected against infective endocarditis with dental procedures. (Refer to American Heart Association Protocol.)
e. Regular cardiac checkups
2. Teach family about the defect and its treatment.
  a. Pathophysiology and natural history
  b. Signs and symptoms of disease progress
  c. Signs and symptoms of complications that might be anticipated
  d. Signs of infection, dehydration
  e. Medications and side effects
  f. Special diets
  g. Emergency precautions related to hypoxic attacks, pulmonary edema, cardiac arrest (if appropriate)
3. Encourage the parents and other persons (teachers, peers, etc.) to treat the child in as normal a manner as possible.
  a. Avoid overprotection and overindulgence

b. Avoid rejection
c. Facilitate performance of the usual developmental tasks within the limits of the child's physiologic state.
  With most congenital cardiac defects it is not necessary to restrict the child's activity; the child will rest when he becomes tired and then resume his play.
d. Prevent adults from projecting their fears and anxieties onto the child.
4. Initiate a community health nursing referral if indicated.
N. *To refer the family to appropriate resources concerned with the financial and/or emotional aspects of caring for a child with congenital heart disease.*

1. Social worker
2. Crippled children's program
3. Parents and organized parent groups
4. American Heart Association

CONGESTIVE HEART FAILURE

Congestive heart failure occurs when the cardiac output is inadequate to meet the metabolic demands of the body and results in accumulation of excessive blood volume in the pulmonary and/or systemic venous system.

Etiology
1. Congenital heart disease (primary cause in the first 3 years of life).
2. Acquired heart disease—rheumatic heart disease, endocarditis, myocarditis.
3. Non-cardiovascular causes—acidosis, pulmonary disease, various metabolic diseases

Clinical Manifestations
1. Dyspnea and tachypnea
2. Tachycardia
3. Orthopnea
4. Peripheral edema—often scrotal or periorbital
5. Feeding difficulties, anorexia
6. Restlessness
7. Easy fatigability
8. Pallor
9. Weight gain
10. Diaphoresis
11. Growth failure
12. Nonproductive, irritative cough
13. Neck vein distention
14. Hepatomegaly

Pathophysiology
1. For any number of reasons, cardiac output is inadequate to meet the oxygenation and nutritional requirements of vital organs.
2. Various compensatory mechanisms occur.
  a. Stroke volume increases and cardiomegaly develops.
  b. Tachycardia occurs in an effort to maintain adequate stroke volume.
  c. Catecholamines are released by the sympathetic venous system that increase systemic vascular resistance and venous tone and decrease cutaneous, splanchnic, and renal blood flow.
  d. Glomerular filtration decreases and tubular reabsorption increases, causing diminished urinary output and sodium retention.
  e. Diaphoresis occurs.
3. Cardiac output decreases further as compensatory mechanisms fail.
4. The pulmonary vascular bed is not emptied efficiently, causing engorgement of the pulmonic system with subsequent pulmonary hypertension and edema.
5. There is diminished blood return to the heart, with venous congestion and a rise in venous pressure.

Diagnostic Evaluation
1. Palpation
  a. May have weak peripheral pulses.
  b. Hepatomegaly (feature of right heart failure).
  c. Abnormal precordial activity may occur.
2. Auscultation
  a. Gallop rhythm (frequent).
  b. Cardiac murmurs may or may not be present.
  c. Rales (infrequent in infants).
3. Chest x-rays—cardiomegaly; pulmonary congestion
4. Laboratory data:
  a. Dilutional hyponatremia
  b. Hypochloremia
  c. Hyperkalemia

Complications
1. Respiratory infections
2. Pulmonary edema
3. Intractable congestive heart failure
4. Myocardial failure

Nursing Objectives and Management
A. *To improve myocardial efficiency*
1. Administer digoxin as prescribed by the physician.
  a. Carefully calculate dosage; digoxin is given to infants and children in very small amounts.

b. Count apical pulse for 1 full minute before administering.
   Be aware of the heart rate at which the physician wants the medication withheld.
c. Report vomiting, which may occur following administration of digoxin, to determine if physician desires dose to be repeated.
d. Observe for the development of premature ventricular contractions when digoxin is initially started; report this to physician.
e. Be aware of signs of digitalis intoxication.
   (1) Altered emotional status, "digitalis blues"
   (2) Decreased appetite
   (3) Bradycardia
   (4) Arrhythmias
   (5) Gastrointestinal symptoms

B. *To reduce energy requirements.*

1. Organize nursing care to provide periods of uninterrupted rest.
2. Avoid unnecessary activities such as frequent complete baths and clothing changes.
3. Prevent excessive crying.
   a. Use pacifier.
   b. Hold baby.
   c. Eliminate sources of distress (e.g., hunger, wet diapers).
4. Explain to the child the need for rest.
5. Provide diversional activities that require limited expenditure of energy.

C. *To remove accumulated sodium and fluid.*

1. Administer diuretics as prescribed by the physician.
   a. Be aware of the side effects of the prescribed medication.
   b. Weigh the child at least daily to observe response.
   c. Maintain an accurate record of intake and output. Record urine specific gravity.
   d. Encourage foods such as bananas and orange juice that have a high potassium content to prevent potassium depletion associated with many diuretics.
      (1) Hypokalemia may cause weakened myocardial contractions and may precipitate digoxin toxicity.
      (2) Oral potassium supplements may be indicated when a child is on diuretics for an extended period of time.
2. Restrict sodium intake
   a. The child is usually placed on a low sodium diet.
   b. Be aware of the prescribed diet and the amount of sodium in foods and fluids offered to the child.
   c. Question the child about his likes and dislikes so that the diet can be made as appealing as possible.
   d. Interpret the diet and its purpose to the child and his parents.
   e. Infants may require low sodium formulas.

D. *To relieve the respiratory distress associated with pulmonary engorgement.*
   Refer to section on Congenital Heart Disease, pp. 1293–1294.

E. *To improve tissue oxygenation.*

1. Administer oxygen therapy—refer to procedure, pp. 1196–2000.
2. Maintain the infant in a neutral thermal environment.

F. *To provide adequate nutrition to meet the caloric requirements of the child.*

1. Provide foods which the child enjoys in small amounts, because he may have a poor appetite due to liver enlargement.
2. Infant feeding:
   a. Feed frequently in small amounts.
   b. Feed slowly in a sitting position, allowing frequent rest periods.
   c. Supplement oral feedings with gavage feeding if the infant is unable to take adequate amount of formula by mouth.
   d. Record the amount of formula taken.
   e. Place the child in an infant seat following feeding to prevent pressure of the viscera on the diaphragm.
   f. Observe for distention and vomiting following feeding.

G. *To decrease the danger of infection.*

1. Practice careful handwashing technique.
2. Avoid exposure to other children with upper respiratory infections, diarrhea, etc.
3. Report such changes as temperature elevation, diarrhea, vomiting, and upper respiratory symptoms promptly.

H. *To observe for signs of disease progress or response to treatment.*

1. Record and report in detail presence or disappearance of signs and symptoms.
2. Monitor vital signs frequently and report any significant changes.

I. *To explain the condition and treatment to the child and family.*

1. Utilize terminology that the child and/or parents can understand.
2. Correct misinterpretations—parents and children frequently interpret congestive heart failure to be synonymous with myocardial infarction, or they may fear that the heart is about to stop beating.

J. *To prepare the parents for the care of the child at home.*

1. Describe symptoms to be aware of and to be reported.
2. Teach them how to administer medications and about the side effects.
3. Explain dietary and/or activity restrictions.
4. Explain methods to prevent infection.
5. Initiate a community health nursing referral if indicated.

NURSING CARE OF THE CHILD UNDERGOING CARDIAC CATHETERIZATION

Cardiac catheterization involves introducing a radiopaque catheter into a vein or artery in the groin or in the arm, either percutaneously or by means of a cutdown. The catheter is advanced into the cardiac chambers and vessels, where pressures are measured and samples for oxygen concentration are obtained. The procedure is usually done in conjunction with angiography, the injection of radiopaque material into various chambers of the heart.

Purpose

1. To establish the diagnosis of cardiovascular defect.
2. To identify the severity of the defect.

3. To evaluate the effects of the defect on cardiovascular function.

Preoperative Nursing Management

1. Reinforce explanations of the procedure to the child and parents.
   a. Provide specific information about:
      (1) Time of the test
      (2) Preparation for the procedure (NPO, sedation, etc.)
      (3) Site of the venipuncture (if known)
      (4) What the child will see (atmosphere of the catheterization room)
      (5) What will be expected of the child during the procedure
      (6) Routines after the procedure
   b. Detail, length, and timing of explanations should be appropriate to the child's age and level of cognitive development.
      (1) Photographs or a miniature replica of the cardiac lab and equipment may facilitate understanding of explanations.
      (2) Older children and parents may benefit from an opportunity to see the room where the procedure will be done.
      (3) It is helpful for some children to handle the mask and other equipment that will be used.
   c. Parents should be provided with an opportunity for private discussion of the anticipated procedure.
2. Maintain adequate hydration (especially important for children with cyanotic heart disease).
   Offer fluids just prior to NPO period.
3. Cleanse proposed catheterization site thoroughly. Clean fingernails and/or toenails.
4. Obtain baseline set of vital signs—including blood pressure—just prior to the time of catheterization.
5. Administer sedation if prescribed.
   a. Raise and secure siderails after child has been medicated.
   b. Observe child closely for depressed respirations.

Postoperative Nursing Management

1. Monitor vital signs frequently and report:
   a. Sudden drop in blood pressure
   b. Changes in pulse rate or rhythm
   c. Increased or depressed respirations
   d. Faintness, weakness
   e. Elevated temperature
2. Observe for complications resulting from damage to the vessels through which the catheter was passed.
   a. Check the dressing or puncture site for bleeding.
   b. Observe site for redness, swelling, pain, or induration.
   c. Observe for numbness, pallor, decreased temperature, decreased motion, cyanosis, or mottling of affected extremity.
   d. Palpate pulses in affected extremity and compare with pulses in the opposite extremity.
3. Keep the child warm to avoid the risk of hypothermia.
   This is especially important for small infants and children who may already be hypoxic because of their cardiac condition.
4. Maintain the child in a reclining position for several hours after catheterization to avoid:
   a. Possibility of sudden drop in blood pressure that may accompany an abrupt assumption of an upright position.
   b. Bleeding at the site of catheter entry.
5. Offer fluids as soon as the child is able to take them to avoid dehydration.
   This is especially important for cyanotic children who are polycythemic and prone to thrombus formation.
6. Reinforce discharge information. Parents should be informed about:
   a. Care of the incision, puncture site
   b. Dressing change (if any)
   c. Activity limitations (if any)
   d. Observation for and reporting of late complications (especially infection)
   e. Follow-up medical care
7. If the child is a candidate for surgery, utilize appropriate opportunities to prepare him and his family for the experience.
   a. Encourage contact with children who are convalescing from surgery.
   b. Answer immediate questions of the parents.

Reference for Teaching

Dee Dee's Heart Test, Children's Hospital of Philadelphia, 34th and Civic Center Blvd., Philadelphia, Pa. 19104

CARDIAC SURGERY

Generally, nursing care of children who require cardiac surgery is the same as that of adults (refer to pp. 303–308). In addition, the following considerations should be kept in mind by the nurse who works with pediatric patients.

Nursing Management

A. *Preoperative*

1. Prepare parents for the experience prior to the day of admission for surgery.
   a. Parents frequently ask questions about:
      (1) What to tell the child
      (2) When to begin preparation
      (3) What to bring to the hospital
      (4) Anticipated sequence of events
      (5) Separation—rooming-in, whether or not to leave at night, etc.
   b. Utilize opportunities for teaching—physician's office, catheterization episode, puppet shows, phone calls, contact with other patients.
2. Prepare child for what he will experience during hospitalization.
   a. Consult with parents prior to beginning explanation. Their desires regarding how much information to give the child should be respected, and they should be active participants in preparation of the child.
   b. Most children need information about:

(1) Preparation for surgery:
  (a) Diagnostic tests
  (b) Antibacterial skin preparation or baths
  (c) NPO period
  (d) Injections—antimicrobials and/or sedatives
  (e) Time of the surgery
  (f) Transportation to operating room
(2) Postoperative expectations:
  (a) Incision (location)
  (b) Chest tube
  (c) Dressings
  (d) Nasogastric tube
  (e) IVs
  (f) Monitors
  (g) Endotracheal tube, ventilator
  (h) Suctioning
  (i) Oxygen equipment
  (j) Pain (ability to relieve)
  (k) Bed scale (may fantasize that it is a stretcher to return child to the OR)
  (l) Appearance of intensive care unit, visiting regulations for parents

c. Have child practice coughing and deep breathing exercises (refer to procedure, p. 1191).
d. Detail, length, and time of explanations should be appropriate to the child's age and level of cognitive development.
  (1) Photographs or a miniature replica of the intensive care unit may facilitate understanding of explanations.
  (2) Older children and parents often benefit from an opportunity to see the intensive care unit.
  (3) It is helpful for some children to have an opportunity to manipulate some of the equipment which will be used.
e. Test the child's comprehension of teaching by asking him simple questions, having him place equipment on a doll, demonstrating coughing and deep breathing, and other similar activities.
f. Allow opportunity for the child to express his concerns, either verbally or in play situations.
3. Provide opportunity for private discussions with the parents about the anticipated surgery.
a. Parents need the same type of information as their child. They also need information about the following:
  (1) Scheduled time of surgery
  (2) Whether or not they can accompany their child to the OR
  (3) Waiting area
  (4) Usual length of surgery
  (5) Intensive care unit expectations and policies
b. Provide emotional support to parents and answer their questions so that they are in the best position to support their child.
  (1) Parents may need help dealing with guilt feelings that they had a role in causing the disease, that they did not seek medical advice soon enough, etc.
  (2) Parents frequently have fears that the child will suffer excessive pain or die.
  (3) Parents may ask technical questions relating to such matters as the heart-lung machine, and the type of material used for patching defects.
4. Observe closely and report any signs of infection or inflammation (upper respiratory infection, hoarseness, elevated temperature, vomiting, diarrhea, skin lesions, etc.).

5. Perform appropriate nursing activities associated with congenital heart disease (refer to pp. 1292–1295).

B. *Postoperative*

1. Send the nursing history and care plan to the intensive care unit and relay information about the child and family to appropriate personnel to insure continuity of care.
2. Refer to:
  Postoperative Nursing Management (adults), pp. 89–92.
  Cardiac Arrhythmias, pp. 313–329.
  Respiratory Procedures, pp. 1189–1201.
  Cardiopulmonary Resuscitation, pp. 1205–1208.
  Managing the Patient Undergoing Water-seal Chest Drainage, p. 226.
  Direct Current Countershock Procedures for Ventricular Fibrillation, p. 277.
  Measuring Central Venous Pressure, p. 271.
  Assisting with Obtaining Blood for Blood Gas Analysis, p. 98.
  Intensive Care, p. 1137.
3. Be aware of specific complications which may occur following surgery for congenital heart disease.
a. Patent ductus arteriosus (rare)
  Recurrent laryngeal nerve injury
b. Coarctation of the aorta
  Paradoxical hypertension
c. Atrial septal defect
  (1) Atrial arrhythmias
  (2) Transient or permanent heart block
d. Ventricular septal defect (VSD)
  (1) Complete heart block
  (2) Recurrent VSD
e. Tetralogy of Fallot
  (1) Low cardiac output
  (2) Pulmonary insufficiency
  (3) Complete heart block
  (4) Recurrent VSD
  (5) Residual pulmonary outflow tract obstruction
f. Transposition of great arteries (Mustard procedure)
  (1) Superior vena cava obstruction
  (2) Pulmonary venous obstruction, pulmonary edema
  (3) Complete heart block
  (4) Residual atrial shunts
  (5) Arrhythmias
g. Aortic stenosis
  Aortic insufficiency
4. Support parents during the time that the child is in the intensive care unit.
a. Accompany parents when they first visit their child following surgery.
  Since this may be traumatic, do not force them to maintain lengthy contact with the child.
b. Address parental concerns and answer questions such as:
  (1) How they should react to their child
  (2) Amount of parental participation that is beneficial
  (3) Fears and fantasies during lengthy periods when they are unable to visit child
  (4) Concern for other children and families
  (5) Technical questions
c. Provide the parents with the phone number of the intensive care unit if they elect to leave.

d. Make certain that parents have a comfortable place to sleep if they elect to stay at the hospital.

e. Reassure parents that it is normal for children to regress following such extensive surgery.

C. *Following Transfer*

The following considerations apply to the child who has been transferred from the intensive care unit.

1. Observe for late complications
   a. Respiratory
      (1) Continue coughing and deep breathing exercises.
      (2) Ambulate child as tolerated.
   b. Infection
      (1) Monitor temperature at regular intervals.
      (2) Observe incision(s) for redness, swelling, drainage.
   c. Congestive heart failure
      Refer to Nursing Management, pp. 1295–1296.
   d. Postpericardiotomy Syndrome
      Symptoms include fever, pericardial friction rub, and pericardial and pleural effusion.
   e. Postperfusion Syndrome
      Symptoms include fever, hepatosplenomegaly, leukocytosis, malaise, and maculopapular rash.
2. Provide emotional support to child and parents:
   a. Explain procedures, medications, special diet to child and parent.
   b. Encourage the child to attend to his personal needs as he is able.
   c. Allow the child to make some decisions in order to give him a feeling of control.
   d. Provide the child with appropriate diversion and play materials.
   e. Encourage parental participation in the child's care.
      (1) Teach parents those aspects of the child's care which they can assume (e.g., coughing and breathing exercises).

(2) Discuss usual convalescent expectations of patient with parents (e.g., fatigue, itching at incision, emotional reactions).

3. Prepare the child and parents for discharge.
   a. Active parental participation in the child's care facilitates discharge teaching.
   b. Provide the family with oral and written discharge recommendations including:
      (1) Activity restrictions
      (2) Care of incision
      (3) Medications—exact amounts and times of administration
      (4) Special diet (low sodium is often indicated)
      (5) Emotional reactions—child may demonstrate:
         (a) Regression in toilet habits, feeding and other learned skills
         (b) Nightmares
         (c) Increased dependency
         (d) Decreased appetite
         (e) Demanding behavior—need to set limits
      (6) Observation for complications:
         (a) Fever
         (b) Increased heart rate
         (c) Chest pain
         (d) Shortness of breath
         (e) Problems with the incision
         (f) Vomiting or diarrhea
         (g) Rash
   c. Provide parents with the names and phone numbers of persons to call for questions and emergencies.

Reference for Teaching

Margaret's Heart Operation, Children's Hospital of Philadelphia, 34th and Civic Center Blvd., Philadelphia, Pa. 19104

ACUTE RHEUMATIC FEVER

Acute rheumatic fever is a systemic disease characterized by inflammatory lesions of connective tissue and endothelial tissue.

Etiology

1. The exact pathogenesis is uncertain.
2. The most important factor in the etiology of rheumatic fever is now accepted to be Group A betahemolytic streptococcus.
3. Most first attacks of rheumatic fever are preceded by streptococcal infection of the throat or upper respiratory tract at an interval of several days to several weeks.
4. There appears to be an inherited tendency or family predisposition toward rheumatic fever.

Altered Physiology

1. The unique pathologic lesion of rheumatic fever is the Aschoff body.
2. The basic changes consist of exudative and proliferative inflammatory reactions in the mesenchymal supporting tissue of the heart, joints, blood vessels, and subcutaneous tissues.

3. The inflammatory process involves all layers of the heart.
4. The inflammation may involve the leaflets and/or chordae tendinae of the heart valves, most frequently the mitral and/or aortic valves.

Clinical Manifestations and Diagnostic Evaluation

No single clinical or laboratory finding is characteristic of rheumatic fever. The diagnosis is based on a combination of manifestations characteristic of this disease and in the absence of other diseases which may mimic it.

1. For this reason, the Jones Criteria, as established by a committee of the American Heart Association, are utilized.
2. The presence of 2 major criteria, or 1 major and 2 minor criteria, plus evidence of a preceding streptococcal infection are required to establish a diagnosis.

A. *Major Manifestations*

1. Carditis—manifested by significant murmurs, signs of pericarditis, cardiac enlargement, or congestive heart failure.

2. Polyarthritis—almost always migratory and manifested by swelling, heat, redness and tenderness, or by pain and limitation of motion of 2 or more joints.
3. Chorea—purposeless, involuntary, rapid movements often associated with muscle weakness.
4. Erythema marginatum—an evanescent, pink rash.
   a. The erythematous areas have pale centers and round or serpiginous (creeping eruption) margins.
   b. They vary greatly in size and occur mainly on the trunk and proximal parts of the extremities, never on the face.
   c. The erythema is transient, migrates from place to place, and may be brought out by the application of heat.
5. Subcutaneous nodules—firm, painless nodules seen or felt over the extensor surface of certain joints, particularly elbows, knees, and wrists, in the occipital region, or over the spinous processes of the thoracic and lumbar vertebrae; the skin overlying them moves freely and is not inflamed.

B. *Minor Manifestations*

1. *Clinical*
   a. History of previous rheumatic fever or evidence of pre-existing rheumatic heart disease
   b. Arthralgia—pain in one or more joints without evidence of inflammation, tenderness to touch, or limitation of motion
   c. Fever—temperature in excess of 38° C. (100.4° F.)
2. *Laboratory*
   a. Erythrocyte sedimentation rate—elevated
   b. C-reactive protein—positive
   c. Electrocardiographic changes—mainly P-R interval prolongation
   d. Leukocytosis

C. *Supporting Evidence of Streptococcal Infection*

1. Increased titer of streptococcal antibodies (antistreptolysin O, or ASO titer)
2. Positive throat culture for Group A streptococci
3. Recent scarlet fever

D. *Other Clinical Features*

1. Abdominal pain
2. Rapid sleeping pulse (tachycardia out of proportion to fever)
3. Malaise
4. Anemia
5. Epistaxis
6. Precordial pain

Nursing Objectives and Management

A. *To become informed as to the child's symptomatology and the medical plan of care.*

1. Discuss with the physician his plan for medical treatment.
2. Make a baseline nursing assessment of the child's condition.
   a. Listen to the child's chest with a stethoscope to become familiar with the murmur or to determine the presence of a murmur not previously heard; listen for a friction rub.
   b. Determine from the child whether he is experiencing any pain or discomfort (also observe the child's facial expression as he moves since children may deny pain thinking they will be able to go home).
   c. Describe the pain as to location, when it occurs,

whether there is any heat, swelling, redness or tenderness.
   d. Examine the knees, elbows, wrists, occipital region and spine for nodules; describe location.
   e. Determine whether the child has any muscle weakness or rapid, purposeless movements.
   f. Assess the child's emotional status.
   g. Report any significant information to the physician.

B. *To initiate specific preventative teaching in order to prevent a recurrence or an additional case of rheumatic fever within the family.*

1. Have all family members screened for streptococcus by referring them for throat cultures.
2. All persons with positive cultures should be treated.
3. Teach the specific symptoms of streptococcal infections.

C. *To treat the precipitating streptococcal infection.*

Administer antibiotics as prescribed by the physician (generally intramuscular penicillin G).

> **NURSING ALERT:** Before administering penicillin, elicit a history for possible drug allergy.

D. *To evaluate the child for evidence of response to treatment or progression of disease.*

1. Observe for the development or disappearance of any major or minor manifestations of the disease.
2. Monitor carditis by careful documentation of the child's pulse, respirations, and blood pressure.
   a. The pulse should be counted for 1 full minute.
   b. The sleeping pulse is a good indicator of the extent of carditis. It should be obtained without waking the child.

E. *To provide symptomatic management of the child's fever.*

1. Refer to section on fever, p. 1148.
2. Antipyretic drugs are usually withheld during the diagnostic period.

F. *To suppress the rheumatic inflammatory process by administering appropriate medications.*

1. Salicylates (generally prescribed for patients without carditis)
   a. Observe for gastrointestinal upsets, ringing in the ears, headaches, bleeding, and disturbances in the mental state.
   b. Administer milk or antacids with salicylates.
   c. Report side effects promptly.
   d. Aspirin therapy should be monitored by salicylate levels.
2. Steroids (generally prescribed for patients with carditis; as steroids are tapered, administration of salicylates is begun).
   a. Prepare the child and his family for the expected side effects of steroid therapy.
      (1) Body appearance may change through rounding facial contour
      (2) Localized fat deposits
      (3) Appearance of acne or excessive hair
      (4) Weight gain with linear markings appearing in the stretched skin
   b. Mental and emotional disturbances may necessitate discontinuance of the medication.
   c. Hypertension and the tendency to accumulate

water and sodium within the tissues may result from steroid therapy.
(1) Provide a low sodium diet.
(2) Weigh child daily—report sudden weight increases.
d. Steroids diminish the child's resistance to infection and may mask symptoms of infection.

> **NURSING ALERT:** Do not place a child with an infectious disease in the room with the child with rheumatic fever.
> Restrict visitors and personnel with infectious diseases from contact with the child on steroid therapy.

e. A combination of steroid therapy and stress may lead to the development of gastric ulcers.
3. Administer medications punctually and at regular intervals to achieve constant therapeutic blood levels.
4. Report signs of increased rheumatic activity as salicylates or steroids are being tapered.

G. *To alleviate the child's anxiety about the functioning of his heart, because anxiety utilizes energy and produces fatigue.*

1. Give the child information about rheumatic fever in terms that he can understand, e.g., "Rheumatic fever is a hard thing to understand because you can't see it. When you scratch yourself, you can see the mark, and you can see the scratch heal. Rheumatic fever is something like that—only you can't see the healing because it happens to the tissue underneath the skin. (And sometimes it happens to the valves in the heart.)"
2. Continually reinforce the teaching and encourage the child to ask questions.
3. Assure the child that physicians know how to treat rheumatic fever.
4. Communicate information about the child's reactions to all staff members in order to provide consistent information.

H. *To decrease the cardiac workload until the acute inflammatory reaction has subsided.*

1. Explain to the child the need for rest (usually prescribed for 4–12 weeks, depending on the severity of the disease and physician's preference).
2. Assure the child that bed rest will be imposed no longer than necessary.
3. Organize nursing care to provide periods of uninterrupted rest.
4. Explain to the child what procedures are going to be performed before they are performed.
5. Assure the child that his needs will be met.
a. Give the child a bell to call the nurse.
b. Answer his calls promptly.
6. Assist the child to resume activity very gradually once he is asymptomatic at rest and indicators of acute inflammation have become normal.
a. Allow the child to participate in decisions about such matters as timing his periods of activity.
b. Monitor the pulse rate carefully after periods of activity in order to assess the degree of cardiac compensation.

I. *To provide frequent and comfortable changes in position to aid in relaxation and to prevent tissue breakdown.*

1. Elevate the back of the bed and support the arms with pillows when child is dyspneic.

2. Position the legs in good body alignment—use a footboard.
3. When the joints are painful, move the child gently, supporting the extremity.
4. Provide meticulous skin care.

J. *To provide nursing care for the child with congestive heart failure.*

Refer to section on congestive heart failure, pp. 1295–1296.

K. *To provide safe, supportive care for the child with chorea.*

1. Place the child in a bed with padded siderails, especially if uncontrolled body movements are severe.
2. Feed the child slowly and carefully because of incoordinate movements of the head, mouth, and swallowing muscles. Avoid the use of sharp eating utensils.
3. Provide frequent feedings that are high in calories, protein, vitamins, and iron, because constant movements cause the child to burn calories at a rapid rate.
4. Spend time talking with the child even though his speech may be defective. If severe, utilize other methods of communication.
5. Administer sedation, if prescribed.
6. Reassure the child about the cause of his instability, and tell him that his symptoms will subside.
7. Encourage positive parent-child relationships which may have been strained if the onset of symptoms was insidious (lack of concentration at school, mood swings, irritability, etc.).
8. Help the child regain his former skills once symptoms begin to subside.
a. Support the child during periods of ambulation.
b. Provide activities which require the use of large muscles and progress to materials which require fine coordination.

L. *To assist the child to develop a realistic attitude toward his illness and encourage him to discuss his concerns.*

1. Help him to realize the restrictions he must face and the fact that progress is slow.
2. Attempt to avoid negative connotations related to activity restrictions. Emphasize what the child is allowed to do—that is, say "You may be up in the chair for 2 hours every day," rather than "You have to stay in bed all day, except for 2 hours."
3. Help him cope with his fears that his playmates may ostracize him or pity him.
4. Alleviate his anxieties about keeping up with his class and school activities.
a. Initiate a referral for a hospital-based school teacher to see him on a regular basis.
b. When this service is not available, encourage the parents to contact his teacher who will prepare lesson plans and short assignments for him—encourage the parents to maintain this contact with the teacher.
c. Plan time each day on a regular basis for the child to complete his assignments.

M. *To provide for diversional activity that will help the child feel a sense of achievement and satisfaction.*

1. Initiate some long-term projects.
2. Refer to section on the hospitalized child, p. 1126.

N. *To help the child to maintain contact with his peers during hospitalization.*

1. Encourage correspondence.
2. Maintain telephone contact, if possible.
3. Place in a room with a child of the same age, sex and interests—preferably a child with a long-term illness.

O. *To assist the family to deal with the emotional and financial stresses caused by the illness and hospitalization.*

1. Assess family's needs in this area and initiate a referral to a social worker if indicated.
2. Refer to section on family-centered care (p. 1131).

P. *To prevent a recurrent attack of rheumatic fever by reinforcing the need for prophylactic antimicrobial therapy.*

1. Penicillin is the drug of choice—either intramuscular benzathine G every 28 days or oral penicillin V or G twice daily.
2. Continuous prophylaxis is recommended throughout the childhood years and well into adult life, often indefinitely.
3. Utilize creativity in recommending methods to remind families about administering the medication.
    a. The child should be taught to assume responsibility for his own medication at an early age so that it becomes habitual.
    b. Some children profit from the use of a calendar or special chart. Others find it useful to associate their medication schedule with other routine tasks, such as brushing their teeth.
4. Be certain that the child receives his prophylactic medication on schedule during his hospitalization and during subsequent hospitalizations (including hospitalization for treatment of other illnesses).

5. When indicated, additional prophylaxis should be utilized for prevention of infective endocarditis.
    The American Heart Association's recommendations for the prevention of endocarditis should be observed for children undergoing certain dental procedures as well as for surgery or instrumentation of the upper respiratory tract, genitourinary tract, or lower gastrointestinal tract.

Q. *To begin to prepare for discharge with the parents in time that sufficient adjustments and preparation may be made.*

1. The child should have a bed of his own and, preferably, a room of his own.
2. A responsible adult must be in the home to care for him.
3. Specific information as to:
    a. Specifically what activity is allowed
    b. When to administer medications, correct amounts —caution about specific side effects
    c. Where to obtain the medication
    d. Specific dietary instruction
    e. Specific symptoms to report:
        Pain
        Malaise
        Anorexia
        Tachycardia (teach to take the pulse)
        Tachypnea
        Weight gain
    f. Telephone number of physician
    g. When to return to clinic
4. Initiate a community nursing referral—this may be done prior to discharge if a home evaluation is desired.

For nursing care of the adult patient with rheumatic heart disease, refer to page 294.

MYOCARDITIS

Myocarditis is an inflammatory disease of the heart. In some instances, the inflammatory process is confined to the myocardium (isolated myocarditis), while in other conditions such as acute rheumatic carditis, myocarditis is part of a pancarditis.

Etiology

1. Often unknown
2. Coxsackie B virus (most common pediatric cause)
3. Rheumatic fever
4. Other infectious agents—viruses, bacteria, fungi, spirochetes, rickettsiae, and parasites
5. Toxic causes—diphtheria, endotoxin, chemotherapeutic agents
6. Various multisystem diseases

Clinical Manifestations

1. Variable, depending on age of child, extent of inflammation, and capacity of myocardium to recover; varies from total absence of clinical manifestations to sudden, unexpected death.
2. Neonate—often presents with sudden onset of congestive heart failure. Signs include respiratory distress, tachycardia, pale skin which is cool and clammy, peripheral cyanosis, diaphoresis, edema, and enlarged liver.

3. Older child:
    a. Onset may be rapid with sudden temperature elevation, dyspnea, and rapid pulse.
    b. Onset may often be insidious, with complaints of fatigue, low-grade fever, respiratory illness, malaise, and gradual development of cardiac findings.

Pathophysiology

1. The inflammatory process interferes with the effectiveness of myocardial contractility.
2. Cardiac enlargement occurs, and congestive heart failure frequently results.
3. Residual myocardial fibrosis may occur, causing subsequent myocardial insufficiency and cardiac enlargement.
4. Prognosis is related to age at onset, extent of inflammation, response to therapy, and presence or absence of recurrences.

Diagnostic Evaluation

1. Auscultation
    a. Heart sounds often indistinct, muffled, or dull.
    b. Systolic murmurs frequently present.
    c. Gallop rhythm possible.
    d. Pulmonary rales may be heard.
2. Palpation

a. Peripheral pulses often rapid, weak, thready.
b. May demonstrate pulsus alternans—a pulse in which there is regular alternation of weak and strong beats.
c. May have hepatomegaly.
3. Chest x-ray—shows generalized cardiomegaly involving all four chambers of the heart. Pulmonary venous congestion is often visualized, and pneumonitis may be present.
4. Electrocardiogram is variable. It may reveal arrhythmias, conduction disturbances, and S–T segment and T-wave changes.
5. Laboratory tests—cultures of blood, stool, nose, and throat; serial antibody testing.

Nursing Objectives and Management

A. *To control the underlying disease causing myocarditis.*

1. Administer specific therapy for treatable conditions such as rheumatic fever, toxoplasmosis, and trichinosis.
2. Administer steroid therapy as prescribed by the physician.
   a. Be aware that steroids are generally not recommended except for the treatment of rheumatic myocarditis with cardiac failure—to suppress the inflammatory process associated with connective tissue disorders, or in situations that are considered life-threatening.
   b. Prepare the child and his family for any expected side effects of steroid therapy:
      (1) Body appearance may change—e.g., rounding of facial contours
      (2) Localized fat deposits
      (3) Appearance of acne or excessive hair
      (4) Weight gain with linear markings appearing in the stretched skin
   c. Be aware of serious side effects of steroid therapy and report promptly:
      (1) Gastrointestinal bleeding, ulcer
      (2) Hypertension and the tendency to accumulate water and sodium within tissues
         (a) Provide a low sodium diet.
         (b) Weigh child daily—report sudden weight gain.

(3) Diminished resistance to infection; may mask symptoms of infection.

> **NURSING ALERT:** Do not place a child with an infectious disease in the room with a child receiving steroid therapy. Restrict visitors and personnel with infectious diseases from contact with the child.

B. *To treat congestive heart failure.*

1. Refer to section on congestive heart failure, page 1295.
2. Be aware that children with myocarditis frequently show increased sensitivity to digitalis and may require a lower dose. Assess for the toxic symptoms.

C. *To observe for the development of cardiac arrhythmias.*

1. Be aware that children with myocarditis are prone to develop arrhythmias.
2. Initiate continuous cardiac monitoring if there is evidence of the development of an arrhythmia. If appropriate, transfer the child to the intensive care unit.
3. Have equipment for resuscitation, cardiac defibrillation, and cardiac pacing available in the event of life-threatening arrhythmia.

D. *To provide supportive nursing care to the severely ill or dying child.*

Refer to section on the dying child, page 1458.

E. *To evaluate the child for evidence of response to treatment or progression of disease.*

1. Observe for the development or disappearance of signs of congestive heart failure.
2. Monitor and record child's pulse, respirations, and blood pressure at frequent intervals.
   a. Count pulse for 1 full minute. Record rate and rhythm.
   b. Monitor the pulse when the child is asleep.

For additional nursing considerations, refer to the section on Nursing Management of Rheumatic Carditis.

INFECTIVE ENDOCARDITIS

Infective endocarditis refers to infection of the endocardial surface of the heart or the intimal surface of certain arterial vessels. It is a rare condition which is usually associated with preexisting cardiovascular disease (congenital or rheumatic) but may develop in a normal heart during a course of septicemia.

For etiology, clinical manifestations, pathophysiology, treatment, and nursing management, refer to discussion on adult, page 294. In addition, the following points of management should be considered by the pediatric nurse.

Nursing Management

1. Although any child with heart disease is at risk for developing endocarditis, those most at risk are children with:
   a. Ventricular septal defect (especially a small VSD).
   b. Surgically created shunts such as Waterston or Blalock shunts.
   c. Patent ductus arteriosus
   d. Semilunar valve stenoses
   e. Coarctation of the aorta
   f. Tetralogy of Fallot
   g. Rheumatic heart disease
2. Long-term (usually at least 4–6 weeks) intravenous administration of antimicrobials is indicated in all cases.
   a. Careful management of intravenous therapy is essential.
      (1) Refer to Intravenous Therapy Procedure, page 1171.
      (2) Drugs must be administered according to schedule to maintain constant therapeutic levels.

(3) The physician should be notified immediately if the IV infiltrates so that it can be restarted.

(4) Heparin locks may be utilized to allow the child freedom of movement between intervals of medication.

b. Appropriate measures should be initiated to help the child maintain his level of development during the lengthy hospitalization.

(1) Refer to The Hospitalized Child, page 1126.

(2) Arrange for continuation of school work.

(3) Facilitate interaction with family, including siblings.

(4) Provide diversional activities that will help the child feel a sense of achievement and satisfaction.

(5) Facilitate contact with peers through written correspondence, telephone, or selected visiting.

3. Prevention is an important nursing responsibility.

a. Procedures which increase the risk of bacteria gaining access to the bloodstream include:

(1) Tooth extraction, oral surgery, and periodontal procedures.

(2) Tonsillectomy and adenoidectomy.

(3) Bronchoscopy

(4) Instrumentation of the genitourinary tract

(5) Surgery or instrumentation of the lower gastrointestinal tract

(6) Childbirth

b. Children with congenital or rheumatic heart disease should receive prophylactic antibiotics in conjunction with these procedures to reduce bacteremia and prevent bacterial implantation. The current recommendations of the American Heart Association for chemoprophylaxis should be observed.

c. The child and family should be instructed regarding the importance of good dental hygiene.

d. Families of children with heart disease should be instructed about prevention of endocarditis, as well as about signs and symptoms of the disease.

ATHEROSCLEROSIS

Atherosclerosis is a condition characterized by fatty deposits on the walls of arteries. It may lead to narrowing and obstruction of major vessels such as the coronary arteries, the arteries of the neck and brain, and those of the lower extremities. It is a cause of coronary heart disease and cerebrovascular disease.

Although the major clinical manifestations of atherosclerosis occur in middle-aged and older adults, the precursors of atherosclerosis may become established in childhood. Thus, the pediatric nurse should be aware of the following factors:

1. Although much is known about the pathology of atherosclerosis and its evolution in adults, there is still much to be learned about its earlier stages.

2. The atherosclerotic process is probably influenced by a variety of inheritance factors, including vascular structure and metabolism as well as environmental factors such as diet.

3. Data indicate that irreversible atherosclerotic changes may occur by 20 years of age. Therefore, the pediatric patient must be identified as being at risk in order for medical treatment to be instituted early enough to meaningfully alter the course of the disease.

Identified Risk Factors

1. Serum lipid disorders—may be genetically determined (e.g., inherited hyperchlolesterolemia) or acquired—probably resulting from an excess intake of saturated fat and cholesterol

2. Hypertension—probably caused by a hereditary predisposition, interacting with environmental factors such as obesity, increased sodium intake, and endogenous and exogenous vasoconstrictors

3. Impaired glucose tolerance

4. Obesity

5. Sedentary living habits, lack of regular exercise

6. Smoking

Nursing Implications

1. Children at risk should be screened for any lipid abnormalities, and these should be corrected by diet or other procedures as indicated.

a. Infants of families with any history of familial hypercholesterolemia or premature cardiovascular disease should be studied for lipid abnormality. If negative, these children should receive periodic reevaluation.

b. All siblings of hyperlipoproteinemic children should be tested.

2. Children should be screened for hypertension at periodic intervals, and appropriate treatment should be initiated.

Refer to Procedure for Taking Blood Pressure, p. 1146 and Normal Vital Sign Values, p. 1145.

3. Initiate diet counseling.

a. Discourage the common habit of adding salt to childhood diets because the habit of adding salt to practically all foods is developed early in life.

b. Teach parents to read labels to learn the sodium content of commercial food products, including baby foods.

c. Counsel parents to provide meals which emphasize skim milk and dairy products derived from skimmed milk, legumes, fruits, starches, lean meats, poultry, and fish. Deemphasize candies, pastries, egg yolks, and animal fats.

d. Discourage overeating and overfeeding.

e. Refer to section on Pediatric Nutrition, p. 1112.

4. Encourage physical activity.

a. Discuss the benefits of physical activity with parents and encourage them to set an example for their children.

b. Encourage participation in physically active games and sports; this helps to establish a pattern for a physically active way of life in adulthood.

5. Discourage cigarette smoking.

a. Discuss the dangers of smoking with parents and encourage them to set a positive example for their children.

b. Make children aware of the dangers of smoking at an early age so that they will be less inclined to develop the habit during adolescence or adult life.

BIBLIOGRAPHY

Books

Anthony C, Arnon R, Fitch C. Pediatric Cardiology. Garden City, Year Book Medical Publishers, 1977

Berenson G. Cardiovascular Risk Factors in Children. The Early Natural History of Atherosclerosis and Essential Hypertension. New York, Oxford University Press, 1980

Berwick D. Cholesterol, Children and Heart Disease. New York, Oxford University Press, 1980

Billig D and Kriedberg M (eds). The Management of Neonates and Infants with Congenital Heart Disease. New York, Grune & Stratton, 1973

Fink BW. Congenital Heart Disease. A Deductive Approach to its Diagnosis. Chicago, Year Book Medical Publishers, 1975

Kaye D. Infective Endocarditis. Baltimore, University Park Press, 1976

Krovetz L, Gessner I, Schieber G (eds). Handbook of Pediatric Cardiology, 2nd ed. Baltimore, University Park Press, 1979

Markowitz M and Gordes L. Rheumatic Fever, 2nd ed. (Vol. II in the series, Major Problems in Clinical Pediatrics.) Philadelphia, WB Saunders, 1972

Moller J. Essentials of Pediatric Cardiology, 2nd ed. Philadelphia, FA Davis 1978

Moss A, Adams F, Emmanouilides G (eds). Heart Disease in Infants, Children and Adolescents. Baltimore, Williams & Wilkins, 1977

Mustard W et al (eds). Pediatric Surgery, Vol I. Chicago, Year Book Medical Publishers, 1979

Petrillo M and Sanger S. Emotional Care of Hospitalized Children, 2nd ed. Philadelphia, JB Lippincott, 1980

Rowe R and Kidd B (eds). The Child With Congenital Heart Disease After Surgery. Mount Kisco, Futura Pub Co., 1975

Strong WB (ed). Atherosclerosis: Its Pediatric Aspects. New York, Grune & Stratton, 1978

Whaley L and Wong D. Nursing Care of Infants and Children. St. Louis, CV Mosby, 1979

Articles

Bindler RM. Home care for a child with a cardiac defect. Issues Compr Pediatr Nurs 1979 Dec; 3:48–60

Chameides L. Congenital heart disease—its effect on the school age child. J Sch Health 1979 Apr; 49(4):205–209

Committee on Rheumatic Fever and Bacterial Endocarditis of the Council on Cardiovascular Disease in the Young of the American Heart Association. Rheumatic Fever Prevention. New York, American Heart Association, 1976

Ebert PA. Conduits—indications, problems and future use. Adv Cardiol 1979, 26:138–139

Ebert PA. Past present and future of palliative shunts. Adv Cardiol 1979; 26:127–128

Ehlers KH. Growth failure in association with congenital heart disease. Pediatr Ann 1978 Nov; 7(11):750–759

Garson A et al. Parental reactions to children with congenital heart disease. Child Psychiatry Hum Dev 1978 Winter; 9(2):86–94

Gildea J et al. Congenital cardiac defects: Pre- and postoperative nursing care. Am J Nurs 1978 Feb; 78(2):273–280

Gottesfeld I. The family of the child with congenital heart disease. MCN 1979 Mar/Apr; 4(2):101–104

Jackson P. Digoxin therapy at home: Keeping the child safe. MCN 1979 Mar/Apr;4(2):105–109

Kitchen LW. Psychological factors in congenital heart disease in children. J Fam Pract 1978 Apr; 6(4):777–783

Lampe RM et al. Brain abscess following dental extraction in a child with cyanotic heart disease. Pediatrics 1978 Apr; 6(4):659–660

Miller W et al. Pediatric cardiology—minimizing the risks of adult heart disease . . . the young cardiac patient: Management considerations. Pediatr Nurs 1980 Jan/Feb; 5(1):29–38

Modrcin MA et al. An update of congenital heart failure in infants. Issues Compr Pediatr Nurs 1979 Dec; 3:5–22

Moss AJ. What every primary physician should know about the postoperative cardiac patient. Pediatrics 1979 Feb; 63(2):320–330

Myers–Vando R et al. The effects of congenital heart disease on cognitive development, illness causality, concepts and vulnerability. Am J Orthopsychiatry 1979 Oct; 49(4):617–625

Nauright L et al. Identifying hypertensive adolescents. Pediatric Nursing 1979 Mar/Apr; 5(2):34–37

Nora JJ et al. The evolution of specific genetic and environmental counseling in congenital heart diseases. Circulation 1978 Feb; 57(2):205–213

Rowland TW. The pediatrician and congenital heart disease—1979. Pediatrics 1979 Aug; 64(2):180–186

Sacksteder S, Gildes J, Dassy D. Common congenital cardiac defects. Am J Nurs 1978 Feb; 78(2):266–272

Shor V. Congenital cardiac defects: Assessment and case finding. Am J Nurs 1978 Feb; 78(2):256–261

Smith K. Recognizing cardiac failure in neonates. MCN 1979 Mar/Apr; 4(2):98–100

Uzark K. A child's cardiac catheterization—avoiding the potential risks. MCN 1978 May/June; 3(3):158–161

Vogel M. Hypertension in children. Pediatric Nursing 1977 Nov/Dec; 3(6):37–39

Agency

American Heart Association, 44 East 23rd Street, New York, New York, 10010

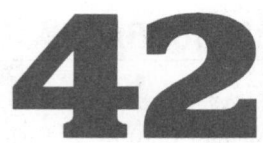
DENTAL CARIES

Dental caries involves loss of tooth structure or the formation of a cavity as a result of bacterial attack—first on the enamel, which is the hard surface of the tooth, and then progressing inward toward the pulp.

Etiology and Pathophysiology

A. *Bacteria*

1. Acidogenic organisms—decalcify the hard tissue by producing acids upon the tooth surface.
2. Proteolytic organisms—digest the product of tooth surface (decalcification thus produces odor and discoloration).
3. Leptotrichae organisms—form structures on the smooth tooth surface which houses acidogenic organisms.

B. *Contributing Factors*

1. Age—most susceptible age groups are children, 4–8 years (primary teeth), and adolescents, 12–18 years (permanent teeth).
2. Diet—large intake of simple sugars between meals, milk-bottle caries in infants and toddlers.
3. Familial tendency to tooth decay.
4. Lack of proper oral hygiene.
5. Poor state of health (illness alters the normal bacteriostatic quality of saliva), chronic disease.

Clinical Manifestations

1. Decay is acute and rapidly penetrates the tooth in children.
2. Caries occurs where food debris collects.
   a. Pits and fissures
   b. Between teeth
   c. At neck of tooth
3. Discoloration of teeth.
4. Decay odor.
5. Pain, abscess, or infection.

Treatment

1. Removal of decay and restoration of tooth surfaces involved.
2. Removal of diseased tooth or teeth that are decayed beyond restoration.

Complications

As a result of missing teeth or multiple caries, the child may experience many problems:
1. Poor nutrition
   a. Refusal to eat foods that need chewing
   b. Teeth drift and cause malocclusion
2. Faulty speech habits and articulation
   a. Weak jaw muscles
   b. Abnormal alveolar bone development
3. Psychological problems
   Embarrassment caused by appearance of teeth and oral odor
4. Oral foci of infection
   Subacute bacterial endocarditis may result in child with congenital heart disease.

Prevention

1. Fluoridation of water supply
2. Biannual topical application of fluoride to teeth
3. Decreased eating between meals
4. Decreased eating of sucrose-containing snacks
5. Removal of plaque and debris from tooth surface with brushing

Nursing Objectives and Health Education

Hospitalization of a child for treatment of dental caries is likely only when special behavior difficulties are anticipated in treatment, when medical problems complicate dental treatment or when extensive repair is necessary.
(See Preventive Pediatrics, Dental Care, p. 1118.)

A. *To prevent dental caries in all patients.*

B. *To know that there is a direct relationship between incidence of dental caries in children and dental health education or knowledge of parents.*

1. Assess parental knowledge and use opportunities to teach parents preventive care.

2. Encourage parental participation with the young child during teeth brushing exercise.

C. *To know the principles of good oral hygiene and practice them when caring for each pediatric patient.*

1. Encourage mouth rinsing or teeth brushing after eating.
   Brush before bedtime to decrease bacteriogenic activity in the warm, undisturbed mouth during sleep.
2. Encourage proper brushing of teeth.
   a. Brush crosswise with a soft bristled brush.
   b. Electric tooth brush cleans teeth and stimulates the gingivae.
3. Supervise brushing in young children. (Dentrifice is not necessary.)

D. *To know the value of good nutrition and its effect in preventing dental caries.*

1. No in-between meal snacking of refined sugar foods. No gum chewing, except of sugarless gum.
   a. Improves appetite at meals.
   b. Substitute fresh fruit for refined sugars. (No lollipops between meals; give after meal before brushing.)
2. Discourage a bottle, other than water, at bedtime or before sleep.
   Residue is left on teeth during long periods of sleep and results in rampant decay.

E. *To know the value of periodic dental examination and preventive measures used to decrease decay.*

1. Encourage patient and parent to participate in regular dentist visits.
   a. Regular visits for cleaning and checking for decay; repair if necessary.

First visit is to familiarize the young child with the dentist and equipment.
   (1) Usually age 18–30 months—or when all primary teeth have erupted
   (2) Should not be when child has toothache
   b. During childhood and adolescence visits are every 3–6 months.
   New decay appears suddenly in multiple areas and advances rapidly.
2. If fluoridation is not supplied in community water, topical application is advisable.
   a. Most effective when applied on newly erupted teeth.
   b. Fluoride makes enamel more resistant to decay as it strengthens calcification of the developing dental tissue.

F. *To keep the adolescent aware of his diet and its effect on dental decay.*

1. Keep in mind diet fads and peer group pressure.
2. Have patient keep a dietary record for 1 week. Then evaluate it against an example of a good nutritious diet. Encourage patient to make his own evaluation.

Parental Education

1. After assessment of parental knowledge has been made, embark on teaching program.
   Main areas of concern:
   a. Proper technique of dental hygiene
   b. Value of good nutrition
   c. Value of fluoridation
   d. Importance of regular visits to the dentist every 3–6 months.
2. American Dental Association, 211 East Chicago Avenue, Chicago, Ill. 60611

CLEFT LIP AND PALATE

Cleft lip and palate results when fusion involving the first brachial arch fails to take place during embryonic development.

Etiology

1. Failure of embryonic development—cause not known
2. Heredity factor

Altered Physiology

1. The lip and palate develop independently; thus, any combination of defects can occur.
   a. Cleft lip—prealveolar cleft
      (1) Varies from a notch in the lip to complete separation of the lip into the nose
      (2) May be unilateral or bilateral
   b. Isolated cleft palate—postalveolar cleft
      (1) Cleft of uvula
      (2) Cleft of soft palate
      (3) Cleft of both soft and hard palate through roof of mouth
      (4) Unilateral or bilateral
   c. Cleft lip and palate combined
      Any degree of involvement
   d. Submucous cleft
      (1) Muscles of soft palate are not joined
      (2) Not recognized until child talks; cannot be seen at birth
2. Associated problems

   a. Eating
      (1) Suction cannot be created for effective sucking
      (2) Food returns through the nose
   b. Nasal speech
   c. Lack of normal dental function and appearance
   d. Repeated bouts of otitis media with subsequent hearing loss

Clinical Manifestations

Physical appearance of cleft lip or palate
1. Incompletely formed lip
2. Opening in roof of mouth

Nursing Objectives and Management

Newborn

A. *To show acceptance of the baby.*

1. The nurse must maintain her composure and not show shock when handling the infant. The manner in which the nurse handles the baby can make a lasting impression on the parents.
   a. The baby with a cleft lip can be unattractive and can cause shock when first seen.
   b. When showing a newborn baby to parents for the first time, support them by accepting both the baby and the parent's feelings. (Parents may be grieving about the perfect infant they did not have and may harbor ambivalent feelings about this baby.)

c. Be supportive of parents by reassuring them that reparative surgery can be done with much success.

   (1) The time when reparative surgery is done depends upon the surgeon, the condition of the baby and the degree to which the parents have accepted the baby.

   (2) Lip surgery may be done several hours after birth or when the infant is 2–3 months of age or has gained 4.54 kg. (10 pounds).

2. Reparative surgery of the palate is done between 12–18 months of age.

   At this age, speech patterns have not been set, yet growth of involved structures allows for improved surgical repair.

B. *To establish and maintain adequate nutrition for growth and development.*

1. Babies with just a cleft lip may feed well if a soft nipple with enlarged holes is used.

2. With certain types and combinations of cleft lips and palates, the baby is unable to create a vacuum and is thus unable to suck. Several types of nipples and feeding devices are available to make feedings easier. A soft base or disposable bottle can be helpful by applying gentle, constant pressure to maintain flow. Feed slowly.

   a. Regular nipple with enlarged holes

   b. Lamb's nipple

   c. Duckey nipple

   d. Brecht feeder

   e. Rubber-tipped asepto syringe or dropper. (Rubber extension should be long enough to extend back into the mouth to prevent regurgitation through the nose.)

3. Feed baby in an upright sitting position to decrease possibility of fluid being aspirated or returned through the nose.

   a. Bubble frequently during feeding, because these babies swallow a great deal of air.

   b. Avoid repeated removal of nipple from infant's mouth because of fear of choking, as this only frustrates the infant, causing him to cry and increasing chances of aspiration.

4. Advance diet as appropriate for age and needs of the baby.

   Eating often improves when solids are introduced, since they are easier for baby to manipulate.

5. Encourage mother to begin feeding infant herself as soon as possible.

C. *To prevent infection in the child so that surgery will not have to be delayed.*

1. Avoid patient contact with anyone who has an infection.

2. Change the baby's position frequently.

3. Clean the cleft after each feeding with clear water and a cotton-tipped applicator.

D. *To support the respiratory efforts and the establishment of adequate nutritional intake and feeding pattern in the infant with Pierre Robin syndrome.* (Features of Pierre Robin syndrome are cleft palate, glossoptosis [tongue falls back on pharynx], and micrognathia [underdeveloped mandible].)

1. Prevent respiratory obstruction, especially on inspiration and when infant is quiet.

   a. Place infant in prone position so that tongue and jaw fall forward.

   b. Tilt head back as best tolerated by infant and slightly elevate upper trunk.

   c. Stockinette cap securely attached to infant's head and suspended from an overhead support may be of some benefit in assisting infant to maintain a position for easy ventilation.

   d. Suction nasopharynx as needed.

   e. The tongue may be sutured to pull it forward; if this is done, observe for slipping, cut tongue, and infection.

2. When this infant is fed, consideration must be given to his respiratory effort, flaccid tongue and cleft palate. Generally, feeding can be done with a nursing bottle (feeding techniques similar to those used for cleft palate).

   a. Use orthopneic position—vertical and slightly forward; this allows infant to push jaw forward to suck and also allows the feeder a clear view of the infant.

   b. Gentle finger pressure by feeder at mandibular attachment can aid in bringing jaw forward.

   c. Feed slowly.

3. By 3–4 months of age, the mandible has grown enough to accommodate the tongue, and respiratory difficulty is greatly diminished.

4. Additional complications associated with Pierre Robin syndrome are slow weight gain and ear infections.

E. *To assist parents in preparing to take the newborn home from the nursery before lip and palate surgery has been done.*

Health Education

1. Prepare mother for home feedings. She should have several days to practice feeding in order to become familiar with the baby's feeding pattern.

   a. Home equipment should be used in the hospital.

   b. Mother should be aware of difficulties with feeding and how to handle them.

     (1) Formula returning through the nose

     (2) Respiratory distress

     (3) Longer time necessary for feeding

   c. Suggest that about a week or so prior to scheduled admission for surgery, mother begin using feeding technique preferred by surgeon for postoperative feeding.

     (1) Side of spoon

     (2) Rubber-tipped dropper

     (3) Toddler cup

2. Encourage parents to prepare siblings at home for the arrival of this baby. (Pictures of the new baby might be suggested.)

3. Initiate a community nurse referral to continue emotional support and teaching program at home.

4. Offer parents available literature about children with cleft lip and palate.*

5. Parents should know what plans have been started for surgical treatment.

6. Social work referral may be indicated.

   a. To listen to mother express her concerns regarding management at home with a handicapped child.

   b. To arrange financial assistance.

    * *The Child with a Cleft Palate.* U.S. Department of Health, Education and Welfare, Social and Rehabilitation Service.
Booklets sponsored by Mead Johnson Laboratories, Evansville, Ind. 47721:
Road to Normalcy for the Cleft Lip and Palate Child
Steps in Habilitation for the Cleft Lip and Palate Child

F. *To be aware of the complexity of long-range care and the importance of the many disciplines involved in the eventual outcome.* The nurse should know all the ramifications and potential problems for this child and his family.

1. The organization of trained professional people from the many disciplines that become involved include: pediatrician, plastic surgeon, otologist, general dentist, orthodontist, prosthodontist, medical-social worker, nurse, speech therapist and psychologist.
2. Long-term follow-up and reparative surgery:
   a. Chronic otitis media and hearing loss (Eustachian tube is abnormally located.)
   b. Lip, palate, and orthodontic repair
   c. Speech therapy
   d. Psychological insult to the child
3. Financial burden on the family
   State programs for crippled children can offer relief.
4. Psychological trauma to the family

G. *To emphasize the importance of the mother's role in caring for the child during outpatient treatment and the many hospitalizations required.*

Mother can offer a great deal of security to the child when he is subjected to the trauma and frightening experiences of treatment.

Preoperative Care of the Child with a Cleft Lip

A. *To prepare the infant for postoperative care so that it will be familiar to him, less frightening and easier for him to accept after surgery.*

1. Practice the feeding method to be used as preferred by the surgeon
   a. Rubber-tipped syringe or asepto syringe
   b. Side of spoon
2. The use of elbow restraints for short periods of time.
   a. Let the child play with them if he is old enough.
   b. Allow mother to become involved in their use.
   c. Jacket restraint may be necessary in the older child to prevent him from rolling over.
3. Help the infant get used to being on his back or propped on his side for long periods of time.

B. *To prepare the mother (parents) as to what to expect when she sees the child postoperatively.*

1. Explain the use of the Logan bow (a curved metal wire that prevents stress on the suture line) and restraints.
2. Encourage mother to be with the infant especially when he wakes up from anesthesia to offer him security and comfort.

Postoperative Care of the Child with a Cleft Lip

A. *To administer good postoperative care based on general principles and to observe for usual postoperative complications.*

B. *To prevent injury to the suture line of the lip.*

1. Elbow restraints are the most effective way to prevent busy hands from reaching the lip, yet still allow some freedom of movement.
   a. Pad restraint and place it from the axilla to inner aspect of the wrist.
   b. Remove restraints occasionally, one at a time, to exercise the arms.
2. Logan bow or Band-Aid placed cheek-to-cheek across top of lip prevents lateral tension.
   Prevent wetting tape, or it will loosen.

3. Prevent baby from crying, because crying also increases tension on the suture line.
   a. Encourage mother to hold and cuddle infant.
   b. Keep the infant dry, fed, and comfortable.
4. Position infant on his back or propped on his side to keep him from rubbing his lip on the sheets. An infant seat may be useful for variation of position, comfort, and entertainment. Provide for appropriate diversional activity, hanging toys, mobiles, etc.

C. *To maintain adequate nutrition and fluid intake for weight gain, growth and prevention of dehydration.*

1. For several days postoperatively feeding will have to be accomplished without tension on the suture line.
   a. Dropper or syringe with a rubber tip, inserted from side to avoid suture line or to avoid stimulating sucking.
   b. Side of spoon (Never put spoon into the mouth.)
   c. Nasogastric gavage—usually last treatment of choice
2. Advance slowly to nipple feeding as indicated by physician preference.
   Baby should be able to suck more efficiently with the lip repaired.
3. Encourage mother to participate as much as possible in the care of the infant. It is good for both infant and mother to continue their relationship.

D. *To keep the suture line clean, to decrease infection and eliminate crust formation which enlarges the resulting scar.* The sutures are removed from 3–14 days after surgery.

   Clean suture line after every feeding.
   a. The cleansing solution used is usually the physician's choice.
      (1) Water
      (2) Hydrogen peroxide
      (3) Saline solution
   b. Gently and frequently wipe with a wet cotton tip applicator.
   c. Gently dry by patting.
      (1) May use antibiotic ointment or petrolatum after drying.
      (2) May be left open to the air.
   d. Water should be given after feeding to clean the mouth.

Preoperative Care of the Child with a Cleft Palate
(Repair may require several operations.)

A. *To be familiar with growth and development as well as the emotional and psychological needs of the toddler, 12–18 months old. (This is the age most common for palate repair.)*

1. Primary objectives for palate repair are to improve speech and to minimize maxillary growth retardation and dental alveolar deformity.
2. This toddler age is selected because the anatomical structures involved are still growing.
3. The toddler finds the hospital strange and frightening. (See p. 1128.)
   a. Encourage mother to stay with the child if possible.
   b. Encourage play.

B. *To prepare the child for postoperative care; if he is familiar with the procedures and routines he will be less frightened and more likely to cooperate.*

1. Use elbow restraints frequently for short periods of time.
2. Do not allow the child to suck from a bottle. Ideally,

he has been taught to drink from a cup. Feed him in the manner in which he will be fed postoperatively.

3. Practice frequent mouth irrigations using the same solution and equipment to be used postoperatively. Allow the child to handle and become familiar with equipment.

C. *To prevent infection by keeping the child away from anyone with infection.*

D. *To prepare the parents as to what to expect when they see the child postoperatively.*

Include the parents in the preparation of the child. Then, with the parents alone discuss in more depth what to expect.

Postoperative Care of the Child with a Cleft Palate

A. *To administer good postoperative care and to observe for possible postoperative complications.*

1. Breathing with a closed palate is different from child's customary way of breathing; the child must also contend with increased mucus production.
2. Note respiratory effort.
3. Croup tent with mist decreases occurrence of respiratory problems and provides moisture to mucous membranes which may become dry because of mouth breathing.
4. Infant may lie on abdomen.

B. *To prevent injury to the suture line in the mouth.*

1. Use elbow restraints.
2. Do not put anything into the mouth. Do not allow the use of straws, eating utensils, fingers.
3. Prevent the child from crying. Blowing, sucking, talking, and laughing put strain on suture line.

C. *To keep the suture line and mouth clean to prevent infection.*

1. Irrigate mouth with normal saline or water.
   a. Direct gentle stream over suture line using ear bulb syringe.
   b. Have child in sitting position with his head forward.
2. Keep mouth moist to promote healing and provide comfort.
3. Rinse mouth after each feeding.

D. *To maintain adequate nutrition for growth and to promote healing.*

1. Diet progresses from clear liquids to full liquids to soft foods.
   Soft foods are usually continued for about 1 month after surgery at which time a regular diet is started, excluding hard food.
2. Check weight periodically to see if adequate nutrition is being maintained.
3. Feed the child in the manner used preoperatively (Cup, side of spoon or rubber-tipped syringe). Never use straw, nipple, plain syringe.

E. *To administer antibiotics as prescribed.*

The mouth and suture line are constantly contaminated.

F. *To provide opportunities for social relationships and play as soon as possible.*

1. While the child must be restrained, he especially needs to have some stimulation and diversional activity.
2. A satisfactory relationship with mother or the nurse can minimize frustration and discomfort from surgery and restraints.

G. *To continue support of parents who have already encountered many frustrations in caring for the child, and to foster continual parental acceptance of the child and his handicap.*

1. Solicit assistance of social worker if appropriate; mother may talk about problems she is having raising a handicapped child.
2. Sincerely compliment the parents for the good work they have already done with this child.
3. Help parents understand that this child can live a normal life in the community.

H. *To begin discharge planning and health teaching soon after admission so parents can learn how to care for the child at home.*

1. Continued protection of the mouth.
   a. May need to use elbow restraints.
   b. Child this age will put everything into mouth—restrict this.
   c. No sucking or blowing.
2. Diet of soft foods will need to be continued. Do not give lollipops.
3. Infection must be prevented.
   Continue to clean mouth after eating.

Parental Education

1. There are 3 specific times when parental teaching is vitally important for continual, effective management of the child:
   a. Management of the child with cleft lip and palate not yet repaired
   b. Preparing for lip or palate surgery.
   c. Preparing for patient's discharge following surgery.
2. In each case specific instructions need to be given in the following areas:
   a. Good nutrition and feeding techniques
   b. Proper oral hygiene
   c. Prevention of injury to operative site
   d. Prevention of infection
   e. Plan for follow-up, especially after surgery
   f. Psychological and social development of child—including speech therapy
3. Other members of the family must be considered.
   a. The child with a cleft lip or palate should not be thought of as sick, but as a child who has special needs, to promote his individual growth and development. But he does not require attention all the time.
   b. The family should be included in his care, but they also must have a life of their own.
   c. The parents need time to themselves.
4. Help the parents realize that even though rehabilitation of the child is long-drawn-out and expensive, the child can live a normal life.
   a. Have the parents discuss the child's problem with the school nurse, the teacher and other responsible adults who will have close contact with the child.
   b. Long-range planning should include detailed communication between the family and various disciplines.
      (1) Collaborative effort between disciplines determines the effectiveness of each discipline.
      (2) Parents may need help in understanding the value of each discipline for the future well-being of their child.
         Speech therapy is often one area where the value is not completely understood.

ESOPHAGEAL ATRESIA WITH TRACHEOESOPHAGEAL FISTULA

Esophageal atresia is failure of the esophagus to form a continuous passage from the pharynx to the stomach during embryonic development. *Tracheoesophageal fistula* is the abnormal connection between the trachea and esophagus.

Etiology

1. Failure of embryonic development
2. Cause unknown in most cases

Clinical Manifestations

Appear soon after birth.
1. Excessive amount of secretions
   a. Constant drooling
   b. Large amount of secretions from nose
2. Intermittent cyanosis
   Aspiration of accumulated saliva in blind pouch
3. Abdominal distention
   Inspired air from trachea passes through fistula into stomach.
4. If fed, the infant will respond violently after first or second swallow.
   a. Infant coughs and chokes.
   b. Fluid returns through nose and mouth.
   c. Cyanosis occurs.
   d. Infant struggles.
5. Inability to pass catheter through nose or mouth into stomach—tip of catheter will stop at blind pouch, or atresia.

NOTE: Be aware of coiling of catheter; coiling may make catheter *appear* to be descending into stomach.

Pathophysiology

A. *Classification of Esophageal Atresia*

Type I —Proximal and distal segments of esophagus are blind; there is no connection to trachea—10–15% of cases.

Type II —Proximal segment of esophagus opens into trachea by a fistula; distal segment is blind—very rare.

Type III—Proximal segment of esophagus has blind end; distal segment of esophagus connects into trachea by a fistula (most common; discussion is limited to this type—80–90% of cases).

Type IV—Esophageal atresia with fistula between both proximal and distal ends of trachea and esophagus—very rare.

Type V —Both proximal and distal segments of esophagus open into trachea by a fistula; no esophageal atresia (H-type)—not usually diagnosed at birth.

B. *Type III—Tracheoesophageal Fistula (TEF)*

1. Child is unable to swallow effectively.
2. Saliva or formula accumulates in upper esophageal pouch and is aspirated into airway from spillover.
3. Regurgitation of gastric acid through distal fistula.
   a. Abdominal distention occurs as a result of air entering the lower esophagus via the fistula and passing into the stomach, especially when child is crying.
   b. Gastric distention may be severe enough to cause respiratory distress by elevation of the diaphragm.

Diagnostic Evaluation

1. Recognize infants at risk for TEF. Two major groups are at risk:
   a. Infants with polyhydramnios
   b. Premature infants
2. Observations of specific symptoms manifested by infant.
3. Inability to pass a stiff, radiopaque 10–14 Fr. catheter into stomach through nose or mouth.
4. X-ray, flat plate of abdomen and chest—reveals presence of gas in stomach and tip of catheter in blind pouch.

Complications Associated with TEF

1. Pneumonitis—secondary to: (a) salivary aspiration, (b) gastric acid reflux
2. Concomitant lesions
   a. Congenital heart disease
   b. Gastrointestinal anomalies, particularly imperforate anus
   c. Skeletal and muscular deformities
3. Prematurity

Treatment

1. Immediate treatment
   a. Propping infant to prevent reflux
   b. Suctioning of upper esophageal pouch with Replogle tube
2. Appropriate treatment of any existing pathologic processes—either acquired complications, such as pneumonitis, or complications from concomitant lesions, such as congestive heart failure.
3. Surgery
   a. Prompt primary repair: division of fistula and esophageal anastomosis of proximal and distal segments.
   b. Short-term delay—subsequent primary repair: used to stabilize infant and to prevent deterioration when patient's condition contraindicates immediate surgery.
   c. Staging: initial fistula division and gastrostomy with later secondary esophageal anastomosis. Approach may be used with very small premature infant, very sick neonate, or when severe congenital anomalies exist.

Nursing Objectives and Management

Preoperative

A. *To position baby with head and chest elevated 20–30 degrees to prevent or decrease reflux of gastric juices into the tracheobronchial tree.*

1. This position may also ease respiratory effort by dropping distended intestines away from the diaphragm.
2. Prone position will allow gastric juices to pool anteriorly away from esophagus. Turn frequently to prevent atelectasis and pneumonia.

B. *To assist in removing nasopharyngeal secretions from esophageal blind pouch and to support infant's respiration.*

1. Intermittent nasopharyngeal suctioning or indwelling Replogle tube (double lumen tube) or sump tube with constant suction is used.

a. Tip of tube is placed in the blind pouch.
b. Replogle or sump tube allows air to be drawn in via a second lumen and prevents tube obstruction by mucous membrane of pouch.
c. Maintain indwelling tube patency by irrigating with 1 ml. normal saline frequently.
d. Change indwelling tube as needed and at least once every 12–24 hours; alternate nostrils. Take care to prevent necrosis of nostrils from pressure by catheter.
2. Place infant in Isolette or radiant warmer with high humidity to aid in liquefying secretions and thick mucus. Give mouth care.
3. Administer oxygen as needed.
4. Be alert for indications of respiratory distress:
a. Retractions
b. Circumoral cyanosis
c. Restlessness
d. Nasal flaring
e. Increased respiration and heart rate

C. *To administer antibiotics and other medications prescribed.*

Give to prevent or treat associated pneumonitis.

D. *To monitor parenteral fluids as prescribed in order to prevent dehydration and electrolyte imbalance* (see p. 1170).

1. Supplies water, caloric and mineral requirements.
2. The infant does not receive oral feedings.

E. *To observe infant carefully for any change in condition; report changes immediately.*

1. Check vital signs, color, amount of secretions, abdominal distention, and respiratory distress.
2. Also be alert for complications that can occur in any neonate or premature infant.

F. *To prevent infection by using the principles of isolation.*

Isolette may be used for environmental isolation.

G. *To be available and to recognize need for emergency care or resuscitation.*

Accompany infant to x-ray or operating room in Isolette with portable oxygen and suction equipment.

H. *To administer supportive nursing care that will prevent any deterioration of infant's condition and will assist in preparation for surgery.*

1. Careful observations, recording and reporting of any signs or symptoms that may indicate additional congenital anomalies or complications.
2. Maintain infant temperature in thermoneutral zone.
3. Gastrostomy tube may be placed prior to definitive surgery to aid in gastric decompression and prevention of reflux. Ensure proper functioning of gastrostomy tube by frequent irrigation with normal saline.

Postoperative Care
There are 2 types of surgery considered for esophageal atresia with tracheoesophageal fistula: (1) fistula division and esophageal anastomosis (called *primary repair*) and (2) palliative surgery temporarily using a gastrostomy and cervical esophagostomy until the infant gains weight so that a bowel transplant or anastomosis can be done. Generally the nursing care is essentially the same for either procedure.

A. *To administer good postoperative care and to observe for signs of possible complications.*

B. *To maintain a patent airway to prevent oxygen starvation, apnea, and aspiration of secretions.*

1. Request that physician mark a suction catheter, indicating how far the catheter can be safely inserted without disturbing the anastomosis.
a. Suction frequently—every 5–10 minutes may be necessary; at least every 1–2 hours.
b. Observe for signs of obstructed airway.
2. Administer chest physiotherapy as prescribed by physician.
a. Change infant's position by turning; stimulate him to cry so that he fully expands his lungs.
b. Head and shoulders elevated 20–30 degrees.
c. Mechanical vibrator (to minimize trauma to anastomosis) may be used 2–3 days postoperatively followed by more vigorous physical therapy after third day. Care should be taken not to hyperextend the neck, this causing stress to operative site.
3. Continue use of Isolette or radiant warmer with humidity. Either device does the following:
a. Provides an environment in which infant can maintain temperature in thermoneutral zone.
b. Provides humidity to liquefy secretions.
c. Allows for observation of and easy access to infant.
4. Be prepared to function in an emergency.
Have emergency equipment available:
(1) Suction machine, catheter
(2) Oxygen
(3) Laryngoscope, endotracheal tubes in varying sizes

C. *To be aware of type of chest drainage present, which may be determined by surgical approach, and provide appropriate care.*

1. Retropleural—small tube in posterior mediastinum; may be left open for drainage.
2. Transthoracic—chest tube placed in pleural space and connected to suction.
a. Keep tubing free from clots; keep it unkinked and without tension.
b. If break occurs in the closed drainage system, clamp tubing close to infant immediately to prevent pneumothorax.

D. *To assist in maintaining adequate nutrition to promote healing, growth, and development.*

Feedings may be given by mouth, by gastrostomy, or—rarely—by a feeding tube into the esophagus, depending upon the type of operation performed and the infant's condition.

1. Gastrostomy feeding
a. Gastrostomy feeding can be started prior to esophageal healing—adequate nutrition is an important factor in healing.
b. Gastrostomy feedings may be continued until infant can tolerate full feedings orally.
c. Care should be taken not to allow air to enter stomach, thereby causing gastric distention and possible reflux.
d. Check with the surgeon before allowing infant to suck on pacifier during gastrostomy feeding.
2. Oral feedings may begin 6–14 days postoperatively following anastomosis.
a. Feed slowly to allow infant time to swallow.
b. Use upright sitting position.
c. Burp frequently.

d. Demand feeding may be more successful and pleasant for the infant than strictly scheduled feeding.

e. Do not allow infant to become overtired at feeding time. Note cardiac rate.

f. Try to make each feeding a pleasant experience for the infant. Use consistent approach and patience.

E. *To care appropriately for cervical esophagostomy.*

1. Keep the area clean of saliva.
   a. Wash with clear water.
   b. Place an absorbent pad over the area.

2. As soon as possible allow infant to suck a few milliliters of milk at the same time gastrostomy feeding is being done. Advance infant to solid foods as appropriate if esophagostomy is maintained for a few months.
   a. Encourage sucking and swallowing.
   b. Familiarize infant with food, so that when he is able to eat orally, he will be used to it.

F. *To be aware of impending complications of esophageal repair.*

1. Leak at the anastomosis (development of mediastinitis, pneumothorax, and saliva in chest tube).
   a. Hypothermia or hyperthermia
   b. Pneumothorax
      (1) Severe respiratory distress
      (2) Cyanosis
      (3) Restlessness
      (4) Weak pulses

2. Stricture at the anastomosis
   a. Difficulty in swallowing
   b. Vomiting or spitting up of ingested fluid
   c. Refusing to eat
   d. Fever—secondary to aspiration and pneumonia

3. Recurrent fistula
   a. Coughing, choking, and cyanosis associated with feeding
   b. Excessive salivation
   c. Difficulty in swallowing associated with abnormal distention
   d. Repeated episodes of pneumonitis
   e. General poor physical condition—no weight gain

4. Atelectasis or pneumonitis
   a. Aspiration
   b. Respiratory distress

G. *To provide for the infant's emotional and social needs.*

The extent of hospitalization and long-term care puts a strain on the normal opportunities in these areas (see ICN, p. 1134).

1. Hold and cuddle infant for feedings and/or after feedings.
2. Encourage mother (parents) to cuddle and love infant.
3. Provide for visual, auditory, and tactile stimulation as appropriate for infant's physical condition and age.

H. *To encourage parental participation in learning to care for and handle the infant and to foster acceptance of the child by his parents and family.*

1. Provide opportunities for the parents to learn all aspects of care of their baby.
2. Initiate a teaching program for the parents early. Offer them available literature and help them become familiar with community resources.
3. Initiate a community nurse referral for continuity of care in the home.
4. Encourage parents to talk about their feelings, fears, and concerns.
5. Help to develop a healthy parent-child relationship.
   a. Frequent visiting
   b. Phone calls
   c. Physical contact of child and parents

Parental Education

1. Teach carefully and thoroughly all procedures to be done at home. Show parents how; then watch return demonstration of the following procedures:
   a. Gastrostomy feedings and care
   b. Esophagostomy care with feeding technique
   c. Suctioning
2. Help parents understand the psychological needs of the infant for sucking, warmth, comfort, stimulation, and love. Suggest that activity be appropriate for age.
3. Encourage parents to continue close medical follow-up and help them learn to recognize possible problems.
   a. Dilatation of esophagus to treat stricture at the site of the anastomosis
   b. Raspy cough for 6–24 months
   c. Eating problems, especially when solids are introduced
   d. Repeated respiratory tract infection
   e. Occurrence of stricture at site of anastomosis weeks to months later—recognized by difficulty in swallowing; spitting of ingested fluid; fever
4. Help parents understand the need for good nutrition and the need to follow the diet regimen suggested by the physician.

CHALASIA

Chalasia is an abnormal, persistent relaxation of the lower end of the esophagus (the cardioesophageal mechanism) causing vomiting in infants (gastroesophageal reflux).

Etiology

1. The cause is undetermined in most patients.
2. Possible causes:
   a. Neuromuscular imbalance; delayed development
   b. Cerebral defects
   c. Obstruction at or just below the pylorus
   d. Physiologic immaturity

Clinical Manifestations

1. Vomiting
   a. Immediately after feeding, especially when infant is placed in prone position
   b. Usually regurgitation rather than projectile vomiting
2. Weight loss or failure to gain weight

3. Dehydration
4. Onset usually soon after birth
5. Relief of vomiting with treatment
   a. Thickened formula
   b. Propping in upright position after feeding

Altered Physiology

Continual relaxation of the cardioesophageal mechanism.
1. Filling of the esophagus from the stomach upon inspiration, leading to vomiting
2. Increased intra-abdominal pressure

Diagnostic Evaluation

1. Upper GI barium x-ray with fluoroscope
   Barium enters stomach but then is regurgitated back into the esophagus.
2. Serum studies
   a. Calcium level—may be lowered
   b. Alkalosis—pH greater than 7.45

Treatment

1. Propping infant in upright position after feeding.
2. Giving thickened formula.
3. Older child—sit or prop at a 50-degree angle.
4. Antacid between feedings if esophagitis is present.
5. Surgical reconstruction of esophagogastric junction—if conservative management does not improve condition.

Complications

1. Aspiration pneumonia
2. Peptic esophagitis
3. Hiatal hernia frequently associated with chalasia

Nursing Objectives and Management

A. *To assist in treatment of dehydration.*
1. Monitor intravenous therapy (see p. 1171).
2. Observe and record accurately urinary output.
   a. Amount, frequency, color and concentration
   b. Specific gravity
3. Promote good skin care to prevent lesions of dry and delicate tissues.
   a. Change position frequently.
   b. Change soiled diapers often.
   c. Apply lotion and gently rub dry any reddened areas.

B. *To maintain adequate nutrition and to prevent vomiting.*
1. Thicken formula for each feeding.

   a. May use cereal.
   b. Enlarge nipple hole so that formula can be more easily extracted.
2. Prop infant in upright position after feeding.
   a. May use infant seat or elevate mattress to 80-degree angle.
   b. Use protective devices or straps to prevent infant from slipping.
   c. Keep infant propped 30–60 minutes after feeding.
3. Handle infant gently, with minimal movement during and after feeding.
4. Bubble frequently during and at completion of feeding.
5. Record accurately activity of infant.
   a. Amount of feeding taken; whether retained
   b. Emesis, estimated amount, type, occurrence in relation to feeding
   c. Any change in behavior as a result of feeding technique

C. *To support family, especially mother, and encourage them to participate in care and feeding of the infant.*
1. Mother may be overly concerned about infant and blame herself and feeding technique for infant's condition.
   a. Help mother understand it is not her fault; she is not a "bad mother."
   b. Let her talk about her concerns.
2. Encourage mother to take an active part in caring for infant—provides a good opportunity to guide mother in correct or preferred methods of handling baby with this condition.

Parental Education

1. Plan a program of intensive parental teaching on how to handle and care for infant. Be certain parents understand why this is being done.
   Help parents understand that it is not necessary to keep infant in infant seat or propped at all times.
   (1) Bathe or play with infant *prior to feeding*
   (2) Change position about 1 hour after feeding
   (3) During the night after feeding, infant can sleep in upright position
   (4) Expect occasional small amounts of vomiting.
2. Help parents to understand that chalasia is self-limited—symptoms usually disappear within 3–6 months.

HYPERTROPHIC PYLORIC STENOSIS

Hypertrophic pyloric stenosis is congenital, progressive hypertrophy of the muscle of the pylorus, causing partial or total obstruction of the stomach outlet.

Clinical Manifestations

Onset is within the first 2 months after birth.
1. Vomiting—onset may be gradual and intermittent or sudden and forceful. The following characteristics may be noted:
   a. Occasional, nonprojectile vomiting at first, gradually increasing in frequency and intensity
   b. Projectile vomiting, not bile-stained

2. Constipation—decreased quantity of stools
3. Loss of weight or failure to gain weight
4. Visible gastric peristaltic waves, left to right
5. Excessive hunger—willingness to eat immediately after vomiting
6. Dehydration—electrolyte disturbance with alkalosis
7. Decreased urinary output
8. Palpable pyloric tumor in upper right quandrant of abdomen

Altered Physiology

1. Increase in size of the circular musculature of the

pylorus with thickening (size and shape of an olive). The pylorus muscle becomes elongated and thickened and is enlarged—about twice the usual size.
2. Hypertrophy of the pylorus musculature occurs with narrowing of the pyloric lumen.
3. Constriction of the lumen of the pyloric canal (at the distal end of the stomach) causes the stomach to become dilated.
4. Gastric emptying is delayed; vomiting after feeding and obstruction also occur.

Diagnostic Evaluation

1. Palpation of pyloric mass ("olive") in conjunction with persistent, projectile vomiting with associated alkalosis
2. Tests for metabolic alkalosis—due to loss of hydrochloric acid and potassium from vomiting
   a. Serum sodium—increases
   b. Serum chloride—decreases
   c. Serum potassium—decreases
   d. Serum pH—increases above 7
   e. Serum CO_2—increases
3. Routine urinalysis—urine becomes alkaline and concentrated
4. Blood hematocrit and hemoglobin—elevated due to hemoconcentration
5. Flat film of abdomen—dilated, air-filled stomach, nondilated pyloric canal
6. X-ray examination with barium
   a. Narrowing of pyloric canal
   b. Delayed gastric emptying time
   c. Enlarged stomach
   d. Increased peristaltic waves
   e. Gas distal to stomach

Nursing Objectives and Management

Preoperative Care

A. *To assist in restoring hydration and electrolyte balance.*

1. Intravenous therapy is usually initiated. (See p. 1171.)
   Electrolytes are added to solution for replacement.
2. Careful observation of output, amount and characteristics.
   a. Urine (Check specific gravity.)
   b. Vomiting
   c. Stools
3. Accurate daily weight—serves as a guide for calculating need for parenteral fluid.

B. *To prevent or decrease the likelihood of vomiting.*

1. Patient may be NPO with indwelling nasogastric tube to remove any residual barium and retained formula.
   Ensure proper functioning of tube and note drainage.
2. Oral feedings may be continued.
   a. Feed small, frequent feedings, given slowly.
   b. Bubble frequently, before, during, and after feeding.
   c. Thickened formula may be prescribed.
3. Proper positioning. (See Figure 42-1.)
   Prop patient in upright position.
   (1) Elevate head of bed, mattress, or infant seat at a 75- to 80-degree angle.
   (2) Place slightly on right side—to aid in gastric emptying.
   (3) Handle gently and minimally after feeding.

C. *To make frequent, accurate observations of the infant's condition.*

1. Dehydration
2. Vomiting
3. Stools and urine output
4. Vital signs
5. Electrolyte imbalance

> **NURSING ALERT:** Respiratory rate may be irregular with apnea when patient is in severe alkalosis.

D. *To provide comfort for the infant.*

1. Mouth care—wet lips
   Let infant suck on pacifier.
2. Physical contact or nearness of the nurse or mother.
3. Audio or visual stimulation may be soothing.
4. Minimal palpation of pyloric olive—will decrease risk of postoperative wound infection from bruising abdominal wall and excoriation of tissue in operative site.

E. *To support parents who are usually very concerned and worried.*

1. Mother may feel guilty, i.e., she may feel she has a poor feeding technique.
   Help her understand that she did not do anything to cause this deformity.
2. Prepare parents for surgery of their child.
   a. Be honest with them.
   b. Inform them of the expected postoperative appearance of the infant.
   c. Show them where the operating room and recovery room are located and where to wait during surgery.
3. Encourage parents to maintain a good relationship with the infant. Allow them to hold infant.
4. Encourage them to get some rest.
   Mother may be tired and frustrated because of the extensive care she has had to give to the child prior to hospitalization.

Postoperative Care

A. *To give good postoperative care and to observe for the usual postoperative complications* (see p. 1140).

B. *To monitor parenteral fluids in order to maintain hydration.*

Intravenous therapy may be continued until adequate oral intake is obtained.

C. *To assist in resuming oral feedings.*

1. Feeding is usually resumed 2–8 hours after surgery.
   a. Feedings usually start with small, frequent feedings of glucose water and slowly advance to full-strength formula and regular diet.
   b. Report any vomiting—the amount and characteristics. Feeding schedule may be withheld 4 hours and then restarted.
   c. Feed slowly and bubble frequently.
   d. Note how feeding is taken and if food is retained.
   e. The amount of feeding is increased as the time interval between feedings is lengthened.
2. Continue to elevate infant's head and shoulders after feeding for 45–60 minutes for several feedings after surgery.

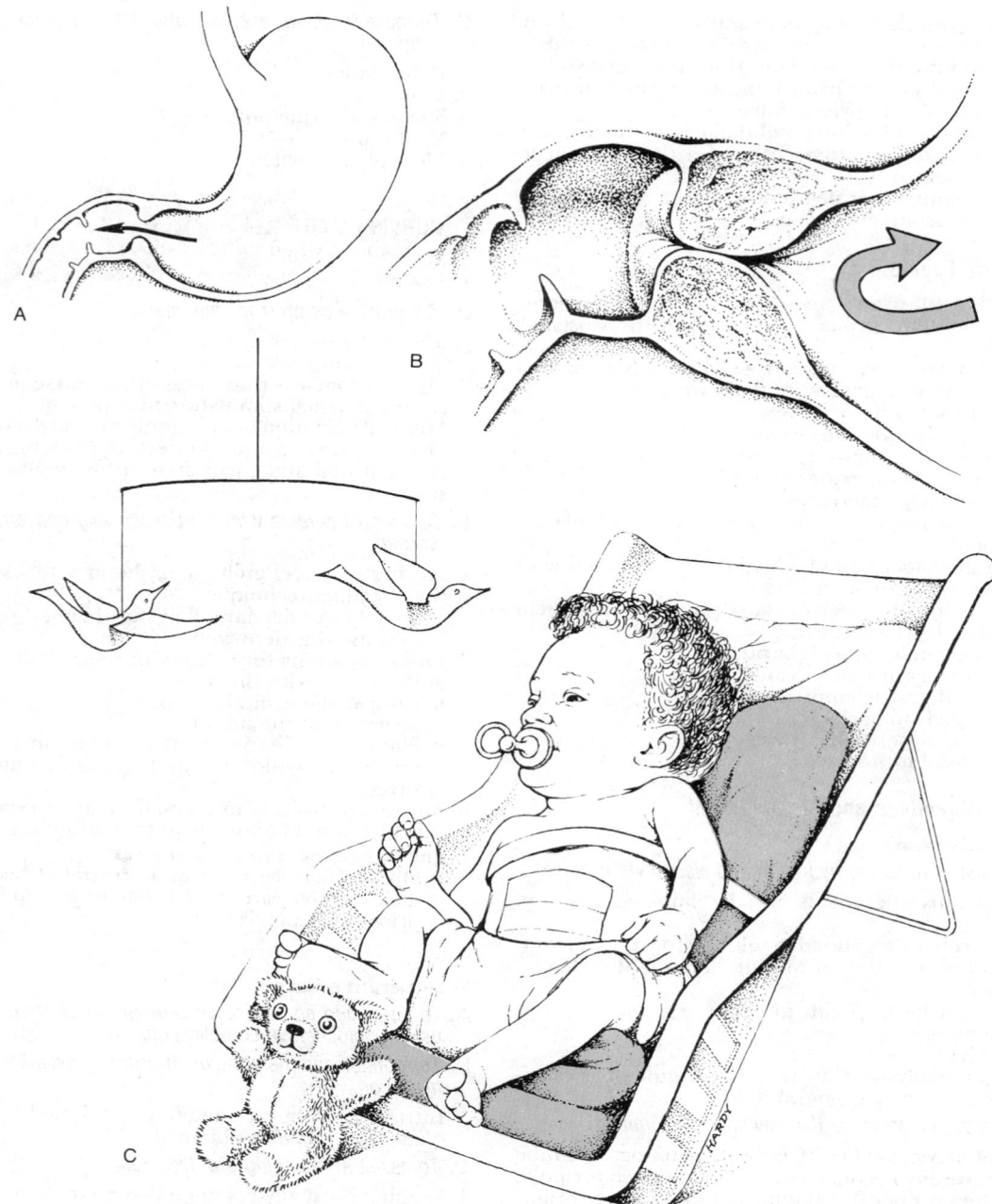

FIGURE 42-1. *Pyloric stenosis. A. Normal passage through pyloric sphincter. B. Stoppage of flow due to stenotic sphincter. C. Postoperative treatment: child propped on right side after feeding to aid gastric emptying.*

Place on right side to aid gastric emptying.

3. Regurgitation may continue for a short period after surgery.

D. *To encourage parents to resume care—especially feeding—of their infant.*

1. This will help to restore their confidence in caring for their baby.

2. This activity provides an opportunity for the nurse to teach.

3. If the mother was breast feeding, resume this as soon as possible.

Parental and Health Education

1. Help parents to understand that surgery has corrected the pyloric stenosis.

a. Discharge of baby will be from 2–5 days after surgery.
b. Proper care of the operative site can be done by the mother.
c. A modified method of feeding technique will be continued at home for only a short period of time.
2. Since this may be a new mother, and the infant may be under 6 weeks of age, the mother may need help with routine infant care.

CELIAC DISEASE

Celiac disease, also called gluten-induced enteropathy, "is a permanent inability to tolerate dietary wheat and rye gluten."*

Etiology

1. Unknown. Although the relationship of gluten to mucosal abnormalities is established, the way in which these mucosal changes occur is not clear.
2. Genetics
   a. Familial incidence
   b. Mode of inheritance is not clear, probably autosomal recessive with incomplete penetrance
3. Environmental inference likely—role of other "allergens" unclear
4. Current theories being investigated include the following:
   a. Immunological (autoimmune vs. specific immune abnormality)
   b. Search to identify deficient enzymes that digest gluten

Clinical Manifestations

The age and mode of presenting signs and symptoms are extremely variable. Diagnosis is most commonly made by 6–24 months of age; however, it can be made in the adult.
1. 3–9 months of age
   a. Acutely ill
   b. Severe diarrhea and vomiting
   c. Failure to thrive
2. 9–18 months of age (age when "typical" celiac appearance is seen)
   a. Impaired growth
      (1) Normal growth during early months of life
      (2) Slackening of weight and weight loss follow
   b. Abnormal stools
      (1) Pale
      (2) Soft
      (3) Bulky
      (4) Having offensive odor
      (5) Greasy—steatorrhea
      (6) May increase in number
   c. Abdominal distention
   d. Anorexia
   e. Muscle wasting—most obvious in buttocks and proximal parts of limbs
   f. Hypotonia
   g. Mood changes—ill humor, irritability, temper tantrums, shyness
   h. Mild clubbing of fingers
   i. Vomiting—often occurring in evening
3. Older child
   a. Signs and symptoms often related to nutritional or secondary deficiencies resulting from disease.
   b. May have abnormal stools and growth impairment.

* Anderson, C. M., and Burke, V.: Paediatric Gastroenterology, p. 175. Oxford, Blackwell Scientific Publications, 1975.

c. May have colicky abdominal pain with constipation and large, pale stools.
4. Manifestations secondary to malabsorption
   a. Anemia, vitamin deficiency
   b. Hypoproteinemia with edema
   c. Hypocalcemia
   d. Hypoprothrombinemia—resulting from impaired vitamin K absorption
   e. Disaccharide intolerance—with acid-sugar containing stools (2° to the altered small bowel mucosa)
5. Celiac crisis—most often seen in very young child and toddler (although rare)
   a. Profound anorexia
   b. Severe vomiting and diarrhea
   c. Weight loss
   d. Marked dehydration and acidosis
   e. Immobility
   f. Grossly distended abdomen
      (1) Fluid rattle is present.
      (2) Abdomen flattens with passage of large liquid stool.
      (3) Patient appears shocklike.
   g. Looks profoundly depressed

Pathophysiology

1. Characteristics of celiac disease include
   a. Impaired intestinal absorption
   b. Histological abnormalities of the small intestine
   c. Clinical and histological improvement with wheat- and rye-free (possibly also barley- and oat-free) diet
   d. Recurrence of clinical manifestations and histological changes after reintroduction of dietary gluten
2. Histological changes in mucosa of small bowel, especially duodenum and jejunum resulting from dietary gluten include
   a. Irregularity of epithelial cells
   b. Loss of normal villous pattern
   c. Obliteration of intervillous spaces which are infiltrated with plasma cells and eosinophils
   d. Loss of epithelial cell brush border
3. This mucosal damage results in
   a. Disaccharidase deficiency
   b. Depression of peptidase activity
4. Subsequent malabsorption probably results from
   a. Decreased area of absorption in small bowel
   b. Impaired enzyme activity
5. The severity of symptoms of the disease depends upon the length of intestine with histologic changes.
   a. The extent of affected intestine is variable.
   b. Generally, proximal small intestine mucosal damage is most severe and condition decreases in severity distally.

Diagnosis

1. Thorough evaluation of history and general status of child

2. Small bowel biopsy—demonstrates abnormal mucosa
3. Determination of fat absorption
4. Measurement of hemoglobin levels—may be reduced
5. Prothrombin time—before intestinal biopsy
6. Radiologic studies—skeletal x-rays commonly show
   a. Demineralization
   b. Retarded bone age
7. Evaluation of clinical and histologic response to withdrawal of and reintroduction of gluten. Reintroduction of gluten is indicated when:
   a. Diagnosis was made on clinical manifestations only.
   b. An infant with milk protein intolerance responded adversely to gluten (temporary gluten intolerance).
8. Sweat test and pancreatic function studies to rule out cystic fibrosis.

Treatment

1. *Life-long* gluten-free diet
   a. Avoid *all* foods containing wheat or rye gluten. The exclusion of barley and oats is controversial; however, it is often wise to err on the safe side or to offer specific challenges and to test with biopsy.
   b. The small intestine mucosa will always respond abnormally to dietary gluten, even though clinical signs may not be immediately evident.
   c. Biopsy reverts to normal with appropriate diet.
   d. Clinical signs of improvement should be seen 1–4 weeks after proper diet is initiated.
2. Adequate caloric intake
3. Supplemental vitamins and minerals
   a. Folic acid for 1–2 months
   b. Vitamin D
   c. Iron for 1–2 months
4. Reduction of fat intake (rare)
5. Possible elimination of lactose from diet for 6–8 weeks—based upon reduced disaccharidase activity
6. Treatment of celiac crisis
   a. IV restoration of electrolyte balance and fluid for replacement of blood volume
   b. Steroids
   c. Parenteral hyperalimentation with amino acids, medium chain triglycerides, and glucose—for short periods of time may be necessary.
   d. Initial oral feedings may need to be disaccharide or completely sugar free.

Complications

1. Recurrence of symptoms if diet is not followed
2. Possible predisposition to malignant lymphoma of small intestine at later age, if diet restrictions are terminated

Nursing Objectives and Management

A. *To follow explicitly the dietary regimen which has been accurately calculated by the physician to include enough calories for weight gain yet to exclude wheat and rye glutens that produce enteropathy.*

1. Initial diet is high in protein, relatively low in fat, and starch-free.
   a. Milk protein or skim milk is sweetened with sucrose or banana powder.
   b. Infants and young children may have a problem in intestinal fat absorption; therefore, fat intake may be reduced.
2. Proteins and sugars should be added gradually.
   a. Individual foods are added one at a time at several-day intervals. Foods included and added are lean meat, cottage cheese, egg white, and raw ground apple.
   b. Starchy foods are added to diet last.
   c. Wheat and rye are never added to diet.
3. The child is given nothing by mouth during the initial treatment of celiac crisis or during diagnostic testing.
4. If the child is ambulatory, take special precautions to ensure that he does not eat restricted foods.
5. Child may have anorexia; feeding him can be difficult.
   a. Make mealtime pleasant.
   b. Serve small, attractive portions.
   c. Do not force him to eat.
6. Note carefully child's reaction to food. Close observation of child's responses to food may reveal other intolerances. Note and record:
   a. Intake, foods refused
   b. Appetite
   c. Change in behavior after eating
   d. Characteristics and frequency of stools
   e. General disposition—behavior improvement often seen within 2–3 days after diet control initiated.
7. New foods may be temporarily eliminated if symptoms increase.

B. *To prevent infection in this child who is malnourished, anemic and very susceptible to respiratory infection, which in turn will increase indigestion.*

1. Avoid exposing the child to anyone with an infection of any kind.
2. Child usually perspires freely and has subnormal temperature with cold extremities.
   a. Keep him dry.
   b. Cover child lightly when room is cool.
3. If child remains quiet in bed, change his position frequently because he is prone to upper respiratory infections.
4. Promote good hygiene.

C. *To be aware of child's behavior or change in behavior and to care for him accordingly.*

1. Diet and eating have a direct effect on behavior. A hungry child may be irritable.
2. Behavior is indicative of how the child is feeling.
3. The child is prone to mood swings—from having temper tantrums to being very timid, nervous, or unstable.
   a. Allow child to express his feelings freely. Provide different types of media for child to express himself.
      (1) Older child talks or complains.
      (2) Baby cries and whines.
   b. The nurse must exhibit patience.
   c. Socialize routine procedures.
4. Record changes in behavior, especially in relation to eating and diet.
5. Avoid conflicts or emotionally upsetting situations; these may precipitate diarrhea, vomiting, and celiac crisis.
6. Teach the older child how to adjust his diet. He can eat buckwheat, millet, corn (maize), and rice.

D. *To meet the child's emotional and psychological needs and to provide diversional activities appropriate for the age of patient and severity of disease.*

1. This child may be withdrawn and indulge in self-play.

Provide opportunity for play with other children, especially when child begins to feel better.
2. Frequently, play is more passive than active. Activity may be very exhausting. Provide appropriate material for constructive activities.
3. The toddler may cling to infantile habits for security. Allow this behavior; it may disappear as his physical condition improves and he feels better.
4. The nurse must show the child she understands his mood swings and irritability by being patient with him. He needs a great deal of emotional satisfaction and support.
5. Offer the child other sensory stimulation to compensate for lack of eating pleasure.

E. *To support the parents and to foster continuing parental acceptance of the child, his disease, and his behavior.*

Help parents maintain a healthy relationship with their child. The most important aspect in working with parents and child is to stress health and family counseling.
1. Encourage parents to visit and care for the child as much as possible. Comforting and holding the child can be very helpful. Child needs much love and understanding, especially from his parents.
2. Start teaching parents early about the disease and how they should care for the child at home.
   a. Acquaint them with available literature, parent groups, and community resources.
   b. Initiate community nurse referral to provide for continued support and teaching at home.
3. Listen to parental concerns and questions.
   a. Give simple, honest answers.
   b. Reinforce what the physician has told them.
4. Allow parents to continue to maintain what other responsibilities they may have outside the hospital. Do not insist they stay at the hospital and attend only to this child.
5. Help parents to understand that after initial rapid weight gain further improvement may be slow.

F. *To be aware of the signs and symptoms of celiac crisis and to attend to the child's care according to medical plans.*

Initial treatment.
   a. Replace fluids and electrolytes by parenteral therapy.
   b. Give nothing by mouth, especially if child is vomiting. Nasogastric tube may be prescribed.
   c. Observe the child carefully.

G. *To be familiar with the medications used in treatment of celiac disease and their implications.*

1. Vitamins A and D—not absorbed well
2. Vitamin B complex and vitamin C—given if child is receiving antibiotics
3. Iron—given if child is anemic
4. Vitamin K—for hypothrombinemia and bleeding
5. Calcium lactate—given if milk is restricted from diet

H. *To assist with gluten-challenge diet, if used, to evaluate histologic and clinical response.*

1. After an extended period of time on dietary regimen, child may dislike gluten-containing foods.
2. Child and parents may be extremely apprehensive about the possible effects of gluten.
3. Child may have mild gastrointestinal symptoms (i.e., loose stools, vague abdominal pain, etc.). These may be related to anxiety.

4. Support the family and provide reassurance. The gluten-challenge diet may last 3–4 months before bowel biopsy is repeated.

Parental Education

1. Help parents to understand what celiac disease is and how it is controlled by diet.
   a. Provide a specific list of restricted foods as well as foods the child is allowed to eat.
   b. Teach mother (parents) how to read labels on foods to identify those containing wheat and rye glutens, thus avoiding them.
   c. Help mother become comfortable and proficient in situation problem-solving (e.g., What can be done when her child is invited to a birthday party where cake will be served? Bake gluten-free cupcakes and take to party).
   d. Provide opportunity for mother, dietician, and nurse to come together and talk about diet. At the same time foster a positive feeling toward dietary controls.
   e. Be certain parents understand the importance of the vitamin regimen.
   f. Help parents understand the importance of continued adherence to diet, even though the child is feeling well, eating well, and has normal stools. Advancing diet too rapidly may result in a setback.
2. Impress upon parents the importance of regular medical follow-up.
   Encourage the parents to seek prompt medical attention if the child has an upper respiratory infection which might trigger celiac crisis if untreated.
3. Encourage parents to practice good hygiene to prevent infection.
   This child is especially prone to infection because of malnutrition and anemia.
4. Help parents to understand that the emotional climate in the home and around the child is vitally important in maintaining the child's medical and physical stability.
   a. Parents must exhibit patience with the child.
   b. Have parents set defined limits of behavior for the child; everyone in the family should know what they are.
   c. Avoid conflicts or any emotional upsets in front of the child.
   d. Social worker may need to become involved if there is domestic disharmony.
   e. Other children and their needs must also be considered in the total family picture.
5. Help parents to understand that the child's physical condition and behavior problems are related to the disease.
   a. Parents may feel guilty or ambivalent toward the child.
   b. Show them how they may avoid becoming overprotective of the child.
6. Help parents to understand that the disorder is lifelong; however, changes in the mucosal lining of the intestine and in general the clinical condition of their child are reversible when dietary gluten is avoided.
7. Offer parents available literature about the American Celiac Society; help them to become familiar with the society and the chapter nearest them.*

* American Celiac Society, 45 Gifford Ave., Jersey City, N.J. 07304.

TABLE 42-1. SOME MALABSORPTION SYNDROMES—BASED ON TYPES OF STOOL*

Disease	Diagnostic Studies	Etiology
A. Watery Stools		
1. Disaccharide intolerance		
a. Lactose	1. Stool pH	Primary—congenital absence of enzyme lactase
(lactose → glucose, galactose)	2. Stool reducing substances	
↑	3. Lactose intolerance test	Secondary—any disease that damages epithelium of small intestine, e.g., gastroenteritis, cow's milk sensitivity, celiac sprue
enzyme: lactase	4. Enzyme assay	
b. Sucrose	1. Stool pH	Primary—congenital absence of enzyme sucrase
(sucrose → glucose, fructose)	2. Stool reducing substances	
↑	3. Sucrose tolerance	Secondary—any disease that damages epithelium of small intestine
enzyme: sucrase	4. Enzyme assay	
2. Monosaccharide intolerance (glucose-galactose)	1. Stool pH	Primary—congenital defect in glucose transport
	2. Stool reducing substances	
	3. Glucose-galactose tolerance tests	Secondary—damage to and decrease of epithelium of intestine from acute gastroenteritis or persistent diarrhea; showing intolerance to fructose and glucose
	4. Trial carbohydrate elimination, using fructose	
3. Cow's milk protein sensitivity	1. Lactose tolerance test	Unknown
	2. Elimination of cow's milk from diet	Sensitivity to cow's milk
	3. Rechallenge with cow's milk will produce same symptoms.	
B. Parasites		
Strongyloidiasis (roundworm)	Examination of intestinal content for rhabtidiform larvae	*Strongyloides*
Giardia lamblia (protozoan)	Stool examination for *Giardia* cysts; duodenal aspirate for trophozoites	Protozoan *Giardia lamblia*
C. Fatty Stool		
Cystic fibrosis, celiac sprue (see above discussion)	Pancreatic enzymes abnormal; sweat test normal; neutropenia	Familial pancreatic enzymes are probably reduced.
Pancreatic insufficiency and bone marrow failure (Schwachman syndrome)		
Short-bowel syndrome		Inadequate absorptive surfaces
		Extensive bowel resection; increase in gastric acidity and production rate (hypersecretion), which in turn may inactivate pancreatic enzymes
Biliary tract obstruction		Biliary atresia
		Choledochal cyst
		Obstructive neonatal hepatitis
D. Normal Stools		
Juvenile pernicious anemia (Vitamin B_{12} malabsorption)		Absence of intrinsic factor activity—cannot absorb vitamin B_{12}

* Adapted from Ament, M. E.: J. Pediatr., 81:685, 1976.
† Nursing care plans can be adapted from discussions on diarrhea, celiac disease, and cystic fibrosis.

DIARRHEA

Diarrhea is an excessive loss of water and electrolytes that occurs with passage of one or more unformed stools. It is a symptom of many conditions and may be caused by many diseases. (Table 42-1.)

Etiology

Often the cause is difficult to determine; occasionally it is unknown. The numerous causes of diarrhea in infants and young children include:
1. Acute and infectious factors
   a. Bacterial
      (1) Enteropathogenic *Escherichia coli*
      (2) *Salmonella*
      (3) *Shigella*
      (4) *Yersinia enterocolitica*
      (5) *Campylobacter fetus*
   b. Viral
      (1) Enteroviruses—ECHO viruses
      (2) Adenoviruses
      (3) Human reovirus-like agent (HRVL)
      (4) *Rotovirus*
   c. Normal intestinal tract inhabitants act as pathogens in certain circumstances, i.e., after ingestion of antibiotics
   d. Fungal—*Candida* enteritis
   e. Parasitic—*Giardia lamblia*
   f. Protozoal
2. Noninfectious factors
   a. Allergy to certain foods—milk, wheat protein
   b. Metabolic disorders
      (1) Celiac disease
      (2) Cystic fibrosis of pancreas
   c. Disaccharidase deficiencies
   d. Infant exposed to overfeeding; displaying emotional excitement and fatigue
   e. Direct irritation of gastrointestinal tract by foods
   f. Inappropriate use of laxatives and purgatives
3. Mechanical disorders
   a. Malrotation
   b. Incomplete small bowel obstruction
   c. Intermittent volvulus
4. Congenital anomalies—Hirschsprung's disease

Signs and Symptoms	Treatment and Nursing Management*†
Infant: watery, acidic diarrhea; vomiting; failure to grow Older child (also): abdominal pain, cramps, abdominal bloating, nausea Fermentative diarrhea when child exposed to lactose in diet	Elimination of all sources of lactose from diet, 1 to several weeks
Infant: watery, acidic diarrhea; vomiting; failure to grow Older child (also): abdominal pain, cramps, abdominal bloating, nausea Fermentative diarrhea when child exposed to lactose in diet	Elimination of sucrose from diet
	Primary: elimination of foods containing glucose from diet; feed foods containing fructose. Secondary: elimination of diet containing fructose and glucose; administration of IV fluid and electrolytes until monosaccharide transport mechanisms are active.
Gradual onset of watery or blood-tinged mucoid diarrhea Steatorrhea Vomiting Fever	Elimination of all sources of cow's milk protein. If sensitivity appears by 6 months of age, tolerance of cow's milk resumes at 1–2 years of age.
Skin red where larvae penetrate Cough, dyspnea, patchy pneumonia for 2–3 weeks Abdominal pain, nausea, vomiting; watery stools	Thiabendazole
Persistent or intermittent watery diarrhea Abdominal distention, poor weight gain, malabsorption syndrome Older child shows celiac picture	Metronidazole (Flagyl)
Frequent infections Poor growth Stools—bulky, loose, and frequent	Exogenous pancreatic enzyme therapy
Steatorrhea Malnutrition	IV alimentation Supplemental oral feedings of predigested formula, advancing slowly Supplemental vitamins A-D-E in water-miscible form Vitamin K, if prothrombin time indicates
Steatorrhea Malabsorption of fat-soluble vitamins	Surgical correction if possible Medical prescription 1. Formula containing medium-chain triglycerides 2. Large doses of vitamins A-D-E in water-miscible form
Megaloblastic anemia Failure to thrive Psychomotor retardation	Monthly vitamin B_{12} injection

Clinical Manifestations

A. Classification of Diarrhea

1. Mild diarrhea—hospitalization may not be indicated.
2. Severe diarrhea with gradual onset.
3. Severe diarrhea with sudden onset—incidence of death is high in infant.

B. Symptoms

All classifications have similar symptoms, the severity of which is dependent upon intensity of diarrhea and type of onset.
1. Fever—low-grade to 41.1° C (106° F)
2. Anorexia
3. Mild and intermittent to severe vomiting
4. Stools
   a. Appearance of diarrhea varies from a few hours to 3 days
   b. Loose and fluid in consistency
   c. Greenish or yellow-green color
   d. May contain mucus, pus, or blood
   e. Frequency varies from 2–20/day
   f. Expelled with force; may be preceded by pain
5. Behavior change
   a. Irritability and restlessness
   b. Weakness/pallor
   c. Extreme prostration
   d. Stupor and convulsions
   e. Flaccidity
6. Respirations
   a. Rapid
   b. Hyperpneic
7. Dehydration
   a. Little to extreme loss of subcutaneous fat
   b. Up to 50% total body weight loss
   c. Urinary output decreases or stops
   d. Poor skin turgor and dry skin
   e. Fontanelles and eyes sunken
   f. Collapse imminent, low blood pressure, high pulse

Pathophysiology

1. The particular etiology of diarrhea does not influence the potentially dangerous cycle of events as much as does the virulence of the organism and the general condition of the child.
2. The effects of diarrhea present more of a threat to infants and young children than to the older child and adult.
   a. Extracellular fluid volume is proportionately larger in the infant and young child.
   b. Nutritional reserves are relatively smaller in the young child.
3. Major alterations in physiology

a. Dehydration—extracellular fluid loss—results from the following:
  (1) Large loss of fluid and electrolytes in watery stools
  (2) Losses with repeated vomiting
  (3) Decreased fluid intake
  (4) Increased insensible fluid losses from skin and lungs resulting from fever and rapid respirations
  (5) Continued urine excretion
b. Electrolyte imbalance
  (1) Potassium—varies
  (2) Chloride; sodium; hypotonic, isotonic, or hypertonic dehydration may occur
c. Acid-base imbalance. Metabolic acidosis may result from
  (1) Large losses of potassium, sodium, and bicarbonate in stools
  (2) Impairment of renal function

Diagnostic Evaluation

1. Thorough history of onset of diarrhea and cause
2. Evaluation of general physical appearance and condition of child, including weight
3. Studies to establish nature of patient's condition
  a. Electrolyte status and kidney function
    (1) Serum sodium
    (2) Serum chloride
    (3) Serum potassium
    (4) BUN (blood urea nitrogen)
  b. Acid-base imbalance
    (1) Serum pH (acidosis)
    (2) Serum CO_2 content or combining power
  c. Plasma volume by hematocrit and hemoglobin; also complete blood count, sedimentation rate, and culture
  d. Urinalysis
  e. Stool pH, reducing substances
4. Studies to determine cause of diarrhea
  a. Bacteriologic cultures of stool
  b. Bacteriologic cultures of rectal swab
  c. Serologic studies for viral pathogens or direct visualization under electron microscope (i.e., HRVL)

Treatment

1. Prevent spread of disease—suspect disease to be communicable until proven otherwise. Isolation; use enteric isolation precautions.
2. Supportive care—maintain hydration and electrolyte balance; record IV fluids, weights, fluid loss from diarrhea, urine, and vomiting.
3. Specific antimicrobial therapy
  Complications:
  (1) Dehydration
  (2) Protracted diarrheal state
  (3) Transient lactase deficiency—lactose intolerance

Complications

1. Direct disturbances caused by diarrhea itself
  a. Dehydration
  b. Acidosis
  c. Hypernatremia
  d. Alterations in potassium levels
2. Infection
  a. Local—i.e., site of cutdown, injection site

b. Respiratory tract
c. Middle ear (otitis media)
3. Nervous system, hemorrhage
4. Iatrogenic
  a. Potassium depletion—"washing out"
  b. Hypernatremia—sodium chloride overload
  c. Edema—excessive amount of parenteral fluids

Nursing Objectives and Management

A. *To monitor intravenous fluid therapy (both amount and rate), which has been appropriately calculated by the physician.*

1. Fluid prescribed as maintenance or replacement depending upon degree of patient's dehydration, must be checked.
2. Fluid is calculated carefully so as not to overload circulatory system.
  a. Check flow rate and amount absorbed hourly and totally.
  b. Check IV site for infiltration or improper flow so site can be changed as necessary.
3. Use appropriate protective devices to prevent patient from moving and injuring himself or causing IV to malfunction.
4. When preparing solution for therapy, use sterile solution and equipment.
5. Weigh patient daily to serve as a guide for specific fluid needs and current patient status.
6. When oral feedings are given in conjunction with IV fluid, careful adherence to prescribed volume is vital to prevent circulatory overload.

B. *To provide physical comfort for the patient.*

1. If protective devices are used, passive range of motion may help to keep patient's joints from stiffening.
2. While the patient is given nothing by mouth, special mouth care should be administered.
  An infant may find comfort in sucking a pacifier. Bubble him frequently to help expel air he has swallowed during sucking.
3. Change position and give good skin care to prevent lesions that may occur because of dehydration.
  Change soiled diapers quickly, because diarrheal stool will cause excoriation. Clean perineum thoroughly after each stool; application of ointment to skin may help protect it from contact with stool. Ointment must be completely removed after each stool. Leave diaper area exposed to air.

C. *To make frequent observations and be constantly alert to the patient's condition.*

Record and report any changes immediately. Careful observations can give clues to improvement or deterioration in the patient's condition and can serve as a guide to medical care.
1. Note any changes in vital signs.
2. Note stool characteristics and number.
  a. Abnormal constituents
  b. Foul odor
  c. Test stool for pH, reducing substances (Clinitest tablets), and occult blood.
3. Note activity, level of consciousness, and neurologic signs.
4. Note vomiting—frequency and characteristics.
5. Record urinary output—amount, frequency, and characteristics.

6. Check for presence of edema, and skin characteristics.
7. Assess child's behavior to determine how he feels.
   a. Eating and restful sleep indicates he feels fairly good.
   b. Crying or legs drawn up to abdomen usually indicates pain.

D. *To prevent spread of infection by using good handwashing and gown techniques as indicated by hospital policy.*

1. Many hospitals use isolation technique for children admitted with diarrhea until the cause has been determined. (Infectious pathogens can spread rapidly and easily among infants and young children.)
2. Follow hospital policy as to care of diapers.

E. *To meet the emotional and psychological needs of the patient.*

1. Hospitalization is frightening—especially when it is sudden, as with diarrhea.
2. Many treatments and procedures are painful—give reassurance to the child before, during, and after them.
   a. Talk to the child.
   b. Hold him and comfort him after the procedure.
   c. Explain to him in language appropriate for his age what is to be done.
3. Provide some means of pleasant stimulation, entertainment, or diversion—especially while he must remain in bed.
   a. Infant—mobile, musical toy
   b. Young child—read to him, something appropriate for age
4. A hungry child is not easily comforted. Physical closeness may be helpful.
   a. Petting, stroking
   b. Holding and rocking

F. *To provide and assist in resuming adequate caloric and volume oral intake.*

1. If diarrhea is mild, oral electrolyte solution may be given. (Do not advance too quickly—base administration of solution on number of stools.)

2. Fluid is usually advanced slowly from clear liquids, such as gelatin-flavored water, to half-strength formula, to regular diet. Older child may advance more rapidly.
3. As diet is advanced, note any vomiting or increase in stools and report it immediately. Oral feedings should not be resumed too early or advanced too rapidly, because diarrhea may occur.

G. *To provide support for the family, especially the mother.*

1. Reassure the mother that she is not the cause of her child's illness.
2. Explain procedures and need for treatment in easy-to-understand language. Be sure family understands the following:
   a. Why infant's hair was shaved off his head for an IV
   b. Reason for not giving the child anything to eat or drink
   c. Need for protective devices
3. Allow mother (parents) to care for and comfort the child as much as possible.
4. Allow her to leave the hospital and attend to other family members and matters. Invite parents to call the hospital when they cannot be there.
5. Initiate a community nurse referral, especially if other children at home are ill or if home conditions have precipitated the diarrhea.

Parental Education

1. After the cause of the diarrhea is determined, it may be necessary to teach proper formula or food preparation, handling, and storage.
   It is especially important to be certain that the mother knows proper formula and bottle sterilization procedures.
2. Parents may need help in understanding the symptoms of a sick child.
3. Help parents understand the importance of medical care and general good hygiene.

HIRSCHSPRUNG'S DISEASE

Hirschsprung's disease (congenital aganglionic megacolon) is a congenital absence of the parasympathetic ganglion nerve cells from within the muscle wall of the intestinal tract, usually at the distal end of the colon.

Etiology

1. An arrest in embryologic development affecting the migration of parasympathetic nerves (innervation) of the intestine, occurring prior to the 12th week of gestation.
2. The cause is unknown—may be familial.

Clinical Manifestations

They vary depending upon degree of involved bowel.
1. Appearing at birth or within first weeks of life.
   a. No meconium passed
   b. Vomiting—bile-stained or fecal
   c. Abdominal distention
   d. Constipation
   e. Overflow-type diarrhea

   f. Anorexia
   g. Temporary relief of symptoms with enema
2. Older child—symptoms not prominent at birth
   a. History may reveal obstipation at birth
   b. Distention of abdomen—progressive enlarging
   c. Thin abdominal wall—superficial veins are visible
   d. Peristaltic activity observable
   e. Constipation
      (1) Never has fecal soiling
      (2) Relieved temporarily with enema
   f. Stool appears ribbonlike, fluidlike or in pellet form
   g. Failure to grow
      (1) Loss of subcutaneous fat
      (2) Appears malnourished; perhaps has stunted growth

Altered Physiology

1. Absence of or reduced number of ganglion cells in the intestinal tract muscle wall, usually the distal end of the colon.

2. No peristalsis occurs in the affected portion of intestine (i.e., spastic and contracted).
    a. This section is usually narrow; therefore no fecal material passes through it.
    b. The intestine above the affected section has an accumulation of fecal material.
3. Proximal to the narrow affected section, the colon is dilated.
    a. Filled with fecal material and gas.
    b. Hypertrophy of muscular coating.
    c. In newborn may see ulceration of mucosa.
4. Abdominal distention and constipation result.

Diagnostic Evaluation

1. Rectal examination—exhibits absence of fecal material
2. Roentgen examination with barium enema
    a. Narrow segment of intestine proximal to anus
    b. Dilated intestine proximal to narrow segment
3. Rectal biopsy—absence or reduced number of ganglion nerve cells

Treatment

Definitive treatment is removal of the aganglionic, nonfunctioning, dilated segment of the bowel, followed by anastomosis.
1. Initially a colostomy or ileostomy is performed to decompress intestine and divert fecal stream.
2. Definitive surgery (abdominoperineal pullthrough) may be delayed until age 9–12 months or until child is 68–69 kg. (15–20 lb.).

Complications

1. Prior to primary surgery
    a. Enterocolitis—a major cause of death
    b. Hydroureter or hydronephrosis
    c. Water intoxication from tap water enemas
    d. Cecal perforation
2. Postoperative
    a. Enterocolitis
    b. Leaking of anastomosis and pelvic abscess
    c. Temporary sudden inability to evacuate colon

Nursing Objectives and Management

Preoperative Care

A. *To assist in emptying the bowel and in preparing for surgery.*
1. Give repeated enemas and colonic irrigations.
    a. Procedure for enema in infant is similar to that in adult, except that less fluid and pressure are used.
    b. Chemotherapeutic agents used to reduce the bacterial flora.
    c. Physiologic saline solution should be used for irrigations.
        Tap water may result in large quantities of water being absorbed and in water intoxication.
    d. Carefully note return from irrigation and degree of abdominal distention.
    e. A continuous rectal tube may be prescribed; ensure that it is properly located and remains in place.
    f. If enema is not expelled, siphoning may be indicated.
2. Note and record frequency and characteristics of stools.(Obstipation is likely to occur.)
3. Prevent injury to mucosa by taking axillary temperature.

B. *To observe for abdominal distention and its effect on patient's condition.*
1. Note any change in degree of distention before and after irrigation. Record if location of distention changes, i.e., upper or lower abdomen.
2. Respiratory embarrassment may result from abdominal distention.
    Elevate head and chest of infant by tilting mattress.
3. Note degree of abdominal tenderness.
    a. Legs of infant drawn up
    b. Chest breathing
4. Note color of abdomen and presence of gastric waves.

C. *To assist in establishing and maintaining hydration and adequate nutrition so that growth and weight gain may take place.*
1. Monitor parenteral fluids appropriately. Measure all output.
2. Feeding may cause additional discomfort because of distention and nausea.
3. Offer small, frequent feedings. (Low-residue diet will aid in keeping stools soft.)
    a. Appetite is poor.
    b. Child must be fed slowly.
    c. Provide as comfortable a position as possible for child during feedings.

D. *To obtain a dietary history regarding food and eating habits.*
1. This will contribute to planning dietary alterations.
2. Eating problems are common with Hirschsprung's disease.

E. *To properly care for patient when nasogastric tube is used to aid in decreasing abdominal distention.*
1. Note drainage from nasogastric tube and chart characteristics.
2. Check for patency.
    a. Saline irrigations may be requested.
    b. Carefully record input and output.
    c. Note increasing distention; measure abdominal girth.
3. Give adequate mouth care.
4. Alternate nares when changing nasogastric tube every 24 hours. (Use minimal amount of tape to prevent skin irritation.)

F. *To provide emotional and psychological support needed by the child.*
1. Encourage mother to visit, even for short periods.
2. Irritable child may be calmed with holding and rocking.
3. Provide suitable diversion appropriate for age.

Postoperative Care

One of 2 surgical procedures may be done in treatment of Hirschsprung's disease: (1) primary resection of aganglionic segment or (2) temporary colostomy above the narrowed section; when condition of child is stabilized or weight is obtained, resection is done and colostomy closed (most common).

A. *To give good postoperative care and to observe for possible postoperative complications.* (See p. 1140.)

B. *To prevent infection.*
1. At the site of surgical wound.
    a. Dressing change, using sterile technique.
    b. Prevent contamination from diaper.
        (1) Apply diaper below dressing.
        (2) Change frequently.

(3) Prevent perianal and anal excoriation by frequent changing, thorough cleansing, and use of ointments.

  c. Use careful handwashing technique.

  d. Report any redness, swelling or drainage, evisceration, or dehiscence immediately.

2. Of the tracheobronchial tree and lungs.
  a. Frequently suction secretions.
  b. Encourage frequent coughing and deep breathing.
     Allow infant to cry for short periods.
  c. Change position frequently to increase circulation and allow for aeration of all lung areas.

C. *To properly care for colostomy and to understand its purpose.*

1. Proper functioning of colostomy.
  a. Note drainage from colostomy—characteristics, frequency, fecal material or liquid drainage.
  b. Note abdominal distention.
  c. Measure fluid loss from colostomy as the amount will affect fluid replacement.

2. Signs of obstruction from peritonitis, paralytic ileus, handling bowel, or swelling.
  a. No output from colostomy
  b. Increased tenderness
  c. Irritability
  d. Vomiting
  e. Increased temperature

3. Good skin care to prevent breakdown around colostomy.
  a. Change soiled dressing or diaper frequently.
  b. Wash skin with clear water.
  c. Use karaya gum, aluminum paste, Maalox or other means to protect skin from contact with secretions.
  d. Keep area open to air occasionally.

D. *To prevent abdominal distention.*

1. Nasogastric tube may be used immediately postoperatively.
  a. Check patency.
  b. Watch for increasing abdominal distention; measure abdominal girth.
  c. Measure fluid loss as amount will affect fluid replacement.

2. Once oral feeding is begun, the nasogastric tube will be removed.
  a. Avoid overfeeding.
  b. Bubble frequently during feeding.
  c. Proper positioning after feeding.

E. *To continue taking axillary temperatures.*

1. Avoids injury.
2. Allows for more accurate reading.

F. *To continue to provide emotional support to the patient.* (See p. 1323, diarrhea.)

1. Recognize the effects of immobility, less handling, and less activity than is generally given the healthy infant.
2. Allow baby to derive some satisfaction from using a pacifier. Hold him often during this time if condition permits.
3. Prepare parents for what they will see postoperatively (i.e., equipment, dressings, stoma).

G. *To help parents understand and accept the child and the disease, as well as all that has happened.*

1. Even a temporary colostomy can be a difficult procedure to accept and to learn to care for.
  a. Support parents when teaching them to care for the colostomy.
  b. Try to help them treat the baby or child as normally as possible.

2. Encourage parents to talk about their fears and anxieties.
    Anticipating future surgery for resection may be confusing and frightening.

3. Initiate community nurse referral to help parents care for child at home away from the comfortable situation of the hospital.

Parental Education

1. Begin early to teach thoroughly and carefully what the colostomy is for, how it works, and how to care for it and the child.
  a. Parents may also need to know gastrostomy feeding techniques as well as procedures for care and dilation of anus.
  b. Allow parents to try these procedures long before infant is to be discharged.
  c. Emphasize the importance of treating the child as normally as possible to prevent behavior problems later.

2. Encourage close medical follow-up and general good health hygiene.
  a. Nutrition
  b. General growth and development
  c. Immunizations

Ostomy Care

Colostomy and ileostomy care in the infant and young child is based on the same principles and is essentially the same as that for an adult (see pp. 426–433) with the following exceptions:

1. Colostomy irrigation is not part of management in small children. Irrigation is primarily for the purpose of regulating the colostomy to empty at regular intervals. Since children have bowel movements at more frequent intervals, this type of control is not feasible. Irrigation should only be done in preparation for tests or surgery and occasionally for the treatment of constipation.

2. Dehydration occurs quickly in the infant or small child; therefore, it is particularly important to observe drainage for amount and characteristics. It should be measured to provide for an accurate basis for computation of fluid replacement.

3. Prevention and treatment of skin excoriation around the stoma is of primary concern and is a nursing challenge. With the advent of better skin shields and equipment that is designed especially for the pediatric patient, keeping an ostomy appliance in place is much less of a problem than it has been in the past. Through careful application and by trying different types of pouches until a proper fit is obtained, most children can be kept clean and dry for at least 24 hours between changes. This is a very significant factor in preventing skin breakdown and subsequent infections in the peristomal area. It is helpful to remember, however, that in the infant, dressings must be checked frequently:
  a. Dressings and collection bags may not adhere well or stay in place.
  b. Skin breakdown is more frequent.
  c. Infant elimination is more frequent than in the older child.

4. Helping agency for parents:

United Ostomy Association, 2001 W. Beverly Boulevard, Los Angeles, Calif. 90057.
5. Some companies manufacturing pediatric size ostomy equipment:
   United Surgical (Division of Howmedia, Inc.), Largo, Fla. 33540

Coloplast, C. R. Bard Inc., 713 Central Ave., Murray Hill, N.J. 07974

Hollister, Inc., 211 E. Chicago Ave., Chicago, Ill. 60611

INTUSSUSCEPTION

Intussusception is the invagination or telescoping of a portion of the intestine into an adjacent, more distal section of the intestine.

Etiology

1. Not usually known
   May be due to increased mobility of intestine and hyperperistalsis present in young children.
2. Possible contributing causes in older child
   a. Meckel's diverticulum
   b. Polyps, cysts in the bowel
   c. Malrotation of intestines
   d. Acute enteritis
   e. Abdominal injury
   f. Abdominal surgery; intestinal intubation
   g. Cystic fibrosis
   h. Celiac disease

Clinical Manifestations

1. Incidence is rare in first month of life.
   a. 4–10 months is most common age of onset (50–70%).
   b. 1–2 years of age—frequency of occurrence is high.
2. Onset is sudden.
   a. Paroxysmal abdominal pain
   b. Currant jelly-like stools
      (1) Blood and mucus present in stool
      (2) One or more stools with this characteristic
      (3) Presence of bloody mucus on finger following rectal examination
   c. Vomiting
   d. Increasing absence of stools
   e. Increasing abdominal distention and tenderness
   f. Sausage-like mass palpable in abdomen
   g. Dehydration and fever
   h. Shock-like state
      (1) Rapid pulse
      (2) Pale skin
      (3) Marked sweating

Altered Physiology

1. Mesentery is pulled into intestine when invagination occurs.
2. Progression to obstruction
   a. Intestine becomes curved, sausage-like—blood supply is cut off.
   b. Bowel begins to swell—hemorrhage may occur.
   c. Complete intestinal obstruction results—necrosis of involved segment.
3. Classification of location.
   a. *Ileocecal* (most common)—ileum invaginates into ascending colon
   b. *Ileocolic*—ileum invaginates into colon
   c. *Colocolic*—colon invaginates into colon
   d. *Ileo-ileo*—(enteroenteric) small bowel invaginates into small bowel

Diagnostic Evaluation

1. General condition and appearance of child; history
2. X-ray examination
   a. Flat plate of abdomen—reveals staircase pattern (invagination appears like stair steps on x-ray)
   b. Barium enema under fluoroscopy—coil-like appearance of bowel

Treatment

1. Hydrostatic reduction of telescoped bowel with barium enema used during first 48 hours after onset.
2. Surgical reduction of intussusception; resection if bowel is gangrenous.

Nursing Objectives and Management

Preoperative Care

A. *To assist in maintaining or restoring hydration and electrolyte balance.*

Monitor parenteral fluids. (See p. 1171, IV Therapy.)

B. *To prevent vomiting and aspiration.*

1. Stomach may be deflated by insertion of nasogastric tube.
2. Maintain patency of nasogastric tube if one is inserted.
   a. Irrigate at frequent intervals.
   b. Note drainage and return from irrigation.
3. Patient is likely to be NPO
   a. Wet lips and give mouth care.
   b. Give infant pacifier to suck.

C. *To be aware of the patient's condition by frequent observations, thereby contributing to the total care of the patient.*

1. Respirations are affected because of abdominal distention.
   a. Grunting
   b. Shallow and rapid if patient is in shock-like state
2. Abdominal distention and unusual appearance of anus—intussusception may look like rectal prolapse.

> **NURSING ALERT:** When anus has an unusual appearance, take axillary temperatures to prevent injury.

3. Behavior
   a. Irritable—very sensitive to handling (Be gentle!)
   b. Lethargic or unresponsive
   c. Behavior indicative of presence or absence of pain

D. *To prepare the patient for surgery when he is shock-like or febrile.*

1. Blood or plasma is given to restore circulating blood volume—observe for transfusion reactions.

2. Observe pulse rate carefully—safe range is below 140/minute.
3. Reduce temperature—fever increases metabolism and makes oxygenation during anesthesia more complicated.

E. *To offer support to parents during this time of crisis and fear.*

1. Encourage parents to verbalize their concerns.
2. Reinforce what the physician has told them.
3. Encourage them to be with child whenever possible.
4. Help them understand the basic defect and the reason for surgery.

Postoperative Care

A. *To give good postoperative care and to observe for possible postoperative complications.* (See p. 1140.)

B. *To be constantly alert for complications arising from surgery for intussusception.*

1. Fever is usually present.
   a. As a result of absorption of foreign protein
   b. Absorption of bacteria through the damaged intestinal wall
2. Diarrhea—from exposure to others who are infected
3. Shock
4. Dehydration
5. Toxicity
6. Peritonitis

C. *To assist in maintaining stomach decompression until first stool is passed.*

1. See that indwelling nasogastric tube is functioning properly.

a. Tube is usually connected to constant intermittent suction.
b. Note returns from drainage and irrigation.
2. Patient is usually given nothing by mouth. Give mouth care.
3. Note passing of flatus or stool and report—indicates peristalsis has returned to normal activity. Oral feedings may start.

D. *To gradually resume full caloric and volume oral intake appropriate for age and weight.*

Progression will vary with physician and will depend upon whether bowel reduction or resection was surgical procedure.

1. Oral fluid is usually begun after the first stool is passed—about 4–5 days after surgery. When only a reduction was performed, oral fluid may be resumed when abdominal peristaltic activity is audible.
2. Give frequent, small feedings.
   a. Start with glucose water or water.
   b. Note and report any abdominal distention or vomiting.

E. *To provide emotional support and meet the psychological needs of the child.*

(See p. 1323, Diarrhea.)

F. *To support parents and to help them to maintain a good relationship with their child.*

1. Encourage them to visit and call. Allow parents to become involved in caring for their child.
2. Help parents to understand that recurrence is rare, but that certain short-term limits must be placed on the child's activity after discharge.

IMPERFORATE ANUS

The term *imperforate anus* is used to describe congenital "abnormalities in the formation of the anorectal canal or in the location of the anus within the perineum."*

Etiology

1. An arrest in embryologic development of the anus, lower rectum, and urogenital tract at the 8th week of embryonic life.
2. Cause unknown.

Types

1. Low imperforate anus—implies that the rectum has descended below the pubococcygeal line (puborectalis muscle) and is in normal anatomical relationship to levator sling and puborectus muscle.
   a. Female
      (1) 90% of females with this condition present with low imperforate anus.
      (2) Fistula is present; rectum ends in fistula which presents in any location from low in vagina to normal position of anus.
   b. Male
      (1) 50% of males with imperforate anus present with this type.
      (2) Perineal fistula is present and is located from anterior or normal position of anus to ventral surface of penis.
2. High imperforate anus—term implies that the rectal

* Gryboski J. Gastrointestinal Problems in the Infant. Philadelphia, W. B. Saunders, 1975, p. 506.

pouch is at or above the pubococcygeal line or the levator musculature.
   a. Male
      (1) 50% of males with imperforate anus present with this type.
      (2) If fistula is present, it will usually communicate with the posterior urethra.
   b. Female
      (1) 10% of females with imperforate anus present with this type.
      (2) Fistula will end high in vagina.

Clinical Manifestations

Condition is usually discovered immediately after birth or within several hours.

1. No anal opening.
2. Thermometer or small finger cannot be inserted into rectum.
3. Absence of meconium stool.
4. Green-tinged urine—if fistula is present (high, male)
5. Progressive abdominal distention.
6. Fistula is likely to be present.
   a. Female—occurs between rectum and vagina or perineum.
   b. Male—occurs between rectum and urinary tract, scrotum or perineum.
7. Other anomalies are likely, especially tracheoesophageal atresia. Other anomalies include those of the gastrointestinal tract, genitourinary system, cardiovascular system, and sacral vertebrae.

Diagnostic Evaluation

1. Visual examination
   a. Presence of perineal fistula
   b. Meconium coming from vagina or presence of meconium-stained urine
2. General examination and/or presence of other associated manifestations
3. Urine examination for presence of meconium and epithelial debris—indicates presence of fistula.
4. Voiding cystourethrogram
5. Wangensteen-Rice x-ray (upside-down position)
   a. Limited accuracy in locating rectal pouch
   b. Useful only after infant is 24 hours of age

Treatment

1. Low—female
   a. Decompression of bowel with catheter irrigations
   b. Dilatation of fistula for 8–12 months thereafter
   c. Definitive repair
2. Low—male
   a. Rectal cutback anoplasty or Y-V plasty
   b. Local dilatation of fistula
3. High—male
   a. Colostomy for decompression
   b. Definitive pull-through surgery—deferred until about 1 year of age or when child attains 6.75–9 kg. (15–20 lbs.)
4. High—female
   a. Colostomy
   b. Definitive repair done when infant is 1 year of age or 6.75–9 kg. (15–20 lbs.)

Complications

1. Rectal stenosis or prolapse, usually confined to mucosa
2. Separation of anastomosis
3. Urethral injury or stricture
4. Urinary retention and infection
5. Recurrent urinary fistulas
6. Fecal impaction or incontinence
7. Small bowel obstruction

Nursing Objectives and Management

Preoperative Care

A. *To assist in maintaining stability in patient's general condition prior to emergency surgery.*

1. Feedings are usually withheld. Note any vomiting, color and amount.
2. Nasogastric tube may be passed to decompress the stomach. Measure abdominal girth.
3. Observe patient carefully for any signs of distress and report these to physician. Check vital signs frequently. Maintain temperature stability.

B. *To observe the infant carefully for any other anomalies or changes in condition.*

1. Use Isolette or radiant warmer.
2. Observe for stool coming from a fistula.
3. Note that urine may be green-tinged.
4. Keep area clean.

Postoperative Care

Depending upon the location of the rectum (see types of imperforate anus), and sex of child, 1 of 3 surgical approaches may be used: (1) anoplasty, (2) temporary colostomy with definitive pull-through at a later time when child is older and larger, or (3) abdominal or sacroperineal pull-through.

A. *To give good postoperative care and to observe for possible postoperative complications.*

(See p. 1140.)
   Especially note any vomiting or stooling.

B. *To provide appropriate care for perineal anoplasty, prevent infection of suture line, and promote healing.*

1. Do not put anything in rectum.
2. Expose perineum to air.
3. Position baby for easy access to perineum for cleansing and minimal irritation to site (ie., place baby on abdomen, possibly with hips elevated, to prevent pressure on perineal surfaces; turn side-to-side).

C. *To provide good colostomy care and to prevent skin breakdown.*

(See p. 1325, Hirschsprung's disease.)

D. *To provide appropriate care for definitive pull-through surgery.*

1. Carry out perineal care as stated above.
2. Provide proper care of gastrostomy or nasogastric tube used to decompress the gastrointestinal tract until peristalsis returns.
3. Provide proper care of bladder catheter, if used, and measure urinary output accurately.
4. Observe carefully for abdominal distention, bleeding from perineum, and respiratory embarrassment.

E. *To maintain adequate nutrition as well as caloric and fluid intake to prevent dehydration and electrolyte imbalance.*

1. Oral feedings are usually started within hours after an anoplasty.
2. Oral feedings are usually withheld until peristalsis returns. When primary repair is done, nasogastric suction may be maintained until feedings are started.
3. Monitor parenteral fluids (see p. 1171).

F. *To foster acceptance of the child and his diagnosis by his parents.*

1. Assure parents that colostomy is temporary.
2. Encourage parents to become involved in care of the child and to give him the emotional security he needs.
3. Support teaching program of surgeon for special care needed at home.
   a. Colostomy care
   b. Anal dilatation to prevent a stricture at site of anastomosis from scar tissue after instructions by physician
4. Initiate referral to community nurse, especially if parents are particularly anxious about caring for the child at home.
5. Encourage parents to talk about their concerns.

Parental Education

1. Provide careful, thorough teaching of special care and procedures to be continued at home—colostomy care, anal dilatation. Develop a plan for return demonstration by mother.
2. Help parents to understand situations that may be encountered as a result of imperforate anus as the baby gets older:
   a. Fecal impaction due to lack of sensation to defecate
   b. Future surgery—if primary repair was not done
   c. Toilet training
   d. Inability to control fecal seepage from rectum

BIBLIOGRAPHY

Books

Anderson CM and Burke J. Paediatric Gastroenterology. Oxford, Blackwell Scientific Publications, 1975

Avery GB. Neonatology. Philadelphia, JB Lippincott, 1981

Lebenthal E (ed). Digestive Diseases in Children. New York, Grune & Stratton, 1978

Postlethwait RW. Surgery of the Esophagus. New York, Appleton–Century–Crofts, 1979

Roberts KB. Manual of Clinical Problems in Pediatrics. Boston, Little, Brown & Co., 1979

Scipien GM et al. Comprehensive Pediatric Nursing, 2nd ed. New York, McGraw–Hill, 1979

Vaughan VC, McKay RJ, Behrman RE. Nelson Textbook of Pediatrics, 11th ed. Philadelphia, WB Saunders, 1979

Articles

Ament ME. Malabsorption syndromes in infancy and childhood. Part I. J Pediatr 1972 Oct; 81:685–697

Edelman R and Levine MM. Acute diarrheal infections in infants: Bacterial and viral causes. Hosp Pract 1980 Jan; 15(1):97–104

Jones KM. Love and lavage: The urgent needs of children with Hirschsprung's disease. Nursing '78 1978 July; 8(7):33–39

Koop CE, Schnaufer L, Broennie AM. Esophageal atresia and tracheoesophageal fistula: Supportive measures that effect survival. Pediatrics 1974 Nov; 54(5):558–564

Ling L and McCamman SP. Dietary treatment of diarrhea and constipation in infants and children. Issues Compr Pediatr Nurs 1978 Oct; 3(4):17–28

Parker SM et al. Gluten challenge in treated celiac disease. Arch Dis Child 1978 June; 53(6):449–455

Sanchez CL. Nursing care of the infant and child with cleft lip and palate. Point of View 1980 Jan; 17(1):14–15

Shah CP and Wong D. Management of children with cleft lip and palate. Can Med J 1980 Jan 12; 122(1):19–24

Trippie R and Jennings R. Nursing bottle syndrome. Keeping Abreast J 1978 Mar 3(2):114

CHILDREN WITH CONDITIONS OF THE KIDNEYS, URINARY TRACT, AND REPRODUCTIVE SYSTEM

43

ACUTE GLOMERULONEPHRITIS

Glomerulonephritis refers to inflammation of the kidneys caused by an antigen-antibody reaction following an infection in some part of the body. Acute glomerulonephritis is predominantly a disease of childhood and is the most common type of nephritis in children.

Etiology

1. Presumed cause—antigen-antibody reaction secondary to an infection elsewhere in the body
2. Initial infection
   a. Usually either an upper respiratory infection or a skin infection
   b. Most frequent causative agent—nephritogenic strains of Group A beta hemolytic streptococcus.
   c. Infrequent causative agents:
      (1) Other bacteria
      (2) Viruses

Altered Physiology

1. The organisms responsible for nephritis contain antigens similar to those of the basement membrane of the renal glomeruli.
2. Antibodies produced to fight the invading organism also react against the glomerular tissue.
3. The antigen-antibody combination results in an inflammatory reaction in the kidney.
   a. There are proliferation and swelling of the endothelial cells of the glomerular capillary wall.
   b. All of the glomeruli are involved, but the extent of proliferation varies among them.
4. Changes in the glomerular capillaries reduce the amount of the glomerular filtrate, allow passage of blood cells and protein into the filtrate, and reduce the amount of sodium and water that is passed to the tubules for reabsorption.
5. General vascular disturbances, including loss of capillary integrity and spasm of arterioles, are secondary to kidney changes and are responsible for much of the symptomatology of the disease.

Incidence

1. Unknown—milder cases are not recognized
2. More common in males than females
3. Most common in preschool and early school age groups
4. Rare in children under 2 years of age
5. Varies with the prevalence of nephritogenic strains of streptococci and the likelihood of cross infection

Clinical Manifestations

A. *Onset*

1. Usually 1–3 weeks after the onset of the initiating infection
2. May be abrupt and severe, or mild and detected only by laboratory measures

B. *Signs and Symptoms*

1. Urinary symptoms
   a. Decreased urine output
   b. Bloody or brown-colored urine
2. Edema
   a. Present in most patients
   b. Usually mild
   c. Often manifested by periorbital edema in the morning
   d. May appear only as rapid weight gain
   e. May be generalized and influenced by posture
3. Hypertension
   a. Present in over 50% of patients
   b. Usually mild
   c. Rise in blood pressure may be sudden
   d. Usually appears during the first 4–5 days of the illness
4. Variable fever
   a. May be high initially
   b. Usually fluctuates at about 37.8°C. (100°F.) for several days
5. Malaise
6. Mild headache
7. Gastrointestinal disturbances, especially anorexia and vomiting

Diagnostic Evaluation

1. Urinalysis
   a. Decreased output—may approach anuria
   b. Microscopic or gross hematuria

c. Specific gravity—moderately elevated
d. Protein
  (1) Variable
  (2) Usually below 3 gm. per day
e. White cells—moderate to many
f. Granular and cellular casts—especially red cell casts

2. Serum complement level—usually reduced
3. BUN and creatinine—often mildly to moderately elevated.
4. ASO or antistreptokinase titer—elevated
5. Sedimentation rate—elevated
6. Chest x-ray—may show pulmonary congestion, cardiac enlargement
7. Renal function studies—normal in 50% of the patients

Prognosis

1. Prognosis is generally good, but variable.
2. Younger children generally have the best prognosis for complete recovery.
3. At least 95% of affected children recover completely.
  a. Acute symptoms usually disappear in 1–3 weeks.
  b. Blood chemistry is usually normal by the end of the second week.
  c. Urine sediment may be abnormal for months or even years following the acute episode.
  d. Sedimentation rate may remain elevated for several months.
4. Death during the acute phase is very uncommon, but may occur due to the effects of hypertensive encephalopathy or heart failure.
5. A small percentage of children develop chronic nephritis.

Complications

(Occur infrequently)

A. *Hypertensive Encephalopathy*

1. Manifestations
  a. Restlessness
  b. Stupor
  c. Convulsions
  d. Vomiting
  e. Severe headache
  f. Visual disturbances
2. Cause—probably ischemia secondary to vasospasm
3. No correlation with the degree of renal impairment or fluid retention
4. Duration
  a. Usually 1–2 days
  b. Ends spontaneously with decreased blood pressure

B. *Congestive Heart Failure*

1. Cardiac failure may occur due to persistent hypertension, hypervolemia, and peripheral vasoconstriction.
2. Manifestations
  a. Dyspnea
  b. Tachycardia
  c. Gallop rhythm
  d. Liver engorgement
  e. Increased venous pressure
  f. Changes in the electrocardiogram
  g. Cardiac enlargement
  h. Pulmonary edema
3. Duration
  a. Variable

b. Usually subsides rapidly with the onset of diuresis and the fall in blood pressure

C. *Uremia* (rare)
Manifestations
  a. Evidence of acidosis
  b. Drowsiness
  c. Coma
  d. Stupor
  e. Muscular twitching
  f. Convulsions

D. *Anemia*
Usually caused by hypervolemia rather than a loss of red blood cells in the urine

Nursing Objectives and Management

A. *To promote healing and prevent disease complications.*

1. No specific measures have been demonstrated to modify the inflammatory process.
2. General measures
  a. Maintain bed rest during the acute phase of the illness, at least until gross hematuria has disappeared and child is no longer hypertensive.
    (1) Organize nursing activities to allow child to have periods of uninterrupted rest.
    (2) Explain to the child why it is necessary for him to stay in bed. (Bed rest is often interpreted by the child as punishment.)
    (3) Administer sedation if required to keep the child quiet and at rest.
    (4) Provide diversion appropriate for the child's age.
    (5) Place the child's bed in a position where he can watch the activities of the unit and other children.
    (6) Provide alternative means of rest for children who are too young to understand the necessity of remaining in bed. (Such children can be held in a chair.)
    (7) Observe the child closely for fatigue once ambulation is begun.
  b. Protect the child from infection.
    (1) Avoid placing the child in a room with patients who have fevers, upper respiratory infections, or any other contagious disease.
    (2) Administer therapeutic doses of antibiotics as prescribed by the physician to eradicate existing infection.
      (a) A 10-day course of intramuscular penicillin is often prescribed.
      (b) Points of emphasis.
        Inject the medication into a large muscle.
        Rotate the site of injection.
        Observe the child closely for adverse reactions such as skin rash, urticaria, serum sickness, and anaphylaxis.
    (3) Protect the child from chilling or overheating.
    (4) Provide scrupulous daily hygiene, including mouth care. Keep the skin clean and dry.
  c. Provide a diet in conformity with the child's age and the recommendation of his physician.
    (1) A regular diet without added salt is usually prescribed during the acute phase in noncomplicated cases.
    (2) A diet restricted in protein and potassium is necessary for children who demonstrate some degree of renal failure.
    (3) Fluids must be restricted in children with

hypertension, edema, congestive failure, or renal failure.

(4) Explain all dietary restrictions to the child and his parents.

(5) Obtain a careful history of dietary preferences and patterns so that the child's meals can be as acceptable as possible.

(6) Place a sign indicating dietary restrictions on the child's bed so that anyone approaching him will be aware of his special needs.

(7) If the child is to be given a restricted amount of fluids, offer small amounts of fluids spaced at regular intervals throughout the day and evening.

Use a cup of appropriate size for the amount of fluid being offered.

(8) Refer to section on nutrition, page 1112.

B. *To observe and record disease progress.*

1. Maintain a complete record of the child's intake and output.
   a. Measure fluids accurately in graduated containers. Do not estimate fluid intake or output.
   b. Place a sign on the child's bed to ensure that no urine is accidentally discarded and that all intake is recorded.
   c. Total the intake and output every 8 hours.
      (1) Notify the physician if output does not appear adequate.
      (2) In children who are not toilet trained, a fairly accurate record of intake and output can be obtained by weighing diapers before and after voiding.
   d. Record other causes of fluid loss such as the number of stools per day, perspiration, etc.
2. Weigh the child daily.
   a. An increase in weight may indicate fluid retention.
   b. Weigh the child on the same scale and at the same time each day.
      (1) It is usually advantageous to weigh the child before breakfast.
      (2) The child should be weighed in a consistent manner, with minimal clothing.
3. Record the blood pressure at frequent intervals.
   a. Refer to the method for determining blood pressure, page 1146.
   b. A diastolic pressure of 100 mm. Hg is an indication of concern and should be reported to the physician immediately.
      Place the child in the bed and observe him closely for cerebral changes.
4. Observe for signs of complications.
   a. Increased blood pressure
   b. Fluid retention or edema
   c. Changes in vital signs, especially more rapid pulse or respirations
   d. Changes in activity status, especially lethargy, restlessness, stupor, or coma
   e. Vomiting
   f. Visual disturbances
   g. Severe headache
   h. Convulsions
5. Record appearance of urine.
   Note the persistence of hematuria or whether the urine appears to be clearing.

C. *To reduce hypertension.*

1. Limit the fluid intake according to the physician's recommendation.

2. Maintain bed rest.
3. Administer antihypertensive drugs as prescribed by the physician.
   a. Reserpine is the drug most frequently employed.
      (1) Route of administration
          Intramuscular or intravenous
      (2) Side effects
          Nasal stuffiness, dryness of mouth, diarrhea
   b. Hydralazine (Apresoline) is often combined with reserpine in refractory cases.
      (1) Route of administration
          (a) Intramuscular.
          (b) This drug may be given orally once initial control of hypertension is established.
      (2) Side effects
          (a) Nausea, vomiting, diarrhea, anorexia
          (b) Headache
          (c) Tachycardia

D. *To provide appropriate nursing care to the child with disease complications.*

1. Encephalopathy
   Refer to the section on care of the child with seizures, page 1402.
2. Congestive heart failure. (Refer to the section on congestive heart failure, p. 1295.)
3. Anemia
   Refer to the section on anemia, page 1277.
4. Renal failure
   a. Maintain strict record of intake and output.
   b. Weigh the child at frequent intervals.
      It may be necessary to weigh the child as often as every 8–12 hours.
   c. Perform all nursing activities as for the care of the child with uncomplicated glomerulonephritis.
   d. Administer fluids as prescribed by the physician.
      (1) Fluid intake is usually restricted to an amount equal to urinary output plus insensible water loss
      (2) Fluid requirements must be recalculated frequently.
          These vary with such factors as the child's activity, sweating, vomiting, body temperature, metabolic rate, etc.
      (3) Some form of carbohydrate is usually prescribed to prevent excessive breakdown of body proteins and to decrease the formation of ketones.
          (a) Fluids, such as ginger ale or syrups, should be offered to the child who can tolerate oral fluids.
          (b) Glucose solutions may be administered intravenously. (Refer to the procedure for the administration of intravenous fluids, page 1171.)
   e. Have appropriate electrolytes available for administration.
      (1) Electrolytes are usually not added to the diet unless indicated by low serum levels or known loss.
          Plasma concentrations of sodium, potassium, chloride, and bicarbonate and also NPN and BUN must be monitored at frequent intervals.
      (2) Replacement of electrolytes is rarely indicated during the oliguric phase.
      (3) Potassium intoxication may occur and is usually counteracted by the administration of calcium gluconate or sodium bicarbonate (rapid but

transient effect) or a cation exchange resin (slower acting, but binds with potassium to remove it from the body).

   (4) Hypocalcemia requires the administration of calcium.

f. Assist with peritoneal or renal dialysis if this is required. (Refer to Guideline, p. 1186.)

E. To provide emotional support to the child and his family during hospitalization.

1. Explain all aspects of the diagnostic tests and treatment in terms that the family can understand.
2. Formulate a nursing care plan which facilitates a consistent approach to the child's care.
3. Allow the child to make some decisions and to participate in his care. He may decide when he wants his bath and should be allowed to make some dietary choices, etc.
4. Maintain discipline. Establish and enforce appropriate limits for the child's behavior.
5. Provide diversion appropriate for the child's age.
6. Arrange for the continued education of the school-age child.

F. To prepare the child and his parents for discharge.

1. Encourage as much family participation as possible during the child's hospitalization. (Refer to section on family centered care, p. 1131.)
2. Help the family plan for adaptation of the child's nursing care to the home environment.
   a. Review the medication schedule.

b. Suggest means of implementing sodium restricted diet.
   (1) Provide the family with a list of commercial foods and fluids which are normally high in sodium content, so that they can avoid these.
   (2) Help the parents to plan sample menus.
   (3) Provide suggestions for low-sodium cooking and baking.

c. Discuss activity and fluid restrictions if appropriate.

3. Make certain that the family has an appointment for continued medical supervision.
4. Initiate appropriate referrals.
   a. Community health nurse
   b. Home tutor

Patient or Parental Education

1. Medical explanation of the disease process should be reinforced.
   a. The need for medical evaluation and culture of all sore throats should be emphasized.
   b. The family should be made aware of signs and symptoms of disease recurrence.
2. Tonsillectomy or other oral surgery is not recommended for several months after the acute phase of glomerulonephritis.
   If this type of surgery is necessary later, penicillin may be recommended before and after the procedure to prevent bacterial infection.

NEPHROSIS

Nephrosis refers to a symptom complex characterized by edema, marked proteinuria, hypercholesterolemia and hypoalbuminemia. Although there are many types of the disease, lipid nephrosis or so-called minimal disease is the most common in children.

Etiology

1. The symptom complex results from large losses of protein in the urine, too great for the body to replenish by albumin synthesis.
2. The exact cause of the protein loss is unknown. The syndrome may be primary or idiopathic, congenital, or secondary to a wide variety of disease states or nephrotoxic agents.

Altered Physiology

1. For unknown reasons the glomerular membrane, usually impermeable to large proteins, becomes permeable.
2. Protein, especially albumin, leaks through the membrane and is lost in the urine.
3. Plasma proteins decrease as proteinuria increases.
4. The colloidal osmotic pressure which holds water in the vascular compartments is reduced owing to decrease in amount of serum albumin. This allows fluid to flow from the capillaries into the extracellular space, producing edema.
5. Accumulation of fluid in the interstitial spaces and peritoneal cavity is also increased by an overproduction of aldosterone, which causes retention of sodium.
6. There is increased susceptibility to infection because of decreased gamma globulin.

7. Generalized edema is responsible for most of the physical characteristics of the disease, including respiratory distress, gastrointestinal symptoms, umbilical and inguinal hernias, rectal prolapse, decreased ambulation, loss of body tissue, and malnutrition.

Incidence

1. Annually afflicts about 2–3 children per 100,000 under the age of 8 years in the United States
2. More common in males than in females
3. Most common age of onset—between 1½ and 3 years

Clinical Manifestations

A. Onset

1. Insidious
2. Edema is often the presenting symptom.
   a. Initially, usually slight and inconstant
   b. Usually first apparent around the eyes

B. Signs and symptoms

1. Irritability and depression
2. Gastrointestinal disturbances, including vomiting and diarrhea
3. Anorexia—malnutrition may become severe
4. Recurrent infections
5. Edema—may be minimal or massive
   a. Ascites may be severe
   b. Intense scrotal edema is common
   c. Peripheral edema is dependent and shifts with the child's position
   d. Striae may appear on the skin from overstretching
6. Profound weight gain; the child may actually double his normal weight

7. Decreased urine output during the edematous phase
8. Wasting of skeletal muscles may occur because of the continuous drain of plasma protein nitrogen into the urine
9. Nephrotic crisis
   a. Abdominal pain
   b. Fever
   c. Erysipeloid skin eruption possible.
   d. Symptoms subside within a few days
   e. Often followed by spontaneous diuresis

Diagnostic Evaluation

1. Urinalysis
   a. Proteinuria—marked
   b. Casts—numerous
   c. Hematuria—absent or transient
2. Renal function tests—variable, often normal
3. Blood
   a. Total serum protein—reduced
   b. Serum albumin—reduced
   c. Total serum globulin—normal or increased
      (1) Alpha and beta fractions—increased
      (2) Gamma fraction—reduced
   d. Amino acid level—decreased
   e. Anemia—absent or slight
   f. Sedimentation rate—elevated
   g. Cholesterol and lipoproteins—increased
4. Blood pressure—usually normal although mild hypertension may be present
5. Ear cartilage—frequently is soft

Clinical Course and Prognosis

1. The severity and duration of the clinical course is variable.
2. Partial or complete remissions occur secondary to spontaneous or induced diuresis.
3. Most children experience a number of remissions and exacerbations over a period of 1–10 years.
4. The majority of affected children eventually have a complete recovery. Some children may have compromised renal function for life.
5. Death may occur from profound sepsis, progressive renal insufficiency, or congestive heart failure.

Nursing Objectives and Management

A. *To relieve edema and other manifestations of the nephrotic state.*

1. Administer steroids as recommended by the physician.
   a. Steroid therapy is the preferred approach to treatment because steroids appear to affect the basic disease process in addition to controlling edema.
   b. Prednisone is usually the drug of choice because it is less apt to induce salt retention and potassium loss.
      There is no standard program of therapy, but most children receive 2–3 mg./kg. until complete remission occurs; this is followed by low-dose maintenance therapy or an intermittent schedule for 8–12 months.
   c. Children with nephrotic syndrome may respond to steroid therapy in several ways:
      (1) Steroid sensitive—children respond to a single short course of steroids without evidence of relapse after cessation of therapy.
      (2) Steroid dependent—children respond incom-

pletely or tend to relapse on lowered dosages of steroids and require additional supportive treatment.
      (3) Steroid resistant—children become resistant to steroid therapy or cannot be maintained in remission without developing serious side effects of treatment.
   d. Observe for evidence of side effects and complications of therapy.
      (1) Cushing's syndrome
         (a) Manifestations include increased body hair (hirsutism), rounding of the face (moon face), abdominal distention, striae, increased appetite with weight gain, and aggravation of adolescent acne.
         (b) The child should have access to a mirror so that he can observe gradual physical changes in his body.
         (c) The child and his parents should be provided with opportunities to discuss their feelings about the child's altered body image. Play therapy may be helpful for the young child.
         (d) It should be stressed that these physical changes are not harmful nor permanent, and will disappear after the steroid treatment is stopped.
      (2) Serious side effects and uncommon complications
         (a) Masking of infections
            The child should be observed very closely for signs of inflammation or infection.
         (b) Peptic ulceration
            1. Give medication with milk or an antacid.
            2. Test all stools with hematest.
         (c) Growth suppression
         (d) Precipitation of diabetes mellitus
         (e) Increased intracranial pressure manifested by headache, anorexia, vomiting, diplopia, and seizures
         (f) Osteoporosis
         (g) Cataracts
         (h) Thromboembolism
         (i) Adrenal suppression and insufficiency

NURSING ALERT: No vaccinations or immunizations should be given during active episodes of nephrosis or while the child is receiving immunosuppressive therapy.

2. Administer immunosuppressive drugs as prescribed by the physician.
   a. Cyclophosphamide is the drug of choice because its efficacy has been most thoroughly documented.
   b. This therapy is generally reserved for children with steroid-dependent or steroid-resistant nephrosis because of severe side effects. It should be administered only with informed consent of the patient or parent.
   c. Observe for complications of therapy.
      (1) Decreased white blood count renders the child very susceptible to infection.
      (2) Hair loss—the child should be prepared for this complication and should be helped to deal with the change in body image. Head scarves or wigs may minimize the child's distress.
      (3) Cystitis—the drug should be given in the morn-

ing and large volumes of fluid given orally to prevent concentration of the drug in the urine.

   (4) Sterility may result in both sexes from long-term use.

3. Administer diuretics as recommended by the physician.

   a. Diuretics are occasionally effective in relieving massive edema.

   b. Be aware of those diuretics which may cause potassium depletion.

      (1) Offer foods high in potassium, such as orange juice or bananas.

      (2) Supplemental potassium chloride may be administered orally if the urine output is adequate.

   c. Plasma expanders, such as salt-poor albumin, are frequently administered in conjunction with diuretic therapy to reduce the danger of hypovolemic shock.

4. Maintain the child on bed rest during periods of severe edema.

   Refer to the section on acute glomerulonephritis, page 1331.

5. Administer a diet low in sodium and high in potassium.

   a. Moderate sodium restriction is usually indicated. Excessively salty foods are excluded and extra salt is eliminated.

   b. Potassium may be provided in juices, fruits, (especially oranges, grapes, and bananas) and milk.

6. Restrict fluids as requested by the physician.

   a. Fluid restriction is usually imposed only during the extreme edematous phases.

   b. Restriction is carefully calculated at frequent intervals, based on the urine output of the previous day plus estimated insensible losses.

   c. Offer small amounts of fluids spaced at regular intervals throughout the day and evening.

      Use a cup of appropriate size for the amount of fluid being offered.

   d. Measure fluids accurately in graduated containers. Do not estimate fluid intake or output.

   e. Place a sign on the child's bed to ensure that no urine is accidentally discarded and that all intake is recorded.

   f. Determine total intake and output every 8 hours.

      In children who are not toilet trained, a fairly accurate record of output can be obtained by weighing diapers before and after voiding.

   g. Record other causes of fluid loss such as the number of stools per day, perspiration, etc.

7. Assist with abdominal paracentesis when this is required because of marked ascites. (See Guidelines, p. 1336.)

B. *To protect the child from infection.*

1. Apply measures stated in the section on acute glomerulonephritis, page 1331.

2. Closely observe the child who is on steroids for signs of infection since this medication masks such symptoms.

3. Provide meticulous skin care to the edematous areas of the body.

   a. Bathe the child frequently and apply powder.

      Areas of special concern are the moist parts of the body and edematous male genitalia.

      Support the scrotum with a cotton pad held in place by a T-binder if necessary for the child's comfort.

   b. Position the child so that edematous skin surfaces are not in contact.

      Place a pillow between the child's legs when he is lying on his side, etc.

   c. Irrigate swollen eyes and cleanse the surrounding area several times daily to remove exudate.

      Elevate the child's head to reduce edema.

4. If possible, avoid femoral venipunctures and intramuscular injections in the buttocks.

   In addition to the risk of infection, the child may be predisposed to thromboembolism because of hypovolemia, stasis, and increased plasma concentration of clotting factors.

C. *To restore lost plasma and tissue proteins.*

1. Offer a high protein, high calorie diet.

   a. Salt restriction is generally not necessary, except during periods of edema and hypertension.

   b. Fluid restriction is of little value in controlling edema in nephrosis.

2. Obtain a complete history of dietary preferences and patterns so that the child's meals can be as acceptable as possible.

3. Place a sign on the child's bed indicating any dietary restrictions, so that anyone approaching him will be aware of his special needs.

4. Offer small amounts of high protein foods at frequent intervals.

   Permit additional amounts of food at the child's discretion.

5. Refer to section on nutrition, page 1112.

D. *To observe for disease progress.*

1. Apply nursing measures outlined in objective B in the section on acute glomerulonephritis, page 1332.

2. Observe the child's entire body at frequent intervals for edema.

   Record areas of transient edema.

3. Measure all urine and test for protein and blood. Record findings:

   a. Decreased urine output

   b. Increased amount of protein

   c. Cloudiness

   d. Hematuria

4. Observe for side effects of all medications.

5. Observe for indications of thrombosis and report these to the physician immediately.

E. *To provide emotional support to the child and his family.*

1. Encourage frequent visiting.

   a. Allow as much parental participation in the child's care as possible.

   b. Refer to section on family centered care, page 1131.

2. Allow the child as much activity as he can tolerate.

   a. Bed rest should be enforced during periods of hypertension.

   b. Balance periods of rest, recreation, and quiet activities during the convalescent phase.

   c. Allow the child to eat his meals with other children.

3. Encourage the child to verbalize his fears.

   a. Young children frequently fear abandonment by their parents or loss of body integrity. (The boy who is unable to visualize his penis because of extensive edema may think that he has been castrated and needs reassurance that his body is intact.)

   b. Refer to section on the hospitalized child, page 1126.

4. Assist parents to verbalize their fears, frustrations, and questions.
   a. Parents often express frustration regarding the uncertainties associated with the cause of the disease, the clinical course, and prognosis.
   b. Parents may question the difference between nephritis and nephrosis.

F. *To prepare for the child's discharge.*

1. Begin discharge planning early.
   a. Have the dietitian discuss special diets with the parents. Encourage them to plan sample menus.
   b. Encourage the parents to administer the child's medication prior to discharge.
   c. Instruct parents about urine testing.
   d. Provide suggestions regarding activity restriction at home.
2. Provide written discharge instructions concerning:
   a. Diet
   b. Prevention of infection
   c. Skin care
   d. Administration of medications
   e. Activity restrictions, if any
   f. Urine testing
   g. Appointment for continued medical supervision.
3. Initiate a community health nursing referral if necessary for reinforcement of teaching.

Parental Education

1. Reinforce medical interpretation of the child's disease. Stress the importance of attention to the details of the child's care and continued medical supervision.
2. Discuss the problem of discipline with the parents. Encourage them to set consistent limits on and expectations of their child's behavior.
3. Emphasize the necessity of taking medication according to the prescribed schedule and for an extended period of time. Discuss complications encountered with steroid therapy.

GUIDELINES: Assisting with Pediatric Abdominal Paracentesis

Purpose   To withdraw fluid from the peritoneal cavity in order to relieve pressure symptoms and respiratory distress.

Equipment

Sterile equipment
  Hypodermic syringe
  Hypodermic and aspiration needles
  Novocain
  Scalpel
  Cannula
  Trocar
  Rubber tubing
  Needle holder
Nonsterile equipment
  Preparation tray
  Test tubes
  Pail for the collection of fluid

Suture needles and sutures
Forceps
Gloves
Towels
Graduated receptacle
Cotton balls
Gauze squares
Abdominal dressing

Abdominal binder
Safety pins

Procedure

NURSING ACTION	RATIONALE/AMPLIFICATION
Preparatory Phase	
1. Explain the procedure to the child in terms he can understand. Stress that he will feel better after the procedure.	1. To allay his fears and assure his cooperation.
2. Have the child void just prior to the procedure.	2. To avoid puncturing the bladder during the procedure.
3. Secure the help of a second person.	3. To observe the child and assist the physician during the procedure.

4. Position the child correctly:
   a. Place him close to the edge of the examining table.
   b. Support his back with your body.
   c. Hold his hands.	

Performance Phase	
1. Maintain the child's position.	1. To avoid injury.
2. Talk to the child frequently and hold his hands. Praise him for his cooperation.	2. To offer emotional support.
3. Observe the child's color and respirations.	3. Symptoms of shock develop if too much fluid is removed.
Follow-up Phase	
1. Apply abdominal binder snugly.	
2. Place the child in bed.	
3. Record the amount and character of the drainage and the child's condition.	
4. Observe frequently for signs of shock and note the drainage on the bandages.	

URINARY TRACT INFECTION

Urinary tract infection refers to an infection within the urinary system. Either the lower urinary tract (urethra, bladder, or the lower portion of the ureters) or the upper urinary tract (upper portion of the ureters or kidney) or both may be involved.

Etiology

1. Causative organisms
   a. E. Coli (most common)
   b. Proteus
   c. Klebsiella
   d. Pseudomonas
   e. Enterobacteriaceae
   f. Staphylococci
   g. Streptococci
   h. Viruses
2. Route of entry
   a. Ascent from the exterior (most common)
   b. Circulating blood
3. Contributing causes
   a. Obstruction, usually congenital
   b. Infections elsewhere in the body
      (1) Upper respiratory
      (2) Diarrhea
   c. Poor perineal hygiene
   d. Short female urethra
   e. Catheterization and instrumentation
   f. Entrance of an irritant into the bladder
   g. Inherent defect in the ability of the bladder mucosa to protect it from microbial invasion.

Altered Physiology

1. Inflammatory changes occur in the affected portions of the urinary tract.
2. Clumps of bacteria may be present.
3. Inflammation results in urinary retention and stasis of urine in the bladder. There may be backflow of urine into the kidneys through the ureters.
4. There are inflammatory changes in the renal pelvis and throughout the kidney when this organ is involved.
5. The kidney may become large and swollen.
6. Scarring of the kidney parenchyma occurs in chronic infection and interferes with kidney function, particularly with the ability to concentrate urine.
7. Eventually, the kidney becomes small, tissue is destroyed and renal function fails.

Incidence

1. Most common renal disease in children.
2. Almost 10 times more common in females than in males, except in the neonatal period.

Clinical Manifestations

A. *Onset*

1. May be abrupt or gradual
2. May be asymptomatic

B. *Signs and Symptoms*

1. Fever
   a. May be moderate or severe
   b. May fluctuate rapidly
   c. May be accompanied by chills or convulsions
2. Anorexia and general malaise
3. Urinary frequency, urgency, dysuria
4. Daytime or nocturnal enuresis
5. Dull or sharp pain in the kidney area
6. Irritability
7. Vomiting
8. Failure to thrive in infancy

Diagnostic Evaluation

1. Urine culture
   a. Documentation of pathogenic organisms in the urine is the only means of definitive diagnosis.
   b. A urine culture demonstrating more than 100,000 bacteria per milliliter indicates significant bacteriuria.
2. Urinalysis
   a. Pus is present in abnormal amounts.
   b. Casts, especially white cell casts, may be present and are indicative of intrarenal infection.
   c. Hematuria—occurs occasionally.
3. Renal concentrating ability—decreased
4. Urologic and radiologic studies:
   A voiding cystourethrogram and IVP should be done after the initial infection subsides to identify abnormalities, which might contribute to the development of infection, and to identify existing kidney changes due to recurrent infection.

Prognosis

1. Generally good in uncomplicated cases.
2. Persistent infection may occur in patients with obstruction or urinary retention and may lead ultimately to renal failure.
3. There is a tendency for recurrence of both treated and untreated infections.

Nursing Objectives and Management

A. *To obtain a clean urine specimen for examination or culture.*

1. A freshly voided early morning specimen is most accurate. (This urine is usually acid and concentrated, which tends to preserve the formed elements.)
2. Refer to the procedure for the collection of urine specimens, page 1166.
3. Catheterization may be necessary to obtain a sterile specimen in older girls.
   Defer this procedure whenever possible in order to avoid emotional trauma and the accidental introduction of additional bacteria.
4. Obtain a midstream specimen whenever possible.
5. The urine should be sent to the lab immediately or refrigerated to avoid a falsely high bacterial count.

B. *To eradicate infective organisms.*

1. Administer antibiotics as prescribed by the physician.
2. Antibiotic therapy is generally determined by the results of urine cultures and sensitivities, and by the child's response to therapy.
3. Most frequently used antibiotics:
   a. Sulfisoxazole (Gantrisin)
      (1) Side effects and toxic effects
         (a) Nausea and vomiting
         (b) Dizziness, headache, drug fever, dermatitis
         (c) Blood dyscrasias
         (d) Oliguria, crystalluria, and anuria—result

from precipitation of the drug in the renal tubules.
    (2) Contraindications
        (a) Drug sensitivity
        (b) Infants under the age of 2–3 months

> **NURSING ALERT:** Keep the child well hydrated to avoid crystallization of the drug in the renal tubules.

    b. Ampicillin
        (1) Side effects
            (a) Diarrhea
            (b) Nausea
            (c) Vomiting
            (d) Epigastric distress
            (e) Mild flatulence
            (f) Pruritis
            (g) Hypersensitivity reactions, including rash, urticaria, angioneurotic edema, and anaphylactic reactions
        (2) Contraindications
            (a) Known hypersensitivity to other penicillins
            (b) Infections caused by penicillinase-producing staphylococci or other penicillinase-producing organisms
        (3) Points of emphasis
            (a) Package circular should be consulted for directions regarding reconstitution, administration, and storage of intramuscular and intravenous preparations.
            (b) Oral preparations should be administered at least two hours after meals to assure maximum absorption.
            (c) Drug must be administered every 6 hours to maintain therapeutic blood levels.
    c. Nitrofurantoin (Furadantin)
        (1) Side effects and toxic effects
            (a) Nausea and vomiting
            (b) Peripheral neuritis
            (c) Hemolytic anemia
            (d) Sensitization
        (2) Contraindications
            (a) Anuria
            (b) Oliguria
            (c) Infants under 1 month of age
        (3) Points of emphasis
            (a) The drug may cause the urine to be amber or brown in color.
            (b) Drug should be administered after meals or with a small amount of food to minimize nausea or vomiting.
            (c) Recommended for prolonged use since resistance develops slowly.

C. *To provide for symptomatic relief of the child's discomfort during the febrile period.*

1. Maintain bed rest.
2. Administer analgesic and antipyretic drugs as recommended by the physician.
3. Encourage fluids to reduce the fever and dilute the concentration of the urine.
    a. Obtain a complete nursing history regarding the child's fluid preferences and method of taking them.
    b. Administer intravenous fluids if necessary. Refer to Guidelines, page 1171.

4. Refer to section on care of the child with fever, page 1148.

D. *To observe for progress of disease.*

Nursing notes should include:
    a. Frequent recording of the child's temperature
    b. Accurate measurement of intake and output
    c. Description of the color and odor of the urine, especially if it is abnormal
    d. Presence of any of the following symptoms
        (1) Frequency of urination
        (2) Burning or pain with voiding
        (3) Enuresis
        (4) Urinary retention
    e. General behavior and activity status of the child
    f. Signs of untoward or toxic effects of drugs
    g. Pain, especially in the kidney area

E. *To provide emotional support to the child and his parents.*

1. Reinforce medical explanations of the disease and its therapy.
2. Explain all diagnostic tests and procedures to the child before they are carried out.
3. Encourage the verbal child to talk about his experience and how he feels about it. Correct any misconceptions he may have, and particularly address concerns that the functioning of the urinary tract is separate from any sexual functions. The child should be reassured that the tests and treatment are for a problem that he did not cause.
4. Provide an environment that is as close to normal as possible during hospitalization. Include opportunities for the child to play.

F. *To prepare the child and his family for discharge.*

1. Discuss any treatment that will be required at home. Provide written discharge instructions regarding:
    a. Rest
    b. Fluid intake
    c. Administration of medications
    d. Appointment for continued medical supervision
2. Communicate or have the parents communicate with the school nurse if it is necessary for the child to receive medications at school.
3. Complete a community nursing referral if reinforcement of discharge teaching appears necessary.

Parental Education

1. Long-term therapy is often prescribed to prevent recurrence of urinary tract infections.
    a. Schedules for prolonged therapy vary from several months to a year.
    b. The infection should not be considered as eradicated until at least 2 negative cultures are obtained 4–6 weeks after cessation of therapy.
2. The child should be kept under continued medical surveillance because of the possibility of disease recurrence.
    a. Emphasis should be placed on the fact that even though this disease may have few symptoms, it can lead to very serious, permanent disability.
    b. Periodic urine cultures are indicated for 2 years following the acute infection.
3. Measures of prevention:
    a. Spread of bacteria from the anal and vaginal areas to the urethra can be minimized in female children by cleansing the perianal area from the urethra back toward the anus.

b. Bubble baths should not be used because of the bladder-irritant effect of these soaps.

c. Encourage adequate fluid intake, especially water.

d. Acidify urine with juices (e.g., cranberry).

e. Encourage child to void frequently and to empty the bladder completely with each voiding.

ABNORMALITIES OF THE GENITOURINARY TRACT WHICH REQUIRE SURGERY

EXSTROPHY OF THE BLADDER

In *exstrophy of the bladder,* the anterior surface of the bladder lies open on the lower part of the abdomen, allowing constant passage of urine to the outside. There are usually associated defects including separation of the pubic rami and epispadias in both sexes: cleft scrotum, undescended testes, and a shortened penis in males; cleft clitoris, separated labia, or shortened vaginal orifice in females.

Etiology

Results from failure of the abdominal wall and its underlying structures to fuse *in utero.*

Clinical Manifestations

1. Constant dribbling of urine excoriates the skin.
2. Infection and ulceration of the bladder mucosa may occur.
3. Genitalia may be ambiguous.
4. Affected children walk with a waddling or unsteady gait.

Management

1. Complete correction by means of plastic and orthopedic surgery is the preferred treatment.
2. Urinary diversion may be necessary in severe cases.

Nursing Management

A. *Preoperative Care*

1. Protect the bladder area from trauma and irritation.
   a. Position the infant on his back or side.
   b. Cleanse the area frequently with mild soap and water. Pat the area dry.
   c. Expose the area to warm, dry air; sunlight; or artificial light at least once or twice each day.
   d. Cover the defect with sterile gauze to which a bland ointment, such as petroleum jelly, has been applied, or with a layer of Saran wrap placed directly over the bladder.
   e. Change the gauze covering and the infant's diaper frequently.
2. Observe the infant closely for signs of infection.
3. Collect urine specimens by holding the infant over an emesis basin in a position that allows urine to drip into the container.
4. Assist parents to deal with their emotional reactions regarding the child's defect.
5. Teach parents how to care for the child at home. Initiate a community nursing referral if reinforcement of teaching or maternal support appears necessary.
6. Prepare the child and his parents for the proposed surgery. Refer to page 1139.

B. *Postoperative Care*

1. Provide care for the ureteral and urethral catheters. Observe and record the amount of urinary drainage, catheter positions, and occurrence of bladder spasms.

2. The child is often placed in a body cast for several weeks. Refer to Guidelines: Care of a Child in a Spica Cast, page 1218.
3. An ileal conduit may be necessary. Refer to page 1342.
4. Observe for complications:
   a. Urinary or incisional infections
   b. Fistulae in the suprapubic or penile incisions
5. Long-term support will be necessary for many children and families to help them deal with such fears as appearance of genitalia, potential inability to procreate, and rejection by peers. Ongoing discussion groups for parents and children may be helpful.

C. *Resource for Parents*

Parents of Children with Exstrophy, Children's Health Center, 2525 Chicago Ave., South, Minneapolis, Minn. 55403

PATENT URACHUS

Patent urachus is persistence of the embryonic connection between the umbilicus and the bladder. In many patients only a cyst persists, located at the upper end of the tract, under the umbilicus.

Clinical Manifestations

1. Urine dribbles from the umbilicus when entire urachus is present.
2. Midline swelling is present in cases of a cyst.
3. Infection of urachal cysts is common.

Treatment

1. Eradication of infection
2. Removal of cysts
3. Surgical obliteration of the patent urachus

OBSTRUCTIVE LESIONS OF THE LOWER URINARY TRACT

Types of Obstruction

1. Urethral valves
   a. Filamentous valves that obstruct urine flow
   b. Most commonly found in males
2. Congenital narrowing of the urethra
3. Bladder neck obstruction
   Most common site of lower urinary tract obstruction
4. Meatal stricture
5. Severe phimosis (rare)
6. Neuromuscular dysfunction (Refer to the section on spina bifida, p. 1391.)

Clinical Manifestations

Abnormal urination
   a. Dysuria
   b. Frequency
   c. Enuresis
   d. Dribbling

e. Reduced force of urine stream
f. Difficulty starting urine stream
g. Straining during urination
h. Abrupt cessation during urination

Altered Physiology

1. Urinary tract becomes distended proximal to the point of obstruction.
2. The bladder dilates and hypertrophies.
3. Stasis of urine occurs.
4. The ureters become elongated, dilated, and tortuous.
5. Hydronephrosis and destruction of kidney tissue inevitably result.

Treatment

1. Eradication and prevention of infection (See section on urinary tract infection, p. 1337.)
2. Dilation of urethral stenosis or stricture
3. Surgical relief of the obstruction

OBSTRUCTIVE LESIONS OF THE UPPER URINARY TRACT

Types of Obstruction

1. Stricture of a ureter
2. Congenital absence of 1 ureter
3. Duplication of the ureter of 1 kidney
4. Compression of a ureter by an aberrant blood vessel

Clinical Manifestations

1. Often asymptomatic. (There is seldom any problem with voiding.)
2. Vague symptoms such as failure to thrive may be present.
3. Urinary tract infections may be frequent.
4. Hypertension may occur.

Treatment

Same as for obstructions of lower urinary tract.

HYPOSPADIAS

Hypospadias is malposition of the urethral opening.

Altered Physiology

A. *Males*

1. The urethra opens on the lower surface of the penis, proximal to its usual site.
2. In severe cases, the urethra may open on the shaft of the penis, at its base, or on the perineum.
3. Frequently associated with congenital chordee in males—cord-like defect which extends from the scrotum up the penis and deflects the penis downward.

B. *Females*

The urethra opens into the vagina (rare).

Clinical Manifestations

1. Inability to void with the penis in the normal elevated position.
2. Severe forms interfere with the ability to procreate.

Treatment

Plastic surgery

CRYPTORCHIDISM (UNDESCENDED TESTIS)

Cryptorchidism is the absence of one or both testes from the scrotum. The testes may be located in the abdominal cavity or inguinal canal.

Etiology

Caused by delayed descent, prevention of descent by some mechanical lesion, or endocrine disorders (rare).

Clinical Manifestations and Altered Physiology

1. Normal development of secondary sex characteristics.
2. Degeneration of the sperm-forming cells occurs after puberty because of the higher temperature of the abdomen compared with the normal location in the scrotum. Sterility results.
3. Emotional disturbances often occur when the child discovers that he is different from his peers.
4. Associated hernias are found in more than 50% of the patients.

Treatment

1. Orchiopexy (placement of the testes in the scrotum) Surgery should be performed by the time the child is 5 years of age to prevent damage to the tissues and to lessen emotional concerns related to body image.
2. Plastic surgery in patients with an absent testis
3. Administration of chorionic gonadotropin—has produced descent of the testes in some children. (Testes would probably have descended spontaneously in these cases.)

Nursing Management

A. *Preoperative Care*

1. Encourage the child and his parents to express their feelings about the condition.
   Expect anxieties regarding sterility and homosexuality and perceptions of the child as defective or inadequate.
2. Discuss the condition and surgery frankly, in terms the child can understand.
   a. Maintain a matter-of-fact attitude.
   b. Clarify any misconceptions the child may have.
3. Provide privacy for medical examinations.

B. *Postoperative Care*

1. Maintain traction.
   a. A suture is placed in the lower portion of the scrotum and is attached to a rubber band which is fastened to the upper aspect of the inner thigh by a piece of adhesive
   b. This traction anchors the testis to the scrotum and is removed in approximately 5–7 days.
2. Prevent contamination of the suture line.
3. Administer antibiotics as prescribed to prevent infection.

AMBIGUOUS GENITALIA

Female Pseudohermaphroditism

1. Most common problem of sexual differentiation.
2. A deficiency of hydrocortisone results in adrenocortical hyperplasia and an overproduction of androgens

3. *Manifestations*—masculinization of the external genitalia in the female infant.
4. *Treatment:*
   a. Close observation for adrenal crisis
   b. Administration of hydrocortisone in children with adrenal hyperplasia
   c. Corrective plastic surgery, if needed
      This should be undertaken as early as possible, before social adjustment becomes a severe problem.

Male Pseudohermaphroditism

See chart below.

True Hermaphroditism

1. May be either genetic males or females.
2. Have both ovarian and testicular tissue.
3. Genitalia are usually ambiguous.
4. Gender choice is based on the infant's anatomy.
   Infant is usually reared as female.

Diagnostic Evaluation

1. Buccal smear to determine the presence or absence of sex chromatin
2. Endoscopy and x-ray studies to reveal presence, absence, and nature of internal genital structures
3. Chromosomal analysis to identify genetic sex
4. Biochemical tests of urinary steroid excretion patterns
5. Laparotomy or gonad biopsy

Nursing Management

1. Recognize the situation as a social emergency.
   Support the parents while they wait for gender assignment for the infant. This should be done as soon as possible, but may require several days or weeks for results of studies.
2. Reinforce medical explanations of the anatomic problems and treatment. Approach the situation matter-of-factly.
3. Initiate appropriate referrals for family support and counseling. These may include:
   a. Social work
   b. Psychiatry
   c. Community health nursing
   d. Child guidance clinic
   e. Genetic counseling

CARE OF THE CHILD REQUIRING UROLOGIC SURGERY

Preoperative Care

1. Determine the child's fantasies regarding his illness and hospitalization. Correct any misconceptions that he reveals.

2. Provide an explanation of the anatomy and physiology of the urinary system in terms that the child can understand.
   a. Use a body outline appropriate for the age of the child.
   b. Explain how the child differs from the normal.
      Relate his defect to his symptoms whenever possible.
3. Explain all diagnostic tests prior to their occurrence. These may include: urinalysis, 24-hour urine collections, intravenous and retrograde pyelography, angiography, and cystoscopy.
   a. Descriptions should include such information as:
      (1) Preparation required—fasting, enemas, etc.
      (2) Location of the test—operating room, radiology department, etc.
      (3) Appearance and attire of personnel
      (4) Positioning
      (5) Anesthesia
      (6) Pain or discomfort
      (7) Expectations following the procedure—diet, rest, urine collections, etc.
   b. Determine the child's understanding of the procedure.
      (1) Ask him simple, direct questions.
      (2) Allow him to perform the procedure on a doll or demonstrate it on a diagram.
4. Explain the surgical procedure.
   a. Explanations should include:
      (1) Preparation required—fasting, enemas, etc.
      (2) Description of the operating room including the appearance of the personnel
      (3) Anesthesia
      (4) Postoperative appearance
         (a) Urinary drainage tubing and collection devices
         (b) Appearance of urine
         (c) Sutures
         (d) Bandages
         (e) Intravenous infusion
   b. Determine the child's understanding of his surgery and reinforce teaching when necessary.
5. Points of emphasis during the preparation:
   a. The child is in no way to blame for his illness.
   b. No other part of the body will be operated on.

Postoperative Care

1. Care for all catheters and urinary tubes according to hospital procedure. Maintain appropriate position of tubes.
2. Observe and record:
   a. Amount and appearance of urinary drainage
   b. Occurrence of bladder spasms
   c. Symptoms of urinary or incisional infection

Male Pseudohermaphroditism

Type	Treatment
1. Normal female genitalia with testes internally.	1. a. Surgical removal of testes. b. Administration of estrogens at puberty. c. Child reared as a girl.
2. Predominantly male genitalia with testes internally.	2. a. Surgical removal of all nonmale structures. b. Child reared as a boy.
3. Ambiguous genitalia due to damaged testes in fetal life.	3. a. Plastic reconstruction. b. Child reared as a boy.

Care of the Child Who Has an Ileal Conduit (Ileoloop)

A. *Definition of the Procedure*

One or both ureters are anastomosed to a segment of ileum, which then serves to carry urine to the external body surface of the abdomen.

B. *Preoperative Care*

1. Refer to the preceding section on the emotional preparation of the child and his family for urologic surgery.
2. Allow the child to try on the ileal conduit apparatus in order to become familiar with it.

   Observe for discomfort and skin reactions to the adhesive or cement.
3. Administer antimicrobials as prescribed by the physician.

   Be aware of the action, side effects, and contraindications of the prescribed therapy.
4. Provide the child and his parents with opportunities to express their fears and ask questions about the procedure.

   Expect worries related to sterility, location and appearance of the stoma, activity restrictions, clothing, and management.
5. Reassure the child and his parents that they will be taught to manage the conduit before leaving the hospital.
6. If appropriate, introduce the family to a rehabilitated individual who has had the same surgery.

   Trained volunteers from the United Ostomy Association may be able to provide valuable psychological support.

C. *Postoperative Care*

1. Maintain the urinary collection apparatus. (A temporary collection bag is usually worn in the immediate postoperative period and may be replaced by a permanent appliance once edema of the stoma subsides.)
   a. Cleanse the area around the stoma with mild soap and water and dry it well.
   b. Keep the skin around the stoma completely dry during application of the appliance to ensure that it will remain attached.
   c. Place the adhesive plate of the appliance securely around the stoma.

      The opening in the adhesive plate should be of a size that fits snugly over the stoma but does not compromise circulation.
   d. Empty the appliance every 2 hours or whenever it contains approximately 100 ml. of fluid. (During the night the appliance may be attached via tubing to a collection bottle.)
   e. Nursing observations related to the appliance.
      (1) Leaking around the appliance
      (2) Skin irritation
      (3) Improper fit of the appliance
   f. Points of emphasis.
      (1) A properly applied apparatus should remain in place 3–5 days. It needs to be changed only when it begins to leak or becomes uncomfortable.
      (2) It is normal for the urine to contain some mucus; it may be blood tinged.
2. Offer generous amounts of fluids to maintain hydration and keep the urine dilute and clear.

   Cranberry juice should be included in the diet because it helps to keep the urine acid.

3. Carefully monitor intake and output.

   Decreased urine output may indicate dehydration, obstruction of ureters, urine drainage into the peritoneal cavity, or compromised kidney function.
4. Observe for complications.
   a. Wound infection
   b. Leaking at the site of anastomosis
   c. Peritonitis
   d. Paralytic ileus
   e. Intestinal obstruction
   f. Stenosis of the stoma
   g. Fluid and electrolyte disturbances
5. Assist the child and his family with problems related to altered body image.
   a. Assume a calm, understanding, and matter-of-fact attitude.
   b. Avoid outward expression of distaste.
   c. Keep equipment used in the management of the conduit out of sight to avoid embarrassment when visitors appear.
   d. Encourage the child to wear his own clothes so he is reassured that the appliance is invisible under clothing.
   e. Take precautions to prevent or eliminate odors, e.g., immediate cleansing of used collection bags, etc.
   f. Help the child and family to achieve control by teaching them to manage the care as soon as possible.
   g. Encourage early resumption of as many normal activities as possible.

D. *Patient or Parental Education*

1. Involve the child and his family in his self-care as soon as possible.

   Teaching should include how to assemble, apply, empty, change, and cleanse the appliance.
2. Explain that appliances can be adapted to meet individual patient's needs.

   Some experimentation will probably be necessary before the most suitable equipment can be identified.
3. Adequate fluid intake (approximately 125 ml./kg. [1.7 oz./lb.] is essential for maintaining good urine flow.
4. Two appliances should be available, one in use and the other as a spare.
5. The appliance should be cleaned and aired regularly to avoid odor or crusting.
   a. A few drops of Lysol to a quart of water whitens and deodorizes the bags.
   b. Crusting can be removed by a solution of white vinegar and water (approximately 1 cup of white vinegar to a quart of water).
   c. A mild soap and warm water should be used to clean the appliance.
6. New appliances should be purchased approximately every 6 months or whenever old ones begin to feel thin or worn.
7. Activity limitations are usually not necessary unless the child has associated physical problems.
8. Clothing may have to be altered slightly to fit over the pouch of the appliance.

E. *Preparation for Discharge*

1. Provide written information regarding the equipment that the child is using and where to obtain it.
2. Provide at least a 2-week supply of equipment for the family to take home.

Advise the parents to order new supplies before the old ones are depleted.
3. Initiate appropriate referrals.
   a. Community nursing agency.
   b. Local "ostomy" clubs.

F. *References for Parents*
Norris C. All About Jimmy. Los Angeles, United Ostomy Association, 1973
United Ostomy Association, 2001 West Beverly Blvd., Los Angeles, Calif. 90057

BIBLIOGRAPHY

Books

Chisholm TC and McParland FA. Exstrophy of the Urinary Bladder. In Ravitch MM (ed). Pediatric Surgery, 3rd ed. Chicago, Year Book Medical Publishers, 1979

Edelmann C (ed). Pediatric Kidney Disease, Vol. 2. Boston, Little, Brown & Co., 1978

Hollerman C. Pediatric Nephrology. Garden City, Medical Examination Pub. Co., 1979

James JA. Renal Disease in Childhood. St. Louis, CV Mosby, 1976

Jeter K. Management of the Urinary Stoma. New York, Department of Urology, College of Physicians and Surgeons of Columbia University Squier Urological Clinic. Columbia Presbyterian Medical Center, 1970

Johnston JH and Goodwin W (eds). Reviews in Pediatric Urology. New York, American Elsevier, 1974

Kelasis PP and King LR (eds). Clinical Pediatric Urology, Vol. 1. Philadelphia, WB Saunders, 1976

Kunin CM. Detection, Prevention and Management of Urinary Tract Infections. Philadelphia, Lea & Febiger, 1979

Lenneberg E and Werner M. The Ostomy Handbook. Los Angeles, United Ostomy Association, 1973

Liberman E. Clinical Pediatric Nephrology. Philadelphia, JB Lippincott, 1976

Petrillo M and Sanger S. Emotional Care of Hospitalized Children, 2nd ed. Philadelphia, JB Lippincott, 1980

Royer P et al. Pediatric Nephrology. Major Problems in Clinical Pediatrics, Vol. 11. Philadelphia, WB Saunders, 1974

Rubin M (ed). Pediatric Nephrology. Baltimore, Williams & Wilkins, 1975

Scipien G et al. Comprehensive Pediatric Nursing, 2nd ed. New York, McGraw–Hill, 1977

Strauss J (ed). Pediatric Nephrology: Current Concepts in Diagnosis and Management, Vol. 5: Nephrotic Syndrome. New York, Stratton Intercontinental Medical Book Corp., 1978

Strauss J (ed). Pediatric Nephrology: Current Concepts in Diagnosis and Management, Vol. 6: Urinary Tract Infection and Tubulo-Interstitial Nephritis, Infectious and Noninfectious. New York, Stratton Intercontinental Medical Book Corp., 1979

Whaley L and Wong D. Nursing Care of Infants and Children. St. Louis, CV Mosby, 1979

Articles

Bergen M et al. Urinary tract infection in the infant: The unsuspected diagnosis. Pediatrics 1978 Oct; 62(4):610–612

Cytryn L et al. Psychological implications of cryptorchidism. J Am Acad Child Psychol 1967 Jan; 6(1):131–165

Dewhurst J. Congenital malformations of the lower urinary tract. J Clin Obstet Gynaecol 1978 Apr; 5(1):51–65

Etkin R et al. Urinary tract infections in school-age girls: Correlations among significant bacteriuria and symptoms, patient history and family history. Pediatrics 1978 Nov; 62(5):544–547

Fine N et al. Long-term results of renal transplantation in children. Pediatrics 1978 Apr; 61(4):641–651

Frauman SAC et al. Habilitation of the pediatric renal transplant patient—the process of assuming a normal lifestyle. Nephrol Nurse 1979 Sept/Oct; 1(5):15–18

Gillenwater JY et al. Natural history of the bacteriuria in schoolgirls. A long-term case-control study. N Engl J Med 1979 Aug; 301(8):396–399

Goldstein LE et al. Exstrophic anomalies: Follow-up of 36 cases. J Urol 1978 Dec; 120(6):738–741

Hendren WH. Some alternatives to urinary diversion in children. J Urol 1978 May; 119(5):652–660

Hetrick A, Frauman A, Gilman C. Nutrition in the renal disease: When the patient is a child. Am J Nurs 1979 Dec; 79(12):2152–2154

Juliana L. When infection leads to acute glomerulonephritis—here's what to do. Nursing '79 1979 Sept; 9(9):40–45

Kunin CM. Epidemiology and natural history of urinary tract infections in school-age children. Pediatr Clin North Am 1971 May; 18(2):509–528

Kunin CM. Priorities in the prevention of pyelonephritis. Am J Dis Child 1977 Nov; 131(11):1281–1282

Lattimer JK et al. The optimum time to operate for cryptorchidism. Pediatrics 1974 Jan; 53(1):96–99

Lewis A and Costellana M. Urinary loop undiversion—a collaborative nursing approach. Pediatric Nursing 1979 July/Aug; 5(4):42–45

Machin GA. Urinary tract malformation in the XYY male. Clin Genet 1978 Dec; 14(6):370–372

McCormick MC. The recognition of urinary tract infections in office-based pediatric practice. Clin Pediatr 1978 Sept; 17(9):713–717

Perry S. Ureteral reimplantation for uretero–vesical reflux. Crit Care Update 1979 Dec; 6:12–16

Randolph MF et al. Home screening for the detection of urinary tract infections in infancy. Am J Dis Child 1979 July; 133(7):713–717

Stann J. Urinary tract infections in children. Pediatric Nursing 1979 July/Aug; 5(4):49–52

Stark J. BUN/Creatinine: Your keys to kidney function. Nursing '80 1980 May; 10(5):33–38

Stevens M and Reinitz M. Nursing a child through exstrophic bladder reconstruction surgery. MCN 1980 July/Aug; 5(4):265–270

Wientzen RL et al. Localization and therapy of urinary tract infections of childhood. Pediatrics 1979 Mar; 63(3):467–474

Resources for Children and Parents

National Kidney Foundation, 116 East 27th Street, New York, N.Y. 10016.

Pamplin H, Light J, Hyman L. Sidney Kidney—A Book for Children and Parents About Renal Disease, Hemodialysis and Transplantation. Washington, D.C., Walter Reed Army Medical Center 20012. Sale by Superintendent of Documents, U.S. Government Printing Office, Washington, D.C. 20402

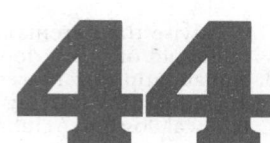
BURNS IN CHILDREN

Burns are a frequent form of childhood injury. A second degree burn of 10% or more of the body surface, 5% or more full thickness, or burns of face, hands, feet or perineum in a child younger than 1 year, or a second degree burn of 15% or more of the body surface in a child over 1 year is considered a very serious injury. The effects of burns are not limited to the burn area.

Incidence and Etiology

1. Burns outnumber all other causes of death during infancy, childhood, and adolescence, with the highest incidence of burns occurring in children under 5 years of age.
2. Causes of burns in children
   a. Burns from hot water
      (1) Child (left unsupervised in tub) turns on the hot water tap
      (2) Child placed in tub of hot water that has not been tested
      (3) Spilling of hot coffee, tea on child; spilling occurs especially when pot handles stick out on top of stove
   b. Burns from open flames
      (1) House fires
      (2) Child climbing up to stove—clothing catches fire
      (3) Child playing with matches
      (4) Playing/working with gasoline
      (5) Gas tank explosion during automobile accident
   c. Electrical burns
      (1) Child playing with electrical outlets or appliances
      (2) Child playing with extension cords
      (3) Child playing on railroad tracks
   d. Caustic acid or alkali burns of mouth and esophagus
      Child ingesting strong household cleaning products
   e. Chemical burns of the skin
      Child playing with gasoline that comes in contact with skin (often the gasoline ignites)
   f. Burns inflicted upon the child as a result of neglect or child abuse

g. Smoke inhalation and inhalation from plastic combustion

Clinical Manifestations

1. The characteristics of burn wounds are classified as follows:
   a. First degree burns (partial thickness—epidermal) involve superficial epidermis; the skin is pink or red in appearance and is painful to touch.
   b. Second degree burns (partial thickness—superficial or deep dermal) involve the entire epidermis; the skin is red, blistered, moist with exudate, and painful to pinprick or touch. Deep dermal injury penetrates deep into corium and may be anesthetic for 1–2 days after burn injury.
   c. Third degree burns (full thickness—subdermal) involve the dermis or underlying fat, muscle, or bone; the skin appears white, dry, or charred and has little pain. Often it is difficult to tell the degree of burn, especially in the young child.
2. Symptoms of shock appear soon after the burn:
   a. Rapid pulse
   b. Subnormal temperature
   c. Pallor
   d. Prostration
   e. Low blood pressure
3. Symptoms of toxemia may develop within 1–2 days after the initial burn:
   a. Prostration
   b. Fever
   c. Rapid pulse
   d. Cyanosis
   e. Vomiting
   f. Edema

NOTE: These symptoms may progress to coma or death.

4. Burns of the respiratory tract result in symptoms of upper airway obstruction resulting from acute edema and inflammation of the glottis, vocal cords, and upper trachea.
   a. Rapid breathing
   b. Dyspnea
   c. Stridor

d. Nasal flaring
e. Restlessness
5. Smoke inhalation may cause no initial symptoms other than mild bronchial obstruction during the initial phase following the burn. Within 6–48 hours the child may develop sudden onset of the following conditions:
a. Bronchiolitis
b. Pulmonary edema
c. Severe airway obstruction
d. Damage from smoke inhalation—can present up to 7 days after the burn injury

Altered Physiology

See section on burns in adults, page 598.

Treatment

See adult section on burns, page 598.
OBJECTIVES: to replace fluid loss from burn surface.
to maintain circulation.
to prevent renal failure.
to prevent or treat infection.
to aim toward early repair of the burn wound.
to restore the child to the best possible state of physical and psychological functioning.
1. Calculation of the burn area
a. Evans' "rule of nine" (used in assessment of extent of burns in adults) has proved quite inexact when applied to young children. May be acceptable to use in child over 10 years of age.
(1) During infancy and early childhood the relative surface area of different parts of the body varies with age.
(2) The younger the child, the greater the proportion of the surface area constituted by the head and the lesser the proportion of the surface area constituted by the legs.
b. Calculation of percentage of burn surface area is based on Lund and Browder's design (Fig. 44-1). This design compensates for the changes in percentage of body surface resulting from growth.
2. Categorization of seriousness of burn is based on
a. Total area injured
b. Depth of injury
c. Location of injury
d. Age of child
e. Condition of patient, i.e., level of consciousness
f. Previous medical history (i.e., chronic disease)

Complications

Depend upon severity of burn injury and are usually the rule rather than exception, especially with severe burn injury.

A. Acute

1. Infection
a. Burn wound sepsis
b. Pneumonia
c. Urinary tract infection
d. Phlebitis
2. Curling's ulcer, GI hemorrhage—most likely to occur in burns >20% body surface area
3. Acute gastric dilation
4. Renal failure
5. Respiratory failure
6. Post-burn seizures
7. Hypertension
8. CNS dysfunction
9. Vascular ischemia
10. Anemia and malnutrition
11. Fecal impaction

B. Long-term

1. Malnutrition
2. Scarring
3. Contractures
4. Psychological trauma

Nursing Objectives and Management

A. *To recognize the symptoms of shock and to use support measures which are initiated to restore and maintain circulation.*
1. Be alert to the symptoms of shock which occur very shortly after a severe burn.
a. Tachycardia
b. Hypothermia
c. Hypotension
d. Pallor
e. Prostration
f. Shallow respirations
2. Monitor the administration of intravenous fluid, since major burns are followed by a reduction in blood volume due to outflow of plasma into the tissues.
a. Maintain the administration of plasma and intravenous fluid—usually lactated Ringer's solution is used during first 24 hours after injury.
b. Obtain weight—this measurement is critical for accurate intravenous fluid volumes to be determined.
Infants and small children: 4 ml./Kg./% burn
Older child: 2–3 ml./Kg./% burn
c. Fluid loss from transcapillary leakage is greatest during the first 12 hours post-injury and diminishes to almost zero 12–24 hours post-injury. Fluid loss after 48 hours is due to vaporization of water from wound.
d. Maintain the administration of other intravenous fluids, including albumin, once the plasma volume is restored.
3. Maintain an accurate record of intake and output.
a. Record time and amount of all fluids given.
b. Measure accurate urinary output every ½ hour to 1 hour.
(1) With severe burn injuries, an indwelling catheter may be used the first 3 days.
(2) Urine flow is a most helpful clinical guide to fluid replacement and kidney function.
(3) Estimate urine output: 1 ml./Kg./hour or
10–20 ml./hour under 2 years of age
20–30 ml./hour 3–5 years of age
30–50 ml./hour over 5 years of age
(4) Check specific gravity.
(5) Report diminishing urinary output.
4. Provide a rich oxygen environment in order to combat hypoxia, as necessary.
5. Provide sedation to relieve pain.
a. Sedatives must be given in very small amounts to children in order to prevent their depressant effect.
b. In severe burn injury, sedation should be given intravenously because of lack of absorption of intramuscular medication during emergency phase.

BURN SHEET

Name _____ Age _____ Number _____

Date of Observation _____

Relative Percentages of Areas Affected by Growth			
Area	Age 0	1	5
A = $\frac{1}{2}$ of head	$9\frac{1}{2}$	$8\frac{1}{2}$	$6\frac{1}{2}$
B = $\frac{1}{2}$ of one thigh	$2\frac{3}{4}$	$3\frac{1}{4}$	4
C = $\frac{1}{2}$ of one leg	$2\frac{1}{2}$	$2\frac{1}{2}$	$2\frac{3}{4}$

	% Burn by Areas			
Probable 3rd burn	Head _____ Neck _____ Body _____ Upper arm _____			
	Forearm _____ Hands _____ Genitals _____ Legs _____			
	Buttocks _____ Thighs _____ Feet _____			
Total burn	Head _____ Neck _____ Body _____ Upper arm _____			
	Forearm _____ Hands _____ Genitals _____ Legs _____			
	Buttocks _____ Thighs _____ Feet _____			
Sum of all areas _____	Probable 3rd _____		Total burn _____	

FIGURE 44-1. *Calculation of burn surface area. (Redrawn from Pascoe, D.J., and Grossman, M: Quick Reference to Pediatric Emergencies. Philadelphia, J.B. Lippincott, 1973; appears in Waechter, E.H., and Blake, F.G.: Nursing Care of Children, 9th ed. Philadelphia, J.B. Lippincott, 1976.)*

6. Provide a source of heat over the child's bed, since additional heat may be necessary to maintain body temperature.
7. Request laboratory results and record on special flow sheet.
   a. Hematocrit or RBC serves as a rough guide to the adequacy of initial treatment, since the loss of plasma results in concentration of red blood cells.
   b. Electrolytes serve as a guide to fluid replacement.
8. Maintain close observation of vital signs in order to evaluate continuously the state of peripheral circulation; check for clear sensorium. Report immediately any significant changes.
9. Observe for additional complaints or circumstances that might suggest associated injury.
   a. GI hemorrhage.
   b. Acute gastric dilatation may occur, especially if child has greater than 20% injury, associated injury, or tachypnea. Nasogastric tube may be inserted to prevent vomiting, aspiration, and paralytic ileus.
   c. Ileus—associated with circulatory problems in small children; may be alleviated with insertion of nasogastric tube.
10. Determine need for tetanus inoculation.

B. *To observe for symptoms of respiratory distress and to initiate measures to alleviate distress.*

Most common form of airway obstruction in young child is from edema of head and neck, glottic and subglottic areas.

1. Be alert for symptoms of respiratory distress:
   a. Dyspnea
   b. Stridor
   c. Rapid respirations
   d. Restlessness
   e. Cyanosis

2. Provide an oxygen source in order to combat anoxia.
3. Report these symptoms.
4. Monitor blood gases.
5. Intubation or tracheostomy may be performed.

C. *To obtain medical history of the child: childhood diseases, immunizations, current medications, and recent infections.*

D. *To provide scrupulous skin care in order to prevent infection and promote healing.*

1. Burn treatment:
   a. Exposure—maintains a dry surface, produces early formation of a protective eschar, and predisposes patient to less infection; usually combined with the use of antibacterial creams and daily soaking in Hubbard tank to remove cream and dead tissue; can allow for increased movement.
   b. Occlusive dressing—burns are kept covered with dressings that have been soaked in a solution, or topical medication is applied followed by dressing. Dressings are changed every 8–24 hours. Burned areas are soaked daily in Hubbard tank. Dressings are often bulky and restrict movement.
   c. Primary excision of burn—necrotic eschar is immediately removed, allowing site to be grafted. Grafting may be postponed 24–48 hours with temporary cover of porcine xenograft.
   d. Escharotomy—incision through eschar to relieve severe constriction and compromised circulation. It is done within first 12–24 hours after injury.
   e. Physicians have their own preferences as to which method is used. The goals remain the same—to prevent infection, to remove dead tissue, and to provide for early closure of wound.
   f. Maintain sterility in working with the burn area regardless of whether the open or closed method is used. Laminar flow units are often used.

2. Cleansing the wound and changing the dressing is critical for preventing infection, preserving tissue, promoting early closure of the wound, and maintaining function.
   a. Hubbard tank is treatment of choice for cleansing.
   b. Use sterile technique—gown, cap, mask, gloves, and plastic apron.
   c. Limit tubbing to 20 minutes to prevent hypothermia, hyponatremia, and hemodilution.
   d. Isotonic solution may be needed for large wounds and small children.
3. The Bradford frame may be used to facilitate skin care.
   a. Provides a method for the collection of urine and feces and maintains cleanliness of the burn areas and dressings.
   b. Contractures may be prevented by maintaining functional position of extremities and good body alignment.
   c. Two Bradford frames may be used to change position of the child from back to stomach and vice versa without having to handle the severely burned child.
4. Position the child and turn him frequently.
5. Apply protective devices to prevent the child from scratching the burn area.
6. Administer antibiotics as prescribed.
   a. Prophylactic penicillin may be used against beta-hemolytic streptococci in the first 5–7 days, especially with autografting.
   b. Specific antibiotic therapy may be necessary for complicating infection.
7. Ensure that serial wound biopsy and quantitative cultures are done if prescribed.
8. Topical antibacterial therapy may include:
   a. 1% silver sulfadiazine cream (Silvadene)—treatment of choice at present; especially for partial thickness burn.
      (1) Easy to apply.
      (2) Does not hurt child upon application.
      (3) Allergic reactions occur very rarely.
   b. Povidone–iodine
      Allergic reaction fairly common.
   c. 10% mafenide acetate (Sulfamylon) cream
      (1) Allergic reaction (rash)—common.
      (2) Painful immediately after application where there is partial thickness burn.
      (3) Metabolically active in kidney as carbonic anhydrase inhibitor resulting in metabolic acidosis and hyperventilation.
      (4) Most effective for extensive burns with thick eschar.
   d. ½% silver nitrate soaks
      (1) Solution is hypo-osmolar, leading to electrolyte deficiencies.
      (2) Soaks are continuous, messy, and turn everything they touch black.
   e. Povidone–iodine
      Allergic reaction fairly common.
9. Heterograft or homografts are used to:
   a. Restore water vapor barrier and decrease protein loss
   b. Decrease pain
   c. Decrease bacterial count at the wound as graft adheres to the site

E. *To monitor parenteral fluids to prevent electrolyte imbalance and dehydration.*

1. Injury-induced fluid loss is greatest up to 48 hours post-burn, at which time reabsorption of these fluids results in diuresis if renal function is intact; accurate urinary output measurement is critical during this time.
2. Decreasing water loss by evaporation can be accomplished by keeping ambient air warm and moist, thus reducing high energy requirements and the chance of metabolic derangements. This, however, sets up an excellent environment for growth of *Pseudomonas*.
3. When parenteral hyperalimentation is used, there is increased risk of infection in the burned patient. Be alert to early signs and symptoms of infection.

F. *To provide a high protein, high calorie diet in order to provide nutrition necessary for healing and for the growth and developmental needs of the child.*

1. Hypernutrition is important, because of the extreme hypermetabolism related to large burn injuries.
   a. High caloric—to support hypermetabolic state; protein synthesis; calories should come from carbohydrates.
   b. High protein—to replace protein lost by exudation; support synthesis of immunoglobulins and structural protein; prevent negative nitrogen balance
   c. Vitamin and mineral supplement—particularly vitamins B and C, iron and zinc
2. Anorexia is common in the burned child.
   a. Tell child why eating is important.
   b. Offer small amounts of food, perhaps 4–5 feedings rather than 3 per day.
   c. Give him a choice of foods; determine his favorite foods.
   d. Offer high protein, high calorie dietary supplements.
   e. Make meals a pleasant time, unassociated with treatments or unpleasant interruptions.
   f. Nasogastric tube feedings may be necessary to supply high nutritive needs.

G. *To maintain a planned physical therapy program in order to achieve the greatest functional capacity for the child.*

1. Carry out physical therapy procedures to minimize joint and skin complications:
   a. Position—position joint in opposite direction of expected contracture.
   b. Splints—aid joint positioning and decrease skin contractures and hypertrophy.
   c. Exercise—gain and maintain optimal range of motion.
   d. Pressure garment—aid circulation, protect newly healed skin, prevent and treat hypertrophic scar formation. It may be necessary to wear pressure garments 12–18 months after injury at which time healed skin has matured and become supple.
2. Plan the time each day for the therapy to be carried out.
3. Utilize play opportunities to help the child accept the program (e.g., tricycle riding may be used as form of exercise).
4. Allow the child to be ambulatory as soon as he is able.

H. *To prepare the child for the many painful surgical and other procedures that he must undergo.*

1. Explain to the child what is going to happen before each procedure.
2. Explain to the child what will happen before he goes

to the operating room, where he will wake up, and who will be there when he does wake up.

3. Explain and demonstrate what equipment will be used following surgery or other procedures.

I. *To provide emotional support for the child who has been very frightened and traumatized by this painful experience.*

1. The child may be suffering from all-encompassing physical pain for which he has no previous experience to prepare him; he becomes confused and frightened and he may regress.
   a. Coupled with physical pain is psychological pain resulting from isolation, separation from parents, reliving the experience of being burned, fear of rejection.
   b. Prepare child for dressing changes and debridement. Provide comfort after procedure.
2. Encourage the child to talk about the way he feels.
   a. The child may feel guilty and think that the burn is punishment for some wrong deed.
   b. Allow the child opportunities at play where he may be able to begin to work out his feelings.
3. The child will be concerned about his appearance.
   a. Continually inform the child that you love him even though he has a bad burn.
   b. Encourage early contact with other children.
   c. Adjustment to disfigurement can be long and painful.
4. Psychiatric consultation is very frequently necessary in order to assist the child to work out his feelings. Signs may include:
   a. Persistent refusal to eat
   b. Resisting all nursing procedures
5. Contact with the child's parents, siblings, and nurse will help him with his feelings of fear, isolation, and rejection.
6. Arrange for services of a schoolteacher for the school-age child as soon as his condition permits.

J. *To support the parents during this very difficult time. They are under extreme stress, because a burned child creates a crisis.*

1. Use knowledge about the family's psychosocial status in planning care.
   a. A medical social worker may offer beneficial psychosocial support to the family.
   b. Be aware of siblings at home and that they may have needs that are being neglected as a result of this crisis.

2. Encourage parents to visit the child often.
   a. Attempt to have them become actively involved in the child's care when they are ready to do so.
   b. If parents are unable to visit, telephone calls and family photographs are helpful.
3. Give the parents the opportunity to discuss their feelings.
   Parents frequently feel very guilty because they feel they did not give the child the appropriate supervision he should have had when the accident occurred.
4. Keep parents informed as to the child's progress.
   a. Begin initial teaching at admission with supportive words and limited technical information.
   b. Education and orientation to the facility and the burn injury will decrease some anxiety and begin to build rapport on which future support can be based.
5. Psychiatric consultation is frequently required in order to assist parents in coping with their feelings.

K. *To prepare child and family for discharge and understanding that rehabilitation is long-term.*

1. Separation from the hospital environment, caretakers, and other patients can produce excessive anxiety. Short-time home passes (over-night, week-end) are helpful prior to final discharge.
2. If child is school age, prepare for school reentry—visit classroom and tell peers what to expect; at the same time teach how to prevent burn injuries.
3. Social reentry can be painful for the child who may have to respond to questions and stares from strangers and rejection by friends.
4. Hospitalization and future scar revisions may be necessary.
5. Special skin care is necessary following burn injury. Give written specific instructions to parents.
   a. Avoid exposure to sunlight.
   b. Treatment for hypertrophic scar and keloid formation—pressure garments.
   c. Use of lotions and creams to prevent drying, cracking and itching.
6. Psychological support of the trauma resulting from the burn injury, the actual event and hospitalization.
7. Physical therapy must be continued.

L. *To provide educational activities in the community to prevent burn injuries.*

ATOPIC ECZEMA (INFANTILE AND CHILDHOOD ECZEMA)

Atopic eczema is a term that describes any inflammatory dermatosis that is characterized by erythema, papulovesiculation, oozing, crusting, and scaling in various phases of resolution.

Etiology and Incidence

1. Infantile eczema usually manifests itself between the 2nd and 6th month of age, up to 2 years.
2. This type of dermatitis is the commonest, earliest manifestation of allergy.
3. Atopic eczema is not a disease but, rather, a reaction state of the skin.
4. The exact etiology is not known. Many infants with eczema have a positive family history of allergy and later develop asthma or hay fever.
5. The following may be triggering factors affecting the day-to-day appearance of the lesions:
   a. Bacterial, viral, or fungal infections
   b. Particulate matter and contactant irritants
   c. Environmental factors
      (1) Temperature and humidity
      (2) Inhalants
   d. Foods
   e. Emotional or physical stress—mother-child relationship
   f. Drugs

Clinical Manifestations

1. Infants—lesions
   a. Erythematous, papular, and weeping lesions develop.
   b. Oozing and crusting of the lesions occur, along with excoriation.
   c. Cheeks, forehead, neck, behind ears and the crawling surfaces of arms and legs are the areas most frequently involved.
   d. Lesions are more concentrated on the head and body than on the extremities; however they may progress to cover body.
2. Older children—lesions
   a. Erythematous, papular, and weeping lesions develop.
   b. Oozing and crusting of the lesions occur.
   c. The flexor surfaces of the upper and lower extremities, antecubital and popliteal fossae, in addition to the face and neck are areas frequently involved.
   d. As the disease becomes chronic, lichenification (leatheriness and hardening of skin) and hyperpigmentation develop.
3. Pruritus—may be mild or severe.
4. Excessive itching may cause restlessness, sleeplessness, and irritability.
5. Excessive scratching may result in an inflammatory reaction and excoriation, bleeding, and subsequent infection.
6. The color of lesions is red (possibly intense red).

Altered Physiology

1. The dermatitis involves the epidermis and the vascular layer of the cutis.
2. The dermatitis goes through a cycle involving areas of erythema, papules, vesicles, wheal reactions, and, ultimately, scaling eruption.
3. With superimposed infection, there is exudation, pustulation, and crust formation.
4. Various stages of the disease can be present on different parts of the child's body.
5. The disease is subject to remissions and exacerbations.
6. Secondary infections may occur from scratching.

Diagnosis

1. Family history of allergies
2. Positive dermal reaction
3. Presence of circulating Prausnitz-Küstner antibodies
4. Tendency to develop blood eosinophilia
5. Clearing of skin with removal of specific allergen and reappearance of dermal reaction upon re-exposure

Treatment

1. Symptomatic and supportive
   a. Trial period of hypoallergenic diet to eliminate any responsible food
   b. Avoidance by patient of any other known allergen; avoid wool clothing, blankets, etc.
   c. Control of any complicating skin infection
   d. Relief of itching and irritability; sedation may be necessary
   e. Measures to improve condition of involved skin:
      (1) Prevent scratching
      (2) Cleansing
2. Preventive—teach mother how to keep condition under control.

Complications

1. Acute infection—pyogenic infection may develop.
2. Long-term—eczema may progress to allergic rhinitis or asthma.

Nursing Objectives and Management

A. *To institute measures which prevent the child from scratching himself when he experiences severe itching in order to prevent further irritation and possible infection of the skin.*

1. Apply protective devices to prevent the child from scratching himself.
   a. Any one or combination of the following protective devices may be used (elbow cuff, ankle and wrist restraint, face mask, jacket restraint).
   b. Apply these protective devices only when absolutely necessary—when scratching cannot be controlled by other methods.
   c. Apply protective devices securely enough to prevent scratching, yet not so tight as to impair circulation. Check circulation frequently when protective devices are used.
   d. When protective devices are used, the device should be removed at frequent intervals.
      (1) Allow for free movement and active range of motion.
      (2) Allow the child to sit on the nurse's or mother's lap.
      (3) Attempt to divert the child's attention by playing with him and reading to him.
      (4) Allow the child to eat his meals free from protective devices; this requires direct supervision.
   e. When the child experiences severe itching and uncontrollable scratching, remove only one protective device at a time so that scratching can be controlled.
   f. Anger and frustration are frequently displayed in violent scratching.
      (1) Keep child comfortable and anticipate his needs.
      (2) Provide as much personal contact and supervision as possible.
      (3) Allow play activities that afford the child the opportunity to act out his anger and frustrations.
      (4) Provide infants with a cradle gym and a pacifier.
2. Cotton hand mitts and booties may be applied to prevent the child from scratching himself.
3. Trim fingernails and toenails and keep them clean.
4. Provide safe toys that will not be used by the child to scratch himself. (Use soft play things made of hypoallergenic material.)
5. Administer prescribed medications.
   a. Sedatives
   b. Antihistamines
   c. The use of local anesthetics to relieve itching is contraindicated because of their potential for skin sensitization.
   d. Antipruritic
   e. Topical steroids

B. *To provide measures which will improve the condition of the involved skin.*

1. Bathe the child by the prescribed method.
   a. Water and soap are often irritating.

b. Starch baths may be used; oil baths may be soothing.

c. Oil may be used if skin is dry and crusted. (Apply oil with a soft cloth.)

d. While giving the child a bath, keep him from scratching himself. (It may be necessary to maintain protective devices at this time.)

2. Local care of the skin is aimed at removing the debris and allaying the inflammatory reaction and pruritus.

a. Wet soaks of Burow's solution may be applied to the affected areas.

(1) These soaks are continuous and must be kept wet. Solution should be at room temperature.

(2) These bulky, wet dressings may serve to immobilize the child sufficiently so that he does not require other protective devices.

b. Lassar's paste or another hydrophilic preparation may be applied to the affected areas.

(1) Local medications must be kept on the skin constantly.

(2) Caution must be exercised to keep ointment out of the child's eyes.

(a) Remove all old ointment before applying new ointment.

(b) Starch bath may be used to remove ointment.

(3) Routine urine examination should be done because of possible toxic effect of medications on kidneys.

(4) Coal tar preparations should be used with caution during the summer when exposure to sun is more likely, because they have a photosensitizing effect.

3. Prevent skin irritation from bed clothing and bed linen.

Padding may be used.

4. Change diapers frequently to prevent skin excoriation.

5. Avoid extreme ambient temperatures.

C. *To promote measures which will prevent contact with dietary and environmental allergens.*

1. Review the child's chart and question the parents regarding known allergies.

a. Note the known allergens on the Kardex and place a tag on the head of the bed to indicate that the child has an allergy.

b. Inform the dietitian as to the child's food allergies.

2. Avoid substances which have a high potential for sensitization.

a. Foods such as milk, eggs, chocolate, wheat cereal, and orange juice are to be avoided.

b. Wool and dust are to be avoided.

3. Observe the child's reactions when an elimination diet is prescribed.

a. A minimal diet is prescribed. Trial diet may be composed of:

(1) Milk substitute

(2) Rice cereal

(3) 2 fruits

(4) 2 vegetables

(5) Beef

(6) Aqueous multivitamins

(7) No egg products

b. A new food is added to the diet every 3–5 days during which time the response to that food is observed.

c. An allergic response occurring during this 3- to

5-day period indicates sensitivity to that food; that particular food is then eliminated from the diet.

d. If no response is apparent, that food is added to the child's diet.

e. Another food substance is then added, and the child is observed for the following 3- to 5-day period. This method is followed until the food allergen is determined.

4. Provide a substitute for cow's milk when the child is allergic to it.

a. Goat's milk may be used.

b. Commercial formulas made from meat or vegetable protein substances are available.

D. *To protect the child from sources of infection.*

1. Protect the child from exposure to sources of infection known to cause exacerbations and severe infections.

a. Contact with other children, visitors, and personnel who have the herpes simplex virus is to be avoided.

> **NURSING ALERT:** If the child needs to be vaccinated against smallpox, it should not be done until his skin has been free from eczema for several months. Use caution with routine immunizations. Skin testing may be advisable.

b. The child should not be exposed to individuals who have a fresh vaccine lesion.

2. When the child is immobilized, his position should be changed frequently to prevent respiratory complications.

E. *To provide the emotional support needed by any child his age who is hospitalized; provide love and attention, and give the child freedom to express his feelings.*

F. *To assist the parents in providing for the child's care following hospitalization.*

1. Explain to parents the usual causes of the problem. Help them to understand that eczema is chronic—that there is no cure—but that a therapeutic regimen can be followed that will control it. Home care is preferred, and a home care program is essential.

2. Demonstrate the application of topical medications and the application of dressings. Explain timing of application of medicine.

a. Weeping and moist areas—cream or lotion

b. Drier areas—paste applied thickly or ointment

3. Give specific information regarding diet. Emphasize the foods which are allowed rather than foods to be avoided.

4. Demonstrate the application of protective devices and the precautions in using them.

5. Additional information in home management may include the following:

a. Launder clothes with a neutral pH soap and double rinse.

b. Control environment.

c. Use apron to cover clothing when holding child.

d. Avoid exposure to extreme heat or cold or to rapid changes in ambient temperature; avoid strenuous activity (can swim), soap, perfume, detergents, and stress.

e. Keep child's fingernails cut short and keep them clean.

f. Do not leave child alone to entertain himself;

prevent play with toys that can be injurious if used to scratch skin.

g. Baths may be effective in relieving itching—Alpha-Keri, Donol, Lubath; give bath using 2 cups cornstarch in tub of tepid water. Lubricate dry skin after bath.

6. Encourage the parents to hold and cuddle the child as much as possible to encourage the body contact that is frequently avoided because of protective devices and ointments.

7. Encourage the parents to discuss their feelings and concerns about the child's illness.
   a. The appearance of the child may be very disturbing to them.
   b. They need to be made to feel adequate in caring for the child at home.
8. A community health nurse referral may be indicated to provide support to the family, especially during initial phases of adjustment.

IMPETIGO

Impetigo is an infectious disease affecting the superficial layers of the skin and is characterized by the formation of vesicles, crusts, or bullae.

Etiology and Incidence

1. Bullous impetigo in neonate and infant—lesions are large, flaccid bullae containing pus and supernatant clear serum that rupture and leave raw edges. Lesions are more prominent in axillae and groin.
2. Impetigo contagiosa in older child—lesions appear with thick, yellow crusts.
3. Impetigo is caused by staphylococci or streptococci.
4. Occurs most frequently where personal hygiene is poor.
5. Occurs most frequently in children under 10 years of age.
6. Spread by contact—easily conveyed from person to person (using same handkerchief, towels, napkins, pencils, toys, etc.); plastic wading pools in summer—when spilled water is replaced and no antiseptic or disinfectant is used.
7. Any abrasion of skin may serve as portal of entry.

Clinical Manifestations

(Impetigo Contagiosa)
1. Incubation period of 1–5 days.
2. Lesion first appears as pink-red macules that quickly change to vesicles which, in turn, enlarge, become pustular, develop crusts, and leave temporary superficial erythematous areas.
3. Face, scalp, and hands are commonly involved, but other areas may be affected.
4. Regional lymphadenopathy—common with secondary infection of insect bites, eczema, poison ivy, scabies.
5. Pruritus may occur.

Diagnosis

1. Aspiration and culture of bullae.
2. Culture after removal of crust.

Treatment

1. Treatment is based on etiology and type of infection.
   a. Local therapy—cleansing skin—including crust removal—and scrubbing with Betadine (povidone-iodine) solution until no new lesions appear.
      (1) Ammoniated mercury 3% or Burow's solution compresses applied to affected area. Best to remove crusts by applying gauze soaked in boric acid or magnesium sulfate; remove crusts when softened and then apply medication.

      (2) The following may be used:
         2% gentian violet
         1:10,000 or 1:15,000 solution of potassium permanganate or bichloride of mercury applied by wet dressings or free application of Mercresin or ointments (Bacitracin, Neomycin, Neosporin, or Garamycin may be used).
   b. Systemic antibiotic—when severe or recurrent.
2. Prevention—avoid contact with sibling(s) of affected child.

Nursing Objectives and Management

A. *To be aware of the appearance of the characteristic lesion of impetigo.*

1. Observe the condition of the child's skin upon admission to the hospital.
2. Report any suspicious-appearing lesions.
3. Record the appearance and location of the lesion.
4. Initiate appropriate measures to prevent the spread of the infection.
   a. Place the child in a single room.
   b. Maintain medical aseptic technique.
5. Watch for the development of new lesions.

B. *To provide measures to prevent secondary infections.*

1. Provide mittens or protective devices to prevent the child from scratching the lesions.
2. Trim the child's fingernails and toenails.
3. Maintain cleanliness of fingernails and toenails.

C. *To provide measures to assure the child's comfort until healing has occurred and the child is free from infection.*

1. Hold child frequently and release from any necessary protective device.
2. Provide diversional therapy.
3. Administer medication and treatment to relieve itching—local medications or packs which relieve itching and promote healing may be used.
4. Provide the child with a diet adequate to meet his growth and development needs.

D. *To practice measures of general health and provide teaching for the child and his parents which will be helpful in preventing spread and further infection.*

1. General measures to improve personal cleanliness should be encouraged.
2. Minor wounds should be adequately cleaned and treated.
3. The child should be isolated if at home.
4. The child should be kept out of school until the lesions have healed.

RINGWORM OF THE SCALP (TINEA CAPITIS)

Ringworm of the scalp is a fungal infection of the scalp and hair follicles.

Etiology

1. Ringworm of the scalp is caused by different species of the *Microsporum canis, Tricophyton tonsurans,* and *Microsporum audouinii.*
2. Ringworm of the scalp is seen primarily in children before puberty.

Clinical Manifestations

1. The lesions usually develop in the occipital, temporal, and parietal areas of the scalp.
2. Pruritus usually occurs in the area.
3. The involved areas of the scalp appear as patches, rounded or oval in outline, covered by scales and lusterless, irregularly broken hairs.
4. Single patches or multiple patches may occur.
5. Systemic manifestations are absent.
6. Evaluation
   a. Wood's lamp—a filtered ultraviolet radiation causes microsporon infections to fluoresce with a brilliant, greenish light.
   b. Microscopic evaluation of infected hair follicles—to identify *Trichophyton* which fluoresces poorly under Wood's lamp—spores visibly coat hair.

Altered Physiology

1. The fungal infection produces an inflammation of the scalp which causes alopecia and broken hairs.
2. The lesions of the scalp may have papulovesicular erythematous borders or may appear only as scaling with a few broken hairs.
3. *Kerion,* an acute inflammation which produces edema, pustules and granulomatous swelling, may occur.
4. The infection may be spread through child-to-child contact, as well as through the common use of towels, combs, brushes, hats. Kittens and puppies may be the source of the infection.

Treatment

1. Griseofulvin—an antifungal antibiotic which is administered orally, 10–14 days.
2. Duration of treatment is generally guided by periodic use of Wood's lamp or cultures.
3. Keratinolytic medication, topical Whitfield's ointment, or salicylanilide ointment may be used in conjunction with griseofulvin.
4. Cut hair short and give daily topical application of antifungal preparation (e.g., miconazole, clotrimazole, or tolnaftate).
5. Keep head and hair clean, and avoid scratching.

Nursing Objectives and Management

A. *To recognize the characteristic lesions of ringworm of the scalp.*
1. Observe the condition of the hair and scalp as a part of the routine assessment of the child on admission to the hospital and at daily bath.
2. Report suspicious-appearing lesions.
3. Record the appearance and location of the lesions.
4. Initiate the appropriate isolation techniques (as per hospital policy).

B. *To be aware of the side effects of the medications used in the treatment of ringworm of the scalp.*
1. Griseofulvin may produce headache, heartburn, nausea, epigastric discomfort, diarrhea, and urticaria.
2. Record and report to the physician any side effects observed.
3. A diet high in fat may be prescribed to enhance intestinal absorption.

C. *To be aware of the case-finding measures to prevent additional cases and to identify the earliest evidence of infection.*
1. All family contacts should be screened.
2. The school should be notified so that appropriate case-finding techniques may be initiated.

D. *To be aware of the psychological trauma associated with loss of hair, especially in a girl, and to provide support as appropriate.*

Use of wigs or scarves may provide some relief of anxiety.

E. *To teach the child and his family methods to prevent further episodes.*
1. Teach general hygiene measures—regular shampooing and bathing.
2. Advise them to avoid the sharing of hats, combs, brushes, etc.
3. Stress the importance of wearing a cap continuously until the infection has been eliminated.
4. All lesions must be dry before child can return to school.

PEDICULOSIS

Pediculosis is the infestation of human beings by lice.

Etiology

1. Three types of lice affect human beings:
   a. *Pediculosis capitis*—head louse
   b. *Pediculosis corporis*—body louse
   c. *Phthirus pubis*—pubic louse/crab louse (seldom found in children) can attach only to curly hair—pubes, axillae, eyebrows
2. Each type of louse generally remains in the area designated by its name, but it may occasionally be seen in other areas of the body.
3. The infestation occurs in areas of filth and poverty, where personal cleanliness is neglected, baths are infrequently taken, and clothing is kept on the body for long periods of time.
4. Lice are transmitted by personal contact with people harboring them or through contact with articles which temporarily harbor them.

Clinical Manifestations

1. Severe itching in the area affected is the primary symptom of pediculosis; scratch marks will be evident in these areas.
2. In children, pubic lice are found most frequently in the eyelashes and eyebrows.
3. Infested scalp areas may become secondarily infected from scratching.
4. Crusts, pediculi, nits and dirt may combine to cause a foul odor and matted hair.
5. Body lice may produce minute red lesions.

Altered Physiology

1. The eggs of lice (nits) are attached to the hair or clothing by a sticky substance which hardens. The eggs hatch within 1 week—the lice reach maturity within 1 month and are then capable of reproducing.
2. The lice on the skin produce itching; the longer the infestation persists, the more severe the skin reaction becomes and the more severe the lesions appear.
3. The lice live on clothing and go to the body for feeding; thus, they produce visible scratch marks and points of puncture.

Treatment

OBJECTIVE: to eliminate and remove nits and pediculi (lice) and to treat the irritated skin.
1. *Pediculosis capitis* may be treated with gamma benzene hexachloride (Kwell), benzyl benzoate emulsion or crotamiton. (See package inserts.)

2. *Pediculosis corporis* may be treated with the above plus chlorophenothane powder.

Nursing Objectives and Management

A. *To maintain technique which will prevent the spread of the infection.*

Institute measures to carry out medical asepsis.

B. *To perform the treatments prescribed to destroy and eliminate the parasite.*

Observe and record the response to treatment.
  a. Note the change in the degree of discomfort caused by itching.
  b. Observe infected areas for changes in the characteristics of the lesions.
  c. Observe for systemic manifestations of infection.

C. *To provide measures to prevent the child from scratching himself.*

1. Provide mittens or protective devices to prevent the child from scratching.
2. Trim fingernails and toenails and keep them clean.
3. Provide the child with diversional therapy to distract him from itching.
4. Hold the child frequently and release him from the protective devices.

D. *To provide appropriate teaching for the family to prevent recurrent attacks.*

E. *To screen the family for parasitic infection.*

SCABIES

Scabies is a disease of the skin produced by the burrowing action of a parasite mite resulting in irritation and the formation of vesicles or pustules.

Etiology

1. Scabies is caused by the itch mite, *Sarcoptes scabiei.*
2. Scabies occurs most frequently in individuals living in areas of poverty, where cleanliness is lacking.
3. Scabies occurs as a result of direct contact with infected persons or by indirect contact through soiled bed linen, clothing, etc.

Clinical Manifestations

1. Itching, particularly at night, is the primary symptom. The itching is usually very severe.
2. Scratching frequently produces secondary skin infection.
3. Systemic manifestations are absent, unless they result from the secondary infection (i.e., fever, leukocytosis).

Altered Physiology

1. Both the male and female parasite live upon the skin.
2. The female parasite burrows into the superficial skin to deposit her eggs.
3. The burrow is seen most commonly between the fingers but may occur in any natural fold of the skin or in pressure areas, e.g., heel of palm, axillary and buttock folds, male genitalia, female breasts.
4. The burrows may occur in any part of the body in infants and small children and are easily identifiable.

5. Pruritus occurs, and the scratching of the skin may produce secondary infection. Scattered follicular eruptions contain immature mites.
6. Inflammation may produce pustules and crusts.
7. Eggs hatch in 4 days. Larvae undergo a series of molts before becoming adult. The life cycle is complete in 1–2 weeks.

Diagnosis

Presence on skin of female mite, ova, and feces.

Treatment

OBJECTIVE: to destroy the parasite, to relieve itching, and to reduce skin irritation.
1. Scrubbing, soaking, use of soap and water bath to remove scaling and crusting debris.
2. Application of a scabicide:
  a. Gamma benzene hexachloride (Kwell)—cream or lotion.
  b. Crotamiton (Eurax) cream or lotion—recommended for use in infants, because Kwell may produce neurotoxic symptoms.
  c. Contagion unlikely 24 hours after treatment.
3. Launder all clothing and bedding with sufficient heat to kill mites.
4. Itching may continue 2–3 weeks after destruction of mites. This can be controlled by using a topical antipruritic.

Nursing Objectives and Management

Same as for pediculosis (see above).

ORAL CANDIDIASIS (THRUSH) AND CANDIDAL DIAPER DERMATITIS

Oral thrush is a mycotic stomatitis characterized by the appearance of white plaques on the oral mucous membrane, the gums, and the tongue.

Candidal diaper dermatitis is a rash characterized by red, scaly, sharply circumscribed but moist patches with pustular satellite lesions.

Etiology

1. Caused by *Candida albicans*.
2. Most frequently seen in newborns, but may be seen in older infants, usually as a complication of antibiotic therapy or underlying disease (malignant neoplasm, immune deficiency disorders).
3. Maternal vulvovaginal candidiasis is the primary source of neonatal thrush.
4. The growth of the organisms is favored by:
   a. Lack of cleanliness
   b. Malnutrition
   c. Diabetes
   d. Antibiotic treatment (destroys normal flora)
   e. Neoplasms
   f. Hyperparathyroidism
5. The infection may be acquired from:
   a. Contaminated hands
   b. Contaminated feeding equipment
   c. Contaminated bedding
   d. Another patient
6. Thrush frequently occurs in children with cleft lip and palate.

Clinical Manifestations

A. Thrush

1. The infant develops small plaques on the oral mucous membrane, tongue, or gums; these plaques appear like curds of milk but cannot be wiped out of the mouth.
2. Thrush often appears to cause the infant no pain or discomfort.
3. The mouth may be dry.
4. Occasionally, the infant may appear to have some difficulty in swallowing, or eat less vigorously.
5. Enteric infection is frequently associated with oral thrush.

B. Diaper Dermatitis

1. Buttock rash consisting of erythematous maculopapular eruption with perianal distribution.
2. Generally causes discomfort, especially with wetting and cleansing.

Altered Physiology

Thrush:

1. Spores lodge between epithelial cells and gradually separate the layers.
2. The infection then spreads to the surface of the mucous membrane.
3. Growth usually begins in several discrete areas of the oral mucous membrane with gradual spreading to the point where a continuous membrane may be formed.

Treatment

A. Thrush

1. Oral administration of nystatin in suspension 3–4 times daily (treatment of choice).
   Apply over affected surfaces of oral cavity after feeding, allowing child to swallow any medication to treat any lesions along the gastrointestinal tract.
2. 1–2% aqueous solution of gentian violet swabbed in the mouth may be used.
   To prevent swallowing of medication and gastrointestinal irritation, place child prone following application.

B. Diaper Dermatitis

1. Keep dry and clean.
2. Topical application of nystatin or miconazole nitrate cream or ointment.
3. Nystatin may be given orally if rash is persistent.

Nursing Objectives and Management

A. *To recognize the appearance of thrush and to be aware of the infant who is particularly susceptible to the development of the condition.*

1. Newborns and infants who have particular susceptibility include:
   a. Sick, debilitated infants
   b. Infants who are on antibiotic therapy
   c. Infants with cleft lip and palate, hyperparathyroidism, and neoplasms
2. Inspect mouth *before* every feeding for presence of thrush.
3. Report the appearance of thrush to the physician and record this information on the nursing record.

B. *To practice measures which prevent the development and spread of thrush.*

1. Practice careful handwashing techniques.
2. Practice techniques which assure that nipples, bottles, or any other object which comes into direct or indirect contact with the infant's mouth is clean.

C. *To recognize the appearance of candidal diaper dermatitis and report to physician immediately.*

D. *To teach mothers (parents) the general principles of preventing diaper dermatitis.*

1. Change diaper as soon as possible after wetting or soiling. Check diaper every hour in newborn.
2. Wash entire diaper area thoroughly and dry area before applying clean diaper.
3. Allow infant to go without a diaper for short periods.
4. Use clean diapers that are soft to the touch and absorbent.
5. Use terminal aseptic rinse when washing diapers to neutralize ammonia produced when infant urinates; use vinegar, Borax, or Diaparene.
6. Avoid powder and oil which tend to clog pores and cake on skin, retaining bacteria.
7. Avoid occlusive plastic coverings, tightly pinned or double diapers, all of which tend to increase production and retention of body heat and moisture.

BIBLIOGRAPHY

Books

Artz CP, Moncrief JA, Pruitt BA. Burns: A Team Approach. Philadelphia, WB Saunders, 1979

Randolph JG et al. The Injured Child: Surgical Management. Chicago, Year Book Medical Publishers, 1979

Sauer GC. Manual of Skin Diseases. Philadelphia, JB Lippincott, 1980

Scipien GM et al. Comprehensive Pediatric Nursing, 2nd ed. New York, McGraw–Hill, 1979

Waley LF and Wong DL. Nursing Care of Infants and Children. St. Louis, CV Mosby, 1979

Practical Approaches to Burn Management. Deerfield, Ethical Communications, Flint Laboratories, Div. Travenol Labs, 1977

Articles

Arneson SW and Triplett JL. How children cope with disfiguring changes in their appearance. MCN 1978 Nov/Dec; 3(6):366–370

Belle AE et al. Hospital epidemic of scabies: Diagnosis and control. Can. J. Public Health 1979 Mar/Apr; 70(2): 133–135

Burgdorf MM. Coping behaviors of a school-age child hospitalized with burns. Maternal-Child Nurs J 1978 Spring; 1(7):11–19

Busby HC. Nursing management of the acute burn patient and nursing management of optimal burn recovery. J. Contin Educ Nurs 1979 July/Aug; 10(4):16–30

Cohen S and Glass GK. Programmed Instruction: Skin rashes in infants and children. Am J Nurs 1978 June; 78(6): 1041–1172

France DM. Atopic eczema and its management. Health Visitor 1978 July; 51(7):294–295

Grebin B and Grebin M. Common pediatric skin conditions. Pediatric Nurs 1978 Nov/Dec; 4(6):41–42 +

Hawkins K. What's Larry got, nurse? Nursing '79 1979 Dec; 9(12):39

Hurwitz S. Newer developments in pediatric dermatology. Pediatr Nurs 1978 Nov/Dec; 4(6):37–41

McGuire A. Prevention of burns. CCQ 1978 Dec; 1(3):1–10

McHugh ML, Dimitroff K, Dinsmore N. Family support group in a burn unit. Am J Nurs 1979 Dec; 79(12):2148–2150

Mieszala P. Postburn psychological adaptation: An overview. CCQ 1978 Dec; 1(3):93–111

Molinard JR. The social fate of children disfigured by burns. Am J Psychiatry 1978 Aug; 135(8):979–980

Orkin M and Mailbach HT. Scabies in children. Pediatr Clin North Am 1978 May; 25(2):371–386

Stoddard JE. Rehabilitation of the burn-injured patient. CCQ 1978 Dec; 1(3):63–76

Weston W, Lane A, Weston J. Diaper dermatitis: Current concepts. Pediatrics 1980 Oct; 66(4):532–536

METABOLIC DISTURBANCES IN CHILDREN

45

JUVENILE DIABETES MELLITUS

Diabetes mellitus is a disorder of carbohydrate metabolism resulting in high serum levels of glucose and the spilling of glucose in the urine. The disease is also associated with abnormal metabolism of fat and protein.

Etiology

1. Believed to be related to inheritance of certain HRA antigens which predispose an individual to autoimmune destruction of pancreatic islets.
   Factors, in addition to genetic ones, are also involved in provoking the clinical manifestations of the disease.
2. Viral etiology for juvenile diabetes has also been suggested.

Altered Physiology

1. The pancreas produces an insufficient amount of insulin.
2. The body is unable to oxidize glucose properly.
3. Protein and fat are oxidized at abnormal rates.
4. Hyperglycemia results from the deficient oxidation of glucose and the inability of tissues to use glucose as fuel.
5 Glycosuria results when the serum level of glucose exceeds the renal threshold.
6. Diuresis is initiated and may progress to dehydration and impaired renal function.
7. Ketones accumulate in the blood when fat is oxidized at abnormal rates.
8. Ketones are excreted in the urine.
9. Acidosis occurs when ketosis is severe enough to lower the CO_2-combining power of the blood. Diabetic coma may result.

Clinical Manifestations

1. Rapid onset (usually over a period of a few weeks)
2. Major symptoms
   a. Increased thirst
   b. Increased urination
   c. Wasting
   d. Easy fatigability
3. Minor symptoms
   a. Skin infections
   b. Dry skin
   c. Monilial vaginitis in adolescent girls
4. Diabetic acidosis
   a. Precomatose state
      Drowsiness
      Dryness of skin
      Cherry red lips
      Increased respirations
      Nausea
      Vomiting
      Abdominal pain
   b. Comatose state
      Extreme hyperpnea (Kussmaul breathing)
      Soft, sunken eyeballs
      Rigid abdomen
      Rapid, weak pulse
      Decreased temperature
      Decreased blood pressure
   c. Circulatory collapse and renal failure may follow, resulting from the combination of lowered pH, electrolyte deficiency, and dehydration.
5. Side effects
   a. Stunting of growth
   b. Failure to develop secondary sex characteristics

Complications

1. Retinopathy and cataracts
2. Neuropathy
3. Renal disease
4. Increased incidence of gangrene, myocardial infarction, and stroke

Nursing Objectives and Management

A. *To recognize signs of diabetic acidosis (see clinical manifestations) and to provide supportive care to the child should this develop.*

1. Be aware of common causes of diabetic acidosis
   a. Untreated diabetes
   b. Inadequate insulin coverage
   c. Failure to adhere to the prescribed diet
   d. Chronic or repeated infections
2. Apply the principles of nursing care of the comatose child. (See nursing the unconscious patient, p. 706.)
3. Maintain intravenous therapy. (See IV procedure, p. 1171.)
   a. Be prepared to administer intravenous sodium bicarbonate if pH <7.2 (use somewhat controversial).
   b. Have intravenous glucose available should the child suddenly become hypoglycemic.

Care is taken to avoid reducing the blood glucose to hypoglycemic levels.

c. Parenteral fluids may need to be changed frequently due to continued polyuria and results of electrolyte determinations.

4. Be prepared to administer relatively large quantities of regular insulin.
    a. A variety of acceptable formulas are available for insulin therapy.
    b. A recent technique involves:
        (1) IV push injection of 0.1 unit of insulin per kg. body weight.
        (2) This is followed by a constant infusion of 0.1 unit per kg. body weight per hour until blood glucose reaches 300 mg./dl.
        (3) Then 5% glucose is started and insulin infusion is halved or subcutaneous insulin is begun.

5. Insert a nasogastric tube to relieve abdominal distention and prevent vomiting.

6. Monitor urine output exactly.
    Test urinary sugar and acetone of each specimen.

7. Provide emotional support to the child and his family.
    a. Respond immediately to the child's needs for physical comfort.
    b. Discuss the child's treatment plan and expected response with his parents to alleviate their anxiety.

8. Reinstitute oral feedings when the child is sufficiently responsive and can tolerate them.
    a. This is usually after 12–16 hours of parenteral therapy.
    b. Begin with a low fat, liquid diet.
        Observe closely for signs of insulin shock or recurrent acidosis once oral feedings are reinstituted.

9. Begin a teaching program with the child as soon as possible to allay his worries concerning his physical status, prognosis, and treatment.

B. *To provide a diet adequate for the child's normal growth and development and sufficient to satisfy his appetite.*

1. The prescribed diet is determined by the child's symptomatology, family and cultural characteristics, and physician preference.
    a. Most prescribed diets are of the unmeasured type. The diet plan eliminates concentrated sweets, follows recommended allowances from all of the 4 basic food groups, but otherwise does not require measuring or rigidity.
    b. Occasionally a more rigid, strictly controlled diet is necessary.
    c. The diet should be composed of 45% carbohydrate, 30–40% fat, and 20% protein.
        (1) Most diets are restricted in carbohydrates, saturated fats, and cholesterol, and may be based on the exchange method as recommended by the American Diabetes Association.
        (2) All diets must supply sufficient caloric intake for activity and growth, sufficient protein for growth, and the required vitamins and minerals.
    d. Foods are distributed throughout the day to accommodate varying peak action of insulin.
        Distribution may be adjusted for increased or decreased amounts of exercise.

2. Determine the child's usual dietary habits so that adherence to his controlled diet will be easier.

3. Include the child and his parents in his meal planning as soon as possible.

4. Allow the child normal activity while hospitalized so that the observed result of his dietary control will be valid.

5. Allow the child to eat with other children.

6. Make certain that the child adheres to his prescribed diet and understands the rationale for this.

C. *To administer insulin in an amount adequate to maintain the child's approximate glycemic equilibrium.*

1. The dose and kinds of insulin are determined from the results of fractional testing of the urine for sugar and acetone.

2. Insulin should be given ½ hour before the morning meal.

3. Be aware of the major types of insulin and their effect (Table 45-1).

4. Develop a systematic plan for injections which emphasizes rotation of sites. In this way, it will be several weeks before it is necessary to return to the same site.
    a. The upper arms and thighs are the most acceptable sites for injection in children, but the outer areas of the abdomen or hips may also be used.
    b. A diagram showing injection sites should be used to maintain the rotation (refer to Figure 45-1).
        The sites can be checked off each day until the routine is familiar.
    c. Injections are begun at an upper corner of the area to be used.
    d. Subsequent injections are given about 2.5 cm. (1 inch) apart, working in rows.
    e. When all rows in one area are completed, injections are begun in the next area.
    f. Guidelines for site location:
        (1) *Arms*—Begin below the deltoid muscle and end one hand breadth above the elbow. Begin at the midline and progress outward laterally using the external surface only.
        (2) *Legs*—Begin one hand breadth below the hip and end one hand breadth above the knee. Begin at the midline and progress outward laterally using only the outer, anterior surface.
        (3) *Abdomen*—Avoid the beltline and 1 inch around the umbilicus.
        (4) *Hips*—Use the upper outer quadrant of the buttocks.

5. Be certain that the measuring scale of the syringe matches the unitage on the bottle of insulin.
    a. Insulin is available in strengths of 40, 80, and 100 units per ml.
    b. U–100 insulin is preferred since it allows the smallest possible amount to be given.
    c. New purified forms of insulin are available but should not be used unless recommended by the physician, as use may require a decrease in insulin dose.

TABLE 45-1. TYPES OF INSULIN AND THEIR EFFECTS

Type of Insulin	Onset (hours)	Maximal Activity (hours)	Duration (hours)
Regular	½–1	2–4	4–6
Semi-Lente	½–1	2–4	12–16
NPH	1–1½	6–8	18–24
Lente	1–2	6–12	24–26
Ultralente	4–6	12–18	24–36

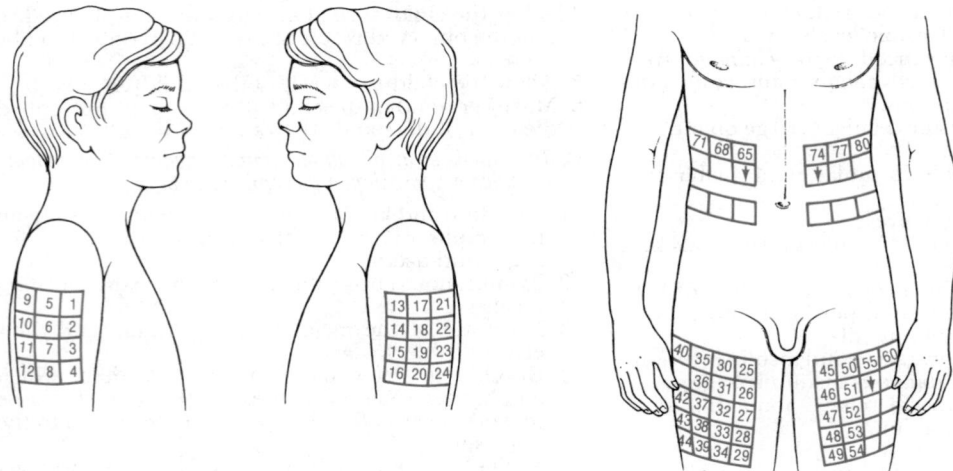

FIGURE 45-1. *Rotating injection sites for insulin in the pediatric patient.*

6. Use insulin that is at room temperature.
   a. The bottle in use may be kept at room temperature without losing appreciable strength.
   b. Extra bottles should be stored in the refrigerator.
7. Mix the solution by rotating the vial between the hands. Do not shake vigorously.
8. Administer insulin subcutaneously and not too near the skin to prevent local skin reactions and to promote absorption.
9. Following injection, exert firm pressure with an alcohol sponge to prevent bleeding; massage the area to aid absorption of the medication.
10. Observe the skin closely for signs of irritation. Avoid the injection site for several weeks if signs of local irritation are observed.
11. Observe the skin for a rash indicating an allergic reaction to the insulin.
12. Be aware of factors which vary the need for and utilization of insulin, particularly exercise and infection.
    a. Exercise
       (1) Tends to lower the blood sugar level.
       (2) Encourage normal activity, regulated in amount and time.
    b. Infection
       (1) Increases the child's insulin requirement.
       (2) Be alert for signs of infection.
13. Encourage the child to express his feelings about the injections.
    The child may be helped to master his fear of injections by gaining control of the situation through play and active participation in the procedure.

D. *To be aware of the symptoms and treatment of insulin shock.*

1. Common causes
   a. Overdose of insulin
   b. Reduction in diet or increased exercise without sufficient caloric coverage
2. Symptoms
   a. Sudden hunger
   b. Weakness
   c. Restlessness
   d. Pallor
   e. Sweating
   f. Tremors
   g. Dizziness
   h. Visual disturbances
   i. Odd behavior
   j. Dilated pupils
   k. Unconsciousness
3. Be prepared to give orange juice or other food containing readily available simple sugars.
4. Have glucose available for intravenous injection or glucagon available for intramuscular or subcutaneous injection.

E. *To test the child's urine regularly for sugar and acetone in order to determine the effectiveness of treatment.*

1. Collect urine specimens 4 times daily, before each meal and before bed.
   a. Because analysis is more accurate if the second voided specimen is used, have the child void from 15–30 minutes before each of the specimens to be tested is obtained.
   b. Discard the first specimen and test the second.
   c. Since obtaining specimens from young children may be difficult, it may be preferable to test the urine with each voiding.
   d. The child should refrain from drinking large amounts of fluid between samples as test results will be inaccurate.
2. Record the results of urine testing accurately.
   a. Use a standard form for recording so that the information will be clear and readily available.
   b. Help the child to understand how his disease is controlled by teaching him to test his own urine, record results, and report information to medical personnel or parents.
   c. Teach parents to look for patterns of spillage rather than individual tests.
3. Be certain that the urine test is done according to the specific instructions for the method being used. Either the 2-drop or the 5-drop Clinitest methods are preferred.
   a. Correct time interval for reading results
   b. Correct color chart for brand of reagent

c. Correct storage, handling, and use of reagent

d. Use of unexpired reagent; check expiration date

F. *To prevent infection.*

1. Bathe daily.
2. Maintain meticulous skin care through such activities as frequent ambulation of the child and application of body lotion.
3. Keep fingernails and toenails clean and well trimmed.
4. Provide prompt treatment for any violations of the skin (bruises, abrasions, lacerations, etc.).

G. *To foster acceptance on the part of the child that he is a normal, healthy person and able to compete with his peers.*

1. Include the child and his parents in the treatment plan in its earliest stages.
2. Emphasize that daily management of his disease can become as routine as matters of personal hygiene.
3. Permit and encourage the development of the child's natural talents. Do not allow him to use his disease as a crutch.
4. Allow the child independence in his care as soon as possible, but provide the necessary direction.
5. Initiate a teaching program for the child and his parents early. Offer them available literature.
6. If appropriate, group diabetic children together on the unit. Initiate group discussions for diabetic adolescents.
7. Invite parents to join a group of parents of diabetic children if such a group is available in the area.
8. Initiate a community nursing referral if the parents or the child appears apprehensive or unsure of themselves.

Patient or Parental Education

Patient or parental education is one of the most important aspects in the nursing care of the diabetic child. Thorough instruction is essential in the following areas:

1. Influence of exercise, emotional stress, and other illnesses on both insulin and diet needs
2. Recognition of the symptoms of insulin shock and diabetic acidosis and knowledge of related emergency management
3. Prevention of infection
   a. Give frequent baths.
   b. Attend to regular body hygiene with special attention to foot care.
   c. Report any breaks in the skin. Treat them promptly.
   d. Report infections promptly to the physician.
   e. Use only properly fitted shoes; do not wear vinyl or plastic, which do not permit ventilation. Avoid calluses and blisters.
   f. Dress the child appropriately for the weather.
   g. See that child receives regular dental check-ups and maintenance.
   h. Follow routine immunizations according to the recommended schedule.
4. Urine testing
   a. Demonstrate the procedure.
   b. Have the child and his parent demonstrate to the nurse.
   c. Allow the child to do the procedure under supervision until his accuracy is certain.
   d. Encourage the child to assume responsibility for his own urine testing.
   e. Help the child to develop an easy method of recording urine results.

A record should be used that includes urine test results, kind and amount of insulin given, and additional remarks, such as child's activity, insulin reactions, etc.

   f. Be certain parents understand what results are desirable for the child and the appropriate action to take when test results are other than those desired.
   g. Warn the parents of the caustic nature of Clinitest tablets if ingested. The agent should be kept away from young children.
5. Administration of insulin
   a. Both the child and his parents should be taught how to do this procedure and what effects the various forms of insulin have.
   b. Give parents an opportunity to express their feelings about the injection.
   c. Explain the procedure simply and demonstrate it.
   d. Discuss the procedure for rotation of sites and the rationale for this method.
   e. Allow the parent and child to practice by injecting normal saline into the nurse.
   f. Have the parent inject his child under supervision.
   g. Have the child inject himself.
      (1) Most children over the age of 8 can be taught to give insulin to themselves.
      (2) Generally, the earlier this responsibility is given to the child, the easier it is for him.
   h. Carefully check the dosage measured by the child and his parent until you are certain of their accuracy.
   i. Complete a community nursing referral for assistance with this procedure at home if indicated.
6. Maintenance and sterilization of insulin equipment
   a. The use of disposable equipment should be encouraged, because it is easier and safer.
   b. Nondisposable syringes and needles must be sterilized before each injection in the following manner:
      (1) Remove the plunger from the barrel of the syringe.
      (2) Place them both into a strainer along with the needle.
      (3) Place the strainer in a saucepan of water and boil for 5 minutes.
         If the family does not have a strainer, the syringe parts and needle should be wrapped in gauze before being placed in water.
      (4) Reassemble the syringe being careful to touch only the outside of the syringe and the knob of the plunger.
      (5) Slip the needle onto the syringe with a twisting motion, being careful to touch only the hub of the needle, never its point.
      (6) Work the plunger back and forth several times to force out any water that remains in it.
      (7) A community nursing referral may also be indicated to assist the family with this procedure until they feel comfortable doing it.
7. Diet
   a. Review the prescribed diet with the family.
   b. Discuss acceptable modifications of exchanges.
   c. Allow the child to manage his own diet as early as possible.

d. Emphasize that the diet is based on normal household foods. The purchase of special, expensive dietetic foods is usually not necessary.

e. Stress that food labels must be scrutinized. A label of "dietetic" or "low-calorie" does not necessarily mean that the food is acceptable for the child.

f. Inform parents and children of the exchange lists which are available from many of the national fast-food restaurants.

8. Precautionary measures
    a. Have the child carry with him an identifying card which states that he has diabetes and includes his name, address, phone number, and his physician's name and phone number.
    b. See that the child has orange juice, a lump of sugar or a bar of candy available in case of insulin reaction.
    c. Have the family discuss the child's disease with the school nurse and with other responsible adults who are in close contact with the child (teachers, scout leaders, etc.).
    d. Advise the parents that vials of insulin should be kept on one's person when traveling, because baggage may be subjected to extreme temperatures and pressures incompatible with the stability of insulin. If necessary, a thermos can be used to keep the insulin at the appropriate temperature.

9. *Teaching materials and Resources for Children and Parents:*

Court J. Helping Your Diabetic Child. New York, Taplinger Publishing Co., 1975

Faro B et al. Diabetic Teaching Manual for Children and Parents. Unpublished manuscript. Rochester, University of Rochester, School of Nursing, 14642.

Kipnis L and Adler S. You Can't Catch Diabetes From A Friend. Gainesville, Triad Scientific Publishers, 1979

Middleton K and Hess M. The Art of Cooking for the Diabetic. Chicago, Contemporary Books, 1978

Travis LB. An Instructional Aid on Juvenile Diabetes Mellitus. Galveston, Dept of Pediatrics, University of Texas, Medical Branch, 1975

Vanderpool S. The Care and Feeding of Your Diabetic Child. New York, Frederick Fell Publications, 1974

10. *Agency:*
American Diabetes Association, 600 Fifth Ave., New York, N.Y. 10020

DIABETES INSIPIDUS

Diabetes insipidus is a disorder of water metabolism caused by a deficiency of vasopressin, the antidiuretic hormone (ADH) secreted by the posterior pituitary.

Etiology

1. Deficient secretion of vasopressin (antidiuretic hormone).
    a. Congenital
        Inherited as an autosomal dominant or X-linked recessive trait.
    b. Acquired
        (1) Brain tumors, especially craniopharyngiomas
        (2) CNS malformation or degenerative disease
        (3) Head trauma or neurosurgery
        (4) Infections of the central nervous system
        (5) Unknown cause
2. Failure of the renal tubules to respond to vasopressin (nephrogenic diabetes insipidus)
    a. Hereditary (dominant) disease
    b. More common in males

Altered Physiology

1. Vasopressin normally acts on the distal tubules and collecting ducts of the kidney to facilitate reabsorption of water.
2. Pathology of the pituitary or hypothalamus results in a deficiency of vasopressin.
3. The kidney is unable to produce a concentrated urine without sufficient vasopressin.
4. Nephrogenic diabetes insipidus
    a. Vasopressin secretion is normal.
    b. The renal tubules do not respond to vasopressin.
    c. The kidney is unable to produce a concentrated urine.

Clinical Manifestations

1. Onset—usually sudden
2. Symptoms
    a. Depend on the age of the child and his primary lesion
    b. Universal symptoms
        (1) Polydipsia (excessive thirst)
        (2) Polyuria (excessive urine output)
        (3) Inability to concentrate urine
    c. Symptoms in infants
        (1) Excessive crying (quieted with water rather than additional milk)
        (2) Hyperthermia
        (3) Vomiting
        (4) Constipation
        (5) Rapid weight loss
        (6) Dehydration
        (7) Growth failure
    d. Symptoms in older children
        (1) Excessive thirst which may interfere with play and sleep
        (2) Enuresis
        (3) Anorexia
        (4) Pale and dry skin
        (5) Reduced sweating
        (6) Viscid saliva

Diagnostic Evaluation

A. *Water Deprivation Test*

1. The child fasts overnight and is served a standard breakfast.
2. No food or drink should be ingested after breakfast until the test is completed.

3. Between 8:30 and 9:30 A.M., a one-hour urine specimen and serum sample are obtained.
4. Between 2:30 and 3:30 P.M., a second urine specimen and serum sample are obtained.
5. Urine and serum osmolality are determined and the ratio of urine to serum osmolality (U/S) ratio are calculated.
6. A final U/S ratio of greater than 1.5 or a change in the U/S of 1.0 or more indicates normal ability to concentrate urine.

B. Vasopressin Sensitivity Test

1. A reduction of urine flow and an increase in urine concentration is observed following the administration of antidiuretic hormone.
2. This test should be used after it has been demonstrated that the child is unable to concentrate urine during the water deprivation test.

Nursing Objectives and Management

A. To prevent dehydration and restore electrolyte balance.

1. Nursing actions when the disorder is caused by a deficiency of vasopressin.
   a. Pitressin tannate in oil is the preparation of choice for replacement therapy.
      (1) Dosage—regulated by trial for each child.
      (2) Route of administration
         (a) Intramuscular
         (b) Never intravenous
      (3) Special precautions
         (a) Careful attention must be given to adequate suspension of the pitressin tannate in oil.
         (b) Hold the ampule under hot water to reduce the viscosity of the suspending medium. (Immersion of the ampule in boiling water destroys the hormone.)
         (c) Shake the ampule vigorously until the active ingredient is smoothly dispersed.
         (d) Inject the medication with a 2.5-cm. (1-inch) No. 20–22 gauge needle.
         (e) Inject the medication deeply into the muscle.
         (f) Following injection, massage the area vigorously to aid absorption of the medication.
         (g) Establish a pattern of systematic rotation of injection sites.
         (h) Water intoxication is a dangerous complication if Pitressin is given too frequently. Its duration of action is usually 24–72 hours.
            Used with caution in patients with vascular disease or epilepsy.
   b. Pitressin may also be administered as a nasal spray, but the duration of its action is so brief that administration is required at 2-hour intervals.
   c. A synthetic analogue of vasopressin (DDAVP) has been developed.
      (1) Administered as a nasal spray, it effectively controls diabetes insipidus using 2 daily doses.
      (2) It is not available for general use in the U.S. at the present time.
2. Nursing actions when the disorder is caused by failure of the kidney to respond to vasopressin.
   a. Administration of pitressin is ineffective.
      These children already produce a sufficient quantity of vasopressin.
   b. Administer water at frequent intervals and in sufficient volume to prevent dehydration.
   c. Administer a low sodium, low solute residue diet to reduce the osmolar load on the kidney.
   d. Administer thiazide therapy as prescribed by the physician.
      This causes sodium diuresis, which acts to promote proximal tubular sodium reabsorption.

B. To observe and record the child's response to therapy.

1. Intake and output
   a. Total the intake and output record every 8 hours.
   b. Record the urine specific gravity of each voiding.
2. Temperature—be alert for the development of fever.
3. Skin turgor—decreased skin turgor is sign of dehydration.
4. Color
5. Appetite—record the child's intake accurately with each meal.

C. To participate in the diagnostic evaluation of diabetes insipidus.

1. Explain the purpose of appropriate laboratory tests and the protocol that the child and family will be asked to follow.
2. Supervise the child closely to avoid surreptitious fluid intake during fasting periods.
3. Observe the child closely for evidence of fluid and electrolyte disturbances while the test is in progress.
   a. Dehydration and shock may occur in severely affected children during the water deprivation test.
   b. Overhydration may occur in patients with primary psychogenic polydipsia during the vasopressin sensitivity test.
4. Collect urine specimens as requested by the physician.
   a. Attempt to collect the urine on schedule.
   b. Record carefully:
      (1) Time of collection
      (2) Fluid intake (including IV fluids), if any
      (3) Volume of urine
      (4) Specific gravity of urine
      (5) Weight of patient

D. To provide emotional support to the family.

Prognosis depends on the underlying condition.
1. Hereditary and idiopathic types—favorable with adequate treatment.
2. Trauma—spontaneous recovery often occurs.
3. Tumor
   a. Varies with the site of the lesion and type of tumor.
   b. Needs of the family accentuated by many problems including surgery and facing the death of the child.

Patient or Parental Education

1. Explain the condition with specific clarification that diabetes insipidus and diabetes mellitus are very different disorders.
2. Teach parents the correct procedure for preparation and administration of injectable vasopressin.
3. Encourage the child to assume full responsibility for his care when he is old enough.
4. The child should wear a medic-alert tag, which identifies his condition.
5. The older child should carry nasal spray for temporary relief of symptoms if necessary.
6. School personnel and other significant adults should be made aware of the child's problem.

HYPOTHYROIDISM

Hypothyroidism is an endocrine disease resulting from deficient production of thyroid hormone. It may be either congenital (cretinism) or acquired (juvenile hypothyroidism).

Etiology

A. *Congenital*

1. Embryonic defect with partial or complete absence of the thyroid gland
2. Defect in the synthesis of thyroid hormone
3. Destruction of fetal thyroid as a result of antigen/antibody reaction
4. Iodide deficiency (endemic cretinism)
5. Toxic substances encountered during pregnancy causing maldevelopment or atrophy of the fetal thyroid gland. These may rarely include some medications administered during pregnancy.

B. *Acquired*

1. Hypoplasia of the thyroid gland
2. Partial defect in synthesis of thyroid hormone
3. Thyroidectomy
4. Medications
   a. Iodides
   b. Cobalt
   c. Propylthiouracil
5. Autoimmune disease
6. Iodine deficiency (rare)

Clinical Manifestations

1. Approximately twice as common in females as in males.
2. Severity of clinical findings depends on the age at onset, extent of thyroid deficiency, and the particular individual.
3. Early signs and symptoms (several days or weeks after birth).
   a. Prolonged physiological jaundice
   b. Nasal obstruction and stuffiness
   c. Feeding difficulties
   d. Hoarse cry
   e. Decreased intestinal activity—constipation
   f. Poor muscle tone—umbilical hernia
   g. Physical and mental sluggishness
   h. Subnormal temperature
4. General appearance
   a. Skin—dry, thick, scaly, coarse, cool, and pale
   b. Facial characteristics
      (1) Bridge of nose—flat, broad, and undeveloped
      (2) Eyes—widely spaced with swollen eyelids
      (3) Anterior fontanelle widely open
      (4) Tongue—thick and protruding
   c. Hair—frequently dry, coarse, brittle, slow-growing
   d. Skeletal
      (1) Short, thick neck
      (2) Broad hands
      (3) Short fingers
      (4) Decrease in linear growth rate
5. Later signs and symptoms
   a. Poor muscle tone
      (1) Protuberant abdomen
      (2) Lumbar lordosis
   b. Delayed dentition
      Teeth decay easily
   c. Delayed skeletal development
      (1) Short stature
      (2) Retarded bone age
      (3) Infantile skeletal proportions
         (a) Large head
         (b) Short extremities
   d. Slow motor and mental development
      (1) Late sitting, standing, walking, talking
      (2) Late attaining normal milestones
      (3) Slow cerebral activity. (If severe hypothyroidism occurs before the age of 2 years, intelligence is often impaired.)
   e. Retarded sexual development
   f. Anemia
   g. Hypersensitivity to cold
   h. Fatigue
6. Clinical manifestations may be delayed in breast-fed infants until the child is weaned because of the thyroid hormone contained in breast milk.

Diagnostic Evaluation

1. X-ray shows retarded bone age.
2. Thyroid function tests are abnormal.
3. Neonatal screening is now possible with a highly sensitive radioimmunoassay for thyroxine or thyroid-stimulating factor.

Prognosis

1. Depends on the child's age at onset and the effectiveness of his therapy.
2. If untreated—mentally deficient dwarf results.
3. When treated:
   a. Normal physical growth and development occur.
   b. Mental development is unpredictable.
      (1) The best results are obtained by giving continuous, full therapy as early as possible (within the first 3–4 months of life).
      (2) The best outlook is for children who have active thyroid tissue during the fetal life, have adequate treatment, and show a high family intelligence quotient.

Altered Physiology

Same as in the adult.

Nursing Objectives and Management

A. *To administer replacement therapy for the deficient hormone.*

Desiccated thyroid or a synthetic hormone such as Sodium Levothyroxine (Synthroid) may be used.

1. Dosage
   a. Initially very low.
   b. Gradually increased to the maximum amount which the child can tolerate without producing signs of toxicity.
2. Route of administration
   a. Always administer thyroid replacement orally.
   b. The tablet may be crushed and mixed with fruit for infants.
3. Special precautions
   a. The total daily requirement is given as a single dose.
   b. Administer the medication at the same time each day.
4. Observe for toxic effects.

a. Excitability
b. Nervousness
c. Tachycardia
d. Tremors
e. Cramps

B. *To provide a complete, well-balanced diet.*

1. Special problems related to nutrition
   a. Anemia
      (1) Increases the child's need for iron.
      (2) Include high quantities of meat, fish, poultry, eggs, enriched breads and cereals in the child's diet.
   b. Increased skeletal development
      (1) Increases the need for additional vitamin D.
      (2) Encourage the child to drink 3–4 glasses of milk daily.
   c. Constipation
      Provide foods which are high in roughage such as raw fruits and vegetables.
2. Determine the child's dietary preferences and use this information to plan his menus.
   a. Include the child in menu planning when this is possible.
   b. Refer to section on nutrition, page 1112.

C. *To prevent tooth decay.*

1. Provide mouth care after each meal.
2. Discourage the intake of sweets, gum, soda, etc.

D. *To provide emotional support to the child and his family.*

1. Assess the child's capabilities and establish realistic expectations and limits.
2. Assist parents to adjust to alterations in their child's behavior as he responds to treatment.
   The child may develop new enthusiasm for the naturally disturbing antics of childhood!
3. Allow parents to discuss their feelings about the child's condition. Parents often feel guilty that they misinterpreted the child's symptoms, resulting in delayed treatment.

E. *To provide support to the parents of a mentally retarded child.*

(Refer to section on mental retardation, p. 1436.)

Patient or Parental Education

A. *Medication*

1. Give the medication conscientiously at the same time every day.
2. Adjust the dosage (by the physician) to the needs of each individual child.
   a. Regular medical follow-up and frequent reevaluation are essential.
   b. Dose may have to be increased during puberty and the reproductive period.
3. The medication must be continued throughout life.
4. Allow the parents to administer the medication during the child's hospitalization so that they will gain confidence in their ability to carry out the procedure.
5. Encourage parents to help the child accept increasing responsibility for his medications as he grows older.

B. *Diet*

1. Discuss the importance of a well-balanced diet.
2. Suggest sample menus. These should be economical and based on the family's normal dietary patterns.
3. Refer the family to an appropriate social service if they are unable to afford sufficient food.
4. Assist the mother of an infant with techniques of feeding.

C. *Dental Care*

1. Teach the child correct techniques for brushing his teeth.
   Stress that he should follow this procedure after each meal.
2. Encourage regular (every 6 months) evaluations by a dentist.
   Refer the family to a dental clinic if necessary.

HYPERTHYROIDISM

Hyperthyroidism is an endocrine disease resulting from an excessive secretion of thyroid hormone. It is frequently characterized by an enlarged thyroid gland (goiter) and prominent eyeballs (exophthalmos).

Etiology

1. Unknown
2. Possible precipitating factors
   a. Autoimmune response
   b. Heredity
   c. Infection
   d. Psychic trauma

Clinical Manifestations

1. Rare and less severe in children as compared to adults.
2. More common in females than males.
3. Onset is usually between 10–15 years of age (usually gradual onset).
4. Signs and symptoms
   a. Enlarged thyroid gland (goiter)
   b. Exophthalmos
   c. Nervousness and motor hyperactivity
      (1) Inability to sit still
      (2) Decreased attention span
      (3) Mood shifts
          Irritable
          Excitable
          Cries easily
      (4) Tremors
   d. Increased appetite and food intake
   e. Weight loss or no weight gain
   f. Heat intolerance
   g. Skin
      Warm
      Moist
      Flushed
   h. Muscular weakness and fatigue
   i. Tachycardia, palpitation and dyspnea
   j. Increased systolic blood pressure
      Increased pulse pressure
   k. Accelerated growth rate
   l. Delayed sexual maturation
   m. Possible amenorrhea in females
   n. Thyroid "crisis" or "storm" (very rare in children)

Diagnostic Evaluation

1. High serum levels of T_4 and T_3
2. T_2 uptake test—elevated
3. Radioactive iodine uptake—rapid
4. Protein-bound iodine—increased
5. Basal metabolic rate—increased
6. Serum cholesterol—low

Prognosis

1. Favorable in children who have passed through the therapeutic phase of hyperthyroidism with good immediate results.
2. Recurrence later in life.
   Recurrence risk cannot be accurately predicted; it depends on various factors in the therapeutic regimen.

Altered Physiology

Same as in the adult.

Nursing Objectives and Management

Nursing care of the child with hyperthyroidism is similar to that of the adult (see section on hyperthyroidism). The following objectives are of special importance in pediatrics:

A. *To avoid excitement.*

1. Provide a quiet environment.
   a. Avoid assigning the child to a large ward or room with several other patients.
   b. Limit the number of playmates that the child has at any one time.
   c. Maintain a fairly constant schedule of daily activities.
   d. Sedate if necessary.
      (1) Barbiturates or tranquilizers are the drugs of choice.
      (2) Sedation may be especially beneficial at bedtime.
2. Encourage quiet rather than strenuous activities.
   Interest the child in diversionary activities which do not require lengthy mental concentration.
3. Maintain constant but gentle discipline.

B. *To provide a diet high in protein, calories and vitamins.*

1. Offer between-meal snacks such as milk shakes.
2. Vitamin supplements may be necessary.
3. Offer foods which can be easily swallowed if the child is experiencing dysphagia.

C. *To administer propylthiouracil or methimazole.*

1. These drugs block the production of T_4 and T_3 by the thyroid, thus controlling the symptoms.
2. Dose
   a. Dosage must be individually regulated for each child.
   b. It is essential to space the dose at regular intervals (every 6–8 hours) throughout a 24-hour period.
      Each dose is fully effective for only a few hours.
3. Observe for clinical response.
   a. It is usually apparent in 2–3 weeks.
   b. Exophthalmos may not reverse, but it should not advance.

c. Record disappearance of symptoms, including decreased enlargement of the thyroid gland.
4. Observe for toxic effects. Report the following:
   a. Fever
   b. Mild, sometimes purpuric, papular rash
   c. Headache
   d. Nausea, abdominal cramps, diarrhea
   e. Sore throat
   f. Signs of overdose, mainly lethargy and somnolence
5. Observe for relapse when the drug is discontinued.
   a. Usually discontinued slowly after 2–3 years of administration.
   b. Relapse usually occurs within 6 months of discontinuing the drug.
   c. Treatment usually continued throughout early adolescence in pubertal children.

D. *To demonstrate understanding of the child's physical and emotional problems.*

1. The disease frequently has its onset during adolescence when the child is very concerned with his body image.
2. Encourage the child to talk about his disease and how he feels about it.
   Correct misinformation and misinterpretations as necessary.
3. Assist the adolescent girl to apply make-up which can significantly reduce the obviousness of her exophthalmos.
4. Discuss the child's disease and treatment with his parents and teachers so that their demands and expectations will be realistic.

E. *To care for the child who requires thyroidectomy.*

(Refer to adult text, p. 634.)
1. Indications for surgery in juvenile hyperthyroid patients include:
   a. Toxicity to antithyroid drugs
   b. Failure to cure after an adequate course of medical therapy
   c. Lack of parent or patient compliance
2. Psychologic preparation for surgery is essential.
   The child may associate death with the thought of cutting his throat at the incisional site.

Patient or Parental Education

A. *Medication*

1. Allow the parent to administer the child's medication under supervision during his hospitalization to ensure accuracy after discharge.
2. Points of emphasis
   a. The medication must be administered in the exact amount that was prescribed.
   b. Daily administration of the drug at regular intervals is essential.
   c. The child must be observed for signs and symptoms of drug toxicity.

B. *Medical supervision*

Close medical follow-up is necessary in order to evaluate the child's progress and regulate his drug dosage.

BIBLIOGRAPHY

Books

Bacon G, Spencer L, Kelch R. A Practical Approach to Pediatric Endocrinology. Chicago, Year Book Medical Publishers, 1975

Gardner L (ed). Endocrine and Genetic Disorders of Childhood. Philadelphia, WB Saunders, 1975

Guthrie DW and Guthrie R (eds). Nursing Management of Diabetes Mellitus. St. Louis, CV Mosby, 1977

Hung W, August G, Glasgow A. Pediatric Endocrinology. Garden City, Medical Examination Pub. Co., 1978

Kruegar JA and Ray JC. Endocrine Problems in Nursing—A Physiologic Approach. St. Louis, CV Mosby, 1976

Laron Z (ed). Pediatric and Adolescent Endocrinology, Vol. 2, Medical Aspects of Balance of Diabetes in Juveniles. Basel, Switzerland, S Karger, 1977

Laron Z (ed). Pediatric and Adolescent Endocrinology, Vol. 3, Psychological Aspects of Balance of Diabetes in Juveniles. Basel, Switzerland, S Karger, 1977

Articles

Bode HH, Vanjonack WJ, Crawford JD. Mitigation of cretinism by breast feeding. Pediatrics 1978 July; 62(1):13–16

Daneman D et al. Postcraniotomy diabetes insipidus: Treatment with DDAVP, a synthetic analog of vasopressin. J Pediatr 1978 Nov; 93(5):879–880

Delange F et al. Transient hypothyroidism in the newborn infant. J Pediatr 1978 June; 92(6):974–976

Fisher DA et al. Recommendations for screening programs for congenital hypothyroidism. Report of a committee of the American Thyroid Association. J Pediatr 1976 Oct; 89(4):692–694

Gogas JG et al. Thyroid disease in children and adolescents. Int Surg 1977 Nov/Dec; 62(11–12):592–594

Guthrie D and Guthrie R. DKA: Breaking a vicious cycle. Nursing '78 1978 June; 8(6):54–61

Guthrie DW. Exercise, diets, and insulin for children with diabetes. Nursing '77 1977 Feb; 7(2):48–54

Guthrie D. Helping the diabetic manage his self-care. Nursing '80 1980 Feb; 10(2):57–64

Guthrie DW, Guthrie RA, Hinnen D. Single vs double void technique for urine testing. Diabetes (Suppl. 1) 1977; 26

Kaufman RV and Hersher B. Body image changes in teenage diabetics. Pediatrics 1971 July; 48(1):123–128

Lee J. Care and management of the adolescent diabetic. Pediatric Nursing 1978 May/June; 4(3):42–45

Miller B and White N. Diabetes assessment guide. Am J Nurs 1980 July; 80(7):1314–1316

Ory M and Kronenfeld J. Living with juvenile diabetes mellitus. Pediatric Nursing 1980 Sept/Oct; 6(5):47–50

Simpson O and Smith M. Lightening the load for parents of children with diabetes. MCN 1979 Sept/Oct; 4(5):293–296

Tarnow JD et al. Juvenile diabetes: Impact on the child and family. Psychosomatics 1978 Aug; 19(8):487–491

Waggoner RW Jr. Improved psychological status of children under DDAVP therapy for central diabetes insipidus. Am J Psychiatry 1978 Mar; 135(3):361–362

Welk D. Preventing insulin-induced lipodystrophies. Nursing '79 1979 Dec; 9(12):42–45

Young LA. Dysthyroid ophthalmology in children. J Pediatr Ophthalmol Strabismus 1979 Mar/Apr; 16(2):105–107

CHILDREN WITH EYE AND EAR CONDITIONS

46

1 CONDITIONS OF THE EYE

THE BLIND CHILD

Impaired vision (blindness) refers to insufficient or inadequate vision in varying degrees.

Etiology

1. Familial factors
    Genetic determination
2. Prenatal or intrauterine factors
    a. Rubella
    b. Toxoplasmosis
    c. Syphilis
3. Perinatal factors
    a. Prematurity
    b. Oxygen toxicity—retrolental fibroplasia
    c. Infections
4. Postnatal factors
    a. Injury or trauma
    b. Infections
    c. Inflammatory disease

Altered Physiology

1. Defective visual fields
2. Impaired color vision
3. Decreased visual acuity
4. No vision—or a small percentage of vision (may have light perception)

Clinical Manifestations

A. *Infant*

1. No eye-to-eye contact, especially with mother
2. Abnormal eye movements
3. Does not follow objects at 2 months of age
4. Failure to locate distant objects at 6–12 months of age
5. Mother senses "something is wrong"

B. *Older Child*

1. Squinting, frequent blinking
2. Bumping into things
3. Frequent rubbing of eyes

Diagnostic Evaluation

1. Legal definition—visual acuity 20/200 or less with correction
2. Tunnel vision—peripheral field of vision has an angular distance not greater than 20 degrees

Treatment

1. Surgical repair of defect
2. Glasses
3. Special training
    a. Language development and acquisition
    b. Mobility-perceptual motor training
    c. Early stimulation therapy

Nursing Objectives and Management

The nurse may become involved with the blind child in the hospital in 3 critical situations: (1) before diagnosis has been made when she may detect a visual loss, usually in an infant, (2) at time of diagnosis, and (3) after diagnosis has been made and she is giving nursing care to the hospitalized child who is blind.

**Detection; Early Care of the Blind Child
After Diagnosis**

A. *To be familiar with the normal pattern of visual development and to be able to recognize deviations as well as manifestations of visual impairment.*

1. Knowing the stages of growth and development can be helpful in recognizing or suspecting visual impairment in the individual child.
2. The appreciation of vision by the infant begins at about 3 months of age.
3. Be alert to and assess the child's response to visual stimulation.

a. Does the infant follow the human face or bright object with his eyes according to his stage of development?
b. Does the infant reach for objects?
c. Does the 9- to 12-month-old child move around?

B. *To be familiar with the causes of visual impairment and blindness in order to recognize from the history whether or not the child is in a high-risk category.*

1. Neonatal and perinatal factors
   a. Prematurity
   b. Oxygen therapy
   c. Infections
2. Past infections—inflammatory diseases

C. *To record observations and report any suspicious behavior by the infant or child indicating visual impairment.*

1. Early diagnosis is the key to successful habilitation and optimal development of the child's capabilities.
2. The complication of complete withdrawal of the child can be avoided by early diagnosis and proper stimulation and emotional support.

D. *To help the family of a newly diagnosed visually impaired child.*

1. Parents must be allowed time to understand and accept what has happened.
2. Their lifestyle will have to change; they will need to find new ways to adjust socially and personally.

E. *To work with physician and parents in helping the child master certain developmental tasks, thus aiding the child in achieving his fullest potential.* Parents need help in recognizing the clues the child presents indicating his need and readiness for new learning experiences. The child must also learn in his own natural way.

1. Continued communication must be fostered between parents, mother, and child.
   a. Mother must learn techniques of touching, handling, and talking to her child.
   b. Mother should make a special effort to help her baby associate her voice and body with receiving pleasure.
   c. Encourage touching by both mother and baby during feeding times, as well as other times. Touch is a good nonverbal form of communication, as it is real.
2. *The child and parents must be helped to develop a discriminating relationship*; specific consistent clues of handling the child can be built into behavior.
   a. Each parent shares some special, individualized activity with the child.
   b. Voice and touch bring parents and child together.
3. The child must be allowed and encouraged to use his hands for exploring his world. Child must also learn appropriate use of hands.
   a. Give child objects of different shapes, sizes, and textures. Use toys that make noise and that are within reach and stay there.
   b. Give finger food to child during meals—when child is about 8 months of age or when he sits up.
   c. Extra tactile opportunities provided for child will compensate to some extent for loss of visual input.
4. The child needs to learn to become mobile.
   a. Mother's voice can encourage child to move toward her.
   b. A favorite toy placed in front of child can encourage him to move toward it.

5. The child needs much help in learning to talk.
   a. Expose the child to sounds that have a specific function—cleaning equipment, dishes.
   b. Mother should talk a great deal to the child. The child cannot benefit from gestures and facial expression used in language.
6. The child needs social exposure to his peers. Nursery school can be very helpful.

F. *To foster continuous acceptance of the child by his parents and to provide support for them.*

1. Evaluate the parents' emotional status and offer them reassurance and explanations.
   a. Parental acceptance and a healthy home atmosphere are vitally important in helping the visually impaired or blind child to accept and adjust to his limitations.
   b. The child can sense his parents' approval or disapproval and the degree to which they love and accept him.
2. Help parents to understand and accept their responsibilities in the care of their child. Parents who have received appropriate information and guidance in handling their child can enrich the time spent with the child and prevent further handicapping and management problems. Indicate that they should do the following:
   a. Provide proper stimulation for the child to learn that which is ordinarily learned through vision. Frustration often occurs when child gives little feedback. Efforts may decrease as a consequence.
   b. The voice is often used to protect the child.
   c. Reinforce that this child has the same needs for growth and development as any child.
3. Help parents understand how they can develop the child's skills in interpreting information through the senses of hearing, touch, smell, and taste. They can learn to understand their blind child.
   a. Hearing
      (1) Help child to determine distance by ringing a bell.
      (2) Familiarize him with appliances, birds, voices.
      (3) Use voice—tone, expression, etc. as nonverbal cues go unnoticed.
   b. Touch
      Allow child to handle different textured materials.
   c. Smell
      Acquaint child with flowers, perfume, kitchen odors.
   d. Taste
      Help child distinguish different kitchen substances.
   e. Memory
      Have child practice retelling stories, his telephone number, address, etc.
4. Initiate referral to the community nurse who can make home visits to reinforce and interpret what mother has heard from the physician and to encourage mother in her efforts.
5. Encourage parents to discuss their feelings about caring for a handicapped child at home.
      Initiate a social worker referral. (The social worker can help parents deal with their feelings.)
6. Help parents understand the problems the child faces and will face as he gets older.
   a. Child will probably be delayed in development. There can be a delay of up to 5 months in creeping and 7 months in walking, even though posture

and balance for such activities are similar to those of sighted child.

b. Child is likely to develop "blindisms"—habits or mannerisms of blind children; these are a manifestation of inadequate impulse control. Child may also show self-stimulatory behavior.

G. *To be familiar with the community resources and the professional team to be involved in habilitation of the visually impaired child.*

Several types of school programs are available to the child, depending upon his confidence and coping abilities.

1. Residential schools.
   a. Used when nothing is available in the local community.
   b. Preferred when the home care of the child would be detrimental to his progress.
2. Day schools for the blind. (Child attends school during day but lives at home.)
3. Public school where blind child is integrated with sighted child. (Child receives special training in braille.)
4. Vocational habilitation programs (training for some occupation).

H. *To evaluate how well the child who was once able to see accepts visual impairment—in terms of his physical abilities and psychologic dependence.* (Vision helps to maintain contact with reality.)

1. A serious impairment in relationships with people can result when the child is unable to express his innermost sentiments.
2. Allow the child to express his feelings, especially those of fear and anger. Talk, play, and certain activities help the child express these feelings.

Hospital Care of the Visually Impaired or Blind Child

Many of the important areas discussed above must be considered when caring for the child in the hospital situation. In addition, emphasis must be placed on the following objectives:

A. *To interview the parents at the time of admission to learn as much as possible about the child and his care and activities at home.*

1. Be aware of the child's schedule and activities during the day. Know what activities he can or cannot do, and what he likes to do.
2. Become familiar with how he is oriented to his new surroundings.
   a. How much does he ambulate?
   b. What precautions are necessary?
3. Be aware of how parents comfort and discipline the child.
   How does he comfort himself or seek security?
4. What special care or treatment must be continued while the child is hospitalized?
5. Share this information with nursing staff in a nursing care plan so continuity of care from home to hospital can minimize fear and frustration in the child.

B. *To attend to the child's needs according to the medical problem that required his hospitalization.*

C. *To plan and provide for the appropriate type of play, activities program and stimulation for the child.*

1. Assess the child's level of growth and development and use the information obtained from parents.

2. Allow the child as much independence as possible in his care, but provide guidance as necessary.
   Orient the ambulatory child thoroughly to his room and surroundings.
3. Encourage the development of the child's abilities. Avoid overprotecting him.
4. Provide activities that will increase his learning and give him pleasure (e.g., talking records).
5. Provide emotional preparation for procedures and surgery, as appropriate.

D. *To meet the psychological and emotional needs of the visually impaired or blind child for protection and security against harm.*

1. The nurse should always speak to the child prior to touching him so as not to frighten or startle him.
2. Always use a warm and gentle touch.
3. Explain strange sounds that may be frightening.
   Tape recording of sounds he may hear help put them into proper perspective.
4. Plan frequent nurse-patient interactions to increase the child's sense of security.
5. Place items he needs and uses within his reach.
   a. Familiar items that give the child security should also be close to him.
   b. Tell him if they are moved.
6. During any procedure, talk to the child the entire time. Explain what is going on around him.

E. *To avoid overemphasizing the child's handicap and to be unobtrusive about meeting his needs.*

Allow the child to explore and learn about his new environment and the hospital.

F. *To provide continual parental support.*

1. Encourage parents to become involved in the care of their child to help maintain or develop a healthy parent-child relationship.
   Separation from parents can be extremely traumatic and has severe implications for the blind child.
2. Encourage parents to talk about their fears and feelings concerning this child. Help them relax.
   Parents can be invaluable in increasing the security and decreasing the fear the child may have as a result of being in a strange place.
3. Discuss realistically long-term and short-term planning for the child, i.e., educational opportunities.
   a. Encourage parents to tell teachers and adults responsible for his care about his special needs.
   b. Avoid overemphasis on educational achievements.
4. Help parents understand that discipline, order and consistency are necessary in the child's environment to give him security.
5. Emphasize that the parents' role is to give this child love and physical care as well as to stimulate and influence him so he may have a satisfactory mental, social and emotional growth.
6. Help parents see that other members of the family must also be considered.
   a. Their handicapped child does need special attention, but he does not need all the attention all the time.
   b. Other members of the family should be included in his care, but they also have a life of their own and need as much attention from parents as they would have if the handicapped child were not present in the family.
   c. Parents need time to themselves. They should be

encouraged to go out alone together and to give time to their marriage.
7. Help parents realize that even though habilitation of their blind child is long, drawn out and expensive, the child may be able to live a normal life in the community.

a. Are parents aware of and do they accept the short- and long-term goals?
b. Many blind people are successful as technicians and professionals.

EYE DEFECTS REQUIRING SURGERY

Eye defects requiring surgery are (1) structural manifestations of the eye present at birth or (2) acquired conditions of the eye. They can be extraocular or intraocular conditions.

Etiology

1. Congenital
   a. Hereditary tendencies
   b. Birth injury
   c. Innervational factors
   d. Intrauterine influences
2. Disease
   a. Metabolic
   b. Infection
3. Trauma to the eye

STRABISMUS

Strabismus is the inability to balance the extraocular muscles; thus the eyes cannot function together at the same time.

Altered Physiology

1. The visual axis of only 1 eye goes to the object being observed. The person appears to be looking in 2 directions at once.
2. Specific Deviations
   a. Paralytic strabismus—muscles of 1 eye are underactive.
   b. Concomitant strabismus—both eyes move, but the deviation between the eyes is always the same.
   c. Hypertropia—eye deviation is upward.
   d. Hypotropia—eye deviation is downward.
   e. Vertical—vertical separation of visual axes.
   f. Esotropia—one eye deviates toward other eye; convergent—"cross-eye."
   g. Exotropia—one eye deviates away from the other eye; divergent—"wall-eye."

Clinical Manifestations

1. Deviations of the eye (constant or intermittent)
2. Squinting
3. Closing one eye to see
4. Tilting head
5. Stumbling or clumsy behavior
6. Inaccuracy in picking up objects
7. Double vision

Complications

1. Amblyopia—poor vision in eye not used.
2. Emotional problems resulting from cosmetic aspect of deformity.
3. Repeated surgery may be necessary.

Treatment

1. Corrective glasses
2. Patching nondiverging eye
3. Surgery
   Lengthening or shortening of extraocular structures
See page 1370 for nursing management.

CATARACT

Cataract is an opacification or milk-white appearance of the eye lens.

Altered Physiology

Inability of light to pass through the clouded lens in adequate amounts—loss of vision as lens becomes more opaque; loss of transparency.

Clinical Manifestations

1. Gradual diminution of visual acuity
2. Strabismus
3. Nystagmus
4. Gray opacities of lens

Diagnostic Evaluation

Ophthalmoscopic examination reveals opacification of the lens.

Treatment

1. Medication—dilation of pupil with mydriatic eye drops
2. Surgery
   a. Optical iridectomy
   b. Lens fragmentation, irrigation, and aspiration

Complications

A. *Untreated Cataract*

1. Bilateral cataract
   a. Nystagmus
   b. Stimulus-deprivation amblyopia
2. Unilateral cataract
   a. Strabismus
   b. Stimulus-deprivation amblyopia

B. *Following surgery for congenital cataract:*

1. Retinal detachment several years later
2. Average vision only 20/70
3. Need for glasses or contact lenses to replace refracting power of lens
See below for nursing management.

TRAUMA

Trauma is injury to the globe, adnexa, and surrounding tissue of the eye as a result of blunt objects (baseball, rock) striking the eye area, or sharp items (scissors, knife) penetrating the eye area.

Altered Physiology

A. *Blunt Injury*
1. Subconjunctival hemorrhage and suffusion of blood into eyelid
2. Secondary hemorrhage days after injury
   a. Accumulation of blood in anterior chamber and blocking of overflow channels
   b. Rapid rise of intraocular pressure (glaucoma)
3. Retinal edema, hemorrhages, and detachment

B. *Penetrating Injury*
1. Loss of aqueous fluid, development of cataract
2. Bleeding into anterior chamber and vitreous
3. Retinal detachment

C. *Corneal Abrasions* (i.e., from fingernail)
   a. Common in young children
   b. Treated for 24 hours with patching and antibiotic ointment

Complications

Sympathetic ophthalmia—inflammation of the uninjured eye probably due to an allergic reaction to pigment released from injured eye. This condition can lead to significant visual loss.

NURSING MANAGEMENT OF THE CHILD UNDERGOING EYE SURGERY

Nursing Objectives and Management

Preoperative Care

A. *To help the child and his parents to know and understand what the surgery entails. (Explanations should be appropriate for the age of the child.)*
1. Take a trip to the operating and recovery rooms if the child is not on bed rest due to trauma.
2. Practice applying eye patches for short frequent periods.
   a. Allow the child to handle the equipment to be used.
   b. Explain that the patches will only be temporary.
3. Help the child become familiar with the protective devices if they are to be used postoperatively.
4. Discuss and practice postoperative exercises if feasible.
5. Relieve child's fears about pain by telling him that there will be a little pain—as if something is in the eye.

B. *To assess the child and his needs according to age and specifically to his eye problem.*
1. Does the child have the ability to read or watch television?
2. Does the child wear glasses? When?
   Help him to learn to protect his glasses when not in use.

C. *To provide as much comfort and reassurance to the child as possible to diminish his fears especially concerning hospitalization and impending surgery.*
1. Room assignment can be significant.
   a. A quiet room with subdued lighting can be more comfortable for trauma patients.
   b. Placement in a room with other children (without infection) may be comforting for elective surgery patients.
2. Allow the child to have familiar tactile and auditory stimulating objects around him.

Postoperative Care

A. *To administer effective postoperative care and to observe for possible postoperative complications.* (See p. 1140.) Be alert to care and consideration for specific eye defect.
1. Strabismus
   a. Frequently child is discharged on the day of surgery, following recovery from anesthesia.
   b. Surgery is extraocular; no postoperative ocular rupture hazards exist.
   c. Activity is not restricted.
   d. Eye bandages may or may not be used.
   e. Eyes will probably be blood-tinged and will drain. Eyes may feel uncomfortable. Black eye is normal, as is postoperative swelling.
   f. Eyes may be difficult to open the morning after surgery. Gently separate lids from above and below. Do not force lids open. Tears will soften secretions.
   g. Child may have photosensitivity.
2. Cataract or intraocular surgery
   a. Child is generally positioned on his back; thus, prevention of aspiration is a concern.
   b. Avoid sudden head movement, crying, and vomiting, because these increase intraocular pressure; they cause strain on sutures and subsequent bleeding.
   c. Avoid surprising patient and making him jump. Avoid noises. Speak gently before touching child.

B. *To prevent the child from pulling off the dressing and causing injury or contamination.*
1. Sedation may be warranted until the child becomes accustomed to having his eye continually bandaged.
2. Protective devices may be used only if necessary. Rest during the immediate postoperative period is necessary and a child struggling because of restraints can defeat their intended purpose.
3. Diet should be increased slowly to prevent vomiting; this could cause possible injury to the eye due to increased pressure.

C. *To provide emotional and psychological reassurance and support to the child who is anxious because his eyes are bandaged preventing him from seeing.*
1. Encourage parents to be with child, especially when he is waking up from anesthesia. If parents are not able to do this, someone should.
   a. Sit with child, stroke him, and speak gently and softly to him.
   b. Let him hold a familiar object.
   c. Hold him if there are no contraindications to his being lifted and held.
2. Always speak to child before touching him so as not to startle him.
   Explain what is going to be done to him before doing it.
3. Tell the child what foods are on his tray.
   Allow him to finger feed himself.
4. Explain sounds. (Sounds in the world without sight can be very frightening.)
5. Reassure child that patches will be removed soon and he will be able to see again (if he is going to see).
6. Provide appropriate diversional activities for the child.
   a. Read him stories.
   b. Provide radio or phonograph.
   c. Talk with him.

D. *To administer appropriate eye medications and change dressing as prescribed.*

1. First dressing change is usually done by physician.
   a. Strabismus—dressing removed day after surgery.
   b. Cataract—dressing may be used for 5–10 days after surgery.
2. Be familiar with types of eye medications used.
   a. Mydriatic—used to dilate pupil.
   b. Miotic—constricts pupil and decreases increased intraocular pressure in early glaucoma.
   c. Anti-inflammatory drugs.
   d. Antibiotics.
3. Be familiar with the principles of instilling eye medications (drops, ointments, and irrigations).
   a. Have room darkened—light may be uncomfortable.
   b. Try to gain the confidence and cooperation of the child and reassure him by talking to him during the procedure.
   c. Assistance may be necessary to stabilize child's head and prevent injury. Have child close eye; drop medication onto inner canthus; open eye and drop will roll in.
   d. Irrigate from inner canthus outward.
   e. To instill drops, pull lower lid down and drop medication onto conjunctiva from dropper parallel to lid. If drops are instilled on conjunctiva and not on cornea, patient tolerates medication better.
   f. Do not force lid open.
   g. Blot away excess fluid with tissue or cotton ball; do not rub eye.
   h. Avoid contaminating dressing.
   i. Always wash hands before and after contact with the eye for any procedure.

E. *To involve parents and child in preparation for discharge.*

1. Teach parents how to instill eye medications. (See above.)
2. Postoperative patches or glasses may be necessary. Help parents and child understand the value and importance of the patching or glasses.
3. Encourage parents to contact the school nurse and other adults responsible for child's care to explain special exercises or specific care for the child.
4. Encourage follow-up as advised by the physician.

Parental Education

Help parents understand what was wrong with the child, what was done to help correct the problem and what the parental responsibilities are in continuing any recommended therapy with the child.

Be certain parents understand what special care is to be given and how it is to be accomplished.

2   CONDITIONS OF THE EAR

OTITIS MEDIA

Otitis media is an infection of the middle ear.

Etiology

1. Bacteriologic
   a. *Haemophilus influenzae*
   b. Beta hemolytic streptococci
   c. Pneumococci
2. Secondary
   a. Cold
   b. Measles
   c. Scarlet fever
3. Eustachian tube dysfunction
   a. Obstruction
   b. Abnormal patency

Altered Physiology

1. Obstruction of the eustachian tube by swelling of mucous membranes.
   a. Air exchange does not take place between the pharynx and middle ear.
   b. Obstruction impedes drainage of secretions to the nasopharynx.
2. Secretions and bacteria become trapped in the middle ear.
   Bacteria multiply rapidly in that environment, spread to mastoid bone or inner ear, and cause permanent damage.
3. Fluid and exudate replace air in the middle ear. Fluid changes from watery secretions to viscous glue-like substance.
   a. Eardrum bulges.
      Otoscope reveals dull gray eardrum.
   b. Tympanic membrane may rupture.

Clinical Manifestations

1. History of cold for several days
2. Fever
3. Older child
   a. Pain in affected ear
   b. Blurred hearing
   c. Headache
   d. Vomiting
4. Infant
   a. May rub ear
   b. Anorexia
   c. Turns head from side to side
   d. Diarrhea

Diagnostic Evaluation

1. Examination will reveal bulging of eardrum, partial or complete obstruction of bony landmarks, and lack of normal luster; ruptured drum may be obscured by secretions. Absence of light reflex, impaired mobility of eardrum when using pneumatic ostoscope.
2. Culture and sensitivity determination of drainage from ruptured drum or through myringotomy in order to select appropriate antibiotic therapy.
3. *Tympanometry*—the use of an electroacoustic impedance bridge with which a tympanogram can be

obtained. The tympanograms produced show the dynamics of the tympanic membrane, middle ear, eustachian tube system.

Treatment

A. *Medical*

1. Antibiotics—appropriate for organism
2. Acetaminophen or aspirin—for fever
3. Analgesic
4. Ear drops for relief of pain
5. Antihistamines and decongestant—to clear nasal pharyngitis and inflammation of eustachian tubes

B. *Surgical*

1. *Myringotomy*—surgical incision of the tympanic membrane to allow drainage and relieve pressure; done when fluid remains in middle ear despite medical treatment, or performed for diagnostic reasons.
2. Tympanostomy ventilating tube. Small plastic tube is inserted into the middle ear through a myringotomy incision, creating an artificial eustachian tube to equalize pressure on both sides of the eardrum.
   a. The tube projects through the drum into the external auditory canal.
   b. This tube is a substitute for the eustachian tube, allowing the following to occur:
      (1) Continuous ventilation of the middle ear
      (2) Drainage of fluid into the external auditory canal
      (3) Promotion of healing of lining membranes
      (4) Prevention of premature closing of incision
   c. The tube may be left in place several weeks to several months. The perforation closes in about a week after the tubes are removed.
   d. Hearing will improve in children with middle ear fluid.
   e. Most common age for treatment is between 2–7 years.
   f. Complications of tympanostomy tube include:
      (1) Recurring otitis media or suppurative otitis media
      (2) Plugging of tube with blood, cerumen, or exudate
      (3) Early spontaneous extrusion of tube
      (4) Permanent perforations
   g. Specific postoperative considerations
      Do not allow water to get into ears (during swimming or bathing) because of the infection potential. Emphasize the advantage—improvement of hearing.

Complications

From untreated or ineffective treatment of acute otitis media
1. Chronic otitis media
2. Mastoiditis
3. Septicemia
4. Meningitis and brain damage
5. Chronic otitis media with mastoiditis and perforated eardrum may lead to impaired hearing or deafness

Nursing Objectives and Management

A. *To administer medications and treatments as prescribed.*

1. Give appropriate antibiotics according to sensitivity of organisms.
   Usual course of treatment is 10 days.

2. Instill nose drops and decongestant.
   May help to shrink mucous membranes and allow drainage from obstructed eustachian tube.
3. Give ear irrigations and instill glycerin or oil for relief of pain.
   a. Child may need to be held, or "mummy" restraint used.
   b. For child under 3 years old—pull auricle down and back.
   c. For child over 3 years old—pull auricle up and back.
   d. Position child so the affected ear is up—allows fluid to run onto the eardrum.

B. *To prevent mixed infection and reduce the chances of complications arising from present infection.*

1. Always wash hands prior to any treatment or contact with the ear.
2. Change position of the child as appropriate.
   a. Position affected ear up to instill medications or to irrigate ear.
   b. Position affected ear down to facilitate drainage when child is resting.
3. Clean any exudate present from myringotomy or perforated drum.
   Prevents excoriation from drainage.

C. *To provide physical comfort for the child while continuing therapy.*

1. Local heat
   a. Use hot water bottle containing water not over 38.9° C. (102° F.).
   b. Place child on side, with affected ear on top of bottle to facilitate drainage.
2. A mild analgesic may be necessary if child is restless and indicates pain.
3. Myringotomy may be done in cases where there is severe pain.
   Small incision of the tympanic membrane to relieve pressure and prevent a jagged opening from a spontaneous rupture. Prepare child for procedure. Use model of ear anatomy for teaching. Show him and let him handle ventilating tubes.
4. Encourage fluid intake to help maintain hydration since the child may have a fever.

D. *To observe for signs of complications and report them.*

1. Mastoiditis
   a. Pain behind affected ear
   b. Increasing irritability
   c. Onset or increase of fever
   d. Tenderness, redness and swelling over mastoid area
2. Meningitis
   a. Sudden onset of high fever
   b. Stiffness of neck
   c. Irritability
   d. Headache
   e. Lethargy
3. Chronic otitis media with perforation of tympanic membrane
   Usually not observed until follow-up care by physician

E. *To provide emotional and psychological support appropriate for child's age and degree of illness.*

1. Encourage child to participate in diversional activities.
2. Reassure child

a. Talk to him gently.
b. Allow child to express his feelings, fears and frustrations by talking, playing and drawing.
c. Hold and rock the younger child.
3. Encourage parental visits and involvement in the child's care.
   a. Ensure that parents understand the diagnosis, pathology involved, and treatment.
   b. Help them to understand the necessity for follow-up and return visit following the episode, and the possible complications.

F. *To help the parents understand that prevention of recurring otitis media is vitally important for the future well-being of the child.*

1. Explain the value of preventing and treating the common cold.
2. Removal of hypertrophied and infected adenoid tissue may be necessary at a later date at the recommendation of the physician.
3. Explain that the child may have decreased hearing for several weeks following this episode of illness.
4. Help parents learn what signs indicate recurrent

otitis media and the need for immediate medical intervention.
   a. Prompt treatment can prevent permanent hearing loss.
   b. Identify the relationship between hearing and language development.

G. *To help parents and child understand treatment and expectations related to ventilating tubes.*

1. Following surgery, antibiotic ear drops may be prescribed to aid in keeping tubes patent.
2. Hearing may not improve for 1–3 weeks postoperatively.
3. Tubes will remain in place from 2–10 months, and are designed to extrude into the external ear canal.
4. When tubes extrude, slight pain and a small amount of bloody drainage may occur. Physician should be notified that the tubes are out.
5. Water should be prevented from entering the external ear canal—use properly fitting ear plugs, cottonballs coated with petroleum, etc.
6. Stress the importance of regular medical follow-up to evaluate proper functioning of tubes.

THE CHILD WITH IMPAIRED HEARING

Impaired hearing occurs when there is a hearing loss in speech frequencies of over 20 decibels, and the child does not learn to talk in the normal way. Speech essentially may have no meaning.

Etiology

1. Unknown
2. Familial factors—genetically transmitted; family history of hearing impairment*
3. Prenatal or intrauterine factors
   a. Rubella*
   b. Preeclampsia or eclampsia
   c. Drugs
   d. Congenital syphilis
4. Perinatal factors
   a. Prematurity*—especially < 1500 gm.
   b. Anoxia at birth
   c. Hyperbilirubinemia*
   d. Erythroblastosis fetalis
   e. Neonatal sepsis*, meningitis
5. Postnatal factors
   a. Ototoxic drugs
   b. Acquired disorders of the central nervous system
   c. Acute infections, otitis media
   d. Injury
   e. Structural defects*
6. Chromosomal anomalies
   a. Trisomy 13-14-15
   b. Trisomy 18

Altered Physiology

A. *Conductive Hearing Loss*

1. Impairment in the mechanism of conducting sound waves to the cochlea
   a. Blockage of sound waves from outer ear, external canal, or middle ear (lack of loudness)
   b. Tympanic membrane damage and scarring
   c. Dislocation or disturbance of tiny ossicular bones in the middle ear

   * Criteria for high risk of impaired hearing.

2. Often recognized in the school-age child

B. *Sensorineural Hearing Loss*

1. Malfunction of inner ear apparatus or 8th cranial nerve—medically irreversible
   a. Lack of loudness
   b. Distorted sounds due to defect of cochlea or neural pathways to temporal lobe of the brain
   c. Problems with discrimination of sound
2. Mixed hearing loss; both sensorineural and conductive hearing loss in some children

Clinical Manifestations

A. *Infant*

1. Little or no interest in sounds of his environment
   a. Does not blink at loud noise
   b. Does not turn eyes toward sound of musical toy or mother's voice at 3 months of age
   c. Does not turn toward whispered voice within 1 meter (3 feet) at 8–12 months of age
   d. Hyperactivity or gesturing may increase.
2. Lack of or minimal vocalization
   a. Does not coo or gurgle
   b. May not smile
   c. Babbling decreases after 6–8 months of age
3. Lack of neonatal startle reflex to noise 1–2 meters (3–6 feet) away

B. *Toddlers*

1. Little or no vocalization
   a. Sounds produced poorly
   b. Will not repeat a word with single stimulus
   c. Uses gestures to express needs
2. Little interest in environmental sounds
   Does not respond to name, doorbell, or telephone

C. *Preschool and School-age Child*

1. Behavioral disturbances
   a. Intense, constant activity
   b. Temper tantrums
   c. Inattentiveness
   d. Slow learner

2. May show abrupt change in social or communicative behavior

D. *Sensorineural vs. Conductive Hearing Loss*

1. Sensorineural
   a. Child may talk more loudly than necessary.
   b. Child may not respond to average loudness but responds to loud sounds.
   c. When intensity of sound is increased above the threshold of sensitivity, child shows some type of response.
2. Conductive
   a. Child has tendency to talk in relatively soft voice.
   b. He hears better in a noisy environment.
   c. Child can hear loud speech and sounds.

Diagnostic Evaluation

1. Otolaryngologic examination (inspection of external ear and tympanic membrane)—to rule out involvement of conductive apparatus.
2. Audiologic examination—to establish the extent of hearing loss and to determine type of hearing aid needed
   a. Observation of child's response to sounds calibrated for intensity and frequency
   b. Objective measuring techniques of hearing loss, i.e., cortical audiometry
3. Hearing loss classification
   Pure tone audiometry hearing threshold level:
   0–25 db—Normal hearing
   26–40 db—Mild hearing impairment
   41–55 db—Moderate hearing loss
   56–70 db—Moderately severe hearing loss
   71–90 db—Severe hearing loss
   91+ db—Profound hearing loss

Complications

1. In childhood when there is a hearing disorder, there is a delay of speech and language development; thus, there is a loss of contact between the individual, his peers, and his environment.
2. Biologic, behavioral and social complications may result when there is a breakdown of the normal communicative process.
3. The seriousness of the total problem depends upon the nature and extent of auditory involvement and upon the age of onset and length of time before the hearing problem is detected.

Treatment

1. Conductive hearing loss
   a. Surgical correction of defect
   b. Hearing aid
2. Sensorineural hearing loss
   a. Hearing aid
   b. Special training
      (1) Language acquisition
      (2) Auditory training
      (3) Speech therapy
      (4) Perceptual motor training

Nursing Objectives and Management

The nurse may become involved with the child with impaired hearing in the hospital in 3 situations: (1) before diagnosis has been made when she may detect a hearing loss, (2) at the time of diagnosis, and (3) after diagnosis has been made when giving nursing care to the hospitalized child.

Detection; Early Care After Diagnosis

A. *To be familiar with the normal pattern of language and learning development and the manifestations of hearing loss in the infant and child.*

1. Knowing the stages of growth and development can be helpful in recognizing and suspecting hearing impairment in the individual child.
2. Be alert to and assess the child's response to auditory stimulation.
   a. Does infant stop activity and listen to vocal sounds?
   b. Does the child respond to his name?
   c. Does the child have unusual visual alertness at age 1 year?
3. The critical period of learning or language development is from birth to 16 months.

B. *To be familiar with the causes of hearing impairment and recognize from the history if the child may be in a high-risk category.*

1. Ensure that follow-up hearing evaluation is planned.
2. Criteria for high risk of impaired hearing (see etiology).

C. *To record observations and report to physician any suspicious behavior by the infant or child that indicates possible hearing loss.*

1. Early diagnosis is the key to successful habilitation and optimal development of the capabilities of the child. Early intervention is aimed toward the child's acquisition of heard and spoken language.
   a. After 16 months of age, habilitation is more difficult.
   b. If hearing loss occurs after the time of critical language development, rehabilitation is less difficult, as the groundwork for verbal communication has been established.
2. The impulse for learning spontaneous speech and acquiring most of the basic verbal skills as well as the structure on which mature use of language and speech is built is reached during the first 3–4 years of life.
3. A current screening device used is the Crib-O-Gram*—an automated method of recording responses of the infant's motor activity before and after test sound.

D. *To be familiar with community resources and the professional team involved in habilitation.*

1. Each child must be treated as an individual.
2. Knowing general philosophies and training techniques of the involved resource can be helpful.
   Help child to capitalize on assets and minimize limitations.

E. *To be familiar with the guidelines and techniques of educating a child with impaired hearing.*

1. The main mode of communication for the child with impaired hearing is visual, supplemented by auditory clues.
   a. Educational task is to develop the child's understanding and expression of language.
   b. Speech can be learned through a multisensory approach, using visual, tactile, kinesthetic and auditory stimulation.
2. The child with a less severe hearing loss uses auditory stimulation, supplemented by visual clues, as his main mode of communication.

* Telesensory System, Inc., Palo Alto, Ca.

Educational task is to develop adequate speech and language and the best use of residual hearing.

3. The 3 basic methods currently used in educating deaf children include:
   a. *Oral Approach*—emphasizes verbal communication, speech reading, and auditory training. Most useful when child has some hearing.
   b. *Manual Communication*—sign language.
   c. *Total Communication Approach*—combines sign language with auditory training and speech reading.
4. The newest concept in education is cued speech, which visually pinpoints a single sound being spoken by using a manual supplement to lip reading of hand shapes used near the mouth to make language sounds look different on the lips or hand.
5. Whatever method of education and communication is used, it is critical for parents to enter the educational process so that they can establish communication with their child.

F. *To help the family cope with and accept a newly diagnosed hearing impairment in their child.*

1. Encourage the physician to have both parents present when he tells them the diagnosis. This allows the parents to support each other.
2. Do not focus all your attention upon the child. Show your concern and interest in the parents.
3. Be aware that parents must be given time to adjust to this usually drastic and unexpected change in their lives before they can deal constructively with meeting the needs of the child.
4. At this time parents need general information—good literature that is specific to their child's problem. Contact with other parents who have made successful adjustments to living with their hearing-impaired children can be helpful to parents. Acquaint them with organizations dealing with deafness (see below).

G. *To be aware of the problems facing the mother (and family) of a hearing-impaired child.* Offer them specific guidance in handling and caring for the child.

1. Problems encountered
   a. Lack of knowledge of principles of parenting methods that govern her child's development.
   b. Does not receive cues from her child that are familiar to most mothers.
   c. Does not get feedback from her child in speech (vocalization), emotional response, or achievement—all of which increase spontaneous mothering. Communicating limitations tend to restrict early mother-child relationships.
      Child is not equipped to show his attachment to his mother.
   d. Parent must be in close contact with the child to control and regulate his behavior.
   e. Her child is infantile in lack of impulse control and is unable to understand and order his world.
   f. Mother may show embarrassment because of her child's behavior.
   g. There is a possible tendency to neglect or deny common childhood conflicts and/or problems.
   h. Frustration—feels she does not know how to help her child.
2. Specific guidance to offer mother:
   a. Allow and encourage her to communicate with her child through mime, gestures, and body language.

There is an increased need for stimulation and physical contact.
   b. Optimize auditory environment.
   c. Teach her how to talk to her child—to use verbal and nonverbal reinforcement of behavior.
   d. Help her baby develop "watching behavior" by rewarding him with pleasure and praise.
   e. Encourage her to look directly into the child's eyes when she talks to him and to use appropriate facial expressions.
   f. Help her to understand that her child is probably unable to express his anxieties; frustration leads to anger and sudden rage or temper tantrums. Help her to gain confidence in her own resourcefulness and care by anticipating child's random behavior through her knowledge of its coincidence with certain situations.
   g. Teach her the stages of language development.

H. *To foster continuous parental acceptance of the child and provide support for family.*

1. Invite parents to become involved in the care of their hospitalized child as much as possible.
2. Help parents to understand the problems the child faces and will face as he gets older.
   a. Although hearing impairment does alter life's experience for the child, it does not limit intelligence or capacity for emotional response and normal growth and development.
   b. Child may not be able to participate in activities in which sounds and verbal commands are used.
   c. Often the referral agency will become very involved in supporting the family.
3. Help parents become aware of their importance in the success of the habilitation of the child.
   a. Parents have the most important educational influence on the child.
   b. Opportunities to use effective ways of stimulating child's awareness and understanding of speech occur daily in the home.
   c. The child needs the warmth and security of a family setting.
4. Help parents to understand what can be accomplished in their child's education to enable him to be a contributing member of society.
5. Stress the importance of close follow-up by the specialists caring for the child.
6. Help parents to understand the use and importance of the hearing aid their child is using.
   a. Most children with a hearing loss have enough residual hearing to respond to and/or recognize sounds with use of an aid.
   b. Use of the aid does not approximate normal hearing; the child receives sounds differently.
   c. Parents must be convinced of the value of the aid but not pay too much attention to it.
   d. Young child does not have much difficulty in adjusting to the hearing aid if the ear mold is comfortable and the sound amplification is not too unpleasant. Place the aid on the child and have him wear it during waking hours.
   e. For the older child who has become used to the aid as a youngster, it is part of his body image and he is dependent upon the sound.
   f. Parents should be sensitive to child's reactions to the aid.
   g. Follow-up care is vital; a malfunctioning aid can cause the child to lose interest in its use.

7. Help shape healthy parental attitudes about their child and guide them through this difficult time.
   a. Prevent denial.
   b. Parents need sympathetic understanding during the time of diagnosis and immediately following when they are bewildered and grieving.
   c. Parental attitudes may be the primary factor in determining the success or failure of the child's progress.
8. Help parents to maintain continued awareness for normal growth and development of their child and the normal stresses and needs during each stage.
9. Encourage parents to write for literature from appropriate agencies.*

Care of the Hospitalized Child Who Has a Hearing Loss

A. *To interview the parents at the time of admission to learn as much as possible about the child and his activities at home.*

1. What is the child's way of communicating his needs? How do parents communicate with the child?
2. Be aware of the child's schedule and activities at home.
   Know what activities he can or cannot do and what he likes to do.
3. Be aware of how parents discipline child and how they comfort him.
4. Does the child wear a hearing aid? When? Any special exercises or training that needs to be continued?
5. Share this information with nursing staff in the

---

* Organizations for parents concerned with hearing problems include the following:
1. Alexander Graham Bell Association for the Deaf, 3417 Volta Place, N.W., Washington, D.C. 20007.
2. The John Tracy Clinic, 806 West Adams Blvd., Los Angeles, California 90007. This clinic offers a free home correspondence course (in English and Spanish) for parents that provides them with information, guidance, and encouragement in training their child.
3. National Association of the Deaf, 814 Thayer Ave, Silver Spring, Maryland 20910.
4. National Easter Seal Society for Crippled Children and Adults, Inc., 2023 W. Ogden Ave., Chicago, Illinois 60612.
5. Bill Wilkerson Hearing and Speech Center, 1114 19th Ave. South, Nashville, Tennessee 37212.
6. American Hearing Society, 919 18th Street, N.W., Washington, D.C. 20006.
7. Gallaudet College, 7th and Florida Ave., N.W., Washington, D.C. 20002 (for information regarding cued speech programs).

nursing care plan to assure continuity of care from home to hospital and to minimize fear and frustration in the child.

B. *To attend to the child's needs according to the medical or surgical problem that required his hospitalization.*

Properly prepare the child for procedures, etc., using increased sense of touch and visual sense.

C. *To plan and provide for the appropriate type of play program and stimulation for the child.*

1. Assess the child's level of development and growth and use information provided by parents.
2. Allow the child as much independence as possible in his care, but provide guidance as necessary—prevent boredom.
3. Encourage the development of the child's abilities.

D. *To meet the emotional needs of the child with impaired hearing for closeness and belonging.*

1. Place the child in a room with a friendly, outgoing child.
2. Plan frequent nurse-patient interactions.
   a. Gentle touch
   b. Games or activities he enjoys
3. Encourage parents, especially mother, to take an active part in his care, thus decreasing fear of desertion.
4. Be aware of coping behaviors seen in the child, including visual information gathering, avoidance, and comfort-seeking measures.

E. *To offer continuous parental support.*

1. Help parents to think of their child as a child first, then as a child with special needs.
2. Emphasize their importance in the habilitation of their child. Point out the value of the home environment in his development.
   a. Talk about the daily routines.
   b. Talk about mother's role in stimulating the child's interest in sounds and speech.
   c. Encourage the use of hearing aids and the learning program set up by specialists in hearing problems in children, as appropriate.
   d. Residential placement may be considered when local facilities are nonexistent or when the home environment would be detrimental to the child's progress.
3. Encourage parents to talk about their fears, frustrations and feelings in caring for the child at home. Initiate a social worker referral, if a social worker is not already involved from the special training center.

BIBLIOGRAPHY

EYE

Books

Bakwin H and Bakwin RM. Behavior Disorders in Children. Philadelphia, WB Saunders, 1972
Feman SS and Reinecke RD. Handbook of Pediatric Ophthalmology. New York, Grune & Stratton, 1978
Halliday C and Kutzhels IW. Stimulating Environments for Children Who Are Visually Impaired. Springfield, Charles C Thomas, 1976
Havener WH, Saunders WH, Keith CF, Prescott AW. Nursing Care in Eye, Ear, Nose, and Throat Disorders. St. Louis, CV Mosby, 1974
Jan JE, Freeman RD, Scott EP. Visual Impairment in Children and Adolescents. New York, Grune & Stratton, 1977
Ulrich S and Wolf AWM. Elizabeth. Ann Arbor, The University of Michigan Press, 1972

Articles

Lewis BJ. Sensory deprivation in young children. Child Care Health Dev 1978 July/Aug; 4(4):229–238
Lovelace BM. The blind child in the hospital. AORN J 1980 Feb; 31(2):256+

Moses S. What's the score on sport and eye injuries? Can Nurs 1980 Apr; 76(4):43–45

Schrader ES. Perioperative nurses reassure ophthalmologic patients. AORN J 1979 Dec; 30(6):1066–1077

Shurtz A. The pediatric strabismus patient in surgery. AORN J 1979 Oct; 30(4):639–646

Stewart LM and Dawson DF. Blind client—sighted therapist: The interface. J. Psychiat Nurs 1979 Nov; 17(11):31–35

Wiley L (ed). Traumatic blindness—nursing grand rounds. Nursing '79 1979 Jan; 9(1):36–41

EAR

Books

Bakwin H and Bakwin RM. Behavior Disorders in Children, 4th ed. Philadelphia, WB Saunders, 1972

Bess FH (ed). Childhood Deafness: Causation, Assessment and Management. New York, Grune & Stratton, 1977

Articles

Barnes B. Cued speech keeps deaf pupils ahead. Children Today 1978 July/Aug; 7(4):28–30

Bloch J. Impaired children: Helping families through the critical period of first identification. Children Today 1978 Nov/Dec; 7(6):2–6

Bluestone CD. Otitis media: Newer aspects of etiology, pathogenesis, diagnosis and treatment. Consultant 1979 Dec; 19(12):66+

Brenman AK et al. Hearing loss—the invisible handicap. Patient Care 1979 Sept 15; 13(15):124+

Brown MS and Grunfeld C. Otitis media. Issues Compr Pediatr Nurs 1978 Aug; 3(2):35–53

Bruch WN. Otitis media. Pediatric Nursing 1979 Jan/Feb; 5(1):9–12

Dahl MO. Early diagnosis in congenital hearing loss. Can Nurs 1979 Jan; 75(1):17–20

Hirshoren A and Schnittjer CJ. Dimensions of problem behavior in deaf children. J Abnormal Child Psychol 1979 June; 7(2):221–228

Holm CS. Deafness: Common misunderstandings. Am J Nurs 1978 Nov; 78(11):1910–1912

Huber HL. Draining the "fluid ear" with myringotomy and tube insertion. Nursing '78 1978 July; 8(7):28–31

Maloney S. A health care protocol for otitis media. In Brandt PA (ed). Current Practice in Pediatric Nursing. Vol 2, pp. 185–202. St. Louis, CV Mosby, 1978

Simmons FB. Identification of hearing loss in infants and young children. Otolaryngol Clin North Am 1978 Feb; 11(1):19–28

Wong D and Shah CP. Identification of impaired hearing in early childhood. Can Med Assoc J 1979 Sept 8; 121(5): 529–546

CONNECTIVE TISSUE DISEASE IN CHILDREN

47

JUVENILE RHEUMATOID ARTHRITIS

Juvenile rheumatoid arthritis (JRA) is a chronic, generalized, systemic disease that involves a wide spectrum of manifestations, including joint, connective tissue, and visceral lesions throughout the body.

Etiology

The cause of juvenile rheumatoid arthritis is unknown.
a. Infection from an unidentified organism
b. Immune process

Modes of Onset and Clinical Manifestations

A. *Acute Febrile-Systemic (Still's Disease)*
1. Highest incidence of onset is in children under 7 years of age; females are affected more often than males.
2. Initially joint involvement is variable—from no joint pain to generalized florid arthritis.
3. Systemic characteristics:
   a. Irritability, anorexia, and malaise
   b. Intermittent fever—1 or 2 spikes a day over 38.9° C. (102° F.); occurrence of subnormal temperature between elevations; possible seizures
   c. Rash consisting of small, discrete, pink macules with pale centers occurring on trunk and extremities; rash may be transient.
   d. Hepatosplenomegaly
   e. Generalized lymphadenopathy
   f. Anemia
   g. Periorbital edema
   h. Carditis—tachycardia (disproportionate to fever), tachypnea, pericarditis, myocarditis
   i. Pleuritis or pneumonitis independent of carditis

B. *Polyarticular Onset*
1. Highest incidence of onset is in child of 6–12 years; higher incidence in females than males.
2. Characterized by arthritis of more than 4 joints.
   a. Acute onset is manifested by painful swelling of joints.
   b. Insidious onset—minimal or no joint pain; however, child may wince on movement or may limp on walking.
   c. Large joints most often involved are knees, wrists, ankles, and elbows.
   d. Other areas often involved

   (1) Rheumatoid foot—metatarsophalangeal joints swollen and tender; pain in heel.
   (2) Cervical spine—tenderness and restricted movement.
3. Systemic manifestation occurs less frequently than in acute febrile onset; may see low-grade fever and general lymphadenopathy.

C. *Oligoarticular Onset*
1. Highest incidence of onset is in children 1–6 years of age, particularly ages 2–3 years. Females are affected more often than males.
2. Characterized by arthritis of 1, or up to 4 joints.
   a. Child under 5 years may be listless and irritable, have low-grade fever, and fail to grow at normal rate.
   b. Older child does not appear ill.
3. Systemic manifestations are few.
   a. May see rash, low-grade fever, lymphadenopathy, and splenomegaly.
   b. There is increased incidence of iridocyclitis.

Generalized Clinical Manifestations

A. *Joints* (changes may occur with or without systemic symptoms)
1. Symptoms may develop gradually with progressive stiffness, swelling and impaired motion of a joint or joints.
2. Symptoms may develop rapidly with sudden appearance of symptomatic arthritis in one or more joints.
3. Knees, ankles, feet, wrists or fingers are usually involved initially.
4. Joints are swollen and warm.
5. Pain and stiffness of joint may appear before objective changes develop.
6. Limitation of motion of inflamed joints occurs.
7. Characteristic posture is one of guarding joints from movement; an anxious pained expression (with polyarthritis) is common.
8. Morning stiffness of joints following periods of inactivity occurs.
9. Atrophy and weakness of muscles near the affected joints may develop.
10. Skin over inflamed joints may be pigmented.
11. Chronically affected joints may become dislocated, deformed or fused.

12. Subcutaneous nodules may appear over pressure points (knees, elbows, etc.).
13. Condition may ultimately affect any joint in the body (knees, ankles, wrists, feet, fingers, toes, shoulders, elbows, neck, jaw, hips and sacroiliac joints are frequently involved).
14. Small, deformed feet result from foot involvement in early childhood.
15. Micrognathia (unusually small lower jaw), as a result of temporomandibular arthritis, is one hallmark of juvenile rheumatoid arthritis.
16. Spindling or fusiform changes of the fingers may occur.

B. *Inflammation of the eye* (unilateral or bilateral uveitis) Child may have no early symptoms. If symptoms occur late, child may develop irreversible eye damage, including scarring and adhesions of the iris and cataracts.
1. Redness
2. Pain
3. Photophobia
4. Decreased visual acuity
5. Nonreactive pupil

C. *Generalized growth retardation*
1. During periods of remission, growth spurts may occur.
2. Treatment with long-term steroid therapy as well as the disease process may contribute to growth failure.

Altered Physiology

1. In early stages one or many joints show signs of inflammation.
2. The inflammation is initially localized in a joint capsule, primarily in the synovium. The tissue becomes thickened from congestion and edema.
3. A characteristic inflammatory response develops in the form of a synovial proliferation which invades the interior of the joint.
4. The inflammatory tissue extends into the interior of the joint along the surface of the articular cartilage to which it may be adherent, so that it deprives the cartilage of nutrition.
5. By starvation and invasion, this inflammatory tissue slowly destroys the articular cartilage.
6. Synovial tissue eventually frees the joint space leading to narrowing, fibrous ankylosis and bony fusion.
7. Growth centers next to inflamed joints may undergo either premature epiphyseal closure or accelerated epiphyseal growth.
8. Tendons and tendon sheaths may develop inflammatory changes similar to the synovial tissues.
9. Inflammation of muscle may occur.
10. Rheumatoid nodules are uncommon in children.

Diagnostic Evaluation

(of limited value)
1. Elevated sedimentation rate
2. Leukocytosis
3. High total serum proteins
4. Positive creatine protein
5. High frequency of serum antinuclear antibodies with oligoarticular onset
6. Possible alteration in serum proteins (increased alpha and gamma; decreased albumin)
7. Changes in bone, demonstrated by x-rays—initially nonspecific

Treatment

OBJECTIVES: to relieve joint inflammation and pain.
to maintain and increase joint range of motion, muscle strength, and tone.
to preserve total growth and development potential.
to support emotional outlook of patient and his family.

1. Although this is a painful disease of long duration, the outlook for remission is good.
2. There is no specific cure; treatment is supportive:
   a. Drug therapy to reduce inflammation, analgesia
   b. Exercise program to promote joint movement

Complications

1. Bony deformities—crippling from progressive polyarthritis
2. Psychological and social reactions to this chronic illness
3. Iridocyclitis—leading to cataracts, glaucoma, or blindness
4. Pericarditis

Nursing Objectives and Management

A. *To offer the patient and his parents realistic encouragement.*
1. Although the response to medication is slow, the recovery is slow, and episodes of acute illness recur, the long-term outlook is generally good.
2. The child may be hospitalized during an acute attack and systemic illness.

B. *To discuss with the parents and the child what they know about the disease and what they expect from treatment.*
1. Determine what information has been given to them by the physician.
2. The child and his family must understand the disease and treatment. This is a chronic disease and has an unpredictable course; however, compliance with prescribed treatment will minimize crippling from progressive polyarthritis and allow child to grow and develop to his potential.

C. *To be an effective member of the special team caring for this patient and his family.*

The team often includes pediatrician, rheumatologist, social worker, physical therapist, occupational therapist, psychologist/psychiatrist, ophthalmologist, hospital nurse, and community health nurse.

D. *To assist in the program of physical therapy in order to maintain or increase joint range of motion and muscle strength and tone.*
1. The parents and child are instructed in the exercises. Encourage development of program (with parental involvement) while patient remains in the hospital.
2. Night splints for the wrists, knees, hip, and ankle may be prescribed to do the following:
   a. Give rest and relief of pain.
   b. Prevent or correct deformity.
   c. Maintain damaged joint in functional position.
   d. Know proper application of splint and help patient to adjust to it.
3. A hot tub bath prior to the exercises and following long rest periods may make the exercises less painful. Whirlpool treatment will aid in decreasing stiffness.
4. Full range of motion exercises should be performed every day.

Encourage child to do his own exercises as soon as possible.

5. Orthopedic surgery may be required to correct some deformities.

E. *To provide the child with the freedom to engage in as much activity as he is able to tolerate.*

1. Children will limit their own activity.
2. Those activities that produce overtiring or cause joint pain should be avoided.
3. Diversional activities should encourage movement based upon child's tolerance.
4. Encourage the child to be as self-sufficient as possible.
5. Allow the child to make some decisions himself (e.g., when he prefers to do his exercises).
6. Limit the use of wheelchairs. Tricycles and pedal cars provide good modes of mobility and exercise.

F. *To use the principles of proper body mechanics and posture whether the child is at rest or is active.*

1. Provide firm mattress to prevent sagging joints.
2. Use thin pillow (not more than 5 cm. [2 inches] thick) to prevent dowager hump. Do not place pillows under joints.
3. Child may attempt to protect joints by assuming a position of flexion to ease discomfort.

G. *To administer medications which are utilized to treat JRA. Know usage, side effects, and screening tests to be done during therapy.*

1. Salicylates
   a. Anti-inflammatory, analgesic, antipyretic
   b. See "Salicylates and Steroids," under Rheumatic Fever, page 1300, for side effects.
2. Water-soluble gold salts (sodium aurothiomalate)
   a. Used in conjunction with salicylates when improvement is not apparent or progression is not halted after several months.
   b. Side effects include: skin rash, nephritis with hematuria or proteinuria, thrombocytopenia, and neurotoxicity.
   c. Monitor urine for protein.
3. Systemic steroids
   a. Used in addition to salicylates when salicylates alone are not effective. Their use does not prevent complications of severe arthritis or influence ultimate prognosis.
   b. See the reference to salicylates and steroids, under Rheumatic Fever.
   c. Tuberculin test should be done prior to starting steroid therapy.
   d. Monitor for glucosuria.

H. *To educate and motivate parents and child in continuing program of treatment at home.* Help parents to understand the needs of the child.

1. Extra rest—but not bed rest, which will contribute to contractures and muscle atrophy.
2. Program of daily exercise—this can be adjusted to fit in with mother's or family's routine.
3. The child should attend school regularly and participate in regular school activities.
   a. This participation will allow child to obtain social and scholastic achievement.
   b. Teachers should be informed of child's condition and needs.
      (1) Child should get out of seat and walk around room every hour.
      (2) Desk and chair should properly fit child, i.e., when child is sitting with his back in the chair, his feet should be on the floor at right angles to legs; the seat should be deep enough to support thighs without pressure on popliteal arteries.
   c. Recreation is important—swimming is a beneficial sport activity.
4. Compensate for activities of daily living—help child understand he must do as much for himself as possible.
   Adapt items he uses to make their use easier (e.g., lift toilet seat several inches).
5. Provide nutritionally balanced diet to eliminate obesity that puts additional weight on joints.
6. Do not force unnecessary restrictions upon child that can produce acute behavioral upsets and interfere with his social development.
7. This disease affects the whole family. Remind parents to devote time to other members of the family and to their marriage. Various agencies can provide pertinent literature and can direct family to helpful local resources.*
8. The child needs continual follow-up after hospitalization.
   a. Community health nurse can assist in home management of exercise program.
   b. Social worker can assist in helping parents work out their emotions and seek financial assistance.
   c. Ophthalmologist—must examine patient every 3–6 months for occurrence of iridocyclitis. Encourage parents to report any eye symptoms that the child may develop.
   d. The physician must be consulted when any new symptoms occur, in an acute attack, or when progression is apparent, as well as for routine care.

   * Contact The Arthritis Foundation, 3400 Peachtree Road, Atlanta, Ga. 30326.

SYSTEMIC LUPUS ERYTHEMATOSUS

Systemic lupus erythematosus (SLE) is a disease of the connective tissue with vascular and perivascular fibrinoid changes that may involve any organ or system.

Incidence and Etiology

1. Incidence higher in females than in males; most common during childbearing period (15–44 years of age.) However, it can affect children 5–15 years of age.
2. Cause is unknown—believed to be an abnormal response of the body against its own connective tissue. Possible causes of this include the following:
   a. Genetic predisposition
   b. Viral—nonspecific antibody rise as part of general immunologic hyperactivity
3. Possible factors that trigger or unmask initial symptoms:
   a. Exposure to sunlight, snow on bright day
   b. Injury
   c. Stress
   d. X-ray therapy
   e. Vaccination
   f. Antitoxins
   g. Other drugs (e.g., anticonvulsants, antibiotics)

Clinical Manifestations

1. General characteristic signs and symptoms may include
   a. Malar erythema which usually spreads over bridge of nose. (Butterfly rash may consist only of an erythematous blush or scaly erythematous papules; rash may be photosensitive.)
   b. Acute polyarthritis
   c. Fever
   d. Fatigue, malaise
   e. Anorexia, weight loss
   f. Pleurisy
   g. Nephritis—at onset or during course of disease
      (1) Hematuria
      (2) Proteinuria
   h. CNS involvement—during course of disease
      (1) Behavior disturbances
      (2) Convulsions
      (3) Coma
   i. Splenomegaly
   j. Hepatomegaly
   k. Lymphadenopathy
   l. Anemia, thrombocytopenia
   m. Hypoglobulinemia
   n. Raynaud's phenomenon
2. Onset may be gradual, with no specific signs and symptoms
   a. Aching joints
   b. Morning stiffness
   c. Butterfly rash
3. Onset may be abrupt, with the development of any of the following:
   a. High fever
   b. Dyspnea, chest pain
   c. Arthritis without severe deformities
   d. Abdominal pain

Altered Physiology

1. Connective tissue in different organs develops nonspecific aberrations such as fibrinoid change in collagen and cellular infiltration, either in the walls of small blood vessels or elsewhere.
2. Alteration of collagen and subendothelial thickening of small blood vessels obstruct the flow of blood. These changes may be widespread or limited in distribution.

Diagnostic Evaluation

1. Thorough physical examination; patient and family history
2. Primary laboratory studies
   a. Fluorescent antinuclear antibody test (FANA) to detect antibodies that react with nucleus of cells
   b. Lupus erythematosus (L.E.) cell test if FANA is positive
   c. Serum sedimentation rate—elevated
   d. Serum complement studies—lowered
   e. CBC—leukopenia and mild to moderate anemia; can be hemolytic anemia
   f. Serum thrombotic accelerator (STA) (serology)—false-positive
3. Kidney function studies
   a. Urine sediment—shows RBCs and granular casts, increased protein, leukocyturia
   b. Serum creatinine—elevated
   c. Urine protein—elevated
   d. Creatinine clearance

   e. Renal biopsy—to identify type and severity of kidney involvement
4. Presence of 4 or more of criteria for SLE proposed by American Rheumatism Association*
   a. Facial erythema
   b. Discoid lupus erythema (uncommon in children)
   c. Photosensitivity
   d. Oral or nasopharyngeal ulceration
   e. Raynaud's phenomenon
   f. Alopecia—focal or diffuse
   g. Arthritis—without severe deformity
   h. L.E. cells
   i. Chronic false-positive serology—syphilis
   j. Profuse proteinuria
   k. Cellular casts in urine
   l. Pleurisy or pericarditis
   m. Psychosis or convulsions
   n. Hemolytic anemia, leukopenia, or thrombocytopenia

Treatment

1. Control of symptoms with medication
   a. Salicylates—relieve joint symptoms, fever, fatigue
   b. Antimalarials such as hydroxychloroquine sulfate (Plaquenil) to relieve joint symptoms and skin rash
   c. Steroids such as prednisone—used when there is renal or neurologic involvement or hemolytic anemia; TB test should be done prior to starting steroid therapy
   d. Immunosuppressive agents such as azathioprine and cyclophosphamide—used in severe disease, especially with nephritis or steroid-resistant patients
   e. Other—ibuprofen (Motrin)—anti-inflammatory preparation
   f. Topical steroid preparations—may help suppress cutaneous lesions
2. Careful and controlled monitoring of drug therapy and reassessment of clinical and laboratory picture
3. Supportive
   a. Rest
   b. Adequate nutrition
   c. Treatment of existing complications
   d. Early identification and treatment of opportunistic infection

Complications

1. Sepsis—primarily resulting from steroid and immunosuppressive therapy
2. Renal involvement; renal failure
3. Neurologic involvement
4. Allergic reactions to drugs
5. Chronic fatigue

Nursing Objectives and Management

a. *To provide opportunities for the patient and the parents to discuss the disease—their understanding of it, their expectations, and their altered living conditions imposed by the disease.*

1. Determine what information has been given to them by the physician.
2. Provide supportive care to help them work out feelings of fear, anxiety, and uncertainty.

* Cohen, A. S., et al. Preliminary criteria for the classification of systemic lupus erythematosus. Bull. Rheum. Dis., 21:643–648, May 1976.

3. Support them in accepting this condition as a long-term illness, with exacerbations and remissions.
   a. They will need continuing support. Initiate early referral to community health nurse and social worker.
   b. Provide available literature and encourage contact with the nearest chapter of the Lupus Erythematosus Foundation.*

B. *To assist the child in developing a realistic attitude about his illness and to assist him in expressing his feelings about his illness.*

1. Provide the child with the opportunity to openly discuss his feelings about illness when he is able to verbalize these feelings.
2. Provide the child with the opportunity to express his feelings; utilize play as a method.
3. Arrange for a visiting teacher so that the child may have the opportunity to continue his education.
4. Encourage the child to continue contact with his peers (i.e., via telephone, letter writing, etc.).
5. Allow the child to make some decisions and become involved in planning his own care.

C. *To be aware of the action and side effects of medications used in the treatment of systemic lupus erythematosus.*

Steroids and salicylates (see section on juvenile rheumatoid arthritis, p. 1300).

D. *To observe closely for the development of symptoms that may indicate development of complications.*

1. Observe for the development of renal symptoms. There is usually some degree of renal involvement.
   a. Record intake and output.
   b. Record specific gravity of urine.
   c. Observe the color and characteristics of urine, especially proteinuria.
   d. Observe for the development of edema.

2. Observe for the development of sepsis.
3. Report to the physician any abnormal findings.

E. *To inform the parents about requirements for caring for the child at home.*

1. Prevent direct exposure to the sun; if exposure to the sun cannot be avoided, a sunscreen lotion should be used.
   a. Child can go outside in early morning or late afternoon.
   b. Avoid snow on bright days, cement, and white buildings because of photosensitivity.
2. Discuss with parents and be certain they are aware of and understand each of the following:
   a. Side effects of any medications being administered at home and what to do about these reactions
   b. Signs of worsening of the disease
   c. Factors that precipitate flare-up or early warning signs of flare-up: chills, fever, anorexia, fatigue
   d. Problems that may be associated with the adolescent—i.e., body image, relationship with peers
3. Provide measures that will be helpful in preventing infection:
   a. Avoid exposure to individuals with infections.
   b. Practice general measures of personal hygiene.
   c. Provide a well-balanced diet.
4. Continual medical follow-up
   a. Disease progress needs reevaluation.
   b. Drug therapy must be strictly controlled and is based on the condition of the child as well as laboratory studies.
   c. Renal function specifically needs to constantly be evaluated.

* Lupus Foundation of America (First National Bank), 100 Federal Steet, Boston, Mass. 02241.
Lupus Erythematosus Foundation, Inc., 44 E. 23rd Street, New York, New York 10010.

SCHÖNLEIN-HENOCH PURPURA (ANAPHYLACTOID PURPURA)

Schönlein-Henoch purpura is a diffuse vascular disease resulting from inflammatory reaction around capillaries and arterioles involving the skin, intestines, joints and kidneys.

Incidence and Etiology

1. Slightly higher incidence in males than in females. Increased incidence of onset is between ages 3 and 7 years.
2. Possible cause is an allergic reaction to a variety of antigenic stimuli such as infection (e.g., Beta streptococci), allergens, insect bites, food, and drugs.
3. Cause is unknown.
4. Disease is usually self-limited.

Clinical Manifestations

1. Rash—sudden onset may precede or follow other manifestations.
   a. Typical rash begins with itching, urticarial wheals and then proceeds to maculopapular erythematous lesions.
   b. These lesions become less raised and more petechial or purpuric in character and do not fade with pressure.
   c. Several stages of the rash may be present at one time.
   d. Rash appears primarily on buttocks, lower back, extensor aspects of arms and legs, and face.
2. Arthritis of knee and ankle joints develops; the condition is moderately severe, with painful swelling due to periarticular edema. Movement is limited.
3. Local edema—especially of scrotum.
4. Colicky abdominal pain—from submucosal hemorrhage.
5. Nausea and vomiting.
6. Proteinuria
7. Microscopic hematuria.

Diagnostic Evaluation

1. Appearance of rash
2. Blood studies—not diagnostic
   a. Platelet count—normal
   b. Erythrocyte sedimentation rate (ESR)—elevated
   c. Anemia possible
   d. Azotemia (with severe kidney involvement)
   e. pH and prothromboplastin tests
3. Urine studies
   a. Proteinuria
   b. Microscopic hematuria
   c. Casts
4. Stool—shows occult blood

Complications

1. Colicky abdominal pain, related to vasculitis and edema of the bowel; steroids may be used.
2. Intussusception.
3. Acute nephritis or nephrosis that may lead to chronic nephritis (urinalysis should be done 6 and 12 months after episode).

Treatment

Treatment is primarily symptomatic and supportive

1. Encourage bed rest until child is able to ambulate and can do so without increasing edema of feet.
2. Remove allergen if it is known.
3. Give antibiotic therapy if acute episode was preceded by infection, especially streptococcal.
4. Manage complicating abdominal or renal involvement:
   a. Steroids (prednisone) may relieve abdominal symptoms and prevent intussusception.
   b. Immunosuppressive therapy (azathioprine or cyclophosphamide) may be given to stabilize persistent renal involvement.

Nursing Objectives and Management

A. *To offer the patient and his parents realistic encouragement.*

The long-term outlook is good when renal involvement is minimal.

B. *To assist child in expressing his feelings about illness and hospitalization.*

1. Provide the child with an opportunity to openly discuss his feelings about illness and his situation when he is able to verbalize these feelings.

2. Provide child with the opportunity to express his feelings; utilize play as a method.
3. Allow child to make some decisions (appropriate for his age), and to become involved in planning his own care.
4. Consider his age and then allow and encourage parental participation.

C. *To provide physical comfort for the child's painful and swollen joints.*

Salicylates are found not to be particularly effective (see Juvenile Rheumatoid Arthritis, p. 1300).

D. *To observe for developing signs and symptoms of complications.*

1. Renal
   a. Record intake and output.
   b. Record specific gravity of urine.
   c. Observe color and characteristics of urine.
   d. Observe development of or increase in edema.
2. Intussusception—sudden onset
   a. Paroxysmal abdominal pain
   b. Currant jelly-like stools
   c. Vomiting
   d. Increasing absence of stools
   e. Increasing abdominal distention and tenderness

E. *To observe and record child's general condition and the current status of the rash.*

F. *To be aware of the action and side effects of medications used in the treatment of anaphylactoid purpura.*

See Juvenile Rheumatoid Arthritis, page 1378.

G. *To encourage parents to return child for follow-up urinalysis 6 and 12 months following acute episode.*

BIBLIOGRAPHY

Books

Brewer EJ. Juvenile Rheumatoid Arthritis, Vol. VI. Philadelphia, WB Saunders, 1979
Gellis SS and Kagan BM. Current Pediatric Therapy, Vol. 9. Philadelphia, WB Saunders, 1980
Hughes JG. Synopsis of Pediatrics. St. Louis, CV Mosby, 1979
Scipien GM et al. Comprehensive Pediatric Nursing, 2nd ed. New York, McGraw–Hill, 1979
Whaley LF and Wong DL. Nursing Care of Infants and Children. St. Louis, CV Mosby, 1979
Vaughan VC, McKay RJ, Behrman RE. Nelson Textbook of Pediatrics. Philadelphia, WB Saunders, 1979

Articles

Ansell BM. Rehabilitation in juvenile chronic arthritis. Rheumatology and rehabilitation. (Suppl) 1979; 74–76
Cohen AS et al. Preliminary criteria for the classification of systemic lupus erythematosus. Bull Rheum Dis 1971 May; 21:643–648
Fink CW. Predicting the outcome of JRA. Consultant 1979 Oct; 19(10):40+

Hartley B. Systemic lupus: A patient perspective. Can Nurs 1978 Feb; 74(2):16–20
Harwitz S. Signals from the skin. Emergency Med 1979 July 15; 11(7):90–95+
Petty RE. Making the diagnosis of Still's disease. Can Med Assoc J 1979 June 23; 120(12):1480–1481
Sisco D. Systemic lupus erythematosus and resultant renal failure. Nephrology Nurse 1979 July/Aug; 1(4):48–49
White JF. Systemic lupus erythematosus. Nursing '78 1978 Sept; 8(9):26–34
Zurier RB. Systemic lupus erythematosus. Hosp Pract 1979 Aug; 14(8):45–54

Booklets

Dubois, E. Information for patients with Lupus Erythematosus. Bonnie Bernard Denn Chapter, American Lupus Society, 4126 Pacific Coast Hwy., Torrance, CA. 90905
Epstein W and Clewley G. Living with SLE. Millberry Union Bookstore, 500 Parnassas Ave. San Francisco, CA. 94143
Lupus and You: A Guide for Patients. St. Louis Park, Minn. 55416

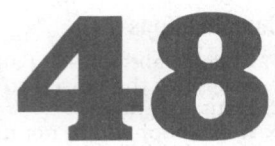
CEREBRAL PALSY

Cerebral palsy is a comprehensive diagnostic term used to designate a group of nonprogressive disorders resulting from malfunction of the motor centers and pathways of the brain. Although there are varying degrees and clinical manifestations of cerebral palsy, it is generally characterized by paralysis, weakness, incoordination and/or ataxia. Cerebral palsy is a major cause of disability among children in the United States.

Etiology

A. *Prenatal Factors*

1. Infection, rubella, toxoplasmosis, herpes simplex, cytomegalic inclusions and other viral or infectious agents
2. Maternal anoxia, anemia, placental infarcts, abruptio placentae
3. Prenatal cerebral hemorrhage, maternal bleeding, maternal toxemia, Rh or ABO incompatibility
4. Prenatal anoxia, twisting or kinking of the cord
5. Miscellaneous—toxins, drugs

B. *Perinatal Factors*

1. Anoxia from any cause
   a. Anesthetic and analgesic drugs administered to the mother may cause anoxia in the infant's brain
   b. Prolonged labor
   c. Placenta previa or abruptio
   d. Respiratory obstruction
2. Cerebral trauma during delivery
3. Complications of birth
   a. "Small for date" babies, prematurity, immaturity, postmaturity
   b. Hyperbilirubinemia
   c. Hemolytic disorders
   d. Respiratory distress
   e. Infections
   f. Hypoglycemia
   g. Hypocalcemia

C. *Postnatal Factors*

1. Head trauma
2. Infections
   a. Meningitis
   b. Encephalitis
   c. Brain abscess
3. Vascular accidents
4. Lead poisoning
5. Anoxia
6. Neoplastic and late neurodevelopmental defects

Clinical Manifestations

A. *Early Signs*—may include one or more of the following:

1. Asymmetry in motion or contour
2. Listlessness or irritability
3. Difficulty in feeding, sucking, or swallowing
4. Excessive or feeble cry
5. Long, thin infants who are slow to gain weight

B. *Later Signs*—may include one or more of the following:

1. Failure to follow normal pattern of motor development
   Delayed gross motor development is a universal manifestation of cerebral palsy.
2. Persistence of infantile reflexes
3. Weakness
4. Apparent preference for one hand before 12–15 months
5. Abnormal postures
6. Delayed or defective speech
7. Evidence of mental retardation

C. *Factors Influencing Symptoms and Degree of Involvement*

(Range—from very mild to severe)
1. Extent and location of cerebral lesion
2. Age at which interruption of brain development occurred
   Intellectual, language, and social skills which were acquired before damage can usually be retained.
3. Status of reflex patterns

D. *Common Associated Findings*

1. Seizures
2. Hearing deficiency
3. Visual defect
4. Perceptual disorders
5. Mental retardation
6. Language disorders

Classification of Cerebral Palsy

A. *Clinical Type*

1. Spasticity—in 50–60% of patients.
   a. Generally appears before 6 months of age.
   b. Motor activity is impaired because of disharmony of muscle movements.
   (1) Arms
      (a) Child often holds his arm pressed against his body with the forearm bent at right angles to the upper arm and the hand bent against the forearm. The fist may be clenched tightly.
      (b) Child with mild involvement may demonstrate an overextended appearance of the fingers and rotation of the wrists when he reaches for things.
   (2) Legs—may be more (usually) or less involved than arms.
      (a) Mild case may only be evident when the child walks, demonstrating wide-based gait (with arms outstretched). The fingers may be alternately clenched and extended.
      (b) Child with moderate involvement may demonstrate slow and labored movements. Walking is jerky and unrhythmic. Balance is poor.
      (c) Child with severe involvement may be unable to sit or walk unsupported.
      (d) When both legs are involved, bilateral contractures may cause "scissoring." (Child crosses his legs and points his toes.)
2. Dyskinesia—in 20–25% of patients.
   a. Characterized by involuntary, extraneous motor activity; accentuated by emotional stress.
   b. Athetosis is the most common manifestation of this group.
   (1) Any or all limbs may be involved.
   (2) Characterized by uncontrollable, jerky, irregular, twisting movements of the extremities, especially the fingers and wrists, except when at rest or asleep.
   (3) If legs are involved, child may walk in a writhing, lurching, stumbling manner with noticeable incoordination of the arms. When calm and well-rested he may walk well.
3. Ataxia—in 1–10% of patients.
   a. Characterized by inability to achieve balance or awkwardness in maintaining it, with associated gross and/or fine motor incoordination.
   b. Gait is often high-stepping, stumbling, or lurching.
   c. Nystagmus is common.
   d. Manifested in varying degrees depending on the pathology.
4. Mixed Types—in 15–40% of patients.
   Consists of various combinations of the above types—most frequently, athetosis combined with spasticity.

B. *Topographical Classification*

1. Hemiplegia—findings are limited to 1 side of the body (35–40% of patients)
2. Diplegia—the legs are involved more than the arms (10–20%); all four extremities involved
3. Paraplegia—the legs only are involved (10–20%)
4. Quadriplegia—all 4 extremities are involved (15–20%); upper and lower limbs equally affected
5. Monoplegia—only 1 limb is involved (rare)
6. Triplegia—3 limbs are involved (rare)

C. *Degree of Severity*

1. Mild—impairment only of fine precision movement.
2. Moderate—gross and fine movements and speech are impaired, but child is able to perform usual activities of living.
3. Severe—inability to perform adequately the usual activities of daily living, i.e., walking, using hands, communicating verbally.

Diagnostic Evaluation

1. History, including prenatal and perinatal factors
2. Neurological examination
3. Laboratory data—pneumoencephalogram is helpful in some instances
4. Psychological testing to determine cognitive functioning
5. Psychosocial assessment, including family adaptation

Prognosis

Factors influencing the prognosis
1. Extent of the manifestations
2. Existence of associated defects, especially mental retardation
3. Ability of the family to cope and to see what is right and normal about their child
4. Type and availability of community resources

Altered Physiology

A. *Spastic Type*

1. Defect in the cortical motor area or pyramidal tract causes abnormally strong tonus of certain muscle groups.
2. Attempt to move a joint causes muscles to contract and block the motion. Permanent contractures develop without muscle training.

B. *Athetotic Type*

Lesions of the extrapyramidal tract and basal ganglia cause involuntary, incoordinated, uncontrollable movements of muscle groups.

C. *Ataxia*

Disturbances of balance result from cerebellar involvement.

Goal and Management

A. *Goal—normalization.* The aim is to help each child reach optimal functional ability in adulthood. Broad aims of therapy include:

1. To gain optimal appearance and integration of motor function.
2. To establish locomotion, communication, and self-help skills.
3. To correct associated defects.
4. To provide opportunities for education appropriate for the individual child's needs and capabilities.

B. *Management*

1. Requires comprehensive evaluation and intervention, including:
   a. General health care.
   b. Correction or alleviation of specific neuromotor deficits and/or associated disabilities.
   c. Developmental enrichment experiences.
   d. Development of prevocational, vocational, and socialization skills.
   e. Emotional, behavioral, and social adjustments.
2. Requires coordination and integration of the con-

tributions of numerous health care professionals as well as societal institutions.
3. The ability of the family to carry out both supportive and participant roles in rehabilitation is a key determinant of the success of any comprehensive management program.

Nursing Management

Like other children, the child with cerebral palsy receives the bulk of his care at home and within his community. The nursing role is no longer confined to care within the hospital setting. Within the expanded role, nurses are involved in working with the family on household routine, integrating the child into the family unit, and helping to "mainstream" the child into regular schools, recreational activities, dating situations, etc.

However, the child with cerebral palsy may experience several hospitalizations for diagnostic evaluation, orthopedic management, and/or medical care. The nurse should consider the following guidelines when caring for the hospitalized child with cerebral palsy.

Nursing Objectives

A. *To assist parents with initial coping and with long-range adaptation to the child's disability.*

1. Encourage the parents to express their feelings about the child and his diagnosis and help them to deal with these feelings.
2. Introduce the concept that the child's potential in large part reflects the quality of parental adaptation.
3. Assist parents to appraise the child's assets so that they may capitalize on these positive features.
   a. Early recognition of the extent of the child's handicap and realistic direction for obtainable goals are essential.
   b. Help parents to recognize immediate needs and identify short-term goals which can be integrated into the long-range plan.
4. Encourage the parents to care for the child during his hospitalization so that they will feel secure about meeting his daily physical needs (feeding, exercise, braces, etc.).
   Refer to section on Family Centered Care, page 1131.
5. Introduce parents to members of the health team who will be involved with the child's care and management.
6. Begin parental teaching about the disability.
   a. Provide parents with appropriate reading material. Encourage their questions and provide them with the information they need.
   b. Refer to Parental Education, which follows this section on nursing objectives.
7. Assist parents in interpreting the child's diagnosis and needs to other family members, teachers, and friends.
8. Initiate appropriate referrals.
   a. Community agencies for disabled children
   b. Community health nurse
   c. Day-care centers
   d. Clinics
   e. Local branch of the United Cerebral Palsy Association
   f. Parent groups

B. *To promote the attainment of developmental milestones as much as possible.*

1. Evaluate the child's developmental level and then assist him to build one skill upon another. (Refer to sections on Growth and Development and the Hospitalized Child, p. 1127.)
2. Provide for continuity of care from home to hospital.
   a. Obtain a thorough history from the mother regarding the child's usual home routines, and use this in planning the child's care during hospitalization.
      (1) Feeding
      (2) Sleeping
      (3) Physical therapy
      (4) Stage of growth and development
      (5) Play
      (6) Special interests, security objects, etc.
   b. Ask the parents to bring to the hospital any special devices or equipment which the child uses in his daily activities.
   c. Encourage the child's parents to participate in the child's care if they so desire and if it is medically feasible. (Refer to section on Family Centered Care, p. 1131.)
3. Be alert for associated defects which could be corrected.
   a. Hearing
   b. Speech
   c. Vision
      (1) Squinting
      (2) Failure to follow objects
      (3) Bringing objects very close to the face

C. *To provide emotional support to parents.*

1. Acknowledge the numerous challenges of daily management and the changes in family life associated with caring for a child with cerebral palsy.
2. Allow the parent(s) to express frustrations they may feel because of the many demands placed on them, with few rewards.
3. Acknowledge parents' feelings of frustration and anger as legitimate and understandable.
4. Provide positive feedback for effective parenting skills and positive approaches to caring for the child.
5. Assist parents to deal with siblings' responses to the disabled child.
6. Assist parents to secure respite from the day-to-day care of the child, as appropriate.

D. *To provide for the child's physical care needs.*

1. Safety
   a. Evaluate the child's need for specific safety measures (suction machine, helmet, seizure precautions, etc.), and modify the environment as appropriate to ensure the child's safety.
   b. Select toys that are safe.
2. Nutrition
   a. Maintain a pleasant environment, free from distractions.
      (1) Provide a comfortable chair.
      (2) Serve the child alone, initially. After he begins to master the task of eating, he may enjoy eating with other children.
      (3) Do not attempt feedings if the child is very fatigued.
   b. Encourage independence, but do not force the child.
      (1) Find the eating position in which the child can do the most for himself.
      (2) Allow the child to hold the spoon even if he has to be fed with another one.

(3) Stand behind the child and reach over his shoulder to guide the spoon from the plate to his mouth.

(4) Serve foods that stick to the spoon, like thick applesauce, mashed potato, etc.

(5) Encourage finger foods that the child can handle alone.

(6) Provide appropriate special equipment for the child to use in feeding himself.

    (a) Spoon and fork with special handles

    (b) Plate and glass holders, etc.

    (c) Feeding chair

(7) Disregard "messy" eating:

    (a) Place newspapers around the feeding chair.

    (b) Use a large plastic bib or towel to protect the child's clothes.

  c. If the child must be fed, do so slowly and carefully. The child may have difficulty sucking and swallowing because he cannot control the muscles of his throat.

(1) Offer foods which the child likes.

(2) Cut solid foods into small pieces.

(3) Place the food back on the tongue for ease in swallowing.

3. Exercise

a. Carry out appropriate exercises under the direction of the physical therapist.

b. Use appropriate appliances to facilitate muscle control and improve body functioning.

(1) Splints

(2) Casts

(3) Braces

c. Encourage active motions that are functionally useful.

d. Use play (games, peg boards, puzzles, etc.) as techniques to improve coordination.

e. Maintain good body alignment to prevent contractures.

4. Rest

a. Avoid exciting events before rest or bedtime.

b. Administer tranquilizing agents or anticonvulsants, etc., as prescribed by the physician.

c. Avoid stress and frustration during the child's program of physical therapy.

E. *To ensure continuity of care.*

1. Communicate with representatives of all of the disciplines involved with the child's management.

2. Communicate with community agencies already involved with the child and his family (school, cerebral palsy center, community health nursing agency, etc.).

3. Formulate a consistent nursing care plan which is well coordinated with the plans and goals of related disciplines and meets the needs of the *entire* child and his family.

4. On discharge, send a report of the child's hospitalization, including a summary of nursing problems, to the appropriate community agencies.

Parental Education

1. Instruct parent in all areas of the child's physical care.

2. Reinforce teaching done by physical therapists. Assist parents to integrate therapy into play activities.

3. Assist parents to modify equipment and activities to facilitate home care.

4. Provide practical suggestions for feeding, holding, bathing, infant stimulation, etc.

5. The child needs regular medical and dental evaluations.

a. It is important for the child to receive his childhood immunizations.

b. He should be taken to the dentist every 6 months starting at the age of 2 years.

c. He may require some adaptations of his toothbrush in order to use it effectively.

(1) The handle can be built up with sponge or a more sophisticated enlarging device.

(2) Brushes with specially bent handles are available.

6. The child needs discipline in order to feel secure and relaxed.

a. He should have realistic limits set, within which he can function successfully.

b. Parents should be firm but not rejecting.

7. References for Parents:

Brightman A. Hollis. New York, Scholastic Book Services, 1978

Napear P. Brain Child, A Mother's Diary. New York, Harper & Row, 1974

Trevarton J. Amy Maura. Syracuse, Human Policy Press, 1975

United Cerebral Palsy Association, 66 E 34th Street, New York, N.Y. 10016

HYDROCEPHALUS

Hydrocephalus is a condition of imbalance between the production of cerebrospinal fluid and its absorption over the surface of the brain into the circulatory system. It is characterized by an abnormal increase in cerebrospinal fluid volume within the intracranial cavity and by enlargement of the child's head.

Etiology and Incidence

1. Obstruction in the system between the source of cerebrospinal fluid production and the area of its reabsorption (the obstruction may be partial, intermittent or complete)

a. The majority of cases are of this type.

b. Causes:

(1) Congenital—etiology largely unknown

(2) Acquired

    (a) Meningitis

    (b) Trauma

    (c) Spontaneous intracranial bleeding

    (d) Neoplasms

2. Failure in the absorption system—cause unknown

3. Excessive production of cerebrospinal fluid—cause unknown (rare)

4. Approximately 3–4 cases per 1000 births, including those associated with spina bifida

Types of Hydrocephalus

A. *Noncommunicating Hydrocephalus*

An obstruction is located within or at the outlets of

the ventricular system, preventing any or all of the cerebrospinal fluid from leaving the ventricles and entering the subarachnoid space.

B. *Communicating Hydrocephalus*
1. There is free communication between the ventricles and the subarachnoid space.
2. Abnormal reabsorption of the cerebrospinal fluid in the subarachnoid space occurs.
3. This is the most common form of hydrocephalus.

Altered Physiology
1. The ventricular system is greatly distended.
2. The increased ventricular pressure results in thinning of the cerebral cortex and cranial bones, especially in the frontal, parietal and temporal areas.
3. The floor of the third ventricle commonly bulges downward, compresses the optic nerves, dilates the sella turcica, and often compresses the hypophysis cerebri.
4. The basal ganglia, brain stem, and cerebellum remain relatively normal but compressed.
5. The choroid plexus is usually atrophied to some degree.

Clinical Manifestations
1. May be rapid, or slow and steadily advancing, or remittent.
2. Clinical signs depend on the age of the child, whether or not the anterior fontanelle has closed, whether the cranial sutures have fused, and the type and duration of hydrocephalus.
   a. Infants
      (1) Excessive head growth (may be seen up to 3 years of age)
      (2) Delayed closure of the anterior fontanelle
         Fontanelle may become tense and elevated above the surface of the skull.
      (3) Signs of increased intracranial pressure include:
         (a) Vomiting
         (b) Restlessness and irritability
         (c) High-pitched, shrill cry
         (d) Alteration in vital signs
            Increased systolic blood pressure
            Decreased pulse
            Decreased and irregular respirations
         (e) Pupillary changes
         (f) Seizures (possible)
         (g) Lethargy
         (h) Stupor
         (i) Coma
      (4) Alteration of muscle tone of the extremities
      (5) Later physical signs
         (a) Forehead becomes prominent.
         (b) Scalp appears shiny with prominent scalp veins.
         (c) Eyebrows and eyelids may be drawn upward, exposing the sclera above the iris.
         (d) Infant cannot gaze upward, causing "sunset eyes."
         (e) Strabismus, nystagmus, and optic atrophy may occur.
         (f) Infant has difficulty in holding head up.
         (g) Child may experience physical and/or mental developmental lag.
   b. Older children who have closed sutures
      (1) Signs of increased intracranial pressure include:

         (a) Headache
         (b) Vomiting
         (c) Lethargy, fatigue, apathy
         (d) Personality changes
         (e) Separation of cranial sutures (may be seen in children up to 10 years of age)
         (f) Double vision, constricted peripheral vision, sudden appearance of internal strabismus, pupillary changes
         (g) Alteration in vital signs similar to those seen in infants
         (h) Difficulty with gait
         (i) Stupor
         (j) Coma

Diagnostic Evaluation
1. Transillumination of the infant's head may show varying degrees of localized glowing indicative of abnormal fluid collection.
2. Percussion of the infant's skull may produce a typical "cracked pot" sound (Macewen's sign).
3. Ophthalmoscopy may reveal papilledema.
4. C.A.T. scan (computerized axial tomography) provides a noninvasive means of diagnosing some types of hydrocephalus by computer analysis of x-ray transmission data.
5. Ventriculography (introduction of air or other contrast media into the lateral ventricles):
   Abnormalities are visualized in the ventricular system or the subarachnoid space
6. Pneumoencephalography (introduction of air into the lumbar subarachnoid space) may show the following:
   a. Dilated ventricles
   b. Extent of the brain damage and the location of the obstruction
7. Radiologic findings show the following:
   a. Widening of the fontanelle and sutures
   b. Erosion of intracranial bone

Prognosis
1. Prognosis is dependent on early diagnosis and prompt therapy.
2. The outcome of treatment depends on the time it is begun, the success of the surgical procedure, good follow-up care, and the child's innate motor and intellectual capabilities.
   a. With improved diagnostic and management techniques, the prognosis is becoming considerably better. Many children experience normal motor and intellectual development.
   b. The severity of neurologic deficits is directly proportional to the interval between onset and the time of diagnosis.
3. Spontaneous arrest sometimes occurs as a result of natural compensatory mechanisms or rupture of the ventricle into the subarachnoid space.
4. A child with postmeningitic hydrocephalus might also undergo spontaneous remission following gradual disappearance of adhesions.
5. Approximately two-third of patients will die at an early age if they are not given surgical treatment.

Surgical Treatment
A. *General Techniques*
1. Direct operation on the lesion causing the obstruction (rarely feasible).

2. Intracranial shunts—useful in selected cases of non-communicating hydrocephalus to divert fluid from the obstructed segment of the ventricular system to the subarachnoid space beyond the block.
3. Extracranial shunts—divert fluid from the ventricular system to an extracranial compartment, frequently the peritoneum or right atrium. Preferred method for treating most cases of communicating hydrocephalus and cases of noncommunicating hydrocephalus not amenable to direct surgery or intracranial shunts.

B. *Common Extracranial Shunt Procedures*

1. Ventriculoperitoneal shunt (V–P Shunt)
   a. Diverts cerebrospinal fluid from a lateral ventricle or the spinal subarachnoid space to the peritoneal cavity.
   b. A tube is passed from the lateral ventricle through an occipital burr hole subcutaneously through the posterior aspect of neck and paraspinal region to the peritoneal cavity through a small incision in the right lower quadrant.
2. Ventriculoatrial shunt (V–A Shunt)
   a. A tube is passed from the dilated lateral ventricle through a burr hole in the parietal region of the skull.
   b. It is then passed under the skin behind the ear and into a vein down to a point where it discharges into the right atrium or superior vena cava.
   c. The tube passes at one point through a one-way pressure sensitive system.
   d. The valve or valves close to prevent reflux of blood into the ventricle and open as ventricular pressure rises, allowing fluid to pass from the ventricle into the bloodstream.
3. *Complications*
   a. Need for shunt revision frequently occurs because of occlusion, infection, or malfunction.
   b. Shunt revision may be necessary because of growth of the child. Newer models, however, include coiled tubing to allow the shunt to grow with the child.
   c. Shunt dependency frequently occurs. The child rapidly manifests symptoms of increased intracranial pressure if the shunt does not function properly.
   d. Children with ventriculoatrial shunts may experience thromboembolism leading to cor pulmonale.
   e. Late complications occur with discouraging frequency the longer an operative series is followed.

Preoperative Nursing Objectives

A. *To observe for and record disease progress.*

1. Measure head.
   a. Measure at the occipitofrontal circumference (OFC)—point of largest measurement).
   b. Measure the head at approximately the same time each day.
   c. Use a centimeter measure for greatest accuracy.
2. Observe for evidence of increased intracranial pressure. Note especially:
   a. Vomiting
   b. Changes in vital signs
      (1) Increased systolic blood pressure
      (2) Decreased pulse
      (3) Decreased or irregular respirations
   c. Pupillary changes

d. Change in level of consciousness
3. Note especially these changes in appearance:
   a. Increased head size, prominent forehead (noticeable over days or weeks)
   b. "Sunset" eyes
   c. Opisthotonic positioning—occurs with brain stem herniation.

B. *To provide adequate nutrition.*

1. Feeding is often a problem because the child may be listless, anorectic, and prone to vomiting.
2. Complete nursing care and treatments before feeding so that the child will not be disturbed after feeding.
3. Hold the infant in a semisitting position with head well supported during feeding. Allow ample time for bubbling.
4. Offer small, frequent feedings.
5. Place the child on his side with his head elevated after feeding to prevent aspiration.

C. *To assist with diagnostic procedures.*

1. Be familiar with the procedure which is being performed. (See diagnostic tests.)
2. Explain the procedure to the child and his parents at their levels of comprehension.
   a. Make certain that they understand what will happen before and after as well as during the procedure.
   b. Play is frequently helpful for explaining the procedure to a young child.
3. Administer prescribed sedatives.
   a. Give the sedative exactly at the prescribed time to ensure its effectiveness.
   b. Organize activities so that the child is permitted to rest after administration of the medications.

NURSING ALERT: Sedatives are contraindicated in many cases because of increased intracranial pressure. If administered, the child should be observed very closely for evidence of respiratory depression.

4. Apply protective measures to limit motion as necessary. (See section on pediatric procedures: restraints, p. 1154, and positioning for a lumbar puncture, p. 1179.)
5. Observe the child closely following the procedure for:
   a. Leaking of cerebrospinal fluid from the sites of subdural or ventricular taps
      These tap holes should be covered with a small piece of gauze or cotton saturated with collodion.
   b. Reactions to the sedative, especially respiratory depression
   c. Changes in vital signs indicative of shock
   d. Signs of increased intracranial pressure which may occur if air has been injected into the ventricles.

D. *To provide supportive nursing care as indicated by the child's condition.* (Without treatment, the child becomes more helpless as head size increases.)

1. Prevent pressure sores and the development of contractures.
   a. Place the child on a sponge rubber or lamb's wool pad or an alternating-pressure mattress to keep his weight evenly distributed.

b. Keep the scalp clean and dry.

c. Turn the child's head frequently; change his position every 2 hours.

   (1) When turning the child, rotate his head and body together to prevent strain on the neck.

   (2) A firm pillow may be placed under the head and shoulders for further support when lifting the child.

d. Provide meticulous skin care to all parts of the body.

   (1) Observe the skin for evidence of pressure sores.

   (2) Pressure sores on the head are a frequent problem.

e. Give passive range of motion exercises to the extremities, especially the legs.

2. Keep the eyes moistened if the child is unable to close his eyelids normally.

   This prevents corneal ulcerations and infections.

3. Provide for the child's emotional needs of love and affection.

a. Hold and cuddle the infant as much as possible.

b. Play with the child according to his mental development.

E. *To provide emotional support to the parents.*

1. Encourage parents to visit and to participate in the child's care as much as possible.

2. Encourage the parents to talk about the child's problem and how they feel about it. Parents are generally fearful of any procedure involving the brain, and may have fears about mental retardation or brain damage.

3. Provide parents with appropriate information concerning the defect. Answer their questions directly and honestly. Correct any misconceptions that they may have such as fear that the child's head may burst.

Postoperative Nursing Objectives

A. *To provide immediate, supportive nursing care.*

1. Monitor the child's temperature, pulse, respiration, blood pressure, and pupillary size and reaction every 15 minutes until fully reactive; then monitor every 1 to 2 hours.

2. Avoid hypothermia or hyperthermia.

a. Provide appropriate blankets or covers as indicated by body temperature.

b. An Isolette or warming cradle may be used for an infant.

c. An older child may profit from use of the hypothermia blanket.

d. Administer a tepid sponge bath or antipyretic medication for temperature elevation. (Refer to section on fever, p. 1149.)

3. Aspirate mucus from the nose and throat as necessary to prevent respiratory difficulty.

4. Turn the child every 2 hours.

5. Use a nasogastric tube if necessary for abdominal distention.

a. This is most frequently used when a ventriculoperitoneal shunt has been performed.

b. Measure the drainage and record the amount and color.

6. Give frequent mouth care to prevent dryness of the mucous membranes.

7. Observe for pallor or mottled condition of the skin, coldness, or clamminess of the body and decreased level of consciousness.

8. Administer prescribed prophylactic antibiotics.

B. *To allow for optimal draining of cerebrospinal fluid through the shunt.*

1. Pump the shunt and position the child as directed by the physician.

a. If pumping is prescribed, carefully compress the valve the specified number of times at regularly scheduled intervals.

b. Report any difficulties in pumping the shunt to the physician.

C. *To prevent the development of pressure sores on the skin overlying the shunt reservoir.*

1. Place cotton behind and over the ears under the head dressing.

2. Avoid positioning the child on the area of the valve or the incision until the wound is well healed.

D. *To maintain fluid and electrolyte balance.*

1. Accurately measure and record total fluid intake and output.

   An external collecting device rather than an indwelling catheter should be used to measure urine output whenever possible as this reduces the danger of an infection ascending from the bladder to the spinal canal. (See procedure for urine collection, p. 1166.)

   Elevate the head of the bed slightly, if the infant's condition permits, to prevent backflow of urine.

2. Administer intravenous fluids as prescribed. (See procedure, p. 1171.)

3. Begin oral feedings once the child is fully recovered from the anesthetic and displays interest.

a. Begin with small amounts of 5% dextrose and water.

b. Gradually introduce formula.

c. Introduce solid foods suitable to the child's age and tolerance. (Refer to section on nutrition, p. 1112.)

d. Encourage a high protein diet.

E. *To observe for signs of complications.*

1. Increased intracranial pressure indicates shunt malfunction. (Refer to listing of symptoms under clinical manifestations.)

2. Dehydration may be manifested in the following ways:

a. Sunken fontanelle (Without additional signs of dehydration, this may only indicate a successful shunt.)

b. Decreased urine output, increased specific gravity

c. Diminished skin turgor and dryness of mucous membranes

d. Lethargy

3. Infection may be manifested by:

a. Fever (Temperature normally fluctuates during the first 24 hours after surgery.)

b. Purulent drainage from the incision

c. Swelling, redness, and tenderness along the shunt tract

F. *To provide continued emotional support to the parents.*

1. Begin discharge planning early. (See Parental Education.)

2. Accompany all instructions with reassurance neces-

sary to prevent the parents from becoming anxious or fearful about assuming the care of the child.

Relay the success that other mothers have had in dealing with similar infants.

3. Encourage the parents to treat the child as normally as possible, providing him with appropriate toys and love.
4. Help the parents with problems of assisting siblings and grandparents to deal with the child's needs.
5. Initiate appropriate referrals.
   a. Social worker
   b. Community health nurse
   c. Parent groups
   d. Community agencies
   e. Specialty clinics and schools

Parental Education

1. Parents should be given complete explanations of the disease, the surgery, the changes that the surgery may produce, and the follow-up care that will be required.
2. Physical nursing care
   a. Special attention should be directed toward specific techniques of supportive nursing care, for example:
   (1) Turning
   (2) Skin care

(3) Play
(4) Exercises to strengthen the child's muscles.
   b. Feeding techniques and patterns
   c. Pumping of shunt

3. Symptoms of increased intracranial pressure, shunt malfunction, infection, and dehydration must be treated.

Parents should be taught not only to recognize these complications (refer to prior listing of signs of complications) but also to report them immediately to the physician.

4. Illnesses which cause vomiting and diarrhea or which prevent an adequate fluid intake are a great threat to the child who has had a shunt procedure. The parents should be instructed regarding:
   a. Prevention of such illnesses
   b. Early recognition of warning symptoms
   c. Necessity of seeking immediate medical care so that the child can receive intravenous therapy to replace fluid and electrolyte loss
5. The child's emotional needs should be stressed. Parents should be encouraged to treat the child as normally as possible. Generally, few restrictions need to be placed on his daily activities.
6. If appropriate, refer to section on mental retardation for additional areas of parent teaching. See page 1437.

SPINA BIFIDA

Spina bifida refers to a malformation of the spine in which the posterior portion of the laminae of the vertebrae fails to close. Several types of spina bifida are recognized of which the following 3 are most common (Fig. 48–1):
1. *Spina bifida occulta,* in which the defect is only in the vertebrae. The spinal cord and meninges are normal.
2. *Meningocele,* in which the meninges protrude through the opening in the spinal canal, forming a cyst filled with cerebrospinal fluid and covered with skin.
3. *Meningomyelocele* (or myelomeningocele), in which both the spinal cord and cord membranes protrude through the defect in the laminae of the spinal canal. Meningomyeloceles are covered by a thin membrane.

Etiology

1. Unknown but generally thought to result from genetic predisposition triggered by something in the environment.
2. Involves an arrest in the orderly formation of the vertebral arches and spinal cord that occurs between the 4th and 6th week of embryogenesis.

Theories of causation:
   (1) There is incomplete closure of the neural tube during the 4th week of embryonic life.
   (2) The neural tube forms adequately but then ruptures.

Incidence

1. Geographical distribution and incidence vary widely.
2. Condition occurs in approximately 1 per 1000 live births in the U.S.
3. Most common developmental defect of the central nervous system.
4. More common in Caucasians than in nonwhite population.

5. Condition may have other congenital anomalies associated with it.
6. Women who have had surgery for spina bifida in infancy have a 3–5% risk of having children with a neural tube defect.
7. The recurrence risks for parents who have had 1 or 2 affected children are about 5% and 10–12%, respectively.

Altered Physiology and Clinical Manifestations

A. *Spina Bifida Occulta*

1. Most common type; may occur in as many as 25% of otherwise normal children.
2. The bony defect may range from a very thin slit separating one lamina from the spinous process to a complete absence of the spines and laminae.
3. A thin fibrous membrane sometimes covers the defect.
4. The spinal cord and its meninges may be connected with a fistulous tract extending to and opening onto the surface of the skin.
5. Most patients have no symptoms.
   a. They may have a dimple in the skin or a growth of hair over the malformed vertebra.
   b. There is no externally visible sac.

B. *Meningocele*

1. An external cystic defect can be seen in the spinal cord, usually in the center line.
   a. The sac is composed only of meninges and filled with cerebrospinal fluid.
   b. The cord and nerve roots are usually normal.
2. The defect may occur anywhere on the cord. Higher defects (from thorax and up) are usually meningoceles.

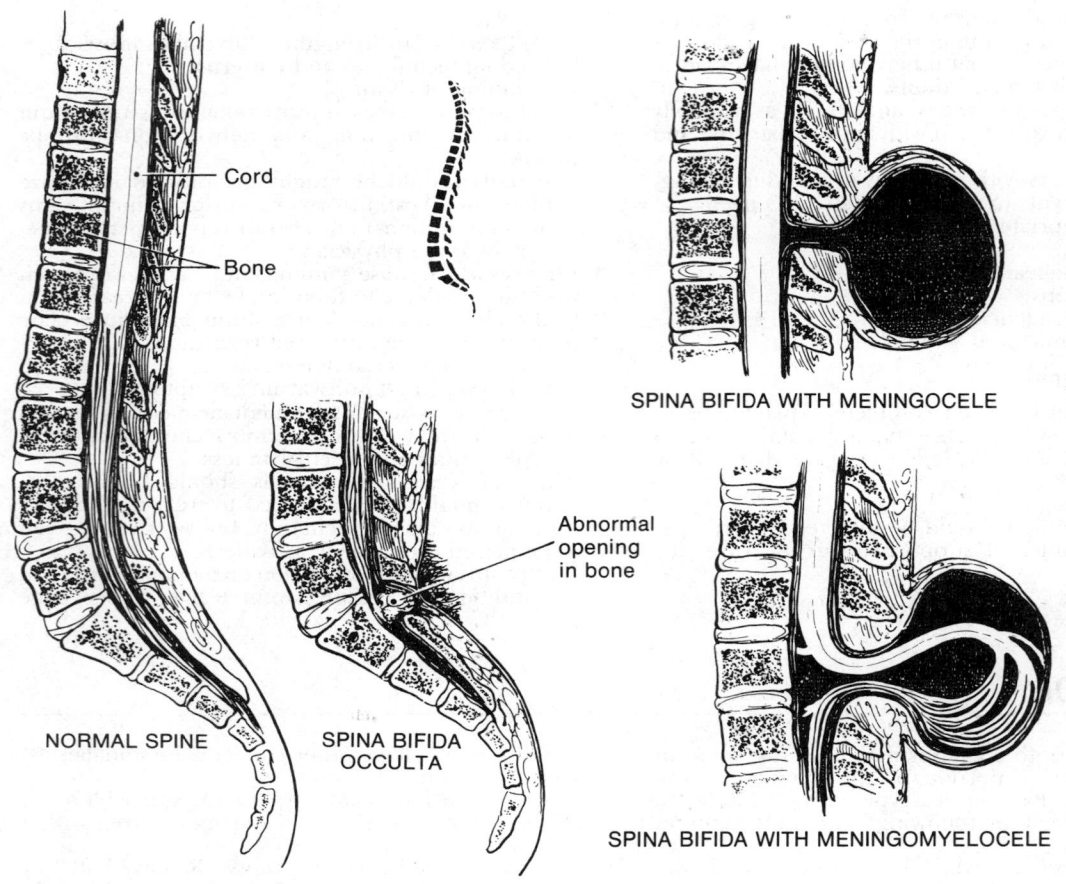

FIGURE 48-1. *Spina bifida. (From Spina Bifida: Hope Through Research. PHS Pub. No. 1023, Health Information Series No. 103, 1970.)*

3. There is seldom evidence of weakness of the legs or lack of sphincter control.
4. Surgical correction is necessary to prevent rupture of the sac and subsequent infection.
5. Hydrocephalus may be an associated finding and may be aggravated after surgery for a meningocele.
   a. Occurs in about 9% of patients.
   b. Usually not associated with the Arnold-Chiari malformation.
6. Prognosis is good with surgical correction.

C. *Meningomyelocele* (Myelomeningocele)

1. Most common type of open spinal defect.
   Occurs 4–5 times more frequently than meningocele.
2. A round, raised, and poorly epithelialized area may be noted at any level of the spinal column. However, the highest incidence of the lesion occurs in the lumbosacral area.
3. The lesion contains both the spinal cord and cord membranes. A bluish area may be evident on the top because of exposed neural tissue.
4. The sac may leak in utero or may rupture after birth, allowing free drainage of cerebrospinal fluid. This renders the child highly susceptible to meningitis.
5. Prognosis

   a. Influenced by the site of the lesion and the presence and degree of associated hydrocephalus. Generally, the higher the defect, the greater the extent of neurological deficit and the greater the likelihood of hydrocephalus.
   b. In the absence of treatment, most infants with meningomyelocele die early in infancy.
   c. Surgical intervention is most effective if it is done early in the neonatal period, preferably within the first few hours of life.
   d. Even with surgical intervention, infants can be expected to manifest associated neurosurgical, orthopedic, and/or urologic problems.
   e. New techniques of treatment, intensive research, and improved services have increased life expectancy and have greatly enhanced the quality of life for most children who receive treatment for the defect.

Common Clinical Problems Associated with Meningomyelocele

A. *Neurologic Problems*

1. Arnold-Chiari malformation
   a. Associated malformation involving the brain stem and cerebellum.
   b. Causes a block in the flow of cerebrospinal fluid

through the ventricles and leads to failure in the reabsorption mechanism of cerebrospinal fluid.

   c. Produces significant hydrocephalus in approximately two-thirds of children with meningomyelocele.

2. Loss of motor control and sensation below the level of the lesion

These conditions are highly variable and depend on the size of the lesion and its position on the cord. For example:

   (1) A low thoracic lesion may cause total flaccid paralysis below the waist.

   (2) A small sacral lesion may cause only patchy spots of decreased sensation in the feet.

B. Mobility and Orthopedic Problems

1. Contractures may occur in the ankles, knees, and/or hips. Hips may be pulled out of the sockets.
   a. Nature and degree of involvement depends on size and location of lesion.
   b. Occurs because some threads of innervation do get through. One side of a hip, knee, or ankle may be innervated and the opposing side may not be. The unopposed side then becomes pulled out of position.
2. Clubfeet are a common accompanying anomaly.
   This anomaly is thought to be related to the position of paraplegic feet in uterus.
3. Scoliosis is common in later years.
   a. Occurs in approximately 50% of patients.
   b. Caused by the congenital lesion in the spinal column.
4. Ambulation and ability to be upright are possible through various types of bracing and equipment.
   Extent of bracing will depend on extent of sensory and motor loss. Children with low sacral lesions can ambulate with small, short, leg braces. Older children with significant loss may choose to use a wheelchair.

C. Urologic Problems

1. Almost all lesions affect the sacral nerves which innervate the bladder. The bladder fails to respond to normal messages that it is time to void, and simply fills and overflows. Usually the bladder does not empty completely, causing two sets of problems:
   a. Susceptibility to urinary tract infections because of constant stasis.
   b. Incontinence, because the bladder is never completely empty and fails to receive signals to void.
2. Management
   a. Children must be followed routinely with IVP, voiding cystoureterogram, urine culture and sensitivity. BUN and creatinine levels must be measured to assess renal status.
   b. Urinary diversions (ileal loop) have been done in the past for infection and continence management.
      (1) Some boys wear external penile devices.
      (2) The newest technique of management is clean, intermittent self-catheterization which has been very effective. Children can generally be taught to catheterize themselves by the age of 6–7 years. Parents can catheterize younger children.
      (3) Research is currently being done to develop mechanical sphincters and electrical bladder-stimulating pacemakers.
   c. Medications
      (1) Antibiotics such as nitrofurantoin (Furadantin,

Macrodantin), Septra, ampicillin, and sulfisoxazole (Gantrisin) are used periodically or prophylactically to prevent urinary tract infections.
      (2) Medications such as imipramine hydrochloride (Tofranil) and ephedrine sulfate are used to help children retain their urine until it can be voided at one time (rather than to dribble continuously). When self-catheterization is used in conjunction with medication, many children can stay dry for 3–4 hours at a time.
   d. Dietary recommendations
      (1) Adequate fluid intake is essential to maintain good urinary flow.
      (2) Foods such as cranberry juice, or medications such as vitamin C are often prescribed to acidify the urine thus preventing stone formation.
   e. The ability to stay dry for reasonable time intervals is one of the greatest factors in enhancing self-esteem and positive body image.

D. Bowel Problems

1. Fecal incontinence and constipation are promoted by poor innervation of the anal sphincter and bowel musculature.
2. To compensate for decreased sensation, children are placed on a toileting schedule and are taught to push. Medications such as stool softeners or suppositories may be utilized to help determine scheduling.
3. Remaining unconstipated is essential to any type of fecal control. High-bulk, high-roughage and/or high-fluid diets as well as medications may be used to increase bulk or soften stool.

E. Skin Problems

1. Areas of decreased sensation have a tendency to break down. Braces and shoes should be checked frequently for rubbing.
2. During hospitalization, the nurse should be particularly watchful for areas of skin breakdown. The use of air mattresses, lamb's wool, and other similar materials may help to prevent skin breakdown in bedridden children.

F. Dietary Problems

1. Many children become overweight because of activity limitations.
2. Dietary control is necessary to prevent obesity.

G. Developmental Problems

1. Most children have average intellectual ability despite hydrocephalus.
   a. There may be an organic origin of the higher incidence of learning disabilities.
   b. Most children are able to learn in a "mainstreamed" normal school, provided they are able to overcome other barriers (architectural and attitudinal).
2. The most significant problems are secondarily handicapping conditions which develop when a child has a disability of this degree.
3. Disabled children need exposure to all activities and to rules and regulations of the nondisabled.

Prevention and Treatment of Meningomyelocele

A. Prenatal Detection

Prenatal detection is now possible through amniocentesis and measurement of alphafetoprotein. This testing should be offered to all women at risk (women who are affected themselves or have had other affected children).

B. *Surgical Intervention*

1. Procedure
Laminectomy and closure of the open lesion and/or removal of the sac can usually be done soon after birth.
2. Purpose
   a. To prevent further deterioration of neural function
   b. To minimize the danger of rupture and infection, especially meningitis
   c. To improve cosmetic effect
   d. To facilitate handling of the infant by parents and nurses

C. *Multidisciplinary Follow-up for Associated Problems*

1. A coordinated team approach will help maximize the physical and mental potential of each affected child.
   a. A group of health care personnel (including a neurologist, neurosurgeon, orthopedic surgeon, urologist, pediatrician, nurse, social worker, and physical therapist) should be available to the child and family.
   b. A continuing, stable relationship with one person on the health care team who is coordinating efforts for the child is of great benefit.
2. Numerous neurosurgical, orthopedic, and urologic procedures and operations may be necessary to help the child achieve his maximum potential.

Preoperative Nursing Objectives for Initial Surgery in the Neonatal Period

A. *To prevent leakage of cerebrospinal fluid or rupture of the sac or lesion.*

1. Position the infant on his abdomen.
   a. Avoid placing the infant on his back, because this would cause pressure on the sac.
   b. A Bradford frame may be used to facilitate positioning. (Refer to procedure for the use of the Bradford frame, p. 1216.)
   c. Check the position of the child at least once every hour.
2. Do not place a diaper or other covering directly over the sac.
3. A doughnut-shaped sterile padding may be placed around the sac.
4. Observe the sac frequently for evidence of irritation or leakage of cerebrospinal fluid.

B. *To prevent infection.*

1. Infection of the sac
   a. This is most commonly caused by contamination by urine and feces.
   b. Keep the buttocks and genitalia scrupulously clean.
      (1) Do not diaper the infant if the defect is in the lower portion of the spine.
      (2) Utilize a divided Bradford frame to allow urine and feces to drain away from the body. (Refer to technique, p. 1216.)
      (3) A small plastic drape taped between the defect and the anus may help to prevent contamination.
   c. A sterile gauze pad or towel or a sterile, moistened

dressing may be applied according to the physician's preference.
   (1) When the sterile covering is used, it should be changed frequently to keep the area free of exudate and to maintain sterility.
   (2) Care must be taken to prevent the covering from adhering to and damaging the sac.
2. Infection of the bladder and urinary tract
   a. Infection is frequently caused by stasis of urine.
   b. Use the Credé method for emptying the bladder if recommended by the physician.
      (1) Apply firm, gentle pressure to the abdomen, beginning in the umbilical area and progressing toward the symphysis pubis.
      (2) Continue the procedure as long as urine can be manually expressed.
      (3) This technique is often contraindicated for infants with vesicoureteral reflux.
   c. Encourage fluid intake to dilute the urine.
   d. Administer prescribed prophylactic antibiotics.

C. *To prevent deformities and ulcerations of lower extremities.*

1. Maintain the infant in the prone position with hips only slightly flexed to decrease tension on the sac.
2. Place a foam rubber pad covered with a soft cloth between the infant's legs to maintain the hips in abduction and to prevent or counteract subluxation. A diaper roll or small pillow may be used in place of the foam rubber pad.
3. Allow the baby's feet to hang freely over the pads or mattress edge to prevent aggravation of foot deformities.
4. Change the infant's position when permissible to relieve pressure.
5. Provide meticulous skin care to all areas of the body—especially ankles, knees, tip of nose, cheeks, and chin.
6. Provide passive range of motion exercises for those muscles and joints which the infant does not use spontaneously. Hip exercises should not be done unless recommended by the physician.
7. Use a foam or fleece pad to reduce pressure of the mattress against the infant's skin.

D. *To provide adequate nutrition and hydration.*

1. Hold the infant for feedings if permissible. This provides the needed position change and affection and facilitates feeding.
   Position the infant in such a way that pressure on the back is eliminated. This may be accomplished by holding the infant in normal feeding position with elbow rotated to avoid touching the sac. Alternatives include feeding the infant on his side or while he is prone on the nurse's lap.
2. The child who must be fed in the prone position should have his head turned to one side and tilted upward.
3. Stop the feeding frequently so that the baby can rest and air can be expelled.
   a. These infants cannot be bubbled in the same way as normal babies.
   b. Small, frequent feedings may be necessary.
4. Monitor the infant's weight pattern to ensure adequate gain.

E. *To provide normal infant stimulation.*

1. Establish eye contact with the infant by sitting at the crib with your face at the level of his.

2. Provide appropriate toys, such as bright mobiles or musical toys.
3. Refer to section on growth and development, page 1093.

F. *To monitor neurological status and observe for signs of complications.*

1. Hydrocephalus
   a. Irritability
   b. Feeding difficulty, vomiting, decreased appetite
   c. Increased head circumference
   d. Tense fontanelle
   e. Temperature fluctuations
   f. Decreased alertness
2. Infection
   a. Oozing of fluid or pus from the sac
   b. Fever
   c. Irritability or listlessness
   d. Convulsions
   e. Concentrated or foul-smelling urine
3. Record the following:
   a. Frequent vital signs
   b. Behavior of the infant
   c. Movement of the legs
   d. Degree of continence
   e. Evidence of urine retention or fecal impaction
   f. Daily head circumference
   g. Evidence of complications

G. *To provide initial emotional support to the family.*

1. Encourage parents to talk about their child and how they feel about the defect.
2. Provide them with basic information about the condition. Answer their questions simply and directly. Reinforce medical interpretations.
3. Encourage them to become involved with the child's care from the beginning.
   a. Demonstrate techniques for holding and feeding the child and for providing routine care.
   b. Emphasize what is *normal* and *well* about their infant.
4. Initiate communication with appropriate members of the multidisciplinary team which manages infants with these problems.

For nursing management of the infant with hydrocephalus or clubfoot, refer to Hydrocephalus, page 1387, and Clubfoot, page 1416, in the pediatric section.

Postoperative Nursing Objectives

A. *To prevent postoperative complications.*

1. Shock
   a. Keep the infant warm by placing him in an Isolette or infant warmer.
   b. Maintain infant in a prone, level position for a few postoperative days.
2. Respiratory Problems
   a. Periodically change infant's position if permitted by his condition and by the extent of surgery.
   b. Have oxygen available if necessary.
   c. Report abdominal distention which may interfere with breathing and feeding.
3. Nutritional Problems
   a. The infant may be fed intravenously for several days or may be fed via gavage if he is unable to take oral feedings (see procedures for intravenous therapy, p. 1171, and gavage feeding, p. 1159).
   b. Apply previously stated principles when bottle-feeding the infant.
4. Infection

   a. Keep the surgical dressing clean and dry.
   b. Observe the dressing frequently for drainage.
   c. Apply previously stated principles to prevent infection.
   d. Administer prescribed antibiotics.
5. Nursing Observations. Record the following:
   a. Frequent measurements of temperature, pulse, and respiration
   b. Color
   c. Neurologic status
   d. Evidence of abdominal distention
   e. Condition of dressing
   f. Evidence of infection
   g. Degree of continence
   h. Behavior of the infant
   i. Evidence of hydrocephalus

B. *To continue appropriate preoperative nursing activities.*

1. Once the infant's back is well healed, he may be placed in a supine position for brief periods, which are gradually increased as the skin tolerates it.
2. The infant may also be positioned on his side at no more than a 45-degree angle for brief periods. This position, however, has the disadvantage of placing the hips in flexion and reduces the desirable use of the arms.
3. Special positioning may be requested by the orthopedic surgeon or the physical therapist.
4. Bikini diapers may be used once the back is well healed.

C. *To provide continued emotional support to the family.*

1. Encourage continued participation by parents in the infant's care.
2. Facilitate communication and interaction with appropriate members of the multidisciplinary clinic for birth defects.
   It is essential that open lines of communication exist between clinic members and the staff that provides daily care for the infant. This ensures that families receive consistent information and facilitates continuity of care.
3. If a multidisciplinary team is not available, initiate appropriate individual referrals—to social worker, clergyman, community health nurse, physical therapist, etc.
4. Foster the goal of helping the child to become as independent as possible.
   a. Emphasize habilation which makes use of the normal parts of the body and minimizes the disabilities.
   b. Focus on immediate planning in such areas as ambulating and bowel and bladder management.
5. Begin discharge teaching early. (See below.)
6. Provide support for dealing with the usual problems of a newborn baby. Answer questions related to formula, bath, problems of growth and development, and discipline.

Parental Education

1. Prepare parents to feed, hold, and stimulate their infant as normally as possible.
   Include information related to the management of the usual neonatal problems such as bathing, feeding, formula preparation, and sleeping. (Refer to section on growth and development, p. 1093.)
2. Teach parents any special techniques which may be required for the infant's physical care. Examples:

a. Methods of holding and positioning the infant
b. Techniques of feeding
c. Care of the incision
d. Provision for adequate elimination:
   (1) Procedure for bladder credé
   (2) Administration of prescribed prophylactic antibiotics
   (3) Signs of constipation and alleviation of the problem through diet regulation
e. Physical therapy exercises if prescribed
f. Skin care
   (1) General measures for avoiding pressure sores, such as frequent position changes
   (2) Perineal care
      (a) Frequent diaper changes
      (b) Careful laundering of diapers, or use of disposable diapers
      (c) Application of protective ointments
   (3) Daily inspection of the skin for such changes as reddened areas and bruises.
3. Safety
   The child with decreased sensation in the extremities should be protected from prolonged pressure, from burns or trauma due to bath water that is too warm, and from contact with hot or sharp objects.
4. Familiarize parents with signs of associated problems, especially signs of increased intracranial pressure or shunt malfunction and signs of infection.
   Instruct parents to notify the physician if a problem does occur.

5. Be certain that a mechanism is developed for the family to receive continued support and teaching following discharge.
   a. This is best provided through a birth defects center.
   b. A community health nursing referral is helpful for many families.
6. References for Parents:
   Allum N. Spina Bifida: The Treatment and Care of Spina Bifida Children. London, George Allen and Unwin, 1975
   Pieper E. The Teacher and the Child With Spina Bifida. Chicago, Spina Bifida Association of America, 1977
   Reid R. My Children, My Children. New York, Harcourt Brace Jovanovich, 1977
   White P. Janet At School. New York, Thomas Y. Crowell, 1978
   Swinyard C. The Child With Spina Bifida. Chicago, Spina Bifida Association of America, 1977
7. Agencies:
   Association for the Aid of Crippled Children, 345 E. 46th St., New York, N.Y. 10017
   National Easter Seal Society for Crippled Children and Adults, 2023 West Ogden Ave., Chicago, Ill. 60612
   National Foundation—March of Dimes, 800 Second Ave., New York, N.Y. 10017
   Spina Bifida Association of America, 343 S. Dearborn St., Chicago, Ill. 60604

BACTERIAL MENINGITIS

Bacterial meningitis is an inflammation of the meninges which follows the invasion of the spinal fluid by a bacterial agent.

Etiology

1. The proportion of cases due to a specific organism varies from year to year; there is also considerable geographic difference.
2. The most common organisms causing bacterial meningitis in different age groups are:
   a. Birth to 2 months
     Escherichia coli
     Streptococcus, group B
     Staphylococcus
   b. 2 months to 3 years
     Hemophilus influenzae
     Diplococcus pneumoniae
     Neisseria meningitidis
   c. 3 to 16 years
     Diplococcus pneumoniae
     Neisseria meningitidis

Altered Physiology

1. Bacterial meningitis is almost always preceded by an upper respiratory infection, which is complicated by bacteremia.
2. Bacteria in the circulating blood then invade the spinal fluid.
3. Bacterial meningitis may occur as an extension of a local bacterial infection such as otitis media, mastoiditis, or sinusitis (less common).

4. Bacteria may also gain direct entry through penetrating wound, spinal tap, surgery, or anatomic abnormalities.
5. The infective process results in inflammation, exudation, and varying degrees of tissue damage in the brain.

Clinical Manifestations

1. Signs and symptoms are variable, depending on the patient's age, the etiologic agent, and the duration of the illness when diagnosed.
   a. Infants less than 1 month of age display the following symptoms:
     (1) Irritability
     (2) Lethargy
     (3) Vomiting
     (4) Lack of appetite
     (5) Seizures
     (6) High-pitched cry
   b. Infants up to 2 years of age manifest symptoms similar to those of the young infant and in addition may have:
     (1) Fever
     (2) Tenseness of the fontanelle
     (3) Neck rigidity
     (4) Positive Kernig's and/or Brudzinski's signs
       (a) Kernig's sign
         With the child in the supine position and knees flexed, the leg is flexed at the hip so that the thigh is brought to a position perpendicular to the trunk. An attempt

is then made to extend the knee. If meningeal irritation is present, this cannot be done and attempts to extend the knee result in pain.
  (b) Brudzinski's sign
    Spontaneous flexion of the lower limbs following passive flexion of the neck.
  c. Children over 2 years of age:
    (1) Common initial symptoms
      (a) Vomiting
      (b) Headache
      (c) Mental confusion
      (d) Lethargy
    (2) Later symptoms
      (a) Neck rigidity within 12 to 24 hours after onset
      (b) Positive Kernig's and/or Brudzinski's sign
      (c) Seizures
      (d) Progressive decline in responsiveness
2. Onset may be insidious or fulminant.
3. Petechiae or purpura may develop.
  a. Characteristic skin lesions are most often observed in cases of meningococcal or *Pseudomonas* infection.
  b. Hemorrhagic rashes may occur in any child with overwhelming bacterial sepsis because of disseminated intravascular coagulation.
4. Septic arthritis suggests either meningococcal or *Hemophilus influenzae* infection.

Diagnostic Evaluation

1. Diagnosis is usually established by performance of a lumbar puncture and examination of the cerebrospinal fluid.
  a. Elevated cerebrospinal fluid pressure
  b. High cell count with mostly polymorphonuclear cells
  c. Low glucose level
  d. Elevated protein level (may also be normal)
  e. Gram stain and cultures positive—to identify the causative organism
2. Additional laboratory studies
  a. Complete blood count (Total white blood cell count is often increased, with a preponderance of young neutrophils in the differential blood count.)
  b. Platelet count
  c. Urinalysis
  d. Blood, urine, and nasopharyngeal cultures
  e. Serum electrolytes—often demonstrate hyponatremia and hypochloremia
  f. Serum glucose
  g. Blood urea nitrogen (BUN) and creatinine
  h. Tuberculin skin test
  i. Skull and chest x-rays

Treatment

1. Intravenous administration of the appropriate antimicrobial agents to promote rapid destruction of the bacteria and to suppress the emergence of resistant strains
2. Recognition and treatment of hyponatremia
3. Supportive management of the comatose child or the child with seizures
4. Appropriate prophylactic treatment provided for contacts when indicated

Complications

1. Seizures
2. Cerebral edema
3. Subdural effusion
4. Hydrocephalus
5. Cerebral infarction or abscess
6. Diffuse residual effects, including slowed development

Nursing Objectives

A. *To practice measures which will prevent the transmission of infection.*

1. Place the child in isolation until at least 24 hours after initiation of antibiotic therapy.
2. Practice careful handwashing technique—to serve as a model of good technique.
3. Personnel with infection should avoid contact with infants.
  a. Seek medical care for infection. (Cultures should be taken.)
  b. Remain out of the nursery.
  c. Wear a mask when it is necessary to enter the nursery.
4. Teach parents and other visitors proper handwashing and gown technique.
5. Maintain sterile technique when procedures demanding this technique are performed.
6. Identify close contacts or high-risk children who might benefit from meningococci vaccination.

B. *To assess the child for evidence of disease progression or response to therapy.*

1. Determine baseline data at admission. Include the following information:
  a. Weight
  b. Head circumference
  c. Vital signs
  d. Blood pressure
  e. Neurologic status
  f. History related to present illness
  g. Usual behavior and feeding patterns
2. Monitor vital signs, blood pressure, and neurologic status at frequent intervals.
3. Monitor intake and output continuously.
4. Monitor weight and head circumference at least daily.
5. Observe for and report the appearance or disappearance of any of the previously listed clinical manifestations.
  a. Be especially alert for vague symptoms which apper early in the course of meningeal irritation in infants:
    (1) Lethargy
    (2) Irritability
    (3) Poor feeding or refusal to feed
    (4) Weight loss
    (5) Temperature changes
  b. Be consistent in planning for the care of infants to provide a means by which these early symptoms may be detected.
    (1) Accurate charting of the infant's previous behavior.
    (2) Assigning the same nurse to care for an infant on successive days.

C. *To administer the prescribed antibiotic therapy to control the infection.*

1. Administer medications at the specified time to achieve optimal serum levels.
2. Since medications are generally administered intravenously for 2 to 3 weeks, restrain the child in a

functional position which safeguards the integrity of the IV. Refer to sections on intravenous therapy, page 1171, and protective devices to limit movement, page 1154.

3. Observe medication sites for evidence of infiltration or development of tissue irritation.
4. Be aware of the actions, proper dilution, and side effects of specific medications.
5. Be aware of drug interactions and incompatibilities.

D. *To observe for evidence of complications of the disease.*

Report the following:
1. Decreased respirations, decreased pulse rate, increased systolic blood pressure, visual disturbances, pupillary changes, or decreased responsiveness, which may indicate increased intracranial pressure.
2. Decreased urine volume and increased body weight, which may indicate inappropriate secretion of antidiuretic hormone.
3. Sudden appearance of a skin rash and bleeding from other sites, which may indicate disseminated intravascular coagulation.
4. Persistent or recurring fever, bulging fontanelle, signs of increased intracranial pressure, focal neurologic signs, seizures, or increased head circumference which may indicate subdural effusion.
5. Hearing disturbances and apparent deafness.

E. *To provide for the nutritional needs of the patient.*

1. During the acute phase of the illness, the patient may be unable to take or tolerate oral feedings.
   a. Carefully monitor the administration of intravenous fluids.
   b. Provide nasogastric feedings if necessary (see section on feeding methods, p. 1156).
   c. Provide for the sucking needs of the infant by offering a pacifier.
2. Initiate oral feedings as soon as the patient's condition improves.
   a. Infants
      (1) Begin by offering small feedings and observe for the following responses:
         (a) Vomiting
         (b) Abdominal distention
         (c) Infant's interest in feeding and ability to suck
         (d) If the infant tires with feeding
      (2) Supplement oral feedings with gavage feedings if necessary.
      (3) Gradually increase amount of feeding.
      (4) Resume regular feeding schedule based on infant's ability to tolerate it.
      (5) Hold the infant for feedings as soon as his condition warrants it.
   b. Older children—refer to section on nutrition, p. 1115.
3. Carefully monitor the child's weight to ensure that caloric needs are being met.

F. *To provide a supportive environment during the stage of irritability.*

1. Reduce the general noise level around the child and shield child from sudden loud noises.
2. Organize nursing care to provide for periods of uninterrupted rest. Disturb only when necessary.
3. Keep general handling of the child at a minimum. When necessary, approach the child slowly and gently.
4. Maintain subdued lighting as much as possible.
5. Speak in a low, well-modulated tone of voice to reduce anxiety.

G. *To provide therapeutic care for the child who experiences seizures.*

(See section on seizures, below.)

H. *To provide therapeutic care for the febrile child.*

(See section on fever, p. 1149.)

I. *To observe for episodes of apnea and initiate measures to stimulate respiration.*

1. Observe the infant closely for apnea or have the infant placed on a respiratory monitor.
2. Stimulate infant when apnea does occur.
   a. Pinch feet and provide more vigorous stimulation if necessary.
   b. When spontaneous respiration does not occur within 15 to 20 seconds, apply hand resuscitator or perform mouth-to-mouth resuscitation.
3. Report frequent periods of apnea to physician.
4. Record length of apnea episode and response to stimulation on nursing record.

J. *To provide supportive care for the child during the convalescent phase of illness.*

1. Record disappearance of symptoms and indications that the child is returning to his normal state.
2. Provide for the emotional needs of the child. (Refer to section on the hospitalized child, p. 1126.)
3. Encourage parental visiting and family-centered care.
4. Note any evidence that the child is developing sequelae of the illness, such as deafness, brain abnormality, or hydrocephalus.

Parental Support and Education

1. Encourage parents to visit the child.
   a. Encourage their participation in the child's care.
   b. Provide them with an opportunity to express their concerns.
   c. Answer questions they may have regarding the infant's progress and care.
2. Discuss symptoms parents should watch for as signs of possible complications.
3. Give specific instruction regarding medications to be administered at home.

CONVULSIVE DISORDERS (SEIZURE DISORDERS, EPILEPSY)

Convulsive disorder is a term used to encompass a number of varieties of episodic disturbances of brain function. Convulsions should not be regarded as one specific disease, but as a symptom of an underlying disorder. They are relatively common in children, being more prevalent during the first 2 years than at any other time in life.

Etiology

(At least 50% of cases)

1. Idiopathic
2. Prenatal factors
   a. Genetic predisposition
   b. Congenital structural anomalies
   c. Fetal infections
   d. Maternal diseases
3. Perinatal factors
   a. Trauma
   b. Hypoxia
   c. Jaundice
   d. Infection
   e. Prematurity
   f. Drug withdrawal
4. Postnatal factors
   a. Primary infection of the central nervous system
   b. Infectious diseases of childhood with encephalopathy
   c. Head trauma
   d. Circulatory diseases
   e. Toxic encephalopathy
   f. Allergic encephalopathy
   g. Metabolic encephalopathy
   h. Degenerative diseases
   i. Cerebral neoplasms
   j. Renal disease

Altered Physiology

1. The basic mechanism for all seizures appears to be prolonged depolarization causing brain cells to become overactive and to discharge in a sudden, violent, disorderly manner.
2. This paroxysmal burst of electrical energy spreads to adjacent areas or may jump to distant areas of the central nervous system. A seizure results.
3. The biochemical basis of seizures is incompletely understood.
4. Some seizures appear to occur under the influence of a triggering factor.
   a. Hormonal factors, such as those related to the menstrual period, menarche, and menopause
   b. Nonsensory factors, such as hyperthermia, hyperventilation, metabolic disorders, sleep deprivation, emotional disturbances, and physical stress
   c. Sensory factors, such as those related to vision, hearing, touch, the startle reaction, and those that are self-induced
5. For international classification of epileptic seizures refer to page 730.

Clinical Manifestations

A. *Grand Mal Epilepsy* (Generalized seizures)

1. Onset
   a. Onset is abrupt.
   b. May occur at night.
   c. An aura (peculiar sensation, often dizziness) occurs in about ⅓ of epileptic children prior to a grand mal seizure.
2. Tonic spasm
   a. The child's entire body becomes stiff.
   b. He usually loses consciousness.
   c. The face may become pale and distorted.
   d. His eyes are frequently fixed in one position.
   e. His back may be arched with his head held backward or to one side.
   f. His arms are usually flexed and his hands clenched.
   g. If standing, the child falls to the ground.

   h. He may utter a peculiar, piercing cry.
   i. He is often unable to swallow his saliva.
   j. Breathing is ineffective and cyanosis results if spasm includes the muscles of respiration.
   k. The pulse may become weak and irregular.
3. Clonic phase
   a. Characterized by twitching movements which follow the tonic state.
   b. Usually start in one place and become generalized, including the muscles of the face.
   c. The child may be incontinent and may bite his tongue or cheek. (This occurs because of sudden forceful contraction of his jaw and abdominal muscles.)
4. Duration
   a. Varies, from a few seconds to 30 minutes or longer.
   b. Usually, convulsions cease after a few minutes.
5. Postconvulsive (postictal) state of child
   a. Usually is sleepy or exhausted.
   b. May complain of headache.
   c. May appear to be in a dazed state.
   d. Often performs relatively automatic tasks without being able to recall the episode.
6. Secondary symptomatology
   a. Represents the patient's response over a long period of time to the injurious attitudes of other people toward the child and the diagnosis.
   b. Child develops a self-image consistent with his perception of how others view him.
7. Electroencephalogram (EEG)
   a. Definite abnormalities can usually be demonstrated in the interval between seizures.
      (1) Random spike discharges
      (2) Diffuse high-voltage slow waves
      (3) Pattern abnormal for child's chronologic age
   b. Multiple high-voltage spike discharges are demonstrated during the seizure.
   c. Asymmetries between the 2 hemispheres and diffuse slowing may be observed after the seizure.

B. *Status Epilepticus*

1. Refers to grand mal seizures which occur in series without the patient's regaining consciousness between attacks.
2. Transient postictal (i.e., period following seizures) signs and symptoms include ataxia, aphasia, and mental sluggishness.
3. Irreversible brain damage may occur secondary to prolonged cellular hypoxia.
4. This condition should be treated as a medical emergency.

C. *Petit Mal Epilepsy*

1. Onset—rarely appears before 3 years of age.
2. Clinical signs
   a. Loss of contact with the environment for a few brief seconds:
      (1) The child may appear to be staring or daydreaming.
      (2) If reading or writing, the child will suddenly discontinue the activity and may resume it when the seizure has ended.
   b. Minor manifestations include rolling of the eyes, nodding of the head, slight hand movements, and smacking of the lips.
3. Duration—usually 5–10 seconds.
4. Frequency—varies from 1 or 2 per month to several hundred each day.

5. Precipitating factors may include hyperventilation, fatigue, hypoglycemia, and stress.
6. Postconvulsive state
   a. Child appears normal.
   b. Is not aware of having had a convulsion.
7. Electroencephalogram (EEG)
   Has characteristic 3-per-second spike and wave pattern during the seizure.

D. Focal Seizures

1. Psychomotor
   a. Occur most frequently in children from 3 years of age through adolescence.
   b. Seizure discharge usually originates in the temporal lobe and may be referred to as "temporal lobe seizures."
   c. Clinical signs:
      (1) Frequently experiences a sense of fullness rising from the abdomen to the thorax.
      (2) Aura, if present, often includes bad odor or taste.
      (3) May experience complex auditory or visual hallucinations, déjà vu feeling, or strong sense of fear and anxiety.
      (4) Perceptual alterations may occur.
      (5) Dysphagia or aphasia may be present.
      (6) Most common motor symptom is drawing or jerking of the mouth and face.
      (7) May perform coordinated but inappropriate movements repeatedly in a stereotyped manner (e.g., clutching, kicking, picking at clothes, walking in circles, chewing, licking, spitting).
      (8) Consciousness may be impaired but is rarely completely lost.
   d. Duration—brief, usually from 30 seconds to 5–10 minutes.
   e. Postconvulsive state—child may be confused after an attack but usually has no memory of what happened.
2. Focal motor
   a. Clinical signs
      (1) Sudden jerking movements occur in a particular area of the body, such as the face, thumb, or toe.
      (2) Consciousness may or may not be disturbed.
      (3) Clonic movements occasionally begin in 1 area of the body and spread to adjacent areas on the same side in a fixed progression (Jacksonian seizures).
   b. Prognosis
      Seizures may become more extensive as the child matures, leading to grand mal seizures.
3. Focal sensory (rare in children)
   Sensations occur, such as numbness, tingling, and coldness in the part of the body controlled by the area of the brain cell overactivity.

E. Infantile Myoclonic Seizures (Massive Myoclonic Spasms)

1. These seizures are peculiar to infants; they are second in incidence only to grand mal seizures in this age group.
2. Peak incidence is in children between 3 and 6 months; onset after 2 years of age is rare.
3. Clinical signs
   a. Sudden, forceful, myoclonic contractions involving the musculature of the trunk, neck, and extremities.
      (1) Flexor type—infant adducts and flexes his limbs, drops his head, and doubles upon himself.
      (2) Extensor type—infant extends neck, spreads arms out, and bends body backward in a position described as "spread eagle."
   b. A cry or grunt may accompany severe attacks.
   c. Infant may grimace, laugh, or appear fearful during or after the attack.
4. Duration—momentary (usually under 1 minute).
5. Frequency—varies from a few attacks per day to hundreds per day.
6. EEG—random, high-voltage slow waves and spikes suggestive of a diffuse disorganized state.
7. Prognosis
   a. Almost always associated with cerebral abnormalities.
   b. Usually this type of seizure disappears spontaneously by the time the child reaches 4 years of age.
   c. Subsequent grand mal or other types of seizures often develop.
   d. Mental retardation usually accompanies this disorder.

Prognosis

1. General prognosis depends on type and severity of seizure disorder, coexisting mental retardation, organic disorders, and the type of medical management.
   a. Medically treated seizures
      Spontaneous cessation of seizures may occur. Drugs may be gradually discontinued when the child has been free from attacks for an extensive period and his EEG pattern has reverted to normal.
   b. Nontreated epilepsy
      Seizures tend to become more numerous.
2. Mental development
   a. Convulsive episodes do not in themselves usually cause irreversible brain damage.
   b. Hypoxia during seizures can cause mental retardation.
   c. Epileptic children with normal mentality can be expected to maintain it with proper control of seizures.

Chemotherapy

A. General Principles Related to the Administration of Medications

1. Selection of the most effective drug(s) depends upon correct identification of the clinical seizure type.
2. A desirable drug level is one which will prevent attacks without producing drowsiness or unsteadiness.
3. Dosages are adjusted according to blood level and clinical signs.
4. Accurate timing is essential to prevent seizures. This is especially true when there is a tendency for the child to have convulsions at a certain period each day.
5. Enteric coated tablets which have a delayed effect should be used for children who are prone to attacks during sleep.
6. Most anticonvulsants are available in liquid form as well as in capsules or tablets.
   Tablets can be crushed and given to infants and small children in coke syrup or applesauce.

7. It may take several months to find the best combination of medications and the best dosages of each to control the child's seizures.
8. One hundred % control of symptoms may not be achieved in every patient.
9. Dosage adjustment may be required from time to time because of the child's growth.
10. Blood counts, urinalyses, and liver-function studies are done at regular intervals in children receiving certain anticonvulsants.
11. Duration of therapy should be prolonged. Medication is usually not discontinued until at least 2–3 years after the last attack.
12. Weaning from medication should always be gradual, with stepwise reduction of dosage and withdrawal of 1 drug at a time.

B. *Common Drugs Used for the Control of Seizures in Children*

1. Phenobarbital
   a. Dosage
      (1) An initial loading dose is usually given intramuscularly or intravenously for an acute, ongoing seizure, because it takes from days to weeks to achieve therapeutic blood levels by the oral route alone.
      (2) The dosage is reduced for maintenance therapy and is generally administered orally.
   b. Indications and advantages
      (1) Drug of choice for initial trial
      (2) One of the safest anticonvulsant drugs
      (3) Relatively inexpensive
   c. Untoward effects
      (1) Excitement, hyperactivity
      (2) Rash
      (3) Gastrointestinal symptoms
      (4) Dizziness, ataxia
      (5) Aggravated psychomotor seizures
      (6) Drowsiness
   d. Toxic effects (rare, except in overdose, accidental ingestion)
      Respiratory, circulatory, or renal depression
   e. Contraindications
      (1) Severe hepatic or renal dysfunction
      (2) Hypersensitivity
2. Phenytoin (diphenylhydantoin, Dilantin)
   a. Route—oral
   b. Indications and advantages
      (1) Does not produce excessive drowsiness
      (2) Safest drug for the management of psychomotor epilepsy
      (3) Often used with phenobarbital
   c. Untoward effects
      (1) May accentuate petit mal seizures
      (2) Hypertrophy of the gums
         Daily gum massage is an important aspect of nursing care for a patient taking phenytoin
      (3) Hirsutism
      (4) Rickets
      (5) Nystagmus
      (6) Ataxia
      (7) Rash
      (8) Nausea and vomiting
   d. Toxic effects—(rare, except in overdose, accidental ingestion)
      (1) Blood dyscrasia
      (2) Liver damage

3. Ethosuximide (Zarontin)
   a. Route—oral
   b. Indications and advantages
      (1) Used for petit mal seizures
      (2) Occurrence of blood dyscrasia is less common following administration of ethosuximide than with trimethadione (Tridione)—the other medication frequently used to control petit mal seizures.
   c. Untoward effects
      (1) Drowsiness
      (2) May increase grand mal seizures
      (3) Gastrointestinal symtoms
         Administer with food
      (4) Headache (rare)
   d. Toxic effects
      (1) Blood dyscrasias
      (2) Psychiatric symptoms
   e. Contraindications
      Hepatic or renal disease
4. Primidone (Mysoline)
   a. Route—oral
   b. Indications and advantages
      (1) Used alone or with other anticonvulsants to control grand mal, psychomotor, or focal seizures.
      (2) May control grand mal seizures not responsive to treatment by other anticonvulsant therapy.
   c. Untoward effects
      (1) More common
         (a) Ataxia
         (b) Vertigo
      (2) Occasional
         (a) GI symptoms
         (b) Fatigue
         (c) Diplopia
         (d) Nystagmus
         (e) Skin eruption
   d. Toxic effects
      (1) Megaloblastic anemia may occur as a rare idiosyncratic response to the drug.
      (2) Drowsiness in nursing newborns of primidone-treated mothers indicates that nursing should be discontinued.
   e. Contraindications
      (1) Patients who are hypersensitive to phenobarbital
      (2) Patients with porphyria
5. Diazepam (Valium)
   a. Route—oral, intravenous, or intramuscular
   b. Indications and advantages
      (1) Intravenous or intramuscular diazepam is indicated in the treatment of status epilepticus and severe recurrent convulsive seizures.
      (2) Oral diazepam may be used adjunctively in maintenance therapy for convulsive disorders.
   c. Special precautions
      (1) If administered intravenously, give slowly over 3 minutes. Avoid intra-arterial administration or extravasation.
      (2) Administer intravenously with caution to children with limited pulmonary reserve, because of the possibility that apnea and/or cardiac arrest may occur.
      (3) Tonic status epilepticus has been precipitated in patients treated with intravenous diazepam for petit mal seizures.
      (4) Concomitant use of barbiturates, alcohol, or

other central nervous system depressants may potentiate the action of diazepam with increased risk of apnea.

    (5) Administer with caution to children with compromised renal function.

  d. Untoward effects

    (1) More common

      (a) Ataxia

      (b) Drowsiness

      (c) Fatigue

      (d) Venous thrombosis and phlebitis at injection site

    (2) Less common

      (a) GI symptoms

      (b) Confusion, depression

      (c) Headache

      (d) Tremor

      (e) Vertigo

      (f) Incontinence or urinary retention

      (g) Visual disturbances

      (h) Skin rash

      (i) Anxiety

      (j) Sleep disturbance

      (k) Neutropenia

      (l) Jaundice

  e. Toxic effects

    (1) Somnolence

    (2) Confusion

    (3) Diminished reflexes

    (4) Hypotension

    (5) Coma

    (6) Apnea

    (7) Cardiac arrest

Nursing Objectives

A. *To control the seizures.*

Administer medications as prescribed.

B. *To protect the child from injury during a convulsive episode.*

1. Preventive Measures

  a. Remove hard toys from the bed. Keep a padded tongue blade or rubber bite block immediately available to put between the child's teeth to prevent him from biting his tongue.

  b. Pad the sides of the crib.

  c. Have a suction machine available to remove secretions during a seizure.

  d. Have an emergency oxygen source in the room in case of sudden respiratory difficulty.

2. Emergency Actions

  a. Clear the area around the child if he is not in bed.

  b. Do not restrain him.

  c. Loosen the clothing around his neck.

  d. If standing, ease the child to his bed or the floor.

  e. Turn the child on his side so that saliva can flow out of his mouth.

  f. Place a small, folded blanket under the head to prevent trauma if the seizure occurs when the child is on the floor.

  g. Place a padded tongue blade or airway between the teeth to prevent damage to the tongue and cheeks and to facilitate respiration if this can be done without difficulty (procedure is controversial). If the teeth have clamped shut, do not attempt to force them open.

  h. Suction the child and administer oxygen as necessary.

  i. Do not give anything by mouth.

  j. After the seizure place the child on his side in bed, if he is not already there.

C. *To accurately record the seizures, include the following:*

1. Significant preseizure events, such as noise, excitement, lethargy

2. Behavior before the seizure, aura

3. Types of movements observed

4. Time seizure began and ended

5. Site where twitching or contraction began

6. Areas of the body involved

7. Movements of the eyes and changes in pupil size

8. Incontinence

9. Amount of perspiration

10. Respiratory changes

11. Color change—pallor, cyanosis, flushing

12. Mouth—teeth clenched, movement, tongue bitten, position, foaming at the mouth

13. Apparent degree of consciousness during the seizure

14. Behavior after the seizure

  a. Degree of memory for recent events

  b. Types of speech

  c. Coordination

  d. Paralysis or weakness

  e. Sleeping after the attack

  f. Pupil reaction

  g. Vital signs

  h. Unusual sensations

D. *To observe the child for recurrent seizures.*

1. Place the child where he can be watched closely.

2. Monitor vital signs and assess neurologic status frequently.

3. Check the child frequently. Report:

  a. Behavior changes

  b. Irritability

  c. Restlessness

  d. Listlessness

E. *To provide emotional support to the child's parents.*

1. Describe completely any examinations, evaluations, treatments that the child is receiving.

  a. EEG

  b. Pneumoencephalogram

  c. Blood studies

  d. Medications

2. Provide information regarding the disease itself.

  a. Orientation should be a continuing process.

  b. Too much information at one time is undesirable.

  c. Points of emphasis:

    (1) Epilepsy is *not* contagious, is seldom dangerous, and does *not* indicate insanity or mental retardation.

    (2) Most children with epilepsy have infrequent seizures and with medications can completely control their convulsions.

    (3) The child may have normal intelligence and can live a useful and productive life.

    (4) The child's medication is not addicting when used as prescribed. It should in no way influence his mental ability or personality or cause him to become a drug addict.

    (5) It is impossible to predict accurately the possibility of the convulsive disorder appearing in siblings or offspring of the affected child.

  d. Refer the family to appropriate community resources and services.

(1) Social worker
(2) Community health nurse
(3) School nurse
(4) Psychiatrist
(5) Parent groups
(6) Voluntary agencies
e. Provide the parents with appropriate literature.
3. Observe the parent-child reaction for evidence of rejection or overprotection.
Offer reassurance and praise for achievements in dealing with the child's problem.
4. Prepare parents for the fact that it may take several months of regulating drug dosages before adequate control is obtained.

F. *To minimize anxiety during the child's hospitalization.*
1. Rationale
The therapeutic value of anticonvulsant drugs is decreased if the child has more anxiety than he can handle.
2. Explain the diagnostic and treatment plan to the child in a manner that he can understand.
a. The use of play is very effective in explaining things to younger children and in allowing them to express their feelings.
b. The older child should be encouraged to ask questions and to talk about his experience.
3. Allow the child as much normal activity as possible. Allow him to be dressed if desired.
4. If the child does have a seizure, stay with him and remain calm.
a. Stay with the child after a convulsion and reassure him and his parents that he is all right.
b. Help the child to adjust to reality if he has difficulty remembering the episode.
c. Older children may require intervention to deal with guilt and embarrassment secondary to incontinence and the loss of body control.
d. Maintain a quiet environment if the child has had a long convulsive period.
5. Provide diversion appropriate for the child's age.
Play equipment should be such that it will not cause injury during a seizure.
6. Avoid unnecessary stimulation.

Parental Education

1. The child should have as normal an environment as possible.
a. Attendance at a regular school with healthy children should be encouraged.
(1) Contact should be made with the school nurse who can help the child's teacher understand his disease, emergency treatment of seizures, etc.
(2) Child should be allowed to participate in organizations and outside activities with limited restrictions.
(a) Each child must be treated individually; the kind of activity depends on the degree of control.
(b) Generally, children with seizure disorders should not be allowed to climb in high places or swim alone.
(c) Responsible adults should be made aware of the child's disease.
(3) Child should not be made to feel that he can never be left alone.
(4) He needs to be disciplined as a normal child.

He should not gain attention directly or indirectly by having seizures.
2. The child should be given appropriate information regarding his diagnosis and treatment. He is less confident of his body and his control over it and therefore less confident of himself.
a. He should be included in conferences with the physician.
b. He needs an opportunity to ask questions which should be answered honestly.
c. He should be aware of his restrictions and helped to deal with them.
d. He should gradually be given responsibility for taking his own medications faithfully.
e. He should be encouraged to wear a medic-alert bracelet.
3. The older child and adolescent should be helped to achieve independence.
a. He should be given the opportunity for privacy to discuss his diagnosis with his physician.
b. He should be allowed to use his own judgment in his daily activities.
c. He should be helped to develop realistic educational and career goals.
(1) The assistance of a social worker or psychiatrist may be invaluable during this period.
(2) Genetic counseling may be indicated in some cases.
(a) People with epilepsy can marry and have children.
(b) There is no proof that epilepsy is hereditary although there may be a tendency to transmit a low convulsive threshold.
(3) Counseling regarding such matters as securing a driver's license and obtaining life, health, and automobile insurance should be available.
d. Any fantasies that "there is nothing wrong with me" or the refusal to take medications require prompt intervention.
4. Factors which may precipitate a convulsive episode should be avoided.
a. The seizures should be treated matter-of-factly. A calm, reassuring attitude is essential during and after a seizure.
The attitude of adults when the child has a seizure influences the attitude of other children toward him.
b. The child should be kept in optimal physical condition with special attention to the status of his teeth and eyes and to the prevention of infection.
c. Excessive fatigue, overhydration and hyperventilation should be avoided.
d. Irregular, fluctuating schedules are detrimental. A routine of daily living should be encouraged.
5. Medical care and supervision to control convulsions are essential.
Instructions regarding medical and nursing care should be stressed.
(1) Administration of medications and side effects of prescribed drugs
(2) Emergency care during a seizure
(3) Observations
(a) Signs of impending seizure
(b) Behavior during and after the seizure
(4) Diet
Ketogenic diets are no longer widely used, except in difficult cases.
6. Parents should be referred to appropriate support

groups for help in dealing with their feelings, concerns, and problems related to their child.
7. References for Parents:
Lagos J. Seizures, Epilepsy and Your Child. New York, Harper & Row, 1974
Sands H and Minters F. The Epilepsy Fact Book. Philadelphia, FA Davis, 1977

Svoboda W. Learning About Epilepsy. Baltimore, University Park Press, 1979
Volle F and Heron P. Epilepsy and You, Springfield, Charles C Thomas, 1978
8. Agency:
Epilepsy Foundation of America, 1828 L. St., N.W., Suite 406, Washington, D.C. 20036

FEBRILE CONVULSIONS

Febrile convulsions refer to seizures which occur in the context of a febrile illness in a previously normal child. The seizures are brief and generalized. They should be distinguished from focal or prolonged seizures which occur in a child with an underlying seizure disorder that is exacerbated by fever.

Etiology

1. Accompany intercurrent infections—especially viral illness, tonsillitis, pharyngitis, and otitis.
2. Appear to occur in a familial pattern, although exact pattern of inheritance is incompletely understood.

Incidence

1. Febrile convulsions occur in approximately 3–5% of all children.
2. The vast majority of first febrile seizures occur in children between the ages of 6 months and 3 years of age.
3. Febrile seizures are unusual after 5 years of age.

Clinical Manifestations

1. Most febrile convulsions consist of generalized tonic-clonic seizures.
2. Seizures generally last less than 20 minutes.
3. Fever is usually high—over 38.8° C.(101.8° F.) rectally.
4. Seizures usually occur near the onset of fever rather than after prolonged fever.

Diagnostic Evaluation

Measures are directed toward delineating the cause of any seizure as precisely as possible so that its implications and prognosis may be discussed with the parents. Diagnostic methods include:
1. Physical examination with special attention to neurologic status
2. Transillumination of the skull
3. Cerebrospinal fluid examination
4. Complete blood count and urinalysis
5. Cultures of nasopharynx, blood, or urine as appropriate to determine cause of fever
6. Blood sugar, calcium, and electrolyte levels
7. Electroencephalogram (EEG)
   (a) Similar to that found during and after a grand mal seizure
   (b) Abnormality frequently persists for as long as a week after the seizure
   (c) Interseizure record—normal
8. Skull films at time of first seizure

Prognosis

1. The likelihood of febrile seizure recurrence is about 40–50% for a second febrile seizure.
2. Factors influencing recurrence rate

a. The younger the child at the time of the first seizure, the greater the risk for additional febrile seizures.
b. Children with a positive family history of febrile convulsions have a greater risk of recurrent febrile convulsions.
3. The risk for development of nonfebrile convulsions is relatively low (about 3%). At risk are those children who demonstrate the following characteristics:
a. Multiple febrile seizures during one day
b. Prolonged febrile seizures
c. Persistent electroencephalographic abnormalities
d. Central nervous system infections

Nursing Objectives

A. *To assess and reduce fever.*
Refer to section on fever, page 1148.

B. *To intervene appropriately during and after the seizure episode(s).*
Refer to objectives A–D in previous section, page 1402.

Parental Education

1. Remain calm and efficient if the child has a seizure in the presence of his parents.
2. Reinforce realistic, reassuring information such as:
a. A convulsion does not necessarily imply that the underlying disease is a serious one.
b. Children rarely die in seizures.
c. The prognosis depends on the cause of the convulsion.
   (1) A single febrile seizure is not indicative of later chronic epilepsy.
   (2) Children who have a tendency to develop febrile convulsions usually lose it as they grow older.
   (3) Occasional, brief convulsions have no adverse effects on the child's ultimate development.
3. Discuss and demonstrate emergency management of seizures.
4. Stress that medical evaluation is indicated as soon as the child develops fever.
a. Review technique of temperature measurement.
b. Prompt administration of antipyretic measures is necessary when the child is febrile.
5. Reinforce medical instructions regarding anticonvulsant therapy.
a. The advisability of long-term anticonvulsant medications in normal children with simple febrile convulsions is currently controversial. Recommendations vary among physicians from no medication to maintenance therapy with phenobarbital.
b. Intermittent therapy with phenobarbital during febrile episodes is apparently of no value because of the length of time required to achieve therapeutic serum levels of the drug.

SUBDURAL HEMATOMA

Subdural hematoma refers to an accumulation of fluid, blood, and its degradation products within the potential space between the dura and arachnoid (subdural space). Subdural hematomas are classified as acute, subacute, or chronic, depending on the time period between injury and the onset of symptoms.

Etiology

1. Direct or indirect trauma to the head.
   a. Birth trauma
   b. Accidental causes
   c. Purposeful violence, as in the battered child syndrome (see p. 1454)
2. Meningitis

Classification*

1. Acute
   a. Syndrome presents as an acute problem within 3 days from the time of presumed injury.
   b. Condition often associated with other intracranial injuries. This connection increases the mortality rate associated with this type of subdural hematoma.
   c. May occur at any pediatric age.
   d. It is the least common type of subdural hematoma.
2. Subacute
   Syndrome presents within 4 to 14 days from the time of presented injury.
3. Chronic
   a. Syndrome presents at 2–4 weeks or more from the time of presumed injury.
   b. Most common type of subdural hematoma in children.
   c. Represents 20% of childhood head injuries.
   d. In 85% of cases, children are 2 years of age or less.
   e. In 80% of infant cases, there is bilateral involvement.
   f. In children over 2 years, subdural hematomas are most frequently unilateral.
   g. It may be difficult or impossible to obtain a history of trauma, since the precipitating episode often appears relatively insignificant and may pass unnoticed or be quickly forgotten.

Altered Physiology

1. Trauma to the head causes tearing of the delicate subdural veins, resulting in small hemorrhages into the subdural space. (Bleeding may be of arterial origin in cases of acute subdural hematoma.)
2. As the blood breaks down, there is an increased capillary permeability and effusion of blood cells and protein into the subdural space.
3. The breakdown products of blood stimulate the growth of connective tissue and capillaries largely from the dura.
4. A membrane is formed which usually extends frontally and laterally over the hemispheres, surrounding the clot.
5. Fluid accumulates within the membrane and increases the width of the subdural space.

   * Classification does not imply any basic differences in the disease process but refers only to the duration of the lesion before it becomes manifest. The classification varies slightly among several sources.

6. Further hemorrhages occur.
7. The lesion enlarges, expanding the skull, and, if unrelieved, ultimately causes cerebral atrophy or death from compression and herniation.
8. The lesion may arrest spontaneously at any point.
9. Further bleeding may occur into an already existing sac and may increase symptoms.
10. In long-standing subdural hematoma, the fluid may disappear, leaving a constricting membrane which prevents normal brain growth.

Clinical Manifestations

A. *Acute*

1. Often present with continuous unconsciousness from the time of injury, but child may present with a lucid interval.
2. Ensuing manifestations include deterioration of level of consciousness, evidence of progressive hemiplegia, and signs of brain stem herniation (pupillary enlargement, changes in vital signs, development of decerebrate state, and respiratory failure).

B. *Chronic*

1. Insidious onset
2. Symptoms are variable and are related to the age of the child.
   a. Infants
      (1) Early signs
          (a) Anorexia
          (b) Difficulty feeding
          (c) Vomiting
          (d) Irritability
          (e) Low grade fever
          (f) Retinal hemorrhages
          (g) Failure to gain weight
      (2) Later signs
          (a) Enlargement of the head
          (b) Bulging and pulsation of the anterior fontanelle
          (c) Tight, glossy scalp with dilated scalp veins
          (d) Strabismus, pupillary inequality, ocular palsies (rare)
          (e) Hyperactive reflexes
          (f) Seizures
          (g) Retarded motor development
   b. Older children
      (1) Early signs
          (a) Lethargy
          (b) Anorexia
          (c) Symptoms of increased intracranial pressure
              (1) Vomiting
              (2) Irritability
              (3) Increased blood pressure
              (4) Decreased pulse
              (5) Decreased or irregular respirations
              (6) Headache
      (2) Later signs (may occur immediately if bleeding takes place rapidly)
          (a) Convulsions
          (b) Coma

Diagnostic Evaluation

1. Complete blood count—anemia of blood loss; low serum protein level

2. X-ray—sutural separation in infants
3. Transillumination of the skull in infants—increased
4. Lumbar puncture—may contain red blood cells, a slight excess of white cells, and increased protein. Procedure may be risky with increased intracranial pressure.
5. Bilateral subdural taps—fluid of any sort in excess of 1–2 ml. or with a protein content significantly higher than that of the cerebrospinal fluid obtained at the same time—required for definitive diagnosis.
6. Electroencephalogram may be abnormal.
7. Carotid angiography shows defect.
8. Cranial Computed Tomography (CCT scan) is the procedure of choice for screening children with suspected subdural hematoma.

Complications

1. Mental retardation
2. Ocular abnormalities
3. Seizures
4. Spasticity
5. Paralysis

Treatment

1. Acute subdural hematoma
   Requires evacuation of the clot through a burr hole or craniotomy.
2. Chronic subdural hematoma
   a. Repeated subdural taps are done to remove the abnormal fluid.
      (1) In infants, the needle can be inserted through the fontanelle or suture line.
      (2) In older children, burr holes into the skull are necessary before the needle can be inserted.
      (3) The subdural taps may be the only treatment required if the fluid disappears entirely and symptoms do not recur.
      (4) Concurrently, treatment is instituted to correct anemia, electrolyte imbalance, and malnutrition.
   b. Shunting procedure may be indicated if repeated taps fail to significantly reduce the volume or protein content of the subdural collections. Shunting is generally to the peritoneal or pleural cavities.

Prognosis

1. Treatment is usually successful when the diagnosis is made early—before cerebral atrophy and a fixed neurologic deficit have occurred. In such cases, subsequent development is normal.
2. Prognosis is dependent on the effect of the initial trauma on the brain as well as the effect of continued fluid collection.
3. Mortality in massive, acute subdural bleeding is very high, even if promptly diagnosed.

Nursing Objectives

A. *To assess the child's neurologic status in order to help evaluate the effectiveness of treatment or to identify disease progress.*
Observe for and document the following:
1. General behavior—especially irritability, lethargy, and evidence of personality changes.
   It is important to obtain a thorough history from the child's parents regarding his normal behavior and level of functioning so that abnormalities can be more easily recognized.
2. Appetite and feeding difficulties, including vomiting.

3. Signs of increased intracranial pressure.
   a. Vital signs, including pulse, respiration, and blood pressure should be monitored frequently.
   b. Be alert for:
      (1) Increased systolic blood pressure
      (2) Increased pulse pressure
      (3) Decreased pulse or irregularities
      (4) Changes in respiratory rate or difficulty breathing
4. Level of consciousness. Describe findings explicitly. The following "levels" may be useful as guidelines:
   a. Alert and responds immediately and appropriately to visual, auditory, and tactile stimuli.
   b. Lethargic, drowsy, and inactive but can be aroused to an alert state.
   c. Lethargic and dull; responds with vigorous stimulation, but quickly returns to lethargic state.
   d. Can be aroused only to a very low level of response with vigorous stimulation.
   e. Moderate coma with rudimentary physiologic or psychomotor responses.
   f. Totally nonresponsive, even to deep pain stimuli.
5. Pupillary changes—especially dilated pupil, double vision, lack of response to light, alterations in visual acuity, and decreased integrity of eye movements.
6. Convulsions.
7. Motor function, including ability to move all extremities.
   The ability to grasp should be checked and compared bilaterally.

B. *To observe for signs of complications.*

1. Infection
   a. Record temperature frequently.
   b. Report purulent drainage from the site of the subdural tap.
2. Recurrent bleeding
   Note rapid changes in vital signs indicating shock or increased intracranial pressure.
3. Paralysis

C. *To avoid additional increase in intracranial pressure.*

1. Maintain a quiet environment.
2. Avoid sudden changes in position.
3. Organize nursing activities to allow for long periods of uninterrupted rest.
4. Administer laxatives or suppositories to prevent straining during a bowel movement.

D. *To assist with subdural taps.*

1. Wrap the infant or young child in a mummy restraint. (See procedure on protective devices to limit motion, p. 1454.)
2. Hold the child securely to avoid injury caused by sudden movement.
3. Apply firm pressure over the puncture site(s) for a few minutes after the tap has been completed to prevent fluid leakage along the needle tract.
4. Observe the child frequently after the procedure for:
   a. Shock
   b. Drainage from the site of the tap
      (1) Note whether this is serous drainage or frank blood.
      (2) Reinforce the dressing, if present, to prevent contamination of the wound.

E. *To provide adequate nutrition.*

Apply principles stated in the section on hydrocephalus, page 1389.

F. *To provide supportive care to the child in coma.*

1. Keep the child's eyes well lubricated to prevent corneal damage.
2. Suction the child as necessary to remove secretions in the mouth and nasopharynx.
3. Provide frequent mouth care.
4. Maintain adequate nutrition and hydration through nasogastric feedings. (Refer to procedure, p. 1159).
5. Carefully regulate fluid administration to avoid danger of rapidly increasing intracranial pressure.
6. Measure urine output and record specific gravity. Observe for bladder distention (indicates fluid retention). Use Credé method to empty bladder or utilize indwelling catheter if child is unable to void.
7. Administer suppositories or enemas as necessary to prevent constipation and impaction.
8. Change the child's position frequently and provide meticulous skin care to prevent hypostatic pneumonia and pressure sores.
9. Prevent contractures.
   a. Apply passive range of motion exercises to all extremities.
   b. Place pillows appropriately to support the child's body in good alignment.
   c. Use a footboard for the older child.
10. Have emergency equipment available for cardiopulmonary resuscitation, respiratory assistance, blood transfusion, subdural tap, etc.
11. Avoid discussing the child's condition near the bedside. Even though comatose, the child may be able to hear.
12. Observe for the development of the following complications:

a. Respiratory problems (infection, aspiration, obstruction, atelectasis)
b. Fluid and electrolyte imbalance
c. Infection (urinary or central nervous system)
d. Bladder and gastrointestinal distention

G. *To care for the child with a craniotomy.*

See section on the postoperative care of the child with a brain tumor, page 1430.

H. *To provide for the child's emotional needs.*

1. Hold and cuddle the infant as much as possible according to his condition.
2. Provide diversion according to the child's age.
   a. Infants—mobiles or musical toys
   b. Older children—quiet games, reading, etc.

I. *To provide emotional support to the parents.*

1. Encourage as much parental participation in the child's care as possible.
2. Reassure the parents that the prognosis is favorable with adequate treatment.
3. Avoid blaming the parents for the child's injury.
   a. Attempt to alleviate their guilt feelings if present.
   b. Refer the parents to a social worker or psychiatrist if this problem is severe.

Parental Education

Reinforce explanations in the following areas:
1. The condition
2. The causes of the child's specific symptoms
3. The need and rationale for treatment
4. Postoperative and recovery expectations
5. Signs of recurrent bleeding
6. Safety measures to prevent accidents in the future

REYE'S SYNDROME

Reye's syndrome is a children's disease which has been clinically characterized as a non-specific "encephalopathy and fatty degeneration of the viscera, mainly affecting the liver, brain, and kidney."*

Etiology and Incidence

1. Unknown
2. Most consistent single factor is an antecedent viral infection
   a. Influenza B—clustered geographically, occurring in older children (mean age is 11 years)
   b. Varicella—sporadic occurrence in younger children (mean age is 6 years)
3. Other related viruses include: adenovirus, coxsackie, ECHO, herpes simplex and zoster, influenza A, reovirus, and polio type I.
4. Other controversial possibilities (contributors)
   a. Genetic make-up of individual child that increases his susceptibility
   b. Environmental factors—incidence higher in suburban–rural areas
   c. Clinical—salicylates and phenothiazines

Altered Physiology

1. Mitochondrial injury or change is primary in all tissues.

*From Reye RD, Morgan G, Barae J. Encephalopathy and fatty degeneration of the viscera—a disease entity in children. Lancet 1963 Oct 12; 2(7310):749

2. Liver—enlarged and bright yellow; fatty infiltration in the form of small lipid droplets; mitochondria are large and swollen with some decrease of enzymatic activity, particularly for ammonia detoxification.
3. Brain—cerebral edema with small ventricles, possible neuronal necrosis, findings consistent with hypoxia, inflammatory reaction absent, grossly enlarged mitochondria; and pervasive watery blebs.
4. Kidney—fatty degeneration of loop of Henle and proximal convoluted tubules with a few lipid droplets in distal tubular cells.
5. Heart—fatty accumulation in fibers; bundle of His, and bundle branches.

Clinical Manifestations

> **NURSING ALERT:** Early diagnosis is critical because of the rapidly fatal course of the disease.

1. Prodromal illness (see etiology) that may be improving
2. Sudden pernicious vomiting—fever usually not present
3. Irrational behavior
4. Altered sensorium—from mild lethargy to progressive stupor and coma
5. Hyperventilation, tachypnea
6. Hepatomegaly

7. Stages

Children with Reye's syndrome advance through definite stages of progression. After diagnosis is made, the child should be categorized as fitting within one of the stages, with any progression noted. Lovejoy's Stages of Progression* follow:

Stage I: Vomiting, lethargy, liver dysfunction, type I EEG†

Stage II: Delirium, combativeness, hyperventilation, hyperactive reflexes, liver dysfunction, type II EEG

Stage III: Obtundent, coma, decerebrate, liver dysfunction, presence of pupillary light reaction, type II EEG

Stage IV: Deepening coma, decerebrate rigidity, costal–caudal progression of brain stem dysfunction, improvement of liver dysfunction, type III EEG

Stage V: Seizures, loss of reflexes, flaccidity, respiratory arrest, correction of liver dysfunction, isoelectric EEG

Diagnosis

1. General condition and appearance of child:
   History of prodromal illness—mild upper respiratory infection or other infection with sudden development of pernicious vomiting, presence of other symptoms.
2. Differential diagnosis—acute toxic encephalopathy, hepatic coma, hepatitis, meningitis, or encephalitis. History to rule out ingestion of medications or toxic materials.
3. Laboratory—essential to obtain:
   Elevated serum ammonia level, elevated serum glutamic–oxaloacetic transaminase (SGOT) level, prolonged prothrombin and partial prothrombin times, serum glucose decreased.
4. Laboratory—optional
   Acid–base imbalance; increased fatty acids (fatty acidemia without ketonemia); elevated uric acid; normal or slightly elevated serum bilirubin jaundice.
5. Lumbar puncture—done if cerebrospinal fluid is needed to rule out other diagnoses. If symptoms of increased intracranial pressure exist, the performance of a lumbar puncture is to be avoided to prevent rapid decompression and herniation of the brain.
6. Liver biopsy—usually done, however the biopsy may not be done unless evidence is insufficient to make a definite diagnosis (shows microvesicular fatty degeneration of liver).

Medical and Nursing Management

1. Because this is a multisystem disease, it must be emphasized that:
   a. Intracerebral integrity is of utmost priority, and if the brain can be supported through the course of the illness, the chances of the other organs running their course uneventfully are very high and are of less concern.
   b. The multidisciplinary team must have a leader who initiates, coordinates, and supervises *all* activities and medical planning. It may be the physician, neurosurgeon, endocrinologist, or the attending pediatrician. However, it should be the person with the knowledge and capability of monitoring and directing care 24 hours a day.

2. Treatment is supportive by maintaining adequate levels of circulating glucose and cerebral perfusion while preventing or controlling IICP (increased intracranial pressure). Supportive intervention includes:**
   a. Admission to an intensive care unit. Multisystem invasive monitoring: complex coordination of care (medical and nursing) of all systems is essential in order to control and reduce IICP.
      (1) It takes many hours to several days after control of the disease process is achieved to begin to withdraw therapy or liberalize intervention without having recurring IICP symptoms.
      (2) The nurse is the most constant and consistent person at the bedside in most institutions and must be alert to all aspects of this very complex critical-care problem.
      (3) The nursing input may have a very significant impact on the morbidity of the patient; a knowledgeable nurse can make very important judgments concerning the timing of interventions and can anticipate problems and needs.
      (4) Nursing responsibilities include assessment, reassessment, anticipation, and documentation of physical status, environmental impacts, and therapeutic interventions.
   b. Administer phytonadione—to combat coagulation defects.
   c. Monitoring blood glucose—IV glucose given to prevent any neurological deterioration (hypertonic solution up to 30% IV drip through a central line).
   d. Limit fluid intake—peripheral IV fluids given at a rate of ⅔'s maintenance because of potential cerebral edema and IICP.
   e. Sedation—(stages I & II) to decrease anxiety and potential for IICP.
   f. Intraventricular pressure catheter or subarachnoid bolt with pressure monitoring and control of IICP.‡
   g. Endo- or naso-tracheal intubation and ventilation—to provide optimum cerebral blood flow. (Auto regulation − $\downarrow$ pCO_2 = $\downarrow$ size blood vessels = $\downarrow$ vol = $\downarrow$ ICP.
   h. Prevent and control IICP wth drugs.
      (1) Muscle relaxation (pancuronium bromide) while on ventilator
      (2) Sedation (Valium, chloral hydrate)
      (3) Osmotic diuretic (mannitol or glycerol)
      (4) Barbiturate therapy (thiopental, phenobarbital)***

---

*From Lovejoy FH et al. Clinical staging in Reye's syndrome. Am J Dis Child 1974 July; 128(1):36–41

†See bibliography for EEG typing references.

** Suggested reading: DeVivo DC, Keating JP, Haymond MW. Reye's syndrome: Results of intensive supportive care, Part I. J Pediatr 1975 Dec; 87(6):875–880

‡ Suggested reading: Hanlon D. Description and uses of intracranial pressure monitoring. Heart Lung 1976 Mar/Apr; 5(2):277–282

*** Suggested reading: Marshall LF, Shapiro HM, Rauscher A, Kaufman NM. Phenobarbital therapy for intracranial hypertension in metabolic coma. Crit Care Med 1978 Jan/Feb; 6(1):1–5

(5) Secondary infection coverage—especially staphylococcus (neuro and lung)

i. When all intensive medical and nursing support has been exhausted and ICP is still uncontrollable or cardiovascular status is unstable, consideration for bilateral decompression craniectomies must be made by the medical team.

Nursing Intervention

1. During the acute phase of the disease, the child should be cared for in an intensive care unit.
2. Refer to:
   Respiratory procedures, page 1189
   Cardiopulmonary resuscitation, page 1205
   Assisting with obtaining blood for gas analysis, page 1165
   Intensive care, page 1137
   Intravenous therapy, page 1171
   Increased intracranial pressure, page 1388
   Care of the comatose patient, page 706
   N/g tube procedures, page 404
   Catheter procedure, page 481
3. Be aware of the medical plan of treatment being used, and be alert to the rapidity of the course of the disease.* Particularly important factors:
   a. Note and report immediately any changes in the child's status or stage of progression (see clinical manifestations).
   b. Therapy is directed at maintaining normal intra-cranial pressure and adequate cerebral perfusion.
   c. Protect the child from complications that may result from the comatose condition or life-saving medical intervention.
   d. Maintain fluid and electrolyte balance.
   e. Before any procedure is done for the child, consider the effects on his intracranial pressure.
4. Support parents during the time that the child may be in the intensive care unit.
   a. Prior to the first visit, explain in detail what the child will look like. Accompany the parents when they first visit their child. Since this may be traumatic, do not force them to maintain lengthy contact with the child.
   b. Address parental concerns and answer questions regarding:
      (1) How they should react to their child
      (2) Amount of parental participation that is beneficial
      (3) Fears and fantasies during lengthy periods when they are unable to visit child
      (4) Concerns for other children and other family members, and their reactions to the illness
      (5) Technical questions
   c. Provide the parents with the phone number of the intensive care unit.
   d. Make sure parents have a comfortable place to sleep if they elect to stay at the hospital.
   e. Help parents who request consults—social service for ICU, chaplain, Reye's Syndrome Foundation parent group (if appropriate and available).

f. Help the family express their feelings about what has happened and how it is affecting them.
   (1) Assess how they are coping; their family support systems.
   (2) Initiate referrals to appropriate social agencies as needed.
   (3) The lack of knowledge and rapid course of the disease from a mild to a critical illness may be difficult for parents to understand. They may have extreme feelings of guilt, and blame themselves or others for not recognizing the seriousness of the illness sooner. They may have other children at home with similar pro-dromal viral infection who may be experiencing guilty feelings about the ill sibling.
5. Provide psychological and emotional support to the child.
   a. Although the child may be heavily sedated, coma-tose, or paralyzed from muscle relaxants, he perceives in varying degrees what is happening to him and to his environment.
   b. Explain procedures to the child while they are being done.
   c. Conversations about the child, his condition, or other children should take place away from the sick child.
   d. Encourage parents to bring in a favorite toy or security object.
   e. Show a constant awareness of any activity, noise, etc. that increases or changes intracranial pressure.
   f. When a sedated or comatose child awakens, he may be disoriented and have no memory of previous events. Provide explanations and reassurance as appropriate.
   g. Parental separation may increase anxiety; support as necessary.
6. Post-transfer to pediatric nursing unit:
   a. Once the child is alert, his condition stable, and he is recovering, he should be transferred to the regular pediatric unit.
   b. The child recovering from Reye's syndrome without any neurologic sequelae, should recover fairly rapidly. Provide support as needed.
   c. When the child has experienced sequelae or complications, attention to his physical manifestations will be needed according to the child's specific deficit (i.e., physical therapy). A multidisciplinary team approach to treatment will continue to provide for optimal functioning.
   d. The child and his family will continue to need emotional support during this period.
   e. A critical role of the nurse is to educate herself, other members of the staff, and the community about Reye's syndrome.†
      (1) Learn to recognize the symptoms that may lead to a diagnosis of the illness.
      (2) Be prepared for the course of the illness, from a mild disease to one that is life-threatening.
      (3) Support parent groups and other community groups to educate parents about Reye's syndrome, and to seek medical consultation when symptoms may indicate the disease.

* Suggested reading: Nikas DC and Konkoly R. Nursing responsibilities in arterial and intracranial pressure monitoring. J Neuro Nur 1975 Dec; 7(2):116–122

† National Reye's Syndrome Foundation, P.O. Box R.S., Benzonia, MI 49616

BIBLIOGRAPHY

Books

Bell W and McCormick W. Neurologic Infections in Children. Philadelphia, WB Saunders, 1975

Buscaglia L. The Disabled and Their Parents: A Counseling Challenge. Thorofare, Charles B Slack, 1975

Conway BL. Pediatric Neurologic Nursing. St. Louis, CV Mosby, 1977

Downey JA and Low NL (eds). The Child with Disabling Illness. Philadelphia, WB Saunders, 1974

Farmer TW (ed). Pediatric Neurology, 2nd ed. New York, Harper & Row, 1975

Freeman J. Practical Management of Meningomyelocele. Baltimore, University Park Press, 1974

Livingston S. Comprehensive Management of Epilepsy in Infancy, Childhood and Adolescence. Springfield, Charles C Thomas, 1972

Lovell W and Winter R (eds). Pediatric Orthopedics, Vol. 1. Philadelphia, JB Lippincott, 1978

McCormick W and Bell W. Increased Intracranial Pressure in Children. Philadelphia, WB Saunders, 1972

Milhorat TH. Hydrocephalus and the Cerebrospinal Fluid. Baltimore, Williams & Wilkins, 1972

Milhorat TH. Pediatric Neurosurgery. In Plum F and McDowell F (eds). Contemporary Neurology Series, Vol. 16. Philadelphia, FA Davis, 1978

O'Brien MS (ed). Pediatric Neurological Surgery. New York, Raven Press, 1978

Svoboda W. Learning about Epilepsy. Baltimore, University Park Press, 1979

Swaiman K and Wright F. Pediatric Neuromuscular Diseases. St. Louis, CV Mosby, 1979

Thompson R and Green J (eds). Pediatric Neurology and Neurosurgery. New York, Spectrum Publications, 1978

Whaley L and Wong D. Nursing Care of Infants and Children. St. Louis, CV Mosby, 1979

Articles

Baum M. I want to be dry! The (almost) carefree way to conquer urinary incontinence. Nursing '78 1978 Feb; 8(2):75–78

Bernardo M. When your caseload includes a hydrocephalic child. Pediatric Nursing 1979 May/June; 5(3):27–29

Bindler R and Howry L. Nursing care of children with febrile convulsions. MCN 1978 Sept/Oct; 3(5):270–273

Carrington EG. A seating position for a cerebral-palsied child. AJOT 1978 Mar; 32(3):179–181

Coughlin M. Teaching children about their seizures and medications. MCN 1979 May/June; 4(3):161–162

Farley J. Valproic acid for children with uncontrolled epilepsy. MCN 1979 May/June; 4(3):163–164

Fishman MA. Febrile seizures: The treatment controversy. J Pediatr 1979 Feb; 94(2):177–184

Freeman JM. Febrile seizures: An end to confusion. Pediatrics 1978 May; 61(5):806–808

Godec CJ et al. Electrical stimulation for incontinence in myelomeningocele. J Urol 1978 Dec; 120(6):729–731

Hall P et al. Scoliosis and hydrocephalus in myelocele patients. The effects of ventricular shunting. J Neurosurg 1979 Feb; 50(2):174–178

Hartman M. Intermittent self-catheterization: Freeing your patient of the foley. Nursing '78 1978 Nov; 8(11):72–74

Hawken M and Ozuna J. Practical aspects of anticonvulsant therapy. Am J Nurs 1979 June; 79(6):1062–1068

Hawley D and Reiser D. Reducing muscle spasms in the child with cerbral palsy. Am J Nurs 1978 July; 78(7):1214–1215

Henderson M and Synhorst D. Bladder and bowel management in the child with myelomeningocele. Pediatric Nursing 1977 Sept/Oct; 3(5):24–31

How to tell if a baby has cerebral palsy . . . and what to tell his parents when he does. Nursing '79 1979 May; 9(5):88–94

Jackson P. Ventriculo-peritoneal shunts. Am J Nurs 1980 June; 80(6):1104–1109

Jones AM. Overcoming feeding problems of the mentally and the physically handicapped. J Hum Nutr 1978 Oct; 32(5):359–367

Jones C. Glasgow coma scale. Am J Nurs 1979 Sept; 79(9):1551–1553

Keane WM et al. Meningitis and hearing loss in children. Arch Otolaryngol 1979 Jan; 104(1):39–44

Langner BE and Schott JR. Nursing implications of central nervous system infections in children. Issues Compr Pediatr Nurs 1977 July/Aug; 2(2)38–53

Lewis A. Ileal loop undiversion: A collaborative nursing approach. Pediatric Nursing 1979 July/Aug; 5(4):42–47

Mills G. Preparing children and parents for cerebral computerized tomography. MCN 1980 Nov/Dec; 5(6): 403–407

Mitchell PH and Mauss NK. Relationship of parent–nurse activity to intracranial pressure variations: A pilot study. Nurs Res 1978 Jan/Feb; 27(1):4–10

Muehl J. Seizure disorders in children: Prevention and care. MCN 1979 May/June; 4(3):154–160

Nelson KB et al. Neonatal signs as predictors of cerebral palsy. Pediatrics 1979 Aug; 64(2):225–232

Nelson KB et al. Prognosis in children with febrile seizures. Pediatrics 1978 May; 61(5):720–727

Ottenbacher K et al. A toilet seat arrangement for children with neuromotor dysfunction. AJOT 1979 Mar; 33(3):193

Owen M. Orthopedic management of a child with a spinal cord disorder. Pediatric Nursing 1977 Sept/Oct; 3(4): 37–40

Park LD. The summer family conference: An adventure in counseling families with handicapped children. Rehabil Lit 1979 Apr; 40(4):108–110

Passo S. Positioning infants with myelomeningocele. Am J Nurs 1974 Sept; 74(9):1658–1660

Robinson L. Phenytoin in anticonvulsant therapy. Pediatric Nursing 1979 May/June; 5(3):57–58

Spitz P and Sweetwood H. Kids in crisis. Part I: Bedside assessment. Special considerations. Nursing '78 1978 Mar; 8(3):70–79

Swift N. Helping patients live with seizures. Nursing '78 1978 June; 8(6):25–31

Teasdale G et al. Observer variability in assessing impaired consciousness and coma. J Neurol Neurosurg Psychiatry 1978 July; 41(7):603–610

Vigliarolo D. Managing bowel incontinence in children with meningomyelocele. Am J Nurs 1980 Jan; 80(1):105–107

Wolf SM et al. Behavior disturbance, phenobarbital and febrile seizures. Pediatics 1978 May; 61(5):728–731

Agency

National Institute of Neurological Diseases and Stroke, National Institutes of Health, Bethesda, Md. 20014

REYE'S SYNDROME

Books

Crocker JF. Reye's Syndrome II. New York, Grune & Stratton, 1979

Levin DC, Morriss FC, Moore GC. A Practical Guide to Pediatric Intensive Care. St. Louis, CV Mosby, 1979

Scipien GM et al. Comprehensive Pediatric Nursing. New York, McGraw-Hill, 1979

Vaughn VC, McKay RS, Behrman RE. Nelson Textbook of Pediatrics, 11th ed. Philadelphia, WB Saunders, 1979

Wright EG. Reye's Syndrome in Current Practice in Pediatric Nursing, Vol. 3, pp. 206–221. Chinn PL and Leonard KB (eds). St. Louis, CV Mosby, 1980

Articles

Aski Y and Lombroso CT. Prognostic value of electroencephalography in Reye's syndrome. Neurology 1973 Apr; 23(4):333–343

Haller J. Intracranial pressure monitoring in Reye's syndrome. Hosp Pract 1980 Feb; 15(2):101–108

Kolata GB. Reye's syndrome: A medical mystery. Science 1980 Mar 28; 207(4438):1453–1454

Lovejoy FC et al. Clinical staging in Reye's syndrome. Am J Dis Child 1974 July 128; 36–41

Nelson DB, Shaywitz BA, Venes SL. Reye's syndrome: Early recognition is vital. Patient Care 1978 Jan 15; 12(1):187+

Reye RD, Morgan G, Barae J. Encephalopathy and fatty degeneration of the viscera—a disease entity in children. Lancet 1963 Oct 12; 2(7310):749–752

Weeks HL. What every ICU nurse should know about Reye's syndrome. MCN 1976 July/Aug; 1:231–238

CHILDREN WITH ORTHOPEDIC CONDITIONS

49

FRACTURES

Generally, nursing care of the child with a fracture is similar to that of an adult. The child is usually hospitalized only for application of a cast (see procedure for cast care, p. 1218) or to be placed in traction (see procedure for traction, p. 1209). The nurse should be aware of the following principles concerning fractures in pediatrics.

General Considerations

1. Bones do not fracture as easily in children as in adults.
      Bones are softer and more pliable.
2. Greenstick fractures in normal bones are unique to children.
    a. The bone breaks at one cortex and bends at the other.
    b. There is no complete loss of bony continuity.
    c. The younger the child, the more likely he is to sustain a greenstick fracture.
    d. The radius, ulna, clavicle, or long bone in the hand are most likely to sustain a greenstick fracture.
3. Comminuted fractures are less common in pediatric patients.
4. Injuries of the epiphyseal plate are unique to children.
    a. The epiphyseal plate is weaker than normal tendons, ligaments or joint capsule.
    b. Injury resulting in a torn ligament or dislocation in the adult is more likely to produce a separation of the epiphysis in a child.
    c. The lower radial epiphysis is more frequently separated than any other.
    d. This type of injury may cause growth disturbance.
5. Fractures in pediatric patients heal more readily than those in adults.
    a. The younger the child, the more rapidly the fracture unites.
    b. The thick periosteum and abundant blood supply make nonunion rare.
6. End-to-end apposition of fracture surfaces is not essential in pediatric patients.
    a. The long bones may be allowed to unite with side-to-side apposition in children up to 11–12 years of age.

    b. Subsequent molding will produce a normal bone by the end of growth.
7. Following injury, the limbs in children are likely to swell much more rapidly and the swelling to disappear more quickly than in an adult.
8. Function is usually restored rapidly and sometimes spontaneously following injury in children.

COMMON FRACTURES IN CHILDREN

Fracture of the Clavicle

A. *Cause*
1. Compression of the shoulders during delivery of a baby
2. Transmitted force caused by falling on an outstretched hand, elbow, or side of the shoulder
3. Direct force (rare)

B. *Treatment*
1. Immobilization with a figure eight bandage or plaster of paris cast
2. Complete fixation by supporting the limb in a triangular sling suspended from the opposite shoulder.
      This treatment is helpful if the child demonstrates associated torticollis or when there is posterior displacement of the distal fragment.

C. *Healing Time*
1. Younger children: 3–4 weeks
2. Older children: 5–6 weeks

Fracture of the Neck of the Humerus

A. *Cause*
1. Indirect force from a fall on an outstretched hand
2. Direct force by blow or fall on the lateral aspect of the shoulder

B. *Treatment*
1. Minimal displacement
      Immobilization of the shoulder and upper limb with stockinette collar and sling.
2. Considerable displacement
    a. Reduction under anesthesia may be done.
    b. Immobilization of the shoulder and upper limb in a collar and cuff sling or a shoulder spica.

c. Dunlop traction followed by use of a shoulder spica cast may be required in severe cases.

C. *Healing Time*

1. Minimal displacement: 3–4 weeks
2. Considerable displacement: 4–6 weeks

Fractures of the Shaft of the Humerus

A. *Cause*

1. Birth injury—most common long bone to be fractured at that time
2. Direct force, such as a fall on the side of the arm
3. Indirect force, such as throwing a ball, grabbing a child's arm to prevent a fall, and pulling an arm in and out of a sleeve roughly

B. *Treatment*

1. Reduction of the fracture
2. Immobilization
   a. Infants and young children
      (1) A U-slab of plaster is used to keep the arm against the chest with the elbow at a 90- to 45-degree angle.
      (2) Skin traction may be necessary for 2–3 weeks if the fracture is unstable or oblique with much overriding of the fragments.
         The arm is then immobilized as described above until healing is complete.
   b. Older children or adolescents
      (1) A shoulder spica cast is used for an unstable fracture.
      (2) Skeletal traction and suspension of the forearm and hand are indicated if the local skin and soft tissue conditions do not permit skin traction.
      (3) A hanging cast may be used for an older adolescent.
         (a) This type of cast permits the child to be ambulatory and active.
         (b) Erect position should be maintained as much as possible during the day.
         (c) The child should sleep in a semirecumbent position.
         (d) There should be no support at the elbow.
         (e) Pressure from clothing or anything that might compress the arm against the body must be avoided as it interferes with traction.

C. *Healing Time*

   4–6 weeks

Supracondylar Fracture of the Humerus

A. *Cause*

   Fall on an outstretched hand with hyperextension of the elbow
   (Most common type of elbow fracture in children and adolescents)

B. *Treatment*

1. Should be managed as an acute emergency because of the danger of neurovascular complications.
2. Minimally displaced fractures—immobilization in a collar and cuff sling.
3. Moderately displaced fractures
   a. Closed reduction under anesthesia
   b. Immobilization in a long arm cast or collar and cuff sling

c. Need for Dunlop skin traction for a period of 5–7 days until swelling subsides and a long arm cast can be applied
   Circulation and neural function should be carefully assessed.
4. Severely displaced fractures
   a. Closed reduction under anesthesia
   b. Skeletal traction with the shoulder abducted 60 degrees and the arm elevated 20 degrees above the horizontal until the fracture is stable
      Circulation and neural function should be carefully assessed.
   c. Continued immobilization in a long arm cast or collar and cuff sling

C. *Healing Time*

1. 3–6 weeks.
2. Several months may be required for complete restoration of function.

D. *Complications*

1. Malunion and changes in carrying angle
2. Vascular complications
   The extremity should be observed for pallor, pain, absent pulse, paresthesia, and paralysis.

Fractures of the Distal Third of the Radius and Ulna

A. *Cause*

1. Fracture may result from indirect force, such as falling on an outstretched hand.
2. Bones may break at different levels, and each fracture may be complete or greenstick.

B. *Treatment*

1. Greenstick fracture
   a. Closed reduction if the degree of angulation exceeds 30 degrees in infants or 15 degrees in children
   b. Immobilization in a long arm cast
2. Complete fracture
   a. Reduction under anesthesia
   b. Immobilization in an above-elbow cast

C. *Healing Time*

   4–6 weeks

Fractures Involving the Distal Radial Physis

A. *Cause*

1. Indirect force by falling on an outstretched hand
2. Most common physical injury

B. *Treatment*

1. Closed reduction
2. Immobilization in a long arm cast

C. *Healing Time*

   3–4 weeks

Fractures of the Phalanges

A. *Cause*

   Direct force to the finger

B. *Treatment*

1. Distal phalanx
   a. Aluminum finger splint
   b. Splinting of adjoining finger
2. Middle phalanx
   a. Manual traction and flexion of the distal fragment

b. Immobilization in a below-elbow plaster cast with a padded aluminum splint

c. Unstable fractures—need for skeletal traction with a pin through the distal phalanx

C. *Healing Time*

2–5 weeks.

Femoral Shaft Fracture

A. *Cause*

1. Major force, either direct or indirect, such as that sustained in automobile accidents or falls from a height
2. Requires treatment as serious injury because of the blood loss and potential shock which may accompany the primary trauma

B. *Treatment*

1. Infants and children under 2 years of age
   a. Bryant's traction for 2–3 weeks until the fracture is stable
   b. Immobilization in a 1½ hip spica cast until solid union occurs
2. Older children and adolescents
   a. Undisplaced fracture
      Immobilization in a hip spica cast
   b. Displaced fracture
      (1) Reduction and traction until fracture is stable.

Traction type depends on location and manner of displacement—usually Russell, split Russell, or balanced traction with Thomas splint and Pearson attachment.

(2) Immobilization in a spica cast until bony union is firm.

C. *Healing Time*

3–12 weeks, depending on the child's age and the type of fracture

D. *Complications*

1. Discrepancy in limb length
2. Angular deformities of the femoral shaft

Fracture of the Tibia or Fibula

A. *Cause*

1. Direct force
2. Indirect rotational twisting force

B. *Treatment*

1. Closed reduction
2. Immobilization in a long leg cast—during the final weeks of healing, partial weight-bearing in a walking cast may be permitted.

C. *Healing Time*

3–6 weeks, depending on the age of the child and the type of fracture

OSTEOMYELITIS

Osteomyelitis is an infection which may involve all parts of a bone.

Etiology

1. Pathogenic bacteria commonly associated with osteomyelitis
   a. *Staphylococcus aureus*—responsible for the majority of cases (up to 90%)
   b. Streptococcal organisms
   c. *Salmonella*
   d. H. influenzae
2. Exogenous osteomyelitis—acquired by direct invasion of the bone by extension from the outside, as from a penetrating wound, fracture, etc.
3. Hematogenous osteomyelitis (more common)—caused by hematogenous spread of organisms from another focus
   Identifiable primary lesions
   (1) Furunculosis
   (2) Impetigo
   (3) Vaccinations
   (4) Infected chicken-pox
   (5) Burns
   (6) Infected scratches, pimples, or boils
   (7) Nose or throat infections
   (8) Abscessed teeth
4. Preconditions favoring development of osteomyelitis in children
   a. Bone regions that have suffered trauma
   b. Bone that suffers from low oxygen tension of sickle cell anemia

Incidence

1. Most frequent occurrence between 5–14 years of age
2. More frequent in males than in females

Altered Physiology

1. Infection starts in the soft, medullary tissues.
2. This causes hyperemia, changes in the capillary permeability and edema of the tissue.
3. Granulocytic leukocytes infiltrate the area and are destroyed by bacteria, liberating a proteolytic enzyme which causes tissue necrosis.
4. The inflammatory reaction causes thrombosis of vessels, producing irregular areas of bone ischemia.
5. Pus forms and spreads toward the diaphysis and extends through the cortex of the bone.
6. A subperiosteal abscess is formed with elevation of the periosteum.
7. There is further interference of blood supply to the bone shaft.
   a. Vascular supply may remain sufficient to maintain life of bone tissue:
      (1) New bone is created.
      (2) Bone healing occurs.
   b. Vascular supply may be diminished below that which is necessary to maintain life of bone tissue.
      (1) Bone dies and becomes inert.
         Small pieces of dead bone may be completely destroyed by granulation tissue from contiguous living tissue.
      (2) Large pieces of dead bone cannot be completely destroyed.
         (a) Central residual remains as a sequestrum composed of cancellous or cortical bone or a combination.
         (b) New bone is laid down beneath the elevated periosteum and tends to form an encasement (involucrum) around the sequestrum.
         (c) The involucrum is punctured by numerous

channels through which pus may escape from the inside.

    (d) Pockets of infection are walled off in which organisms can lie dormant for long periods of time.

    (e) Chronic sinuses may form which eventually reach the surface and drain.

    (f) Drainage continues until infection quiets once more.

        Channels become plugged up with granulations and remain closed until the pressure of the pus builds up and causes the sinuses to reopen or reach the surface via new channels (chronic osteomyelitis).

    (g) Complete healing takes place only when all of the dead bone has been destroyed, discharged, or excised.

Clinical Manifestations

A. *Onset*

1. Usually abrupt
2. May be altered when osteomyelitis follows an infection which has been treated by antimicrobials.

B. *Initial Symptoms*

1. Pain in the involved area
2. Fever
3. Malaise

C. *Later Symptoms*

1. Swelling, redness, and warmth over the affected bone
2. Weakness
3. Irritability
4. Generalized signs of sepsis

D. *Common Sites of Infection in Children*

1. Large, cylindrical bones of the extremities
   a. Femur
   b. Tibia
   c. Humerus
   d. Radius
2. Primary focus is usually in the metaphysis of a bone at the end of the area of most rapid growth.
   a. Knee region
   b. Lower end of the femur
   c. Upper end of the tibia

Diagnostic Evaluation

1. Leukocytosis
2. Blood culture—usually positive
3. Sedimentation rate usually elevated
4. X-ray data
   a. Progressive findings
      (1) Periosteal reaction
      (2) Areas of radiolucency secondary to bone destruction
      (3) Evidence of the formation of involucrum (reactive, living bone)
   b. Progress of the disease not seen on x-ray for at least 5 days in small children; as long as 8–10 days in older children.
5. Tomography may reveal bone changes at an early stage.

Treatment

1. Intravenous administration of antimicrobial therapy
2. Immobilization of the affected extremity

3. Surgical decompression of the infected bony area may be necessary with insertion of drains.

Prognosis

1. Mortality rate markedly improved with the advent of modern antimicrobial agents
2. Depends on early institution of appropriate therapy and adequate continuation

Nursing Objectives

A. *To treat the infection with antimicrobial therapy.*

1. Administer intravenous antimicrobials as prescribed by the physician.
   a. Administer medication exactly on schedule in order to maintain consistent blood levels.
   b. Monitor intravenous infusion carefully.
      (1) Notify physician if infiltration is suspected, so that the IV can be restarted.
      (2) A venous cutdown is often necessary, especially for a small child.
      (3) A constant infusion pump may be helpful if the infusion rate is slow.
      (4) A heparin lock may be useful because it allows the child to be more active between medication doses.
2. Perform irrigations of the infected area with antimicrobial solutions as prescribed by the physician.
3. Be alert for evidence of drug reactions.
4. Consider drug stability and compatability with other intravenous antibiotics when planning schedule for administration.

B. *To increase the child's comfort.*

1. Administer analgesics as prescribed by the physician.
2. Rest the affected extremity.
   a. Traction or splints may be used to reduce pain and prevent contractures in the soft tissues.
   b. Avoid excessive handling of the infected extremity, because this is very painful and may spread infection.
      (1) Bed linens should be changed only when necessary.
      (2) When it is necessary to move the extremity, support the joints above and below the affected part as well as the area itself.
      (3) Move the extremity in a smooth, unhurried, and gentle manner.

C. *To protect other patients and personnel from the infectious organism.*

1. Isolate children with draining wounds.
2. Utilize careful handwashing procedure.
3. Utilize strict aseptic technique when performing irrigations, changing dressings, and handling drainage.

D. *To facilitate wound healing.*

Maintain adequate nutrition and hydration.

1. Offer abundant fluids according to the child's preference.
2. Provide a diet which is rich in protein and vitamin C.
3. Allow the child to participate in selection of foods and preparation of his meal tray.
4. Refer to section on nutrition, p. 1112.

E. *To observe for evidence of response to treatment or progress of disease.*

1. Monitor the child's temperature at frequent intervals and record the pattern.

Notify the physician of a sudden increase in temperature.
2. Monitor and record the extent of swelling, redness, pain, and limitation of movement in the affected extremity.
3. Monitor and record the amount and nature of drainage if the infection has been drained.

F. *To provide emotional support to the parents.*

1. Parents often feel guilty if they did not recognize early signs of the disease.
2. Assist parents to express and deal with their feelings. Initiate a social service referral if appropriate.
3. Refer to section on family-centered care, p. 1131.

G. *To assist the child to maintain many of his normal activities during the lengthy hospitalization.*

1. Allow the child to be dressed during the convalescent period.
2. Encourage the child to attend playroom activities, even if he must be moved in his bed.
3. Initiate plans for the child's continuing education, and provide time each day for his school work.

4. Encourage liberal visiting by family and friends.

H. *To provide for continuity of care following the child's discharge from the hospital.*

1. Encourage parents to participate in all aspects of the child's care during hospitalization.
   a. Parents should be instructed and should have an opportunity to practice (under nursing supervision) all procedures which will be required at home. (Procedures often include changes of dressing, application of a splint, or use of appliances such as crutches.)
   b. The child should not be discharged until both the parents and the nurse are satisfied with the parents' level of competency.
2. Instruct parents to observe for evidence of complications, such as deformity, stiffness of joints, fracture, and disease recurrence.
3. Initiate a community health nursing referral if appropriate.

CONGENITAL DISLOCATION OF THE HIP

Congenital dislocation of the hip refers to a malposition of the head of the femur in the acetabulum. The head of the femur is usually dislocated posterosuperiorly. Dislocation may be either partial or complete and may be either unilateral or bilateral.

Etiology

1. Unknown
2. Possible causes
   a. Abnormal development of the joint caused by:
      (1) Fetal position
      (2) Genetic factors
   b. Abnormal relaxation of the capsule and ligaments of the joint caused by hormonal factors
   c. Environmental factors such as breech delivery

Altered Physiology

1. Acetabulum tends to be shallow and extremely oblique.
2. Head of the femur tends to be smaller than normal.
3. Ossification centers are delayed in appearance.

Incidence

1. More common in female infants than in males.
2. Recurrence risk among siblings is greater when one child in the family has been affected.

Clinical Manifestations

(May not be observed until 1–2 months of age)
1. Asymmetry of the gluteal folds with deeper creases apparent on the affected side
2. Limited ability to abduct the hip when the infant is lying on his back with his knees and hips flexed to 90 degrees
   Normally, the hips will abduct at least 65 degrees.
3. Trendelenburg's sign
   Pelvis drops on the normal side if the child stands on his abnormal leg.
4. Apparent shortening of the thigh on the affected side

5. Knee joint on the affected side appears higher than the normal joint
6. Delayed walking
7. Limp
   a. Trunk dips when the child puts weight on his involved leg.
   b. Waddling gait is observed in children with bilateral dislocation.

Diagnostic Evaluation

1. Barlow's maneuver
   a. With the infant on a firm surface, the examiner grasps the symphysis pubis in front and the sacrum in back with one hand. The second hand grasps the thigh on the side of the hip being tested.
   b. Slight outward pressure is applied over the proximal thigh by the thumb while longitudinal pressure is applied in an effort to dislocate the hip out of its socket.
   c. Sensation of abnormal movement indicates a dislocation.
2. Ortolani's maneuver
   a. The examiner positions his hands in the same manner as for Barlow's maneuver.
   b. The thigh is brought away from the midline of the body into a position of abduction.
   c. A sensation or sound of a clicking or jerking into place may be detected with reduction of the head into the socket.
3. X-ray data (helpful only after the age of 4–5 months, when the hip bones are sufficiently developed).
   a. Acetabular angle greater than 40 degrees
   b. Upward and outward displacement of the femoral head.

Treatment

1. Varies with age and extent of the defect.
2. Early stages
   a. Reduction by gentle manipulation
   b. Splinting the hip in abduction by means of double

or triple diapers, an abduction splint, or a cloth harness
3. Later stages
   a. Preliminary traction
   b. Closed reduction
   c. Immobilization in a hip spica cast or splint
4. Older child
   a. Preliminary traction
   b. Possible need for open reduction or osteotomy
   c. Immobilization in a hip spica cast

Prognosis

1. Depends on the age of the child when the condition is diagnosed.
2. Delay in diagnosis prolongs treatment and may preclude formation of a normal hip.

Nursing Management

Generally, nursing care of the child with congenital dislocation of the hip is provided in a convalescent hospital or by the mother at home. Nursing activities during hospitalization are those related to the child's care when he is in traction or after application of a hip spica cast (refer to p. 1218). In addition, the following considerations are important:
1. If the child is to be treated with an abduction splint, explain its purpose and demonstrate its application to the parents.
   a. Allow parents to practice application of the splint with nursing supervision.
   b. Clarify with parents the times that the splint is to be worn and how long it can be removed for bathing, dressing, diaper changes, etc.
   c. Demonstrate handling of the child in such a way that the hips are kept abducted.
2. Encourage family-centered care (refer to p. 1131).

CONGENITAL CLUBFOOT (TALIPES EQUINOVARUS)

Congenital clubfoot refers to a deformity in which the affected foot and leg have a clublike appearance. Talipes equinovarus is one of the most common congenital deformities of the foot, occurring in approximately one in 1000 live births.

Etiology

1. Exact cause unknown.
2. Evidence indicates a mixed genetic and environmental causation.
3. Tends to recur in families already having 1 affected child.
4. Males are affected twice as often as females.

Pathophysiology

1. Pathologic anatomy
   a. Inversion and adduction of the forepart of the foot
   b. Inversion of the heel
2. Soft tissue changes are adaptive in nature, conforming to the skeletal deformity.
   The soft tissues on the medial and posterior aspect of the foot and ankle are shortened.

Clinical Manifestations

1. Varies in severity from a mild deformity to one in which the toes touch the medial side of the lower leg.
   a. Rigid type
      (1) Very severe deformity
      (2) Corrected only minimally by passive manipulation
      (3) Usually accompanied by moderate atrophy of the leg
   b. Flexible type
      The condition can be readily corrected to neutral position by passive manipulation.
2. Deformity increases progressively, and contractures become more rigid if the deformity is untreated.
   a. Child bears weight on the lateral border of the foot.
   b. Ambulation is difficult and gait is awkward.
   c. Callosities and bursae may develop over the lateral side of the foot.

Diagnostic Evaluation

1. Diagnosis is determined by clinical manifestations.
2. X-ray valuable for the following:
   a. Determination of the degree of varus and equinus deformity
   b. Demonstration of the deranged mechanics of the hindfoot
   c. Accurate assessment of the amount of correction obtained with treatment

Treatment and Nursing Management

1. Passive stretching exercises to manipulate the foot into normal position
   a. Technique of manipulation should be demonstrated to the nurse and parents by the physician, because there are many variations in the manner of performing the manipulation.
   b. The foot should be grasped well below the malleoli with 1 hand while the ankle is held rigid and stable with the other hand to avoid displacement of the epiphysis.
   c. The midfoot should not be stretched by forced dorsiflexion of the forefoot, or a "rocker-bottom" foot will result.
   d. The corrected position should be maintained to the count of 10.
   e. The exercises should be continued for 10 to 15 minutes several times each day.
   f. Manipulation should be done before feedings, because it may cause some discomfort for the baby.
2. Manipulation and casting
   a. A plaster of paris cast is applied from the toes to the groin with the knee flexed.
      Casts are changed frequently; with each cast change the foot is manipulated to obtain further correction.
   b. Once the deformity is fully corrected, the foot is held in an overcorrected position in a solid cast for 3 to 6 weeks.
      (1) Parents should be instructed in cast care. (Refer to p. 1218.)
      (2) Parents should be alerted that if the foot

portion of the cast becomes thin or worn, the cast should be reapplied.

(3) Parents can be taught to soak off old casts prior to clinic visits by immersing the cast in a solution of 1 part vinegar to 4 parts water and then unwrapping the plaster.

3. Denis Browne splint
   a. The splint is composed of a flexible horizontal bar attached to a pair of footplates.
      (1) The infant's feet are attached to the footplates by means of special shoes or adhesive tape.
      (2) The desired position of the foot is controlled by positioning the abduction bar and the footplates.
      (3) The infant provides his own corrective manipulation by his normal activity.
   b. Parents should be instructed in the following details of care:
      (1) Application and removal of the splint
      (2) Times the splint is to be worn
      (3) Protection of the feet by socks
      (4) Skin care

(5) Use of splint key to tighten the shoes against the bar if they become loose

4. Continued treatment
   a. Treatment is continued until the child is able to walk normally and until the wear on several pairs of shoes demonstrates that there has been no recurrence of deformity.
   b. Foot is held in an overcorrected position at night by means of bivalved casts or a Denis Browne splint.
   c. A prewalker clubfoot shoe with valgus strap may be prescribed for the infant's use during the day.
   d. An older child may require special shoes which promote walking in the overcorrected position.
   e. Passive stretching exercises are continued.

5. Indications for surgical measures
   a. Failure of conservative methods to correct the deformity
   b. In older children severe and rigid deformities which will obviously not respond to nonsurgical measures

LEGG-CALVÉ-PERTHES DISEASE (COXA PLANA)

Legg-Calvé-Perthes disease is an aseptic necrosis of the capital femoral epiphysis secondary to ischemia.

Etiology

Unknown

Incidence

1. Males between the ages of 4–10 years of age are most frequently affected.
2. Condition tends to recur in families.
3. White children are affected 10 times more frequently than black children.

Clinical Manifestations

(May be intermittent initially)
1. Synovitis causing limp and pain in the hip.
2. Referred pain to the knee, inner thigh, and groin
3. Limited abduction and internal rotation of the hip
4. Mild to moderate muscle spasm
5. Atrophy of the muscles of the mid and upper thigh
6. Bilateral involvement is infrequent

Altered Physiology

A. *Stage I (Avascularity)*
1. Spontaneous interruption of the blood supply to the upper femoral epiphysis occurs.
2. Bone-forming cells in the epiphysis die and bone ceases to grow.
3. Slight widening of the joint space occurs.
4. Swelling of the soft tissues around the hip occurs.

B. *Stage II (Revascularization)*
1. Growth of new vessels supplies the area of necrosis; both bone resorption and deposition take place.
2. The new bone is not strong, and pathologic fractures occur.
3. Abnormal forces on the weakened epiphysis may produce progressive deformity, including lateral epiphyseal fracture and extrusion of the femoral head laterally from the acetabulum.

C. *Stage III (Reossification)*
1. The head of the femur gradually reforms.
2. Nucleus of the epiphysis breaks up into a number of fragments with cyst-like spaces between them.
3. New bone starts to develop at the medial and lateral edges of the epiphysis which becomes widened.
4. Dead bone is removed and is replaced with new bone which gradually spreads to heal the lesion.

D. *Stage IV (Postrecovery Period)*
1. Without treatment
   a. Head of the femur flattens and becomes mushroom shaped.
   b. Incongruity between the head of the femur and the acetabulum persists.
   c. Degenerative changes develop later in life.
2. Complete recovery
   a. Head of the femur remains spherical.
   b. Acetabulum appears normal.
   c. Width of the neck of the femur is normal.

Diagnostic Evaluation

X-ray findings are related to the stage of the disease.
1. Incipient period
   a. Swelling of the capsular shadows about the hip
   b. Widening of the joint space
   c. Demineralization of the femoral metaphysis in the neck
   d. Evidence of growth cessation of the proximal femoral epiphysis
2. Period of necrosis
   Increased density of the femoral head is observed in addition to the above changes.
3. Regenerative period
   a. Radiolucent areas—indication of revitalization of the femoral head
   b. Considerable flattening and widening of the femoral head
   c. Regeneration of the femoral head occurring until the head is filled in completely

Treatment

(Depends on type of involvement)
1. First goal—to restore full range of motion of the hip joint by alleviating synovitis and muscle spasm.
   Bed rest with or without traction
2. Second goal—to locate the femoral head deep in the acetabulum, thereby protecting it while revascularization and growth occur.
   a. Non-weightbearing abduction cast or brace.
   b. Weightbearing abduction casts or braces may be used once full range of motion has been restored except in older children with major femoral head involvement.
   c. Femoral osteotomy—indicated in cases of severe involvement of the femoral head.
3. Final goal—return to unassisted weightbearing.
   a. Unassisted weightbearing can be resumed once the increased density in the femoral head disappears, usually 6–15 months.
   b. The child's time out of the brace is gradually increased and his hip motion is evaluated frequently. Loss of motion is an indication that a longer period of bracing is necessary.

Prognosis

1. Depends on the stage at which the disease was diagnosed and treatment was instituted, and the age of the child at the time of onset.
   a. Treatment is more effective when it is begun early in the disease.
   b. Treatment is considered successful if the contour of the hip joint allows normal function after resolution of the disease.
   c. The younger the child at the onset of the disorder, the more complete recovery can be anticipated.
2. The disease may be present for 2–4 years, after which time it spontaneously resolves.
3. Limitation of motion and incongruity of joint surfaces may result if treatment is ineffective; condition may lead to degenerative joint disease in later life.

Nursing Objectives and Management

A. *To care for the child requiring traction or a spica cast.*

Refer to procedures, pages 1209 and 1218.

B. *To evaluate the home and provide guidance to the family regarding the child's home care.*

1. This guidance is important, because treatment may be continued in the home for an extended period.
2. The family should be made aware of convalescent facilities as an alternative to home care.

The family should be helped to make the decision between these alternatives and should be supported in its decisions.
3. Encourage family participation in the child's care so that members can become familiar with the details of his management. (Refer to section on family-centered care, p. 1131.)
4. A firm mattress is necessary.
5. Appropriate referrals may include the following:
   a. Community health nurse
   b. Social service
   c. Home teacher
   d. Physical therapy
   e. Occupational therapy

C. *To enable the child to participate in as many normal activities of life as possible.*

1. Plans must be made for continuing education.
2. Diversion is an extremely important consideration.
3. Play should include exercise for uninvolved extremities.
4. Special activities with peers should be arranged.

D. *To provide emotional support to the child and his family because of the long-term nature of the illness.*

1. Provide the family with frequent opportunities to express their feelings and concerns.
   Techniques of therapeutic play should be used with the child.
2. Point out even small indications of the recovery process.
3. Introduce the family to other families with similarly affected children, if available.

Patient and Parental Education

1. General techniques of home nursing
   a. Bathing and skin care
   b. Maintenance of good muscle tone, proper body alignment and prevention of contractures
   c. Provision for elimination
   d. Nutritional considerations
   e. Bedmaking
   f. Special equipment (e.g., traction, casts)
2. Pathology of the disease and rationale of treatment
   a. Reinforce medical explanations and clarify interpretations as necessary
   b. Allow the child to view his own x-rays with his parents, to increase his knowledge of the disease.
   c. Emphasize that complete recovery can occur only with strict adherence to the treatment regimen.
3. Necessity of regular medical follow-up for evaluation of the child's progress.

STRUCTURAL SCOLIOSIS

Structural scoliosis is a lateral curvature of the spine characterized by a defect in the bones and surrounding tissues of the spine.

Classification

1. According to the spinal segment involved
   a. Thoracic
   b. Lumbar
   c. Thoracolumbar
2. According to age group
   a. Infantile—birth to 3 years
   b. Juvenile—4 to 9 years

c. Adolescent—10 years to cessation of growth (usually found in females, with a right thoracic curve most common)

Etiology

1. Idiopathic
   a. Accounts for 80% of cases
   b. Possible familial incidence
2. Congenital
   a. Failure of vertebral formation
   b. Failure of segmentation
3. Neuropathic

Results from conditions such as poliomyelitis, cerebral palsy, paralysis, and neurofibromatosis.
4. Myopathic
   Associated with conditions such as muscular dystrophy and myopathies.
5. Osteopathic
   Results from conditions such as fractures, bone disease, arthritis, and infection.
6. Trauma such as fractures, burns, thoracoplasty.
7. Irritative phenomena such as spinal cord tumor or nerve root irritation.
8. Miscellaneous—Marfan's syndrome, postirradiation, metabolic, nutritional, or endocrinic factors.

Clinical Manifestations

1. Presenting complaints (See Pediatric Physical Examination, p. 1066.)
   a. Poor posture
   b. One shoulder higher than the other
   c. Hemline hanging unevenly
   d. One hip that seems more prominent
   e. Crooked neck
   f. Lump on back
   g. Waistline uneven
   h. One breast appearing larger
2. Visualization of deformity
3. Back pain

Pathophysiology

1. Lateral flexion of a scoliotic spine causes the trunk to shift away from the midline, altering the center of gravity and causing shortening of the spine.
2. Simultaneously, the spine rotates on its longitudinal axis, contributing to many of the clinical manifestations.
3. The vertebrae become permanently wedge-shaped.
4. The scoliosis is increased by additional factors:
   a. The weight of the trunk itself.
   b. The muscles on the concave side, being contracted, have a mechanical advantage over the lengthened muscles on the convex side.
   c. Disturbed forces on active growing vertebral elements bring about structural changes in the bone.
5. Changes occur in the shape of the rib cage.
   a. The thoracic cavity narrows.
   b. The ribs do not move in a plane which allows normal expansion of the lungs.
6. Untreated scoliosis may cause back pain, degenerative arthritis, and disturbances in cardiopulmonary function in later life.

Diagnostic Evaluation

1. Detailed history from patient, parent, and other family members
2. Thorough examination of the back with patient first in the forward bent position and then standing erect
3. Assessment of the neurologic status of the lower extremities
4. Inclusion of clinical photographs in the record for future reference
5. X-rays of the spine to identify and measure primary and compensating curves
6. Pulmonary function studies for children who require surgery to predict risk of postoperative respiratory complications
7. Intravenous pyelography for children with congenital scoliosis because of a high evidence of associated renal anomalies.

Treatment

1. Milwaukee brace and exercises
   May eliminate the need for surgery or may prevent a curvature from becoming worse.
2. Casts—used preoperatively to correct a curvature or postoperatively to maintain correction
   a. Localizer cast—utilizes cephalopelvic traction as well as pressure directly over the major curves to provide correction
   b. Cotrel's E.D.F. (elongation, derotation, and flexion) cast—used to correct the rib hump of severe thoracic curves
   c. Surcingle cast—also provides correction of the rib hump
3. Traction—used preoperatively to stretch out soft tissue structures or correct spinal curvature
   a. Cotrel traction—used for soft tissue stretching around moderate curves
   b. Halofemoral and halopelvic traction—used to correct severe and resistant curves
      The child may be returned to traction postoperatively.
4. Surgery
   a. Harrington instrumentation and posterior spinal fusion
      (1) Indications:
         (a) Thoracic curves of from 40–70 degrees
         (b) Double major curves
         (c) Paralytic scoliosis in which the whole spine is involved, necessitating fusion from the upper thoracic spine, possibly to the sacrum
      (2) A localizer plaster of paris jacket is usually required for 6 months to 1 year postoperatively to maintain correction, depending on the age of the child and the type of scoliosis.
   b. Dwyer instrumentation and anterior spinal fusion
      (1) Indications:
         (a) Severe lumbar or thoracolumbar lordosis
         (b) Problems such as myelomeningocele that preclude a posterior approach
         (c) When maximum correction is essential
         (d) For effective derotation of rotated spines
         (e) When previous posterior approaches have failed
      (2) A full plaster of paris jacket is usually required postoperatively for 3–4 months to maintain correction.

Prognosis

Best when curve is mild at the time of initial diagnosis and effective treatment is initiated early.

Nursing Objectives and Management

A. *To care for the child who is using a Milwaukee brace.*

1. Educate the child and parents concerning the brace and supplemental exercise program.
   a. Clarify goals of therapy with the family.
   b. Exercises are prescribed to increase muscle strength of the torso to counteract the effects of splinting and to assist actively in correcting the abnormal curves and rib deformities.
   c. Offer incentives for compliance with the recommended treatment program.
2. Prevent break in tissue integrity.
   a. Provide meticulous skin care to areas in contact with the brace.

b. Use a smooth-fitting undershirt or stockinette under the brace to protect the skin.

c. Examine skin surfaces for evidence of pressure areas.

d. Have brace adjusted if skin breakdown occurs because of improper fit.

3. Assist child and family to modify normal activities such as bathing and dressing to accommodate the brace.

a. Clothing must be loose or must be purchased in larger sizes to fit over the outside of the appliance.

b. Underpants should be worn over the brace to facilitate toileting.

B. *To care for the child in Cotrel traction.*

Refer to section on traction, page 1209.

C. *To care for the child in halopelvic/femoral traction.*

Refer to section on traction, page 1209.

D. *To prepare the child for surgical correction (spinal fusion).*

1. Explain to the child and his parents the nature of the care immediately before surgery, the anesthesia, postoperative care, and appearance.

2. Introduce the child and his parents to a nurse from the intensive care unit if the child will be transferred there postoperatively.

3. Have the child practice aspects of the anticipated therapy, such as deep breathing and other respiratory routines, leg exercises, logrolling, use of the Stryker frame or CircOlectric bed, and use of the fracture bedpan.

E. *To provide postoperative care to the child following spinal fusion.*

1. Observe for signs of hypotension.

a. Monitor fluid balance.

b. Maintain blood pressure at desired level; report changes.

2. Observe wound for bleeding, hematoma, or infection.

a. Maintain aseptic technique when caring for the wound.

b. Report any redness, swelling, drainage, or heat in the incisional area.

3. Relieve pain.

a. Identify causes of pain through discussion with patient and through observation.

b. Administer analgesic therapy as prescribed by the physician.

4. Maintain tissue integrity.

a. Turn patient as prescribed. (Usually patient is turned by logrolling at 2-hour intervals.)

b. Provide skin care with each turning maneuver.

c. Use sheepskin under pressure areas.

5. Prevent respiratory complications

Utilize breathing exercises, blow bottles, and/or intermittent positive pressure to increase respiratory exchange.

6. Observe for neurologic deficits.

Assess neurologic status each nursing shift, including dorsiflexion, mobility of legs, perineal sensation, and bladder function.

7. Observe for evidence of urinary retention which may develop as an effect of anesthesia, neurologic trauma, hypovolemia, or drugs.

a. Maintain careful record of intake and output.

b. Notify physician if patient does not void within 8 hours following surgery.

c. Care for the urethral catheter if present. (Refer to procedure, pp. 484–485.)

8. Observe for signs of paralytic ileus.

Note hypoactive and hyperactive bowel sounds, nausea, vomiting, or abdominal pain as diet is gradually increased.

9. Prevent development of thrombophlebitis.

a. Have patient do leg exercises.

b. Apply elastic stockings.

c. Observe for leg swelling, redness, or pain upon dorsiflexion; also note chest symptoms such as dyspnea, chest pain, or hemoptysis.

10. Prevent displacement of the rod or hook.

a. Do not lift patient under the axillae.

b. Use turning sheet.

c. Instruct patient not to lift hands over head.

11. Maintain adequate nutrition and hydration.

a. Be aware of normal requirements for size and age.

b. Evaluate nutritional value of diet and provide appropriate supplements.

12. Provide a safe environment for the patient.

a. Place the bed so that it is not easily jolted.

b. Be certain that all equipment is in good working order and that personnel are instructed in its use.

F. *To care for the child following application of a jacket cast.*

1. Stay with the patient during the casting procedure to provide emotional support because of the unfamiliar, frightening, and embarrassing nature of the experience.

2. Observe for evidence of compromised circulation.

Report changes in color, sensation, temperature of extremities, respiratory compromise, or abdominal distress.

3. Prevent potential trauma.

a. Help patient to accept the realities of activity limitation by providing safe alternatives.

b. Facilitate patient's getting in and out of bed by use of a hospital bed.

c. Teach patient safe methods of becoming mobile.

4. Instruct patient about how to arrange for cast changes as required either by growth of the patient or by soiling of the cast.

5. For additional information related to cast care, refer to section on casts, page 1218.

G. *To provide emotional support for the child.*

1. Allow the child to continue as many of his normal activities as possible.

a. Continue schooling.

b. Encourage peer visiting or telephone contact.

2. Provide diversional activities.

a. Assess patient's interests and provide things that he can do within the limits of his position.

b. Use prism glasses, mirrors, bedboards, and easels.

c. Bring others into the patient's room and transport the patient in his bed to the recreation room as soon as his condition allows.

d. Establish schedules and make each day meaningful.

3. Be sensitive to the patient's concerns about body image and intervene appropriately.

a. Many adolescent girls express concerns that the cast will prevent growth or change the shape of their breasts, or that menstruation will temporarily cease while they are in the cast.

b. Patients may feel vulnerable because of the restrictions imposed by casts or traction.

4. Provide as much privacy as possible especially during bathing, toileting, and cast changing.

5. Refer to section on the hospitalized adolescent, page 1130.

H. *To prepare the patient and family for discharge.*

1. Have patient and family practice cast care during hospitalization.
2. Demonstrate techniques of personal hygiene, including such matters as special skin care and hair washing.
3. Assist patient to develop an exercise program within limitations but adequate to maintain tonicity.
4. Provide dietary instructions, including basic nutritional needs for age and necessary modifications because of immobilization.
5. Provide assistive devices to facilitate physical care needs.
6. Prearrange home equipment with available services.

7. Provide continuity by referral to appropriate community agencies.
8. Arrange for transportation and/or social service assistance if needed.
9. Act as a liaison between the patient and his school to encourage the school nurse to supervise patient compliance after return to school and to provide support for the child with adjustment problems.
10. References for Patients and Parents:

    Brower E. Children Should Be Seen . . . . A Handbook for Teachers. University Youth Spine Center, 2074 Abington Road, Cleveland, Ohio 44106

    Scoliosis—A Handbook for Patients. Scoliosis Research Society, 430 N. Michigan Ave., Chicago, Ill. 60611

    Schatzinger L. What if You Need An Operation for Scoliosis and Brace Yourself—Scoliosis and the Milwaukee Brace. University Youth Spine Center, 2074 Abington Road, Cleveland, Ohio 44106

BIBLIOGRAPHY

Books

Blount W and Moe J. The Milwaukee Brace, 2nd ed. Baltimore, Williams & Wilkins, 1975
Ferguson A. Orthopedic Surgery in Infancy and Childhood, 4th ed. Baltimore, Williams & Wilkins, 1975
Hilt N and Schmitt E. Pediatric Orthopedic Nursing. St. Louis, CV Mosby, 1975
Keim H. The Adolescent Spine. New York, Grune & Stratton, 1976
Larson C and Gould M. Orthopedic Nursing, 9th ed. St. Louis, CV Mosby, 1978
Lovell W and Winter R (eds). Pediatric Orthopedics, Vols. 1 and 2. Philadelphia, JB Lippincott, 1978
Rang M. Children's Fractures. Philadelphia, JB Lippincott, 1974
Riseborough EJ and Herndon JH. Scoliosis and Other Deformities of the Axial Skeleton. Boston, Little, Brown & Co., 1975
Rothman RH and Simeone FA. The Spine. Philadelphia, WB Saunders, 1975
Sharrard WJW. Pediatric Orthopaedics and Fractures, Vols 1 and 2. London, Blackwell Scientific Publications, 1978
Specht WT. Special orthopedic problems. In Behrman RE (ed). Neonatal–Perinatal Medicine: Diseases of the Fetus and Infant, 2nd ed. St. Louis, CV Mosby, 1977
Whaley L and Wong D. Nursing Care of Infants and Children. St. Louis, CV Mosby, 1979.

Articles

Anderson B. Carole, a girl treated with bracing. Am J Nurs 1979 Sept; 79(9):1592–1597
Barrett M. Surviving adolescence in a back brace: Laura's experience. MCN 1977 May/June; 2(3):160–163
Bover E and Nash C. Evaluating growth and posture in school-age children. Nursing '79 1979 Apr; 9(4):58–63
Bunch W. Common deformities of the lower limb. Pediatric Nursing 1979 July/Aug; 5(4):18–22

Carroll NC et al. The pathoanatomy of congenital clubfoot. Orthop Clin North Am 1978 Jan; 9(1):225–232
DePaz AC Jr et al. Talipes equinovarus: Pathiomechanical basis of treatment. Orthop Clin North Am 1978 Jan; 9(1):171–185
DeToledo C. The patient with scoliosis. The defect: Classification and detection. Am J Nurs 1979 Sept; 79(9):1588–1591
Hawkins RW et al. Skeletal trauma in skateboard injuries. Am J Dis Child 1978 Aug; 132(8):751–752
Hill P and Romm L. Screening for scoliosis in adolescents. MCN 1977 May /June; 2(3):156–159
Ishii Y et al. Long-term results of closed reduction of complete congenital dislocation of the hip in children under one year of age. Clin Orthop 1978 Nov/Dec; 137:167–174
Keim H. Scoliosis. Clin Symp 1972 Jan; 24(1):1–32
Micheli L, Magin M, Rouvales R. The patient with scoliosis. Surgical management and nursing care. Am J Nurs 1979 Sept; 79(9):1599–1607
Mignogna S. Scoliosis. Nursing '77 1977 May; 7(5):50–55
Neff J. Feminine identity concerns of girls undergoing correction for scoliosis. Matern Child Nurs J 1972 Spring; 1(1):9–18
Palmer EE et al. Supracondylar fracture of the humerus in children. J Bone Joint Surg 1978 July; 60(5):653–656
Pous JG et al. Neonatal surgery in clubfoot. Orthop Clin North Am 1978 Jan; 9(1):233–240
Rang MC et al. Fractures and sprains. Pediatr Clin North Am 1977 Nov; 24(4):749–773
Schatzinger L, Brower E, Nash C. Spinal fusion: Emotional stress and adjustment. Am J Nurs 1979 Sept; 79(9):1608–1612
Septimus EJ et al. Osteomyelitis: Recent clinical and laboratory aspects. Orthop Clin North Am 1979 Apr; 10(2):347–359
Sharrard WJ. Neonatal diagnosis of congenital dislocation of hip. Dev Med Child Neurol 1978 June; 20(3):389–390
Wedge JH et al. The natural history of congenital dislocation of the hip: A critical review. Clin Orthop 1978 Nov/Dec; 137:154–162

PEDIATRIC ONCOLOGY

GENERAL CONSIDERATIONS

Incidence

1. Cancer is the leading cause of death from disease in children from 1–14 years of age.
2. Cancer affects approximately 10 per 100,000 children annually.
3. Mortality rate is approximately 5.3 per 100,000 children annually.

Types

A. *Common Types of Cancer in Children* (in order of frequency)

1. Leukemia
2. Cancer of the central nervous system
3. Lymphoma
4. Neuroblastoma
5. Rhabdomyosarcoma
6. Wilms' tumor
7. Bone tumor
8. Retinoblastoma

B. *Less Common Central Nervous System Neoplasms*

1. Craniopharyngiomas
2. Cerebral tumors
3. Optic nerve gliomas
4. Pineal tumors

Warning Signals of Cancer in Children

1. Marked change in bowel or bladder habits; nausea and vomiting for no apparent cause
2. Bloody discharge of any kind; failure to stop bleeding in the usual time
3. Presence of swelling, lump, or mass anywhere in the body
4. Any change in the size or appearance of moles or birthmarks
5. Unexplained stumbling in the child
6. Generally run-down condition
7. Unexplained pain or persistent crying of an infant or child

Treatment Modalities*

A. *Surgery*

B. *Radiation Therapy*

Nursing Considerations:
a. Prepare the child and his family for the procedure.
b. Do not wash off any marks placed by the radiologist to indicate the area to be treated.
c. Initiate comfort and support measures when the child demonstrates any side effects of treatment.
  (1) General malaise and headache
  (2) Nausea and vomiting
  (3) Diarrhea
  (4) Anorexia
  (5) Skin irritation and breakdown
  (6) Lethargy
d. Refer to adult text, section on radiation in diagnosis and therapy, page 853.

C. *Chemotherapy*

Nursing Considerations:
a. Be aware of the chemotherapeutic agents most frequently used to treat childhood cancer, their side-effects, and precautions for administration. Refer to Table 50-1, page 1423.
b. Care for the child who develops side-effects of chemotherapy.
  (1) Prepare the child and his family for the possible side effects of the chemotherapeutic agents he is receiving.

    Explain to the child that the medicine is to help him feel better but that when he first begins to take the medicine he may feel sicker. By explaining this prior to the development of symptoms, the child will be more trusting and less frightened.
  (2) Nausea and vomiting

* For additional information, refer to Chapter 21, Nursing Patient with Cancer (Adult), page 842.

TABLE 50-1. DRUGS COMMONLY USED IN THE TREATMENT OF CHILDHOOD CANCER

Drug/Category	Administration	Side Effects/Toxicity	Specific Nursing Implications
Prednisone: Adrenocorticosteroid	Oral	Increased appetitie, weight gain, fluid retention, hypertension, Cushing's syndrome, striation, growth arrest, immunosuppression, psychosis, GI tract ulceration	1. Avoid excessive sodium intake. 2. Observe for evidence of GI bleeding. 3. Protect from infection.
Vincristine (Oncovin): Periwinkle alkaloid	IV	Alopecia, constipation, peripheral neuropathy, hyponatremia, mild myelosuppression. Causes chemical irritation on extravasation.	1. Use different needles to withdraw and inject. Check patency of IV line with saline flush before injecting. Inject cautiously, observing for signs of infiltration. Follow injection with saline flush. 2. Observe for constipation; report condition promptly. Keep well hydrated. Administer laxatives or stool softeners as prescribed. 3. Alter activities appropriately if weakness of hands, feet, or legs occurs or if patient becomes easily fatigued. 4. Prepare children and parents for the possibility of numbness and tingling of fingers and toes.
Adriamycin: Antibiotic	IV	Nausea and vomiting, alopecia, stomatitis, myelosuppression, cardiotoxicity, red urine. Causes chemical irritation on extravasation.	1. Utilize the same precautions when administering this medication as with vincristine.
L-Asparaginase: Enzyme	IV	Hypersensitivity reaction, nausea and vomiting, lethargy, somnolence, fever, hepatotoxicity, coagulopathy, pancreatitis, hyperproteinemia, convulsions.	1. Observe for hypersensitivity reaction. Have epinephrine and resuscitation equipment available. 2. Observe for confusion, irritability, convulsions, and other neurologic signs. 3. Do not shake vial. 4. Use clear solution only.
Daunomycin: Antibiotic	IV	Cardiotoxicity, myelosuppression, nausea and vomiting, abdominal pain, fever, skin rash, red urine. Causes chemical irritation on extravasation.	1. Utilize the same precautions when administering this medication as those followed with vincristine.
6-Mercaptopurine: Antimetabolite: Purine antagonist	Oral	Nausea and vomiting, myelosuppression, anorexia, dermatitis, mucous membrane ulceration, hepatotoxicity, abdominal pain.	1. Dosage should be reduced to one-third of the usual dosage if a child is also receiving allopurinol, since this drug inhibits the degradation of 6-mercaptopurine.
Methotrexate: Antimetabolite; Folic acid antagonist	Oral, IV, IM, IT (intrathecal)	Nausea and vomiting, GI mucosal ulceration, myelosuppression, pneumonitis, osteoporosis, hepatotoxicity, hyperpigmentation.	1. Avoid side effects of meningeal irritation during IT injection by diluting the drug in a preservative-free vehicle, bringing it to room temperature and filtering it through a 0.22 millimicron Millipore filter. 2. Do not enter vial twice for IT use. 3. Method of IT injection a. A lumbar puncture is performed. b. A volume of spinal fluid equal to the volume of drug to be injected is removed. c. Without aspiration, the medication is injected in a continuous infusion (15–30 seconds/10 ml. of solution). d. The stylet is reinserted and the needle is removed. e. The child may be required to remain in the Trendelenburg position for 30 minutes after the injection to insure optimal circulation of the medication throughout the central nervous system.

TABLE 50-1. DRUGS COMMONLY USED IN THE TREATMENT OF CHILDHOOD CANCER (continued)

Drug/Category	Administration	Side Effects/Toxicity	Specific Nursing Implications
Cyclophosphamide (Cytoxan): Alkylating agent	Oral or IV	Alopecia, nausea and vomiting, myelosuppression, hemorrhagic cystitis, mucous membrane ulceration, immunosuppression, infertility, hyperpigmentation.	1. To prevent exposure of the bladder to chemical irritants, maintain liberal hydration for 48 hours after weekly dose and then continuously when given daily. Have the child empty his bladder frequently after the drug is administered, including at least once during the night. 2. Protect child from infection.
Cytosine arabinoside (Cytosar): Antimetabolite; Pyrimidine antagonist	IV, IM, SC, or IT	Nausea and vomiting, myelosuppression, mucous membrane ulcerations, hepatotoxicity, immunosuppression.	1. Anticipate severe nausea and vomiting during or soon after administration. 2. May require premedication with antiemetics. 3. Protect child from infection. 4. Do not enter vial twice for IT use.
Carmustine: Nitrosurea	IV	Facial burning and flushing on infusion, burning pain along IV infusion, nausea and vomiting, bone marrow depression	1. Avoid extravasation.
Lomustine: Nitrosurea	PO	Nausea and vomiting, bone marrow depression	1. Administer 4 hours after meals on an empty stomach.
Procarbazine.	PO	Severe nausea and vomiting, lethargy, dermatitis, arthralgia, bone marrow depression, stomatitis	1. Central nervous system depressants (phenothiazines and barbiturates) enhance CNS symptoms. 2. Acts as an MAO inhibitor—sympathomimetic drugs and natural foods such as yogurt, aged cheese, and bananas should be avoided.
Dacarbazine	IV	Nausea and vomiting (especially after the first dose), flulike syndrome, bone marrow depression	1. Used with caution in children with renal dysfunction.

(a) Administer antiemetics as prescribed.

(b) Plan activities and meals according to the medical schedule.

Many children prefer to receive chemotherapeutic agents that cause nausea and vomiting during the evening so that they can sleep through the hours of greatest nausea.

(c) Carefully observe the sleeping child who is prone to vomiting. Position him in a manner which prevents aspiration.

(d) Offer foods and fluids which are most appealing to the child (e.g., warm tea, carbonated beverages, soups).

(e) Record the nature of the nausea and vomiting.

(f) Report any prolonged or delayed nausea or vomiting which may be an indication that the medication should be withheld or that the dosage should be reduced.

(3) Anorexia

(a) Create a pleasant eating environment that is free of sights, sounds, and odors that cause nausea or that discourage or distract the child.

(b) Encourage the child to eat in the playroom with other children.

(c) Give good mouth care prior to eating.

(d) Provide frequent small meals.

(4) Extreme fluctuations in appetite

Be aware that this is temporary and that eventually, normal eating patterns will be established. Reassure parents of this fact.

(5) Gastrointestinal mucosal cell damage causing stomatitis, gastrointestinal ulceration, rectal ulceration, diarrhea, or bleeding

(a) Provide meticulous oral hygiene. Local anesthetics may be prescribed for painful mouth ulcers.

(b) If diarrhea or rectal ulcers occur, keep the skin clean and dry to prevent maceration and secondary infection.

(c) These signs of toxicity are generally indications for temporary discontinuation of therapy or a reduction of dosage.

(6) Alopecia

(a) Assist the family in obtaining wigs or caps in preparation for hair loss.

(b) Reassure the child and family that the hair will grow back, although it might be of a different color and texture.

(7) For side effects and nursing interventions associated with specific drugs refer to Table 50-1, Drugs Commonly Used in the Treatment of Childhood Cancer.

Prevention

1. Children and adults should be educated regarding the hazards of known carcinogens, especially cigarette smoking, and excessive exposure to sunlight or radiation.
2. Female adolescents should be instructed concerning the method of breast self-examination. Males should be taught to do testicular self-examination. Periodic examinations should be encouraged for cancer screening.
3. Parents should be taught the warning signals of childhood cancer.

ACUTE LYMPHOCYTIC LEUKEMIA

Acute lymphocytic leukemia is a primary disorder of the bone marrow in which the normal marrow elements are replaced by immature or undifferentiated blast cells. When the quantity of normal marrow is depleted below the level necessary to maintain peripheral blood elements within normal ranges, anemia, neutropenia, and thombocytopenia occur.

Incidence and Classification

1. Acute leukemia is the most common malignancy in children, occurring in nearly 4 per 100,000 children under 15 years of age.
2. Acute leukemia is classified according to the cell type involved.
   a. Approximately 85% of pediatric cases are of the acute lymphocytic leukemia (ALL) type.
   b. The remainder are primarily cases of acute myelogenous leukemia (AML).
3. The clinical pictures of ALL and AML are similar, but the response of the child to therapy is markedly different.
   The percentage of children achieving remission is smaller with AML (approximately 40% as compared to 90–95% with ALL), and the mean survival time is shorter with AML.
4. The incidence of ALL is more common among Caucasian children.

Etiology

1. The exact cause of acute leukemia is unknown.
2. Environmental causes, infectious agents (especially viruses), genetic factors, and chromosomal abnormalities are suspected in some cases.

Clinical Manifestations

1. Manifestations depend on the degree to which the bone marrow has been compromised and the location and extent of extramedullary infiltration.
2. Presenting symptoms
   a. Fatigability
   b. General malaise, listlessness
   c. Persistent fever of unknown cause
   d. Recurrent infection
   e. Prolonged bleeding following simple surgical procedures (e.g., dental extractions and tonsillectomy)
   f. Tendency to bruise easily
   g. Pallor
   h. Enlarged lymph nodes
   i. Abdominal pain due to organomegaly
   j. Bone and joint pain
   k. Headache and vomiting (with CNS involvement)
3. Presenting symptoms may be isolated or in any combination or sequence.

Altered Physiology

1. Acute lymphocytic leukemia results from the growth of an abnormal type of nongranular, fragile leukocyte in the blood-forming tissues, particularly in the bone marrow, spleen, and lymph nodes.
2. The abnormal cell has little cytoplasm and a round, homogenous nucleus which resembles that of a lymphoblast.
3. Normal bone marrow elements may be displaced or replaced in this type of leukemia.
4. The changes in the blood and bone marrow result from the accumulation of leukemic cells and from the deficiency of normal cells.
   a. Red cell precursors and megakaryocytes from which platelets are formed are decreased, causing anemia, prolonged and unusual bleeding, and tendency to bruise easily.
   b. Normal white cells are markedly decreased, predisposing the child to infection.
   c. The bone marrow is hyperplastic with a uniform appearance due to the presence of leukemic cells.
5. Leukemic cells may infiltrate into lymph nodes, spleen, and liver, causing diffuse adenopathy and hepatosplenomegaly.
6. Expansion of marrow or infiltration of leukemic cells into bone results in bone or joint pain.
7. Invasion of the central nervous system by leukemic cells may cause headache, vomiting, cranial nerve palsies, convulsions, and coma.
8. Weight loss, muscle wasting, and fatigue may occur when the body cells are deprived of nutrients because of the immense metabolic needs of the proliferating leukemic cells.

Diagnostic Evaluation

A. *Physical Findings*
1. Pallor, especially of the mucous membranes
2. Scattered petechiae and ecchymoses
3. Generalized lymphadenopathy
4. Enlarged liver and spleen
5. Unexplained bruising
6. Continued bone and joint pain
7. Fever

B. *Laboratory Evaluation*
1. May have altered peripheral blood counts. Blood studies may show the following:
   a. Low hemoglobin, red cell count, hematocrit, and platelet count
   b. Decreased, elevated, or normal white cell count
2. Stained peripheral smear and bone marrow examination show large numbers of lymphoblasts and lymphocytes.

3. Lumbar puncture—to determine if there is central nervous system involvement.
4. Renal and liver function studies—to determine any contraindications or precautions for chemotherapy.

Complications

1. Infection—most frequently occurs in the lungs, gastrointestinal tract, or skin
2. Hemorrhage—usually due to thrombocytopenia
3. Central nervous system involvement
4. Bony involvement
5. Testicular involvement
6. Urate nephropathy

Treatment

A. *Supportive Therapy*—to control disease complications such as hyperuricemia, infection, anemia, and bleeding.

B. *Specific Therapy*—to eradicate malignant cells and to restore normal marrow function.

1. Chemotherapy is utilized to achieve complete remission with restoration of normal peripheral blood and physical findings.
2. There is no universally accepted standard therapy for the treatment of children with acute leukemia, but most centers have similar protocols which utilize the same drugs alone or in combination (refer to Table 50-1).
3. Components of therapy
   a. Induction—course of therapy designed to achieve a complete remission
   b. Central nervous system prophylaxis—treatment begun early in the course of the illness to destroy leukemic cells that have infiltrated the central nervous system. It generally consists of cranial irradiation and intrathecal methotrexate.
   c. Maintenance or continuation therapy—to maintain remission and to continue reducing the number of leukemic cells. Includes periodic doses of intrathecal methotrexate to maintain the CNS prophylaxis.
   d. Reinduction therapy to reinduce remission if relapse occurs.
   e. Extramedullary disease therapy.
4. Research is continuing to determine the optimal method of inducing and maintaining remission with the least risk to the patient.
5. Two modes of therapy—bone marrow transplantation and immunotherapy—are currently under investigation and may hold promise for the future.

Prognosis

1. Uncertain.
2. The life span of children with ALL has been lengthened.
3. At least 90% of children with ALL can be expected to achieve an initial remission if treated in a specialty center.
4. In about 50% of the cases, the disease will remain in remission for at least 5 years.
5. Many children who have not been in continuous remission survive 5 years or more.
6. The prognosis becomes poorer with each relapse the child experiences.
7. The term "cure" is difficult to define because later relapses still occur after long remissions.
8. Prognosis appears to be related to the child's age

and white blood count on diagnosis, and the exact cell type of the leukemia.

Nursing Objectives and Management

A. *To provide emotional support to the parents when the diagnosis of leukemia is made known to them.*

1. Be available to the parents when they feel that they want to discuss their feelings.
2. Kindness, concern, consideration, and sincerity toward the child and his parents help to serve as a source of consolation.
3. Contact the family's clergyman or the hospital chaplain if the parents desire this.
4. Utilize the services of a social worker as appropriate to help the family work out their feelings.
5. Avoid discussing life expectancy in terms of the time element—offer the hope that therapy will be effective and will prolong life.
6. Allow the parents to participate in the child's care so that they will feel that they are actually doing something for the child. This also helps the family feel more secure. (Refer to section on family-centered care, p. 1131.)
7. Assess family dynamics and coping mechanisms and plan intervention accordingly.

B. *To give skillful, supportive care in the early stages of treatment and to sustain life until antileukemic agents have had a chance to become effective.*

1. Initiate nursing activities associated with anemia. (Refer to p. 1276.)
2. Provide adequate hydration.
   a. Maintain parenteral fluid administration.
   b. Offer small amounts of oral fluids if tolerated.
   c. Record and report vomiting if this occurs.
3. Observe renal function carefully.
   a. Measure and record urinary output.
   b. Check specific gravity.
   c. Observe the urine for any evidence of gross bleeding.
4. Provide a highly nutritious diet if the child can tolerate it.
   a. Determine the child's likes and dislikes.
   b. Offer small, frequent meals.
   c. Offer supplemental feedings which are high in calories and protein.
   d. Encourage parents to assist at mealtime.
   e. Allow the child to eat with a group at a table if his condition allows this.
5. Protect the child from sources of infection.
   a. Family, friends, personnel, and other patients who have infections should not visit or care for the child.
   b. Do not place a child with an infection in the room with a child with leukemia.
   c. Reverse isolation procedure may be utilized (a protective technique that provides the child with protection from those people with whom he has contact—gowns and masks are worn by any person with whom the child has contact).
      Explain to both the child and his parents the purpose of this protective technique.
   d. Observe the child closely and be alert to signs of impending infection.
      (1) Observe any area of broken skin or mucous membrane for signs of infection.
      (2) Report any febrile incidents.
   e. Teach preventive measures at discharge (i.e.,

handwashing, isolation from children with communicable disease).

C. *To be alert for the symptoms of hemorrhage which may occur when the platelet count is diminished or may appear as side effects of antileukemic therapy.*

1. Record vital signs and report any changes which may be indicative of hemorrhage.
   a. Tachycardia
   b. Lowered blood pressure
   c. Pallor
   d. Diaphoresis
   e. Increasing anxiety and restlessness
2. Give careful oral hygiene since the gums and mucous membranes of the mouth bleed easily.
   a. Use a soft toothbrush.
   b. If the child's mouth is bleeding or painful, clean the teeth and mouth with a moistened cotton swab.
   c. Use a nonirritating rinse for the mouth (e.g., hydrogen peroxide).
   d. Apply petroleum jelly to cracked, dry lips.
3. Observe for gastrointestinal bleeding.
   a. Hematemesis.
   b. Tarry stools or bloodstained stools.
4. Move and turn the child gently since hemarthrosis may occur and cause movement to be very painful.
   a. Handle child in a gentle manner.
   b. Turn frequently to prevent pressure sores.
   c. Place the child in proper body alignment, in a position comfortable for him.
   d. Allow child to be out of bed in a chair if this position is more comfortable for him.
5. Avoid intramuscular injections if possible.
6. Handle catheters as well as drainage and suction tubes carefully to prevent mucosal bleeding.
7. Protect the child from injury by monitoring his activities and environmental hazards.
8. Be aware of emergency procedures for control of bleeding:
   a. Careful application of local pressure so as not to interfere with clot formation.
   b. Administration of blood and blood components. (Refer to section on anemia, p. 1276.)

D. *To prepare the child for diagnostic and treatment procedures.*

1. Utilize knowledge of growth and development to prepare the child for such procedures as bone marrow aspirations, blood transfusions, and chemotherapy. (Refer to section on the hospitalized child, p. 1126.)
2. Provide a means for talking about the experience. Play, storytelling, or role-playing may be helpful.
3. Convey to the child an acceptance of his fears and anger.

E. *To control hyperuricemia which may occur because of rapid cell turnover and tumor lysis.*

1. Administer allopurinal as prescribed to neutralize the effects of uric acid on the kidney.
2. Provide liberal oral and/or IV hydration.
3. Administer sodium bicarbonate or acetazolamide (Diamox) as prescribed to alkalize the urine.
4. Collect urine specimens to monitor urinary excretion of uric acid.

F. *To be aware of the chemotherapeutic agents and the side effects of these agents which are capable of inducing remissions in children with acute leukemia.*

1. Induction—Usually includes a combination of vincristine and prednisone. A third drug, such as 6-Mercaptopurine, L-Asparaginase, Daunorubicin, Adriamycin, or Cytosine Arabinoside, may be added.
2. Maintenance—usually includes methotrexate, used in alternating sequence with the same drugs used to induce remission. Also includes periodic CNS prophylaxis.
3. Reinduction—remissions can often be reinduced using the same initial drugs or with other agents.
4. Refer to Table 50-1, Drugs Commonly Used in the Treatment of Childhood Cancer.

G. *To provide symptomatic care for the child who develops side effects of chemotherapy.*

Refer to section on chemotherapy, page 1422.

H. *To observe for the possibility of CNS involvement.*

Report changes in behavior or personality: persistent nausea and vomiting, headache, lethargy, irritability, dizziness, ataxia, convulsions, or alteration in state of consciousness.

I. *To provide supportive nursing care to the child receiving cranial irradiation.*

Refer to section on radiation therapy, page 1422.

J. *To provide pain relief.*

1. Position the child so that he is most comfortable. Water beds and beanbag chairs are often helpful.
2. Administer medications on a preventive schedule before pain becomes severe. Individualize medication schedule for each patient.
3. Manipulate the environment as necessary to increase the child's comfort and minimize unnecessary exertion.

K. *To provide emotional support to the child.*

1. Provide for continuity of care.
2. Encourage family-centered care (refer to p. 1131).
3. Prepare the child for potential changes in his body image (alopecia, weight loss, wasting, etc.) and help him cope with related feelings.
4. Facilitate play activities for the child and utilize opportunities to communicate with him through play.
5. Maintain some discipline, placing calm limitations on unacceptable behavior.
6. Provide appropriate diversional activities.
7. Encourage independence and provide opportunities which allow the child to control his environment.
8. Avoid exposing the child to activities that he will be unable to accomplish.

L. *To provide continued emotional support to the parents throughout the course of hospitalization.*

1. Assist parents to feel comfortable on the unit.
2. Provide guidelines concerning how parents and the treatment team can work together most profitably.
3. Encourage parental participation in care—to the extent that they feel comfortable.
4. Suggest tasks that the parents may do to reduce their feelings of helplessness and anxiety.
5. Provide for continuity of care so that parents are able to establish trusting relationships with a few nurses.
6. Assist parents to deal with anticipatory grief.
7. Assist parents to deal with other family members, especially siblings and grandparents and friends.
8. Encourage parents to discuss concerns about limiting their child's activities, protecting him from

infection, disciplining him, and having anxieties about the illness.

9. Answer parental questions related to such matters as home management, the purpose of periodic tests, treatments and clinic visits, side effects of medications, and indications for medical intervention.

10. Facilitate communication with the clinic nurse and/ or clinical specialist who may interact with the child during the entire course of illness.

11. Initiate appropriate referrals (e.g., to social worker, parent group, clergy, and community health nurse).

M. *To provide supportive care to the terminally ill or dying child.*

Refer to section on care of the dying child, page 1458.

N. *References for Children and Parents*

Baker L.S. You and Leukemia—A Day At A Time. Philadelphia, WB Saunders, 1978

Sherman M. The Leukemic Child, DHEW Pub No (NIH) 78-863 National Cancer Program, National Cancer Institute, Bethesda, Md. 20014

Leukemia Society of America, 211 East 43rd St., New York, N.Y. 10017

BRAIN TUMORS IN CHILDREN

Brain tumors are expanding lesions within the skull. About 20% of the malignant tumors which occur in children are brain tumors.

Etiology

The etiology of brain tumors is unknown.

Clinical Manifestations

(Signs and symptoms are directly related to the location and size of the tumor.)

1. Headache
   a. May occur at any time, but usually is more severe in early morning hours.
   b. May be intermittent and disappear for days or weeks—may be due to yielding of the sutures.
2. Nausea or vomiting
   a. May occur at any time, but frequently occurs in early morning hours.
   b. Vomiting may be projectile.
3. Visual disturbances
   a. Nystagmus
   b. Diplopia
   c. Blurred vision
   d. Loss of peripheral vision
   e. Significant loss of visual acuity
4. Muscular problems
   a. Lack of balance
   b. Incoordination
   c. Deficits in muscle functioning—eyes, face, extremities
   d. Paralyis
   e. Spasticity
5. Behavioral changes
   a. Arrest or regression in development
   b. Irritability or lassitude
   c. Lack of attentiveness
   d. Deterioration in school performance
   e. Personality changes.
   f. Loss of sphincter control
   g. Disturbances in sleep and eating patterns
6. Slow cerebration
   a. Child answers questions after a considerable delay.
   b. Child appears to talk slowly.
   c. Child responds to any stimulus in a slow manner.
7. Seizures—usually focal, psychomotor, or generalized

Diagnostic Evaluation

(Determined by the type of tumor that is suspected; usually includes many or all of the following procedures):

1. Thorough neurological examination
   a. Fundoscopic examination
   b. Tests for cerebral function (level of consciousness, orientation, intellectual performance, mood, behavior, etc.)
   c. Assessment of cranial nerves
   d. Tests for cerebellar function (e.g., balance and coordination)
   e. Evaluation of the motor system—especially muscle size, tone, strength, and abnormal muscle movements
   f. Evaluation of the sensory system
   g. Assessment of reflexes
2. Electroencephalogram—of limited value, but possibly useful when seizures are manifested
3. Skull x-ray
4. Computed tomography (EMI scan or CAT scan)
   a. Safe, noninvasive procedure using a combination of sophisticated electronic and computer technology
   b. Scanning of head by a slit x-ray beam passing through at a multitude of angles
   c. Absorption values, varying with the density of tissues and fluids, are calculated and analyzed. This allows for differentiation of normal and abnormal brain tissue and ventricular sizes and configurations.
5. Isotopic brain scanning
6. Angiography
7. Air-contrast studies

Treatment

1. Surgery is performed to determine the type of the tumor, the extent of invasiveness, and to excise as much of the lesion as possible.
2. Radiation therapy is usually initiated as soon as the diagnosis is established and the surgical wound healed.
3. Chemotherapy is used to induce remissions in recurrent brain tumors, especially astrocytomas and medulloblastomas. The role of chemotherapy for treatment of primary tumors is currently being investigated. Commonly used drugs include nitrosoureas, vincristine, methotrexate, procarbazine, and steroids.

Prognosis

1. Prognosis is improved in cases involving early diagnosis and adequate therapy.
2. Prognosis is related to completeness of surgical

removal, extent of invasion, and rate of tumor growth.
3. Approximately 50% of children with brain tumors will survive more than 1 year.
4. Five-year survivors are increasing, especially in children with medulloblastoma or higher-grade astrocytoma.

CEREBELLAR ASTROCYTOMA

Cerebellar astrocytoma is a slow-growing, often cystic type of tumor of the cerebellum.

Incidence

1. Most common type of brain tumor.
2. The peak incidence occurs at 5–8 years of age.

Clinical Manifestations

Insidious onset and slow course
1. Evidence of increased intracranial pressure—especially headache, visual disturbances, papilledema, and personality changes
2. Cerebellar signs—ataxia, dysmetria, (inability to control the range of muscular movement), nystagmus
3. Behavioral changes

Pathophysiology

1. The tumor produces slowly increasing intracranial pressure.
2. Condition classified according to its malignancy—from Grade I (least malignant) to Grade IV (most malignant).

Treatment

Surgical removal—the tumor can often be removed with few sequelae.

MEDULLOBLASTOMA

Medulloblastoma is a highly malignant, rapidly growing tumor usually found in the cerebellum.

Incidence

1. Medulloblastomas account for nearly 20% of brain tumors in children.
2. The peak incidence occurs in children from 2–6 years of age.
3. About 75% of medulloblastomas occur in males.

Clinical Manifestations

1. Similar to manifestations of cerebellar astrocytoma, but condition develops more rapidly.
2. The child may present with unsteady gait, anorexia, vomiting, and early morning headache and later develop ataxia, nystagmus, papilledema, and drowsiness.

Pathophysiology

1. The tumor grows rapidly and produces evidence of increased intracranial pressure progressing over a period of weeks.
2. As the tumor grows, it seeds along cerebrospinal fluid (CSF) pathways.

Treatment

1. Partial excision or decompression of the posterior fossa (complete removal is rarely possible)
2. Radiation of site and spinal canal
3. Chemotherapy
4. Shunt to relieve CSF obstruction

BRAIN STEM GLIOMA

Brain stem glioma is a tumor of the brain stem. It accounts for approximately 10% of brain tumors in children.

Incidence

1. Brain stem gliomas occur almost exclusively in children.
2. The peak age at onset is 6–7 years.

Clinical Manifestations

1. Cranial nerve palsies
   a. Strabismus
   b. Weakness, atrophy and fasciculations of the tongue
   c. Swallowing difficulties
2. Hemiparesis
3. Cerebellar ataxia
4. Signs of increased intracranial pressure (rare)

Altered Physiology

Through its growth this type of tumor interferes early with the function of cranial nerve nuclei, pyramidal tracts, and cerebellar pathways.

Treatment

1. Surgical removal is not possible
2. Radiation of site

EPENDYMOMA OF THE FOURTH VENTRICLE

Ependymoma refers to a tumor derived from the ependyma, or lining, of the central canal of the spinal cord and cerebral ventricles. It frequently arises on the floor of the fourth ventricle, causing obstruction of the flow of cerebrospinal fluid.

Incidence

Not related to age or sex of child.

Clinical Manifestations

1. Nausea or vomiting
2. Headache
3. Unsteady gait
4. Signs of increased intracranial pressure

Altered Physiology

1. Tumors grow with varying speed.
2. Because of location, tumors can invade the cardiorespiratory center, cerebellum, and spinal cord.

Management

1. Partial surgical removal.
2. Radiation therapy, including the entire craniospinal axis

CARE OF THE CHILD UNDERGOING SURGERY FOR BRAIN TUMOR

Nursing Objectives

A. *To assess the child's neurologic status in order to help locate the site of the tumor and the extent of involvement; to identify signs of disease progress.*

1. Obtain a thorough nursing history from the child and his parents—particularly data related to normal behavioral patterns and presenting symptoms.
2. Perform portions of the neurologic examination as appropriate.
   Assess muscle strength, coordination, gait, and posture.
3. Observe for the appearance or disappearance of any of the clinical manifestations previously described. Report these to the physician and record each of the following in detail:
   a. Headache—duration, location, severity
   b. Vomiting—time occurring, whether or not projectile
   c. Convulsions—activity prior to seizure; type of seizure; areas of body involved; behavior during and after seizure
4. Monitor vital signs frequently, including blood pressure and pupillary reaction.
5. Monitor occular signs.
   Check pupils for size, equality, reaction to light, and accommodation.
6. Observe for signs of brain stem herniation—should be considered a neurosurgical emergency.
   a. Attacks of opisthotonos
   b. Tilting of the head; neck stiffness
   c. Poorly reactive pupils
   d. Increased blood pressure; widened pulse pressure
   e. Change in respiratory rate and nature of respirations
   f. Irregularity of pulse or lowered pulse rate
   g. Alterations of body temperature

B. *To provide the parents and child with emotional support during the very stressful preoperative period.*

1. Assess the family unit and its coping mechanisms.
2. Allow parents to ask questions and encourage them to discuss their fears and concerns.
   Many parents feel guilty for not seeking help earlier because they either did not recognize or dismissed symptoms.
3. Deliver nursing care to the child in a manner that provides support.
   a. Assume a gentle, concerned attitude toward both parents and child.
   b. Make the child as comfortable as possible.
4. Utilize knowledge of growth and development to provide emotional care for the child. (Refer to section on the hospitalized child, p. 1126.)
5. Prepare child and parents for what to expect during hospitalization (e.g., nursing routines and diagnostic tests).

C. *To provide appropriate nursing care for the child undergoing diagnostic tests.*

1. Prepare the child and parents for each procedure.
2. If prescribed, administer preliminary sedative on time. (If child is not adequately sedated, completion of the test may be impossible.)
3. Refer to adult text, page 701, for nursing care related to specific procedures.

D. *To prepare the child and parents for surgery.*

1. Refer to section on preparation for surgery, page 1139.
2. Determine physician's plans regarding shaving the head, bandages, and other procedures, and prepare the child accordingly.
   a. Encourage the child to express his feelings regarding the threat to his body image.
   b. Reassure the child that he will be able to wear a wig or hat after recovery.
   c. If the area is to be shaved, allow the child and parents the option of saving the hair.
3. Prepare parents for the postoperative appearance of their child and for the fact that he might be comatose immediately following surgery.
4. If appropriate, introduce the child and his family to intensive care nursing personnel and arrange a tour of the unit.
5. Prepare the child for postoperative expectations (i.e., he may feel sleepy or have a headache and will need to remain quiet).

E. *To provide an adequate diet for the child preoperatively.*

1. Re-feed the child when he vomits. (Vomiting is not usually associated with nausea.)
2. Allow the child to participate in the selection of foods and the preparation of his tray.
3. Maintain IV hydration if indicated.

F. *To provide care for the child during the immediate postoperative period.* (This is usually provided in an intensive care unit.)

1. Position the child according to physician's request—usually on his unaffected side with his head level.
   a. Raising the foot of the bed may increase intracranial pressure and bleeding.
   b. Post a sign above the bed noting the exact position of the head.
2. Check the dressing for bleeding and for drainage of cerebrospinal fluid.
3. Monitor the child's temperature closely.
   a. A marked rise in temperature may be due to trauma, to disturbance of the heat-regulating center, or to intracranial edema.
   b. If hyperthermia occurs, utilize appropriate measures to reduce it. (Refer to section on fever, p. 1148.)
      Temperature should not be reduced too rapidly.
4. Observe child closely for signs of shock, increased intracranial pressure, and alterations in level of consciousness.
5. Assess the child for edema of the head, face, and neck.
   a. Edema may inhibit respirations and impair circulation of lacrimal secretion.
   b. Apply cold compresses to the affected areas, being careful not to dampen the dressing.
   c. Apply methylcellulose drops to the eyes to prevent corneal damage.
6. Carefully regulate fluid administration in order to prevent increased cerebral edema.
7. Change the child's position frequently and provide meticulous skin care to prevent hypostatic pneumonia and pressure sores.
   a. Move the child carefully and slowly, being certain to move the head in line with the body.
   b. Support paralyzed or spastic extremities with pillows, rolls, or other means.

8. Avoid discussing the child's condition in his presence, even if he appears to be unconscious.
9. Have equipment readily available for cardiopulmonary resuscitation, respiratory assistance, oxygen-inhalation, blood transfusion, ventricular tap, and other potential emergency situations.
10. Continue to support parents who may be very frightened and upset by the appearance of their child and necessary emergency procedures.

G. *To provide care for the child during the convalescent phase.*

1. Maintain adequate nutrition and hydration.
   a. Encourage the child to eat increasingly larger meals.
   b. Provide tube feedings if the child is unable to eat.
2. Allow and encourage the child to regain his independence as his condition improves.
3. Facilitate the return of normal parent-child relationships.
   a. Parents may tend to be overprotective.
   b. Help parents to see the child's increasing capabilities and encourage them to foster independence.
4. Make provisions for play activities.
   a. Allow the child to meet and play with other children.
   b. Provide the child with quiet play activities when it is necessary to encourage rest.
   c. Be careful that the child does not hit his head or fall until he is completely healed.
      A head dressing, football helmet, or wig may be used to prevent trauma should the child fall.

5. Assist the child to adjust to his altered body image.
   a. Utilize stocking caps, surgical caps, head scarves, hats, or wigs as appropriate.
   b. If the child's hair has not been totally shaved, it may be combed so that the area of baldness is not evident.
   c. Reassure the child that his hair will grow back.
6. For care of children with residual effects from surgery, refer to adult text, section on rehabilitation concepts, page 54.

H. *To care for the child receiving radiation therapy.*

Refer to section on radiation therapy, page 1422.

I. *To care for the child receiving chemotherapy.*

Refer to section on chemotherapy, page 1422.

J. *To prepare the child and his family for discharge.*

1. Provide parents with written information regarding the child's needs—medications, activity, care of incision, follow-up appointments, etc.
2. Initiate a referral to a community health nurse to reinforce teaching and to maintain therapeutic support for the family.
3. Encourage the parents to contact the child's teacher and the school nurse before the child returns to school so that they can prepare his classmates for his return and help them to deal with their feelings.
4. Provide parents with the phone number of the nursing unit so that they may call if questions occur to them after discharge.

K. *To provide supportive care to the terminally ill child.*

Refer to section on the dying child, page 1458.

NEUROBLASTOMA

Neuroblastoma refers to a malignant tumor arising from the sympathetic nervous system.

Etiology

Unknown

Incidence

1. Most common extracranial solid tumor of childhood.
2. Occurs in approximately 1 per 10,000 live births.
3. Primarily affects infants and young children; almost 75% of cases occur in children less than 2 years of age.
4. Accounts for about 8% of all deaths from cancer in children each year.

Clinical Manifestations

1. Symptoms depend on the location of the tumor and the stage of the disease.
2. Most tumors are located within the abdomen and present as firm, nontender, irregular masses that cross the midline.
3. Other common signs:
   a. Bowel or bladder dysfunction resulting from compression by a pelvic tumor
   b. Neurologic symptoms because of compression by the tumor on nerve roots or because of tumor extension
   c. Supraorbital ecchymosis, periorbital edema, and exophthalmos resulting from metastasis to the skull bones and retrobulbar soft tissue
   d. Lymphadenopathy, especially in the cervical area
   e. Bone pain with skeletal involvement
   f. Swelling of the neck or face, and cough with thoracic masses
   g. General symptoms of pallor, anorexia, weight loss, and weakness with widespread metastasis

Pathophysiology

1. Tumors arise from embryonic neural crest cells anywhere along the craniospinal axis.
2. Histologic picture varies greatly from tumor to tumor and even within the same tumor.
3. Tumors are staged primarily on the basis of the extent of disease, from Stage I (tumor is confined to the organ or structure of origin) to Stage IV (there is remote disease involving the skeleton, parenchymal organs, soft tissue, or distant lymph glands). Stage IV-S refers to cases with remote disease confined to only 1 or more sites, either the liver, skin, or bone marrow without x-ray evidence of skeletal metastasis.
4. Neuroblastoma is one of the few tumors that may demonstrate spontaneous regression.

Diagnostic Evaluation

To document the extent of the disease:
1. X-rays of the chest, skull, abdomen, and long bones
2. Intravenous pyelogram
3. Bone marrow aspiration
4. Complete blood count with platelet count
5. Urinary catecholamine determination (VMA)

6. Bone scan
7. Histologic confirmation
8. Additional studies
   a. Myelogram
   b. Liver/spleen scan
   c. Oblique films of spine
   d. Inferior venacavography

Medical/Surgical Management

1. Management is controversial and depends on the stage of the child's disease at the time of diagnosis.
2. When complete surgical resection of a Stage I tumor is possible, this may be the only treatment required.
3. Children with other than Stage I disease generally receive a combination of surgery, radiation therapy, and chemotherapy.
   Drugs of choice include vincristine, dacarbazine, and cyclophosphamide.

Prognosis

1. Overall survival rate is about 30 to 35%, with almost all recurrences or deaths occurring within the first 2 years after diagnosis.
2. Influencing factors:
   a. Stage of disease—the earlier the stage, the better the prognosis.
   b. Age—infants under 1 year of age demonstrate the best survival.
   c. Pattern of metastasis—children with metastases to the bone marrow, liver, and skin have better prognoses than those with radiographic bone involvement.
   d. Site of primary tumor—children with tumors of

the thorax, pelvis, or neck appear to do better than children with abdominal tumors.
3. Neuroblastoma is one of few childhood tumors that has not responded dramatically to modern antitumor therapy.
4. The use of newer chemotherapeutic drugs and other techniques, such as immunotherapy, may improve survival rates for these children.

Nursing Management

Nursing care for children with neuroblastoma is similar to that of children with other types of cancer.
Points of emphasis:
1. The child must be prepared for diagnostic tests and treatments in ways that are appropriate for his age and level of development.
2. General principles of preoperative and postoperative care should be applied for children who require abdominal, thoracic, or cranial surgery. Refer to sections on Wilms' tumor, below, cardiovascular surgery, page 1297, or brain tumor, page 1430.
3. For nursing care of the child receiving chemotherapy, refer to page 1422.
4. For nursing care of the child receiving radiation therapy, refer to page 1422.
5. Parents should be encouraged to express their feelings about the child's disease, and should be supported in their efforts to cope with the child's illness.
   Many parents feel guilty for not recognizing or reporting early signs of the illness. They may express anger toward health professionals or place blame on one another.
6. For nursing care of the terminally ill child, refer to page 1458.

WILMS' TUMOR

Wilms' tumor is a malignant renal tumor.

Etiology

1. The etiology of Wilms' tumor is not known.
2. Current evidence implicates unknown genetic factors.

Incidence

1. Wilms' tumor is the most common neoplasm involving the retroperitoneal space in children.
2. It constitutes approximately 30% of all pediatric renal masses and 7% of all childhood tumors.
3. 75% of cases occur before the child is 5 years of age.
4. Average age at time of diagnosis is 3 years.

Clinical Manifestations

1. A firm, nontender upper quadrant abdominal mass is usually the presenting sign; it may be on either side. (It is frequently observed by the parents.)
2. Abdominal pain, which is related to rapid growth of the tumor, may occur. As the tumor enlarges, pressure may cause constipation, vomiting, abdominal distress, anorexia, weight loss, and dyspnea.
3. Less common: hypertension, fever, hematuria, anemia.
4. Associated anomalies:
   a. Hemihypertrophy
   b. Aniridia (absence of the iris)
   c. Genitourinary anomalies

Pathophysiology

1. Wilms' tumor has a capacity for very rapid growth and usually grows to a large size before it is diagnosed.
2. The effect of the tumor on the kidney depends on the site of the tumor.
3. In most cases, the tumor expands the renal parenchyma, and the kidney becomes stretched over the surface of the tumor.
4. The covering of the tumor may be very thin and easily torn.
5. The tumor is often exceedingly vascular, soft, mushy, or gelatinous in character.
6. Wilms' tumors present various histological patterns from patient to patient.
7. The neoplasms metastasize early, either by direct extension or by way of the bloodstream. May invade perirenal tissues, lymph nodes, the liver, the diaphragm, abdominal muscles, and the lungs. Invasions of bone and brain are less common.
8. Staging of Wilms' tumor is done on the basis of clinical and anatomical findings. It ranges from Group I (tumor is limited to the kidney and is completely resected) to Group IV (metastases are present in the liver, lung, bone, or brain). Group V includes those cases in which there is bilateral involvement either initially or subsequently.

Diagnostic Evaluation

1. Abdominal x-ray
2. IVP—to demonstrate the tumor and to assess the status of the opposite kidney
3. X-ray of chest and skeletal survey to identify metastases
4. CBC and peripheral smear
5. Urinalysis
6. Blood chemistries, especially serum electrolytes, uric acid, renal function tests (BUN and creatinine), and liver function tests (bilirubin, SGOT, SGPT, LDH, total protein, albumin and alkaline phosphatase)
7. Coagulation studies—PT, PTT, and fibrinogen
8. Urinary VMA
9. Bone marrow examination—for tumor cells
10. Radioisotope scans and tomography to rule out metastasis (often postponed until after surgery)

Treatment

1. Determined by the stage of the tumor.
2. Includes a combination of surgery, radiation therapy, and chemotherapy.

Prognosis

1. Guarded, but encouraging.
2. High cure rate associated with early diagnosis and optimal treatment.
3. Prognosis best in children whose tumor is classified as Group I or II and who receive multimodal therapy.

Nursing Objectives and Management

A. *To support the family and the child at the time the diagnosis is made.*

1. Discuss with the physician what specific information has been given to the parents.
2. Provide the parents with the opportunity to express their concerns.
3. Provide the parents with a place where they may have some privacy when they wish to be alone.
4. Convey a compassionate attitude to the parents in talking with them, and assure them that their child's needs will be met.
5. Refer to section on family-centered care, page 1131.

B. *To exercise caution in the manipulation of the child in order to avoid inadvertently increasing the danger of metastasis.*

1. Bathe the child carefully, avoiding manipulation of the abdomen.
2. Hold the child carefully to prevent abdominal pressure.
3. Communicate the need for this caution to all staff members.
4. Place a sign on the child's bed to reduce indiscriminate palpation.

C. *To explain to the child and his parents the elements of preoperative and postoperative care.*

1. Utilize knowledge of growth and development to plan a teaching program for the child that will include diagnostic tests, preoperative care, and postoperative care. (Refer to section on the hospitalized child, p. 1126.)
2. Involve the parents in the teaching plan and encourage them to support the child at this time.

D. *To provide preoperative and postoperative care for the child.*

1. Refer to section on the child undergoing surgery, page 1139.
2. Many children require gastric suction postoperatively to prevent distention or vomiting.
   a. Refer to Guidelines: Nasogastric Intubation, page 392.
   b. Monitor gastric output accurately and replace it with appropriate IV fluids as prescribed by the physician.
   c. When oral feedings are resumed, begin with small amounts of clear fluids.
3. Continue to avoid abdominal manipulation, because cells may have escaped locally from the excised tumor.

E. *To care for the child receiving radiation therapy.*

1. Radiation therapy is given to the tumor bed postoperatively to render nonviable all cells that have escaped locally from the excised tumor. It is usually indicated for all children with Wilms' tumor except those under 18 months of age with Stage I disease.
2. Alterations in the growth and development of bones, joints, and musculature may occur as a result of radiation therapy.
3. Be aware that acute skin reactions occasionally occur when dactinomycin is given concomitantly with or follows administration of radiation therapy.
4. Refer to section on radiation therapy, page 1422.

F. *To care for the child receiving chemotherapy.*

1. Chemotherapy is initiated postoperatively to achieve maximal killing of tumor cells.
2. The usual chemotherapeutic agents employed are dactinomycin, vincristine, and Adriamycin.
3. Prepare the child and his family for chemotherapy.
4. Refer to section on chemotherapy, page 1422.

G. *To provide diversional therapy for the child.*

Provide the child with the opportunity for play as his condition permits.

H. *To provide supportive care appropriate for the dying child when the tumor metastasizes and the child's condition deteriorates.*

See section on the dying child, page 1458.

OSTEOGENIC SARCOMA

Osteogenic sarcoma is a malignant tumor of the bone.

Etiology

Unknown

Incidence

1. Most frequent malignant bone cancer in children.
2. Peak incidence between 10 and 25 years of age.

a. Most common at the peak of the adolescent growth spurt.
b. Males are affected more often than females, with a ratio of 1.5:1.

3. Common sites of occurrence—distal end of the femur or knee (over 50% of cases), proximal humerus, distal radius, and distal tibia.

Clinical Manifestations

1. Pain in the affected site, frequently causing limp or limitation of motion
2. Palpable, tender, fixed bony mass
3. Additional symptoms related to site of metastasis, if present

Pathophysiology

1. Presumably arises from bone-forming mesenchyme tissue.
2. Produces malignant spindle-cell stroma, which gives rise to malignant osteoid tissue.
3. Most osteogenic sarcomas are fully malignant but may appear in relatively nonmalignant forms.
4. Most commonly metastasizes to lungs and other bones.

Diagnostic Evaluation

1. X-ray examination—to visualize the tumor.
2. Serum alkaline phosphatase—often elevated.
3. Bone scan—helpful in detecting initial extent of malignancy, planning therapy, and evaluating effects of treatment.
4. Biopsy of lesion—to confirm the diagnosis and provide histologic data for the selection of a treatment plan.
5. Chest x-ray and tomography—to identify lung metastasis.
6. Renal and liver function tests—to screen for problems prior to initiating chemotherapy.

Medical/Surgical Management

1. Radical amputation of the affected limb, and often the joint proximal to the involved area, is required in most cases.
2. Newer techniques include transmedullary amputation and limb-salvaging surgery, such as total femur replacement.
3. Chemotherapy is advocated for 1–3 years following surgery. It is also used preoperatively for patients undergoing resectional surgery and for metastatic disease.

a. High-dose methotrexate with citrovorum factor rescue is the drug of choice.
b. Other drugs include doxorubicin, cyclophosphamide, derivatives of nitrogen mustard, bleomycin, and dactinomycin.

Prognosis

1. Survival has greatly improved with the aggressive use of multimodal therapy.
2. Approximately 50–60% of patients who undergo surgery followed by chemotherapy can expect to be disease-free after 3 years.
3. Limb-saving surgery has improved the quality of life for many survivors.

Nursing Management

Nursing care of the child with osteogenic sarcoma is essentially the same as care of the adult. Refer to page 789.
Points of emphasis:
1. The child must be prepared for diagnostic tests, surgery, and chemotherapy in ways that are appropriate for his age and level of development.
2. Radical body alterations caused by surgery and chemotherapy are especially upsetting for adolescents.
   a. They need time and support to accept the diagnosis and surgery, and to grieve for their lost body part.
   b. They can be helped to select clothing that camouflages the prosthesis yet is sexually appealing.
   c. Wigs, scarves, or hats are useful for children experiencing hair loss.
3. Discharge planning should be done to promote normalcy and resumption of appropriate presurgical activities.
   a. Accessibility of home and school should be assessed and environmental handicaps alleviated.
   b. The school nurse should be contacted to facilitate re-entry into school.
   c. Visits by peers should be encouraged, and the child should be helped to deal with questions and reactions from peers.
   d. A tutor should be arranged for students who must remain out of school for lengthy periods.
   e. A community health nursing referral should be initiated if appropriate.
4. For nursing care of the hospitalized adolescent, refer to page 1130.
5. For nursing care of the child receiving chemotherapy, refer to page 1422.

BIBLIOGRAPHY

Books

Alexander M and Brown M. Pediatric History Taking and Physical Diagnosis for Nurses. New York, McGraw–Hill, 1978
Jones PG and Campbell PE. Tumors of Infancy and Childhood. Philadelphia, JB Lippincott, 1976
Peterson BH and Kellogg CJ (eds). Current Practice in Oncologic Nursing. St. Louis, CV Mosby, 1976
Petrillo M and Sanger S. Emotional Care of Hospitalized Children. Philadelphia, JB Lippincott, 1978
Pochedly C. Neuroblastoma. Acton, Publishing Sciences Group Inc., 1976

Pochedly C (ed). Pediatric Cancer Therapy. Baltimore, University Park Press, 1979
Pochedly C and Miller D (eds). Wilms' Tumor. New York, John Wiley & Sons, 1976
Scipien G et al. Comprehensive Pediatric Nursing, 2nd ed. New York, McGraw–Hill, 1979
Sutow WW, Vietti TJ, Fernbach DJ. Clinical Pediatric Oncology, 2nd ed. St. Louis, CV Mosby, 1979
Van Eys J (ed). The Normally Sick Child. Baltimore, University Park Press, 1979
Whaley L and Wong D. Nursing Care of Infants and Children. St. Louis, CV Mosby, 1979

Articles

Barlock A, Howser D, Hubbard S. Nursing management of adriamycin extravasation. Am J Nurs 1979 Jan; 79(1):94–96

Belle–Isle J et al. Report of a discussion group for parents of children with leukemia. Matern Child Nurs J 1979 Spring; 8(1):49–58

Brand WN. Malignant diseases of infancy, childhood and adolescence: Radiotherapy. Major Probl Clin Pediatr 1978; 18:89–101

Brown N. The child with acute lymphocytic leukemia. MCN 1978 Sept/Oct; 3(5):290–295

Cotter JM et al. Malignant diseases of infancy, childhood and adolescence: Psychological and social support for the patient and family. Major Probl Clin Pediatr 1978; 18:120–127

DeLamerans SA. Management of Wilms' tumor. Pediatr Ann 1978 Aug; 7(8):52–71

Filler RM et al. Parenteral feeding in the management of children with cancer. Cancer (Suppl) 1979 May; 43:2117–2120

Fortunato RP et al. Death at home for children with acute lymphoblastic leukemia. Va Med 1979 Feb; 106(2):125–126

Gardner GG, August CS, Githens J. Psychological issues in bone marrow transplantation. Pediatrics 1977 Oct; 60(4):625–631

Gogan JL. Pediatric cancer survival and marriage: Issues affecting adult adjustment. Am J Orthopsychiatry 1979 July; 49(3):423–430

Gold E et al. Risk factors for brain tumors in children. Am J Epidemiol 1979 Mar; 109(3):309–319

Hvizdala AV et al. A summer camp for children with cancer. Med Pediatr Oncol 1978; 4(1):71–75

Klopovich P. Immunosuppression in the child who has cancer. MCN 1979 Sept/Oct; 4(5):288–292

Lansky SB. Childhood cancer: Nonmedical costs of the illness. Cancer 1979 Jan; 43(1):403–408

Lansky SB. Childhood cancer: Parental discord and divorce. Pediatrics 1978 Aug; 62(2):184–188

Leventhal BG. Immunotherapy in childhood cancer. Pediatr Ann 1978 Aug; 7(8):570–574

Mackey C and Hopefl A. Keeping infections down when risks go up. Nursing '80 1980 June; 80(6):69–73

Manchester P et al. The child with cancer—A plan of care. Pediatric Nursing 1978 Sept/Oct; 4(5):72–76

Maxwell M. Scalp tourniquets for chemotherapy-induced alopecia. Am J Nurs 1980 May; 80(5):900–902

Ostchega Y. Preventing and treating cancer chemotherapy's oral complications. Nursing '80 1980 Aug; 10(8):47–52

Pfefferbaum B. Pediatric bone marrow transplantation: Psychosocial aspect. Am J Psychiatry 1977 Nov; 134(11):1299–1301

Pochedly C. Acute lymphoid leukemia in children. Am J Nurs 1978 Oct; 78(10):1714–1716

Pochedly C. Guinea pigs get the best treatment—cooperative children's cancer therapy research. Pediatric Nursing 1978 Sept/Oct; 4(5):64–67

Powell K. Host defense mechanisms—the immune compromised host. Pediatric Nursing 1978 Sept/Oct; 4(5):13–16

Ritchie JA. Nursing the child undergoing limb amputation. MCN 1980 Mar/Apr; 5(2):114–121

Satterwhite B. What to do when adriamycin infiltrates. Nursing '80 1980 Feb; 10(2):37

Toal D. Tumor cell kinetics and cancer chemotherapy. Am J Nurs 1980 Oct; 80(10):1802–1804

Welch D. and Lewis K. Chemotherapy and alopecia. Am J Nurs 1980 May; 80(5):903–905

Wolf W and Bancroft B. Early detection of childhood malignancies. Pediatric Nursing 1980 Jan/Feb; 5(1):43–46

Additional References for Children and Parents

Diet and Nutrition: A resource for parents of children with cancer. U.S. Dept. of HEW, PHS, National Institutes of Health, Pub. No. 80–2038, Dec., 1979

Shilman R. Day by Day. California, Scrimshaw Press, 1977

There is A Rainbow Behind Every Dark Cloud. Center for Attitudinal Healing, 19 Main St., Tiburon, Ca. 94920

MENTAL RETARDATION

Mental retardation refers to significantly subaverage general intellectual functioning existing concurrently with deficits in adaptive behavior and manifested during the developmental period.*

Etiology

A. *General*

1. Congenital lack of brain cells
2. Later destruction of cells originally present

B. *Prenatal Factors*

1. Heredity
2. Fetal irradiation
3. Infection—maternal or fetal
4. Kernicterus due to Rh or ABO incompatibility
5. Anoxia
6. Cranial anomalies
   a. Hydrocephalus
   b. Craniosynostosis
7. Chromosomal abnormalities
8. Disorders of metabolism

C. *Natal Factors*

1. Anoxia
   a. Maternal
   b. Placental
   c. Respiratory obstruction
2. Breech delivery with delay in delivery of the head
3. Cerebral injury
   a. Trauma
   b. Cephalopelvic disproportion
   c. Precipitate delivery
   d. Prematurity
4. Infection
5. Intracranial hemorrhage

D. *Postnatal Factors*

1. Central nervous system infection
2. Brain injury, hemorrhage, or tumor
3. Cerebral degenerative disease
4. Anoxia
5. Poisoning
6. Vascular disorders
7. Social and cultural factors

E. *Unknown*

1. No identifiable organic or biologic cause for 65–75% of retardation in children.
2. Suspected causes include sociocultural or environmental deprivation or poverty.
3. Generally, these children are more mildly retarded than children with associated organic and physical defects.

Incidence

1. It is estimated that approximately 100,000–200,000 infants born each year in the U.S. will at some time in their lives be classified as mentally retarded.
2. A decrease in infant deaths, a longer life span, and improved case finding have caused a rise in the total number of persons classified as mentally retarded.

Classification**

1. In the past, the IQ score has been used to separate retarded children into 4 convenient categories:
   a. Mildly retarded (educable)—IQ 52–68
   b. Moderately retarded (trainable)—IQ 36–51
   c. Severely retarded—IQ 20–35
   d. Profoundly retarded (custodial)—IQ 19 and below
2. It is now known that although the IQ score may be helpful in assessing and planning for retarded children, low IQ itself is not sufficient to make a diagnosis of mental retardation.
3. Both intellectual level and adaptive behavior level (the effectiveness or degree with which the individual meets the standards of personal independence and social responsibility expected of his age and cultural

* Definition of the American Association on Mental Deficiency. In Heber R (ed). A Manual on Terminology and Classification in Mental Retardation. (Monograph Supplement). Am J Ment Defic 64:3, 1958

** Source: Grossman HJ. Manual on Terminology and Classification in Mental Retardation (A publication of the American Association on Mental Deficiency), pp. 15–33. Baltimore, Garamond/Pridemark Press, 1973

group) should be considered when one makes the classification.

4. Scales have been developed for measuring and classifying adaptive behavior based on the following expectations:
   a. *Infancy and early childhood*
      (1) Sensory-motor skills development
      (2) Communication skills (including speech and language)
      (3) Self-help skills
      (4) Socialization
   b. *Childhood and early adolescence*
      (1) Application of basic academic skills in daily life activities
      (2) Application of appropriate reasoning and judgment in mastery of environment
      (3) Social skills, group activities
   c. *Late adolescence and adult life*
      Vocational and social responsibilities and performances

5. Only those children who demonstrate deficits in both intellectual level and adaptive behavior should be classified as mentally retarded.

Clinical Manifestations

1. Developmental delay—Failure to meet normal motor, mental, and/or social milestones for age
2. Physical
   a. Approximately 75% of retarded individuals have no obvious physical stigma.
   b. Mentally retarded children have a greater percentage of sensory defects, language disorders, neuromuscular impairment, seizures, and physical anomalies than the general population.

Diagnostic Evaluation

1. Diagnosis is difficult and is most reliable when the determination is made by a comprehensive team that offers medical, psychological, social, and educational examinations.
2. Care must be taken to ensure that no child is mislabeled as mentally retarded.

Prognosis

1. Factors which influence the prognosis
   a. Degree of retardation
   b. Existence of additional, physical defects
   c. Family and community resources available to help the child to use his mental resources
2. Factors which favor improvement in intelligence
   a. Modification of the environment to eliminate stress and deprivation
   b. Improvement in learning opportunities
   c. Increased social acceptance
   d. Early intervention
3. The prognosis is best for the mildy retarded child without a coexistent physical defect.

Nursing Objectives

A. *To support parents during the initial period of diagnosis.*

1. Provide time for the parents to comprehend the extent of their problem and to mobilize their resources to work on its solution.
   a. When parents appear ready, offer counseling and verbal support at a slow pace, one step at a time.
   b. Be sensitive to clues concerning the type of support that is most helpful to each family.

2. Encourage both parents to talk about the diagnosis and how they feel about it.
   a. The parents' reaction will be individually determined by such factors as the nature of the diagnosis, the manner in which the family is told of the diagnosis, the perceived attitude of health professionals, the parents' previous life experiences, their attitudes toward retardation, their marital relationship, and their personal aspirations.
   b. Expect attitudes of guilt, shame, and self-pity; feelings of grief, hostility, and ambivalence; expressions of denial; thoughts that they might be unable to care for the child.
   c. Provide privacy for discussions.
   d. Express sympathetic understanding of the family's problems and show acceptance of their attitudes.
      Reassure them that many parents react to the diagnosis with grief and sorrow.
3. Assure the family that their child has had the benefit of the best diagnostic procedures and has been given any treatment that is indicated.
4. If appropriate, initiate a referral to a social worker, a psychiatrist, or any other professional who may assist the family to deal with their immediate reactions and may plan for the child's long-term care.
      Many parents benefit from the continuous or intermittent support of a variety of health professionals.
5. Communicate a genuine concern for the parents as individuals and an understanding of the responsibilities they have outside the hospital, i.e., care of other children, work, etc.

B. *To foster acceptance of the child by his parents and family, and to increase feelings of self-worth and self-confidence in parents.*

1. Serve as a role model by interacting with the child in a manner which conveys acceptance, respect, and love.
2. Help parents to develop a fundamental understanding of what has happened to their child and what this means in terms of his future development.
   a. Clarify and support medical speculations regarding the cause of the retardation.
      (1) Genetic counseling is indicated, especially in familial types of retardation.
      (2) Answer parental questions sensitively but directly.
      (3) Provide explanations in terms they can understand.
      (4) Avoid vague generalities, such as "the child is slow," and demoralizing words, such as "moron" or "imbecile."
   b. Provide as much specific information as possible. Parents have the right to know what diagnostic tests have been done, what positive or negative conclusions have been made, what uncertainties remain, and what general prognosis can be made.
3. Involve both parents in the child's care so that they may gain a realistic concept of his ability.
   a. Point out the child's areas of strengths and weaknesses and show how these can be considered in his management.
   b. Emphasize the *well* part of the child and that he has the same needs as a normal child for love and security.
4. Include the family as soon as possible with other

members of the health team in planning for the child's future care.

   a. The plan should be based on the degree of the child's retardation, the reaction of the family to the diagnosis, and the availability of community resources.

   b. The family should be supported in the decisions they make.

   c. The family should be guided to make decisions for the child's care which will allow for maximum utilization of his capabilities.

5. Discuss with parents their plans for dealing with the siblings of the retarded child.

   a. Adequate explanations and information should be given to siblings early to avoid any misconceptions later.

   b. Siblings often need help in explaining the retarded child's abnormality to their friends.

   c. Caution parents to guard against intense sibling rivalry; the other children often feel neglected because of the amount of time devoted to the retarded child.

6. If appropriate, initiate a community health nursing referral for assistance with planning and implementing home care.

C. *To provide mental and motor stimulation.*

1. Assess the child's functional level of development, and define and implement plans to help him achieve the next developmental tasks. (Refer to section on growth and development, p. 1093.)

2. Play is an essential part of the child's care.

   Select toys on the basis of functional level, not on the age group for which they were intended.

3. Expose the child to a variety of materials and toys which stimulate all of his senses.

   a. Equipment such as rocking chairs, musical instruments, record players, blocks, art materials, and simple picture books are indispensable.

   b. Toys should be accessible for the child to use when he desires.

4. An educational specialist or occupational therapist may be able to provide invaluable guidance in this area.

D. *To teach the child basic skills with the long-range goal of developing independent behavior at the highest level possible according to the child's potential.*

1. Determine the child's care plan according to his individual areas of strengths and weaknesses and coordinate it with the plans of the related health professionals.

2. Because a retarded child has a limited attention span, present a smaller amount of material to him at a slower rate and over a longer period of time than to a normal child.

3. Provide organized, consistent, and repetitive experiences.

4. Employ techniques of positive reinforcement.

   a. Give rewards for positive responses so that the probability of recurrence of that response will be strengthened.

     Rewards should be given consistently and immediately after the approved response.

   b. Do not reward unacceptable behaviors.

5. Break complex behaviors down into small steps which the child can easily achieve.

   a. This is very important in the areas of feeding, dressing, and toilet training.

   b. Do not expect the child to transfer learning from one situation to another.

6. Base expectations for the child on his mental ability, *not* on his chronological age.

7. Maintain a relaxed learning environment.

E. *To reduce destructive behavior and encourage that which is socially acceptable.*

1. Establish a routine of daily living so that the child knows precisely what is expected of him.

2. Employ consistent discipline.

   a. Use language that the child understands so that he can comprehend his misdeed.

   b. When punishment is necessary, it should follow the misdeed immediately.

3. Provide immediate reinforcement for positive behaviors and ignore undesirable behaviors.

F. *To prepare the mentally retarded individual so that he may cope successfully (within his potentiality) with the problems and adjustments of adult life.*

1. Help parents identify areas of home responsibilities which may be delegated to the retarded child.

2. In the child's early learning activities, provide habits which are essential to his later vocational life.

   a. Getting to places on time

   b. Cooperating

   c. Focusing and holding attention on the task at hand

   d. Establishing acceptable interpersonal relationships

3. Help the child to develop a set of attitudes and behaviors that will motivate him to work.

4. Identify attainable occupational goals early in the child's educational experience.

   Early education should tie into later social and vocational programs.

G. *To be aware of nursing activities associated with hospitalization of a child previously diagnosed as mentally retarded.*

1. Apply all of the previously outlined principles.

2. Obtain a thorough nursing history from the parent and/or child regarding the child's usual home routines.

   a. Feeding

   b. Sleeping

   c. Toilet habits

   d. Learning activities

   e. Play

   f. Vocabulary

   g. Discipline

3. Utilize the information obtained to develop a nursing care plan which provides for continuity of care from home to hospital in order to maintain the child's sense of security and minimize his regression.

   Counsel the mother that some regression can be anticipated even in normal children who require hospitalization.

4. Encourage parental participation to the extent that it is therapeutic for both the child and the parent(s).

5. Provide a safe environment according to the child's needs.

   a. This environment is best determined by observing the child and from information obtained during the admission interview.

   b. If possible, use the type of bed with which the child is familiar.

   c. Remove any objects that are potentially injurious to the child.

6. Whenever possible, assign consistent nursing personnel to care for the child.
7. Explain procedures to the child using communication methods appropriate for his level of cognitive development.

H. *To help modify existing social attitudes toward retardation.*

1. Assess and work through your own feelings about the retarded, including personal attitudes and defenses which are used to avoid personal involvement in the care of retarded children and their families.
2. Utilize opportunities to influence the attitudes of other hospitalized children and their families.
   a. Serve as a role model in your own interactions with retarded children.
   b. Encourage hospitalized children to socialize with the retarded child during play programs or other activities, and help them to understand and accept the child.
   c. Provide opportunities for other parents to discuss their feelings about retardation and to ask questions. Correct any misconceptions they may have.
3. Initiate and/or support community educational and service programs.
4. Support federal legislation relating to funding for research and services for the mentally retarded.

Parental Education

1. The mentally retarded child may require more medical supervision than the healthy child. Regular dental care is also essential.
   a. The child is often more susceptible to infections.
   b. He may eat poorly.
   c. He may be underweight or overweight.
   d. He may have poor motor coordination.
   e. He often has speech and language problems.
2. Secondary handicaps such as visual or hearing problems should be treated.
3. The child's environment has a great influence on his behavior, growth, and development. It should provide experiences which contribute to a positive self-concept of a person who is loved, wanted, valued, and respected.
4. Parents need to be helped to recognize their child's method of communicating so that they can respond to his needs.
5. Parents should be assisted to identify learning readiness in their child in order to help him achieve his maximum level of development without subjecting him to unnecessary experiences of failure and frustration.
6. Practical, tangible suggestions relative to everyday living should be offered to the parents.
   a. Selection of toys

   b. Techniques of feeding
   c. Patterns for toilet training
   d. Methods of discipline
7. Special precautions may be necessary to provide a safe environment for the child.
   His delayed motor, intellectual, and social development make him more vulnerable to the usual childhood accidents.
8. The child should have the opportunity of participating in social, religious, and recreational activities.
   a. Organizations should be selected in which the probability of success is the highest.
   b. The parent should discuss the situation with the group leader and the leader should have an opportunity to meet the child so that both child and leader can assess each other.
9. Available literature should be offered to parents; they should also be made aware of community resources.
   a. Community nursing agencies
   b. Day care centers
   c. Foster grandparent programs
   d. Nursery groups
   e. Special schools
   f. Parent groups
   g. Volunteer organizations
   h. Specialized diagnostic facilities
   i. Recreational programs
   j. Vocational training
   k. Residential settings
   l. National associations
10. Parents need to know that they are important as people. They each should be encouraged to lead a normal life. They should be helped to feel that they are not their child's only resource, but that others care and are willing to help.
11. Parents should be assisted in making decisions regarding residential placement.
   a. Alternatives to home care and reasons for placement should be discussed as appropriate.
   b. Parents should be helped to select the best alternative to home care and establish ways to maintain contact with the child.
12. References for Parents:
   American Association on Mental Deficiency, 5201 Connecticut Ave. N.W., Washington, D.C. 20015
   Joseph P. Kennedy Jr. Foundation, 200 Park Ave., New York, N.Y. 10017
   National Association for Retarded Children, 420 Lexington Ave., New York, N.Y. 10017
   National Recreation Association, Consulting Service on Recreation for the Ill and Handicapped, 8 West 8th St., New York, N.Y. 10011

DOWN'S SYNDROME

Down's syndrome is a chromosomal abnormality involving an extra chromosome (number 21), characterized by a typical physical appearance and mental retardation.

Etiology

A. *Trisomy 21*

1. The abnormality is an error in cell division.
   a. Both number 21 chromosomes in the pair instead of just one of the pair migrate to one daughter cell during meiosis.
   b. 47 chromosomes are present in the new individual rather than the normal 46.
   c. There are 3 number 21 chromosomes, thus extra genetic material.
2. Occurrence is associated with advanced maternal age.
   a. Risk is increased after maternal age of 35.

b. Occurrence in the same set of parents is rare, but dependent upon maternal age.

3. This form of Down's syndrome is not inherited.

B. *Translocation*

1. Chromosome number 21 attaches to another chromosome, usually the 13–15 group.
2. This abnormal attachment occurs in the parent.
   a. Parent passes on to the offspring an extra dose of chromosome 21, plus a normal chromosome 21.
   b. The child with this type of Down's syndrome has 46 chromosomes.
3. This form of Down's syndrome is inherited.
   In most cases it is a fresh occurrence, and for chromosomally normal parents there is small risk of a future child with Down's syndrome. In one-third of the cases, one parent is a balanced trans-location carrier; thus, there is risk of recurrence.

Altered Physiology

1. The normal person, without Down's syndrome, has 46 chromosomes (23 pairs).
   a. One pair of chromosomes is sex-determining.
   b. 22 pairs of chromosomes are non-sex-determining and are called *autosomes*.
2. The individual with Down's syndrome has an extra chromosome—number 21. He carries extra genetic material.
3. Abnormalities that are present at birth occurred during fetal growth.
   a. Normal fetal growth has been interfered with.
   b. This interference affects mainly the heart, brain, eyes, hands, and general growth.

Clinical Manifestations

1. Physical stigmata recognized at birth:
   a. Marked hypotonia and floppiness
   b. Joint hyperextension or hyperflexibility
   c. Tendency to keep mouth open with tongue protruding; high, arched palate; furrowed tongue
   d. Brachycephaly with relatively flat occiput
   e. Eyes slant upward and outward with internal epicanthal folds
   f. Excess skin on back of neck
   g. Flattened nasal bridge and flat facial profile
   h. Small ears, often incompletely developed
   i. Spade-like hands; there is inward curving of distal phalanx of fifth finger; simian crease
   j. Short, broad feet; there is a wide separation between first and second toe (plantar furrow)
   k. Small male genitalia
   l. Absence of Moro reflex. (Response to sudden loud noise, causing body to stiffen and arms to go up and out, then forward and toward each other. Thumb and index finger will assume "C" shape.)
2. Complications most likely to be present at birth:
   a. Congenital cardiac defects, especially atrial septal defect
   b. Duodenal stenosis and other intestinal obstruction
3. Later findings in the child (up to 1 year of age):
   a. Slow intellectual development (IQ 20–75; mean: 50)
   b. Slow motor development

Complications

1. Recurrent infection of upper respiratory tract
2. Skin infections
3. Complications secondary to physical anomalies present at birth:

a. Eye problems—strabismus; error in refractions
b. Elevated leukocyte enzymes
   (1) Small percentage of affected children born with fatal leukemia
   (2) Leukemia—acute type developing in first 2–3 years
4. Serious behavioral problems

Diagnostic Evaluation

Chromosomal analysis (karyotyping) will show how the third chromosome, number 21, is attached to another autosome in translocation or nondisjunction.

Nursing Objectives and Management

Newborn

A. *To establish and maintain adequate nutrition to allow for growth and development.*

1. The diet is calculated according to infant's needs.
2. Due to poor muscle tone and protruding tongue, the infant may be a poor eater with a weak and ineffective suck.
   a. Provide the appropriate nipple so that minimal sucking effort is needed to feed.
   b. Allow adequate time for feeding. Do not allow the infant to become overly tired.
   c. Note and report poor eating and insufficient sucking.

B. *To observe carefully for any signs of physical complications that may occur with Down's syndrome. Record and report them immediately.*

1. Intestinal obstruction (duodenal stenosis)
   a. Observe for abdominal distention and its association with feeding.
   b. Note vomiting—what is vomited and when.
      (1) Bile-stained emesis indicates lower tract obstruction.
      (2) Partially digested milk indicates upper tract obstruction.
   c. Note absence of stools.
2. Congenital cardiac defect
   a. When taking vital signs, note any irregularity of the heart rate. Murmurs may not be evident to the untrained ear. Note any respiratory distress or labored respirations.
   b. Note any cyanosis and when it occurs—with crying, feeding, or all the time.
   c. Be particularly alert to the infant tiring easily during feeding.

C. *To provide a safe environment for the infant.*

1. Infant is usually very floppy due to poor muscle tone. When handling the infant, support him well with a firm grasp.
2. Position infant in such a manner that if vomiting should occur he will not aspirate.
   a. If he is on his abdomen, be certain that he can turn his head to the side.
   b. Prop him with a diaper roll so that position will be maintained.
   c. This infant is not usually very active; thus, his position will need to be changed frequently.

D. *To provide proper stimulation according to the child's age.*

1. Be aware that this infant needs stimulation from the very start to begin to help him develop to his potential. Develop a plan of stimulation so that your activity and actions lead toward this goal.

a. Babies with Down's syndrome who are quiet and undemanding tend to be understimulated, so they do not reach their full potential.

b. Begin a program of mental stimulation early— one that can be continued at home.

(1) Program should include exercises built around existing reflexes; these can reduce hypotonia.

(2) Encourage exercises to develop eye-hand co-ordination and later finger-thumb grasp.

2. Offer positive and effective sensory stimulation. Hold and fondle infant, especially during feeding.

3. When the infant is awake, the adult face in his visual field is good stimulation and should interest him for a few seconds.

4. The gentle sound of talking or music can provide a pleasant auditory experience. The infant should stop activity and listen.

E. *To encourage parental participation in caring for and handling the infant and to foster acceptance of the child by his parents and family.*

1. Provide opportunities for the parents to learn all aspects of caring for their baby. The basic needs of the baby with Down's syndrome are the same as those of other infants.

Emphasize the need for parents to appreciate the child for his unique attributes; he can be lovable and can be enjoyed as a person, but he demands special attention.

2. All the support and help given the parents during hospitalization will make home care easier. Early intervention and support should strengthen and support the parental role.

a. Encourage physician to have both parents present, possibly with the infant, when he tells them of child's diagnosis. In this way they can turn to each other for support.

b. Make special efforts to involve the father. Respond to his needs—he may require special attention, support, and guidance.

c. Adaptation by both parents is critical for the continual improvement of the child's functioning and to foster optimal growth and development.

d. Encourage parents to tell siblings about their "special" baby early. Openness with the family can provide mutual support and communication.

e. Help parents to be honest in their thoughts and emotions concerning the baby.

f. Help parents to accept the fact that their child has Down's syndrome and to accept the child for himself.

3. Assist parents in learning what Down's syndrome is and how it alters a child's mental and physical development.

a. Provide appropriate literature. (See bibliography for some suggestions.)

b. Inform them of local or national organizations.

c. Alert parents to some common physical deviations that occur with Down's syndrome and the consequent effect of these deviations on behavior. If possible, provide an adjusted time table of development which takes into account the child's retardation.

4. Initiate community nurse referral. A community nurse can be helpful to the family in planning home care.

5. Initiate social work referral. The social worker can help parents to better understand their family situation and their feelings about their child.

6. Invite parents to join a group of parents who have children with Down's syndrome. Counseling can also alleviate the parents' loss of self-concept and feeling of self-worth.

7. Be aware of problems that new parents of a Down's syndrome baby may encounter.

a. Grief for the loss of the expected normal child.

b. Poor communication with the baby's physician.

c. Difficulty in telling family and friends.

8. Emphasize the infant's need for love, affection, consideration, and individual attention.

F. *To work effectively with parents.*

To accomplish this, health professionals relating to parents must:

1. Recognize and understand their own feelings about the infant.

2. Have an objective approach to each family situation.

3. Discuss all information with both parents.

The Older Child

The older child with Down's syndrome is usually admitted to the hospital because of some medical complication, such as an acute respiratory infection.

A. *To interview the parents thoroughly at the time of admission to learn as much as possible about the child and his activities at home.*

1. What is the child's vocabulary? What words or sounds does he use for elimination, certain foods, etc.?

2. Be aware of the child's schedule and activities at home.

a. This patient usually functions better in a familiar environment. He may react adversely to the new situation.

b. Know what activities the child can or cannot do and what he likes to do.

3. Be familiar with the child's eating habits and pattern.

a. Give him foods he likes and avoid foods he dislikes.

b. Adjust his mealtimes to those he is used to as much as possible and know at which mealtime he eats best.

4. Be aware of how parents discipline the child.

5. Share this information with nursing staff to assure continuity of care from home to hospital to minimize fear and frustration in the child.

6. Plan the child's day according to what he is used to as much as possible.

B. *To attend to the child's needs according to the medical problem that required his hospitalization.*

C. *To provide a safe environment for the child according to his needs.*

1. This can best be judged by observing the child and by obtaining information during the parental interview.

2. If possible, use the type of bed with which the child is familiar.

3. Remove any objects which might be injurious to the child should he play with them.

D. *To plan and provide for the appropriate type of play program and stimulation for the child.*

1. Assess the child's level of growth and development and consider this in the plan.

2. Do not try to teach the child new or different things as he may react adversely to the newness.

3. Allow the child as much independence as possible in his care, but provide guidance as necessary.

4. Permit the development of the child's abilities. Minimize frustrating situations.

E. To foster continuing parental acceptance of the child and to provide support for them.

1. Invite parents to care for their child as much as they can. Rooming-in may be advisable.
2. Help the parents to understand why the child behaves as he does.
3. Encourage parents to talk about their feelings or problems they have with the child. Reemphasize the need for parents to appreciate their child for his unique attributes and special characteristics, such as sociability and sensitivity to feelings of others.
4. Initiate a teaching program for the child and his parents early. Continued educational experiences are vital. Offer the family available literature and help them to become familiar with community resources.
   a. Parents can provide positive and effective sensory training.
   b. Help child to socialize with other children and provide an environment that will stimulate him mentally.
5. Allow parents to continue to maintain what other responsibilities they may have outside the hospital, i.e., other children, work.

   Do not insist they stay at the hospital and attend only to this child.

Parental Education

Parental education is one very important aspect in the nursing care of a child with Down's syndrome, especially in the following areas:

1. The environment has an influence on the rate of the child's progress in performance, behavior, growth, and development.
   a. The role of the parents is critical. A nurturing and loving environment gives the child the best chance to develop to his full potential.
   b. Encourage the entire family to be included in the child's care.
   c. The child will usually be lovable and quiet, affectionate, and socially responsive if he is loved and if individual attention is given to his specific needs.
   d. Patience and understanding must be developed by parents and family.
2. The child learns best in the play situation.
   a. The child is slower at learning and will require more time to learn each new skill.
   b. The child tends to mimic, which later results in learning.
   c. He may have a sensitivity to rhythmic stimulation and usually likes music.
   d. Social development is more advanced than the level of mental development.
3. Provide a safe environment.
   Because he may be less sensitive to heat, cold and pain, attention should be directed toward eliminating these hazards.
4. Help parents to understand that in spite of signs of slow mental growth, the child can make steady progress. In early life, the child with Down's syndrome should not be stereotyped in behavior. His behavior is similar to the norm when mental age is considered. Help parents not to lower their expectations.
   a. The child needs a great deal of repetition in all areas of learning.

b. He usually has a good memory, can acquire a fairly large vocabulary and can learn to spell. Arithmetic may be more difficult for him.
c. Speech may lag behind walking by 1–2 years. He may encounter trouble in pronouncing certain words. Stammering may occur if the child is under pressure.
d. Parents need help in learning to recognize the child's readiness to learn these skills.
e. A general decrease of IQ score occurs with increasing age and should be an expected occurrence because of the increasing verbal and abstract content of test materials at the higher mental age.

5. The child's motor development is slow. The degree of hypotonia probably greatly influences the early motor development; genetic potential and environmental stimulation of the child also influence motor development.
   a. Encourage motor coordination. It will take time for the child to learn to sit. At age 5 or 6 years, he may still walk like a 2-year-old child. Toilet training can generally be accomplished.
   b. He may always have trouble with fine motor skills.
   c. Encourage child to do as much for himself as he can.
6. Precautionary measures should be taken.
   a. Discuss the importance of good nutrition for growth. Supply available literature for a balanced diet appropriate for age.
   b. Obtain prompt treatment for any medical problems that may occur. This child is particularly prone to infection. Good nutrition, proper exercise, appropriate dress, and good general hygiene can help prevent infection.
   c. The child with Down's syndrome needs discipline. Limits need to be set so he knows what he can or cannot do.
7. Other members of the family must be considered.
   a. The child should not be thought of as a sick child, but as a child who needs special handling to promote his individual growth and development. But he does not need all the attention all the time.
   b. The family should be included in his care, but they also must have a life of their own and as much parental attention as they would receive if the child were not present in the family.
   c. Parents need time to themselves. They should be encouraged to go out alone together and to give time to their marriage.
   d. Encourage parents to be open with the family and to discuss concerns. Children are sensitive to parental distress. Lack of communication can create and increase parental isolation and can cause unrealistic concerns.
   e. Sibling reactions generally reflect the parent's reactions toward the child with Down's syndrome.
   f. Assist parents to assess their family situation to promote healthy family relationships. Do the following situations exist?
      (1) Are older siblings frequent caretakers of the child with Down's syndrome?
      (2) Is there excessive parental attention to afflicted child at expense of other siblings?
      (3) Do the parents show hostility toward the child?
      (4) Are there excessive expectations of other children?
      (5) Is the family dominated by the destructiveness or overactivity of child with Down's syndrome?

8. Future in society
   a. The child with Down's syndrome should go to school. He learns by copying. Have parents discuss the child's problem with the school nurse, the teacher, and other adults who have close contact with the child.
   b. Education enables the child with Down's syndrome to be productive to some extent in society, to have a fuller life, and to take pride in his accomplishments. Such children can learn routine housework, gardening, or farming. They can run errands, learn to obey traffic rules, and ride buses.
   c. Help parents to discuss their feelings or plans regarding continued home care or placement in an institution. Alternatives to complete home life are the following:
      (1) Day care centers or special preschool programs
      (2) Special education programs in public schools
      (3) Sheltered workshops
      (4) Foster home
      (5) Institutionalization (preferably not before age 5–6)

Agencies

American Association on Mental Deficiency, 5201 Connecticut Ave. N.W., Washington, D.C. 20015

Caring—a national organization for parents of children with Down's syndrome. P.O. Box 196, Milton, Washington 98354. (Publishes *Sharing and Caring* 5 times per year.)

Closed Look Box 1492, Washington, D.C., 20013 (A parent information service operated by the National Information Center for the Handicapped; provides information on services for the handicapped.)

Joseph P. Kennedy Jr. Foundation, Room 3021, 200 Park Ave., N.Y., N.Y. 10017

National Association for Retarded Children, 420 Lexington Ave., N.Y., N.Y. 10017

National Association for Retarded Citizens, Inc., 2709 Ave. E East, Arlington, Texas 76011

National Recreation Association, Consulting Service on Recreation for the Ill and Handicapped, 8 West 8th St., N.Y., N.Y. 10011

State Department of Mental Health

MINIMAL BRAIN DYSFUNCTION

Minimal brain dysfunction (MBD) is a general term used to refer to children of normal intelligence who have learning or behavioral disabilities which are associated with deviations of function of the central nervous system.

Etiology

1. Unknown.
2. Multiple causes, including psychosocial factors, may be involved.
3. Contributing factors:
   a. Genetic variations
   b. Some insult, usually mild, during the early developmental months
   c. Bio-chemical irregularities
   d. Dietary sensitivity to specific foods or food additives

Incidence

1. Estimated to occur in as many as 15% of children.
2. Males are affected more frequently than females.
3. Most important cause of school underachievement.

Clinical Manifestations

The child usually demonstrates a constellation of the following features:
1. Behavioral Characteristics
   a. Hyperactivity—stimulus-bound behavior which lacks consistent direction and frequently shifts focus. Usually manifested in mild to moderate degrees.
   b. Short attention span—inability to focus on the task at hand because of low threshold to distracting stimuli.
   c. Impulsivity—inability to delay gratification. Difficulty restraining impulses to move or speak.
   d. Labile emotions—poorly modulated emotional response. Results in extreme reactions of pleasure and displeasure triggered by relatively minor stimuli.
   e. Perseveration—inability to shift attention appropriately from one activity to another.
   f. Impaired interpersonal relations and antisocial behavior.
   g. Hypoactivity—much less common than hyperactivity.
2. Learning Disability
   Specific deficit of learning, such as of listening, thinking, reading, writing, or arithmetic.
3. Neurological Features
   a. Poor motor integration or coordination.
   b. Perceptual deficits—difficulty with perception of time, space, form, sound, and sequence resulting in confusion of right to left, before and after, etc.

Diagnostic Evaluation

1. Detailed medical, developmental, and behavioral history.
2. Neurologic examination to detect abnormalities.
3. Psychologic testing to determine the exact nature of cognitive or perceptual dysfunctions that may be present.
4. Additional testing depends on the child's symptomatology and frequently includes EEG and hearing evaluation.

Management

A multi-faceted approach involving some or all of the following aspects is necessary:

1. Family education and counseling concerning MBD
2. Medication
   Central nervous system stimulants such as Benzedrine, Dexedrine, and Ritalin used alone or in combination are effective in reducing many of the symptoms of some children with MBD.
3. Environmental manipulation to decrease external stimuli and encourage desirable behavior patterns
4. Remedial education focused on the specific area(s) of deficit
5. Psychiatric or psychologic therapies

Nursing Objectives and Management

A *To identify minimal brain dysfunction.*

1. Be aware of the clinical features of MBD.
2. Observe the child's behavior for evidence of abnormality.
3. Include developmental and behavioral components in the nursing history.
4. Make appropriate referrals for diagnosis in suspected cases of MBD.

B. *To provide emotional support to the family.*

1. Provide parents with opportunities to express their feelings and concerns about the diagnosis.
2. Expect such reactions as guilt, disbelief, relief, anger, and frustration. Reassure parents that these feelings are normal and acceptable.
3. Provide factual information about the disorder and treatment plan.
4. Assist parents to deal with identified problems, and provide them with positive feedback when appropriate.
5. Help parents anticipate and deal with the reactions and needs of siblings.
6. Assist the family to find appropriate programs to meet the child's special needs.
7. Serve as coordinator of services between family, school, physician, and other agencies.
8. Refer to a parent support group if one is available.

C. *To reduce symptoms.*

1. Administer prescribed medications.
   a. The child is usually started on a small dose, which is gradually increased until the desired response is achieved.
   b. Evaluate the child's response to medication by direct observation and consultation with others, such as parents and teachers.
   c. Observe for side-effects, including appetite suppression, sleep disturbance, stomach upset, and blurred vision.
      These usually disappear after a few weeks of therapy or with alteration of dosage.
2. Provide controlled diet if prescribed.

D. *To provide a therapeutic physical environment.*

1. Assist parents to manipulate the home environment to reduce stimulation and stress.
   a. Maintenance of regular sleeping, eating, working, and playing routines is helpful.
   b. Provide a minimum of external stimuli and alternatives.
   c. Set firm but reasonable limits on behavior, and carry through with consistent discipline.

d. Avoid situations that cause excessive excitement, stimulation, or fatigue.
2. Evaluate the environment for safety hazards and eliminate them.
3. Provide for energy release.
   a. Plan for periods of physical activity, vocal outlet, and outdoor play.
   b. Channel need for movement into safe, appropriate activities.

E. *To care for the hospitalized child previously diagnosed with MBD.*

1. Elicit a detailed history emphasizing management techniques currently used by the family.
2. Continue home management techniques during the hospitalization as much as possible.
3. Manipulate the hospital environment to reduce unnecessary stimulation and stress.
4. Eliminate any safety hazards.
5. Observe the child for response to hospitalization and his therapeutic regimen.
6. Provide continued support to parents.

F. *To participate in community programs.*

1. Take advantage of opportunities to teach about MBD.
2. Assist with related screening programs.

Parental Education

1. Provide factual information about the disorder, clearly differentiating MBD from mental retardation, autism, and other disabilities.
2. Teach parents regarding all aspects of the management program.
   a. Medication
      (1) Parents should be instructed concerning the dosage and schedule, desired effects and side-effects of medication.
      (2) They should be helped to think of the use of medication for MBD as a necessity, much as insulin is used for the diabetic, rather than as a tranquilizer.
      (3) They can be assured that there is no evidence that the drugs produce any euphoric effect or addiction in children.
   b. Diet
      Parents may need help in locating sources for the proper foods.
   c. Environmental manipulation to reduce stimulation and stress
   d. Consistent and appropriate disciplinary techniques
   e. Remedial education
      Assist parents to understand, select, and demand the best alternatives for their child's education.
3. Caution parents about unproven approaches which profess a single solution to the problem of MBD.
4. Resources for Parents:
   Fisher J. A Parents' Guide To Learning Disabilities, New York, Charles Scribner's, 1978
   Association for Children With Learning Disabilities, 4156 Library Road, Pittsburgh, Pa. 15234

GENETIC COUNSELING

Genetic counseling is the process of providing families with information about hereditary and congenital disorders. It involves determining the risk of occurrence or recurrence, interpreting the findings, and assisting the family in making a reasonable decision.

Indications for Prenatal Diagnosis of Genetic Disorders

1. Increased risk of chromosomal disorders
   a. Advanced maternal age—woman 35 years of age and older
   b. Parent known to be a carrier of chromosomal disorder
   c. Previous pregnancy resulting in child with chromosomal disorder
2. Known risk for significant metabolic disorders
3. Known risk for significant sex-linked genetic disorders
4. Willingness to consider termination of the pregnancy if an abnormal fetus is detected

Prenatal Diagnosis of Genetic Disorders

A. *Amniocentesis* (see Obstetrics, p. 1002)

1. Method of obtaining amniotic fluid of a pregnant woman by inserting a needle transabdominally through the uterus.
2. Examination is made of amniotic fluid, amniotic fluid cells, and cultured amniotic fluid cells.
3. Procedure done at 12–16 weeks gestation.
4. Useful in diagnosing some inborn errors of metabolism.

B. *Roentgenography*

1. Useful in diagnosing anencephaly, hydrocephaly, achondroplasia, osteogenesis imperfecta congenita, myelomeningocele, and bilateral cleft palate.
2. Many diagnoses are established only in the last trimester.
3. Risk of radiation exposure to fetus is high if done prior to third trimester.

C. *Amniography-Fetography*

1. A technique of intra-amniotic injection of a contrast material which opacifies the fluid and displaces the fetal soft tissue parts.
2. Useful in diagnosing soft tissue and gastrointestinal malformations, intrauterine growth retardation, and multiple gestation.

D. *Ultrasonography*

1. Used in conjunction with other clinical, laboratory, and sometimes radiologic studies in diagnosing malformations of the central nervous system.
2. Used to determine the size of the fetus and the fetal head.
3. Useful when an amniocentesis is to be done.

E. *Fetoscope*

Visualization of fetus in utero by endoscopic instruments (experimental).

Diagnostic Studies Performed from Amniocentesis

A. *Amniotic Fluid*

1. Steroid levels
2. Enzyme studies
3. Mucopolysaccharide determinations
4. Alpha-fetoprotein levels

B. *Amniotic Cells*

1. Enzyme studies
2. Sex chromatin and Y-body fluorescence

C. *Amniotic Fluid Cells, Cultured*

1. Cytogenetic studies (karyotype)
2. Enzyme studies
3. Autoradiographic studies
4. Histochemistry

Major Genetic Disorders

See Table 51-1.

Goals of Genetic Counseling

1. To provide clients with information about the genetic defect in question.
2. To communicate to clients the risk of transmitting the defect to subsequently conceived children.
3. To enable individuals and couples to make informed decisions regarding marriage and/or parenthood (e.g., having children, adopting children, continuing or terminating an existing pregnancy).
4. To provide psychological support to assist clients with their decision-making process and the necessary reordering of their lives.
5. To reduce the number of individuals affected by genetic disease.
6. To alert other health professionals involved with the family of the possibility of genetic disease in family background.

Nursing Objectives Related to Genetic Counseling

A. *To identify families who need genetic counseling and to whom the service should be offered.*

1. Be alert to information in the family history which would indicate referral for genetic counseling.
2. Be aware of evidence of deviation from normal growth and development and of other abnormalities (e.g., a single umbilical artery, low-set ears, or defects of the genitalia) which may indicate genetic problems.
3. Offer the opportunity for counseling to any family that has a child with a known genetic problem.

B. *To assist families to acquire sufficient and correct information about the genetic problem in question.*

1. Be aware of local and regional centers for genetic counseling and other available resources.
2. Be knowledgeable about the types of genetic disorders and their probability of occurrence (see Table 52-1), genetic principles, and genetic diagnostic methods.

C. *To serve as a liaison between the genetic counselor and the family.*

NOTE: In some situations, the nurse acts as the counselor.

1. Prepare parents for the experience of counseling.

TABLE 51-1. COMMON GENETIC DISORDERS

Types	Incidence	Characteristics	Risk	Discussion
Chromosomal Disorders				Chromosomal disorders result from:
1. Autosomal Abnormalities Down's syndrome (Trisomy 21) (See p. 1439)	1 in 600 live births; varies with maternal age; meiotic nondisjunction Young mother: 1 in 1000 live births Mother over 35: 1 in 300 live births	Brachycephalic skull; oblique palpebral fissures; epicanthal folds; Brushfield's spots; multiple eye defects; flat nasal bridge; protruding, fissured tongue; growth retardation; short extremities; dry, scaly skin; clinodactyly and simian line; mental retardation; congenital heart disease	Insufficient data	1. Failure of a chromosome to separate at cell division (nondisjunction), causing loss or gain of genetic material. 2. Cell division error causing a chromosomal imbalance or rearrangement of genetic material. Error is associated with major structural changes.
2. Monosomy (autosomal)	Product of conception rarely survives		Spontaneous abortion rates are high (10–60%)	Most of the variations and abnormalities are directly transmitted to offspring from parent.
3. Sex chromosome abnormalities Klinefelter's syndrome (XXY abnormality)	1 in 400 male live births	Diagnosis is rare before puberty; mentally retarded; body may be tall, slim, and underweight; small testes; pubertal development delayed; azoospermia and infertility; psychosocial, learning, or school adjustment problems		
Turner's syndrome (X abnormality, also monosomy sex chromosome, applies to phenotype female with genotype 45,XO)	1 in 2500–3000 female live births	Face is heart-shaped; premature aging of face; multiple eye defects; micrognathia; short stature; webbed neck; infantile external genitalia; underdeveloped breasts; lymphedema of hands and feet during infancy; mentally retarded		
Mendelian Disorders—Single Gene				Mendelian inheritance: A single deleterious gene can cause multiple anomalies or isolated malformations.
1. Autosomal Dominant Achondroplasia, classic	1 in 10,000 live births	Brachycephaly; frontal bossing; depressed nasal bridge; dwarfism; short extremities; lumbar lordosis; bowed legs; pelvic tilt	Usually sporadic occurrence. Affected parent has a 50% chance of having affected offspring with each pregnancy.	
Skeletal disorders (e.g., syndactyly)				

Disorder	Incidence	Clinical Features	Genetic Risk / Counseling	Comments
2. Autosomal Recessive			Risk of affected parent having affected offspring is 25% per pregnancy; 50% carrier state	
Sickle cell anemia*	1 in 625 live births of blacks			
Cystic fibrosis*	1 in 2000 live births (predominantly white)			Carrier can be identified
Tay-Sachs disease	50 live births per year (occurs mainly in Jewish children)	Lack of CNS maturation; impaired motor development; cherry-red spot on eyes; early death		
Inherited metabolic disorders (e.g., galactosemia)				
3. Sex-Linked Recessive			Sex-linked disorders occur mainly in males, although the female is the carrier. Most sex-linked disorders are recessive.	
Glucose-6-phosphate dehydrogenase (G6PD)	12% of male live births in blacks 24% of female live births in blacks			
Hemophilia, classic*	1 in 10,000 male live births		If affected male reproduces, offspring will be as follows. Males are normal; females are carriers. Unaffected female carrier offspring: 50% male affected 50% male normal 50% female carrier 50% female normal	
Duchenne's muscular dystrophy		Onset in early childhood; muscles seem well-developed but weak; slow to walk and climb—no gross motor milestones; Gower's sign (when in sitting position will climb up legs to stand); mental retardation		
4. Sex linked Dominant (rare) Vitamin D-resistant rickets		Lateral bowing deformity of legs; frontal bossing; costochondral beading; enlarged wrists; dental defects; hyphosphatemia; short stature	Transmitted from affected male to all female offspring. Male offspring are normal. Affected female—50% of all offspring will be affected.	
Multifactorial-Polygenic Disorders				
Neural tube defects* (myelomeningocele)	1 in 500–1000 live births		Risk varies with racial background. Recurrence risk is usually 2–7% but is related to outcome of previous pregnancies.	Polygenic disorders are probably the result of several deleterious genes combined with environmental factors.
Cleft lip and cleft palate*	1 in 1000 live births			These disorders are difficult to prove, because they are mainly the result of slight variations at multiple gene loci.
Pyloric stenosis*	1 in 200 male live births 1 in 1000 female live births			

* See text under the specific subject.

Help them know what to anticipate to lower their anxiety level and to make the counseling sessions a better experience.

2. If possible, attend the counseling session. This facilitates reinforcement of information and makes it easier to answer questions adequately.
3. Assess the family's need for additional counseling sessions, and initiate these if the need is recognized.

D. *To help families handle the information received and to guide them in coping with this crisis in their lives.*

1. Utilize interviewing skills to facilitate discussion regarding parental feelings.
   Consider such factors as timing and privacy.
2. Alleviate parental feelings of guilt and shame.
   a. If a recessive trait is involved, both parents may blame themselves. A parent who is a carrier of a dominant anomaly may blame himself, and the other parent may blame him as well even if she (or he) does not outwardly express these feelings.
   b. Emphasize that a person has no choice or responsibility in acquiring the genes that cause the problem.
   c. Reassure parents that information gathered is important for determining an accurate diagnosis and the nature of inheritance; assure them that it will be kept confidential.
   d. It may be helpful to inform parents that many other people have hidden, recessive genes.
3. Anticipate parental questions and areas of difficulty and conflict.
   a. Many parents are afraid to ask questions. They may fear they will sound stupid; they may not know what to ask—much less how to ask questions.
   b. Listen carefully for parental areas of unanswered or unasked questions.
   c. Help parents formulate questions. Utilize statements such as, "Many parents have questions about _____."
   d. Be available to parents when they have something to ask.
   e. Listen carefully to parents' questions and answer them whenever possible.
4. Remain objective.
   a. Be aware of personal feelings about specific genetic disorders.
   b. Come to terms with your own emotional difficulty related to genetic disorders and to issues such as abortion.
   c. Avoid letting personal reactions affect your attitude toward counseling and behavior toward the family.
      (1) If the nurse avoids the situation, parents are tacitly given professional sanction to do the same thing.
      (2) A nurse who conveys the impression that he/she cannot cope with the fact of genetic disease is unlikely to convey assurance that a family should be able to cope with the consequences of the disease.
5. Reinforce information about the genetic disorder, probability, possible interventions to correct the defect or minimize the disability, self-care goals, and limitations requiring adaptation.
   a. Frequently parents do not understand the mean-

ing of the risk ratio quoted to them, or they may attach too much or too little importance to it.
   b. Be certain that parents understand specifically what the predictions imply.
6. Clarify understanding of all family members.
   Have both parents present for discussions as frequently as possible to prevent misinterpretations and distortions from being passed from one to the other. Include grandparents and siblings as appropriate.
7. Assist parents to evaluate the total situation and to see the ramifications of any decision they may make.
   Facilitate realistic assessment of the expected burden to the parents, the child, and society; have them evaluate their capacity for dealing with the situation and expected problems.
8. Provide psychological support to allow parents to make and carry out decisions.
   a. Parents who decide against having children should be given information about contraception, sterilization.
   b. Parents who elect pregnancy should be informed about appropriate techniques of prenatal diagnosis of genetic disorders.
   c. Parents who elect adoption should be given the opportunity for additional advice when the adoption is being undertaken.

E. *To assure continued and comprehensive nursing care for the affected child and the family.*

1. Continue to educate parents about the defect the child may have. Even though they may have received genetic counseling, if they have a child with the defect they may not fully understand what it is and what it means.
2. In order to be more effective in supporting parents after the birth of a defective baby, it is important to understand the phases of adjustment they go through.
   a. Shock and disorganization—denial of the infant's defect while dealing with their own emotions
   b. Adjustment—partial acceptance along with anger
   c. Reintegration—resumption of effective and realistic functioning
3. Complete necessary referrals to appropriate professionals and to community resources. These may include infant stimulation programs, preschool programs, parent groups, social service agencies, and other similar resources.

F. *To provide information regarding known genetic risk factors to the general public. ***

1. Support the concept of premarital counseling.
2. Support prenatal counseling to increase awareness of potential hazards of infections such as rubella, to the impact of drugs on the fetus, and to pollution of water and foodstuffs by pesticides and fertilizers.

---

* Professional Education Department, The National Foundation/March of Dimes, Box 2000, White Plains, N.Y. 10602 (for information on location of genetic services)
   National Clearinghouse for Human Genetic Diseases, 1776 East Jefferson Street, Rockville, Md. 20852 (for information on Clinical Genetic Service Centers—a directory of institutions in the United States providing services for a range of genetic conditions)

POISONING

INGESTED POISONS

Poisoning by ingestion refers to the oral intake of a harmful substance which, even in a small amount, can damage tissues, disturb bodily functions, and cause possible death. In the pediatric population, poisoning is often caused by the ingestion of medications as well as toxic household substances such as furniture polish, charcoal lighter, kerosene, paint remover, cleansers, and lye.

Etiology

1. Improper or dangerous storage
2. Poor lighting—causes errors in reading
3. Human factors
   a. Failure to read label properly
   b. Failure to return poison to its proper place
   c. Failure to recognize the material as poisonous

Clinical Manifestations

1. Gastrointestinal symptoms (common in metallic, acid, alkali, and bacterial poisonings)
   a. Anorexia
   b. Abdominal pain
   c. Nausea
   d. Vomiting
   e. Diarrhea and/or intestinal cramping
2. Central nervous system symptoms
   a. Convulsions—common in poisoning due to ingestion of central nervous system stimulants such as camphor and strychnine.
   b. Coma—common in poisoning due to ingestion of central nervous system depressants such as alcohol, atropine, chloral hydrate, barbiturates.
   c. Dilated pupils—common in poisoning due to atropine, nicotine, cocaine, ephedrine.
   d. Pinpoint pupils—common in poisoning due to opiates.
3. Skin symptoms
   a. Rashes
   b. Burns
   c. Eye inflammation
   d. Skin irritation
   e. Stains around the mouth or lesions of the mucous membranes
   f. Cyanosis—cyanide and strychnine poisoning
4. Cardiopulmonary symptoms
   a. Dyspnea
   b. Cardiopulmonary depression or arrest

Diagnostic Evaluation

Analysis reveals presence of toxic substances in:
1. Blood
2. Urine
3. Gastric washings
4. Vomitus

Nursing Objectives

A. *To assist the family by telephone management.*

1. Calmly secure and record the following information:
   a. Name, address, and telephone number of caller.
   b. Age and condition of the child.
   c. Name of the ingested product, approximate amount ingested, and time of ingestion.

2. Instruct the caller regarding appropriate emergency actions (refer to section on patient and parental education).
3. Direct the patient to the nearest emergency room. Dispatch an ambulance if necessary.
4. Instruct parents to save vomitus, unswallowed liquid or pills, and the container, and then to bring them to the hospital as aids in identifying the poison.

B. *To identify the poison.*

1. Determine the nature of the ingested substance from the child's history or by reading the label on the container.
2. If necessary, call the nearest poison control center or toxicology section of the medical examiner's office to identify the toxic ingredient and obtain recommendations for emergency treatment.
3. Save vomitus and urine output for analysis once the child reaches the hospital.

C. *To remove the poison from the body.*

1. Induce vomiting.
   a. For children over 1 year of age, administer syrup of ipecac according to the directions on the label. (The usual dose is 15 ml. [about 1 tablespoon] mixed in a glass of warm water.)

> **NURSING ALERT:** Do not use tincture of ipecac; it is much stronger than the syrup and is itself a poison.

   b. Stimulate posterior pharynx with finger.
   c. Position child with his head down or on his side to prevent aspiration of vomitus.

> **NURSING ALERT:** Do *not* induce vomiting if:
> 1. Child is convulsing, semiconscious, or comatose.
> 2. Poison is known to be a strong acid or alkali, strychnine, or a hydrocarbon (e.g., lighter fluid, gasoline, kerosene, paint remover, or fingernail polish remover). Strong acids or alkalis may damage the esophagus for a second time during emesis, and hydrocarbons can cause severe pneumonia if aspirated.

2. Administer gastric lavage. (This is indicated when vomiting is impossible because of the child's condition, age, or when induction of vomiting has been unsuccessful.) Refer to Guidelines, page 890.
   a. A cuffed endotracheal tube may be inserted prior to lavage to protect the child from aspiration.
   b. Use the largest size tube that can be passed orally—preferably one with a double lumen.
   c. Place the child on his left side with his head lower than his stomach.
   d. Aspirate the stomach.
   e. Lavage with small, repeated introductions and withdrawals of normal saline, ½ normal saline, or special lavage solution.
   f. Do not leave a large amount of water in the child's stomach.
   g. Follow lavage with a cathartic to hasten removal of the poison from the gastrointestinal tract.

h. Be aware of the dangers associated with lavage:
  (1) Esophageal perforation—may occur in corrosive poisoning
  (2) Gastric hemorrhage
  (3) Impaired pulmonary function resulting from aspiration
  (4) Cardiac arrest
  (5) Convulsions—may result from stimulation in strychnine ingestion

D. *To reduce the effect of the poison by administering an antidote.*

1. An antidote may either react with the poison to prevent its absorption or counteract the effects of the poison after its absorption.
2. Not all poisons have specific antidotes.
3. Information regarding appropriate antidotes for specific poisons is available through all poison control centers and in many pediatric textbooks.
    Antidotes for the most common poisons should be listed in the emergency room of the hospital.
4. Effectiveness of the antidote usually depends on the amount of time which elapses between ingestion of the poison and administration of the antidote.
5. Activated charcoal absorbs all poisons except cyanide. Administer orally, after vomiting has occurred, in a dose of 5–10 grams per gram of ingested poison in 177–237 ml. (6–8 oz.) of water.

E. *To eliminate the absorbed poison.*

1. Force diuresis.
    a. Administer large quantities of fluid either orally or intravenously.
    b. Carefully monitor intake and output.
2. Assist with kidney dialysis which may be necessary if the child's own kidneys are not functioning effectively.
3. Assist with exchange transfusion if this method is indicated for removing the poison.

F. *To observe the child for progression of symptoms and to provide supportive care should these develop.*

1. Central Nervous System Involvement
    a. Observe for:
        Restlessness, confusion, delirium, convulsions, lethargy, stupor, coma
    b. Administer sedation with caution—in order to avoid depression and masking of symptoms.
    c. Avoid excessive manipulation of the child.
    d. See nursing care of the child with seizures, page 1402.
    e. See nursing care of the unconscious patient, page 706.
2. Respiratory Involvement
    a. Observe for:
        Respiratory depression, obstruction, pulmonary edema, pneumonia, tachypnea
    b. Have an artificial airway available.
    c. Be prepared to administer oxygen and provide artificial respiration.
    d. Other nursing concerns.
        (1) Nursing care of the child on a ventilator, page 1200.
        (2) Procedures for administration of oxygen, page 1196.
        (3) Procedure for cardiopulmonary resuscitation, page 1205.
3. Cardiovascular Involvement
    a. Observe for:

Peripheral circulatory collapse, disturbances of heart rate and rhythm, cardiac failure
    b. Maintain intravenous therapy of saline and glucose solution, plasma or blood.
        See procedure for the administration of intravenous fluids, page 1171.
    c. Be prepared for cardiac arrest.
        See procedure for cardiopulmonary resuscitation, page 1205.
4. Gastrointestinal Involvement
    a. Observe for:
        Nausea, pain, abdominal distention, and difficulty in swallowing
    b. Maintain intravenous therapy to replace water and electrolyte loss.
        See procedure for intravenous therapy, page 1171.
    c. Offer a diet which is easily swallowed and digested.
        (1) Begin with clear liquids.
        (2) Progress to full liquids, soft foods and then a regular diet as the child's condition improves.
5. Kidney Involvement
    a. Observe the child for decreased urine output. Record urine output exactly.
    b. Observe for hypertension.
    c. Insert indwelling catheter if necessary for urinary retention.
    d. Administer appropriate amounts of fluids and electrolytes.
    e. See nursing care of the child with renal failure, page 1332.
6. General Considerations
    a. Maintain adequate caloric, fluid and vitamin intake.
        Oral fluids are preferable if they can be retained.
    b. Avoid hypo- or hyperthermia.
        (1) Control of body temperature is impaired in many types of poisoning.
        (2) Monitor the child's temperature frequently.
    c. Observe closely for infection.
        (1) This is especially important in ingestion of kerosene or other hydrocarbons, which cause chemical pneumonitis.
        (2) Isolate the patient from other children, especially those with respiratory infections.
        (3) Administer antibiotics as prescribed by the physician.

G. *To provide emotional support for the child and his family.*

1. Remain calm and efficient while working rapidly.
2. Discourage anxious parents from handling, caressing, and overstimulating their child.
3. Counsel parents who often feel guilty about the accident.
    a. Encourage parents to talk about the poisoning.
    b. Emphasize how their quick action in getting treatment for their child has helped.
    c. Discuss ways that they can be supportive to their child during his hospitalization.
    d. Do not allow prolonged periods of self-incrimination to continue.
        Refer the parents to a social worker or psychiatrist for assistance in resolving these feelings if necessary.
4. Involve the young child in therapeutic play to determine how he views the situation.

a. The child often sees nursing measures as punishments for his misdeed involving the poisoning.

b. Explain the child's treatment and correct his misinterpretations in a manner appropriate for his age.

H. *To help prevent further poisoning episodes.*

1. Initiate patient and parental teaching once the acute episode is over.
2. Initiate a community health nursing referral.
   A home assessment should be made so that underlying problems are recognized and appropriate help is provided.

Patient and Parental Education

A. *Prevention*

1. Information concerning poison prevention should be available on any hospital pediatric unit.
   a. Many free booklets and home safety checklists are available from such sources as insurance companies and drug companies.
   b. Teaching may be done with any parent regardless of the reason for the child's hospitalization.
2. General Precautions
   a. Keep medicines and poisons out of the reach of children.
   b. Provide locked storage for highly toxic substances.
   c. Do not store poisons in the same area as foods.
   d. Be certain all containers are properly marked and labeled. Keep medicines, drugs and household chemicals in their original containers.
   e. Do not discard poisonous substances in receptacles where children can reach them.
   f. Teach children not to taste or eat unfamiliar substances.
   g. Medications
      (1) Clean out medicine cabinets periodically.
         (a) Dispose of old medications in containers out of the reach of children.
         (b) Prescription medications should be discarded when the illness for which they were prescribed has run its course.
         (c) Keep medications in "child-proof" containers that are securely closed.
      (2) Read all labels carefully before each use.
         (a) Follow exact directions on the label.
         (b) Never take a drug from an unlabeled bottle.
      (3) Do not give medicines prescribed for one child to another child.
      (4) Never refer to drugs as candy or bribe children with such inducements.
      (5) Never give or take medications in the dark.
   h. Never puncture or burn aerosol containers.
   i. Store lawn and garden pesticides in a separate place under lock and key outside of the house.
   j. Keep a 30-ml. (1-ounce) bottle of ipecac syrup and a can of activated charcoal available in the home.
   k. Keep a list of emergency phone numbers including the poison control center, physician's number, nearest hospital, and ambulance service.

l. Be prepared to act in cases of poisoning. Keep a list of emergency actions readily available.

B. *Emergency Actions*

1. Suspect poisoning with the occurrence of sudden, bizarre symptoms or peculiar behavior in toddlers and preschoolers.
2. Read the label on the ingested product or call physician, hospital, or poison control center for instructions regarding treatment for the poisoning. Give all relevant information about the child, his condition, and the substance he took.
3. Maintain an adequate airway in a child who is convulsing or who is not fully conscious.
4. Dilute the poison.
   a. For ingestion of alkali (drain cleaner, bleach, ammonia, any lye product) administer citrus juice or water.
   b. For acidic substances (toilet bowl cleaner, rust remover, etc.) administer milk.
   c. If nature of substance is unknown (whether acid or alkali), give water or milk.

NURSING ALERT: Be careful not to administer such large quantities of fluid that the poison is forced through the pylorus.

5. Make the child vomit if so directed. Do not induce vomiting if any of the following occurs:
   a. Child is unconsious or convulsing.
   b. Ingested poison was a strong corrosive such as lye or drain cleaner.
   c. Ingested poison contains gasoline, kerosene, or other petroleum distillates.
6. Directions for making the child vomit:
   a. Administer 1 tablespoon of ipecac syrup with at least 250 ml. (about 1 cup) of warm water.
   b. If vomiting does not occur in 20 minutes, this dose may be repeated once only.
   c. Vomiting may also be induced by touching the back of the throat with a finger to stimulate the gag reflex.
7. Transport the child promptly to the nearest medical facility.
   a. Wrap the child in a blanket to prevent chilling.
   b. Bring the container and any vomitus or urine to the hospital with the child.
8. If transportation to a medical facility is impossible, do the following:
   a. Continue to induce vomiting until vomitus is a clear liquid.
   b. Administer activated charcoal between vomiting episodes.
9. Avoid excessive manipulation of the child.
10. Act promptly but calmly.
11. Do not assume the child is safe simply because the emesis shows no trace of the poison or because child appears well. The poison may produce a delayed reaction or may have reached the small intestine, where it is still being absorbed.

LEAD POISONING

Lead poisoning (plumbism), is a relatively common disease in young children that results from the consumption of lead in some form. Each year it causes the death of approximately 200 children and leaves others with chronic neurologic handicaps, mental deficiency, and/or behavioral problems.

Etiology

1. Ingestion of substances containing lead
   a. Toys, furniture, windowsills, household fixtures, and plaster painted with lead-containing paint may be ingested. (New legislation stipulates that toys, children's furniture, and the interior of homes be painted with lead-free paint; however, the problem may continue if the deeper layers of paint and plaster are contaminated with lead.)
   b. Lead toys
   c. Oil paints
   d. Acidic juices or foods served in pottery made with lead glazes
   e. Paints used in newspapers, magazines, children's books, matches, and playing cards
   f. Water from lead pipes
   g. Fruit covered with insecticides
   h. Dirt containing lead fallout from automobile exhaust
   i. Antique pewter, particularly when used to serve acidic juices or foods
   j. Lead weights (curtain weights, fishing sinkers)
2. Inhalation of fumes containing lead (less common cause in children)
   a. Motor fuel
   b. Burning storage batteries
   c. Dust-containing lead salts
   d. Dust in the air at shooting galleries and in enclosed firing ranges with poor ventilation

Altered Physiology

1. Lead salts are absorbed by the blood from the respiratory tract or the intestines.
2. A large portion of the absorbed lead enters the portal circulation and is excreted by the liver.
3. Lead that reaches the systemic circulation is deposited in soft tissues, causing damage primarily to the nervous system, the blood, and the kidneys.
   a. Nervous system
      (1) Brain—edema, vascular damage; destruction of brain cells, causing convulsive disorders; neurological deficits; learning difficulties
      (2) Peripheral nerve palsies
   b. Blood
      (1) Increases in the concentration of hemoglobin precursors in body fluids.
      (2) Inhibition of a number of steps in the biosynthesis of heme, thus reducing the number of red blood cells, increasing fragility, and reducing half-life
   c. Kidneys
      Injury to the cells of the proximal tubules, causing abnormal excretion of amino acids, protein, glucose, and phosphate
4. Lead is slowly transferred from soft tissues to bone.
   a. It is deposited in insoluble form with calcium.
   b. The deposition causes increased thickness and density of long bones.
   c. Decalcification is associated with the release of lead from bone.

Epidemiologic Factors

1. Slums and old neighborhoods are high-risk areas because of old, deteriorating housing.
2. Pica (a habit of eating nonfood items such as paint chips, often involving a craving type of behavior) is a common precondition.
   a. Poisoning associated with pica is a chronic process.
   b. Clinical manifestations appear after 3–6 months of fairly steady lead ingestion.

Incidence

1. Highest in children between 1–6 years of age, especially those between 1–3 years
2. High in Blacks and Spanish-speaking individuals living in old homes or slum areas
3. No significant difference in sex
4. High among siblings
5. Symptomatic lead poisoning usually occurs in the summer months
6. Recurrence rate is high

Clinical Manifestations

1. Gastrointestinal symptoms
   a. Vomiting
   b. Vague abdominal pain
   c. Colic
   d. Constipation
   e. Loss of appetite
   f. Weight loss
2. Central nervous system symptoms (common in children)
   a. Falling, clumsiness, loss of coordination
   b. Irritability
   c. Dispositional changes
   d. Convulsions with or without local paralysis
   e. Drowsiness, coma
   f. Peripheral nerve palsies
3. Hematological symptoms
   a. Anemia
   b. Pallor
4. Cardiovascular symptoms
   a. Hypertension
   b. Bradycardia
5. Symptoms depend on the amount of lead in the soft tissues and blood:
   a. Onset is insidious.
   b. Usually progresses from mild to severe manifestations as the lead slowly accumulates.
   c. Infants and toddlers may present severe manifestations initially.
   d. Symptoms may be intermittent for several months.

Diagnostic Evaluation

1. Detailed history with emphasis on the presence or absence of clinical symptoms, evidence of pica, family history of lead poisoning, possible source of exposure to lead, recent change in behavior, developmental delay, or behavior problems.
2. Erythrocyte–protoporphyrin (EP) level—often used as the initial screening test. Children with values ≥ 50 µg/dl should have a blood–lead determination done.
3. Blood–lead level—values above 50–60 µ/100 ml. often indicate need for treatment, depending on the results of a more complete medical and laboratory examination of the individual child.
4. Hematologic evaluation for anemia.
5. Flat plate of abdomen—may reveal radiopaque material if lead has been ingested during the preceding 24–36 hours.
6. X-ray of long bones—may show increased density at the epiphyseal lines.
7. Calcium disodium EDTA mobilization test—dem-

onstrates increasing levels of lead in the urine over a 24-hour period following injection of calcium disodium EDTA.

8. Urinary coproporphyrin (UCP) level—elevated with high blood–lead levels.

9. Urinary delta—aminolevulinic acid (ALA) level— >3 mg./m^2 for 24 hours is considered abnormal.

Prognosis

1. Improving with increased emphasis on prevention and screening.

2. Children with central nervous system involvement have a poor prognosis for normal development. Residual effects on the nervous system are permanent and progressive.

   Late symptoms of mental retardation may appear 3–9 years after treatment. Specific intellectual defect may interfere with the child's progress at school.

Nursing Objectives

A. *To collect a urine specimen as a diagnostic tool.*

A 24-hour specimen is more accurate than a single voided specimen. (See section on specimen collection.)

B. *To prevent absorption of lead.*

1. Administer cleansing enemas if radiopaque lead particles are observed on abdominal x-rays.

2. Make certain that all sources of lead are removed from the child's environment, including the hospital environment.

C. *To increase excretion of lead from the body.*

Administer appropriate chelating agents (refer to Table 51-2).

   a. Action—React with lead to form nontoxic compounds which are excreted by the body.

   b. Dosage—Depends on individual drug, child's weight, severity of poisoning, prior history, and whether or not other chelating agents are being used simultaneously.

   c. Needle play should be used when appropriate to prepare the child for the injections, and as an outlet for the pain and anger he feels.

D. *To provide supportive care to the child with encephalopathy.*

1. Observe for:
   a. Rising blood pressure
   b. Papilledema
   c. Slow pulse
   d. Convulsions
   e. Unconsciousness

2. See section on pediatric neurological problems, page 1384.

3. Plan nursing care around periods when medications must be given.

TABLE 51-2. CHELATING AGENTS USED TO TREAT LEAD POISONING IN CHILDREN

	Calcium EDTA (ethylenediamine tetra-acetic acid, Versenate)	Dimercaprol (BAL)
Route of Administration	1. IM injection is the preferred route in children. 2. Rapid IV infusion may be lethal by suddenly increasing intracranial pressure in patients with cerebral edema.	IM injection
Excretion of Lead	Urinary excretion increased 20–50 times.	Urinary and fecal output increased. Produces greater total excretion than calcium EDTA alone.
Untoward Reactions	1. Rash, vomiting, tetany, lethargy, transient fever. 2. Usually appear with IV rather than IM administration of calcium EDTA.	1. Symptoms begin within 10 to 15 minutes after injection of BAL and subside within 1–2 hours. 2. Symptoms Increased lacrimation, salivation, sweating, nausea and vomiting, headache, pain in teeth, burning sensation of lips, mouth, throat. Tachycardia, increased blood pressure, muscular ache, fever.
Toxic Reactions	Renal Toxicity 1. Do not administer to dehydrated patients. 2. Check urine daily for protein and blood. Transient Hypercalcemia Monitor serum calcium	Renal Toxicity 1. Encourage fluids to maintain adequate excretion of the lead via the urine. 2. Check urine daily for protein and abnormalities of urinary sediment.
Special Considerations/Precautions	1. Usual course of treatment is 5 days. A second course of therapy may be necessary after an interval of 2 days if signs and symptoms of lead poisoning persist or if serum level remains elevated. 2. Injections are very painful. 3. Minimize the pain at the injection site. a. A small amount of local anesthetic, such as procaine, may be added to the syringe. It should be drawn up last and not mixed. b. Inject the medication deep into the muscle. c. Establish a pattern for the rotation of injection sites. d. Record the site of each injection. e. Apply warm compresses or allow the child to soak in a warm bath to alleviate muscular soreness. 4. Encourage ambulation to facilitate absorption of the medication.	1. Often given in combination with calcium EDTA. In children with very high lead levels, BAL is often given initially in order to lower the blood level before calcium EDTA is given, which may actually raise the blood lead level temporarily when therapy is initiated. When administering with calcium EDTA, use a separate site. 2. Monitor vital signs for 15 minutes after giving BAL, because of the potential for causing tachycardia and increased blood pressure. 3. Do not administer iron to children receiving BAL, since BAL forms a toxic complex with iron.

E. *To observe for factors associated with lead poisoning.*

1. Pica
   a. Observe and record the child's eating habits and food preferences.
   b. Report any attempted eating of nonfood substances.
   c. Provide regular meals and make mealtime a pleasurable time for the child.
   d. Discourage oral activity and substitute activity that contributes to play, social skills, and ego development.
   e. Refer the family for additional social or psychiatric casework if indicated to reduce the psychological or cultural factors which result in pica in the child.
2. Strained parent-child relationships
   Record when family members visit as well as the nature of their interaction with the child.

F. *To provide the child with social and motor stimulation.*

1. Assess the child's level of development. The DDST (Denver Developmental Screening Test) may be useful for this purpose. (Refer to Chapter 26, pp. 1090–1091.)
2. Provide and encourage activities that will help the child to learn and progress from his present developmental state. (Refer to section on growth and development, p. 1093.)
3. Initiate appropriate referrals in cases of obvious developmental delays. Such referrals may be to such professionals as psychologists, psychiatrists, and specialists in early child education.
4. Share the results of developmental testing with the parent(s) and discuss ways to provide stimulation for the child at home.

G. *To provide emotional support to the parent(s) and/or caretakers.*

1. Utilize sensitivity in interviewing and teaching to avoid causing or increasing guilt feelings about the poisoning and to establish a positive, trusting relationship between the family and the health care facility.
2. Explain the treatment and its purpose, since parents are frequently faced with putting an asymptomatic child through painful treatments.

H. *To prevent reexposure of the child to lead.*

1. Instruct parents regarding the seriousness of repeated exposure to lead.
2. Initiate a referral to a community health nurse to determine if exposure to lead is continuing and to provide continuing support to the family.
3. Advise parents to require landlord to remove lead paint from the walls; assist them with this process.
   a. Refer the parents to the housing authority.
   b. Do not allow the child in the home while lead paint is being removed. Place the child temporarily in a convalescent home or foster home if necessary.
4. When it is impossible to eliminate lead hazards from the home:

a. Scrape loose or chipped paint and plaster from the window sills, woodwork, moldings, etc., and tape the areas with masking tape or contact paper.
b. Remove all crumbling plaster and replaster or cover the area with wallboard or contact paper.
5. Make certain that the family is able to provide close supervision of the child or assist them to make arrangements to ensure that the child is adequately supervised at home.

I. *To participate in the prevention of lead poisoning.*

1. Initiate and support educational campaigns through schools, day care centers, and news media to alert parents and children to hazards and symptoms of lead poisoning.
2. Provide in clinics, waiting rooms, and other appropriate settings literature stressing the hazards of lead, sources of lead, and signs of lead intoxication.
3. Inquire about the presence of pica in all children under 6 years of age.
4. Screen siblings of known cases immediately.
5. Screen all children from high-risk areas.
6. Provide follow-up to all children suffering from lead poisoning as well as to those in the early stage of undue lead absorption to prevent their becoming poisoned.
7. Support legislation to study the nature and extent of the lead poisoning problem, to detect and treat such poisoning, and to eliminate the causes of lead poisoning.

Patient or Parental Education

Parent education is an extremely important part of the nursing care of a child with lead poisoning. It should include the following points of emphasis:

1. Long-term medical follow-up is essential.
   a. Residual lead is liberated gradually after treatment.
      (1) May result in the renewal of symptoms.
      (2) May increase serum lead to a dangerous level.
      (3) Additional damage to the central nervous system may become apparent for several months (after discharge from the hospital).
   b. Acute infections must be recognized and treated promptly. (These may reactivate the disease.)
   c. Some children are placed on D-penicillamine for long-term chelation. If this drug is used, it should be given on an empty stomach, 2 hours before breakfast.
2. Reexposure to lead must be prevented.
3. Siblings and playmates should be screened for lead poisoning.
4. Literature stressing the causes and prevention of lead poisoning should be provided.*

* Literature is available from the Lead Industries Association, 292 Madison Avenue, N.Y., N.Y. 10017 and from the U.S. Dept. of Health, Education, and Welfare, Superintendent of Documents, U.S. Government Printing Office, Washington, D.C. 20402.

THE ABUSED CHILD (CHILD ABUSE AND NEGLECT)

Child abuse and neglect refers to "a child under the age of 18 who is suffering from physical injury (inflicted upon him by other than accidental means), or sexual abuse, or malnutrition, or suffering physical or emotional harm or substantial risk thereof by reason of neglect. Reporting of neglect shall take into account the accepted child-rearing practices of the culture of which he or she is part."*

Child abuse and neglect includes the following conditions:
1. Battering—physical injury
2. Nutritional neglect—deliberate omission of adequate nutrition. "Failure to thrive" results when child's weight is below 3rd percentile for age and sex and child has no predisposing physical abnormality.
3. Drug abuse—intentional administration of harmful drugs
4. Medical neglect—intentional omission of basic preventive-medicine practices or specific treatment for medical problems
5. Sexual abuse—sexual assault or molestation
6. Safety neglect—intentional omission of safety precautions appropriate for age of child
7. Emotional abuse—scapegoating, belittling, humiliating, lack of mothering
8. Child neglect—lack of providing the child with basic needs of survival: shelter, clothing, stimulation, development of trust, etc.

Etiology

Child abuse is not a uniform phenomenon with one set of causal factors, but a multidimensional phenomenon. The phenomenon may be related to:

The combined presence of 3 factors: special kind of child, special kind of parent, special circumstances of crisis;
   a. Psychopathology of the abuser,
   b. Cultural, social, and economic factors, and
   c. Specific child characteristics, i.e., premature, debilitated, child needing special care.

Contributing Factors

1. Incidents of child abuse may develop as a result of disciplinary action taken by the abuser who responds in uncontrolled anger to real or perceived misconduct of the child. Parents may confuse punishment with discipline. "Good parenting" may be equated with physical contact to eradicate undesirable child behavior.
2. Incidents of child abuse may develop from a general attitude of resentment or rejection on the part of the abuser toward the child.
3. Atypical child behavior (e.g., hyperactivity) may provoke the abuser. This may be child-initiated or child-provoked abuse.
4. Incidents of child abuse may develop out of a quarrel between the caretakers. The child may come to the aid of one parent, may find himself in the midst of the quarrel, or may object to the quarrel.
5. The abuser may be a stern, authoritarian disciplinarian.
6. The abuser may be under a great deal of stress because of life circumstances (debt, poverty, illness) and may thus resort to child abuse. Crisis and stress may be ongoing. The abuser may have a low frustration tolerance level and may not have a well-developed means of coping with stress in general.
7. The abuser may be intoxicated with alcohol or drugs at the time of the abuse.
8. Child abuse frequently occurs while the mother is

out of the home and the child is left in the care of a babysitter or boyfriend.
9. Lack of early mothering, inappropriate mother-child bonding, and punitive treatment as a child may contribute to child neglect.
10. Specific characteristics evident in many abusing parents include:
    a. Low self-esteem—a sense of incompetence in role; unworthiness; unimportance
    b. Unrealistic attitudes and expectations of child; little regard for child's own needs and age-appropriate abilities
    c. Fear of rejection—a deep need to feel wanted and loved, but a feeling of rejection when love is not obvious. A crying infant may elicit a feeling of rejection.
    d. Inability to accept help—isolation from the community; loneliness
    e. Unhappiness due to unsatisfactory relationships; may look to child for satisfaction of own emotional needs.
11. The abused or neglected child may be seen by the parent as "special." The premature infant or one having a serious illness may have resulted in failure of emotional-bonding. Parents perhaps could not provide special care to the child because of their own psychological variables or situation.

Clinical Manifestations

A. *Physical characteristics utilized as an index of suspicion.*

1. Child usually under 3 years of age. School age child is also subject to abuse, however.
2. General health of the child indicates neglect (diaper rash, poor hygiene, malnutrition)
3. Characteristic distribution of fractures (scattered over many different parts of body)
4. Disproportionate amount of soft tissue injury
5. Evidence that injuries occurred at different times (healed and new fractures, resolving and fresh bruises)
6. Cause of recent trauma in question
7. History of similar episodes in past
8. No new lesions occurring during the child's hospitalization
9. The child may develop behaviors through interaction with parents and peers that place him at risk for abuse.

B. *Injuries or types of abuse that may occur:*

1. Bruises, welts (most common)
2. Abrasions, contusions, lacerations (most common)
3. Wounds, cuts, punctures
4. Burns (cigarette, radiator, etc), scalding
5. Bone fractures (including skull)
6. Sprains, dislocations
7. Subdural hemorrhage or hematoma
8. Brain damage
9. Internal injuries
10. Drug intoxication
11. Malnutrition (deliberately inflicted)
12. Freezing, exposure
13. Whiplash-type injury
14. Eye injuries
15. Periorbital injuries

C. *Possible characteristics of the child suspected of being abused or neglected:*

1. May show a wide range of reactions—may be either

---

* Clinical Proceedings. Washington, D.C. Children's Hospital National Medical Center, Vol. 30, No. 2, Feb. 1974, p. 38

very withdrawn or overactive. Child may be anxious, tense, or nervous.
2. Avoids physical contact with parents; does not look to parents for comfort; shows distinct preference for one parent, while fearfully withdrawing from the other.
3. Is fearful, constantly alert for danger; seeks information as to what is going to happen next; is mistrustful of environment.
4. May show unusual affection for strangers or may be overly fearful of adults and avoid any physical contact with them.

D. *Identifying behavior common in abusing or neglecting parent(s):*
(Be aware that not all abusing parents exhibit these behaviors.)
1. Anxiously volunteers information or withholds information.
2. Gives an explanation of the injury that does not fit the condition or gets story confused concerning the injury.
3. Shows inappropriate reaction to severity of injury.
4. Becomes irritable about questions being asked.
5. Seldom touches or speaks to child; does not respond to him. May be critical of child or indicate unreal expectations of him.
6. Delays seeking medical help; refuses to sign permit for diagnostic studies. Frequently changes hospitals of physicians.
7. Shows no involvement in care of the hospitalized child; does not inquire about child.
8. The problem of abuse is a total family problem—family dysfunction.

Nursing Objectives

A. *To inspect every child's body upon admission to the hospital for evidence of abuse.*
1. Describe on nursing record all bruises, lacerations, etc., as to location and state of healing. Look carefully at areas generally covered with clothing, i.e., buttocks, underarms, behind knees, bottom of feet. Be alert for abuse of school-age child. Most often the child's injury is not severe enough to require medical attention, but the child may be hospitalized for some other medical problem.
2. Discuss with the physician the case of any child suspected of being abused.
   a. Every state (as well as District of Columbia) has mandatory reporting laws. All states provide statutory immunity for those who report real or suspected child abuse. There is no immunity from civil or criminal liability for failure to report such.
   b. Every nurse is morally and legally responsible to report and provide protective services for the abused child.
   c. Become familiar with laws, procedures, and protective services in your community and state.

B. *To be prepared to effectively care for the sexually assaulted child.*
1. Sexual abuse should be suspected when the young, prepubital child presents with:
   a. Trauma not readily explained
   b. Gonorrhea, syphilis, or other venereally related organisms
   c. Blood in urine or stool
   d. Painful urination or defecation

e. Penile or vaginal infection or itch
f. Penile or vaginal discharge
g. Report of increased, excessive masturbation
h. Report of increased, unusual fears
2. Establish a relationship with the child based upon mutual respect, empathy, and sensitivity.
   a. The child may be extremely calm or hysterical. She/he may verbally express a desire to talk about the incident. Take into consideration the different ways emotions are expressed by children at different developmental stages.
   b. Consideration of the child's emotions in conjunction with a good relationship may encourage the child to express his or her feelings either verbally or through drawings or play.
   c. Prepare the child both physically and psychologically for the necessary physical and pelvic examination.
   d. Talk with the child without the presence of the parents, especially when incest is possible.
3. Know the state laws regarding the reporting of suspected child abuse, as well as the legal definition of sexual deviation. In 1974, Public Law #93–237 established a National Center on Child Abuse and Neglect* to provide financial assistance for prevention, identification, and treatment of child abuse and neglect.
   a. Document any physical findings—bruises, abrasions, telltale secretions in mouth or pharynx, on hair or skin, in and around buttocks, clothes.
   b. Collect any necessary specimens for identification of organisms, sperm, or semen.
   c. Take colored photographs.
4. Participate in the therapeutic approach.
   a. Talk with the child and parents alone. Be honest with the mother.
   b. Prevent venereal disease, pregnancy, and tetanus. Prophylactic treatment should be given for penile penetration of any orifice.
   c. Support the parents who may have feelings of guilt, anger, and helplessness. Explain to them the extent of trauma and educate them regarding pediatric gynecology; allow them to ventilate their feelings. Support their parental role in handling the child (i.e., allow child to talk about or play out the incident, but do not force it).
   d. Encourage compliance with the treatment selected for the child, parents, and family (i.e., group counseling, psychiatry).

C. *To observe and record pertinent information regarding the parent-child relationship.*
1. Do the parents visit the child? Do parents become involved in caring for child?
2. How does the parent(s) respond to the child? Does the parent talk to the child, touch him, hold him, play with him?
3. How does the child react to the parent? Is he excited when the parent arrives? Does he appear frightened and withdrawn? Does he cry when the parent leaves?
4. What does the parent expect of the child? Are his expectations appropriate for child? Is there role-reversal between parent and child?

* National Center on Child Abuse and Neglect, Children's Bureau, Office of Child Development, U.S. Dept. of Health, Education, and Welfare, Washington, D.C. 20013

D. *To obtain a thorough nursing history in order to establish a nursing care plan that is individualized to meet specific needs of the child.*

1. Information should be obtained relating to the child's sleeping habits, toilet habits, favorite foods and eating habits, favorite toy or security objects, play habits and favorite playmate, names and ages of siblings, nickname, previous hospital experience, developmental assessment, and persons who will visit child.
2. Care and good judgment must be used in obtaining this information from parents, because they undoubtedly have already been asked many questions by many people. Use chart information already obtained to eliminate repetition.
3. Obtaining a nursing history in a nonthreatening, nonjudgmental manner can convey to parents that you have a genuine interest in caring for their child, and that you respect the knowledge they have as parents of their child. Getting the history will also allow you to assess the parents' knowledge and expectations of their child and will set a positive atmosphere for a continued relationship.

E. *To provide for the child a milieu to reduce trauma similar to that of any hospitalized child placed in the strange and frightening environment of the hospital by implementing the principles of emotional support. (See p. 1126.)*

The child must be treated as an individual. He may need extra help in the following areas:
1. Having ambivalent feelings toward his parent or parents
2. Overcoming his low self-image and the fear that something is wrong with him
3. Fearing future abuse upon his return home
4. Satisfying his strong need for attention, affection, and having a trusting relationship with an adult
5. Learning alternate ways of expressing his needs and feelings

F. *To foster a trusting relationship with the child who may be fearful of adults.*

1. Assign 1 nurse to care for the child over a period of time. Select the right nurse for the right patient.
2. Make no threatening moves toward the child. The child will indicate his readiness and awareness of the environment by his verbal or facial expressions.
3. Touch the child gently.
4. Provide nonthreatening physical contact (hold the child frequently and cuddle him). Pick him up and carry him around; encourage any exploration of your face, hair, etc.
5. Enlist the cooperation of volunteers to provide additional mothering.
6. Provide appropriate opportunities for play.
7. Set limits for him.

G. *To come to grips with your own feelings of anger, disgust, and contempt for the parents.*

A critical part of working in this area is learning to recognize, examine and work with these feelings. It may help to do the following:
1. Realize that most abusing parents do love their child and want the best for him in spite of their ambivalent feelings for him.
2. Understand the dynamics of child abuse and neglect. This crisis is due to the stress with which the parents are unable to cope and to the deprivations they have themselves suffered in their past.

3. Focus on the needs of the parents rather than on the injuries of the child. Treatment is aimed at helping parents reach their maximum potential as parents.
4. Expect repeated rejection from the parents who lack self-esteem and trust.
5. Understand that these parents are often difficult to like under ordinary conditions. They are experiencing terror, guilt, and remorse; they are fearful and yet expect criticism and condemnation.

H. *To foster a relationship with the parents that will encourage them to accept guidance and will help in dealing with the problem.*

1. Assume a nonjudgmental attitude that is neither punitive nor threatening. The desire to help must be conveyed.
2. Refrain from questioning them about the incident of abuse. (The suspected abuser will be interviewed by the physician, the social worker, and the authority who investigates the case.)
3. Include parents in the hospital experience—i.e., orient them to the unit and to any procedure to be done to the child. Serve as role model in the management of the child's behavior as well as their own. Try to give the parents as much information as possible about the care of their child. Listen to what they are saying.
4. Refrain from challenging all the information they may give.
5. Express appropriate concern and kindness. Remain objective yet empathetic. This will help foster the parents' self-respect and improve their self-image and dignity.

I. *To foster a healthy mother-child relationship.*

1. Build a relationship by working with the mother's strengths rather than her weaknesses. Use compliments as positive reinforcement.
2. Serve as a role model of appropriate methods of child care in areas such as feeding, bathing, and play.
3. Provide the mother with psychological support and reinforcement for appropriate mothering behaviors she does exhibit.
4. Work with the mother in planning for the child's future care.
5. Determine in what areas the mother needs help: Does the baby cry a lot? How does this make her feel? How does she comfort him? When she is alone, is there someone she can call for help? Does she feel the child understands what she expects of him?
6. By forming a helping relationship with the mother, the nurse will strengthen the protective ability of the mother and bind her to her child.

J. *To teach the parents about normal growth and development.*

(See section on growth and development, p. 1094).
1. Give specific information and examples as to the type of behavior to expect at the various stages of development. Point out in a nonthreatening way normal behavior exhibited by their child.
2. Give specific information on dealing with this behavior.
3. Serve as role model and teacher; minimize intensity when parents become threatened.

K. *To teach the parents how to use discipline without resorting to physical force.*

1. Discipline must be consistent. Offer suggestions for alternative ways of handling undesirable behavior.
2. Rewards may be used for acceptable behavior (e.g., a trip to the zoo, staying up later than usual for a special TV show, a special treat).
3. Rewards are withheld for unacceptable behavior.

L. *To support the parent and the child when a decision is made to have the child removed from the home.*

1. The decision is made for the safety and protection of the child.
2. The parents are afforded the opportunity to have counseling to help them learn to deal with their problem.
3. The child must be prepared for his removal from the home and placement plans. He must be allowed time to work through his feelings.

M. *To support the parents and child in preparation for discharge to home.*

1. Both parents and child (if age is appropriate) need to know and understand any specific instructions relative to injury and follow-up care.
2. Parents need to be made aware of the most common posthospitalization behavior children may have. (See p. 1127.)
3. Make known to parents your continued concern and your availability as a source of help. Stress need for follow-up care. Help them to use community resources available, i.e., homemaker, community health nurse, therapy for parents, etc.

N. *To be aware of the child who has the potential for being abused and to provide anticipatory guidance toward prevention of abuse.*

1. The premature infant, the hyperactive child, the chronically ill child, the retarded child, the child who requires a great deal of care and confines the mother to the home, the child involved in a disturbed mother-infant bond all have the potential for being abused.
2. Encourage early participation of mother (parents) in the care of the child during hospitalization.
3. Prepare the mother for the fact that the child does require a great deal of care, but encourage her to find outlets for her frustrations.
4. Provide her with the name and telephone number of someone at the hospital to whom she can look for help (e.g., social worker).
5. Initiate a community nursing referral.

O. *To be aware of the entire scope of nursing responsibilities in dealing with the abused and neglected child.*

1. Case finding—identify the potential (or suspected) abused and neglected child. Be a participating and contributing member of the multidisciplinary team in treating the abused child and his family.
2. Nurse-parent relationships—develop therapeutic, trusting relationships that will help parents develop to their full potential.
3. Support community assistance programs to help parents overcome isolation—crisis nurseries, parent aids, Parents Anonymous, foster care facilities, and day care centers.
4. Support public reeducation to enhance the parenting capabilities of every man and woman: Education for Parenting, Home Start, and adolescent parenthood programs.

P. *To be aware that the goal of treatment of the parents is to assure the physical and emotional safety of the child.*

1. It is estimated that 90% of abusing parents can be rehabilitated.
2. The ideal approach is to return the child to his biologic parents.
3. Treatment is offered to help parents to do the following:
   a. Understand and redirect their anger.
   b. Develop an adequate parent-child relationship.
   c. See their child as an individual with his own needs and differences.
   d. Enjoy their child.
   e. Develop realistic expectations of their child.
   f. Decrease their use of criticism.
   g. Increase their own sense of self-esteem and confidence.
   h. Establish supportive relationships with others.
   i. Improve economic situation (if appropriate).
   j. Show progress toward physical, emotional, and intellectual development.
4. Inform parents of organizations designed to help them:
   a. Parents Anonymous, 2810 Artesia Blvd., Redondo Beach, Ca. 90278. This is a private organization of self-help groups for parents who have abused or fear they might have abused their children. *Frontiers* is their publication.
   b. The National Center for the Prevention and Treatment of Child Abuse and Neglect, 1205 Oneida St., Denver, Colo. 80220

THE DYING CHILD

Nursing Objectives

A. *To work out one's own feelings about death and to develop a philosophy which enables the nurse to be a source of support to the dying child and his family.*

1. Become familiar with literature in the area of death and dying and use of a resource in planning and developing nursing care.
2. Recognize that the goal is to assist the child and his family to cope with this pain and grief in such a way that the experience will promote growth rather than destroy family integrity and emotional well-being.
3. Share personal feelings about death and dying with colleagues. It is not unusual for the nurse to experience personal feelings of anger, frustration, helplessness, and guilt.

B. *To recognize the stages of dying as identified by E. Kübler-Ross and to utilize this knowledge in planning and implementing care.* (Refer to table: Stages of Dying as Identified by Dr. Elizabeth Kübler-Ross, p. 1459.)

1. Be aware that dying children, their families, and the staff will all progress through these stages, not necessarily at the same time.
2. Children experience the stages with much variation. They tend to pass more quickly through the stages and may merge some of these stages.
3. The nursing goal is to be aware of one's own feelings

and to accept the child and family wherever they are, not to push them through the stages.

C. *To understand the meaning of illness and death to the child at the various stages of growth and development and to utilize this information in planning and implementing care.*

1. Refer to table: Stages in the Development of A Child's Concept of Death, page 1460.
2. Be aware of other factors that influence a child's personal concept of death. Of particular importance are:
   a. The amount and type of direct exposure a child has had to death.
   b. Cultural values, beliefs, and patterns of bereavement.
   c. Religious beliefs about death and afterlife.

D. *To utilize the knowledge about children's interpretation of the meaning of death at the various stages of growth and development in talking to the child about his illness and in answering questions concerning death.*

1. Research indicates that children generally can cope with more than adults will allow, and that children appreciate the opportunity to know and understand what is happening to them.
2. It is important that the child's questions be answered simply, but truthfully, and that they be based on his particular level of understanding.
3. The following responses have been suggested by Eassom in *The Dying Child* and may be useful as a guide.
   a. Preschool-age Child
      (1) When the child at this age is comfortable enough to ask questions about his illness, he should be told what he asks. When death is anticipated at some future time and the child asks "Am I going to die?" a response might be, "We will all die someday but you are not going to die today or tomorrow."
      (2) When death is imminent and the child asks, "Am I going to die?" the response might be, "Yes, you are going to die, but we will take care of you and stay with you."
      (3) The parents should be allowed to stay with the child to provide him with protection and support.
      (4) When the child asks "Will it hurt?" the response should be truthful and factual. Death may be described as a form of sleep—a sleep where he will be secure in the love of those around him. (Some children may fear sleep as the result of this type of explanation.)
      (5) Parents can express to the child the fact that they do not want him to go and that they will miss him very much; they feel sad too that they are going to be separated.
   b. School-age Child
      (1) Responses to the school-age child's questions about death should be answered truthfully. The child looks for support from those he trusts.
      (2) The school-age child should be given a simple explanation of his dagnosis and its meaning; he should also receive an explanation of all treatments and procedures.
      (3) The child should be given no specific time in

Stages of Dying as Identified by Dr. Elizabeth Kübler-Ross

Stage	Nursing Implications
I. Denial. Shock. Disbelief.	Accept denial, but function within a reality sphere. Do not tear down the child's (or family's) defenses. Be aware that denial usually breaks down in the early morning when it may be dark and lonely. Be certain that it is the child or family who is using denial, not the staff.
II. Anger. Rage. Hostility.	Accept anger and help child express it through positive channels. Be aware that anger may be expressed toward other family members, nursing staff, physicians, and other persons involved. Help families to recognize that it is normal for children to express anger for what they are losing.
III. Bargaining (from "No, not me." to "Yes, me, but . . .")	Recognize this period as a time for the child and family to regain strength. Encourage the family to finish any unfinished business with the child. This is the time to do such things as take the promised trip or buy the promised toy.
IV. Depression. (The child and/or family experiences silent grief and mourns past and future losses.)	Recognize this as a normal reaction and expression of strength. Help families to accept the child who does not want to talk and excludes help. This is a usual pattern of behavior. Reassure the child that you can understand his feelings.
V. Acceptance.	Assist families to provide significant loving human contact with their child.

Stages in the Development of a Child's Concept of Death

Age of Child	Stage of Development
Child up to 3 years	At this stage the child cannot comprehend the relationship of life to death, since he has not developed the concept of infinite time. The child fears separation from protecting and comforting adults. The child perceives death as a reversible fact.
Preschool-age Child	At this age the child has no real understanding of the meaning of death; he feels safe and secure with his parents. The child may view death as something that happens to others. The child may interpret his illness as a type of punishment for real or imagined wrongdoing. The child may interpret the separation that occurs with hospitalization as punishment; the painful tests and procedures that he is subjected to support this idea. The child may become depressed because he is not able to correct these wrongdoings and regain the grace of adults. The concept may be connected with magical thoughts and mystery.

School-age Child	The child at this age sees death as the cessation of life; he understands that he is alive and that he can become "not alive"; he fears dying.
	The child differentiates death from sleep. Unlike sleep, the horror of death is in pain, progressive mutilation, and mystery.
	The child is vulnerable to guilt feelings related to death because of difficulty in differentiating between death wishes and the actual event.
	The child learns the meaning of death from his own personal experiences.
	    Pets
	    Death of family members, political figures, etc.
	Television and movies have contributed to his concepts of death and understanding of the meaning of illness.
	    Develops more knowledge in the meaning of diagnosis
	    Death may occur violently

Adolescent	The adolescent comprehends the permanence of death much as the adult does, although he may not comprehend death as an event occurring to persons close to himself. He wants to live—he sees death as thwarting pursuit of his goals: independence, success, achievement, physical improvement, and self-image. He fears death before fulfillment. The adolescent may become depressed and resentful because of bodily changes which may occur, dependency, and the loss of his social environment. The adolescent may feel isolated and rejected, since his own adolescent friends may withdraw when faced with his impending death. The adolescent may express rage, bitterness and resentment. He especially resents the fact that he is fated to die.

terms of days or months since each individual and each illness is different.

(4) When the school-age child asks "Am I going to die?" and death is inevitable, he should be told the truth. The school-age child does have the emotional ability to look to his parents and those he trusts for comfort and support.

(5) The school-age child believes in his parents. He should be allowed to die in the comfort and security of his family.

(6) The school-age child knows death means final separation and he knows what he will miss. He must be allowed to mourn this loss as he dies. He may be sad and bitter and demonstrate aggressive behavior. He must be allowed the opportunity to verbalize this if he is able to do so.

  c. Adolescent

(1) The adolescent should be given an explanation of his illness and all necessary treatment procedures.

(2) The adolescent feels deprived and reasonably resentful regarding his illness because he wants to live and reach fulfillment.

(3) As death approaches, the adolescent becomes emotionally closer to his family.

(4) The adolescent should be allowed to maintain his emotional defenses—he may deny absolutely. The adolescent will indicate by his questions what kind of answer he wants.

(5) If the adolescent states "I am not going to die" he is pleading for support. Be truthful and state "No, you are not going to die right now."

(6) The adolescent may ask "How long do I have to live?" He is able to face reality more directly and can tolerate more direct answers. No

absolute time should be given since that absolutely blocks all hope. If an adolescent has what is felt to be a prognosis of approximately 3 months, the response might be "People with an illness like yours may die in 3 to 6 months, but some may live much longer."

(7) The bitterness and resentment of the fact that he is fated to die may interrupt necessary procedures and treatments. This behavior must be appropriately handled.

E. *To confer with the parents regarding feelings about discussing the illness with the child and to give them information which will be helpful in allowing them to play a more supportive role.*

1. Determine what information they have given the child about his illness, and how the child reacted to this information.
2. Determine what specific questions the child has asked about his illness and how the parents have responded.
3. Share with parents your assessment of what the child knows about his illness and what he wants to know.
4. Discuss with the parents how children of various age levels interpret the meaning of death and offer suggestions as to how children's questions regarding death may be answered.
5. Provide parents with helpful literature about explaining death to children. (See references for parents, p. 1462.)
6. Assist parents to explain the child's illness to siblings and to answer their questions. If appropriate, help parents to identify ways that siblings can share in the child's care.

F. *To assist the parents in dealing with their adaptation to their child's illness and anticipated death.*

1. Develop a plan of care that includes the following approach:
   a. The primary responsibility for communicating with the parents should be designated to one nurse.
   b. Information regarding the parents' concerns should be communicated to all staff members.
2. Accept parental feelings about the child's anticipated death and help parents deal with these feelings.
   a. It is not unusual for parents to reach the point of wishing the child dead and to experience guilt and self-blame because of this thought.
   b. Parents may withdraw emotional attachments to the child if the process of dying is lengthy. This occurs because parents complete most of the mourning process before the child reaches biological death. They may relate to the child as if he were already dead.
3. Be aware of factors which affect the family's capacity to cope with fatal illness, especially social and cultural features of the family system, previous experiences with death, present stage of family development, and resources available to them.
4. Recognize the various stages that the parents will go through during the child's illness.

G. *To perform the nursing measures which provide the child with both physical and emotional care during illness.*

1. Provide physical care that makes the child as comfortable as possible.
   Deliver care in a calm, assured, gentle manner.
2. Talk to the child and answer his questions truthfully.

3. Provide an atmosphere that offers the child the greatest security (e.g., room with another child, room near nurse's station, etc.).
4. Provide opportunities for play therapy as the child's condition permits.
5. Plan for consistency of assignment so that the child can experience continuity of contact with a few nurses who inspire confidence and trust.
6. Encourage active involvement in living to the extent that the child is able (e.g., participation in activities of daily living, play, schooling, socialization).
7. Observe children carefully during play for clues to their symbolic language. Watch carefully what they do and listen to what they say. Drawings and self portraits may also help the child to express his feelings.
8. Communicate caring through touch. The child is comforted by being held, especially by his parents.
9. Allow the child opportunity to direct activities and to let his wishes be known.
10. Set realistic limits for the child when necessary, and enforce them consistently.

H. *To encourage the parents to spend as much time as possible with the child and allow the opportunity to participate in the child's care.* (Refer to section on Family-Centered Care, p. 1131.)

1. Allow the parents to bathe the child and to do procedures within their ability and desire. This allows the parents the feeling that they are doing something for their child.
2. Provide the parents with the opportunity to learn how to care for the child and assure them that he will be cared for in their absence.
3. Provide the parents with a place to stay and be comfortable. They should be told where they can find privacy when they want to be alone.

I. *To utilize appropriate services and resources in planning the care of the child and family.*

1. Team members often include:
   a. Physician
   b. Nurse
   c. Child
   d. Family
   e. Social worker
   f. Psychiatrist
   g. Clergyman
   h. Community health nurse
   i. School nurse
   j. Parent groups
2. Teamwork is essential because:
   a. Terminally ill children and their families may require different kinds of assistance at different points in time.
   b. They face many problems that are nonmedical in nature.
   c. The child's need for assistance may be very different from that required by his family.
   d. Team members may support one another.
3. To be effective team members, nurses must:
   a. Communicate, collaborate, and cooperate with other members of the team.
   b. Accept responsibility for their contribution to the plan of care and be accountable for the outcome.

J. *To provide emotional support to parents following the death of the child.*

1. Allow families who wish it the opportunity to spend some time alone with the child after death.

2. Provide privacy for parents to express their grief in whatever manner they choose.
3. If appropriate, compliment parents on the excellent care they gave their child.
4. Be aware that your compassionate silence may be more helpful to families than small talk.
5. Assist families to contact other relatives and funeral home as appropriate.
6. Make certain that families have a safe and comfortable means to get home.
7. Invite parents to call if they have lingering questions or concerns that they wish to discuss.
8. References for Parents:

Grollman E. Explaining Death to Children. Boston, Beacon Press, 1967

Grollman E. Talking About Death: A Dialogue Between Parent and Child. Boston, Beacon Press, 1967

McBride M. Children's literature on death and dying. Pediatric Nursing 1979 May/June; 5(3):31–33

Mills G. Books to help children understand death. Am J Nurs 1979 Feb; 79(2):291–295

Schiff H. The Bereaved Parent. New York, Crown Publishers, 1977

BIBLIOGRAPHY

MENTAL RETARDATION

Books

Accardo PJ and Capute AJ. The Pediatrician and the Developmentally Delayed Child. Baltimore, University Park Press, 1979

Barnard KE and Erickson ML. Teaching Children With Developmental Problems—A Family Care Approach, 2nd ed. St. Louis, CV Mosby, 1976

Chinn P, Drew C, Logan D. Mental Retardation: A Life Cycle Approach. St. Louis, CV Mosby, 1979

Clarke A and Clarke A. Mental Deficiency: The Changing Outlook. New York, The Free Press, 1974

Curry JB and Peppe KK (eds). Mental Retardation: Nursing Approaches to Care. St. Louis, CV Mosby, 1978

Johnston RB and Magrab PR (eds). Developmental Disorders: Assessment, Treatment, Education. Baltimore, University Park Press, 1976

Robinson NM and Robinson H. The Mentally Retarded Child. New York, McGraw-Hill, 1976

Articles

Attwood T. The Croydon workshop for parents of pre-school mentally handicapped children. Child Care Health Dev 1978 Mar/Apr; 4(2):79–97

Barlow C. Mental retardation and related disorders. In Plum F and McDowell F (eds). Contemporary Neurology Services. Philadelphia, FA Davis, 1978

Berry P et al. Social interactions and communication patterns in mentally retarded children. Am J Ment Defic 1978 July; 83(1):44–51

Ellis D. Methods of assessment for use with the visually and mentally handicapped: a selective review. Child Care Health Dev 1978 Nov/Dec; 4(6)397–410

Erickson MP. Care approaches to the child with mental retardation in a hospital setting. Clin Pediatr 1978 July; 17(7):539–547

Erickson MP. Hospital care of the ill child with mental retardation. Dev Med Child Neurol 1978 Oct; 20(5):674–677

Foley JM. Effect of labeling and teacher behavior on children's attitudes. Am J Ment Defic 1979 Jan; 83(4):380–384

Harris J. Working with parents of mentally handicapped children on a long term basis. Child Care Health Dev 1978 Mar/Apr; 4(2):121–130

Hetherington RW et al. Evaluation of a regional resource center for multiply handicapped retarded children. Am J Ment Defic 1979 Jan; 83(4):367–379

Nelson KB et al. Perinatal risk factors in children with serious motor and mental handicaps. Ann Neurol 1977 Nov; 2(5):371–377

Pipes PL. Nutrition and feeding of children with developmental delays and related problems. In Pipes PL. Nutrition in Infancy and Childhood. St. Louis, CV Mosby, 1977

Salomon MK et al. Use of play materials in treating a severely handicapped child. Child Care Health Dev 1978 Mar/Apr; 4(2):131–140

DOWN'S SYNDROME

Books

Canino FJ and Reeve RE. General issues in working with parents of handicapped children. In Abidin RR (ed). Parent Education and Intervention Handbook. Springfield, Charles C Thomas, 1980

Scipien G et al. Comprehensive Pediatric Nursing. New York, McGraw-Hill, 1979

Wacht MA. The Mentally Disabled Child. In Johnson SH (ed). High-Risk Parenting. Philadelphia, JB Lippincott, 1979

Articles

Bears S. Children with Down's syndrome. Health Visitor 1979 July; 52(6):266–268

Buckhalt JA, Rutherford RB, Goldberg KE. Verbal and nonverbal interaction of mothers with their Down's syndrome and nonretarded infants. Am J Ment Defic 1978 Jan; 82(4):337–343

Erickson MP. Responding to the needs of sick children with mental retardation. Children Today 1980 Jan/Feb; 9(1):24–25

Harris SR. Transdisciplinary therapy model for the infant with Down's syndrome. Phys Ther 1980 Apr; 60(4):420–423

MINIMAL BRAIN DYSFUNCTION

Books

Johnston RB and Magrab PR (eds). Developmental Disorders: Assessment, Treatment, Education. Baltimore, University Park Press, 1976

Meir J. Developmental and Learning Disabilities: Evaluation, Management and Prevention in Children. Baltimore, University Park Press, 1976

Peters JE et al. Physician's Handbook, Screening for MBD. Summit, Ciba Medical Horizons, 1973

Rie HE and Rie ED (eds). Handbook of Minimal Brain Dysfunction. New York, John Wiley & Sons, 1980

Safer D and Allen R. Hyperactive Children: Diagnosis and Management. Baltimore, University Park Press, 1976

Articles

Drabman RS and Jarvie G. Counseling parents of children with behavior problems: The use of extinction and time-out techniques. Pediatrics 1977 Jan; 59(1):78–85

Lazor A et al. Criteria for early diagnosis of brain dysfunction. Can Psychiatr Assoc J 1978 Aug; 23(5):317–324

Saccar CL. Drug therapy in the treatment of minimal brain dysfunction. Am J Hosp Pharm 1978 May; 35(5):544–552

GENETICS

Books

Butnarescu G, Tillotson DM, Villarreal PP. Perinatal Nursing, Vol. 2. Reproductive Risk. New York, John Wiley & Sons, 1980

Siggers DC. Prenatal Diagnosis of Genetic Disease. London, Blackwell Scientific Publications, 1978

Vaughn VC, McKay RJ, Behrman RE. Nelson Textbook of Pediatrics, 11th ed. Philadelphia, WB Saunders, 1979

Whaley LF and Wong DC. Nursing Care of Infants and Children. St. Louis, CV Mosby, 1979

Articles

Epstein CS et al. Risk, communication, and decision making in genetic counseling. The Natl Found/March of Dimes Birth Defects: Original Article Series, 1979, 10(5): entire issue

Goldbus MS and Hall BD. Diagnostic approaches to the malformed fetus, abortus, stillborn and deceased newborn. The Natl Found/March of Dimes Birth Defects: Original Article Series 1979; 10(5A): entire issue

Kaback MM (guest ed). Symposium on medical genetics. Pediatr Clin North Am 1978 Aug; 25(3)

Miller L. Toward a greater understanding of the parents of the mentally retarded child. J Pediatr 1968 Nov; 73(5):699–705

Myrianthopoulus NC and Bergsma D. Recent advances in the developmental biology of central nervous system malformations. The Natl Found/March of Dimes Birth Defects: Original Article Series 1979; 10(3): entire issue

O'Donnell JJ and Hall BD. Penetrance and variability in malformation syndromes. The Natl Found/March of Dimes. Birth Defects: Original Article Series 1979 10(5B).

Townes BD, Priest SR, Ellison RM. Hierarchy of birth planning values: An aid in genetic counseling. J Psychiatr Nurs 1979 Sept; 17(9)37–41

Townes BD, Priest SR, Ellison RM. Early warning systems for genetic risk. Emergency Medicine 1978 Nov; 10(11):124–131+

Townes BD, Priest SR, Ellison RM. The need to know? Can Nurs 1980 May; 76(5):30–32

POISONING

Books

Dube S (ed). Immediate Care of the Sick and Injured Child. St. Louis, CV Mosby, 1978

Pascoe DJ and Grossman M. Quick Reference to Pediatric Emergencies, 2nd ed. Philadelphia, JB Lippincott, 1978

Preventing Lead Poisoning in Young Children. U.S. Dept. of HEW Public Health Service, Center for Disease Control, Bureau of State Services, Environmental Health Services Division, Atlanta, Georgia 30333, April 1978

Reece RM and Chamberlain JW. Manual of Emergency Pediatrics. 2nd ed. Philadelphia, WB Saunders, 1978

Articles

Braden BT. Validation of a poison prevention program. Am J Public Health 1979 Sept; 69(9):942–944

Charney E, Sayre J, Coulter M. Increased lead absorption in inner city children. Where does the lead come from? Pediatrics 1980 Feb; 65(2):226–237

Chisholm JJ et al. Recognition and management of children with increased lead absorption. Arch Dis Child 1979 Apr; 54(4):249–262

Ford P. Update on first aid management. Pediatric Nursing 1980 Sept/Oct; 6(5):35–36

Gilles C. Management of pediatric poisoning—the role of the nurse practitioner. Pediatric Nursing 1980 Sept/Oct; 6(5):33–35

Godwin RH. Child-resistant locks in poison control. Pediatrics 1978. May; 61(5):750–752

Ipecac syrup and activated charcoal for treatment of poisoning in children. Med Lett Drugs Ther 1979 24 Aug; 21(17):70–72

Lovejoy F. Management of pediatric poisoning: Part I. Pediatric Nursing 1980 Sep/Oct; 6(5):37–39

Mofenson HC et al. Poisoning—an update. Clin Pediatr 1979 Mar; 18(3):144–146

Sachs HK et al. IQ following treatment of lead poisoning: A patient–sibling comparison. J Pediatr 1978 Sept; 93(3):428–431

Sachs HK et al. Lead poisoning with encephalopathy. Effect of early diagnosis on neurologic and psychologic salvage. Am J Dis child 1979 Aug; 133(8):786–790

Temple A. Management of pediatric poisoning: Part II. Pediatric Nursing 1980 Sept/Oct; 6(5):40–43

THE ABUSED CHILD

Books

Fontana VJ. Somewhere a Child is Crying. New York, Macmillan, 1973

Fontana VJ and Besharow DJ. The Maltreated Child, 4th ed. Springfield, Charles C Thomas, 1979

Gorin LL. The nurse and the sexually assaulted child. In Chinn PL and Leonard KB (eds). Current Practice in Pediatric Nursing, pp. 155–176. St. Louis, CV Mosby, 1980

Helfer RE and Kemp CH (eds). Helping the Battered Child and His Family. Philadelphia, JB Lippincott, 1972

Helfer RE and Kemp CH. Child Abuse and Neglect—The Family and the Community. Cambridge, Mass., Ballinger, 1976

Helfer RE and Kemp CH. The Battered Child, 2nd ed. Chicago, University of Chicago Press, 1974

Kauffman C and Neill MK. The abused child. In Johnson SH (ed). High Risk Parenting, pp. 227–242. Philadelphia, JB Lippincott, 1980

Articles

Cael T. Child abuse: Hospital team and public agencies help patients and parents. Hospitals 1978 Nov 16; 52(22):135–136

Carr JL. Communicating with the child-abusing family. Topics in Clinical Nursing 1979 Oct; 1(3):41–48

Cicchetti D, Taraldson BJ, Egeland B. Perspective in the treatment and understanding of child abuse. In Goldstein AP (ed). Prescriptions for Child Mental Health and Education. New York, Pergamon Press, 1978

Coolsen P. Community involvement in the prevention of child abuse and neglect. Children Today 1980 Sept/Oct; 9(5):5–8

Cooney KM. Nursing care of emotionally abused and deprived children. Issues Compr Pediatr Nurs 1978 Sept; 3(3):54–62

Copans S et al. The stresses of treating child abuse. Children Today 1979 Jan/Feb; 8(1):22–27+

Fitzpatrick L. A team approach to child abuse. Can Nurs 1979 Jan; 75(1):36–39

Foster PH, Lanier MW, Whitworth JM. Expanding the role of nurses in child abuse, protection and treatment. J Psychiatr Nurs 1980 Feb; 18(2):24–28

Hall NM. Group treatment for sexually abused children. Nurs Clin North Am 1978 Dec; 13(4):701–705

Holter JC. Child abuse. Nurs Clin North Am 1979 Sept; 14(3):417–427

Hunter RS, Kilstrom N, Kraybill EN, Loda F. Antecedents of child abuse and neglect in premature infants: A prospective study in a newborn intensive care unit. Pediatrics 1978 Apr; 61(4):629–635

McDonald AE and Reece RM. Child abuse: Problems of reporting. Pediatr Clin North Am 1979 Nov; 26(4):785–791

McFadden EJ. Fostering the battered and abused child. Children Today 1980 Mar/Apr; 9(2):13–15+

Ortman E. Attachment behaviors in abused children. Pediatric Nursing 1979 July/Aug; 5(4):25–29

Press-Rigler M, Kent JT, Croot P, Finnila M. Parent aides: An intervention program in cases of child abuse and neglect. J Assoc Care Children in Hospitals 1980 Winter; 8(3):64–68

Scharer K. Nursing intervention with abusive and neglectful families within the community. Matern Child Nurs J 1979 Summer; 8(2):85–94

Scharer K. Nursing therapy with abusive and neglectful families. J Psychiatr Nurs 1979 Sept; 17(9):12–21

Tomlinson A, Dumore S, Bradander T: Child abuse. J Canadian Psychiatr Nurs 1979 Mar/Apr; 20(2):9+

Tomlinson A, Dunmore S, Bradander T. Beyond child abuse. Emergency Medicine 1979 Jan 15; 11(1):226–228+

Films

The Nurse in Child Abuse Prevention.
   The American Journal of Nursing, Educational Services Division Dept., PMH–6A, 555 W. 57th Street, New York, N.Y. 10019
   30 minutes, 16 mm and videocassettes
   The child abuse syndrome is examined together with the nurse's role in detecting, treating, and preventing this serious disorder.

THE DYING CHILD

Books

Bluebond–Langer M. The Private Worlds of Dying Children. Princeton, Princeton University Press, 1978

Easson W. The Dying Child: The Management of the Child or Adolescent Who is Dying. Springfield, Charles C Thomas, 1970

Garfield C. Stress and Survival: The Emotional Realities of Life Threatening Illness. St. Louis, CV Mosby, 1979

Grollman E. Explaining Death to Children. Boston, Beacon Press, 1967

Grollman E. Talking About Death: A Dialogue Between Parent and Child. Boston, Beacon Press, 1967

Kübler–Ross E. On Death and Dying. New York, Macmillan, 1970

Martinson I. Home Care for the Dying Child, Professional and Family Perspectives. New York, Appleton–Century–Crofts, 1976

Sahler OJ. The Child and Death. St. Louis, CV Mosby, 1978

Schiff H. The Bereaved Parent. New York, Crown Publishers, 1977

Schoenburg B et al (eds). Psychosocial Aspects of Terminal Care. New York, Columbia University Press, 1972

Schulmann J. Coping With Tragedy: Successfully Facing the Problem of a Seriously Ill Child. Chicago, Follett Pub. Co., 1978

Articles

Elliot BA et al. Neonatal death—reflections for parents. Pediatrics 1978 July; 62(1):100–102.

Elliott BA et al. Neonatal death—reflections for physicians. Pediatrics 1978 July; 62(1):96–100

Farley FH. The hypostatization of death in adolescence. Adolescence 1979 Summer; 14(54):341–350

Ferguson F. Children's cognitive discovery of death. JACCH 1978 Summer; 7(2):8–14

Helmrath TA et al. Death of infant: Parental grieving and the failure of social support. J Fam Pract 1978 Apr; 6(4):785–790

Kerner J et al. The impact of grief: A retrospective study of family function following loss of a child with cystic fibrosis. J Chronic Dis 1979; 32(3):221–225

Lascari AD. The dying child and the family. J Fam Pract 1978 June; 6(6):1279–1286

Lewis E. Mourning by the family after a stillbirth or neonatal death. Arch Dis Child 1979 Apr; 54(4):303–306

Lewis N. I probably won't have all the luxuries in the world. JACCH 1978 Summer; 7(1):28–32

Martinson I. Home care for the dying child. Am J Nurs 1977 Nov; 77(11):1816–1818

McBride M. Children's literature on death and dying. Pediatric Nursing 1979 May/June; 5(3):31–33

Mills G. Books to help children understand death. Am J Nurs 1979 Feb; 79(2):291–295

Rowe J et al. Follow-up of families who experience a perinatal death. Pediatrics 1978 Aug; 62(8):166–170

Schreiner RL et al. Physician's responsibility to parents after death of an infant: Beneficial outcome of a telephone call. Am J Dis Child 1979 July; 133(7):723–736

Smialek Z. Observations on immediate reactions of families to sudden infant death. Pediatrics 1978 Aug; 62:160–165

Vernick J. Meaningful communication with the fatally ill child. In Anthony EJ, and Koupernick C (eds). The Child in His Family: The Impact of Disease and Death. New York, John Wiley & Sons, 1973

APPENDIXES AND INDEX

APPENDIX I:
DIAGNOSTIC STUDIES AND THEIR MEANING

TABLE OF ABBREVIATIONS

kg. = kilogram	L. = liter	mm. = millimeter
gm. = gram	dl. = 100 milliliters	μ. = micron or micrometer
mg. = milligram	ml. = milliliter	mm. Hg = millimeters of mercury
μg. = microgram	cu.mm. = cubic millimeter	mU = milliunit
$\mu\mu$g. = micromicrogram	nM. = nanomolar	μU = microunit
ng. = nanogram		mEq. = milliequivalent
pg. = picogram		IU = International Unit
		mIU = milliInternational Unit

NORMAL VALUES—HEMATOLOGY*

Determination	Normal Value	Clinical Significance
A$_2$ hemoglobin	1.90–3.86%	Increased in certain types of thalassemia
Bleeding time	30 sec.–6 min.	Prolonged in purpura hemorrhagica, in which platelets are reduced, and in chloroform and phosphorus poisoning
Clotting time	5–10 min.	Prolonged in hemorrhagic disease and in various coagulation factor deficiencies
Factor V assay	75–125%	Pro–accelerin factor
Factor VIII assay (antihemophiliac factor)	50–150%	Deficient in classical hemophilia
Factor IX assay (plasma thrombo plastin component)	75–125%	Deficient in Christmas disease (pseudohemophilia)
Factor X (Stuart factor)	75–125%	Stuart clotting defect
Fibrinogen	200–400 mg./dl.	Increased in pregnancy, pneumonia, infections accompanied by leukocytosis, and nephrosis. Decreased in acute yellow atrophy of liver, cirrhosis, typhoid fever, chloroform poisoning, abruptio placentae
Fibrinolysins (whole blood clot lysis time)	No lysis in 24 hrs.	Increased activity associated with massive hemorrhage, extensive surgery, and transfusion reactions
Partial thromboplastin time (activated)	20–45 sec.	Prolonged in Factor VIII, IX, and X deficiency
Prothrombin consumption	Over 20 sec.	Impaired in factor VIII, IX, and X deficiency
Prothrombin time	60–100% of control	Prolonged in factor X deficiency and other hemorrhagic diseases, and in cirrhosis, hepatitis, and acute toxic necrosis of the liver
Erythrocyte count	Males: 4,600,000–6,200,000 per cu. mm. Females: 4,200,000–5,400,000 per cu. mm.	Increased in severe diarrhea and dehydration, polycythemia, secondary polycythemia, acute poisoning, pulmonary fibrosis, and Ayerza disease. Decreased in all anemias, in leukemia, and after hemorrhage, when blood volume has been restored.
Erythrocyte indices Mean corpuscular volume (MCV)	80–94 (cu. microns)	Increased in macrocytic anemias, decreased in microcytic anemia
Mean corpuscular hemoglobin (MCH)	27–32 $\mu\mu$g. per cell	Increased in macrocytic anemias, decreased in microcytic anemia
Mean corpuscular hemoglobin concentration (MCHC)	33–38%	Decreased in severe hypochromic anemia
Reticulocytes	0.5–1.5% of red cells	Increased with any condition stimulating increase in bone marrow activity, i.e., infection, blood loss (acute and chronic); following iron therapy in iron deficiency anemia, polycythemia rubra vera. Decreased with any condition depressing bone marrow activity, acute leukemia, late stage of severe anemias.
Erythrocyte sedimentation rate	Males: 0–9 mm./hr. Females: 0–20 mm./hr.	Increased in tissue destruction, whether inflammatory or degenerative, and during menstruation, pregnancy, and in acute febrile diseases.

*Laboratory values vary according to the techniques used in different laboratories.

NORMAL VALUES—HEMATOLOGY* (continued)

Determination	Normal Value	Clinical Significance
Hematocrit	Males: 42–50% Females: 40–48%	Decreased in severe anemias, anemia of pregnancy, acute massive blood loss. Increased in erythrocytosis of any cause, and in dehydration or hemoconcentration associated with shock
Hemoglobin	Males: 13–16 gm./dl. Females: 12–14 gm./dl.	Decreased in various anemias, pregnancy, severe or prolonged hemorrhage, and with excessive fluid intake. Increased in polycythemia, chronic obstructive pulmonary diseases, failure of oxygenation because of congestive heart failure, and normally, in people living at high altitudes
Hemoglobin F	Less than 2%	Increased in infants and children, in thalassemia and many anemias
Leukocyte alkaline phosphatase	Score of 40–100	Decreased in chronic myelocytic leukemia and chronic lymphocytic leukemia. Increased in nonleukemic leukocytosis and myeloproliferative diseases
Leukocyte count Neutrophils Eosinophils Basophils Lymphocytes Monocytes	Total: 5,000–10,000 cu. mm. 60–70% 1–4% 0–0.5% 20–30% 2–6%	Elevated in acute infectious diseases—predominantly in the neutrophilic fraction with bacterial diseases, and in the lymphocytic and monocytic fractions in viral diseases. Eosinophils elevated in collagen diseases, allergy, intestinal parasitosis. Elevated in acute leukemia, following menstruation, and following surgery or trauma. Depressed in aplastic anemia, agranulocytosis, and by toxic agents, such as chemotherapeutic agents used in treating malignancy
Osmotic fragility of red cells	Increase if hemolysis occurs in over 0.5% NaCl Decrease if hemolysis is incomplete in 0.3% NaCl	Increased in congenital spherocytosis, idiopathic acquired hemolytic anemia, isoimmune hemolytic disease, ABO hemolytic disease of newborn. Decreased in sickle-cell anemia, thalassemia
Platelet count	200,000–350,000 per cu. mm.	Increased with chronic granulocytic leukemia, hemoconcentration. Decreased in thrombocytopenic purpura, acute leukemia, aplastic anemia, and during cancer chemotherapy.

NORMAL CHEMISTRIES—SERUM, PLASMA, WHOLE BLOOD

Determination	Normal Adult Values	Clinical Significance (Increased)	(Decreased)
Acetoacetate and acetone	0.3–2.0 mg./dl.	Diabetic acidosis Fasting Toxemia of pregnancy Carbohydrate-free diet High-fat diet	
Adrenocorticotropic hormone (ACTH) (plasma), RIA*	Less than 100 pg./ml.	Pituitary-dependent Cushing's syndrome Ectopic ACTH syndrome Primary adrenal atrophy	Adrenocortical tumor Adrenal insufficiency secondary to hypopituitarism
Aldolase	0.5–3.1 mU/ml.	Hepatic necrosis Granulocytic leukemia Myocardial infarction Skeletal muscle disease	
Aldosterone (plasma), RIA	Supine: 3–10 ng./dl. Upright: 5–30 ng./dl. Adrenal vein: 200–800 ng./dl.	Primary (Conn's syndrome) Secondary aldosteronism	Addison's disease
Alpha amino nitrogen	3.0–5.5 mg./dl.	Phosphorus, arsenic, chloroform, carbon tetrachloride poisoning Infectious hepatitis Eclampsia	Bacterial pneumonia Administration of anterior pituitary extracts Administration of insulin
Alpha-1-antitrypsin	200–400 mg./dl.	Early inflammatory processes Pneumonia Abscess formations Arthritis	Chronic lung disease
Alpha-1-fetoprotein	None detected	Hepatocarcinoma Metastatic carcinoma of liver Germinal cell carcinoma of the testis or ovary	
Alpha-hydroxybutyric dehydrogenase	up to 140 mU/ml.	Myocardial infarction Granulocytic leukemia Hemolytic anemias Muscular dystrophy	
Ammonia (plasma)	5–70 μg./dl.	Severe liver disease Hepatic decompensation	
Amylase	15–200 units/dl.	Acute pancreatitis Mumps Duodenal ulcer Carcinoma of head of pancreas Prolonged elevation with pseudocyst of pancreas	Chronic pancreatitis Pancreatic fibrosis and atrophy Cirrhosis of liver Acute alcoholism Toxemias of pregnancy
Androstenedione, RIA	Females: 0.6–3.0 ng./ml.	Increases in many cases of hirsutism and virilization	

* By radioimmunoassay

NORMAL CHEMISTRIES—SERUM, PLASMA, WHOLE BLOOD (continued)

Determination	Normal Adult Values	Clinical Significance	
		(Increased)	*(Decreased)*
Arsenic	6–20 µg./dl.	Accidental or intentional poisoning Excessive occupational exposure	
Ascorbic acid (vitamin C)	0.4–1.5 mg./dl.	Large doses of ascorbic acid as a pro- phylactic against the common cold	Rheumatic fever Collagen diseases Deficient vitamin C intake Renal and hepatic disease Congestive heart failure
Bilirubin	Total: 0.1–1.0 mg./dl. Direct: 0.1–0.2 mg./dl. Indirect: 0.1–0.8 mg./dl.	Hemolytic anemia (indirect) Biliary obstruction Hepatocellular damage Pernicious anemia Hemolytic disease of newborn Eclampsia	
Bromsulphalein (BSP)	Less than 5% retention in 45 minutes	Acute hepatic disease	
Calcitonin	Basal: Nondetectable (below 400 pg./ml.)	Medullary carcinoma of the thyroid Some nonthyroid tumors Zollinger-Ellison syndrome Pernicious anemia Chronic renal failure	
Calcium	8.5–10.5 mg./dl.	Tumor or hyperplasia of parathyroid Hyperparathyroidism Hypervitaminosis D Multiple myeloma Nephritis with uremia	Hypoparathyroidism Diarrhea Celiac disease Rickets Osteomalacia Malnutrition Nephrosis After parathyroidectomy
CO_2 content	Adults: 24–32 mEq./L. Infants: 18–24 mEq./L.	Tetany Respiratory disease Intestinal obstruction Vomiting	Acidosis Nephritis Eclampsia Diarrhea Anesthesia
Carcinoembryonic antigen (CEA), RIA	0–2.5 ng./ml.	The repeatedly high incidence of this an- tigen in cancers of the colon, rectum, pancreas, and stomach suggest that CEA levels may be a useful adjunct in the diagnosis of these conditions	
Carotene, beta	70–250 µg./dl.	Carotenemia Hypothyroidism Diabetes Hyperlipemia	Malabsorption syndromes Hepatic disease Dietary deficiencies
Catecholamines, plasma, RIA	Recumbent: 200–600 ng./L. Upright: 300–1000 ng./L.	Pheochromocytoma	
Cephalin flocculation	Negative to 1 +	Severe liver disease Atypical viral pneumonia Malaria Syphilis Infectious mononucleosis Congestive heart failure	
Ceruloplasmin	Males: 29–80 mg./dl. Females: 32–156 mg./dl.	Pregnancy Myocardial infarction Hepatic cirrhosis	Wilson's disease (hepatolenticular de- generation)
C_1 Esterase inhibitor	50–100% of normal control		Hereditary angioneurotic edema Lymphoproliferative disorders
Chloride	95–105 mEq./L.	Nephritis Urinary obstruction Cardiac decompensation Anemia Ether anesthesia	Diabetes Diarrhea Vomiting Pneumonia Heavy metal poisoning Cushing's syndrome Burns Intestinal obstruction Febrile conditions
Cholesterol	150–300 mg./dl.	Lipemia Obstructive jaundice Diabetes Hypothyroidism	Pernicious anemia Hemolytic anemia Hyperthyroidism Severe infection Terminal states of debilitating disease
Cholesterol esters	60–70% of total		The esterified fraction decreases in liver disease
Cholinesterase	Serum: 0.61–1.50 delta pH Red cells: 0.60–1.00 delta pH	Nephrosis Exercise	Nerve gas intoxication (greater effect on red cell activity) Insecticides, organic phosphates (greater effect on plasma activity)
Chorionic gonadotrophin, beta subunit, RIA	0–5 IU/L.	Pregnancy Hydatidiform mole Choriocarcinoma	

NORMAL CHEMISTRIES—SERUM, PLASMA, WHOLE BLOOD (continued)

Determination	Normal Adult Values	Clinical Significance (Increased)	Clinical Significance (Decreased)
Chorionic somatomammo-trophin	None detectable	Pregnancy	
Complement, Human C$_3$	Males: 88–252 mg./dl. Females: 88–206 mg./dl.	Some inflammatory diseases	Acute glomerulonephritis Disseminated lupus erythematosus with renal involvement
Complement, C$_4$	14–51 mg./dl.	Some inflammatory diseases	Often decreased in immunological diseases, especially with active SLE Hereditary angioneurotic edema
Complement, total (hemolytic)	90–94% complement	Some inflammatory diseases	Acute glomerulonephritis Epidemic meningitis Subacute bacterial endocarditis
Congo red	60–100% retained in bloodstream		Deposits of amyloid in tissue absorb congo red. In amyloid disease, less than 40% of the dye will remain in the plasma. In severe cases, less than 10% is retained.
Copper	70–165 µg./dl.	Cirrhosis of liver Pregnancy	Wilson's disease
Cortisol, RIA	8 A.M.: 7–25 µg./dl. 4 P.M.: 2–9 µg./dl.	Stress: infectious disease, surgery, burns, etc. Pregnancy Cushing's syndrome Pancreatitis Eclampsia	Addison's disease Anterior pituitary hypofunction
C-peptide Reactivity	1.5–10 ng./ml.	Insulinoma	Diabetes
Creatine	0.2–0.8 mg./dl.	Biliary obstruction Pregnancy Nephritis Renal destruction Trauma to muscle Pseudohypertrophic muscular dystrophy	
Creatine phosphokinase (CPK)	Males: 50–325 mU/ml. Females: 50–250 mU/ml.	Myocardial infarction Skeletal muscle diseases Intramuscular injections Crush syndrome Hypothyroidism Delirium tremens Cerebrovascular disease	
Creatine phosphokinase isoenzymes	MM band present (skeletal muscle): MB band absent (heart muscle)	MB band increased in myocardial infarction	
Creatinine	0.7–1.4 mg./dl.	Nephritis Chronic renal disease	
Creatinine clearance	100–150 mls. of blood cleared of creatinine/min.		Kidney diseases
Cryofibrinogen, qualitative (plasma)	Negative	Neoplasms Acute rheumatic fever Acute glomerulonephritis Ulcerative colitis Thromboembolic states	
Cryoglobulins, qualitative	Negative	Multiple myeloma Chronic lymphocytic leukemia Lymphosarcoma Systemic lupus erythematosus Rheumatoid arthritis Subacute bacterial endocarditis Some malignancies	
Cyclic AMP (plasma), RIA	Males: 17–33 nM./L. Females: 11–27 nM./L.	Has proved valuable in differentiating nephrogenic diabetes insipidus from that of primary hypothalamic diabetes insipidus. Administration of ADH appears to be incapable of eliciting an increase of cyclic AMP in nephrogenic diabetes insipidus.	
11-Desoxycortisol	0–2 µg./dl.	Hypertensive form of virilizing adrenal hyperplasia due to an 11-beta hydroxylase defect.	
Dibucaine number	Normal: 70–85% inhibition Heterozygote: 50–65% inhibition Homozygote: 16–25% inhibition		Important in detecting carriers of abnormal cholinesterase activity who are susceptible to succinyldicholine anesthetic shock
Dihydrotestosterone	Males: 50–210 ng./dl. Females: None detectable		Testicular feminization syndrome
Erythropoietin	7–36 milli-immuno-chemical units/ml.	Many red blood cell anemias Some cases of "secondary" polycythemia	Polycythemia vera Some types of renal disease

NORMAL CHEMISTRIES—SERUM, PLASMA, WHOLE BLOOD (continued)

Determination	Normal Adult Values	Clinical Significance	
		(Increased)	*(Decreased)*
Erythropoietin (continued)		Possible as an early manifestation of kidney transplant rejection	

Estradiol, RIA	Females:
	  Menstruation: 1.5–7.5 ng./dl.
	  Follicular phase: 2.0–20 ng./dl.
	  Midcycle: 12–40 ng./dl.
	  Luteal phase: 10–30 ng./dl.
	  Postmenopausal: 1.0–5.0 ng./dl.
	Males: 0.5–5.0 ng./dl.
		Pregnancy	Depressed or failure to peak—ovarian failure

Estriol, RIA	Nonpregnant females: less than 0.5 ng./ml.
	Pregnant females:
	  1st trimester—up to 1.0 ng./ml.
	  2nd trimester—0.8 to 7.0 ng./ml.
	  3rd trimester—5.0 to 25.0 ng./ml.
	Males: less than 0.5 ng./ml.
		Pregnancy	Depressed or failure to peak—ovarian failure

Estrogens, total, RIA	Females:
	  Menstrual flow: 43–67 ng./dl.
	  Follicular phase: 40–103 ng./dl.
	  Ovulation peak: 75–139 ng./dl.
	  Luteal phase: 47–113 ng./dl.
	Males: 47–74 ng./dl.
		Pregnancy
		Measured on a daily basis can be used to evaluate response of hypogonadotrophic, hypoestrogenic women to human menopausal or pituitary gonadotropin
			Fetal distress
			Ovarian failure

Estrone, RIA	Females:
	  Day 1–10: 4.3–18.0 ng./dl.
	  Day 11–20: 7.5–19.6 ng./dl.
	  Day 21–30: 13.0–20.0 ng./dl.
	Males: 2.5–7.5 ng./dl.
		Pregnancy	Depressed or failure to peak—ovarian failure

Fatty acids	Total: 250–300 mg./dl.	Diabetes Anemia Nephrosis Hypothyroidism Nephritis	Hyperthyroidism
Ferritin, RIA	Males: 10–270 ng./ml. Females: 5–100 ng./ml.	Hemochromatosis Certain neoplastic diseases Acute myelogenous leukemia Multiple myeloma	Iron deficiency
Fibrinogen degradation products (FDP)	Less than 10 µg./ml. (negative in the 1:5 dilution)	Thrombotic episodes of any kind, including myocardial infarction, postoperative deep vein thrombosis, and certain pregnancy disorders	
Folic acid, RIA	4–16 ng./ml.		Megaloblastic anemias of infancy and pregnancy Inadequate diets Liver disease Malabsorption syndrome Severe hemolytic anemia

Follicle stimulating hormone (FSH), RIA	Normal Females:
	  Follicular phase: 5–20 mIU/ml.
	  Peak of middle cycle: 12–30 mIU/ml.
	  Luteinic phase: 5–15 mIU/ml.
	Menopausal Females: 40–200 mIU/ml.
	Normal Males: 5–25 mIU/ml.
		Menopause and primary ovarian failure	Pituitary failure

Galactose-1-phosphate uridyl transferase	Above 18 units of activity per gram of hemoglobin 0.05–1.5: Possibly galactosemic 0–0.05: Galactosemic		Galactosemia
Gamma glutamyl transpeptidase	Males: less than 45 IU/L. Females: less than 30 IU/L.	Hepatobiliary disease Anicteric alcoholics Drug therapy damage	
Gastrin, RIA	Fasting: 50–155 pg./ml. Postprandial: 80–170 pg./ml. Zollinger-Ellison syndrome: 200–over 2000 pg./ml.	Zollinger-Ellison syndrome Peptic ulceration of the duodenum Pernicious anemia	

NORMAL CHEMISTRIES—SERUM, PLASMA, WHOLE BLOOD (continued)

Determination	Normal Adult Values	Clinical Significance	
		(Increased)	*(Decreased)*
Gastrin, RIA (continued)	Pernicious anemia: 130–2260 (mean 912) pg./ml.		
Glucose	Fasting: 60–110 mg./dl. Postprandial (2 hour): 65–140 mg./dl.	Diabetes Nephritis Hyperthyroidism Early hyperpituitarism Cerebral lesions Infections Pregnancy Uremia	Hyperinsulinism Hypothyroidism Late hyperpituitarism Pernicious vomiting Addison's disease Extensive hepatic damage
Glucose tolerance (oral)	Features of a normal response: 1. Normal fasting between 60–125 mg./dl. 2. No sugar in urine 3. The upper limits of normal are: fasting—125 1 hour—190 2 hours—140 3 hours—125	(Flat or inverted curve) Hyperinsulinism Adrenal cortical insufficiency (Addison's disease) Anterior pituitary hypofunction Hypothyroidism Sprue and celiac disease	(High or prolonged curve) Diabetes Hyperthyroidism Primary adrenal cortical tumor or hyperplasia Severe anemia Certain central nervous system disorders
Glucose–6–phosphate dehydrogenase (red cells)	Screening: Decolorization in 20–100 minutes Quantitative: 1.86–2.50 IU/ml. RBC		Drug induced hemolytic anemia Hemolytic disease of newborn
Glycoprotein	110–140 mg./dl.	Neoplasm Tuberculosis Diabetes complicated by degenerative vascular disease Pregnancy Rheumatoid arthritis Rheumatic fever Infectious liver disease Lupus erythematosus	
Growth hormone, RIA	Males: up to 3 ng./ml. Females: up to 5 ng./ml.	Acromegaly	Failure to stimulate with arginine or insulin—hypopituitarism
Haptoglobin	50–200 mg./dl.	Pregnancy Estrogen therapy Chronic infections Various inflammatory conditions Tissue destruction or necrosis	Hemolytic anemia Hemolytic blood transfusion reaction
Hemoglobin (plasma)	2–7 mg./dl.	Transfusion reactions Paroxysmal nocturnal hemoglobinuria Intravascular hemolysis	
Hexosaminidase, total	Controls: 333–375 nM./ml./hr. Heterozygotes: 288–644 nM./ml./hr. Tay-Sachs disease: 284–1232 nM./ml./hr. Diabetics: 567–3560 nM./ml./hr.	Diabetes Tay-Sachs disease	
Hexosaminidase A	Controls: 49–68% of total Heterozygotes: 26–45% of total Tay-Sachs disease: 0–4% of total Diabetics: 39–59% of total		Tay-Sachs disease and heterozygotes
High density lipoprotein Cholesterol (HDL cholesterol)	Age (years) / Males (mg./dl.) / Females (mg./dl.) 0–19 30–65 30–70 20–29 35–70 35–75 30–39 30–65 35–80 40–49 30–65 40–85 50–59 30–65 35–85 60–69 30–65 35–85		HDL cholesterol is lower in patients with increased risk for coronary heart disease
17-Hydroxyprogesterone, RIA	Males: 0.4–4.0 ng./ml. Females: 0.1–3.3 ng./ml. Children: 0.1–0.5 ng./ml.	Congenital adrenal hyperplasia Pregnancy Some cases of adrenal or ovarian adenomas	
Icterus index	1–6 units	Biliary obstruction Hemolytic anemias	Secondary anemias
Immunoglobulin A	Adult Males: 60–297 mg./dl. Adult Females: 48–295 mg./dl. (In children the normals are lower and vary with age.)	Gamma A myeloma Wiscott-Aldrich syndrome Autoimmune disease Hepatic cirrhosis	Ataxia telangiectasis Agammaglobulinemia Hypogammaglobulinemia, transient Dysgammaglobulinemia Protein-losing enteropathies

NORMAL CHEMISTRIES—SERUM, PLASMA, WHOLE BLOOD (continued)

Determination	Normal Adult Values	Clinical Significance	
		(Increased)	(Decreased)
Immunoglobulin D	0–30 mg./dl.	IgD multiple myeloma Some patients with chronic infectious diseases	
Immunoglobulin E	20–740 ng./ml.	Allergic patients and those with parasitic infestations	
Immunoglobulin G	Adult Males: 635–1400 mg./dl. Adult Females: 645–1300 mg./dl.	IgG myeloma Following hyperimmunization Autoimmune disease states Chronic infections	Congenital and acquired hypogammaglobulinemia IgA myelomas, Waldenstrom's (IgM) macroglobulinemia Some malabsorption syndromes Extensive protein loss
Immunoglobulin M	Adult Males: 41–248 mg./dl. Adult Females: 59–280 mg./dl.	Waldenstrom's macroglobulinemia Parasitic infections Hepatitis	Agammaglobulinemias Some IgG and IgA myelomas Chronic lymphatic leukemia
Insulin, RIA	5–25 μU/ml.	Insulinoma Acromegaly	Diabetes mellitus
Iodine, protein-bound	4.0–8.0 μg./dl.	Hyperthyroidism	Hypothyroidism
Ionized calcium	2.04–2.44 mEq./L.	Ionized calcium is a much more sensitive indicator of disease states than the total calcium. Useful in diagnosing hyperparathyroidism in patients with normal and near normal total calcium levels. Also a necessary protocol in management of hemodialysis patients	Hypothyroidism
Iron	65–170 μg./dl.	Pernicious anemia Aplastic anemia Hemolytic anemia Hepatitis Hemochromatosis	Iron deficiency anemia
Iron binding capacity	IBC: 150–235 μg./dl. TIBC: 250–420 μg./dl. % Saturation: 20–50	Iron deficiency anemia	Chronic infectious diseases
Isocitric dehydrogenase	50–180 units	Hepatitis, cirrhosis Obstructive jaundice Metastatic carcinoma of the liver Megaloblastic anemia	
Lactic acid (whole blood)	9–16 mg./dl.	Increased muscular activity Congestive heart failure Hemorrhage Shock Some varieties of metabolic acidosis Some febrile infections May be increased in severe liver disease	
Lactic dehydrogenase (LDH)	100–225 mU/ml.	Untreated pernicious anemia Myocardial infarction Pulmonary infarction Liver disease	
Lactic dehydrogenase isoenzymes			
Total lactic dehydrogenase LDH–1 LDH–2 LDH–3 LDH–4 LDH–5	100–225 mU/ml. 20–35% 25–40% 20–30% 0–20% 0–25%	LDH–1 and LDH–2 are increased in myocardial infarction, megaloblastic anemia, and hemolytic anemia LDH–4 and LDH–5 are increased in pulmonary infarction, congestive heart failure, and liver disease	
Lead (whole blood)	up to 40 μg./dl.	Lead poisoning	
Leucine aminopeptidase	1–3 micromoles/hr./ml.	Liver or biliary tract diseases Pancreatic disease Metastatic carcinoma of liver and pancreas Biliary obstruction	
Lipase	0.2–1.5 units/ml.	Acute and chronic pancreatitis Biliary obstruction Cirrhosis Hepatitis Peptic ulcer	
Lipids, total	400–1000 mg./dl.	Hypothyroidism Diabetes Nephrosis Glomerulonephritis	Hyperthyroidism

NORMAL CHEMISTRIES—SERUM, PLASMA, WHOLE BLOOD (continued)

Determination	Normal Adult Values	Clinical Significance	
		(Increased)	(Decreased)
Lipoprotein phenotype			

SUMMARY OF FINDINGS IN THE PRIMARY HYPERLIPOPROTEINEMIAS

Type	Appearance	Triglyceride	Cholesterol	Lipoprotein Staining				Secondary Causes
				Beta	Pre-Beta	Alpha	Chylo-microns	
Normal	Clear	Normal	Normal	Moderate	Zero to moderate	Moderate	Weak	
I	Creamy	Markedly increased	Normal to moderately increased	Weak	Weak	Weak	Markedly increased	Dysglobulinemia
II	Clear	Normal to slightly increased	Slightly to markedly increased	Strong	Zero to strong	Moderate	Weak	Hypothyroidism, myeloma, hepatic disease, nephrotic syndrome, macroglobulinemia, and high dietary cholesterol
III	Clear, cloudy or milky	Increased	Increased	Broad intense band	Extends into beta	Moderate	Weak	
IV	Clear, cloudy or milky	Slightly to markedly increased	Normal to slightly increased	Weak to moderate	Moderate to strong	Weak to moderate	Weak	Hypothyroidism, diabetes mellitus, pancreatitis, glycogen storage diseases, nephrotic syndrome, myeloma, pregnancy, and oral contraceptives
V	Cloudy to creamy	Markedly increased	Increased	Weak	Moderate	Weak	Strong	Diabetes mellitus, pancreatitis, and alcoholism

Types I and II are fat induced; III and IV are carbohydrate induced; type V is fat and carbohydrate induced.

Determination	Normal Adult Values	(Increased)	(Decreased)
Lithium	Usual maintenance level: 0.5–1.0 mEq./L.		
Low density lipoprotein cholesterol (LDL cholesterol)	Age (years) / mg./dl. 0–19 50–170 20–29 60–170 30–39 70–190 40–49 80–190 50–59 80–210	LDL cholesterol is higher in patients with increased risk for coronary heart disease.	
Luteinizing hormone, RIA	Males: 6–30 mIU/ml. Females: Follicular phase: 2–30 mIU/ml. Ovulatory Peak: 40–200 mIU/ml. Luteal Phase: 0–20 mIU/ml. Postmenopausal: 35–120 mIU/ml.	Pituitary tumor Ovarian failure	Depressed or failure to peak—pituitary failure
Lysozyme (muramidase)	2.8–8.0 µg./ml.	Certain types of leukemia (acute monocytic leukemia) Inflammatory states and infections	Acute lymphocytic leukemia
Magnesium	1.3–2.4 mEq./L.	Ingestion of Epsom salts Parathyroidectomy	Chronic alcoholism Toxemia of pregnancy Severe renal disease
Manganese	0.08–0.26 µg./dl.		Defective growth
Mercury	up to 10 µg./dl.	Mercury poisoning	
Myoglobin, RIA	up to 85 ng./ml.	Myocardial infarction	
Nonprotein nitrogen	20–35 mg./dl.	Acute nephritis Polycystic kidneys Obstructive uropathy Peritonitis Congestive heart failure Pregnancy	
5' Nucleotidase	3.2–11.6 IU/L.	Hepatobiliary disease	
Osmolality	280–300 milliosmoles/kg.	Useful in the study of electrolyte and water balance	Inappropriate secretion of antidiuretic hormone
Oxygen saturation arterial (whole blood)	96–100%	Polycythemia Anhydremia	Anemia Cardiac decompensation Chronic obstructive pulmonary disease
pCO_2 (whole blood) arterial	35–45 mm. Hg	Respiratory acidosis Metabolic alkalosis	Respiratory alkalosis Metabolic acidosis
pH (whole blood) arterial	7.35–7.45	Vomiting Hyperpnea	Uremia Diabetic acidosis

NORMAL CHEMISTRIES—SERUM, PLASMA, WHOLE BLOOD (continued)

Determination	Normal Adult Values	Clinical Significance	
		(Increased)	(Decreased)
pH (whole blood) arterial (continued)		Fever Intestinal obstruction	Hemorrhage Nephritis
pO₂ (whole blood) arterial	95–100 mm. Hg	Directly related to oxygen saturation	
Parathyroid hormone	163–347 pg./ml.	Hyperparathyroidism	
Pepsinogen	200–425 units/ml.		Conditions which decrease gastric acidity Pernicious anemia Achlorhydria
Phenylalanine	0–6 mg./dl. first week 0.7–3.5 mg./dl. thereafter	Phenylketonuria Oasthouse urine disease	
Phosphatase, acid, total	0–11 IU/L.	Carcinoma of prostate Advanced Paget's disease Hyperparathyroidism	
Phosphatase, acid, prostatic, RIA	0–10 ng./ml. Borderline: 2.5–3.3 IU/L.	Carcinoma of prostate	
Phosphatase, alkaline	Adults: 30–115 mU/ml.	Conditions reflecting increased osteoblastic activity of bone Rickets Hyperparathyroidism Liver disease	
Phosphatase, alkaline, thermostable fraction	Thermostable fraction greater than 35%: hepatic disease and combined disease with predominant hepatic component. Thermostable fraction between 25–35%: combined hepatic and skeletal disease. Thermostable fraction less than 25%: skeletal disease with increased osteoblastic activity.	Hepatic disease	
Phosphohexose isomerase	20–90 IU/L.	Malignancy Diseases of heart, liver, and skeletal muscles	
Phospholipids	125–300 mg./dl.	Diabetes Nephritis	
Phosphorus, inorganic	2.5–4.5 mg./dl.	Chronic nephritis Hypoparathyroidism	Hyperparathyroidism
Potassium	3.5–5.0 mEq./L.	Addison's disease Oliguria Anuria Tissue breakdown or hemolysis	Diabetic acidosis Diarrhea Vomiting
Progesterone, RIA	Follicular phase: up to 0.8 ng./ml. Luteal phase: 10–20 ng./ml. End of cycle: less than 1 ng./ml. Pregnant: up to 50 ng./ml. in 20th week	Useful in evaluation of menstrual disorders and infertility and the evaluation of placental function during pregnancies complicated by toxemia, diabetes mellitus, or threatened miscarriage.	
Prolactin, RIA	Females: 6–24 ng./ml. Males: 7–18 ng./ml.	Pregnancy Functional or structural disorders of the hypothalamus Pituitary stalk section Pituitary tumors Primary hypothyroidism	
Protein, total Albumin Globulin	6.0–8.0 gm./dl. 3.5–5.0 gm./dl. 1.5–3.0 gm./dl.	Hemoconcentration Shock Multiple myeloma (globulin fraction) Chronic infections (globulin fraction) Liver disease (globulin)	Malnutrition Hemorrhage Loss of plasma from burns Proteinuria
Electrophoresis (Cellulose acetate) Albumin Alpha₁ globulin Alpha₂ globulin Beta globulin Gamma globulin	3.3–5.0 gm./dl. 0.2–0.4 gm./dl. 0.6–1.0 gm./dl. 0.6–1.2 gm./dl. 0.7–1.5 gm./dl.		
Protoporphyrin, erythrocyte (whole blood)	15–100 µg./dl.	Lead toxicity Erythropoietic porphyria	
Pyridoxine	3.6–18 ng./ml.		A wide spectrum of clinical conditions such as mental depression, peripheral neuropathy, anemia, neonatal seizures, and reactions to certain drug therapy

NORMAL CHEMISTRIES—SERUM, PLASMA, WHOLE BLOOD (continued)

Determination	Normal Adult Values	Clinical Significance	
		(Increased)	(Decreased)
Pyruvic acid (whole blood)	0.3–0.7 mg./dl.	Diabetes Severe thiamine deficiency Acute phase of some infections, possibly secondary to increased glycogenolysis and glycolysis	
Renin (plasma), RIA	*Normal Diet:* Supine: 0.3–1.9 ng./ml./hr. Upright: 0.6–3.6 ng./ml./hr. *Low Salt Diet:* Supine: 0.9–4.5 ng./ml./hr. Upright: 4.1–9.1 ng./ml./hr.	Renovascular hypertension Malignant hypertension Untreated Addison's disease Primary salt-losing nephropathy Low-salt diet Diuretic therapy Hemorrhage	Frank primary aldosteronism Increased salt intake Salt-retaining steroid therapy Antidiuretic hormone therapy Blood transfusion
Riboflavin (whole blood)	0.9–1.31 (activity coefficient)		Riboflavin deficiency
Sodium	135–145 mEq./L.	Hemoconcentration Nephritis Pyloric obstruction	Alkali deficit Addison's disease Myxedema
Sulfate	0.5–1.5 mg./dl.	Nephritis Nitrogen retention	
Testosterone, RIA	Females: 25–100 ng./dl. Males: 300–800 ng./dl.	Females: Polycystic ovary Virilizing tumors	Males: Orchidectomy for neoplastic disease of the prostate or breast Estrogen therapy Klinefelter's syndrome Hypopituitarism Hypogonadism Hepatic cirrhosis
Thymol turbidity	1–4.5 units/ml.	Liver disease Infectious diseases with antibody production	
T_3 uptake	25–35%	Hyperthyroidism TBG deficiency Androgens and anabolic steroids	Hypothyroidism Pregnancy TBG excess Estrogens and antiovulatory drugs
T_3, Triiodothyronine (total circulating), RIA	75–200 ng./dl.	Pregnancy Hyperthyroidism	Hypothyroidism
T_4, Thyroxine, RIA	4.5–11.5 µg./dl.	Hyperthyroidism Thyroiditis Cases of elevated thyroxine-binding proteins caused by oral contraceptives Pregnancy	Primary and pituitary hypothyroidism Idiopathic involvement Cases of diminished thyroxine-binding proteins caused by androgenic and anabolic steroids Hypoproteinemia Nephrotic syndrome
T_4, Thyroxine, free	1.0–2.2 ng./dl.	Euthyroid patients with normal free thyroxine levels may have abnormal T_3 and T_4 levels caused by drug preparations	
Thyroid stimulating hormone (TSH), RIA	0–10 µIU/ml.	Primary hypothyroidism	
Thyroid binding globulin	10–26 µg./dl.	Hypothyroidism Pregnancy Estrogen therapy Oral contraceptives Genetic and idiopathic	Androgens and anabolic steroids Nephrotic syndromes Marked hypoproteinemia Hepatic disease
Transaminase (SGOT) (Aspartate aminotransferase)	7–40 mU/ml.	Myocardial infarction Skeletal muscle disease Liver disease	
Transaminase (SGPT) (Alanine aminotransferase)	10–40 mU/ml.	Same conditions as SGOT, but increase is more marked in liver disease than SGOT	
Transferrin	230–320 mg./dl.	Pregnancy Iron-deficiency anemia due to hemorrhaging Acute hepatitis Polycythemia Oral contraceptives	Prenicious anemia in relapse Thalassemic and sickle cell anemia Chromatosis Neoplastic and hepatic diseases
Transketolase (whole blood)	Pentose utilization: 9.66–15.50 micromoles/hr./ml. or 1.70–3.04 micromoles/hr./10^9 red blood cells		Thiamine deficiency
Triglycerides	10–150 mg./dl.	See lipoprotein phenotype	
Tryptophan	1.4–3.0 mg./dl.		Tryptophan-specific malabsorption syndrome
Tyrosine	0.5–4.0 mg./dl.	Hyperthyroidism Tyrosinosis	

NORMAL CHEMISTRIES—SERUM, PLASMA, WHOLE BLOOD (continued)

Determination	Normal Adult Values	Clinical Significance (Increased)	Clinical Significance (Decreased)
Urea nitrogen (BUN)	10–20 mg./dl.	Acute glomerulonephritis Obstructive uropathy Mercury poisoning Nephrotic syndrome	Severe hepatic failure Pregnancy
Uric acid	2.5–8.0 mg./dl.	Gouty arthritis Acute leukemia Lymphomas treated by chemotherapy Toxemia of pregnancy	Xanthinuria Defective tubular reabsorption
Viscosity	1.4–1.8 relative to water at 37°C. (98.6°F.)	Patients with marked increases of the gamma globulins	
Vitamin A	50–220 μg./dl.	Hypervitaminosis A	Vitamin A deficiency Celiac disease Sprue Obstructive jaundice Cystic fibrosis Giardiasis Parenchymal hepatic disease
Vitamin B$_1$ (thiamine)	1.6–4.0 μg./dl.		Anorexia Beriberi Polyneuropathy Cardiomyopathies
Vitamin B$_6$ (pyridoxal phosphate)	3.6–18.0 ng./ml.		Chronic alcoholism Malnutrition Uremia Neonatal seizures Malabsorption, such as celiac syndrome
Vitamin B$_{12}$ RIA	130–785 pg./ml.	Hepatic cell damage and in association with the myeloproliferative disorders (the highest levels are encountered in myeloid leukemia)	Strict vegetarianism Alcoholism Pernicious anemia Total or partial gastrectomy Ileal resection Sprue and celiac disease Fish tapeworm infestation
Vitamin E	0.5–2.0 mg./dl.		Vitamin E deficiency
Water content	92.6–94.3 gm./dl.	Useful in the study of electrolyte and water balance	
Xylose absorption test	2 hr. 30–50 mg./dl.		Malabsorption syndrome
Zinc	55–150 μg./dl.	Zinc is essential for the growth and propagation of cell cultures and the functioning of several enzymes	
Zinc turbidity	2–12 units/ml.	Same clinical significance as thymol turbidity	

NORMAL VALUES—URINE CHEMISTRY

Determination	Normal Value	Clinical Significance (Increased)	Clinical Significance (Decreased)
Acetone and acetoacetate	Zero	Uncontrolled diabetes Starvation	
Acid mucopolysaccharides	Negative	Hurler's syndrome Marfan's syndrome Morquio-Ulrich disease	
Aldosterone	*Normal salt:* Normal: 4–20 μg./24 hr. Renovascular: 10–40 μg./24 hr. Tumor: 20–100 μg./24 hr. *Low salt:* Normal: 10–40 μg./24 hr. Renovascular: 20–100 μg./24 hr. Tumor: 20–100 μg./24 hr.	Primary aldosteronism (adrenocortical tumor) Secondary aldosteronism Salt depletion Potassium loading ACTH in large doses Cardiac failure Cirrhosis with ascites formation Nephrosis Pregnancy	
Alpha amino nitrogen	64–199 mg./24 hr.	Leukemia Diabetes Phenylketonuria Other metabolic diseases	
Amylase	35–260 units excreted/hr.	Acute pancreatitis	
Arylsulfatase A	Greater than 2.4 units/ml.		Metachromatic leukodystrophy
Bence-Jones protein	None detected	Myeloma	
Bile melanin	Zero	Advanced melanoma Ochronosis	
Calcium	Less than 150 mg./24 hr.	Hyperparathyroidism Vitamin D intoxication Fanconi syndrome	Hypoparathyroidism Vitamin D deficiency

NORMAL VALUES—URINE CHEMISTRY (continued)

Determination	Normal Value	Clinical Significance (Increased)	(Decreased)
Catecholamines	Total: 0–275 µg./24 hr. Epinephrine: 10–40% Norepinephrine: 60–90%	Pheochromocytoma Neuroblastoma	
Chloride	70–250 mEq./24 hr.	Urine chloride levels vary with excretion of sodium, potassium, ammonia, and bicarbonate	
Chorionic gonadotrophin, qualitative (pregnancy test)	Negative	Pregnancy Chorionepithelioma Hydatidiform mole	
Copper	20–70 µg./24 hr.	Wilson's disease Cirrhosis Nephrosis	
Coproporphyrin	50–300 µg./24 hr.	Poliomyelitis Lead poisoning Porphyria hepatica Porphyria erythropoietica Porphyria cutanea tarda	
Cortisol, free	20–90 µg./24 hr.	Cushing's syndrome	
Creatine	0–200 mg./24 hr.	Muscular dystrophy Fever Carcinoma of liver Pregnancy Hyperthyroidism Myositis	
Creatinine	0.8–2.0 gm./24 hr.	Typhoid fever Salmonella infections Tetanus	Muscular atrophy Anemia Advanced degeneration of kidneys Leukemia
Creatinine clearance	100–150 mls. of blood cleared of creatinine/min.		Measures glomerular filtration rate Renal diseases
Cystine	10–100 mg./24 hr.	Cystinuria	
Delta amino-levulinic acid	0.00–0.54 mg./dl.	Lead poisoning Porphyria hepatica Hepatitis Hepatic carcinoma	
11-Desoxycortisol	20–100 µg./24 hr.	Hypertensive form of virilizing adrenal hyperplasia due to an 11-beta hydroxylase defect	
Diagnex blue	Greater than 0.6 mg. Presumptive evidence for hypochlorhydria: 0.3–0.6 mg. Presumptive evidence for achlorhydria: less than 0.3 mg.		Hypochlorhydria Achlorhydria
Estriol (placental)	*Weeks of pregnancy* *mg./24 hr.* 12 less than 1 16 2–7 20 4–9 24 6–13 28 8–22 32 12–43 36 14–45 40 19–46		Decreased values occur with fetal distress of many conditions, including preeclampsia, placental insufficiency, and poorly controlled diabetes mellitus
Estrogens, total (fluorimetric)	Females: Onset of menstruation: 4–25 µg./24 hr. Ovulation peak: 28–99 µg./24 hr. Luteal peak: 22–105 µg./24 hr. Menopausal: 1.4–19.6 µg./24 hr. Males: 5–18 µg./24 hr.	Hyperestrogenism due to gonadal or adrenal neoplasm	Primary or secondary amenorrhea
Etiocholanolone	Males: 1.9–6.0 mg./24 hr. Females: 0.5–4.0 mg./24 hr.	Adrenogenital syndrome Idiopathic hirsutism	
Follicle stimulating hormone, RIA	Females: Follicular: 5–20 IU/24 hr. Luteal: 5–15 IU/24hr. Midcycle: 15–60 IU/24 hr. Menopausal: 50–100 IU/24 hr. Males: 5–25 IU/24 hr.	Menopause and primary ovarian failure	Pituitary failure
Glucose	Negative	Diabetes mellitus	

NORMAL VALUES—URINE CHEMISTRY (continued)

Determination	Normal Value	Clinical Significance	
		(Increased)	*(Decreased)*
Glucose (continued)		Pituitary disorders Intracranial pressure Lesion in floor of 4th ventricle	
Hemoglobin and myoglobin	Negative	Extensive burns Transfusion of incompatible blood Myoglobin increased in severe crushing injuries to muscle	
Homogentisic acid, qualitative	Negative	Alkaptonuria Ochronosis	
Homovanillic acid	Up to 15 mg./24 hrs.	Neuroblastoma	
17-hydroxycorticosteroids	2–10 mg./24 hr.	Cushing's syndrome	Addison's disease Anterior pituitary hypofunction
5-hydroxyindoleacetic acid, qualitative	Negative	Malignant carcinoid tumors	
Hydroxyproline	25–77 mg./24 hr.	Paget's disease Fibrous dysplasia Osteomalacia Neoplastic bone disease Hyperparathyroidism	
17-ketosteroids, alpha-beta fractionation	Alpha concentration 85% or more	Adrenal carcinomas (in beta fraction)	
17-ketosteroids, total	Males: 10–22 mg./24 hr. Females: 6–16 mg./24 hr.	Interstitial cell tumor of testes Simple hirsutism, occasionally Adrenal hyperplasia Cushing's syndrome Adrenal cancer, virilism Arrhenoblastoma	Thyrotoxicosis Female hypogonadism Diabetes mellitus Hypertension Debilitating disease of mild to moderate severity Eunuchoidism Addison's disease Panhypopituitarism Myxedema Nephrosis
Kynurenic and xanthurenic acids	Kynurenic acid: up to 18.0 mg./24 hr. Xanthurenic acid: up to 4.0 mg./24 hr.	Vitamin B_6 deficiency Acute typhoid fever Sandfly fever Tularemia	
Lead	up to 150 μg./24 hr.	Lead poisoning	
Lipase	0.1–0.75 units/ml.	Pancreatitis	
Luteinizing hormone	Males: 5–18 IU/24 hr. Females: Follicular phase: 2–25 IU/24 hr. Ovulatory peak: 30–95 IU/24 hr. Luteal phase: 2–20 IU/24 hr. Postmenopausal: 40–110 IU/24 hr.	Pituitary tumor Ovarian failure	Depressed or failure to peak—pituitary failure
Metanephrines, total	Less than 1.3 mg./24 hr.	Pheochromocytoma, a few patients with pheochromocytoma may have elevated urinary metanephrines but normal catecholamines and VMA	
Osmolality	Males: 390–1090 millimoles/kg. Females: 300–1090 millimoles/kg.	Useful in the study of electrolyte and water balance	
Oxalate	up to 40 mg./24 hrs.	Primary hyperoxaluria	
Phenolphthalein (PSP)	At least 25% excreted in 15 min., 40% by 30 min., and 60% by 120 min.	Primarily measures renal tubular function	Delayed in renal diseases Low in nephritis, cystitis, pyelonephritis, congestive heart failure
Phenylpyruvic acid, qualitative	Negative	Phenylketonuria	
Phosphorus, inorganic	0.8–1.3 gm./24 hr.	Fever Nervous exhaustion Tuberculosis Rickets Chronic lead poisoning	Acute infections Nephritis Chlorosis Pregnancy
Porphobilinogen, qualitative	Negative	Acute porphyria Liver disease	
Porphobilinogen, quantitative	0.00–0.03 mg./dl.	Acute porphyria Liver disease	
Porphyrins, qualitative	Negative	See porphyrins, quantitative	
Porphyrins, quantitative (Coproporphyrin and Uroporphyrin)	Coproporphyrin: 50–300 μg./24 hr. Uroporphyrin:	Porphyria hepatica Porphyria erythropoietica Porphyria cutanea tarda	

NORMAL VALUES—URINE CHEMISTRY (continued)

Determination	Normal Value	Clinical Significance	
		(Increased)	(Decreased)
Porphyrins, quantitative (Coproporphyrin and Uroporphyrin) (continued)	up to 50 μg./24 hr.	Lead poisoning (only coproporphyrin increased)	
Potassium	40–65 mEq./24 hr.	Hemolysis	
Pregnanediol	Females: Proliferative phase: 0.5–1.5 mg./24 hr. Luteal phase: 2–7 mg./24 hr. Menopause: 0.2–1.0 mg./24 hr. Pregnancy: *(Weeks of* *gestation)* *mg./24 hr.* 10–12 5–15 12–18 5–25 18–24 15–33 24–28 20–42 28–32 27–47 Males: 0.1–2.0	Corpus luteum cysts When placental tissue remains in the uterus following parturition Some cases of adrenocortical tumors Pregnancy	Placental dysfunction Threatened abortion Intrauterine death
Pregnanetriol	0.4 mg./24 hr.	Congenital adrenal androgenic hyperplasia	
Protein	up to 100 mg./24 hr.	Nephritis Cardiac failure Mercury poisoning Bence-Jones protein in multiple myeloma Febrile states Hematuria Amyloidosis	
Sodium	130–200 mEq./24 hr.	Useful in detecting gross changes in water and salt balance	
Titratable acidity	20–40 mEq./24 hr.	Metabolic acidosis	Metabolic alkalosis
Urea nitrogen	9–16 gm./24 hr.	Excessive protein catabolism	Impaired kidney function
Uric acid	250–750 mg./24 hr.	Gout	Nephritis
Urobilinogen	Random urine: less than 0.25 mg./dl. 24 hr. urine: up to 4 mg./24 hr.	Liver and biliary tract disease Hemolytic anemias	Complete or nearly complete biliary obstruction Diarrhea Renal insufficiency
Uroporphyrins	up to 50 μg./24 hr.	Porphyria	
Vanillylmandelic acid (VMA)	0.7–6.8 mg./24 hr.	Pheochromocytoma Neuroblastoma Coffee, tea, aspirin, bananas, and several different drugs	
Xylose absorption test (5 hour)	16–33% of ingested xylose		Malabsorption syndromes
Zinc	0.15–1.2 mg./24 hr.	Zinc is an essential nutritional element	

NORMAL VALUES—CEREBROSPINAL FLUID

Determination	Normal Value	Clinical Significance	
		(Increased)	(Decreased)
Albumin	15.5–32.0 mg./dl.	Certain neurological disorders Lesion in the choroid plexus or blockage of the flow of CSF Damage to the blood-CNS barrier	
Cell count	0–5 mononuclear cells/cu. mm.	Bacterial meningitis Neurosyphilis Anterior poliomyelitis Encephalitis lethargica	
Chloride	100–130 mEq./L.	Uremia	Acute generalized meningitis Tubercular meningitis
Colloidal gold	0000000000	Acute meningitis Neurosyphilis	
Glucose	50–75 mg./dl.	Diabetes mellitus Diabetic coma Epidemic encephalitis Uremia	Acute meningitides Tuberculous meningitis Insulin shock
Glutamine	6–15 mg./dl.	Hepatic encephalopathies, including Reye's syndrome Hepatic coma Cirrhosis	

NORMAL VALUES—CEREBROSPINAL FLUID (continued)

Determination	Normal Value	Clinical Significance	
		(Increased)	*(Decreased)*
IgG	0–6.6 mg./dl.	Damage to the blood-CNS barrier Multiple sclerosis Neurosyphilis Subacute sclerosing panencephalitis Chronic phases of CNS infections	
Lactic acid	Less than 24 mg./dl.	Bacterial meningitis Hypocapnia Hydrocephalus Brain abscesses Cerebral ischemia	
Lactic dehydrogenase	One tenth that of serum	CNS disease	

Protein
  Lumbar
  Cisternal
  Ventricular
	
	15–45 mg./dl.
	15–25 mg./dl.
	5–15 mg./dl.
		Acute meningitides
		Tubercular meningitis
		Neurosyphilis
		Poliomyelitis
		Guillain-Barré syndrome	

Protein Electrophoresis
  (Cellulose acetate)
  Prealbumin
  Albumin
  Alpha$_1$ globulin
  Alpha$_2$ globulin
  Beta globulin
  Gamma globulin
	% of total
	
	3.0–7.0
	56.0–74.0
	2.0–6.5
	3.0–12.0
	8.0–18.5
	4.0–14.0
		An increase in the level of albumin alone can be the result of a lesion in the choroid plexus or a blockage of the flow of CSF. An elevated gamma globulin value with a normal albumin level has been reported in multiple sclerosis, neurosyphilis, subacute sclerosing panencephalitis, and the chronic phase of CNS infections. If the blood-CNS barrier has been severely damaged during the course of these diseases, the CSF albumin level may also be elevated.	

MISCELLANEOUS VALUES

Determinations	Normal Value	Clinical Significance	
Acetaminophen	Zero	Therapeutic level = 10–20 μg./ml.	
Aminophylline (theophylline)	Zero	Therapeutic level = 10–20 μg./ml.	
Bromide	Zero	Therapeutic level = 5–50 mg./dl.	
Carbon monoxide	0–2%	Symptoms with over 20% saturation	
Digitoxin	Zero	Therapeutic level = 5–30 ng./ml.	
Digoxin	Zero	Therapeutic level = 0.5–2.0 ng./ml.	
Dilantin (phenytoin)	Zero	Therapeutic level = 10–20 μg./ml.	
Ethanol	0–0.01%	Legal intoxication level = 0.10% or above 0.3–0.4% = marked intoxication 0.4–0.5% = alcoholic stupor	
Gentamicin	Zero	Therapeutic level = 4–10 μg./ml.	
Librium (chlordiazepoxide)	Zero	Therapeutic level = 1–3 μg./ml.	
Methanol	Zero	May be fatal in concentrations as low as 10 mg./dl.	
Mysoline (primidone)	Zero	Therapeutic level = 5–12 μg./ml.	
Phenobarbital	Zero	Therapeutic level = 15–40 μg./ml.	
Quinidine	Zero	Therapeutic level = 0.2–0.5 mg./dl.	
Salicylate	Zero	Therapeutic level = 2–25 mg./dl. Toxic level = over 30 mg./dl.	

Sulfonamide	Zero	Therapeutic levels:
		  Sulfadiazine 8–15 mg./dl.
		  Sulfaguanidine 3–5 mg./dl.
		  Sulfamerazine 10–15 mg./dl.
		  Sulfanilamide 10–15 mg./dl.	

Valium (diazepam)	Zero	Therapeutic level: 0.5–2.5 μg./dl.	
Gastric Analysis		*(Increased)*	*(Decreased)*
Free HCl	0–30 mEq./L.	Neuroses	Pernicious anemia
Total acidity	15–45 mEq./L.	Peptic ulcer	Gastric carcinoma
Combined acid	10–15 mEq./L.	Zollinger-Ellison syndrome	Chronic atrophic gastritis Decreases normally with age

APPENDIX II: CONVERSION TABLES

METRIC UNITS AND SYMBOLS

Quantity	Unit	Symbol	Equivalent
Length	millimeter	mm.	1000 mm. = 1 m.
	centimeter	cm.	100 cm. = 1 m.
	decimeter	dm.	10 dm. = 1 m.
	meter	m.	1000 m. = 1 km.
Volume	cubic centimeter	cc. or cm.^{3}	$1000 \begin{cases} \text{cc. or dm.}^3 \\ \text{ml.} \end{cases} = 1 \text{ cm.}^3 \text{ or liter}$
	milliliter	ml.	
	cu. decimeter	dm.^{3}	$1000 \begin{cases} \text{dm.}^3 \\ 1 \end{cases} = 1 \text{ m.}^3$
	liter	L.	
Mass	microgram	μg.	1000 μg. = 1 mg.
	milligram	mg.	1000 mg. = 1 g.
	gram	g.	1000 g. = 1 kg.
	kilogram	kg.	1000 kg. = 1 metric ton (t)

TABLE OF METRIC AND APOTHECARIES' SYSTEMS*

(Approved *approximate* dose equivalents are enclosed in parentheses. Use *exact* equivalents in calculations.)

Conversion Factors

Metric	Apothecaries	Metric	Apothecaries
1 milligram (mg.)	¹⁄₆₄ grain	3.888 cubic centimeters or grams	1 dram (4 cc. or grams)
64.79 milligrams	1 grain (65 mg.)	31.103 cubic centimeters or grams	1 ounce (30 cc. or grams)
1 gram	15.43 grains (15 grains)	473.167 cubic centimeters	1 pint (500 cc.)
1 cubic centimeter (cc.)	16 minims		

WEIGHTS

Metric	Apothecaries	Metric		Apothecaries
0.0001 gram—0.1 mg.	¹⁄₆₄₀ grain (¹⁄₆₀₀ grain)	0.057 gram —57	mg.—⅞	grain
0.0002 gram—0.2 mg.	¹⁄₃₂₀ grain (¹⁄₃₀₀ grain)	0.06 gram —60	mg.—⁹⁄₁₀	grain (1 grain)
0.0003 gram—0.3 mg.	¹⁄₂₁₀ grain (¹⁄₂₀₀ grain)	0.065 gram —65	mg.—1	grain (60 mg.)
0.0004 gram—0.4 mg.	¹⁄₁₅₀ grain	0.07 gram —70	mg.—1¹⁄₂₀	grains
0.0005 gram—0.5 mg.	¹⁄₁₂₀ grain	0.08 gram —80	mg.—1⅕	grains
0.0006 gram—0.6 mg.	¹⁄₁₀₀ grain	0.09 gram —90	mg.—1⅓	grains
0.0007 gram—0.7 mg.	¹⁄₉₀ grain	0.097 gram —97	mg.—1½	grains (0.1 gram)
0.0008 gram—0.8 mg.	¹⁄₈₀ grain	0.12 gram —120	mg.—2	grains
0.0009 gram—0.9 mg.	¹⁄₇₅ grain	0.2 gram —200	mg.—3	grains
0.001 gram—1 mg.	¹⁄₆₄ grain (¹⁄₆₀ grain)	0.24 gram —240	mg.—4	grains (0.25 gram)
0.0011 gram—1.1 mg.	¹⁄₆₀ grain	0.3 gram —300	mg.—4½	grains
0.0013 gram—1.3 mg.	¹⁄₅₀ grain (1.2 mg.)	0.33 gram —330	mg.—5	grains (0.3 gram)
0.0014 gram—1.4 mg.	¹⁄₄₈ grain	0.4 gram —400	mg.—6	grains
0.0016 gram—1.6 mg.	¹⁄₄₀ grain (1.5 mg.)	0.45 gram —450	mg.—7	grains
0.0018 gram—1.8 mg.	¹⁄₃₆ grain	0.5 gram —500	mg.—7½	grains
0.0020 gram—2 mg.	¹⁄₃₂ grain (¹⁄₃₀ grain)	0.53 gram —530	mg.—8	grains
0.0022 gram—2.2 mg.	¹⁄₃₀ grain	0.6 gram —600	mg.—9	grains
0.0026 gram—2.6 mg.	¹⁄₂₅ grain	0.65 gram —650	mg.—10	grains (0.6 gram)
0.003 gram—3 mg.	¹⁄₂₀ grain	0.73 gram —730	mg.—11	grains
0.004 gram—4 mg.	¹⁄₁₆ grain (¹⁄₁₅ grain)	0.80 gram —800	mg.—12	grains (0.75 gram)
0.005 gram—5 mg.	¹⁄₁₂ grain	0.86 gram —860	mg.—13	grains
0.006 gram—6 mg.	¹⁄₁₀ grain	0.93 gram —930	mg.—14	grains
0.007 gram—7 mg.	⅑ grain	1. gram —1000	mg.—15	grains
0.008 gram—8 mg.	⅛ grain	1.06 grams—1060	mg.—16	grains
0.009 gram—9 mg.	⅐ grain	1.13 grams—1130	mg.—17	grains
0.01 gram—10 mg.	⅙ grain	1.18 grams—1180	mg.—18	grains
0.013 gram—13 mg.	⅕ grain (12 mg.)	1.26 grams—1260	mg.—19	grains
0.016 gram—16 mg.	¼ grain (15 mg.)	1.30 grams—1300	mg.—20	grains
0.02 gram—20 mg.	⅓ grain	1.50 grams—1500	mg.—22	grains
0.025 gram—25 mg.	⅜ grain	2 grams—2000	mg.—30	grains (½ dram)
0.03 gram—30 mg.	⅖ grain (½ grain)	4 grams	—1	dram (60 grains)
0.032 gram—32 mg.	½ grain (30 mg.)	5 grams	—75	grains
0.04 gram—40 mg.	⅗ grain (⅔ grain)	8 grams	—2	drams (7.5 grams)
0.043 gram—43 mg.	⅔ grain (40 mg.)	10 grams	—2½	drams
0.05 gram—50 mg.	¾ grain	15 grams	—4	drams
		30 grams	—1	ounce

LIQUID MEASURES**

Metric	Apothecaries	Metric	Apothecaries
0.03 cubic centimeter —½ minim		8 cubic centimeters—2 fluid drams	
0.05 cubic centimeter —¾ minim		10 cubic centimeters—2½ fluid drams	
0.06 cubic centimeter —1 minim		15 cubic centimeters—4 fluid drams	
0.1 cubic centimeter —1½ minims		20 cubic centimeters—5½ fluid drams	
0.2 cubic centimeter —3 minims		25 cubic centimeters—⅚ fluid ounce	
0.25 cubic centimeter —4 minims		30 cubic centimeters—1 fluid ounce	
0.3 cubic centimeter —5 minims		50 cubic centimeters—1¾ fluid ounces	
0.5 cubic centimeter —8 minims		60 cubic centimeters—2 fluid ounces	
0.6 cubic centimeter —10 minims		100 cubic centimeters—3½ fluid ounces	
0.75 cubic centimeter —12 minims		120 cubic centimeters—4 fluid ounces	
1 cubic centimeter —15 minims		200 cubic centimeters—7 fluid ounces	
2 cubic centimeters—30 minims		250 cubic centimeters—8 fluid ounces	
3 cubic centimeters—45 minims		360 cubic centimeters—12 fluid ounces	
4 cubic centimeters—1 fluid dram		500 cubic centimeters—1 pint	
5 cubic centimeters—1¼ fluid drams		1000 cubic centimeters—1 quart	

* (From Culver, V. M.: Modern Bedside Nursing. Philadelphia, W. B. Saunders, 1969.)
** Note: A cubic centimeter (cc.) is the approximate equivalent of a milliliter (ml.). The terms are used interchangeably in general medicine.

24-HOUR CLOCK

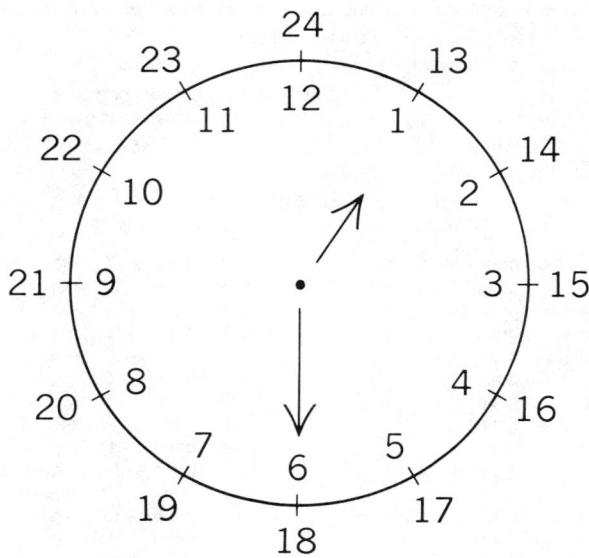

From midnight to noon—12-hour time ⎱ identical
24-hour time ⎰

From noon to midnight—Add 12 to P.M. time = 24-hour time

12-hour Time		24-hour Time
12:00 midnight	....	24:00
12:01 A.M.	....	00:01
12:59 A.M.	....	00:59
1:00 A.M.	....	01:00
12:00 noon	....	12:00
12:01 P.M.	....	12:01
1:00 P.M.	....	13:00
5:30 P.M.	....	17:30
10:08 P.M.	....	22:08
12:00 midnight	....	24:00

A useful clock for avoiding confusion about A.M. and P.M. designations.

NOMOGRAM FOR ESTIMATING SURFACE AREA OF INFANTS AND YOUNG CHILDREN

HEIGHT		SURFACE AREA	WEIGHT	
feet	centimeters	in square meters	pounds	kilograms

HEIGHT
feet — centimeters

3' — 95
34" — 90
— 85
32" — 80
30" — 75
28" — 70
26" — 65
2' — 60
22" — 55
20" — 50
18" — 45
16" — 40
14" — 35
1' — 30
10" —
9" — 25
8" —
— 20

SURFACE AREA
in square meters

.8
.7
.6
.5
.4
.3
.2
.1

WEIGHT
pounds — kilograms

65 — 30
60
55 — 25
50
45 — 20
40
35 — 15
30
25
20 — 10
15
10 — 5
— 4
— 3
5 — 2
4
3
— 1

To determine the surface area of the patient draw a straight line between the point representing his height on the left vertical scale to the point representing his weight on the right vertical scale. The point at which this line intersects the middle vertical scale represents the patient's surface area in square meters. (Courtesy, Abbott Laboratories.)

NOMOGRAM FOR ESTIMATING SURFACE AREA OF OLDER CHILDREN AND ADULTS

HEIGHT		SURFACE AREA	WEIGHT	
feet	centimeters	in square meters	pounds	kilograms

HEIGHT (feet / centimeters):
7' — 220, 215, 210
10" — 210
8" — 205
6" — 200
4" — 195
2" — 190
6' — 185
10" — 180
8" — 175
6" — 170
4" — 165
2" — 160
5' — 155
150
10" — 145
8" — 140
6" — 135
4" — 130
2" — 125
4' — 120
10" — 115
8" — 110
6" — 105
4" — 100
2" — 95
3' — 90
10" — 85
8" — 80
6" — 75

SURFACE AREA (square meters):
3.00, 2.90, 2.80, 2.70, 2.60, 2.50, 2.40, 2.30, 2.20, 2.10, 2.00, 1.95, 1.90, 1.85, 1.80, 1.75, 1.70, 1.65, 1.60, 1.55, 1.50, 1.45, 1.40, 1.35, 1.30, 1.25, 1.20, 1.15, 1.10, 1.05, 1.00, .95, .90, .85, .80, .75, .70, .65, .60

WEIGHT (pounds / kilograms):
440 — 200
420 — 190
400 — 180
380 — 170
360 — 160
340 — 150
320 — 140
300
290 — 130
280
270 — 120
260
250
240 — 110
230
220 — 100
210 — 95
200 — 90
190 — 85
180 — 80
170
160 — 75
150 — 70
140 — 65
130 — 60
120 — 55
110 — 50
100 — 45
90 — 40
80 — 35
70 — 30
60 — 25
50 — 20

(Courtesy, Abbott Laboratories.)

CELSIUS (CENTIGRADE) AND FAHRENHEIT TEMPERATURES

Celsius (Centigrade)	Fahrenheit
0	32
36.0	96.8
36.5	97.7
37.0	98.6
37.5	99.5
38.0	100.4
38.5	101.3
39.0	102.2
39.5	103.1
40.0	104.0
40.5	104.9
41.0	105.8
41.5	106.7
42.0	107.6

F A H R E N H E I T

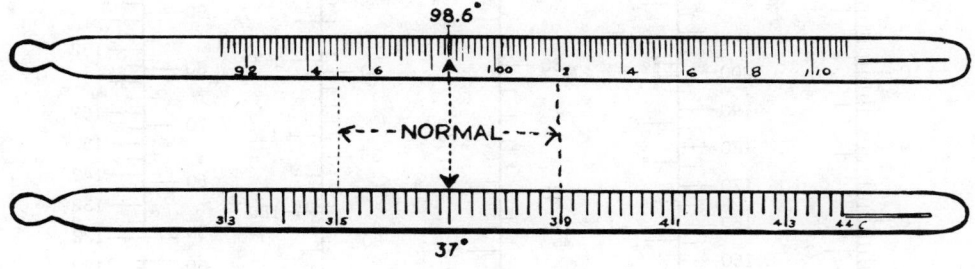

C E L S I U S

To convert degrees F. to degrees C.
    Subtract 32, then multiply by 5/9

To convert degrees C. to degrees F.
    Multiply by 9/5, then add 32

COMPARATIVE SCALES OF MEASURES, WEIGHTS, AND TEMPERATURES*

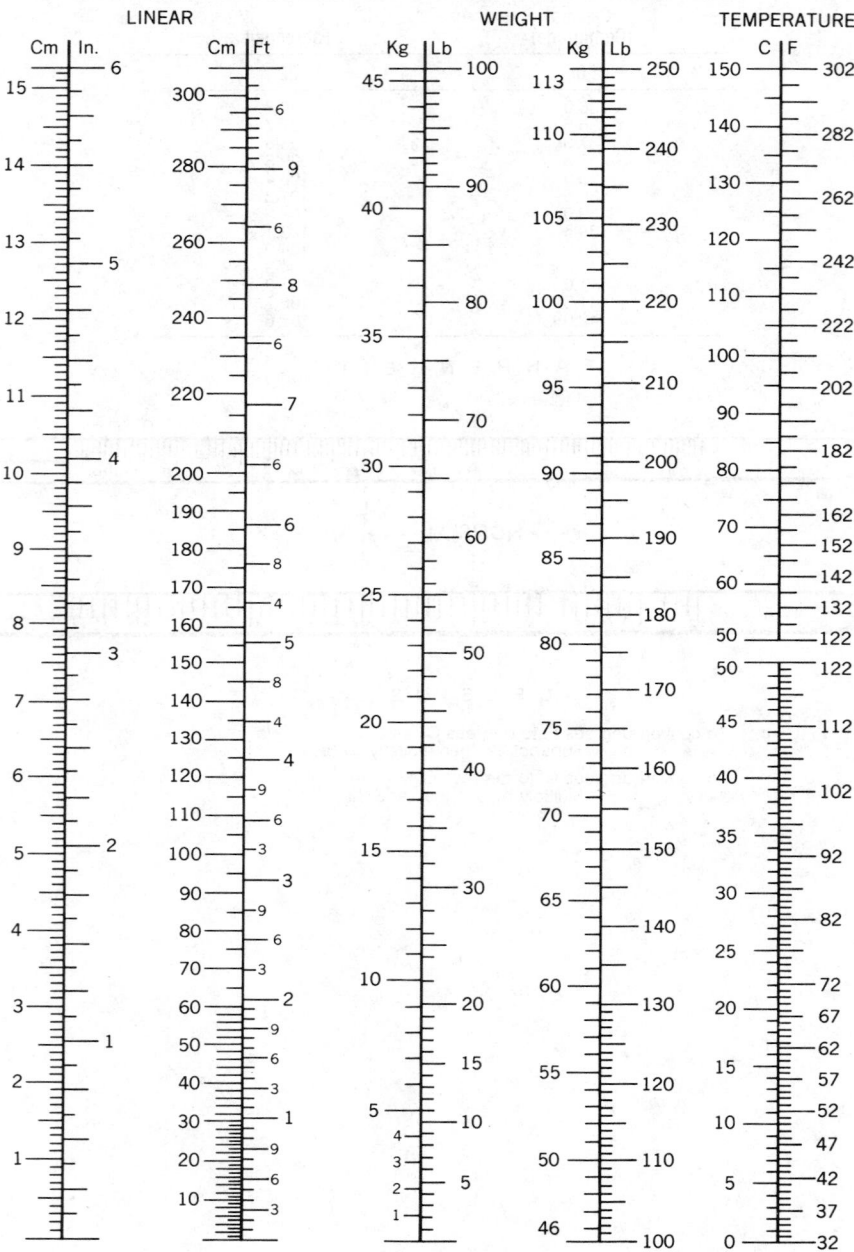

LINEAR WEIGHT TEMPERATURE

* 2.5 cm = 1 in.   1 kg. = 2.2 lb.

RECOMMENDED DAILY DIETARY ALLOWANCES

FOOD AND NUTRITION BOARD, NATIONAL ACADEMY OF SCIENCES–NATIONAL RESEARCH COUNCIL
RECOMMENDED DAILY DIETARY ALLOWANCES,[a] Revised 1980

Designed for the maintenance of good nutrition of practically all healthy people in the U.S.A.

	Age (years)	Weight (kg)	Weight (lb)	Height (cm)	Height (in)	Protein (g)	Vitamin A (µg RE)[b]	Vitamin D (µg)[c]	Vitamin E (mg α-TE)[d]	Vitamin C (mg)	Thiamin (mg)	Riboflavin (mg)	Niacin (mg NE)[e]	Vitamin B-6 (mg)	Folacin (µg)[f]	Vitamin B-12 (µg)	Calcium (mg)	Phosphorus (mg)	Magnesium (mg)	Iron (mg)	Zinc (mg)	Iodine (µg)
Infants	0.0–0.5	6	13	60	24	kg × 2.2	420	10	3	35	0.3	0.4	6	0.3	30	0.5[g]	360	240	50	10	3	40
	0.5–1.0	9	20	71	28	kg × 2.0	400	10	4	35	0.5	0.6	8	0.6	45	1.5	540	360	70	15	5	50
Children	1–3	13	29	90	35	23	400	10	5	45	0.7	0.8	9	0.9	100	2.0	800	800	150	15	10	70
	4–6	20	44	112	44	30	500	10	6	45	0.9	1.0	11	1.3	200	2.5	800	800	200	10	10	90
	7–10	28	62	132	52	34	700	10	7	45	1.2	1.4	16	1.6	300	3.0	800	800	250	10	10	120
Males	11–14	45	99	157	62	45	1000	10	8	50	1.4	1.6	18	1.8	400	3.0	1200	1200	350	18	15	150
	15–18	66	145	176	69	56	1000	10	10	60	1.4	1.7	18	2.0	400	3.0	1200	1200	400	18	15	150
	19–22	70	154	177	70	56	1000	7.5	10	60	1.5	1.7	19	2.2	400	3.0	800	800	350	10	15	150
	23–50	70	154	178	70	56	1000	5	10	60	1.4	1.6	18	2.2	400	3.0	800	800	350	10	15	150
	51+	70	154	178	70	56	1000	5	10	60	1.2	1.4	16	2.2	400	3.0	800	800	350	10	15	150
Females	11–14	46	101	157	62	46	800	10	8	50	1.1	1.3	15	1.8	400	3.0	1200	1200	300	18	15	150
	15–18	55	120	163	64	46	800	10	8	60	1.1	1.3	14	2.0	400	3.0	1200	1200	300	18	15	150
	19–22	55	120	163	64	44	800	7.5	8	60	1.1	1.3	14	2.0	400	3.0	800	800	300	18	15	150
	23–50	55	120	163	64	44	800	5	8	60	1.0	1.2	13	2.0	400	3.0	800	800	300	18	15	150
	51+	55	120	163	64	44	800	5	8	60	1.0	1.2	13	2.0	400	3.0	800	800	300	10	15	150
Pregnant						+30	+200	+5	+2	+20	+0.4	+0.3	+2	+0.6	+400	+1.0	+400	+400	+150	h	+5	+25
Lactating						+20	+400	+5	+3	+40	+0.5	+0.5	+5	+0.5	+100	+1.0	+400	+400	+150	h	+10	+50

[a] The allowances are intended to provide for individual variations among most normal persons as they live in the United States under usual environmental stresses. Diets should be based on a variety of common foods in order to provide other nutrients for which human requirements have been less well defined. See text for detailed discussion of allowances and of nutrients not tabulated.

[b] Retinol equivalents. 1 retinol equivalent = 1 µg retinol or 6 µg β carotene. See text for calculation of vitamin A activity of diets as retinol equivalents.

[c] As cholecalciferol. 10 µg cholecalciferol = 400 IU of vitamin D.

[d] α-tocopherol equivalents. 1 mg d-α tocopherol = 1 mg α-TE. See text for variation in allowances and calculation of vitamin E activity of the diet as α-tocopherol equivalents.

[e] 1 NE (niacin equivalent) is equal to 1 mg of niacin or 60 mg of dietary tryptophan.

[f] The folacin allowances refer to dietary sources as determined by *Lactobacillus casei* assay after treatment with enzymes (conjugases) to make polyglutamyl forms of the vitamin available to the test organism.

[g] The recommended dietary allowance for vitamin B-12 in infants is based on average concentration of the vitamin in human milk. The allowances after weaning are based on energy intake (as recommended by the American Academy of Pediatrics) and consideration of other factors, such as intestinal absorption; see text.

[h] The increased requirement during pregnancy cannot be met by the iron content of habitual American diets nor by the existing iron stores of many women; therefore the use of 30–60 mg of supplemental iron is recommended. Iron needs during lactation are not substantially different from those of nonpregnant women, but continued supplementation of the mother for 2–3 months after parturition is advisable in order to replenish stores depleted by pregnancy.

Recommended Dietary Allowances 9th ed. The National Research Council National Academy of Sciences, Washington D.C. 1980.

* Refer to Recommended Dietary Allowances, 9th ed. Washington, D.C., The National Research Council National Academy of Sciences, 1980.

APPENDIX III:
PEDIATRIC LABORATORY VALUES

(It should be noted that laboratory determinations vary from hospital to hospital depending on the techniques used by individual laboratories.)

BLOOD CHEMISTRIES

These values are compiled from the published literature, *Pediatric Clinical Chemistry,* and the Johns Hopkins Hospital Department of Laboratory Medicine. They are the most widely accepted normal values. Normal values, however, vary with the analytic method used. If any doubt exists, you should consult your laboratory for its analytical method and normal range of values. *Ref.:* Ed., Meites S., *Pediatric Clinical Chemistry,* Columbus, Ohio: Abbott Laboratories, 1975.

Acid phosphatase:
Newborn	7.4–19.4 IU/ml
2–13 years	6,4–15.2 IU/ml
Adult	0.2–11.0 IU/ml

Aldolase:
Adult	<11 IU/L
Children	2×–4× Adult Values

Alkaline phosphatase:
Newborn	20–266 IU/L
1 month–1 year	50–260 IU/L
1–2 years	146–477 IU/L
2–6 years	70–160 IU/L
7–10 years	45–273 IU/L
Puberty	56–258 IU/L
Adult	13–40 IU/L

Alpha 1-Antitrypsin:
PI type M (normal)	>75% normal pool
PI type MZ	55–75% normal pool
PI type SZ	30–50% normal pool
PI type Z or null	<40% normal pool

Alpha fetoprotein: <10 mg/dl

Ammonia Nitrogen (Venous Sample):
Newborn	90–150 micrograms/dl
0–2 weeks	70–129 micrograms/dl
>1 month	20–79 micrograms/dl
Infant-child	29–80 micrograms/dl
Adult	13–48 micrograms/dl

Amylase: 60–160 Somogyi units/dl

Bicarbonate: 22–30 mEq/L

Bilirubin (total):
Cord	<1.8 mg/dl
24 hours	Premature 1–6 mg/dl
	Full term 2–6 mg/dl
48 hours	Premature 6–8 mg/dl
	Full term 6–7 mg/dl
3–5 days	Premature 10–15 mg/dl
	Full term 4–12 mg/dl
1 month–Adult	1 mg/dl
Conjugated:	<0.4 mg/dl

Bromsulphalein Retention:
Newborn:	up to 20%
Thereafter:	less than 5%

Calcium (total):
Premature <1 week	6–10 mg/dl
Full term <1 week	7.0–12.0 mg/dl
Child	8–11.0 mg/dl
Adult	8.5–11.0 mg/dl

Calcium (ionized): 4.4–5.4 mg/dl

Carotenoids (carotenes):
Birth	70 micrograms/dl
<1 year	70–340 micrograms/dl
>3 years	100–150 micrograms/dl

Ceruloplasmin: 20–40 mg/dl
(280–570 units)

Chloride: 94–106 mEq/L

Cholesterol (total):
Full term	50–120 mg/dl
1–2 years	70–190 mg/dl
2–16 years	135–250 mg/dl
Adult	130–270 mg/dl

Copper:
0–6 months	70 micrograms/dl
6 months–5 years	27–153 micrograms/dl
5–17 years	94–234 micrograms/dl
Adult	70–155 micrograms/dl

Creatine Kinase (Creatine Phosphokinase):
Newborn	30–100 U/L
Child	15–50 U/L
Adult	5–40 U/L

Creatinine (Serum):
1–18 months	0.2–0.5 mg/dl
2–12 years	0.3–0.8 mg/dl
13–20 years	0.5–1.2 mg/dl
Adults	0.8–1.5 mg/dl

Ferritin:
Children	10–150 nanograms/ml
Females (Adult)	10–60 nanograms/ml
Males (Adult)	30–100 nanograms/ml

Fibrinogen: 200–400 mg/dl

Folic Acid (Folate):   5–21 nanograms/ml

Glucose (Serum):
Children	60–100 mg/dl
Premature	>30 mg/dl
Full term	>40 mg/dl

Haptoglobins:
Newborn	Detectable in only 10–20%
>1 year	400—1800 mg of Hb bound/L

Iron (Iron binding capacity):

	Iron (micrograms/dl)	Iron Binding Capacity (micrograms/dl)	Approximate Percent Saturation (micrograms/dl)
Newborn	110–270	59–175	65%
4–10 months	30–70	250–400	25%
3–10 years	53–119	250–400	30%
Adult	87–279	250–400	35%

Ketones:
Qualitative:	negative
Quantitative:	up to 3 mg%

Lactate:
Venous	0.5–1.6 mEq/L
Arterial	0.3–1.0 mEq/L

Lactate Dehydrogenase:
Birth	290–501 U/L
1 day–1 month	185–404 U/L
1 month–2 years	110–244 U/L
<4 years	60–170 U/L
3–17 years	85–165 U/L
Adult	30–90 U/L

Lactate Dehydrogenase Isoenzymes (% total):
LD_1 Heart	24–34%
LD_2 Heart, Erythrocytes	35–45%
LD_3 Muscle	15–25%
LD_4 Liver, trace muscle	4–10%
LD_5 Liver, muscle	1–9%

Lead: <40 micrograms/dl

Lipids (Total):   450–1000 mg/dl

Lipoproteins:
Alpha	286–450 mg/dl
Pre-Beta	22–72 mg/dl
Beta	276–438 mg/dl

Magnesium:
Newborn	1.52–2.33 mEq/L
Child	1.4–1.9 mEq/L
Adult	1.3–2.5 mEq/L

Methemoglobin: <0.3 g/dl or <3% of total Hb

5' Nucleotidase: <1.6 U/L

Osmolarity: 285–296 mOsm/kg
     (270–285 mOsm/L plasma)

Phenylalanine: <3 mg/dl

Phospholipids:
Cord blood	0.48–1.6 gms/L
2–13 years	1.66–2.47 gms/L
3–20 years	1.93–3.38 gms/L

Phosphorus (Inorganic):
Newborn	4.0–10.5 mg/dl
1 year	4.0–6.8 mg/dl
5 years	3.6–6.5 mg/dl
Adult	3.0–4.5 mg/dl

Porcelain: 8–20 mEq/L

Porphyrins: <7.0 micrograms/dl

Potassium:
<10 days of age	3.5–7.0 mEq/L
>10 days of age	3.5–5.5 mEq/L

Proteins Average (Range) in Grams/dl

Age	Total	Albumin	Globulin	Gamma Globulin
Premature	5.5 (4.0–7.0)	3.7 (2.5–4.5)	1.8 (1.2–2.0)	0.7 (0.5–0.9)
FT Newborn	6.4 (5.0–7.1)	3.4 (2.5–5.0)	3.1 (1.2–4.0)	0.8 (0.7–0.9)
1–3 months	6.6 (4.7–7.4)	3.8 (3.0–4.2)	2.5 (1.0–3.3)	0.3 (0.1–0.5)
3–12 months	6.8 (5.0–7.5)	3.9 (2.7–5.0)	2.6 (2.0–3.8)	0.6 (0.4–1.2)
1–15 years	7.4 (6.5–8.6)	4.0 (3.2–5.0)	3.1 (2.0–4.0)	0.9 (0.6–1.2)

Pyruvate: 0.05–0.14 mEq/L

Serotonin:
Child	127–187 nanograms/dl
Adult	119–171 nanograms/dl

Sodium:
Premature	130–140 mEq/L
Older	135–145 mEq/L

Transaminase (SGOT):
1–3 days	16–74 U/L
<6 months	20–43 U/L
6 months–1 year	16–35 U/L
1 year–5 years	6–30 U/L
5 years–adult	19–28 U/L
Adult	Male 8–46 U/L
	Female 7–34 U/L

Transaminase (SGPT):
Infants	<54 U/L
Children	1–30 U/L
Adults	0–19 U/L

Triglycerides: 29–154 mg/dl

Urea Nitrogen: 6–23 mg/dl

Uric Acid: 2.5–8.0 mg/dl

Vitamin A Retinol:
<6 months	20–90 micrograms/dl
1–5 years	30–100 micrograms/dl
5–16 years	60–100 micrograms/dl
Adult	20–80 micrograms/dl

Vitamin B_{12}:   330–1025 micrograms/dl

Vitamin C: 0.4–1.5 mg/dl

Vitamin E:
Newborn	>0.3 micrograms/dl
Child–Adult	0.5–1.2 micrograms/dl

Zinc:
0–1 year	Range:	74–146 micrograms/dl
2–10 years		72–128 micrograms/dl
11–18 years		65–125 micrograms/dl
Adult		60–120 micrograms/dl

TERM INFANTS—NORMAL BLOOD CHEMISTRY VALUES

Determination	Sample Source	Cord	1–12 hr.	12–24 hr.	24–48 hr.	48–72 hr.
Sodium, mmol/l*	Capillary	147 (126–166)	143 (124–156)	145 (132–159)	148 (134–160)	149 (139–162)
Potassium, mmol/l.		7.8 (5.6–12)	6.4 (5.3–7.3)	6.3 (5.3–8.9)	6.0 (5.2–7.3)	5.9 (5.0–7.7)
Chloride, mmol/l		103 (98–110)	100.7 (90–111)	103 (87–114)	102 (92–114)	103 (93–112)
Calcium, mg./dl		9.3 (8.2–11.1)	8.4 (7.3–9.2)	7.8 (6.9–9.4)	8.0 (6.1–9.9)	7.9 (5.9–9.7)
Phosphorus, mg./dl		5.6 (3.7–8.1)	6.1 (3.5–8.6)	5.7 (2.9–8.1)	5.9 (3.0–8.7)	5.8 (2.8–7.6)
Blood urea, mg./dl		29 (21–40)	27 (8–34)	33 (9–63)	32 (13–77)	31 (13–68)
Total protein, gm./dl		6.1 (4.8–7.3)	6.6 (5.6–8.5)	6.6 (5.8–8.2)	6.9 (5.9–8.2)	7.2 (6.0–8.5)
Glucose, mg./dl		73 (45–96)	63 (40–97)	63 (42–104)	56 (30–91)	59 (40–90)
Lactic acid, mg./dl		19.5 (11–30)	14.6 (11–24)	14.0 (10–23)	14.3 (9–22)	13.5 (7–21)
Lactate, mmol/l†		2.0–3.0	2.0			

(From Avery, GB. Neonatology. JB Lippincott, 1981. Original data from:
* Acharya, PT and Payne, WW. Arch Dis Child, 40:430, 1965.
† Daniel, SS, Adamsons, K Jr, James, LS. Pediatrics, 37:942, 1966)

LOW BIRTH WEIGHT INFANTS—NORMAL BLOOD CHEMISTRY VALUES
(CAPILLARY BLOOD, FIRST DAY)

Determination	<1000	1001–1500	1501–2000	2001–2500
Sodium, mmol/l	138	133	135	134
Potassium, mmol/l	6.4	6.0	5.4	5.6
Chloride, mmol/l	100	101	105	104
Total CO_2, mmol/l	19	20	20	20
Urea, mg./dl	22	21	16	16
Total protein, g/dl	4.8	4.8	5.2	5.3

(From Avery, GB. Neonatology. Lippincott, 1981. Original data from Pincus, JB et al. Pediatrics, 18:39, 1956)

ACID-BASE STATUS

VIGOROUS TERM INFANTS

Determination	Vaginal Delivery	Birth	1st Hr.	3rd Hr.	24 Hr.	2 Days	3 Days
pH	Umbilical artery	7.26					
	Umbilical vein	7.29					
pCO2 torr	Arterial	54.5	38.8	38.3	33.6	34	35
	Venous	42.8					
O2 sat.	Arterial	19.8	93.8	94.7	93.2		
	Venous	47.6					
pH	Left atrial		7.30	7.34	7.41	7.39 (temp. artery)	7.38 (temp. artery)
CO2 content, mmol/l			20.6	21.9	21.4		

PREMATURE INFANTS

	Capillary						
pH	<1250 g					7.36	7.35	7.35
pCO2 torr						38	44	37
pH	>1250 g					7.39	7.39	7.38
pCO2 torr						38	39	38

(From Avery, GB. Neonatology. Lippincott, 1981. Data of Weisbort, LM et al. J. Pediatr, 52:395, 1958; and Bucci, E et al. Biol Neonate, 8:81, 1965)

NORMAL VALUES—HEMATOLOGY

Age	Hgb (gm %)	Hct (%)	MCV (fl)	MCHC (gm/dl RBC)	Retic (%)	WBC per mm³ × 100 range (avg)	% Neutrophils
28 week gestation	14.5	45	120	31	—	—	
32 week gestation	15.0	47	118	32	—	—	
Full term							
1 day +	16.8–21.2	57–68	110–128	29.7–33.5	1.8–4.6	7–35 (18)	45–85
1 week +	15.0–19.6	46–62	107–129	30.4–33.6	0.1–0.9	4–20 (10)	30–50
1 month +	11.1–14.3	31–41	93–109	33.3–36.5	0.1–1.7	6–18 (10)	30–50
3–5 months	10.4–12.2	33	80–96	31.8–36.2	0.4–1.0	6–17 (10)	30–50
6–11 months	11.8	35	77	33	0.7–2.3	6–16 (10)	30–50
1 year	11.2	35	78	32	0.6–1.7	6–15 (10)	30–50
2–10 years	12.8	37	80	34	0.5–1.0	7–13 (9)	35–60
11–15 years	13.4	39	82	34	0.5–1.0	5–12 (8.5)	40–60
Adult							
Male	16.0 ± 2.0	47 ± 7	91 (82–101)	34 (31.5–36)	0.8–2.5	4.3–10 (7)	25–62
Female	14.0 ± 2.0	42 ± 5			0.3–4.1		

+ Under 1 month of age, capillary Hgb exceeds venous: 1 hour—3.6 gm difference
　5 days—2.2 gm difference
　3 weeks—1.1 gm difference

Absolute eosinophil count: avg 250/mm³ (100–600/mm³)
Ref.: Am. J. Dis. Child 93:486, 1957; Acta Paed. (Stockholm) 60:317, 1971; Wintrobe, Clinical Hematology 7th ed. Lea and Febiger, Phila, 1974; Mauer, Pediatric Hematology, McGraw-Hill, N.Y. 1969; Oski and Naiman, Hematologic Problems in the Newborn Infant, W.B. Saunders, Phila., 1972
(Reproduced with permission from Johns Hopkins Hospital: The Harriet Lane Handbook, 8th edition, Kenneth C. Schubert and Basil J. Zitelli (editors). Copyright © 1978 by Year Book Medical Publishers, Inc., Chicago.)

URINALYSIS

Determination		Age/Sex	Normal Range		
Addis count	Leukocytes		<10		
	Erythrocytes		< 5		
	Casts		occasional hyaline		
Colony count, colonies/ml urine (fresh specimen)			Clean Catch, Midstream*	Catheterization	Suprapubic Bladder Puncture
		Infant/Child	< 1,000	100	0
		Thereafter	<10,000	100	0
Microscopic	Leukocytes		0–4 per high-power field		
	Erythrocytes		rare per high-power field		
	Casts		rare per high-power field		
Osmolarity		Premature/Newborn	50– 600 mOsm/l		
		Thereafter	50–1400		
		Thereafter	>850 (after fluid restriction)		
pH		Newborn/Neonate	5.0–7.0		
		Thereafter	4.8–7.8		
Protein	qualitative		Negative		
	quantitative		10–100 mg/d (higher after strenuous exercise)		
Specific gravity, random		Newborn/Infant	1.001–1.020		
		Thereafter	1.001–1.030		
		Thereafter	>1.025 (after fluid restriction)		
Sugar, qualitative (including glucose)			Negative		
Volume		Newborn/Neonate	50– 300 ml/d		
		Infant	350– 550		
		Child	500–1000		
		Adolescent	700–1400		
		Thereafter: M	800–2000		
		F	800–1600		

* Pure cultures with colony counts >100,000 are considered diagnostic in adults, whereas colony counts of >10,000 are usually considered diagnostic in children. Intermediate counts must be interpreted relative to the clinical situation. For females, the physician must be aware of the cleanliness and care used in collecting the specimen. Urine obtained by means of a plastic collection device or by voiding into a container without prior preparation of the patient is usually contaminated, and has limited usefulness in evaluating the possibility of urinary tract infections.
(From Vaughan, V.C., McKay, R.J., and Behrman, R.E.: Nelson's Textbook of Pediatrics. Philadelphia, W.B. Saunders, 1979.)

NORMAL SEROLOGIC REFERENCE VALUES

Anti-Streptolysin O Titer
  Preschool   <1:85
  School ages and adults   <1:170
  Older adults   <1:85
Anti-Hyaluronidase   <1:256
Anti-Nuclear Antibody   <1:40
C-Reactive Protein   Negative
C'_3 70–176 mg/dl
C'_4 16–45 mg/dl
Chorioembryonic
  Antigen (CEA)   <2.5 nanograms/ml
Febrile Agglutinins   <1:80 or <four fold rise in titer
Mononucleosis Screen   Negative
Proteus OX-19 Agglutinins   <1:80 or <four fold rise in titer
Rheumatoid Latex Titer   1:80–1:160 Doubtful
    1:40-Negative
Rheumatoid Screen   Negative
Tularemia Agglutinins   <1:80 or <four fold rise in titer
W. Rose Titer   1:10 Negative
    1:20–1:40 Doubtful
    >1:80 Positive

Complement Fixation Tests should be negative or <1:8
  Brucellosis
  Cytomegalic Inclusion Disease
  Eastern and Western Equine Encephalitis
  Epidemic Typhus
  Influenza Type A (F.M.I. and P.R. 8)
  Influenza Type B (Lee)
  Lymphocytic Choriomeningitis
  Lymphogranuloma Venereum
  Mumps
  Psittacosis
  Q Fever (American)
  Rickettsial Pox
  Rocky Mountain Spotted Fever
  St. Louis Encephalitis
  Toxoplasmosis
  Tularemia

CEREBROSPINAL FLUID

Cell Count   % PMN's
  Preterm mean: 9.0   (0–25.4 WBC/mm³)   57%
  Term mean: 8.2   (0–22.4 WBC/mm³)   61%
  >1 month   0–7   0
Glucose
  Preterm   24–63 mg/dl   (mean 50)
  Term   34–119 mg/dl   (mean 52)
  Child   40–80 mg/dl
CSF Glucose/Blood Glucose (%)
  Preterm   55–105
  Term   44–128
  Child   ~50%
Lactic Acid Dehydrogenase   Mean: 20 U/ml (range 5–30 U/ml)
Pandy   Negative, May be + in newborn
Pressure: Initial L.P.
  Newborn   80–110 <110 mm H_2O
  Infant/Child   <200 Lateral recumbent positions
  Respiratory movements   5–10 mm/H_2O
Protein
  Preterm   (mean 115)   65–150 mg/dl
  Term   (mean 90)   20–170 mg/dl
  Children   Ventricular   5–15 mg/dl
    Cisternal   5–25 mg/dl
    Lumbar   5–40 mg/dl
Specific Gravity   1.005–1.009

Ref.: Sarff, L.D., et al. J. Peds. 88:473–477, 1976.

CONVERSION OF POUNDS AND OUNCES TO GRAMS

POUNDS	0	1	2	3	4	5	6	7	8	9	10	11	12	13	14	15
0	—	28	57	85	113	142	170	198	227	255	283	312	340	369	397	425
1	454	482	510	539	567	595	624	652	680	709	737	765	794	822	850	879
2	907	936	964	992	1021	1049	1077	1106	1134	1162	1191	1219	1247	1276	1304	1332
3	1361	1389	1417	1446	1474	1503	1531	1559	1588	1616	1644	1673	1701	1729	1758	1786
4	1814	1843	1871	1899	1928	1956	1984	2013	2041	2070	2098	2126	2155	2183	2211	2240
5	2268	2296	2325	2353	2381	2410	2438	2466	2495	2523	2551	2580	2608	2637	2665	2693
6	2722	2750	2778	2807	2835	2863	2892	2920	2948	2977	3005	3033	3062	3090	3118	3147
7	3175	3203	3232	3260	3289	3317	3345	3374	3402	3430	3459	3487	3515	3544	3572	3600
8	3629	3657	3685	3714	3742	3770	3799	3827	3856	3884	3912	3941	3969	3997	4026	4054
9	4082	4111	4139	4167	4196	4224	4252	4281	4309	4337	4366	4394	4423	4451	4479	4508
10	4536	4564	4593	4621	4649	4678	4706	4734	4763	4791	4819	4848	4876	4904	4933	4961
11	4990	5018	5046	5075	5103	5131	5160	5188	5216	5245	5273	5301	5330	5358	5386	5415
12	5443	5471	5500	5528	5557	5585	5613	5642	5670	5698	5727	5755	5783	5812	5840	5868
13	5897	5925	5953	5982	6010	6038	6067	6095	6123	6152	6180	6209	6237	6265	6294	6322
14	6350	6379	6407	6435	6464	6492	6520	6549	6577	6605	6634	6662	6690	6719	6747	6776
15	6804	6832	6860	6889	6917	6945	6973	7002	7030	7059	7087	7115	7144	7172	7201	7228
16	7257	7286	7313	7342	7371	7399	7427	7456	7484	7512	7541	7569	7597	7626	7654	7682
17	7711	7739	7768	7796	7824	7853	7881	7909	7938	7966	7994	8023	8051	8079	8108	8136
18	8165	8192	8221	8249	8278	8306	8335	8363	8391	8420	8448	8476	8504	8533	8561	8590
19	8618	8646	8675	8703	8731	8760	8788	8816	8845	8873	8902	8930	8958	8987	9015	9043
20	9072	9100	9128	9157	9185	9213	9242	9270	9298	9327	9355	9383	9412	9440	9469	9497
21	9525	9554	9582	9610	9639	9667	9695	9724	9752	9780	9809	9837	9865	9894	9922	9950
22	9979	10007	10036	10064	10092	10120	10149	10177	10206	10234	10262	10291	10319	10347	10376	10404

OUNCES (column headers) / POUNDS (row labels)

Index